Critical Care Nursing

5e

Critical Care Nursing

5e

Leanne Aitken
RN, PhD, GCertMgt, GDipScMed(ClinEpi), GCertAcadPrac, BHSc(Nurs)Hons,
FACCCN, FACN, FAAN, Life Member – ACCCN
Professor of Critical Care and Associate Dean – Research, Enterprise & Global Engagement,
School of Health & Psychological Sciences, City University of London, UK
Honorary Professorial Fellow, Faculty of Medicine, Dentistry and Health Sciences,
University of Melbourne, VIC, Australia
Honorary Professor, William Harvey Research Institute,
Queen Mary University of London, UK

Andrea Marshall
RN, PhD, MN(Research), Grad Cert Ed Studies (Higher Ed),
BN, IC Cert, FACCCN, FACN, Life Member – ACCCN
Professor of Intensive Care Nursing,
School of Nursing and Midwifery and
Menzies Health Institute Queensland,
Griffith University, QLD, Australia
Intensive Care Unit, Gold Coast Health,
QLD, Australia

Thomas Buckley
RN, PhD, GradCertHPol, MN(Research), BSc(Health)Hons,
Cert(ICU), Member ACCCN
Associate Professor Acute and Critical Care Nursing,
and Deputy Head of School, Susan Wakil School of Nursing and Midwifery,
University of Sydney, Australia
Adjunct Professor, School of Health and Human Sciences,
Southern Cross University, Lismore, Australia.

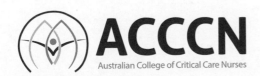

Australian College of Critical Care Nurses

ELSEVIER

Elsevier Australia. ACN 001 002 357
(a division of Reed International Books Australia Pty Ltd)
Tower 1, 475 Victoria Avenue, Chatswood, NSW 2067

ISBN: 978-0-7295-4446-7

Notice

National Library of Australia Cataloguing-in-Publication Data

 A catalogue record for this book is available from the National Library of Australia

---

Content Strategists: Natalie Hunt and Dorothy Chiu
Content Project Managers: Kritika Kaushik and Shubham Dixit
Edited by Chris Wyard
Proofread by Tim Learner
Cover by Georgette Hall
Internal design: Non-Standard
Index by Straive
Typeset by GW Tech
Printed in Malaysia by Papercraft

Last digit is the print number: 9   8   7   6   5   4   3   2   1

Contents

Preface

Critical care as a clinical specialty is over half a century old. With every successive decade, advances in the education and practices of critical care nurses have been made. Over the past four years since the last edition and through the COVID-19 pandemic, we have seen enormous growth in the interest and recognition of critical care nursing, as well as an explosion of the body of evidence informing practice. Today, critical care nurses are some of the most knowledgeable and highly skilled nurses in the world, and ongoing professional development and education are fundamental elements in ensuring we deliver the highest quality care to our patients and their families.

This book is intended to encourage and challenge nurses to further develop their critical care nursing practice. Since the first edition in 2007, with a focus on Australasian practice, we have now expanded the text to reflect international practice and expertise in the field. Our authors come from many countries including Australia, Canada, England, Greece, the Netherlands, New Zealand, Northern Ireland, Scotland, Sweden, Switzerland and the USA.

This fifth edition of Critical Care Nursing has 29 chapters that reflect the collective talent and expertise of 56 contributors – a strong mix of clinicians and academics with a passion for critical care internationally. All contributors were carefully chosen for their current knowledge, clinical expertise and strong professional reputations.

The book has been developed primarily for use by practising critical care clinicians, managers, researchers and graduate students undertaking a specialty critical care qualification. In addition, senior undergraduate students studying high-acuity nursing subjects will find this book a valuable reference tool, although it may go beyond the learning needs of these students. The aim of the book is to be a comprehensive evidence-informed resource, as well as a portal to an array of other important resources, for critical care nurses. The nature and timeline of book publishing dictate that the information contained in this book reflects a snapshot in time of our knowledge and understanding of the complex world of critical care nursing. We therefore encourage our readers to continue to search also for the most contemporary sources of knowledge to guide their clinical practice. A range of website links have been included in each chapter to facilitate this process.

This fifth edition is divided into three broad sections: the scope of critical care nursing, core components of critical care nursing and specialty aspects of critical care nursing. Revisions to existing chapters were based on our reflections and suggestions from colleagues and reviewers as well as on evolving practices and emerging evidence in critical care.

Section 1 introduces a broad range of professional issues related to practice that are relevant across critical care. Initial chapters provide contemporary information on the scope of practice, systems and resources and ethical issues, with expanded information on quality and safety, and recovery and rehabilitation in critical care.

Content presented in Section 2 is relevant to the majority of critical care nurses, with a focus on concepts that underpin practice such as essential physical, psychological, social and cultural care. Remaining chapters in this section present a systems approach in supporting physiological function for a critically ill person. This edition has multiple linked chapters for some of the major physiological systems – four chapters for cardiovascular, three for respiratory and two for neurological. Chapters on support of renal function; nutrition assessment and therapeutic management; gastrointestinal, metabolic and liver alterations; management of shock; and multiorgan dysfunction complete this section.

Section 3 presents specific clinical conditions such as emergency presentations, trauma, resuscitation, postanaesthesia recovery, paediatric considerations, pregnancy and postpartum considerations and organ donation, by building on the principles outlined in Section 2. This section enables readers to explore some of the more complex or unique aspects of specialty critical care nursing practice.

Chapters have been organised in a consistent format to facilitate identification of relevant material. Where appropriate, each chapter commences with an overview of the relevant anatomy and physiology and the epidemiology of the clinical states. Nursing care of the patient, delivered independently or provided collaboratively with other members of the healthcare team, is then presented. Pedagogical features include a case study that elaborates relevant care issues and a critique of a research publication that explores a related topic. Tables, figures and practice tips have been used extensively throughout each chapter to identify areas of care that are particularly pertinent for readers. Each chapter also has specific learning activities, and model responses to these questions to further support learning can be found online. It is not our intention that readers progress sequentially through the book, but rather explore chapters or sections that are relevant for different episodes of learning or practice.

The delivery of effective, high-quality critical care nursing practice is a challenge in contemporary healthcare with a constantly evolving body of evidence. We trust that this book will be a valuable resource in supporting your care of critically ill patients and their loved ones.

Leanne **Aitken**
Andrea **Marshall**
Tom **Buckley**

About the editors

Leanne Aitken is Professor of Critical Care and Associate Dean – Research, Enterprise & Global Engagement at City University of London, United Kingdom. She holds honorary professorial appointments at both the University of Melbourne, Australia and Queen Mary University of London, United Kingdom. She has had a long career in critical care nursing, including practice, education and research roles. In all her roles, Leanne has been inspired by a sense of enquiry, pride in the value of expert nursing and a belief that improvement in practice and resultant patient outcomes is always possible. Research interests include developing and refining interventions to improve long-term recovery of critically ill and injured patients, decision-making practices of critical care nurses and a range of clinical practice issues within critical care, such as sedation management.

Leanne has been active in the Australian College of Critical Care Nurses (ACCCN) for more than 35 years and was made a Life Member and Fellow of the College in 2006 after holding positions on a range of state and national boards, panels and working groups; she has also been an Associate Editor with Australian Critical Care. Leanne is an Ambassador for the World Federation of Critical Care Nurses.

Leanne is a Fellow of both the American Academy of Nursing and the Australian College of Nursing. She is also a Fulbright Alumnus after receiving a Fulbright Senior Scholarship to undertake research at the University of Pennsylvania, Philadelphia, USA. Leanne has published more than 170 original publications in peer-reviewed journals. She is also a peer reviewer for a number of national and international journals and reviews grant applications for a range of organisations internationally.

Andrea Marshall is Professor of Intensive Care Nursing at Griffith University and Gold Coast Health, Queensland, Australia. She has been working in critical care as a clinician, educator and researcher for more than two decades. Andrea has a strong interdisciplinary focus on research, translation of research into clinical practice and implementing patient- and family-centred approaches to clinical care and research. Her program of research focuses on improving nutrition delivery to acute and critically ill patients during hospitalisation and following discharge.

Andrea has been actively involved with the ACCCN for over two decades in a variety of state- and nationally-based leadership roles. In 2014 her contribution to the College was recognised with Life Membership. She is currently Editor-in-Chief of Australian Critical Care and has played a key editorial role with this journal since 2003. She has published over 180 peer reviewed publications, is an active contributor to grant reviews for a number of national and international funding bodies and serves as a reviewer on several international journals, many of which have an interdisciplinary focus.

Thomas Buckley (Tom) is Associate Professor of Acute and Critical Care Nursing at the University of Sydney. He has been a critical care clinical nurse, educator and researcher for almost three decades and has served as an editor with Australian Critical Care over the past 7 years.

Tom is an active researcher with a strong focus on the interaction between psychological stressors and adverse health risk, as well as end-of-life care practices in intensive care. In addition to his research, Tom has a track record in nurse practitioner education and has served as the Chair of the Australian Nursing and Midwifery Accreditation Council (ANMAC) Nurse Practitioner Accreditation Committee (2015-2019). In addition, he contributed as co-investigator on research that informed the Australian Nurse Practitioner Standards for Practice (2014) and Registered Nurse Standard for Practice (2016) and led the development of the ACCCN Position Statement on Advanced Practice in Critical Care in 2021.

Reviewers

Melissa J Bloomer
PhD, MN(Hons), MPET, MNP, GCDE, Crit Care Cert,
BN, RN
Griffith University & Princess Alexandra Hospital
Brisbane, QLD, Australia

Rand Butcher
MClinSc (Intensive Care Nursing), GradDipN (Nurse
Education), Int Care Cert, BHlthSci (Nursing), DipAppSci
(Nursing)
Chief Executive Officer, Australian College of Critical
Care Nursing
Clinical Nurse Consultant, Critical Care, The Tweed
Hospital
Honorary Adjunct Associate Professor, Bond University
Cudgen, NSW, Australia

Steven Hardman
RN Adult, DPSN, BSc Hon, PGCert Critical Care,
PGCert Education, MSc, PhD
Senior Lecturer & National Undergraduate Program
Coordinator
University of Notre Dame Australia
Fremantle, WA, Australia

Alison Hodak
Masters Health Service Management, Grad Dip Critical
Care Nurs, Bachelor of Nursing
National President, ACCCN
Canberra, ACT, Australia

Rebecca Jarden
PhD, MN, RN
The University of Melbourne / Austin Health
Melbourne, Victoria, Australia

Kate Leutert
MN(Ed), MN(PeadCritCare), GCert (Pead ICU), GCert
(Paed Neo & Youth Health), BSc(Nu), RN
Nurse Educator PICU
The Children's Hospital at Westmead
Sydney, NSW, Australia

Sarah Mills
RN, BN, (Hon), MN, GradCertTEd, MACN
Associate Lecturer in Nursing
College of Nursing & Midwifery
Charles Darwin University
Brisbane, QLD, Australia

Naomi Morick
Director of Nursing Midwifery Education Research and
Training
Alice Springs Hospital
Central Australia Health Service
The Gap, NSW, Australia

Kaye Rolls
RN, BAppSc, DNurs
Lecturer
School of Nursing
University of Wollongong
Wollongong, NSW, Australia

Julia Muller Spiti
GCert ICUNsg, GDip CardiacNsg, MCSc
Lecturer
Faculty of Health and Medical Sciences
Adelaide Nursing School
The University of Adelaide
Adelaide, SA, Australia

Pre-proposal Reviewers

Steven Hardman
RN Adult, DPSN, BSc Hon, PGCert Critical Care,
PGCert Education, MSc, PhD
Senior Lecturer & National Undergraduate Program
Coordinator
University of Notre Dame Australia
Fremantle, WA, Australia

Rosemary Turner
RN, MA, Grad DipNur (Critical Care), Grad CertNur
(Critical Care)
Lecturer, Nursing
Division of Medicine, Dentistry, and Health Sciences
The University of Melbourne
Parkville, VIC, Australia

Acknowledgements

A project of this nature and scope requires many talented and committed people to see it to completion. The decision to publish this fifth edition was supported enthusiastically by Elsevier Australia. To our chapter contributors for this edition, both those returning from the previous editions and our new collaborators – thank you for accepting our offer to write, for having the courage and confidence in yourselves and us to be involved in the text, and for being committed in meeting writing deadlines while developing the depth and quality of content that we had planned. This is particularly appreciated given the enormously challenging environment within critical care over recent years, and we acknowledge the wide range of competing demands that many of you were dealing with.

Our heartfelt thanks go to our colleague and friend, Wendy Chaboyer, who has been on this journey with us since the first edition. Wendy has contributed an enormous amount to the dream of this text, and we thank her for the time, effort and memories in working with us to make it a reality. We also acknowledge the work of chapter contributors from our previous edition – Jane Bancroft, Suzanne Bench, Lina Bergman, Maureen Coombes, Fiona Coyer, Susan Dirkes, Ruth Endacott, Anne Flodén, Paula Foran, Deb Friel, Janice Gullick, Alister Hodge, Anastasia Hutchinson, Ruth Kleinpell, Leila Kuzmiuk, Frances Lin, Marion Mitchell, DaiWai M Olson, Mona Ringdal, Karen Smith and Teresa Williams.

We acknowledge support from the staff at Elsevier Australia, our publishing partner. Thanks to our Content Strategist, Natalie Hunt, for guiding this major project, our Content Development Specialist, Kritika Kaushik, and to Chris Wyard, our editor. To others who produced the high-quality figures, developed and executed the marketing plan and undertook myriad other activities, without which a text such as this would never come to fruition, thank you. We acknowledge our external reviewers who devoted their time to provide insightful suggestions in improving the text and contributed to the quality of the finished product. We also acknowledge the role of ACCCN in reviewing the chapters and endorsing this text as a valuable resource for critical care nurses.

Finally, and most importantly, to our respective loved ones – Steve; David, Abi and Hannah; and Natalie, Liam and Callum – thanks for your belief in us, and your understanding and commitment in supporting our careers.

Leanne **Aitken**
Andrea **Marshall**
Tom **Buckley**

Abbreviations

6MWT	6 minute walk test
AACN	American Association of Critical-Care Nurses
AAST	American Association for the Surgery of Trauma
ABCDEF	awakening and breathing coordination, choice of sedatives and analgesic exposure, delirium monitoring and management, early mobility, family engagement
ABG	arterial blood gas
ABIC	age, serum bilirubin, INR and serum creatinine score
A/C	assist control ventilation
ACCCN	Australian College of Critical Care Nurses
ACCESS	assistance, coordination, contingency, education, supervision, support
ACEI	angiotensin-converting enzyme inhibitor
ACEP	American College of Emergency Phsyicians
ACh	acetylcholine
ACLF	acute-on-chronic liver failure
ACS	abdominal compartment syndrome
ACS	acute coronary syndrome
ACT	activated clotting time
ADH	antidiuretic hormone
ADL	activities of daily living
ADVOS	advanced organ support
AE	adverse event
AED	automatic external defibrillator
AF	atrial fibrillation
AFE	amniotic fluid embolism
AGREE II	Appraisal of Guidelines for Research and Evaluation II
AHF	acute heart failure
AIDS	acquired immune deficiency syndrome
AIMS–ICU	Australian Incident Monitoring Study–ICU
AIS	Abbreviated Injury Score
AKI	acute kidney injury
ALARP	as low as reasonably possible
ALF	acute liver failure
ALI	acute lung injury
ALS	advanced life support
AMI	acute myocardial infarction
AMR	antimicrobial resistance
AMS	automatic mode switching
ANLH	acute native lung hyperinflation
ANP	atrial natriuretic peptide
ANS	autonomic nervous system
ANZ	Australia and New Zealand
ANZBA	Australia and New Zealand Burns Association

AODR	Australian Organ Donor Register
AOTA	Australian Organ and Tissue Authority
AP	anteroposterior
APACHE	Acute Physiology And Chronic Health Evaluation (score)
APH	antepartum haemorrhage
APRV	airway pressure release ventilation
APSIC	Asia Pacific Society of Infection Control
APTT	activated partial thromboplastin time
ARAS	ascending reticular activating system
ARB	angiotensin receptor blocker
ARC	Australian Resuscitation Council
ARDS	acute respiratory distress syndrome
ARF	acute renal failure
ARF	acute respiratory failure
ARP	absolute refractory period
ASV	adaptive support ventilation
AT	atrial tachycardia
ATC	automatic tube compensation
ATLS	advanced trauma life support
ATN	acute tubular necrosis
ATP	adenosine triphosphate
ATS	Australasian Triage Scale
AUD	Australian dollar
AV	atrioventricular
AVNRT	atrioventricular nodal re-entry tachycardia
AVRT	atrioventricular re-entrant tachycardia
AWS	alcohol withdrawal syndrome
BACCN	British Association of Critical Care Nurses
BCL	bandage contact lenses
BE	base excess
βHCG	beta-human chorionic gonadotropin
BiPAP	bi-phasic positive airways pressure
BLS	basic life support
BMI	body mass index
BP	blood pressure
BPS	Behavioural Pain Scale
BSLTx	bilateral sequential lung transplantation
BURP	backwards, upwards, rightward pressure
CABG	coronary artery bypass graft
CACCN	Canadian Association of Critical Care Nurses
CALD	culturally and linguistically diverse
CAM-ICU	Confusion Assessment Method for the Intensive Care Unit
CAP	community-acquired pneumonia
CAPD	Cornell Assessment for Pediatric Delirium
CAUTI	catheter-associated urinary tract infection
CAVH	continuous arteriovenous haemofiltration
CBF	cerebral blood flow
CBT	cognitive behavioural therapy
CBV	cerebral blood volume

CCRN	critical care registered nurse
CCU	coronary/cardiac care unit
CDC	Centers for Disease Control and Prevention
CHB	complete heart block
CHD	congenital heart disease
CHD	coronary heart disease
CHF	congestive heart failure
CHF	chronic heart failure
CHG	chlorhexidine gluconate
CI	cognitive impairment
CI	cardiac index
CIM	critical illness myopathy
CINM	critical illness neuromyopathy
CIP	critical illness polyneuropathy
CIRCI	critical illness-related corticosteroid insufficiency
CIWA-Ar	Clinical Institute Withdrawal Assessment of Alcohol Scale
CK	creatine kinase
CKD	chonic kidney disease
CLABSI	central line associated blood stream infection
CLL	chronic lymphocytic leukaemia
cLMA	classic laryngeal mask airway
CMV	controlled mandatory ventilation
CN	cranial nerve
CNC	clinical nurse consultant
CNE	clinical nurse educator
CNM	clinical nurse manager
CNS	central nervous system
CO	carbon monoxide
CO	cardiac output
CO_2	carbon dioxide
COPD	chronic obstructive pulmonary disease
CoV-2	coronavirus 2
COVID-19	coronavirus disease 2019
COX	cyclo-oxygenase
CPAP	continuous positive airway pressure
CPAx	Chelsea critical care physical assessment tool
CPB	cardiopulmonary bypass
CPE	carbapenemase-producing Enterobacteriaceae
CPG	clinical practice guidelines
CPOE	computerised provider order entry
CPOT	Critical-care Pain Observation Tool
CPP	cerebral perfusion pressure
CPR	cardiopulmonary resuscitation
CQR	clinical quality registries
CR	cardiac rehabilitation
CRP	C-reactive protein
CRRT	continuous renal replacement therapy
CRS	cytokine release syndrome
CRT	cardiac resynchronisation therapy
CSF	cerebral spinal fluid
CT	computerised tomography
CTA	computed tomography angiography
CTAS	Canadian Triage and Acuity Scale
CTG	cardiotocograph
CTI	cavotricuspid isthmus
CTPA	computerised tomography pulmonary angiogram
CUSP	comprehensive unit-based safety program
CVAD	central venous access device
CVC	central venous catheter
CVD	cardiovascular disease
CVP	central venous pressure
CVVH	continuous venovenous haemofiltration
CVVHDf	continuous venovenous haemodiafiltration
CX	circumflex coronary artery
CXR	chest X-ray
DAOH	days alive and out of hospital
DCDD	donation after circulatory determination of death
DCR	damage-control resuscitation
DCS	damage-control surgery
DDD	dual-chamber pacing, dual-chamber sensing and dual responses
DEMMI	De Morton Mobility Index
DES	dry eye syndrome
DIC	disseminated intravascular coagulation
DKA	diabetic ketoacidosis
DLT	double-lumen endotracheal tubes
DNA	deoxyribonucleic acid
DNS	Dependence Nursing Scale
DPL	diagnostic peritoneal lavage
DRG	diagnostic related groups
DVT	deep vein thrombosis
E	expiration
EAST	Eastern Association for the Surgery of Trauma
EBP	evidence-based practice
EC	extracorporeal circuit
ECC	external cardiac compressions
ECG	electrocardiography
ECLS	extracorporeal life support
ECMO	extracorporeal membrane oxygenation
ED	emergency department
EDD-f	extended daily dialysis filtration
EEG	electroencephalogram/electroencephalography
EfCCNa	European federation of Critical Care Nursing associations
EM	early mobilisation
EMDR	eye movement desensitisation and reprocessing
EMR	electronic medical records
EMS	emergency medical service
EMSB	early management of severe burns
EN	enteral nutrition
EoL	end of life
EPAP	expiratory positive airway pressure
EQ-5D	EuroQol Five dimension
ERAS	early/enhanced recovery after surgery
ERC	European Resuscitation Council
ESI	emergency severity index
ESRD	end-stage renal disease
ETT	endotracheal tube
EVD	external ventricular drain

F	frequency
FAST	focused assessment with sonography in trauma
FBC	full blood count
FCC	family-centred care
FEES	flexible endoscopic evaluation of swallowing
FES	fat embolism syndrome
FEV1	forced expiratory volume in one second
FFP	fresh frozen plasma
FH	fetal heart
FICM	Faculty of Intensive Care Medicine
FIM	Functional Independence Measure
FiO_2	fraction of inspired oxygen
FLACC	Faces Legs Activity Cry Consolability
FRC	functional residual capacity
FSS	functional status score
FTE	full-time equivalent
FTND	Fagerström Test for Nicotine Dependence
f/V_T	frequency/tidal volume
FVC	forced vital capacity
GABA	gamma-aminobutyric acid
GAH	Glasgow Alcoholic Hepatitis
GCS	Glasgow Coma Scale
GEDV	global end-diastolic volume
GEDVI	global end-diastolic volume index
GFR	glomerular filtration rate
GIT	gastrointestinal tract
GRADE	grading of recommendations, assessment, development and evaluation
GRV	gastric residual volume
H^+	hydrogen ion
H_2CO_3	carbonic acid
H2RA	histamine-2 receptor antagonist
HAC	hospital-acquired complication
HADS	Hospital Anxiety and Depression Scale
HAI	hospital-acquired/healthcare-acquired infection
Hb	haemoglobin
HBV	hepatitis B virus
HCM	hypertrophic cardiomyopathy
HCO_3^-	bicarbonate ion
HCV	hepatitis C virus
HD	haemodialysis
HDU	high-dependency unit
HE	hepatic encephalopathy
HELLP	haemolysis, elevated liver enzymes and low platelets
HEMS	helicopter emergency medical service
HEPA	high-efficiency particulate air
HFNC	high-flow nasal cannulae
HFO	high-flow oxygen
HFOV	high-frequency oscillation ventilation
HFpEF	heart failure with preserved ejection fraction
HFrEF	heart failure with reduced ejection fraction
HHFNC	humidified high-flow oxygen via nasal cannulae
HHS	hyperosmolar hyperglycaemic state
Hib	*Haemophilus influenzae* type b
HIV	human immunodeficiency virus
HME	heat and moisture exchanger
HMGB1	high-mobility group box 1
HPA	hypothalamic–pituitary–adrenal
HPIV	human parainfluenza virus
HOB	head of bed
HR	heart rate
HRO	high-reliability organisation
HRQOL	health-related quality of life
HRS	hepatorenal syndrome
HRS-AKI	hepatorenal syndrome acute kidney injury
HRS-NAKI	hepatorenal syndrome non-acute kidney injury
HSV	herpes simplex virus
Hz	frequency, hertz
I	inspiration
IABP	intra-aortic balloon pump
IAD	incontinence-associated dermatitis
IAH	intraabdominal hypertension
IAP	intraabdominal pressure
ICC	intercostal catheter
ICC	intraclass correlation coefficient
ICD	implantable cardioverter defibrillator
ICDSC	Intensive Care Delirium Screening Checklist
ICF	International Classification of Functioning, Disability and Health
ICN	International Council of Nurses
ICP	intracranial pressure
ICS	Intensive Care Society (UK)
ICTRP	International Clinical Trial Registry Platform
ICU	intensive care unit
ICU-AW	intensive care unit-acquired weakness
IDC	indwelling catheter
I:E	inspiratory/expiratory ratio
IESR	Impact of Event Scale Revised
IHPA	Independent Hospital Pricing Authority
ILCOR	International Liaison Committee on Resuscitation
ILV	independent lung ventilation
IMD	invasive meningococcal disease
IMS	ICU Mobility Scale
IMT	inspiratory muscle training
INR	international normalised ratio
IP	inflation point
IPAP	inspiratory positive airway pressure
IPC	infection prevention and control
IPC	intermittent pneumatic compression
IPH	interventional patient hygiene
IPV	intimate partner violence
ISTAP	International Skin Tear Advisory Panel
ITBV	intrathoracic blood volume
ITBVI	intrathoracic blood volume index
IV	intravenous
IVC	inferior vena cava
JVP	jugular venous pressure

KDIGO	Kidney Diseases Improving Global Outcomes		**NEWS**	National Early Warning Score
KT	knowledge translation		**NFR**	not for resuscitation
LAD	left anterior descending		**NGAL**	neutrophil gelatinase-associated lipocalin
LAP	left atrial pressure		**NHMRC**	National Health and Medical Research Council
LBBB	left bundle branch block		**NHPPD**	nursing hours per patient day
LMA	laryngeal mask airway		**NHS**	National Health Service (UK)
LMICs	low- and middle-income countries		**NICE**	National Institute for Health and Care Excellence (UK)
LOS	length of stay		**NICU**	neonatal intensive care unit
LP	lumbar puncture		**NIPPV**	non-invasive positive pressure ventilation
LSD	lysergic acid diethylamide		**NIPSV**	non-invasive pressure support ventilation
LV	left ventricle		**NIPT**	non-invasive prenatal testing
LVAD	left ventricular assist device		**NIV**	non-invasive ventilation
LVEDV	left ventricular end-diastolic volume (preload)		**NMBA**	Nursing and Midwifery Board of Australia
LVEF	left ventricular ejection fraction		**NMBA**	neuromuscular blockade agent
LVF	left ventricular failure		**NMES**	neuromuscular electrical stimulation
LVSWI	left ventricular stroke work index		**NO**	nitric oxide
MAP	mean arterial pressure		**NOC**	nurses' observation checklist
MARSI	medical adhesive-related skin injuries		**NP**	nurse practitioner
MASD	moisture-associated skin damage		**NPC**	nurse practice coordinator
MCS	mechanical circulatory support		**NPWT**	negative pressure wound therapy
MDR-TB	multi-drug-resistant TB		**NRT**	nicotine replacement therapy
MDT	multidisciplinary team		**NSAID**	non-steroidal anti-inflammatory drug
MELD	model of end-stage liver disease		**NTS**	National Triage Scale
MELD-NA	model of end-stage liver disease-sodium		**NTS**	non-technical skills
MERS	Middle East respiratory syndrome		**Nu-DESC**	Nursing DElirium Symptom Checklist
MERS-CoV	Middle East respiratory syndrome coronavirus		**NUM**	nursing unit manager
MET	medical emergency team		**NUTRIC**	NUTritional RIsk in the Critically ill score
MEWS	modified early warning score		O_2	oxygen
MI	myocardial infarction		**OECD**	Organisation for Economic Co-operation and Development
MIS-C	multisystem inflammatory syndrome in children		**ONS**	oral nutrition supplements
MI-E	mechanical insufflation: exsufflation		**OSA**	obstructive sleep apnoea
mmHg	millimetres of mercury		**OT**	operating theatre
MMP	matrix metalloproteinase		**OUD**	opioid use disorder
MoCA	Montreal Cognitive Assessment		ΔP	driving pressure
MODS	multiple organ dysfunction syndrome		*Pa*	arterial pressure
MP	mechanical power		*PA*	alveolar pressure
MRC	Medical Research Council		**PA**	phlebostatic axis
MRI	magnetic resonance imaging		**PA**	posterioanterior
MRO	multi-resistant organism		**PA**	*Pseudomonas aeruginosa*
MRSA	methicillin-resistant *Staphylococcus aureus*		**PAC**	pulmonary artery catheter
MSCT	multi-slice CT		$PaCO_2$	partial pressure of carbon dioxide in arterial blood
MTS	Manchester Triage Scale		**PACU**	post-anaesthesia care unit
MV	mechanical ventilation		PaO_2	partial pressure of oxygen in arterial blood
MV	minute ventilation		**PAOP**	pulmonary artery occlusion pressure
MVA/C	motor vehicle accident/collison		**PAP**	pulmonary artery pressure
MVE	Murray Valley encephalitis		**PAPR**	powered air purifying respirators
nAchR	nicotinic acetylcholine receptor		**PAT**	Paediatric Assessment Triangle
NAM	National Academy of Medicine		**PAV**	proportional assist ventilation
NAS	Nursing Activities Score		*Paw*	airway pressure
NASA-TLX	NASA Task Loading Index		**PAWSS**	Prediction of Alcohol Withdrawal Severity Scale
NAVA	neurally adjusted ventilatory assist		**PCA**	patient-controlled analgesia
NEMS	Nine Equivalents of nursing Manpower use Score		**PCI**	percutaneous coronary intervention
NETS	newborn emergency transfer service			

PCP	phencyclidine	**PVR**	pulmonary vascular resistance
PCR	polymerase chain reaction	**QD**	qualitative description
PCV	pressure-controlled ventilation	**QOL**	quality of life
PCWP	pulmonary capillary wedge pressure	**qSOFA**	quick Sequential Organ Failure Assessment
PD	peritoneal dialysis	**QTc**	corrected QT
PDSA	plan–do–study–act	**R**	respiration
PE	pulmonary embolism	**RAP**	right atrial pressure
PEA	pulseless electrical activity	**RASS**	Richmond Agitation Sedation Scale
PEEP	positive end-expiratory pressure	**RAT**	rapid antigen test
PELD	paediatric end-stage liver disease	**RBANS**	Repeatable Battery for the Assessment of
PER	passive external re-warming		Neuropsychological Status
PEST	political, economic, social, technical	**RBC**	red blood cell
PetCO$_2$	partial pressure of end-tidal carbon dioxide	**RCA**	right coronary artery
PEth	phosphatidylethanol	**RCA**	root cause analysis
PFIT	Physical Function ICU Test	**RCSQ**	Richards–Campbell Sleep Questionnaire
P/F ratio	ratio of PaO$_2$ to FiO$_2$	**RCT**	randomised controlled trial
PGD	primary graft dysfunction	**REBOA**	resuscitative endovascular balloon
pH	acid–alkaline logarithmic scale		occlusion of the aorta
PICC	peripherally inserted central venous catheter	**REE**	resting energy expenditure
PICO	population, intervention, comparator,	**REM**	rapid eye movement
	outcome	**RHD**	rheumatic heart disease
PiCCO	pulse-induced contour cardiac output	**RIFLE**	risk, injury, failure, and outcome criteria
PICS	post-intensive care syndrome		of loss and end-stage disease
PICS-F	post-intensive care syndrome – family	**RM**	recruitment manoeuvres
PICS-p	post-intensive care syndrome – paediatrics	**RN**	registered nurse
PICU	paediatric intensive care unit	**ROM**	range of motion
PICU-MAPS	paediatric intensive care unit	**ROMPIS**	Reaper Oral Mucosa Pressure Injury Scale
	Multidimensional Assessment Pain Scale	**ROSC**	return of spontaneous circulation
PIMS-TS	paediatric inflammatory multisystem	**ROTEM**	rotational thromboelastometry
	syndrome temporally associated with	**RR**	relative risk, risk ratio
	COVID-19	**RR**	respiratory rate
PIP	peak inspiratory pressure	**RRP**	relative refractory period
Pinsp	inspiratory pressure	**RRS**	rapid response system
PIRO	predisposition, infection, response, and	**RRT**	rapid response team
	organ failure (score)	**RRT**	renal replacement therapy
PMCS	perimortem caesarean section	**RSV**	respiratory syncytial virus
pMDI	pressurised metered-dose inhalers	**RV**	right ventricular
PMT	pacemaker-mediated tachycardia	**RVEDV**	right ventricular end-diastolic volume
PN	parenteral nutrition	**RVEDVI**	right ventricular end-diastolic volume index
PNS	peripheral nervous system	**RVEF**	right ventricular ejection fraction
POD	postoperative delirium	**RVESV**	right ventricular end-systolic volume
POUR	postoperative urinary retention	**RVF**	right ventricular failure
PP	prone positioning	**RVSWI**	right ventricular stroke work index
PPE	personal protective equipment	**SA**	sinoatrial node
PPH	postpartum haemorrhage	**SaO$_2$**	saturation of oxygen in arterial blood
PPI	proton pump inhibitors	**SAPS**	Simplified Acute Physiology Score
PPlat	plateau pressure	**SARS**	severe acute respiratory syndrome
PR	pulse rate	**SATS**	South African Triage Scale
PRISMA	Preferred Reporting Items for Systematic	**SBP**	systolic blood pressure
	Reviews and Meta-Analyses	**SBS**	State Behavioural Scale
PS	pressure support	**SBT**	spontaneous breathing trial
PSG	polysomnography	**SCA**	sudden cardiac arrest
PSI	Pneumonia Severity Index	**SCD**	sudden cardiac death
PSV	pressure support ventilation	**SCI**	spinal cord injury
PTSD	post-traumatic stress disorder	**SCUF**	slow continuous ultrafiltration
PTSS	post-traumatic stress symptoms	**SD**	standard deviation
PV	per vagina	**SEIPS**	Systems Engineering Initiative for Patient
Pv	venous pressure		Safety

SGA	supraglottic airway
SGLT2	sodium–glucose cotransporter-2
SIADH	syndrome of inappropriate antidiuretic hormone
SIMV	synchronised intermittent mandatory ventilation
SIRS	systemic inflammatory response syndrome
SLED	slow low-efficiency dialysis
SLTx	single lung transplantation
SNS	sympathetic nervous system
SOFA	sequential organ failure assessment
SOMANZ	Society of Obstetric Medicine of Australia and New Zealand
SOS-PD	Sophia Observation withdrawal Symptoms-Paediatric Delirium
SpO_2	saturation of oxygen in peripheral tissues
SR	sinus rhythm
SSD	subglottic secretion drainage
SSRI	selective serotonin reuptake inhibitors
ST	sinus tachycardia
STEMI	ST-elevation myocardial infarction
SUP-ICU	stress ulcer prophylaxis in the intensive care unit
SV	stroke volume
SVG	saphenous vein graft
SvO_2	saturation of oxygen in venous system
SVR	systemic vascular resistance
SVT	supraventricular tachycardia
SWAN	Subjective Workload Assessment for Nurses
SWOT	strengths, weaknesses, opportunities, threats
SWS	slow wave sleep
TAD	thoracic aortic dissection
TAP	transverse abdominis plane
TAP	treatment action plan
TBI	traumatic brain injury
TBSA	total body (or burn) surface area
TBW	total body weight
TdP	torsades de pointes
TEAM	treatment with early activity and mobilisation
TEG	thromboelastograph
TEVAR	thoracic endovascular aortic repair
TIA	trans-ischaemic attack
TICS-M	Telephone Interview of Cognitive Status – Modified version
TIPSS	transjugular intrahepatic portosystemic shunt/stent
TISS	Therapeutic Intervention Scoring System
TNF-α	tumour necrosis factor alpha
TOE	transoesophageal echocardiography
TRALI	transfusion–related acute lung injury
TST	total sleep time
TTE	transthoracic echocardiography
TURP	transurethral resection of the prostate
UK	United Kingdom
URTI	upper respiratory tract infection
USA	United States of America
VA	venoarterial
VAD	ventricular assist device
VAD	voluntary assisted dying
VAE	ventilator-associated event
VAP	ventilator-associated pneumonia
VAS	visual analogue scale
VAS-A	visual analogue scale – anxiety
VATS	video-assisted thorascopic surgery
VCA	vascularised composite allotransplantation
VCV	volume-controlled ventilation
VE	expired minute volume
VEES	videoendoscopic swallowing study
VF	ventricular fibrillation
VILI	ventilator-induced lung injury
V/Q	ventilation/perfusion
VRE	vancomycin-resistant enterococci
V_T	tidal volume
VT	ventricular tachycardia
VTE	venous thromboembolism
VV	venovenous
VVIR	Ventricular pacing, Ventricular activity, Inhibiting pacing, Rate responsiveness
VOO	Ventricular pacing, no (O) sensing capability, no (O) capability to respond
WAT-1	Withdrawal Assessment Tool
WBC	white blood cell
WBCT	whole-body CT
WEST	Western Association for the Surgery of Trauma
WCC	white cell count
WFCCN	World Federation of Critical Care Nurses
WFSICCM	World Federation of Societies of Intensive and Critical Care Medicine
WHO	World Health Organization
WHODAS 2.0	World Health Organization Disability Assessment Scale 2.0
WSACS	World Society of Abdominal Compartment Syndrome

Scope of critical care

Chapter 1

Scope of critical care practice

Leanne Aitken, Andrea Marshall, Thomas Buckley

Learning objectives

After reading this chapter you should be able to:

- discuss the influences on the development of critical care nursing as a discipline and the professional development of individual nurses
- discuss the education and professional development of critical care nurses
- outline the various roles available to nurses within critical care areas or in outreach services and examine how these roles influence the standard of care
- discuss the role of research in the development of critical care nursing, including strategies to achieve evidence-based practice
- analyse the leadership attributes and strategies that are likely to be effective in the critical care practice setting.

Introduction

For over 50 years, critical care services have been supporting the sickest of patients and today they are available in most countries in the world.[1] Although the focus was originally at local, regional and national levels, there is now an imperative for a strong international focus for the delivery of critical care services. National and international collaborations are necessary for responding to events that result in a sudden increased need for critical care services, including pandemics and disasters.[2,3] This need has been witnessed during the worldwide response to the COVID-19 pandemic more than ever before.[4,5] The term 'critical care' is used in different ways in different contexts; although critical care can be considered to include practice in the emergency department in some contexts, in this text we are primarily focusing on practice in intensive care (including all specialties) and coronary care settings.

There is unprecedented demand for critical care services globally. Increasing population sizes, extended life expectancies and disease patterns mean that the projected need for critical care beds will continue to increase.[6] The effect of limited intensive care unit (ICU) bed capacity has been witnessed over the past 2 years during the COVID-19 pandemic, with evidence that strain on ICU bed capacity affects hospital mortality rates.[7] The number of critical care nurses available has been noted as the primary limiting factor in bed availability.[8]

The number of ICU beds available varies between countries. When considering only Organisation for Economic Co-operation and Development (OECD) countries, a range of 3.3 beds per 100,000 population in Mexico up to 33.9 beds per 100,000 in Germany has been reported (https://www.oecd.org/coronavirus/en/data-insights/intensive-care-beds-capacity). Similar data related to non-OECD countries are not available, but it is recognised far fewer resources exist. These figures frequently do not include patients admitted to coronary care, paediatric or other specialty units, so the overall clinical activity for 'critical care' is much higher in many countries.

Survival in critically ill patients is high, with approximately 80% of patients surviving to be discharged out of acute hospital,[9] although this figure has reduced to between 60 and 70% during the COVID-19 pandemic.[10] Importantly, critical care treatment is a high-expense component of hospital care. Various cost estimates have been conducted, with European costs estimated to be between €1000 and €1500 per day for direct ICU costs,[11] and with slightly higher costs reported in the USA at US$2636 per ICU day.[12] Approximately two-thirds of daily costs are for staff, with the remainder spread between clinical consumables, diagnostic procedures, hotel and nutritional costs.[13] In developing countries such as India the daily cost of ICU is substantially less (approximately US$200 per day),[14] although this continues to represent a substantial cost relative to the cost of living. The true cost of critical care is, however, difficult to compare because there is no internationally agreed methodology, there is a wide variation in resource consumption by patients in different settings, and there are different models of care. Further, survivors of critical illness continue to require healthcare resources at a higher rate than non-critically ill hospitalised patients for up to 5 years, and this ongoing cost to individuals and the healthcare system is not always recognised.[15]

This chapter provides a context for subsequent chapters, outlining some key principles and concepts for studying and practising nursing in a range of critical care areas. Development of the specialty is discussed, along with the professional development and evolving roles of critical care nurses in contemporary healthcare. The scope of critical care nursing is described including advanced practice roles and, specifically, the nurse practitioner role. Leadership, as it pertains to the practice and development of critical care nursing, is also reviewed.

Critical care nursing

Critical care as a specialty in nursing has developed significantly since its inception.[16] Importantly, the development of the specialty has occurred alongside intensive care medicine as a defined clinical specialty.[17]

Critical care nursing is defined by the World Federation of Critical Care Nurses as:

> *Specialised nursing care of critically ill patients who have manifest or potential disturbances of vital organ functions and who need assistance, support and restoration to health or the delivery of pain management preparation for a dignified death.*[18]

Critically ill patients are those at high risk of actual or potential life-threatening health problems and may be cared for in a number of different locations in the hospital. Broadly, the term critical care is generally considered to incorporate subspecialty areas of emergency, coronary care, high-dependency, cardiothoracic, paediatric, surgical, neurological and general intensive care units.

Developing critical care nursing knowledge and practice

Critical care as a specialty emerged in the 1950s and 1960s in Australasia, North America, Europe and South Africa.[16,19-22] During these early stages, critical care consisted primarily of coronary care units for the care of cardiology patients, cardiothoracic units for the care of postoperative patients, and general intensive care units for the care of patients with respiratory compromise. Later developments in renal, metabolic and neurological management led to the principles and context of critical care that exist today, and technological advances in critical care have continued to require expanded nursing knowledge, skills and critical thinking.[23]

The role of adequately educated and experienced nurses in these units was recognised as essential from an early stage,[22] and led to the development of the nursing specialty of critical care. Today, evidence-based workforce standards have been identified and adherence to these can have a positive impact on patient outcome.[24] In Australia, standards are specifically set to address case mix and unit design; nursing knowledge, education, skills and qualifications; support for bedside nurses, equipment and specialist roles, such as the liaison nurse and nurse researcher in relation to workforce requirements.[25]

As the practice of critical care nursing evolved, so too have the associated areas of critical care education and specialty professional organisations, of which there are over 50 from across six continents.[26] The combination of adequate nurse staffing, observation of the patient and the expertise of nurses to consider the complete needs of patients and their families is essential to optimise the outcomes of critical care. As critical care continues to evolve, the challenge remains to combine excellence in nursing care with judicious use of technology to optimise patient and family outcomes.

Research

Research is fundamental to the development of nursing knowledge and practice. Research is a systematic inquiry using structured methods to understand an issue, solve a problem or refine existing knowledge. *Qualitative research* involves in-depth examination of a phenomenon of interest, typically using interviews, observation or document analysis, to build knowledge and enable depth of understanding. Qualitative data analysis is in narrative (text) form and involves some form of content or thematic analysis, with findings generally reported as narrative (words rather than numbers describe the research findings). In contrast, *quantitative research* involves the measurement (in numeric form) of variables of interest and the use of statistics to test hypotheses. Results of quantitative research are often reported in tables and figures, identifying statistically significant findings. One particular type of quantitative research, the randomised controlled trial (RCT), is used to test the effect of a new nursing intervention on patient outcomes. In essence, RCTs involve:

1 randomly allocating patients to receive either a new intervention (the experimental or intervention group), or an alternative or standard intervention (the control group)

2 delivering the intervention or alternative treatment measuring an a priori identified patient outcome

3 statistical analyses are used to determine whether the new intervention is better for patients than the alternative treatment.

Mixed methods research has now emerged as an approach that integrates data from qualitative and quantitative research at some stage in the research process.[27] In mixed-method approaches, researchers decide on both the priority and sequence of qualitative and quantitative methods. In terms of priority, equal status may be given to both approaches. Priority is indicated by using capital letters for the dominant approach, followed by the symbols + and → to indicate either concurrent or sequential data collection, for example:

- QUAL + QUANT: both approaches are given equal status and data collection occurs concurrently.

- QUAL + quant: qualitative methods are the dominant approach and data collection occurs concurrently.

- QUAL → quant: the qualitative study is given priority and qualitative data collection will occur before quantitative data collection.

There are other mixed-methods classifications used. For example, Pluye and Hong[28] describe terms such as sequential exploratory, sequential explanatory and convergent mixed methods designs. For more details, refer to their publication.

Irrespective of which type of research design is used, there are several common steps in the research process (Table 1.1), consisting of three phases: planning for the research, undertaking the research, and analysing and reporting the research findings.

While not all nurses are expected to conduct research, it is a professional responsibility to use research in practice.[29] Each chapter in this text contains a critical care research critique to assist nurses in developing critical appraisal skills, which will help to determine whether research evidence should change practice.

Evidence-based nursing

Evidence-based practice (EBP) involves explicitly using good judgement in the integration of high-quality research in nursing practice, taking into consideration patient values, clinical expertise and the strength of the evidence when making clinical decisions.[30] Research evidence, however, is only one of four considerations in making a clinical decision. Three other considerations include: (1) knowledge of patients' conditions (i.e. preferences and symptoms); (2) the nurses' clinical expertise and judgement; and (3) the context in which the decision is taking place (i.e. setting, resources). Fig. 1.1 provides a schematic representation of evidence-based nursing, using an example of a decision about weaning a patient from a mechanical ventilator. EBP has emerged as a way to improve nursing practice by considering the care that nurses give to patients, and whether this care results in the best possible outcomes for patients. Over the past few decades, recognition has emerged that EBP is more complex than simply focusing on knowledge to inform clinical decision making. This has led to a focus on better understanding about the challenges in changing clinical practice in order to use this evidence including approaches to teaching EBP,[31] competencies[32] and the importance of nursing leadership in promoting and sustaining EBP.[33] As a result, knowledge translation has emerged as a means to bridge the evidence–practice gap.

Knowledge translation

Clinicians, quality improvers and researchers have identified that, despite high-quality evidence, it is very difficult to get this evidence into practice (i.e. change clinicians' behaviour). As a result of this, knowledge translation (KT) and implementation science have developed as approaches to research and practice to try to guide this process. KT has been defined by the Canadian Institutes of Health Research as a dynamic and iterative process that includes the synthesis, dissemination, exchange and ethically sound application of knowledge to improve health, provide more effective health services and products, and strengthen the healthcare system.[34] This definition has been widely adopted including by the World Health Organization. KT is recognised as integral to incorporate evidence into clinical practice. Some authors distinguish between KT and implementation science, the latter having been defined as the scientific study of methods to promote the systematic uptake of research findings and other evidence-based practices into routine practice, and hence to improve the quality and effectiveness of health services and care.[35] Thus, KT is often viewed as the process used to bridge the evidence–practice gap, and implementation science is viewed as the formal study of how this can be done.

TABLE 1.1

Steps in the research process

PHASE	STEP	DESCRIPTION
Planning the research	Identify a clinical problem or issue	Clinical experience and practice audits are two ways that clinical issues or problems can be identified.
	Review the literature	A comprehensive literature review is vital to ensure that the issue or problem has not yet been solved and that the proposed research builds on what is already known, and extends it to fill a gap in knowledge.
	Develop a clear research question	A precise question may follow either of two approaches: 1 PICO (population, intervention, comparator, outcome) 2 SPIDER (sample, phenomenon of interest, design, evaluation, research type).
	Write a research proposal	Write a clear description of the proposed research design and sample and a plan for data collection and analysis. Ethical considerations and the required resources (i.e. budget and personnel) for the research should be identified.
	Secure resources	Resources such as funding for supplies and research staff, institutional support and access to experienced researchers are needed to ensure a study can be completed. Plans for how to access the relevant type and number of study participants should also be considered.
	Obtain ethics and governance approvals	Approval of the proposed research by a human research ethics committee (HREC) is required before the study can commence. Some jurisdictions also require institutional governance approval.
Undertaking the research	Conduct the research	Adequate time for recruitment of participants, data collection and analysis are crucial to ensure that valid and relevant data are obtained.
Analysing and reporting the research	Data analysis	Ensure the analyst has the appropriate skills to conduct the analysis. The data analysis plan developed in the first phase (write the research proposal) should be followed. If there are deviations, there should be a clear rationale for these deviations.
	Disseminate the research findings	Discussion of the results and implications for practice with clinicians within the study site should occur as soon as possible. Distribution of a brief summary of the results is also frequently provided to study participants. Conference presentations and journal publications are two additional ways that research findings are disseminated and are vital to ensure that both nursing practice and nursing knowledge continue to be developed.

Over the past 10–15 years, there has been a plethora of theories, models and frameworks developed to guide KT[36] and these can be used to help guide, understand or explain the translation of research evidence (or other knowledge) into practice.[37] Some have come from disciplines such as psychology, sociology and marketing, while others have been developed by researchers focusing their work on KT and implementation science. Using structured approaches to implementing clinical practice change is important for both success and sustainability of the new practice. Effectively facilitating implementation and knowledge translation requires capacity building of clinical staff; however, few formal training programs in this area currently exist.[38] An example approach is provided in Table 1.2.[39]

Education

Appropriate preparation of specialist critical care nurses is a vital component in providing quality care to patients and their families. A central tenet within this framework

FIGURE 1.1 Schematic representation of evidence-based nursing including an example of weaning from mechanical ventilation.

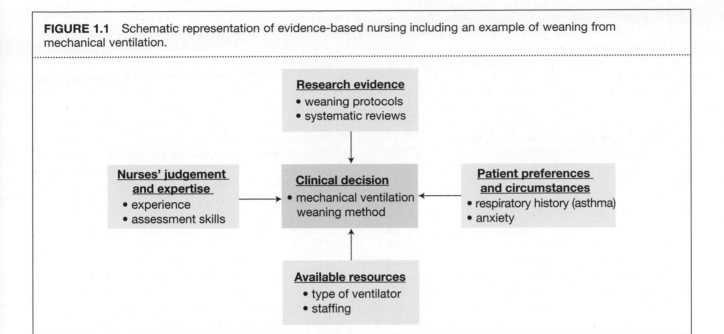

TABLE 1.2

Steps for developing a theory-informed implementation intervention[39]

STEP	TASKS
STEP 1: Who needs to do what differently?	• Identify the evidence–practice gap. • Specify the behaviour change needed to reduce the evidence–practice gap. • Specify the health professional group in which behaviour needs changing.
STEP 2: Using a theoretical framework, which barriers and enablers need to be addressed?	• From the literature, and experience of the development team, select which theory(ies), or theoretical framework(s) are likely to inform the pathways of change. • Use the chosen theory(ies), or framework, to inform the pathways of change and the possible barriers and enablers to that pathway. • Use qualitative and/or quantitative methods to identify barriers and enablers to behaviour change.
STEP 3: Which intervention components (behaviour change techniques and model(s) of delivery) could overcome the modifiable barriers and enhance the enablers?	• Use the chosen theory, or framework, to identify potential behaviour change techniques to overcome the barriers and enhance the enablers. • Identify evidence to inform the selection of potential behaviour change techniques and modes of delivery. • Identify what is likely to be feasible, locally relevant and acceptable, and combine identified components into an acceptable intervention that can be delivered.
STEP 4: How can behaviour change be measured and understood?	• Identify mediators of change to investigate in the proposed pathways of change. • Select appropriate outcome measures. • Determine feasibility of outcomes to be measured.

Source: Reproduced with permission from French SD, Green SE, O'Connor DA, et al. Developing theory-informed behaviour change interventions to implement evidence into practice: a systematic approach using the Theoretical Domains Framework. Implement Sci 2012;7(1):38. doi: 10.1186/1748-5908-7-38.

of preparation is the formalised education of nurses to practise in critical care areas.[40] Formal education – in conjunction with experiential learning, continuing professional development and training and reflective clinical practice – is required to develop competence in critical care nursing, although how this is achieved across different international contexts is inconsistent and not well understood.[41] The knowledge, skills and attitude necessary for quality critical care nursing practice have been articulated in competency statements[42–46] and within certification processes that recognise the knowledge and expertise of critical care nurses.[47,48]

Critical care nursing education developed in unison with the advent of specialist critical care units. Initially, this consisted of ad hoc training developed and delivered in the work setting, with nurses and medical officers learning together. For example, medical staff brought expertise in physiology, pathophysiology and interpretation of electrocardiographic rhythm strips, while nurses brought expertise in patient care and how patients behaved and responded to treatment.[49] Formalised, post-registration critical care nursing courses were subsequently developed from the early 1960s in both Australasia and the UK.[16,22] Today there are a number of different approaches to educating critical care nurses. Workplace learning can be facilitated through transition programs designed to provide support for newly graduate or novice nurses who may be working in critical care settings.[50] In some countries, education is provided in universities at a postgraduate level,[41] while, in others, self-directed learning is formally assessed through an accreditation and examination process such as the Critical Care Registered Nurse (CCRN) exam offered by the American Association of Critical Care Nurses.[47] Although variability within these programs is recognised, many incorporate clinical components and are conducted in conjunction with healthcare providers.

The diversity of critical care programs internationally has led to significant variability in programs and outcomes.[41] The recent development of the Standard of Practice and Evaluation of Critical-Care-Nursing Tool (SPECT) may be one strategy for assessing outcomes of critical care programs internationally by means of standardising minimum criteria for critical care qualifications,[51] although further international validation of this tool is required.

In more recent times, education in critical care nursing practice has focused on targeted education programs to prepare a critical care workforce that was rapidly expanding in response to the coronavirus disease 2019 (COVID-19) pandemic.[52] There was also a need to rapidly educate existing critical care nurses regarding the disease and the rapidly evolving treatment strategies, with multidisciplinary education frequently featuring in recommendations for preparing for and managing a pandemic response.[53,54]

The intent of critical care specific education programs for nurses is to improve outcomes for critically ill patients and their families; yet, to date, consumer consultation to inform curricula development has been rare.[55] Both the impact of post-registration education on practice and the most appropriate level of education that is required to underpin specialty practice remain controversial, with no universal acceptance internationally.[41] Globally, the Declaration of Madrid, which was endorsed by the World Federation of Critical Care Nurses, provides a baseline for critical care nursing education. Originally developed in 1993 and subsequently updated in 2005 and again in 2020, the Declaration of Madrid presents guidelines accepted worldwide by critical care professionals to guide education of critical care nurses. The central principles underpinning the Declaration of Madrid are provided in Table 1.3.[56]

A range of factors continue to influence critical care nursing education provision, including government policies at national and state levels, funding mechanisms and resource implications for organisations and individual students, education provider and healthcare sector partnership arrangements, and tensions between workforce and professional development needs.[41,57]

Continuing education for critical care nurses is an imperative to maintaining high-quality clinical care. Innovations in health professional education such as interprofessional and interdisciplinary learning, simulated learning[58] and use of innovative technologies including social media[59] are strategies to consider in the delivery of ongoing education to critical care nurses. The advances in technology and normalisation of online learning, communication and information sharing during the pandemic has resulted in a wide range of online learning resources which are easily accessible, allow for tailored independent learning and allow flexibility of access. One example is Continulus (https://www.continulus.com), an online learning platform featuring some of the world's leading experts in critical care nursing and practice that supports education through freely accessible lectures.

Specialist critical care competencies

Critical care nursing involves a range of skills, classified as psychomotor (or technical), cognitive or interpersonal and performance of these skills requires special training and practice to enable proficiency. Clinical competence is a combination of personal traits, professional clinical practice, legal and ethical practice, ensuring safety and quality, communication, management of nursing care, leadership, teaching–coaching, cooperation and therapeutics practice, critical thinking and innovation, and professional development.[60] Although the concepts of competence are broad, they do need to be applied to the specific context in which the nurse is working.[61] Assessing the level of competency of a critical care nurse is challenging, although ways of measuring competency are being explored.[62] All elements comprising the notion of competence are equally important in promoting quality critical care nursing practice.

Worldwide there are a number of practice standards published which are specific to critical care nursing.[43–46]

TABLE 1.3
Central principles underpinning the provision of critical care nurse education[56]

PRINCIPLE	DESCRIPTION
1	Critically ill patients and families have the right to receive individualised, evidence-based critical care from qualified professionally registered nurses.
2	Critical care registered nurses must possess advanced knowledge and skills to effectively meet the needs of critically ill patients.
3	Basic nursing education programs do not typically include advanced theory and practice curriculum related to the specialised knowledge required of critical care nurses. Access to initial and ongoing professional development opportunities must be provided to registered nurses responsible for the care of critically ill patients and their families.
4	Registered nurses with specialised knowledge and expertise in the provision of care to critically ill patients should play an integral part in the education and preparation of critical care nurses.
5	The preparation of critical care nurses must be accessible, evidence based and include a sufficient experiential component (e.g. high-fidelity simulation and preceptorship in the critical care unit).
6	Professional certification or postgraduate qualification in critical care nursing is recommended and demonstrates achievement of specialised knowledge that meets national and international standards required for delivery of the safest nursing care to critically ill patients.

Most practice standards build upon respective national registered nurse entry-to-practice standards[41] and, although there are some differences in approaches, the common tenet of each set of practice standards is the goal of promoting the delivery of quality care to critically ill patients and their family. Common elements include patient- and family-focused care, recognition of scope of practice and reflection, professional development, planning of care, leadership and evidence-based practice.[41]

Professional organisations

Professional leadership of critical care nursing has undergone considerable development in the past three decades. On an international level, the World Federation of Critical Care Nurses (WFCCN) was formed in 2001 to provide professional leadership for the specialty, so as to strengthen the influence and contribution that critical care nurses make globally through improved nursing practice.[18] Professional bodies that represent critical care nurses around the world are eligible to join the WFCCN. The role of the WFCCN is supported by regional bodies such as those that exist in Europe, South America, Asia and Africa.

At the country level, more than 40 organisations exist to represent the interests of critical care nurses through improving education, communication and professional standards. The first of these professional organisations was formed in 1969 in the USA with the formation of the American Association of Cardiovascular Nurses, which, 2 years later, changed its name to the Association of Critical-Care Nurses (AACN).[63]

Within Australia, the Australian College of Critical Care Nurses (ACCCN, formerly the Confederation of Australian Critical Care Nurses) was formed from a number of preceding state-based specialty nursing bodies (e.g. the Australian Society of Critical Care Nurses, the Clinical Nurse Specialists Association) that had provided professional leadership for critical care nurses since the early 1970s. Similar organisations that have been formed for many years include the British Association of Critical Care Nurses (BACCN) and the Canadian Association of Critical Care Nurses, (CACCN).

The professional bodies that exist to represent critical care nurses also have strong links with professional bodies representing their medical and allied health colleagues, including the World Federation of Societies of Intensive and Critical Care Medicine (WFSICCM) and various regional and country specific bodies. (See Online resources for further details about professional bodies and activities.)

Advanced practice nursing

The concept of advanced practice nursing has been developing for over three decades with considerable debate, which at times highlights the lack of clarity or confusion around the term used to describe practice or roles at an advanced level. In the revised Nurse practitioner standards for practice published by the Nursing and Midwifery Board of Australia in 2021, advanced practice was defined as:

where nurses incorporate professional leadership, education, research and support of systems into their practice. Their practice includes relevant expertise, critical thinking, complex decision-making, autonomous practice and is effective and safe. They work within a generalist or specialist context and they are responsible and accountable in managing people who have complex healthcare requirements. Advanced practice in nursing is demonstrated by a level of practice and not by a job title or level of remuneration.[64]

The International Council of Nurses, Guidelines on Advanced Practice Nursing 2020 defines an advanced practice nurse as: *'One who has acquired, through additional education, the expert knowledge base, complex decision-making skills and clinical competencies for expanded nursing practice, the characteristics of which are shaped by the context in which they are credentialed to practice'.*[65]

The ICN notes that the education of nurse practitioners/advanced practice nurses is at an advanced level and is accredited or approved, with some form of licensure, registration, certification or credentialling.

The ICN describes the nature of practice of nurse practitioners/advanced practice nurses as including a high degree of autonomy and independent practice.[65] While the ICN acknowledges country specific regulation, it suggests nurse practitioners/advanced practice nurses will be able to diagnose, prescribe medications and treatments, refer clients to other health professionals and admit patients to hospital. Skills such as advanced health assessment and decision making are required.

In response to the revised ICN advanced practice guidelines, in 2021 the ACCCN released a position statement on advanced practice in critical care,[66] which states that nurses working at an advanced practice level in critical care:

- are registered nurses providing safe and competent patient care to critical or potentially critically ill patients
- have roles or levels of practice which require formal education in critical care nursing beyond the preparation of the registered nurse (minimum required level is a Master's degree or equivalent)
- have roles or levels of practice with increased levels of competency and capability that are measurable, beyond that expected of the specialist critical care nurse
- demonstrate advanced clinical expertise, competency in leadership and facilitate translation of research to practice
- have acquired the ability to explain and apply the theoretical, empirical, ethical, legal and professional development required for advanced practice nursing
- have defined competencies and standards which are periodically reviewed for maintaining currency in practice, and
- are influenced by the global, social, political, economic and technological milieu.

Nurse practitioners

There is a growing body of research on the nurse practitioner (NP) role, which is generally distinguished by the authority right to diagnose, prescribe medications and treatments, refer clients to other health professionals and in some contexts admit patients to hospital. In Australia, standards for practice for NPs came into effect in 2014, and were most recently updated in 2021.[64] These standards encompass assessment using diagnostic capabilities, planning of care and engaging others in this planning, prescribing and implementing therapeutic interventions and supporting health systems.[64] In addition to the requirements for defining advanced practice among all nurses, the NMBA state that *'Advanced practice for the purpose of the nurse practitioner endorsement requires 5,000 hours of clinically-based advanced practice in the past six years'*,[64] reflective of the mandatory requirements for endorsement as a NP in the Australian context, where the title 'Nurse Practitioner' is a legislatively protected title, similar to other countries such as Canada and the USA.

Leadership in critical care nursing

Effective leadership within critical care nursing is essential at several organisational levels, including the unit and hospital levels, as well as within the specialty on a broader professional scale. The leadership required at any given time and in any specific setting reflects the surrounding environment and the prevailing culture. Regardless of the setting, effective leadership involves having and communicating a clear vision – particularly one that represents excellence, motivating a team to achieve a common goal, communicating effectively with others, being approachable, good decision making, role modelling, meaningful recognition, creating and sustaining the critical elements of a healthy work environment, and implementing change and innovation.[67,68] Many of these same characteristics have been described as essential during the recent COVID-19 pandemic,[69] with additional desirable characteristics including presence, transparency and empathy.[70]

Leadership at the unit and hospital levels is essential to ensure excellence in practice, retention of a skilled and satisfied body of staff and adequate clinical governance. In addition to the generic strategies described above, it is essential for leaders in critical care units and hospitals to demonstrate a patient focus, establish and maintain excellence in standards of practice, and foster collaboration with other members of the multidisciplinary healthcare team. There is also recognition of the need for clinical leaders to have strong knowledge of the evidence base, and to use that knowledge to inform decisions and practices within the clinical environment.[71]

Leadership is essential to achieve growth and development in our specialty and is demonstrated through such activities as conducting research, producing publications, delivering conference presentations, representation on relevant government and healthcare councils and committees, and participation in organisations such as the WFCCN, ACCCN, BACCN, AACN and the European federation of Critical Care Nursing associations (EfCCNa). As outlined earlier, we have seen the field of critical care grow in the course of a generation from early ideas and makeshift units to a well-developed and highly organised international specialty able to deal with a dramatic pandemic. Such development would not have been possible without the vision, enthusiasm and commitment of many critical care leaders throughout the world.

Leadership styles vary and are influenced by the mission and values of the organisation as well as the values and beliefs of individual leaders. These styles of leadership are described in many different ways, sometimes by using theoretical underpinnings such as 'transactional' and 'transformational' and sometimes by using leadership values and characteristics. More recently, 'authentic leadership' has been described as developing from transformational leadership and it particularly focuses on the personal characteristics of a leader.[72] Regardless of the terminology in use, some common principles can be expressed. Desired leadership characteristics include the ability to:

- articulate a personal vision and expectations
- inspire a shared vision that represents excellence
- act as a catalyst for change and be prepared to challenge the status quo
- establish and implement organisational standards
- model effective leadership behaviours through both change processes and stable contexts
- show interest for team well-being and take the time to discuss team concerns
- monitor practice in relation to standards and take corrective action when necessary
- recognise the characteristics and strengths of individuals, and stimulate and support individual development and commitment
- empower staff to act independently and interdependently.[67,73,74]

Personal characteristics of an effective leader, regardless of the style, include honesty, integrity, respect, commitment, credibility, courage, self-awareness and wisdom, as well as the ability to be approachable and supportive.[68,71] Effective leaders inspire their team members to take the extra step towards achieving the goals articulated by the leader and to feel that they are valued, independent, responsible and autonomous individuals within the organisation. Members of teams with effective leaders are not satisfied with maintaining the status quo, but believe in the vision and goals articulated by the leader and are prepared to work towards achieving a higher standard of practice.

Although all leaders share common characteristics, some elements vary according to leadership style. Different styles – for example, transactional, transformational, authoritative or laissez faire – incorporate different characteristics and activities. Having leaders with different styles or a range of strengths and characteristics ensures that there is leadership for all stages of an organisation's

operation or a profession's development. A combination of leadership styles also helps to overcome team member preferences and problems experienced when a particularly visionary leader leaves. The challenges often associated with the departure of a leader from a healthcare organisation are generally reduced in the clinical critical care environment, where a nursing leader is usually part of a multidisciplinary team, with resultant shared values and objectives.

Clinical leadership

Clinical leaders are those who provide leadership specifically within a clinical area; such leadership is an essential component of any effective team. It is generally accepted that effective clinical leaders require a combination of clinical expertise and leadership characteristics to perform this role to a high level.[75,76] Leadership characteristics that are considered particularly important for clinical leaders include creating a culture of collaboration, role modelling, good decision making and creating a work environment that is conducive to delivering the highest quality of care to patients and their family.[68,71,77] Clinical leaders may or may not have formal authority vested in them, but are ultimately responsible for the quality and safety of patient care that is delivered within their clinical area. It is therefore essential that clinical leaders work within an effective interdisciplinary model, so that all aspects of patient care and family support, as well as the needs of all staff, are met.[76,78] Effective clinical leadership of critical care is essential in achieving:

- effective and safe patient care
- high-quality, evidence-based healthcare
- satisfied patients and family members
- satisfied staff, with a high level of retention
- development of staff through an effective coaching and mentoring process.[71,79]

Effective clinical leaders build cohesive and adaptive work teams, and improve interdisciplinary collaboration.[78] They also promote the intellectual stimulation of individual staff members, which encourages the analysis and exploration of practice that is essential for evidence-based nursing.[79] We have witnessed how important effective clinical leadership is over the past 2 years of the COVID-19 pandemic, with the need for ongoing change and development essential. Throughout the development of critical care, we have witnessed significant changes in the organisation and delivery of care, with the development of new roles such as the nurse practitioner (see this chapter) and liaison nurse (see Chapter 3), the introduction of services such as rapid response systems, including medical emergency teams (see Chapter 3) and the extension of activities across the care continuum (see Chapter 8). Effective clinical leadership ensures that:

- critical care personnel are aware of, and willing to fulfil, their changing roles

- personnel in other areas of the hospital or outside the hospital recognise the benefits and limitations of developments, are not threatened by the developments and are enthusiastic to use the new or refined services provided by critical care
- staff are satisfied in their work setting, improving staff retention and reducing the need for high levels of staff turnover and the challenges associated with orientating large numbers of new staff
- patients receive optimal quality of care.[80,81]

The need to provide educational opportunities to develop effective clinical leadership skills is recognised. A range of programs that focus on personal development, teamwork and leadership skills development are available, with evaluation suggesting that essential characteristics of these programs include team-based approaches to improve clinical leadership competencies.[82] These programs might be delivered within the clinical environment and in partnership with higher education institutions. Factors that influence leadership ability include the external and internal environment, demographic characteristics such as age, experience, understanding, stage of personal development including self-awareness capability and communication skills.[67,83] In relation to clinical leadership, at least some of the development of these factors must be in a clinical setting, so the development of clinical leaders should be based in that environment. Development programs based on mentorship, with strong academic support, are superbly suited to developing those that demonstrate potential for such capabilities.[84,85]

Mentorship has received significant attention in the healthcare literature and has been specifically identified as a strategy for clinical leadership development.[84,85] Although many different definitions of mentoring exist, common principles include a relationship between two people that incorporates mutual sharing, learning and acquisition of knowledge, usually for the purpose of helping one person in the relationship to develop new skills related to their career. A related process might also be referred to as coaching.[84] Mentoring programs can be either formal or informal and either internal or external to the work setting. Mentorship involves a variety of activities directed towards facilitating new learning experiences for the mentee, guiding professional development and career decisions, providing emotional and psychological support and assisting the mentee in the socialisation process both within and outside the work organisation to build professional knowledge and networks.[84,85] Role modelling of occupational and professional skills and characteristics is an important component of mentoring that helps develop future clinical leaders.

Summary

This chapter has provided a context for subsequent chapters, outlining some key issues, principles and concepts for practising and studying nursing in a range of critical care areas. Critical care nursing now encompasses a broad and ever-expanding scope of practice. The previous focus on patients in an ICU only has given way to a broader concept of caring for an individual located in a variety of clinical locations across a continuum of critical illness.

The discipline of critical care nursing, in collaboration with multidisciplinary colleagues, continues to develop to meet the expanding challenges of clinical practice in today's healthcare environment. Critical care clinicians also continue their professional development individually, focusing on education and training and on practice improvement and research activities, to facilitate quality patient and family care during a time of acute physiological derangement and emotional turmoil. The principles of decision making and clinical leadership at all levels of practice serve to enhance patient safety in the critical care environment.

RESEARCH VIGNETTE

Kleinpell R, Grabenkort WR, Kapu A, et al. Nurse practitioners and physician assistants in acute and critical care: a concise review of the literature and data 2008–2018. Crit Care Med 2019;47(10):1442–9.

Abstract

Objectives: To provide a concise review of the literature and data pertaining to the use of NPs and physician assistants (PAs), collectively called advanced practice providers, in ICU and acute care settings.

Data sources: Detailed search strategy using the databases PubMed, Ovid MEDLINE and the Cumulative Index of Nursing and Allied Health Literature for the time period from January 2008 to December 2018.

Study selection: Studies addressing nurse practitioner, physician assistant or advanced practice provider care in the ICU or acute care setting.

Data extraction: Relevant studies were reviewed, and the following aspects of each study were identified, abstracted and analysed: study population, study design, study aims, methods, results and relevant implications for critical care practice.

Data synthesis: Five systematic reviews, four literature reviews and 44 individual studies were identified, reviewed and critiqued. Of the research studies, the majority were retrospective, with others being observational, quasi-experimental or quality improvement, along with two randomised control trials. Overall, the studies assessed a variety of effects of advanced practice provider care, including on length of stay, mortality and quality-related metrics, with a majority demonstrating similar or improved patient care outcomes.

Conclusions: Over the past 10 years, the number of studies assessing the impact of advanced practice providers in acute and critical care settings continue to increase. Collectively, these studies identify the value of advanced practice providers in patient care management, continuity of care, improved quality and safety metrics, patient and staff satisfaction, and on new areas of focus including enhanced educational experience of residents and fellows.

Critique

The role of the NP in the ICU environment has evolved greatly in the last decade and NPs now practise in many ICUs worldwide. The results of this literature review provide insights into the roles and outcomes associated with nurse practitioner practices in the ICU environment. Fifty-three English language publications originating from the United States of America, Canada, Australia, United Kingdom and Europe were included in the review, of which five were systematic reviews, four were literature reviews and 44 were individual research studies.

Studies highlighted the role of NPs and PAs in ICU, collectively referred to as advanced practice providers (APPs) in the review.

Comparison of APPs with resident/fellows or house staff, where similar patient mortality outcomes were reported, found that in several studies APP-led care was associated with lower length of stay, improved physician and nursing satisfaction, higher rates of discharge destinations to home, decreased emergency department time to transfer to ICU, decreased costs of care related to laboratory test use, decreased re-admission rates, increased discharges by noon, decreased costs of care for heart failure patients, and indirect economic and patient care impacts such as decreased time to the operating room and operative time, and decreased complications. The review highlights a number of studies reporting that the role that the APP is associated with improved quality of care, enhanced patient safety and greater continuity of care. Studies identified the impact of APP care on reducing UTI rates, increasing deep vein thrombosis prophylaxis rates, and early identification of patients with sepsis. Studies also reported that generally critical care physicians, residents and fellows were satisfied with the APP role and perceived that patient care was positively affected by APP care owing to continuity of care and enhanced communication with families. Interestingly, the APP role is reported to be associated with reductions in resident doctors' workload and enhanced medical trainee training.

Although the findings of this review report favourable outcomes related to APPs in ICUs, there are a few limitations that need to be considered. Many studies cited were either observational, pre–post design or retrospective comparisons so, therefore, were not controlling for potential confounders. Additionally, studies from the USA and Canada mostly did not report data on NP-led care separately from PA-led care, making it difficult to understand the models of care related to findings reported. However, despite these limitations, this review does offer insight into the past decade of research related to APPs in ICU and outcomes and, based on the results of the review, the authors proposed that APP positions should be further developed in such a way that their roles are accepted, understood and beneficial to patients.

Learning activities

1 As the nurse educator in an ICU, you have recently become aware of the high-quality research evidence for the benefits of early mobilisation of mechanically ventilated patients. But, in your unit, this does not occur. Describe a process you could use to try to bridge this evidence–practice gap.

2 Your hospital is expanding the number of NPs and the nursing leadership team has asked for you to identify a team who can develop a proposal for one position to be linked to the ICU. Who do you think should be on this team and how would you establish the value-add for this position?

3 Your mixed medical–surgical ICU has recently expanded the number of available beds and new staff members are currently being hired. Several of the new staff members have ICU experience in much smaller units where predominantly medical patients were admitted. As an intensive care nurse educator, what advice would you provide to support their ongoing professional development?

4 Observe the leaders within your critical care practice environment and reflect on the attributes they have and strategies they use to provide leadership to the team. Consider what you think are their strengths and how you could develop similar characteristics and abilities.

Online resources

American Association of Critical-Care Nurses, https://www.aacn.org

ANZICS/ACCCN Annual Scientific Meeting on Intensive Care, www.intensivecareasm.com.au

ANZICS Clinical Trials Group, www.anzics.com.au/clinical-trials-group

Australia and New Zealand Intensive Care Society, https://www.anzics.com.au

Australian College of Critical Care Nurses, www.acccn.com.au

British Association of Critical Care Nurses, baccn.org.uk

Canadian Association of Critical Care Nurses, https://caccn.ca

Canadian Critical Care Trials Group, https://www.ccctg.ca

College of Intensive Care Medicine (CICM), https://www.cicm.org.au

Continulus, https://www.continulus.com

European federation of Critical Care Nursing associations (EfCCNa), https://www.efccna.org/

European Society of Intensive Care Medicine, https://www.esicm.org

Intensive Care Foundation (Australia and New Zealand), https://www.intensivecarefoundation.org.au

Intensive Care National Audit and Research Centre, https://www.icnarc.org

Intensive Care Society, https://ics.ac.uk

Life in the FastLane, https://litfl.com

NHS Leadership Academy, The Healthcare Leadership Model, https://www.leadershipacademy.nhs.uk/resources/

New Zealand College of Critical Care Nurses, https://www.nzno.org.nz/groups/colleges_sections/colleges/new_zealand_college_of_critical_care_nurses

Scottish Intensive Care Society, https://www.scottishintensivecare.org.uk

World Federation of Critical Care Nurses, https://wfccn.org

World Federation of Societies of Intensive and Critical Care Medicine, https://www.world-critical-care.org

Further reading

Rapport F, Clay-Williams R, Braithwaite J, editors. Implementation science: the key concepts. Oxford: Routledge; 2022.

Paine N. Workplace learning. London: Kogan Page; 2019.

Greenhalgh TM, Bidewell J, Crisp E, et al., editors. Understanding research methods for evidence-based practice in health. 2nd ed. Chichester, UK: John Wiley and Sons; 2019.

References

1. Murthy S, Wunsch H. Clinical review: international comparisons in critical care – lessons learned. Crit Care 2012;16(2):218.

2. Sprung CL, Zimmerman JL, Christian MD, et al. Recommendations for intensive care unit and hospital preparations for an influenza epidemic or mass disaster: summary report of the European Society of Intensive Care Medicine's Task Force for intensive care unit triage during an influenza epidemic or mass disaster. Intensive Care Med 2010;36(3):428–43.

3. Devereaux AV, Tosh PK, Hick JL, et al. Engagement and education: care of the critically ill and injured during pandemics and disasters: CHEST consensus statement. Chest 2014;146(4 Suppl.):e118S–33S.

4. Dichter JR, Devereaux AV, Sprung CL, et al. Mass critical care surge response during COVID-19: implementation of contingency strategies – a preliminary report of findings from the task force for mass critical care. Chest 2022;161(2):429–47.

5. Al Mutair A, Amr A, Ambani Z, et al. Nursing surge capacity strategies for management of critically ill adults with COVID-19. Nurs Rep 2020;10(1):23–32.

6. Rhodes A, Moreno RP. Intensive care provision: a global problem. Rev Bras Ter Intensiva 2012;24(4):322–5.

7. Wilcox ME, Rowan KM, Harrison DA, et al. Does unprecedented ICU capacity strain, as experienced during the COVID-19 pandemic, impact patient outcome? Crit Care Med 2022;50(6):e548–56.

8. Litton E, Huckson S, Chavan S, et al. Increasing ICU capacity to accommodate higher demand during the COVID-19 pandemic. Med J Aust 2021;215(11):513–17.

9. Intensive Care National Audit & Research Centre (ICNARC). Key statistics from the Case Mix Programme: 1 April 2019 to 31 March 2020. London: ICNARC; 2020.

10. Intensive Care National Audit & Research Centre (ICNARC). ICNARC report on COVID-19 in critical care: England, Wales and Northern Ireland, 10 April 2022. London: ICNARC; 2022.

11. Kaier K, Heister T, Wolff J, et al. Mechanical ventilation and the daily cost of ICU care. BMC Health Serv Res 2020;20(1):267.

12. Gershengorn HB, Garland A, Gong MN. Patterns of daily costs differ for medical and surgical intensive care unit patients. Ann Am Thorac Soc 2015;12(12):1831–6.

13. Tan SS, Bakker J, Hoogendoorn ME, et al. Direct cost analysis of intensive care unit stay in four European countries: applying a standardized costing methodology. Value Health 2012;15(1):81–6.

14. Shweta K, Kumar S, Gupta AK, et al. Economic analysis of costs associated with a Respiratory Intensive Care Unit in a tertiary care teaching hospital in Northern India. Indian J Crit Care Med 2013;17(2):76–81.

15. Lone NI, Gillies MA, Haddow C, et al. Five-year mortality and hospital costs associated with surviving intensive care. Am J Respir Crit Care Med 2016;194(2):198–208.

16. Wiles V, Daffurn K. There's a bird in my hand and a bear by the bed – I must be in ICU. The pivotal years of Australian critical care nursing. Melbourne, VIC: Australian College of Critical Care Nurses; 2002.

17. Vincent JL, Shehabi Y, Walsh TS, et al. Comfort and patient-centred care without excessive sedation: the eCASH concept. Intensive Care Med 2016;42(6):962–71.

18. World Federation of Critical Care Nurses (WFCCN). Constitution of the World Federation of Critical Care Nurses. Brighton le Sands, NSW: WFCCN; 2016.

19. Prien T, Meyer J, Lawin P. Development of intensive care medicine in Germany. J Clin Anesth 1991;3(3):253–8.

20. Scribante J, Schmollgruber S, Nel E. Perspectives on critical care nursing: South Africa. Connect: The World of Critical Care Nursing 2005;3(4):111–15.

21. Grenvik A, Pinsky MR. Evolution of the intensive care unit as a clinical center and critical care medicine as a discipline. Crit Care Clin 2009;25(1):239–50, x.

22. Gordon IJ, Jones ES. The evolution and nursing history of a general intensive care unit (1962-1983). Intensive Crit Care Nurs 1998;14(5): 252–7.

23. Bellomo R, Stow PJ, Hart GK. Why is there such a difference in outcome between Australian intensive care units and others? Curr Opin Anesthesiol 2007;20(2):100–5.

24. Penoyer DA. Nurse staffing and patient outcomes in critical care: a concise review. Crit Care Med 2010;38(7):1521–8; quiz 1529.

25. Chamberlain D, Pollock W, Fulbrook P; Group AWSD. ACCCN Workforce standards for intensive care nursing: systematic and evidence review, development, and appraisal. Aust Crit Care 2018;31(5):292–302.

26. World Federation of Critical Care Nurses (WFCCN). Our current members. Brighton le Sands, NSW: WFCCN; 2022. Available from: https://wfccn.org/our-current-members/. [Accessed 10 February 2023].

27. Molina-Azorin JF, Fetters MD. Building a better world through mixed methods research. J Mixed Methods Res 2019;13(3):275–81.

28. Pluye P, Hong QN. Combining the power of stories and the power of numbers: mixed methods research and mixed studies reviews. Annu Rev Public Health 2014;35:29–45.

29. Melnyk BM, Gallagher-Ford L, Zellefrow C, et al. The First U.S. study on nurses' evidence-based practice competencies indicates major deficits that threaten healthcare quality, safety, and patient outcomes. Worldviews Evid Based Nurs 2018;15(1):16–25.

30. Christenbery TL. Nursing's commitment to best clinical decisions. In: Christenbery TL, editor. Evidence-based practice in nursing: foundations, skills and roles. New York: Springer; 2017, p. 3–20.

31. Wu Y, Brettle A, Zhou C, et al. Do educational interventions aimed at nurses to support the implementation of evidence-based practice improve patient outcomes? A systematic review. Nurse Educ Today 2018;70:109–14.

32. Saunders H, Gallagher-Ford L, Kvist T, et al. Practicing healthcare professionals' evidence-based practice competencies: an overview of systematic reviews. Worldviews Evid Based Nurs 2019;16(3):176–85.

33. Bianchi M, Bagnasco A, Bressan V, et al. A review of the role of nurse leadership in promoting and sustaining evidence-based practice. J Nurs Manag 2018;26(8):918–32.

34. Straus SE, Tetroe J, Graham I. Defining knowledge translation. CMAJ 2009;181(3-4):165–8.

35. Eccles MP, Mittman BS. Welcome to implementation science. Implement Sci 2006;1(1):1.

36. Strifler L, Cardoso R, McGowan J, et al. Scoping review identifies significant number of knowledge translation theories, models, and frameworks with limited use. J Clin Epidemiol 2018;100:92–102.

37. Nilsen P. Making sense of implementation theories, models and frameworks. Implement Sci 2015;10:53.

38. Moore JE, Rashid S, Park JS, et al. Longitudinal evaluation of a course to build core competencies in implementation practice. Implement Sci 2018;13(1):106.

39. French SD, Green SE, O'Connor DA, et al. Developing theory-informed behaviour change interventions to implement evidence into practice: a systematic approach using the Theoretical Domains Framework. Implement Sci 2012;7:38.

40. Gullick J, Lin F, Massey D, et al. Structures, processes and outcomes of specialist critical care nurse education: an integrative review. Aust Crit Care 2019;32(4):331–45.

41. Gill FJ, Leslie GD, Grech C, et al. A review of critical care nursing staffing, education and practice standards. Aust Crit Care 2012;25(4): 224–37.

42. Gill FJ, Kendrick T, Davies H, et al. A two phase study to revise the Australian practice standards for specialist critical care nurses. Aust Crit Care 2017;30(3):173–81.

43. Henriksen KF, Hansen BS, Woien H, et al. The core qualities and competencies of the intensive and critical care nurse, a meta-ethnography. J Adv Nurs 2021;77(12):4693–710.

44. Zhang X, Meng K, Chen S. Competency framework for specialist critical care nurses: a modified Delphi study. Nurs Crit Care 2020;25(1): 45–52.

45. Deacon KS, Baldwin A, Donnelly KA, et al. The national competency framework for registered nurses in adult critical care: an overview. J Intensive Care Soc 2017;18(2):149–56.

46. Endacott R, Scholes J, Jones C, et al. Development of competencies for advanced nursing practice in intensive care units across Europe: a modified e-Delphi study. Intensive Crit Care Nurs 2022;71:103239.

47. American Association of Critical-Care Nurses (AACN). Get certified. Aliso Viejo, CA: AACN; 2022. Available from: https://www.aacn.org/certification/get-certified. [Accessed 10 February 2023].

48. Canadian Association of Critical-Care Nurses(AACN). Certification. Aliso Viejo, CA: AACN; 2022. Available from: https://caccn.ca/education-certification-resources/certification/. [Accessed 10 February 2023].

49. Fairman J, Lynaugh JE. Critical care nursing: a history. Philadelphia: University of Pennsylvania Press; 1998.

50. Innes T, Calleja P. Transition support for new graduate and novice nurses in critical care settings: an integrative review of the literature. Nurse Educ Pract 2018;30:62–72.

51. Gill FJ, Leslie GD, Grech C, et al. Developing and testing the Standard of Practice and Evaluation of Critical-Care-Nursing Tool (SPECT) for critical care nursing practice. J Contin Educ Nurs 2014;45(7):312–20.

52. Marks S, Edwards S, Jerge EH. Rapid deployment of critical care nurse education during the COVID-19 Pandemic. Nurse Lead 2021;19(2):165–9.

53. Marshall AP, Austin DE, Chamberlain D, et al. A critical care pandemic staffing framework in Australia. Aust Crit Care 2021;34(2):123–31.

54. Griffin KM, Karas MG, Ivascu NS, et al. Hospital preparedness for COVID-19: a practical guide from a critical care perspective. Am J Respir Crit Care Med 2020;201(11):1337–44.

55. Gill FJ, Leslie GD, Grech C, et al. Health consumers' experiences in Australian critical care units: postgraduate nurse education implications. Nurs Crit Care 2013;18(2):93–102.

56. Goldsworthy S, Alexandrov A, Bloomer M, et al. Position statement: provision of critical care education. Brighton le Sands, NSW: WFCCN; 2020. Available from: https://wfccn.org/wp-content/uploads/2020/07/WFCCN-Education-PS_secured.pdf. [Accessed 10 February 2023].

57. Rose L, Goldsworthy S, O'Brien-Pallas L, et al. Critical care nursing education and practice in Canada and Australia: a comparative review. Int J Nurs Stud 2008;45(7):1103–9.

58. Leclair LW, Dawson M, Howe A, et al. A longitudinal interprofessional simulation curriculum for critical care teams: eExploring successes and challenges. J Interprof Care 2018;32(3):386–90.

59. O'Connor S, Jolliffe S, Stanmore E, et al. A mixed study systematic review of social media in nursing and midwifery education: protocol. J Adv Nurs 2017;73(8):1989–96.

60. Liu Y, Aungsuroch Y. Current literature review of registered nurses' competency in the global community. J Nurs Scholarsh 2018;50(2):191–9.

61. Lakanmaa RL, Suominen T, Perttilä J, et al. Basic competence in intensive and critical care nursing: development and psychometric testing of a competence scale. J Clin Nurs 2014;23(5-6):799–810.

62. Franklin N, Melville P. Competency assessment tools: an exploration of the pedagogical issues facing competency assessment for nurses in the clinical environment. Collegian 2015;22(1):25–31.

63. American Association of Critical-Care Nurses (AACN). History of AACN. Aliso Viejo, CA: AACN; 2022. Available from: https://www.aacn.org/About%20AACN/Complete%20History%20AACN. [Accessed 10 February 2023].

64. Nursing and Midwifery Board of Australia (NMBA). Nurse practitioner standards for practice. Melbourne, VIC: NMBA; 2021. Available from: https://www.nursingmidwiferyboard.gov.au/codes-guidelines-statements/professional-standards/nurse-practitioner-standards-of-practice.aspx. [Accessed 2 August 2023].

65. International Council of Nurses (ICN). Guidelines on advanced practice nursing 2020. Geneva: ICN; 2020. Available from: https://www.icn.ch/system/files/documents/2020-04/ICN_APN%20Report_EN_WEB.pdf. [Accessed 10 February 2023].

66. Australian College of Critical Care Nurses (ACCCN). Position statement: advanced practice in critical care. Surrey Hills, VIC: ACCCN; 2021. Available from: https://acccn.com.au/publications/position-statements/. [Accessed 10 February 2023].

67. Hargett CW, Doty JP, Hauck JN, et al. Developing a model for effective leadership in healthcare: a concept mapping approach. J Healthc Leadersh 2017;9:69–78.

68. Brewster DJ, Butt WW, Gordon LJ, et al. Leadership in intensive care: a review. Anaesth Intensive Care 2020;48(4):266–76.

69. Spivack LB, Spivack M. Understanding and adapting to leadership challenges: navigating the COVID-19 crisis in the Bronx. Am J Crit Care 2021;30(1):80–2.

70. Hayes MM, Cocchi MN. Critical care leadership during the COVID-19 pandemic. J Crit Care 2022;67:186–8.

71. Larsson IE, Sahlsten MJ. The staff nurse clinical leader at the bedside: Swedish registered nurses' perceptions. Nurs Res Pract 2016;2016:1797014.

72. Blake N. Authentic leadership: how does it differ from transformational leadership? AACN Adv Crit Care 2020;31(2):196–7.

73. Cosentino C, De Luca E, Sulla F, et al. Leadership styles' influence on ICU nurses' quality of professional life: a cross-sectional study. Nurs Crit Care 2021;Dec 28. doi: 10.1111/nicc.12738. Online ahead of print.

74. Lima EC, Bernardes A, Baldo PL, et al. Critical incidents connected to nurses' leadership in intensive care units. Rev Bras Enferm 2017;70(5):1018–25.

75. Stanley D, Stanley K. Clinical leadership and nursing explored: a literature search. J Clin Nurs 2018;27(9-10):1730–43.

76. Richardson J, West MA, Cuthbertson BH. Team working in intensive care: current evidence and future endeavors. Curr Opin Crit Care 2010;16(6):643–8.

77. Chávez EC, Yoder LH. Staff nurse clinical leadership: a concept analysis. Nurs Forum 2015;50(2):90–100.

78. Bender M, Connelly CD, Brown C. Interdisciplinary collaboration: the role of the clinical nurse leader. J Nurs Manag 2013;21(1):165–74.

79. Wilson L, Orff S, Gerry T, et al. Evolution of an innovative role: the clinical nurse leader. J Nurs Manag 2013;21(1):175–81.

80. Kiwanuka F, Nanyonga RC, Sak-Dankosky N, et al. Nursing leadership styles and their impact on intensive care unit quality measures: an integrative review. J Nurs Manag 2021;29(2):133–42.

81. Shanafelt TD, Noseworthy JH. Executive leadership and physician well-being: nine organizational strategies to promote engagement and reduce burnout. Mayo Clin Proc 2017;92(1):129–46.

82. Mianda S, Voce A. Developing and evaluating clinical leadership interventions for frontline healthcare providers: a review of the literature. BMC Health Serv Res 2018;18(1):747.

83. Dierckx de Casterle B, Willemse A, Verschueren M, et al. Impact of clinical leadership development on the clinical leader, nursing team and care-giving process: a case study. J Nurs Manag 2008;16(6):753–63.

84. McNamara MS, Fealy GM, Casey M, et al. Mentoring, coaching and action learning: interventions in a national clinical leadership development programme. J Clin Nurs 2014;23(17-18):2533–41.

85. Leggat SG, Balding C, Schiftan D. Developing clinical leaders: the impact of an action learning mentoring programme for advanced practice nurses. J Clin Nurs 2015;24(11–12):1576–84.

Chapter 2

Systems and resources

Ged Williams, Natalie Pattison

Learning objectives

After reading this chapter, you should be able to:

- describe historical influences on the development of critical care and the way this resource is currently viewed and used
- explain the organisational arrangements and interfaces that may be established to govern a critical care unit
- identify resources and supports that assist in the governance and management of a critical care unit
- describe factors that impact on planning for the physical design and equipment requirements of a critical care unit
- describe the human resource requirements, supports and training necessary to ensure a safe and appropriate workforce
- explain common risks and the appropriate strategies, policies and contingencies necessary to support staff and patient safety
- discuss leadership and management principles that influence the quality, efficacy and appropriateness of the critical care unit
- discuss critical care considerations in responding to the threat of a pandemic.

Introduction

In 1966 Dr B Galbally, a hospital resuscitation officer at St Vincent's Hospital, Melbourne, published the first article on the planning and organisation of an intensive care unit (ICU) in Australia.[1] He identified that critically ill patients who have a reasonable chance of recovery require life-saving treatments and constant nursing and medical care, but this intensity of service delivery *does not necessarily continue until the patient dies, and it should not continue after the patient is considered no longer recoverable*.[1]

The need for prudent and rational allocation of limited financial and human resources was as important in the 1960s as it is for today. This chapter explores the influences on the development of critical care and the way this resource is currently viewed and used; describes various organisational, staffing and training arrangements that need to be in place; considers the planning, design and

KEY WORDS

budget

business case

competence

critical care

governance

pandemic

patient dependency

resource management

risk management

skill mix

staff

equipment needs of a critical care unit (CCU); covers other aspects of resource management including the budget and financial modelling; and finishes with a description of how critical care staff may respond to a pandemic or other acute and dramatic demands on resources. First, however, the principles of ethical decision making when managing resources at the unit level is no less important than ethical decision making at the individual patient level.

Practice tip

The principles of ethical decision making when managing resources at the unit level is no less important than ethical decision making at the individual patient level. Open and transparent communication is key.

Ethical allocation and utilisation of resources

In management, as in clinical practice, careful consideration of the pros and cons of various decisions must be made on a daily basis. The interests of the individual patient, extended family, treating team, the organisation and the broader community are not always congruent, nor are they always consistent. Decisions surrounding the provision of critical care services are often governed by a compromise between conflicting interests and ethical theories. Two main perspectives on ethical decision making, *deontological* and *utilitarian*, are explored briefly.[2]

The *deontological* principle suggests that a person has a fundamental duty to act in a certain way – for example, to provide full, active medical treatment to all persons. The rule of rescue, or the innate desire to do something – anything – to help those in dire need, may be a corollary to the deontological principle. These two concepts, the duty to act and the rule of rescue, tend to sit well with many trained and skilled clinicians and the Hippocratic Oath. In critical care there are some families and some clinicians who, for personal and/or religious reasons, take a strong stand and demand treatments and actions based on a deontological view (i.e. the fundamental belief that a certain action is morally obligatory).

At the other end of this spectrum is the *utilitarian* view, which suggests an action is right only if it achieves the greatest good for the greatest number of people. This concept tends to sit well with pragmatic managers and policy makers. An example of a utilitarian view might be to ration funding allocated to heart transplantation and to utilise any saved money for prevention and awareness campaigns. A heart disease prevention campaign lends a greater benefit to a greater number in the population than does one transplant procedure.

The appropriate provision and allocation of critical care services and resources tends to sit somewhere between these two extreme ethical principles. This dilemma is true of all health services, but critical care – because of its high-technology, high-cost, low-volume outputs – is under particular scrutiny to justify its resource usage within a healthcare system. Therefore, critical care managers not only need to be prudent, responsible and efficient guardians of this precious resource, they also need to be seen as such if they are to retain the confidence of, and legitimacy with, the broader community values of the day.

Historical influences

The 1960s and early 1970s saw the development of the first critical care units in many parts of the developed world. If a hospital was to be relevant, it had to have one. In fact, what distinguished a tertiary referral teaching hospital from other hospitals was at its fundamental conclusion, the existence of a critical care unit.[3] Over time, practical reasons for establishing critical care units have led to their spread to most acute hospitals with more than 100 beds, at least in well-resourced countries. Reasons for the proliferation of critical care services include, but are not limited to:

- economies of scale by cohorting critically ill patients in one area
- development of expertise in doctors and nurses and other healthcare professionals who specialise in the care and treatment of critically ill patients
- an ever-growing body of research demonstrating that critically ill patient outcomes are better if they are cared for in specifically equipped and staffed critical care units.[4]

Funding for critical care services has evolved over time to be somewhat separate from mainstream patient funding, owing to the unique requirements of critical care units. Critical care is unique because patients are at the severe end of the disease spectrum. For instance, the funding provided for a patient admitted for chronic obstructive airway disease in an ICU on a ventilator is very different from that provided for a patient with the same diagnosis but treated in a medical ward only. Each country/jurisdictional health department tends to create its own unique approach to funding ICU services. For instance, the Research and Development Corporation study[4] examined funding methods in many countries and concluded that there was no obvious example of 'best practice' or a dominant approach used by a majority of systems. Each approach had advantages and disadvantages, particularly in relation to the financial risk involved in providing intensive care. While the risk of underfunding intensive care may be highest in systems that apply Australian Refined Diagnostic Related Groups (AR-DRGs) to the entire episode of hospital care, including intensive care, concerns about potential underfunding were voiced in all systems reviewed. Arrangements for additional funding in the form of co-payments or surcharges may reduce the risk of underfunding critical care episodes of care. However, these approaches also face the difficulty of determining the appropriate co-payment amount to be paid.[4]

Australia has established the Independent Hospital Pricing Authority (IHPA) whose task it is to harmonise the variations in funding processes across all states and territories and to establish a common, consistent and transparent funding process to be agreed by all.[5] But agreement on a common funding model for intensive care services has been difficult.

The National Efficient Price (NEP), which is a single national price based on costing information from all states and territories, was developed by the IHPA and intended to provide a consistent and transparent method to determine Commonwealth growth funding to states and territories for health services provided by hospitals. This average price is applied to admitted services, emergency and non–admitted services. All price weights are expressed as a single unit of measure, being the national weighted activity unit (NWAU). It provides a scale that identifies the relative measure of resource use of each public hospital service and guides the Commonwealth contribution to funding such services. In 2022–3, NEP per NWAU is AU\$5797.[6]

Critical care is an area that requires significant resources to the treatment of patients, which an AR-DRG alone does not reflect. Therefore, additional funding over and above the acute inpatient payment is made where a patient is admitted to an eligible ICU, neonatal intensive care unit (NICU) or paediatric intensive care unit (PICU).[5] The IHPA has developed a list of ICUs that are eligible to receive an ICU adjustment based on a measure of the size of the ICU and the overall complexity mix of patients.[5] The application of the model for ICU funding is based on an hourly rate of $0.0471 \times$ NWAU.[5] Therefore (in theory) the ICU receives AU\$273 (AU\$5797 $\times$ 0.0471) for every hour the patient remains in the ICU, however the national ICU bed rate has been set at AU\$250/hour.[6] This figure is over and above the AR-DRG funding for the underlying diagnosis that brought the patient to hospital in the first place.

At the hospital level, most critical care units have capped and finite budgets that are linked to 'available beds' – that is, beds that are equipped, staffed, funded and ready to be occupied by a patient, regardless of whether they are actually occupied.[7] This is one crude yet common way that hospitals can control costs emanating from the critical care unit. The other method is to limit the number of trained and experienced nurses available to the specialty; consequently, a shortage of qualified critical care nurses results in a shortage of critical care beds, resulting in a rationing of the service available. The capping of beds and qualified critical care nurse positions can be a convenient mechanism to ration access and expense in critical care.

Practice tip

The capping of beds and qualified critical care nurse positions can be a convenient mechanism to ration access and expense in critical care.

Funding based on achieving positive patient outcomes would be ideal, as it would ensure that critical care units were using their resources only for those patients who were most likely to achieve positive outcomes in terms of morbidity and mortality. However, funding based on health outcomes alone raises the risk of encouraging clinicians to 'cherry pick' only the most 'profitable' or 'successful' patient groups at the expense of others. In private (for-profit) hospitals or countries with very poor health systems, 'cherry picking' only those patients for whom a successful outcome is guaranteed is likely to be more common, whereas in the public hospitals of most high-income countries an educated and informed guess/ risk is often applied to the decision as to whether a patient should enter the critical care unit or not.

It is vital to note the very important role played by rural and isolated health services and, in particular, critical care units and outreach services in these regions. Many of the contemporary activity-based funding formulas are difficult to apply to rural and isolated settings. There are diseconomies of scale in such settings as a result of small bed numbers, limited but highly skilled nurses and doctors, and unpredictable peaks and troughs in demand, which make workforce planning and the management of call-in/overtime and fatigue difficult for small teams to manage. The professional isolation and limited access to education, training and peer support can also create morale problems for some members of the team. Furthermore, the diseconomies and isolation require empathetic funding processes to recognise the difficulties unique to rural and isolated critical care services. If such units are to remain viable and capable of delivering safe and effective care equivalent to those expected in larger metropolitan hospitals, then additional support is required to compensate for the cost and limitations that result from being remote and isolated. To compensate further for these challenges, the use of tele-ICU,[8] artificial intelligence[9] and robotics[10] is beginning to show promise in helping to improve the quality and sustainability of treatment options in rural and isolated settings, and these are areas of contemporary research that hope to overcome the tyranny of distance and isolation.

Economic considerations and principles

One early comprehensive study of costs found that 8% of patients admitted to the ICU consumed 50% of resources but had a mortality rate of 70%, while 41% of patients received no acute interventions and consumed only 10% of resources.[11] More-recent studies show that critical care services are increasingly being provided to patients who are older and with a higher severity of acute and chronic illnesses, despite higher mortality rates compared with matched younger patients.[12-14] However, a global snapshot of ICU services in 730 centres across 84 countries showed that, on average, mortality in ICUs remains at around 16% and total in-hospital mortality of ICU patients is 22%. The scrutiny on the cost–benefit analysis of ICU remains vigilant and in need of explaining/ justifying on an almost daily basis![15]

Some authors provide scenarios as examples of poor economic decision making in critical care and argue for less extreme variances in the types of patients ICUs choose to treat in order to reduce the burden of cost on the health dollar.[16,17] Others have suggested that, if all the healthcare provided were appropriate, rationing would not be required.[18,19] Defining what is 'appropriate' can be subjective, although not always. The Research and Development Corporation[4] group suggests that there are at least three approaches that can be used to assess appropriateness of care. These include the benefit–risk, benefit–cost and implicit approaches. The first two approaches are considered to be explicit approaches, while the third tends to be subjective. However, all approaches have a subjective element. While the implicit approach is considered to be subjective in nature, the medical practitioner must contemplate 'benefit–risk' and 'benefit– cost' considerations but should also involve the patient/ family in the contemplation and ultimate decision. Similar discussions have been advocated by the Taskforce on Values, Ethics and Rationing in Critical Care, which suggests rationing is not only unavoidable but also essential to ensuring the ethical distribution of medical goods and services.[20,21] In end-of-life care situations, medical emergency teams and ICU outreach nurses can facilitate early intervention, discussion and decision making to reflect the views of family, patient and the care team.[22]

What is best for the patient is not just the opinion of the treating clinical team, but also needs to be considered in much broader terms such as the patient's previous expressed wishes and the family's opinion as de-facto patient representatives.[23] The quality of the decision and the quality of the expected outcome require many competing considerations.

Practice tip

What is best for the patient is not just the opinion of the treating doctor and needs to be considered in much broader terms such as the patient's previous expressed wishes and the family's opinion as de-facto patient representatives.

Proponents of the 'quality' agenda in healthcare have argued for 'best practice' and 'best outcomes' in the provision of health services, although it may be more pragmatic to consider 'value' when discussing what is and what is not an appropriate decision in critical care. The following equation expresses the concept 'value' simply:

$$\text{Value} = \frac{\text{Quality}}{\text{Cost}} = \frac{\text{Benefit} \times \text{Sustainability}}{\text{Price} \times \text{Suffering}}$$

The quality of the outcome is a function of the benefit to be achieved and the sustainability of the benefit. The *benefit* of critical care is associated with such factors as survival, longevity and improved quality of life (e.g. greater functioning capacity and less pain and anxiety). The benefit is enhanced by sustainability: the longer the benefit is maintained, the better it is.[24]

Cost is separated into two components: monetary (price) and non-monetary (suffering). Non-monetary costs include such considerations as morbidity, mortality, pain and anxiety in the individual, or broader societal costs and suffering (e.g. opportunity costs to others who might have used the resources but for the current occupants, and what other health services might have been provided but for the cost of this service).[24]

Ethico-economic analyses of services like critical care and expensive treatments like organ transplantation are the new consideration of this century and are as important to good governance as are discussions of medico-legal considerations. Sound ethical principles to inform and guide human and material resource management and budgets ought to prevail in the management of limited health resources.[2]

Budget and finance

This section provides information on types of budget: the budgeting process, and how to analyse costs and expenditure to ensure resources are utilised appropriately and in line with the service management plan – that is, the operational and service goals of the critical care team expected by the hospital and broader community. As noted by one author, *'Nothing is so terrifying for clinicians accustomed to daily issues of life and death as to be given responsibility for the financial affairs of their hospital division!'*[18] Yet, in essence, developing and managing a budget for a critical care unit follows many of the same principles as managing a family budget. Consideration of value for money, prioritising needs and wants, and living within a relatively fixed income is common to all. This section in no way attempts to undermine the skill and precision provided by the accounting profession, nor will it enable clinicians to usurp the role of hospital business managers. Rather, the aim is to provide the requisite knowledge to empower clinicians to manage the key components of budget development and budget setting, and to know what questions to ask when confronted by this most daunting responsibility of managing a service budget.

Practice tip

Nothing is so terrifying for clinicians accustomed to daily issues of life and death as to be given responsibility for the financial affairs of their hospital division![18]

Types of budget

There are essentially three types of budget that a manager must consider: personnel, operational and capital. Within these budget types, there are two basic cost types: fixed and variable. Fixed costs are those essential to the service and are relatively constant, regardless of the fluctuations in workload or throughput (e.g. nurse unit manager salary, security, ventilators). Variable costs change with changing throughput (e.g. nurse agency, medicines or other clinical consumable items).

Personnel budget

Healthcare is a labour-intensive service, and critical care epitomises this fact, with personnel costs being the most expensive component of the unit's budget. The staffing requirement for critical care generally follows a formula of x nurses per open (funded) bed. This figure is expressed in full-time equivalents (FTEs) (i.e. the equivalent of a person working a 40-hour week if the standard full-time working week is 40 hours). This may equate to 5×8-hour shifts per week or 20×12-hour shifts in a 6-week period, or any other variable measure as determined by local employment law and custom.

Personnel costs include productive and non-productive hours. Productive hours are those utilised to provide direct work. A manager will determine the minimum or optimum number of nurses to be scheduled per shift and then calculate the nursing hours per day, multiplied by the hourly rate of pay and any penalties that are to be attributed to work done during the after-business-hours period. Non-productive hours include sick leave, holiday leave, education hours, maternity leave and any other paid time away from the actual job that staff are employed to do.

Personnel budgets tend to be fixed costs, in that the majority of staff members are employed permanently, based on an expected or forecast demand. Prudent managers tend to employ 5–10% less than the actual forecast demand and use casual staff to 'flex-up' the available FTE staff establishment in periods of increasing demand, hence contributing a small but variable component to the personnel budget.

Operational budget

All other non-personnel costs (except major capital equipment) tend to be allocated to the operational budget. This includes fixed costs such as minor equipment, maintenance contracts, utility costs (e.g. electricity) and variable costs that fluctuate with patient type and number (e.g. pharmaceuticals, meals, consumable supplies such as gloves and dressings, laundry).

Compared with personnel costs, operational costs in critical care tend to be relatively small, but they can be managed and rationed with the help of good information and cooperation. For example, there is a range of dressing materials available on the market, and a simple dressing that requires less expensive materials should always be used unless a more expensive product is indicated, and a protocol exists to inform staff of this clinical need/ justification.

Practice tip

Compared with personnel costs, operational costs in critical care tend to be relatively small and can be managed and rationed with the help of good information and cooperation.

Fixed costs can also be turned into variable costs and hence encourage efficient usage. For example, pressure-reduction mattresses, traditionally purchased as a fixed asset with variable (and unpredictable) repair and maintenance costs, can now be leased on a per-day or per-week basis, with no need for storage, cleaning or maintenance costs (these are built into the daily or weekly hire cost). Further, critical care managers can work with other hospital managers to create 'purchasing power' by cooperating to standardise the range and volume of products used so as to obtain a better price for a product that will benefit all users – the 'economies of scale' principle.

Capital budget

Capital budget items are generally expensive and/or large fixed assets that are considered long-term investments, such as building extensions, renovations and large equipment purchases such as computed tomography (CT) scanners or electronic medical record installation. Capital budget items tend to be considered as assets that are depreciated over time. Most hospitals consider these items as a global asset – that is, as a group of investment items and activities for the hospital – rather than attributing these costs to an individual unit or department.

To request a capital budget item, a written proposal (business case – see later in this chapter) is generally required describing the item, its expected benefits, whether it replaces an existing item's service or function, the cost, the possible revenue and the cost-mitigating benefits. This analysis does not always have to demonstrate a profit, although the value and benefit of the service would need to be established/justified through a business case.

Budget process

The budget includes three fundamental steps: budget preparation and approval, budget analysis and reporting, and budget control and action.

Practice tip

The budget includes three fundamental steps: budget preparation and approval, budget analysis and reporting, and budget control and action.

Budget preparation and approval

A budget plan essentially runs in parallel with a unit or service management plan, forecasting likely activity and resulting financial costs. In most circumstances, the preceding year's activity and costs are a good benchmark on which to base the next year's budget. However, hospital expectations in terms of new services, greater patient throughput or changes to staff salary entitlements will need to be factored into the new budget.

The budget period is generally a financial year, but developing monthly budgets (cash flowing) to coincide with predictable variations allows for a more realistic representation of how costs are incurred and paid throughout the financial year period. If the budget plan is well constructed, one always hopes and expects the final budget allocation (i.e. the approved budget) to be close to achievable.

Budget analysis and reporting

Most critical care managers analyse their expenditure against budget projections on a monthly basis to identify variances from planned expenditure. Information should not merely be financial: a breakdown of the monthly and year-to-date expenditures for personnel (productive and non-productive) and operational (fixed and variable) costs should be matched against other known measurable indicators of activity or productivity (e.g. patient bed-days, patient diagnosis types/groups and staffing hours, including overtime and other special payments).[18] Ideally, such measures should be matched against other quality outcome measures such as pressure injuries, CLABSI, CAUTI, LOS and mortality indices, etc.

One common management maxim is: if it cannot be measured, then it cannot be controlled. Clinical managers therefore need to work closely with finance managers to develop consistent data measurements and reports to inform themselves and staff about where they should focus their efforts to achieve the approved budget target.

Budget control and action

When signs of poor performance or financial overrun are evident, managers cannot merely analyse the financial reports, hoping that things will sort themselves out. Every variance of a sizeable amount requires an explanation. Some will be obvious: an outbreak of community influenza among staff will increase sick leave and casual staff costs for a period of time; concurrently the same epidemic may increase demands on ICU beds. Other overruns can be insidious but no less important: overtime payments, although sometimes unavoidable, can also reflect poor time management or a culture of some staff wanting to boost their income surreptitiously.

An effective method of controlling the budget is to actively engage staff in the process of managing costs. Managers can explain to staff how the budget has been developed and how their performance against budget is progressing, and identify areas for potential improvement. Seeking ideas from staff on how to improve efficiency and productivity and giving them some responsibility for the budget performance can encourage an esprit de corps and

improvements from the whole team that a single manager cannot achieve alone.[25]

Developing a business case

The most common reason for writing a business case is to justify the resources and capital expenditure to gain the support and approval for a change in service provision and/or purchase of a significant new piece of equipment/technology. This section provides an overview of a business case and a format for its presentation. The business case can be a valuable tool in the strategic decision-making process, particularly in an environment of constrained resources.[26]

A business case is a management tool that is used in the process of explaining and meeting a strategic goal of an organisation. Within a setting such as healthcare, the business case is required to clearly outline the clinical need and implications to be understood by leaders. Financial imperatives, such as return on investment (ROI), must also be defined and identified.[27,28] A business case is a document in which all the facts relevant to the case are identified and linked cohesively. Various templates are available (see Online resources) to assist with the layout. Key questions are generally the starting point for the response to a business case: why, what, when, where, who and how, with each question's response adding additional information to the process (Table 2.1). Business cases can vary in length from just a couple of pages to many pages. Most organisations will have standardised headings and formats for the presentation of these documents. If the document is lengthy, inclusion of an executive summary is recommended to summarise the salient points of the business case (Box 2.1).

Practice tip

A goal without a plan is a wish!

Antoine de Saint-Exupéry

In summary, the business case is an important tool that is increasingly required at all levels of an organisation to clearly define a proposed service change or equipment purchase. This document should include clear goals and outcomes, a cost–benefit analysis, quality and safety considerations and timelines for achievement of the solution. While such a document is often developed towards the end of a formal multiprofessional collaboration, the questions at Table 2.1 can also be used to structure early discussions about changes in nursing practices or roles in ICU.

Critical care environment

A critical care unit is a distinct unit within a hospital that has easy access to the emergency department, operating

---

TABLE 2.1

Key questions in writing a business case

QUESTION	EXAMPLE
Why?	What is the background to the project, and why is it needed: PEST (political, economic, sociological, technological) and SWOT (strengths, weaknesses, opportunities and threats) analysis?
What?	Clearly identify and define the project and the purpose of the business case and outline the solution. Clearly defined goals, outcomes and measurable benefits should be documented.
What if?	A risk assessment of the current situation, including any controls currently in place to address/mitigate the issue, and a risk assessment following the implementation of the proposed solution.
When?	What are the timelines for the implementation and achievement of the project/solution?
Where?	What is the context within which the project will be undertaken, if not already included in the background material?
Who?	Who will be affected by this change, positively and negatively? Who will be responsible for overseeing and managing of the project/change?
How?	How much money, people and equipment, for example, will be required to achieve the benefits? A clear cost–benefit analysis should be included in response to this question.

BOX 2.1

Business case: sample headings
- Title
- Purpose
- Background
- Key issues
- Cost–benefit analysis
- Recommendations
- Risk assessment

---

theatre and medical imaging. It provides care to patients with a life-threatening illness or injury and concentrates the clinical expertise, technological and therapeutic resources required. In Ontario, Canada there are six levels of critical care,[29] while the Australian College of Intensive Care Medicine[7] and the UK Faculty of Intensive Care Medicine[30] define three levels of intensive care to support the role delineation of a particular hospital, dependent upon staffing expertise, facilities and support services. Critical care facilities vary in nature and extent between hospitals and are dependent on the operational policies of each individual facility. In smaller facilities, the broad spectrum of critical care may be provided in combined units (intensive care, high-dependency, coronary care unit) to improve flexibility and aid the efficient use of available resources.[31]

Environmental design

The functional, organisational and unit designs are governed by available finances, an operational brief and the building and design standards of the state or country in which the hospital is located. A critical care unit should have access to minimum support facilities, which include staff station, clean utility, dirty utility, storeroom(s), education and teaching space, staff amenities, patients' ensuites, patients' bathroom, linen storage, disposal room, pathology area and offices. Most notably, the actual bed space/care area for patients needs to be well designed.[31,32]

The design of the patient's bed space has received considerable attention in recent years. Most governments have developed guidelines of minimum standards to assist in the design process. Each bed space should be a minimum of 20–25 square metres and provide for visual privacy from casual observation. At least one hand basin per single room or per two beds should be provided to meet minimum infection control guidelines.[31–33] Each bed space should have piped medical gases (oxygen and air), suction, adequate electrical outlets (essential and non-essential), data points and task lighting sufficient for use during the performance of bedside procedures. Further detailed descriptions are available in various health department documents.[31,32]

Equipment

Since the advent of critical care units, healthcare delivery has become increasingly dependent on medical technology to deliver that care. Equipment can be categorised into several funding groups: capital expenditure (generally in excess of AU$10,000 or £6000), equipment expenditure (all equipment less than AU$10,000 or £6000), and the disposable products and devices required to support the use of equipment. This section examines how to evaluate, procure and maintain that equipment.

Initial set-up requirements

Critical care units require baseline equipment that allows the unit to deliver safe and effective patient care. The list of specific equipment required by each individual unit will be governed by the scope of that unit's function. For example, a unit that provides care to patients after neurosurgery will require the ability to monitor intracranial pressure. Changes in practice such as early mobilisation[34] have an impact on both equipment requirements and storage space, although financial modelling has demonstrated considerable cost savings.[35] Table 2.2 lists the basic equipment requirements for a critical care unit. Information technology and communications options and requirements are growing rapidly in health and in the critical care environment, with instant access to patient's physiological data at the bedside becoming standard practice. The rapid pace of innovation and change in this area requires the managers to think carefully when setting up information technology infrastructure and to be careful not to overcapitalise on technology that might not be easily upgradeable when new and more efficient or more-effective substitutes come on to the market. Envisioning what might be available in the future is difficult, but it is important to consider such matters carefully to avoid very expensive upgrades in the future.[36] Further detail regarding information and communication technology can be found in Chapter 3.

> **Practice tip**
>
> Envisioning what might be available in the future is difficult but it is important to consider such matters carefully to avoid very expensive upgrades in the future.

TABLE 2.2
Basic equipment requirements

MONITORING	THERAPEUTIC
Monitors (including central station)	Ventilators (invasive and non-invasive)
End-tidal CO_2 monitoring	Infusion pumps
Arterial blood gas analyser (±electrolytes)	Syringe drivers
	CVVHDF
Invasive monitoring (including transport)	EDD-f
• arterial	Resuscitators
• central venous pressure	Temperature control device
• intracranial pressure	Bronchoscopy/laryngoscopy
• cardiac output	Temporary pacemaker
Access to image intensifier	Defibrillator
Ultrasound	Suctioning apparatus
Access to CT/MRI	

CT = computed tomography; CVVHDF = continuous venovenous haemodiafiltration; EDD-f = extended daily diafiltration; MRI = magnetic resonance imaging.

Purchasing

The procurement of any equipment or medical device requires a rigorous process of selection and evaluation. This process should be designed to select functional, reliable products that are safe, cost effective and environmentally conscious[37] and that promote quality of care while avoiding duplication or rapid obsolescence. In most healthcare facilities, a product (or medical devices) evaluation committee exists to support this process.

The product evaluation committee should include members who have an interest in the equipment being considered and should comprise, for example, biomedical engineers and representatives from the central sterile supply unit administration, infection control, end users and other departments that may have similar needs. Once a product evaluation committee has been established, clear, objective criteria for the evaluation of the product should be determined (Box 2.2). Ideally, the committee will screen products and medical devices before a clinical evaluation is conducted to establish its viability, so avoiding any unnecessary expenditure in time and money.

BOX 2.2
Example criteria for product evaluation
- Safety
- Performance
- Quality
- Use
  - purpose
  - ease of
- Cost–benefit analysis
  - include disposables
- Cleaning
  - central sterilising supply unit
  - infection control
- Regulatory control
  - Therapeutic Goods Administration
  - Australian standards
- Adaptability to future technological advancements
- Service agreements
- Training requirements

Source: Adapted from Association of Operating Room Nurses. Recommended practices for product selection in perioperative practice settings. AORN J 2004;79:678–82, with permission;
Elliott D, Hollins B. Product evaluation: theoretical and practical considerations. Aust Crit Care 1995;8(2): 14–19, with permission.

The decision to purchase or lease equipment will, to some extent, be governed by the purchasing strategy approved by the hospital or health authority. The advantages of leasing equipment include the capital expenditure being defrayed over the life of the lease, with ongoing servicing and product upgrades built into the lease agreement and price structure. Any final presentation from the product evaluation committee should, therefore, include a recommendation to purchase or lease, based on a cost–benefit analysis of the ongoing expenditure required to maintain the equipment.

Replacement and maintenance

The process for replacement of equipment is closely aligned with the process for the purchase of new equipment. The stimulus for the process to begin can be either the condemning of equipment by biomedical engineers or the planned replacement of equipment nearing the end of its life cycle. In general, most capital equipment is deemed to have a life cycle of 5 years. This time frame takes into account both the longevity of the physical equipment and its technology.

Ongoing maintenance of equipment is an important part of facilitating safety in the unit. Maintenance may be provided in-house by individual facility biomedical departments or as part of a service contract arrangement with the vendor company. The provision of a maintenance/ service plan should be clearly identified during the procurement phase of the equipment purchase process. While equipment maintenance is not the direct responsibility of the nurses in charge of the unit, they should be aware of the scheduled maintenance plan for all equipment and ensure that timely maintenance is undertaken.

Routine ongoing care of equipment is outlined in the product information and user manuals that accompany devices. This documentation clearly outlines routine care required for cleaning, storage and maintenance. All staff involved in the maintenance of clinical equipment should be trained and competent to carry it out. As specialist equipment is a fundamental element of critical care, effective resourcing includes consideration of the purchase, set-up, maintenance and replacement of equipment. Equipment is therefore an important aspect of the budget process.

> **Practice tip**
>
> The provision of a maintenance/service plan should be clearly identified during the procurement phase of the equipment purchase process.

Staff

Staffing critical care units is an important human resource consideration. The focus of this section is on nursing staff, although the important role that multiprofessional team members provide is acknowledged, particularly in relation to impact on nursing. It is important to consider the definition of a critical care nurse, whose core attributes include caring for the high-acuity patients in critical care areas requiring intensive monitoring and organ support therapies (without a need for direct supervision), and applying knowledge, skills and critical thinking to holistic patient and family care.[38–40]

Staffing is key to quality and safety in critical care and, along with other staff salaries, consumes a considerable proportion of critical care budgets. Nurses' salaries often account for the largest cost incurred in critical care provision owing to prescribed staffing ratios to provide continual care for patients. Numerous studies, some of which will be discussed later, demonstrate how nurse staffing levels influence at different levels to directly and indirectly influence patient, system (hospital and unit) and staff outcomes. These influences include the initiation of appropriate nursing care strategies and mediation and implementation of the care strategies of other members of the multidisciplinary healthcare team.[41] Therefore, ensuring an appropriate skill mix is an important aspect of unit management and strategy. This section considers how appropriate staffing levels are determined and explores these through system- (organisational and higher), unit- and individual-level factors.

Staffing roles

The role of critical care nurses and their contribution to these factors is a key issue here. There are a number of different nursing roles in the critical care nursing team, and various guidelines determine the requirements of these roles. Some critical care nursing organisations have documented position statements surrounding the critical care workforce and staffing.[38,42–45] The advent of the COVID-19 pandemic has also challenged these statements, with some organisations re-issuing them in light of the profound changes required as a result of surge activity during the pandemic. A designated nursing manager (nursing unit manager/nurse practice coordinator/clinical nurse manager, or equivalent title) is required for each unit to direct and guide clinical practice. The nurse manager must possess a post-registration qualification in critical care or in the clinical specialty of the unit.[29,30,38,42,46] A clinical nurse educator (CNE) should be available in each unit.[4] In Australia, the Australian College of Critical Care Nurses (ACCCN) recommends a minimum ratio of one full-time equivalent CNE for every 50 nurses on the roster, to provide unit-based education and staff development.[43] This varies in other parts of the world; for example, the UK recommends one per unit (or 1 per 75 staff), in line with World Federation of Critical Care Nursing guidelines.[30,46] Registered nurses within the unit are generally nurses with formal critical care post-registration qualifications and varying levels of critical care experience. However, this varies across countries, with the UK specifying a minimum of 50% of registered nurses who hold a critical care nursing qualification.[46]

In many developed economies, specialist critical care nurse education has moved from largely hospital-based certificates[43] into the tertiary education sector, or provision at a regional/network level. A Europe-wide survey identified wide variation in the regulation, assessment, program duration and qualification awarded for specialist critical care nurse education.[47] Since the move to tertiary education, postgraduate, university-based programs at the graduate certificate, postgraduate diploma or Master's level have become available, although some hospital-based or regional/critical care network (where they apply in certain countries, such as the UK) courses that are seen as equitable to formal university programs may also be accessible. Board certification may additionally be required in some countries, such as the US. Some critical care organisations have developed position statements on the provision of critical care nursing education.[30,33,48] Various support staff are also required to ensure the efficient functioning of the department, including, but not limited to, administrative/clerical staff, clinical support workers, domestic assistant staff, clinician scientists, technicians and biomedical engineering staff.

Staffing levels

Staffing establishments refer to the number of nurses required to provide safe, efficient, quality care to patients on any given unit. This can be considered as a whole staff establishment (total number of nurses employed to staff a unit overall) and daily establishment (number of nurses required to fulfil the staffing requirements for that day/shift). Staffing levels are influenced by many factors, including the economic, political and individual characteristics of the unit in question and patient case mix, alongside adherence to centralised guidelines. Other factors, such as the population served, the fluctuations in services provided by the hospital and the region, and the subspecialties of medical staff working at each hospital, also influence staffing. Specific issues to be considered include nurse-to-patient ratios, nursing competencies and skill mix.

The starting point for most units in the establishment of minimum, or base, staffing levels is the patient census approach. Determining what the numbers are for sufficient staff to provide care to those patients (based on an average estimate of need, such as historical use of ICU beds) and meet daily rosters is a key factor here.[49] The number and classification (ICU or high-dependency unit (HDU), sometimes referred to as level 2 and level 3 patients[44]) of patients within the unit determine the number of nurses required to be scheduled on duty on any given shift. In many countries a registered nurse-to-patient ratio of 1:1 for ICU patients and 1:2 for HDU patients has been accepted for many years.[30,42–45] Other countries, such as the USA, have lower nurse staffing levels, but in those countries the nursing staff is augmented by other types of clinical or support staff, such as dialysis and respiratory technicians,[50] and in the UK these roles include clinician scientists, physician assistants (also in the US) and associates,

and other non-registered clinical support workers.[51–54] The limitations of alternative staffing approaches are discussed later in this chapter. The unit manager is required to calculate the number of FTEs that are required to implement the roster, additionally calculating baseline staffing numbers per shift. One FTE is equivalent to the number of hours worked in 1 week by a full-time employee (see earlier in this chapter). Factors such as 'headroom' (planned numbers of unavailable staff that are on study leave, annual leave and projected sickness) also need accounting for. Hospitals often underestimate indirect time (where staff are unavailable because of leave), with highly variable and unrealistic targets for planned unavailability.[55]

The development of the nursing establishment is dependent on many factors. Historical data from previous years of patient throughput, planned expansions (at local, regional and national levels), and average and fluctuating patient acuity and case mix assist in the determination of future requirements.

Nurse-to-patient ratios

Nurse-to-patient ratios refer to the number of nursing hours required to care for a patient with a particular set of needs. This is calculated on a *per diem* basis as nursing hours per patient day (NHPPD). Depending on the acuity of patients, unit configuration (environmental layout and design) and other factors, such as skill mix, different nurse-to-patient ratios are required for these often-diverse groups of patients. It is important to note that nurse-to-patient ratios may be provided merely as a guide to staffing levels, and implementation should depend on patient acuity, local knowledge and expertise.

Australia and New Zealand have several documents that guide nurse-to-patient ratios. The World Federation of Critical Care Nurses (WFCCN) states that critically ill patients require one registered nurse to be allocated at all times.[43] The College of Intensive Care Medicine in Australia and the Faculty of Intensive Care Medicine in the United Kingdom also identified the need for a minimum nurse-to-patient ratio of 1:1 for intensive care patients and 1:2 for high-dependency patients.[29,44] The ACCCN 2018 workforce standards emphasise that, in addition to minimum standards, units should be able to determine additional staffing requirements based on case mix, design and environment (e.g. numbers of single rooms).[43]

Practice tip

The WFCCN states that critically ill patients require one registered nurse to be allocated at all times.

The ACCCN,[43] the British Association of Critical Care Nurses,[44] the UK Critical Care Nursing Alliance[56] and the Critical Care Nurses Section – New Zealand Nurses Organisation[45] have outlined the appropriate

TABLE 2.3

Ten key points of intensive care nursing staffing[44]

POINT	DESCRIPTION
1. Ventilated patients and any other patient that the nurse-in-charge deems to be clinically unstable or at risk	Require a standard nurse-to-patient ratio of at least 1:1.
2. Patients requiring a high complexity level of care (e.g. non-ventilated patients recovering from critical illness)	Require a standard nurse-to-patient ratio of at least 1:2.
3. Clinical coordinator (team leader)	There must be a designated critical-care-qualified senior nurse per shift who is supernumerary and whose primary role is responsibility for the logistical management of patients, staff, service provision and resource utilisation during a shift.
4. ACCESS nurses	These are nurses in addition to the bedside nurses, clinical coordinator, unit manager, educators and non-nursing support staff. They provide Assistance, Coordination, Contingency, Education, Supervision and Support.
5. Nursing manager	At least one designated Master's-prepared nursing manager (NUM/CNC/NPC/CNM or equivalent) who is formally recognised as the unit nurse leader is required per ICU.
6. Clinical nurse educator	At least one designated Master's-prepared CNE should be available in each unit. The recommended ratio is one FTE CNE for every 50 nurses on the ICU roster.
7. ICU liaison nurse services	A liaison nurse service must be provided to optimise the use of the ICU within the hospital, with one liaison nurse per 10 ICU beds.
8. Critical care nurses	The ACCCN recommends an optimum specialty qualified critical care nurse proportion of 75%.
9. Resources	These are allocated to support nursing time and costs associated with quality assurance activities, nursing and multidisciplinary research, and conference attendance.
10. Support staff	ICUs are provided with adequate administrative staff, ward assistants, manual handling assistance/equipment, cleaning and other support staff to ensure that nursing staff can focus on the delivery of care for critically ill patients.

ACCCN = Australian College of Critical Care Nurses; CNC = clinical nurse consultant; CNE = clinical nurse educator; CNM = clinical nurse manager; NUM = nursing unit manager; NPC = nurse practice coordinator.

Source: Chamberlain D, Pollock W, Fulbrook P; ACCCN Workforce Standards Development Group. ACCCN workforce standards for intensive care nursing: systematic and evidence review, development, and appraisal. Aust Crit Care 2018;31(5):292–302.[43]

nurse staffing standards for ICUs within the context of accepted minimum national standards and evidence that supports best practice. The ACCCN statement identifies key principles to meet the expected standards of critical care nursing[43] (Table 2.3).

These recommendations are aimed as a guide to determining nurse-to-patient ratios, as extraneous factors such as the clinical practice setting (design/environment), patient acuity and case mix, and the skill mix, knowledge and expertise of available staff will influence final staffing patterns and may need to be adapted to suit the requirements of individual countries or units.

Tools to determine staffing remain poorly evidence based.[57–59] These centre on the following areas to guide these staffing decisions: patient-based tools, which are predicated on the condition and needs of the patient, including dependency scoring models; activity/bed-based models, including professional judgement (focused on time and number of nurses needed for activities/tasks); and those focused on other factors such as psychosocial (risk and mental demand).[57] The differences between these approaches are discussed below.

Patient-based tools/models

Patient dependency refers to an approach to quantify the care needs of individual patients, matching these needs to the nursing staff workload and skill mix.[57] These are also sometimes referred to under the umbrella of acuity–quality models.[57] Historically, patient census was the commonest method for determining the nursing workload within an ICU. That is, the number of patients dictated the number of nurses required to care for them, based on the accepted nurse-to-patient ratios of 1:1 for ICU patients and 1:2 for HDU patients. This reflects the unit-based workload, and is also the common funding approach for ICU bed-day costs and establishment funding.

The nursing workload at the individual patient level, however, is also reflective of patient acuity and case mix, the complexity of care required, the variation in types of patients (e.g. elective surgical versus emergency patients) and clinical (including psychological) status of the patient, and the likely course of illness. Strict adherence to the patient census model leads to the inflexibility of matching nursing resources to demand. For example, some ICU patients receive care that is so complex that more than one nurse is required (nursing patients receiving extracorporeal membrane oxygenation treatment is an example of where 2:1 is a norm),[60] and an HDU patient may require less medical care than an ICU patient, but conversely may require more than 1:2 nursing care level secondary to such factors as physical care requirements, acute delirium and agitation, anxiety and pain.[61,62] A patient-census approach, therefore, does not allow for the varying nursing hours required and variations in need (i.e. a level 2 patient moving to become a level 3 patient) for individual patients over a shift, nor does it allow for unpredicted peaks and troughs in activity, such as multiple admissions or multiple discharges, or indeed unit design (for example, within-shift unit reconfiguration may be rapidly required because of infection outbreaks).

Activity-based models

Activity-based models calculate the time spent by nurses on patient and family activities. The prime purpose of these models is to classify patients into groups requiring similar nursing care and to attribute a numerical score that indicates the amount of nursing care required. Assumptions are based on the fact that sicker patients require more nursing resource[57] and activities. Patients may also be classified according to the severity of their illness. There are several key approaches to activity-based models such as those based on nursing interventions and tasks; these include the Nursing Activities Score (NAS),[63] a weighted scoring system developed to address missing nursing elements in the Therapeutic Intervention Scoring System (TISS)[64] (which was originally developed to determine severity of illness in order to establish nurse-to-patient ratios and to assess current bed utilisation,[50] but failed to sufficiently capture the breadth of the ICU nursing role) and the Dependence Nursing Scale (DNS),[65] both of which are task activity-based methods. The Nine Equivalents of nursing Manpower use Score (NEMS)[66] is a professional judgement method based on an acuity–quality framework. Other professional judgement methods include the Nursing Interventions Classification (NIC)[67] and the American Association of Critical Care Nurses (AACN) Synergy Model for Patient Care,[68,69] which incorporated patient/family judgements alongside objective data (including

staff competency levels) to create a weighted scoring system. Generic tools such as the Safer Nursing Care Tool[58] are also used in critical care areas, although not specifically intended for these areas. Each of these models attributes a score to either the clinical condition of the patients or the number of procedures/interventions performed, with the premise that the greater the acuity or number of nursing procedures performed, the higher the score, and in turn the higher the severity of illness, the greater is the intensity of nursing care needed.[57,58] While tools such as the NAS capture a greater portion of nurses' time than the TISS-28[63,64] and have been used to examine workload of different shifts,[54] the subjective nature of some items affect reliability.[59] Indeed, a systematic review examining staffing tools in ICU iterated that no single tool was likely to be applicable to all ICUs, and many were deemed country or continent specific, such as the NAS.[57] Therefore, while these scoring systems may provide valuable information on the acuity of the patients within the ICU, they are not accurate indicators of total nursing workload.

Other specific measures have been developed and applied to ICU nursing, including those that incorporate risk management (Managing Risk Instrument)[70] and the NASA Task Loading Index (NASA-TLX),[71,72] which examines different psychosocial factors such as mental demand. In both cases, the usability and reliability applied to critical care nursing was questionable, so these have not been pursued in practice. The Subjective Workload Assessment for Nurses (SWAN tool), based on nurses' subjective perception of workload, similarly was not found to be useful in practice. The limited evidence base underpinning all of these tools mean they have limited clinical applicability and are not widely accepted in practice.[57]

Skill mix

Skill mix refers to the ratio of caregivers with varying levels of skill, training, and experience in a clinical unit. In critical care, skill mix also refers to the proportion of registered nurses possessing a formal specialist critical care qualification, and non-registered nursing support staff. In parts of the world such as the UK, there are roles allied to nursing, for example nursing associates who are not registered nurses but are higher skilled than clinical support workers and who complete a training program.[73] The ACCCN recommends an optimum qualified critical care nurse to unqualified critical care nurse ratio of 75%.[43] In Australia and New Zealand, approximately 55% of the nurses employed in critical care units currently have some form of critical care qualification.[45]

> **Practice tip**
>
> Unit-specific orientation should be a formal, structured program of assessment, demonstration of competence and identification of ongoing educational needs, and should be developed to meet the needs of all staff new to the unit.

Debate continues to determine the optimum skill mix required to provide safe, effective nursing care to patients in critical care.[39,57,74,75] Much of the original research fuelling this debate was undertaken in the general ward setting, but evidence is now mounting of the impact of ICU nurse staffing on patient outcomes. Quality of care outcomes that have been shown to worsen with lower numbers of registered nurses in ICU include nosocomial (healthcare acquired) infection, length of stay (both ICU and hospital) and adverse incidents, as well as reduced ventilation and weaning time and reduced multiorgan failure. Similar findings are reported in a systematic review in acute care, with improved outcomes where there was better skill mix in the following areas: hospital length of stay; ulcer, gastritis and upper gastrointestinal bleeds; acute myocardial infarction; restraint use; failure to rescue; pneumonia; sepsis; urinary tract infection; mortality/30-day mortality; pressure injury; infections and shock/cardiac arrest/heart failure.[76]

Researchers have examined the substitution of one grade of staff with a lesser skilled, trained or experienced grade of staff, using adverse events as the outcome measure. Study results demonstrate that a rich registered nurse skill mix reduces the occurrence of adverse events.[77–79] Taking this further, things like intravenous (IV) drug administration skills can also be modelled, as in a recent UK study[80] where once 60% of registered nurses were IV trained the rate of shifts deemed to be understaffed (using the Safer Nursing Care Tool) was low. Another study modelled the effect of increasing non-registered nursing numbers (dilution of registered nursing skill mix) on general wards, demonstrating this would lead to worse outcomes and increased costs.[81] A recent systematic review of longitudinal studies of hospital nurse staffing and patient outcomes supported the proposition that higher levels of registered nurse staffing are likely to lead to better patient outcomes.[82] Studies have examined aspects of workload such as patient turnover and the number of life-sustaining procedures undertaken for the patient, and their subsequent impact on mortality. One prospective study conducted in eight French ICUs over a calendar year found both of these indicators were associated with increased ICU mortality.[83] Further, researchers undertook a retrospective analysis of nursing workload, severity of illness and hospital survival in two ICUs in Hong Kong and found that patients exposed to a higher workload/nurse ratio for ≥1 day had lower risk-adjusted odds of survival to hospital discharge than patients who were never exposed to a high ratio.[84]

While there has not been a formal examination of skill mix in the critical care setting in Australia and New Zealand, two older publications,[85,86] which continue to be cited as evidence of the relationship between nurse skill mix and adverse outcomes, emerged from the Australian Incident Monitoring Study–ICU (AIMS–ICU). Of note, 81% of the reported adverse events resulted from inappropriate numbers of nursing staff or inappropriate skill mix.[87] Furthermore, nursing care without expertise could be harmful for the patient, as studies have shown that the rate of errors by experienced critical care nurses was likely to rise during periods of staffing shortages, when inexperienced nurses required supervision and assistance.[41,85] A Queensland study emphasised how staffing shortages and poor skill mix led to implicit healthcare rationing.[88] In the UK, recent qualitative work across the UK outlined the importance of skill mix and its influence on ICU staffing, with a staffing decision made throughout the shifts and adoption of a whole multidisciplinary team (MDT) approach to mitigate nurse staffing shortfalls.[89] Factors including fluctuating patient and family needs, staff well-being, ICU design (layout/environment of ICU) and MDT experience and availability all impacted on staffing planning.[90,91]

Professional organisations have developed position statements on the use of staff other than registered nurses in the critical care environment.[42,43,45] The British Association of Critical Care Nurses asserts that healthcare assistants employed in a critical care setting must undertake only direct patient care activities for which they have received training and for which they have been assessed as competent and under the supervision of a registered nurse.[44]

Staffing levels and skill mix within critical care units should therefore be based on individual unit needs (e.g. unit size, layout and location) and patient clinical presentations/acuity, and be guided by the best available evidence to ensure safe, quality care for their patients within the context of national standards, expectations and resources.

In addition, there is increasing evidence that nurse outcomes are also worse in poor staffing conditions,[91,92] including increased burnout (emotional exhaustion, depersonalisation, stress) and fatigue, specifically in ICU nursing.[93]

Rostering

Once the nursing establishment for a unit is determined and the skill mix considered, the rostering (rota) format is decided. In times of nursing shortages, one of the factors identified as affecting the retention of staff is the ability to provide flexibility in rostering practices.[94,95] To some extent, rostering practices are governed by government, hospital and human resources policies and these should be considered when deciding the roster format for individual units.

The traditional shift patterns are based on 3 × 8-hour shifts per day (Fig. 2.1) or 2 × 12-hour (or variations of 12.5- and 13-hour) shifts. The implementation of a 12-hour roster requires careful consideration of its risks and benefits, with full consultation of all parties, unit staff, hospital management and the relevant nurses' union. Perceived benefits of working a 12-hour roster include improvement in personal/social life, reduced carbon emissions, enhanced work satisfaction, improved patient care continuity and a better recovery time between shifts.[96] An Australian survey also noted the popularity of 12-hour shifts for improving family life and reducing sick time, without compromising patient outcomes.[97] Perceived risks, such as an alteration in the level of sick-leave hours,

---

FIGURE 2.1   Calculating staff requirements.

The following example is for a 6-bed intensive care unit. A roster has been determined to employ 6 nurses using a 3-shift/day approach (morning, evening, night [10 h]). A 2-hour morning (a.m.) to afternoon (p.m.) shift handover period and a 30-minute afternoon to night (ND) shift handover period are included. Local shift times and practices can be substituted.

Step 1 Calculate the number of working hours needed:

a.m. shift	0700 to 1530	= 7.6 h × 6 nurses × 7 days	319.2 h
p.m. shift	1330 to 2200	= 7.6 h × 6 nurses × 7 days	319.2 h
Night shift	2130 to 0730	= 10 h × 6 nurses × 7 days	420 h
Total			1058.4 h

These initial figures do not include sick leave or annual leave. An additional adjustment is therefore required to factor in paid, unpaid, sick and study leave. A 22% 'leave allowance' is included to accommodate these aspects. A locally derived figure may be substituted here, usually available from the finance or personnel department.

Step 2 Add the leave allowance:
1058.4 h × 1.22 (leave allowance) = 1291.2 h/38 h (1 FTE) = 33.9 FTEs

With a staffing pattern of 6 staff per shift, this unit requires an establishment of 33.9 full-time equivalents (FTEs) to meet the needs of this roster. This figure does not include positions such as the nurse unit manager, team leader/shift coordinator and clinical nurse educator, as outlined in the ACCCN guidelines[41]

---

decreased reaction times and reduced alertness during the longer shift, have not been found to be significant, and a review of the evidence showed there was no clear evidence for implementing or withdrawing 12-hour shifts.[98] However, significant fatigue, worsening with cumulative shifts, has been reported.[99,100] A mix of short and long shifts has also been found to worsen outcomes in terms of perceived care left undone and staffing shortfalls,[101] along with missed care, such as observations.[102] A reported disadvantage of 12-hour shifts is the loss of the shift overlap time, which has traditionally been used for providing in-unit educational sessions. A consideration, therefore, for units proposing the implementation of a 12-hour shift pattern is to build formal staff education sessions into the roster proposal. Sufficient break time should also be considered, and even nap times have been suggested in recent research to improve fatigue in ICU nurses on 12-hour shifts.[103]

Rostering may also need to take account of additional staffing requirements to allow early rehabilitation and to staff recovery clinics, which are frequently staffed through ICU nursing rotas. Staff availability has been reported as a key barrier to implementing or sustaining early rehabilitation for critically ill patients,[104] and in another study rehabilitation therapy was not provided for 50% of ICU days per patient because of limited staffing.[105]

Education and training

During the latter half of the 20th century, specialist critical care nursing education made the transition from hospital-based courses to the tertiary education sector. While some hospitals maintain in-house critical care courses, these are generally designed to meet the tertiary requirements of postgraduate education and to articulate with higher-level university programs.

Some organisations and regional networks (where these exist), including professional bodies, and private and public organisations, continue to offer a variety of short continuing education courses as well. These vary in the level of knowledge and skills and do not generally reach tertiary education standards, nor are accredited at that level. These do, however, play a role in providing an introduction for a novice practitioner.[43] Position statements on the preparation and education of critical care nurses have been developed by professional societies.[43,48,106] These present frameworks to ensure that the course curricula provide adequate content to prepare nurses for this specialist nursing role.

Nursing has always been a profession that has required currency of knowledge and clinical skills through continuing education input, because of the rapidly changing knowledge base and innovative treatment regimens. These changes are occurring at an increasingly rapid rate, particularly in critical care. The need for critical care nurses to maintain current, up-to-date knowledge across a broad range of clinical states has, therefore, never been more important. In addition, these curricula need to be underpinned by relevant and up-to-date research, as in the Australian clinical practice outcome standards in critical care nurse education.[107] Specific issues related to orientation and continuing education programs are briefly discussed below.

Orientation and competencies

The term orientation reflects a range of activities, from a comprehensive unit-based program, attendance at a hospital induction program covering the mandatory educational requirements of that facility, through to familiarisation with the layout of a department. The aim of an orientation program is the development of safe and effective practitioners, but a study evaluating an orientation program for new RN graduates in critical care also reported significantly improved retention rates at 3, 6 and 12 months, and financial savings as a result of reduced nurse turnover.[108]

Unit-specific orientation should be a formal, structured program of assessment, demonstration of competence and identification of ongoing educational needs, and should be developed to meet the needs of all staff members who are new to the unit. Competency-based orientation is learner focused and based on the achievement of core skills that reflect unit needs and enable new employees to function in their role at the completion of the orientation period.[109] A number of countries have developed core competency standards for specialist critical care nurses,[48,110–113] which may be used as a framework on which to build competency-based orientation programs. In the UK, for example, there are nationwide competencies for adult critical care nurses to progress through, with the aim of introducing nurses to critical care and developing critical care nursing to a high (advanced practitioner/nurse-in-charge) standard.[106]

Practice tip

The ACCCN recommends an optimum qualified critical care nurse ratio of 75%.

Continuing education

In 2003, both the Royal College of Nursing Australia and the College of Nursing implemented systems of formally recognising professional development, with the awarding of continuing education points. While professional development has always been a requirement of continuing practice, this process is becoming more formalised. The Australian Health Practitioner Regulation Agency (AHPRA) mandated a formal requirement for continuing education or professional development in 2010. The Nursing and Midwifery Board of Australia (NMBA), a subgroup of the above agency, clearly identifies the standard for continuing professional development of nurses and midwives.[114] In New Zealand there is a requirement for nurses to complete a minimum of 60 hours professional development and 450 hours of clinical practice over a 3-year period for the purposes of registration renewal.[115] Similarly, in the UK and Europe, mandatory professional development hours and evidence of learning are required for registration renewal.[110,111] Conversely, North American nursing associations have for many years had formal programs for recognising continuing education and awarding continuing education points. These continuing education points have often been required to support continued registration.

Risk management

Managing risk is a high priority in health, and critical care is an important risk-laden environment in which the manager needs to be on the lookout for potential error, harm and medico-legal vulnerability. The Sentinel Events Evaluation study[116] has given an indication of this risk for critical care patients. The authors undertook a 24-hour observational study of 1913 patients in 205 ICUs worldwide; 584 errors were identified, causing harm or potential harm to 391 patients. The study authors concluded there was an urgent need for development and implementation of strategies for prevention and early detection of errors.[116] A second study by the same team specifically targeted errors in administration of parenteral drugs in ICUs.[117] In this study, 1328 patients in 113 ICUs worldwide were studied for 24 hours; 861 errors affecting 441 patients occurred, or 74.5 parenteral drug administration errors per 100 patient days. The authors concluded that organisational factors such as error reporting systems and routine checks would reduce the risk of such errors.[117]

What is more alarming is that many health practitioners do not acknowledge their own vulnerability to error. In one study airline flight crews (30,000) and health professionals (1033 ICU/operating room doctors and nurses, of whom 446 were nurses) from five different countries were asked a simple question, 'Does fatigue affect your (work) performance?', with fascinating results.[118] Of those responding, the following replied in the affirmative to the question: pilots and flight crew, 74%; anaesthetists, 53%; surgeons, 30% (a figure for nurses' responses to this question was not provided in the study). The study also found that only 33% of hospital staff thought errors were handled appropriately in their hospital and that over 50% of ICU staff found it hard to discuss errors.[119]

Practice tip

It is alarming that many health practitioners do not acknowledge their own vulnerability to error.

Assessing risk in any setting requires an assessment of the problem, the cause and the solution. The problem requires a specific definition (e.g. power outage in ICU). Multiple approaches have been developed to examine risks in hospitals, the most common being the matrix

FIGURE 2.2 Risk matrix example.

		Consequence				
		Negligible 1	Minor 2	Moderate 3	Major 4	Catastrophic 5
Likelihood	5 Almost certain	Moderate 5	High 10	Extreme 15	Extreme 20	Extreme 25
	4 Likely	Moderate 4	High 8	High 12	Extreme 16	Extreme 20
	3 Possible	Low 3	Moderate 6	High 9	High 12	Extreme 15
	2 Unlikely	Low 2	Moderate 4	Moderate 6	High 8	High 10
	1 Rare	Low 1	Low 2	Low 3	Moderate 4	Moderate 5

Source: From https://www.repository.cam.ac.uk/bitstream/handle/1810/273747/Kaya-2018-PhD.pdf?sequence=1&isAllowed=y

approach where the likelihood and consequences of a risk occurring are examined to determine whether the risk is low, medium, high or extreme, as shown in Fig. 2.2.[119] At one end of the spectrum, if the likelihood is rare and the consequence of the risk occurring is negligible or minor then the risk is categorised as low. However, if the likelihood is likely or almost certain and the consequence is major or catastrophic then the risk is extreme.

Other important elements to the risk assessment will be cause and preventative controls (i.e. how to reduce likelihood of risk occurring) and mitigating controls (i.e. how to reduce consequence/harm should the risk event occur). More specifically, treatment action plans (TAPs) to mitigate the risk will be developed and documented with a named TAP owner and due-by date. Finally, an ALARP (as low as reasonably possible) rating will be calculated suggesting the most likely risk rating one could expect if all TAPs are successfully implemented.[120]

Governance and management of the critical care environment requires a MDT of senior clinician managers who understand both the clinical risk and the quality cycles of the environment as well as the executive requirements for financial and organisational viability. An astute and careful balance between good clinical governance (patient care and clinician practices) and good corporate governance (hotel, finance, IT and other support services) is required to ensure sustainable and appropriate healthcare for all users. The take-home message in all this is that managers in hospitals manage enormous risks with patients, staff and visitors but often do not appreciate their own level of vulnerability to error and risk. Yet claims of negligence and charges of incompetence can be as threatening to the manager as they are to the clinician.

Negligence

Negligence is a legal term that can be proven only in a court. In tort law, four aspects to the charge of negligence are generally accepted:

1 The provider owed a duty of care to the recipient.

2 The provider failed to meet that duty, resulting in a breach of care.

3 The recipient sustained damages (loss) as a result.

4 The breech by the provider caused the recipient to suffer reasonably foreseeable damages.[121]

Since the introduction of Civil Liability legislation in most states and territories of Australia, courts use a multifactorial assessment of all the facts to determine the level of liability or otherwise of the defendant. However, the case of UK *GMC vs Bawa-Garba* has demonstrated two important facts: that hospital staff are vulnerable to charges of manslaughter should they make an unintended mistake or omission that results in the death of a patient and that nurses should not try to represent themselves in court under such circumstances.[122]

Critical to reducing liability in this area is the need for health services and managers to have in place current policies, procedures and supervision processes to ensure contemporary and safe practices among its workforce.[123]

The role of leadership and management

Managers must also be leaders, and the need to have good leaders and managers is as relevant to critical care as it is to any other business or clinical entity. Seminal research studies on organisational structures in ICUs across the USA in the 1980s[124] and 1990s[125] demonstrated the important role leadership plays in patient care and risk management in the ICU. Using APACHE (Acute Physiology And Chronic Health Evaluation) scoring, organisational efficiency and risk-adjusted survival were measured. High-performing ICUs demonstrated that actual survival rates exceeded predicted survival rates.[124,125]

Further investigation and analysis of the higher-performing units noted that these units had well-defined protocols, a medical director to coordinate activities, well-educated nurses and collaboration between nurses and doctors.[124,125] Clear and accessible policies and procedures to guide staff practice in the ICU setting were also highlighted. These policies and procedures need to be in written form, simple to read and in a consistent format, evidence-based, easy to understand and easy to apply.

The later study by Zimmerman et al[125] showed similar characteristics: they had a patient-centred culture, strong medical and nursing leadership, effective communication and coordination, and open and collaborative problem solving and conflict management. One cannot underestimate the value of strong, dedicated and collaborative leadership from managers as the key to organisational success in the critical care setting. These factors are as pertinent now as they were when first studied over 30 years ago and they remind us of the important role of leadership to ensure the safety of patients, visitors and staff alike in this complex health setting. Chapter 1 contains a discussion about leadership.

Managing injury: staff, patient or visitor

When staff members are injured, the response must be swift and deliberate. Injury can come in many forms, involving physical injuries, biological exposures or psychological distress, for example. More often, the problems are grievances, such as missing out on an opportunity afforded to others (e.g. a promotion), feeling marginalised by others or not getting a preferred roster.

For patients, an injury can be physical, such as a drug error or an iatrogenic infection; however, the injury can

---

> **BOX 2.3**
>
> **Defensive principles to minimise risk after an incident (patient or staff)**
>
> - Those persons encouraged to participate in decision making are more inclined to 'own' the decisions made; therefore, involve them in deciding how the issue is to be tackled and help to make the expectations realistic.
> - Education of the person in the various aspects of the incident/activity will reduce fear and anxiety.
> - Explain the range of possible outcomes and where the affected person is currently situated on that continuum.
> - Provide frequent and accurate updates on the person's situation and what is being done to improve that situation.
> - Maintain a consistent approach and as far as possible the same person should provide such information/feedback.
>
> *Source: Williams G. Quality management in intensive care. In: Gullo A, editor. Anesthesia, pain, intensive care and emergency medicine. Berlin:Springer-Verlag; 2003. p. 1239–50.*[24]

---

also be non-physical and can affect patients, visitors and staff members, as with complaints about lack of timely information, misinformation or rudeness of staff. In all circumstances a manager needs to intervene proactively to minimise or contain the negativity or harm felt by the 'victim'. Regardless of the cause of the injury, the principles governing good risk management are common to many situations and are summarised in Box 2.3.

If an incident does occur, it is always prudent to document the event as soon as possible afterwards and when it is safe to do so. The clinician who discovers and follows up an incident must document the event, asking the questions that a manager, family member, police officer, lawyer or judge might wish to ask. The written account provided soon after the event or incident by a person closely involved in it, or witness to it, will form a very important testimonial in any subsequent investigation. Key points to document are identified in Table 2.4.

> **Practice tip**
>
> If an incident does occur, it is always prudent to document the event as soon as possible afterwards and when it is safe to do so.

Contemporary wisdom in modern health agencies advocates open disclosure: telling the truth to the patient or family about why and how an adverse event has occurred.[126,127] This practice may be contrary to informed

TABLE 2.4

Key points when documenting an incident in a patient's file notes

QUESTION	EXPLANATION
Where did the incident occur?	For example, bedside, toilet, drug room.
Were there any pre-event circumstances of significance?	For example, short-staffed, no written protocol, medications with side effects that could have contributed.
Who witnessed the event?	Including staff, patient, visitors.
What was done to minimise negative effects?	For example, extra staff brought in to assist, spill wiped up, sign placed on front of patient chart warning of reaction/sensitivity, etc.
Who in authority was notified of the incident?	Involving a senior, experienced manager/authority should help expedite immediate and effective action.
Who informed the victim of the event? What was the victim told? What was the response?	Clear, concise and non-judgemental explanations to victim or representative are necessary as soon as possible, preferably from a credible authority (manager/director).
What follow-up support, counselling and revision occurred?	This is important for both victim and perpetrator; ascertain when counselling occurred and who provided it.
What review systems were commenced to limit recurrence of the event?	Magistrates and coroners in particular want to know what system changes have occurred to limit the recurrence of the event.

Source: Williams G. Quality management in intensive care. In: Gullo A, editor. Anesthesia, pain, intensive care and emergency medicine. Berlin:Springer-Verlag; 2003. p. 1239–50.[24]

legal advice and may not preclude legal action against the staff or institution.[128–130] However, openly informing the patient/family of what has occurred can regain trust and respect and may help to resolve anger and frustration. The open disclosure process can also provide learning and education on how such events can be prevented in the future and provide consumers and their advocates with greater confidence and trust in the healthcare system.[131–133]

The process of root cause analysis (RCA) can also assist the team to explore in detail the sequence of events and system failures that precipitated an incident and help to inform future system reforms to minimise harm. A RCA is a generic method of 'drilling down' to identify hospital system deficiencies that may not immediately be apparent, and that may have contributed to the occurrence of a 'sentinel event'. The general characteristics of an RCA are that it:[134]

- focuses on systems and processes, not individual performance
- is fair, thorough and efficient
- focuses on problem solving
- uses recognised analytical methods
- uses a scale of effectiveness to develop recommendations.

Despite more than two decades of human error studies in health, and critical care specifically, the incidence of error, omission and patient harm continues to plague our industry and requires ongoing vigilance, commitment, research and focus.

Management of disease outbreaks and pandemics

The World Health Organization (WHO) defines a pandemic as the worldwide spread of a new disease.[135] A disease outbreak, on the other hand, is the occurrence of cases of disease in excess of what would normally be expected in a defined community, geographical area or season. An outbreak may occur in a restricted geographical area or may extend over several countries. It may last for a few days or weeks, or for several years. A single case of a communicable disease long absent from a population, or caused by an agent (e.g. bacterium or virus) not previously recognised in that community or area, or the emergence of a previously unknown disease, may also constitute an outbreak and should be reported and investigated.[136] Importantly, defining an outbreak as a pandemic has significant implications for the public health response and pandemic preparedness.[137] The advent of the COVID-19 pandemic in 2019, continuing in waves with peaks over several years, has been a stark reminder of the scale and devastating impact of such pandemics.

Planning for the impact, or potential impact, of a disease outbreak/pandemic is required at the global (WHO), national (federal government), regional (state/province), organisational (hospital), departmental (ICU) and individual (health professional) level. This section highlights the areas and responsibilities to be considered at the individual facility (i.e. hospital) and regional (in case of staffing transfers, as we saw in the COVID-19 pandemic with inter-state working in some countries as part of the national response) levels, with an emphasis on ICU-specific considerations in a pandemic.

Intensive care beds and their associated resources (e.g. space, equipment and staffing) are finite resources and coordinated national, regional and organisational responses are required to maximise potential ICU capacity during outbreaks. Lessons learnt from the global H1N1 pandemic in 2009 and the Australian disease outbreak of H3N2 in 2017[104] informed the COVID-19 pandemic response, particularly with regards vaccination planning.[138] However, this was not universal, with many OECD countries failing to learn from H1N1,[139] with the International Panel for Pandemic Preparedness and Response describing a global failure on the responses to COVID-19, and with an overhaul of health systems required to address future pandemics.[141,142] The need to plan for the potential increased demand on critical care services in the face of a pandemic was not fully understood in terms of scale, with many countries resorting to increased expansion through the use of temporary structures (tents or repurposed alternative facilities) and redeployment of staff, and cessation of what were deemed non-essential services (such as elective surgery) in order to provide resources to mount the response. Low- and middle-income countries (LMICs) in particular have been hit hard by the recent COVID-19 pandemic, exacerbating global health inequalities.[140,141] Numerous critiques of the critical care response to the COVID-19 pandemic have outlined comprehensive failures at a systems level, compounded by a pre-existing global shortage of critical care staff, beds and infrastructure.[142–145] Analysis of the four S's – Space, Staff, Supplies, Systems – evidenced key deficits,[146] including insufficient personal protective equipment (PPE) in many parts of the world, that subsequently had a devastating impact on people, both staff members and ICU patients. An international Delphi of global experts has since defined the minimum specifications needed for critical care in a pandemic, including drugs, human resources, training, equipment, routines, guidelines and infrastructure required.[144] While it is beyond the scope of this chapter to cover this subject comprehensively, the aim is to outline the areas for further examination, touching on the concept of the development of a surge plan. Chapter 14 contains a description of critical care clinical responses to respiratory pandemics.

In earlier experiences,[147–152] critical care units played a key role in an organised response to a pandemic, particularly an airborne one such as influenza, where critical care units are more often severely affected than other clinical areas of a hospital. As has been evidenced throughout the COVID-19 pandemic, demand for these services will often exceed normal supply.

Development of surge plans

The WHO,[146] in response to COVID-19, adapted Barbisch et al's[153] 'four S's', outlined above and used frequently in surge activity to highlight where pandemic responses could be strengthened, and we draw on these here in terms of developing a surge plan in critical care. We will include 'command and communication' under Systems. The resources required are examined under these headings.

Staff (human resources)

The ability to provide additional staff for a potentially expanded critical care bed base should examine the following:

- staff with critical care skills who do not currently work in this area
- staff from other areas with critical care-based skills, such as recovery, anaesthetics, coronary care
- cessation of other services in order to facilitate staff redeployment to critical care
- deployment and ability of critical care staff in allied roles (such as physiotherapists) to carry out critical care nursing duties *in extremis*
- provision of comprehensive training and education to support less experienced staff, including non-registered nursing staff and people with no healthcare experience at all
- development of critical care teams in which critical care expertise is spread across the teams to manage the patient load appropriately, for example using a range of critical care professionals to provide team-based care and creation of task teams and support of those in satellite units
- planning for critical care staff sick leave
- consideration of cessation of study/planned leave
- planning for fluctuations in staffing requirements in the longer term as public health intelligence emerges at a national, regional and local level, and knowledge is consolidated through pandemic experience
- provision to redeploy staff who are at increased risk from the cause of the pandemic, for example pregnant staff, staff with chronic health conditions and/or emotionally vulnerable staff
- consideration of inter-state/region transfer of patients and inter-state/region staff transfers (including training and indemnity requirements) to deal with localised outbreaks/surges
- emotional support in the form of team debriefing, and occasionally individual counselling. This is essential during and after the event. Anxiety, panic, burnout, compassion fatigue and post-traumatic stress are clearly associated with an intense and sustained pandemic. One cannot underestimate the importance of experienced, emotionally intelligent, visible leadership during such events.

Practice tip

Staff well-being must be a staff-planning priority for managers, with allocated time for staff well-being and restorative supervision to be incorporated into roster planning.

Supplies

The ability to manage supplies at times of uncertain demand is a key element for examination, as is the knowledge and understanding of the processes for accessing additional equipment such as ventilators and medications from international/state emergency stockpiles, for example:

- Ensure supplies of appropriate personal protective equipment and planning for PPE supplies based on public health intelligence (so that stockpiling in one area does not occur and that there is agility to move supplies across areas/organisations as required).

- Develop plans/policies for the rational use of personal protective equipment, based on clear and up-to-date evidence.

- Ensure supplies, and access to supplies, of required medications, using pharmacy/manufacturing networked intelligence and medical professional bodies to underpin this and ensure contingency plans are published and shared widely.

- Plan ability to boost ventilator capacity, such as with increased use of bi-phasic positive airways pressure/continuous positive airway pressure (BiPAP/CPAP) or accessing state/regional/national emergency stockpiles, or short-term leasing options with company providers, and manufacturers if greater scaling is required to produce new ventilators.

- Plan to increase renal replacement therapy capacity by looking at alternative options to, for example, continuous venovenous haemodiafiltration (CVVHDF) in the event of potential shortages, such as using sustained low-efficiency dialysis (SLED).

Space

Examine and plan strategies to functionally increase the available critical care bed capacity, as follows:

- Defer elective surgery and other elective procedures.
- Explore the ability of local private hospitals to assist with service provision for non-deferrable surgical cases.
- Identify alternative clinical areas within the hospital that may provide additional critical care beds as a satellite unit, such as recovery and coronary care.
- Identify non-clinical areas that can be rapidly transformed into critical care areas (e.g. office blocks/conference centres/temporary structures such as tents)
- Triage access to limited ventilation and/or critical care resources.[154–158]

Systems

Where there are well-connected critical care units, through national networks and bodies, the responses can be better coordinated. A systems approach is needed to address coordination to:

- maintain essential services during a pandemic, while freeing up capacity for, for example, a COVID response[146]

- mobilise financial and logistical support at a national and local level, and remove usual barriers (including consideration of rapid law changes to allow organisational data sharing without the usual hurdles, for example)

- anticipate barriers for vulnerable people in terms of healthcare access (e.g. people with intellectual disabilities who may be frightened of attending an emergency department)

- ensure role clarity (and make this visible, through publishing on organisational webpages/internal communications) across organisations and at regional/national levels in critical care and in wider healthcare

- protect the physical health of frontline workers[146] (see above), and consider vulnerability in certain populations such as black and ethnic minority staff, which became particularly evident in the COVID-19 pandemic in terms of genetic susceptibility, using evidence to underpin this

- consolidate existing and implement new rapid decision-making structures to streamline clinical processes and services

- ensure that teamwork, shared decision making (where possible) and respect is at the forefront of all interaction in order to maximise collaborative working.

Command and communication

- Identification of a clear chain of command is essential to facilitate fast and efficient decision making, communication and action. The person in command must have authority, experience and maturity to guide and decide during very dynamic changing circumstances. In addition they must be precise in their communication, ensuring orders are correct, understandable and implementable. Whilst these qualities are essential in all leadership roles, they are particularly necessary during intense situations such as these.

- Hospital signage and communication to (a) restrict visitor entrance, (b) minimise person-to-person contact (social distancing may be required) and (c) appropriate use of PPE. Consideration should be given to the use of international symbols as well as common languages in the community.

- Provision of training and education of all staff to avoid panic and concern and to communicate appropriate messaging to others. For example, domestic and catering staff can play an important role in containing spread of disease/panic if informed and confident in their knowledge and role during an outbreak.

- Regular information circulars to keep all staff and the community abreast of what is being done to contain the disease and to keep people safe.

Critical care surge plan

Templates to assist in the development of critical care surge plans are now widely available, particularly since the advent of COVID-19.[159–161] A 2020 survey demonstrated that Australian ICUs had the capacity to triple capacity *in extremis*,[162] but noted that this would require an increase in nursing workforce of an additional 42,720 registered nursing staff (365% above baseline staffing); however, this was variable depending on where surge capacity increase would take place (e.g. beds in or outside ICU). Most COVID-19 surge plans in critical care adopted team-based care approaches, which were found in one study to be the most flexible way team skills could be shared.[90] The following example from New South Wales is predicated on staged levels of capacity increase with recommendations for staffing:

Level 0 – business as usual, minimal impact, prepare to surge workforce

- A standard workforce model is used with experienced intensive care staff as per the Australian and State workforce standards and guidelines[43,164]

Level 1 – moderate compromise and impact on workforce

- Supplement standard workforce model with non-ICU critical care staff (e.g. in anaesthetics, emergency, operating theatres, recovery and coronary care units, nurses who have been part of an ICU refresher model)
- Where possible, maintain 1 FTE physiotherapist for 4 ICU beds and other allied health staffing at recommended levels[165,166]

Level 2 – severe compromise and impact on workforce

- The model will move to a MDT-based model, which groups staff members into role- or experience-based tasks (e.g. intubation teams, proning and turning teams, transfer teams, medication teams, IV access teams, hygiene teams or 'expert senior' support teams, etc.).
- It is important that senior nursing roles are available as supernumerary and work in teams to provide support, review nursing management and maintain safe standards:
  - 1 × nursing manager (NM)/ nursing unit manager (NUM) 24/7 across all unit/pods.
  - 1 × NP or clinical nurse consultant (CNC) 24/7 across all unit/pods.
  - 1 × 24/7 NUM1 per unit/pod.
  - 1 × 24/7 nurse educator (NE)/clinical nurse educator (CNE) per unit/pod.
  - 1 × 24/7 ACCESS (assistance, coordination, contingency, education, supervision, support) nurse per unit/pod.
  - 1 × 24/7 ICU registered nurse (RN) team leader per unit/pod.
  - 1 × experienced ICU RN to supervise 2 critical care RNs.
  - Critical care RNs to supervise 2 × non-ICU nurses caring for ICU2-type patients.
  - 1 × infection control coordinator across all units/pods.
- It is important to increase allied health staffing across all professions to accommodate increased demand and maintain multidisciplinary care, where possible.

Level 3 – extreme compromise and overwhelming impact with local workforce exhausted

- Team-based model
  - 1 × whole of hospital duty intensive care consultant with other medical specialists to support intensive care triage and decision making on resuscitation and goals of care.
  - 1 × intensive care nurse co-ordinator per 28 beds.
  - 2 × senior intensive care nurses per 28 beds.
  - 2 × anaesthetic or refresher ICU nurses per 28 beds.
  - 1 × intensive care or critical care RN to supervise 4 nurses and/or other staff.
  - 1 × infection control coordinator across all units/pods.

Sources: Adapted from https://aci.health.nsw.gov.au/__data/assets/pdf_file/0007/594772/Adult-intensive-care-workforce-report.pdf,[163] and NSW Ministry of Health Demand Escalation Framework 2016.[165]

The use of such a template, which can be populated with locally appropriate definitions and information, can provide the basis for a comprehensive unit/facility specific response to the requirement for a graduated response to a pandemic. Comprehensive models for redeployment of staff from non-critical care areas into critical care, based on experiences in COVID-19, are also available.[167,168] However, COVID-19 has provided salient lessons that surge plans must be applied alongside plans to support staff well-being, which was adversely affected by COVID-19,[169–172] to allow for initiatives like restorative supervision,[173] and to provide structural support (e.g. adequate rest facilities), also felt by staff to be key.[174] Contingencies must also account for the high levels of staff sickness that are likely to accompany pandemics. Planning for events such as a pandemic require a coordinated, collaborative approach, informed by the latest evidence, with input from all members of the healthcare team from management to delivery staff. Clear planning is key to developing scalable, flexible plans that are underpinned by national and state structures, and local management structures/policies, and that support clear and transparent communication. De-escalation plans are also important for staff well-being and resource management.[175]

Summary

The management of all resources in the critical care unit is key to meeting the needs of the patients in a safe, ethical, timely and cost-effective manner. Many factors influence not only the resources available but also how these resources are allocated. Managers of critical care units are required to be knowledgeable in the design and equipping of units; human resource management, including the constitution of the nursing workforce; and the fundamentals of the budget – how it is determined, monitored and managed. Understanding the principles of risk management and tools such as those that measure nursing workload help nurse managers in their planning and decision making. Having good structures and processes in place that place staff as a priority alongside patients helps facilitate the delivery of care during times of crisis, such as that experienced when pandemics occur.

Case study

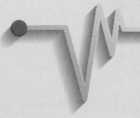

The Nightingale Hospital is a 650-bed, metropolitan, general teaching public hospital that is planning to expand their intensive care unit from 35 to 45 beds. The additional 10 beds will have negative pressure/isolation capacity in 5 of the rooms. Your task as the NUM is to plan what additional nursing and equipment resources are required to make this a functional unit once it is fully commissioned. The hospital also has a separate 20-bed CCU, 30-bay post-anaesthetic care unit (PACU) and a 10-bed PICU. The hospital is geographically co-located to a 300-bed private hospital and 15 kilometres from a large international airport that receives direct flights from all over the world.

Among other things, you must consider the following tasks and make recommendations to the Director of Nursing of the Nightingale Hospital (see Learning activities 1–4 below). Utilise information contained in this chapter to inform your work and recommendations.

CASE STUDY QUESTIONS

1 Calculate the additional staffing numbers in FTEs that you will require to staff the increase in beds. Determine the estimated cost of these additional staff, including a breakdown of both productive and non-productive FTEs required.

2 Identify the major equipment needs for the additional 10 beds and develop an estimated budget plan for these items based on your knowledge of costs in your region. List the criteria that should be included in the evaluation of new consumable products for this expansion.

3 Identify the three fundamental steps in the budget process and the important considerations for each in this project.

4 In preparation for writing a critical care surge plan, calculate the surge capacity required for an additional 25-ICU-patient capacity beyond the capacity of the new expanded (45-bed) ICU.

RESEARCH VIGNETTE

Rae P, Pearce S, Greaves PJ, et al Outcomes sensitive to critical care nurse staffing levels: a systematic review. Intensive Crit Care Nurs 2021;67:103110[76]

Abstract

Objective: To determine associations between variations in registered nurse staffing levels in adult critical care units and outcomes such as patient, nurse, organisational and family outcomes.

Methods: We published and adhered to a protocol, stored in an open access repository and searched for quantitative studies written in the English language and held in CINAHL Plus, MEDLINE, PsycINFO, SCOPUS and NDLTD databases up to July 2020. Three authors independently extracted data and critically appraised papers meeting the inclusion criteria. Results are summarised in tables and discussed in terms of strength of internal validity. A detailed review of the two most commonly measured outcomes, patient mortality and nosocomial infection, is also presented.

Results: Our search returned 7960 titles after duplicates were removed; 55 studies met the inclusion criteria. Studies with strong internal validity report significant associations between lower levels of critical care nurse staffing and increased odds of both patient mortality (1.24 to 3.50 times greater) and nosocomial infection (3.28 to 3.60 times greater), increased hospital costs, lower nurse-perceived quality of care and lower family satisfaction. Meta-analysis was not feasible because of the wide variation in how both staffing and outcomes were measured.

Conclusions: A large number of studies including several with strong internal validity provide evidence that higher levels of critical care nurse staffing are beneficial to patients, staff and health services. However, inconsistent approaches to measurement and aggregation of staffing levels reported makes it hard to translate findings into recommendation for safe staffing in critical care.

Critique

This systematic review drew together available literature to determine how variations in staffing levels in adult critical care had a bearing on outcomes at a patient, staff and organisational level. In accordance with systematic review methods, the review was registered a priori on an open, publicly available database, articles were independently screened and data were abstracted via an extraction tool. The quality of studies and the heterogeneity of outcomes did not permit pooled analysis in a meta-analysis, and the aim of the review was to capture the range of outcomes; therefore, this was appropriate. The authors assessed the internal validity of studies in order to provide estimates of confidence in their review findings; these were organised into categories of low, medium and high validity (which only 23 of the 55 studies achieved). Although interpretations of validity were agreed between the authors, these were subjective and relied on individual interpretations of validity. The 55 studies reviewed most often constituted cross-sectional studies, with only 14 longitudinal studies, and the studies were a mix of retrospective and prospective, but no interventional studies met the eligibility criteria for the review, emphasising the difficulties in conducting interventional studies in nurse staffing. Outcomes measured included family satisfaction ($n = 4$), nurse staffing as the key outcome ($n = 44$), care process outcomes ($n = 13$) and only one focused on nurse outcomes.

Clear evidence from studies spanning a single ICU to one including 1265 ICUs, and 30 to 159,400 patients, was found for higher levels of nurse staffing being beneficial for patient outcomes (patient survival was improved). Evidence for family satisfaction and nurse well-being, patient incidents and hospital costs was weak, in part due to the small number of studies examining these factors. The authors acknowledge the limitations of the review in their discussion, namely that risk-adjustment methods were not accounted for in the review; risk adjustments were frequently applied to various variables in each of the studies in the review, e.g. unit and patient/nurse risk adjustments (particularly those in those studies with high reported validity), with a high degree of heterogeneity of adjustment methods. The authors outline how these adjustments included level of critical care nursing experience and training and type of patient admission, alongside many more. While this approach is reasonable in systematic reviews, it is possible that unaccounted-for reasons may have been present that influenced the findings at both study and review level. The authors also draw attention to the ongoing problem of inconsistent approaches to measuring staffing, defining staff groups and combining staffing data for wider interpretation. Detail in the review allows replication of the review and sufficient information is provided to permit interpretation of the results. Overall, this is a high-quality review that provides a clear account of a range of outcomes and their relationship to nurses staffing in ICU.

Online resources

ACSQH Business template. https://www.safetyandquality.gov.au/sites/default/files/migrated/BusinessCaseTemplate.pdf

Ettelt S, Nolte E. Funding intensive care: approaches in systems using diagnosis-related groups, https://www.rand.org/content/dam/rand/pubs/technical_reports/2010/RAND_TR792.pdf

IHI. Optimizing a business case for safe health care: an integrated approach to safety and finance, https://www.ihi.org/resources/Pages/Tools/Business-Case-for-Safe-Health-Care.aspx

NHS General business case guidelines, https://www.england.nhs.uk/publication/general-business-case-process-guidance/

Further reading

Durbin CG. Team model: advocating for the optimal method of care delivery in the intensive care unit. Crit Care Med 2006;34(3 Suppl.):S12–17.

Gill FJ, Leslie GD, Grech C, et al. An analysis of Australian graduate critical care nurse education. Collegian 2015;22:71–81.

Manojlovich M, Saint S, Forman J, et al. Developing and testing a tool to measure nurse/physician communication in the intensive care unit. J Patient Saf 2011;7(2):80–4.

Parker MM. Critical care disaster management. Crit Care Med 2006;34(3 Suppl.):S52–5.

Redden PH, Evans J. It takes teamwork ... the role of nurses in ICU design. Crit Care Nurs Q 2014;37(1):41–52.

Robnett MK. Critical care nursing: workforce issues and potential solutions. Crit Care Med 2006;34(3 Suppl.):S25–31.

Valentin A, Ferdinande P. Recommendations on basic requirements for intensive care units: structural and organizational aspects. Intensive Care Med 2011;37:1575–87.

References

1. Galbally B. The planning and organization of an intensive care unit. Med J Aust 1966;1(15):622–4.
2. Johnston MJ. Bioethics: a nursing perspective. 7th ed. Sydney, NSW: Elsevier; 2019.
3. Wiles V, Daffurn K. There is a bird in my hand and a bear by the bed – I must be in ICU. Sydney, NSW: Australian College of Critical Care Nurses; 2002.
4. Ettelt S, Nolte E. Funding intensive care – approaches in systems using diagnosis-related groups. Santa Monica, CA: RAND; 2010. Available from: https://www.rand.org/content/dam/rand/pubs/technical_reports/2010/RAND_TR792.pdf. [Accessed 10 February 2023].
5. Independent Hospital Pricing Authority (IHPA). National efficient price determination 2022–23. Sydney, NSW: IHPA; 2022. Available from: https://www.ihacpa.gov.au/resources/national-efficient-price-determination-2022-23. [Accessed 10 February 2023].
6. Independent Hospital Pricing Authority (IHPA). National pricing model technical specifications 2022–23. Sydney, NSW: IHPA; 2022. Available from: https://www.ihacpa.gov.au/resources/national-pricing-model-technical-specifications-2022-23. [Accessed 10 February 2023].
7. College of Intensive Care Medicine (CICM). Minimum standards for intensive care units. Prahran, VIC: CICM; 2016. Available from: https://cicm.org.au/CICM_Media/CICMSite/Files/Professional/IC-1-Minimum-Standards-for-Intensive-Care-Units.pdf. [Accessed 10 February 2023].
8. Kleinpell R, Barden C, Rincon T, et al. Assessing the impact of telemedicine on nursing care in intensive care units. Am J Crit Care 2016; 25(1):e14–e20.
9. Gutierrez G. Artificial intelligence in the intensive care unit. Crit Care 2020;24(1):101. doi: 10.1186/s13054-020-2785-y.
10. Halpern NA, Anderson DC, Kesecioglu J. ICU design in 2050: looking into the crystal ball! Intensive Care Med 2017;43(5):690–2.
11. Oye RK, Bellamy PE. Patterns of resource consumption in medical intensive care. Chest 1991;99(3):685–9.
12. Blot, S, Koulenti D, Dimopoulos G, et al. Prevalence, risk factors, and mortality for ventilator-associated pneumonia in middle-aged, old, and very old critically ill patients. Crit Care Med 2014;42(3):601–9.
13. Nguyen YL, Angus, DC, Boumendil A, et al. The challenge of admitting the very elderly to intensive care. Ann Intensive Care 2011;1:29. doi: 10.1186/2110-5820-1-29.
14. Sim YS, Jung H, Shin TR, et al. Mortality and outcomes in very elderly patients 90 years of age or older admitted to the ICU. Respir Care 2015;60(3):347–55.
15. Vincent JL, Marshall J, Ñamendys-Silva SA, et al. Assessment of the worldwide burden of critical illness: the Intensive Care Over Nations (ICON) audit. Lancet Respir Med 2014;2(5):380–6.
16. Anesi GL, Wagner J, Halpern SD. Intensive care medicine in 2050: toward an intensive care unit without waste. Intensive Care Med 2019;43(4): 554–6. doi: 10.1007/s00134-016-4641-8.
17. Pastores SM, Dakwar J, Halpern NA. Costs of critical care medicine. Crit Care Clin 2012; 28(1):1–10.
18. Lawson JS, Rotem A, Bates PW. From clinician to manager. Sydney, NSW: McGraw-Hill; 1996.
19. Strosberg MA, Wiener J, Baker R. Rationing America's medical care: the Oregon plan and beyond. Washington DC: Brookings Institute Press; 1992.
20. Truog RD, Brock DW, Cook DJ, et al. Rationing in the intensive care unit. Crit Care Med 2006;34(4):958–63, quiz 971.
21. Supady A, Brodie D, Curtis JR. Ten things to consider when implementing rationing guidelines during a pandemic. Intensive Care Med 2021;47:605–8.
22. Guo C, Elliot S, Soso M. The role of Medical Emergency Team in end of life care planning for hospitalised patients. Aust Crit Care 2018;31(2):118.
23. Harvey SV, Adenwala AY; Lane-Fall MB. Defining familial interactions and networks: an exploratory qualitative study on family networks and surrogate decision-making. Crit Care Explor 2021;3(8):e0504. doi: 10.1097/CCE.0000000000000504.
24. Williams G. Quality management in intensive care. In: Gullo A, editor. Anesthesia, pain, intensive care and emergency medicine. Berlin: Springer-Verlag; 2003. p. 1239–50.
25. Donahue L, Rader S, Triolo PK. Nurturing innovation in the critical care environment: transforming care at the bedside. Crit Care Nurs Clin North Am 2008;20(4):465–9.

26. Carter H. How to write a robust business case for service development. Nurs Times [online] 2017;113(7):25–8.

27. Weaver DJ, Sorrells-Jones J. The business case as a strategic tool for change. J Nurs Adm 2007;37(9):414–19.

28. James Cook Univeristy. How to write a business case: tips, resources and examples. North QLD; 2020. Available from: https://online.jcu.edu.au/blog/how-to-write-business-case. [Accessed 10 February 2023].

29. Critical Care Services Ontario (CCSO). Adult critical care levels of care. Toronto: CCSO; 2022. Available from: https://criticalcareontario.ca/wp-content/uploads/2020/11/Adult-LoC-Guidance-Document-Final.pdf. [Accessed 10 February 2023].

30. Faculty of Intensive Care Medicine/Intensive Care Society (FICM/ICS). Guidelines for the provision of intensive care services. 2nd ed, version 2.1. FICM/ICS; 2022. Available from: https://www.ficm.ac.uk/sites/ficm/files/documents/2021-10/gpics-v2.pdf. [Accessed 10 February 2023].

31. Australian Health Infrastructure Alliance (AHIA). Australasian health facility guidelines: part B – health facility briefing and planning 360-intensive care-general. North Sydney, NSW: AHIA; 2016. Available from: https://aushfg-prod-com-au.s3.amazonaws.com/HPU_B.0360_6_0.pdf. [Accessed 10 February 2023].

32. Department of Health (DOH). Health building note 04-02. Critical care units. London: HMSO; 2013. Available from: https://www.england.nhs.uk/wp-content/uploads/2021/05/HBN_04-02_Final.pdf. [Accessed 10 February 2023].

33. International Health Facility Guideline (iHFG). Part B: health facility briefing & design. 130. Intensive care unit – general. Version 5, Milsons Point, NSW: iHFG; 2017. Available from: https://www.healthfacilityguidelines.com/ViewPDF/ViewIndexPDF/iHFG_part_b_intensive_care_unit_general. [Accessed 10 February 2023].

34. Hodgson CL, Schaller SJ, Nydahl P, et al. Ten strategies to optimize early mobilization and rehabilitation in intensive care. Crit Care 2021;25:324. doi: 10.1186/s13054-021-03741-z.

35. Escalon MX, Lichtenstein AH, Posner E, et al. The effects of early mobilization on patients requiring extended mechanical ventilation across multiple ICUs. Crit Care Explor 2020;2(6):e0119. doi: 10.1097/CCE.0000000000000119.

36. Meissen H, Gong MN, Wong AI, et al, on behalf of the Society of Critical Care Medicine's Future of Critical Care Taskforce. The future of critical care: optimizing technologies and a learning healthcare system to potentiate a more humanistic approach to critical care. Crit Care Explor 2022;4(3):e0659. doi: 10.1097/CCE.0000000000000659.

37. Huffling K, Schenk E. Environmental sustainability in the intensive care unit: challenges and solutions. Crit Care Nurs 2014;37(3):235–50.

38. New Zealand College of Critical Care Nurses (NZCCCN). New Zealand College of Critical Care Nurses position statement (2019) on the definition of critical care nursing. Wellington, New Zealand: NZCCCN; 2019.

39. Pattison N. An ever-thorny issue: defining key elements of critical care nursing and its relation to staffing. Nurs Crit Care 2021;26(6):421–4.

40. Royal College of Nursing (RCN). Guidance for nurse staffing in critical care. London: RCN; 2003.

41. Kelly DM, Kutney-Lee A, McHugh MD, et al. Impact of critical care nursing on 30-day mortality of mechanically ventilated older adults. Crit Care Med 2014;42(5):1089–95.

42. UK Critical Care Nursing Alliance (UKCCNA). Position statement: critical care nurse staffing during surge. London: UKCCNA; 2021. Available from: https://www.ficm.ac.uk/sites/ficm/files/documents/2022-01/UKCCNA%20position%20Sep%202021%20FINAL.pdf. [Accessed 10 February 2023].

43. Chamberlain D, Pollock W, Fulbrook P; ACCCN Workforce Standards Development Group. ACCCN workforce standards for intensive care nursing: systematic and evidence review, development, and appraisal. Aust Crit Care 2018;31(5):292–302.

44. British Association of Critical Care Nurses (BACCN). Standards for nurse staffing in critical care. London: BACCN; 2008. Available from: https://www.baccn.org/static/uploads/resources/BACCN_Staffing_Standards.pdf. [Accessed 10 February 2023].

45. Critical Care Nurses' Section: New Zealand Nurses Organisation (NZ CCCN). New Zealand standards for critical care staffing. Wellington: NZ CCCN ; 2020. Available from: https://www.nzno.org.nz/Portals/0/Files/Documents/Groups/Critical%20Care%20Nurses/2020%20NZ%20Standards%20for%20Critical%20Care%20Nurse%20Staffing%20DRAFT.pdf. [Accessed 10 February 2023].

46. Bloomer M, Fulbrook P, Goldsworthy G, et al. World Federation of Critical Care Nurses 2019 position statement: provision of a critical care nursing workforce. Connect: The World of Critical Care Nursing 2019;13:3–7.

47. Endacott R, Jones C, Bloomer MJ, et al. The state of critical care nursing education in Europe: an international survey. Intensive Care Med 2015 Dec;41(12):2237–40.

48. New Zealand College of Critical Care Nurses. Position statement on critical care nurse education. Wellington: NZNO; 2017.

49. Griffiths P, Saville C, Ball J, et al. Performance of the Safer Nursing Care Tool to measure nurse staffing requirements in acute hospitals: a multicentre observational study. BMJ Open 2020;10(5):e035828.

50. Haupt MT, Bekes CE, Brilli RJ, et al. Guidelines on critical care services and personnel: Recommendations based on a system of categorization of three levels of care. Crit Care Med 2003;31(11):2677–83.

51. National Health Service (NHS). Critical care science is about caring for patients who are critically ill. London: HMSO; 2022. Available from: https://www.healthcareers.nhs.uk/explore-roles/healthcare-science/roles-healthcare-science/physiological-sciences/critical-care-science. [Accessed 10 February 2023].

52. Royal College of Physicians (RCP). Who are physician associates? London: RCP; 2022. Available from: https://www.fparcp.co.uk/about-fpa/who-are-physician-associates. [Accessed 10 February 2023].

53. Halter M, Wheeler C, Pelone F. Contribution of physician assistants/associates to secondary care: a systematic review. BMJ Open 2018;8(6):e019573. Available from: https://bmjopen.bmj.com/content/8/6/e019573. [Accessed 10 February 2023].

54. Bakshi V. The role of the physician assistant in critical care. ICU Manag Pract 2019;19(1). Available from: https://healthmanagement.org/c/icu/issuearticle/the-role-of-the-physician-assistant-in-critical-care. [Accessed 10 February 2023].

55. Drake R. Staff unavailability and safe staffing: are headroom allowances 'realistic'? Br J Nurs 2020;29(7):406–13.

56. UK Critical Care Nursing Alliance (UKCCNA). UKCCNA position statement: critical care nursing workforce post COVID-19. London: UKCCNA; 2021. Available from: https://www.ficm.ac.uk/sites/ficm/files/documents/2021-10/ukccna_position_statement_critical_care_nursing_workforce_post_covid_05.05.2020.pdf. [Accessed 10 February 2023].

57. Greaves J, Goodall D, Berry A, et al. Nursing workloads and activity in critical care: a review of the evidence. Intensive Crit Care Nurs 2018;48:10–20.

58. Griffiths P, Saville C, Ball J, et al. Nursing workload, nurse staffing methodologies and tools: a systematic scoping review and discussion. Int J Nurs Stud 2020;103:103487.

59. Wynendaele H, Willems R, Trybou J. Systematic review: association between the patient–nurse ratio and nurse outcomes in acute care hospitals. J Nurs Manag 2019;27:896–917.

60. Van Kiersbilck C, Gordon E, Morris D. Ten things that nurses should know about ECMO. Intensive Care Med 2016;42:753–5.

61. D'Lima DM, Murray EJ, Brett SJ. Perceptions of risk and safety in the ICU: a qualitative study of cognitive processes relating to staffing. Crit Care Med 2018 Jan;46(1):60–70.

62. Adomat R, Hewison A. Assessing patient category/dependence systems for determining the nurse/patient ratio in ICU and HDU: a review of approaches. J Nurs Manag 2004;12(5):299–308.

63. Reis Miranda DR, Nap R, de Rijk A, et al. Nursing activities score. Crit Care Med 2003;31:374–82.

64. Reis Miranda, D. The Therapeutic Intervention Scoring System: one single tool for the evaluation of workload, the work process and management? Intensive Care Med 1997;23(6):615–17.

65. Clini E, Vitacca M, Ambrosino N. Dependence nursing scale: a new method to assess the effect of nursing work load in a respiratory intermediate intensive care unit. Respir Care 1999;44:29–37.

66. Reis Miranda D, Moreno R, Iapichino G. Nine equivalents of nursing manpower use score (NEMS). Intensive Care Med 1997;23(7):760–5.

67. Butcher HK, Bulechek GM, Dochterman JMM, et al. Nursing interventions classification (NIC), 7th ed. (E-book) St Louis: Mosby/Elsevier Health Sciences; 2018.

68. Kaplow, R. Reed, K. The AACN synergy model for patient care: a nursing model as a force of magnetism. Nurs Econ 2008;26(1):17–25.

69. Cohen SS, Crego N, Cuming RG, et al. The synergy model and the role of clinical nurse specialists in a multihospital system. Am J Crit Care 2002;11(5):436–46.

70. Ball C, McElligott M. 'Realising the potential of critical care nurses': an exploratory study of the factors that affect and comprise the nursing contribution to the recovery of critically ill patients. Intensive Crit Care Nurs 2003;19:226–38.

71. Hart SG, Staveland LE. Development of NASA-TLX (Task Load Index): results of empirical and theoretical research. Adv Psychol 1988;52:139–83.

72. Hoonakker P, Carayon P, Gurses A, et al. Measuring workload of ICU nurses with a questionnaire survey: the NASA Task Load Index (TLX). IIE Trans Healthc Syst Eng 2011;1:131–43.

73. Kessler I, Steils N, Samsi K, et al. NIHR Policy Research Unit in Health and Social Care Workforce. Evaluating the introduction of the nursing associate role in health and social care: interim report. London: NIHR/Kings College; 2020 Available from: https://www.kcl.ac.uk/business/assets/PDF/covid-research-papers/interim-report-evaluating-the-introduction-of-the-nursing-associate-role-in-health-and-social-care.pdf. [Accessed 10 February 2023].

74. Australia and New Zealand Intensive Care Society (ANZICS). Centre for Outcome and Resource Evaluation 2019 report. Camberwell, VIC: ANZICS; 2020. Available from: https://www.anzics.com.au/wp-content/uploads/2020/11/2019-CORE-Report.pdf. [Accessed 10 February 2023].

75. Rae P, Pearce S, Greaves P, et al. Outcomes sensitive to critical care nurse staffing levels: a systematic review. Intensive Crit Care Nurs 2021;67:103110.

76. Twigg DE, Kutzer Y, Jacob E, et al. A quantitative systematic review of the association between nurse skill mix and nursing-sensitive patient outcomes in the acute care setting. J Adv Nurs 2019;75(12):3404–23.

77. Cho E, Sloane DM, Kim EY, et al. Effects of nurse staffing, work environments, and education on patient mortality: an observational study. Int J Nurs Stud 2015;52(2):535–42.

78. Aiken LH, Sloane DM, Bruyneel L, et al. Nurse staffing and education and hospital mortality in nine European countries: a retrospective observational study. Lancet 2014;383(9931):1824–30.

79. Duffield C, Roche M, Diers D, et al. Staffing, skill mix and the model of care. J Clin Nurs 2010;19(15-16):2242–51.

80. Griffiths P, Ball Griffiths P, Saville C, et al. The Safer Nursing Care Tool as a guide to nurse staffing requirements on hospital wards: observational and modelling study. Health Services and Delivery Research 8.16. Southampton, UK: NIHR Journals Library; 2020. Available from: https://www.ncbi.nlm.nih.gov/books/NBK555320/. [Accessed 10 February 2023].

81. Griffiths P, Ball J, Bloor K, et al. Nurse staffing levels, missed vital signs and mortality in hospitals: retrospective longitudinal observational study. Health Services and Delivery Research 6.38. Southampton, UK: NIHR Journals Library; 2018. doi: 10.3310/hsdr06380. Available from: https://www.ncbi.nlm.nih.gov/books/NBK534527/. [Accessed 10 February 2023].

82. Dall'Ora C, Saville C, Rubbo B, et al. Nurse staffing levels and patient outcomes: a systematic review of longitudinal studies. Int J Nurs Stud 2022;134:104311. doi: 10.1016/j.ijnurstu.2022.104311.

83. Neuraz A, Guérin C, Payet C, et al. Patient mortality is associated with staff resources and workload in the ICU: a multicenter observational study. Crit Care Med 2015;43(8):1587–94.

84. Lee A, Cheung YS, Joynt GM, et al. Are high nurse workload/staffing ratios associated with decreased survival in critically ill patients? A cohort study. Ann Intensive Care 2017;7(1):46.

85. Beckmann U, Baldwin I, Durie M, et al. Problems associated with nursing staff shortage: an analysis of the first 3600 incident reports submitted to the Australian Incident Monitoring Study (AIMS-ICU). Anaesth Intensive Care 1998;26(4):396–400.

86. Morrison AL, Beckmann U, Durie M, et al. The effects of nursing staff inexperience (NSI) on the occurrence of adverse patient experiences in ICUs. Aust Crit Care 2001;14(3):116–21.

87. Australian College of Critical Care Nurses. Position statement on the use of healthcare workers other than division 1 registered nurses in intensive care. Melbourne, VIC: ACCCN; 2006. Available from: https://acccn.com.au/wp-content/uploads/Use-of-Healthcare-Workers-Other-than-Division-1-Registered-Nurses-in-ICU.pdf. [Accessed 10 February 2023].

88. Hegney DG, Rees CS, Osseiran-Moisson R, et al. Perceptions of nursing workloads and contributing factors, and their impact on implicit care rationing: a Queensland, Australia study. J Nurs Manag 2019;27(2):371–80.

89. Endacott R, Pattison N, Dall'Ora C, et al. SEISMIC study team. The organisation of nurse staffing in intensive care units: a qualitative study. J Nurs Manag 2022;30(5):1283–94. doi: 10.1111/jonm.13611.

90. Endacott R, Pearce S, Rae P, et al; SEISMIC Study Team. How COVID-19 has affected staffing models in intensive care: a qualitative study examining alternative staffing models (SEISMIC). J Adv Nurs 2022;78(4):1075–88.

91. Ausserhofer D, Zander B, Busse R, et al. Prevalence, patterns and predictors of nursing care left undone in European hospitals: results from the multicountry cross-sectional RN4CAST study. BMJ Qual Saf 2014;23(2):126–35.

92. Griffiths P, Ball J, Murrells T, et al. Registered nurse, healthcare support worker, medical staffing levels and mortality in English hospital trusts: a cross-sectional study. BMJ Open 2016;6(2):e008751.

93. Bae SH. Intensive care nurse staffing and nurse outcomes: a systematic review. Nurs Crit Care 2021 Nov;26(6):457–66.

94. Timewise. Flexible working in the NHS – the case for action. 2018. Available from: https://timewise.co.uk/wp-content/uploads/2018/07/Flexible-working-in-the-NHS-the-case-for-action.pdf. [Accessed 10 February 2023].

95. Timewise. Improving nurses' work–life balance with team-based rostering. London: Timewise; 2019. Available from: https://timewise.co.uk/article/improving-nurses-work-life-balance/. [Accessed 10 February 2023].

96. Costa G, Anelli MM, Castellini G, et al. Stress and sleep in nurses employed in "3 × 8" and "2 × 12" fast rotating shift schedules. Chronobiol Int 2014;31(10):1169–78.

97. Webster J, McLeod K, O'Sullivan J, et al. Eight-hour versus 12-h shifts in an ICU: comparison of nursing responses and patient outcomes. Aust Crit Care 2019;32(5):391–6.

98. Harris R, Sims S, Parr J, et al. Impact of 12h shift patterns in nursing: a scoping review. Int J Nurs Stud 2015;52(2):605–34.

99. Johnston DW, Allen J, Powell D, et al. Why does work cause fatigue? A real-time investigation of fatigue, and determinants of fatigue in nurses working 12-hour shifts. Ann Behav Med 2019;53(6):551–62.

100. Yu F, Somerville D, King A. Exploring the impact of 12-hour shifts on nurse fatigue in intensive care units. Appl Nurs Res 2019;50:151191.

101. Saville C, Dall'Ora C, Griffiths P. The association between 12-hour shifts and nurses-in-charge's perceptions of missed care and staffing adequacy: a retrospective cross-sectional observational study. Int J Nurs Stud 2020;112:103721. doi: 10.1016/j.ijnurstu.2020.103721.

102. Dall'Ora C, Griffiths P, Redfern O, et al; the Missed Care Study Group. Nurses' 12-hour shifts and missed or delayed vital signs observations on hospital wards: retrospective observational study. BMJ Open 2019;9:e024778. doi: 10.1136/bmjopen-2018-024778.

103. Han K, Hwang H, Lim E, et al. Scheduled naps improve drowsiness and quality of nursing care among 12-hour shift nurses. Int J Environ Res Public Health 2021;18(3):891.

104. Dafoe S, Stiller K, Chapman M. Staff perceptions of the barriers to mobilizing ICU patients. Internet J Allied Health Sci Practice 2015;13(2):Article 8.

105. Zanni JM, Korupolu R, Fan E, et al. Rehabilitation therapy and outcomes in acute respiratory failure: an observational pilot project. J Crit Care 2010;25:254–62.

106. Critical Care Networks – National Nurse Leads (CC3N). Step competency framework. 2018. Available from: https://www.cc3n.org.uk/step-competency-framework.html. [Accessed 10 February 2023].

107. Gill FJ, Leslie GD, Grech C, et al. An analysis of Australian graduate critical care nurse education. Collegian 2015;22,71–81.

108. Friedman MI, Cooper AH, Click E, et al. Specialized new graduate RN critical care orientation: retention and financial impact. Nurs Econ 2011;29(1):7.

109. Harper JP. Preceptors' perceptions of a competency-based orientation. J Nurses Staff Dev 2002;18(4):198–202.

110. European Commission (EC). Report of the High Level Group on health services and medical care. Brussels: EC; 2006. Available from: https://ec.europa.eu/health/archive/ph_overview/co_operation/mobility/docs/highlevel_2005_013_en.pdf. [Accessed 10 February 2023].

111. Nursing and Midwifery Council (NMC). Revalidation. London: NMC; 2022. Available from: https://www.nmc.org.uk/revalidation/. [Accessed 10 February 2023].

112. American Association of Critical-Care Nurses (AACN), Institute for Credentialing Excellence (ICE), National Commission for Certifying Agencies (NCCA). Scope and standards for progressive and critical care nursing practice. Aliso Viejo, CA: AACN; 2014. Available from: https://www.aacn.org/nursing-excellence/standards/aacn-scope-and-standards-for-acute-and-critical-care-nursing-practice. [Accessed 10 February 2023].

113. European federation of Critical Care Nursing associations (EfCCNa). EfCCNa Competency tool for European critical care nurses. Amsterdam: EfCCNa; 2013. Available from: http://efccna.org/images/stories/publication/competencies_cc.pdf. [Accessed 10 February 2023].

114. Nursing and Midwifery Board of Australia (NMBA). Registration standard: continuing professional development. Melbourne, VIC: NMBA; 2016. Available from: http://www.nursingmidwiferyboard.gov.au/Registration-Standards/Continuing-professional-development.aspx. [Accessed 10 February 2023].

115. Nursing Council of New Zealand. Guidelines for competence assessment. Wellington: NZNO; 2008. Available from: https://www.nursingcouncil.org.nz/Public/Nursing/Continuing_competence/NCNZ/nursing-section/Continuing_Competence.aspx?hkey=6542ac27-9b56-4e89-b7ae-db445c5cb952. [Accessed 10 February 2023].

116. Valentin A, Capuzzo M, Guidet B, et al. Patient safety in intensive care: results from the multinational Sentinel Events Evaluation (SEE) study. Intensive Care Med 2006;32(10):1591–8.

117. Valentin A, Capuzzo M, Guidet B, et al. Errors in administration of parenteral drugs in intensive care units: multinational prospective study. BMJ 2009;338:b814.

118. Sexton JB, Thomas EJ, Helmreich RL. Error, stress, and teamwork in medicine and aviation: cross sectional surveys. BMJ 2000;320(7237):745–9.

119. Paladin. Do we need a risk matrix? Mitchell, ACT: Paladin; 2018. Available from: https://paladinrisk.com.au/do-we-need-a-risk-matrix/. [Accessed 10 February 2023].

120. Health and Safety Executive (HSE). ALARP at a glance. London: HSE; 2023. Available from: https://www.hse.gov.uk/managing/theory/alarpglance.htm. [Accessed 10 February 2023].

121. MacFarlane PJM, Reid SJ. Queensland health law book, 16th ed. Brisbane: Federation Press; 2006.

122. Hodson N. Regulatory justice following gross negligence manslaughter verdicts: Nurse/doctor differences. Nurs Ethics 2020;27(1):247257. doi: 10.1177/0969733019833124.

123. Cheluvappa R, Selvendran S. Medical negligence – key cases and application of legislation. Ann Med Surg (Lond) 2020;57:205–11. doi: 10.1016/j.amsu.2020.07.017.

124. Knaus WA, Draper EA, Wagner DP, et al. An evaluation of outcome from intensive care in major medical centers. Ann Intern Med 1986;104(3):410–18.

125. Zimmerman JE, Shortell SM, Rousseau DM, et al. Improving intensive care: observations based on organizational case studies in nine intensive care units: a prospective, multicenter study. Crit Care Med 1993;21(10):1443–51.

126. Australian Commission on Safety and Quality in Healthcare (ACSQHC). Australian Open Disclosure Framework. Sydney, NSW: ACSQHC; 2013. Available from: https://www.safetyandquality.gov.au/sites/default/files/migrated/Australian-Open-Disclosure-Framework-Feb-2014.pdf. [Accessed 10 February 2023].

127. Iedema RA, Mallock NA, Sorensen RJ, et al. The national open disclosure pilot: evaluation of a policy implementation initiative. Med J Aust 2008;188(7):397–400.

128. Gold M. Is honesty always the best policy? Ethical aspects of truth telling. Intern Med J 2004;34(9-10):578–80.

129. Madden B, Cockburn T. Bundaberg and beyond: duty to disclose adverse events to patients. J Law Med 2007;14(4):501–27.

130. Johnstone M. Clinical risk management and the ethics of open disclosure. Part I. Benefits and risks to patient safety. Austral Emerg Nurs J 2008;11(2):88–94.

131. Olazo K, Wang K, Sierra M, et al. Preferences and perceptions of medical error disclosure among marginalized populations: a narrative review. UCSF; 2022. Available from: https://escholarship.org/uc/item/238915ds. [Accessed 10 February 2023].

132. Uveges MK, Milliken A, Afi A. Role of the critical care nurse in disclosing difficult news. AACN Adv Crit Care 2019;30(3):287–93. doi: 10.4037/aacnacc2019436.

133. Byju AS, Mayo K. Medical error in the care of the unrepresented: disclosure and apology for a vulnerable patient population. J Med Ethics 2019;45:821–3.

134. Department of Health Victoria. Clinical incident invesigations – root cause analysis. Melbourne, VIC: DOH; 2021 Available from: https://www.health.vic.gov.au/quality-safety-service/clinical-incident-investigations-root-cause-analysis. [Accessed 10 February 2023].

135. World Health Organization (WHO). What is a pandemic? Geneva: WHO; 2010.

136. World Health Organization (WHO). Disease outbreaks. Geneva: WHO; n.d.

137. Singer BJ, Thompson RN, Bonsall, MB. The effect of the definition of 'pandemic' on quantitative assessments of infectious disease outbreak risk. Sci Rep 2021;11:2547.

138. Fraser, M, Blumenstock, J. Lessons relearned? H1N1, COVID-19, and vaccination planning. J Public Health Manag Pract 2021;27(Suppl. 1):S106–10.

139. Organisation for Economic Co-operation and Development (OECD). Policy responses to coronavirus (COVID-19). First lessons from government evaluations of COVID-19 responses: a synthesis. Paris: OECD; 2022. Available from: https://www.oecd.org/coronavirus/policy-responses/first-lessons-from-government-evaluations-of-covid-19-responses-a-synthesis-483507d6/. [Accessed 10 February 2023].

140. Kupferschmidt, K. 'A toxic cocktail': panel delivers harsh verdict on the world's failure to prepare for pandemic. Report proposes major overhaul of health systems to fight future threats. Washington DC: AAAS; 2021. Available from: https://www.science.org/content/article/toxic-cocktail-panel-delivers-harsh-verdict-world-s-failure-prepare-pandemic. [Accessed 10 February 2023].

141. The Lancet Respiratory Medicine. Future pandemics: failing to prepare means preparing to fail. Lancet Respir Med 2022;10(3):221–2.

142. Rednor, S. Eisen L, Cobb P, et al. Critical care response during the COVID-19 pandemic. Crit Care Clin 2022;38(3):623–37.

143. Kodama C, Kuniyoshi G, Abubakar A. Lessons learned during COVID-19: building critical care/ICU capacity for resource limited countries with complex emergencies in the World Health Organization Eastern Mediterranean Region. J Glob Health 2021;11:03088.

144. Schell CO, Khalid K, Wharton-Smith A, et al; The EECC Collaborators. Essential emergency and critical care: a consensus among global clinical experts. BMJ Global Health 2021;6:e006585.

145. Ma X, Vervoort D. Critical care capacity during the COVID-19 pandemic: global availability of intensive care beds. J Crit Care 2020;58:96–7.

146. World Health Organization (WHO). Strengthening the health systems response to COVID-19. Geneva: WHO; 2020. Available from: https://apps.who.int/iris/bitstream/handle/10665/332562/WHO-EURO-2020-670-40405-54163-eng.pdf?sequence=1&isAllowed=y. [Accessed 10 February 2023].

147. Hota S, Fried E, Burry L, et al. Preparing your intensive care unit for the second wave of H1N1 and future surges. Crit Care Med 2010;38(4 Suppl.):e110–19.

148. Daugherty EL, Branson RD, Deveraux A, et al. Infection control in mass respiratory failure: preparing to respond to H1N1. Crit Care Med 2010;38(4 Suppl.):e103–9.

149. Funk DJ, Siddiqui F, Wiebe K, et al. Practical lessons from the first outbreaks: clinical presentation, obstacles, and management strategies for severe pandemic (H1N1) 2009 influenza pneumonitis. Crit Care Med 2010;38(4 Suppl.):e30–7.

150. Duggal A, Pinto R, Rubenfeld G, et al. Global variability in reported mortality for critical illness during the 2009-10 Influenza A(H1N1) pandemic: a systematic review and meta-regression to guide reporting of outcomes during disease outbreaks. PLoS One 2016;11(5):e0155044. doi: 10.1371/journal.pone.0155044.

151. World Health Organization (WHO). Pandemic influenza risk management – interim guidance. Geneva: WHO; 2013. Available from: https://cdn.who.int/media/docs/default-source/documents/pandemic-influenza-risk-management.pdf?sfvrsn=4e530456_2&download=true. [Accessed 10 February 2023].

152. New South Wales Health. Influenza pandemic – providing critical care: PD2010_28. Sydney: NSW Health; 2010. Available from: https://www1.health.nsw.gov.au/PDS/pages/doc.aspx?dn=PD2010_028. [Accessed 10 February 2023].

153. Barbisch DF, Koenig KL. Understanding surge capacity: essential elements. Acad Emerg Med 2020;13:1098–102. doi: 10.1197/j.aem.2006.06.041.

154. Barros LM, Pigoga JL, Chea S, et al. Pragmatic recommendations for identification and triage of patients with COVID-19 in low- and middle-income countries. Am J Trop Med Hyg 2021;104(3 Suppl.):3-11. doi: 10.4269/ajtmh.20-1064.

155. Fiest KM, Krewulak KD, Plotnikoff KM, et al. Allocation of intensive care resources during an infectious disease outbreak: a rapid review to inform practice. BMC Med 2020;18(1):404. doi: 10.1186/s12916-020-01871-9.

156. Downar J, Smith MJ, Godkin D, et al. A framework for critical care triage during a major surge in critical illness. Un algorithme pour le triage aux soins intensifs lors d'une augmentation majeure des maladies graves. Can J Anaesth 2022;69(6):774–81. doi: 10.1007/s12630-022-02231-2.

157. White DB, Lo B. Mitigating inequities and saving lives with ICU triage during the COVID-19 pandemic. Am J Respir Crit Care Med 2021;203(3):287–95. doi: 10.1164/rccm.202010-158 3809CP.

158. Maves RC, Downar J, Dichter JR, et al. Triage of scarce critical care resources in COVID-19 an implementation guide for regional allocation: an expert panel report of the Task Force for Mass Critical Care and the American College of Chest Physicians. Chest 2020;158(1):212–25.

159. South Australia Government Nursing and Midwifery Office. The 2020/2021 critical care surge nursing workforce strategy COVID-19. Adelaide, SA: SA Health; 2021.

160. Marshall AP, Austin DE, Chamberlain D, et al. A critical care pandemic staffing framework in Australia. Aust Crit Care 2021;34(2):123–31.

161. Ridley EJ, Freeman-Sanderson A, Haines KJ. Surge capacity for critical care specialised allied health professionals in Australia during COVID-19. Aust Crit Care 2021;34(2):191–3.

162. Litton E, Bucci T, Chavan S, et al. Surge capacity of intensive care units in case of acute increase in demand caused by COVID-19 in Australia. Med J Aust 2020;212(10):463–7.

163. New South Wales Government. Adult intensive care workforce report in COVID-19 pandemic. Available from: https://aci.health.nsw.gov.au/__data/assets/pdf_file/0007/594772/Adult-intensive-care-workforce-report.pdf. [Accessed 27 September 2023].

164. New South Wales Agency for Clinical Innovation (ACI). NSW adult intensive care services pandemic response planning. Sydney, NSW: ACI; 2020.

165. New South Wales. Ministry of Health. NSW Ministry of Health demand escalation framework. Sydney, NSW: Ministry of Health; 2016.

166. NSW Ministry of Health. Koff, E. Letter from Secretary, 31 March 2020. Sydney: NSW Ministry of Health; 2020.

167. NHS England and NHS Improvement with Health Education England. Advice on acute sector workforce models during COVID-19. NHS – coronavirus guidance for clinicians and NHS managers. London: NHS; 2020.

168. Royal College of Nursing UK (RCN). RCN guidance on redeployment – COVID-19. London: RCN; 2020.

169. COVID-19 Critical Intelligence Unit. In brief: COVID-19 pandemic and wellbeing of critical care and other healthcare workers. Sydney, NSW: NSW Government; 2022. Available from: https://aci.health.nsw.gov.au/__data/assets/pdf_file/0014/706010/Evidence-Check-COVID-19-pandemic-and-wellbeing-of-workers.pdf. [Accessed 10 February 2023].

170. Montgomery CM, Humphreys S, McCulloch C, et al. Critical care work during COVID-19: a sociological analysis of staff experiences. BMJ Open 2021;11(5):e048124.

171. Sumner, S. Impact of the COVID-19 pandemic on the work environment and mental health of intensive care unit nurses: reflections from the United States. Nurs Crit Care 2022;10.1111/nicc.12759.doi: 10.1111/nicc.12759. Online ahead of print.

172. Greenberg N, Weston D, Hall C, et al. Mental health of staff working in intensive care during Covid-19. Occup Med (Lond) 2021;71(2):62–7.

173. NHS England. Professional nurse advocate. London: NHS; 2021. Available from: https://www.england.nhs.uk/nursingmidwifery/delivering-the-nhs-ltp/professional-nurse-advocate/. [Accessed June 2022].

174. Vera San Juan N, Aceituno D, Djellouli N, et al. Mental health and well-being of healthcare workers during the COVID-19 pandemic in the UK: contrasting guidelines with experiences in practice. BJPsych Open 2020;7(1):e15. doi: 10.1192/bjo.2020.148.

175. Clark SE, Chisnall G, Vindrola-Padros C. A systematic review of de-escalation strategies for redeployed staff and repurposed facilities in COVID-19 intensive care units (ICUs) during the pandemic. EClinicalMedicine 2022;44:101286.

Chapter 3

Quality and safety

Elizabeth Scruth, Amy Spooner

Learning objectives

After reading this chapter, you should be able to:

- describe different approaches to quality and safety monitoring
- identify the steps in developing clinical practice guidelines
- explain the role care bundles and checklists have in promoting quality and safety in critical care practice
- discuss the use of national quality indicators in intensive care
- describe the use of information and communication technologies in critical care
- identify techniques used to understand situations that place patients at risk of adverse events in critical care
- discuss rapid response systems used to respond to deteriorating patients
- explain the safety culture in ICUs
- identify strategies to improve the non-technical skills in critical care.

Introduction

Today's critical care units are fast paced and complex, where nurses, physicians and other health professionals use their knowledge, expertise and available technology to provide patient care. The National Academy of Medicine (NAM) in the USA, formerly called the Institute of Medicine until 2015, defines quality of health as *'the degree to which health services for individuals and populations increase the likelihood of desired health outcomes and are consistent with current professional knowledge'*. NAM aims to improve health and health equity through providing trusted advice nationally and globally.[1]

Critical care nurses are acknowledged for their skills in ongoing surveillance of a patient's condition, enabling the nurse to be ideally positioned to prevent, discover, assess and mitigate healthcare errors.[2] Thus, nurses play a key role in improving quality and safety in critical care, the focus of this chapter. First, approaches to quality are considered. Included in this section are the topics of quality monitoring, quality indicators, clinical practice guidelines (CPGs), care bundles, checklists and information and communication technologies. Finally, patient safety is described, including the noteworthy problem of medication errors, safety culture, rapid response systems and non-technical skills. In Chapter 2, risk management, clinical governance and the role of clinical leaders and managers in delivering critical care services were addressed; this information is complementary to what is discussed in this chapter.

Approaches to quality

Healthcare quality is commonly described in terms of Donabedian's three major domains:[3]

1 structure – the way the healthcare setting and/or system is organised to deliver care (e.g. staffing, beds, equipment)

2 process – the practices involved in the delivery of care (e.g. pressure ulcer prevention strategies)

3 outcomes – the results of care in terms of recovery, restoration of function and/or survival (e.g. mortality, health-related quality of life).

In addition to Donabedian's quality model, the Systems Engineering Initiative for Patient Safety (SEIPS) model has been developed.[4-6] The model provides a framework for understanding how the above-described domains (e.g. structures, processes and outcomes) and their relationships, can be used in clinical practice and research. Fig. 3.1 graphically presents the SEIPS model. The general structure of the model is that the work system (left), in which care is provided, affects clinical processes (middle), which further influence patient, employee and organisational outcomes (right).[4] Specifically, it expands Donabedian's first domain 'structure' (e.g. how care is organised) to include five components, referred to as the 'work system'.[4] The SEIPS model defines five work system components as: (a) person(s) (i.e. patient, healthcare provider or the team), (b) tasks, (c) tools and technologies, (d) environment and (e) organisation. Accordingly, a *person* performs *tasks* using *tools and technologies*. These performances occur in a physical *environment* influenced by *organisational* conditions.[6] The SEIPS model was updated (SEIPS 3.0) to expand the processes component and increase attention to the journey of the patient over time.[7] The SEIPS model has been applied in various healthcare settings to guide quality and safety assessments, often providing recommendations for safety improvements[4] including analysing the use of barcode medication administration technology errors[8] and evaluating the intra-hospital transfer process of critically ill patients.[9]

The overall aim of quality improvement in healthcare is to improve the safety of interventions and to ensure that the patient and family are always considered part of the process. Crossing the Quality Chasm in the United States identifies and recommends improvements in six dimensions of healthcare, and Crossing the Global Quality Chasm takes it one step further to address defects in the quality of care globally, focusing on the front-line delivery of safe, effective and equitable healthcare[10,11] Quality improvement activities identify and address gaps between knowledge and practice. Importantly, these activities need to reflect the most recent and robust clinical evidence to improve patient care and reduce harm. A common approach used for rapid improvement in healthcare is the plan–do–study–act (PDSA)[12] method, where four essential steps are carried out in a repeated sequence to ensure processes are continually improved:

1 *Plan* – identify a goal, specify aims and objectives to improve an area of clinical practice, and how that might be achieved (i.e. how to test the intervention).

FIGURE 3.1   Systems Engineering Initiative for Patient Safety Improvement model 3.0.[7]

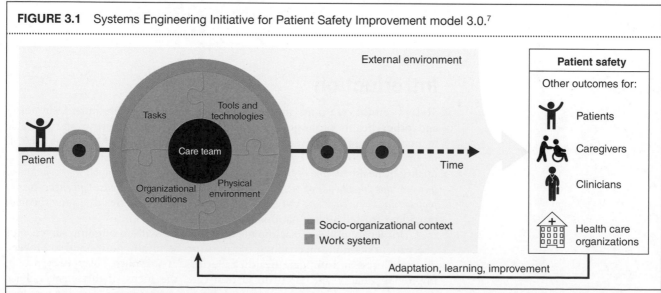

Source: Carayon P, Wooldridge A, Hoonakker P, et al. SEIPS 3.0: human-centered design of the patient journey for patient safety. Appl Ergon 2020;84:103033. doi: 10.1016/j.apergo.2019.103033.

2 *Do* – implement the plan of action, collect relevant information that will inform whether the intervention was successful and in what way, taking note of problems and unexpected observations that arise.

3 *Study* – evaluate the results of the intervention, particularly its impact on practice improvement, noting any strengths and limitations of the intervention.

4 *Act* – determine whether the intervention should be adopted, abandoned or adapted for further rapid cycle testing recommencing at the plan phase.

All quality improvement methods require constant reviewing and updating to ensure they remain relevant to the changing environment of healthcare. Quality monitoring includes measurement of, and response to, the incidence and patterns of adverse events (AEs). The rate of AEs varies greatly; in a recent meta-analysis exploring AEs the incidence of hospital AEs was 8.6 per 100 patient admissions of which half were preventable, and one-third resulted in moderate to significant harm.[13] In critical care settings during nursing procedures, up to 30% of patients had an associated AE.[14] A 2021 observational study exploring AEs during bed baths in 24 ICUs revealed that 56% of patients experienced at least one serious event. The study defined serious adverse events as: cardiac arrest, unintentional extubation, desaturation, hypotension, cardiac arrhythmias, acute pain, accidental disconnection of equipment, and any patient falls.[15]

Clinical practice guidelines

The development and use of CPGs is one strategy to improve the quality and safety of healthcare.[16,17] Clinical practice guidelines are an essential resource aiding nursing and medical decision making based on scientific evidence. They are systematically developed to assist clinicians, consumers and policy makers in healthcare decisions and provide critical summaries of available evidence on a particular topic.[16] There are a number of benefits of using CPGs. They represent the highest level of evidence and aim to standardise care, ensuring quality of care is maintained. There are some concerns with CPCs that have been identified in the literature including difficulty in locating them. Poorly developed guidelines may not improve care and may actually result in substandard care, suggesting there is need for improvement in the overall score of guidelines and rigour of development.[17] In Australia, the Intensive Care Coordination and Monitoring Unit of the New South Wales Department of Health has led the development of CPGs associated with a number of common nursing interventions that are available online including: (1) tracheostomy care, (2) central venous access device care, (3) eye care, (4) non-invasive ventilation guidelines, (5) physical activity and movement, (6) pressure injury prevention, (7) suctioning an adult ICU patient and (8) temperature measurement.[18] Other examples of recently developed ICU CPGs include those for family-centred care, which are updated every 5 years using a robust evidence-based methodology,[19] ICU admission,

discharge and triage,[20] management of sepsis and septic shock,[21] safe medication use,[22] and the provision and assessment of nutrition support therapy.[23]

Clinical audits are often used to establish the need to develop new CPGs and protocols at the local unit level. Clinical audits usually involve several stages including preparing staff, assessing practice, analysis, feedback and decisions on actions to improve upon.[24] Clinical audits reveal variations in the standard of practice that are without adequate justification. If clinical audits or other methods establish a need for improving practice then adopting, adapting or developing CPG is one approach that is used.

Developing, implementing and evaluating clinical practice guidelines

A number of steps are undertaken when developing CPGs. Organisations such as the Australian National Health and Medical Research Council (NHMRC) provide detailed descriptions for various aspects of the CPG development and reporting process.[25] The NHMRC has recently published a set of standards that guidelines must adhere to, in order to be approved by this national organisation. These standards are identified in Table 3.1.[26] As shown in this table, it is important to consider the appropriate membership of the guideline development team, including the role of end users such as patients and health professionals, and how to manage conflicts of interest. It is important to recognise that developing CPG takes a lot of time, expertise and resources.

While research and systematic reviews form the foundation for CPGs, the quality of evidence must be assessed. One appraisal method – Grading of Recommendations, Assessment, Development and Evaluation (GRADE) – is recommended in the Cochrane handbook for systematic reviews of interventions.[27] The GRADE approach specifies four levels of the certainty for a body of evidence for a given outcome: high, moderate, low and very low.

GRADE assessments of certainty are assessed with risk of bias, inconsistency, indirectness, imprecision and any publication bias. Overall summaries of the evidence with some quality assessment such as GRADE is essential. These summaries are used to develop the guidelines, which generally include a series of statements about the care to be provided, a rationale for this care and both the quality of evidence and strength of the recommendation.

Once the guidelines are developed, a group of experts and users should assess the guidelines for accuracy, clinical utility and comprehension. A commonly used appraisal tool is the one that international experts developed and have subsequently revised termed the Appraisal of Guidelines for Research and Evaluation II (AGREE II). The tool comprises of 23 appraisal criteria organised within six domains and two overall assessments: (1) scope and purpose of the CPG (three items), (2) stakeholder involvement in CPG development (three items), (3) rigour of development (eight items), (4) clarity of presentation

TABLE 3.1

National Health and Medical Research Council standards for guidelines

STANDARD	SUB-ITEMS
1 To be relevant and useful for decision making guidelines will:	1.1 Address a health issue of importance 1.2 Clearly state the purpose of the guideline and the context in which it will be applied 1.3 Be informed by public consultation 1.4 Be feasible to implement.
2 To be transparent guidelines will make publicly available:	2.1 The details of all processes and procedures used to develop the guideline 2.2 The source evidence 2.3 The declarations of interest of members of the guideline development group and information on how any conflicts of interest were managed 2.4 All sources of funding for the guideline.
3 The guideline development group will:	3.1 Be composed of an appropriate mix of expertise and experience, including relevant end users 3.2 Have clearly defined, documented processes for reaching consensus.
4 To identify and manage conflicts of interest guideline developers will:	4.1 Require all interests of all guideline development group members to be declared 4.2 Establish a process for determining if a declared interest represents a conflict of interest, and how a conflict of interest will be managed.
5 To be focused on health and related outcomes guidelines will:	5.1 Be developed around explicitly defined clinical or public health questions 5.2 Address outcomes that are relevant to the guideline's expected end users 5.3 Clearly define the outcomes considered to be important to the person/s who will be affected by the decision, and prioritise these outcomes.
6 To be evidence-informed guidelines will:	6.1 Be informed by well-conducted systematic reviews 6.2 Consider the body of evidence for each outcome (including the quality of that evidence) and other factors that influence the process of making recommendations including benefits and harms, values and preferences, resource use and acceptability 6.3 Be subjected to appropriate peer review.
7 To make actionable recommendations guidelines will:	7.1 Discuss the options for action 7.2 Clearly articulate what the recommended course of action is, and when it should be taken 7.3 Clearly articulate what the intervention is so it can be implemented 7.4 Clearly link each recommendation to the evidence that supports it 7.5 Grade the strength of each recommendation.
8 To be up-to-date guidelines will:	8.1 Ensure that the recommendation is based on an up-to-date body of evidence 8.2 Propose a date by which the evidence and the guideline should be updated. This may be specific to each recommendation.
9 To be accessible guidelines will:	9.1 Be easy to find 9.2 Ideally be free of charge to the end user 9.3 Be clearly structured, easy to navigate and in plain English 9.4 Be available online.

Source: National Health and Medical Research Council. Standards for guidelines, 2016. https://www.nhmrc.gov.au/ guidelinesforguidelines/standards.

(three items), (5) applicability (four items) and (6) editorial independence (two items).[28] Instruments such as AGREE II can be used to assess the quality of CPGs.

Based on the assessment of the CPG, revisions may be required. Next, strategies for disseminating and implementing the guidelines should be developed along with a plan for their future updates. Importantly, simply publishing and circulating CPGs will have a limited impact on clinical practice, so specific activities must be undertaken to promote CPG adherence.[29] A recent qualitative synthesis analysis during the COVID surge, exploring the adherence to infection prevention and control (IPC) guidelines for respiratory infectious diseases, resulted in several factors being identified. Issues with the IPC around the implementation included: how it was communicated to staff, support from the management, training during the implementation of the IPC, workplace culture, and access to and trust in the personal protective gear. The study emphasised the need to include all staff in the development of CPGs.[29]

Finally, a process for regularly evaluating and updating the guidelines must be developed, which may involve quality improvement activities or clinical research and include perspectives of patients and other stakeholders.[30] In summary, by developing, using and evaluating CPGs, nurses may improve patient care and outcomes. Additionally, the use of CPGs should ensure that nursing practice is based on the most recent evidence available.

Quality indicators

The true incidence of both errors and AEs has been found to be higher than what was reported.[29] A culture of safety is essential to improve the quality of care and for reporting of all errors in ICUs. Long-term engagement of the whole healthcare team is needed for sustainability of a blame-free reporting system that promotes a safety culture, reducing harm and adoption of high-reliability organisation (HRO) principles.[31] High-reliability organisations have been defined as: *'organisations that operate in complex, high-hazard domains for extended periods without serious accidents or catastrophic failures'*.[32] A variety of frameworks and evaluation metrics have been published to support HRO implementation and evaluation, with the Joint Commission's HRHCM/Oro 2.0 standing out as robust and externally validated.[33] Fortunately, most healthcare errors do not result in patient harm because of safety-net processes including a culture of safety in hospitals.[34] To improve the culture of safety in hospitals, the following need to be explored in depth: reporting of errors and increased safety awareness, gender and demographics, experience of the clinical and non-clinical staff, and the staffing levels. In the last two decades, there has been growing emphasis placed on healthcare performance indicators to measure quality of care.[35] Quality performance indicators is a specified quantitative measure to assess clinical performances (on a hospital or unit level). One of the aims with quality performance indicators is to identify and prevent differences in quality of care, and also to initiate and facilitate quality improvement projects.[35]

Quality performance indicators measuring structural prerequisites include how the ICU is integrated into the hospital, the type and amount of technology available, and the number, roles and responsibilities of ICU staff. Process-related quality performance indicators refer to what we do, or fail to do, for patients and their families – for example, adherence to guidelines or transfers of patients between ICUs. Outcome-related quality performance indicators focus on the results achieved, such as standardised mortality ratios, AEs and patient satisfaction.[35] Moreover, quality performance indicators should be valid (i.e. both empirical research and clinical expertise support that the indicator measures quality of care), reliable, responsive, interpretable and feasible.[35]

Another method for continually evaluating quality performance is the use of clinical quality registries (CQRs).[36] These are repositories of routinely collected healthcare information that is analysed, and the results communicated back to the healthcare team with the aim of improving the safety and quality of patient care on a constant basis. There is evidence in the literature that this system of audit and feedback is very effective in improving healthcare processes and patient outcomes.[36]

The choice of quality performance indicators varies among countries. Comparing quality performance indicators in eight countries, the most commonly used domains in performance frameworks were safety, effectiveness and access. Cardiovascular, surgery and mental health were the most frequently reported disease groups among all countries.[37]

Earlier in 2016, Flaatten identified that those most commonly used were standardised mortality ratio followed by the availability of an intensivist in the ICU.[38] Some countries, for example Sweden, provide open access to the results even at individual hospital level. This enhances comparison between hospitals as well as benchmarking. Table 3.2 provides a list of examples of quality indicators used in intensive care.[39]

Adhering to the practices included in a ventilator care bundle (where appropriate) may lead to improved patient and service efficiency outcomes.

Care bundles

One quality improvement approach to the optimal use of best-practice guidelines at the bedside is the development of 'care bundles'.[40] A care bundle is a set of evidence-based interventions or processes of care applied to selected patients in order to standardise and ensure appropriate delivery of care. Bundles are designed to facilitate implementation of the care outlined in CPGs and are refined over time.[41] A number of bundles have been developed for critical care (Table 3.3).[42–46] A national study including 15,000 adult ICU patients evaluated outcomes from the use of the ABCDEF (**A**ccess; **B**oth awakening and breathing coordination of daily sedation and ventilator removal trials; **C**hoice of sedatives and analgesic exposure; **D**elirium monitoring and management; **E**arly mobility and exercise; and **F**amily) bundle. Results demonstrated that complete bundle performance was associated with: lower hospital death within 7 days, lower next-day mechanical ventilation, less delirium, lower use of restraints, reduced ICU re-admissions and lower likelihood of being discharged anywhere other than home.[41] Evaluating the effect of an early care bundle on severe sepsis and septic shock in patients with suspected sepsis in US hospitals, the study results demonstrated that there was an immediate increase in lactate testing but no change in short-term mortality rates. The study recommended other approaches to decrease sepsis mortality may be warranted in addition to care bundles.[47]

TABLE 3.2

Examples of global quality performance indicators used in intensive care

INDICATOR	INPUT/ PROCESS/ OUTPUT
ICU mortality	Output
ICU length of stay	Output
Rate of re-admission to ICU	Output
Rate of healthcare-associated infections	Output
Percentage of use of structure checklists	Process
Rate of ventilator-associated pneumonia (VAP)	Output
Hand hygiene compliance	Process
Nursing hours per patient per day in the ICU	Input
Staff burnout rate	Process
Rate of patient satisfaction	Process
Rate of patient participation in hospital education	Process
The use of a pain scale	Process
Availability of intensivists (per hour)	Output
Rate of delirium	Output
Rate of discharge within 48 hours	Output
Rate of adverse events	Output
Daily sedation status	Output
Return to the hospital within 48 hours after discharge	Process
Early enteral nutrition	Process
Balanced budget	Input

Source: Nouira H, Ben Abdelaziz A, Kacem M, et al. Which indicators use to assess quality performance in intensive care units: a systematic review of medical literature. Anaesth Crit Care Pain Med 2018;37(6):583–7. doi: 10.1016/j.accpm.2018.06.003.

Checklists

Checklists have long been used in other industries, such as aviation, to ensure the safety and operability of complex systems, reducing the likelihood of human errors. Checklists in healthcare elevate quality and safety especially in the ICU.[48] A checklist typically contains a list of action items or criteria arranged in a systematic way, addressing specific topics related to health quality and efficiency, allowing the person completing it to record the presence or absence of individual items in order to ascertain that all are considered or completed.[49]

In critical care settings, checklists have been used to facilitate staff training, detect errors, check compliance with safety standards and evidence-based processes of care (such as those outlined previously), increase knowledge of patient-centred goals and prompt clinicians to review certain practices on morning rounds in the ICU. Studies suggest checklists contributed to improved outcomes such as reduced AEs, improved patient and care partner satisfaction,[50] and improved delivery of essential daily care processes (such as pain management and physical therapy).[51,52] However, one randomised, multicentre study including 118 ICUs in Brazil, which tested the effectiveness of checklist, daily goals assessment and clinical prompts as a multifaceted quality improvement, found the intervention did not reduce in-hospital mortality.[53] Careful consideration of both checklist design and implementation is required when planning to incorporate checklists into the clinical setting, as checklists can be problematic when applied to clinical problems that require non-linear responses, and are not well suited to clinical scenarios that require multiple adaptive responses.[54,55] Based on the results of a qualitative multicentre study in 32 ICUs in the USA, a framework for adapting a checklist in clinical practice has been developed. It suggests that development of a checklist should include attention to brevity and relevance to the specific ICU. Consistent and integrated use is needed when implemented. Moreover, review of the checklist should include updates in accord with changes in ICU practice, including item reduction, item rotation and revisiting goals.[49]

> **Practice tip**
>
> When developed in line with published guidelines, and all stakeholders, checklists may improve practice delivery by serving as an *aide mémoire*.

Information and communication technologies

Health departments continue to develop systems and processes that will result in a complete electronic medical record. Critical care is at the forefront of these developments, with bedside clinical information systems, order-entry strategies, decision support, handheld technologies and telehealth initiatives continuing to evolve and influence practice. Digital innovations are changing medicine – for example, the way in which information is delivered, where graphical displays and visualisation make it possible to absorb large amounts of

TABLE 3.3
Examples of care bundles

BUNDLE NAME	AIM	BUNDLE COMPONENTS
CLABSI (central line-associated blood stream infection) management of sepsis and septic shock	Reduce blood stream infections from central lines. The bundles are to provide guidance for the clinician treating adult patients with sepsis or septic shock in the hospital setting. Early identification and appropriate treatment in the early hours after the onset of sepsis to improve outcomes.	(see components below)

1. Use appropriate hand hygiene.
2. Use chlorhexidine for skin preparation.
3. Use full-barrier precautions during central venous catheter insertion.
4. Avoid using the femoral vein for catheters in adult patients.
5. Remove unnecessary catheters.

Updates to CLABSI recommendations in 2022 by the Society for Healthcare Epidemiology of America (SHEA)

Before insertion:
1. Provide easy access to an evidence-based list of indications for CVC use.
2. Require education and competency assessment of healthcare clinician involved in insertion, care, and maintenance of CVCs about CLABSI prevention.
3. Bath IC patient aged >2 months with a chlorhexidine preparation daily.

At insertion:
1. In ICU – a process should be in place – checklist.
2. Hand hygiene prior to insertion and whenever the catheter is being touched.
3. Subclavian is the preferred site.
4. Use an all-inclusive catheter cart.
5. Use ultrasound-guided approach.
6. Use maximum sterile barrier.
7. For skin preparation, use an alcoholic chlorhexidine antiseptic.

After insertion:
1. Ensure appropriate nurse to patient ratio – limit the use of nurses who are not regularly in the ICU.
2. Use chlorhexidine-containing dressing for CVCs in patients over 2 months of age.
3. For non-tunnelled CVCs, change transparent dressings and perform site care at least every 7 days.
4. Disinfect catheter hubs before use.

Remove non-essential catheters.
Perform surveillance for CLABSI in ICU.
The emphasis is on early recognition of sepsis/septic shock and early administration of antimicrobials and target mean arterial pressure of 65 mmHg.

In the 2021 revision of the guidelines, several new recommendations were made:

Screening for sepsis or septic shock:
1. Use a screening tool – National Early Warning Score (NEWS), Modified Early Warning Score (MEWS), Systemic Inflammatory Response Syndrome (SIRS); do not use quick Sequential Organ Failure Assessment (qSOFA) by itself.

Initial resuscitation:
1. Treat as medical emergencies and begin treatment immediately.
2. For patients with sepsis induced hypoperfusion or septic shock we suggest that at least 30 mL/kg of IV crystalloid fluid be administered within 3hrs of resuscitation.
3. For adults with sepsis or septic shock, use dynamic measures as well as physical assessment and static parameters to guide fluid resuscitation.
4. For adults with sepsis or septic shock, resuscitation should be assessed to decrease serum lactate when it is elevated.
5. For adults with septic shock, use capillary refill as well as other assessments to measure perfusion.

Mean arterial pressure:
For adults with septic shock on vasopressors – aim for initial MAP of 65 mmHg.

Admission to intensive care:
Adults with sepsis or septic shock – admit to ICU within 6 hours.

Continued

TABLE 3.3

Examples of care bundles—cont'd

BUNDLE NAME	AIM	BUNDLE COMPONENTS
		Infection: Antimicrobials within 1 hour of recognition of sepsis/septic shock. *Ventilation:* 1 Low tidal volume (LTV) for sepsis-associated acute respiratory distress syndrome (ARDS). 2 Prone positioning in moderate to severe ARDS. *Goals of care:* *In the revised guidelines, emphasis is placed on involving families in the goals of care, long-term recovery of sepsis/septic shock – focusing on the sequelae such as cognitive and mobility issues.*
ICU liberation bundle – ABCDEF	This bundle implements all the components of the prevention and management of pain, agitation/sedation, delirium, immobility and sleep disruption in adult patients.	1 Assess, prevent, and manage pain – using evidence-based assessment tools to assess pain (A). 2 For ventilated patients assess SAT – spontaneous awakening trial and SBT – spontaneous breathing trial (B). 3 Assess level of sedation and use the right sedation for the right patient (C). 4 Assess for delirium (using an evidence-based tool). Prevent delirium by understanding risk factors. Treat delirium when present (D). 5 Mobilise every patient after assessing readiness to mobilise (E). 6 Involve family in the care of every ICU patient (F).

Sources: Agency for Healthcare Research and Quality. CLABSI. https://www.ahrq.gov/hai/cusp/index.html; *Buetti N, Marschall J, Drees M, et al. Strategies to prevent central line-associated bloodstream infections in acute-care hospitals: 2022 update. Infect Control Hosp Epidemiol. 2022;43(5):553-69; Evans L, Rhodes A, Alhazzani W, et al. Surviving sepsis campaign: international guidelines for management of sepsis and septic shock 2021. Crit Care Med 2021;49(11):e1063-143. doi: 10.1097/CCM.0000000000005337; ICU Liberation bundle:* https://www.sccm.org/iculiberation/abcdef-bundles; *Devlin JW, Skrobik Y, Gélinas C, et al. Clinical practice guidelines for the prevention and management of pain, agitation/sedation, delirium, immobility, and sleep disruption in adult patients in the ICU. Crit Care Med 2018;46(9):e825-73.*

data quickly.[56] Clinical decision support algorithms are now integrated into the electronic medical record to assist clinicians and to reduce human error and omissions in care.[57] This section examines the current and future impacts that these technologies will have on patient care and safety, and on clinician workflows and practices, as clinical information fully assimilates with evidence-based practice and clinical decision support systems.

Clinical information systems

Clinical information systems may enable improved data collection, storage, retrieval and reporting of patient-based information, and facilitate unit-based outcomes research and quality improvement activities. Continuous monitoring systems technology have been shown to improve cost outcomes.[56] Patient-based bedside clinical information systems offer increasingly sophisticated functionality and device interfaces, enabling real-time data capture, trending and reporting and linkage to relational databases.[58] A recent systematic review identified computerised clinical decision support systems that were associated with better patient outcomes.[59]

The introduction of intravenous 'smart pump' technology is one application aimed at reducing adverse drug events and improving patient care by supporting evidence-based guidelines for medication management.[60] The operator-error prevention software is based on a device-based drug library with institution-established concentrations/dosage limits incorporated into the function of the pump. Resulting software functions include clinician alerts (for keystroke errors)[60] and transaction log data (post-incident analysis).[60] Medication errors and adverse drug events can be detected by this software. There is evidence to suggest, however, that, despite the use of smart pumps, errors related to administration of intravenous medication remain.[60] A large medical centre implemented smart pump technology across 45 departments over 3 months. Describing the implementation, the authors stressed that an effective approach involves a strong partnership with the vendor, extensive planning and collaboration among the advance practice nurses and educators and consultants from both organisations to ensure that quality improvement is achieved.[60] To enhance efficiency and accountability in the implementation, the authors also utilised lean principles. This highlights the need for promotional and quality improvement activities targeting compliance in using smart pumps, including actions to increase usability such as upgrading drug libraries, decreasing the number of unnecessary warnings and developing approaches to minimise workarounds.[60]

Although the proportion of ICUs using a clinical information system is not known, there are indications that uptake is on the increase. Numerous benefits to healthcare systems that lead to enhanced quality of care have been reported such as improved documentation, legibility, increased access to data, evidence-based decision support, interdisciplinary communication and reduced duplication and medical errors.[61] Throughout Australia many hospitals have implemented hospital-wide electronic medical records (EMRs) with varying degrees of functionality. However, few have implemented end-to-end digital systems with the ability to completely transform clinical care.[62] In intensive care they have reduced documentation time and increased the proportion of time spent on direct care activities.[63] Moreover, they facilitate the use of real-time measurements of care processes and can be used for continuous quality improvements.[63] End-user support has been identified as an important factor in the success of clinical information system implementation, and supporting end users is one aspect that requires dedicated resources to manage effectively.[64] Barriers that have been identified include integration issues with other software systems, poor usability, insufficient technical support, lack of knowledge and training, limited experience and confidence in using clinical information systems, time issues due to increased work demands, and lack of consultation with end users.[64]

Clinical alert functions are designed to improve delivery of care; however, they may compromise patient safety when used excessively in clinical settings.[65] Alarm fatigue in the ICU is well documented in the literature. A recent appraisal of current research on how an alarm management program impacts alarm fatigue among registered nurses (RN) revealed that, despite extensive literature highlighting the astronomical prevalence of alarm fatigue in RNs, there was a lack of current high-quality data related to implementing alarm management programs.[65] Researchers examining factors influencing ICU nurses' response to alarms concluded that visual access to physiological data, experience, teamwork and false alarms are important determinants.[66] A systematic review revealed improvements in prescribing behaviours as a result of computerised alerts and prompts; however, among those studies investigating patient outcomes, no significant improvements were found.[67] A recent study on the usability testing of physiological monitors revealed major ineffectiveness and inefficiencies in the current nurse–monitor interactions.[68] The study demonstrated the potential for safety issues when performing routine tasks related to adjusting alarms and using physiological monitors. Training on monitor use should include critical monitoring functions that are necessary for safe, effective, efficient and appropriate monitoring.

Computerised order entry and decision support

Computerised provider order entry (CPOE) is a system that allows orders for medications, intravenous fluids, diagnostic tests and procedures to be entered and then rapidly communicated to pharmacies. It can also be used for results management, treatment orders and clinical decision support.[69] CPOE is viewed as an important innovation in reducing medical errors, through minimising transcribing, dispensing and administration errors.[69]

A systematic review and meta-analysis of the impact of CPOE and clinical decision support systems on medication errors, length of stay and mortality in ICU found that the transition from paper-based ordering to CPOE systems was associated with an 85% reduction in medical prescribing errors and a 12% reduction in ICU mortality rates. However, no significant changes in hospital mortality and length of stay were found.[69] Furthermore, implementation of CPOE and related clinical decision support systems demonstrates significant reductions in redundant or unnecessary order requests.[70] A systematic review exploring the use of clinical decision support systems on clinical decision making for pressure ulcer treatment by nurses resulted in no significant effects found on nurses' knowledge following the integration of clinical decision support systems into the workflow, with assessments made for a brief period of up to 6 months.[71] More studies are needed that prioritise better adoption and interaction by nurses. Decision support systems interface with hospital databases to retrieve patient-specific and other relevant clinical data to support medical decisions and other tasks. Importantly, clinical decision making at the bedside can be enhanced by providing clinicians with a readily available tool that incorporates relevant clinical information and evidence-based medicine. Clinician alerts (e.g. allergies or interaction effects) or prompts (e.g. to check coagulation when prescribing warfarin) can be generated. Yet, there is limited evidence that these systems reduce errors that are system related over time.[72] This might be explained by implementation issues, failure to adequately tailor alarms resulting in alert fatigue, or system design problems. Further studies are needed focusing on when system-related errors occur and what the causative factors are for the future prevention and mitigation of the errors.[72]

Additional developments involving wireless communication, handheld technologies and closed-loop delivery systems may improve the efficiency, effectiveness and adoption of this innovation in clinical practice. A 2020 survey of ICU clinicians exploring improvements and the future of ICU technology resulted in the following recommendations: information technology departments and medical device manufacturers should focus on reducing false-alarm fatigue, implementing hospital alarm standard operating procedures and improvements in wireless technology, educating all staff on the use of artificial intelligence, and improving all clinicians' knowledge of digital technology.[73]

Closed-loop delivery systems offer automated treatment using feedback principles and are designed to maintain a given variable around a desired set point (e.g. inotropic dosages adjusted to a range for mean arterial pressure). Compared with manual control, automated systems can improve stability of target parameters and reduce workload in clinical practice.[74] An example in ICU settings is automated weaning systems using closed-loop controls to adapt ventilator output to the individual need of the patient. Closed-loop ventilation modes are increasingly being used in ICUs to ensure more automaticity. A study comparing visual behaviour between experienced and non-experienced ICU nurses while using a closed-loop ventilation system demonstrated gaze patterns of intensive care nurses were mainly focused on numeric values and settings. More visual attention to oxygenation Intellivent and ventilation Intellivent by experienced nurses implied more routine and familiarity with closed-loop modes. The findings of the study highlighted the need for repeated and ongoing training and education with new technology in the ICU.[75] Compared with non-automated weaning strategies, it significantly decreased weaning time and length of stay in the ICU.[76]

Handheld technologies

Wireless applications enable clinical information access, portability and mobility within a critical care environment at the point of care. Handheld computers and devices use operating systems and pen-like styluses that enable touchscreen functionality, handwriting recognition and synchronisation with other hospital-based computer systems. Handheld devices provide easy access to information and enable timely documentation. They can provide healthcare professionals with evidence-based decision support and improve information seeking, adherence to guidelines and clinical decision making.[77]

In critical care, handheld devices have been used to document clinical activities such as logging critical care procedures, which was demonstrated as feasible and useful – for example, a smartphone application for assessing delirium in the ICU.[78] They have also been used to improve communication and pain assessment of critically ill patients with mechanical ventilation through the use of videoconferencing platforms, especially during the recent COVID pandemic.[79] Communication and shared decision making between surrogates and healthcare professionals is further enhanced through teleconferencing and use of handheld electronic devices.[79,80]

An increasing array of clinical applications and content is available for downloading to these devices. Specific applications for healthcare professionals in the ICU have been developed – for example, an application for delirium assessment and decision-making assistance as described above,[78] and one for pressure injury/ulcer lesion

monitoring and decision making in patients with mechanical ventilation.[81]

The benefits of this mobile computing also create concerns over confidentiality, however. Health services, designers and developers therefore need policies that recognise individuals' rights regarding information collected on them. Researchers and developers should design new methods that address security issues such as authentication, identification, data anonymisation and software assurance.[82] The issue with protecting health data is also of concern to the patient. In a systematic review exploring understanding the patient privacy perspective demonstrated there may be an oversimplification of the amount of concern and its impact due to the amount of patient privacy research being conducted and published. The patient–healthcare provider relationship could be affected if the patient has a concern about their medical data being widely accessible.[82] As these issues are addressed, these technologies will form an integral component of routine clinical practice in critical care.

> **Practice tip**
>
> Although handheld devices can assist nurses in their practice, with a range of helpful clinical applications now available, it is necessary to ensure that patient confidentiality is not compromised and the devices are secure.

Telehealth initiatives

Remote critical care management (tele-ICU) using telemedicine/telehealth technologies is expanding as the necessary high bandwidths for transmitting large amounts of data and digital imagery become available between partner units or hospitals. Videoconferencing functions enable direct visualisation and communication of patients and on-site staff with the 'virtual' critical care clinician or team. Review of real-time physiological data, patient flowcharts and other documents (e.g. electrocardiograms, laboratory results) or images (e.g. radiographs) provides a comprehensive data set for patient assessment and management.

One systematic review of telemedicine and clinical decision support for ICU found a reduction in hospital mortality. However, they concluded that most studies investigating tele-ICU were of poor methodological quality, highlighting the need for further studies to determine the effectiveness of tele-ICU.[83] Another systematic review and meta-analysis of the literature concluded that tele-ICU may reduce ICU and hospital mortality and shorten ICU length of stay. But no significant effect was found in hospital length of stay, and its long-term cost effectiveness is still unclear.[84] A recent systematic review and meta-analysis exploring decision making authority during tele-ICU demonstrated reduction in mortality and length of stay. The study highlighted the need for evidence-based ICU telemedicine guidelines for all tele-ICUs to consider adopting.[85]

There are also characteristics of tele-ICU that are likely to impact on both the process and the outcomes of care. Benefits are likely to be generated from the availability of extra resources and the ability of the tele-ICU to serve as a quality improvement trigger (e.g. checking compliance with evidence-based medicine), and to provide medication management support, software alerts and prompts and real-time patient monitoring by camera.[86] For these benefits to be realised, however, the technology needs to be accepted and used appropriately by ICU staff. Further studies that include detailed descriptions of system implementation are required to determine the most-effective elements of this technology in critical care settings as well as their impact on care processes and outcomes.[87] For instance, one study examining how tele-ICU nurses and organisational characteristics influenced trust and satisfaction among bedside ICU nurses concluded that optimised communication is an important aspect to establish trust between tele-ICU and bedside nurses.[88]

In addition to remote patient assessment and management, telecommunications have been used to deliver continuing education to rural healthcare professionals for many years via audio, video and computer. E-learning, defined as education mediated electronically via the internet, has steadily increased among healthcare professionals.[89] One Cochrane review, including 16 randomised trials, concluded that there were little or no differences in patient outcomes or healthcare professionals' behaviours, skills and knowledge between e-learning and traditional learning.[89] E-learning training platforms and tools have been used, for example, to increase the use of tools for neurological monitoring in ICU,[90] to prevent healthcare-associated infections,[91] and to increase nurses' skills in assessing and classifying pressure injuries.[92] The potential impact of online communities and social media in nursing education and clinical practice has also been systematically examined.[93] Online professional development courses are also available, but more trials are needed to assess the superiority of e-learning over traditional learning methods.[89]

Further exploring the benefits of tele-ICU interventions in a scoping review, the study results showed excellent benefits for centralised systems extending critical care services in a community setting and improving care compliance in tertiary level hospitals. There was not strong evidence to support reduction of patient transfers following tele-ICU intervention.[94]

Patient safety

The signing of the Declaration of Vienna in 2009[95] committed critical care organisations around the world, including the World Federation of Critical Care Nurses, to patient safety. Patient safety is viewed as a crucial component of quality.[96] Over the years, numerous definitions of patient safety have emerged in the literature. The Institute of Medicine described it as the absence of preventable harm to a patient during the process of healthcare.[10] The World Health Organization (WHO) has focused its patient safety efforts on providing global leadership and fostering collaboration, developing guidelines and tools and building capacity, and engaging patients and families for safer healthcare and monitoring improvements in patient safety.[96] It has also established global safety challenges such as medication without harm,[96] and more recently launched the first-ever World Patient Safety Day in 2019 to promote patient safety through increasing public awareness and engagement and encouraging people (patients, families, healthcare professionals, researchers, etc.) to show their commitment to making healthcare safer.[97]

Three techniques used to understand patient risk are: (1) analysing reports of clinical incidents and AEs, (2) root cause analyses (RCAs) and (3) failure mode and effect analysis. Research on AEs in critical care has helped practitioners to better understand patient risks and target improvement activities. For example, medications, indwelling lines and equipment failure were the three most frequent types of AEs in a study of 205 ICUs worldwide.[98] Focusing on analysing the narratives written about AEs is viewed as an important way to learn from errors. However, a systematic review of incident and reporting systems in the ICU found that none of the 36 papers reviewed completely met the WHO's criteria for AE reporting.[99] RCA is a structured process generally used to analyse catastrophic or sentinel events.[100] In RCA, the various situations that led to the event are documented and analysed in order to identify contributing factors to the event and make recommendations for system changes to prevent the event from occurring again. Learning from both incident reporting and RCAs is based on the premise that the information they contain is of sufficient quality to allow accurate analysis, interpretation and detection of the root causes of problems and, even more importantly, the formulation and implementation of corrective actions. In one recent publication, the Veterans Health Administration in the United States analysed 70 ICU RCAs and found that delays in care and medication errors were the most common types of events, with the root causes identified as predominantly related to policies and procedure processes, equipment or supply issues and knowledge deficit.[101] To further strengthen the recommendations reported from RCAs, the incorporation of human factors and independent investigators has been suggested to gain greater understanding of the work environment (e.g. task complexity, workforce, process design, fatigue, stress) and reduce bias in order to improve the sustainability and efficiency of RCA recommendations.[102] Failure mode and effect analysis identifies potential failures and their effects, calculating their risk and prioritising potential failure modes based on risk.[103] A recent Spanish study used failure mode and effect analysis as part of their approach to improving the use of strategies to prevent venous thromboembolic disease in ICU patients.[104] In addition to examining patient risk, another strategy has focused on understanding the safety culture of a unit or organisation, with subsequent activities aimed at improving components of this culture. Therefore, it appears that contemporary techniques to understand patient safety risks are being used in critical care.

Practice tip

By undertaking a root cause analysis, the contributing factors to the event can be identified and strategies to mitigate future AEs can be implemented.

Medication errors

Medication administration is the most common intervention in healthcare, but the medication management process in the acute hospital setting is complex and creates risk for patients. As a result, medication-related events are one of the most common AEs for critically ill patients[98] and the rationale for a focus on it. A Spanish study of adverse drug events in a 30-bed ICU found 53 AEs occurred in 142 patients over a 4-month period.[105] Although the rates of medication errors and adverse drug events vary greatly between settings despite geographical location, they are common in critical care units,[106] with higher rates of harmful errors than in non-ICU settings, and those errors are more likely to be associated with requiring life-sustaining intervention, permanent harm or death.[107]

How medication incidents are defined and measured impacts on reported error/adverse event rates and their interpretation. The way in which medication errors, for example, are calculated requires careful consideration of both the numerator (e.g. count of any error in the medication process) and the denominator (this could be the number of patients, patient days, medication days, administered doses – depending on the aim or purpose of the measure).[108]

One observational study found that an average of 2.9 preventable or potential adverse drug events occurred in each ICU admission[109] and, in Australia, research suggests that errors occur in 9% of all medications administered in hospitals.[110] Although it is estimated that only one out of 10 medical errors results in AEs,[108] such errors can lead to costly additional treatments and prolonged hospital stays as well as other implications for patients, families and healthcare providers.[108,111] Approximately 5% of medication errors relate to infusion pumps. These pumps are used to administer high-impact medications, such as inotropes, heparin or antineoplastics.[55] Analysis of a database describing 537 hospitals with ICUs showed the main medication errors were errors of omission, improper dose or quantity and incorrect administration technique.[107] The leading sources of errors

that caused harm in ICUs were knowledge and performance deficits (57%), not following procedure or protocol (26%), faulty communication (15%) and dispensing device errors (14%).[107] Using the SEIPS model, one literature review revealed that human factors (i.e. stress, high workload, knowledge and performance deficits) were associated with medical errors in the ICU.[112] Factors contributing to medication errors were frequent interruptions, communication problems and poor usability of health information technologies.[112] The occurrence of medical errors in ICUs has also been linked to increased task volume with increased workload for nurses.[113] In response to this body of evidence pertaining to medication error, a number of strategies have been instituted; for example, in Australia under the auspices of the National Medicines Policy, the Quality Use of Medicines map is a searchable online database of related projects to assist health practitioners and researchers plan and carry out their work, and to help policy makers evaluate quality use of medicines activity for potential use in policy development (see Online resources).

It is important to evaluate interventions that can reduce the incidence and impact of adverse intravenous drug events, particularly in critical care settings.[114] As most medication errors in the ICU occur in the administration phase,[107] critical care nurses play a key role in detection and prevention of errors before patient harm results. Evidence suggests that nurses who are interrupted while administering medications may have an increased risk of making medication errors.[115] Reducing interruptions to medication administration in ICU requires interventions that consider the complexity of working in an imperfect environment, in multidisciplinary teams and under uncertain circumstances.[116]

Practice tip

Given the high frequency and consequences of medication errors, it is important to be cognisant of the potential for error and be aware of strategies that can be used to prevent such errors, such as limiting interruptions.

Safety culture

Measurement of the baseline safety culture facilitates an action plan for improvement. Safety culture has been defined as *'the product of individual and group values, attitudes, perceptions, competencies, and patterns of behaviour that determine the commitment to, and the style and proficiency of, an organisation's health and safety management'*.[117] It is commonly referred to as 'the way we do things around here'.[118] A systematic review found evidence for a relationship between safety culture and patient outcomes at both the hospital and unit level.[119] In addition to patient outcomes, researchers have studied the association between safety culture and staff outcomes. For example, in a study of

ICU nurses in six Norwegian hospitals, researchers showed a positive safety culture was associated with lower burnout scores and a stronger sense of coherence, a construct reflecting how people cope with stressful situations.[120]

A widely used instrument to measure safety culture, the Safety Attitudes Questionnaire (SAQ), focuses on six domains: teamwork climate, safety climate, job satisfaction, perceptions of management, working conditions and stress recognition.[121] Interestingly, studies in Canada,[122] Iran,[123] Africa[124] and 10 ICUs in Australia[125] showed that nurses and doctors differed in their perceptions of safety culture. The Australian study also identified some differences between bedside nurses and nursing leaders.[125] Using the SAQ, a Palestinian neonatal ICU study found a wide variation in the perceptions of the safety culture held by 164 nurses and 40 physicians in 16 hospitals.[126] Another European study of 378 patients in 57 ICUs showed a relationship between positive safety culture and fewer errors.[127] A recent study conducted in Brazil found that ICU staff in adult, paediatric and neonatal ICUs scored job satisfaction and teamwork climate high on a SAQ; both of these are considered excellent markers of patient safety.[128]

> **Practice tip**
>
> A positive safety culture is associated with better patient outcomes.

One strategy to improve the safety culture has been to identify factors that make organisations safe, which in turn allows initiatives to be developed that target areas of specific need. For example, five characteristics of organisations that have been able to achieve high reliability include:[129]

1 safety viewed as a priority by leaders
2 flattened hierarchy that promotes speaking up about concerns
3 regular team training
4 use of effective methods of communicating
5 standardisation.

There are a number of other resources available to those interested in improving patient safety. For example, WHO has published a patient safety curriculum guide to assist organisations in this endeavour.[130] Leadership, teamwork and behavioural change strategies provide a foundation for improvements in safety culture[131] (see Further reading for more detail on behaviour change). In the USA, the Comprehensive Unit-based Safety Program (CUSP) has emerged as one specific safety intervention.[132] Recent publications about the CUSP program support its benefits.[133,134] Another American critical care quality improvement program found that a nurse-led safety program that included executive walkarounds and a

multidisciplinary team tasked with identifying and resolving safety issues was effective.[135] The three top safety issues identified related to nursing, supplies and daily unit operations, with 36–70% of the issues being resolved. In summary, understanding the various dimensions of safety culture in a unit can be used as a foundation for the development and implementation of programs targeted at specific aspects that may benefit from improvements. To be successful, safety programs have to be supported by the leaders as well as other members of the unit.[121,136]

Rapid response systems

Rapid response systems (RRSs) have been developed to recognise and provide emergency response to patients who experience acute deterioration.[137] In 2014, at least 95% of Australian hospitals with an ICU had implemented an RRS.[138] A 2020 review and meta-analysis of 10 studies of RRSs found that there was moderate evidence linking the implementation of an RRS with decreased mortality and non-ICU cardiac arrests.[139] While papers about RRS often reflect experiences in Australia, the USA and the UK, the 2020 review included studies from Canada, Pakistan, Portugal, Saudi Arabia, South Korea, Sweden and The Netherlands. One study not included in this review, which was set in 12 hospitals in The Netherlands, found an RRS had positive effect on the composite outcome of cardiopulmonary arrest, unplanned ICU admission and death.[140] More recently, following statewide adoption of the 'Between the Flags' RRS in New South Wales, Australia, a prospective observational study of the RRS registry across 35 hospitals with an ICU showed significant reduction in cardiac arrests in hospitals and ICU admissions secondary to cardiac arrests.[141]

Although there has been a proliferation of papers on RRS, one recent and promising US innovation has been the development of an airway RRS, which focuses on airway emergencies.[142] The Australian Commission on Safety and Quality in Health Care identified nine essential elements in an RRS (Table 3.4).[143] Further, McGaughey and colleagues' realist review of over 270 papers on RRS identified that they were beneficial when there was a sufficient skill mix of experienced staff, when a scoring system for the identification of the deteriorating patient was used flexibly alongside clinical judgement, and when staff had access to ongoing, multiprofessional competency-based education.[144] Realist reviews focus on understanding the underlying theory of an intervention like RRS, including how the context, mechanism of action and outcomes interact. McGaughey and colleagues' theory, which underpins the RRS, is displayed in Fig. 3.2.

RRSs were originally conceptualised to have three components.[145] First, there are the criteria and a system for identifying and activating the rapid response team, often referred to as the afferent limb.[137] Second, there is the response, also termed the efferent limb.[145] Finally, there is an administrative and quality improvement component,[145] which is now referred to as two separate

TABLE 3.4

Essential elements of a rapid response system (RRS)

DOMAIN	ELEMENT	DESCRIPTION
Clinical processes	Measurement and documentation	Regular measurement and documentation of vital signs and other physiological observations is essential for recognising acute deterioration.
	Diagnosis	The underlying cause of a patient's deterioration may need to be tailored to the specific circumstances of the patient, e.g. implementation of algorithms, protocols and pathways specific to the patient's diagnosis such as stroke or sepsis.
	Escalation of care	A protocol for the organisation's response in dealing with abnormal physiological measures and observations including appropriate modifications to nursing care, increased monitoring, medical review and calling for emergency assistance.
	Rapid response systems	When severe deterioration occurs, medical emergency teams or nurse-led rapid response teams liaison nurses are available to respond.
	Communicating for safety	Structured communication protocols are used to hand over information about the patient and provide ongoing management of the patient.
Organisational prerequisites	Leadership and governance	Executive and clinical leadership and organisational governance are aligned with the NSQHS standards.
	Education and training	Education should cover clinical observation, measurement and interpretation, diagnostics, escalation protocols, communication strategies, teamwork and initiating early interventions.
	Evaluation, audit and feedback	Ongoing monitoring and evaluation are required to track changes in outcomes over time and to check that the RRS is operating as planned.
	Systems to support high-quality care	As relevant technologies are developed, they should be incorporated into service delivery, after considering evidence of their efficacy and cost as well as potential unintended consequences.

Source: Adapted from Australian Commission on Safety and Quality in Health Care. National consensus statement: essential elements for recognising and responding to acute physiological deterioration. Sydney, NSW: ACSQHC; 2021.

limbs: administrative and quality improvement.[146] Each of these limbs is briefly described.

Afferent limb

Recognising the deteriorating patient, the afferent limb has focused on measuring clinical signs including vital signs, level of consciousness and oxygenation as well as acting on abnormalities in these measurements.[145] They may also include concerns expressed by clinicians[147] and families.[148] Various scoring systems to identify ward patients with clinical deterioration have evolved as part of the development of critical care outreach[149] and the medical emergency team (MET).[147] Authors of a 2017 scoping review of 21 studies on the use of early-warning and track-and-trigger systems noted that a combination of parameters including respiratory rate, oxygen saturation, supplementary oxygen flow rates, systolic blood pressure,

heart rate, temperature and level of consciousness continue to be used.[150] Two recent variations of early-warning scoring systems are HOTEL (**h**ypotension, **o**xygen saturation, **t**emperature, **e**lectrocardiograph abnormalities, **l**oss of independence) and TOTAL (**t**achypnoea, **o**xygen saturation, **t**emperature, **a**lert, **l**oss of independence); both were found to be better for their particular populations than the modified early-warning system (MEWS).[150] All systems identify abnormalities in commonly measured parameters. There is also emerging research indicating that machine learning models (artificial intelligence) have the potential to more accurately and cost effectively predict in-hospital cardiac arrests compared with MEWS.[151] Continued research is needed to test the translation of these models into larger clinical practice settings.

Early-warning systems include calling criteria for contacting the admitting medical team, ICU staff, the

FIGURE 3.2   Rapid response program theory.

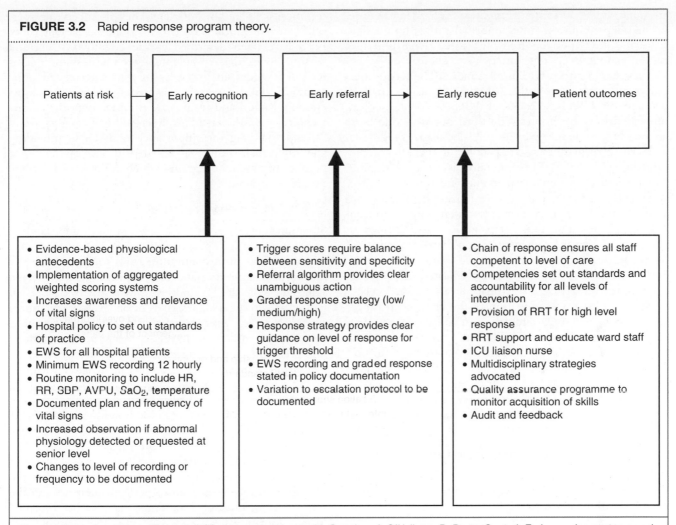

| Patients at risk | Early recognition | Early referral | Early rescue | Patient outcomes |

- Evidence-based physiological antecedents
- Implementation of aggregated weighted scoring systems
- Increases awareness and relevance of vital signs
- Hospital policy to set out standards of practice
- EWS for all hospital patients
- Minimum EWS recording 12 hourly
- Routine monitoring to include HR, RR, SBP, AVPU, SaO$_2$, temperature
- Documented plan and frequency of vital signs
- Increased observation if abnormal physiology detected or requested at senior level
- Changes to level of recording or frequency to be documented

- Trigger scores require balance between sensitivity and specificity
- Referral algorithm provides clear unambiguous action
- Graded response strategy (low/medium/high)
- Response strategy provides clear guidance on level of response for trigger threshold
- EWS recording and graded response stated in policy documentation
- Variation to escalation protocol to be documented

- Chain of response ensures all staff competent to level of care
- Competencies set out standards and accountability for all levels of intervention
- Provision of RRT for high level response
- RRT support and educate ward staff
- ICU liaison nurse
- Multidisciplinary strategies advocated
- Quality assurance programme to monitor acquisition of skills
- Audit and feedback

Source: Reproduced from Figure 2: RRS programme theory; McGaughey J, O'Halloran P, Porter S, et al. Early warning systems and rapid response to the deteriorating patient in hospital: a systematic realist review. J Adv Nurs 2017;73(12):2877–91, with permission.

critical care outreach team or the MET, depending on the severity of the patient's clinical deterioration and the resources available in the local clinical environment. In a 2017 review of 30 papers, activation of the RRS was influenced by perceptions and clinical experiences of ward nurses and physicians, accuracy of the activation criteria and monitoring technology.[152] Other barriers include education level and cultural and traditional hierarchical models that inhibit staff from activating response teams efficiently.[139] Impediments included seeking further justification, deliberating overreactions from the RRT and the impact of workload and staffing.[152] In an Australian study of factors that influenced RRS in one hospital, organisational barriers were identified: that RRT medical responsibility was inversely proportional to clinical experience, system flexibility contributed to protocol deviation, misdistribution of resources led to perceptions of inadequate staffing, which prevented full optimisation of the RRS, and poor communication and documentation increased clinician workload.[153] Patients and/or families

calling the RRT is becoming more commonplace. In Australia, various models have been implemented with different labels and activation processes: Call and Respond Early in Western Australia,[154] Recognise, Engage, Act, Call, Help (REACH) is on its way in New South Wales[155] and Ryan's Rule (RR) in Queensland.[156] These models provide pathways for patient and families to escalate care when they are concerned, resulting in an independent clinical review. A 2016 review of 10 studies focusing on family initiation of escalation of care for deteriorating patients found all of the 436 calls were appropriate, and stemmed from communication or system breakdowns.[148] Families viewed this calling positively, but staff found the introduction of family activation to be stressful.[148]

Efferent limb

The efferent limb involves the team responding to clinical deterioration.[145] Some teams will include physicians and nurses, known as the MET or RRT, whereas others such as critical care outreach teams[145] and ICU liaison nurses are nurse led.[157] In some organisations, a graded response occurs, depending on how abnormal the early-warning score is. One paper reported on a three-tiered response system as follows.[153] The first tier is a clinical review by two registered nurses within 30 minutes. The second tier is a rapid response by the patient's admitting medical team/medical registrar and an RRS resident medical officer within 30 minutes. The third tier is a code blue attended to immediately by an ICU-led team of registrars and critical care nurses. Irrespective of the title of the model used, the RRTs generally assess deteriorating patients and then initiate emergency treatments. A 2014 systematic review of critical care transition programs in general found that they were associated with a reduced risk of ICU re-admission.[158] This positive association was also found when the only service considered was an ICU liaison nurse.[158] One group reported that nurses on the MET undertake technical tasks related to airway (suctioning, inserting naso-pharyngeal airways, etc.), breathing (physical examination of the chest, increasing/adding oxygen, etc.), circulation (clinically examining circulation, performing ECGs, etc.), nervous system (assessing with the Glasgow Coma Scale, etc.) and various other tasks.[159] Non-technical tasks performed include reviewing investigations, contributing to information about patient history and plans for care, reassuring other healthcare professionals, educating staff, documenting care, applying monitoring equipment and supervising patient transport.[159] This study indicates the wide variety of activities that nurse members of a RRT undertake, which suggests the need for advanced knowledge and skills in a number of areas. Chapter 1 provides an overview of advanced nursing practice.

Administrative and quality improvement limbs

The third and fourth components of an RRS focus on administration and quality improvement.[145] Generally, this involves both a governance plan and the collection and analysis of RRS data including the reason for the call, the treatments administered and patient outcomes. Analysing RRS data provides managers, clinicians and policy makers with guidance for future improvements. These activities are linked to previous information in this chapter on clinical audits, the PDSA cycle, etc. In summary, RRSs have evolved to provide emergency care to patients whose condition is deteriorating, and who are not already in the critical care unit. RRSs involve a mechanism to identify these patients and call for help, as well as a response team. They also generally involve some administrative and quality improvement components to improve the service. RRTs rely on team members working together, which leads to the next section, on non-technical skills.

Non-technical skills

Nurses need to have current knowledge and skills in critical care to ensure safe, high-quality care, but these technical skills are not sufficient. They also need to possess other, non-technical skills (NTS) to ensure patient safety. NTS have been described as the cognitive, social and personal skills that complement technical skills.[160] This section provides an overview of four interrelated non-technical skills: situational awareness, decision making, communication and teamwork. Another important non-technical skill, leadership, is described in Chapters 1 and 2. Understanding the importance of NTS in providing safe, high-quality care has led to the development of a number of training programs, which are briefly described in this section.

Situational awareness

Situational awareness is the awareness and understanding of a situation and its possible outcomes.[161] Situations may be categorised on a continuum from routine and easily managed to confusing and dangerous, requiring specific skills and expertise.[162] Endsley,[163] whose work has been particularly influential, describes three levels of situational awareness. Level 1, *perception*, involves gathering data about the current situation. Level 2, *comprehension*, reflects interpretation and understanding the data. Level 3, *projection*, is concerned with predicting what can happen in the future. Fig. 3.3 demonstrates application of these three levels of situational awareness using the scenario of a postoperative patient whose blood pressure has dropped. Importantly, situational awareness is viewed as a necessary precursor for good-quality decision making.[161]

Team situational awareness is a term applied to teams and reflects the notion that team members possess the situational awareness needed to perform their tasks in the team.[161] Team situational awareness has also been termed 'shared situational awareness'.[163] In the critical care environment, nurses and physicians will have some unique but related tasks to undertake, including during procedures such as central line insertions, intubations and bronchoscopies, and these tasks will require both complementary and shared situational awareness. For example, a paediatric cardiac ICU implemented a huddle process during the COVID-19 pandemic to create situational awareness among staff by preparing stuff for major patient events such as intubation or extracorporeal membrane oxygenation cannulation. Shared cognition was extremely effective in mitigating staff anxiety and preparing staff for potential and actual events.[164] The extent of team or shared situational awareness will influence the quality of decisions and subsequent team performance.[161]

> **Practice tip**
>
> Team briefings before undertaking a complex procedure can help to develop team situational awareness.

One review identified that both individual factors and interpersonal behaviours influenced situational awareness.[165] Lapses in situational awareness can occur

FIGURE 3.3 Situational awareness model.[163]

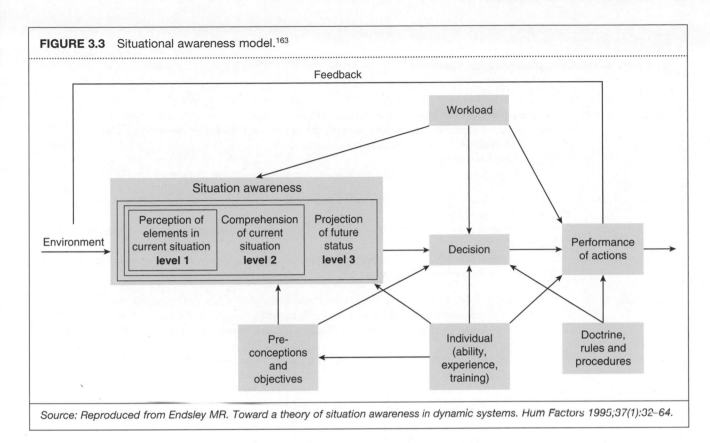

Source: Reproduced from Endsley MR. Toward a theory of situation awareness in dynamic systems. Hum Factors 1995;37(1):32–64.

because of issues such as distractions, fatigue, time pressures and team dynamics such as assertive authority figures. A number of strategies are recommended to overcome these lapses. They include having thorough briefings about the nature and risk of a given activity, minimising distractions and interruptions during critical tasks, receiving regular updates, instituting good time management, being physically and mentally fit for work, and speaking up when not sure of a goal, procedure or next step.[163,166,167]

Decision making

Decision making involves a judgement or choosing an option (i.e. a course of action) to meet the needs of a given situation.[163] In critical care, multiple, complex decisions are made in rapid succession.[168] Decision making entails defining a problem, generating and considering one or more alternatives, selecting and implementing an option and reviewing the outcome. Clinical decision making is a complex process and is influenced by a number of factors. For example, nursing experience along with additional factors such as organisation and unit culture influences, education, understanding the condition of the patient, situation awareness and autonomy underpin the decision-making process.[169] Individual factors such as fatigue, affective state interruption in work and distractions can also influence decision making.[170,171] Authors of a systematic review on cognitive biases associated with medical decision making describe a decision-making framework that suggests two ways decisions are made.[172] In the first, unconscious, automatic or intuitive decisions

are made quickly and effortlessly. In the second, decisions are deliberate, made more slowly and require effort. Overreliance on the first method can lead to cognitive biases, which influence decision making.[172]

Critical care nursing practice has been the focus of many studies on decision making in the early to mid 2000s. One study demonstrated that critical care nurses generate one or more hypotheses about a situation prior to decision making.[168] Other studies indicated that experienced and inexperienced nurses differ in their decision-making skills,[170,171,173] and that role models or mentors are important in assisting to develop decision-making skills.[174] A Greek study classified ICU nurses' decisions as urgent or non-urgent, and as independent or dependent.[175] The researchers observed that 75% (962/1281) of decisions were non-urgent and 60% (220/368) were independent.[175] It is clear that good-quality clinical decisions, irrespective of what they are about, will probably improve patient care and outcomes.

Recommendations for developing clinical decision-making skills

Strategies to help critical care nurses develop their clinical decision-making abilities are identified in Table 3.5.[176,177] These strategies can be used by nurses at any level to develop their own decision-making skills or by educators in planning educational sessions. It is important to note, however, that a review of interventions to improve decision making concluded that most studies in this area were of relatively poor quality.[178]

TABLE 3.5

Strategies to develop clinical decision making

STRATEGY	DESCRIPTION
Iterative hypothesis testing	Description of a clinical situation for which the clinician has to generate questions and develop hypotheses; with additional questioning the clinician will develop further hypotheses. Three phases are: 1 asking questions to gather data about a patient 2 justifying the data sought 3 interpreting the data to describe the influence of new information on decisions.
Interactive model	Schema (mental structures) used to teach new knowledge by building on previous learning. Three components are: 1 advanced organisers – blueprint that previews the material to be learned and connects it to previous materials 2 progressive differentiation – a general concept presented first is broken down into smaller ideas 3 integrative reconciliation – similarities and differences and relationships between concepts explored.
Case study	Description of a clinical situation with a number of cues followed by a series of questions. Three types are: 1 stable – presents information, then asks clinicians about it 2 dynamic – presents information, asks the clinicians about it, presents more information, asks more questions 3 dynamic with expert feedback – combines the dynamic method with immediate expert feedback.
Reflection on action	Clinicians are asked to reflect on their actions after a particular event. This pondering focuses on clinical judgements made, feelings surrounding the actions and the actions themselves. Reflection on action can be undertaken as an individual or group activity and is often facilitated by an expert.
Thinking aloud	A clinical situation is provided and the clinician is asked to 'think aloud' or verbalise their decisions. Thinking aloud is generally facilitated by an expert and can be undertaken individually or in groups.

Sources: Narayan S, Corcoran-Perry S. Teaching clinical reasoning in nursing education. In: Higgs J, Jones MA, Loftus S, et al, editors. Clinical reasoning in the health professions. 3rd ed. Philadelphia: Butterworth-Heinemann; 2008, p. 405–30; Rivett DA, Jones MA. Using case reports to teach clinical reasoning. In: Higgs J, Jones M, editors. Clinical reasoning in the health professions. Philadelphia: Butterworth-Heinemann; 2008, p. 477–84.

Communication

Communication has been described as *'the exchange of information, feedback or response, ideas and feelings'*.[160] Good-quality communication is viewed as a two-way sharing of information, whereby the sender encodes some idea into a message and transmits it to a receiver. The receiver then decodes the message to gain an understanding of it. Next, the receiver becomes the sender, encoding and transmitting a subsequent message.[160] There are various types of communication, including verbal and non-verbal. Non-verbal communication includes written communication and body cues or gestures.

Reason,[179] a well-known safety researcher, suggests that there are three kinds of communication failure that contribute to incidents. The first, *system failure*, occurs when there are either no channels of communication or the channels that exist are not working or are not used. The second, *message failure*, happens when necessary information is not communicated. Finally, *reception failure* occurs when the information is misinterpreted or arrives too late.

> **Practice tip**
>
> Using closed-loop communications, where the receiver acknowledges the message was heard, can prevent miscommunication.

Experts recommend that communication be explicit, efficient and closed loop.[180] By being explicit, a person is being clear in what they are saying. Being efficient means that the message is conveyed using only as many words as necessary. And closed-loop communication is a term used to signify that a receiver acknowledges or responds to the sender of information. This response lets the initiator know that the message was heard. Other strategies to improve communication include ensuring that it is timely and assertive.[180] Timely communication means that the sender is cognisant of the other activities that the receiver may be doing and, because of this, provides information at a relevant time. Assertiveness involves standing up for yourself while respecting others.

In the critical care setting, two specific communication situations have been the focus of recent research: clinical handover and rounds. Handover is more than the transfer of patient information; it has been described as the transfer of professional responsibility and accountability for some or all aspects of care for a patient, or group of patients, from one care provider to another.[181] Besides sharing patient information, handovers provide nurses with opportunities for social bonding, coaching and educating, and team building.[182,183] One Australian study focused on the content of ICU nursing handover.[184] The researchers found that, while >95% of observed handovers included identifying nursing care needs, vital sign observations, changes in patient condition and the medical management of the patient, <40% included a discussion of discharge or long-term plans, cross-checking and reporting on resuscitation status.[184] A second study of 157 nursing shift-to-shift handovers conducted in seven ICUs in three countries (Australia, Israel and the UK)[185] found that handovers were more comprehensive when: (1) the oncoming nurse did not know the patient, (2) the patient was expected to die during the shift, or (3) the family were present. Over 70% of nurses in Israel had cared for the patient in the previous 48 hours, in comparison with only 29% of UK and 20% of Australian nurses. Over 75% of the handover communication included the goals for care and 73% included pain management, but legal issues such as advance directives and identification of a health proxy were mentioned in less than 10% of the handovers. In recent years there have been many other studies of ICU handovers. For example, research focuses on shift-to-shift nursing[186] or medical handover,[187,188] handover from ICU to the wards[189,190] or the operating room,[191] and handover from the operating room to the ICU.[192] A recent systematic review of eight studies of the handover from the ICU to the ward identified that most studies were conducted in Australia, and examined various processes and interventions including the use of the ICU liaison nurse or critical care outreach service as a handover tool.[193] However, all but one meta-analysis was at a moderate or high risk of bias, suggesting there is a need for high-quality research in this area.

A 2013 review identified three important features of good quality handover including: (1) face-to-face, two-way communication, (2) standardised templates or checklists that incorporate a minimum dataset, and (3) content that includes the patient's current diagnosis and clinical situation.[194] In order to improve the quality of handovers, a group of Australians has developed an interactive, 3D computer simulation (virtual world) for training intensive care nurses in shift-to-shift handover.[195]

Multidisciplinary rounds are seen to be one way to promote shared situational awareness. A 2016 review identified that multidisciplinary rounds utilising a structured communication tool may improve staff satisfaction,[196] while a 2013 systematic review of ICU rounds concluded that *'rounds conducted using a standardised structure and a best practice checklist by a multidisciplinary group of providers, with explicitly defined roles and a goal-orientated approach, had the strongest supporting evidence'.*[194] Table 3.6 provides more specific details of the recommendations from this review. One notable cluster-randomised study undertaken in 118 Brazilian ICUs tested the effect of the use of a checklist and daily goal setting during multidisciplinary rounds.[53] Over 6750 patients were enrolled in the trial. The researchers found no difference in in-hospital mortality between the intervention and control groups, although significant improvements were found in some specific secondary outcomes such as the use of low tidal volumes, avoidance of heavy sedation, use of central venous and urinary catheters, and perceptions of teamwork and safety climate.

Teamwork

Teams have been described as two or more individuals with specialised roles and responsibilities who act interdependently to achieve some common goal,[197] although in their systematic review Dietz and colleagues noted that teamwork is a broad term with varying definitions.[198] High-performing teams share an understanding of the activity they are working on, they understand the aim or mission of that activity and they know each other's roles and expectations. They are also trained and skilled in leadership, conflict resolution, back-up behaviour and closed-loop communication. Important aspects of leadership include coordinating the team, distributing workloads equitably and monitoring the team's performance. Conflict resolution often requires clarification of roles and responsibilities, fostering useful debate and assertive communication. Back-up behaviour is when one team member can step in to assist another in their role, providing support to other team members. In essence, teamwork is dependent on each member being able to anticipate the needs of others, adjust to others' actions and the changing environment and have a shared understanding of how a task should be performed. Dietz and colleagues found that standardised protocols (such as using checklists), implementing daily rounds and training were the three main solutions used to improve ICU teamwork.[198] The findings from a more-recent study focused on ICU teamwork in North America suggested it was more accurate to describe this work as interprofessional work, rather than teamwork.[199] They found that various relational factors, such as professional cultures, medical dominance and hierarchies, both within and between professions, influenced how work was undertaken. In another recently published grounded theory study of ICU teamwork in Sweden, balancing intertwined responsibilities was the core category identified.[200] Contextual conditions associated with this core category included the dynamic nature of the ICU and the number of team members in the ICU. Conditions that resulted in this balancing act included the need to be prepared and flexible, and the interdependence with others associated with overlapping roles. Intervening conditions that influenced team processes included the

TABLE 3.6

Recommendations for ICU rounds

BEST PRACTICE	STRENGTH OF RECOMMENDATION
Implement multidisciplinary rounds (including at least a medical doctor, registered nurse and pharmacist).	Strong – definitely do it
Standardise location, time and team composition.	Strong – definitely do it
Define explicit roles for each HCP participating on rounds.	Strong – definitely do it
Develop and implement structured tool (best practices checklist).	Strong – definitely do it
Reduce non-essential time-wasting activities.	Strong – definitely do it
Minimise unnecessary interruptions.	Strong – definitely do it
Focus discussions on development of daily goals and document all discussed goals in health record.	Strong – definitely do it
Conduct discussions at bedside to promote patient-centredness.	Weak – probably do it
Conduct discussions in conference room to promote efficiency and communication.	Weak – probably do it
Establish open collaborative discussion environment.	Weak – probably do it
Ensure clear visibility between all HCP.	Weak – probably do it
Empower HCP to promote team-based approach to discussions.	Weak – probably do it
Produce visual presentation of patient information.	No specific recommendation

HCP = healthcare professional.
Source: Adapted from Lane D, Ferri M, Lemaire J, et al. A systematic review of evidence-informed practices for patient care rounds in the ICU. Crit Care Med 2013;41(8):2015–29.

organisational and workplace culture and staff characteristics. As a result, staff adopted both active and passive approaches to clinical activities. Another term closely related to teamwork is interprofessional care, which in the ICU is described as: *'care provided by a team of healthcare professionals with overlapping expertise and an appreciation for the unique contribution of other team members as partners in achieving a common goal'*.[201]

Non-technical skills training

Increasing recognition of the importance of NTS has led to the development of a number of training programs. These programs recognise that, while human error cannot be eliminated, it can be minimised, trapped or mitigated.[160] A systematic review of NTS training to enhance patient safety documented both the content of and training methods used in NTS training.[201] Fig. 3.4 demonstrates the content covered in the team-training studies reviewed by Gordon and colleagues.[202] In addition to the core NTS described in this section, the review also identified training programs focused on understanding error and systems such as the human/technology interface. Two

well-known teamwork experts noted that factors such as how the team training is implemented, the method of its delivery and leadership all influence the effectiveness of team training on both processes and outcomes.[203]

Fig. 3.4 provides an overview of these training methods.[202] Most of the team-training studies reviewed took a multidisciplinary approach, reflecting contemporary clinical practice. Simulation has attracted a lot of attention recently as a team-training strategy. It allows clinicians to practise skills and reflect on their performance in a simulated environment. That is, it increases both knowledge and performance. In their 2013 systematic review, Schmidt and colleagues[204] asserted that simulation as a patient safety strategy had four purposes: (1) education, (2) assessment, (3) research and (4) health system integration. It is evident that teamwork and NTS team training are core components of patient safety. One study of the use of a 2-day team-training intervention, called crew resource management, in six ICUs in The Netherlands identified that participants were positive about the training, and that participants recognised the importance of situational awareness.[205] Compared with the control group, participants reported

FIGURE 3.4 Analysis of non-technical skills training teaching methods.

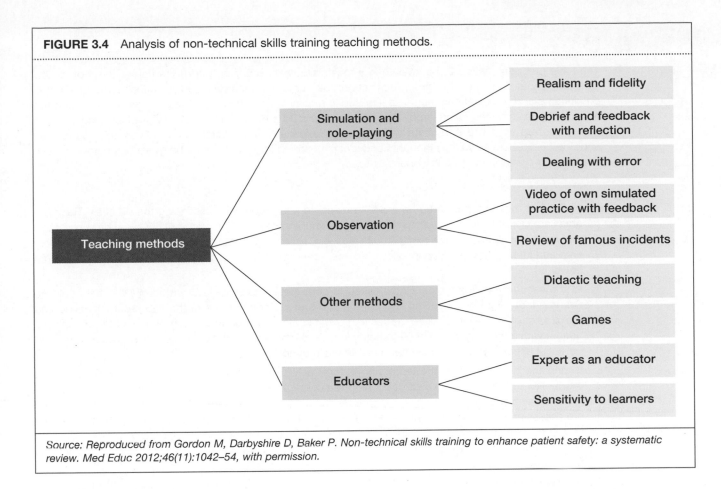

Source: Reproduced from Gordon M, Darbyshire D, Baker P. Non-technical skills training to enhance patient safety: a systematic review. Med Educ 2012;46(11):1042–54, with permission.

enacting situational awareness and teamwork more, but there was no statistically significant difference in communication between the two groups and no changes in patient outcomes were identified. In another study undertaken in two ICUs in Hong Kong, blended learning (both online and in person) and the flipped-classroom approach, where didactic teaching occurs prior to face-to-face teaching, were used to improve patient safety culture.[206] The researchers found that in the intervention site there were significant improvements in both perceptions of teamwork and perceptions of management support for patient safety. Intervention participants also reported greater improvements than control participants in other aspects of patient safety. In summary, patient safety involves understanding the risks to patients and developing strategies to minimise these risks. Safety culture and non-technical skills are two important aspects of patient safety, with a number of strategies and programs available to enhance both.

Summary

In summary, this chapter has provided an overview of safety and quality in critical care. The development and use of evidence-based CPGs is an important foundation to standardise and promote a high standard of care. The use of care bundles, checklists and information and communication technologies may also improve the quality of care by promoting continuity and standardisation of care. Quality and safety monitoring enables decision makers to identify critical gaps in practice and to mitigate safety risks in critical care. Techniques including analysis of clinical incidents, root cause analysis and failure mode and effects analysis help to identify situations that place patients at risk of AEs. For example, RRSs have been implemented to mitigate high-risk scenarios associated with the deteriorating patient. Not only do nurses require current knowledge and skills to practise in critical care, they also require a high level of non-technical skills (e.g. situational awareness, decision-making skills, effective communication, teamwork and leadership skills) to ensure patients are safe. Various initiatives are being introduced to promote positive safety cultures in critical care such as simulation and interprofessional NTS training. This chapter provides a foundation for critical care nurses to develop their knowledge and skills in quality and safety principles, so that they can identify and effectively manage risk and provide quality care.

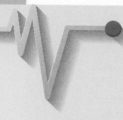

Case study

You have just been asked to participate in a multidisciplinary group to perform a risk analysis of clinical care delivery at your ICU. The group consists of the nurse unit manager, senior critical care nurses, ICU consultants and a critical care nurse specialised in quality improvement. The team is assigned to perform a risk analysis using the failure mode and effect analysis (FMEA) model. As a newly graduated critical care nurse, you are asked to contribute with your own experiences of clinical care delivery (e.g. suctioning endotracheal tubes) as well as thoughts and ideas regarding improvements. The questions below ask you to plan your contribution to this working group.

CASE STUDY QUESTIONS

1   At the first meeting, the group begins with mapping and graphically describing the process. The main areas are identified (e.g. preparing the patient for endotracheal (ETT) suctioning), followed by sub-areas – that is, all steps performed within the main area (e.g. assessing breath sounds). Choose one care delivery area and identify the main areas followed by sub-areas in the clinical care delivery process by making a flowchart.

2   At the second meeting, you are now asked to consider all possible failure modes (i.e. what could go wrong?) that might occur during each of the sub-areas. Choose three of the sub-areas identified and make a list of all possible failure modes (e.g. what could go wrong in the sub-process of preparing the patient within the main areas of ETT suctioning). Also, consider each failure mode's possible cause and potential effect (e.g. what would happen if the failure mode occurred).

3   During the third meeting, the team will perform a hazard analysis for each failure mode. Rate the probability that the failure would occur (1 = remote, 2 = unlikely, 3 = likely, 4 = frequent). Thereafter, rate the severity of harm (1 = minor, 2 = moderate, 3 = major, 4 = catastrophic). When all failure modes are assessed, calculate each failure mode's 'hazard score' by multiplying the probability by the severity (e.g. 2 (unlikely probability) × 3 (major severity) = 6 (hazard score)). Rank all failure modes from the ones with the highest score to those with the lowest. This will give you an overview and might guide the group's decision on how to prioritise areas of improvements.

4   Now it is time for the group to review all failure modes and decide whether to accept the failure mode as it exists or to redesign the process. Choose three of your identified failure modes and consider *how* the process could be redesigned to either eliminate the failure or mitigate potential patient harm.

5   Make a brief outline of your risk analysis of the three clinical care delivery processes you chose. The report should include:
   - the aim of the risk analysis
   - a short description of methods used and how the analysis was performed
   - a flowchart of the process and results of the risk analysis (questions 1–4)
   - suggested areas of improvement (including scientific evidence that supports your findings)
   - a short plan on how to implement and evaluate suggested areas of improvement.

Recommended reading for this case study:

Roohollah A, Shafii, M. Failure mode and effect analysis: improving intensive care unit risk management processes. Int J Health Care Qual Assur 2017;30(3):208–15.

RESEARCH VIGNETTE

Sun J, Han W, Cui N, et al. Effect of nurse-led goal-directed lung physical therapy on the prognosis of pneumonia in sepsis patients in the ICU: a prospective cohort study. J Intensive Care Med 2022;37(2):258–66.
doi: 10.1177/0885066620987200.

Abstract

Background: Pneumonia poses a significant burden on healthcare systems. However, few studies have focused on nurse-led goal-directed lung physical therapy (GDLPT) for pneumonia in sepsis patients in the ICU.

Objectives: This study aimed to investigate the effects of nurse-led GDLPT on the prognosis of pneumonia in sepsis patients in the ICU.

Methods: We performed a prospective two-phase (before-and-after) study over 3 years. After an observational phase (phase 1, $n = 188$), we designed, implemented and evaluated a nurse-led GDLPT protocol (phase 2, $n = 359$) for pneumonia in sepsis patients in the ICU. The primary outcome was 28-day mortality.

Results: We evaluated 742 critically ill patients with sepsis from January 2017 to January 2020. Among the 742 sepsis patients, 609 were diagnosed with pneumonia and 547 who met the inclusion criteria were enrolled in the study. Compared with patients in phase 1, patients in phase 2 had significantly shorter mechanical ventilation duration (5 (4, 6) days vs 5 (4, 8) days, $P = 0.037$), shorter ICU stay (9 (4, 16) days vs 9 (6, 20) days, $P = 0.010$), lower ICU mortality (15.0% (54/359) vs 25.5% (48/188), $P = 0.003$), and lower 28-day mortality (16.7% (60/359) vs 27.1% (51/188), $P = 0.004$). Multivariate logistic regression analysis revealed that nurse-led GDLPT (odds ratio (OR) 0.540, 95% confidence interval (CI) 0.345–0.846, $P = 0.007$), clinical pulmonary infection score (OR 1.111, 95% CI 1.012–1.221, $P = 0.028$), and ventilation day (OR 1.160, 95% CI, 1.058–1.240, $P < 0.001$) were independent predictors of 28-day mortality for pneumonia in sepsis patients, and that nurse-led GDLPT was a protective factor.

Conclusions: Nurse-led GDLPT improved the outcomes of pneumonia in sepsis patients and was particularly associated with shortened mechanical ventilation duration and ICU stay, and reduced ICU mortality and 28-day mortality.

Critique

This study investigated the effects of a nurse-led goal-directed lung physical therapy (GDLPT) on the prognosis of pneumonia in sepsis patients in the ICU. The researchers have provided a clear rationale for undertaking the study, which is supported by the existing literature, on sepsis and its high mortality rates if not treated and managed early in the critically ill patient with pneumonia as the underlying cause. The authors used a prospective two-way phased study design (before and after), with the first phase lasting 1 year and the second phase 2 years. The study was conducted in an ICU in a large hospital in China. Between the two phases the researchers designed the GDLPT protocol and educated and trained the nursing staff in the ICU before enacting phase 2. A before-and-after study design is ideal when studying the effects of an intervention and reduces any ethical issues that would arise if a randomised control trial were conducted, as with the latter there would be patients who would not receive the intervention designed to improve outcomes. Inclusion and exclusion criteria for enrolling the patients included using evidence-based international definitions for sepsis and pneumonia, which provide feasibility for the study to be replicated in other countries. The sample size was appropriate: 547 patients (188 in observation group and 359 in the treatment group). The authors did not state the power analysis that determined what the sample size should be. Primary outcome of the study was 28-day mortality and secondary outcomes included mechanical ventilation duration and ICU length of stay. These are standard outcomes reported in most ICU studies. In the univariate analysis all variables with a $P < 0.05$ were entered into the multivariate logistic regression to determine the independent 28-day mortality risk factors. The results of the study demonstrated that nurse-led GDLPT was a protective factor and ventilator days was an independent predictor of 28-day mortality. Limitations of the study included one hospital from which the sample of patients was chosen and in one country, which limits the generalisability of the study results. The responsibility of physical therapy in ICUs is also different outside China and it is not always the ICU nurse that performs that function. The study results demonstrate the value of nursing observation and easy-to-apply non-pharmacological interventions to improve outcomes in the critically ill patient.

Learning activities

1   Using each domain of quality and safety as headings (i.e. structure, process, outcome), list some of the key considerations for a quality improvement project targeting shift-to-shift nursing handover in your unit.

2   After identifying a CPG that guides nurses in providing care in your unit, assess it against the NHMRC standard displayed in Table 3.1.

3   Examine the patterns of frequent adverse events in your unit over the past 12 months. What were the causes of incidents? What targeted strategies could be used to reduce the incidence of these AEs?

4   Identify and provide a rationale for the use of a checklist for the prevention of catheter-associated urinary tract infections in your unit. Develop some specific checklist items that you think should be included.

5   Describe how technology is used in your unit to improve care delivered to patients. Using the information outlined in the section on information and communication technologies, identify the benefits to using digital checklists to improve care delivery in comparison with paper checklists. Use examples specific to your unit.

6   Describe the role of nurses, doctors, allied health staff and pharmacists in the conduct of multidisciplinary rounds in the ICU.

7   Consider the NTS skills training teaching methods identified in Fig. 3.4 (simulation and role playing, observation, other methods such as didactic teaching and gaming and the use of educators) and reflect on the ways you think you learn best. Then identify three recent education/training sessions you have attended and comment on the extent to which the teaching methods were congruent with how you learn.

Online resources

Agency for Healthcare Research and Quality, https://www.ahrq.gov

Australian Commission on Safety and Quality in Health Care (ACSQHC), https://www.safetyandquality.gov.au

Australian Council on Healthcare Standards (ACHS), https://www.achs.org.au

Institute for Healthcare Improvement (IHI), USA, https://www.ihi.org

Joint Commission (USA), https://www.jointcommission.org

National E-Health Transition Authority, https://www.digitalhealth.gov.au/

National Health and Medical Research Council, https://www.nhmrc.gov.au

National Institute for Health and Care Excellence, https://www.nice.org.uk/

National Quality Forum, https://www.qualityforum.org

Patient Safety Network, https://psnet.ahrq.gov/

Quality Use of Medicines, https://www.safetyandquality.gov.au/our-work/medication-safety/quality-use-medicines

Society of Critical Care Medicine, https://www.sccm.org/Home

World Health Organization Patient Safety, https://www.who.int/news-room/fact-sheets/detail/patient-safety

Further reading

Alrabae YMA, Aboshaiqah AE, Tumala RB. The association between self-reported workload and perceptions of patient safety culture: a study of intensive care unit nurses. J Clin Nurs 2021;30(7–8):1003–17. doi: 10.1111/jocn.15646.

Australian Commission on Safety and Quality in Health Care. Safety and Quality Improvement Guide Standard 9: recognising and responding to clinical deterioration in acute health care. Sydney, NSW: ACSQHC; 2021.

Donabedian A. Evaluating the quality of medical care. Milbank Mem Fund Q 2005;44(3):691–729.

Edward KL, Galletti A, Huynh M. Enhancing communication with family members in the intensive care unit: a mixed-methods study. Crit Care Nurse 2020;40(6):23–32. doi: 10.4037/ccn2020595.

Francis JJ, O'Connor D, Curran J. Theories of behaviour change synthesised into a set of theoretical groupings: introducing a thematic series on the theoretical domains framework. Implementation Sci 2012;7(1):1–9.

Johnson MJ, May CR. Promoting professional behaviour change in healthcare: what interventions work, and why? A theory-led overview of systematic reviews. BMJ Open 2015;5:1–13. doi: 10.1136/bmjopen-2015-008592.

Khurrum M, Asmar S, Joseph B. Telemedicine in the ICU: innovation in the critical care process. J Intensive Care Med 2021;36(12):1377–84. doi: 10.1177/0885066620968518.

Reason JT. The human contribution: unsafe acts, accidents and heroic recoveries. Aldershot, Hants: Ashgate; 2008.

Ryan L, Jackson D, Woods C, et al. Intentional rounding – an integrative literature review. J Adv Nurs 2019;75(6):1151–61. doi: 10.1111/jan.13897.

Srigley JA, Corace K, Hargadon DP, et al. (2015) Applying psychological frameworks of behaviour change to improve healthcare worker hand hygiene: a systematic review. J Hosp Infect 91:202–10. doi: 10.1016/j.jhin.2015.06.019.

Vincent C. Patient safety. 2nd ed. Chichester, Sussex: Wiley-Blackwell; 2010.

Winterbottom FA. The role of tele-critical care in rescue and resuscitation. Crit Care Nurs Clin North Am 2021;33(3): 357–68. doi: 10.1016/j.cnc.2021.05.010.

World Health Organization (WHO). Patient safety tool kit. Cairo: WHO Regional Office for the Eastern Mediterranean; 2015.

References

1. National Academy of Medicine (NAM). An equity agenda for the field of health care quality improvement. Washington DC: NAM; 2022. Available from: https://nam.edu/. [Accessed 15 February 2023].

2. Gaffney TA, Hatcher BJ, Milligan R. Nurses' role in medical error recovery: an integrative review. J Clin Nurs 2016;25(7–8):906–17.

3. Donabedian A. Evaluating the quality of medical care. 1966. Milbank Q 2005;83(4):691–729.

4. Holden RJ, Carayon P, Gurses AP, et al. SEIPS 2.0: a human factors framework for studying and improving the work of healthcare professionals and patients. Ergonomics 2013;56(11):1669–86.

5. Lumley C, Ellis A, Ritchings S, et al. Using the Systems Engineering Initiative for Patient Safety (SEIPS) model to describe critical care nursing during the SARS-CoV-2 pandemic (2020). Nurs Crit Care 2020;25(4):203–5.

6. Holden RJ, Carayon P. SEIPS 101 and seven simple SEIPS tools. BMJ Qual Saf 2021;30(11):901–10.

7. Carayon P, Wooldridge A, Hoonakker P, et al. SEIPS 3.0: human-centered design of the patient journey for patient safety. Appl Ergon 2020;84:103033.

8. Mulac A, Mathiesen L, Taxis K, et al. Barcode medication administration technology use in hospital practice: a mixed-methods observational study of policy deviations. BMJ Qual Saf 2021;30(12):1021–30.

9. Bergman LM, Pettersson ME, Chaboyer WP, et al. Safety hazards during intrahospital transport: a prospective observational study. Crit Care Med 2017;45(10):e1043–9.

10. Institute of Medicine. Crossing the Quality Chasm: a new health system for the 21st century. Washington DC: National Academy Press; 2001.

11. National Academy of Sciences, Engineering, and Medicine. Crossing the Global Quality Chasm: improving health care worldwide. Washington, DC: The National Academies Press; 2018.

12. Knudsen SV, Laursen HVB, Johnsen SP, et al. Can quality improvement improve the quality of care? A systematic review of reported effects and methodological rigor in plan-do-study-act projects. BMC Health Serv Res 2019;19(1):683.

13. Sauro KM, Machan M, Whalen-Browne L, et al. Evolving factors in hospital safety: a systematic review and meta-analysis of hospital adverse events. J Patient Saf 2021;17(8):e1285–95.

14. Lesny M, Conrad M, Latarche C, et al. Adverse events during nursing care procedure in intensive care unit: the PREVENIR study. Intensive Crit Care Nurs 2020;60:102881.

15. Decormeille G, Maurer-Maouchi V, Mercier G, et al. Adverse events in intensive care and continuing care units during bed-bath procedures: the prospective observational NURSIng during critical carE (NURSIE) Study. Crit Care Med 2021;49(1):e20–30.

16. Agency for Healthcare Research and Quality. Guidelines and measures updates. Rockville, MD; 2018. Available from: https://www.ahrq.gov/gam/updates/index.html. [Accessed 15 February 2023].

17. O'Shaughnessy SM, Lee JY, Rong LQ, et al. Quality of recent clinical practice guidelines in anaesthesia publications using the Appraisal of Guidelines for Research and Evaluation II instrument. Br J Anaesth 2022;128(4):655–63.

18. Intensive Care Coordination and Monitoring Unit. Clinical practice guides. HSNet – human services network. Sydney, NSW: New South Wales Department of Health; 2014. Available from: https://www.aci.health.nsw.gov.au/networks/icnsw/intensive-care-manual/statewide-guidelines. [Accessed 15 February 2023].

19. Davidson JE, Aslakson RA, Long AC, et al. Guidelines for family-centered care in the neonatal, pediatric, and adult ICU. Crit Care Med 2017;45(1):103–28.

20. Nates JL, Nunnally M, Kleinpell R, et al. ICU Admission, discharge, and triage guidelines: a framework to enhance clinical operations, development of institutional policies, and further research. Crit Care Med 2016;44(8):1553–602.

21. Evans L, Rhodes A, Alhazzani W, et al. Surviving sepsis campaign: international guidelines for management of sepsis and septic shock 2021. Intensive Care Med 2021;47(11):1181–247.

22. Kane-Gill SL, Dasta JF, Buckley MS, et al. Clinical practice guideline: safe medication use in the ICU. Crit Care Med 2017;45(9):e877–915.

23. Compher C, Bingham AL, McCall M, et al. Guidelines for the provision of nutrition support therapy in the adult critically ill patient: The American Society for Parenteral and Enteral Nutrition. J Parenter Enteral Nutr 2022;46(1):12–41.

24. Sykes M, Thomson R, Kolehmainen N, et al. Opportunities to enhance ward audit: a multi-site qualitative study. BMC Health Serv Res 2021;21(1):226.

25. National Health and Medical Research Council (NHMRC). Information for guideline developers. Canberra, ACT: Commonwealth of Australia; 2017. Available from: https://nhmrc.gov.au/research-policy/guideline-development. [Accessed 15 February 2023].

26. National Health and Medical Research Council (NHMRC). Standards for guidelines. Canberra, ACT: Commonwealth of Australia; 2016. Available from: https://www.nhmrc.gov.au/guidelinesforguidelines/standards. [Accessed 15 February 2023].

27. Higgins J, Thomas J. Cochrane handbook for systematic reviews of interventions. Cochrane Collaboration; 2022. Available from: https://training.cochrane.org/handbook. [Accessed 15 February 2023].

28. Hoffmann-Esser W, Siering U, Neugebauer EA, et al. Guideline appraisal with AGREE II: systematic review of the current evidence on how users handle the 2 overall assessments. PLoS One 2017;12(3):e0174831.

29. Houghton C, Meskell P, Delaney H, et al. Barriers and facilitators to healthcare workers' adherence with infection prevention and control (IPC) guidelines for respiratory infectious diseases: a rapid qualitative evidence synthesis. Cochrane Database Syst Rev 2020;4:CD013582.

30. Montero-Odasso MM, Kamkar N, Pieruccini-Faria F, et al. Evaluation of clinical practice guidelines on fall prevention and management for older adults: a systematic review. JAMA Netw Open 2021;4(12):e2138911.

31. Veazie S, Peterson K, Bourne D, et al. Implementing high-reliability organization principles into practice: a rapid evidence review. J Patient Saf 2022;18(1):e320–8.

32. Agency for Healthcare Research and Quality (AHRQ), Patient Safety Network. Patient safety 101: high reliability. Rockville, MD: AHRQ; 2019. Available from: https://psnet.ahrq.gov/primer/high-reliability. [Accessed 15 February 2023].

33. Joint Commission Center for Transforming Healthcare. Oro 2.0 high reliability assessment: Oakbrook Terrace, IL: The Joint Commission; 2022. Available from: https://www.centerfortransforminghealthcare.org/products-and-services/oro-2/. [Accessed 15 February 2023].

34. Azyabi A, Karwowski W, Davahli MR. Assessing patient safety culture in hospital settings. Int J Environ Res Public Health 2021;18(5):2466.

35. Barbazza E, Klazinga NS, Kringos DS. Exploring the actionability of healthcare performance indicators for quality of care: a qualitative analysis of the literature, expert opinion and user experience. BMJ Qual Saf 2021;30(12):1010–20.

36. Litton E, Guidet B, de Lange D. National registries: lessons learnt from quality improvement initiatives in intensive care. J Crit Care 2020;60:311–18.

37. Braithwaite J, Hibbert P, Blakely B, et al. Health system frameworks and performance indicators in eight countries: a comparative international analysis. SAGE Open Med 2017;5:2050312116686516.

38. Flaatten H. National ICU quality indicators revisited. ICU Manage Pract 2016;16(4):202–3.

39. Nouira H, Ben Abdelaziz A, Kacem M, et al. Which indicators used to assess quality performance in intensive care units? A systematic review of medical literature. Anaesth Crit Care Pain Med 2018;37(6):583–7.

40. Alvarez-Maldonado P, Reding-Bernal A, Hernandez-Solis A, et al. Impact of strategic planning, organizational culture imprint and care bundles to reduce adverse events in the ICU. Int J Qual Health Care 2019;31(6):480–4.

41. Pun BT, Balas MC, Barnes-Daly MA, et al. Caring for critically ill patients with the ABCDEF bundle: results of the ICU liberation collaborative in over 15,000 adults. Crit Care Med 2019;47(1):3–14.

42. Buetti N, Marschall J, Drees M, et al. Strategies to prevent central line-associated bloodstream infections in acute-care hospitals: 2022 update. Infect Control Hosp Epidemiol 2022;43(5):553–69.

43. Devlin JW, Skrobik Y, Gelinas C, et al. Clinical practice guidelines for the prevention and management of pain, agitation/sedation, delirium, immobility, and sleep disruption in adult patients in the ICU. Crit Care Med 2018;46(9):e825–73.

44. Evans L, Rhodes A, Alhazzani W, et al. Surviving Sepsis campaign: international guidelines for management of sepsis and septic shock 2021. Crit Care Med 2021;49(11):e1063–143.

45. Agency for Healthcare Research and Quality (AHRQ). Toolkit for preventing CLABSI and CAUTI in ICUs. Rockville MD: AHRQ; 2022. Available from: https://www.ahrq.gov/hai/tools/clabsi-cauti-icu/index.html. [Accessed 15 February 2023].

46. Society of Critical Care Medicine (SCCM). ICU liberation. Mount Prospect, IL: SCCM; 2020. Available from: https://www.sccm.org/iculiberation/abcdef-bundles. [Accessed 15 February 2023].

47. Rhee C, Yu T, Wang R, et al. Association between implementation of the severe sepsis and septic shock early management bundle performance measure and outcomes in patients with suspected sepsis in US Hospitals. JAMA Netw Open 2021;4(12):e2138596.

48. Dippel KS, Duli L, Keckeisen M. The use of checklists among new graduate nurses in a surgical intensive care unit to improve patient safety and outcomes. J Nurses Prof Dev 2022;38(1):7–18.

49. Hallam BD, Kuza CC, Rak K, et al. Perceptions of rounding checklists in the intensive care unit: a qualitative study. BMJ Qual Saf 2018;27(10):836–43.

50. Dykes PC, Rozenblum R, Dalal A, et al. Prospective evaluation of a multifaceted intervention to improve outcomes in intensive care: the Promoting Respect and Ongoing Safety Through Patient Engagement Communication and Technology Study. Crit Care Med 2017;45(8):e806–13.

51. Ali R, Cornelius PJ, Herasevich V, et al. Effect of daily use of electronic checklist on physical rehabilitation consultations in critically ill patients. J Crit Care 2017;38:357–61.

52. Conroy KM, Elliott D, Burrell AR. Testing the implementation of an electronic process-of-care checklist for use during morning medical rounds in a tertiary intensive care unit: a prospective before-after study. Ann Intensive Care 2015;5(1):60.

53. Writing Group for the C-ICUI, the Brazilian Research in Intensive Care N, Cavalcanti AB, et al. Effect of a quality improvement intervention with daily round checklists, goal setting, and clinician prompting on mortality of critically ill patients: a randomized clinical trial. JAMA 2016;315(14):1480–90.

54. Delaney A, Hammond N, Litton E. Checklists and protocols in the ICU: less variability in care or more unnecessary interventions? Intensive Care Med 2020;46(6):1249–51.

55. Burian BK, Clebone A, Dismukes K, et al. More than a tick box: medical checklist development, design, and use. Anesth Analg 2018;126(1):223–32.

56. Dykes PC, Lowenthal G, Lipsitz S, et al. Reducing ICU utilization, length of stay, and cost by optimizing the clinical use of continuous monitoring system technology in the hospital. Am J Med 2022;135(3):337–41.e1.

57. Sarti AJ, Zheng K, Herry CL, et al. Feasibility of implementing Extubation Advisor, a clinical decision support tool to improve extubation decision-making in the ICU: a mixed-methods observational study. BMJ Open 2021;11(8):e045674.

58. Carra G, Salluh JIF, da Silva Ramos FJ, et al. Data-driven ICU management: using big data and algorithms to improve outcomes. J Crit Care 2020;60:300–4.

59. Varghese J, Kleine M, Gessner SI, et al. Effects of computerized decision support system implementations on patient outcomes in inpatient care: a systematic review. J Am Med Inform Assoc 2018;25(5):593–602.

60. Lehr J, Vitoux RR, Evanovich Zavotsky K, et al. Achieving outcomes with innovative smart pump technology: partnership, planning, and quality improvement. J Nurs Care Qual 2019;34(1):9–15.

61. NSW Government. Electronic record for intensive care (eRIC) 2018. Available from: http://www.ehealth.nsw.gov.au/programs/clinical/eric. [Accessed 15 February 2023].

62. Scott IA, Sullivan C, Staib A. Going digital: a checklist in preparing for hospital-wide electronic medical record implementation and digital transformation. Aust Health Rev 2019;43(3):302–13.

63. Mills S. Electronic health records and use of clinical decision support. Crit Care Nurs Clin North Am 2019;31(2):125–31.

64. Kiepek W, Sengstack PP. An evaluation of system end-user support during implementation of an electronic health record using the model for improvement framework. Appl Clin Inform 2019;10(5):964–71.

65. Dee SA, Tucciarone J, Plotkin G, et al. Determining the impact of an alarm management program on alarm fatigue among ICU and telemetry RNs: an evidence based research project. SAGE Open Nurs 2022;8:23779608221098713.

66. Despins LA. Factors influencing when intensive care unit nurses go to the bedside to investigate patient related alarms: a descriptive qualitative study. Intensive Crit Care Nurs 2017;43:101–7.

67. Page N, Baysari MT, Westbrook JI. A systematic review of the effectiveness of interruptive medication prescribing alerts in hospital CPOE systems to change prescriber behavior and improve patient safety. Int J Med Inform 2017;105:22–30.

68. Sowan AK, Staggers N, Berndt A, et al. Improving the safety, effectiveness, and efficiency of clinical alarm systems: simulation-based usability testing of physiologic monitors. JMIR Nurs 2021;4(1):e20584.

69. Prgomet M, Li L, Niazkhani Z, et al. Impact of commercial computerized provider order entry (CPOE) and clinical decision support systems (CDSSs) on medication errors, length of stay, and mortality in intensive care units: a systematic review and meta-analysis. J Am Med Inform Assoc 2017;24(2):413–22.

70. Curtis CE, Al Bahar F, Marriott JF. The effectiveness of computerised decision support on antibiotic use in hospitals: a systematic review. PLoS One 2017;12(8):e0183062.

71. Araujo SM, Sousa P, Dutra I. Clinical decision support systems for pressure ulcer management: systematic review. JMIR Med Inform 2020; 8(10):e21621.

72. Kinlay M, Zheng WY, Burke R, et al. Medication errors related to computerized provider order entry systems in hospitals and how they change over time: a narrative review. Res Social Adm Pharm 2021;17(9):1546–52.

73. Poncette AS, Mosch L, Spies C, et al. Improvements in patient monitoring in the intensive care unit: survey study. J Med Internet Res 2020;22(6):e19091.

74. Brogi E, Cyr S, Kazan R, et al. Clinical performance and safety of closed-loop systems: a systematic review and meta-analysis of randomized controlled trials. Anesth Analg 2017;124(2):446–55.

75. Buehler PK, Herling A, Bienefeld N, et al. Differing visual behavior between inexperienced and experienced critical care nurses while using a closed-loop ventilation system – a prospective observational study. Front Med (Lausanne) 2021;8:681321.

76. Burns KE, Lellouche F, Nisenbaum R, et al. Automated weaning and SBT systems versus non-automated weaning strategies for weaning time in invasively ventilated critically ill adults. Cochrane Database Syst Rev 2014;2014(9):CD008638.

77. Mickan S, Atherton H, Roberts NW, et al. Use of handheld computers in clinical practice: a systematic review. BMC Med Inform Decis Mak 2014;14:56.

78. Tang E, Laverty M, Weir A, et al. Development and feasibility of a smartphone-based test for the objective detection and monitoring of attention impairments in delirium in the ICU. J Crit Care 2018;48:104–11.

79. Rose L, Yu L, Casey J, et al. Communication and virtual visiting for families of patients in intensive care during the COVID-19 pandemic: a UK national survey. Ann Am Thorac Soc 2021;18(10):1685–92.

80. Ernecoff NC, Witteman HO, Chon K, et al. Key stakeholders' perceptions of the acceptability and usefulness of a tablet-based tool to improve communication and shared decision making in ICUs. J Crit Care 2016;33:19–25.

81. Loudet CI, Marchena MC, Maradeo MR, et al. Reducing pressure ulcers in patients with prolonged acute mechanical ventilation: a quasi-experimental study. Rev Bras Ter Intensiva 2017;29(1):39–46.

82. Shen N, Bernier T, Sequeira L, et al. Understanding the patient privacy perspective on health information exchange: a systematic review. Int J Med Inform 2019;125:1–12.

83. Mackintosh N, Terblanche M, Maharaj R, et al. Telemedicine with clinical decision support for critical care: a systematic review. Syst Rev 2016; 5(1):176.

84. Chen J, Sun D, Yang W, et al. Clinical and economic outcomes of telemedicine programs in the intensive care unit: a systematic review and meta-analysis. J Intensive Care Med 2018;33(7):383–93.

85. Kalvelage C, Rademacher S, Dohmen S, et al. Decision-making authority during tele-ICU care reduces mortality and length of stay – a systematic review and meta-analysis. Crit Care Med 2021;49(7):1169–81.

86. Rincon TA, Manos EL, Pierce JD. Telehealth intensive care unit nurse surveillance of sepsis. Comput Inform Nurs 2017;35(9):459–64.

87. Goedken CC, Moeckli J, Cram PM, et al. Introduction of tele-ICU in rural hospitals: changing organisational culture to harness benefits. Intensive Crit Care Nurs 2017;40:51–6.

88. Hoonakker PLT, Pecanac KE, Brown RL, et al. Virtual collaboration, satisfaction, and trust between nurses in the tele-ICU and ICUs: results of a multilevel analysis. J Crit Care 2017;37:224–9.

89. Vaona A, Banzi R, Kwag KH, et al. E-learning for health professionals. Cochrane Database Syst Rev 2018;1:CD011736.

90. Mistraletti G, Umbrello M, Anania S, et al. Neurological assessment with validated tools in general ICU: multicenter, randomized, before and after, pragmatic study to evaluate the effectiveness of an e-learning platform for continuous medical education. Minerva Anesthesiol 2017;83(2):145–54.

91. Labeau SO, Rello J, Dimopoulos G, et al. The value of e-learning for the prevention of healthcare-associated infections. Infect Control Hosp Epidemiol 2016;37(9):1052–9.

92. Bredesen IM, Bjoro K, Gunningberg L, et al. Effect of e-learning program on risk assessment and pressure ulcer classification – a randomized study. Nurse Educ Today 2016;40:191–7.

93. Asiri H, Househ M. The impact of Twitter and Facebook on nursing practice and education: a systematic review of the literature. Stud Health Technol Inform 2016;226:267–70.

94. Guinemer C, Boeker M, Furstenau D, et al. Telemedicine in intensive care units: scoping review. J Med Internet Res 2021;23(11):e32264.

95. Moreno RP, Rhodes A, Donchin Y, et al. Patient safety in intensive care medicine: the Declaration of Vienna. Intensive Care Med 2009; 35(10):1667–72.

96. World Health Organization (WHO). Patient safety: making health care safer. Geneva, Switzerland: WHO; 2017.

97. World Health Organization (WHO). World patient safety day. Geneva, Switzerland: WHO; 2019. Available from: https://www.who.int/multi-media/details/speak-up-for-patient-safety—-world-patient-safety-day-2019. [Accessed 15 February 2023].

98. Valentin A, Capuzzo M, Guidet B, et al. Patient safety in intensive care: results from the multinational Sentinel Events Evaluation (SEE) study. Intensive Care Med 2006;32(10):1591–8.

99. Brunsveld-Reinders AH, Arbous MS, De Vos R, et al. Incident and error reporting systems in intensive care: a systematic review of the literature. Int J Qual Health Care 2016;28(1):2–13.

100. Bagian JP, Gosbee J, Lee CZ, et al. The Veterans Affairs root cause analysis system in action. Jt Comm J Qual Improv 2002;28(10):531–45.

101. Corwin GS, Mills PD, Shanawani H, et al. Root cause analysis of ICU adverse events in the Veterans Health Administration. Jt Comm J Qual Patient Saf 2017;43(11):580–90.

102. Hibbert PD, Thomas MJW, Deakin A, et al. Are root cause analyses recommendations effective and sustainable? An observational study. Int J Qual Health Care 2018;30(2):124–31.

103. McDonough JE. Proactive hazard analysis and health care policy. New York: Milbank Memorial Fund; 2002.

104. Viejo Moreno R, Sanchez-Izquierdo Riera JA, Molano Alvarez E, et al. Improvement of the safety of a clinical process using failure mode and effects analysis: prevention of venous thromboembolic disease in critical patients. Med Intensiva 2016;40(8):483–90.

105. Suclupe S, Martinez-Zapata MJ, Mancebo J, et al. Medication errors in prescription and administration in critically ill patients. J Adv Nurs 2020;76(5):1192–200.

106. Garrouste-Orgeas M, Timsit JF, Vesin A, et al. Selected medical errors in the intensive care unit: results of the IATROREF study: parts I and II. Am J Respir Crit Care Med 2010;181(2):134–42.

107. Latif A, Rawat N, Pustavoitau A, et al. National study on the distribution, causes, and consequences of voluntarily reported medication errors between the ICU and non-ICU settings. Crit Care Med 2013;41(2):389–98.

108. Moyen E, Camire E, Stelfox HT. Clinical review: medication errors in critical care. Crit Care 2008;12(2):208.

109. Carayon P, Wetterneck TB, Cartmill R, et al. Characterising the complexity of medication safety using a human factors approach: an observational study in two intensive care units. BMJ Qual Saf 2014;23(1):56–65.

110. Roughead EE, Semple SJ, Rosenfeld E. The extent of medication errors and adverse drug reactions throughout the patient journey in acute care in Australia. Int J Evid Based Healthc 2016;14(3):113–22.

111. Foster MJ, Gary JC, Sooryanarayana SM. Direct observation of medication errors in critical care setting: a systematic review. Crit Care Nurs Q 2018;41(1):76–92.

112. Frith KH. Medication errors in the intensive care unit: literature review using the SEIPS model. AACN Adv Crit Care 2013;24(4):389–404.

113. Xu J, Reale C, Slagle JM, et al. Facilitated nurse medication-related event reporting to improve medication management quality and safety in intensive care units. Nurs Res 2017;66(5):337–49.

114. Plutínská Z, Plevová I. Measures to prevent medication errors in intensive care units. Cent Eur J Nurs Midw 2019;10(2):1059–67.

115. Colligan L, Bass EJ. Interruption handling strategies during paediatric medication administration. BMJ Qual Saf 2012;21(11):912–17.

116. Bower RA, Coad JE, Manning JC, et al. A qualitative, exploratory study of nurses' decision-making when interrupted during medication administration within the paediatric intensive care unit. Intensive Crit Care Nurs 2018;44:11–17.

117. Sorra JS, Nieva VF. Hospital survey on patient safety culture. Rockville, MD: Westat; 2004.

118. Davies HT, Nutley SM, Mannion R. Organisational culture and quality of health care. Qual Health Care 2000;9(2):111–19.

119. DiCuccio MH. The relationship between patient safety culture and patient outcomes: a systematic review. J Patient Saf 2015;11(3):135–42.

120. Vifladt A, Simonsen BO, Lydersen S, et al. The association between patient safety culture and burnout and sense of coherence: a cross-sectional study in restructured and not restructured intensive care units. Intensive Crit Care Nurs 2016;36:26–34.

121. Dunstan E, Coyer F. Safety culture in two metropolitan Australian tertiary hospital intensive care units: a cross-sectional survey. Aust Crit Care 2020;33(1):4–11.

122. Dodek PM, Wong H, Jaswal D, et al. Organizational and safety culture in Canadian intensive care units: relationship to size of intensive care unit and physician management model. J Crit Care 2012;27(1):11–17.

123. Abdi Z, Delgoshaei B, Ravaghi H, et al. The culture of patient safety in an Iranian intensive care unit. J Nurs Manag 2015;23(3):333–45.

124. Tlili MA, Aouicha W, Sahli J, et al. Assessing patient safety culture in 15 intensive care units: a mixed-methods study. BMC Health Serv Res 2022;22(1):274.

125. Chaboyer W, Chamberlain D, Hewson-Conroy K, et al. CNE article: safety culture in Australian intensive care units: establishing a baseline for quality improvement. Am J Crit Care 2013;22(2):93–102.

126. Hamdan M. Measuring safety culture in Palestinian neonatal intensive care units using the Safety Attitudes Questionnaire. J Crit Care 2013;28(5):886.e7–14.

127. Steyrer J, Schiffinger M, Huber C, et al. Attitude is everything? The impact of workload, safety climate, and safety tools on medical errors: a study of intensive care units. Health Care Manage Rev 2013;38(4):306–16.

128. Santiago TH, Turrini RN. Organizational culture and climate for patient safety in intensive care units. Rev Esc Enferm USP 2015;49:123–30.

129. Clarke JR, Lerner JC, Marella W. The role for leaders of health care organizations in patient safety. Am J Med Qual 2007;22(5):311–18.

130. World Health Organization (WHO). Patient safety curriculum guide: multi-professional edition. Geneva: WHO; 2001. Available from: https://www.who.int/publications/i/item/9789241501958. [Accessed 15 February 2023].

131. Weaver SJ, Lubomksi LH, Wilson RF, et al. Promoting a culture of safety as a patient safety strategy: a systematic review. Ann Intern Med 2013;158(5 Pt 2):369–74.

132. Morello RT, Lowthian JA, Barker AL, et al. Strategies for improving patient safety culture in hospitals: a systematic review. BMJ Qual Saf 2013;22(1):11–18.

133. Hsu YJ, Marsteller JA. Influence of the comprehensive unit-based safety program in ICUs: evidence from the Keystone ICU Project. Am J Med Qual 2016;31(4):349–57.

134. Thornton KC, Schwarz JJ, Gross AK, et al. Preventing harm in the ICU – building a culture of safety and engaging patients and families. Crit Care Med 2017;45(9):1531–7.

135. Saladino L, Pickett LC, Frush K, et al. Evaluation of a nurse-led safety program in a critical care unit. J Nurs Care Qual 2013;28(2):139–46.

136. Hsu YJ, Marsteller JA. Who applies an intervention to influence cultural attributes in a quality improvement collaborative? J Patient Saf 2020;16(1):1–6.

137. Winters BD, Weaver SJ, Pfoh ER, et al. Rapid-response systems as a patient safety strategy: a systematic review. Ann Intern Med 2013;158(5 Pt 2):417–25.

138. The Joint College of Intensive Care Medicine and Australian and New Zealand Intensive Care Society Special Interest Group on Rapid Response Systems. Resource use, governance and case load of rapid response teams in Australia and New Zealand in 2014. Crit Care Resusc 2016;18(4):275–82.

139. Hall KK, Lim A, Gale B. The use of rapid response teams to reduce failure to rescue events: a systematic review. J Patient Saf 2020;16(3S Suppl. 1):S3–7.

140. Ludikhuize J, Brunsveld-Reinders AH, Dijkgraaf MG, et al. Outcomes associated with the nationwide introduction of rapid response systems in The Netherlands. Crit Care Med 2015;43(12):2544–51.

141. Bhonagiri D, Lander H, Green M, et al. Reduction of in-hospital cardiac arrest rates in intensive care-equipped New South Wales hospitals in association with implementation of Between the Flags rapid response system. Intern Med J 2021;51(3):375–84.

142. Atkins JH, Rassekh CH, Chalian AA, et al. An airway rapid response system: implementation and utilization in a large academic trauma center. Jt Comm J Qual Patient Saf 2017;43(12):653–60.

143. Australian Commission on Safety and Quality in Health Care (ACSQHC). National consensus statement: essential elements for recognising and responding to acute deterioration Sydney, NSW: ACSQHC; 2021. Available from: https://www.safetyandquality.gov.au/publications-and-resources/resource-library/national-consensus-statement-essential-elements-recognising-and-responding-deterioration-persons-mental-state. [Accessed 15 February 2023].

144. McGaughey J, O'Halloran P, Porter S, et al. Early warning systems and rapid response to the deteriorating patient in hospital: a systematic realist review. J Adv Nurs 2017;73(12):2877–91.

145. DeVita MA, Braithwaite RS, Mahidhara R, et al. Use of medical emergency team responses to reduce hospital cardiopulmonary arrests. Qual Saf Health Care 2004;13(4):251–4.

146. DeVita M, Hillman KM. Expanding the scope of the rapid response system. Jt Comm J Qual Patient Saf 2017;43(12):651–2.

147. Lee A, Bishop G, Hillman KM, et al. The medical emergency team. Anaesth Intensive Care 1995;23(2):183–6.

148. Gill FJ, Leslie GD, Marshall AP. The impact of implementation of family-initiated escalation of care for the deteriorating patient in hospital: a systematic review. Worldviews Evid Based Nurs 2016;13(4):303–13.

149. Morga R, Lloyd-Williams F, Wright M, et al. An early warning scoring system for detecting developing critical illness. Clin Intens Care 1997;8:100.

150. Le Lagadec MD, Dwyer T. Scoping review: the use of early warning systems for the identification of in-hospital patients at risk of deterioration. Aust Crit Care 2017;30(4):211–18.

151. Moffat LM, Xu D. Accuracy of machine learning models to predict in-hospital cardiac arrest: a systematic review. Clin Nurse Spec 2022;36(1):29–44.

152. Chua WL, See MTA, Legio-Quigley H, et al. Factors influencing the activation of the rapid response system for clinically deteriorating patients by frontline ward clinicians: a systematic review. Int J Qual Health Care 2017;29(8):981–98.

153. Rihari-Thomas J, DiGiacomo M, Phillips J, et al. Clinician perspectives of barriers to effective implementation of a rapid response system in an academic health centre: a focus group study. Int J Health Policy Manag 2017;6(8):447–56.

154. Western Australia South Metropolitan Health Service Freemantle Hospital and Health Service. Care and respond early (CARE) – patient, carer activated escalation at Freemantle Hospital. Freemantle, WA: Government of Western Australia; 2017. Available from: https://www.fhhs.health.wa.gov.au/About-us/News/Call-and-Respond-Early-CARE. [Accessed 15 February 2023].

155. Clinical Excellence Commission. REACH. Sydney, NSW: NSW Government; 2022. Available from: https://www.cec.health.nsw.gov.au/improve-quality/quality-improvement-toolkits/reach. [Accessed 15 February 2023].

156. Clinical Excellence Queensland. Ryan's rule. Brisbane, QLD: Queensland Government; 2014. Available from: https://clinicalexcellence.qld.gov.au/priority-areas/safety-and-quality/ryans-rule. [Accessed 15 February 2023].

157. Eliott S, Chaboyer W, Ernest D, et al. A national survey of Australian intensive care unit (ICU) liaison nurse (LN) services. Aust Crit Care 2012;25(4):253–62.

158. Niven DJ, Bastos JF, Stelfox HT. Critical care transition programs and the risk of readmission or death after discharge from an ICU: a systematic review and meta-analysis. Crit Care Med 2014;42(1):179–87.

159. Topple M, Ryan B, Baldwin I, et al. Tasks completed by nursing members of a teaching hospital medical emergency team. Intensive Crit Care Nurs 2016;32:12–19.

160. Flin RH, O'Connor P, Crichton M. Safety at the sharp end: a guide to non-technical. Burlington: Ashgate Publishing; 2008.

161. Wright MC, Endsley M. Building shared situation awareness in healthcare settings. In: Nemeth CP, editor. Improving healthcare team communication: building on lessons from aviation and aerospace. Burlington, VT: Ashgate Publishing; 2008, p. 97–116.

162. Bucknall TK. Critical care nurses' decision-making activities in the natural clinical setting. J Clin Nurs 2000;9(1):25–35.

163. Endsley M. Toward a theory of situation awareness in dynamic systems. Hum Factors Hum Factors 1995;37(1):32–64.

164. Christensen K, Colman N, Van Voorhis K, et al. Situational awareness huddles in a pediatric cardiac intensive care unit during the COVID-19 pandemic. Crit Care Nurse 2021:e1–8.

165. Stubbings L, Chaboyer W, McMurray A. Nurses' use of situation awareness in decision-making: an integrative review. J Adv Nurs 2012;68(7):1443–53.

166. Croskerry P, Singhal G, Mamede S. Cognitive debiasing 1: origins of bias and theory of debiasing. BMJ Qual Saf 2013;22 (Suppl. 2):ii58–64.

167. Sendelbach S, Funk M. Alarm fatigue: a patient safety concern. AACN Adv Crit Care 2013;24(4):378–86; quiz 387–8.

168. Aitken LM. Critical care nurses' use of decision-making strategies. J Clin Nurs 2003;12(4):476–83.

169. Nibbelink CW, Brewer BB. Decision-making in nursing practice: an integrative literature review. J Clin Nurs 2018;27(5–6):917–28.

170. Currey J, Botti M. The influence of patient complexity and nurses' experience on haemodynamic decision-making following cardiac surgery. Intensive Crit Care Nurs 2006;22(4):194–205.

171. Thompson C, Dalgleish L, Bucknall T, et al. The effects of time pressure and experience on nurses' risk assessment decisions: a signal detection analysis. Nurs Res 2008;57(5):302–11.

172. Saposnik G, Redelmeier D, Ruff CC, et al. Cognitive biases associated with medical decisions: a systematic review. BMC Med Inform Decis Mak 2016;16(1):138.

173. Hoffman KA, Aitken LM, Duffield C. A comparison of novice and expert nurses' cue collection during clinical decision-making: verbal protocol analysis. Int J Nurs Stud 2009;46(10):1335–44.

174. Hough MC. Learning, decisions and transformation in critical care nursing practice. Nurs Ethics 2008;15(3):322–31.

175. Karra V, Papathanassoglou ED, Lemonidou C, et al. Exploration and classification of intensive care nurses' clinical decisions: a Greek perspective. Nurs Crit Care 2014;19(2):87–97.

176. Narayan S, Corcoran-Perry S. Teaching clinical reasoning in nursing education. In: Higgs J, Jones MA, Loftus S, et al, editors. Clinical reasoning in the health professions. Philadelphia: Butterworth-Heinemann; 2008. p. 405–30.

177. Rivett DA, Jones MA. Using case reports to teach clinical reasoning. In: Higgs J, Jones M, editors. Clinical reasoning in the health professions. Philadelphia: Butterworth-Heinemann; 2008. p. 477–84.

178. Thompson C, Stapley S. Do educational interventions improve nurses' clinical decision making and judgement? A systematic review. Int J Nurs Stud 2011;48(7):881–93.

179. Reason JT. Managing the risks of organizational accidents. Aldershot, Hants: Ashgate Publishing; 1997.

180. Orasanu J, Fischer U. Improving healthcare communication: lessons from the flightdeck. In: Nemeth CP, editor. Improving healthcare team communication: building on lessons from aviation and aerospace. Burlington, VT: Ashgate Publishing; 2008. p. 23–46.

181. Australian Commission on Safety and Quality in Health Care (ACSQHC). OSSIE guide to clinical handover improvement. Sydney, NSW: ACSQHC; 2010. Available from: https://www.safetyandquality.gov.au/publications-and-resources/resource-library/ossie-guide-clinical-handover-improvement. [Accessed 15 February 2023].

182. Chaboyer W, McMurray A, Wallis M. Bedside nursing handover: a case study. Int J Nurs Pract 2010;16(1):27–34.

183. Halm MA. Nursing handoffs: ensuring safe passage for patients. Am J Crit Care 2013;22(2):158–62.

184. Spooner AJ, Chaboyer W, Corley A, et al. Understanding current intensive care unit nursing handover practices. Int J Nurs Pract 2013; 19(2):214–20.

185. Ganz FD, Endacott R, Chaboyer W, et al. The quality of intensive care unit nurse handover related to end of life: a descriptive comparative international study. Int J Nurs Stud 2015;52(1):49–56.

186. Spooner AJ, Aitken LM, Corley A, et al. Developing a minimum dataset for nursing team leader handover in the intensive care unit: a focus group study. Aust Crit Care 2018;31(1):47–52.

187. Lane-Fall MB, Collard ML, Turnbull AE, et al. ICU attending handoff practices: results from a national survey of academic intensivists. Crit Care Med 2016;44(4):690–8.

188. Nanchal R, Aebly B, Graves G, et al. Controlled trial to improve resident sign-out in a medical intensive care unit. BMJ Qual Saf 2017;26(12): 987–92.

189. Bunkenborg G, Bitsch Hansen T, Holge-Hazelton B. Handing over patients from the ICU to the general ward: a focused ethnographical study of nurses' communication practice. J Adv Nurs 2017;73(12):3090–101.

190. Graan SM, Botti M, Wood B, et al. Nursing handover from ICU to cardiac ward: standardised tools to reduce safety risks. Aust Crit Care 2016;29(3):165–71.

191. Caruso TJ, Marquez JLS, Gipp MS, et al. Standardized ICU to OR handoff increases communication without delaying surgery. Int J Health Care Qual Assur 2017;30(4):304–11.

192. Wibrandt I, Lippert A. Improving patient safety in handover from intensive care unit to general ward: a systematic review. J Patient Saf 2020 Sep;16(3):199–210. doi: 10.1097/PTS.0000000000000266.

193. Salzwedel C, Mai V, Punke MA, et al. The effect of a checklist on the quality of patient handover from the operating room to the intensive care unit: a randomized controlled trial. J Crit Care 2016;32:170–4.

194. Lane D, Ferri M, Lemaire J, et al. A systematic review of evidence-informed practices for patient care rounds in the ICU. Crit Care Med 2013;41(8):2015–29.

195. Brown R, Rasmussen R, Baldwin I, et al. Design and implementation of a virtual world training simulation of ICU first hour handover processes. Aust Crit Care 2012;25(3):178–87.

196. Mercedes A, Fairman P, Hogan L, et al. Effectiveness of structured multidisciplinary rounding in acute care units on length of stay and satisfaction of patients and staff: a quantitative systematic review. JBI Database System Rev Implement Rep 2016;14(7):131–68.

197. Brannick MT, Prince C. An overview of team performance measurement. In: Brannick MT, Salas E, Prince C, editors. Team performance assessment and measurement: theory, methods, and applications. Mahwah, NJ: Lawrence Erlbaum Associates; 1997.

198. Dietz AS, Pronovost PJ, Mendez-Tellez PA, et al. A systematic review of teamwork in the intensive care unit: what do we know about teamwork, team tasks, and improvement strategies? J Crit Care 2014;29(6):908–14.

199. Alexanian JA, Kitto S, Rak KJ, et al. Beyond the team: understanding interprofessional work in two North American ICUs. Crit Care Med 2015;43(9):1880–6.

200. Bjurling-Sjoberg P, Wadensten B, Poder U, et al. Balancing intertwined responsibilities: a grounded theory study of teamwork in everyday intensive care unit practice. J Interprof Care 2017;31(2):233–44.

201. Donovan AL, Aldrich JM, Gross AK, et al. Interprofessional care and teamwork in the ICU. Crit Care Med 2018;46(6):980–90.

202. Gordon M, Darbyshire D, Baker P. Non-technical skills training to enhance patient safety: a systematic review. Med Educ 2012;46(11):1042–54.

203. Salas E, Rosen MA. Building high reliability teams: progress and some reflections on teamwork training. BMJ Qual Saf 2013;22(5):369–73.

204. Schmidt E, Goldhaber-Fiebert SN, Ho LA, et al. Simulation exercises as a patient safety strategy: a systematic review. Ann Intern Med 2013;158(5 Pt 2):426–32.

205. Kemper PF, de Bruijne M, van Dyck C, et al. Crew resource management training in the intensive care unit. A multisite controlled before-after study. BMJ Qual Saf 2016;25(8):577–87.

206. Ling L, Gomersall CD, Samy W, et al. The effect of a freely available flipped classroom course on health care worker patient safety culture: a prospective controlled study. J Med Internet Res 2016;18(7):e180.

Chapter 4

Ethical issues in critical care

Carol Grech, Jayne Hewitt

Learning objectives

After reading this chapter, you should be able to:

- understand key ethical and legal principles in healthcare and how to apply them in everyday practice as a critical care nurse
- appreciate the complex ethical challenges inherent within contemporary critical care nursing practice
- identify and access additional resources that may inform and support ethical and professional conduct in critical care
- discuss ethical decision making when complex clinical situations arise during admission and discharge, end-of-life care, working with families and collaborating as a member of a multidisciplinary clinical team
- describe the ethical conduct of human research in critical care, in particular issues of patient risk, protection and privacy, and how to apply ethical principles within research practice.

KEY WORDS

admission and
  discharge to
  critical care

autonomy

consent

ethical principles

end-of-life care

family

human research
  ethics
  committees

justice

privacy

quality of life

team perspectives

Introduction

Nursing work, regardless of the context, will always involve an ethical dimension, and therefore nursing care should be guided by ethical principles. This has long been recognised, with the International Council of Nurses (ICN) adopting a Code of ethics for nurses,[1] which, since its development in 1953, has undergone many iterations, in many languages. This code informs the ethical standards and guidelines developed by nursing authorities across the world. As a result, nurses are expected to provide compassionate and ethically coherent care, meet professional standards as stated by their regulatory authority and act in accordance with relevant codes of ethics at all times (see Box 4.1). In March 2018, the Nursing and Midwifery Board of Australia (NMBA) adopted the ICN Code of ethics for nurses in recognition that the Code is contextually relevant for all nurses and has been widely adopted internationally.

Why is ethics so important and relevant to critical care? Critical care nurses regularly encounter clinical situations that require them to employ ethical reasoning. However, the application of ethical reasoning to inform clinical decision making can be challenging and demanding. Some of the routine challenges encountered in critical care include: developing clinical care plans for unconscious patients who lack decision-making capacity, working with family members who may be surrogate decision makers, managing conflict about the use, withdrawal or withholding of life-sustaining technologies, and making decisions about the equitable allocation of resources. Identifying the 'best' course of action in the face of opposing choices requires nurses to use rational and logical reasoning.

Working in contemporary healthcare, where health technology is constantly evolving and life expectancy increasing, requires increasingly complex decisions to be made about patient and health resource management. This was exemplified during the worldwide coronavirus pandemic (COVID-19) where insufficient resources, even in well-resourced health systems, posed unprecedented challenges and elevated the need for ethical decision making. It demonstrated that difficult situations can arise for health professionals where no previous consensus has been established to assist in ethical decision making or where all alternatives in a given situation have shortcomings. These types of situations are referred to as 'ethical dilemmas'.[2] It is in this world of ethical dilemmas that critical care nurses often find themselves.

This chapter, therefore, seeks to provide a resource to understand some of the current ethical issues across the continuum of critical care services. The chapter has three sections. The first section outlines the broad principles that underpin ethical decision making. The distinction between ethics, morality and values, and key ethical concepts, is explored. In linking ethics with the law, legal positions that inform healthcare are also described. The second section describes the application of ethical principles in critical care, with particular emphasis on decision-making processes that inform admission and discharge to critical care and end-of-life care. The challenges of making decisions with others and developing resilience to maintain professional and ethical competence are also explored. The third and final section examines key ethical issues that arise from clinical research in the context of critical care.

Ethics, morality and values

Ethical reasoning in critical care, while fundamental to competent practice, can challenge even the most experienced clinicians. Hence, clinicians need to understand the differences and intersections between ethics, morality and human values. In the context of applied ethics in health service delivery, clinicians are often concerned with clinical situations that invite reflection and raise questions about health professionals' inherent values informing decision making, as distinct from specific diagnostic or technical questions. *Ethics* involves the study of rational processes to inform a course of action in response to a particular situation where conflicting options exist.[3] On the other hand, *morality* can be understood as the norms widely shared by a community or among a professional group.[4] *Values* are the beliefs and attitudes that individuals hold about what is important and therefore influence actions and decision making. It is important that critical care nurses remain attuned to, and reflect on, their personal and professional ethical, moral and value positioning to understand how they will approach ethical decision making in clinical practice.

Where *personal ethics* can be described as a personal set of moral values that an individual chooses to live by, *professional ethics* refer to agreed standards and behaviours expected of members of a particular professional group.[5] The value statements developed to underpin nursing and medical practice were originally informed by the moral traditions of Western civilisations, with the resultant standards intended to guide and justify professional conduct. Interest in ethical practice in healthcare has now developed to such an extent that bioethics has emerged as a subject area concerned with moral issues raised by biological science developments and health service delivery.

Although this section has delineated the differences in definitions of ethics and morality, these concepts are sometimes used interchangeably when professional organisations articulate codes of professional conduct, for example in the Code of conduct for nurses in Australia.[6] Such codes exist globally and identify legal requirements, professional behaviour and conduct expectations for all nurses. Cultural safety is integral to such codes and establishes the way for nurses to contribute to better health outcomes and experiences for First Nations peoples.

Ethical and legal dimensions

When critical care practice calls into question how, as a health practitioner, one should or ought to respond, the need to consider the legal and ethical dimensions of the situation inevitably arises. Ethics and law are fundamental components of nursing and medical education and practice internationally. However, it is important to recognise that, while most ethical theories and principles have universal currency, laws and societal norms may differ between countries. Despite their differences, laws seek to provide a benefit to society by making explicit what is considered morally right. This includes taking steps to protect the public and those in society that are vulnerable. In healthcare, this is achieved through laws that regulate who can practise, for example, as a nurse, doctor or allied health professional and setting professional standards of behaviour and conduct. In some circumstances, such as when a person is critically unwell and lacks decision-making capacity, they may also prescribe who is authorised to make health-related decisions.

It is beyond the scope of this chapter to cover health laws pertaining to all countries and jurisdictions. However, it is recognised that, increasingly, the relationship between ethics and the law affecting health professionals in the workplace is shifting and adapting globally.

Practice example

During the COVID-19 pandemic, public health laws sought to protect the public through a system of monitoring and action to promote the prompt identification, investigation and confirmation of an outbreak or case of contamination.[7] These measures effectively limited the movement of people during the pandemic; they also necessitated an increase in the use of technologies such as telehealth so that people could connect with their healthcare providers. While this may have been empowering for some patients, lawmakers were aware of the need for regulatory standards to ensure service quality.[8]

Ethical principles

There are many different ethical frameworks that can help guide ethical decision making.[9,10] One of the most common frameworks is known as *principlism,* which promotes ethical decision making based on sound moral principles. This perspective features the work of American philosophers Beauchamp and Childress, who use the principles of autonomy, non-maleficence, beneficence and justice as a foundation for ethical decision making.[4] Other principles that feature in healthcare include fidelity and veracity. All are applicable to critical care practice. These are explored individually in the following paragraphs or incorporated as part of the discussion of clinical issues, such as treatment withdrawal.

Autonomy

An autonomous person is an individual who is capable of deliberation, self-determination and action without the influence of external coercion. To respect autonomy is to give weight to, and respect, the autonomous person's considered opinions and choices and to not obstruct their actions unless these are detrimental to themselves or others.[4] To show a lack of respect for an autonomous agent, or to withhold information necessary for that person to make a considered judgement when there are no reasons to do so, is to reject that person's judgement. To deny a competent individual their autonomy is to treat that person paternalistically. All individuals, including critical care patients, should be treated as autonomous agents and be able to self-determine unless otherwise indicated. However, individuals with diminished autonomy – for example, an unconscious person – are entitled to protection and, depending on the risk of harm and likely benefit of protecting them, paternalism may be considered justifiable.[4] In such cases, healthcare professionals should act to respect the autonomy of the individual as much as possible – for example, by attempting to discover what the patient's preferences and decisions would have been in the circumstances.

Beneficence and non-maleficence

The principle of beneficence (i.e. to do good) requires that actions are undertaken to promote the well-being of another person. This incorporates the actions of doing no harm and maximising possible benefits while minimising possible harm (non-maleficence).[4] In healthcare practice, treatment is focused on 'doing no harm'. However, there may be times where, to 'maximise benefits' for health outcomes, it may be ethically justifiable to expose the patient to a 'higher risk of harm'. For example, consider a common clinical situation in the intensive care unit (ICU) where a patient requires a central venous catheter (CVC) to optimise fluid and drug therapy. This intervention is not without inherent risks (e.g. infection, pneumothorax on insertion). To minimise possible harm to the patient, evidence-based procedures are therefore developed to ensure safe insertion and subsequent care.

Justice

Justice may be defined as fair, equitable and appropriate treatment considering what is due or owed to an individual. The fair, equitable and appropriate distribution of healthcare, as determined by justified rules or 'norms', is termed distributive justice.[4] There are well-regarded theories of justice in healthcare including egalitarian theories that propose people are provided with an equal distribution of particular goods or services. However, it is recognised that justice does not always require equal sharing of all possible social benefits. In situations where there are insufficient resources to be equally distributed, guidelines (e.g. ICU admission policies) may be developed in order to ensure treatment is as fair and equitable as possible. This became evident during the COVID-19 pandemic where a proliferation of triage guidelines triggered researchers to conduct ethical analyses of international guidelines for allocating ICU resources.[11–13] One of these studies found that justice and maximising benefit were the two normative foundations of the guidelines they reviewed.[13]

Conditions of scarcity and competition for resources often lead to problems associated with fair and equitable allocation of resources (distributive justice). For example, a shortage of intensive care beds may result in critically ill patients having to 'compete' for access to the ICU. There is considerable debate about ICU admission criteria that varies across institutions, jurisdictional boundaries and countries with different health funding structures. Such resource limitations can impact distributive justice if decisions about access are influenced by economic factors as distinct from clinical need.[4]

Veracity and fidelity

The principle of veracity is concerned with telling the truth and is based on respect for persons and the concept of autonomy. To provide the opportunity for patients, or those authorised by law to act on their behalf, to make informed decisions about treatment options, they must be provided with full and honest disclosure so that they can weigh up the risks and benefits of treatments. It is also important to note that the principle of veracity can be violated through the omission of important information – deliberately withholding information or using medical jargon or language that may camouflage or mislead the patient or their legal guardian. Critical care environments are highly complex, as are the technologies and procedures that patients are exposed to. Patients and their families can easily feel overwhelmed by the critical care environment and the choices they may face during critical illness.[14] Ensuring that patients and families are informed and fully involved in the decision making is pivotal. Nurses and medical staff need to be vigilant in ensuring they convey information to patients and their families using language that can be readily understood and ensuring support services are drawn upon (e.g. social workers, religious and spiritual advisers) to provide additional help to augment understanding so that patients or their legal guardian can make informed choices about care.

The intersection of ethics and the law in critical care

Although distinct, ethics and the law overlap in many important ways. Moral rightness or wrongness may be quite distinct from legal rightness or wrongness and, while ethical decision making will always require consideration of the law, there may be conflict about the morality of the law. Consider, for example, apartheid laws that segregated a population based on their race,[15] or those that permitted people suffering from genetic diseases to be forcibly sterilised.[16] In contrast, other legal requirements underpinning healthcare practice, such as respect for human rights, confidentiality and consent, are consistent with ethical nursing practice.[5,17]

The law enforces rules that are desirable for the social good in every country. Laws passed by parliament are referred to as Acts of Parliament, statutes or legislation. A general distinction can be made between civil law jurisdictions (e.g. in France, Germany, Spain), which codify laws and in which the law is almost entirely based on legislative enactments and considered binding for all, and common law systems (e.g. in England, the USA, Australia and New Zealand (NZ)), where the law continually evolves in addition to being amended by laws passed by parliament.[3] In some countries, religion informs law, such as Sharia or Islamic law that specifically influences the legal code in some Muslim countries.

In some countries such as Australia, each state and territory has many different Acts pertaining to healthcare practices, and this can be confusing when practitioners work across jurisdictional borders. This is less problematic in countries such as NZ, where legislation applies across the whole country. Therefore, when sourcing laws relevant to healthcare in specific countries or jurisdictions, it is important to use validated sources such as government websites.

Privacy and confidentiality

Western democratic societies value individual autonomy highly. This includes deciding what is done to their body, and who has access to their personal information. The principle of autonomy extends to concepts such as privacy and confidentiality. These are fundamental human entitlements recognised in all major treaties and agreements on human rights. The constitutions of most countries acknowledge that their citizens have a right to privacy either explicitly or implicitly. The right to privacy has been involved in new areas of debate given technology's increasing erosion of privacy, for example via video surveillance cameras, the internet and harvesting and sharing of data captured from social media sites. There is a growing trend towards comprehensive privacy and data protection legislation around the world. Many countries are adopting such laws to ensure compatibility with international standards developed by the European Union, the Council of Europe and the Organization for Economic Cooperation and Development. In NZ, privacy legislation is described in the *Privacy Act 1993*[18] and in Australia in the Commonwealth *Privacy Act 1988*.[19] In addition, each state and territory in Australia has additional jurisdictional regulatory guidelines that apply to privacy matters and disclosure of health information.

Although there is a presumption that information patients provide to their healthcare professionals will remain confidential, this obligation is not absolute. It is common and necessary for health information to be shared among healthcare professionals caring for the patient. Health information may be disclosed to another person if the patient consents. Confidential health information must be disclosed during legal proceedings, and where there is a mandatory obligation to report it. This generally occurs in relation to certain infectious diseases so that steps may be taken to contain an outbreak, or in relation to some types of cancer so that appropriate public health policies and programs can be implemented.[20]

Patients' rights

Patients' rights arise from human rights law that universally recognises that everyone is born free and with equal rights irrespective of nationality, place of residence, gender, ethnic origin, race or religion.[21] Statements with a focus on patients' rights relate to the particular moral interests that a person might have in a healthcare context and any particular protection required when a person assumes the role of a patient.[5] Institutional-based charters (position statements), such as those in hospitals, are helpful in developing a shared understanding among patients/consumers, families and carers of the rights of people receiving healthcare and of the entitlements and special interests to be respected. Such charters also emphasise to health professionals that relationships with patients are constrained ethically and bound by certain associated duties.[5] The World Federation of Critical Care Nurses has recognised the importance of this and developed a position statement on the rights of the critically ill patient (see the World Federation of Critical Care Nurses website, https://wfccn.org).

To further protect patients' rights, attention should be paid to cultural differences in the provision of healthcare and to ensure cultural safety of both patients and the healthcare team. Clinical situations are culturally safe when patients and their families feel that cultural and spiritual needs are acknowledged and that those needs are met without prejudice.[22,23] In Australia, the impact of colonisation on the cultural, social and spiritual lives of Aboriginal and Torres Strait Islander peoples has contributed to significant health inequities in this population. Therefore, cultural safety has been enshrined in the Registered nurse standards for practice[24] and other key documents relevant to healthcare delivery.[25,26] Professional codes of conduct also incorporate an understanding of patients' rights and acknowledge that nurses accept the rights of individuals to make informed choices about their treatment and care. Box 4.2 provides some useful tips to ensure that the needs of diverse populations in critical care may be met.

Consent

Another way that a person's autonomy is protected is through the ethical and legal obligation to obtain consent prior to providing healthcare. All people have a legal right to bodily integrity, which means they should not be subject to intentional touching without their consent. A clinician must not assume that a patient provides their consent purely on the basis that the individual has been admitted to a hospital.[17] Responsibility for obtaining consent rests with the clinician undertaking the treatment or procedure. However, as advanced practice nurse roles develop in specialties like critical care, delegated consent for some procedures are being explored through position

---

BOX 4.2

Needs of diverse population groups in critical care

To cater for the needs of diverse population groups in critical care it is important to:

- organise and use qualified interpreters and cultural advisers when required
- create care environments that facilitate optimal patient and family control of decisions
- work collaboratively with other healthcare workers in a culturally sensitive and competent manner to ensure optimal outcomes
- identify and address bias, prejudice and discrimination in healthcare service delivery
- integrate measures of patient satisfaction into improvement programs.

BOX 4.3

Criteria for consent

For consent to meet the legal requirements of being valid, the person providing consent must:

- have the decision-making capacity to make the determination
- give their consent freely and voluntarily without coercion or undue influence
- give their consent to the specific procedure or treatment proposed
- have sufficient information about their condition, treatment options, the benefits and risks relevant to them, possible alternative options, and what to anticipate before and after the procedure. It is essential that clinicians apply a systematic approach when gaining consent that centres the person in the decision-making process. This includes explicitly establishing the goals of care, prioritising them in the context of the person's other life goals, providing ample opportunity for them to ask questions and discuss concerns.

Additional information can be found at the Australian Commission on Safety and Quality in Health Care, Fact sheet for clinicians: Informed consent in health care. Sydney, NSW: ACSQHC; 2020. https://www.safetyandquality.gov.au/publications-and-resources/resource-library/informed-consent-fact-sheet-clinicians.

---

statements.[27] Practitioners who provide treatment without valid consent may be liable for the civil action of battery. Box 4.3 lists key criteria for valid consent.

In some circumstances, providing treatment or undertaking a procedure without ensuring that the patient has sufficient information about their diagnosis and proposed treatment, including any potential risks and benefits, and other feasible options, can result in the practitioner being guilty of civil negligence. It is a legal obligation that clinicians take reasonable care to ensure the patient is aware of any material risks.[28] A risk is 'material' if, in the circumstances of a particular case, a reasonable person in the patient's position would be likely to attach significance to it, or the practitioner should reasonably be aware that the particular patient would likely attach significance to the risk.[28]

To provide safe care where patients can make choices with informed consent, clear systems and processes are required. Critical care nurses need to be aware of relevant professional, organisational and unit-based policies and understand their obligations and responsibilities in this area. While the treating medical practitioner is most often legally regarded as the person who informs the patient about material risks,[28] it is incumbent on all critical care nurses to be aware of the potential risks in critical care and ensure that informed consent is obtained. Nurses should also be aware of the circumstances where consent is not required – that is, where treatment is required in an emergency and is necessary to avoid the immediate risk of substantial harm.[29]

Consent issues in critical care may be concerned with health treatment or, as discussed later, participation in human research and the use and disclosure of personal health information. To provide consent, an adult must have decision-making capacity. This means they must understand the nature and effect of their decision, make the decision freely and voluntarily, and be able to communicate their decision in some way.[30] Many critical care patients lack decision-making capacity and therefore cannot provide consent. How this is addressed through the law is described next.

Practice tip

Make sure that informed consent is consistently applied in every healthcare encounter. As such, consent is required for turning a patient and making them comfortable, for making sure that the patient understands the procedure that they are undergoing or that they understand what is involved in the research study that they have recently enrolled in. If a patient does not understand, stop and ensure appropriate information is given by the person whose responsibility it is before continuing your intervention further.

Consent to treatment

An adult with decision-making capacity has the right to decline or accept healthcare treatment. This right is enshrined in common law in Australia, New Zealand and the UK. With the introduction of human rights acts (e.g. in the UK),[31] there is global awareness of the individual rights of patients in healthcare and of patients being actively encouraged to participate in treatment decisions. An adult must have decision-making capacity to provide consent, but it is important to recognise that this is an assessment that is decision specific. For example, a person may have decision-making capacity for a simple decision, such as whether they want to sit out of bed, but not for other more complex decisions. Where the outcome of a decision is particularly grave, such as a decision to refuse life-sustaining treatment, the person's decision-making capacity must be commensurate with the decision. Where decision-making capacity is impaired, adults should be provided with the support they need to make the decision. This may include support provided by another person, such as a nurse, to assist the patient by providing explanations, or ensuring they have the time needed to decide. If a patient lacks decision-making capacity for a decision, for example if they have an altered level of consciousness, legislation will set out who has authority to make decisions and provide consent for them. This will

include decisions that are made in an advance health directive, those made by a person appointed by the patient (medical decision maker or attorney), or those by a spouse or adult child. It may even be a close friend or carer. Nurses must be aware of who is authorised, by the law in the jurisdiction where they work, to provide consent for a patient they are caring for, if the patient cannot provide it themselves (see Online resources at the end of this chapter).

Consent assures that patients and others are neither deceived nor coerced in decision making; this recognises the person's autonomy. Consent procedures should minimise the potential for deception and coercion, and should be designed to give patients control over the amount of information received and the opportunity to rescind consent already given.[17] However, clinical information can be complex and confusing for patients, and obtaining informed consent can be problematic. Improved communication skills for clinicians go some way towards resolving this problem. Shared decision making in clinical care can best be achieved by framing the relevant information in a comprehensible way to the patient, while understanding that some patients may not wish to make such choices themselves, preferring to have decisions made by clinicians.[32]

Disclosure

It is important for all health professionals to recognise their obligations for disclosing information that may put the public at risk. This may include physical illnesses, mental health or addiction conditions that call into question a practitioner's fitness to practise safely and effectively. Codes of conduct like those in the UK for nurses and midwives[33] identify what good nursing (and midwifery) practice looks like and clearly outline the obligation for disclosure of self and others when patient safety is at risk. In Australia and NZ this is outlined within legislation governing health practitioners.[34–36]

Nurses working in critical care may undertake exposure-prone procedures; however, the risk for transmission can be minimised when correct infection control protocols are followed (see Chapter 5). Nevertheless, in the case of blood-borne viruses (BBVs) there are mutual obligations by health practitioners and patients concerning the risk of transmission treatments and therefore reasonable disclosure policies must be in place to protect health workers and the public.[37] It is also the responsibility of employers and health workers to operate in a way that minimises the risk of occupational exposure to BBVs and ensure that the use of the information must comply with relevant anti-discrimination, privacy, industrial relations and equal employment opportunity legislation.

During the COVID-19 pandemic, additional public health directions were initiated across many jurisdictions regarding disclosure of vaccination status for health workers. Furthermore, hospitals and health services were required to provide and report additional training support provided to staff on infection control and the use of PPE (including the setting for the use of N95 masks) and surveillance measures of staff exposed to COVID-19.

Application of ethical principles to the care of the critically ill

Any health professional working with critically ill patients knows that the number and complexity of decisions made about clinical interventions are ever increasing. Given this, questions raised about medical and nursing care must be underpinned by consideration of the ethical dimensions involved.

With the expanding number of technological developments, critical care nursing has evolved in scope and practice. Critical care nurses are more autonomous in their role, using more-developed assessment and diagnostic skills, and managing more-advanced patient interventions. With such increased autonomy comes increased responsibility; this reinforces the need for greater ethical awareness in practice. As demonstrated in findings from an international study,[37] ethical issues now pervade many aspects of critical care nursing practice from admission to critical care (equality, distributive justice) through to end-of-life decision making (respecting autonomy). Faced with operating in such a difficult environment, nurses in clinical practice can feel vulnerable managing their ethical responsibilities.[38] This is an important issue to recognise, as the ongoing challenge of navigating practice while upholding professional values, responsibilities and duties can lead to nurses experiencing moral distress. This can result in increased levels of emotional distress, withdrawal from patient care, decreased job satisfaction and, ultimately, increased attrition in nursing.[39] This section explores some of the key ethical challenges current in critical care practice, namely: admission and discharge decisions in critical care, end-of-life decision making, making decisions with others and developing resilience to maintain professional and ethical competence.

Admission and discharge decisions in critical care

Critical care is an expensive healthcare resource.[40] Given the changing population health needs, the increased profile of chronic health illnesses and greater use of technological diagnostics and interventions, it is not unreasonable to expect greater demand for use of critical care services. It is therefore likely that clear decision-making processes about the use of critical care facilities – that is, who will be admitted into and who will be discharged from critical care – will become even more important in the future.[41] Chapter 2 describes the ethical allocation and utilisation of critical care resources but, when practitioners are faced with excessive demand on critical care beds, patients who would benefit most from critical care are generally admitted. Indeed, this is the

model most frequently cited during discussions on meeting unprecedented need during the COVID-19 pandemic.[42]

Another area prompting debate regarding critical care admission concerns the age of the referred patient. Admitting very premature babies into neonatal care,[43] or very elderly patients[44] into critical care, has always been challenging, raising ethical issues related to justice, the value or quality of life, and care that is in the patient's best interest. There are many examples of neonatal unit admission policies, electronically available, that state prematurity and weight of the neonate as key considerations for referral to a neonatal unit. There is also evidence that a decision to admit an elderly patient to critical care should be based on factors such as patient comorbidities, the severity of illness and pre-hospital functional status, rather than chronological age.[45] However, decision making about admission to critical care should be based on more than physiological variables. We would suggest that a combination of a clear understanding of the ethical challenges raised, comprehension of the current evidence on patient management and outcomes, and an awareness of what are the patient/family wishes will enable full appreciation of the context and consequences for each case.

Less attention has been focused on the discharge of patients from critical care to other units, or to ward areas. Although decisions are based on the best interest of the patient, the subject of which patient to discharge is often raised when critical care areas are at full bed capacity and referrals for admission are being made. To date, literature in this area mainly focuses on family needs/experiences during discharge or tools to facilitate decision making,[46] with little exploration of the ethical challenges that discharge from critical care can invoke. However, there is an ethical challenge for patients and staff in the premature or suboptimal discharge from intensive care.[47] Misunderstandings and irritation can occur between intensive care and general ward during discussions about transferring patients out of intensive care. Ward staff members perceive that intensive care staff overestimate the technical capabilities of ward staff, as well as the amount of time ward staff can give each patient. Clinical areas can operate independently and use 'lifeboat' ethics,[48] a metaphor for resource distribution, to prioritise care. Staff across clinical areas need to come together to understand how they can make decisions interdependently with each other, cognisant of the full pressures experienced in the system.

Admission to critical care will continue to challenge healthcare and so it is important to use the best clinical and ethical evidence to inform the development of policies, and guide decision making.[45] Finally, it must be recognised that much of our understanding of critical care has historically been informed by the Western world and by developed countries. Globally, not all countries have the same level of critical care provision, and this brings its own unique ethical and resource challenges with regard to admission and discharge in ways that some of us may find difficult to comprehend.[45]

End-of-life decision making

With advances in healthcare, it is now possible to restore, sustain and prolong life with the use of technology – for example, extracorporeal oxygenation and ventricular assist devices. Each new medication or treatment on the market seems to promise added benefits to patients with improved outcomes and fewer side effects. However, critical care remains more concerned with the provision of supportive therapies until recovery occurs (or does not occur), rather than offering curative treatments.[40]

While this leads to many patients surviving their critical illness, it also results in some patients receiving life-sustaining therapies for prolonged periods with limited evidence about survival rates or impact on long-term quality of life. Therefore, a common ethical dilemma experienced by doctors and nurses in critical care concerns how to work through the opposing decision-making positions of 'maintaining life at all costs' and 'relieving suffering associated with the prolongation of life'. These are complex, emotive and much-debated areas that often surface during decision making about withdrawal and withholding of life-supporting treatment.[49]

While the following section explores these through the lens of intensive care, similar end-of-life challenges occur in emergency departments,[50] high-dependency units and ward areas where critically ill patients may deteriorate, requiring support from critical care practitioners.[51] While the contexts are different, the ethical principles and key decision-making approaches apply across all environments.

Withdrawing and withholding treatment

The incidence of withholding and withdrawal of life support from critically ill patients has increased to the extent that these practices now precede many deaths in intensive care.[52] Withholding or withdrawal of life-sustaining therapies such as ventilator support, inotropic support or antibiotics occurs in the knowledge that the patient will most probably die from their underlying disease. This is considered ethically acceptable and clinically desirable if it reduces unnecessary patient suffering for those who will not recover from their illness and the ongoing provision of treatment would not provide a benefit. A worldwide study seeking consensus on principles of end-of-life care for the critically ill found that, if there is a low chance of survival, therapy may be withheld or withdrawn from the patient, but participants were not able to agree on how this should be undertaken.[53] In practice, generally, there is a preference for withholding life-sustaining treatments, rather than withdrawing them, but this can vary according to country, religion and culture.[54]

There are marked differences in the foregoing of life-sustaining treatments between countries, and even within states. What may be adopted legally and ethically in one country may not be acceptable in another. Further, complexities in care arise owing to the differing views held internationally on whether withdrawal of treatment is ethically the same as withholding treatment.[55] In Australasia, the same legal and ethical principles apply whether active treatment is withdrawn or withheld. The Australian and New Zealand Intensive Care Society (ANZICS) and College of Intensive Care Medicine (CICM) of Australia and New Zealand recommend that, when treatment withdrawal or withholding has been discussed and agreed with the family, an 'alternative care plan' with a focus on dignity and patient comfort be implemented. It is suggested that such discussions are recorded in the patient notes including the basis for the decision, those involved in the discussions and the specifics of treatment(s) being withheld or withdrawn.[56]

Given that universal consensus on withdrawing and withholding life-sustaining treatment has been difficult to achieve, country-specific strategies that focus on quality end-of-life care have been developed. For example, Australia's consensus statement on the essential elements for safe and high-quality end-of-life care acknowledges the importance of keeping the goals of the patient at the centre of care and ensuring clear, open communication in relation to treatment decisions.[57] Similarly, in the UK, end-of-life care guidelines no longer refer to withdrawing or withholding treatment; rather, they focus on treatment and care at the end of life, and good practice in decision making.[58]

Although guidelines can support treatment-limiting decisions, they cannot address the full range of factors that influence these decisions. A US study exploring physicians' views about the types of treatments that are likely to provide a benefit found there was poor consensus and that treatment decisions may be affected by factors unrelated to the patient's illness, including the presence of family members and the availability of resources.[59] As decision makers must account for a range of factors, it is not surprising that gaining consensus on these complex clinical situations can be difficult. However, variability in end-of-life decision making is ethically problematic and can be disconcerting for nurses and other members of the intensive care team.[60] In cases where there is uncertainty about the efficacy or appropriateness of life-sustaining treatment, it may be considered preferable to commence treatment, with an option to withdraw treatment after broad consultation has occurred.

Critical care nurses can actively contribute to supporting the processes of decision making at end of life. However, research has consistently shown that it is common for nurses to be excluded from these decisions. In 2003 the Ethicus study was conducted to compare and contrast differences in end-of-life care across 37 ICUs in 17 European countries.[61] Ethicus 2 was conducted in 2019 and included 199 ICUs worldwide. Analysis of the data revealed a decrease in the frequency of end-of-life discussions with nurses. The study authors suggested that this may be due to fewer decisions about withdrawing treatment being made, or that an increase in the number of published recommendations and guidelines has resulted in less ambiguity, dilemmas and conflict obviating the need to involve nurses in these discussions.[62] Another explanation is that doctors and nurses approach end-of-life decision making from different perspectives. For doctors, meeting the needs of the family may take precedence, while nurses seek to advocate on behalf of the patient and what they interpreted as the patient's best interest.[63] In these circumstances both professions are acting in line with their respective ethical and professional obligations; however, the differing perspectives can hinder collegial end-of-life decision making.[63] Interdisciplinary end-of-life communication can be enhanced with the support of clear organisational processes, and the leadership of senior clinicians.[64] Additional educational opportunities where communication skills can be developed are also required.[64]

Although all members of the critical care team must contribute to such discussions, legal responsibility and accountability for the decision lie with the senior treating doctor. Where conflict arises with family members, especially if a family member has the authority to act as a substitute decision maker, the doctor must consider this and respect the rights of any patient legal representative. It is unlikely that withdrawal of treatment will occur until a consensus decision is reached. This is a different situation to that of a person who is legally declared brain dead,[56] where different ethical challenges are posed[65] (see Chapter 29).

Once a decision to limit or withdraw treatment has been agreed upon, a plan is made as to how this will occur, which treatments will be withdrawn/withheld, when and by whom. Critical care nurses play an important role in managing end-of-life care at this time.[66] Concepts of caring for the dying patient in a critical care unit are no different to those in a hospital ward or hospice. The principles of care encompass privacy, dignity, relief of pain, provision of comfort and support for patients and relatives. Recognising and being respectful of the religious, spiritual and cultural needs of the patient and family are also important. The care given at this time continues beyond the moment of the patient's death, with particular attention placed on how the death of the person is pronounced, how the family is notified of this death and the immediate bereavement support offered to the family, including discussions about a possible autopsy. Compassionate care to the family at this time is essential.

Decision-making principles

Despite significant advances in critical care medicine, approximately 16% of patients over the age of 16 admitted to ICUs do not survive. This rises to nearly 26% in patients admitted with sepsis.[67] The majority of patients who die in critical care do so after planned withdrawal of life-prolonging therapies, as opposed to dying after unexpected and unsuccessful cardiopulmonary resuscitation.[68] Given the complex nature of the decisions made at end of life, it

is unsurprising that key ethical challenges arise. These mainly focus on arguments about quality of life, best interest and whether treatment is futile.

Although debate about *quality of life* is often engaged with when justifying the continuation or discontinuation of life-sustaining treatment in critical care,[5] there is no single agreed definition of quality of life. When making decisions about medical treatments based on quality-of-life arguments, it is important, therefore, that consideration is given to the personal preferences and well-being of the individual together with a review of the person's independent health and welfare status.[17]

Best interest is a further guiding principle for making decisions in, and about, healthcare. It is defined as acting in a way that optimally promotes good for the individual and is referred to when one person makes a decision on behalf of another. The best-interest principle is often invoked in situations where the patient may be assessed as unable to participate in the decision-making process. The best-interest principle relies on decision makers holding an understanding of, and knowing the views held by, the person in question (e.g. critically ill patient). The best-interest principle poses particular challenges including how assumptions are made about what quality of life means for individuals, and whether those views are current – that is, have been recently communicated to a significant other, and therefore not been changed over time.[69]

The third ethical position often explored at end of life is whether ongoing medical treatment is *futile* or non-beneficial. In other words, whether the treatment has no apparent physical benefit to the patient (physiological futility) or where the benefit of recovery of the patient is outweighed by the burden of survival – that is, the person survives but with the potential of physical or mental incapacity.[4] Treatment is considered futile if the medical therapy will never enable the person to achieve a state beyond permanent unconsciousness or that it is unlikely that the person will ever be discharged alive from intensive care.[70] This acknowledges that physiological decay of the body due to old age and/or illness will exceed the body's response to medical treatments.[71] Futility is a concept in widespread use in healthcare ethics and poses clinical challenges and international debate.[72] Futility is often used by critical care doctors and nurses as a rationale for why life-saving or life-sustaining medical treatments are considered to be not in the patient's best interest. While this is logical, the concept of futility should not be used unethically – for example, to coerce relatives into agreeing to cease a patient's treatment.[73]

Clinicians usually reflect on past clinical experiences, experiential knowledge gained from colleagues and reported empirical data to conclude that treatments are futile.[74] To help clinicians, patients and families better understand what futile or non-beneficial treatment involves, the Society of Critical Care Medicine Ethics Committee developed the following definition. It seeks to support a collective understanding of the goals of intensive care, so that treatment that does not align with these goals may be considered non-beneficial or futile.[75]

> *ICU interventions should generally be considered appropriate when there is no reasonable expectation that the patient will improve sufficiently to survive outside the acute care setting, or when there is no reasonable expectation that the patient's neurological function will improve sufficiently to allow the patient to perceive the benefits of treatment.* (p. 1771)

Futile interventions are seen to cause pain and discomfort at end of life, give false hope to patients and family, delay palliative care and expend limited medical resources. While the ethical requirement to respect patient autonomy entitles a patient to choose or reject the medically acceptable treatment options, it does not entitle patients to receive whatever treatments they want, including futile treatments. Clinicians are required only to offer treatment consistent with professional standards and that benefits the patient. With respect to the law governing withholding and withdrawing treatment, there have been few cases internationally where courts have been consistent in concluding that there is no duty to provide life-sustaining treatment that is futile.[76] Fig. 4.1 outlines factors influencing ethical decision-making processes in healthcare delivery.

Understanding patient preferences at end of life: advance directives

The principle of autonomy underpins decision making in healthcare. However, this can be challenging when adults have impaired decision-making capacity. To address this challenge, it is possible for adults to make their wishes for treatment known in an advance directive. The directive must be completed when the adult had decision-making capacity, and takes effect when capacity is impaired. Because they are also seen as a way of limiting non-beneficial treatment, significant steps have been taken to support their acceptance and use.[77] For example, the National Institute for Health and Care Excellence in the UK and Advance Care Planning Australia provide a range of resources for healthcare professionals and the public.[78,79] In many jurisdictions, directions provided in an advance directive are legally binding, which means that healthcare professionals are obliged to comply with these instructions. However, research demonstrates that non-adherence is common.[80] Reasons for this include instructions in a directive being ambiguous or in conflict with what is perceived to be clinically indicated for the patient.[80] Globally, there are significant gaps in clinicians' knowledge and understanding of advance directives, and this also impacts their uptake.[81]

Advance directives set out patient preferences for care and treatment should they lose decision-making capacity for a specific decision. Although a person may request all treatment available to maintain life, there is no obligation for doctors to provide treatment they consider non-beneficial or not in the patient's best interest.[76] This includes the provision of cardiopulmonary resuscitation (CPR) in the event of a cardiac arrest. Should treating doctors believe that CPR is unlikely to have a positive outcome for the patient, then a decision to withhold CPR should invite broader inclusive conversations around

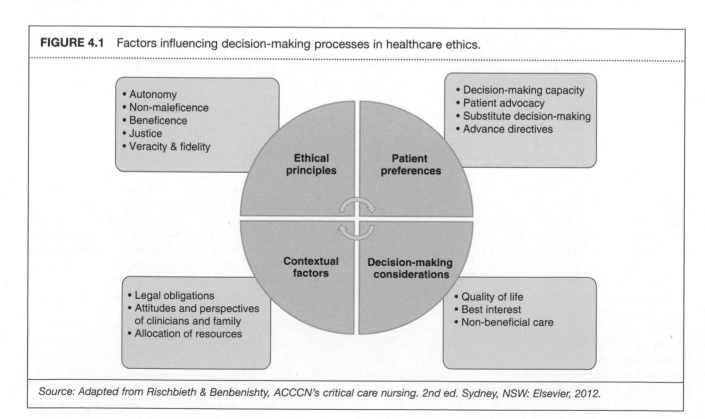

FIGURE 4.1   Factors influencing decision-making processes in healthcare ethics.

• Autonomy
• Non-maleficence
• Beneficence
• Justice
• Veracity & fidelity

• Decision-making capacity
• Patient advocacy
• Substitute decision-making
• Advance directives

Ethical principles

Patient preferences

Contextual factors

Decision-making considerations

• Legal obligations
• Attitudes and perspectives of clinicians and family
• Allocation of resources

• Quality of life
• Best interest
• Non-beneficial care

Source: Adapted from Rischbieth & Benbenishty, ACCCN's critical care nursing. 2nd ed. Sydney, NSW: Elsevier, 2012.

goals of treatment or care.[82] As each patient case is considered on its merit, any decisions or outcomes from these discussions must be well documented in the patient's notes or on the appropriate forms so that misinterpretations do not occur. Clear discussion and broad consultation across the clinical team(s) and patient/family must occur. A management plan that incorporates assessment of patient and family understanding, disclosure of the patient's situation, and discussion and consensus gaining with the patient and family can be particularly useful.[79]

Understanding patient preferences: substitute decision makers and patient advocates

Patient advocacy has, at its heart, a focus on patient rights, values and interests. It seeks to promote autonomy when patients are unable or incapable of participating in making decisions about their healthcare. If a person does not have the decision-making capacity to make medical decisions, a surrogate decision maker should be identified. Substituted judgement is where an appropriate surrogate attempts to determine what the patient would have wanted in his/her present circumstances[70] by referring to the values and preferences of the patient. Making a substituted judgement is a relatively informal process, in the sense that the patient has not formally appointed the proxy decision maker. Rather, the role of proxy tends to be assumed on the basis of an existing relationship between the proxy and the patient. However, this informal arrangement means that making an accurate substituted judgement can be difficult[83] and that the proxy might not be the most appropriate person for this role.

There are more formally recognised patient advocate and substitute decision maker roles that are created by laws in different jurisdictions. Internationally, there are many different terms for these roles including 'medical or healthcare agent', 'medical power of attorney' and 'enduring guardian'. A substitute decision maker for healthcare decisions is someone chosen by the individual (e.g. a partner, child, friend over 18 years of age) to make medical decisions and provide consent for healthcare treatment on their behalf if they lack decision-making capacity. Generally, this is recorded on a designated form and may need to be witnessed. If a patient has not appointed a substitute decision- maker, or there is no one available to act in this role, then a statutory decision maker may be appointed. The legislation that sets out the process to be followed varies between jurisdictions, and therefore it may be pertinent to consult with your legal team if you are uncertain about who has the correct legal authority to act as a substitute decision maker for your patient.

Voluntary assisted dying in critical care

Voluntary assisted dying (VAD), otherwise termed euthanasia, physician-assisted dying or medical assistance in dying, is a controversial and contested topic that creates much international debate. Euthanasia is generally understood as the termination of a person's life to relieve their irremediable suffering. There is an increasing number of jurisdictions, including Australia, New Zealand, Canada and several states in the US, where VAD or its equivalent is legal.[84] In all jurisdictions, the criteria that make a person eligible for VAD are set out in legislation. Doctors (or nurse practitioners in Canada) are authorised to assess whether a person meets these criteria.[84] Once assessed as eligible, a person can access the VAD medication and choose when (and to some extent where) it is administered. Different laws have different requirements in relation to administration. For example, in US states where VAD is legal, the person must self-administer the substance. In Canada, self-administration or practitioner administration is permitted, but most people choose to have a doctor or nurse practitioner administer it.[84] Importantly, the primary objective of all VAD legislation is to enable people who are dying and suffering the choice about when their life ends.

As discussed above, decisions to withdraw treatment are among the end-of-life decisions frequently made in ICU. In these circumstances, it is recommended that nurses assess their patient's need for pain relief. If required, opioids and/or benzodiazepines may be prescribed and administered.[85] Research demonstrates, however, that nurses may be reluctant to administer adequate pain relief because they fear hastening the person's death.[86] The British Medical Association guidelines on the use of analgesics at the end of life reinforce that the provision of medications that may hasten death is ethical and lawful when it is in the patient's best interest, and the intention is to relieve the patient's suffering and not to intentionally hasten their death.[87] This essentially restates the *doctrine of double effect*, a long-standing Catholic doctrine that argues:[88]

> *where certain criteria are met, a person acts ethically when acting to bring about a good or morally neutral effect, even if her [sic] action also has certain foreseen, though not intended or desired, bad effects.* (p. 266)

In the case of withdrawing treatment from a person who is suffering at the end of life, the relief of pain is an ethically good effect. The other criteria the doctrine requires are that there must be no other means of bringing about the good effect and that the nurse administering the medication intends to relieve the pain, and not hasten death. It is the intentionality of the nurse that attracts the protection of the doctrine.[5] Intention also differentiates the provision of pain-relieving medication, including opioids, at the end of life from VAD. In VAD, medication is being administered, or self-administered, with the intention of ending life. The intention when administering opioids is not to end life, but to relieve suffering.

Making decisions with others: patient, family and clinical team perspectives

Critical care nurses aim to bring the ethical principles of patient autonomy, beneficence and non-maleficence to their daily bedside practices. Discussions can be held directly with patients to determine their treatment wishes. However, there are times in critical care where it can be difficult to uphold patient autonomy – for example, when patients are unconscious or sedated with no advance directives. For many patients, family members then become surrogate decision makers, and the patient's wishes are known through them.

However, communication can be a complicated process, especially when challenging information is exchanged over a short time frame. Communication can become even more complex if doctors and nurses lack communication skills,[89] or are fearful of holding discussions with family members because of concerns about litigation.[90] Collectively, these factors can lead to misunderstandings and confusion about what the patient wants, what the family wish for and what critical care staff feel is achievable. Indeed, upholding patient autonomy and working with surrogate decision makers have been identified as frequent ethical situations challenging nurses daily.[91] This is despite the fact that nurses at the bedside are well placed to support the patient/family make choices congruent with their values and wishes.[92]

Critical care doctors and nurses often receive requests from family members for potentially inappropriate treatment for a critically ill relative.[93] Such situations need careful management to ensure that open communication channels are maintained between healthcare staff and family members. Asking questions to understand whose perspectives and ethical principles are being used to inform the requests can be helpful. Fear of loss can make distressed families focus on what is best for them as a family, rather than what may be best for the patient. Careful use of appropriate language can help families understand the gravity of situations, especially at end of life.[94] Talking about withdrawal of treatment, rather than withdrawal of care, can ensure that family members are clear about what is and what is not being offered for their family member, and this may ease ethical and moral distress.

Some situations in critical care can be ambiguous for families – for example, a patient who is brain dead, but who looks to be pink and 'breathing'. Nursing staff may continue to talk to the patient while providing care, despite the family being informed that the patient is brain dead with no possibility of recovery. This may be confusing for some family members, while others may be comforted by staff talking to their family member. There is no right and wrong here, rather that such situations reinforce the need for all staff to be sensitive to how their words and actions may be perceived, and to be clear with families as to what is informing these. Cultural sensitivity also needs to be demonstrated, given that some families (e.g. traditional Chinese) prefer to keep information about death and dying away from patients in order to protect their loved one from any distress during end of life.[95] What is important is that doctors and nurses have a heightened awareness of the emotional distress that families may be under at this time, and to ensure that communication with families is sensitive, timely, clear and compassionate.

Critical care is delivered by a team, and yet team members may have different perspectives on what 'good' critical care looks like; this is informed by different professional ethical decision-making frameworks. While the values of patients' rights, justice and quality of life are central to medicine's ethical framework, empirical work demonstrates that patient dignity, comfort and respect for patients' wishes are central to nurses' ethical framework.[96] Despite the contribution that nurses can make to decision making in critical care, the nursing voice can be silent. Several studies demonstrate the lack of engagement by nurses during decision making.[62] While there may be specific cultural challenges in sensitive areas such as end of life, it is generally recommended that open communication occurs with all doctors and nurses involved.

Practice is made more challenging for doctors and nurses when further ethical conflicts result from organisational ethical issues – for example, allocation of funding and resources, and administration support, or lack of it.[97] In situations where complex ethical dilemmas are faced, access to debriefing, interdisciplinary education or a clinical ethicist/clinical ethics committee[98] may help in bringing together those involved and offer an ethical review to mediate the problem.

Developing moral resilience to maintain ethical competence

In reading through the preceding sections, the many aspects of critical care nursing that hold moral and ethical challenges are clearly visible. Ethical issues in practice range from the 'big' subjects, such as assisted dying or when treatment should, or should not, be offered, through to the 'everyday' ethical challenges of nursing practice, such as the use of chemical versus physical restraints for patients.[99] While professional codes of conduct exist to highlight ethical values that should inform the actions of nurses, the reality of upholding these values in practice is more challenging.

If decisions are made where nurses' professional or personal ethical views have not been considered, this can result in a perception that unsatisfactory decisions have been made,[100] with nurses experiencing the despair and hopelessness associated with moral distress. Moral distress occurs when nurses face ethical conflicts but are unable to respond to them in a way that maintains their personal or professional integrity.[100] The impact of this is felt by the individual nurse (e.g. burnout) and by organisations (e.g. increased turnover, shortage of workforce, staff becoming increasingly disengaged).[100]

The development of moral resilience is one way to mitigate moral distress. Moral resilience is described as an ability to choose how one responds to ethical challenges in ways that preserve integrity and minimise one's own suffering. As individuals, nurses can foster greater self-awareness to become more familiar with their moral values and their own strengths and limitations. They can develop self-regulatory capacities so that they are able to uphold their moral position in the face of external approval,[101] and develop ethical competence in developing a moral vocabulary and an openness to understanding the values of others.[100]

Healthcare organisations also need to develop fair and transparent ethical decision-making processes, at every level.[102] Traditionally strategies to address moral distress have focused on improving understanding, awareness and communication between individuals and included education to build skills in ethical decision making, conflict resolution and interdisciplinary collaboration.[103] To address moral distress and build moral resilience requires an organisational and professional commitment to develop practice areas as moral communities[104] where ethically-driven practice is central. This will be essential to address the moral and ethical challenges that critical care nurses face in the future.

Ethics in research

When conducting research studies involving humans, all researchers must follow ethical codes of conduct that ensure valid consent and mitigation of harm to participants. There are various ethical guidelines for the conduct of research globally – for example, the Declaration of Helsinki is regarded as an authoritative source.[105] In the UK, the General Medical Council provides guidance to researchers in the form of its good medical practice statement.[106] Healthcare research in Australia is performed in accordance with guidelines issued by the National Health and Medical Research Council (NHMRC), while in NZ the guidelines are issued by the Health Research Council (HRC).

Most countries now have national guidelines in place that are used to inform researchers conducting research with human participants, members of an ethics review committee reviewing/approving research, those involved in research governance, and potential research participants. Such guidelines will also set up the expected composition of local level (site-specific) research and ethics bodies.[107] In Australia and NZ the NHMRC and HRC respectively hold statutory authority, and health service and university human research ethics committees (HRECs) are required to consider research proposals in accordance with the relevant recommended processes and procedures outlined by these councils (see Online resources for a list of relevant resources).

Application of ethical principles

When considering human clinical research in the context of critical care, the concept of *respect for persons* is linked to the ethical principle of autonomy.[107] In human research, respect for persons demands that participants receive adequate information and choose to participate voluntarily in the research without coercion. Similar criteria as for consent to treatment should be applied by researchers

seeking to recruit participants into their study. Although there may be some variation between organisations and jurisdictions, Box 4.4 provides the type of information that potential participants should be provided with to meet ethical requirements for consent in medical

---

BOX 4.4

Information requirements for participant consent in medical research

Consent to medical research documentation should include:

- a statement that the study involves research
- an explanation of the purposes of the research
- the expected duration of the subject's participation
- a description of the procedures to be followed
- identification of any procedures that are experimental
- a description of any reasonably foreseeable risks or discomforts to the subject
- a description of any benefits to the subject or to others that may reasonably be expected from the research
- a disclosure of appropriate alternative procedures or courses of treatment, if any, that might be advantageous to the subject
- a statement describing the extent, if any, to which confidentiality of records identifying the subject will be maintained
- for research involving more than minimal risk, an explanation as to whether any compensation, and as to whether any medical treatments are available, if injury occurs and, if so, what they consist of, or where further information may be obtained
- an explanation of whom to contact for answers to pertinent questions about the research and research subjects' rights, and whom to contact in the event of a research-related injury to the subject
- a statement that participation is voluntary, refusal to participate will involve no penalty or loss of benefits to which the subject is otherwise entitled, and the subject may discontinue participation at any time without penalty or loss of benefits, to which the subject is otherwise entitled.

....

Source: National Health and Medical Research Council, Australian Research Council, Australian Vice-Chancellors' Committee. National statement on ethical conduct in human research. Canberra, ACT; Commonwealth of Australia, 2007 (updated May 2018). Available from: https://www.nhmrc.gov.au/about-us/publications/national-statement-ethical-conduct-human-research-2007-updated-2018.

research.[108] When research studies are being considered in critical care areas, surrogate consent may be applicable.[109]

Other important and relevant ethical principles for consideration in human research are beneficence and non-maleficence. *Beneficence* in the research context is expressed by the researcher's responsibility to act to promote well-being, and *non-maleficence* by minimise the risk of harm or discomfort to research participants.[107] Research protocols should be designed to ensure that respect for dignity and well-being takes precedence over any expected knowledge benefits from the research. With regard to *justice* in research, this requires that within a population there is a fair distribution of 'benefits and burdens' for research participation. In using this concept, it is the scientific objective, as opposed to membership of either a privileged or vulnerable population, that should determine the participants for a study, and the sample population should be selected to share most equitably the risks and benefits of the research.

When recruiting research participants, under the principles of respect and autonomy, it is important to ensure that any initial approach is taken appropriately. When the study involves recruitment of hospital inpatients including those in critical care settings, this approach should be made by someone directly involved in their care, with the aim of seeking permission from the patient or legal guardian in strict accordance with approval provided by a duly constituted ethics committee. Another guiding value in ethical research is that of *integrity*. This requires that the researcher be committed to the search for knowledge and to the principles of ethical research, conduct and results dissemination.[107]

Human research ethics committees

HRECs play a central role in the ethical supervision of research involving humans. Individual research institutes/centres, universities, regional/local health authorities and hospitals will have an HREC (or equivalent body) and articulate requirements for research to be conducted in their institution. The HREC will review proposals for research involving humans to ensure that the research is soundly designed and conducted according to high ethical standards such as those articulated in Australia in the National statement on ethical conduct in human research 2007 (known as the National statement), which incorporates updates as of May 2015.[107] Individual HRECs have protocols for submission of ethics applications, compliance, monitoring and complaints-handling processes. Importantly, no research study involving humans can be commenced until ethical clearance has been formally given by the relevant HREC(s).

The role of an HREC should not be confused with another form of clinical ethics committee that has been established in some hospitals and health services to provide closed forums for clinicians to raise ethical and legal concerns associated with particular clinical treatments or decisions. These are advisory committees that can also take into account patients' and/or their families' wishes when this raises complex decision making with clinicians.

In addition to providing clinicians with advice on particular cases, these committees may also assist with the development of organisational policies on patient care and facilitate staff and patient education about ethical issues.

Research involving unconscious persons

The question of whether it is justifiable to include an unconscious patient in a research project without his or her consent is a problematic issue that most critical care researchers and HRECs must attend to.[107,109] Paramount in these considerations is the careful weighing up of potential risks and benefits by a competent individual. However, analysis of these risks and benefits by a surrogate on behalf of an incompetent individual poses a range of ethical difficulties. Most national and international guidelines concur that such research is justified as long as safeguards are in place. Both the National statement[107] and the Operational standards[110] outline categories of vulnerable persons and the relevant ethical considerations that apply to these groups. The governing bodies recommend careful consideration of these highly vulnerable groups. Of note, the New Zealand Operational standards[110] recognise that research on unconscious patients is appropriate but emphasises the need for communication with the family or other legal representatives wherever possible. These standards do note that, in emergency situations, consultation with the family/legal representatives may not be possible, but that the 'healthcare practitioner must always act in the best interests of the consumer'.[110]

Clinical trials

Clinical trials are a specific type of research study that explores whether a medical treatment, drug or device is safe and effective for humans. As these trials use people/patients as subjects in the study, these studies must follow strict scientific standards that are set within each country. The Therapeutic Goods Administration (TGA) in Australia has adopted the Guidelines for good clinical research practice,[111] but, at the same time, note there is some overlap with the National statement, which prevails. The TGA has published an annotated version for the Australian regulatory context. The Guidelines for good clinical practice[111] is an internationally accepted standard for the designing, conducting, recording and reporting of clinical trials.

The Australian government, through the NHMRC, has funded and established the Australian Clinical Trial Registry (ACTR) at the NHMRC Trials Centre in Sydney, which complies with these requirements. Clinical trials must be registered online prior to subject recruitment, as there are important implications for future research publication in journals. The World Health Organization (WHO) has developed the International Clinical Trial Registry Platform (ICTRP)[112] as a global project to facilitate access to information about controlled trials and their results. The Clinical Trials Search Portal provides access to a central database containing the trial registration data sets provided by the registries listed. It also provides links to the full original records. To facilitate the unique identification of trials, the search portal bridges (groups together) multiple records about the same trial.[112]

Ethics in publication

One of the key ways research findings are disseminated is through publication in peer-reviewed journals. Many international high-quality journals, including Australian Critical Care, support the implementation of the Committee of Publication Ethics (COPE) Core practices[113] for journal editors and publishers. These guidelines recognise the important roles of editors, editorial boards and publishers in promoting and supporting ethical practices in reporting research. Therefore, journal editors are increasingly requiring that researchers demonstrate evidence of their ethics review process before a manuscript/ study is considered for publication.

In Australia, the NHMRC Australian code for the responsible conduct of research (2018)[114] provides guidance on the minimum requirements for authorship of research. Authorship is defined as substantial participation, where all the following conditions are met:

- conception and design, or data collection or analysis/ interpretation of data
- drafting the article, or revising it critically for important intellectual content
- final approval of the version to be published.[114]

Authors must also ensure that all those who have contributed to the work are recognised and acknowledged. Acquisition of research funding or general supervision of a research group is not considered sufficient for authorship. Intellectual honesty should be paramount and used to inform publication ethics and to prevent misconduct.[114] Furthermore, under best-practice guidelines, journals should ensure processes whereby researchers are obliged to disclose any potential competing interests before a manuscript is published and ensure all published reports and reviews of research papers have been peer reviewed by suitably qualified persons and, where needed, publish corrections, clarifications, retractions and apologies.[113]

Summary

Managing ethical issues in any healthcare setting can be complex and, at times, contentious. As has been explored in this chapter, the critical care environment provides some unique challenges where the patient is particularly vulnerable; decision making is potentially complex; and resource utilisation is challenging. Critical care nurses, therefore, need to use ethical principles to guide the care of the critically ill and inform the conduct of clinical human research. As nurses provide a continuous presence at the bedside and a key voice heard in clinical management and leadership discussions across critical care, it is important that nurses develop and maintain a strong ethical and moral compass to guide care delivered.

Case study

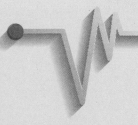

Joanna is a critical care nurse who has worked in the intensive care unit (ICU) of a large metropolitan teaching hospital for 5 years. The hospital she works in is a quaternary referral centre designated for the treatment of patients with COVID-19. As the number of patients admitted to the ICU with COVID-19 increased, Joanne was often allocated to one of the 'Class N' negative pressure rooms (with an antechamber for applying PPE) to care for the most critically ill or she was deployed as a member of the dedicated intubation and 'proning' team in the unit.

Since completing her postgraduate critical care qualification 3 years ago, Joanna worked 12-hour shifts, three days a week. As the number of patients in the ICU with COVID-19 increased, Joanne made a request to her manager to reduce her working hours to 8.5-hour shifts over a 7-day/fortnight roster. She found the infection control protocols, including donning and doffing PPE and wearing an N95 mask and face-shield during a 12-hour shift, uncomfortable and her exhaustion level at the end of each shift profound. Her overall quality of life was being impacted by her work and, for the first time, Joanne was questioning her career choice.

Her request was approved by the nurse manager and, initially, Joanne found that her energy levels were increasing. However, she was frequently being contacted on her days off to work extra shifts due to workforce shortfalls and was feeling remorseful and guilt-ridden when she declined. Joanne was also finding it difficult to cope at work with the distress experienced by family members, who under the hospital's strict policies for patients with suspected or confirmed COVID-19, could not visit their loved one. This was particularly the case for dying patients. In these situations, two family members could visit the ICU, but neither was allowed to enter the patient's room to say goodbye requiring the nursing staff to often be the conduit of final, highly personal messages to the patient.

When a 79-year-old retired engineer, Tom Jons, was admitted to the ICU from a residential aged care facility, Joanne found his case particularly distressing. Mr Jons was widowed with one adult son living interstate. Mr Jons had a history of hypertension and, while experiencing a CVA 2 years ago, he had generally recovered well and required assistance only for showering and dressing. When initially admitted to the ICU with COVID-19, Mr Jons' hypoxia was managed with high-flow nasal oxygen. He was able to relay to staff that while he didn't have an advanced care directive in place, he felt that he had had a good life and did not wish to be intubated and ventilated. He specifically told Joanne that he was lonely, his son rarely visited him and he did not want to go back to the aged care facility.

Later in the day, Mr Jons' condition deteriorated and, following a conversation with his son, the medical staff decided to intubate and ventilate him. Joanne related to the medical team Mr Jons' wishes not to be intubated and ventilated; however, the medical staff responded that his son wished him to be ventilated and without an advanced care directive in place there was no other option. Mr Jons died 3 days later in the ICU. Joanne was caring for Mr Jons' on the day he died and had called his son to ascertain if he wished to visit the ICU. His son declined and stated that he couldn't travel interstate and that he and his father 'weren't that close'.

CASE STUDY QUESTIONS

1　Are the experiences of Joanne reflective of other ICU nurses working during the pandemic and, if so, what actions should be taken by managers to support and relieve moral distress experienced by staff?

2　What ways can nurses develop moral resilience and how does moral resilience support nurses when faced with ethical challenges?

3　Consider the issues of mental capacity raised in Mr Jons' case and answer the following questions:

　a　How are assessments about someone's decision-making capacity made in your clinical area?
　b　What legal, professional and organisational processes and guidance are in place to assist this?
　c　What actions would you take if your assessment of a patient's capacity were not reflective of others in your team?

4　If there were a similar set of circumstances at your hospital, how would it be managed and what factors would guide the approach to be taken?

5　In your practice, are there decisions made by adult patients with decision-making capacity that challenge your thinking about the limits to someone's autonomy? What are those circumstances and how are these managed in practice?

6　Ethically, is there a difference between a person with decision-making capacity making a well-thought-through request and such a person making an irrational one?

RESEARCH VIGNETTE

Flannery L, Peters K, Ramjan, L. The differing perspectives of doctors and nurses in end-of-life decisions in the intensive care unit: A qualitative study. Aust Crit Care 2020;33:311-16.

Abstract

Background: End-of-life (EoL) decision making in the ICU can be emotionally challenging for both doctors and nurses, who are sometimes placed in difficult positions where they are required to make decisions on behalf of patients. With an ageing population and advances in medical technology, there is an increase in such decisions being made in ICUs.

Objectives: The objective of this study was to explore the perspectives of doctors and nurses involved in the EoL decision-making process in an ICU.

Methods: This study used a qualitative methodology based on naturalistic inquiry. Intensive care nurses and doctors from a large Sydney metropolitan public hospital were purposively selected, and data saturation was reached after a total of eight nurses and four doctors were interviewed. Data were collected through semi-structured interviews, either face-to-face or over the telephone. Interviews were then transcribed verbatim, and themes were identified and coded through a line-by-line analysis of each transcript (manual thematic analysis).

Findings: The findings revealed two main themes: 'Doctors' and nurses' roles in decision making' and 'Managing family expectations'. These themes highlighted key differences in decision-making processes, in that doctors tended to aim to meet the family's needs, while the nurses tended to advocate on behalf of the patient and what they interpreted as the patient's best interests. Furthermore, nurses tended to feel undervalued in decision making during family conferences, when, in reality, the doctors were making decisions based on all information obtained, primarily from nursing staff.

Conclusions: EoL decision making is complex and affects doctors and nurses involved in different ways. More emphasis on interprofessional education and collaboration between the two disciplines may enhance future decision-making processes.

Critique

This qualitative Australian study explores the perspectives of doctors and nurses involved in EoL decision-making processes in an ICU. The paper begins with a succinct outline of the study's context. The current state of knowledge with regards to the EoL decision making is highlighted including the importance of open communication with family members, the need for collaborative interdisciplinary team working and organisational support for staff (education and emotional support). The aim of the study is clearly stated, and the underpinning research question is described. A particular strength of this section is the provision of the types of decisions that constitute an EoL decision. These details, which researchers often assume a shared understanding of, enhance the integrity of the research.

This qualitative study collected data using semi-structured interviews with intensive care doctors and nurses to gain an in-depth understanding of their perspectives on EoL decision making. It is stated that ethics approval was given by the participating university and hospital human research ethics committee. It is usual for ethical approval to be granted by a recognised HREC, for example a university-based or health agency HREC at local, state or national jurisdictional level. For this study, arrangements were in place for review of the research proposal to ensure that the study met the requirements for ethical conduct and that study participants were protected. There is limited information provided about the setting; however, given that the focus of the study was describing perspectives, this does not affect the validity of the findings.

The sampling strategy is well described, outlining purposeful sampling and the criteria for selection. Recruitment was undertaken by advertising the study in locations frequented by potential study participants. Those who were interested in participating were asked to contact the researchers, which limits the potential for coercion.

The questions that formed the basis of the semi-structured interviews were provided, and the authors report the use of prompts to elicit further information. There is no indication, however, of how frequently the prompts were used or the extent to which they enhanced data collection. The potential for researcher bias based on their 'preconceived' ideas about the subject matter was reported, along with the steps taken to mitigate this. Data management was well described, and the process of thematic data analysis was outlined.

Clear tabulated information summarised the demographic and qualification characteristics; however, the relevance of some of this data was not apparent. For example, data were collected in relation to participants' first language and training, but these results did not feature in the analysis.

Generally, the reader would expect to see reference to the process used to code the data, as this helps with the identification of themes and increases the credibility of the findings. This aspect was missing in the manuscript.

The findings are presented under two themes, the first of which has two subthemes. While the link between the first theme on the first subtheme was clear, the second subtheme was labelled 'inconsistencies in the decision-making process' and did not appear to relate to the roles assumed by doctors and nurses in the decision-making process. Rather it recounted the effect of decisions made by different doctors, mostly due to the way they were rostered for duty. The second theme related to families' expectations. However, much of the analysis highlighted the different ways that doctors and nurses approached the decision-making process, rather than families per se. This analysis was novel and insightful and could have been better reflected in a more suitable label. The themes were well supported by data extracts. The discussion section of the paper explores all key points raised by the data, with a particular focus on the need for improved communication, interdisciplinary collaboration and decision-making skills. The study authors did not address any of the limitations of their study.

The paper concludes by recommending more interprofessional education and collaboration between doctors and nurses, which is supported by the study findings. The study was published in a peer-reviewed, clinical journal and adds to the body of knowledge about EoL decision-making processes in ICU.

Learning activities

1 Consider the decision-making challenges reported in the Research vignette paper by Flannery and colleagues. Reflect on your experiences in this area of EoL. What are some of the actions that you could take to improve collaboration in care?

2 You are on duty when a patient who has ingested a poisonous substance is admitted. The patient does not want medical intervention and only wants pain relief. What ethical and legal issues need consideration for this person? How can these be managed?

3 There is a colleague at work who frequently refuses to care for long-term patients and who appears to be getting more stressed and anxious at work. Think about the section on moral distress in this chapter. What could you do to offer support?

4 What are the ethical principles involved in clinical research? How can you safeguard the rights of patients who are involved in clinical trials?

Online resources

AFRICA

Egyptian Network of Research Ethics Committees, www.enrec.org/

Health Professions Council of South Africa, Guidelines for good practice in the health care professions general ethical guidelines for health researchers, https://www.up.ac.za/media/shared/6/files/hpcsa-ethical-guidelines-for-researchers.zp158370.pdf

Nigerian Federal Ministry of Health, Department of Health Planning and Research National Health Research Ethics Committee of Nigeria 2007, www.nhrec.net/nhrec/NCHRE_10.pdf

ASIA

China's Ethical Review System, n.d., http://trust-project.eu/wp-content/uploads/2016/03/Chinese-Ethics-Review-System.pdf

Indian Council of Medical Research, National ethical guidelines for biomedical and health research involving human participants 2017, https://ethics.ncdirindia.org/asset/pdf/ICMR_National_Ethical_Guidelines.pdf

Japanese Ministry of Health, Labor and Welfare, Ethical guidelines for clinical research, 2003, https://www.niph.go.jp/wadai/ekigakurinri/guidelines.pdf

Malaysian code of responsible conduct in research, 2021, https://www.akademisains.gov.my/asm-publication/the-malaysian-code-of-responsible-conduct-in-research-2nd-edition/

Singapore statement of research integrity, n.d., https://www.jsps.go.jp/english/e-kousei/data/singapore_statement_EN.pdf

AUSTRALIA

Australian state and territory privacy principles, https://www.oaic.gov.au/privacy/privacy-in-your-state/privacy-in-the-act/territory-privacy-principles

National Health and Medical Research Council (NHMRC), An ethical framework for integrating palliative care principles into the management of advanced chronic or terminal conditions, https://pallcarevic.asn.au/wp-content/uploads/2015/11/Ethical-Framework-for-Integrating-Palliative-Care-Principles-.pdf

National Health and Medical Research Council (NHMRC), Challenging ethical issues in contemporary research on human beings, https://www.nhmrc.gov.au/about-us/publications/challenging-ethical-issues-contemporary-research

National Health and Medical Research Council (NHMRC), Ethics and integrity, https://www.nhmrc.gov.au/research-policy/ethics-and-integrity

National Health and Medical Research Council (NHMRC), National statement on ethical conduct in human research, https://www.nhmrc.gov.au/about-us/publications/national-statement-ethical-conduct-human-research-2007-updated-2018

EUROPE

Council for International Organisations of Medical Sciences (CIOMS), International ethical guidelines for health-related research involving humans. 4th ed. 2016. https://cioms.ch/publications/product/international-ethical-guidelines-for-health-related-research-involving-humans/

European Network of Research Ethics Committees – EUREC, www.eurecnet.org/index.html

European Commission – Public Health, https://ec.europa.eu/health/home_en

UK National Health Service, UK policy framework for health and social care research, 2020, https://www.hra.nhs.uk/planning-and-improving-research/policies-standards-legislation/uk-policy-framework-health-social-care-research/

World Health Organization, List of ethics committees, 2015, http://apps.who.int/ethics/nationalcommittees/NEC_full_web.pdf

World Health Organization, Operational guidelines for ethics committees that review biomedical research, 2000, https://apps.who.int/iris/handle/10665/66429

World Medical Association, Declaration of Helsinki – ethical principles for medical research involving human subjects, updated 2018, https://www.wma.net/policies-post/wma-declaration-of-helsinki-ethical-principles-for-medical-research-involving-human-subjects/

NEW ZEALAND

Health Act 1956 (NZ), https://www.legislation.govt.nz/act/public/1956/0065/latest/DLM305840.html

Health Research Council of New Zealand (HRCNZ), The role of ethics, https://www.hrc.govt.nz/grants-funding/role-ethics

Health Research Council of New Zealand (HRCNZ), HRC research ethics guidelines, https://hrc.govt.nz/sites/default/files/2021-04/HRC%20Research%20Ethics%20Guidelines-%20April%202021_1.pdf

National Ethics Advisory Committee NZ, https://neac.health.govt.nz/

New Zealand Privacy Commissioner website, https://www.privacy.org.nz/

Public Health and Disability Act 2000 (NZ), Amended as NZ Public Health and Disability Amendment Bill 2010, https://www.parliament.nz/en/pb/bills-and-laws/bills-digests/document/49PLLawBD17731/new-zealand-public-health-and-disability-amendment-bill

NORTH AMERICA

Government of Canada, Navigating the ethics of human research, https://ethics.gc.ca/eng/policy-politique_tcps2-eptc2_2022.html

Medical Research Council of Canada (MRC), Tri council policy statement, ethical conduct for research involving humans – TCPS 2 (2022), https://ethics.gc.ca/eng/policy-politique_tcps2-eptc2_2022.html

US Department of Health & Human Services, National Institutes of Health, Human subjects research, https://humansubjects.nih.gov/

US Department of Health and Human Services, Office for Human Research Protections, https://www.hhs.gov/ohrp/

US Department of Health and Human Services, Federal policy for the protection of human subjects ('common rule'), https://www.hhs.gov/ohrp/regulations-and-policy/regulations/common-rule/index.html

OTHERS

International Committee of Medical Journal Editors (ICMJE), Recommendations (the uniform requirements), https://www.icmje.org

Committee of Publication Ethics (COPE), Code of conduct and best practice guidelines for journal editors, 2011, https://academic.oup.com/DocumentLibrary/journals/Code_of_conduct_for_journal_editors_1.pdf

Further reading

Asadi N, Royani Z, Maazallahi M, et al. Being torn by inevitable moral dilemma: experiences of ICU nurses. BMC Med Ethics 2021;22:159. doi: 10.1186/s12910-021-00727-y.

DeAngelis CD, Drazen JM, Frizelle FA, et al. Clinical trial registration: a statement from the International Committee of Medical Journal Editors. JAMA 2004;292:1363–4.

Farrugia L; WASP (Write a Scientific Paper). The ongoing process of ethical decision-making in qualitative research: Ethical principles and their application to the research process. Early Hum Dev 2019;133:48–51. doi: 10.1016/j.earlhumdev.2019.03.011.

Nicoli F, Cummins P, Raho JA, et al. If an acute event occurs, what should we do? Diverse ethical approaches to decision-making in the ICU. Med Health Care Philos 2019;22:475–86. doi: 10.1007/s11019-019-09887-6.

Obeidat AS, Komesaroff PA. Clinical ethics from the Islamic perspective: a qualitative study exploring the views of Jordanian doctors. Bioeth Inq 2021;18:335–48. doi: 10.1007/s11673-021-10108-0.

Variath C, Peter E, Cranleyl, et al. Health care providers' ethical perspectives on waiver of final consent for Medical Assistance in Dying (MAiD): a qualitative study. BMC Med Ethics 2022;23:8. doi: 10.1186/s12910-022-00745-4.

Young MJ, Bodien YG, Edlow BL. Ethical considerations in clinical trials for disorders of consciousness. Brain Sci 2022;12:211. doi: 10.3390/brainsci12020211.

References

1. International Council of Nurses (ICN). The ICN code of ethics for nurses. Revised 2021. Available from: https://www.icn.ch/sites/default/files/inline-files/ICN_Code-of-Ethics_EN_Web.pdf. [Accessed 10 February 2023].

2. Rainer J, Schneider JK, Lorenz RA. Ethical dilemmas in nursing: an integrative review. J Clin Nurs 2018 Oct;27(19-20):3446–61.

3. McIlwraith J, Madden B. Health care and the law. 6th ed. Sydney, NSW: Thomson Reuters (Professional) Australia; 2014.

4. Beauchamp TL, Childress JF. Principles of biomedical ethics. 8th ed. New York: Oxford University Press; 2019.

5. Johnstone M-J. Bioethics: a nursing perspective. 8th ed. Sydney, NSW: Elsevier; 2023.

6. Nursing and Midwifery Board of Australia (NMBA). Professional codes and guidelines. Melbourne, VIC: NMBA; 2018. Available from: https://www.nursingmidwiferyboard.gov.au/codes-guidelines-statements/professional-standards.aspx. [Accessed 10 February 2023].

7. Griffith R. Using public health law to contain the spread of COVID-19. Br J Nurs 2020;29(5):326–7.

8. Fisk M, Livingstone A, Pit S. Telehealth in the context of COVID-19: changing perspectives in Australia, the United Kingdom, and the United States. J Med Internet Res 2020;22(6):e19264. doi: 10.2196/19264.

9. Pollard CL. What is the right thing to do: use of a relational ethic framework to guide clinical decision-making. Int J Caring Sci 2015;8(2):362–8.

10. Clement G. Care, autonomy, and justice: feminism and the ethic of care. London: Routledge; 2018.

11. Antommaria AH, Gibb TS, McGuire AL, et al. Ventilator triage policies during the COVID-19 pandemic at US hospitals associated with members of the association of bioethics program directors. Ann Intern Med 2020;173(3):188–94. doi: 10.7326/M20-1738.

12. Romney D, Fox H, Carlson S, et al. Allocation of scarce resources in a pandemic: a systematic review of US state crisis standards of care documents. Disaster Med Public Health Prep 2020;14(5):677–83. doi: 10.1017/dmp.2020.101.

13. Jöbges S, Vinay R, Luyckx VA, et al. Recommendations on COVID-19 triage: international comparison and ethical analysis. Bioethics 2020;34(9):948–59. doi: 10.1111/bioe.12805.

14. Nelson JE, Puntillo KA, Pronovost PJ, et al. In their own words: patients and families define high-quality palliative care in the intensive care unit. Crit Care Med 2010;38(3):808–18.

15. Fenton HN. State and local anti-apartheid laws: misplaced response to a flawed national policy on South Africa. NYUJ Int Law Pol 1986;19:883.

16. Freckelton I. Bioethics, biopolitics and medical regulation: learning from the Nazi doctor experience. J Law Med 2009;16(4):555–67.

17. Staunton P, Chiarella M. Law for nurses and midwives. 8th ed. Sydney, NSW: Elsevier; 2017.

18. Privacy Act 1993 (NZ). Available from: https://www.legislation.govt.nz/act/public/1993/0028/latest/DLM296639.html. [Accessed 10 February 2023].

19. Privacy Act 1988 (Cth). Available from: https://www.oaic.gov.au/privacy-law/privacy-act/. [Accessed 10 February 2023].

20. White B, McDonald FJ, Willmott L. Health law in Australia. 3rd ed. Pyrmont, NSW; Thomson Reuters (Lawbook Co); 2018.

21. United Nations (UN). The universal declaration of human rights 1948. New York: UN; 2014. Available from: https://www.un.org/en/about-us/universal-declaration-of-human-rights. [Accessed 10 February 2023].

22. Grech C. Factors affecting the provision of culturally congruent care to Arab Muslims by critical care nurses. Aust Crit Care 2008;21(3):167–71.

23. Bloomer MJ, Al-Mutair A. Ensuring cultural sensitivity for Muslim patients in the Australian ICU: considerations for care. Aust Crit Care 2013;26(4):193–6.

24. Nursing and Midwifery Board of Australia. Registered nurse standards for practice. Sydney, NSW: NMBA;2016. Available from: http://www.nursingmidwiferyboard.gov.au/Codes-Guidelines-Statements/Professional-standards/registered-nurse-standards-for-practice.aspx. [Accessed 10 February 2023].

25. National Health and Medical Research Council (NHMRC). Cultural competency in health: a guide for policy, partnerships and participation. Canberra, ACT: Australian Government; 2006. Available from: https://www.nhmrc.gov.au/about-us/publications/cultural-competency-health. [Accessed 10 February 2023].

26. Commonwealth of Australia Department of Health. Aboriginal and Torres Strait Islander health curriculum framework. Canberra, ACT: 2014. Available from: https://www.health.gov.au/sites/default/files/documents/2020/12/aboriginal-and-torres-strait-islander-health-curriculum-framework.pdf. [Accessed 10 February 2023].

27. Queensland Health. Delegated consent position statement. Brisbane, QLD: Queensland Government; 2013. Available from: https://www.health.qld.gov.au/__data/assets/pdf_file/0022/156082/delegated_consent_pos_sta.pdf. [Accessed 10 February 2023].

28. *Rogers v Whitaker* (1992) 175 CLR 479. Available from: https://staging.hcourt.gov.au/assets/publications/judgments/1992/051—ROGERS_v._WHITAKER—(1992)_175_CLR_479.html. [Accessed 10 February 2023].

29. Faunce T. Disclosure of material risk as systems-error tragedy: *Wallace v Kam* (2013) 87 ALJR 648; [2013] HCA 19. J Law Med 2013;21:53–65.

30. *Guardianship and Administration Act 2000* (Qld) sch 4. Available from: https://www.legislation.qld.gov.au/view/pdf/2013-08-29/act-2000-008. [Accessed 10 February 2023].

31. *Human Rights Act 1998* (UK). Available from: http://www.legislation.gov.uk/ukpga/1998/42. [Accessed 10 February 2023].

32. Kon AA, Davidson JE, Morrison W, et al. Shared decision making in intensive care units: an American College of Critical Care Medicine and American Thoracic Society policy statement. Crit Care Med 2016;44(1):188–201.

33. Nursing and Midwifery Council (NMC). The Code: professional standards of practice and behaviour for nurses and midwives. London: NMC; 2015. Available from: https://www.nmc.org.uk/standards/code/. [Accessed 10 February 2023].

34. *Health Practitioner Regulation National Law Act 2009* (Qld). Available from: https://www.legislation.qld.gov.au/view/html/inforce/current/act-2009-045. [Accessed 10 February 2023].

35. *The Health Practitioners Competence Assurance Act 2003* (NZ). Available from: https://www.legislation.govt.nz/act/public/2003/0048/latest/whole.html. [Accessed 10 February 2023].

36. Australian Government Department of Health. Australian national guidelines for the management of health care workers known to be infected with bloodborne viruses. Canberra, ACT: Australian Government; 2018. Available from: https://www.health.gov.au/resources/collections/cdna-national-guidelines-for-healthcare-workers-on-managing-bloodborne-viruses?utm_source=health.gov.au&utm_medium=callout-auto-custom&utm_campaign=digital_transformation. [Accessed 10 February 2023].

37. Van den Bulcke B, Metaxa V, Reyners AK, et al. Ethical climate and intention to leave among critical care clinicians: an observational study in 68 intensive care units across Europe and the United States. Int Care Med 2020;46(1):46–56. doi: 10.1007/s00134-019-05829-1.

38. Langeland K, Sørlie V. Ethical challenges in nursing emergency practice. J Clin Nurs 2011;20(13–14):2064–70.

39. Pauly BM, Varcoe C, Storch J. Framing the issues: moral distress in healthcare. HEC Forum 2012;24:1–11.

40. Thompson K, Taylor C, Forde K, et al. The evolution of Australian intensive care and its related costs: a narrative review. Aust Crit Care 2018;31(5):325–30.

41. Persad G, Wertheimer A, Emanuel EJ. Principles for allocation of scarce medical interventions. Lancet 2009;373(9661):423–31.

42. Jaziri R, Alnahdi S. Choosing which COVID-19 patient to save? The ethical triage and rationing dilemma. Ethics Med Public Health 2020;15:100570. doi: 10.1016/j.jemep.2020.100570.

43. Liu J, Chen XX, Wang XLJ. Ethical issues in neonatal intensive care units. J Matern Fetal Neonatal Med 2016;29(14):2322–6.

44. Nguyen Y-L, Angus DC, Boumendil A, et al. The challenge of admitting the very elderly to intensive care. Ann Intensive Care 2011;1(29):1–7.

45. Nates JL, Nunnally M, Kleinpell R, et al. ICU admission, discharge, and triage guidelines: a framework to enhance clinical operations, development of institutional policies, and further research. Crit Care Med 2016;44(8):1553–602.

46. Stelfox HT, Lane D, Boyd JM, et al. A scoping review of patient discharge from intensive care: opportunities and tools to improve care. Chest 2015;147(2):317–27.

47. Oerlemans AJM, van Sluisveld N, van Leeuwen ESJ, et al. Ethical problems in intensive care unit admission and discharge decisions: a qualitative study among physicians and nurses in the Netherlands. BMC Med Ethics 2015;16(9):1–10.

48. Kraus CK, Levy F, Kelen GD. Lifeboat ethics: considerations in the discharge of inpatients for the creation of hospital surge capacity. Disaster Med Public Health Prep 2007;1(1):51–6.

49. Taylor IH, Dihle A, Hofsø K, et al. Intensive care nurses' experiences of withdrawal of life-sustaining treatments in intensive care patients: a qualitative study. Intensive Crit Care Nurs 2020;56:102768.

50. George NR, Kryworuchko J, Hunold KM, et al. Shared decision making to support the provision of palliative and end-of-life care in the emergency department: a consensus statement and research agenda. Acad Emerg Med 2016;23(12):1394–402.

51. Downar J. Rapid response teams and end-of-life care. Can Respir J 2014;21(5):268.

52. Mark NM, Rayner SG, Lee NJ, et al. Global variability in withholding and withdrawal of life-sustaining treatment in the intensive care unit: a systematic review. Intensive Care Med 2015;41(9):1572–85.

53. Sprung CL, Truog RD, Curtis JR, et al. Seeking worldwide professional consensus on the principles of end-of-life care for the critically ill. The consensus for Worldwide End-of-Life Practice for Patients in Intensive Care Units (WELPICUS) study. Am J Resp Crit Care Med 2014;190(8):855–66.

54. Avidan A, Sprung CL, Schefold JC, et al. Variations in end-of-life practices in intensive care units worldwide (Ethicus-2): a prospective observational study. Lancet Resp Med 2021;9(10):1101–10.

55. Wilkinson D, Savulescu J. A costly separation between withdrawing and withholding treatment in intensive care. Bioethics 2014;28(3):127–37.

56. Australian and New Zealand Intensive Care Society (ANZICS), College of Intensive Care Medicine of Australia and New Zealand. The ANZICS statement on withholding and withdrawing treatment. Camberwell, VIC: ANZICS; 2013. Available from: https://cicm.org.au/CICM_Media/CICMSite/CICM-Website/Resources/Professional%20Documents/IC-14-Statement-on-Withholding-and-Withdrawing-Treatment.pdf. [Accessed 10 February 2023].

57. Australian Commission on Safety and Quality in Health Care. National consensus statement: essential elements for safe and high-quality end-of-life care. Sydney, NSW: ACSQHC; 2015. Available from: https://www.safetyandquality.gov.au/publications-and-resources/resource-library/national-consensus-statement-essential-elements-safe-and-high-quality-end-life-care. [Accessed 10 February 2023].

58. UK General Medical Council. Treatment and care towards the end-of-life: good practice in decision making. London: GMC; 2022. Available from: https://www.gmc-uk.org/ethical-guidance/ethical-guidance-for-doctors/treatment-and-care-towards-the-end-of-life. [Accessed 10 February 2023].

59. Valley TS, Admon AJ, Zahuranec DB, et al. Estimating ICU benefit: a randomized study of physicians. Crit Care Med 2019;47(1):62–8. doi: 10.1097/CCM.0000000000003473.

60. Wilkinson DJ, Truog RD. The luck of the draw: physician-related variability in end-of-life decision-making in intensive care. Int Care Med 2013;39(6):1128–32.

61. Sprung CL, Cohen SL, Sjokvist P, et al; Ethicus Study Group. End-of-life practices in European intensive care units: the Ethicus Study. JAMA 2003:290(6):790–7.

62. Benbenishty J, Ganz FD, Anstey MH, et al. Changes in intensive care unit nurse involvement in end of life decision making between 1999 and 2016: descriptive comparative study. Int Crit Care Nurs 2022;68:103138.

63. Flannery L, Peters K, Ramjan LM. The differing perspectives of doctors and nurses in end-of-life decisions in the intensive care unit: a qualitative study. Aust Crit Care 2020;33(4):311–16.

64. Brooks LA, Manias E, Nicholson P. Communication and decision-making about end-of-life care in the intensive care unit. Am J Crit Care 2017;26(4):336–41. doi: 10.4037/ajcc2017774.

65. National Health and Medical Research Council (NHMRC). Organ and tissue donation after death, for transplantation: guidelines for ethical practice for health professionals. 2007. Available from: https://www.nhmrc.gov.au/guidelines-publications/e75. [Accessed 10 February 2023].

66. Long-Sutehall T, Willis H, Palmer R, et al. Negotiated dying: a grounded theory of how nurses shape withdrawal of treatment in hospital critical care units. Int J Nurs Stud 2011;48(12):1466–74.

67. Vincent JL, Marshall JC, Ñamendys-Silva SA, et al. Assessment of the worldwide burden of critical illness: the intensive care over nations (ICON) audit. Lancet Resp Med 2014;2(5):380–6.

68. Connolly C, Miskolci O, Phelan D, et al. End-of-life in the ICU: moving from 'withdrawal of care' to a palliative care, patient-centred approach. Br J Anaesth 2016;117(2):143–5.

69. Chaet D. The AMA code of medical ethics' opinions relevant to patient- and family-centered care. AMA J Ethics 2016;18(1):45–8.

70. Loretta MK. The best interests standard for incompetent or incapacitated persons of all ages. J Law Med Ethics 2007;35(1):187–96.

71. Morgan J. End-of-life care in UK critical care units – a literature review. Nurs Crit Care 2008;13(3):152–61.

72. Coombs M, Long-Sutehall T, Shannon S. International dialogue on end of life: challenges in the UK and USA. Nurs Crit Care 2010;15(5):234–40.

73. Haynes LI. Palliative care: attitudes and practices of trauma care providers. Tucson, AZ: University of Arizona; 2017.

74. Aghabarary M, Dehghan Nayeri N. Medical futility and its challenges: a review study. J Med Ethics Hist Med 2016;9(11):1–13.

75. Kon AA, Shepard EK, Sederstrom NO, et al. Defining futile and potentially inappropriate interventions: a policy statement from the Society of Critical Care Medicine Ethics Committee. Crit Care Med 2016;44(9):1769–74.

76. Willmott L, White B, Downie J. Withholding and withdrawal of 'futile' life-sustaining treatment: unilateral medical decision-making in Australia and New Zealand. J Law Med 2013;20(4):907–24.

77. Solis GR, Mancera BM, Shen MJ. Strategies used to facilitate the discussion of advance care planning with older adults in primary care settings: a literature review. J Am Assoc Nurs Pract 2018;30(5):270–9. doi: 10.1097/JXX.0000000000000025.

78. National Institute for Health and Care Excellence (NICE). Advance care planning. London: NICE; 2022 Available from: https://www.nice.org.uk/about/nice-communities/social-care/quick-guides/advance-care-planning. [Accessed 10 February 2023].

79. Austin Health. Advance care planning Australia. Kew, VIC: Austin Health; 2021. Available from: https://www.advancecareplanning.org.au/. [Accessed 10 February 2023].

80. Craig DP, Ray R, Harvey D, Shircore M. Factors which influence hospital doctors' advance care plan adherence. J Pain Sympt Mgmt 2020;59(5):1109–26.

81. Dowling T, Kennedy S, Foran S. Implementing advance directives – an international literature review of important considerations for nurses. J Nurs Mgmt 2020;28(6):1177–90.

82. Perkins GD, Griffiths F, Slowther AM, et al. Do-not-attempt-cardiopulmonary-resuscitation decisions: an evidence synthesis. Southampton, Hants: NIHR Journals Library; 2016.

83. Phillips J. Clarifying substitute judgement: the endorsed life approach. J Med Ethics 2015;41(9):723–30.

84. Mroz S, Dierickx S, Deliens L, et al. Assisted dying around the world: a status quaestionis. Ann Palliat Med 2021;10(3):3540–53.

85. Durán-Crane A, Laserna A, López-Olivo MA, et al. Clinical practice guidelines and consensus statements about pain management in critically ill end-of-life patients: a systematic review. Crit Care Med 2019;47(11):1619–26.

86. Gerber K, Willmott L, White B, et al. Barriers to adequate pain and symptom relief at the end of life: A qualitative study capturing nurses' perspectives. Collegian 2022;29(1):1–8.

87. British Medical Association (BMA) Board of Science. Improving analgesic use to support pain management at the end of life. London: BMA; 2017. Available from: https://www.bma.org.uk/media/2102/analgesics-end-of-life-1.pdf. [Accessed 10 February 2023].

88. Symons X. Does the doctrine of double effect apply to the prescription of barbiturates? Syme vs the Medical Board of Australia. J Med Ethics 2018;44(4):266–9.

89. Brighton LJ, Koffman J, Hawkins A, et al. A systematic review of end-of-life care communication skills training for generalist palliative care providers: research quality and reporting guidance. J Pain Symptom Manag 2017;54(3):417–25.

90. Ha JF, Longnecker N. Doctor patient communication: a review. Ochsner J 2010;10(1):38–43.

91. Ulrich CM, Taylor C, Soeken K, et al. Everyday ethics: ethical issues and stress in nursing practice. J Adv Nurs 2010;66(11):2510–19.

92. Price D, Knotts S. Communication, comfort, and closure for the patient with cystic fibrosis at the end of life: the role of the bedside nurse. J Hosp Palliat Nurs 2017;19(4):303–4.

93. Bosslet GT, Kesecioglu J, White DB. How should clinicians respond to requests for potentially inappropriate treatment? J Intensive Care Med 2016;42:422–5.

94. Curtis JR, Sprung CL, Azoulay E. The importance of word choice in care of critically ill patients and their families. J Intensive Care Med 2014;40:606–8.

95. Cheng F, Ip M, Wong KK, et al. Critical care ethics in Hong Kong: cross-cultural conflicts as East meets West. J Med Philos 1998;23(6):616–27.

96. Flannery L, Ramjan LM, Peters K. End-of-life decisions in the intensive care unit 9 (ICU) – exploring the experiences of ICU nurses and doctors – a critical literature review. Aust Crit Care 2016;29(2):97–103.

97. Gaudine A, LeFort SM, Lamb M, et al. Ethical conflicts with hospitals: the perspective of nurses and physicians. Nurs Ethics 2011;18(6):756–66.

98. Hall RM. Ethical consultations in the ICU: by whom and when? Crit Care Med 2014;42(4):983–4.

99. Holt J, Convey H. Ethical practice in nursing care. Nurs Stand 2012;27(13):51–6.

100. Rushton CH. Moral resilience: a capacity for navigating moral distress in critical care. AACN Adv Crit Care 2016;27(1):111–19.

101. O'Connell C. Gender and the experience of moral distress in critical care nurses. Nurs Ethics 2015;22(1):32–42.

102. Rushton CH, Schoonover-Shoffner K, Kennedy MS. A collaborative state of the science initiative: transforming moral distress into moral resilience in nursing experts recommend strategies to develop moral resilience and support ethical practice. Am J Nurs 2017;117(2):S2–6.

103. Grace P, Robinson E, Jurchak M, et al. Clinical ethics residency for nurses: an education model to decrease moral distress and strengthen nurse retention in acute care. J Nurs Adm 2014;44(12):640–6.

104. Austin W. The ethics of everyday practice: healthcare environments as moral communities. ANS Adv Nurs Sci 2007;30(1):81–8.

105. World Medical Association (WMA). The WMA Declaration of Helsinki – ethical principles for medical research involving human subjects. Ferney-Voltaire, France: WMA; 2013. Available from: https://www.wma.net/policies-post/wma-declaration-of-helsinki-ethical-principles-for-medical-research-involving-human-subjects/. [Accessed 10 February 2023].

106. General Medical Council. Consent: patients and doctors making decisions together. London: GMC; 2008. Available from: https://www.gmc-uk.org/-/media/documents/gmc-guidance-for-doctors---decision-making-and-consent-english_pdf-84191055.pdf. [Accessed 10 February 2023].

107. National Health and Medical Research Council (NHMRC). National statement on ethical conduct in human research 2007 (updated May 2018). Canberra, ACT: NHMRC; 2007. Available from: https://www.nhmrc.gov.au/guidelines/publications/e72. [Accessed 10 February 2023].

108. Rischbieth A, Blythe D. Ethics handbook for researchers, Australian and New Zealand Intensive Care Society (ANZICS) Clinical Trials Group (CTG). Melbourne, VIC: Wakefield Press; 2005.

109. Council for International Organizations of Medical Sciences (CIOMS). International ethical guidelines for biomedical research involving humans. 4th ed. Geneva: CIOMS; 2016. Available from: https://cioms.ch/wp-content/uploads/2017/01/WEB-CIOMS-EthicalGuidelines.pdf. [Accessed 10 February 2023].

110. New Zealand Ministry of Health. Operational Standard for ethics committees: updated edition. Wellington: Ministry of Health; 2006. Available from: https://www.parliament.nz/resource/0000162273. [Accessed 10 February 2023].

111. Australian Therapeutic Goods Administration (TGA). ICH guidance for good clinical practice (ICH E6(R2)) Annotated with TGA comments. Woden, ACT: TGA; 2018. Available from: https://www.tga.gov.au/resources/publication/publications/ich-guideline-good-clinical-practice. [Accessed 10 February 2023].

112. World Health Organization (WHO). International clinical trials registry platform (ICTRP). Geneva: WHO; 2018. Available from: http://www.who.int/ictrp/en/. [Accessed 10 February 2023].

113. Committee on Publication Ethics (COPE). Core practices. Eastleigh, Hants: COPE; 2022. Available from: https://publicationethics.org/core-practices. [Accessed 10 February 2023].

114. National Health and Medical Research Council (NHMRC). Australian code for the responsible conduct of research. Canberra, ACT: NHMRC; 2018. Available from: https://www.nhmrc.gov.au/sites/default/files/documents/attachments/grant%20documents/The-australian-code-for-the-responsible-conduct-of-research-2018.pdf. [Accessed 5 February 2023].

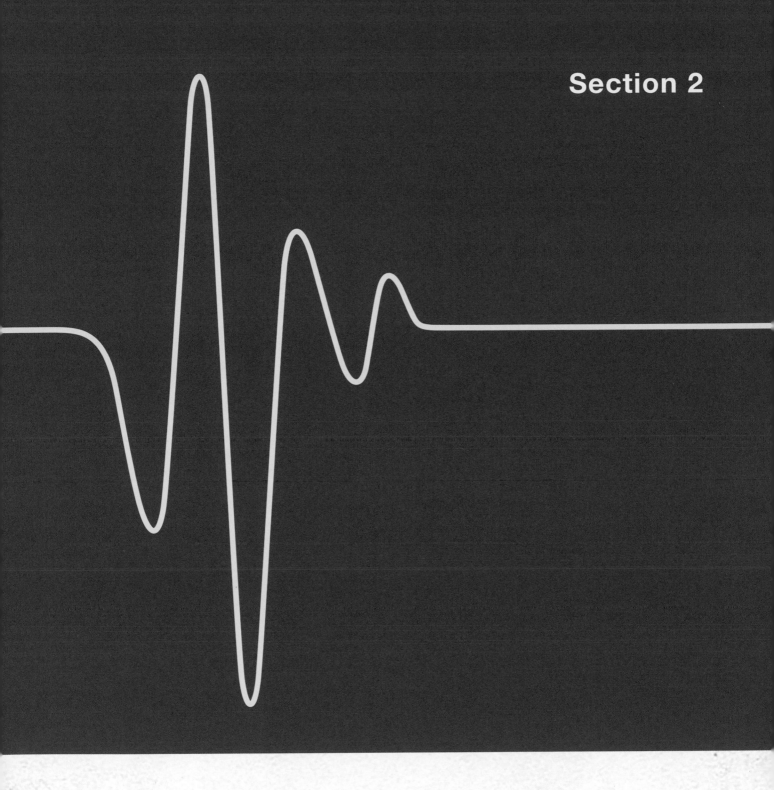

Principles and practice of critical care

Chapter 5

Essential nursing care of the critically ill patient

Bernadette Grealy, Lotta Johansson

Learning objectives

After reading this chapter, you should be able to:

- describe best practice for the provision of physical care and hygiene
- identify risks posed to critically ill patients relating to ineffective physical care and hygiene
- describe eye- and oral-related risks associated with critical illness and mechanical ventilation
- describe factors of importance in the care of critically ill patients with special needs, such as older adults and overweight patients
- describe nursing care measures necessary for critically ill patients to prevent hospital-related infections and incidences
- understand the key elements of safe transport of critically ill patients within the hospital setting
- understand the principles of infection control risk identification and management for critically ill patients
- understand the effective use of personal protective equipment.

Introduction

This chapter is about essential nursing care and its role in the care and management of the critically ill patient. Sometimes referred to as basic nursing, it may not be considered a priority. Yet, how well patients are cared for has a direct effect on their sense of well-being, the prevention of complications and their recovery. This chapter focuses on physical care, infection control, preventive therapies and transport of critically ill patients. The recent worldwide experience of the COVID-19 pandemic has acutely brought into focus all the key elements of infection risk, prevention and control. How well patients' physical care and preventive therapies are managed directly impacts their risk for hospital related complications or infections. The essential features of critical care nursing within this chapter relate to every critically ill patient.

TABLE 5.1
Principles of practice

REDUCING RISKS TO PATIENTS	PROVISION OF QUALITY CARE
• Recognition of the specific needs of critically ill patients, particularly those who are unconscious, sedated or immobile	• Development of knowledge and skills for practice
• Recognition of specific complications that may require special observation or treatment	• Evidence-based practice
	• Optimal use of protocol-driven therapy
• Vigilant monitoring and early recognition of signs of deterioration	• Competent, efficient and safe practice
• Selection, implementation and evaluation of specific preventive measures	• Selection and application of appropriate nursing interventions
• Management of potentially detrimental environmental factors that may affect the patient	• Monitoring the consequences of nursing interventions
	• Review and evaluation of nursing practices
	• Continuity of care
	• Effective critical care team functioning

Comfort is a paramount concern in intensive care. Two key aspects of care – reducing risk and providing quality care – are closely related and served by a series of principles (Table 5.1). Implementing evidence-based essential nursing care is a key strategy to reduce avoidable errors and improve patient outcomes.[1] 'Interventional patient hygiene' (IPH) is a systematic, evidence-based approach to nursing actions designed to improve patient outcomes using a framework of hygiene, catheter care, skin care, mobility and oral care.[1] Patients are assessed thoroughly and on a regular basis to detect problems and treated early, thereby preventing the development of unnecessary complications. Although this chapter focuses on the physical dimension of nursing care, patients' psychosocial care is also of paramount importance (see Chapters 6 and 7). Further, while this chapter describes essential nursing care, care bundles encompassing groups of activities are described in Chapter 3.

Practice tip

Ensure patients and their support persons know your name when you are caring for them; introducing yourself is professionally appropriate and reassuring to patients and their support persons.

Skin integrity

One of the most basic needs of patients is to maintain healthy skin. Intact skin is the body's first line of defence against the invasion of microorganisms, provides protection from numerous environmental threats, and facilitates retention of moisture. Maintaining the critically ill patient's skin integrity is one of the most fundamental yet critical goals of nursing practice.

Personal hygiene

Poor hygiene may increase the risk of bacterial colonisation and subsequent infection in the critically ill patient.[2,3] Daily bed baths, plus intermittent as needed, or freshening washes are usually provided for most critically ill patients. Bed baths provide an opportunity to achieve other clinical goals such as skin assessment, comfort and stimulating circulation.[1] Personal hygiene is closely related to an individual's esteem and sense of well-being. It may also influence family members' perception of the quality of care the patient is receiving and the confidence they have in the staff. Reports of the benefits in reducing hospital-acquired bloodstream infections[3] and reducing the microbial load on a patient's skin[2] through the use of chlorhexidine gluconate (CHG)-impregnated washcloths for bathing in intensive care, along with the convenience of the washcloths versus the questionable cleanliness of basins for soap and water washes, have contributed to this change in many ICUs.[3] The correlation of CHG washcloths relating to reduction of multi-resistant organism (MRO) colonisation, hospital-acquired bloodstream infections or line-associated bloodstream infections is still being tested.[2,4] When water washes are used, consideration of the wash product and need for rinsing should be given along with good practices for basin cleanliness.[4] Following the wash with use of a skin moisturiser or protective lotion is also helpful to maintain skin integrity.[4]

Assessment of personal hygiene

Assessment of critical care patients' personal hygiene needs should be undertaken on two levels: first, determining what patients are able, and want, to do for themselves and second, the nurse's assessment of what is required. As with all aspects of care, the patient has the right to refuse personal hygiene measures. Where critically ill patients are unable to participate in decision making, it is then the nurse's responsibility to determine what level of care is necessary.[1] Consideration of the patient's specific condition or therapy needs may influence when and how personal hygiene is performed. For example, the patient may have to be moved slowly when changing bed linen because of their cardiovascular instability, or they may require a blanket while bathing if they are hypothermic. Equally, the timing of personal hygiene interventions related to other therapy needs can be helpful to the comfort of the patient, and promoting optimal rest. There are a number of areas to consider when assessing the skin (Table 5.2).

TABLE 5.2

Skin and tissue assessment

FACTOR	OBSERVATIONS
Colour of the skin	• Jaundice, erythema, pallor, cyanosis
Condition of the skin	• Skin turgor (elasticity): evidence of oedema (taut skin), dehydration (dryness, tenting of the skin), age-related or steroid-related damage (thin, papery, easily torn skin), skin tears • Presence of: rash, cellulitis, irritation, bruising, swelling
Tissue perfusion	• Hypoperfusion: capillary refill time, cool extremities, pulse strength and volume, blanching of the skin • Hyperaemia: very warm, red areas of skin • Thrombus formation: warm, red, swollen areas (especially calves)
Moisture	• Excessive sweating • Skin damage caused by moisture, especially in skinfolds: under the breasts, in the groin, between the buttocks
Wounds, drains, cannulae, catheters	• Evidence of inflammation, infection, pressure damage, skin excoriation caused by leaking exudates, correct positioning of drains, need to redress wounds

Essential hygiene care

A daily complete bed bath with intermittent washes of the face and hands is standard care; however, the following key points should be considered:

- Patients who are sweating, incontinent, bleeding or with leaking wounds should be promptly washed and their bed linen changed as often as necessary.

- It may be appropriate to give prophylactic pain relief before commencing a bed bath.

- Timing should be based on patient preference, clinical stability and to avoid disruption to other therapies and patients' sleep.

- Planning ahead to coordinate patient repositioning helps avoid unnecessary delays and interruptions that may affect the dignity of the patient.

- Privacy for the patient should be of paramount concern.

- Perform the bed bath promptly to prevent patient shivering.

- Use of a low-pH skin cleanser is recommended and no-rinse pH balanced cleansers is preferred to alkaline soaps where washing and then rinsing is required.[4]

- Normal shampoo can be used to wash the patient's hair; however, hair caps and washing products are available that are easier to use for patients in bed.

- Facial hair should be managed as per the patient's normal routine, such as maintaining a beard or shaving.

- Ears should be gently inspected for debris or injury.

- Clean nails should be maintained. Care should be taken if nails require trimming, especially if the patient has brittle nails or is diabetic.

Practice tips

Personal grooming is a factor in how we see ourselves and how others identify with us. With the many changes that come with illness and therapies applied in critical care, it is important to keep the patient's 'look' as normal as possible – simple things such as styling hair or trimming beards – if not for the patients themselves, who might be unaware, then for their families. Referring to a recent photo of the patient prior to their illness is an easy way to get this right.

Privacy is of paramount importance for the patient, especially when managing personal and hygiene care. Unit/team practices where the privacy of closed doors or curtains of patient bedsides are respected and not breached are helpful.

Impaired skin integrity

Managing skin integrity for patients is another essential part of nursing care. The processes used: screening patients for risk factors, assessing skin condition and current risks, prevention strategies, determining type of conditions, implementing treatments and monitoring effectiveness are similar for all patients.[5] This section will relate these processes to the critically ill patient, with some of their particular risk factors and prevention strategies employed. Impaired skin integrity in the critically ill patient encompasses a number of conditions; pressure injuries, moisture–associate skin damage (MASD), medical adhesive-related skin injuries (MARSI) and skin tears. Information about each of these conditions is provided.

Pressure injury

The terms 'pressure injury' and 'pressure ulcer' are both commonly used depending upon local terminology. The majority of pressure injuries are considered preventable hospital adverse events.[5] The risk of developing a pressure injury is considerably greater in intensive care patients compared with other hospitalised patients. An international point prevalence study found a pressure injury rate of 26%, of which 16.2% were ICU aquired.[6] The most-prominent pressure injury sites were the sacrum at 37% and heels at 19.5%.[6] Pressure injury can develop from pressure damage at skin level deteriorating through to deeper tissue, or to pressure damage at soft tissue layers rising to skin surface.[7] Pressure injury risk for critically ill patients can be attributed to their relative immobility, lack of sensory protective mechanisms, suboptimal tissue perfusion and oxygenation, and environmental factors that cause pressure and friction.[5] Significant risk factors include age, number of days since admission, anaemia, need for vasoactive medication or cardiovascular mechanical support,[7,8] and subsequent risk from medical devices, malnutrition and delays in the use of pressure-relieving mattresses and other prevention strategies[5] and the additional impact of the presence of multiple risk factors concurrently in critically ill patients.[8] The commonest locations for pressure injuries in critical care are the sacrum, the heels and the head.[8]

Pressure injury risk assessment, using the designated facility tool to identify at-risk patients, should be undertaken as soon as possible after the patient's admission.[5] There are many pressure injury risk assessment tools available such as the Braden score, the Conscious level-Mobility-Haemodynamics-Oxygenation-Nutrition (COMHON) index and the Critical Care Pressure Ulcer Assessment Tool Made Easy (CALCULATE).[9,10] The latter two were designed specifically for use in intensive care patients and they identify many factors that need to be considered and monitored prior to and during procedures for pressure injury prevention[9] and specific physiological risks in the critically ill patient.[10] A comprehensive head-to-toe skin assessment for pressure should be completed at least daily, particularly examining any sites at risk due to patient position or therapy. At the same time, review the effectiveness of any in use pressure-relieving devices. Skin should be inspected at each episode of patient repositioning. Skin assessment should include testing for blanching response and checking for areas of oedema, induration, redness or localised heat.[5] Pressure injury prevention practices include the use of alternating pressure-relief mattresses, low-pressure mattresses and air-flow mattresses. For bariatric patients (usually those heavier than 150 kg), specialist beds and mattresses are best used.[5] Optimising the functions of the mattress surface or system and bed-positioning options enhance effective management.

Intensive care patients are at risk of pressure injuries and injury from medical devices in common ICU use, such as endotracheal tubes (ETTs), nasogastric tubes and non-invasive ventilation masks (Table 5.3).[11] Detailed and frequent observation of the patient, the patient's position and the presence and location of equipment is required to prevent skin damage.[12] It is imperative to choose the correct size of the device for the patient, and cushion and protect the skin with dressings without applying additional pressure where appropriate. Inspect the skin in contact with the device regularly and be aware of the presence of oedema under devices and the potential for skin injury. It is also important to remove aids such as compression stockings and cervical collars to assess the skin. Vulnerable patients, such as those with poor tissue perfusion, anaemia, oedema, diaphoresis and poor sensory perception, can develop pressure injuries relatively quickly. These very same conditions may impede healing of pressure injuries, so prevention is always paramount. Even in the most critically unstable patients, prevention of pressure injuries caused by equipment is entirely avoidable. Regular repositioning of patients unable to move themselves is a fundamental practice undertaken by nurses to assist in the prevention of pressure injuries. All patients, including those who are unstable, may benefit for comfort and pressure prevention from frequent mini-movements or minor repositioning by using bed features to adjust angles when patients themselves can't be turned.

Prone positioning, recently used more frequently in the treatment of patients with respiratory failure from COVID-19 virus, has highlighted the gaps in effective pressure injury prevention for this therapy.[12] Table 5.4 outlines the type and cause of potential skin damage related to prone positioning. Things to consider are the securement of medical devices where oedema may occur, such as endotracheal tubes and facial oedema and the sheer and friction effects from mattresses and linen and gravitational pull from bed position changes.[12]

All pressure points and any pressure injuries should be examined closely and monitored frequently as the critically ill patient transitions through risks associated with their changing condition and treatments (e.g. dehydration, peripheral ischaemia, fluid therapy, vasopressors, renal failure, oedema). The key areas of monitoring are identified in Table 5.5. It is important to use standardised methods to objectively assess pressure injuries and their response to therapy. If a patient develops one pressure injury, there is a high likelihood another could develop. Nursing intervention includes the placing of patients in positions that avoid pressure on the affected area(s), positioning the patient securely to prevent sheer injury, and employing measures such as good fluid management to improve tissue perfusion, using a more protective mattress system, reducing the risk of infection and promoting tissue granulation with the use of appropriate dressings. The use of prophylactic layered silicone foam dressings has been shown to have a positive impact in reducing sacral pressure injury incidence in critically ill patients.[11,13] Similar foam dressing used on heels[13] and 'off-loading' of heels are recommended.[12]

TABLE 5.3

Risk of pressure injuries from commonly used equipment

RISK FACTOR	COMMENTS
Endotracheal tubes	The ETT should be repositioned from one corner of the mouth to the other on a daily basis to prevent pressure on the same area of oral mucosa and lips. Care should also be taken when positioning and tying ETT tapes: friction burns may be caused if they are not secure; pressure sores may be caused if they are too tight (particularly above the ears and in the nape of the neck). Moist tapes exacerbate problems and harbour bacteria.
Oxygen saturation probes	Repositioning of oxygen saturation probes 1–2-hourly prevents pressure on potentially poorly perfused skin. If using ear probes, these must be positioned on the lobe of the ear and not on the cartilage, as this area is very vulnerable to pressure and heat injury.
Blood pressure cuffs	Non-invasive blood pressure cuffs should be regularly reattached and repositioned. If left in position without reattachment for long periods of time, they can cause friction and pressure damage to skin. Care should be taken to ensure that tubing is not caught under the patient, especially after repositioning.
Urinary catheters, central lines and wound drainage	The patient should be checked often to ensure that invasive lines are not trapped under the patient. In addition to causing skin injury, they may function ineffectively.
Bed frame or bed accessories	Limbs should not press against bed frames or bed accessories such as transport tables, bed rails or bed cradles; good positioning prevents this but pillows should be used if the patient's position or size makes this likely.
Oxygen masks	Use correct-sized mask and hydrocolloid protective dressing on the bridge of the nose to assist with prevention of pressure from non-invasive or CPAP masks, especially when these are in constant or frequent use.
Splints, traction and cervical collars	Devices such as leg/foot splints, traction and cervical collars can all cause direct pressure when in constant use and friction injury if they are not fitted properly. ICU patients often have rapid body mass loss (especially muscle) following admission, so daily assessment is required.

CPAP = continuous positive airway pressure; ETT = endotracheal tube.

TABLE 5.4

Skin damage and prone positioning

TYPE OF SKIN DAMAGE	CONTRIBUTING FACTORS
• High risk of PI development • Facial PI/MASD • Oral PI/mucosal/medical/device injury • Pelvic PI/MASD/medical device injury • Skin tears	• Patient immobile for extended time • Body weight on bony areas with soft tissue or in presence of facial oedema, e.g. chin, forehead and ears. • Moisture from oral/pharyngeal/respiratory secretions related to endotracheal tubes • Bony areas, moisture in lower abdominal and pelvic skin folds, urinary catheter malpositioning • Mechanical injury from positioning

MASD = moisture-associate skin damage; PI = pressure injury.

Source: Adapted from Fourie A, Ahtiala, M, Black J, et al. Skin damage prevention in the prone ventilated critically ill patient: A comprehensive review and gap analysis (PRONEtect study). Journal of Tissue Viability, 2021;30:466-477.

TABLE 5.5

Monitoring pressure injuries

FACTOR	ACTIONS
Size	• Measure length, width and depth.
Stage/grading	• Use a standardised measure to grade the injury.
PI status	• Note the absence/presence/location of PIs on admission and discharge. • Keep a record of nursing interventions and treatments used to treat PIs.
Treatment	• Monitor response to therapy by assessing the size and stage/grade of the PI on a daily basis and use of photos with permission.
Observing other at-risk sites	• Dependent areas of the body are susceptible: sacrum, heels, back of the head, hips, shoulders, elbows, knees. • Areas of the body where equipment is causing pressure are susceptible: nose, ears, corners of the mouth, fingertips. • Areas of the body where tissue perfusion is poor are susceptible: extremities.

PI = pressure injury.

The International Pressure Ulcer Classification System[5] is summarised as follows:

- stage I: non-blanchable redness of intact skin (dark pigmented skin may not blanch but differ from surrounding area)
- stage II: partial thickness skin loss or blister (not skin tear, dermatitis, excoriation)
- stage III: full-thickness skin loss (subcutaneous fat may be visible)
- stage IV: full-thickness tissue loss (muscle/bone visible)
- unstageable pressure injury: depth unknown
- suspected deep tissue injury: depth unknown
- mucosal injury.[13]

Skin injuries are differentiated from mucosal injuries. Mucosal pressure injuries are defined as injuries found on mucous membranes with a history of a medical device in use at the location of the injury.[13] Ventilated patients in ICU are at significant risk of medical device-related mucosal pressure injury from endotracheal tubes and enteral tubes. Beyond presence of medical devices, some other risk factors for mucosal pressure injury are dry mucosa, oedema, friction, poor sensory perceptions, low body mass index, anaemia, low blood albumin and vasoactive medications.[13] Staging of mucosal injuries can be done via the Reaper Oral Mucosa Pressure Injury Scale (ROMPIS).[13]

> **Practice tip**
>
> It is worthwhile knowing the key features of the beds and mattresses commonly used in your area so that you can use them effectively to match patient requirements for bed functions, bed type (e.g. bariatric suitability) and pressure prevention (e.g. high-, medium- or low-risk mattress systems).

Moisture-associated skin damage (MASD)

MASD is an umbrella term for skin damage due to excess moisture or prolonged exposure to moisture. This includes: peristomal dermatitis, where healthy skin around the stoma is exposed to stomal effluent; peri-wound dermatitis, where healthy skin surrounding a wound is exposed to wound exudate; intertriginous dermatitis, where sweat trapped in skin folds (e.g. under the breasts, in the armpits or under the abdominal pannus) causes skin inflammation; and incontinence-associated dermatitis (IAD), where the skin has prolonged exposure to urine, stool or both.[14] A point-prevalence study across 23 Norwegian ICUs found occurrence of MASD (not IAD) to be 9%, the predominant site of MASD being the pelvic area.[15]

Incontinence-associated dermatitis (IAD)

IAD, a type of MASD, is a preventable skin condition that occurs when the skin has prolonged or repeated exposure to urine, stool or both. It is characterised by patchy or consolidated inflammation of the epidermis, observed as erythema. Repeated exposure to the irritants results in denudation of the skin's superficial layers, which may present as erosion with vesicles or bullae and clear exudates.[16] The patient may experience itching or burning sensations and often severe pain.[14] Complications of IAD include increased risk of developing an associated pressure injury or a perineal skin infection.[14] It is recognised that IAD development is influenced by the type of incontinence, with the presence of frequent liquid faeces placing a patient at the highest risk.[14] The potential for faecal incontinence in the ICU is high, with significant risk and occurrence of IAD.[15] Prevention and treatment of IAD involves removing or reducing skin exposure to urine and faeces, or both, and management of urinary and faecal incontinence is described later in this chapter.[15] Prevention and management of IAD should include a skin protection product designed to form a barrier between the skin and the irritant. Although prevention and treatment regimens include cleansing and protection, treatment may also require the management of a possible skin infection.[14]

Medical adhesive-related skin injuries (MARSI)

Medical adhesives are used commonly in the intensive care setting, yet patient skin injuries caused by medical adhesive remain an overlooked and underestimated problem, according to Hitchcock and colleagues.[17] Skin injury occurs when skin to adhesive attachment is stronger than the skin cell to skin cell attachment, causing the epidermal layers to separate or complete separation of the epidermis from the dermis.[17] This can be categorised into three types: mechanical, dermatitis and other. Skin stripping, tension injuries or blisters and skin tears are of the mechanical type. Dermatitis is irritant contact or allergic dermatitis, while maceration or folliculitis fall into the other type.[17] A history of patient allergies and sensitivities should be obtained and documented. The skin underneath adhesives should be assessed at least daily for evidence of damage, and a comprehensive assessment performed to determine injury severity. Prevention of MARSI includes identification of at-risk patients, for example older adult critically ill patients, and patients with dermatological conditions, gross oedema, malnutrition or dehydration. Care of these patients includes the use of gentler adhesives, barrier products and medical adhesive removers.[17]

Skin tears

Skin tears result from routine activities such as dressing, positioning and transferring.[18] At greatest risk are dependent patients who require total care, older adults, those with fragile skin (particularly those with a history of previous skin tears), those who require the use of devices to assist lifting, those who are cognitively or sensorially impaired and those who have skin problems such as oedema, purpura or ecchymosis. Most skin tears occur on the upper and lower limbs, with the back of hands a prime site. The International Skin Tear Advisory Panel (ISTAP) classification system[18] uses three categories to describe skin tears: type 1 is no skin/flap loss, type 2 is partial skin/flap loss and type 3 is total skin/flap loss.[19] As defined by Van Tiggelen and colleagues,[19] a flap in skin tears is a portion of the skin (epidermis/dermis) that is unintentionally separated partially or fully from its original place due to shear, friction and/or blunt force. Further, it is noted that this flap is not to be confused with skin-grafting surgical flaps.[19]

Skin tears can be prevented by careful handling of patients to reduce skin friction and shear during repositioning and transfers. Padded bed rails, pillows and blankets can be used to protect and support arms and legs. Paper-type or non-adherent dressings should be used on frail skin and should be removed gently and slowly. Wraps or nets can be used instead of surgical tape to secure dressings and drains in place. Application of a moisturising

TABLE 5.6
Treatment of skin tears

FACTOR	INTERVENTIONS
Control bleeding	• Apply gentle pressure and elevate limb to control initial bleeding from skin tear.
Cleansing	• Gently clean skin with saline or non-toxic wound cleaner. • Allow to dry or pat dry carefully.
Skin flap	• Very carefully debride *only* necrotic tissue. • Re-align the skin tear flap if present, back into place as closely as possible, using a gloved finger, dampened cotton tip or forceps.
Dressing	• Provide appropriate wound dressing according to wound bed condition: dry, moist, inflamed or exudate. • Secure non-adherent dressing with a light wrap or tubular non-adhesive wrap. • Limit dressing changes to accessed need or the manufacturer's recommendations. • Remove any product with an adhesive backing with utmost care to avoid further trauma.
Monitor	• Record details of skin tear, describe or photograph wound, record details of dressings and implementation of measures to reduce the risk of further occurrences.

lotion to dry skin helps to keep it adequately hydrated. Treatment of skin tears is outlined in Table 5.6.[18] The focus of nursing care should be on careful cleansing and protection of the skin tear so as to prevent further damage and documentation of interventions and healing progress.

> **Practice tip**
>
> Monitor any bruising regularly, as these areas may be at risk of developing skin tears.

Eye care

The eyes are one of the most sensitive parts of the human body, and careful eye assessment and eye care in critically ill patients are important because many of the mechanisms normally involved in protecting the eye from infection and injury are compromised.[20] When patients are critically ill, mainly four types of injuries are found: exposure keratopathy (including dry eyes), chemosis (conjunctival swelling), microbial conjunctivitis and keratitis, and direct injury to the cornea. These types can occur separately, but can also be related to each other and present at the same time.[21,22]

The ability to produce tears, to blink and to close the eyes with rest or sleep is essential for protecting and keeping the eyes healthy. Exposure keratopathy is defined as corneal damage from prolonged exposure to the external environment,[23] and dry eye syndrome (DES) is a multifactorial disease caused by inadequate tear production and/or the fast evaporation of tears.[21] Both conditions adversely affect the eye's protective mechanisms and may result in complications, such as keratopathy, inflammatory diseases in the cornea and, in the worst case, ulcerations and perforations. All of these complications are painful and affect the patient's quality of life.[21] The extent of DES is influenced by both intrinsic and extrinsic factors. Intrinsic factors could be hormonal imbalance, autoimmune diseases (rheumatoid arthritis, lupus, myasthenia gravis, Sjögren's syndrome), systemic diseases (stroke, hyperlipidaemia, diabetes mellitus, systemic arterial hypertension) and infections such as HIV and hepatitis.[21] Patients who are exposed to extrinsic factors, such as high flows of air/oxygen and continuous positive airway pressure (CPAP) systems, may be at risk of DES. Other factors for patients in the ICU that can precede the occurrence of DES are the presence of drugs (diuretics, beta-blockers, antidepressants, antihistamines, anxiolytics and eye drops for glaucoma), the incomplete or defective closure of the eyelids (lagophthalmia), sedation, insufficient blinking periodicity, length of admission, frequent use of health technological devices, use of mechanical ventilation (MV) and environmental factors such as low humidity and colder temperatures.[21]

Conjunctival oedema (chemosis), or 'ventilator eye', is a common problem in the ICU because it inhibits eyelid closure and proper blinking responses.[22,23] Chemosis is common in patients who are ventilated, those who are in prone position and those with generalised oedema. Incomplete eyelid closure can also predispose patients to chemosis. Conjunctival oedema can lead to subconjunctival haemorrhage, and it is also associated with positive pressure ventilation, positive end-expiratory pressure (PEEP), fluid overload and systemic inflammatory response syndromes.[22,23]

Infections

Serious infections with bacteria can progress rapidly, resulting in blindness if not treated promptly.[24] A majority of ventilated patients are colonised by at least one abnormal bacterial species and are at risk of infections such as microbial conjunctivitis and/or keratitis.[22] *Pseudomonas aeruginosa*, *Acinetobacter* species and *Staphylococcus epidermidis* are some examples of isolated organisms that might be found in critically ill patients' eyes.[25,26] These infections are thought to occur from respiratory secretions, for example from direct contact with the tracheal suction catheter.[24]

Microbial keratitis occurs when there is a defect in the cornea that becomes infected, and the eye will be sticky and usually red. The cause is usually bacterial, but herpes simplex keratitis may be present in immunosuppressed patients in intensive care.[24]

Direct injury to the cornea

Corneal abrasion is a superficial scratch that removes the surface epithelium, causing the eye to become red. Corneal injury may occur in up to 10–20% of critically ill patients.[27,28] The risk of corneal abrasion or iatrogenic trauma is greatest when patients are unable to close their eyes spontaneously. Severe damage to the cornea can result in irreversible blindness, necessitating the need for a corneal transplant.[29] When the eyes are exposed, they are at greater risk of injury and infection. For the intensive care patient, who often has multiple intravenous lines, nasogastric tubes and ventilation tubes and their various connections, there is potential to unintentionally damage one of the eyes with one of these devices during position changes.[28]

Eye assessment

Eye assessment should be undertaken, and findings documented, as soon as possible after admission and thereafter at least every 12 hours, even for conscious patients who are able to blink spontaneously.[29] Patients should be checked if they wear contact lenses, and if the lenses are in situ they should be removed in order to reduce the risk of corneal surface infections. If a patient normally wears glasses, it should be documented, and if the glasses are present but not being used, they should be labelled and stored safely.

The general principles of eye assessments are shown in Table 5.7, including a full examination of the eye's external structure, colour and response. A flashlight can be used to inspect if the eyelids are closed because small openings can otherwise be hidden by the eyelashes. Various assessment tools have been developed for this purpose; however, a universally accepted protocol for the protection of eyes in the ICU does not exist. Thorough eye assessment should assess appearance (which may provide indications of disease or trauma) and physical and neurological functions. When a red eye is identified, with or without exudate, bilateral swabs for cultures should be taken and an ophthalmologist referral should be completed.[22]

If there is concern about any aspect of a patient's eyes, medical staff must be informed and ophthalmic help sought. Conjunctivitis in the ICU setting is usually bacterial and can be highly infectious and virulent.[22] Without due care, it can spread to other patients and staff. Note that if the eye is very red but not sticky this might not indicate conjunctivitis and referral for assessment should be made to an ophthalmologist.[22]

Essential eye care

The goals of eye care are to provide comfort and protect the eyes from injury and infection. The recommendation is to implement an eye care protocol, as it has been found to reduce the incidence of corneal injury[22,27] and positively impact patients' rehabilitation and quality of life after intensive care.[29] Great care should be taken with hand hygiene. The general consensus is that eye care should be performed under sterile conditions, cleansing the eye from the outside towards the nose, usually with saline or sterile

TABLE 5.7
Assessment of the eyes

EXTERNAL STRUCTURE	COLOUR	REACTION
• Is it bulging or misshapen? • Is the pupil circular? • What size are the pupils? • Are both pupils the same size? • Is the pupil clear? • Is there any visible trauma? • Is it weeping? • Does it look dry or moist?	• Is the sclera its normal off-white colour or is there evidence of jaundice or haemorrhage? • Does it look red and inflamed?	• Is the blink reflex present? • Do both pupils react to light with equal speed? • Is there a composite reaction to light in the opposite eye?

water and gauze, twice daily or more if needed. However, eye care regimens have not been rigorously researched. Cotton wool is not recommended because of the presence of particulates that may cause corneal abrasions.

Eye care and the administration of artificial tears should be provided as required if the patient complains of sore or dry eyes or if there is visible evidence of encrustation. If a patient is receiving high-flow oxygen therapy via a mask, they may benefit from regular 4-hourly administration of artificial tears or artificial tear ointment to lubricate the eyes; this may be unnecessary while they are sleeping. Regular scheduled eye care with an ocular lubricant is used to reduce the potential for corneal abrasions or subsequent corneal ulceration or infection. Ointments are preferred over eye drops as they remain on the ocular surface for a longer period of time.[29] An evidence-based eye care guideline for critically ill patients is outlined in Table 5.8.[30] Further recommendations relate to regular monitoring, reporting and timely referral if ophthalmological complications develop.

Eye drops or ointments should be administered gently, inserting the drop in the uppermost part of the opened eye and as close to the eye as possible without touching it. Sometimes eye drops can sting, so it is advisable to warn the patient of this possibility. In patients who are unable to close their eyes, for example if they are either paralysed or heavily sedated, most research states that eye closure be maintained by polyethylene covers and artificial tear drops at first hand.[31–33] An alternative to keeping the eyes closed is applying a wide piece of adhesive tape horizontally to the upper part of the eyelid. If taping is required, ointment should first be applied to the eye.[29] However, the use of tape may be inappropriate for patients whose skin is very fragile. Soft, extended-wear contact lenses composed of fluorosilicone hydrogel, so called bandage contact lenses (BCL), might be another way to protect corneal damage in critically ill patients with dry eyes. One pilot study suggested that the use of BCLs and punctal plugs was more effective in preventing worsening of corneal damage compared with standard eye care with ocular lubricants in mechanically ventilated and sedated critically ill patients.[34] Further research is needed, however, before this method can be recommended.

TABLE 5.8
Eye care in the critically ill

Assessment	• Patients must be assessed for risk factors for iatrogenic eye complications. • Daily assessment of the ability of the patient to maintain eyelid closure. • Weekly assessment of iatrogenic eye complication (at the microepithelial level) using instillation or fluorescein or a cobalt blue pen torch.
Management	• Eyelid closure should be maintained either passively or mechanically. • All patients who cannot achieve eyelid closure should receive 2-hourly eye care. • Eye care should be cleaning with saline-soaked gauze and administration of an eye-specific lubricant.

Source: Adapted from Marshall A, Elliott R, Rolls K, et al. Eye care in the critically ill: clinical practice guideline. Aust Crit Care 2008;21(2);97–109, with permission.[30]

Practice tip

A source of irritant to the eyes can be the constant air flow from air-conditioning vents or fans, making it vital for you to check that your at-risk patient is not positioned directly in line with these vents or fans.

Inform the patient that blurred vision may occur temporarily. Inform relatives of the reason in cases where the eye needs to be plasticised/taped/covered.

Oral hygiene

Oral care aims to ensure healthy oral mucosa, prevent halitosis, maintain a clean and moist oral cavity, prevent pressure sores from devices such as ETTs,[35] prevent trauma caused by teeth grinding or biting of the tongue and reduce bacterial activity that can lead to local and systemic infections such as ventilator-associated pneumonia (VAP).[36] Keeping the mucosa moist is the basic rule for oral care. Oral care requires time, preparation and competence.

Preparation

Oral care for a non-intubated, conscious patient with a healthy mouth generally involves daily observation of the mucosa and tooth brushing twice a day. Oral care should generally be performed every 2 hours on unconscious patients, although the evidence is inconclusive and the recommended frequency ranges from every 2 to every 12 hours. If the mouth is unhealthy, it may be necessary to provide oral hygiene even more frequently. Performing oral care in MV adults is a complex procedure. It is painfully discomforting and emotionally distressing for the patient, and it is difficult for the staff.[37,38]

A correct assessment is important and, therefore, an established assessment tool should be used. See Box 5.1 for characteristics of a healthy mouth. Making an assessment when the patient is in a prone position (PP) is difficult, while the risks of, for example, pressure ulcers in the mouth are greater.[39]

The procedure requires the right equipment and a good light source available. Good hand hygiene and a visor should be maintained throughout the procedure. The basic method for oral care is to use a soft toothbrush and non-irritant fluoride toothpaste (even for intubated patients) to remove plaque, which will assist with gum care as well as cleaning the teeth.[40,41] Dental plaque contains pathogens that can be harmful, so need to be removed regularly.[42] Brush the teeth, tongue and ETT if present twice daily for a minimum of two minutes. If the patient has a bone-anchored bridge, extra careful brushing in the gap between the jawbone and the tooth to prevent infection in the jawbone is essential. The oral cavity needs to be rinsed with sterile water, as toothpaste dries the oral mucosa.

Some kind of suction, such as a suction toothbrush or ordinary suction, while the teeth are being brushed should be used. Between brushings, a swab is recommended for cleaning and moistening the oral cavity every 2–4 hours. If oral foam head swabs are used, the manufacturers' recommendations should be followed.[43]

It has been debated, but not yet fully explored, if and to what degree surfactant sodium lauryl sulfate (SLS), which is found in many toothpastes, interferes with chlorhexidine.[44] Choose a toothpaste without SLS to prevent a reduced effect of chlorhexidine.[45] It is important to be aware that some toothpastes can also contain small amounts of allergens, such as milk proteins and eggs, which could be problematic for some patients. Ensuring that all toothpaste is rinsed away properly can also assist with keeping the oral mucosa moistened. Toothbrushes are frequently contaminated with potentially pathogenic bacteria and need to be cleaned properly by rinsing them under hot running water.[46] Using mouth swabs only for oral hygiene is ineffective. Toothbrushes perform substantially better than foam swabs in removing plaque. Thirst is one of the most distressing symptoms critically ill patients suffer from, and it does not disappear after oral care and must be frequently assessed and treated.[47,48] Regular sips of fluid or mouth washing with water is recommended. Immunosuppressed patients or those on high-dose antibiotics may also require antifungal treatment to treat oral thrush.

CHG mouthwashes have long been, and are still, used as a part of the oral hygiene care to prevent VAP in critically ill adult patients who are receiving MV.[41,49] Chlorhexidine may induce bacterial resistance,[50] hypersensitivity[51] and in high concentrations tooth discoloration and mucosal ulcerations, so caution must be taken when using it.[52] The extent to which chlorhexidine is beneficial for patient outcomes is not clear and requires further investigation, as recent studies found only moderate evidence of significant effects.[53–56]

BOX 5.1

Characteristics of a healthy mouth

- Pink moist oral mucosa and gums; absence of coating, redness, ulceration or bleeding
- Pink, moist tongue; no coating, cracking, blisters or areas of redness
- Clean teeth/dentures; free of debris, plaque and dental caries
- Well-fitting dentures
- Adequate salivation
- Smooth and moist lips; no cracking, bleeding or ulceration
- No difficulties eating or swallowing

Practice tips

If patients object to the taste of the CHG mouthwash, consider a follow-up rinse of water.

Performing oral hygiene with toothbrush and toothpaste in an intubated patient and ensuring the mouth is rinsed well may be assisted by the use of a dental sucker, which is flexible. This disposable device attached to a continuous suction system can be positioned in the mouth to aid in the continual removal of fluids while brushing and rinsing is performed.

Patient positioning and mobilisation in the ICU

Positioning and mobilising patients correctly, at the right time and at appropriate intervals, have long been considered as important for critically ill patients. Research has shown that a critical illness, combined with immobility, increases the risk of pressure injuries, venous thromboembolism (VTE) and pulmonary dysfunction.[57–59] Some recent studies have indicated that early mobilisation (EM) and rehabilitation may also have a positive effect on other healthcare areas, such as ICU length of stay (LoS), time spent on mechanical ventilation, health status and ICU delirium increasing the interest in EM in the ICU.[59–65] However, at present, randomised trials demonstrate mixed results regarding these outcomes.[59,60,64,66–68] Furthermore, the definition of 'early' is debated in the literature.[69,70] One definition of EM is operationalised as 'positioning and early mobilisation in prophylaxis or therapy of pulmonary disorders' within 72 hours of admission to an ICU.[69] This refers to the implementation of a physiotherapy program (passive mobilisation, active mobilisation and respiratory muscle training) or new mobilisation techniques (ergometry cycle or neuromuscular electrical stimulation) at an early stage of a patient's stay at the hospital.[71] This means that the optimal timing, type and duration of the activities and interventions have still not been fully investigated.[70]

In this section, why, how and when repositioning and/or activity should be performed in the ICU are discussed.

Immobility in the ICU

Many patients who are cared for in the ICU move to a limited extent, or not at all, on their own. One study found that patients recovering from critical illnesses spend less than 5% of the day being physically active.[72] There are many reasons for immobility, however. Unstable patients whose status is compromised when they are moved, patients who are in critical care for a long time, older adults and frail or malnourished patients and patients who are unable to move themselves (e.g. due to sedation, trauma, surgery or obesity) are all at risk of immobility. Even previously fit patients who experience critical illnesses can develop severe limitations in their mobility in the ICU. There are many physiological risks associated with immobility in critically ill patients in the ICU. As mentioned earlier, pressure injuries, VTE and pulmonary dysfunction are three examples of complications related to physical inactivity.[57–59] ICU-acquired muscle weakness (ICUAW) – a loss of muscle mass in critically ill patients, caused by myopathy, polyneuropathy, or both, in the absence of another plausible aetiology – is another post-intensive care complication that may occur as early as a few hours from the onset of immobility.[73] The 'gold standard' for the diagnosis of ICUAW remains electromyography,[74] which measures muscle response or electrical activity in response to a nerve's stimulation of the muscle. Patients with multiple morbidities, prolonged

MVs, extended length of ICU stays (ICU-LoS), sepsis on admission, renal replacement therapies (RRT) and organ failure have an increased risk of developing ICUAW.[74] ICUAW may contribute to prolonged ventilation and longer ICU-LoS, as well as a delayed return to physical normality.[74]

Assessment of body positioning

Table 5.9 offers a simple guide to assessment, which includes visual and physical assessment of all limbs and joints. Provided there are no contraindications (see Table 5.10 for factors to consider), function should be stimulated by regular passive then active movements of all limbs and joints in order to maintain both flexibility and comfort.

A big challenge with mobilisation in the ICU is to know when, in what way and with what intensity a seriously ill patient should engage in physical activity.[70,75] It is known that everyday nursing bedside procedures such as patient position change may generate physiological changes in critically ill patients – for example, blood oxygen desaturation, ventilatory distress and hypotension.[76,77] However, recent reviews have concluded that mobilisation can be safely initiated in most patients on the first day of ICU admission and even during MV, administration of vasopressors and continuous renal replacement therapy (CRRT).[78,79] There are few reported adverse events associated with mobilisation in the ICU and, when there are, the events tend to be minor in nature.[78,80]

The key is, therefore, to individualise all physical activity and to understand and take into account the patient's physiological, as well as psychological, preferences before starting EM.[81] Two groups of safety factors need to be considered prior to mobilising the critically ill patient: those specific to the patients and their physical and physiological conditions and those extrinsic to the patients such as the environment, staffing and devices.[80,82] Cardiovascular stability, respiratory function, cerebral or spinal function, nausea and pain are all factors that influence the positioning of patients in critical care areas.[80] Other risk factors exist, such as age, ICU-LoS, use of adrenaline (epinephrine) and/or noradrenaline

---

TABLE 5.9

Musculoskeletal assessment

MUSCLES AND JOINTS	MOBILITY
• Power/strength • Range of movement • Symmetry • Tenderness and pain • Inflammation, swelling, wasting	• Degree of independence • Need for assistance • Adherence/compliance with physiotherapy/mobility regimen • Need for planned rest periods • Use of splints or collar

TABLE 5.10

Factors to consider when positioning patients

FACTOR	COMMENTS
Haemodynamic and cardiopulmonary responses	• Placing patients in the left lateral position can cause a (usually harmless) fall in oxygenation for a few minutes
Timing	• Position the patient to avoid clashes with treatment/ investigations such as chest physiotherapy or chest X-ray • Consider the need for the patient to rest
Method	• The need to use lifting devices • The availability of staff to perform a safe manoeuvre • The placement of pillows to support limbs, to facilitate both comfort and respiratory efficiency • Use of bed adjustments to create 'chair' positions to prepare patients to sit out of bed
Restrictions on positioning	• The need for spinal alignment • Cerebral injury • Haemodynamic instability • Respiratory compromise • Access to devices for therapies • Body size

(norepinephrine) infusions, and comorbidities such as cardiovascular disease and diabetes. Regular musculoskeletal assessment should be done, focusing on the patient's major muscles and joints and the degrees of mobility. A physiotherapist's knowledge and advice should be sought regarding the correct range of movement (ROM) and the frequency of passive exercises. This is particularly important for burn injury patients. The patient's pain and the location and extent of the burn injury affect how and when mobilisation can be done.[83,84] In terms of equipment safety, it is important to consider any weight restrictions of the equipment, the physical space available for patient mobilisation, the number of available staff and infection control considerations (need for protective equipment).[81] Checking that all devices are set up to accommodate the repositioning before anyone begins to move the patient is also an important preliminary step.

The psychological preferences of the patient are more difficult to assess and, hence, more difficult to respond to. Patient participation, cooperation and a trust between all involved are key concepts when it comes to EM.[85] When a patient can trust the healthcare team, it increases their motivation to change position and exercise. Many patients have reported that lying in bed for long periods is a painful experience both because of the primary injury or disease and because of the physical position they need to lie in.[86] This means that any type of mobilisation may take considerable effort, exhausting the patient quickly. Patients describe that they are frightened, especially during the first mobilisation attempts, but many also find mobilisation stimulating.[85–87] When the patient is ready to engage in active exercises, they must be carefully informed about how the procedure works and what is expected of them. The patient also needs to be assured that the staff members are used to the task and that everything is well prepared.[86] Family members should be involved if possible.[85]

Mobilisation in the ICU

Given the potential complications of immobilisation, activity and/or repositioning in any form and as early as possible is of importance for all critically ill patients in the ICU. Mobilisation for a critically ill patient can be described as a graduated increase in a range of activities from positioning, through passive movements, sitting upright in bed, sitting in a chair to actually ambulating. Furthermore, mobilisation can be divided into passive and active exercises. Passive exercises are performed when patients are either too weak or incapable of active exercise. Active exercises are those that can be performed by the patient with no, or minimal, assistance – for example, resistive ROM exercises, sitting on a bed or chair, bed exercises (e.g. cycling), dangling, transfers or tilting up. For an extensive discussion of approaches to mobilising within and beyond the ICU, see Chapter 8.

Position changes and passive exercise

Positioning a patient and employing passive exercises regularly are important nursing activities. Positioning a patient aims to achieve maximum comfort, therapeutic benefit and pressure area relief. Positioning and repositioning (1) promote comfort, relaxation and rest, (2) help inflate the lungs, (3) improve oxygenation and help mobilise airway secretions, (4) orient the patient to their surroundings and for a change of view and (5) improve circulation to the limbs. Position changes can be made with the help of advanced beds or mattresses, or manually with the help of healthcare professionals. There are pressure-relieving mattresses that can be adjusted according to the patient's comfort and needs. The mattress type is chosen based on the patient's physique and weight, whether the patient can move independently and whether pressure ulcers have already developed. Furthermore, new materials and types of positioning equipment are constantly being developed – for example, pillows filled with a viscous fluid mix that can be moulded by hand to adjust to the body of each patient.[88]

Provided there are no specific contraindications, an immobile patient should be positioned at the head of bed (HOB) raised by 30 degrees semirecumbent or more, as research has demonstrated that it helps reduce VAP.[89] The routine standard for immobilised patients in the ICU is

2–3-hourly body repositionings, although the optimal interval for turning critically ill patients is unknown. Patients at high risk of developing a pressure ulcer should, if possible, be assisted with a change of position more often than that. Passive exercises may improve functional exercise capacity, perceived functional status and quadriceps muscle strength and decrease pain scores.[71] Passive exercises put the main joints through their ROM, which helps reduce joint stiffness and maintains muscle integrity, preventing contractures. Shoulders, hands, hips and ankles are particularly at risk of stiffness and muscle contracture. It is important, however, to ensure that joints and muscles are not overstretched, as this is painful for patients and can cause permanent injury. Splints may be used when the patient is resting to keep joints in a neutral passive position. See Chapter 8 for discussion of active mobilisation.

Mobilisation in neurological ICUs

Concern has been expressed about both passive and active EM in neurological ICUs.[90,91] Common diagnoses of patients admitted to the neurological ICU include acute ischaemic and haemorrhagic strokes, subdural hematomas, subarachnoid or intracranial haemorrhages, hydrocephalus, status epilepticus, neuromuscular disorders, brain tumours and traumatic brain injuries. Here, consideration must be given to intracranial pressure (ICP) levels, altered motor control, reduced motor tone, and alterations in perception and cognition as nursing interventions such as repositioning may increase the risk of secondary insults.[77] Olkowski and Shah[91] recommended a safety checklist specific to EM in the neurological ICU before initiating mobilisation. The checklist involves factors to be considered before EM, such as diagnosis, external ventricular drain (EVD), ICP, ICU delirium and use of intravenous drugs. Further discussion of processes to ensure patient safety during mobilisation can be found in Chapter 8.

Practice tip

Movement of the lower legs, ankles and feet can be done in conjunction with a gentle massage or application of moisturiser. Family members may wish to undertake this, giving them an opportunity to provide the patient with care and touch.

Practice tip

Even small readjustments in positioning may improve patient comfort and often can be made without much effort by the nurse or disturbance to the resting patient. Most electric beds provide for adjustments to the backrest angle, knee bend and bed tilt, and adjustments can be easily made. In addition to comfort, these adjustments will aid in pressure changes between repositionings of the patient.

Prone position (PP)

PP is a highly recommended intervention for critically ill patients in the ICU with severe acute respiratory distress syndrome (ARDS).[92] The described length of PP varies, but PP for more than 16 hours has been found to have a positive impact on respiratory mechanics and gas exchange, potentially decreasing the risk of the development of ventilation-induced lung injury.[93,94] Positioning a seriously ill patient into and out of the PP is a resource-intensive measure that requires careful planning and an adequate number of care staff. Absolute contraindications to prone ventilation include patients with spinal instability or at risk of spinal instability, unstable fractures (especially facial and pelvic), anterior burns and open wounds, shock, pregnancy, recent tracheal surgery and elevated ICP. However, adverse events are rare in other patients.

Before the patient is turned to the PP, careful planning is required. All staff involved must have theoretical knowledge and practical skills about PP, and at least five staff members are needed for the procedure. A checklist, including the following elements, should be available to prevent anything significant being missed or overlooked: (a) optimise pain relief and sedation; (b) administer eye ointment and apply narrow tape horizontally over the eyes to keep them closed while patients are in PP; (c) check the endotracheal tub, fixation, cuff pressure, tube position, aspirate in the extra lumen, and change the inner cannula; (d) suction out the intubation tube and throat; (e) disconnect enteral nutrition and aspirate into the gastric tube; (f) check that the arterial line and other intravenous lines are well fixed, untangled and positioned appropriately for the move; (g) place the urinary catheter and its tube between the patient's knees, placing the container on the footboard; and (h) check that the ventilator hoses and other hoses are long enough during the entire turning step.[93] All hoses should be placed upwards, towards the head. The change of position itself can be carried out in different ways and will vary according to the team and equipment available.

Since patients have to lie in PP for many hours, the upper body must change position every 2 hours. To do this, both of the patient's arms should be placed down along the body. Then the patient's upper body should be lifted in the sheet with their head facing the other direction. Lastly, it is important to change the position of the arms, with the arm on the face side being up. Team communication and a coordinated approach is key in reducing complications associated with a significant move. Patients requiring PP often have cardiovascular and respiratory instability making the move more complex. If the team has knowledge and practical experience of PP and everything is carefully prepared, the measure is safe. Facial oedema and facial pressure ulcers are the most common adverse events; whereas enteral nutrition is generally well tolerated even during long-term PP.[95]

Rotational therapy

Continuous lateral rotation therapy or kinetic bed therapy is an intervention in which the patient is rotated continually on a specialised bed through a set number of degrees. This helps to relieve pressure areas and can significantly improve oxygenation. Continuous lateral rotation therapy may also reduce the prevalence of VAP in patients requiring long-term ventilation.[96–98] Most studies in this area are old and, therefore, a clear definition of the patient group that benefits from continuous lateral rotation therapy is still lacking.[98] Appropriate evaluation of the benefits and suitability of the patient for continuous lateral rotation therapy should be undertaken by the team, and the therapy should be implemented according to local protocols.

In summary, mobilisation in the ICU is a multiprofessional task involving physicians, physiotherapists, nurses and nurse assistants.[99] Rehabilitation and mobilisation, especially as part of the ABCDEF bundle[100] (A – Assess, prevent and manage pain; B – Both spontaneous awakening trials and spontaneous breathing trials; C – Choice of analgesia and sedation; D – assess, prevent, and manage Delirium; E – Early mobility and exercise; and F – Family engagement and empowerment) require team communication and coordination.[99] However, nurses are central figures, as they are present all hours of the day and should have an overall picture of the patients' conditions and daily form.

Venous thromboembolism (VTE) prophylaxis

Venous thromboembolism can be defined as deep vein thrombosis (DVT), pulmonary embolism (PE), or both, diagnosed after more than 24 hours after ICU admission and confirmed by ultrasound, CT or nuclear medicine imaging.[101] DVT and PE are separate conditions but are collectively referred to as venous VTE. Blood clots form in major veins of the lower body owing to poor venous flow, endothelial injury to the vein, trauma, venous stasis or coagulation disorders. VTE is a major risk factor for hospitalised patients in general and critically ill patients in particular. VTE ICU-related risk factors include sepsis, vasopressor use, central catheters, mechanical ventilators and respiratory, cardiac or renal failure.[102] Patients with VTE may also develop post-thrombotic syndrome, where tissue injury occurs leading to pain, paraesthesia, pruritus, oedema, venous dilatation and venous ulcers.[103] PEs occur when a part of a thrombosis moves through the circulatory systems and lodges in the lungs.

It is important to consider the individual patient (age, body mass index) and their history (previous VTE, coagulation disorders) along with their current condition, whether it be surgical or medical and features of their treatment (immobilisation) when determining the risks for VTE.[102] Both the risk assessment and the patient's current condition will determine the most appropriate VTE prophylaxis strategy.[102] Prophylaxis consists of a combination of pharmacological and mechanical interventions that may be used together or separately

depending on the level of risk for VTE and/or contraindications to particular therapies. However, the effects of combined therapies compared with either pharmacological therapy alone or compression therapy alone in the prevention of DVT are unclear.[104–106] More research in the area is needed. The National Safety and Quality Health Service (NSQHS) clinical practice guidelines for the prevention of VTE (DVT and PE) in patients admitted to Australian hospitals provides a comprehensive guide to the risks and management relating to VTE for critical care in Australia.[107]

Low-molecular-weight heparin or unfractionated heparin is the most common pharmacological therapy prescribed, while other medications could be prescribed for patients depending on individual factors.[101] Mechanical prophylaxis is provided through a range of graduated compression stockings and various pneumatic venous pump or sequential compression devices.[108,109] The compression stockings decrease the diameter of venous vessels, improve venous flow velocity, avoiding venous stasis, and overall improve venous return from the extremities to which they are applied. However, these effects are related to muscular activity of the limb and may be less efficacious in an immobile patient. Furthermore, poor fit and excessive compression can cause complications, such as skin marking, blistering, ulceration, pain, discomfort and peroneal palsy.[109] The intermittent pneumatic compression device (IPC) has fewer of these kinds of complications and is thereby preferred in comparison with graduated compression stockings. IPC helps prevent VTE in two ways. First, the compression accelerates blood forwards and facilitates venous emptying while decreasing stasis. Second, this increase in the arterial–venous pressure gradient also increases arterial blood flow and decreases peripheral vascular resistance.[109] Along with pharmacological and mechanical venous thromboembolism prophylaxis, maintaining patients' hydration and implementing early mobilisation are key components of care in preventing VTE.[101,110] Given the risks of VTE for critically ill patients, it is medically important that nurses contribute to lowering the risks by knowing the range of risk factors for their patients, along with the appropriate pharmacological prophylaxis that may be prescribed. It is also important to know how to appropriately implement and manage the mechanical prophylactic devices and, most importantly, to facilitate the EM of the patient.[111]

Bowel management

Supporting patients and monitoring and managing disruptions to normal bowel action is an essential nursing care function, but only part of the effect of critical illness on potential gastrointestinal dysfunction in intensive care, including abdominal distention, gastrointestinal bleeding, residual gastric volumes and intra-abdominal hypertension. This section will be addressing management of bowel actions. Maintaining good bowel care in the critically ill patient can have changing foci from promoting defecation to containing diarrhoea, as throughout critical illness the gut function, upper and lower motility and microbiota are influenced by changing therapies, medications, nutrition, hydration and mobility of the patient.[112] Ultimately, good bowel care promotes patient comfort and reduces the risks of associated problems such as nausea, vomiting and abdominal/pelvic discomfort. Enteral feeding is sometimes attributed as a cause of diarrhoea; however, poor gastric fluid intake causes constipation, and improved gut motility decreases the risk of aspiration and subsequent pneumonia. Early enteral nutrition is associated with improved outcomes and return to normal gut functioning.[112] Additional to the need to manage faecal incontinence, the two spectrums of constipation and diarrhoea are particular challenges for nurses to provide patient-specific, effective management in a sensitive and dignified way for their critically ill patient.

Often patients find bowel care to be awkward and embarrassing, and the routines that individuals may have developed, especially the older adult, to sustain effective bowel function in their daily lives are then interrupted by their illness, and their loss of control over their body for this function can be particularly distressing. Sensitive nursing care that respects the dignity of the patient is paramount.

Bowel assessment

Initial bowel assessment should be undertaken to determine the patient's usual bowel habits, as a daily bowel action is not common for most of the population. In general, older patients are more susceptible to constipation. Use of the neurogenic bowel dysfunction score may be helpful for assessment in relevant patients. As with other system assessments in intensive care, gut function should be assessed at the start of each nursing shift (Box 5.2). The use of a bowel protocol is common in intensive care. Protocols usually address both constipation and diarrhoea and may include rectal examination or testing for *Clostridium difficile*[113,114] and alternative therapies as determined from assessment and investigation results. Objective monitoring of the quality of faecal stools can be via tools such as the Bristol stool form scale, which uses a 7-point grading system to assess stool consistency (Table 5.11).[115] Establishing the cause of faecal incontinence is important, as this will direct the treatment

TABLE 5.11
Bristol stool form scale

GRADE	DESCRIPTION
0	No bowel movement
1	Separate hard lumps; like nuts; hard to pass
2	Sausage-shaped but lumpy
3	Like a sausage but with cracks on the surface
4	Like a sausage or snake but smooth and soft
5	Soft blobs with clear-cut edges; easily passed
6	Fluffy pieces with ragged edges; a mushy stool
7	Watery; no solid pieces; entirely liquid

Source: Lewis SJ, Heaton KW. Stool form scale as a useful guide to intestinal transit time. Scand J Gastroenterol 1997;32 (9):920–4.[115] Reprinted by permission of the publisher, Taylor & Francis Ltd, https://www.tandfonline.com.

and management plan. Faecal incontinence may occur in the presence of certain medications like antibiotics or sedatives, and in conditions such as neurological and spinal conditions, intestinal diseases such as Crohn's and cognitive impairment such as dementia, or may be the result of anal sphincter or rectal injury or dysfunction, or intestinal impaction and overflow.[116]

Practice tip

When undertaking bowel assessment consider the patient's normal diet and any laxatives or probiotics routinely taken, as this information may influence any bowel regimen developed for the patient.

Essential bowel care

Nursing care is based on providing privacy, managing patient embarrassment and providing therapies that promote effective gut function. Where bowel care is concerned, it is always appropriate to first explain to patients what is to be done, and to gain their consent if they are conscious. Constant reassurance is important so that patients feel safe and secure in the knowledge that their privacy will be maintained to the greatest degree possible.

Peristaltic movement of the gut is stimulated by exercise. Although difficult in the intensive care setting, many patients are awake, and even those who require sedation should be sedated with the minimal amount

BOX 5.2

Assessment of gut function

- Observation of nasogastric aspirate volume
- Visual inspection and palpation of abdomen, noting any tenderness, pain or distention
- Recording the frequency, nature and quantity of bowel actions
- The presence or absence of bowel sounds

necessary for their safety, enabling some degree of movement. Promoting patient mobility, especially voluntary movement, helps to improve gut motility.

Ensuring the appropriate administration of fluid and an adequate dietary fibre intake[117] helps to prevent constipation and maintain normal bowel function. Although enteral feeding increases faecal bulk and provides gastric fluid, which helps to maintain gut motility, Bishop and colleagues[118] found a higher rate of enteral nutrition was strongly associated with a looser type of stool. Choice of enteral formula is important, and Chapter 19 contains an in-depth discussion on the principles of enteral feeding.

The use of sedatives is often an ascribed cause of constipation in critically ill patients. This is not due to their direct effect, but rather to the subsequent immobility of patients when sedatives are used. Opiates, which are often used to control pain, slow propulsive gut contraction. The main drugs that cause constipation in critical care settings are analgesics, anaesthetic agents, anticonvulsants, diuretics and calcium channel blockers. Although it is difficult to avoid giving these drugs, their judicious use in tandem with other preventive measures will help avoid constipation. Laxatives, antiemetic and prokinetic agents can also be used in critical care patients and Bishop and colleagues[118] found the administration of ondansetron was a significant predictor of defecation on that day in their critical care patient cohort.

Constipation

Constipation is common in critically ill patients; its incidence varies from 20% to 83%.[119] Variations in incidence may be attributed to the lack of a consistent definition for constipation. Constipation is described as fewer than three bowel movements per week, incomplete evacuation, hard or difficult-to-pass stools or the requirement of manual faecal removal, according to the American Gastroenterological Association.[120]

Causes of constipation in critically ill patients range from shock and reduced gut motility to changes in nutrition and lack of mobility. The consequences of constipation in critically ill patients are not well defined but can include increased abdominal distention and resulting impedance of lung function, inability to establish adequate enteral nutrition and increased acquired bacterial infections.[120] The prevention of constipation is particularly important for patients with high cervical spinal injuries, as if left untreated it may cause potentially fatal autonomic dysreflexia.[121] De Azevedo and colleagues[117] discussed the need to determine whether constipation is a marker of severity and poor prognosis in critically ill patients or if it is a dysfunction contributing to a worsening clinical condition. However, the need for effective prevention and management of constipation in critically ill patients is clear.

Non-pharmacological methods to reduce constipation include exercise or moving, increasing fluid intake and adding dietary fibre.[112] These means should be implemented routinely before the need to use laxatives arises. There are many types of laxatives available, which can be given to prevent or treat constipation. Bulk-forming agents work by increasing faecal size; stimulants, such as senna, increase peristalsis; and osmotic agents draw fluid into the gut. A recent study on the use of a prophylactic laxative bowel regimen reported an increased risk of diarrhoea, but use didn't reduce risk of constipation.[119] Faecal impaction should be treated with enemas, not stimulant laxatives. Common bowel protocols indicate treatment of constipation, commencing with senna administration and progressing to lactulose if ineffective.[113]

Diarrhoea

Incidences of diarrhoea for intensive care patients are reported ranging from 3% to 78%.[119] In severe cases it may lead to electrolyte imbalances, dehydration, malnutrition (see also Chapter 19) and skin breakdown. Furthermore, it can be very distressing for the patient, who may also suffer from abdominal distention, nausea and cramp-like pain. Investigations should be implemented to determine the cause of the diarrhoea, and if the cause is infectious then the patient should be managed with appropriate precautions to prevent cross-contamination. If laxatives are being administered they should be stopped, and a stool specimen should be obtained for microbiological examination. Antimotility drugs may be used, except with bloody diarrhoea or proven infection with *E. coli*.[113] Appropriate rehydration should be implemented. If patients are being fed enterally, there may be a reduction in episodes of diarrhoea if fibre-enriched feed is used.[112]

Faecal containment devices, sometimes referred to as faecal diversion systems, or just rectal tubes or an anal pouch[122] and drainage system may be used in severe cases of diarrhoea when other control measures have failed and in conjunction with other measures to support the patient's comfort.[122,123] Broadly, indications for use of a faecal containment device are persistent incontinent diarrhoea, diagnosis of *C. difficile* infection, perianal wound or incontinence-associated dermatitis,[122] plus the patient must have anal sphincter tone to enable securement if using a balloon device.[122,123] Along with assessing patient suitability for using the incontinence system against the manufacturer's guidelines, it is vital that there is a careful review of any conditions or factors preventing safe use of the device for individual patients, such as allergy to the materials in the product, risk of autonomic dysreflexia in spinal cord injury patients, or rectal and anal conditions.[122,123] It is imperative that both medical and nursing consultation occurs, along with patient consent before use of such devices, as the potential for complications ranges from discomfort, dislodgement and re-insertions and balloon or device failure through to infection and rectal and bowel injuries. Faecal management devices and associated serious events of rectal mucosal ulceration, perforation and haemorrhage, or development of recto-urethral and ano-vaginal fistulas have been reported.[122–126] An appropriate bowel therapy regimen and close monitoring of these systems should be implemented so as to optimise functioning and reduce risk.

Urinary catheter care

Urinary catheters are frequently required in critically ill patients in ICU. Catheter-associated urinary tract infections (CAUTI) form approximately 26% of device-related healthcare-associated infections (HAIs).[127] CAUTI in intensive care is associated with increased mortality and length of stay in the ICU.[128] Monitoring the incidence of CAUTI is a requirement in many jurisdictions.[128,129] Alvarez Lerma and colleagues[129] raised the prospect of a national 'Zero UTI' project in Spain to address CAUTI, following success of Spain's 'Zero bacteraemia', 'Zero Pneumonia' and 'Zero Resistance' healthcare improvement projects. In principle, urinary catheters should be inserted only when deemed clinically necessary, and they should be removed as soon as they are no longer required clinically. Alternatives to urinary catheterisation should be considered; however, most critically ill patients require accurate monitoring of their urinary output and fluid balance, and a catheter is required for this reason.[128] CAUTI are primarily caused by contamination during insertion or management of the catheter/drainage system, reflux of contaminated urine or breaks in the closed drainage system.[128] While routine screening for urinary tract infection is not required,[128] as the primary clinicians responsible for urinary catheter care in the ICU, critical care nurses should be mindful of the risk factors for CAUTI such as prolonged catheterisation, older age, impaired immunity and any breaches in good practices related to the insertion and maintenance of urinary catheters and drainage.[128,129] In partnering with patients, they should be advised of the reasons for and care requirements of urinary catheters.[127] Remember that the consequences of poor urinary catheter care and management are not only distressing to the patient but very detrimental to their health.

Urinary catheterisation assessment

The rationale for urinary catheter insertion outlined in Table 5.12 should be carefully considered and a portable ultrasound to evaluate the volume of bladder urine may help with the assessment.[128] Once it is established that a urinary catheter is necessary, the type of catheter should be determined. While the primary purpose of urinary catheters is management of urine drainage, the choice of catheter type may be influenced by the concurrent need for urinary temperature monitoring or continuous irrigation. The smallest-size catheter possible is used to reduce bladder neck and urethral damage[128] although narrow-bore tubes flex easily, which can be problematic in male catheterisation. Larger-diameter catheters may be required to drain haematuria and clots. The routine use of antibiotic-impregnated catheters or silver alloy catheters is not currently recommended.[128]

Urinary catheterisation essential care

Catheter insertion and maintenance should be according to facility policies and undertaken by people appropriately trained in the procedures.[128] To reduce the risk of infection, effective aseptic techniques and hand hygiene should be adhered to during catheter insertion and during any manipulation of the catheter or drainage system.[128]

The urine drainage system should be sterile and continuously closed with an outlet designed to avoid contamination.[128] It should have a sample port for taking urine samples. Where appropriate, patients should be given a choice of system suited to their needs. For example, a shorter drainage tube with a leg-bag may be more comfortable for a patient who is mobile. All procedures involving the catheter and drainage system should be documented in the clinical notes, including size and type of catheter, balloon size and the date of insertion. An anticipated date of removal should also be documented at the time of insertion in order to trigger staff to remove the catheter as soon as possible.

Catheter maintenance

Daily assessment of the requirement for a urinary catheter should be made and justification for requirement documented to encourage a focus on early removal. Criteria that enable registered nurses to remove catheters without a medical review may result in early removal and subsequent reduction in catheter-related infections. Routine hygiene at appropriate intervals for patient comfort is adequate for urethral meatal care.[128]

Urinary catheters should be changed only if there is a breach in the closed system or according to manufacturer's guidelines. Urinary catheters and closed drainage systems are changed together for clearly defined clinical reasons. Bladder washout should be avoided and closed continuous irrigation implemented only to prevent likely obstruction from clots of debris. Contamination of the drainage system outlet must be avoided during emptying.[128] An aseptic technique and sterile equipment must be used when taking a urine sample via the sample port.[128]

The whole drainage system should be maintained with patient comfort in mind, and care should be taken to ensure that the patient is not lying on the drainage tube, which can cause blockage to flow or pressure injury. Furthermore, the catheter itself should be positioned and then secured so that it is not pulling on the urethra or kinked. The drainage bag should be kept below the level of the bladder at all times to maintain an unobstructed

TABLE 5.12
Urinary catheter quick reference

COMPONENT OF CARE	CONSIDERATIONS
Criteria for insertion and/or continuing use *Re-evaluate continuing use daily against rationale and remove catheter as soon as possible when no longer required.*	• Acute urinary retention or bladder obstruction. • Need for accurate measurement of urinary output in critically ill patients. • Perioperative use for selected surgical procedures. • Assist in healing of open sacral or perineal wounds in incontinent patients. • Patient requiring prolonged immobilisation, e.g. spinal injury. • Patient admitted with chronic indwelling catheter. • Management of acute urinary retention and urinary obstruction. • Exceptional circumstances such as to improve end-of-life care.
Insertion *Use principles of aseptic non-touch technique.*	• Follow documented facility policy on urinary catheter insertion. • Staff performing procedure follow policy and are trained in technique. • Use sterile equipment, including sterile drape. • Use aseptic technique when inserting catheter and connecting to sterile drainage system. • Clean meatus with sterile normal saline before catheter insertion. • Use smallest diameter catheter to minimise urethral trauma. • Use appropriate sterile, single-use lubricant or anaesthetic gel. • Secure catheter after insertion to prevent movement and urethral traction. • Document insertion information in patient record.
Maintenance *Consider each shift:* • *How long has the catheter been in situ?* • *Is the catheter still required?* • *Are there any indications of infection or complications?* • *Is the drainage system being managed appropriately?*	• Maintain aseptic continuously closed system drainage. • Perform hand hygiene and use non-sterile gloves prior to any manipulation of the drainage system. • Position drainage bag to prevent backflow or contact with floor. • Empty drainage bag frequently to maintain urine flow and prevent reflux and empty before patient transport. • Use separate urine collection container for each patient, avoiding contact between drainage bag and container. This collection container should be discarded if single use, or cleaned and sterilised if reusable. • Obtain urine sample from sampling port using sterile syringe after disinfecting port. • Change drainage bags with catheter changes or according to manufacturers' guidelines without clamping as it is unnecessary. • Daily meatal hygiene via routine hygiene. • Avoid use of bladder irrigation, instillation or washouts as routine measures to prevent catheter-associated infections. • Document all related assessment and procedures for the catheter and drainage system. • Document daily justification for continual catheter use.

Source: Adapted from National Health and Medical Research Council (2019) Australian Guideline for the Prevention and Control of Infection in Healthcare. Canberra: Commonwealth of Australia. Available at: https://www.nhmrc.gov.au/about-us/publications/australian-guideline-prevention-and-control-infection-healthcare-2019.

flow of urine,[128,129] and it should be emptied into a disinfected or single-use container. The drainage system should be replaced if it is leaking, if there has been a break in the closed system or whenever the catheter is changed.[128]

Practice tip

Use a catheter support device or bandage on the leg to secure the urinary catheter. It lessens tension and irritation from catheter movement, patient comfort is improved, and it also promotes effective drainage and, in restless patients, may prevent accidental catheter removal as well.

Care of the older adult

Older adults are being admitted to the ICU in greater numbers as this section of the population continues to grow. There are no absolute definitions of 'older persons', but the United Nations describes 60 plus years as older, while many developed countries use 65 plus years as older.[130] Another term used in the context of the elderly is 'frail'. Frailty is an age-related syndrome that reduces physiological and cognitive reserves, which in turn increases people's vulnerability to insults such as infection and trauma.[131] It is found that about 40% of ICU patients in Australia and New and Zealand aged 80 years or more are frail, or 6.1% of all adults admitted to ICUs.[132]

There are a multitude of physiological changes that result from ageing.[133] Common causes of anaemia in older persons are iron deficiency and the presence of chronic disease or inflammation followed by chronic kidney dysfunction. In critical illness, anaemia may contribute to the older patient's fatigue, so careful consideration should always be given to planning activities such as hygiene and mobilisation.[134] Some older patients are quite fragile, because of anorexia of ageing and, after 65 years of age, a person may have less body fat and lower weight as a consequence of reduced food intake.[135] Acute illness or injury risks increasing the extent of malnutrition.[133] Other consequences of ageing include impaired muscle function and decreased bone mass, which impair mobility and lead to increased falls. Mobility problems are exacerbated by both loss of muscle mass and function and degenerative joint disease.[136] However, early mobilisation is as important for older adults as it is for younger persons with critical illness in order to prevent ICU-acquired weakness and reduce duration of mechanical ventilation.[137] Older adults' functional and cognitive status should be assessed and documented as soon as possible after admission, either through an evaluation tool or from the patient's family to identify patients at high risk of cognitive disabilities. In addition, daily monitoring should be performed to pay attention to potential changes. In ventilated patients, it is important to optimise sedation and pain management strategies in order to reduce the incidence of intensive care-associated delirium.[138]

Loss of muscle mass and then muscle activity reduces metabolic function and subsequently causes loss of body heat, so care should be taken to ensure the older adult is well covered at all times with additional lightweight warming devices available to be used as required.[139]

Skin, the biggest organ, is often the most visible sign of age in the older patient.[140] The epidermis atrophies, especially in exposed areas of the body, and once over 65 years, blistered skin takes longer to repair than in a young adult.[141] From fragile to easily bruised skin or moist skin folds in those who are overweight, careful hygiene care is required and consideration should be given to the use of specific products for these patients. Symptoms of urinary tract infection, such as dysuria and frequency, are less likely to be as obvious in the older adult as in the young, as the capacity of the bladder decreases with age and especially if the patient suffers from stress incontinence already. As with other functions, ageing blunts the immune system response, which results in increased susceptibility of the older adult to infection. This, along with the additional deterioration in skin integrity and likely increased exposure to antibiotics over time, means that this group of patients may be at greater risk of hospital-acquired infections and MROs.[133,141]

Consideration should be given to a suitable environment for the older patients, such as increased sound proofing, more comfortable and supportive chairs, cutlery and utensils that are easy to grip, enableing meals that are more comfortable. Music for short periods during the day may be calming and prevent ICU delirium as it addresses pathophysiological mechanisms that contribute to delirium such as neurotransmitter imbalance, inflammation and acute physiological stressors.[142] Do not forget issues related to vision (glasses) and hearing (hearing aids).[130] Above all, nurses should adjust some of their behaviours with the older person, such as speaking clearly, listening carefully without interruption, anticipating frequent personal care needs and allowing time to enable mobilisation without haste, all of which may help to facilitate feelings of independence and control of their circumstances for these patients.[143]

Bariatric considerations

Obesity continues to be a major health issue around the world; an even higher proportion of obese patients in the ICU exists compared with a normal population.[144,145] Total body weight (TBW) in kg and body mass index (BMI) (weight (kg)/lengths (m^2)) are two common methods to classify underweight, overweight and obesity in adults. While BMI is widely used, it has limitations as age and muscle mass are not included in the calculation.[146] Lean body weight, a descriptor of weight devoid of all adipose tissue, and predicted normal body weight that takes into account gender, height and weight to estimate the fractional fat mass, are two other measures used. What applies to all bariatric care is that each patient is unique, and all measures and treatments must be decided in relation to the individual patient's conditions and needs.

People who are obese contend with a negative bias but this same negative bias from health professionals including nurses may then interfere with their ability to obtain quality healthcare.[147,148] The key to providing quality, patient-centred, sensitive care to the bariatric patient is R-E-S-P-E-C-T: **R**apport, **E**nvironment/**e**quipment, **S**afety, **P**rivacy, **E**ncouragement, **C**aring/**c**ompassion and **T**act.[149] Simple things such as an appropriately sized gown and suitable bed linen that provide the patient with adequate covering are often not well organised for this patient group, unless the nurse takes the time to arrange specific supplies if they are not routinely available.[150]

Respiratory considerations

Obese patients may have increased intra-abdominal pressure and decreased chest wall compliance resulting in a decrease in low functional residual capacity and expiratory reserve volume. Obstructive sleep apnoea is common in the obese population. It is a state characterised by short episodes of apnoea (breathing cessation), accompanied by nocturnal oxygen desaturation and fragmented sleep, and results in impaired pulmonary gas exchange both at rest and with exercise.[151,152] These significant changes in static and dynamic respiratory mechanics adversely affect the patient in the form of changes in breathing such as increased respiratory rate, increased oxygen consumption, increased work of breathing and decreased tidal volumes.

As a result, more oxygen is required and time to desaturation is decreased.[153] Lowered functional residual capacity increases the risk of atelectasis and therefore non-invasive ventilation and CPAP are tools necessary to help derecruitment (alveolar closing). Ventilation mode should be oriented on ideal body-weight tidal volume 6–8 mL/kg. An individually adapted PEEP level is important. PEEP levels that are too low may result in atelectasis, while excessive tidal volumes and high PEEP may generate higher autoPEEP and shear force and thus lung damage. Unfortunately, optimal PEEP level in obese critically ill patients is still unknown. As weaning often takes a longer time in bariatric patients, post-extubation non-invasive ventilation should be considered. Although there are risks with tracheostomy, this should be discussed early as well as a no-sedation strategy. Ensure there is a secure fit of tracheostomy support device – adjustment for increased neck circumference may be needed.

To help obese patients in their work of breathing, positioning is important, and a continuous active mobilisation regimen may be necessary. When the airway is secured, the patient should be positioned in a reversed Trendelenburg position (head up, feet down), or 'beach chair position'.[154] This position decreases pressure on the diaphragm and therefore decreases intrathoracic pressure and as a result improves respiratory compliance and gas exchange.[155] If possible, the patient should be mobilised to bedside and standing as early as possible.[156] Prone position in severe hypoxaemic obese patients with ARDS is feasible without increased complications compared with non-obese patients when performed by a trained team.[157]

Circulation

Obesity affects the circulatory system in various ways through increased blood volume, decreased fibrinolysis and increased blood viscosity.[146] Close glucose-monitoring regimens should be implemented and appropriately calculated dosages for medications prescribed. As obese persons often have venous stasis disease, VTE prophylaxis is recommended with weight-adjusted dosing of medications.[158,159] Combining pharmacological and mechanical prophylaxis is recommended for this high-risk group.[102] Care must be taken with measuring the limb to obtain the correct size legging or stocking. Early mobilisation is important as it assists in reducing the incidence of VTE. Extra consideration must be given to the patient's skin.[160] Observe the entire skin costume several times daily. Be extra observant for exposed places like breast and lumps and keep the skin dry and clean.

Drugs and diets

There are many factors affecting the distribution, binding and elimination of drugs in obesity (Box 5.3). Drug doses are not necessarily administered according to the actual body weight, but more often are based on other dosing approaches.[161] Sedation in the bariatric patient needs to be carefully managed so as to avoid the resultant risk of respiratory failure and the need for ventilation. Reducing narcotic usage through use of combinations of other analgesia along with sedatives will also reduce the risk of respiratory failure. Therefore, drug doses must be individually adjusted to provide effects based on the patient's characteristics, thereby minimising side effects.[161,162]

Equipment

Adapted techniques to enhance patient assessment may be required, such as auscultating over the left lateral chest wall to hear heart sounds while the patient is positioned towards their left side, or using a thigh or regular blood pressure cuff on the patient's forearm. The use of arterial monitoring rather than non-invasive blood pressure measurements should be considered, because of the difficulty in obtaining accurate readings if the cuff is not sized or positioned correctly. Use specific bariatric equipment and techniques to move patients safely for both the patient and the staff involved.[163] It is important to be aware of the weight capacities of various facilities, such as lifts and equipment, which may be required in the care of the bariatric patient. Overweight patients can be challenging in any setting, and it is important to consider the health and safety of the staff involved in lifting and moving patients.[164] Equally important is maintaining the patient's dignity and feeling of safety and minimising their self-consciousness during repositioning, irrespective of the method required. Lifts and hoists and other equipment that are designed for heavier people should be used. A well-thought-out strategy by an interdisciplinary group can work through the local issues within a hospital or unit and produce a bariatric kit, containing a range of equipment appropriate to the needs of the bariatric patients in various settings including the ICU.

BOX 5.3

Pharmacological concerns in obesity

- Greater than normal amount of adipose tissue
- Increased lean body mass
- Increased blood volume
- Smaller than normal fraction of total body water
- Increased cardiac output
- Decreased pulmonary function
- Increased proteins, free fatty acids
- Increased renal blood flow
- Increased glomerular filtration rate
- Abnormal liver function

Practice tip

Ensure adequate equipment for obese patients is available including beds and wheelchairs. Identify and document weight capacity of equipment, such as how much weight beds and lifts can handle to ensure safe care.

General principles of infection prevention and control in critical care

The importance of infection control as a public health measure as well as in healthcare settings has been emphasised throughout the COVID-19/SARS CoV-2 pandemic which was declared by the World Health Organization (WHO) on 11 March 2020.[165] In an epidemic (unexpected increase in the number of disease cases in a specific geographical location) or pandemic (worldwide spread of a new disease), specific infection control measures based on the principles of infection control are enacted. Depending on the type of disease outbreak, local or national governments or the WHO will provide public health instructions and healthcare worker guidelines, freely available online from official government health sites, often with all relevant information and resources available from a single portal – for example, the Australian COVID-19 site at https://www.health.gov.au/health-alerts/covid-19.[166] As has happened with the COVID-19 pandemic, these instructions, guidelines and standards have been frequently updated in response to new experiences, healthcare practices, treatment information or variants of the disease.[167] So far, the SARS CoV-2 virus has had five variants of concern: alpha identified in the United Kingdom, beta identified in South Africa, gamma identified in Brazil, delta identified in India and, the most recent to date, omicron identified in South Africa.[165] All these variants had some changes to transmission rates, symptoms or predominant symptoms and contagiousness, which required adaption to public health instructions or healthcare practice guidelines. During epidemics or pandemics, it is easy to be overwhelmed by the volume of information, as sharing of information electronically between colleagues, local and international and professional organisations, and other health and well-being sites is easy. Effective care and safety for the patients in intensive care is reliant on the ICU team acting in unison, from endorsed information sources and using health practices that meet authorised guidelines, and these same factors are crucial in epidemic or pandemic situations.

This infection section will outline general principles of infection prevention and control in critical care under normal circumstances. Effective infection prevention and control is vital in the critical care setting to prevent further health risks such as HAIs[168] to critically ill patients already compromised by their disease or trauma. Factors that increase patient susceptibility to infection are: a compromised immune status, being a neonate or elderly, having comorbidities, the virulence and transmissibility of the pathogen, and having portals for access of pathogens such as invasive devices or surgical procedures. Critically ill patients often require multiple invasive devices and therapies to manage their illness and, while vital to patient management, they are not without risks, such as the increased potential for infection. VAP, CAUTIs and central line-associated bloodstream infection (CLABSI) are all aligned with invasive device use and form a significant source of HAIs within critical care.[168] Critical care staff themselves need to protect against contracting infections while providing care for their patients.

When patients are admitted to intensive care, their history, symptom development and presentation will provide indicators for risk of infection. It is impossible to identify whether or not they are newly colonised with microorganisms, or are carrying an infection, without further investigation.

To protect against infection transmission in healthcare settings, 'standard precautions' are applied in the management of all patients regardless of the reason for their admission. Standard precautions are the first step in protecting the patient against the chain of infection transmission in healthcare settings, which includes a causative pathogen, reservoir, exit portal, transmission method, entry portal and a susceptible host.[168] Standard precautions include: hand hygiene, respiratory hygiene and cough etiquette; the use of appropriate personal protective equipment; safe handling of sharps, waste and used linen; appropriate cleaning and environmental controls; appropriate reprocessing of reusable equipment; and the use of aseptic non-touch techniques during procedures.[168]

Continuing emphasis on respiratory hygiene, cough etiquette and effective hand hygiene to limit respiratory illnesses is vital.[168] Further 'transmission-based precautions' are implemented as required in response to suspicion (while awaiting confirmation from tests) or diagnosis of a condition in which standard precautions may not be sufficient to control the transmission of microorganisms.[168] Transmission-based precautions appropriately applied to specific microorganisms disrupt their method of transmission to other patients, visitors and healthcare workers. Transmission-based precautions include continuation of standard precautions, the use of personal protective equipment specific to the risk of transmission, use of individual patient equipment where possible and specific cleaning protocols for shared equipment, placement of patients in single rooms (or cohorted if appropriate) and specific air filtration or circulation and environmental-cleaning protocols.[168]

There are three types of transmission-based precautions recommended to counteract the various infectious agents: 'contact precautions', 'droplet precautions' and 'airborne precautions'[168] (Table 5.13). These types of precautions are applied with refinement to the use of personal protective equipment, room requirements and recommendations for visitors specific to the mode of transmission of the organism. The WHO 2016 guideline on infection prevention and control programs outlines eight core components for acute healthcare facilities.[169] These are broad topics of national programs, national and facility level guidelines, education and training, HAI surveillance, strategies for implementing prevention and control strategies, monitoring, workload and occupancy and environment, materials and equipment at facility level.[169] Critical care nurses should be knowledgeable about both facility and national guidelines and protocols for infection control in order to provide safe care to all their patients. Failure to consistently apply standard precautions and,

TABLE 5.13

Transmission-based precautions in healthcare settings

TRANSMISSION-BASED PRECAUTIONS	EXAMPLES OF INFECTIOUS CONDITIONS
Contact Remember contact transmission may be direct (person to person) or indirect (person to equipment to person)	• MROs: MRSA, MRGN, VRE, ESBL, CRE • Gastrointestinal pathogens: *C. difficile* • Norovirus • Highly contagious skin infections
Droplet Particles >5 micrometre. Usually travel distance of 1 m or less	• Influenza • RSV • Meningococcal
Airborne Particles <5 micrometre. Dispersed widely e.g. via air condition systems = HEPA filters in situ	• Pulmonary TB • Chickenpox (varicella), measles (rubella) • SARS, MERS

CRE = carbapenem-resistant Enterobacteriaceae; ESBL = extended-spectrum beta-lactamase-producing (Enterobacteriaceae); MERS = Middle East respiratory syndrome coronavirus; MRGN = multi-resistant Gram-negative bacilli; MRO = multi-resistant organism; MRSA = methicillin-resistant *Staphylococcus aureus;* RSV = respiratory syncytial virus; SARS = severe acute respiratory syndrome; TB = tuberculosis; VRE = vancomycin-resistant enterococcus.

Source: Adapted from NHMRC Australian guidelines for the prevention and control of infection in healthcare 2019, https://www.nhmrc.gov.au/about-us/publications/australian-guidelines-prevention-and-control-infection-healthcare-2019.

when implemented, transmission-based precautions, adds to the patient's risk of HAIs, especially in those who are critically ill. Key components of effective infection prevention and control and their application in critical care are now described in more detail.

Prevention

Within healthcare settings a prime goal is to protect the patient, staff and visitors from risk of infection transmission as well as to prevent the development of MROs. Healthcare facility environment maintenance, cleaning, hand hygiene facilities, equipment use and reprocessing are aimed at meeting these goals. Health services should apply designated guidelines and operate within clearly defined infection control procedures, which are based on standard precautions for all patients and situations with transmission-based precautions applied in response to patient condition and infection risk.[168] Critical care nurses should refer to their specific hospital infection control policies and transmission based precaution guidelines for specific procedural details. Consistent application of procedures and processes by all personnel is a key component of their effectiveness in keeping patients, visitors and health personnel safe.

Risk management in infection control

When presented with new procedures or infection outbreaks, a clear process is needed to ensure infection prevention controls can be established. Using a risk model provides a process to describe the infection related situation or event, identify the hazards, analyse the likelihood or consequences of the infection, evaluate strategies and control the infection risks, such as modification of the procedure, workflow or work practices, providing education and monitoring compliance.[167] Where the ability or potential to prevent cross-infection is not possible, risk mitigation actions are employed, such as limiting persons in an area during aerosol-generating procedures such as intubation are occurring.

Surveillance

ICU patients may be colonised or infected with an MRO prior to admission,[168] so routine screening is recommended in order to detect the presence of pathogens of concern.[168] Surveillance for respiratory virus commonly occurs during seasonal outbreaks or pandemics so as to determine both the patient infectious status and the ICU 'load' of like patients. COVID-19 pandemic has required surveillance of patients, staff and visitors within healthcare settings.[167] Local conditions, risk factors and protocols will provide guidance, but commonly critically ill patients will be screened for MROs such as *Staphylococcus aureus* (MRSA) and vancomycin-resistant *Enterococcus* (VRE) on admission.[168,169] In the 1980s, a landmark study established that HAIs may be reduced by around one-third if surveillance and prevention programs are implemented.[170] Reporting surveillance data to the clinical team regularly can aid with infection control strategy compliance.

Control

Once an organism has been identified, the goal is to limit its spread. Colonisation refers to the presence of microorganisms in any amount, whereas infection means that pathological tissue injury or disease has occurred as a result of the invasion and multiplication of the microorganism.[168] Typically, surveillance measures identify many patients who are colonised with MRSA or VRE and, although they themselves are not infected, it is important to stop the spread of bacteria to patients more vulnerable and hence more susceptible to opportunistic infection, by implementing transmission-based precautions.[168,169] Key measures demonstrated to be effective in managing multi-resistant bacterial infections in ICUs include early identification of infected patient and use of contact precautions, along with containment of equipment such as stethoscopes and thermometers for exclusive use of a single patient. When the organism is spread by droplet or aerosol transmission such as in influenza or COVID-19 and the number of affected patients is high, additional controls of cohorting patients and healthcare teams to reduce transmission opportunities may be implemented.[167]

Due to the vulnerable nature of critically ill patients, management of environmental cleanliness is a key factor in infection control. This extends to cleaning standards and frequency, waste management, water quality, air quality and circulation, the changing of bed linen and its handling for disposal or removal for cleaning. During the COVID-19 pandemic, specific recommendations for alterations to existing environmental, personnel and workflow features in intensive care occurred, such as cohorting clinical teams, limits to the use of shared facilities and changes to patient transport and staff and visitor traffic flows.[171,172]

Hand hygiene

At the core of standard precautions is effective hand hygiene, which reduces the spread of bacteria and is the most effective and least expensive method of preventing healthcare-associated or nosocomial infection.[167,168] The 'five moments for hand hygiene' were created by the WHO in 2009.[169] Constant diligence is required to ensure good hand hygiene, as compliance can be variable.[165,166] However, regular education programs, feedback and reminders are known to support improvement, hence the annual world hand hygiene day.[169] Due to its accessibility, alcohol-based hand rub is the preferred method for hand hygiene unless the hands are soiled or in the presence of *C. difficile* or Norovirus.[169] Clinicians should monitor their hand skin integrity and be alert to any product irritation, given the frequency of hand hygiene required in clinical settings and for their personal safety. Hand hygiene has been a prominent feature of public health measures during the COVID-19 pandemic.

> **Practice tip**
>
> Good hand hygiene is vital before and after all interventions with patients. There are multiple objects within a ward or unit that are touched by many people within a day. Movement of contaminants from inanimate objects to patients and the reverse is possible if adherence to good hand hygiene is not upheld. Remember the five moments for hand hygiene.

> **Practice tip**
>
> Compliance with local protocols for surveillance, isolation and use of personal protective equipment (PPE) for MROs and infectious conditions is vital to the safe management of all patients, and the safety of personnel and visitors in critical care units.[170–172]

Personal protective equipment (PPE)

PPE may include any and all of the following: plastic aprons, gowns (single use or sterile), gloves (single use or sterile), masks ranging from surgical to particulate filter N95 or PPF3 masks or P2 respirators, and eye protection such as goggles or face shields that also protect mucous membranes of the mouth and nose.[167,168] Mask fit testing helps identify the most appropriate type and size mask for healthcare personnel. Subsequently, each time a mask is worn a 'fit check' should be performed by the user to eliminate leaks.[173] Powered air-purifying respirators (PAPRs) may be required for extended period use. Personnel should be trained in PAPR checks and use.[173] The specific sequences for putting on PPE (hand hygiene, gown, mask, eye protection or face shield, gloves) and removing it (gloves, hand hygiene, gown (or gloves and gown then hand hygiene), eye protection or face shield, mask then finish with hand hygiene) minimise the risk of contamination and should be familiar to all healthcare personnel.[167,168] In critical situations, or when knowledge of the pathogen is limited, having a 'buddy' or support person to observe correct donning and doffing of PPE can aid safety. When PPE is required by visitors, clear instructions and assistance by staff should be provided to keep them safe.

History tells us of many local and regional infectious epidemics, such as malaria, poliomyelitis, cholera, dengue fever, ebola and measles, all of which require specific applications of PPE. In the last 20 years there have been epidemic outbreaks of various infectious respiratory conditions which threatened many populations across the world. Epidemic outbreaks of the severe acute respiratory syndrome (SARS) coronavirus initially occurred in China then, via travel to Canada, Hong Kong, Singapore and Vietnam in 2003, cases were reported subsequently in over 25 countries.[174] SARS was transmitted between patients, healthcare workers and hospital visitors, and large within-hospital outbreaks were associated with aerosol-generating procedures such as bronchoscopy, endotracheal intubation and the use of aerosol therapy,[167] which are commonplace in critical care areas. In Hong Kong more than 20% of cases were healthcare workers.[174,175] Because of the high level of morbidity and mortality associated with SARS,[174] the risk to healthcare staff was considerable and so, during the Hong Kong SARS outbreak, healthcare workers wore full head covers with a visor.[175]

The SARS outbreaks emphasised the need for effective infection control procedures, especially for airborne pathogens. With airborne pathogens such as pulmonary tuberculosis or the Middle East respiratory syndrome coronavirus (MERS-CoV),[176,177] airborne precautions[168] using properly fitted N95 masks (face mask with 95% or greater filter efficiency), gowns and gloves are implemented to reduce the spread of the organism. In addition, the use of airborne infection isolation rooms or negative air pressure rooms with room exhaust via high-efficiency particulate air (HEPA) filtration and strict control of family visiting may be needed.[168] Additional measures may include the use of high-efficiency bacterial filters to filter patients' expired air, closed suction systems and ventilator scavenging systems.[168]

MERS-CoV was first reported in 2012 in Saudi Arabia, which has been primarily affected with the majority of cases and associated deaths from MERS. Countries near to the Arabian Peninsula were the next affected through travellers. However, a large outbreak in North Korea was reported in 2015, where 186 persons were affected and linked to a single traveller back from the Middle East.[176] As of November 2022, 2600 cases and 935 deaths have been reported from 27 countries, with 84% within Saudi Arabia.[177] In Saudi Arabia nearly 100 healthcare workers contracted MERS in 2015 and the infection continues to linger, with five MERS cases reported there in May of 2022.[177] In the early period of the COVID-19 pandemic, when knowledge of the virus was still growing, the intensive care community reflected on lessons from these relatively recent viral epidemics, and PPE and healthcare worker safety was a primary focus which led to specific guidance on PPE in the context of COVID-19.[173]

Both influenza A and B circulate as seasonal flu, but influenza A is a regular reminder of the changing nature of virus. In the 20th century there was the 1918 'Spanish flu' influenza pandemic, which was an influenza A virus subtype H1N1.[178] In 1957 the influenza A virus pandemic was subtype H2N2, the flu pandemic in 1968 was subtype H3N2, whereas in 1977 an epidemic of influenza A was again subtype H1N1.[178,179] The use of 'droplet precautions' is the main feature of infection control for influenza, along with early testing. In the 21st century we have already experienced epidemics of 'avian' influenza A subtype H5N1 from 2003 and subtype H7N9 from 2013.[178,179] Additionally, there was the 'swine flu' pandemic of influenza A subtype H1N1 in 2009, referred to as H1N1pdm09 virus,[178,179] which again alerted everyone to the need for vigilance in infection control, and the critical roles of contact and droplet transmission precautions, early testing and vaccinations in the control of influenza. Currently, both the influenza A H1N1 and H3N2 subtypes are known to be circulating globally.[165] Influenza vaccines are redeveloped as the influenza virus changes. Vaccines for COVID-19 were developed as a series of vaccinations was recommended to protect against the virulence of the virus. All healthcare workers and especially those in critical care should be knowledgeable of the vaccinations that may be available to them through their employers

and those that are recommended by local jurisdictions because of endemic diseases as well as epidemic outbreaks.

Multi-resistant organisms (MROs)

MROs, or multi-drug-resistant organisms, are collective terms for a number of infections with antimicrobial resistance (AMR). Antimicrobials include antibiotic, antiviral, antifungal and antiparasitic medications.[180] While the early diagnosis of an MRO and immediate implementation of organism-specific 'transmission-based precautions' is key to management, there are increasing numbers of multi-resistant bacteria such as methicillin-resistant *Staphyloccocus aureus* (MRSA), extended-spectrum beta-lactamase-producing Enterobacteriaceae (ESBL-E) and *Pseudomonas aeruginosa* (PA). VRE has become a serious health issue, as well as carbapenemase-producing Enterobacteriaceae (CPE) and *Acinetobacter* spp.[180] *Escherichia coli* (*E. coli*) is a common cause of urinary tract infections and is reportedly increasing in resistance to ciprofloxacin and fluoroquinolone.[180] *Klebsiella pneumoniae* resistance to carbapenem antibiotics is reportedly in all world regions,[180] and multi-drug-resistant TB (MDR-TB) is occurring in both new and previously treated TB patients.[180]

Risk factors for MROs include antimicrobial use, compromised skin integrity, contaminated surfaces, shared items and suboptimal cleanliness. Transmission of MROs is associated with contact. MRO management includes routine screening on and during ICU admission and employing transmission-based precautions for reducing their spread. As with any screening process, it is important to distinguish between colonisation and infection. Combating growing AMR is a WHO top 10 global health priority[180] and this can be aided with effective infection prevention and control and prescribing antimicrobial medications only when required.

Practice tip

In critical situations, antibiotics are sometimes prescribed broadly to cover a potential range of pathogens. Early microbiological testing and resultant adjustment of antibiotics to target specific organisms found should occur.

Healthcare-acquired infection (HAI)

HAI is a subset of hospital-acquired complications (HACs), which encompass adverse events and complications of treatments; it is a significant issue for critically ill patients.[168,169] HAI can occur in up to 15% of hospitalised patients and this can increase to 37% of patients admitted to ICUs.[181] WHO recommends a multimodal approach to addressing HAI.[169] This includes monitoring acquired infection incidence, education and training, process and procedure reviews and the use of focused 'care bundles'.

Critically ill patients with sepsis often require significant antimicrobial medications. The presence of

MROs complicates management and clinicians need to have a focus on antimicrobial stewardship for the optimal use of antibiotics.[182] Antimicrobial stewardship facilitates a factual review of prescribing, provision of guidance and education to support best practice among other activities. Countries may have a national body to provide governance or reports for healthcare providers on this important topic, such as the Australian report AURA,[182] which provides factual updates on the national surveillance data and trends for AMR and use and prescribing appropriateness of antimicrobials.[182]

The extensive use of medical devices and therapies within critical care heightens the potential risk of patients in ICU acquiring a HAI. Risk of infection may occur during the insertion procedure or subsequent maintenance care of the medical device, unless appropriate techniques are used. The use of an aseptic technique during insertion of a device is a feature of infection control, asepsis being the elimination of pathogens. Aseptic non-touch technique is a format for guiding practice in standard or surgical application.[168] The principles of avoidance of touch, and protective measures, assist the prevention of contamination during invasive procedures. Standard aseptic non-touch technique involves standard hand hygiene, a general aseptic field and non-sterile or sterile gloves and is used for minor procedures that are simple and of short duration – that is, less than 20 minutes. Examples of procedures include simple wound dressings and intravenous cannulation or urinary catheterisation by proficient practitioners. Surgical aseptic non-touch technique is used for complex or lengthy procedures such as insertion of a central venous catheter and involves the use of full barrier precautions (sterile gown and gloves, face mask), extensive drapes and a critical aseptic field.[168] Box 5.4 provides some basic points to guide management of the use of medical devices in critical care.

The commonest HAIs occur at surgical sites and in the urinary tract, lower respiratory tract and bloodstream. For the critically ill patient, intravascular cannulas including central venous catheters, urinary catheters, enteral or nasogastric tubes and artificial airways and ventilation circuits are some of the healthcare devices associated with risk. Extracorporeal life support (ECLS) is another potential risk for HAI, but the complexities of patients requiring ECLS often with infectious conditions and limited direct ECLS linked HAI data make this a topic for further research.[183] Information follows on VAP and CLABSI and the section on urinary catheters provides information regarding CAUTI. A recent multicentre study in Italy confirmed the positive impact a hand hygiene program can have on reducing healthcare-associated respiratory infections.[181]

Ventilator-associated pneumonia (VAP)

VAP is a common complication of mechanical ventilation; it is considered preventable and hence subject to extensive efforts to prevent. Although VAP incidence is monitored in intensive care, the diagnosis of VAP or infection-related

BOX 5.4

Invasive device management

- Does the patient need the invasive device for effective management of their condition?
- Is the chosen device the most suitable for the individual patient, e.g. size and type of device?
- Are the healthcare professional/s trained to safely insert and manage the device?
- Use the appropriate aseptic procedure for device insertion.
- Follow management protocols to minimise the risk of infection while the device is in situ.
- Monitor the patient for signs and symptoms of infection.
- Review the need for the device in the management of the patient daily and remove as early as possible.

Source: Adapted from NHMRC. Australian guidelines for the prevention and control of infection in healthcare. 2019. https://www.nhmrc.gov.au/about-us/publications/australian-guidelines-prevention-and-control-infection-healthcare-2019.

ventilator conditions remains variable and comparisons subsequently difficult.[184,185] The use of ventilator bundles or projects such as the Spanish 'Pneumonia Zero' strategy[186] assist ICU team cohesion in the implementation of effective care strategies for the ventilated patient and reduction of VAP within an ICU. Table 5.14 outlines common VAP prevention strategies. Two of the simplest and most effective are raising the head of the bed and frequent effective oral hygiene, although even these are not without variations. Positioning the ventilated patient with the head of bed elevated to between 30 and 60 degrees helps avoid gastroesophageal reflux and respiratory aspiration, but the optimal angle is a continuing discussion.[89,184] The use of CHG mouthwash was a part of VAP oral hygiene protocol, but reports of associated oral mucosal lesions have reduced chlorhexidine concentrations or eliminated its use, replaced by tooth brushing.[53] Good analgesia and minimising sedation plus avoidance of muscle-relaxant medications along with early mobilisation are some of the other strategies that may contribute to the reduction of VAP. Using a heat and moisture exchanger limits the need to change ventilator circuits, while a closed ventilator circuit with closed suction system avoids potential circuit contamination. Maintaining effective endotracheal cuff pressures and eliminating subglottic secretions with ETT above a cuff drainage port both reduce respiratory aspiration.

Selective digestive decontamination continues to be studied extensively. In theory, the use of antimicrobial agents to reduce gut flora in intubated intensive care patients reduces the risk of pneumonia due to

TABLE 5.14

Strategies to prevent VAP

MEASURE	INTERVENTIONS
Infection control measures	• Hand hygiene • Active surveillance • Appropriate PPE when managing ventilation-related devices, e.g. ETT, ventilator circuits, tracheal suctioning
Gastrointestinal tract	• Oral hygiene protocol • Stress ulcer prophylaxis • Avoiding gastric overdistention • Enteral nutrition
Patient position	• Semirecumbent with head raised to >30 degrees • Rotational bed therapy
Artificial airway	• Respiratory airway care • Avoiding unplanned extubations • Securing tracheal airway cuff/maintaining cuff pressure • Inline continuous or intermittent subglottic secretion removal
Mechanical ventilation	• Maintenance of ventilation equipment, heat and moisture exchangers, safe removal of condensate from circuits • Minimisation of ventilation time • Daily interruption to sedation and/or assessment for readiness to wean therapy and/or extubate • Non-invasive mechanical ventilation

ETT = endotracheal tube; PPE = personal protective equipment; VAP = ventilator-associated pneumonia.

Source: Adapted from NHMRC. Australian guidelines for the prevention and control of infection in healthcare 2019. https://www.nhmrc.gov.au/about-us/publications/australian-guidelines-prevention-and-control-infection-healthcare-2019.

microaspiration (see Chapter 19). Related information on respiratory failure, VAP and ventilation can be found in Chapters 14 and 15.

Central line-associated bloodstream infection (CLABSI)

The use of central venous lines is common in critical care areas for purposes of fluid and medication administration, pressure monitoring and delivery of therapies. CLABSI is determined when a positive laboratory-confirmed bloodstream infection not related to infection at another site occurs within 48 hours of central line insertion.[187]

CLABSI is one of the most severe infections that can occur in ICU and patients with renal failure may be at significant increased risk.[167] Implementation of quality improvement measures to ensure adherence to evidence-based guidelines, such as the Asia Pacific Society of Infection Control (APSIC) guidelines for prevention of CLABSI,[127] results in a significant reduction of catheter-related bloodstream infection.[168,187]

After implementing strategies to reduce CLABSI, staff engagement and diligent adherence to protocols are required to maintain success. Typically, strategies will address the stages of catheter use: insertion, catheter site dressing, line management, therapy management and then catheter removal as early as possible. Application of infection prevention and control principles is required for all stages.[167] Some key points will be addressed here, and Chapter 3 contains more-detailed information on central-line care bundles and checklists.

Use of antibiotic-impregnated catheters can aid in reduction of bacteraemia,[188] but should be used according to manufacturer guidelines. Current strategies include the use of hand hygiene for every single intervention related to the catheter, lines or therapies.[168,188] Additionally, full-barrier precautions (head cap, face mask, sterile body gown, sterile gloves and full-size body drape) are employed during insertion of central venous catheters by appropriately trained personnel using ultrasound guidance to reduce insertion attempts.[168,188] Chlorhexidine solutions are recommended for skin preparation, but be aware that solution concentrations and therefore their effectiveness may vary.

Nurses are responsible for the maintenance of central venous catheters once inserted, including care of the insertion site dressing and infusion line management. Catheter insertion site dressings provide an infection barrier and security of the catheter to prevent migration or accidental removal. Nurses monitoring the catheter dressing should assess whether it is clean, dry and intact. Additionally, they should assess the surrounding skin for signs of irritation or moisture-associated skin damage. Dressings should be replaced if they are not intact or every 7 days.[189] Consider the catheter position and insertion site anatomy when applying a new dressing to ensure good seal and line security. CHG-impregnated dressings are known to be effective in reducing intravascular catheter infections.[168,189] These dressings may be CHG gel or CHG-impregnated sponges. The gel dressing allows for greater visualisation of the insertion site.[189] For security of catheter and lines to prevent pulling, additional tape may be used.[189] Catheter hubs are sites at risk of colonisation from microorganisms such as *Staphylococcus epidermidis*, and effective hand hygiene should be implemented, including use of chlorhexidine or alcohol disinfection swabs along with non-touch aseptic techniques when accessing the catheter hub.[189] Hub connectors and intravenous administration sets are changed at the same time as per local protocols, usually between 96 hours and 7 days.[189] Infusion lines containing blood products or lipids or parenteral nutrition infusions are changed either when the infusion completes or daily, while infusion lines for medications such as propofol or nitroglycerine follow manufacturer guidelines for set changes, but are usually frequent.[188]

After removal of the catheter, and once homeostasis has been established, the site should be covered with an occlusive dressing, which should be left in place for 48 hours to minimise the risk of infection. The catheter should be examined after removal and any damage reported. It may be hospital or unit policy to send the catheter tip for culture and sensitivity; however, a single-centre study showed that colonisation is heaviest at the intravascular proximal segment compared with the distal tip of the catheter.[190]

> ### Practice tip
>
> Unless contraindicated in a specific patient, a central venous catheter dressing should be changed whenever there is evidence of fluid accumulation or loss of the dressing's occlusive seal.

Transport of critically ill patients: general principles

The transport of critically ill patients may occur for several reasons, such as from an accident site, categorised as pre-hospital transport, or to move a patient to another facility for treatment, which is known as inter-hospital transport, or within a hospital from one department to another, this being intra-hospital transport.[191] This section will focus on intra-hospital transport, while inter-hospital transport is described in Chapter 23. There are three groups of critically ill patients undergoing intra-hospital transport. First, there are those unstable patients transported from the emergency department (ED)[191] to the ICU or radiology, cardiac intervention unit or the operating theatres. Another significant group are those deteriorating patients within a hospital ward or persons attended to by a medical emergency response team, who require emergency transfer to the ICU. Finally, patients within the ICU often require transport to and from imaging departments for scans or operating theatres for procedures or cardiac catheterisation laboratory for angiography.

Guidelines for the transport of critically ill patients are available in many countries including Australia and New Zealand,[191] with the principles applying to intra-hospital and other transport.[191,192] Specific guidelines may need to be observed for certain groups of patients – for example, those with head injury. While the patients from the emergency department or from medical emergency calls are generally being moved to facilities where more treatment or care can be provided, the decision to transport an intensive care patient for diagnostic tests or interventions not possible within the ICU is given careful consideration as to the benefits to be gained, as transporting such patients

is not without risk and the goal should be no reduction in care during transport.[191–198] To reduce the risk of adverse events during transport, various diagnostic tests or surgical procedures should be evaluated in terms of their potential to be undertaken in the critical care unit.

Considerations

A diversity of adverse events during intra-hospital transport have been reported in various studies, with rates of up to 70% depending on the criteria used to determine the adverse event.[194,196,197] In a recent systematic review, Murata and colleagues found the pooled frequency of equipment-related adverse events to be between 10% and 44%, serious adverse events at around 10% and pooled frequency of life-threatening adverse events low.[197] Bergman and colleagues identified categories of hazards pre-, during and post-intra-hospital transport as: team, tasks, tools and technologies, environment and organisation.[193] Recognition of the risk of adverse events during intra-hospital transports has long been a concern in critical care and remains so today.[194–197] The primary focus should be on patient safety and the prevention of adverse events. A transport 'event' can be any event that has an adverse impact and can be patient, staff or equipment related.[193,194] The patient may be affected during transport, ranging from anxiety or pain to respiratory or cardiovascular compromise.[197] Staff may have difficulty with managing the patient's needs during transport and equipment-related problems during transport of critically ill patients are a major consideration along with device dislodgement.[193,194] Risk–benefit assessment is helpful to identify patients with a high risk of complications.[193] For example, the potential risk of moving a severely head-injured patient with unstable ICP may outweigh the potential benefit of a CT scan. Parmentier-Decrucq and colleagues[194] found that sedation of the patient before transport, PEEP >6 cmH$_2$O and the need for fluid infusion for transport to be risk factors for any adverse event during intra-hospital transport. Meticulous planning for all aspects of the transport, based on a thorough assessment of the patient's anticipated needs, is the key to safe intra-hospital transport.[191,192] Consideration of specific patient needs, such as the availability of lifting devices for transferring bariatric patients from bed to CT table or appropriate warming devices for the use of older adult patients during lengthy interventional radiological procedures, need to be communicated to the procedural areas prior to transport commencing so that no delays occur. A comprehensive guide of information addressing key components of intra-hospital transport of critically ill patients should be available to personnel at every hospital.[191]

Safe transport requires accurate assessment and stabilisation of the patient before transport.[191] Key elements are identified in Box 5.5.[192] Securing vascular accesses should be essential, while consideration may be given to having two intravenous accesses in situ. All equipment should be checked for functionality prior to transport and, while it is vital to ensure that sufficient equipment is taken to maintain the patient, unnecessary equipment complicates

---

BOX 5.5

Key elements of safe transfer

- Experienced staff
- Appropriate equipment
- Full assessment and investigation
- Extensive monitoring
- Careful stabilisation of patient
- Reassessment
- Continuing care during transfer
- Direct handover
- Documentation and audit

Source: Reproduced from Wallace PGM, Ridley SA. ABC of intensive care: transport of critically ill patients. BMJ 1999;319(7206):368–71,[192] with permission.

---

the logistics of managing the transport efficiently. Specifically constructed transport beds or attachments such as equipment tables designed to support and secure equipment safely during transfer are useful and protect the patient from equipment misplacement injuries.[191,193] The transport time should be as short as possible, although safety should not be sacrificed for speed. Pre-planning the route of transport and good dialogue between department staff can help to maximise the efficiency of transport and reduce unnecessary delays.[195] At all times, the team must be confident that all safety considerations have been made. Both 'haste' and 'pressure to proceed' with transport are contributing factors in adverse events.[193] Adverse events are described in various studies relating to poor preparation and decisions, lack of situational awareness, deficits in skill and ad-hoc work-arounds or non-compliance with designated procedures or practices.[193]

Additionally, in circumstances of intra-hospital transport of COVID-19 or other potentially highly infectious patients, Yousuf and colleagues describe the inclusion of extra items such as transparent drapes for the patient and transparent equipment covers, as well as important considerations of coordinating the transport route for clear passage, PPE, disinfection of equipment and arranging for housekeeping staff suitably attired in PPE to decontaminate the transfer route if necessary.[195]

Practice tip

Transport preparation should include: (1) establishing the need and purpose of transport; (2) time duration relating to the route to be taken, length of procedure and return journey; (3) necessary equipment; (4) patient assessment and preparation; (5) appropriately skilled and numbers of staff; (6) supplies required to continue therapies during transport event; and (7) consideration of emergency and contingency plans.

Essential nursing care during transport

Essential care during transport involves major components: the patient, the team, the monitoring and therapy equipment, and the preparation. Importantly, the patient and their family should be given an explanation of why the transport is necessary, how long the procedure is expected to take and that the transport process includes a team accompanying the patient to continue monitoring and provide required treatment.

The level of experience and specialty of personnel involved in the transport of critically ill patients are factors influencing safe transport.[191] Staff should be trained in the various aspects of patient transport,[191,198] including competent management and troubleshooting of all equipment required for particular patient needs (e.g. intra-aortic balloon pump). Team members should be aware of their specific roles, the expected standards to be maintained and promotion of excellent communication both within the team and with associated department personnel throughout the transport procedure. Nursing responsibilities during transport of the patient include all aspects of patient and therapy monitoring, comfort and maintaining appropriate documentation. Documentation may relate to a transport checklist[198] or notation of patient-related events or observations on a paper or digital record. Continuous or frequent monitoring of the patient's vital signs and physiological parameters and equipment alarms and parameters should be undertaken throughout the transport event, and all equipment should be regularly checked for correct functioning. Gas reserves of oxygen cylinders and battery time of all devices require pre-transport calculation before being used and vigilant attention during transport. Patient safety is paramount and close attention to detail is required. Throughout the transport, patients should be reassured regarding their condition and the progress of the purpose of the transport.

Practice tip

Staff involved in patient transport should be knowledgeable about the most efficient route to take as well as the facilities at their destination such as power and gas supplies.

Equipment

Equipment used during patient transport must be robust, lightweight and battery powered,[193] and must adhere to relevant national manufacturing and safety standards. Equipment-related complications occur in around a third of transports.[196] All equipment must be adequately secured during transport, and must be available continuously to the operator.[191] Oxygen requirements should be calculated in advance (or it should be established that piped oxygen is available at the destination department) to ensure an adequate supply, both for the journey and for the duration

TABLE 5.15
Standard equipment for intra-hospital transport

RESPIRATORY SUPPORT EQUIPMENT	CIRCULATORY SUPPORT EQUIPMENT	OTHER EQUIPMENT	PHARMACOLOGICAL AGENTS
• Airway management equipment, including intubation set, range of ETTs and laryngeal mask airways, hand ventilation set with PEEP valve and emergency surgical airway set • Oxygen, masks, nebuliser • Pulse oximeter and capnography • Sufficient oxygen supply • Suction equipment • Portable ventilator with disconnect and high-pressure alarms • Pleural drainage equipment	• Monitor/defibrillator/ external pacer combined unit • Non-invasive blood pressure device • IV cannula, IV fluids, pressure infusion set, infusion pumps • Arterial cannulae and arterial monitoring device • Syringes and needles, sharps' disposal container • Pericardiocentesis equipment	• Nasogastric tube and bag • Dressings, antiseptic lotions, bandages, tape, • Torch • Thermal insulation and temperature monitor • PPE for transport team	• Checked and clearly labelled drugs: standard resuscitation drugs and those specific to the patient's condition

ETT = endotracheal tube; IV = intravenous; PEEP = positive end-expiratory pressure; PPE = personal protective equipment.

Source: Adapted from College of Intensive Care Medicine Australia and New Zealand (CICM). Guidelines for transport of critically ill patients. 2015. https://www.cicm.org.au.

of the investigation/procedure. Staff responsibility for the safe management of the patient during transport extends to competence with troubleshooting equipment and responsiveness to unexpected equipment, environmental or logistical situations of varying degrees of seriousness.[198] Standard equipment for inter-hospital transport is identified in Table 5.15[191] and, while some items may be unnecessary for all intra-hospital transport, this table provides a useful checklist so that all necessary equipment is taken. Development of an institutional checklist[198] to aid the safe transport of critically ill patients may be common; however, not all may contain all the relevant aspects of the transport such as pre-transport (preparation), during transport and post-transport with each component informed by analysis of local events and factors such as transport routes and logistical challenges.[199] Additional specialist equipment may be required for certain patients, such as spare tracheostomy tubes in case of accidental extubation.

Practice tip

To ensure safe equipment preparation, especially during emergency transport events, have two nurses perform independent checks against a transport checklist that includes battery life and gas cylinder data for equipment in your unit as a standard transport preparation practice. Consider additional length infusion lines and ventilation circuits if the destination requires, such as for magnetic resonance imaging (MRI) scans.

Before transport, equipment should be prepared and checked, including the function of visible and audible alarms. All non-essential therapy should be discontinued or simplified during the transport, such as enteral nutrition or completed infusion administration sets from intravenous lines. The patient's physical safety should be maintained, and care should be taken to ensure that bed rails are used and the patient's limbs are secure and not likely to be injured by equipment. All vital monitoring and therapy equipment should be transferred to portable equipment, and the patient should be stabilised before being moved. Some transport equipment ventilators may not provide identical parameters or functioning to a ventilator the patient is already using, so time must be taken to adjust the transport ventilator to effective ventilation for the patient. If the patient is being transported for MRI, it is important to ensure that all equipment is compatible.

Practice tip

If ceasing nutrition during patient transport, make sure that the patient is not at risk of hypoglycaemia from concurrent insulin therapy.

Monitoring

The need for monitoring relates to both patient and equipment, as identified in Table 5.16.[191] Some monitoring should be continuous, such as cardiac, oxygen saturation, capnography if the patient is intubated and arterial, pulmonary artery and intracranial monitoring if the

TABLE 5.16
Monitoring during transport

CLINICAL PATIENT MONITORING	EQUIPMENT MONITORING
• Circulation	• Pulse oximeter and capnography
• Respiration	
• Oxygenation	• Breathing system alarms
• Neurological	• Electrocardiograph
• Pain score	• Physiological pressures
• Patient comfort	• Other clinically indicated equipment
	• Audible and visual equipment alarms

Source: Adapted from Australasian College for Emergency Medicine (ACEM), Australian and New Zealand College of Anaesthetists (ANZCA), College of Intensive Care Medicine Australia and New Zealand (CICM). Guidelines for transport of critically ill patients; 2015. Available at: https://www.cicm.org.au/.

respective devices are in situ. There are particular complexities of transport for patients with traumatic brain injuries, from the clamping of external ventricular drains during transport and potential intracranial haemodynamic complications[199] to the potential for secondary insults due to instability,[198] to the rise in ICP observed in one series of patients during vertical movement in an elevator.[200] Other intermittent clinical monitoring should be undertaken as indicated by the patient's condition.[191]

A complete record should be made on one of either the ICU chart, specific transport form or electronic record of all details of the patient's condition, personnel involved, clinical events, observations and therapy given during transport. Predetermining minimum documentation and observation standards during transport will enhance patient safety and ongoing management. The transporting team should hand over directly to the receiving team providing continuing care for the patient[196,198] or should remain during the intervention/procedure to manage the patient's care.

Enhancing intra-hospital transport safety

There are many aspects to improving patient safety in intra-hospital transports including the use of guidelines, checklists, team training, incident reviews and team debriefs. Bergman and colleagues identified, from clinician interviews of adverse events during intra-hospital transport, 3 categories (organisational prerequisites, professional skills, attributes and behaviours and actions to perform transfer safely) and 12 subcategories of practices occurring during the events.[201] In the same study, 3 themes (hazardous procedure, performing when it matters and towards safe practices) and 10 subthemes related to clinician experiences of intra-hospital transport critical incidents evolved from the interviews.[201] In a subsequent study, the same authors tested a new instrument for measuring patient safety during intra-hospital transport.[202] This took the form of a structured questionnaire using the topics of: organisation, tools and technology, transport tasks, environment and teamwork to enable a review of each intra-hospital transport.[202] These recent studies are two of many which focus on improving practice in this challenging critical care practice area.

Summary

In the management of critically ill patients, there is always an initial focus on assessing and treating the patient's most life-threatening and immediate problems. Early attention should then be given to the implementation of preventive therapies such as VTE prophylaxis and pressure injury prevention, along with a thorough assessment of physical care needs and a subsequent plan of management. Recovery for patients to normal functioning after a critical illness is dependent upon a multitude of factors and is a dynamic process over time; however, much of the essential nursing care given to critically ill patients assists in reducing both deficits associated with their episode of illness and the time taken to achieve normal functioning.

Diligently attending to personal hygiene, including eye and oral care and positioning, is not only therapeutic but also provides comfort to patients in their stressful condition or situation of being in ICU. When patients are critically ill, the development of preventable complications such as constipation and urinary tract infection may have significant consequences for them, especially in the older patients. All critically ill patients are at risk of infection, and essential nursing care requires effective application of surveillance, prevention and control measures that should be applied equally to all patients. This principle is embedded in the recommended use of standard precautions. Critically ill patients are often transported to and from ICU; all transports pose a potential risk to patients, particularly if they are unstable. The essential nursing care topics discussion in this chapter are vital to the critically ill patient's well-being and recovery without unwelcome healthcare-related preventable complications.

This chapter has provided a comprehensive overview of the general but essential nursing care of critically ill patients. It offers a guideline for nurses that is relevant for most patients, most of the time. As with all other aspects of nursing practice, nursing care and intervention should be based on a thorough assessment of each individual patient's needs and risks and tailored to their preferences and other care requirements.

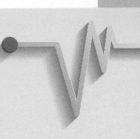

Case study

Mr L (Jack) is a widowed gentleman in his late seventies living independently in a retirement community. He was found collapsed at home by friends after missing a golf game. The friend who found him and called the ambulance said that, at his golf game 2 days prior, he had complained of a headache and sinus congestion and feeling quite tired. The ambulance team found him quietly sitting on the floor wedged up against a couch. He was cradling his left arm and wrist against his body. He was rousable and coherent, saying that he had been sitting on the couch yesterday afternoon and 'blacked out' for a short time so decided to just rest. A bit later, when getting up off the couch, he felt dizzy and a bit breathless and slipped and hurt his arm. He was unable to get up because of the extreme pain in his arm, so went to sleep where he was.

Observations were: temperature 37.6°C, respiratory rate 30, heart rate 92 and oxygen saturation SpO_2 91% via pulse oximetry, blood pressure (BP) 145/86 and pain score 4 when still and 9 when moving. The ambulance team applied nasal specs with 4 L oxygen, stabilised his arm and wrist in a sling and administered an analgesic via Penthrox (methoxyflurane) inhaler before transporting Mr L to the hospital.

On arrival at the ED, the triage nurse took the history and performed a rapid antigen test (RAT) for COVID-19 immediately. This was negative but, given Mr L's respiratory symptoms, a nasal pharyngeal swab for COVID-19 PCR (polymerase chain reaction) was taken, as the RAT result may be a false negative, being less sensitive than the PCR test.

Mr L was moved to a single room in the ED with staff wearing PPE. His vital signs were: respiratory rate 30, heart rate 84, oxygen saturation 90% despite 4 L oxygen via nasal specs, BP 157/82. Oxygen was increased to 6 L/minute via a non-rebreather face mask. A CXR showed bilateral diffuse changes and fractured clavicle but no malpositioning. The arm and wrist X-ray showed a fracture of the distal radius but again the wrist was aligned. A splint was applied to the left wrist and forearm to stabilise it, and his arm was placed back into the sling to limit shoulder and arm movement.

An intravenous cannula was inserted and intravenous fluids given to rehydrate Mr L. Neurological observations were normal but were to be repeated hourly. Neurovascular observations of the left arm and hand were also normal and to be repeated to observe for signs of numbness (nerve damage) or paleness (vascular/blood flow damage).

Mr L had been most anxious that someone contacted his daughter, who lives with her family 2 hours from the city. She provided the following information. Mr L manages all his own shopping, cooking, personal care and business needs. He is a keen golfer playing twice a week, though due to arthritic joints and some intermittent breathlessness, which he attributes to his large belly, he sometimes uses a golf cart rather than walking the entire course. Mr L's medical history includes moderate hypertension managed with antihypertensive medication, chronic lymphocytic leukaemia (CLL) (not requiring active treatment) and osteoarthritis in joints managed with paracetamol.

Mr L had continuing tachypnoea and little improvement in oxygen saturations despite the 6 L oxygen via non-rebreather mask. An arterial blood gas (ABG) analysis found pH 7.32, $PaCO_2$ 45 mmHg, PaO_2 77 mmHg, HCO_3 25 Eq/L. There was decreased air flow, crackling and a slight wheeze on breathing detected on lung auscultation.

Following review by the intensive care team for admission for respiratory support, a CT head scan was arranged during transport to ICU, as while Mr L continued to be generally orientated, the description of 'blacking out' and subsequent unwitnessed fall led to concerns of potential transient ischaemic attack (TIA) and to rule out head injury.

Mr L was transferred to ICU via a CT in the ED radiography department, which limited his transition through other areas of the hospital. All appropriate transmission-based precautions and staff used full PPE during the transport. Mr L was transported with full monitoring, still on the non-rebreather mask now at 8 L oxygen. During the transport and CT, close monitoring of Mr L's clinical condition, particularly his breathing and orientation, and constant reassurance were priorities of care.

Soon after arrival in ICU, it was noted the provisional result of the head CT scan was clear for injury from the fall and the COVID-19 PCR was negative. Therefore, causes of respiratory disease other than SARS-CoV2 needed to be considered. Standard precautions with respiratory hygiene were initiated, along with single room placement to enable contact, droplet and airborne precautions until the respiratory viral panel results were known.

Full assessment of Mr L was performed and appropriate vascular access (arterial catheter and a peripherally inserted central venous catheter (PICC)) was secured. Mr L had tried unsuccessfully to void in ED and again in ICU and shared that he sometimes had problems with voiding. His distended bladder was verified on portable bladder scanner and a urinary catheter was inserted aseptically. Ongoing monitoring and management of lines and catheters to prevent HAI was a nursing focus.

Routine laboratory assessments (serum electrolytes, complete blood screen), respiratory viral screen (nasal/pharyngeal swab – influenza A + B, rhinovirus, coronavirus, respiratory syncytial virus (RSV), human metapneumovirus, human parainfluenza virus (HPIV) 1, 2, 3, 4, adenovirus) and sputum specimen (for bacterial infection) were obtained.

It was found that Mr L was visited by his 3 grandchildren the previous weekend, one of whom had some mild cold-like symptoms. This was likely RSV and fitted with timelines for Mr L's exposure to the virus and the subsequent development of his own symptoms (RSV exposure to symptoms = 2–8 days and symptoms last around 3–7 days with a peak on day 5). Mr L's results from the respiratory viral panel subsequently tested positive for RSV. The infectious diseases team was consulted and ribavirin antiviral therapy was prescribed intravenously. Monitoring for ribavirin's potential side effects included: itching, rash, fatigue, headache, nausea, muscular pain, fever, insomnia and depression.

Mr L is a tall man with a large abdomen, which meant it can be difficult to breathe deeply when sitting up in bed. The nurses adjusted his bed to extend the length and then to simulate a chair. His injured arm was supported on a pillow. Mr L was nursed in a reverse Trendelenberg position (head up and feet down). This position decreases pressure on the diaphragm and improves respiratory compliance and gas exchange. The risk associated with this position is the potential for shear injury from sliding down the bed. To avoid this, the bed itself was tilted to enable Mr L to maintain the position. Despite these measures, Mr L remained tachypnoeic with borderline oxygen saturations and so non-invasive ventilation (NIV) was commenced. Mr L was still able to communicate verbally and eat and drink when appropriate. Mr L was using a full-face mask so the problem of increased pressure across the bridge of his nose was avoided. Fortunately, Mr L did not have a beard, and his cheeks were not sunken, so after selecting the appropriate size full-face mask the nurse was able to fit it without leaks. While the mask is in use, monitoring for facial pressure injury from mask edges is important.

Regular eye care and administration of artificial tears or ointment to lubricate the eyes when tolerated by Mr L were implemented to prevent potential DES from high-gas-flow leaks in NIV. Oral care was performed at least twice daily using toothpaste and brushing. His mouth was rinsed thoroughly to remove all residual toothpaste as this can be drying. Moistening the mouth with moist swabs, sips of water or mouth rinses regularly were provided for mucosal health and patient comfort.

As with all oxygen and ventilation therapy, essential monitoring included Mr L's airway (signs of obstruction, work of breathing), breathing (respiratory rate and breath sounds, bilateral chest symmetry, use of intercostal muscles), gas exchange (continuous pulse oximetry and as needed arterial blood gas sampling) and therapy (system intact with no leaks, parameters correct, mask well fitting).

Mr L's skin, especially his face, limbs and hands, could be described as 'weathered' from his frequent outside activities. On admission his skin was intact other than bruising and a skin tear on his left arm from the fall. He also had four small bruised areas on his neck, right hand and elbow area and left lower abdomen that may be related to his CLL. His coagulation profile was: INR slightly elevated (normal 0.8–1.1 ratio), APTT slightly elevated (normal 25–37 s), fibrinogen low end of normal (2.0–4.5 g/L), and low platelets (normal 150–450). CLL symptoms are anaemia with potential for shortness of breath, high lymphocyte count (that is less effective than normal against infections), abdominal discomfort from enlarged liver or spleen and low platelets.

Silicone dressings were applied to his sacrum and heels to prevent pressure injuries. The skin tear was carefully cleaned, realigned and lightly bandaged in place and monitored for signs of infection.

Mr L's bed was fitted with a pressure-relieving mattress and he was assisted in turning for regular skin assessment by a group of nurses, while they ensured they moved slowly given Mr L's restrictions from breathing and left clavicle and arm pain and for their own safety as he was a tall man and unable to assist much. Significant repositioning of Mr L was limited in the first 48 hours, but careful attention to small adjustments to the angles of the bed enabled some comfort and pressure prevention strategies to be implemented frequently.

Mr L was prescribed low-molecular-weight heparin for VTE prophylaxis and changed from graduated compression stockings to an IPC device because the initial compression stockings were ill fitting, causing skin indentation. Nurses carefully monitored for issues from the IPC device such as discomfort, warmth or sweating beneath the leggings, skin breakdown, rare nerve damage or rare pressure injury. The leggings were removed for only a short time each day (30 minutes) to allow for bathing and skin and neurovascular assessment prior to reapplication of the therapy. Mr L was encouraged to move his limbs frequently along with deep breathing and coughing. He became constipated on day 3, probably from dehydration pre-admission. He was administered senna without success, then lactulose, which worked well.

Over the following days, Mr L's care was focused on close monitoring of his respiratory function and any imminent fatigue. In addition, close attention was given to the prevention of complications such as pressure injury due to the limitations in patient repositioning and further infections due to invasive devices and therapies. To promote rest, the nurses scheduled groups of care activity and ensured regular rest periods with lights lowered and quiet room. Visitors were limited to his daughter's once-daily visits in full PPE (due to COVID-19 in the community).

On day 4, Mr L's respiratory function had improved and he was transitioned to a nasal high-flow oxygen system and was assisted to sit on the side of the bed. This was day 11 since he first had symptoms of RSV and so his contagious period was finishing. PPE was still required by staff in order to protect themselves and other unit patients. Following gradual weaning of oxygen and flow and assistance to sitting out of bed daily, on day 6 Mr L was placed on 2 L oxygen via nasal specs and transferred to the medical ward for ongoing recovery.

CASE STUDY QUESTIONS

1   What respiratory viruses does your healthcare facility routinely test for? How do you implement appropriate protective measures while waiting for the results?

2   What bed and mattress features does your unit/ward have available for patients with complex needs? What other strategies could be used to supplement these features?

3   How can you facilitate early mobilisation and what are the potential benefits of early mobilisation?

RESEARCH VIGNETTE

Dale CM, Carbone S, Gonzalez AL, et al. Recall of pain and discomfort during oral procedures experienced by intubated critically ill patients in the intensive care unit: a qualitative elicitation study. Can J Pain 2020;4(3):19-28.[38]

Abstract

Background: Intubated and mechanically ventilated patients in the ICU may experience pain during routine oral procedures such as oral suctioning and tooth brushing. Despite the importance of pain prevention and management, little is known about patients' experiences of procedural oral pain.

Aims: The aim of this study was to explore patients' recollections and recommendations for pain and discomfort during routine oral procedures.

Methods: A qualitative descriptive design was used. Adult patients were recruited from a mixed medical–surgical–trauma ICU in an academic hospital in Toronto, Canada. Participants were interviewed using object elicitation methods within 7 days of discharge from the ICU. Data were analysed using directed content analysis methods.

Results: We recruited 33 participants who were primarily male (23, 70%), with an average age of 54 (standard deviation (SD) = 18) years, admitted with a medical (13, 39%), trauma (11, 33%) or surgical (9, 27%) diagnosis and dentate (27, 82%). Most participants described oral procedures as painful, discomforting and emotionally distressing. Identified sources of pain included dry, inflamed oral tissues and procedural technique. Procedural pain behaviours were perceived to be frequently misinterpreted by clinicians as agitation, with consequences including physical restraint and unrelieved suffering. Participants advocated for greater frequency of oral care to prevent oral health deterioration, anticipatory procedural guidance and structured pain assessment to mitigate the dehumanising experience of unmanaged pain.

Conclusions: Patients described routine oral care procedures as painful and recalled suboptimal management of such pain. Procedural oral pain is an important target for practice improvement.

Critique

Oral care is performed several times a day for all patients cared for in ICUs, and if patients have sores, diseases or injuries in their mouths, oral care may generate pain several times a day. Examples of oral diseases are mucositis (inflammation, ulceration and haemorrhage of mucosal tissues), candidiasis (yeast/fungal infection of the mucous membranes), odynophagia (painful swallowing), gingivitis (gum inflammation) and tube-related (e.g. endotracheal, orogastric) pressure injuries. Since studies investigating patient recollection and recommendations for oral pain are lacking, this study fills an important gap in the literature.

A qualitative description (QD) design was employed in this study to better understand patient experiences of oral care. The study was conducted in a mixed medical–surgical–trauma ICU in a university-affiliated hospital in Canada. In that ICU, the patients received a unit-based oral hygiene regimen, including tooth brushing every 12 hours, suctioning of oral secretions every 1–4 hours and topical oral application of an antimicrobial solution (CHG 0.12%) using a swab every 6 hours. This regimen is in line with the literature and medical recommendations. Patients were included in the study if they were: (1) ≥18 years of age, (2) orally intubated in the ICU for ≥48 hours, (3) able to recall having an endotracheal tube, (4) competent to provide informed consent, (5) able to verbalise or communicate by other means, and (6) available to participate in an interview within 7 days of ICU discharge. Participants were prospectively recruited from a cohort of patients observed in another parent study following discharge from the ICU. Unfortunately, precisely how the patients were recruited and by whom was not described, making it challenging to replicate or generalise their findings. However, this was also noted in their limitations' section by the authors themselves.

A total of 33 patients met the inclusion criteria and were interviewed within 7 days of discharge. Interviewing patients so soon after discharge from the ICU could produce limited data, as patients are often exhausted after having critical illnesses. During the interviews, participants were allowed to see the devices that were used during their ICU stays, such as endotracheal tubes, Yankauer oral suction devices, toothbrushes and sponge-tipped swabs. The participants were also invited to rate their highest recollected procedural pain score on a 0 to 10 numeric rating scale. Giving patients the opportunity both to see the equipment and to share their experiences in their own words is a strength, as it may have helped patients better recall their oral care and pain levels during their ICU stays. Numeric pain intensity data and patient characteristics were presented in tables. Means and standard deviations or medians were used for continuous variables, and frequencies and percentages were used for categorical variables.

Content analysis was used to process and analyse the qualitative data. The analysis process is well described and resulted in four categories: descriptors of pain and emotional distress in participants' own words, perceived sources or contributors to pain, examples of unrecognised suffering and recommendations for professional care and support. Furthermore, words describing oral pain were counted and presented in a table. The four categories were clearly presented with short quotations related to the text, which can be seen as a strength. Eldh and colleagues[203] stated that quotations might be used in qualitative research to illustrate the analysis process and/or findings, the main purpose being to bring the text to life – or bring life to the text. In summary, this is a well-written important, relevant and innovative study that should be read by healthcare professionals working in ICUs.

Learning activities

1 List the benefits and risks of faecal containment devices.

2 Outline ICU patient preparation for transfer to the operating theatre.

3 What criteria do you use to evaluate the positioning in bed of your patients?

4 Name some of the significant infection risks for patients in ICU.

5 Summarise circulatory and respiratory challenges in the care of obese patients.

6 Describe how patients in intensive care are at risk of eye damage.

Online resources

Australian Department of Health and Aged Care, https://www.health.gov.au

Cochrane Library/Database of Systematic Reviews, https://cochranelibrary.com/cdsr/about-cdsr

College of Intensive Care Medicine of Australia and New Zealand (CICM), https://www.cicm.org.au

European Pressure Ulcer Advisory Panel, https://epuap.org

International Skin Tear Advisory Panel, https://www.skintears.org

US Centers for Disease Control and Prevention, https://www.cdc.gov

World Health Organization, https://www.who.int

Further reading

Dykes PC, Rozenblum R, Dalal A, et al. Prospective evaluation of a multifaceted intervention to improve outcomes in intensive care: the promoting respect and ongoing safety through patient engagement communication and technology study. Crit Care Med 2017;45(8):e806–13.

Dale CM, Tran, J, Herridge MS. Leaving a mark: pressure injury research in the intensive care unit. Intensive Care Med 2021;47:222–4.

References

1. El-Soussi AH, Asfour HI. A return to the basics; nurses' practices and knowledge about interventional patient hygiene in critical care units. Intensive Crit Care Nurs 2017;40:11–17. doi: 10.1016/j.iccn.2016.10.002.

2. Urbancic KF, Martensson J, Glassford N, et al. Impact of unit-wide chlorhexidine bathing in intensive care on bloodstream infection and drug-resistant organism acquisition. Crit Care Resusc 2018;20:109–16.

3. Afonso E, Blot K, Blot S. Prevention of hospital-acquired bloodstream infections through chlorhexidine gluconate-impregnated washcloth bathing in intensive care units: a systematic review and meta-analysis of randomised crossover trials. Euro Surveill 2016; 21. doi: 10.2807/1560–7917.ES.2016.21.46.30400.

4. Martin ET, Haider S, Palleschi M, et al. Bathing hospitalized dependent patients with prepackaged disposable washcloths instead of traditional bath basins: A case-crossover study. Am J Infect Control 2017;45:990–4. doi: 10.1016/j.ajic.2017.03.023.

5. European Pressure Ulcer Advisory Panel, National Pressure Injury Advisory Panel, Pan Pacific Pressure Injury Alliance (EPUAP/NPIAP/PPPIA). Haesler E, editor. Prevention and treatment of pressure ulcers/injuries: clinical practice guideline. EPUAP/NPIAP/PPPIA; 2019. Available from: https://internationalguideline.com/guideline.

6. Labeau SO, Afonso E, Benbenishty J, et al. Prevalence, associated factors and outcomes of pressure injuries in adult intensive care unit patients: the DecubICUs study. Intensive Care Med 2021;47:160–9. doi: 10.1007/s00134-020-06234-9.

7. Kottner J, Cuddigan J, Carville K, et al. Pressure ulcer/injury classification today: an international perspective. J Tissue Viability 2020;29:197–203. doi: 10.1016/j.jtv.2020.04.003.

8. Nowicki JL, Mullany D, Spooner A, et al. Are pressure injuries related to skin failure in critically ill patients? Aust Crit Care 2018;31:257–63. doi: 10.1016/j.aucc.2017.07.004.

9. Fulbrook P, Anderson A. Pressure injury risk assessment in intensive care: comparison of inter-rater reliability of the COMHON (Conscious level, Mobility, Haemodynamics, Oxygenation, Nutrition) Index with three scales. J Adv Nurs 2016;72:680–92. doi: 10.1111/jan.12825.

10. de Souza GKC, Kaiser DE, Morais PP, et al. Assessment of the accuracy of the CALCULATE scale for pressure injury in critically ill patients. Aust Crit Care 2022; S1036–7314(22)00001–7. doi: 10.1016/j.aucc.2021.12.010.

11. Lovegrove J, Fulbrook P, Miles S, et al. Effectiveness of interventions to prevent pressure injury in adults admitted to intensive care settings: a systematic review and meta-analysis of randomised controlled trials. Aust Crit Care 2022;35:186–203. doi: 10.1016/j.aucc.2021.04.007.

12. Fourie A, Ahtiala M, Black J, et al. Skin damage prevention in the prone ventilated critically ill patient: a comprehensive review and gap analysis (PRONEtect study). J Tissue Viability 2021;30:466–77. doi: 10.1016/j.jtv.2021.09.005.

13. Fitzgerald S, McTier L, Whitehead C, et al. Inter-rater reliability of descriptors for the classification of mucosal pressure injury: a prospective cross-sectional study. Aust Crit Care 2022;S1036-7314(21):00178–8. doi: 10.1016/j.aucc.2021.12.004.

14. Beeckman D. A decade of research on Incontinence-Associated Dermatitis (IAD): evidence, knowledge gaps and next steps. J Tissue Viability 2017;26:47–56. doi: 10.1016/j.jtv.2016.02.004.

15. Johansen E, Lind R, Sjobo B, et al. Moisture associated skin damage (MASD) in intensive care patients: a Norwegian point-prevalence study. Intensive Crit Care Nurs 2020;60:102889. doi: 10.1016/j.iccn.2020.102889.

16. Coyer F, Campbell J. Incontinence-associated dermatitis in the critically ill patient: an intensive care perspective. Nurs Crit Care 2018;23: 198–206. doi: 10.1111/nicc.12331.

17. Hitchcock J, Haigh DA, Martin N, et al. Preventing medical adhesive-related skin injury (MARSI). Br J Nurs 2021;30:S48–56. doi: 10.12968/bjon.2021.30.15.S48.

18. LeBlanc K, Campbell KE, Wood E, et al. Best practice recommendations for prevention and management of skin tears in aged skin: an overview. J Wound Ostomy Continence Nurs 2018;45:540–2. doi: 10.1097/WON.0000000000000481.

19. Van Tiggelen H, LeBlanc K, Campbell K, et al. Standardizing the classification of skin tears: validity and reliability testing of the International Skin Tear Advisory Panel Classification System in 44 countries. Br J Dermatol 2020;183:146–54. doi: 10.1111/bjd.18604.

20. Plaszewska-Zywko L, Sega A, Bukowa A, et al. Risk factors of eye complications in patients treated in the intensive care unit. Int J Environ Res Public Health 2021;18:11178. doi: 10.3390/ijerph182111178.

21. Fernandes APNdL, Araújo JNdM, Botarelli FR, et al. Dry eye syndrome in intensive care units: a concept analysis. Rev Bras Enferm 2018;71:1162–9. doi: 10.1590/0034-7167-2016-0582.

22. Hearne BJ, Hearne EG, Montgomery H, et al. Eye care in the intensive care unit. J Intensive Care Soc 2018;19:345–50. doi: 10.1177/1751143718764529.

23. Parekh PH, Boente CS, Boente RD, et al. Ophthalmology in critical care. Am Thorac Soc 2019;16:957–66. doi: 10.1513/AnnalsATS.201812-848CME.

24. Small J, Robertson E, Runcie C. Care of the eye during anaesthesia and intensive care. Anaesth Intensive Care Med 2019;20:731–4. doi: 10.1016/j.mpaic.2019.10.008.

25. Hilliam Y, Kaye S, Winstanley C. Pseudomonas aeruginosa and microbial keratitis. J Med Microbiol 2020;69:3–13. doi: 10.1099/jmm.0.001110.

26. Mela EK, Drimtzias EG, Christofidou MK, et al. Ocular surface bacterial colonisation in sedated intensive care unit patients. Anaesth Intensive Care 2010;38:190–3. doi: 10.1177/0310057X1003800129.

27. Kousha O, Kousha Z, Paddle J. Incidence, risk factors and impact of protocolised care on exposure keratopathy in critically ill adults: a two-phase prospective cohort study. Crit Care (London, England) 2018;22:5. doi: 10.1186/s13054-017-1925-5.

28. Silva Carneiro e Silva R, Raphael Escobar Gimenes F, Pimentel Moreno Mantilla N, et al. Risk for corneal injury in intensive care unit patients: a cohort study. Intensive Crit Care Nurs 2021;64:103017. doi: 10.1016/j.iccn.2021.103017.

29. Sansome SG, Lin PF. Eye care in the intensive care unit during the COVID-19 pandemic. Br J Hosp Med (Lond) 2020;81:1–10. doi: 10.12968/hmed.2020.0228.

30. Marshall AP, Elliott R, Rolls K, et al. Eyecare in the critically ill: clinical practice guideline. Aust Crit Care 2008;21:97–109. doi: 10.1016/j.aucc.2007.10.002.

31. Khatiban M, Moradi Amin H, Falahinia G, et al. Polyethylene eye-cover versus artificial teardrops in the prevention of ocular surface diseases in comatose patients: a prospective multicenter randomized triple-blinded three-arm clinical trial. PloS one 2021;16:e0248830. doi: 10.1371/journal.pone.0248830.

32. Kocaçal Güler E, Eşer İ, Eğrilmez S. Nurses can play an active role in the early diagnosis of exposure keratopathy in intensive care patients: exposure keratopathy in intensive care units. Jpn J Nurs Sci 2018;15:31–8. doi: 10.1111/jjns.12165.

33. Nikseresht T, Rezaei M, Khatony A. The effect of three eye care methods on the severity of lagophthalmos in intensive care patients: a randomized controlled clinical trial. J Ophthalmol 2021;2021:1–7. doi: 10.1155/2021/6348987.

34. Bendavid I, Avisar I, Serov Volach I, et al. Prevention of exposure keratopathy in critically ill patients: a single-center, randomized, pilot trial comparing ocular lubrication with bandage contact lenses and punctal plugs. Critical Care Med 2017;45:1880–6. doi: 10.1097/CCM.0000000000002681.

35. Choi BK, Kim MS, Kim SH. Risk prediction models for the development of oral-mucosal pressure injuries in intubated patients in intensive care units: a prospective observational study. J Tissue Viability 2020;29:252–7. doi: 10.1016/j.jtv.2020.06.002.

36. El-Rabbany M, Zaghlol N, Bhandari M, et al. Prophylactic oral health procedures to prevent hospital-acquired and ventilator-associated pneumonia: a systematic review. Int J Nurs Stud 2015;52:452–64. doi: 10.1016/j.ijnurstu.2014.07.010.

37. Dale CM, Angus JE, Sutherland S, et al. Exploration of difficulty accessing the mouths of intubated and mechanically ventilated adults for oral care: a video and photographic elicitation study. J Clin Nurs 2020;29:1920–32. doi: 10.1111/jocn.15014.

38. Dale CM, Carbone S, Gonzalez AL, et al. Recall of pain and discomfort during oral procedures experienced by intubated critically ill patients in the intensive care unit: a qualitative elicitation study. Can J Pain 2020;4:19–28. doi: 10.1080/24740527.2020.1732809.

39. Hockova B, Riad A, Valky J, et al. Oral complications of ICU patients with COVID-19: case-series and review of two hundred ten cases. J Clin Med 2021;10:581. doi: 10.3390/jcm10040581.

40. de Lacerda Vidal CF, Vidal AKdL, Monteiro JJGdM, et al. Impact of oral hygiene involving toothbrushing versus chlorhexidine in the prevention of ventilator-associated pneumonia: a randomized study. BMC Infect Dis 2017;17:112. doi: 10.1186/s12879-017-2188-0.

41. Hua F, Zhao T, Wu X, et al. Oral hygiene care for critically ill patients to prevent ventilator-associated pneumonia. Cochrane Database Syst Rev 2020;12(12):2020:CD008367. doi: 10.1002/14651858.CD008367.pub4.

42. Sands KM, Wilson MJ, Lewis MAO, et al. Respiratory pathogen colonisation of dental plaque, the lower airways and endotracheal tube biofilms during mechanical ventilation. J Crit Care 2016;37:30–7. doi: 10.1016/j.jcrc.2016.07.019.

43. Collins T, Plowright C, Gibson V, et al. British Association of Critical Care Nurses: evidence-based consensus paper for oral care within adult critical care units. Nurs Crit Care 2021;26:224–33. doi: 10.1111/nicc.12570.

44. Elkerbout TA, Slot DE, Bakker EWP, et al. Chlorhexidine mouthwash and sodium lauryl sulphate dentifrice: do they mix effectively or interfere? Int J Dent Hyg 2016;14:42–52. doi: 10.1111/idh.12125.

45. Sälzer S, Graetz C, Dörfer CE, et al. Contemporary practices for mechanical oral hygiene to prevent periodontal disease. Periodontology 2020;84:35–44. doi: 10.1111/prd.12332.

46. Unahalekhaka A, Butpan P, Wongsaen R, et al. Contamination of antimicrobial-resistant bacteria on toothbrushes used with mechanically ventilated patients: a cross sectional study. Intensive Crit Care Nurs 2022;68:103120. doi: 10.1016/j.iccn.2021.103120.

47. Doi S, Nakanishi N, Kawahara Y, et al. Impact of oral care on thirst perception and dry mouth assessments in intensive care patients: an observational study. Intensive Crit Care Nurs 202166:103073. doi: 10.1016/j.iccn.2021.103073.

48. Kjeldsen CL, Hansen MS, Jensen K, et al. Patients' experience of thirst while being conscious and mechanically ventilated in the intensive care unit. Nurs Crit Care 2018;23:75–81. doi: 10.1111/nicc.12277.

49. Rabello F, Araújo VE, Magalhães SMS. Effectiveness of oral chlorhexidine for the prevention of nosocomial pneumonia and ventilator-associated pneumonia in intensive care units: Overview of systematic reviews. Int J Dent Hygiene 2018;16:441–9. doi: 10.1111/idh.12336.

50. Hughes C, Ferguson J. Phenotypic chlorhexidine and triclosan susceptibility in clinical *Staphylococcus aureus* isolates in Australia. Pathology 2017;49:633–7. doi: 10.1016/j.pathol.2017.05.008.

51. Chiewchalermsri C, Sompornrattanaphan M, Wongsa C, et al. Chlorhexidine allergy: current challenges and future prospects. J Asthma Allergy 2020;13:127–33. doi: 10.2147/JAA.S207980.

52. Winning L, Lundy FT, Blackwood D, et al. Oral health care for the critically ill: a narrative review. Crit Care (London, England) 2021;25:353. doi: 10.1186/s13054-021-03765-5.

53. Dale CM, Rose L, Carbone S, et al. Effect of oral chlorhexidine de-adoption and implementation of an oral care bundle on mortality for mechanically ventilated patients in the intensive care unit (CHORAL): a multi-center stepped wedge cluster-randomized controlled trial. Intensive Care Med 2021;47:1295–302. doi: 10.1007/s00134-021-06475-2.

54. Deschepper M, Waegeman W, Eeckloo K, et al. Effects of chlorhexidine gluconate oral care on hospital mortality: a hospital-wide, observational cohort study. Intensive Care Med 2018;44:1017–26. doi: 10.1007/s00134-018-5171-3.

55. Jackson L, Owens M. Does oral care with chlorhexidine reduce ventilator-associated pneumonia in mechanically ventilated adults? Br J Nurs 2019;28:682–9. doi: 10.12968/bjon.2019.28.11.682.

56. Blot S. Antiseptic mouthwash, the nitrate-nitrite-nitric oxide pathway, and hospital mortality: a hypothesis generating review. Intensive Care Med 2021;47:28–38. doi: 10.1007/s00134-020-06276-z

57. Chaboyer WP, Thalib L, Harbeck EL, et al. Incidence and prevalence of pressure injuries in adult intensive care patients: a systematic review and meta-analysis. Crit Care Med 2018;46:e1074–81. doi: 10.1097/CCM.0000000000003366.

58. Minet C, Potton L, Bonadona A, et al. Venous thromboembolism in the ICU: main characteristics, diagnosis and thromboprophylaxis. Crit Care (London, England) 2015;19:287. doi: 10.1186/s13054-015-1003-9.

59. Waldauf P, Jiroutkova K, Krajcova A, et al. Effects of rehabilitation interventions on clinical outcomes in critically ill patients: systematic review and meta-analysis of randomized controlled trials. Crit Care Med 2020;48:1055–65. doi: 10.1097/CCM.0000000000004382.

60. Arias-Fernandez P, Romero-Martin M, Gomez-Salgado J, et al. Rehabilitation and early mobilization in the critical patient: systematic review. J Phys Ther Sci 2018;30:1193–201. doi: 10.1589/jpts.30.1193.

61. Lai CC, Chou W, Chan KS, et al. Early mobilization reduces duration of mechanical ventilation and intensive care unit stay in patients with acute respiratory failure. Arch Phys Med Rehabil 2017;98:931–9. doi: 10.1016/j.apmr.2016.11.007.

62. Paton M, Lane R, Paul E, et al. Mobilization during critical illness: a higher level of mobilization improves health status at 6 months, a secondary analysis of a prospective cohort study. Crit Care Med 2021;49:E860–9. doi: 10.1097/CCM.0000000000005058.

63. Schaller SJ, Scheffenbichler FT, Bose S, et al. Influence of the initial level of consciousness on early, goal-directed mobilization: a post hoc analysis. Intensive Care Med 2019;45:201–10. doi: 10.1007/s00134-019-05528-x.

64. Zang K, Chen B, Wang M, et al. The effect of early mobilization in critically ill patients: a meta-analysis. Nurs Crit Care 2020;25:360–7. doi: 10.1111/nicc.12455.

65. Schaller SJMD, Anstey MMPH, Blobner MP, et al. Early, goal-directed mobilisation in the surgical intensive care unit: a randomised controlled trial. Lancet (British edition) 2016;388:1377–88. doi: 10.1016/S0140-6736(16)31637-3.

66. Doiron KA, Hoffmann TC, Beller EM, et al. Early intervention (mobilization or active exercise) for critically ill adults in the intensive care unit. Cochrane Database Syst Rev 2018;3(3):CD010754. doi: 10.1002/14651858.CD010754.pub2.

67. Menges D, Seiler B, Tomonaga Y, et al. Systematic early versus late mobilization or standard early mobilization in mechanically ventilated adult ICU patients: systematic review and meta-analysis. Crit Care 2021;25:16. doi: 10.1186/s13054-020-03446-9.

68. Tipping CJ, Harrold M, Holland A, et al. The effects of active mobilisation and rehabilitation in ICU on mortality and function: a systematic review. Intensive Care Med 2016;43:171–83. doi: 10.1007/s00134-016-4612-0.

69. Bein T, Bischoff M, Bruckner U, et al. S2e guideline: positioning and early mobilisation in prophylaxis or therapy of pulmonary disorders : Revision 2015: S2e guideline of the German Society of Anaesthesiology and Intensive Care Medicine (DGAI). Anaesthesist 2015;64(Suppl. 1): 1–26. doi: 10.1007/s00101-015-0071-1.

70. Lang JK, Paykel MS, Haines KJ, et al. Clinical practice guidelines for early mobilization in the ICU: a systematic review. Crit Care Med 2020;48:e1121–8. doi: 10.1097/CCM.0000000000004574.

71. Cameron S, Ball I, Cepinskas G, et al. Early mobilization in the critical care unit: a review of adult and pediatric literature. J Crit Care 2015;30:664–72. doi: 10.1016/j.jcrc.2015.03.032.

72. Rollinson TC, Connolly B, Berlowitz DJ, et al. Physical activity of patients with critical illness undergoing rehabilitation in intensive care and on the acute ward: An observational cohort study. Aust Crit Care 2022;35(4):362–8. doi: 10.1016/j.aucc.2021.06.005.

73. Frade-Mera MJ, Zaragoza-García I, Gallart E, et al. Care and treatments related to intensive care unit–acquired muscle weakness: a cohort study. Aust Crit Care 2021;34(5):435–45. doi: 10.1016/j.aucc.2020.12.005.

74. Zorowitz RD. ICU-acquired weakness: a rehabilitation perspective of diagnosis, treatment, and functional management. Chest 2016;150:966–71. doi: 10.1016/j.chest.2016.06.006.

75. Krupp AE, Ehlenbach WJ and King B. Factors nurses in the intensive care unit consider when making decisions about patient mobility. Am J Crit Care 2019;28:281–9. doi: 10.4037/ajcc2019624.

76. Engström J, Bruno E, Reinius H, et al. Physiological changes associated with routine nursing procedures in critically ill are common: an observational pilot study. Acta Anaesthesiol Scand 2017;61:62–72. doi: 10.1111/aas.12827.

77. Nyholm L, Steffansson E, Fröjd C, et al. Secondary insults related to nursing interventions in neurointensive care: a descriptive pilot study. J Neurosci Nurs 2014;46:285–91. doi: 10.1097/jnn.0000000000000077.

78. Nydahl P, Sricharoenchai T, Chandra S, et al. Safety of patient mobilization and rehabilitation in the intensive care unit. Systematic review with meta-analysis. Ann Am Thorac Soc 2017;14:766–77. doi: 10.1513/AnnalsATS.201611-843SR.

79. Pradalier F, Jourdan C, Laffont I, et al. Safety of early rehabilitation in neuro-intensive care units: How far can we go? Scoping review and meta-analysis of adverse events. Ann Phys Rehabil Med 2018;61:e273. doi: 10.1016/j.rehab.2018.05.636.

80. Boyd J, Paratz J, Tronstad O, et al. When is it safe to exercise mechanically ventilated patients in the intensive care unit? An evaluation of consensus recommendations in a cardiothoracic setting. Heart Lung 2018;47:81–6. doi: 10.1016/j.hrtlng.2017.11.006.

81. Hodgson CL, Schaller SJ, Nydahl P, et al. Ten strategies to optimize early mobilization and rehabilitation in intensive care. Crit Care 2021;25: 324. doi: 10.1186/s13054-021-03741-z.

82. Yang R, Zheng Q, Zuo D, et al. Safety assessment criteria for early active mobilization in mechanically ventilated ICU subjects. Respir Care 2021;66:307–15. doi: 10.4187/respcare.07888.

83. Cambiaso-Daniel J, Parry I, Rivas E, et al. Strength and cardiorespiratory exercise rehabilitation for severely burned patients during intensive care units: a survey of practice. J Burn Care Res 2018;39:897–901. doi: 10.1093/jbcr/iry002.

84. Kim E and Drew PJ. Management of burn injury. Surgery (Oxford) 2022;40:62–9. doi: 10.1016/j.mpsur.2021.11.006.

85. van Willigen Z, Ostler C, Thackray D, et al. Patient and family experience of physical rehabilitation on the intensive care unit: a qualitative exploration. Physiotherapy 2020;109:102–10. doi: 10.1016/j.physio.2020.01.003.

86. Soderberg A, Karlsson V, Ahlberg BM, et al. From fear to fight: patients' experiences of early mobilization in intensive care. a qualitative interview study. Physiother Theory Pract 2020:1–9. doi: 10.1080/09593985.2020.1799460.

87. Corner EJ, Murray EJ, Brett SJ. Qualitative, grounded theory exploration of patients' experience of early mobilisation, rehabilitation and recovery after critical illness. BMJ Open 2019;9:e026348. doi: 10.1136/bmjopen-2018-026348.

88. Sousa I, Kapp S, Santamaria N. Positioning immobile critically ill patients who are at risk of pressure injuries using a purpose-designed positioning device and usual care equipment: An observational feasibility study. Int Wound J 2020;17:1028–38. doi: 10.1111/iwj.13365.

89. Pozuelo-Carrascosa DP, Cobo-Cuenca AI, Carmona-Torres JM, et al. Body position for preventing ventilator-associated pneumonia for critically ill patients: a systematic review and network meta-analysis. J Intensive Care 2022;10:9. doi: 10.1186/s40560-022-00600-z.

90. Newman ANL, Gravesande J, Rotella S, et al. Physiotherapy in the neurotrauma intensive care unit: a scoping review. J Crit Care 2018;48: 390–406. doi: 10.1016/j.jcrc.2018.09.037.

91. Olkowski BF and Shah SO. Early mobilization in the neuro-ICU: how far can we go? Neurocrit Care 2016;27:141–50. doi: 10.1007/s12028-016-0338-7.

92. Guérin C. Prone position. Curr Opin Crit Care 2014;20:92–7. doi: 10.1097/MCC.0000000000000059.

93. Díaz-Bohada L, Segura-Salguero JC, Garzón-Beltrán NF, et al. Considerations of invasive mechanical ventilation in prone position. A narrative review. Colombian J Anesthesiol 2021;50:e1013. doi: 10.5554/22562087.e1013.

94. Langer T, Brioni M, Guzzardella A, et al. Prone position in intubated, mechanically ventilated patients with COVID-19: a multi-centric study of more than 1000 patients. Crit Care 2021;25:128. doi: 10.1186/s13054-021-03552-2.

95. Rodriguez-Huerta MD, Diez-Fernandez A, Rodriguez-Alonso MJ, et al. Nursing care and prevalence of adverse events in prone position: characteristics of mechanically ventilated patients with severe SARS-CoV-2 pulmonary infection. Nurs Crit Care 2021;27(4):493–500. doi: 10.1111/nicc.12606.

96. Schieren M, Piekarski F, Dusse F, et al. Continuous lateral rotational therapy in trauma – a systematic review and meta-analysis. J Trauma Acute Care Surg 2017;83:926–33. doi: 10.1097/TA.0000000000001572.

97. Schieren M, Wappler F, Klodt D, et al. Continuous lateral rotational therapy in thoracic trauma – a matched pair analysis. Injury 2020;51:51–8. doi: 10.1016/j.injury.2019.11.009.

98. Störmann P, Marzi I and Wutzler S. Rotational therapy in thoracic injuries: what is the evidence? Curr Opin Crit Care 2017;23:527–32. doi: 10.1097/MCC.0000000000000467.

99. Parry SM, Nydahl P, Needham DM. Implementing early physical rehabilitation and mobilisation in the ICU: institutional, clinician, and patient considerations. Intensive Care Med 2018;44:470–3. doi: 10.1007/s00134-017-4908-8.

100. Ely EW. The ABCDEF bundle: science and philosophy of how ICU liberation serves patients and families. Crit Care Med 2017;45:321–30. doi: 10.1097/CCM.0000000000002175.

101. Viarasilpa T, Panyavachiraporn N, Marashi SM, et al. Prediction of symptomatic venous thromboembolism in critically ill patients: the ICU-Venous Thromboembolism Score. Crit Care Med 2020;48:e470–9. doi: 10.1097/CCM.0000000000004306.

102. Ejaz A, Ahmed MM, Tasleem A, et al. Thromboprophylaxis in intensive care unit patients: a literature review. Curēus (Palo Alto, CA) 2018;10:e3341. doi: 10.7759/cureus.3341.

103. Galanaud J-P, Monreal M, Kahn SR. Epidemiology of the post-thrombotic syndrome. Thromb Res 2018;164:100–9. doi: 10.1016/j.thromres.2017.07.026.

104. Alisha S, Mary S, Vijay S, et al. Deep venous thrombosis prophylaxis practices in surgical intensive care unit patients: a cross-sectional study. J Clin Diag Res 2021;15:UC11–13. doi: 10.7860/JCDR/2021/46724.14495.

105. Arabi YM, Al-Hameed F, Burns KEA, et al. Adjunctive intermittent pneumatic compression for venous thromboprophylaxis. N Engl J Med 2019;380:1305–15. doi: 10.1056/NEJMoa1816150.

106. Fernando SM, Tran A, Cheng W, et al. VTE prophylaxis in critically ill adults. Chest 2022;161:418–28. doi: 10.1016/j.chest.2021.08.050.

107. Australian Commission on Safety and Quality Health Service (ACSQHS). Hospital-acquired complication – 7. Venous thromboembolism. In: Selected best practices and suggestions for improvement for clinicians and health system managers. Available from: https://www.safetyandquality.gov.au/sites/default/files/migrated/SAQ7730_HAC_Factsheet_VenousThromboemolism_LongV2.pdf. [Accessed 11 February 2023].

108. Greenall R, Davis RE. Intermittent pneumatic compression for venous thromboembolism prevention: a systematic review on factors affecting adherence. BMJ Open 2020;10:e037036. doi: 10.1136/bmjopen-2020-037036.

109. Weinberger J, Cipolle M. Mechanical prophylaxis for post-traumatic VTE: stockings and pumps. Curr Trauma Rep 2016;2:35–41. doi: 10.1007/s40719-016-0039-x.

110. Lin T-L, Dhillon NK, Conde G, et al. Early positive fluid balance is predictive for venous thromboembolism in critically ill surgical patients. Am J Surg 2021;222:220–6. doi: 10.1016/j.amjsurg.2020.08.032.

111. Qin X, Yu P, Li H, et al. Integrating the "best" evidence into nursing of venous thromboembolism in ICU patients using the i-PARIHS framework. PloS One 2020;15:e0237342. doi: 10.1371/journal.pone.0237342.

112. Heinonen T, Ferrie S, Ferguson C. Gut function in the intensive care unit – what is 'normal'? Aust Crit Care 2020;33:151–4. doi: 10.1016/j.aucc.2018.12.007.

113. Wanik J, Teevan C, Pepin L, et al. Implementation of a bowel protocol to improve enteral nutrition and reduce Clostridium difficile testing. Crit Care Nurse 2019;39:e10–18. doi: 10.4037/ccn2019304.

114. Dionne JC, Sullivan K, Mbuagbaw L, et al. Diarrhoea: interventions, consequences and epidemiology in the intensive care unit (DICE-ICU): a protocol for a prospective multicentre cohort study. BMJ Open 2019;9:e028237. doi: 10.1136/bmjopen-2018-028237.

115. Lewis SJ, Heaton KW. Stool form scale as a useful guide to intestinal transit time. Scand J Gastroenterol 1997;32:920–4. doi: 10.3109/00365529709011203.

116. Bianchi J S-GT. The dangers of faecal incontinence in the at-risk patient. Wound Int 2012;3:15–21. doi: Available from: https://www.woundsinternational.com. [Accessed 11 February 2023].

117. de Azevedo RP, Machado FR. Constipation in critically ill patients: much more than we imagine. Rev Bras Ter Intensiva 2013;25:73–4. doi: 10.5935/0103-507X.20130014.

118. Bishop S, Young H, Goldsmith D, et al. Bowel motions in critically ill patients: a pilot observational study. Crit Care Resusc 2010;12:182–5.

119. Hay T, Bellomo R, Rechnitzer T, et al. Constipation, diarrhea, and prophylactic laxative bowel regimens in the critically ill: a systematic review and meta-analysis. J Crit Care 2019;52:242–50. doi: 10.1016/j.jcrc.2019.01.004.

120. Locke GR, 3rd, Pemberton JH, Phillips SF. American Gastroenterological Association Medical position statement: guidelines on constipation. Gastroenterology 2000;119:1761–6. doi: 10.1053/gast.2000.20390.

121. Gacouin A, Camus C, Gros A, et al. Constipation in long-term ventilated patients: associated factors and impact on intensive care unit outcomes. Crit Care Med 2010;38:1933–8. doi: 10.1097/CCM.0b013e3181eb9236.

122. Zhang Y, Leng M, Guo J, et al. The effectiveness of faecal collection devices in preventing incontinence-associated dermatitis in critically ill patients with faecal incontinence: A systematic review and meta-analysis. Aust Crit Care 2021;34:103–12. doi: 10.1016/j.aucc.2020.04.152.

123. Wilson N, Bellomo R, Hay T, et al. Faecal diversion system usage in an adult intensive care unit. Crit Care Resusc 2020;22:152–7.

124. Bright E, Fishwick G, Berry D, et al. Indwelling bowel management system as a cause of life-threatening rectal bleeding. Case Rep Gastroenterol 2008;2:351–5. doi: 10.1159/000155147.

125. A'Court J, Yiannoullou P, Pearce L, et al. Rectourethral fistula secondary to a bowel management system. Intensive Crit Care Nurs 2014;30:226–30. doi: 10.1016/j.iccn.2013.12.003.

126. Massey J, Gatt M, Tolan DJ, et al. An ano-vaginal fistula associated with the use of a faecal management system: a case report. Colorectal Dis 2010;12:e173–4. doi: 10.1111/j.1463-1318.2009.01945.x.

127. Mangal S, Pho A, Arcia A, et al. Patient and family engagement in catheter-associated urinary tract infection (CAUTI) prevention: a systematic review. Jt Comm J Qual Patient Saf 2021;47:591–603. doi: 10.1016/j.jcjq.2021.05.009.

128. Lo E, Nicolle LE, Coffin SE, et al. Strategies to prevent catheter-associated urinary tract infections in acute care hospitals: 2014 update. Infect Control Hosp Epidemiol 2014;35:464–79. doi: 10.1086/675718.

129. Alvarez Lerma F, Olaechea Astigarraga P, Nuvials X, et al. Is a project needed to prevent urinary tract infection in patients admitted to Spanish ICUs? Med Intensiva (Engl ed.) 2019;43:63–72. doi: 10.1016/j.medin.2017.12.003.

130. Flaatten H, de Lange DW, Artigas A, et al. The status of intensive care medicine research and a future agenda for very old patients in the ICU. Intensive Care Med 2017;43:1319–28. doi: 10.1007/s00134-017-4718-z.

131. Athari F, Hillman KM, Frost SA. The concept of frailty in intensive care. Aust Crit Care 2019;32:175–8. doi: 10.1016/j.aucc.2017.11.005.

132. Darvall JN, Bellomo R, Paul E, et al. Frailty in very old critically ill patients in Australia and New Zealand: a population-based cohort study. Med J Aust 2019;211:318–23. doi: 10.5694/mja2.50329.

133. Guidet B, Vallet H, Boddaert J, et al. Caring for the critically ill patients over 80: a narrative review. Ann Intensive Care 2018;8:114–15. doi: 10.1186/s13613-018-0458-7.

134. Palmer K, Vetrano DL, Marengoni A, et al. The relationship between anaemia and frailty: a systematic review and meta-analysis of observational studies. J Nutr Health Aging 2018;22:965–74. doi: 10.1007/s12603-018-1049-x.

135. Tsutsumimoto K, Doi T, Makizako H, et al. Aging-related anorexia and its association with disability and frailty. J Cachexia, Sarcopenia Muscle 2018;9:834–3. doi: 10.1002/jcsm.12330.

136. Larsson L, Degens H, Li M, et al. Sarcopenia: aging-related loss of muscle mass and function. Physiol Rev 2019;99:427–511. doi: 10.1152/physrev.00061.2017.

137. Brummel NE, Balas MC, Morandi A, et al. Understanding and reducing disability in older adults following critical illness. Crit Care Med 2015;43:1265–75. doi: 10.1097/CCM.0000000000000924.

138. Reznik ME, Slooter AJC. Delirium management in the ICU. Curr Treat Options Neurol 2019;21:1–18. doi: 10.1007/s11940-019-0599-5.

139. Strøm C, Rasmussen LS, Steinmetz J. Practical management of anaesthesia in the elderly. Drugs Aging 2016;33:765–77. doi: 10.1007/s40266-016-0413-y.

140. Serra R, Ielapi N, Barbetta A, et al. Skin tears and risk factors assessment: a systematic review on evidence-based medicine. Int Wound J 2018;15:38–42. doi: 10.1111/iwj.12815.

141. Chambers ES, Vukmanovic-Stejic M. Skin barrier immunity and ageing. Immunology 2020;160:116–25. doi: 10.1111/imm.13152.

142. Johnson K, Fleury J, McClain D. Music intervention to prevent delirium among older patients admitted to a trauma intensive care unit and a trauma orthopaedic unit. Intensive Crit Care Nurs 2018;47:7–14. doi: 10.1016/j.iccn.2018.03.007.

143. Thiolliere F, Allaouchiche B, Boyer H, et al. Association between out-of-bed mobilization during the ICU stay of elderly patients and long-term autonomy: a cohort study. J Crit Care 2022;68:10–15. doi: 10.1016/j.jcrc.2021.11.007.

144. Dennis DM, Bharat C, Paterson T. Prevalence of obesity and the effect on length of mechanical ventilation and length of stay in intensive care patients: a single site observational study. Aust Crit Care 2017;30:145–50. doi: 10.1016/j.aucc.2016.07.003.

145. Grossschaedl F and Bauer S. The relationship between obesity and nursing care problems in intensive care patients in Austria. Nurs Crit Care 2022;27(4):512–18. doi: 10.1111/nicc.12554.

146. Carbone S, Canada JM, Billingsley HE, et al. Obesity paradox in cardiovascular disease: where do we stand? Vasc Health Risk Manag 2019;15:89–100. doi: 10.2147/VHRM.S168946.

147. Tomiyama AJ, Carr D, Granberg EM, et al. How and why weight stigma drives the obesity 'epidemic' and harms health. BMC Med 2018;16:123. doi: 10.1186/s12916-018-1116-5.

148. Flint SW, Leaver M, Griffiths A, et al. Disparate healthcare experiences of people living with overweight or obesity in England. EClinicalMed 2021;41:101140. doi: 10.1016/j.eclinm.2021.101140.

149. Bejciy-Spring S. R-E-S-P-E-C-T: a model for the sensitive treatment of the bariatric patient. Bariatr Nurs Surg Patient Care 2008;3(1):47–56.

150. Robstad N, Söderhamn U, Fegran L. Intensive care nurses' experiences of caring for obese intensive care patients: a hermeneutic study. J Clin Nurs 2018;27:386–95. doi: 10.1111/jocn.13937.

151. Roesslein M, Chung F. Obstructive sleep apnoea in adults: peri-operative considerations: a narrative review. Eur J Anaesthesiol 2018;35:245–55. doi: 10.1097/EJA.0000000000000765.

152. Wang R, Mihaicuta S, Tiotiu A, et al. Asthma and obstructive sleep apnoea in adults and children – an up-to-date review. Sleep Med Rev 2022;61:101564. doi: 10.1016/j.smrv.2021.101564.

153. De Jong A, Chanques G, Jaber S. Mechanical ventilation in obese ICU patients: from intubation to extubation. Crit Care 2017;21:63. doi: 10.1186/s13054-017-1641-1.

154. Hassan EA and Baraka AAE. The effect of reverse Trendelenburg position versus semi recumbent position on respiratory parameters of obese critically ill patients: a randomised controlled trial. J Clin Nurs 2021;30:995–1002. doi: 10.1111/jocn.15645.

155. Fischer AJ, Kaese S, Lebiedz P. Management of obese patients with respiratory failure – a practical approach to a health care issue of increasing significance. Respir Med 2016;117:174–8. doi: 10.1016/j.rmed.2016.06.002.

156. Rees M, Collins CE, De Vlieger N, et al. Non-surgical interventions for hospitalized adults with class ii or class iii obesity: a scoping review. Diabetes Metab Syndr Obes 2021;14:417–29. doi: 10.2147/DMSO.S280735.

157. De Jong A, Verzilli D, Jaber S. ARDS in obese patients: specificities and management. Crit Care (London, England) 2019;23:74. doi: 10.1186/s13054-019-2374-0.

158. Berrios LA. The ABCDs of managing morbidly obese patients in intensive care units. Crit Care Nurse 2016;36:17–26. doi: 10.4037/ccn2016671.

159. Lee YR, Blanco DD. Efficacy of standard dose unfractionated heparin for venous thromboembolism prophylaxis in morbidly obese and non-morbidly obese critically ill patients. J Thromb Thrombolysis 2017;44:386–91. doi: 10.1007/s11239-017-1535-8.

160. Hirt PA, Castillo DE, Yosipovitch G, et al. Skin changes in the obese patient. J Am Acad Dermatol 2019;81:1037–57. doi: 10.1016/j.jaad.2018.12.070.

161. Erstad BL, Barletta JF. Drug dosing in the critically ill obese patient – a focus on sedation, analgesia, and delirium. Crit Care (London, England) 2020;24:315–18. doi: 10.1186/s13054-020-03040-z.

162. May M, Schindler C, Engeli S. Modern pharmacological treatment of obese patients. Ther Adv Endocrinol Metabol 2020;11:2042018819897527. doi: 10.1177/2042018819897527.

163. Wiggermann N, Smith K, Kumpar D. What bed size does a patient need? The relationship between body mass index and space required to turn in bed. Nurs Res (New York) 2017;66:483–9. doi: 10.1097/NNR.0000000000000242.

164. Hales C, Coombs M, de Vries K. The challenges in caring for morbidly obese patients in intensive care: a focused ethnographic study. Aust Crit Care 2018;31:37–41. doi: 10.1016/j.aucc.2017.02.070.

165. World Health Organization (WHO). Coronavirus disease (COVID-19) pandemic. Available from: https://www.who.int/emergencies/diseases/novel-coronavirus-2019. [Accessed 11 February 2023].

166. Australian Government Department of Health. Coronavirus (COVID-19) pandemic. Online: Available from: https://www.health.gov.au/health-alerts/covid-19. [Accessed 11 February 2023].

167. Australian Commission on Safety and Quality in Health Care. COVID-19 infection prevention and control risk management – Guidance. Available from: https://www.safetyandquality.gov.au/publications-and-resources/resource-library/covid-19-infection-prevention-and-control-risk-management-guidance. [Accessed 11 February 2023].

168. National Health and Medical Research Council (NHMRC). Australian guideline for the prevention and control of infection in healthcare (2019). Available from: https://www.nhmrc.gov.au/health-advice/public-health/preventing-infection. Canberra, ACT: NHMRC; 2019. [Accessed 11 February 2023].

169. World Health Organization (WHO). Guidelines on core components of infection prevention and control programs at the national and acute health care facility level. Geneva: WHO; 2016. Available from: https://www.who.int/publications/i/item/9789241549929. [Accessed 11 February 2023].

170. Haley RW, Culver DH, White JW, et al. The efficacy of infection surveillance and control programs in preventing nosocomial infections in US hospitals. Am J Epidemiol 1985;121:182–205. doi: 10.1093/oxfordjournals.aje.a113990.

171. Australian and New Zealand Intensive Care Society (ANZICS). ANZICS COVID-19 guidelines version 4. Available from: https://www.anzics.com.au/anzics-covid-19-guidelines-version-4/. [Accessed 11 February 2023].

172. Marshall AP, Austin DE, Chamberlain D, et al. A critical care pandemic staffing framework in Australia. Aust Crit Care 2021;34:123–31. doi: 10.1016/j.aucc.2020.08.007.

173. Australian Government Infection Control Expert Group. Guidance on the use of personal protective equipment (PPE) for health care workers in the context of COVID-19. Available from: https://www.health.gov.au/resources/publications/guidance-on-the-use-of-personal-protective-equipment-ppe-for-health-care-workers-in-the-context-of-covid-19. [Accessed 11 February 2023].

174. Gamage B, Moore D, Copes R, et al. Protecting health care workers from SARS and other respiratory pathogens: a review of the infection control literature. Am J Infect Control 2005;33:114–21. doi: 10.1016/j.ajic.2004.12.002.

175. Chan D. Clinical management of SARS patients in ICU. Connect (London, England: 2001) 2003;2:76–9. doi: 10.1891/1748–6254.2.3.76.

176. Centers for Disease Control and Prevention (CDC). Middle East respiratory syndrome (MERS). Available from: http://www.cdc.gov/coronavirus/MERS/index.html. [Accessed 11 February 2023].

177. Middle East respiratory syndrome: global summary and assessment of risk, 16 November 2022. WHO-MERS-RA-2022.1-eng.pdf at https://www.who..int/publications/i/item/WHO-MERS-RA-2022.1. [Accessed 12 May 2023].

178. Centers for Disease Control and Prevention (CDC). Past pandemics. Washington DC: CDC; 2018. Available from: https://www.cdc.gov/flu/pandemic-resources/basics/past-pandemics.html. [Accessed 11 February 2023].

179. World Health Organization (WHO). Disease outbreak news (DONs). Geneva: WHO; n.d. Available from: https://www.who.int/emergencies/disease-outbreak-news. [Accessed 11 February 2023].

180. World Health Organization (WHO). Antimicrobial resistance. Geneva: WHO; n.d. Available from: https://www.who.int/health-topics/antimicrobial-resistance. [Accessed 11 February 2023].

181. Finco G, Musu M, Landoni G, et al. Healthcare-associated respiratory infections in intensive care unit can be reduced by a hand hygiene program: a multicenter study. Aust Crit Care 2018;31:340–6. doi: 10.1016/j.aucc.2017.10.004.

182. Australian Commission on Safety and Quality in Health Care (ACSQHC). AURA 2021. Fourth Australian report on antimicrobial use and resistance in human health. Available from: https://www.safetyandquality.gov.au/publications-and-resources/resource-library/aura-2021-fourth-australian-report-antimicrobial-use-and-resistance-human-health. [Accessed 11 February 2023].

183. Abrams D, Grasselli G, Schmidt M, et al. ECLS-associated infections in adults: what we know and what we don't yet know. Intensive Care Med 2020;46:182–91. doi: 10.1007/s00134-019-05847-z.

184. Colombo SM, Palomeque AC, Li Bassi G. The zero-VAP sophistry and controversies surrounding prevention of ventilator-associated pneumonia. Intensive Care Med 2020;46:368–71. doi: 10.1007/s00134-019-05882-w.

185. Harward M, Smith A, Aitken LM. Inconsistent VAP definitions raise questions of usefulness. Aust Crit Care 2018;31:54–55. doi: 10.1016/j.aucc.2017.01.004.

186. Alvarez-Lerma F, Palomar-Martinez M, Sanchez-Garcia M, et al. Prevention of ventilator-associated pneumonia: the multimodal approach of the Spanish ICU "Pneumonia Zero" program. Crit Care Med 2018;46:181–8. doi: 10.1097/CCM.0000000000002736.

187. Hallam C, Jackson T, Rajgopal A, et al. Establishing catheter-related bloodstream infection surveillance to drive improvement. J Infect Prev 2018;19:160–6. doi: 10.1177/1757177418767759.

188. Ling ML, Apisarnthanarak A, Jaggi N, et al. APSIC guide for prevention of central line associated bloodstream infections (CLABSI). Antimicrob Resist Infect Control 2016;5:16. doi: 10.1186/s13756-016-0116-5.

189. Buetti N, Rickard CM, Timsit JF. Catheter dressings. Intensive Care Med 2022;48(8):1066–8. doi: 10.1007/s00134-022-06734-w.

190. Koh DB, Robertson IK, Watts M, et al. Density of microbial colonization on external and internal surfaces of concurrently placed intravascular devices. Am J Crit Care 2012;21:162–71. doi: 10.4037/ajcc2012675.

191. Australasian College for Emergency Medicine (ACEM), Australian and New Zealand College of Anaesthetists (ANZCA), College of Intensive Care Medicine Australia and New Zealand (CICM). Guidelines for transport of critically ill patients IC-10. Available from: https://www.cicm.org.au/CICM_Media/CICMSite/CICM-Website/Resources/Professional%20Documents/IC-10-Guidelines-for-Transport-of-Critically-Ill-Patients.pdf. [Accessed 11 February 2023].

192. Wallace PG, Ridley SA. ABC of intensive care. Transport of critically ill patients. BMJ 1999;319:368–71. doi: 10.1136/bmj.319.7206.368.

193. Bergman L, Pettersson M, Chaboyer W, et al. Safety hazards during intrahospital transport: a prospective observational study. Crit Care Med 2017;45:e1043–9. doi: 10.1097/CCM.0000000000002653.

194. Parmentier-Decrucq E, Poissy J, Favory R, et al. Adverse events during intrahospital transport of critically ill patients: incidence and risk factors. Ann Intensive Care 2013;3:10. doi: 10.1186/2110-5820-3-10.

195. Yousuf B, Sujatha KS, Alfoudri H, et al. Transport of critically ill COVID-19 patients. Intensive Care Med 2020;46:1663–4. doi: 10.1007/s00134-020-06115-1.

196. Jia L, Wang H, Gao Y, et al. High incidence of adverse events during intra-hospital transport of critically ill patients and new related risk factors: a prospective, multicenter study in China. Crit Care 2016;20:12. doi: 10.1186/s13054-016-1183-y.

197. Murata M, Nakagawa N, Kawasaki T, et al. Adverse events during intrahospital transport of critically ill patients: A systematic review and meta-analysis. Am J Emerg Med 2022;52:13–19. doi: 10.1016/j.ajem.2021.11.021.

198. Williams P, Karuppiah S, Greentree K, et al. A checklist for intrahospital transport of critically ill patients improves compliance with transportation safety guidelines. Aust Crit Care 2020;33:20–4. doi: 10.1016/j.aucc.2019.02.004.

199. Chaikittisilpa N, Lele AV, Lyons VH, et al. Risks of routinely clamping external ventricular drains for intrahospital transport in neurocritically ill cerebrovascular patients. Neurocrit Care 2017;26:196–204. doi: 10.1007/s12028-016-0308-0.

200. Trofimov A, Kalentiev G, Yuriev M, et al. Intrahospital transfer of patients with traumatic brain injury: increase in intracranial pressure. Acta Neurochir Suppl 2016;122:125–7. doi: 10.1007/978-3-319-22533-3_25.

201. Bergman L, Pettersson M, Chaboyer W, et al. Improving quality and safety during intrahospital transport of critically ill patients: a critical incident study. Aust Crit Care 2020;33:12–19. doi: 10.1016/j.aucc.2018.12.003.

202. Bergman L, Chaboyer W, Pettersson M, et al. Development and initial psychometric testing of the Intrahospital Transport Safety Scale in intensive care. BMJ Open 2020;10:e038424. doi: 10.1136/bmjopen-2020-038424.

203. Eldh AC, Årestedt L, Berterö C. Quotations in qualitative studies: reflections on constituents, custom, and purpose. Int J Qual Methods 2020;19:1. doi: 10.1177/1609406920969268.

Chapter 6

Patient comfort and psychological care

Rosalind Elliott, Leanne Aitken, Julia Pilowsky

Learning objectives

After reading this chapter, you should be able to:

- implement appropriate evidence-based strategies to manage patient anxiety and depression
- describe the subtypes of delirium
- discuss strategies to potentially prevent, or reduce the duration and severity of, delirium in the critically ill patient
- implement and evaluate delirium assessment screening instruments for the critically ill
- implement screening strategies to identify patients at risk of substance dependence
- implement alcohol withdrawal assessment monitoring instruments
- integrate best practice into pain assessment and management
- describe the different instruments available to assess sedation needs in critically ill patients and discuss the benefits and limitations of each
- determine methods to promote rest and sleep for critically ill patients.

Introduction

Promotion of comfort, psychological health and well-being of patients is an essential aspect of care for critically ill patients. Patients experience significant discomfort and ongoing compromise of their psychological health both while in the critical care environment and beyond. Effective management of both patients' comfort and their psychological health also influences their physical health. Aspects of patient comfort and psychological health that are most relevant in the care of the critically ill include the recognition and management of anxiety, depression, delirium, withdrawal from alcohol or other substances, pain, sedation and sleep. Inclusion of the patient's family in promoting comfort and psychological health is an important consideration. Despite widespread recognition of the need for regular assessment using validated instruments and targeted management to achieve patient comfort, there are repeated reports indicating absent or infrequent and incomplete assessment, with a lack of subsequent care, internationally.[1–4]

Although each of the concepts of anxiety, depression, delirium, pain, sedation and sleep are reviewed sequentially through this chapter, in reality it is often difficult to separate them as their effects are additive or synergistic. While it is important to ensure that assessment incorporates each of the individual concepts, management may often target multiple aspects concurrently.

Anxiety and depression

Patients may experience anxiety and depression both during and following a period of critical illness. Anxiety has been defined as an unpleasant emotional arousal or condition caused by a perceived threat or stressor.[5] It can be classified as an underlying mental health disorder, as well as a transient emotional state, known as state anxiety, which manifests as 'subjective feelings of tension, apprehension, nervousness, and worry'.[6] Depression is characterised by a persistent low mood and loss of interest in general activities, and may also be accompanied by sleep disturbances and cognitive changes.[7]

Factors contributing to symptoms of anxiety or depression include:[8–14]

- pre-existing high trait anxiety
- current or previous dependence on alcohol or illicit substance/opioids
- previous mental illness
- unwanted symptoms such as pain, sleeplessness, thirst, and discomfort and immobility
- interventions including mechanical ventilation, invasive devices, repositioning and suctioning
- increased severity of illness
- use of certain medications such as vasopressors and benzodiazepines
- adverse and unfamiliar environmental conditions such as noise and light

- extended ICU length of stay
- concerns about current illness together with underlying chronic disease and the ongoing impact of illness on recovery.

Anxiety has been identified in approximately half of critically ill patients, and symptoms of depression in approximately one-third.[7,8,15–17] Patterns of anxiety vary widely; high levels of anxiety early or later in the ICU stay are frequent.[18] The prevalence of anxiety in critically ill patients appears to be similar across countries and cultures.[10,16,19]

Both anxiety and depression can lead to negative outcomes for critical care patients during and after their stay in ICU. Physiological and psychological responses to anxiety reflect a stress response and incorporate avoidance behaviour, increased vigilance and arousal, activation of the sympathetic nervous system and release of cortisol from the adrenal glands.[20] The humoral response, mediated by the hypothalamic–pituitary–adrenal (HPA) axis, regulates this activity. Physiological changes occur to multiple body systems, with the most relevant including constriction of blood vessels, increased heart rate, relaxation of airways, increased secretion of adrenaline (epinephrine) and noradrenaline (norepinephrine), as well as increased glucose production,[20] and result in behavioural, psychological/cognitive and social manifestations (Table 6.1).[21–23] Symptoms of depression such as low mood and motivation can result in these patients not participating in beneficial therapies during the ICU admission, such as early mobilisation and physiotherapy.[24] Depression is also associated with significantly higher mortality rates after patients have been discharged from ICU.[7,25,26]

Anxiety and depression assessment

The importance of psychological and emotional assessment, with the aim of ameliorating the adverse effects of anxiety and depression, is widely accepted.[27] However, recognition

---

TABLE 6.1

Clinical indicators of anxiety

PHYSIOLOGICAL	BEHAVIOURAL	PSYCHOLOGICAL/COGNITIVE	SOCIAL
Heart rate	Restlessness	Confusion	Seeking reassurance
Blood pressure	Agitation	Anger	Need for attention/
Chest pain	Sleeplessness	Negative thinking	companionship
Respiratory rate	Hypervigilance	Verbal expression of stress/anxiety	Limiting interaction
Shortness of breath	Fighting ventilator	Crying	
Altered O$_2$ saturation	Facial grimacing/tension	Inability to retain and process	
Coughing/choking feeling	Uncooperative	information	
Diaphoresis	Rapid speech		
Pallor	Difficulty verbalising		
Cold and clammy	Distrustful/suspicious		
Dry mouth	Avoidance/desire to leave stressful area		
Pain			
Headache			
Nausea and vomiting			
Swallowing difficulty			

and interpretation of anxiety and depression is complex, particularly when signs and symptoms are masked by critical illness and its treatment. History and previous experience are vital adjuncts to patient assessment and diagnosis and often provide information that is vital to effective care and treatment.[28] Alterations in levels of biochemical markers, such as cortisol and catecholamines, that are frequently associated with anxiety may also be attributed to physiological stress.[23] Hence, validated rating scales are advocated and may offer benefits not found with unstructured clinical assessment.[29]

> **Practice tip**
>
> Remember, a patient's history and previous experiences are vital to 'knowing the person' so if a patient is unable to communicate then ask their family and friends about past experiences of illnesses, hospitalisations, phobias, likes and dislikes and usual coping strategies.

A structured approach to assessment is needed to accurately and consistently understand patients' psychological problems. A number of self-report scales are available to assess anxiety and depression (Table 6.2).[6,22,30–38] These scales require a degree of cognitive acumen and an ability to communicate responses – a challenge for many critically ill patients. In addition, some scales have up to 21 items, making them both time consuming and unmanageable for routine use. Patients with visual and auditory impairments may require additional assistance, such as larger print, hearing aids or glasses, in order to complete the forms.

The visual analogue scale for anxiety (VAS-A) is a single-item measure which is fast and simple to complete, and has been shown to have good reliability and validity.[35] It comprises a 100-millimetre vertical line, with the bottom marker labelled 'not anxious at all' and the top marker labelled 'the most anxious I have ever been'.

Similarly, the Faces Anxiety Scale, another single-item self-reporting scale which was developed by Australian researchers, accurately detects anxiety in critically ill patients.[22] There are five possible responses to assess anxiety (Fig. 6.1).

Anxiety and depression management

The detrimental short- and long-term effects of anxiety and depression, and importance of ameliorating or managing these unpleasant psychophysiological states, are widely accepted.[29,39,40] Although pharmacological interventions such as anxiolytic medications and analgesia are well recognised and frequently used, non-pharmacological treatments (i.e. environmental and nurse-initiated interventions) are also useful.

Non-pharmacological treatments

An advantage of non-pharmacological treatments is that they can be nurse initiated. Environmental aspects may be implemented when units are designed or refurbished (Table 6.3).[41–51] Although the benefits of some complementary therapies may be widely accepted in the community, use of them in critical care is dependent on their acceptance, safety, efficacy and patient consent. While the level of evidence is low, beneficial effects for some complementary therapies such as music therapy and massage have been reported and include lowered blood pressure, heart rate and respiratory rate; improved sleep; and

---

TABLE 6.2

Anxiety and depression self-report assessment scales

SCALE	NUMBER OF ITEMS	COMMENTS
Hospital Anxiety and Depression Scale (HADS)[30]	14	Easy and fast to complete Extensively used and therefore international comparisons are available Demonstrated validity
Depression Anxiety and Stress Scale 21 (DASS 21)[31]	21	Items measured on scale of 0 (did not apply to me at all) to 3 (applied to me very much or most of the time) Demonstrated validity in clinical populations[32]
Spielberger State Anxiety Inventory (SAI)[33]	20	Items measured on a scale of 1 (not at all) to 4 (very much so) Validity demonstrated in various populations[6] Too long for routine clinical use, but may be useful in associated research; attempts to shorten the SAI have provided inconsistent results[6,34]
Visual Analogue Scale – Anxiety (VAS-A)[35]	1	10 cm/100 mm line from 'not at all anxious' to 'very anxious' Demonstrated validity[35]
Faces Anxiety Scale[22]	1	5 possible responses or 'faces' to reflect anxiety Fast and easy to use Validity has been demonstrated in a small number of ICU cohorts[22,36–38]

FIGURE 6.1 Faces Anxiety Scale.[22]

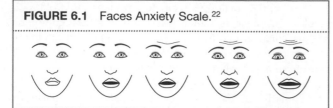

Source: Adapted from McKinley S, Coote K, Stein-Parbury J. Development and testing of a Faces Scale for the assessment of anxiety in critically ill patients. J Adv Nurs 2003;41(1):73–9, with permission.

TABLE 6.3

Non-pharmacological measures to reduce anxiety

NURSE-INITIATED TREATMENTS	ENVIRONMENTAL FACTORS
Patient massage[41,42]	Provision of natural light[45]
Aromatherapy[48,49]	Calming wall colours such as blue, green and violet
Music therapy[43,44,50]	Noise reduction with consideration of alarms, paging systems, talking, etc.[51]

reduced stress (and concomitant sedative medication requirements), anxiety and pain.[41–45] More-structured non-pharmacological therapies, such as cognitive behavioural therapy, have also been reported to reduce the symptoms of anxiety as well as potentially having other effects such as a reduction in duration of mechanical ventilation.[46,47] As with any therapy, each non-pharmacological treatment may have different effects on individual patients; consequently, ongoing assessment is essential. In addition, the safety of these therapies during critical illness has not been well demonstrated, necessitating thorough monitoring and caution throughout administration.

Other strategies to improve patients' psychological health include communication and information sharing by the healthcare team and inclusion of family members in care processes.[27] The presence of a family member can provide additional reassurance and inner strength (see Chapter 7). In addition, the very presence of the nurse has been reported to be a great source of security, reducing feelings of vulnerability.[53]

Pharmacological treatments

Treatment for pain and other reversible physiological causes of anxiety and agitation should be a priority. If anxiety and agitation continue, despite the incorporation of non-pharmacological interventions, pharmacological treatment with relevant medications may be initiated. A brief overview of these medications in the treatment of unrelieved anxiety is provided in Table 6.4.[54–57] Generally, non-benzodiazepine sedative medications such as propofol are recommended in preference to benzodiazepines.[54] A thorough medication history should also be conducted, as the abrupt cessation of outpatient psychoactive medications in the ICU may increase agitation or lead to withdrawal symptoms.[55] If the patient is medically stable, it may be more appropriate to restart medications they were previously taking rather than commencing other therapies to treat agitation.[56]

Delirium

Delirium is a significant concern for critically ill patients and clinicians. It is a central nervous dysfunction in which behaviours and physiological responses are not conducive to healing and recovery. Arguably, the condition has been underrecognised and undertreated[58] and is only recently receiving the attention it deserves. Early detection and treatment of delirium is vital, as it is associated with adverse clinical outcomes such as prolonged duration of ventilation and hospitalisation and higher rates of morbidity and mortality.[59–61] Furthermore, long periods of delirium have been associated with long-term cognitive impairment[62] and an increase in delusional memories.[63, 64]

There are three subtypes of delirium: *hypoactive*, *hyperactive* and *combined* (a combination of both).[65] Disturbances in attention (e.g. reduced ability to direct,

TABLE 6.4

Pharmacological treatment for anxiety[54, 57]

DRUG GROUP	DRUG/DOSE RANGE	ACTION	SIDE EFFECTS	COMMENT
Sedative hypnotic agent	Propofol 10–100 micrograms/kg/min (infusion)	General anaesthetic agent	Hypotension Respiratory depression Myocardial depression when given as bolus Reported to affect memory May cause dreams	Dedicated intravenous line Infusions recommended High metabolic clearance Patient's conscious level increases more quickly once drug is ceased Expensive
Non-benzodiazepine sedative	Dexmedetomidine 0.2–0.7 micrograms/kg/h (infusion)	Highly selective alpha-2-adrenoceptor agonist	Initial hypertension may be experienced Hypotension Bradycardia may persist Hyperglycaemia	Minimal respiratory depression Rapid onset Infusions preferred Not suitable when deep sedation is required May reduce incidence of delirium
Benzodiazepine sedative	Diazepam 5–10 mg bolus	Block encoding on GABA receptors	Long-acting metabolites Hypotension Respiratory depression	No analgesia properties Used to treat alcohol withdrawal
	Midazolam 0.5–10 mg/h (infusion) 1–2 mg (bolus)		Less likely to have above side effects, but they may still occur	Useful as continuous infusion Rapid onset No analgesia properties Amnesic effect
	Lorazepam 0.01–0.1 mg/kg/h (≤10 mg/h)		Less likely to have above side effects, but they may still occur	Not licensed for use in some countries Strong anxiolytic

Sources: Devlin JW, Skrobik Y, Gelinas C, et al. Clinical practice guidelines for the prevention and management of pain, agitation/sedation, delirium, immobility, and sleep disruption in adult patients in the ICU. Crit Care Med 2018;46:e825–73; Zaal Zaal IJ, Devlin JW, Peelen LM, et al. A systematic review of risk factors for delirium in the ICU. Crit Care Med 2015;43:40–7. doi: 10.1097/CCM.0000000000000625.

focus, sustain and shift attention) and awareness (e.g. reduced orientation to the environment) that develop over a short period of time (e.g. hours to a few days) are characteristic of all subtypes of delirium.[66] This contrasts with dementia, in which cognitive decline occurs over months and years. Cognitive and perceptive ability often fluctuates through the day, worsening at night. A change in an additional cognitive domain such as memory deficit, disorientation or language disturbance that is not better accounted for by a pre-existing, established or evolving other neurocognitive disorder and does not occur in the context of a severely reduced level of arousal such as coma is diagnostic of delirium. There should also be evidence from the patient's history, physical examination or laboratory findings that the disturbance is a direct physiological consequence of another medical condition or substance intoxication or withdrawal.[67] Alcohol, nicotine or illicit substance/opioid dependence is more common than many clinicians suspect and this is often a result of history taking that lacks detail.[68] This topic is explored more thoroughly in the next section.

Lethargy, slow quiet speech and reduced alertness are typical behaviours of hypoactive delirium. This is the most common type of delirium; however, given that many patients with hypoactive delirium appear 'quietly' confused, it may not be recognised and treated.[65] Behaviours evident in hyperactive delirium such as hyperactivity and agitation cannot go unnoticed by clinicians and present overt risks of self-injury such as unintentional extubation/decannulation and intravenous/arterial device removal. Combined delirium is characterised by fluctuations in activity and attention levels including the behaviours of both hyperactive and hypoactive subtypes.

Delirium occurs in approximately one-third of ICU patients, although reports from individual studies vary widely,[61,65] an unsurprising finding given that it is notoriously difficult to diagnose in patients who are unable to communicate verbally. The prevalence in other critical care areas such as emergency departments is generally reported to be lower,[69] probably because the patients' severity of illness varies.

The exact pathophysiology of delirium is not yet fully understood; however, imbalances in brain cholinergic and dopaminergic neurotransmitter systems are thought to be responsible.[70,71] Many predisposing and precipitating risk factors have been identified (Table 6.5)[49,54,70,72–75] and current opinion suggests that there is an additive effect: patients with more than one predisposing factor will require less noxious precipitating factors to develop delirium than patients who have none.[72] Predisposing risk factors are those that exist prior to the occurrence of critical illness, while precipitating risk factors occur during the course of critical illness and may be disease-related or iatrogenic. Prevention and therapeutic management of risk factors is the mainstay delirium treatment.

Practice tip

Perform a patient assessment to identify predisposing and contributing risk factors for delirium (see Table 6.5). Interview the family if the patient is unable to provide a history. Discuss your findings with the multidisciplinary healthcare team and develop a plan for prevention (using the strategies suggested in this chapter). Document and evaluate.

TABLE 6.5

Risk factors for delirium

PREDISPOSING RISK FACTORS	PRECIPITATING RISK FACTORS[54,57,73–75]
Advanced age	Increased severity of illness
Dementia	Emergency surgery or
Illicit substance use	multitrauma
Excessive intake of	Metabolic, fluid and electrolyte
alcohol	disturbance (particularly
Smoking	uraemia)
Sensory deficits	Systemic inflammatory
Renal insufficiency	response (particularly infection)
Previous cerebral	Hypoxia
damage	Acute injury affecting the CNS
Hypertension	Medications that affect
Congestive heart failure	acetylcholine transmission, e.g.
History of depression	atropine, fentanyl
Genetic propensity	Psychoactive medications, e.g.
Functional dependence	benzodiazepines
and frailty	Prolonged pain
	Excessive noise
	Sleep deprivation
	Immobility
	Blood transfusion administration

Assessment of delirium

The increased morbidity and mortality associated with delirium make it imperative to incorporate reliable and valid assessment in routine care.[76] A practical delirium assessment screening instrument for the critically ill cannot be reliant on patient–assessor verbal communication. Both the Intensive Care Delirium Screening Checklist (ICDSC)[76] (Fig. 6.2) and the Confusion Assessment Method for the Intensive Care Unit (CAM-ICU)[77] (Fig. 6.3) have been shown to fulfil these requirements, although clinical judgement should also be retained in the screening process.[54,78,79]

The ICDSC contains eight items based on the Diagnostic and statistical manual of mental disorders (DSM-IV) criteria for delirium and was validated in a study conducted within ICU.[76] It is also simple to use and easily integrated into patient documentation. All features of delirium are incorporated such as sleep pattern disturbances and hypo- or hyperactivity. The first step in using the ICDSC is an assessment of conscious level using a five-point scale (A–E). Only patients whose conscious level is sufficient for them to respond to moderate physical stimuli (C–E on the scale) are able to be assessed. The eight items of the ICDSC are rated present (1) or absent (0). A score of four or higher is considered to be indicative of delirium.[76]

The CAM-ICU was also validated for screening delirium in the ICU population (see Further reading for more information).[77,80] Acute onset of mental status changes or fluctuating course is assessed using neurological observations conducted over the previous 24 hours. Inattention is tested in patients who are unable to communicate verbally by using either picture recognition or a random letter test. Disorganised thinking is assessed by listening to the patient's speech and, for patients who are unable to verbally communicate, a simple command is provided such as 'hold up the same number of fingers as me' (while the assessor holds up their fingers). Any conscious level other than 'alert' is considered 'altered'. An overall score is not derived from the CAM-ICU; delirium is either present or absent.[77]

Prevention and treatment of delirium

Although the causes of delirium are thought not to be strictly 'psychological' in nature, many interventions and preventative strategies focus on reducing anxiety, maintaining safety and providing a calming and low stimulus environment together with ameliorating or eliminating risk factors. Individual patient risk factors should be identified and where possible modified (even in the absence of delirium). Potential preventative measures include:

- adequate pain relief
- reassurance to reduce anxiety
- judicious use of sedative medications, particularly benzodiazepine medications (avoidance of continuous infusions)

FIGURE 6.2 Intensive Care Delirium Screening Checklist (ICDSC).[76]

PATIENT EVALUATION	DAY 1	DAY 2	DAY 3	DAY 4	DAY 5
Altered level of consciousness* (A–E)					
If A or B do not complete patient evaluation for the period					
Inattention					
Disorientation					
Hallucination – delusion – psychosis					
Psychomotor agitation or retardation					
Inappropriate speech or mood					
Sleep/wake cycle disturbance					
Symptom fluctuation					
TOTAL SCORE (0–8)					

		Score
Level of consciousness*:	A: no response	none
	B: response to intense and repeated stimulation (loud voice and pain)	none
	C: response to mild or moderate stimulation	1
	D: normal wakefulness	0
	E: exaggerated response to normal stimulation	1

SCORING SYSTEM:
The scale is completed based on information collected from each entire 8-hour shift or from the previous 24 hours. Obvious manifestation of an item = 1 point. No manifestation of an item or no assessment possible = 0 point. The score of each item is entered in the corresponding empty box and is 0 or 1.

1. Altered level of consciousness:
A) No response or B) the need for vigorous stimulation in order to obtain any response signified a severe alteration in the level of consciousness precluding evaluation. If there is coma (A) or stupor (B) most of the time period then a dash (-) is entered and there is no further evaluation during that period.
C) Drowsiness or requirement of a mild to moderate stimulation for a response implies an altered level of consciousness and scores 1 point.
D) Wakefulness or sleeping state that could easily be aroused is considered normal and scores no point.
E) Hypervigilance is rated as an abnormal level of consciousness and scores 1 point.

2. Inattention: Difficulty in following a conversation or instructions. Easily distracted by external stimuli Difficulty in shifting focuses. Any of these scores 1 point.

3. Disorientation: Any obvious mistake in time, place or person scores 1 point.

4. Hallucination, delusion or psychosis: The unequivocal clinical manifestation of hallucination or of behaviour probably due to hallucination (e.g, trying to catch a non-existent object) or delusion. Gross impairment in reality testing. Any of these scores 1 point.

5. Psychomotor agitation or retardation: Hyperactivity requiring the use of additional sedative drugs or restraints in order to control potential dangerousness (e.g. pulling out IV lines, hitting staff), hyperactivity or clinically noticeable psychomotor slowing. Any of these scores 1 point.

6. Inappropriate speech or mood: Inappropriate, disorganised or incoherent speech. Inappropriate display of emotion related to events or situation. Any of these scores 1 point.

7. Sleep/wake cycle disturbance: Sleeping less than 4 hours or waking frequently at night (do not consider wakefulness initiated by medical staff or loud environment). Sleeping during most of the day. Any of these scores 1 point.

8. Symptom fluctuation: Fluctuation of the manifestation of any item or symptom over 24 hours (e.g. from one shift to another) scores 1 point.

Source: Adapted from Bergeron N, Dubois MJ, Dumont M, et al. Intensive care delirium screening checklist: evaluation of a new screening tool. Intensive Care Med 2001;27(5):859–64.

- correction of the physiological effects of critical illness (e.g. hypoxia, hypotension, infection and fluid and electrolyte imbalance)
- optimisation of the sleep cycle
- early mobilisation
- treatment of the underlying illness
- family participation and involvement in patient care.

Research investigating the prevention and management of delirium in ICU is growing; however, evidence for the majority of interventions is low. There is emerging evidence that intervention bundles directed towards preventing delirium among other aspects of care in ICU patients may be beneficial.[51,81–83] Given the hypothesised underlying pathophysiology of delirium, it is not surprising that strategies to promote and maintain good-quality

FIGURE 6.3 Confusion Assessment Method – Intensive Care Unit (CAM-ICU).[80]

CAM-ICU Worksheet

		Positive	Negative
Feature 1: Acute Onset or Fluctuating Course Positive if you answer 'yes' to either 1A or 1B.		Positive	Negative
1A: Is the patient different than his/her baseline mental status? Or 1B: Has the patient had any fluctuation in mental status in the past 24 hours as evidenced by fluctuation on a sedation scale (e.g. RASS), GCS, or previous delirium assessment?		Yes	No
Feature 2: Inattention Positive if either score for 2A or 2B is less than 8. Attempt the ASE letters first. If patient is able to perform this test and the score is clear, record this score and move to Feature 3. If patient is unable to perform this test or the score is unclear, then perform the ASE Pictures. If you perform both tests, use the ASE Pictures' results to score the Feature.		Positive	Negative
2A: ASE Letters: record score (enter NT for not tested) Directions: Say to the patient, "*I am going to read you a series of 10 letters. Whenever you hear the letter 'A', indicate by squeezing my hand.*" Read letters from the following letter list in a normal tone. SAVEAHAART Scoring: Errors are counted when patient fails to squeeze on the letter "A" and when the patient squeezes on any letter other than "A".		Score (out of 10):_____	
2B: ASE Pictures: record score (enter NT for not tested) Directions are included on the picture packets.		Score (out of 10):_____	
Feature 3: Disorganised Thinking Positive if the combined score is less than 4		Positive	Negative
3A: Yes/No Questions (Use either Set A or Set B, alternate on consecutive days if necessary): Set A Set B 1. Will a stone float on water? 1. Will a leaf float on water? 2. Are there fish in the sea? 2. Are there elephants in the sea? 3. Does one pound weigh more than 3. Do two pounds weigh more than two pounds? one pound? 4. Can you use a hammer to pound a nail? 4. Can you use a hammer to cut wood? Score___(Patient earns 1 point for each correct answer out of 4) 3B: Command Say to patient: "Hold up this many fingers" (Examiner holds two fingers in front of patient) "Now do the same thing with the other hand" (Not repeating the number of fingers). (If patient is unable to move both arms, for the second part of the command ask patient "Add one more finger") Score___(Patient earns 1 point if able to successfully complete the entire command)		Combined Score (3A + 3B): _____ (out of 5)	
Feature 4: Altered Level of Consciousness Positive if the Actual RASS score is anything other than "0" (zero)		Positive	Negative
Overall CAM-ICU (Features 1 and 2 and either Feature 3 or 4):		Positive	Negative

Source: © E. Wesley Ely, MD, MPH. Pulmonary and Critical Care and Health Services Research. Vanderbilt University and VA-GRECC. https://www.icudelirium.org.

sleep and avoidance of benzodiazepines are emphasised in these 'bundles'. Regardless of the efficacy of the interventions[84] to date, the creation of environmental conditions that are conducive to rest and sleep, in particular sound reduction and adjusting light levels appropriate for the time of day, as well as sedation minimisation, delirium monitoring and early mobilisation, have not been shown to cause harm and therefore represent good practice.

In cases where non-pharmacological strategies are not successful, antipsychotic medications (e.g. olanzapine) or the selective alpha-2-adrenoceptor agonist dexmedetomidine may be considered.[54] Although frequently used, there is little evidence showing the efficacy of haloperidol and atypical antipsychotics in reducing the duration of delirium in adult ICU patients (and humans generally).[85,86] Evidence is inconsistent,[87] but dexmedetomidine has shown promise in reducing both the duration and the incidence of delirium in critically ill patients.[88–90] It should also be noted that any medication designed to enhance cognition has the potential to make delirium worse and there are many potential unwanted side effects (e.g. Q–T interval prolongation for some antipsychotics[91] and bradycardia and hypotension for alpha-2-adrenoceptor agonists[88]); therefore these medications should be used judiciously in the critically ill.

Alcohol, benzodiazepine, nicotine and opioid withdrawal

Patients who are dependent on alcohol (ethanol), benzodiazepines, nicotine or opioids are at risk of developing a withdrawal syndrome in the initial stages of treatment in ICU. Withdrawal from opioids may also occur later in the illness trajectory for patients who receive large doses of analgesics for painful injuries and conditions ('iatrogenic dependency'). Unrecognised and therefore untreated withdrawal from any substance may lead to prolonged length of stay and duration of mechanical ventilation and increased risk of infection and delirium, and even mortality.[92] Opioid and nicotine withdrawal is unpleasant but rarely physiologically dangerous. However, sudden cessation of ethanol or benzodiazepines in the setting of prolonged use and neurobiological adaptation may lead to alcohol withdrawal syndrome (AWS) or benzodiazepine withdrawal and serious complications.[93] Therefore, early identification of the possibility of withdrawal (within 24 hours for alcohol) is essential to ensure timely treatment.

As ethanol mimics gamma-aminobutyric acid (GABA) in the brain, regular and excessive intake of ethanol leads to changes in the inhibitory GABA and excitatory glutamate systems, decreased endogenous GABA levels, fewer and less-sensitive GABA receptors and glutamate system activation.[93] Postsynaptic N-methyl-D-aspartate (NMDA) receptors are more reactive and glutamate concentration increases. Therefore, cessation of ethanol may lead to unopposed neuronal excitation and resulting autonomic hyperactivity.

Criteria for classifying withdrawal are based on history of heavy alcohol use, symptoms and effect of symptoms on physical and mental functioning which cannot be accounted for by another mental disorder.[94] Frequency and quantity of alcohol consumption, together with other factors including previous detoxification episodes and withdrawal seizures and structural brain lesions, are thought to be predictive of AWS symptom severity.[92, 95] Withdrawal may occur 6–24 hours after cessation or significant reduction in intake. The physiological basis of benzodiazepine withdrawal is similar, resulting in autonomic hyperactivity. The severity is in part dependent on the half-life of the type of benzodiazepine. The most severe form of AWS, delirium tremens, occurs from 12 to 72 hours after cessation and is characterised by fluctuating consciousness level, including attention and cognitive deficits (hallucinations,

confusion and delirium), and severe hyperthermia and hypertension. The result of untreated delirium tremens may be withdrawal seizures, cardiovascular and respiratory failure, multiorgan dysfunction and death.[93]

The international estimation of opioid use disorder (OUD) in the population is approximately 5%.[96–98] Given the concomitant adverse health effects of OUD, a significant number of people with OUD who are at risk of opioid withdrawal are treated in an ICU. Data for nicotine withdrawal in critical care are also likely to reflect population rates for daily tobacco smoking, which range from 11% in Australia, North America and parts of Europe[99–101] to over 30% in parts of Asia.[102] The underlying physiology of withdrawal symptoms is similar for these chemicals. Opioids act on the dopaminergic mesolimbic system. Dependency results in lower levels of endogenous opioids and down-regulation of the dopaminergic system[103] so withdrawal produces unpleasant symptoms such as dysphoria, anxiety, joint pain, diarrhoea and vomiting.[104] Similarly nicotine dependency results in neurological adaptation that is desensitisation to nicotine which causes up-regulation of nicotinic acetylcholine receptors (nAchRs). The nAchRs modulate many mood-enhancing neurotransmitters, dopamine and acetylcholine causing a physiological 'need' and nicotine-seeking behaviour. Withdrawal symptoms related to reduced levels of neurotransmitters are unpleasant. Neither opioid nor nicotine withdrawal is life threatening but may result in delirium or agitation, which increases the risk of self-injury.

It is estimated that up to 33% of patients treated in ICU with continuous infusions of opioids for an extended time experience iatrogenic opioid withdrawal.[92, 105] The incidence of iatrogenic benzodiazepine withdrawal is estimated to be 8%,[100] although opioid and benzodiazepine withdrawal often occurs simultaneously and the signs are non-specific so the exact incidence for either iatrogenic withdrawal is unclear. The risk of withdrawal can be reduced by using all opioids and sedative medications judiciously based on individual patient needs (to maintain comfort and a calm and cooperative patient).[54] It is also recommended that medications are tapered for patients who require continuous opioid and sedative infusions for several days or a program of methadone replacement is instituted to facilitate a gradual reduction (5–10% per day) of the infusion doses.[92]

Screening for and assessment of withdrawal symptoms

Identification of withdrawal is challenging because symptoms may be the same for the underlying illness unless the reason for treatment in ICU is related to alcohol, benzodiazepine or opioid consumption (in which case the likelihood of withdrawal is high).[92] Hence no screening or assessment scales have been specifically validated for use in ICU and history taking is a vital adjunct to assessment and diagnosis. As highlighted earlier, history taking regarding alcohol and substance use often lacks detail. A brief interview schedule such as the 4-item CAGE questionnaire[106] (administered to the patient's proxy if the patient is unable to participate, ensuring confidentiality is maintained) is a recommended approach to guide history taking. Screening questions pertain to previous intentions to 'Cut down' drinking, Annoyance about being criticised for drinking, previous Guilty feelings about drinking and need to drink first thing in the morning ('Eye opener'). The presence of two or more of these features indicates that alcohol dependency is likely and requires further investigation. An alternative is the Prediction of Alcohol Withdrawal Severity Scale (PAWSS).[95] Although the frequency and amount of a substance consumed is important, it should also be noted that the definition of 'excessive intake' of any substance varies and is dependent on factors such as gender, body size and fat composition, liver function and genetic composition.

In cases in which alcohol withdrawal is suspected, it is recommended that withdrawal assessment scales (Table 6.6) are used to guide treatment and monitor progress particularly in the first 24–48 hours.[92] Although not necessarily tested in ICU, both the Clinical Institute Withdrawal Assessment of Alcohol Scale, revised (CIWA-Ar) and the AWS Scale have been shown to perform well in clinical practice[107] so the context and patient specifics should dictate choice of scale.[108–110] To overcome the limitations of using the CIWA-Ar with non-verbal patients (e.g. mechanically ventilated),[92,108,110] clinicians recommend using it with a sedation or agitation scale. The AWS[109,110] scale overcomes the difficulty of requiring a verbal response and may be more appropriate for the ICU population.

The Fagerström Test for Nicotine Dependence (FTND) is a commonly used validated tool to assess likelihood of nicotine withdrawal.[111] The score ranges from 0 to 10; higher scores indicate higher dependency. The FTND relies on self-report so has some limitations for use in the ICU. Recent pack-year history (packs per day × number of years smoking) may also provide the clinician with useful information about the likelihood of withdrawal.

Withdrawal screening and assessment tools specifically designed for other substances such as opioids have poor validity and reliability.[112] Clinical judgement is primarily used to monitor and guide treatment.

Practice tip

The CAGE ('Cut down' drinking, Annoyance about being criticised for drinking, previous Guilty feelings and need to drink first thing in the morning ('Eye opener')) screening approach can be adapted for use for detecting dependence to other substances such as benzodiazepines. Practise using the adapted screening approach next time you care for a patient who is suspected of being dependent on benzodiazepines and opioids.

Management of withdrawal

Comprehensive supportive care underpins the management of any withdrawal syndrome. Withdrawal from many substances does not necessarily require pharmacological

---

TABLE 6.6
Widely used alcohol withdrawal assessment scales

SCALE	DESCRIPTION	COMMENT
The Clinical Institute Withdrawal Assessment for Alcohol (CIWA-Ar) scale[110]	10-item scale. Maximum score 67; higher scores indicate more severe withdrawal; <8 = mild withdrawal; 8–15 = moderate withdrawal; >20 = severe withdrawal. Administer a minimum of every hour until symptoms subside.	Widely used in ICU setting. Patient must be able to verbally communicate to complete 4 items (7–10). Best used together with the sedation-agitation scale to guide treatment. Scores <8–10 indicate that pharmacological treatment probably not necessary.
Alcohol Withdrawal Syndrome (AWS) Scale[110]	Consists of two subscales; somatic symptoms = s, and mental symptoms = m. S subscale: pulse rate, diastolic blood pressure, temperature, breathing rate, sweating, tremor. M subscale: agitation, contact, orientation, hallucination, anxiety. Maximum score: 55; higher scores indicate more severe withdrawal; 5 = mild; 6–9 = moderate; and ≥10 = severe. Administer every hour until symptoms subside.	Allows separate assessment of somatic and mental withdrawal symptoms. Developed specifically for patients with severe withdrawal or delirium (but not for ICU patients); does not need verbal response from patient.

treatment and depends on the substance and the severity of withdrawal. Supportive care (e.g. maintenance of fluid and electrolyte balance and serum thiamine levels) may be all that is required for minor alcohol withdrawal. Clinicians should be aware that the psychological 'need' for alcohol or any other substance may continue beyond the period of physiological withdrawal. People with a pre-existing substance dependency may require ongoing psychological support and understanding; the involvement of specialist 'drug and alcohol' healthcare teams is advised.

Treatment for alcohol withdrawal comprises pharmacological agents guided by symptom severity. A loading dose of benzodiazepine followed by tapering doses should be used. Diazepam is the conventional approach; however, other medications such as barbiturates, dexmedetomidine, clonidine, ketamine and propofol (often in combination with benzodiazepines) have been explored.[113] Barbiturates are indicated in the setting of severe withdrawal requiring escalating benzodiazepine doses.[114] Further research is required before recommendations for treatment of AWS with other pharmacological agents can be made. Wernicke's encephalopathy is a potential catastrophic consequence of AWS caused by overwhelming metabolic demands on brain cells with depleted intracellular thiamine. Thiamine and B vitamin complex supplementation is an essential component of treatment, reducing mortality and morbidity.[115]

As the underlying pathophysiology of benzodiazepine withdrawal is the same as that in AWS, a similar treatment regimen of a tapering dose of a long-acting benzodiazepine is advised together with supportive therapy. 'Benzodiazepine-sparing' treatment regimens incorporating dexmedetomidine are also recommended.[54] It should be noted that there is an increased risk of mortality for younger patients (<65 years) associated with a dexmedetomidine sedation regimen early during mechanical ventilation,[116] and continuous infusion of dexmedetomidine over several days may result in dependency. Low-dose flumazenil is an approach provided as multiple bolus intravenous doses together with or without benzodiazepine tapering to reduce withdrawal symptoms.[117] Efficacy and safety has largely been tested in ambulatory care settings; guidelines for use during critical illness are not available.

Mild opioid withdrawal may be treated with supportive therapy alone, but moderate-to-severe withdrawal is treated with tapering doses of methadone.[118] More recently, buprenorphine has been found to control withdrawal symptoms better than methadone and may reduce long-term dependence.[119] The first dose of buprenorphine is administered when withdrawal symptoms are moderate, reducing the risk of precipitated withdrawal.[118] Other anxiolytic medications such as clonidine, dexmedetomidine and benzodiazepines may also play a role in reducing somatic withdrawal symptoms.[120]

Nicotine replacement therapy (NRT) has been associated with adverse outcomes, consequently universal use of NRT is not recommended for the critically ill.[121, 122] It should be reserved for patients for whom the risk of not providing NRT (e.g. severe agitation or anxiety attributable to nicotine withdrawal) outweighs potential harms.[123] The usual regimen for NRT comprises transdermal administration of tapering doses of 24-hour-release nicotine-impregnated patches.

Comprehensive guidance for all substance withdrawal syndromes is beyond the scope of this textbook. The reader is advised to consult papers published in journals such as Alcohol and Alcoholism and the Journal of Chemical Dependency and relevant textbooks (Erickson, 2011; Mack, 2016; see Further reading) as well as local practice guidelines.

Practice tip

Next time you care for a patient who has experienced alcohol withdrawal, ask them about the symptoms and strategies other than medications that helped reduce their discomfort.

Pain

Pain is an unobservable, inherently subjective, experience. The nebulous multifaceted nature of pain has led to significant difficulties in not only understanding the mechanisms underlying the experience but also assessing and managing the phenomenon.

Pain is a sensation widely experienced by critical care patients and is one of the stressors most commonly reported by former and current ICU patients.[63,124] In particular, apparently innocuous procedures such as turning or positioning may cause mild or moderate pain while invasive procedures (e.g. chest drain removal) are often severely painful.[125] Arguably, pain management is not always afforded the same emphasis as more 'life-threatening' conditions such as haemodynamic instability. However, its alleviation is an essential element of critical care nursing and should be emphasised in order to reduce potential suffering and the need for sedative medication. Myths such as the possibility that patients may become dependent on analgesics, that the very young and elderly have higher tolerance for pain, and our cultural tendency to reward high pain tolerance may lead to inadequate pain management. In critical care, nurses assume a fairly autonomous role in titrating analgesic medication. With this increased autonomy comes a responsibility to be knowledgeable and aware of effective pain management and assessment of the 'fifth vital sign'.

Pathophysiology of pain

Pain is transmitted to the central nervous system via one of two pathways. The fast pain pathway occurs when the stimuli are carried by small myelinated A-delta fibres, producing a sharp, prickling sensation that is easily localised. The slow pathway acts in response to polymodal nociceptors, is carried by small unmyelinated C fibres and produces a dull, aching or burning sensation. It is difficult to locate, acts after fast pain, and is considered to be more unpleasant than fast pain.[126]

Perceptions of pain are thought to occur in the thalamus, whereas behavioural and emotional responses occur in the hypothalamus and limbic system.[126] Perceptions of pain are influenced by prior experience, and by cultural and normative practices, which helps to explain individual reactions to pain.[126]

There are negative physiological effects of pain that include a sympathetic response with increased cardiac work, potentially compromising cardiac stability.[127] Respiratory function may be impaired in the critically ill undergoing surgical procedures when deep breathing and coughing is limited by increased pain, reducing airway movement and increasing the retention of secretions and the possibility of nosocomial pneumonia.

Adverse psychological sequelae of poorly treated pain include diminished feelings of control and self-efficacy and increased fear and anxiety. An inability to engage in rehabilitation and health-promoting activities may transpire. The long-term effects of undertreated pain are not clearly understood, but almost certainly impact on recovery and may even lead to worsening chronic pain.[128] When these unwanted outcomes are considered alongside the physiological effects of poorly treated pain, the vital importance of pain management is evident.

Pain assessment

Pain is whatever the experiencing person says it is, existing whenever he [sic] says it does.[129]

The nebulous quality and subjective nature of the pain experience lead to considerable problems in its assessment. This is compounded in critically ill patients, who often have insufficient cognitive acumen to articulate their needs and an inability to communicate verbally. A common language and process in which to assess pain is essential in ameliorating some of these challenges. Furthermore, accurate assessment and consistent recording are fundamental aspects of pain management. Without these vital components, it is impossible to evaluate interventions designed to reduce pain. Despite the importance of assessing pain, there is evidence to suggest that timely and rigorous assessment does not occur.[1,130]

Since the pain experience is subjective, all attempts should be made to facilitate patient communication of the nature, intensity, body part affected and characteristics of their pain. The patient's usual communication aids, such as glasses and hearing aid, should be used. Whenever patients cannot verbally communicate, other strategies must be established and used consistently. For example, strategies involving nodding, hand movements, facial expressions, eye blinks, mouthing answers and writing can be highly effective. In cases when there is limited motor function but the patient is cognitively able, the speech pathologist may be able to advise on alternative communication strategies.

When possible, a patient's health history (from the family if the patient is unable), including any existing painful conditions, should be taken. Quite apart from the presenting condition, which may be painful, critical care patients may have significant comorbidities such as rheumatoid/osteoarthritis and chronic back pain. It is imperative that the patient's usual pain management strategies are identified and implemented if possible. For example, factors that relieve the pain or increase its intensity should be recorded, along with its relationship to daily activities such as sleep, appetite and physical ability.

Regardless of the patient's communication capability, strategies to ensure consistent objective assessment and management should be implemented. Laminated cards displaying body diagrams, words to describe pain and pain intensity measures (including visual analogues and numerical scales) are useful instruments in meeting these requirements. Verbal numerical reporting scales and visual analogue scales are commonly used. These are outlined in Table 6.7.[131,132] VAS can be difficult to administer to critically ill patients; however, a combined VAS and numerical reporting scale includes the benefit of a visual cue with the ability to quantify pain intensity.

Other physiological and behavioural pain indicators may be used to assess pain in less-responsive or unconscious patients.[133] A large range of instruments have been developed and validated for use in the critically ill adult patient. The Behavioural Pain Scale (BPS) (Fig. 6.4)[131] and the Critical Care Pain Observation Tool (CPOT)[132] (http://ajcc.aacnjournals.org/content/15/4/420/T1.expansion.html) are the most robust scales for assessing pain in critically ill adults.[54] Briefly, scores are assigned to categories such as altered body movements, restlessness and synchronisation with the ventilator, providing a global score for comparison after pain relief interventions. The CPOT offers several benefits over the BPS, including use of an indicator assessing muscle tension where resistance to passive movement is assessed as 0 = relaxed, 1 = tense or rigid, 2 = very tense or rigid, and an alternative indicator to compliance with ventilation that can be used in extubated patients – assessments include whether the patient is talking in normal tone or no sound = 0; sighing, moaning = 1; crying out, sobbing = 2.

Nurses should not rely solely on changes in physiological parameters, including cardiovascular (elevated blood pressure and heart rate) and respiratory recordings to assess pain intensity, as other pathophysiological or treatment-related factors may be responsible.[134,135] Classic reactions to stressors (e.g. pain), such as increased heart rate and blood pressure, do not always occur in critically ill patients and are therefore unreliable pain assessment methods.[134] A potential explanation is that autonomic tone may be dysfunctional in a large proportion of ICU patients.[136] In haemodynamically stable long-term critical patients, vital signs may be useful if used in conjunction with other forms of assessment.[54] Where necessary, for example when the patient is unable to self-report their pain experience, it may be appropriate to involve the family.[54] Although

TABLE 6.7
Pain scales

SCALE	DESCRIPTION	COMMENT
Verbal numeric reporting scale	Self-rating scale. Single-item scale. Scale from 0 (no pain) to 10 (worst pain ever).	Patient must be able to communicate verbally. Needs to understand concept of rating pain. Dependent on prior pain experiences. Simple, easy to use.
Visual analogue scale	Self-rating scale. Single-item. A horizontal line with equal divisions is used for the patient to rate current pain level (no pain is on far left and worst pain is far right).	Patient can communicate by pointing. Needs to understand concept of rating pain. Dependent on patient's prior pain experiences. Simple, easy to use.
Behavioural Pain Scale (see Fig. 6.4)[131]	Based on pain-related behaviours: the sum of three items. Higher scores indicate higher pain intensity (range: 3–12).	Patient does not have to communicate. Simple, easy to use. Includes 'ventilator compliance' (may no longer be relevant for pain assessment when using modern ventilators).
Critical Care Pain Observation Tool (CPOT)[132]	Based on previously developed instruments using pain-related behaviour to assess pain, e.g. BPS 4 items: facial expression, body movements, muscle tension and compliance with ventilator or vocalization. Higher scores indicate more pain (range: 0–8).	Patient does not have to communicate. Simple, easy to use. Includes 'ventilator compliance' (may no longer be relevant for pain assessment when using modern ventilators) or vocalisation in extubated patients

FIGURE 6.4   Behavioural Pain Scale.[131]

Item	Description	Score
Facial expression	Relaxed	1
	Partially tightened (e.g. brow lowering)	2
	Fully tightened (e.g. eyelid closing)	3
	Grimacing	4
Upper limbs	No movement	1
	Partially bent	2
	Fully bent with finger flexion	3
	Permanently retracted	4
Compliance with ventilation	Tolerating movement	1
	Coughing but tolerating ventilation for most of the time	2
	Fighting ventilator	3
	Unable to control ventilation	4

Source: Payen JF, Bru O, Bosson JL, et al. Assessing pain in critically ill sedated patients by using a behavioral pain scale. Crit Care Med 2001;29(12):2258–63.

family reports have been found to be closer to the patients than clinical staff, these reports should not be taken ahead of self-report by the patient.

In addition, it is particularly important to regularly consider and search for potential sources of pain in unresponsive patients and those who are unable to communicate. Nurses should assume pain is present if there is a reason to suspect pain; an analgesic trial may assist in identifying this. As a general rule, analgesia medication should be administered to patients who are heavily sedated or receiving muscle relaxants as a precaution.

Pain management

Although pain management is discussed here independently, in practice it is often combined with sedative administration to reduce anxiety. However, pain management should always be the first goal for achieving overall patient comfort (the so-called analgosedation approach[137]). Efforts to improve patient comfort for intubated patients often favour the concurrent use of both sedative and analgesic medications.[54] This practice therefore makes it difficult to assess the single effect of each medication on the patient's pain and highlights its multidimensional properties. In addition to pharmacological treatment of pain, non-pharmacological strategies can be effective as an adjunct to drug therapy or as an alternative.

Pain relief may be required for pre-existing injuries or prior to specific procedures to prevent pain. Being turned is often cited as a painful procedure; however, wounds, drain removal, tracheal suction, femoral catheter removal, placement of a central venous catheter and wound dressings and coughing may also cause considerable discomfort.[124] Guidelines and written protocols for procedures such as femoral sheath removal and insertion of a central venous catheter can significantly reduce pain intensity as they often contain reminders to provide analgesia. Some procedures, such as insertion of invasive devices, require additional pain management such as local anaesthetics. This highlights the potential need for additional pain protocols linked to key standard procedures (e.g. patient turning) to reduce patients' pain experience.

Pain-relieving medication can be administered via a number of routes, including oral, enteral feeding tube, intravenous, rectal, topical, subcutaneous, intramuscular, epidural and intrathecal. For all routes of administration, assessment of the patient's suitability and contraindications for use are an essential part of the decision-making process. Patient-controlled analgesia for intravenous and, more recently, epidural analgesia is commonly part of critical care nursing.

Epidural pain management requires additional evaluation, including sensory and functional assessment, because both local anaesthetic and opioid medications are used. Sensory function should be regularly checked using a dermatome chart to gauge segments that are blocked by the local anaesthetic agent. In addition to sensory blockade, regular assessment for lower-limb motor deficit is required to detect changes in motor response, which may impair the ability to mobilise safely. Sudden or subtle changes may also indicate a complication such as epidural haematoma. The Bromage Assessment Scale is often used to assess motor response. The catheter site must be regularly checked to identify complications such as bleeding, haematoma and infection early and to ensure catheter patency. Intrathecal administration of analgesic medications has similar contraindications and complications to epidural analgesia and requires similar precautions. It is important to note that intrathecal (as compared with intravenous) administration does not eliminate all opioid side effects (see Further reading).

Non-pharmacological treatment for pain

Non-pharmacological strategies to reduce pain are linked to some key strategies to reduce stress. Excessive pain may lead to stress as the body attempts to maintain homeostasis and stress may exacerbate pain. Strategies to reduce stress and pain include both comfort measures and diversional interventions, which require the nurse to individualise and adapt strategies to match the patient's needs and preferences. Diversional methods may include distraction strategies, and aim to refocus the patient's thinking away from the pain and on to other more pleasant thoughts or activities. Research has highlighted the importance patients place on the presence of family members in the facilitation of emotional and physical strategies of pain management.[138,139] Some interventions that may be effective are listed in Table 6.8.[140,141]

Non-pharmacological interventions have the benefit of being nurse initiated, non-invasive and able to be personalised. These strategies may not reduce pain intensity significantly on their own but have the capacity to enhance the effects of analgesic medication and humanise the critically ill patient's experience.

Pharmacological treatment for pain

Pharmacological treatment for pain in critically ill patients centres on opioid medications, which act as opioid agonists binding to the mu-receptors in the brain, central nervous system and other tissues.[54] Opioid medications have a rapid action and are readily titrated, and their metabolites, if present, are less likely to accumulate. Morphine sulfate and fentanyl are routinely used in critical care, and their properties, side effects and nursing implications are outlined in Table 6.9.

TABLE 6.8
Non-pharmacological treatment for pain

COMFORT MEASURES	DIVERSIONAL MEASURES
Repositioning[54]	Relaxation
Oral and endotracheal suctioning	Breathing exercises
Mouth, oral and/or wound care	Visual imagery
Reassurance and information	Music therapy[50, 140]
Massage	Family presence[141]
Cold therapy[54]	

TABLE 6.9

Analgesics

DRUG/DRUG DOSE	PROPERTIES	SIDE EFFECTS	NURSING IMPLICATIONS
Morphine sulfate 1–10 mg/h (IV infusion), 1–4 mg (IV bolus).	Water-soluble. Peak effect 30 min. Half-life: 3–7 h. Sedative effect and release of histamines.[54]	Vasodilatory effect. Decreased gastric motility. Respiratory depression. Nausea and vomiting.[126]	Intermittent doses, rather the need for continuous infusions.[54]
Fentanyl 25–200 micrograms/h (IV infusion), 25–100 micrograms (IV bolus).	Lipid-soluble Synthetic opioid 80–100 times more potent than morphine. Peak effect in 4 min. Half-life: 1.5–6 h.[54]	Respiratory depression. Bradycardia. Muscular rigidity.	Useful where: hypotension or tachycardia needs to be avoided; gastric and/or histamine side effects occur with morphine.
Tramadol hydrochloride 100 mg (IV bolus), then 50–100 mg 4–6/24 h. Provide orally/enterally when able.	Centrally acting opioid-like analgesic for moderate to severe pain.	Better side effect profile than opioids; however, nausea, vomiting, dizziness and dry mouth are possible. Headache. Sweating.	Intermittent doses only. Do not administer in combination with MAOIs. Do not administer in the setting of seizures or epilepsy. Adjust dose for the elderly. Monitor hepatic function.
Tapentadol immediate release 50–100 mg/3 or 4/24. Tapentadol sustained release 50–250 mg 2/24 h (do not exceed 500 mg/24 h).	Centrally acting opioid analgesic for moderate or severe pain (immediate release for acute pain and sustained release for chronic pain). First-line analgesic for intolerance to other opioids.	Opioid-related side effects such as respiratory depression, nausea. Considered to have a better opioid side effect profile than other opioids.	Not recommended in the setting of severe renal or hepatic impairment. Monitor renal and liver function. Do not administer in combination with MOAIs.
Paracetamol (acetaminophen) 1 g 4–6/24 h (max 4 g and 3 g/24 h for over 80 years, <50 kg body weight and hepatic impairment) given IV, orally/enterally or per rectum.	Centrally acting analgesic suitable for mild to moderate pain.	Liver impairment.	Monitor hepatic function.
NSAIDs IV, oral/enteral or rectal routes.	Analgesia and antipyretics.	Gastrointestinal. Some have anticoagulant side effects.	Not used routinely but may be used for procedural pain. Renal clearance.
Ketamine 0.5 micrograms/kg IV bolus then 1 micrograms/kg/min infusion.	Analgesic and dissociative anaesthetic for painful procedures. Onset of action 1–2 min. Analgesic/anaesthetic effects last 5–15 min. Half-life 3 h.	Hypertension and respiratory depression (administer slowly). Increased intracranial pressure. Hallucinations.	Use for painful procedures, e.g. wound dressings or as an adjuvant to opioid therapy. Administer 2 mg of midazolam at the start of the procedure or continue midazolam infusion to minimise the dysphoric and hallucinogenic side effects.

The table above contains an overview only. Consult local drug formulary and guidance before prescribing and administering. MOAI = monoamine oxidase inhibitor, NSAIDs = non-steroidal anti-inflammatory drugs.

(For ischaemic chest pain management see Chapter 10.) There is growing evidence of improved effectiveness of pain relief with combination therapy – for example, the addition of paracetamol, ketamine or neuropathic pain medications to opioid therapy.[54]

Although non-steroidal anti-inflammatory drugs (NSAIDs) are not recommended as an adjuvant to opioid therapy, they can be considered as an alternative to opioids to manage pain during specific procedures in critical care.[54] NSAIDs act by inhibition of an enzyme within the inflammatory cascade, and may produce analgesia (especially when combined with opioids) for bone and soft tissue injuries. As with all medication, side effects and contraindications can be serious and, in the case of NSAIDs, include gastrointestinal bleeding, renal insufficiency and exacerbation of asthma.

Pain relief is a primary goal for critical care nursing and requires regular assessment of pain intensity. No single medication is ideal for all patients, and clinicians need to carefully select, monitor and titrate the doses of any agent. In the case of major thoracic or abdominal surgery, patient-controlled analgesia may provide the most effective pain management strategy (see Chapter 12). Non-pharmacological strategies add to the relief of pain and come under the domain of nursing care. Without adequate pain management, patients will be unable to achieve adequate rest and sleep, both essential for healing and well-being.

Sedation

Maintaining appropriate levels of sedation is a core component of care during critical illness, when patients are treated with invasive and difficult-to-tolerate procedures and interventions. Some critically ill patients will require no sedation to be comfortable, while others may require significant amounts to both be comfortable and maintain optimal physiological status. Individualising sedation management is crucial to effective treatment, with accurate assessment a core requirement. Adequate sedation is paramount for those patients receiving muscle relaxants. In association with sedation management, it is essential that adequate pain relief and anxiolysis are provided to all critically ill patients.

There is growing evidence of the detrimental effects of sedation on outcomes in critically ill patients, although the evidence linking level of sedation to outcomes is inconsistent.[142] A light, rather than deep, level of sedation has been associated with shorter duration of mechanical ventilation and hospital length of stay, as well as reduced incidence of ventilator-associated pneumonia in some studies.[142] Strategies to achieve light sedation are now the mainstay of sedation assessment and management for the critically ill. In short-term sedation there is also a growing recognition that the use of benzodiazepines should be minimised.[54]

Assessment of sedation

Assessment of the effect of all sedative treatments is essential. When pharmacological agents are used there is always a risk of over- or undersedation, and both can have significant negative effects on patients.[143] Oversedation may lead to detrimental physiological effects including cardiac, renal and respiratory depression and can result in longer duration of mechanical ventilation, associated complications and recovery. Undersedation has the opposite effect on the cardiac system, with hypertension, tachycardia, arrhythmias, ventilator dyssynchrony, agitation and distress, with the potential for accidental self-harm.

Objective sedation scales provide an effective method of assessing and monitoring consciousness or arousal level, as well as evaluating parameters such as cognition, agitation and patient–ventilator synchrony. Although a number of sedation scales have been developed, only the Richmond Agitation–Sedation Scale (RASS)[144] and the Riker Sedation–Agitation Scale (SAS)[145] have been validated appropriately for use in intensive care (Figs 6.5 and 6.6). Even though clinicians are frequently concerned about the reliability of sedation assessment in patients with neurological compromise, there is evidence that the RASS is reliable.[146]

Bispectral index monitoring provides an objective measurement of sedation level. A self-adhesive electrode pad is secured to the patient's forehead to continuously record cortical activity, which is scored on a scale from 0 (absence of brain activity) to 100 (completely aware). There is not yet consensus on the most appropriate brain activity level for intensive care patients or what role bispectral index monitoring can offer in their care,[147,148] although there is growing belief that it may be helpful in optimising sedation titration. More studies to evaluate the efficacy of bispectral index are required.

Sedation protocols

Patients' sedation needs are complex. There is growing awareness of the need to ensure optimal pain management prior to considering sedation, with the knowledge that sedation will not always be required once adequate pain management has been implemented (see Pain above).

In situations where sedation is required, one of the strategies used is a sedation protocol. The aim of sedation protocols is to improve sedation management by encouraging regular discussion of sedation goals among the healthcare team, while enabling nurses to manage ongoing sedative needs. Not all patients' sedative needs will be met within the sedation protocol; in these instances, specific care should be planned and implemented by the multidisciplinary healthcare team.

Sedation protocols offer a framework, or algorithm, within which clinicians can manage specific patient care with prearranged outcomes. Aspects of sedation management that should be incorporated into sedation protocols include:

- the sedation scale to be used, as well as frequency of assessment
- an algorithm-based process for selecting the most appropriate sedative agent
- the range of sedative agents that might be considered and associated administration guidelines

FIGURE 6.5 Richmond Agitation–Sedation Scale (RASS).[144]

Richmond Agitation Sedation Scale (RASS)

Sore	Term	Description	
+4	Combative	Overtly combative, violent, immediate danger to staff	
+3	Very agitated	Pulls or removes tube(s) or catheter(s); aggressive	
+2	Agitated	Frequent non-purposeful movement, fights ventilator	
+1	Restless	Anxious but movements not aggressive vigorous	
0	Alert and calm		
–1	Drowsy	Not fully alert, but has sustained awakening (eye-opening/eye contact) to *voice* (≥10 seconds)	Verbal Stimulation
–2	Light sedation	Briefly awakens with eye contact to *voice* (<10 seconds)	Verbal Stimulation
–3	Moderate sedation	Movement or eye opening to *voice* (but not eye contact)	
–4	Deep sedation	No response to voice, but movement or eye opening to *physical* stimulation	Physical Stimulation
–5	Unarousable	No response to *voice* or *physical* stimulation	

Procedure for RASS Assessment

1. Observe patient
   a. Patient is alert, restless, or agitated. (score 0 to +4)
2. If not alert, state patient's name and *say* to open eyes and look at speaker.
   b. Patient awakens with sustained eye opening and eye contact. (score –1)
   c. Patient awakens with eye opening and eye contact, but not sustained. (score –2)
   d. Patient has any movement in response to voice but no eye contact. (score –3)
3. When no response to verbal stimulation, physically stimulate patient by shaking shoulder and/or rubbing sternum.
   e. Patient has any movement to physical stimulation. (score –4)
   f. Patient has no response to any stimulation. (score –5)

Source: Reprinted with permission of the American Thoracic Society. Copyright © 2019 American Thoracic Society. Sessler CN, Gosnell M, Grap MJ, et al. The Richmond Agitation–Sedation Scale: validity and reliability in adult intensive care patients. Am J Respir Crit Care Med 2002;166:1338–44. The 'American Journal of Respiratory and Critical Care Medicine' is an official journal of the American Thoracic Society.

FIGURE 6.6 Riker Sedation–Agitation Scale (SAS).[145]

Riker Sedation-Agitation Scale (SAS)

Score	Term	Description
7	Dangerous agitation	Pulling at ET tube, trying to remove catheters, climbing over bedrail, striking at staff, thrashing side-to-side
6	Very agitated	Requiring restraint and frequent verbal reminding of limits, biting ETT
5	Agitated	Anxious or physically agitated, calms to verbal instructions
4	Calm and cooperative	Calm, easily arousable, follows commands
3	Sedated	Difficult to arouse but awakens to verbal stimuli or gentle shaking, follows simple commands but drifts off again
2	Very sedated	Arouses to physical stimuli but does not communicate or follow commands, may move spontaneously
1	Unarousable	Minimal or no response to noxious stimuli, does not communicate or follow commands

Guidelines for SAS Assessment

1. Agitated patients are scored by their most severe degree of agitation as described.
2. If patient is awake or awakens easily to voice ('awaken' means responds with voice or head shaking to a question or follows commands), that's a SAS 4 (same as calm and appropriate – might even be napping).
3. If more stimuli such as shaking is required but patient eventually does awaken, that's SAS 3.
4. If patient arouses to stronger physical stimuli (may be noxious) but never awakens to the point of responding yes/no or following commands, that's a SAS 2.
5. Little or no response to noxious physical stimuli represents a SAS1.

Source: Riker RR, Picard JT, Fraser GL. Prospective evaluation of the Sedation–Agitation Scale for adult critically ill patients. Crit Care Med 1999;27(7):1325–9.

- a target sedation score
- when to commence, increase, decrease or cease sedative agents
- when to seek review by a medical officer.

Sedation protocols usually also incorporate an analgesia component, frequently with an emphasis on pain assessment and management as the first step to achieve patient comfort.

Although sedation protocols have widespread support, there is mixed evidence regarding the benefits of their implementation.[54] It is likely that sedation protocols provide most benefit in settings where ratios of critical care nurses and medical officers to patients are low (that is, are not available or limited in numbers).

> **Practice tip**
>
> Assessing and managing pain first, prior to providing any sedation, will improve comfort and reduce the need for sedation in many patients.

Nurse-led sedation protocols

Nurse-led sedation protocols are usually ordered by a doctor or advanced practice nurse with prescribing rights, contain guidance regarding sedation management and are usually used by nurses although they may have input from pharmacists or other members of the healthcare team. While some studies show benefits associated with nurse-led sedation protocols, particularly in relation to hospital length of stay, others do not.[149] Until further research is undertaken, sedation protocols should be considered on a local basis where current practice conditions indicate potential benefit from care standardisation. Appropriate evaluation of the impact of protocol implementation should be undertaken.

> **Practice tip**
>
> Patients should be kept 'calm and cooperative' unless there is a reason for deeper sedation. Strategies to minimise sedation include discussion and agreement of a target sedation score, and regular assessment of pain, agitation and delirium.

Sedation minimisation protocols

A range of multidimensional protocols have been developed for use by all the multidisciplinary team for the purpose of minimising the amount of sedation delivered and the patients' sedation level. Some of these have been incorporated into bundles such as the Wake Up and Breathe Program[150] or the expanded ABCDEF bundle.[151]

Like nurse-led sedation protocols, benefits have been demonstrated in some settings but not all.[152] Despite these inconsistent results, the lack of adverse effects associated with these multidimensional protocols means implementation of such a protocol should be considered, although any plans to implement such a protocol should take into account local practice and ensure continuous evaluation of the benefits as well as adverse events.

Daily interruption of sedation

A specific form of sedation protocol is the daily interruption of sedation. Although the initial study in this area found benefits in reduced duration of mechanical ventilation and ICU length of stay,[153,154] these benefits have not been demonstrated subsequently. In both a meta-analysis of data from nine studies including 1282 patients and a multicentre study of 423 patients in 16 centres across Canada and the USA, no improvement was seen in duration of mechanical ventilation, ICU or hospital length of stay or rates of delirium.[155,156] Further, in the multicentre study, patients who received daily interruption of sedation required higher daily doses of some sedative and analgesic agents, and greater nurse workload was required for patients in this group.[156] From a practical perspective there are growing reports of clinicians' concerns regarding patient comfort such as agitation and pain, as well as adverse events such as device removal during sedation interruption.[157,158] Given this evidence, daily interruption of sedation cannot be recommended. Instead, the mainstay of achieving good practice in this setting is maintaining appropriate targets for sedation levels that are as light as possible and based on individual patient needs.

Sleep

The function of sleep is not yet fully understood; however, it is considered to be required for many bodily functions.[159] It is vital for well-being, and sleep disruption or deprivation leads to physical illness[160] and premature mortality.[161] Good-quality sleep is associated with better psychological health.[162] Hence sleep is considered to be physically and psychologically restorative and essential for healing and recovery from illness. Arguably, critically ill people are in greater need of undisrupted sleep, given their need for healing and recovery, but are more likely to experience poor-quality sleep.[163]

Sleep in the healthy adult comprises one consolidated period of 6–8 hours (mean 7.5 hours) in each 24-hour period occurring at night according to natural circadian rhythms.[164] There are two main sleep states: rapid eye movement sleep (REM) (approximately 25% of total sleep time (TST)) and non-rapid eye movement sleep (non-REM) (approximately 75% of TST). Non-REM sleep is composed of three stages: stages 1 and 2 or light sleep and stage 3 or slow-wave sleep (SWS), which must be completed in sequence in order to enter REM sleep.

The consolidated sleep period consists of four to six sleep cycles: stages 1–3 followed by REM sleep, which lasts 60–90 minutes.[165] All sleep stages are important to health and, unfortunately, critically ill patients commonly experience little SWS or REM sleep.

Evidence suggests that, although critically ill patients may experience normal sleep quantities, the quality is poor, with very few experiencing SWS or REM sleep.[166] Sleep is highly disrupted and distributed across 24 hours, with roughly equal amounts occurring in the day and at night.[167,168] These findings, obtained using polysomnography (PSG), have been corroborated by patients' self-reports of their sleep in critical care.[169] Patients consistently rate their overall sleep quality as poor and, more specifically, they report light sleep with frequent awakenings.[170] Many factors are thought to affect the patient's ability to sleep, including those intrinsic to the patient such as abnormal temperature and pain, others that are environmental such as noise and light, and those that are treatment related such as medications, tubes and mechanical ventilation.[171,172]

There are changes in sleep architecture over the adult lifespan that require consideration in the context of critical care nursing. TST and the percentage of SWS decline with age (TST by 10 minutes and SWS by 2% per decade) and light sleep increases slightly (by 5% between 20 and 70 years).[173] REM sleep remains fairly constant, with an approximate 0.6% decline per decade until age 70 years, when REM increases with a simultaneous decrease in TST.[174] Time spent awake after sleep onset increases with age by 10 minutes per decade after age 30 years.[173]

Sleep assessment/monitoring

The patient's sleep history should be taken as soon as possible after admission. The person closest to the patient (ideally living in the same home) may be willing to provide a sleep history if the patient is unable to communicate verbally. The requirement for nocturnal non-invasive ventilation or sleep medication should be considered with the multidisciplinary team. Particular attention should be paid to reports of daytime sleepiness, dissatisfaction with sleep and bed partner reports of excessive snoring as these may indicate an undiagnosed sleep disorder. Usual sleep habits such as 'going to bed', 'getting up' and shower times should be accommodated while the patient is treated in critical care whenever possible.

Unfortunately, few objective methods of assessing sleep reliably in critically ill patients are available. PSG, a method of recording electroencephalography, electrooculography and electromyography, is the 'gold standard' for assessing sleep. PSG data are analysed according to Rechtschaffen and Kales' (R & K)[175] criteria to provide TST and sleep stage times. Difficulties in applying standard R & K sleep criteria to critically ill patients' sleep data and the need for a trained operator to undertake analysis preclude its routine clinical use in critical care. Actigraphy is another method of recording sleep that has been attempted in the critically ill. Modern actigraphs are small wristwatch devices (they may also be located on the ankle) containing accelerometers that detect motion in a single axis or multiple axes.[176] Although actigraphy has been shown to be feasible in the critically ill population,[176,177] there is some evidence that actigraphy provides an overestimation of sleep time given that critically ill patients are typically immobile for long periods regardless of sleep state. The other objective method that has been attempted in critical care is bispectral index monitoring.[178] At present, considerable algorithm development using comparisons with PSG data are required before it is a viable option to measure sleep accurately in any setting, although there is some early evidence of feasibility.[179]

The most reliable option for the critical care clinician to assess sleep is a patient self-report (in any case, the patient is best placed to judge the adequacy of their sleep if they are able). Two instruments have been specifically developed for use in critical care: the Richards–Campbell Sleep Questionnaire (RCSQ)[180] and the Sleep in Intensive Care Questionnaire (SICQ) (Table 6.10).[181] The RCSQ comprises five 100-mm VASs: sleep depth, latency, awakenings, time awake and quality of sleep. It was validated in 70 male patients where there was a moderate correlation between total RCSQ score and PSG sleep efficiency index, r = 0.58, ($P < 0.001$).[180] The SICQ is better suited for use when assessing a unit/organisation-wide change in practice rather than an individual patient's sleep (see Table 6.10).

Up to 50% of patients treated in critical care may be unable to complete a sleep self-assessment, in which case the only remaining option is nurse assessment. The Nurses' Observation Checklist (NOC)[182] can be used to obtain the bedside nurses' assessments of the patient's sleep quantity. It is a relatively simple instrument to use. However, evidence from many studies suggests that nurses tend to overestimate sleep time, so sleep time derived from the NOC may be better used as a trend rather than a definitive report for an individual night's sleep.[183,184]

Sleep promotion and maintenance

There is a growing, although still small and often low-quality, body of evidence of interventions that are effective in promoting sleep for patients in ICU. These interventions include optimising patient comfort and adapting the environment to be more conducive to normal sleep routines. Multidimensional interventions that incorporate a number of strategies have been found to be beneficial.[51] Individualised approaches to all aspects of care are best and this is particularly important when promoting and maintaining sleep in the critically ill. The following information, based on research and expert opinion, provides some general advice that may promote and maintain sleep and, at the very least, create conditions conducive to rest.

TABLE 6.10
Sleep assessment instruments

INSTRUMENT	DESCRIPTION	COMMENTS
Richards–Campbell Sleep Questionnaire[180]	Five VAS (0–100 mm). Total score derived from average of the five scales (high scores indicate good sleep).	Patient does not need to be able to write (nurse can mark the line as instructed by patient). Patient requires sufficient level of cognitive function to use it.
Sleep in Intensive Care Questionnaire[181]	Seven questions (some have more than one item). Likert scales 1–10. No global score. Good for organisational changes in practice.	Patient does not need to be able to write (nurse can circle the response as instructed by patient). Patient requires sufficient level of cognitive function to use it. Not yet validated.
Nurses' observation checklist[182]	Tick box table. Assignment of a category: 'awake', 'asleep', 'could not tell' and 'no time to observe' every 15 min.	No training required. Typically, nurses tend to overestimate sleep. Better for trend over several nights.

Comfort measures

- Ensure pain relief is offered and administered if pain is suspected.
- Reduce anxiety by providing information and the opportunity to have questions answered. Anxiolytics such as low-dose benzodiazepines may also be required (recognising that these may adversely affect sleep quality).
- Avoid night-time sedation (unless the patient took this prior to hospitalisation). Sedatives and hypnotics rarely improve the quality and quantity of sleep and when prescribed in hospital are likely to continue beyond hospital,[185] predisposing the patient to the risk of dependency and long-term sleep difficulties (and fall injuries particularly in the elderly[186]).
- Consider providing a light massage or music therapy unless contraindicated to encourage relaxation.[187]
- Provide an extra cover for warmth (metabolic rate typically drops during sleep).
- Request the patient's family to provide some of the patient's own personal belongings such as pillows and toiletries.
- Ear plugs and eye covers may assist some patients,[150,187] and have been shown to reduce the risk of delirium, although patients provided with ear plugs and eye covers should have the ability to remove them without assistance if they wish.

Care activities

- Attend to nursing care at the beginning of the night to reduce the likelihood of disturbing sleep during the night, for example:
  - redress wounds and empty drainage bags
  - wash, clean teeth and change gown and sheets
  - reposition with suitable pressure support measures
  - level the transducer at the phlebostatic axis to ensure accurate haemodynamic monitoring so you do not need to disturb the patient again later
  - ensure intravenous lines and drains are accessible.
- Plan care activities to allow the patient 1.5–2-hour periods of undisturbed time during the night. Negotiate with other healthcare personnel to allow these uninterrupted periods at night and during daytime rest times. 'Cluster care', for example, time medication administration, planned ETT suctioning and pressure area care to coincide.
- Provide the daily bath to suit patient needs rather than organisational needs (either before settling for the night or during normal waking hours).

> **Practice tip**
>
> Enabling the patient to experience good quality and quantities of sleep should be a major priority for critical care nursing. Demonstrate your commitment to improving rest and sleep for intensive care patients by incorporating sleep into the treatment reminder system used in the unit you work in (e.g. FASTHUG becomes FASSTHUG).

Environmental

- Reduce sound levels especially during rest times and at night, which may require a unit-wide change in practice as several critical care studies highlight the association between noise levels and sleep disruption.[188,189] Sound levels in adult critical care areas consistently exceed hospital standards; for example, the World Health Organization guidelines that recommend sound levels during the night inside a hospital should not exceed 40 dB, with particular attention given to sound levels in the ICU.[190]

- Ensure that lights are sufficiently dimmed and window blinds drawn during rest times and at night and that lighting is bright and blinds opened at all other times. It is known that critically ill patients' melatonin metabolism is often non-circadian so it is particularly important to attempt to use lighting that encourages normal circadian rhythm.[191,192] Generally, critical care areas contain fluorescent lights that may emit up to 600 lux. It is well known that artificial lights emit light with sufficient short-wave content to affect melatonin secretion, but research indicates that it is contemporary practice to provide sufficiently low light levels at night although daytime light may be inadequate to entrain circadian rhythms.[193,194]

> **Practice tip**
>
> Ask your patient (or their relatives) about their usual night-time 'settling routine' for sleep. Try to emulate the routine as closely as possible. Then check whether this improved their sleep.

Treatments

- Discuss the need for alternative mechanical ventilation settings at night with the medical team. Hyperventilation caused by inappropriately high inspiratory pressure can cause hypocapnia, which may lead to central apnoeas and sleep disturbance.[195]
- Many medications administered in critical care affect sleep architecture. Even vasoactive medications such as adrenaline have the capacity to affect the quality of sleep. Sedatives, especially benzodiazepines and opioids, reduce time in stage 3 and REM, so reduce the quantity and quality of sleep.[196–198] Pain relief and anxiolysis may be essential for sleep to occur, but an awareness of potential adverse medication reactions is important in the prevention of escalating sleep disturbances.
- Administration of specific medications to promote sleep are not recommended in hospital and ICU.[54,199,200]

> **Practice tip**
>
> Next time you are at work in the ICU, take the time to consider the sound level. At an appropriate time and position in the ICU, close your eyes for 1 minute and consider whether you would be able to rest. In addition, find a patient who is well enough to be discharged to the hospital ward and ask them about the factors that they found most disruptive to rest and sleep while they were being treated in ICU.

> **Practice tip**
>
> If after interviewing the patient or their family about their usual sleep and assessing their sleep in ICU you suspect they might have an existing untreated sleep disorder, request the treating medical team to make a sleep medicine referral. Untreated sleep problems long term may be associated with increased risk of cardiovascular disease and cancer.

Melatonin

This naturally occurring hormone is both sleep promoting and sleep maintaining. Melatonin is used for the short-term alleviation of secondary sleep disorders (e.g. insomnia and shift-work-induced circadian disruption).[201] There is some evidence to suggest it is useful for improving self-reported sleep quality for people with chronic diseases.[202] Several small-scale studies have been undertaken to examine whether melatonin improves either sleep or delirium in the critically ill, and, although there are some promising signs, evidence remains limited, conflicting and inconclusive.[203] Difficulties occur in emulating the typical endogenous pulsatile secretion of the hormone and, together with its short half-life, these probably explain why the evidence is inconclusive. The high doses required to achieve an adequate plasma level overnight when administered once at the beginning of the night are likely to persist in the body and may disrupt circadian rhythm. The typical dose is 3–5 mg once or twice a day.

The current advice of the authors based on evidence available to date is that conditions that encourage the normal circadian secretion of endogenous melatonin (i.e. provide lighting and activity levels appropriate for the time of day) may be more effective than administering exogenous melatonin. However, the risk profile of exogenous melatonin is low so it may considered as a useful adjunct to improve sleep.

Summary

Meeting the psychological needs of patients is essential in the care of critically ill patients. In this chapter the various methods that are available to assess and then effectively manage aspects of patient care related to anxiety, delirium, pain, sedation and sleep are outlined. Assessment of these aspects of the patient's condition require thorough clinical assessment, with a range of validated instruments available to help improve consistency over time and between clinicians, as well as to inform decisions regarding the most appropriate interventions. Although these aspects of care have been reviewed sequentially in this chapter, in reality they are closely interrelated and should be considered concurrently.

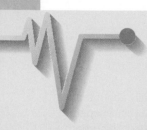

Case study

A 44-year-old man, Ian, was brought to hospital with 'difficulty breathing' by ambulance after a 5-day history of a flu-like illness. Ian had a positive polymerase chain reaction (PCR) COVID-19 test 2 days previously. On arrival in the emergency department, Ian was hypoxic and hypercapnic, his respiratory rate was 40 per minute and his Glasgow Coma Scale score was 7. He was transferred to the ICU for emergency intubation in the negative pressure room.

Ian was reported by his wife, Maddy, via video conference to be healthy with no underlying physical health conditions and rarely saw his GP. She also added that Ian worked long hours in information technology and was occasionally stressed and 'down in the dumps' but rarely complained of sleeping badly. Ian was a non-smoker and rarely drank alcohol but occasionally ate marijuana cookies with some old school friends. He weighed 85 kg and was 185 cm tall (BMI: normal). The couple had two sons: an 8-year-old and a teenager. At the time of Ian's admission Maddy reported than none of the family were vaccinated against COVID-19. Ian was admitted to hospital during a COVID-19 pandemic wave.

Ian was mechanically ventilated on pressure control and required FiO_2 1.00 to maintain his oxygenation. High doses of steroids and immunomodulating therapy were given. He was placed in a prone position for the first five consecutive nights of his stay in ICU. High doses of fentanyl and midazolam were used and cisatracurium was used at night. Cisatracurium was withheld during the day. Target sedation level on the Richmond Agitation–Sedation Scale (RASS) was −5 (during muscle relaxant hold). Despite all efforts, Ian remained difficult to oxygenate and ventilate. By day 7 his lung compliance was so poor his tidal volumes were <40 mL. Therefore, extracorporeal membrane oxygenation (ECMO) was started and continued until his lung function improved sufficiently 14 days later. When the ECMO was removed (day 21 ICU) the cisatracurium infusion was stopped and the sedative medication infusion rates were reduced.

On day 22 Ian was stable enough to be transferred to a room with windows facing outside the building. His lung function remained poor; he required FiO_2 0.5 and high inspiratory pressures to ventilate him and maintain normocapnia. Quantitative PCR testing revealed that his viral load was still high. He was physically weak and delirious.

By ICU day 24, Ian had sufficient strength to move his head vigorously from side to side greatly jeopardising his airway and frequently causing the ventilator tubing to disconnect from his endotracheal tube. Given his obvious discomfort and the anticipated protracted nature of his lung disease he was tracheostomised on ICU day 27. Despite this he remained agitated and required large doses of sedatives to maintain his safety. Infection prevention and control for the COVID-19 infection required healthcare workers to use full PPE, to minimise time in the room and to keep the room door closed. In addition, demands on the nursing workforce, including a high number of patients and high acuity patients and a limited number of nurses with sufficient expertise, lead to difficulties maintaining continuity of care. Ian was delirious (Confusion Assessment Method-ICU positive), appeared fearful and withdrawn most of the time. He was awake all night and seemed unable to stay awake during the day.

TREATMENT

From ICU day 28 an ICU nurse practitioner case managed Ian's early recovery with input from the entire multidisciplinary team including physiotherapy, dietitian, social work and speech pathology. A daily routine was developed with input from Maddy (Ian was still too delirious to provide input), which included set 'wake up' and 'lights out' times. In-depth information about Ian's personality, his interests and likes and dislikes were obtained and documented in a care plan. Instructions about the daily routine were placed in prominent places in Ian's room. A low-dose dexmedetomidine infusion was administered at night if Ian was delirious and he was ventilated using pressure control at night and pressure support during the day. The speech pathologist helped find strategies to improve communication. Regular video conferences were scheduled for Maddy and Ian and their sons to see each other (until visiting restrictions were reduced and Ian had two negative PCR tests towards the end of his ICU stay).

When Ian was no longer delirious, he was asked about his goals for the future. He simply wanted to 'breathe without the ventilator' and 'go home'. Therefore, rehabilitation started with an emphasis on developing respiratory function to address these goals. At times he was despondent and discouraged by the lack of progress, especially in relation to his respiratory function.

- Ian was encouraged to express his feelings using the communication strategies available (at first picture boards containing faces of different emotions were used and Ian was asked to point at these).

- Ian's lists of interests were consulted by nurses and other healthcare professionals before they entered the room and used as 'conversation starters' and he was encouraged to watch his favourite TV programs.

- Within the constraints of the COVID-19 infection prevention and control, non-pharmacological interventions were used to manage delirium as much as possible with the addition of nocturnal dexmedetomidine.

- Nurses were encouraged to ensure the room was well lit during the day to ensure circadian entrainment.

- When COVID-19 infection prevention and control visiting restrictions were relaxed, Ian was visited each day by Maddy.

- Maddy was provided with support and advice about carer support.

- A summary of his day's achievements, however small, were written on a whiteboard in the room.

Ian was treated in ICU for 6 weeks and was discharged to an inpatient rehabilitation facility 2 weeks later. His frailty and impaired respiratory function were the main reasons for his continued need for inpatient treatment.

RECOVERY

Ian's physical recovery was uneventful; however, he continued to experience severe low mood. While treated in the inpatient rehabilitation facility he saw a psychologist as he was experiencing the symptoms of post-traumatic stress disorder (PTSD). He saw his GP after returning home in the community, who prescribed a mood stabiliser and antidepressant. Three months after he returned home, he visited the ICU and expressed his gratitude for his treatment. He reported that he had experienced repeated flashbacks about not being able to breathe and that this contributed to his low mood.

DISCUSSION

Ian's recovery was complicated by significant challenges associated with delirium and frailty. It is possible, given his history of low moods, that he had experienced depression prior to this hospitalisation and this contributed to the challenges he faced. His 'unproblematic' use of marijuana may have been a method of self-treatment. Many patients have unrecognised mental health disorders which may manifest more strongly during recovery from critical illness. For the large proportion of his ICU stay, Ian's psychological care needs were greater than his physical needs. The situation was compounded by the pandemic-related restrictions on visiting, continuity of care and usual care provided for delirium. However, technology (video conferencing), expert nursing (nurse practitioner) and his main supporter and advocate, Maddy, resulted in a good outcome.

CASE STUDY QUESTIONS

1 List Ian's risk factors for delirium (other than sedative medications) and the non-pharmacological nursing interventions that were used in caring for him, as well as any additional strategies that might have been used.

2 One of the interventions used to assist Ian's to sleep was to ensure the room was brightly lit during the day. Explain the underlying rationale for this intervention.

RESEARCH VIGNETTE

Kusi-Appiah E, Karanikola M, Pant U, et al. Tools for assessment of acute psychological distress in critical illness: a scoping review. Aust Crit Care 2021;34(5):460-72.

Abstract

Objectives: Patients' experience of psychological distress in the ICU is associated with adverse effects, reduced satisfaction and delayed physical and psychological recovery. There are no specific guidelines for the assessment and management of acute psychological distress during hospitalisation in the ICU. We reviewed existing tools for the assessment of acute psychological distress in ICU patients, examined evidence on their metric properties and identified potential gaps and methodological considerations.

Method: A scoping review based on literature searches (Cumulative Index to Nursing and Allied Health Literature, Medical Literature Analysis and Retrieval System Online, Excerpta Medica Database, PsycINFO, Scopus, Health and Psychosocial Instruments, Dissertations and Theses Global, and Google Scholar) and predefined eligibility criteria was conducted as per current scoping review guidelines.

Findings: Overall, 14 assessment tools were identified having been developed in diverse ICU settings. The identified tools assess mainly anxiety and depressive symptoms and ICU stressors, and investigators have reported various validity and reliability metrics. It was unclear whether available tools can be used in specific groups, such as non-communicative patients and patients with delirium, brain trauma, stroke, sedation and cognitive impairments.

Conclusion: Available tools have methodological limitations worth considering in future investigations. Given the high prevalence of psychiatric morbidity in ICU survivors, rigorously exploring the metric integrity of available tools used for anxiety, depressive and psychological distress symptom assessment in the vulnerable ICU population is a practice and research priority.

Relevance to clinical practice: These results have implications for the selection and implementation of psychological distress assessment methods as a means for promoting meaningful patient-centred clinical outcomes and humanising ICU care experiences.

Critique

The importance of assessing psychological distress in critically ill patients is increasingly recognised. Use of valid and reliable instruments is essential to optimise the value of the information gained in such assessments. The search in this scoping review was extensive and covered relevant databases with no date or language limits applied at the time of the search, although non-English papers were subsequently excluded.

Fourteen tools for assessing psychological distress were identified, with initial development work conducted in a range of countries including the USA ($n = 6$), the UK ($n = 2$), Australia ($n = 2$), China ($n = 2$) and 1 in each of Brazil, India and Iran (total = 15 as 1 development study was conducted across 2 countries). Some instruments were designed to assess anxiety alone or in combination with depression, or alternatively a broader construct of psychological distress; there was a mix of instruments designed for self-assessment by the patient or use by clinical/research staff to assess the patient.

The number of items on each instrument range from 1 to 61, with half having 35 items or more. The length of the instruments was identified by the review authors as a feasibility consideration, with 20 items or more considered to create significant test burden, fatigue and frustration for the patients.

Development of the psychological distress instruments rarely involved adequate blinding and the new instruments were frequently not compared with a 'gold standard'. Despite the limitations of the development, adequate validity and reliability measurements were reported on the parameters that have been assessed for many of these instruments. A number of the instruments have also been tested by other author groups to determine applicability in additional settings.

Given the growing recognition of the importance of assessment within critical care, and the challenges involved in assessing psychological constructs such as anxiety, distress and depression in patients who are not completely alert, it is essential that further development work is undertaken to establish reliability and validity in larger sample sizes and multiple settings. Interventions to reduce psychological distress are relevant for all patients, but specific targeting towards patients with greater levels of distress will probably promote improved outcomes.

Despite the limited rigour in the development of these assessment instruments to date, this review offers the best summary of instruments available and provides some guidelines for those in clinical areas redesigning care protocols to incorporate assessment of psychological distress.

Learning activities

1 The assessment of anxiety and pain is integral to critical care nursing:

   a Discuss the assessment strategies you would use to differentiate between anxiety and pain.

   b List any special considerations associated with your choices.

2 Outline some non-pharmacological strategies that could be employed to reduce pain.

3 Discuss how family could help with the management of the patient's anxiety.

4 Critically ill patients who experience delirium require highly skilled and informed nursing. The following exercises may enhance your ability to manage patients with delirium:

   a Identify risk factors for the patient and think of ways to ameliorate them (in practice always discuss with the multidisciplinary team).

   b Highlight nursing interventions that may reduce the potential for delirium. Describe the rationale for your selection of nursing interventions using current research.

5 Outline the differences between delirium and dementia.

6 Effective treatment for alcohol and substance withdrawal is dependent on identifying symptoms early. Outline the strategies to identify patients at risk of alcohol withdrawal in critical care.

7 Why is thiamine and complex B vitamin supplementation considered a vital component of treatment for alcohol dependence?

8 Compare and contrast the various pain assessment instruments and discuss the relative merits and disadvantages of using each of these instruments. Now repeat the exercise for each of the instruments for sedation assessment and for delirium assessment.

9 Using the references provided in this chapter:

   a Highlight the importance of good quality sleep in health and illness.

   b Identify theories that explain the function of sleep.

10 Think about the last time you experienced fragmented sleep or insufficient sleep and describe how you felt in terms of your:

   a mood

   b cognitive function

   c physical function

   d appetite

   e motivation.

Online resources

Australasian Sleep Association, www.sleep.org.au

Healthtalk.org (Former patients talk about their experience), http://www.healthtalk.org/peoples-experiences/intensive-care/intensive-care-patients-experiences/topics.

ICU Delirium and Cognitive Impairment Study Group, www.icudelirium.org

Further reading

Devlin JW, Skrobik Y, Gelinas C, et al. Clinical practice guidelines for the prevention and management of pain, agitation/sedation, delirium, immobility, and sleep disruption in adult patients in the ICU. Crit Care Med 2018;46:e825–73.

Erickson CK. Addiction essentials: the go-to guide for clinicians and patients. New York: WW Norton; 2011.

Kampman K, Jarvis M. American Society of Addiction Medicine (ASAM) national practice guideline for the use of medications in the treatment of addiction involving opioid use. J Addict Med 2015;9:358–67.

Kyranou M, Puntillo K. The transition from acute to chronic pain: might intensive care unit patients be at risk? Ann Intensive Care 2012;2:36.

Mack AH. Clinical textbook of addictive disorders. New York: Guilford Press; 2016.

NSW Therapeutic Advisory Group Inc. Getting it right for sleep at night: Guidance for promoting sleep and reducing harm from inappropriate pharmacologic management of sleep disturbance and insomnia in hospitalised patients. Darlinghurst: NSW TAG; 2021. Available from: nswtag.org.au/wp-content/uploads/2021/12/1.-Guidance_Getting-it-right-for-sleep-at-night_21Dec2021.pdf.

Seo Y, Lee HJ, Ha EJ, et al. 2021 KSCCM clinical practice guidelines for pain, agitation, delirium, immobility, and sleep disturbance in the intensive care unit. Acute Crit Care 2022;37(1):1–25. doi: 10.4266/acc.2022.00094.

References

1. Elliott D, Aitken LM, Bucknall TK, et al. Patient comfort in the intensive care unit: a multicentre, binational point prevalence study of analgesia, sedation and delirium management. Crit Care Resusc 2013;15:213–19.

2. Kotfis K, Zegan-Baranska M, Zukowski M, et al. Multicenter assessment of sedation and delirium practices in the intensive care units in Poland – is this common practice in Eastern Europe? BMC Anesthesiol 2017;17:120. doi: 10.1186/s12871-017-0415-2.

3. Richards-Belle A, Canter RR, Power GS, et al. National survey and point prevalence study of sedation practice in UK critical care. Crit Care 2016;20:355. doi: 10.1186/s13054-016-1532-x.

4. Aragon RE, Proano A, Mongilardi N, et al. Sedation practices and clinical outcomes in mechanically ventilated patients in a prospective multicenter cohort. Crit Care 2019;23:130. doi: 10.1186/s13054-019-2394-9.

5. Spielberger CD. Anxiety: current trends in theory and research: I. New York: Academic Press, 1972.

6. Abed MA, Hall LA, Moser DK. Spielberger's state anxiety inventory: development of a shortened version for critically ill patients. Issues Ment Health Nurs 2011;32:220–7. doi: 10.3109/01612840.2010.546493.

7. Wewalka M, Warszawska J, Strunz V, et al. Depression as an independent risk factor for mortality in critically ill patients. Psychosom Med 2015;77:106–13. doi: 10.1097/PSY.0000000000000137.

8. Castillo MI, Cooke M, Macfarlane B, et al. Factors associated with anxiety in critically ill patients: a prospective observational cohort study. Int J Nurs Stud 2016;60:225–33. doi: 10.1016/j.ijnurstu.2016.05.007.

9. Lamas DJ, Owens RL, Nace RN, et al. Opening the door: the experience of chronic critical illness in a long-term acute care hospital. Crit Care Med 2017;45:e357–62. 2016/09/16. doi: 10.1097/ccm.0000000000002094.

10. Oh J, Sohn JH, Shin CS, et al. Mutual relationship between anxiety and pain in the intensive care unit and its effect on medications. J Crit Care 2015;30:1043–8. doi: 10.1016/j.jcrc.2015.05.025.

11. Tate JA, Devito Dabbs A, Hoffman LA, et al. Anxiety and agitation in mechanically ventilated patients. Qual Health Res 2012;22:157–73. doi: 10.1177/1049732311421616.

12. Vesz PS, Costanzi M, Stolnik D, et al. Functional and psychological features immediately after discharge from an intensive care unit: prospective cohort study. Rev Bras Ter Intensiva 2013;25:218–24. doi: 10.5935/0103-507x.20130038.

13. Wade DM, Howell DC, Weinman JA, et al. Investigating risk factors for psychological morbidity three months after intensive care: a prospective cohort study. Crit Care 2012;16:R192. doi: 10.1186/cc11677.

14. Gezginci E, Goktas S, Orhan BN. The effects of environmental stressors in intensive care unit on anxiety and depression. Nurs Crit Care 2022;27:113–19.

15. Chung CR, Yoo HJ, Park J, et al. Cognitive impairment and psychological distress at discharge from intensive care unit. Psychiatry Investig 2017;14:376–9. doi: 10.4306/pi.2017.14.3.376.

16. Fink RM, Makic MB, Poteet AW, et al. The ventilated patient's experience. Dimens Crit Care Nurs 2015;34:301–8. doi: 10.1097/DCC.0000000000000128.

17. May AD, Parker AM, Caldwell ES, et al. Provider-documented anxiety in the ICU: prevalence, risk factors, and associated patient outcomes. J Intensive care Med 2021;36:1424–30.

18. Chlan L, Savik K. Patterns of anxiety in critically ill patients receiving mechanical ventilatory support. Nurs Res 2011;60:S50–7. doi: 10.1097/NNR.0b013e318216009c.

19. De Jong MJ, Chung ML, Roser LP, et al. A five-country comparison of anxiety early after acute myocardial infarction. Eur J Cardiovasc Nurs 2004;3:129–34.

20. Bear MF, Connors BW, Paradiso MA. Neuroscience exploring the brain. Philadelphia: Lippincott Williams & Wilkins; 2007.

21. Frazier SK, Moser DK, Riegel B, et al. Critical care nurses' assessment of patients' anxiety: reliance on physiological and behavioral parameters. Am J Crit Care 2002;11:57–64.

22. McKinley S, Coote K, Stein-Parbury J. Development and testing of a Faces Scale for the assessment of anxiety in critically ill patients. J Adv Nurs 2003;41:73–9.

23. Porth C. Essentials of pathophysiology: concepts of altered health states. Philadelphia: Lippincott Williams & Wilkins; 2011.

24. Dubb R, Nydahl P, Hermes C, et al. Barriers and strategies for early mobilization of patients in intensive care units. Ann Am Thorac Soc 2016;13:724–30.

25. Hatch R, Young D, Barber V, et al. Anxiety, depression and post traumatic stress disorder after critical illness: a UK-wide prospective cohort study. Crit Care 2018;22:310. doi: 10.1186/s13054-018-2223-6.

26. McPeake J, Quasim T, Henderson P, et al. Multimorbidity and its relationship with long-term outcomes after critical care discharge: a prospective cohort study. Chest 2021;160:1681–92. doi: 10.1016/j.chest.2021.05.069.

27. King J, O'Neill B, Ramsay P, et al. Identifying patients' support needs following critical illness: a scoping review of the qualitative literature. Crit Care 2019;23:187. doi: 10.1186/s13054-019-2441-6.

28. Jackson JC, Santoro MJ, Ely TM, et al. Improving patient care through the prism of psychology: application of Maslow's hierarchy to sedation, delirium, and early mobility in the intensive care unit. J Crit Care 2014;29:438–44. doi: 10.1016/j.jcrc.2014.01.009.

29. Mikkelsen ME, Still M, Anderson BJ, et al. Society of Critical Care Medicine's international consensus conference on prediction and identification of long-term impairments after critical illness. Crit Care Med 2020;48:1670–9.

30. Zigmond AS, Snaith RP. The hospital anxiety and depression scale. Acta Psychiatr Scand 1983;67:361–70.

31. Lovibond SH, Lovibond PF. Manual for the Depression Anxiety Stress Scales. 2nd ed. Sydney: Psychology Foundation: 1995.

32. Ng F, Trauer T, Dodd S, et al. The validity of the 21-item version of the Depression Anxiety Stress Scales as a routine clinical outcome measure. Acta Neuropsychiatr 2007;19:304–10. doi: 10.1111/j.1601-5215.2007.00217.x.

33. Spielberger CD, Gorsuch R, Lushene R, et al. Manual for the state-trait anxiety inventory. Palo Alto, CA: Consulting Psychologist Press; 1983.

34. Chlan L, Savik K, Weinert C. Development of a shortened state anxiety scale from the Spielberger State-Trait Anxiety Inventory (STAI) for patients receiving mechanical ventilatory support. J Nurs Meas 2003;11:283–93.

35. Hornblow AR and Kidson MA. The visual analogue scale for anxiety: a validation study. Aust N Z J Psychiatry 1976;10:339–41.

36. Gustad LT, Chaboyer W, Wallis M. Performance of the Faces Anxiety Scale in patients transferred from the ICU. Intensive Crit Care Nurs 2005;21:355–60. doi: 10.1016/j.iccn.2005.06.006.

37. McKinley S, Madronio C. Validity of the Faces Anxiety Scale for the assessment of state anxiety in intensive care patients not receiving mechanical ventilation. J Psychosom Res 2008;64:503–7. doi: 10.1016/j.jpsychores.2008.02.002.

38. McKinley S, Stein-Parbury J, Chehelnabi A, et al. Assessment of anxiety in intensive care patients by using the Faces Anxiety Scale. Am J Crit Care 2004;13:146–52.

39. Milton A, Bruck E, Schandl A, et al. Early psychological screening of intensive care unit survivors: a prospective cohort study. Crit Care 2017;21:273. doi: 10.1186/s13054-017-1813-z.

40. Nikayin S, Rabiee A, Hashem MD, et al. Anxiety symptoms in survivors of critical illness: a systematic review and meta-analysis. Gen Hosp Psychiatry 2016;43:23–9. doi: 10.1016/j.genhosppsych.2016.08.005.

41. Alves da Silva T, Stripari Schujmann D, Yamada da Silveira LT, et al. Effect of therapeutic Swedish massage on anxiety level and vital signs of intensive care unit patients. J Bodyw Mov Ther 2017;21:565–8. doi: 10.1016/j.jbmt.2016.08.009.

42. Boitor M, Gelinas C, Richard-Lalonde M, et al. The effect of massage on acute postoperative pain in critically and acutely ill adults post-thoracic surgery: systematic review and meta-analysis of randomized controlled trials. Heart Lung 2017;46:339–46. doi: 10.1016/j.hrtlng.2017.05.005.

43. Chlan LL, Weinert CR, Heiderscheit A, et al. Effects of patient-directed music intervention on anxiety and sedative exposure in critically ill patients receiving mechanical ventilatory support: a randomized clinical trial. JAMA 2013;309:2335–44. doi: 10.1001/jama.2013.5670.

44. Davis T, Jones P. Music therapy: decreasing anxiety in the ventilated patient: a review of the literature. Dimens Crit Care Nurs 2012;31:159–66. doi: 10.1097/DCC.0b013e31824dffc6.

45. Rashid M. Two decades (1993-2012) of adult intensive care unit design: a comparative study of the physical design features of the best practice examples. Crit Care Nurs Q 2014;37:3–32. doi: 10.1097/cnq.0000000000000002.

46. Hosey MM, Wegener ST, Hinkle C, et al. A cognitive behavioral therapy-informed self-management program for acute respiratory failure survivors: a feasibility study. J Clin Med 2021;10:872.

47. Cohen JN, Gopal A, Roberts KJ, et al. Ventilator-dependent patients successfully weaned with cognitive-behavioral therapy: a case series. Psychosomatics 2019;60:612–19. doi: 10.1016/j.psym.2019.02.003.

48. Halm MA. Essential oils for management of symptoms in critically ill patients. Am J Crit Care 2008;17:160–3.

49. Lytle J, Mwatha C, Davis KK. Effect of lavender aromatherapy on vital signs and perceived quality of sleep in the intermediate care unit: a pilot study. Am J Crit Care 2014;23:24–9. doi: 10.4037/ajcc2014958

50. Mofredj A, Alaya S, Tassaioust K, et al. Music therapy, a review of the potential therapeutic benefits for the critically ill. J Crit Care 2016;35:195–9. doi: 10.1016/j.jcrc.2016.05.021.

51. Patel J, Baldwin J, Bunting P, et al. The effect of a multicomponent multidisciplinary bundle of interventions on sleep and delirium in medical and surgical intensive care patients. Anaesthesia 2014;69:540–9. doi: 10.1111/anae.12638.

52. Chlan L, Heiderscheit A. A tool for music preference assessment in critically ill patients receiving mechanical ventilatory support. Music Ther Perspect 2009;27:42–7. doi: 10.1093/mtp/27.1.42.

53. McKinley S, Nagy S, Stein-Parbury J, et al. Vulnerability and security in seriously ill patients in intensive care. Intensive Crit Care Nurs 2002;18:27–36.

54. Devlin JW, Skrobik Y, Gelinas C, et al. Clinical practice guidelines for the prevention and management of pain, agitation/sedation, delirium, immobility, and sleep disruption in adult patients in the ICU. Crit Care Med 2018;46:e825–73. doi: 10.1097/ccm.0000000000003299.

55. Kelly JM, Rubenfeld GD, Masson N, et al. Using selective serotonin reuptake inhibitors and serotonin-norepinephrine reuptake inhibitors in critical care: a systematic review of the evidence for benefit or harm. Crit Care Med 2017;45:e607–16.

56. La MK, Bastin MLT, Gisewhite JT, et al. Impact of restarting home neuropsychiatric medications on sedation outcomes in medical intensive care unit patients. J Crit Care 2018;43:102–7.

57. Zaal IJ, Devlin JW, Peelen LM, et al. A systematic review of risk factors for delirium in the ICU. Crit Care Med 2015;43:40–7. doi: 10.1097/CCM.0000000000000625.

58. Spronk PE, Riekerk B, Hofhuis J, et al. Occurrence of delirium is severely underestimated in the ICU during daily care. Intensive Care Med 2009;35:1276–80. doi: 10.1007/s00134-009-1466-8.

59. Han JH, Shintani A, Eden S, et al. Delirium in the emergency department: an independent predictor of death within 6 months. Ann Emerg Med 2010. doi: 10.1016/j.annemergmed.2010.03.003.

60. Karnatovskaia LV, Johnson MM, Benzo RP, et al. The spectrum of psychocognitive morbidity in the critically ill: a review of the literature and call for improvement. J Crit Care 2015;30:130–7. doi: 10.1016/j.jcrc.2014.09.024.

61. Salluh JIF, Wang H, Schneider EB, et al. Outcome of delirium in critically ill patients: systematic review and meta-analysis. BMJ 2015;350:h2538.

62. Wilcox ME, Brummel NE, Archer K, et al. Cognitive dysfunction in ICU patients: risk factors, predictors, and rehabilitation interventions. Crit Care Med 2013;41:S81–98. doi: 10.1097/CCM.0b013e3182a16946.

63. Roberts BL, Rickard CM, Rajbhandari D, et al. Factual memories of ICU: recall at two years post-discharge and comparison with delirium status during ICU admission – a multicentre cohort study. J Clin Nurs 2007;16:1669–77.

64. Svenningsen H, Tonnesen EK, Videbech P, et al. Intensive care delirium – effect on memories and health-related quality of life – a follow-up study. J Clin Nurs 2014;23:634–44. doi: 10.1111/jocn.12250.

65. Krewulak KD, Stelfox HT, Leigh JP, et al. Incidence and prevalence of delirium subtypes in an adult ICU: a systematic review and meta-analysis. Crit Care Med 2018;46:2029–35.

66. Meagher DJ, Leonard M, Donnelly S, et al. A longitudinal study of motor subtypes in delirium: Relationship with other phenomenology, etiology, medication exposure and prognosis. J Psychosom Res 2011;71:395–403. doi: 10.1016/j.jpsychores.2011.06.001.

67. American Psychiatric Association. Diagnostic and statistical manual of mental disorders (DSM-5-TR®). Washington DC: APA; 2022.

68. Broyles LM, Colbert AM, Tate JA, et al. Clinicians' evaluation and management of mental health, substance abuse, and chronic pain conditions in the intensive care unit. Crit Care Med 2008;36:87–93. doi: 10.1097/01.CCM.0000292010.11345.24.

69. Mariz J, Santos NC, Afonso H, et al. Risk and clinical-outcome indicators of delirium in an emergency department intermediate care unit (EDIMCU): an observational prospective study. BMC Emerg Med 2013;13:2. doi: 10.1186/1471-227x-13-2.

70. Maldonado JR. Acute brain failure: pathophysiology, diagnosis, management, and sequelae of delirium. Crit Care Clin 2017;33:461–519. doi: 10.1016/j.ccc.2017.03.013.

71. Wilson JE, Mart MF, Cunningham C, et al. Delirium. Nat Rev Dis Primers 2020;6(1):90. doi: doi: 10.1038/s41572-020-00223-4.

72. Boogaard Mvd, Pickkers P, Slooter AJC, et al. Development and validation of PRE-DELIRIC (PREdiction of DELIRium in ICu patients) delirium prediction model for intensive care patients: observational multicentre study. BMJ 2012;344:e420. doi: 10.1136/bmj.e420.

73. Girard TD, Ely EW. Delirium in the critically ill patient. Handb Clin Neurol 2008;90:39–56. doi: 10.1016/S0072-9752(07)01703-4.

74. Girard TD, Pandharipande PP, Ely EW. Delirium in the intensive care unit. Crit Care 2008;12(Suppl. 3):S3. doi: 10.1186/cc6149.

75. Ruppert MM, Lipori J, Patel S, et al. ICU delirium-prediction models: a systematic review. Crit Care Explor 2020; 2(12):e0296.

76. Bergeron N, Dubois MJ, Dumont M, et al. Intensive Care Delirium Screening Checklist: evaluation of a new screening tool. Intensive Care Med 2001;27:859–64.

77. Ely EW, Inouye SK, Bernard GR, et al. Delirium in mechanically ventilated patients: validity and reliability of the confusion assessment method for the intensive care unit (CAM-ICU). JAMA 2001;286:2703–10. doi: 10.1001/jama.286.21.2703.

78. Neto AS, Nassar AP, Jr., Cardoso SO, et al. Delirium screening in critically ill patients: a systematic review and meta-analysis. Crit Care Med 2012;40:1946–51. doi: 10.1097/CCM.0b013e31824e16c9.

79. Shi Q, Warren L, Saposnik G, et al. Confusion assessment method: a systematic review and meta-analysis of diagnostic accuracy. Neuropsychiatr Dis Treat 2013;9:1359–70. doi: 10.2147/NDT.S49520.

80. Ely EW, Margolin R, Francis J, et al. Evaluation of delirium in critically ill patients: validation of the Confusion Assessment Method for the Intensive Care Unit (CAM-ICU). Crit Care Med 2001;29:1370–79.

81. Kamdar BB, King LM, Collop NA, et al. The effect of a quality improvement intervention on perceived sleep quality and cognition in a medical ICU. Crit Care Med 2013;41(3):800–9. doi: 10.1097/CCM.0b013e3182746442.

82. Smith CD, Grami P. Feasibility and effectiveness of a delirium prevention bundle in critically ill patients. Am J Crit Care 2016;26:19–27. doi: 10.4037/ajcc2017374.

83. Liang S, Chau JPC, Lo SHS, et al. Effects of nonpharmacological delirium-prevention interventions on critically ill patients' clinical, psychological, and family outcomes: a systematic review and meta-analysis. Aust Crit Care 2021;34:378–87.

84. Flannery AH, Oyler DR, Weinhouse GL. The impact of interventions to improve sleep on delirium in the icu: a systematic review and research framework. Crit Care Med 2016;44:2231–40. doi: 10.1097/CCM.0000000000001952.

85. Neufeld KJ, Yue J, Robinson TN, et al. Antipsychotics for prevention and treatment of delirium in hospitalized adults: a systematic review and meta-analysis. J Am Geriatr Soc 2016;64:705–14. doi: 10.1111/jgs.14076.

86. Weaver CB, Kane-Gill SL, Gunn SR, et al. A retrospective analysis of the effectiveness of antipsychotics in the treatment of ICU delirium. J Crit Care 2017;41:234–9. doi: 10.1016/j.jcrc.2017.05.034.

87. Kawazoe Y, Miyamoto K, Morimoto T, et al. Effect of dexmedetomidine on mortality and ventilator-free days in patients requiring mechanical ventilation with sepsis: a randomized clinical trial. JAMA 2017;317:1321–8. doi: 10.1001/jama.2017.2088.

88. Cruickshank M, Henderson L, MacLennan G, et al. Alpha-2 agonists for sedation of mechanically ventilated adults in intensive care units: a systematic review. Health Technol Assess 2016;20:1–118. doi: 10.3310/hta20250.

89. Reade MC, Eastwood GM, Bellomo R, et al. Effect of dexmedetomidine added to standard care on ventilator-free time in patients with agitated delirium: a randomized clinical trial. JAMA 2016;315:1460–8. doi: 10.1001/jama.2016.2707.

90. Burry LD, Cheng W, Williamson DR, et al. Pharmacological and non-pharmacological interventions to prevent delirium in critically ill patients: a systematic review and network meta-analysis. Intensive Care Med 2021;47.943–60. doi: 10.1007/s00134-021-06490-3.

91. Hale GM, Kane-Gill SL, Groetzinger L, et al. An evaluation of adverse drug reactions associated with antipsychotic use for the treatment of delirium in the intensive care unit. J Pharm Pract 2016;29:355–60. doi: 10.1177/0897190014566313.

92. Awissi DK, Lebrun G, Coursin DB, et al. Alcohol withdrawal and delirium tremens in the critically ill: a systematic review and commentary. Intensive Care Med 2013;39:16–30. doi: 10.1007/s00134-012-2758-y.

93. Schuckit MA. Recognition and management of withdrawal delirium (delirium tremens). N Engl J Med 2014;371:2109–13. doi: 10.1056/NEJMra1407298.

94. American Psychiatric Association. Substance-related and addictive disorders. In: DSM-5 – TR: diagnostic and statistical manual of mental disorders. 5th ed. Washington DC: APA;2022.

95. Maldonado JR, Sher Y, Ashouri JF, et al. The "Prediction of Alcohol Withdrawal Severity Scale" (PAWSS): systematic literature review and pilot study of a new scale for the prediction of complicated alcohol withdrawal syndrome. Alcohol 2014;48:375–90. doi: 10.1016/j.alcohol.2014.01.004.

96. Australian Institute of Health and Welfare (AIHW). Non-medical use of pharmaceuticals: trends, harms and treatment, 2006–07 to 2015–16. Canberra: AIHW; 2017.

97. US Department of Health and Human Services (HHS). Facing addiction in America: the Surgeon General's report on alcohol, drugs, and health. Washington DC: HHS; 2016. Available from: https://health.gov/healthypeople/tools-action/browse-evidence-based-resources/facing-addiction-america-surgeon-generals-report-alcohol-drugs-and-health. [Accessed 12 February 2023].

98. United Nations Office on Drugs and Crime. World drug report 2017. New York: UN; 2017.

99. Banks E, Joshy G, Weber MF, et al. Tobacco smoking and all-cause mortality in a large Australian cohort study: findings from a mature epidemic with current low smoking prevalence. BMC Med 2015;13:38. doi: 10.1186/s12916-015-0281-z.

100. Greenhalgh EM, Bayly M, Winstanley MH. 1.2 Overview of major Australian data sets. In: Scollo MM, Winstanley MH, editors. Tobacco in Australia: facts and issues. Melbourne, VIC: Cancer Council Victoria; 2015. Available from: https://www.tobaccoinaustralia.org.au/chapter-1-prevalence/1-2-overview-of-major-australian-data-sets. [Accessed 12 February 2023].

101. Australian Institute of Health and Welfare (AIHW). National drug strategy household survey. Canberra, ACT: AIHW; 2019. Available from: https://www.aihw.gov.au/reports/illicit-use-of-drugs/national-drug-strategy-household-survey-2019/contents/summary. [Accessed 12 February 2023].

102. Ng M, Freeman MK, Fleming TD, et al. Smoking prevalence and cigarette consumption in 187 countries, 1980–2012. JAMA 2014;311:183–92. doi: 10.1001/jama.2013.284692.

103. Koob GF, Volkow ND. Neurobiology of addiction: a neurocircuitry analysis. Lancet Psychiatry 2016;3:760–73. doi: 10.1016/S2215-0366(16)00104-8.

104. Donroe JH, Tetrault JM. Substance use, intoxication, and withdrawal in the critical care setting. Crit Care Clin 2017;33:543–58. doi: 10.1016/j.ccc.2017.03.003.

105. Wang PP, Huang E, Feng X, et al. Opioid-associated iatrogenic withdrawal in critically ill adult patients: a multicenter prospective observational study. Ann Intensive Care 2017;7:88. doi: 10.1186/s13613-017-0310-5.

106. Ewing JA. Detecting alcoholism. The CAGE questionnaire. JAMA 1984;252:1905–7.

107. Mirijello A, D'Angelo C, Ferrulli A, et al. Identification and management of alcohol withdrawal syndrome. Drugs 2015;75:353–65. doi: 10.1007/s40265-015-0358-1.

108. Sutton LJ, Jutel A. Alcohol withdrawal syndrome in critically ill patients: identification, assessment, and management. Crit Care Nurse 2016;36:28–38. doi: 10.4037/ccn2016420.

109. Wetterling T, Kanitz RD, Besters B, et al. A new rating scale for the assessment of the alcohol-withdrawal syndrome (AWS scale). Alcohol Alcohol 1997;32:75360.

110. Sullivan JT, Sykora K, Schneiderman J, et al. Assessment of alcohol withdrawal: the revised clinical institute withdrawal assessment for alcohol scale (CIWA-Ar). Br J Addict 1989;84:1353–7.

111. Heatherton TF, Kozlowski LT, Frecker RC, et al. The Fagerström test for nicotine dependence: a revision of the Fagerström Tolerance Questionnaire. Br J Addict 1991;86:1119–27.

112. Chiu AW, Contreras S, Mehta S, et al. Iatrogenic opioid withdrawal in critically ill patients: a review of assessment tools and management. Ann Pharmacother 2017;51:1099–111. doi: 10.1177/1060028017724538.

113. Dixit D, Endicott J, Burry L, et al. Management of acute alcohol withdrawal syndrome in critically ill patients. Pharmacotherapy 2016;36: 797–822. doi: 10.1002/phar.1770.

114. Perry EC. Inpatient management of acute alcohol withdrawal syndrome. CNS Drugs 2014;28:401–10. doi: 10.1007/s40263-014-0163-5.

115. Thomson AD, Cook CC. Parenteral thiamine and Wernicke's encephalopathy: the balance of risks and perception of concern. Alcohol Alcohol 1997;32:207–9.

116. Shehabi Y, Serpa Neto A, Howe BD, et al. Early sedation with dexmedetomidine in ventilated critically ill patients and heterogeneity of treatment effect in the SPICE III randomised controlled trial. Intensive Care Medi 2021;47:455–66. doi: 10.1007/s00134-021-06356-8.

117. Hood SD, Norman A, Hince DA, et al. Benzodiazepine dependence and its treatment with low dose flumazenil. Br J Clin Pharmacol 2014;77:285–94. doi: 10.1111/bcp.12023.

118. Kampman K, Jarvis M. American Society of Addiction Medicine (ASAM) national practice guideline for the use of medications in the treatment of addiction involving opioid use. J Addict Med 2015;9:358–67. doi: 10.1097/ADM.0000000000000166.

119. Gowing L, Ali R, White JM, et al. Buprenorphine for managing opioid withdrawal. Cochrane Database Syst Rev 2017;2(2):CD002025. doi: 10.1002/14651858.CD002025.pub5.

120. Srivastava AB, Mariani JJ, Levin FR. New directions in the treatment of opioid withdrawal. Lancet 2020;395:1938–48. doi: 10.1016/S0140-6736(20)30852-7.

121. Kowalski M, Udy AA, McRobbie HJ, et al. Nicotine replacement therapy for agitation and delirium management in the intensive care unit: a systematic review of the literature. J Intensive Care 2016;4:69. doi: 10.1186/s40560-016-0184-x.

122. Ng K, Gillies M, Griffith D. Effect of nicotine replacement therapy on mortality, delirium, and duration of therapy in critically ill smokers: a systematic review and meta-analysis. Anaesth Intensive Care 2017;45:556–61.

123. Wilby KJ, Harder CK. Nicotine replacement therapy in the intensive care unit: a systematic review. J Intensive Care Med 2014;29:22–30. doi: 10.1177/0885066612442053.

124. Puntillo KA, Max A, Chaize M, et al. Patient recollection of ICU procedural pain and post ICU burden: the memory study. Crit Care Med 2016;44:1988–95.

125. Puntillo KA, Max A, Timsit JF, et al. Determinants of procedural pain intensity in the intensive care unit. The Europain(R) study. Am J Respir Crit Care Med 2014;189:39–47. doi: 10.1164/rccm.20130-1174OC.

126. Fishman S, Ballantyne J, Rathmell JP. Bonica's management of pain. 4th ed. Philadelphia: Lippincott Williams & Wilkins; 2009.

127. Milgrom LB, Brooks JA, Qi R, et al. Pain levels experienced with activities after cardiac surgery. Am J Crit Care 2004;13:116–25.

128. Dunwoody CJ, Krenzischek DA, Pasero C, et al. Assessment, physiological monitoring, and consequences of inadequately treated acute pain. J Perianesth Nurs 2008;23:S15–27. doi: 10.1016/j.jopan.2007.11.007.

129. McCaffery M. Understanding your patient's pain. Nursing (Lond) 1980;10:26–31.

130. Kerbage SH, Garvey L, Lambert GW, et al. Pain assessment of the adult sedated and ventilated patients in the intensive care setting: a scoping review. Int J Nurs Stud 2021;122:104044. doi: 10.1016/j.ijnurstu.2021.104044.

131. Payen JF, Bru O, Bosson JL, et al. Assessing pain in critically ill sedated patients by using a behavioral pain scale. Crit Care Med 2001;29:2258–63.

132. Gélinas C, Fillion L, Puntillo KA, et al. Validation of the critical-care pain observation tool in adult patients. Am J Crit Care 2006;15:420–7.

133. Herr K, Coyne PJ, Key T, et al. Pain assessment in the nonverbal patient: position statement with clinical practice recommendations. Pain Manag Nurs 2006;7:44–52. doi: 10.1016/j.pmn.2006.02.003.

134. Arbour C, Gelinas C. Are vital signs valid indicators for the assessment of pain in postoperative cardiac surgery ICU adults? Intensive Crit Care Nurs 2010;26:83–90. doi: 10.1016/j.iccn.2009.11.003.

135. Azevedo-Santos IF, DeSantana JM. Pain measurement techniques: spotlight on mechanically ventilated patients. J Pain Res 2018;11: 2969–80. doi: 10.2147/JPR.S151169.

136. Frazier SK, Moser DK, Schlanger R, et al. Autonomic tone in medical intensive care patients receiving mechanical ventilation and during a CPAP weaning trial. Biol Res Nurs 2008;9:301–10. doi: 10.1177/1099800408314707.

137. Wiatrowski R, Norton C, Giffen D. Analgosedation: improving patient outcomes in icu sedation and pain management. Pain Manag Nurs 2016;17:204–17. doi: 10.1016/j.pmn.2016.02.052.

138. Gosselin É, Richard-Lalonde M. Role of family members in pain management in adult critical care. AACN Advanced Critical Care 2019;30:398–410. doi: 10.4037/aacnacc2019275.

139. Gelinas C, Puntillo KA, Joffe AM, et al. A validated approach to evaluating psychometric properties of pain assessment tools for use in nonverbal critically ill adults. Semin Respir Crit Care Med 2013;34:153–68. doi: 10.1055/s-0033-1342970.

140. Richard-Lalonde M, Gélinas C, Boitor M, et al. The effect of music on pain in the adult intensive care unit: a systematic review of randomized controlled trials. J Pain Symptom Manage 2020;59:1304–19. doi: 10.1016/j.jpainsymman.2019.12.359.

141. Gelinas C, Arbour C, Michaud C, et al. Patients and ICU nurses' perspectives of non-pharmacological interventions for pain management. Nurs Crit Care 2013;18:307–18. doi: 10.1111/j.1478-5153.2012.00531.x.

142. Aitken LM, Kydonaki K, Blackwood B, et al. Inconsistent relationship between depth of sedation and intensive care outcome: systematic review and meta-analysis. Thorax 2021;76:1089. doi: 10.1136/thoraxjnl-2020-216098.

143. Jackson DL, Proudfoot CW, Cann KF, et al. A systematic review of the impact of sedation practice in the ICU on resource use, costs and patient safety. Crit Care 2010;14:R59.

144. Sessler CN, Gosnell M, Grap MJ, et al. The Richmond Agitation–Sedation Scale: validity and reliability in adult intensive care patients. Am J Respir Crit Care Med 2002;166:1338–44.

145. Riker RR, Picard JT, Fraser GL. Prospective evaluation of the Sedation–Agitation Scale for adult critically ill patients. Crit Care Med 1999;27:1325–9.

146. Yu A, Teitelbaum J, Scott J, et al. Evaluating pain, sedation, and delirium in the neurologically critically ill-feasibility and reliability of standardized tools: a multi-institutional study. Crit Care Med 2013;41:2002–7. doi: 10.1097/CCM.0b013e31828e96c0.

147. Anderson J, Henry L, Hunt S, et al. Bispectral index monitoring to facilitate early extubation following cardiovascular surgery. Clin Nurse Spec 2010;24:140–8. doi: 10.1097/NUR.0b013e3181d82a48.

148. Weatherburn C, Endacott R, Tynan P, et al. The impact of bispectral index monitoring on sedation administration in mechanically ventilated patients. Anaesth Intensive Care 2007;35:204–8.

149. Aitken LM, Bucknall T, Kent B, et al. Protocol-directed sedation versus non-protocol-directed sedation to reduce duration of mechanical ventilation in mechanically ventilated intensive care patients. Cochrane Database Syst Rev 2015;1:Cd009771. doi: 10.1002/14651858. CD009771.pub2.

150. Hu RF, Jiang XY, Hegadoren KM, et al. Effects of earplugs and eye masks combined with relaxing music on sleep, melatonin and cortisol levels in ICU patients: a randomized controlled trial. Crit Care 2015;19:115. doi: 10.1186/s13054-015-0855-3.

151. Tainter CR, Levine AR, Quraishi SA, et al. Noise levels in surgical ICUs are consistently above recommended standards. Crit Care Med 2016;44:147–52. doi: 10.1097/ccm.0000000000001378.

152. Balas MC, Tan A, Pun BT, et al. Effects of a national quality improvement collaborative on ABCDEF bundle implementation. Am J Crit Care 2022;31:54–64. doi: 10.4037/ajcc2022768.

153. Kress JP, Gehlbach B, Lacy M, et al. The long-term psychological effects of daily sedative interruption on critically ill patients. Am J Respir Crit Care Med 2003;168:1457–61. doi: 10.1164/rccm.200303-455OC.

154. Kress JP, Pohlman AS, O'Connor MF, et al. Daily interruption of sedative infusions in critically ill patients undergoing mechanical ventilation. N Engl J Med 2000;342:1471–7.

155. Burry L, Rose L, McCullagh IJ, et al. Daily sedation interruption versus no daily sedation interruption for critically ill adult patients requiring invasive mechanical ventilation. Cochrane Database Syst Rev 2014;2014(7):CD009176. doi: 10.1002/14651858.CD009176.pub2.

156. Mehta S, Burry L, Cook D, et al. Daily sedation interruption in mechanically ventilated critically ill patients cared for with a sedation protocol: a randomized controlled trial. JAMA 2012;308:1985–92.

157. Rose L, Fitzgerald E, Cook D, et al. Clinician perspectives on protocols designed to minimize sedation. J Crit Care 2015;30:348–52. doi: 10.1016/j.jcrc.2014.10.021.

158. Sneyers B, Laterre PF, Bricq E, et al. What stops us from following sedation recommendations in intensive care units? A multicentric qualitative study. J Crit Care 2014;29:291–7. doi: 10.1016/j.jcrc.2013.11.004.

159. Zielinski MR, McKenna JT, McCarley RW. Functions and mechanisms of sleep. AIMS Neurosci 2016;3:67–104. doi: 10.3934/Neuroscience.2016.1.67.

160. Cappuccio FP, Miller MA. Sleep and cardio-metabolic disease. Curr Cardiol Rep 2017;19:110. doi: 10.1007/s11886-017-0916-0.

161. Cappuccio FP, D'Elia L, Strazzullo P, et al. Sleep duration and all-cause mortality: a systematic review and meta-analysis of prospective studies. Sleep 2010;33:585–92. doi: 10.1093/sleep/33.5.585.

162. Scott AJ, Webb TL, Martyn-St James M, et al. Improving sleep quality leads to better mental health: a meta-analysis of randomised controlled trials. Sleep Med Rev 2021;60:101556. doi: 10.1016/j.smrv.2021.101556.

163. Pisani MA, D'Ambrosio C. Sleep and delirium in adults who are critically ill: a contemporary review. Chest 2020;157:977–84. doi: 10.1016/j.chest.2019.12.003.

164. Kryger MH, Roth T, Goldstein CA. Principles and practice of sleep medicine. 7th ed. Philadelphia: Elsevier; 2021.

165. Iber C, Ancoli-Israel S, Chesson A, et al. AASM Manual for the scoring of sleep and associated events: rules, terminology and technical specification. Westchester, IL: American Academy of Sleep Medicine: 2007.

166. Watson PL, Pandharipande P, Gehlbach BK, et al. Atypical sleep in ventilated patients: empirical electroencephalography findings and the path toward revised ICU sleep scoring criteria. Crit Care Med 2013;41(8):1958–67. doi: 10.1097/CCM.0b01e1828af75.

167. Drouot X, Cabello B, d'Ortho M-P, et al. Sleep in the intensive care unit. Sleep Med Rev 2008;12(5):391–403. doi:10.1016/j.smrv.2007.11.004.

168. Elliott R, McKinley S, Cistulli P, et al. Characterisation of sleep in intensive care using 24-hour polysomnography: an observational study. Crit Care 2013;17:R46. doi: 10.1186/cc12565.

169. Ritmala-Castren M, Axelin A, Kiljunen K, et al. Sleep in the intensive care unit – nurses' documentation and patients' perspectives. Nurs Crit Care 2017;22:238–46. 2014/10/02. doi: 10.1111/nicc.12102.

170. Rood P, Frenzel T, Verhage R, et al. Development and daily use of a numeric rating score to assess sleep quality in ICU patients. J Crit Care 2019;52:68–74. doi: 10.1016/j.jcrc.2019.04.009.

171. Aitken LM, Elliott R, Mitchell M, et al. Sleep assessment by patients and nurses in the intensive care: an exploratory descriptive study. Aust Crit Care 2017;30(2):59–66. doi: 10.1016/j.aucc.2016.04.001.

172. Honarmand K, Rafay H, Le J, et al. A systematic review of risk factors for sleep disruption in critically ill adults. Crit Care Med 2020;48:1066–74. doi: 10.1097/ccm.0000000000004405.

173. Ohayon MM, Carskadon MA, Guilleminault C, et al. Meta-analysis of quantitative sleep parameters from childhood to old age in healthy individuals: developing normative sleep values across the human lifespan. Sleep 2004;27:1255–73.

174. Floyd JA, Janisse JJ, Jenuwine ES, et al. Changes in REM-sleep in percentage over the adult lifespan. Sleep 2007;30:829–36.

175. Rechtschaffen A, Kales A. A manual of standardized terminology: techniques and scoring system for sleep stages of human subjects. Los Angeles, CA: UCLA Brain Information Service/Brain Research Institute; 1968.

176. Kamdar BB, Kadden DJ, Vangala S, et al. Feasibility of continuous actigraphy in patients in a medical intensive care unit. Am J Crit Care 2017;26:329–35. doi: 10.4037/ajcc2017660.

177. Raj R, Ussavarungsi K, Nugent K. Accelerometer-based devices can be used to monitor sedation/agitation in the intensive care unit. J Crit Care 2014;29:748–52. doi: 10.1016/j.jcrc.2014.05.014.

178. Nieuwenhuijs D, Coleman EL, Douglas NJ, et al. Bispectral index values and spectral edge frequency at different stages of physiologic sleep. Anesth Analg 2002;94:125–9.

179. Giménez S, Romero S, Alonso JF, et al. Monitoring sleep depth: analysis of bispectral index (BIS) based on polysomnographic recordings and sleep deprivation. J Clin Monit Comput 2017;31:103–10. doi: 10.1007/s10877-015-9805-5.

180. Richards KC, O'Sullivan PS, Phillips RL. Measurement of sleep in critically ill patients. J Nurs Meas 2000;8:131–44.

181. Freedman NS, Kotzer N, Schwab RJ. Patient perception of sleep quality and etiology of sleep disruption in the intensive care unit. Am J Respir Crit Care Med 1999;159:1155–62.

182. Edwards GB, Schuring LM. Pilot study: validating staff nurses' observations of sleep and wake states among critically ill patients, using polysomnography. Am J Crit Care 1993;2:125–31.

183. Beecroft JM, Ward M, Younes M, et al. Sleep monitoring in the intensive care unit: comparison of nurse assessment, actigraphy and polysomnography. Intensive Care Med 2008;34:2076–83.

184. Richardson A, Crow W, Coghill E, et al. A comparison of sleep assessment tools by nurses and patients in critical care. J Clin Nurs 2007;16:1660–8.

185. Bourcier E, Baptiste A, Borowik A, et al. Sedative–hypnotic initiation and renewal at discharge in hospitalized older patients: an observational study. BMC Geriatr 2018;18:278. doi: 10.1186/s12877-018-0972-3.

186. Donnelly K, Bracchi R, Hewitt J, et al. Benzodiazepines, Z-drugs and the risk of hip fracture: a systematic review and meta-analysis. PLoS One 2017;12:e0174730. doi: 10.1371/journal.pone.0174730.

187. Hu RF, Jiang XY, Chen J, et al. Non-pharmacological interventions for sleep promotion in the intensive care unit. Cochrane Database Syst Rev 2015;2015(10):CD008808. doi: 10.1002/14651858.CD008808.pub2.

188. Darbyshire JL, Young JD. An investigation of sound levels on intensive care units with reference to the WHO guidelines. Crit Care 2013;17:R187. doi: 10.1186/cc12870.

189. Lewis SR, Schofield-Robinson OJ, Alderson P, et al. Propofol for the promotion of sleep in adults in the intensive care unit. Cochrane Database Syst Rev 2018;1:CD012454. doi: 10.1002/14651858.CD012454.pub2.

190. Berglund B, Lindvall T, Schwela DH. Guidelines for community noise. Geneva: World Health Organization; 1999.

191. Engwall M, Fridh I, Johansson L, et al. Lighting, sleep and circadian rhythm: an intervention study in the intensive care unit. Intensive Crit Care Nurs 2015;31:325–35. doi: 10.1016/j.iccn.2015.07.001.

192. Korompeli A, Muurlink O, Kavrochorianou N, et al. Circadian disruption of ICU patients: a review of pathways, expression, and interventions. J Crit Care 2017;38:269–77. doi: 10.1016/j.jcrc.2016.12.006.

193. Lusczek ER, Knauert MP. Light levels in ICU patient rooms: dimming of daytime light in occupied rooms. J Patient Exp 2021;8:23743735211033104. doi: 10.1177/23743735211033104.

194. Durrington HJ, Clark R, Greer R, et al. 'In a dark place, we find ourselves': light intensity in critical care units. Intensive Care Med Exp 2017;5:9. doi: 10.1186/s40635-017-0122-9.

195. Cabello B, Thille AW, Drouot X, et al. Sleep quality in mechanically ventilated patients: comparison of three ventilatory modes. Crit Care Med 2008;36:1749–55.

196. Bourne RS, Mills GH. Sleep disruption in critically ill patients – pharmacological considerations. Anaesthesia 2004;59:374–84.

197. Hardin KA. Sleep in the ICU: potential mechanisms and clinical implications. Chest 2009;136:284–94. doi: 10.1378/chest.08-1546.

198. Roehrs T, Roth T. Drug-related sleep stage changes: functional significance and clinical relevance. Sleep Med Clin 2010;5:559–70. doi: 10.1016/j.jsmc.2010.08.002.

199. Sateia MJ, Buysse DJ, Krystal AD, et al. Clinical practice guideline for the pharmacologic treatment of chronic insomnia in adults: an American Academy of Sleep Medicine clinical practice guideline. J Clin Sleep Med 2017;13:307–49. doi: 10.5664/jcsm.6470.

200. NSW Therapeutic Advisory Group Inc. Getting it right for sleep at night: guidance for promoting sleep and reducing harm from inappropriate pharmacologic management of sleep disturbance and insomnia in hospitalised patients. Darlinghurst: NSW TAG; 2021. Available from: nswtag.org.au/wp-content/uploads/2021/12/1.-Guidance_Getting-it-right-for-sleep-at-night_21Dec2021.pdf.

201. Li T, Jiang S, Han M, et al. Exogenous melatonin as a treatment for secondary sleep disorders: a systematic review and meta-analysis. Front Neuroendocrinol 2019;52:22–8. doi: 10.1016/j.yfrne.2018.06.004.

202. Fatemeh G, Sajjad M, Niloufar R, et al. Effect of melatonin supplementation on sleep quality: a systematic review and meta-analysis of randomized controlled trials. J Neurol 2022;269:205–16. doi: 10.1007/s00415-020-10381-w.

203. Lewis SR, Pritchard MW, Schofield-Robinson OJ, et al. Melatonin for the promotion of sleep in adults in the intensive care unit. Cochrane Database Syst Rev 2018;5:CD012455. doi: 10.1002/14651858.CD012455.pub2.

Chapter 7

Family and cultural care of the critically ill patient

Denise Wilson, Judy E Davidson

Learning objectives

After reading this chapter, you should be able to:

- describe models of care and evaluate how they meet patient and family needs
- recognise appropriate resources to enhance communication
- develop an understanding of the needs of families and patients who die in the ICU
- evaluate and implement appropriate strategies for working with families from a diversity of cultures
- recognise and implement the unique needs of the critically ill and/or dying patient from a lens of diversity and inclusion
- meet the diverse spiritual and religious needs of families and their patients who are dying or who have died.

Introduction

Care of critically ill patients is complex and multifactorial. Although management of the haemodynamic parameters and healthcare interventions is an essential component of effective care of the critically ill, the psychosocial health and well-being of patients and their families are intimately related to their wellness and eventual illness outcome. There is a tendency, due to the technologically complex nature of nursing in critical care areas, for novice critical care nurses to focus their attention on the management of medical treatment regimens. This is an important part of the learning trajectory. However, nurses need to be guided to see beyond the waveforms and physical parameters to provide holistic care for the patient/family dyad attending to their unique spiritual and cultural needs and value-driven preferences. The previous chapter examined specific aspects of the psychological well-being of the critically ill with strategies to improve patient outcomes. This chapter extends the focus to incorporate the family into the caring paradigm and introduces the concept of person-centred, patient-centred and patient, family-centred care. The word family in this chapter is defined as whomever the patient considers to be their family and will generally incorporate those who have a

KEY WORDS

bereavement

communication

continuity of care

cultural care

cultural humility

cultural responsiveness

cultural safety

diversity

end-of-life care

equity

family care

inclusion

models of care

patient, family-centred care

post-intensive care syndrome

social justice

spiritual care

underserved and marginalised groups

lasting and intergenerational relationship with the patient irrespective of legal or familial/genetic ties. Nursing practices that incorporate the patient's family into the care of the critically ill acknowledge, support and promote the vital part that families play in the illness continuum.

The assessment, understanding and incorporation of the patient's and family's cultural needs are essential elements of nursing the critically ill, and involve the entire interdisciplinary team. These elements are important for both the recipients of the care (the patient and family) and the critical care nurse; they bring humanity and holistic aspects of the patient's well-being into the critical care nurse's focus. Cultural factors include social factors and human behaviours associated with emotional and spiritual needs. In this chapter, models of nursing are examined with particular reference to the philosophy of patient, family-centred care, which may be an appropriate nursing model for use within critical care settings. The specific needs of the families of critically ill patients as well as the implications for critical care nursing are discussed. Differing world views on health and illness are highlighted for consideration of appropriate care. Many of the populations for whom we provide care exhibit diversity of gender and sexual identity, sexuality, ethnicity, country of origin and cultural practices. Effective communication is crucial to meet patient and family needs. Communication with patients and families is addressed to include the added complexity of caring for the linguistically diverse population. End-of-life care is discussed in general terms and specific cultural considerations are highlighted with particular reference to racial or ethnic groups and other underserved and marginalised groups (such as transgendered youth).

Overview of models of care

Nurses manage their daily activities and patient care in response to both the critical care unit's model of care delivery and the individual nurse's personal philosophy of what and how nursing is constructed. These are both influenced by broader hospital, national and international priorities together with guidance from professional organisations.[1-3]

Alternative models of care are examined in this section and their use in critical care areas discussed. Nursing models define shared values and beliefs that guide practice. Various philosophies and models of nursing care delivery have evolved over the decades and contrast with the 'medical model', which focuses on the diagnosis and treatment of disease.[4]

Primary nursing

Models such as primary nursing and team nursing have organisational and management properties, focused on the skill mix and consistency of assignment making. In primary nursing a single nurse is assigned to be the facilitator of nursing care for that patient, and is assigned to the patient on each day of work. The consistency is thought to establish improved rapport with the patient and family while gaining a better understanding of their unique needs and values. The primary nurse refines the plan of care for others to follow in their absence.

Team nursing

Team nursing, on the other hand, is an approach focused on optimising use of skills and allows nurses and unlicensed assistive personnel to work at the top of scope of their practice. Teams are formed each shift, with one or more registered nurses and unlicensed assistive personnel designated to care for a patient assignment together. The lead registered nurse delegates to the other nurses and unlicensed personnel. Due to the complexity and technology-driven care required in the ICU, team nursing is used less often because of the volume of tasks that cannot be delegated. However, during the COVID-19 pandemic, when crisis standards were being enacted or considered, the use of team nursing was revisited and updated to include creating teams of ICU nurses and non-ICU nurses to care for ICU patients. In this situation, non-ICU nurses delivered care within their scope of practice (e.g. administering medications), while the ICU nurse retained ownership of the care requiring technology (e.g. advanced haemodynamic monitoring or ventricular assist devices).

Patient-centred care

Patient-centred practice is a model where a partnership is developed between health professionals and the patient and their family, and decisions are made collaboratively to align with patient goals.[4-6] Patient-centred care shifts control in health-related decisions from the healthcare professional to the patient – the recipient of care – hence challenging existing paradigms.[7] This model has patient empowerment as the core element. To facilitate empowerment, patients need to be well informed in such a way that they can understand the information to help with their decisions.[8] It is incumbent upon critical care nurses to have a conversation with patients about their illness perceptions, priorities and future plans. Having a clear understanding of patients' concepts of illness, their cultural beliefs and intent is vital.[8] Treating patients with respect and providing care that is responsive to individual patient preferences, needs and values is fundamental to acknowledging patient identity and empowerment.[6]

Implementation of patient-centred care requires a culture change and therefore needs support at an individual, professional and organisational level.[9,10] A study in the USA examined how critical care nurses communicate with patients and families within a patient-centred care framework that was operating within their unit. They found that nurses predominantly communicated information related to the patient's acute biophysical status.

Although the nurses in the study supported the importance of shared power and responsibility, they exhibited few examples in practice. They reflected that they felt sharing power fell within the domain of intensivists' discussions with patients and families rather than theirs.[11] Nurses deferring responsibility for communication in such a way highlights the importance of a whole-of-team approach to patient-centred care, where healthcare professionals share the responsibility of meaningfully involving patients and their families in decisions and care options. Nurses need to have adequate support to meet the intense demands that come with caring for the critically ill for them to overcome the barriers to achieving optimum patient-centred care.[5,9]

Person-centred care

Person-centred care is similar to patient-centred care. The Oxford English dictionary defines 'patient' in passive terms as the receiver of care whereas a 'person' is acknowledged as being an individual in their own right.[12] Those who read about patient-centred care (as outlined above) will understand that the word 'patient' in the context of patient-centred care is far from the passive role in this dictionary definition. However, if consumers are to understand healthcare organisations' working paradigms, semantics and first impressions are important. The term 'person-centred care' emphasises the individual nature of the person with the illness. It promotes the perception of equal power and a shared partnership between the person and healthcare provider/s. Here, the person is an acknowledged expert in their own health values and goals. The partnership is both collaborative and respectful and highlights the importance of knowing the person behind the patient and understanding that the patient is more than their illness.[13]

There is a scarcity of evaluations of person-centred care in critical care areas.[14] However, some evidence, outside the critical care environment, has been reported by the Centre for Person-Centred Care in the University of Gothenburg in Sweden where improved patient outcomes have been reported.[14] In one in-hospital study of chronic heart failure patients, length of stay was reduced by a third with no compromise in their perceived quality of care when person-centred care was compared with usual care. The individualised care plan based on understanding each patient's needs was seen to be a major contributing factor in reducing hospital stay.[15] In another study of patients with chronic heart failure in five wards of a single organisation in the USA,[11] person-centred care was evaluated in relation to how it reduced patients' uncertainty about their illness.[11] The differing organisational and operational features of the ward were examined. In wards where goal setting, planning, control and stability were evident, patients' uncertainty in illness was reduced, which the authors linked to a person-centred approach to care.[11] Within an ICU environment, however, a truly shared partnership with the patient may be problematic, where critical illness restricts a patient's involvement in decision making and care planning. In reality, it is generally family members who provide the link between the patient and the healthcare team.

During the 1980s, the role of the family was one focus of nursing debate and discussion. Friedman believed that families were the greatest social institution influencing individuals' health in our society.[16] A worldwide trend is for health professionals to value the role of family members in providing ongoing, post-acute care,[17] with the reality being that families provide considerable support during rehabilitation phases of critical illnesses. The family is strongly incorporated within these philosophies and, whichever model is selected, it must be practical and understood in the clinical setting for which it is intended. There are entire organisations, such as Plaintree, that provide resources for patients, families and organisations on how to implement strategies to enhance the philosophy of person-centred care.[18]

Patient, family-centred care

Patient, family-centred care is a third term you may see used. This is intended to describe sharing of responsibility of patient care decisions with the family, where appropriate, and therefore highlights the importance of family in critical care areas. This developed during the early 1990s, primarily in North America in the area of children's nursing, where incorporating the family was considered fundamental to the care of the patient.[19] Over the past decades, the scope and extent of family-centred care has broadened and the Institute for Family-Centered Care now defines family-centred care more broadly to patient, family-centred care, which it describes as *'an innovative approach to the planning, delivery, and evaluation of healthcare that is governed by mutually beneficial partnerships among healthcare providers, patients and families'*.[20] Patient, family-centred care applies to patients of all ages, and it may be practised in any healthcare setting.[21]

Patient, family-centred care is founded on mutual respect and partnership among patients, families and healthcare providers. It incorporates all aspects of physical and psychosocial care, from assessment to care delivery and evaluation.[20] Five elements of patient and family participation include: (1) a physical presence, (2) having needs met, (3) effective communication, (4) decision making and (5) contributing to care.[22] Healthcare providers that value the family/patient partnership during a critical illness strive to facilitate relationship building and provide amenities and services that facilitate families being connected and physically near their hospitalised relative.[17] Parent and nurse perceptions on the quality of patient, family-centred care have been examined in a study of 11 neonatal ICUs in Europe where innovative text-messaging data collection methods were used. Although parents perceived high levels of patient and family-centred care, there were areas for improvement such as providing emotional support to parents, including parents in decision making and encouraging fathers to participate in their infant's care.[23] Many nurses also value family involvement in the care of their own sick relative.[24,25] Other strategies to improve patient, family-centred care within adult critical care areas include involving family members in partnering with the nursing staff to consider the involvement they, and the patient, would like them to have, which may include providing fundamental care to their sick relative.[26] Family members can decide in consultation and negotiation with the direct care nurse the care that they want, and are able to provide that aligns with the patient's preferences.

Direct care provided by the family may vary from moisturising their relative's skin to a full sponge and will require negotiation. Such acts of caring allow family members to connect in what they see as a meaningful way with their sick relative. In addition, it can also improve communication with critical care nurses and facilitate close physical and emotional contact with their relative.[27] An independent nursing intervention such as partnering with family to provide care constitutes an example of how to operationalise a patient, family-centred care model in the clinical setting and assists in the evaluation of other future interventions directed to improve patient, family-centred approaches.

To date, there have been limited quality evaluation studies assessing the efficacy of patient, family-centred interventions. However, some have shown a reduction in length of ICU stay and improved patient and family satisfaction scores and psychological symptoms.[28] Patient and family experience would probably benefit from a whole-of-unit approach where there is a cultural shift to a patient, family-centred care philosophy rather than the current research that predominantly focuses on single elements of patient, family-centred care in isolation.[8,28,29] It is acknowledged that taking care of critically ill patients requires considerable knowledge and skill. When family members are incorporated into the caring paradigm, as advocated within patient, family-centred care, health professionals equally need specific knowledge and skills. This information should be initiated in foundation degrees, continued within postgraduate studies and via ongoing professional development opportunities.[11,30] Internationally, it is recognised that the benefits of involving families extends to the promotion of safe practice.[9,31,32]

Professional critical care associations in both USA and Australia have shown leadership by providing guidelines with multiple recommendations for practice[8] and a position statement on partnering with families in critical care.[3] These documents are based on low levels of evidence highlighting the need for future evaluation research. The family knows the patient best, has their best interest foremost and is the one constant throughout the illness. Importantly, family members frequently provide ongoing care beyond the ICU, and involving them during the critical illness phase supports their ability to provide immediate feedback and prolonged care to their relative. Partnering with families is not necessarily time consuming but, to be able to do this, an understanding of their needs is required.[16,33]

Though there is ample evidence for engaging in family-centred care (FCC) including open flexible family presence, family communication through presence on rounds and in routine family care conferences and family diaries, implementing these strategies where they do not exist is not without challenge. Despite the evidence, there is widespread variation in the implementation of recommendations. A review of 365 hospitals across the US found 99 (18.5%) practised unrestricted visiting.[34] An international survey encompassing feedback from 43 countries found that enhancing factors to provision of FCC included support and visible encouragement from leaders, an environment conducive to family presence, and clear role expectations in the form of policies and guidelines. Staff education is also needed as communicating with families and engaging families in care is a developed skill that is just as important as inserting lines and catheters. Creating a culture that embraces FCC facilitates its success and nurtures junior staff in developing positive relationships with families. Lastly, staff members are less likely to embrace FCC if policies regarding preventing, mitigating or administratively dealing with violence against staff have not been effective.[35]

Public health emergencies of international concern such as the COVID-19 pandemic wreak havoc with even the most well-established programs of FCC. Decision making during a pandemic shifts from a shared model to crisis standards where decisions are made by a command or crisis centre, organisational leadership or the government. Additionally, family presence will be limited when contagion is a concern. Knowing that family health is adversely affected without FCC, forethought needs to be given to how to accommodate family needs and include those actions in disaster planning. Past pandemics prompted the development of guidance by the Society of Critical Care Medicine to consider when attempting to navigate a public health crisis while maintaining FCC approach to care. These recommendations included informing the public regarding the changes in decision making: who is making decisions and why, and how that affects normal hospital operations. In addition, practitioners should directly increase electronic communication with family, assess family needs and be creative in allowing families to engage in care and communication with the patient through electronic means. When building or remodelling the healthcare environment, family viewing windows in isolation rooms should be considered.[36] During the COVID-19 pandemic, family presence in the ICU halted globally. It was theorised that this disruption in the social structure would increase post-intensive care syndrome-family (PICS-F) to include stress disorders and complicated grief. Soon thereafter, reports did appear validating the negative family impact the void in services created in the presence of the pandemic: stress disorders, depression, physical decompensation and inability to return to baseline working status.[37–39]

Stellar organisations reported strategies that they found effective to fill the gap to include assigning a family liaison team tasked to provide telephonic family communication.[40] In a UK-wide study of 117 hospitals, 50% used a family liaison strategy successfully during the pandemic to improve family communication.[41] Tele-ICU phone conferencing was also reported to be largely satisfying to family members while eliciting feelings of relief, gratitude and joy.[42] However, care should be taken with these reports as they were retrospective in nature, and outcomes were limited to satisfaction and emotion.

Needs of the family during critical illness

Family members of critically ill patients have little time to prepare or adapt to the demands of an ICU admission, resulting in anxiety, worry and stress. Critical care nurses have a responsibility to support family members through this confronting period of their lives.[43] Understanding their needs is fundamental to being able to provide appropriate support measures. Consistently, family needs include the need for assurance, information, proximity, comfort and support and, although there will always be the need to individualise care, assurance and information needs are paramount.[44] Assurance needs are closely related to information needs, where family members want to know the diagnosis, treatment options, plan of care and short- and longer-term goals.[43] Written and other forms of sharing information with families are important considerations for ensuring their needs are met. Be mindful that families are receiving information in a high-stress situation, which may impair their capacity to process what they hear. Having something they can refer to following conversations that includes information is helpful for families. The manner in which family needs are met is directly related to family members' satisfaction with the care their relative receives[44] and is considered a legitimate quality indicator in many hospitals.[45,46]

On a very practical level, family members are often the decision makers on treatment options owing to the impaired cognitive state of the patient. Their contribution to healthcare decisions is sought in both acute and ongoing care situations as they have insight and knowledge of the patient on an entirely different level to that of health professionals.[47] Importantly, family members provide not only support in the critical illness situation, but also continuity of care through rehabilitation. This responsibility together with the often-sudden critical illness may create stress, anxiety, depression and/or post-traumatic stress disorder (PTSD) for family members.[48,49] A primary outcome of patient, family-centred care is to reduce the risk of stress-related reactions to the ICU experience, which is often traumatic for family members.[50,51]

Practice tip

Suggest to a family member that they might like to provide some care to their relative with your help. This will need some discussion, as you will want to gain an understanding of their relationship with the patient and what they feel the patient might want and what is possible in the situation. They might want to comb their hair or massage their hands. Alternatively, they might like to read something to them that they know will be of interest. By giving the family member permission to do these things, you will be making them feel involved, helpful and contributing to the patient's care. It will also give you insight into the person your patient really is – their likes and dislikes.

The term 'post-intensive care syndrome family' is used to describe the cluster of symptoms that may evolve from family exposure to critical illness.[52] Stress and anxiety associated with having a critically ill relative can hinder a family's coping ability, adaptation, decision making[53] and long-term health, with the possibility that post-traumatic stress disorder (PTSD) may develop in family members of ICU patients.[54–57] Families that experience stress before the critical illness do not cope as well, and may need additional assistance.[58] As many as half of family members report symptoms of anxiety and depression, indicating that it is a very real problem.[56,59] These figures are concerning, particularly when symptoms continue beyond 6 months post ICU.[54,60] Early identification and prevention strategies are an important area for further research. Physical health may deteriorate because of the caregiver burden, including new sleep disturbances. Social issues such as financial instability and marital/family strain are also common.[61] The nurse can advocate for appropriate referrals when these issues are identified. Meeting the needs of families during this stressful and demanding time has the capacity to reduce their stress, promote positive coping strategies and reduce the aftermath of exposure to critical illness.[56]

A combined healthcare team approach is needed to meet the family's needs, as differing perceptions among the healthcare team can result in non-unified approaches that are potentially confusing. The needs of families with critically ill relatives are complex and multifactorial, reinforcing the need for an all-of-team approach.[62] Family members' needs were recognised in Molter's influential study in 1979, in which she researched the specific needs of ICU patients' family members.[63] Although Molter's sample was small ($n = 40$), 45 potential needs of family members were identified and ranked in order of importance. Family needs continue to be researched[48,57,64,65] and can be generally grouped into the need for: (1) information, (2) reassurance, (3) proximity, (4) support and (5) comfort.[53] More specifically, families' needs include the following:[53]

- to know their relative's progress and prognosis
- to have their questions answered honestly
- to speak to a doctor at least once a day
- to be given consistent information by staff
- to feel their relative is looked after by competent and caring people
- to feel confident that staff will call them at home if changes occur in their relative's condition
- to be given a sense of hope
- to know about transfer plans as they are being made.

Meeting information needs

Families' needs for information and reassurance are paramount during a critical illness, which is often unexpected or unexplained. Seven out of the top 10 requirements of families are related to information needs.[66] When information is provided, it is important to spend sufficient time with family members to ascertain understanding. A self-designated family member can act as the primary receiver of information and take the responsibility of relaying the information to others. It is not sufficient to think, 'But I told them all that yesterday'. Communication is a two-way process and as such needs to be received in a meaningful way as well as given appropriately. Repeating information in different ways, multiple times may be necessary. In a case study report of a mother and her adult war-injured son, the mother tells how she tried to remember things the staff told her. She said,[48] 'I loved how my questions would be answered when we asked (except for the daily one about his brain damage) and how most people did not take offense at me writing down everything. I know that I was scared to death most of the entire time' (p. 18).

Strategies to improve communication with family members can include conversations around their current concerns and needs.[43] Once the needs have been identified, specific strategies can be developed to meet those needs. Some critical care areas may choose to have an additional strategy of a designated nursing position that focuses on family advocacy within a patient, family-centred care philosophy.[67]

Interdisciplinary patient rounds that meaningfully include the family demonstrate an inclusive and open communication process that values all contributors as they collectively make an individual plan of care for the patient.[8,48] Our paediatric critical care colleagues lead the way and are trialling ways not just to introduce but also to improve patient rounds that routinely include the family. Beck and colleagues trialled a revised process that focused the objectives of the round to one of advancing the care of the patient in a time-efficient manner. They successfully implemented a standard plan-of-day template that included a checklist for review of quality and safety indicators. They reported a culture of improvement together with halving of the rounding time from 4 to 2 hours.[68]

New ways to practise can be daunting and we know that our attitudes and perceptions are one of the greatest influences on our behaviour. Canadian researchers surveyed their medical and nursing staff on their perceptions of family-centred rounds in order to gain an understanding of their staff's views.[69] Just one-third of the nurses and two-thirds of the medical staff felt comfortable with the idea or thought that family should be given an option to attend family rounds. Experienced nurses held greater reservations and less comfort with the thought than did less-experienced nurses (58% vs 26%).[69] The promotion of patient, family-centred care has led to family presence at rounds as not being considered discretionary but rather recognised as a gold standard.[70] Understanding unit culture and individual clinicians' perceptions provides a foundation for future strategies to progress achieving this standard of care.

In addition, routine family meetings may be a useful way to improve communication and understanding.[64]

Frequently, however, family meetings are called when the family is needed to make critical decisions about the ongoing care of their relative rather than as a proactive and positive strategy that allows for patient and family preferences to be integrated into patient care.[64] Family conferences with the interdisciplinary team should be organised in a staged and planned manner, with the first occurring within the first 48 hours of admission, the second after around 3 days and a third when there is a significant change in treatment goals.[66,71] Fundamental topics for the interdisciplinary meetings with the family could include the patient's condition and prognosis together with short- and long-term treatment goals.[45,71,72] Family conferences provide time for discussion among family members with the healthcare team as a resource, and also for the team to make an assessment of the family's understanding of the situation. Importantly, they provide an opportunity to develop an awareness of specific family needs that can be addressed by the healthcare team.[45] Unhurried family conferencing allows opportunities for families to pose questions and longer family conferences can result in families feeling greater support and significantly reduce PTSD symptoms.[73] Providing family members, prior to the meeting, with an outline of the purpose of the meeting and points for discussion can be helpful. This meeting guide prompts family members to jot down their questions beforehand and ensures their questions are discussed,[74] as it is well recognised that families forget or are hesitant to ask their questions. Although family conferencing has been found beneficial, it is advocated that multiple modes of communication and information sharing are required. Individualised and/or general information via leaflets, brochures and internet-based information and support strategies are also helpful.[45,73,75] To promote communication, nurses can discuss with the family whether they would like a phone call or text message at night updating them on their relative's condition. It is important to follow through on prearranged strategies. Alternatively, nurses can give them a time to phone before change of shift. This will help to allay anxiety and promotes positive communication and trust. When patients are transferred from critical care, families and patients may become anxious or concerned by the reduced level of care in the new ward area. This can be alleviated by providing families with verbal and individualised written transfer information as a means to help prepare them for transfer.[76] In addition, a structured transferring plan helps critical care nurses feel better equipped to ensure they give families the information they need at this important time of transfer.[76]

Inclusive decision making

All patient, person-centred and patient/family-centred care models rely on the flexibility to engage in shared decision making versus defaulting to a patriarchal approach of directing care. In shared decision making, decisions are made by the clinicians, patients and/or their surrogates together aligned to patients' goals and values while using the best available evidence. Shared decision making is endorsed formally by critical care societies as evidence supports that most patients and families prefer to be included in decision making. However, an individual assessment needs to be made prior to adopting the model for each patient/family as there is variation in the desire to be included in decision making. If shared decision making is used when not desired, it can cause unnecessary stress on the patient and/or family. When using a shared decision-making model the clinician is not beholden to deploy patient or family decisions that are not indicated by sound evidence. Options of acceptable decisions are presented to the family with a lay description of the pros and cons of each approach. Usually these decisions are limited to those that centre around value-laden constructs where one person might decide differently from another based upon their personal values. Nurses are encouraged to be present when physicians engage in decision making with patients and families so that they can clarify and support the process after the physician leaves. Surrogates need to be taught 'best-interest' principles when making decisions for the incapacitated patient. The surrogate is instructed to make the decision that the patient would have if they were able to make it on their own. This diminishes the burden of decision making from the surrogate as they are answering purely from the space of 'what would your family member have wanted in this situation?'[77] The nurse is in a unique position to help families prepare for a session of decision making with the multi-disciplinary team by exploring their concerns and questions in advance of rounds or a family meeting and helping the family to generate questions and provide meaningful input about the patient's known baseline, goals and values.

Family presence – fostering inclusion and belonging

For many years, advocates of family-centred care have promoted the use of the term 'presence' versus 'visitation' to connote that family members are not visitors, but instead an integral part of patient healing. Now, efforts are made to move past mere presence to a sense of inclusion and belonging, which brings a sense of purpose to families. It is known that when we look back on crises we evaluate our response by what we did during these times. To create a sense of purpose and belonging, families need to have the freedom to be present and participate in care in meaningful ways. The mid-range theory of facilitated sensemaking outlines an approach that nurses can use to fulfill this vision.[78,79] The theory is grounded in the fact that families need to make sense out of their new situation and that nurses can help them develop adaptive coping through fostering of caring relationships, optimal communication, and encouraging presence and involvement in decision making.[80]

Patients find that family provides a link to who they were before their illness and that they provide support and comfort.[81] This, together with the families' need to be physically close to their critically ill relative, supports the concept of unrestrictive family presence. Central to family presence is the need for due consideration of patient confidentiality and privacy.[8,82,83]

Family-friendly policies with few restrictions that centre on genuine patient care issues require the support of critical care nurses, medical officers and others.[8] Flexibility is particularly relevant for families who live long distances from the hospital and have to travel for many hours in order to be with there for their relative. Unrestrictive family presence, though advocated, is not common. In the UK, approximately 80% of 206 surveyed ICUs restricted both the visit duration and number of visitors.[84] A similar situation was found to be the case in the USA, where, from 606 hospitals, 90% restricted family presence.[85] Sweden reports the least restrictive policies, with only 30% of surveyed units having some restrictions.[85] The disparity has been addressed by clear practice guidelines from critical care associations in the USA and Australia that guide clinicians to support family members and patients by recommending open or flexible family presence at the bedside.[3,8]

Family-friendly policies have been found to have an unintended but positive outcome in that they improve quality indicators, with higher patient satisfaction levels.[68] An Australian study found that ICU staff reported satisfaction with the policy change, once introduced. Interestingly, the vast majority of families chose to be with their relative between 11 o'clock in the morning and 8 o'clock at night.[81] Family members are not just 'visitors': they have an intimate relationship with the patient which helps to form crucial components of the patient's identity.[86,87] There are often different meanings or interpretations of 'family', with family often meaning more than just the immediate nuclear family but rather inclusive of wider family networks (e.g. aunties, uncles, cousins). Examples of people whose families are a wider collective group are gypsy Roma travellers, Indigenous peoples (such as New Zealand Māori, Australian First Nations people and US Native Americans), and people from nations like India, Italy or Greece, who may be immigrants in some countries. The notable difference from these family constellations in comparison with nuclear families is that each of its members has responsibilities and obligations not only to the other members but also to the family as a collective group. Negotiation of family presence processes that consider these cultural understandings is imperative.

After decades of building family-friendly approaches to the practice of critical care, the worldwide COVID-19 pandemic brought an abrupt halt to the progress and further caused a regression in practice caused by fear of spreading the virus. For nearly 2 years, families were not allowed physical presence in the ICU. At the time of writing (2023), most organisations have not reverted back to baseline. Families have suffered from this forced separation.[88,89] It will take hard work and diligence to restore family-centred care to its fragile yet necessary foothold as a standard of practice. Working with families at the bedside can be challenging for those who are not skilled in communication and navigating family emotions.[90] To complicate matters further, nurses entering the workforce now are generationally less equipped to have face-to-face discussions with family members. They have lived their entire lives with 'smart' technology, texting and cellphones. It is known that this reliance on technology for communication has had a negative impact on the ability to skillfully navigate face-to-face discussions, an essential skill for critical care nurses. It is, therefore, suggested that nurses are provided with practice through simulations dealing with family situations in the same way that they might be given the opportunity to simulate resuscitation in training.

Practice tip

Sometimes the number of 'close' family members can be overwhelming for critical care nurses. Remember that, for those families comprising extended family networks, identifying each family's needs in terms of providing the patient support and negotiating a system of communication through one or two spokespersons is helpful.

There is a genuine concern by some parents or carers that children should not come to see family members who are critically ill as they may find the ICU environment and presence traumatic. However, this needs to be balanced against a child who experiences separation anxiety, which can be intense and have a negative impact on their adaptive functioning. In addition, when children are appropriately supported, they are more likely to not be frightened but rather curious about their surroundings.[33] Children may have questions and it is recommended that they be prepared well with adequate information before, during and after their time with their relative in the critical care area.

Patients, however, may want visiting restricted as some patients find the presence of others stressful or tiring. Contrary to popular belief, unrestricted visiting hours are not associated with long visits. In three separate studies where unrestricted family presence was introduced, the number of hours that family members spent with the patient varied and usually family came during the day. This suggests that when family members have free access to their sick relative they do not perceive a sense of duty to be there all day and night.[15,91,92] Participating in patient care is one way for family members to feel closer to their critically ill family member and at the same time promotes family integrity.[93,94] Most family members, however, will not ask if they can help with care,[25] as this is seen as the nurses' domain in adult critical care areas.[8] Nurses, therefore, should invite family members to be part of the patient's care, with massaging and helping to wash the patient being popular activities.[26] Creating a list of

activities for family members to choose from has been demonstrated to reduce family anxiety within a structured environment of family engagement in care.[95] Providing care allows the family members to feel connected emotionally with their relative and provides a means to get to know and communicate with the nurses, which families consider important. Family members appreciate invitations from nurses as this allows them to feel more in control[23] in a situation where family members do not often experience this.[96,97] For family participation to work effectively and safely, a number of guiding principles should be incorporated, as outlined in Table 7.1. It is useful for critical care nurses to explore their beliefs and practices concerning family participation, as many support family participation but do not always implement these beliefs in their practice.

Communication

The ability to communicate effectively is an underlying tenet of nursing practice and a fundamental need for people. As mentioned previously in the context of caring for family members, for communication to occur there needs to be a two-way passage of ideas, thoughts and messages. It is a basic requirement to be able to comprehend what is being conveyed before one can interpret, internalise and respond. This is referred to as *health literacy* and is defined by the Institute of Medicine as *'the degree to which individuals have the capacity to obtain, process, and understand basic health information and services needed to make appropriate health decisions'*.[98] Families with deficient health literacy will misunderstand medical terminology around their relative's care or illness and this is problematic.[99] In addition to health literacy issues, patients have physical impediments to communication that cause, or add to, anxiety, frustration, stress and depression as they lose control over their life and healthcare decisions.[100] It is therefore imperative for healthcare professionals to find ways to communicate with patients in simple non-technical everyday language that is understandable and is targeted at their health literacy level. Critically ill patients commonly have communication difficulties due to mechanical devices (e.g. endotracheal tubes), cognitive impairment from the disease and/or pharmacological medications or language difficulties. Therefore, effective communication is challenging, and critical care nurses and other staff need additional knowledge and understanding of these complex situations to assist in meeting the key communication needs of patients and families. With the objective for minimal levels of patient sedation in mechanically-ventilated patients, the need to find effective communications strategies is more relevant than ever.[100] It is equally important to continue speaking to critically ill patients who are unconscious as it has been known for decades that sedated and unconscious patients can hear and recall some verbal communication once they regain consciousness.[101,102]

Mobile applications to enhance communication with critically ill patients are continually being developed and have been tested. These products include digital voice

TABLE 7.1

Family participation in patient care

PRINCIPLE	PROCEDURE
Consent	Gain patient consent beforehand where possible. For some cultures, beliefs about illness mean families take on the decision making to relieve patients of this burden. Hence, consent may be devolved to a family member.
Building of trust	Relationships are important for building trust. Introduce the concept of family members' involvement in care after a period during which a rapport is developed, which includes agreeing on roles and expectations.
Individualise for patient and family	Offer suitable options from which family members can choose; for example, massaging feet and hands, cleaning teeth and feeding may be appropriate options for short-term patients, whereas additional options may exist for long-term patients.
Safety	The registered nurse should remain physically close by at all times.
Promote achievement of goals	Provide sufficient information to the family member to support successful completion of the care.
Reflect on outcomes	Provide feedback to family members on how they performed the task.
Continuity of care	Document the care the family members participated in and any relevant information, especially information shared by family members.

automation and finger-drawing capacity so that patients with limited fine motor ability can generate their own messages to the provider.[103] The use of mobile applications to improve communication between family and patient can decrease family stress and frustration.[104] Because these tools change so rapidly, readers are encouraged to search availability at regular intervals so that updates can be made to products encouraged for use in your organisation or department.

It is important to focus communication with critically ill patients on what is important to them as they fatigue easily and have difficulty maintaining concentration. Medications may blunt or block memory formation, making it necessary to repeat basic instructions. Asking patients for their needs and assessment of pain and comfort is critical. Providing reassurance, with both speech and touch, contributes to a sense of empathy and feelings of safety for the patient within an environment that takes into consideration the cultural perspective.[105] Role modelling these techniques with the family present demonstrates concern while teaching the family how to communicate despite endotracheal intubation.

Communicating empathy is further supported by family members' presence and interaction with their relative. In addition, constructive strategies should be identified to overcome difficulties with patient communication. Augmentative and alternative communication methods are advocated.[106] The following methods may be used individually or together to enhance communication, and many can readily be initiated by nurses:[106,107]

- body language
- lip reading
- writing
- alphabet boards
- communication boards
- pictures
- gestures, including nodding and blinking of the eyes
- tablets, e.g. iPads and smartphones
- speaking tracheostomy tube with inflated cuff
- electrolarynx
- mobile applications specifically designed for patient communication, e.g. Vidatak™
- eye-tracking devices as used with spinal cord injury patients in the outpatient area.

Practice tip

When you are meeting your patient's relatives for the first time that day, ask them about how they think their relative is progressing. You will get a better understanding of their comprehension of the illness situation and health literacy than if you provide information to them. This understanding will enable you to structure the way you communicate for the rest of your shift. Check with them when they last spoke to the doctor and see if that is a priority for them that day. If they want to speak with the doctor, try to plan ahead so this can be achieved during their time in the unit.

An effective strategy to promote good communication is for health professionals to seek and maintain eye contact (if culturally appropriate). Sit down on a chair beside the bed to facilitate face-to-face communication. This act also conveys a sense of the importance the health professional is placing on the interaction by taking time to ensure they understand each other. Associated with this is the need to use commonly understood language. A quiet environment reduces extraneous noise and potential interruptions, and may promote communication and concentration. Check the patient history to see whether eyeglasses or hearing aids are needed to effectively communicate and use when indicated by need and condition. Adjust the plan of care to add specific communication strategies that have been found effective so that they can be used from shift to shift by others. Communication methods that are found to be effective, such as facial expression, head nods and eye blinks used to respond to questions, should be passed on to the next nurse and recorded in the patient's notes to promote continuity of care.

> **Practice tip**
>
> Check with the patient's family whether they wear glasses or hearing aids. Ask them to bring them in next time they come, ensuring the cases are clearly named with the patient's identification label. Ask for extra batteries for the hearing aids. These will assist communication.

Language barriers may necessitate the assistance of an interpreter, as miscommunication is detrimental to the development of trust and impacts on decision making. Interpreters require some knowledge of healthcare terminology to ensure the content is adequately translated. An independent person ensures that the patient receives the message in its entirety from the health professional but, in practice, interpreters are not always available.[108–111] Though convenient, translating through family members can invoke a breach of confidentiality and place undue burden on family members for being the bearer of bad news. The requirement to provide information in the preferred language of the patient may be regulated.[112]

It is widely acknowledged that communicating with critically ill and/or mechanically ventilated patients is challenging for the healthcare professional, the patient and their family. Specific communication skills workshops for ICU nurses have been advocated.[113,114] In addition, skill acquisition on different ways to communicate needs to be a feature of postgraduate and unit level education programs to support critical care nurses in their ability to successfully use appropriate communication strategies, mechanical devices and technology in order to connect meaningfully with our patients.[113] Effective communication with the patient or their family is vital in determining their cultural beliefs and practices to further enhance appropriate communication and promote understanding.[115]

Equity, diversity and inclusion

Critical nurses must be aware of and understand that effective communication and responsive cultural care are underpinned by the notions of social justice, equity, diversity and inclusion. Like other health professionals, critical care nurses have biases and assumptions about people belonging to underserved or marginalised groups in our community. Unchecked, these biases and beliefs can influence critical care nurses' practice and contribute to disparities in the access to and quality of care.

The inverse care law refers to people who do not receive the level of healthcare they need, which leads to inequalities in their health outcomes compared with those who receive expected care.[116] Social justice refers to people having the right to '…*full participation in society and the balancing of benefits and burdens by all citizens, resulting in equitable living and a just ordering of society*'.[117] Fairness and equity are at the heart of social justice to optimise people's well-being through participation in society, such as through healthcare services.[118] Differences in avoidable health outcomes are unfair and unjust. Thus, diversity and inclusion – that is, being aware of affirming people's uniqueness and differences and inclusion in care plans – is fundamental to avoiding failing to understand the patient's and family's voices.

Critical care nurses who recognise that people have differing levels of advantage are more likely to achieve equitable outcomes through responding to each patient and family's needs.[119] In this way, critical care nurses who are equity informed remain sensitive to their practice's role in achieving equity. They recognise the realities and needs of people belonging to the underserved and marginalised groups and the necessity to adjust usual practice approaches to achieve equity in outcomes.[120] Culturally responsive care requires responding to patients' and families' diverse ways of thinking, knowing and understanding that influence how they process information.

Cultural care

The challenge for critical care nurses is to establish positive working relationships with the patient (when possible) and family so that their important values, beliefs and practices can be shared and incorporated into plans of intervention and treatment. It is not always possible to 'know' another person's culture in any great depth, or 'know' all cultural beliefs and practices of the patients and families a critical care nurse will encounter. Therefore, establishing relationships with the patient and their family during their critical care experience is crucial. It also demonstrates both respect for, and the value of, patients and their families and the cultural beliefs and practices they hold. This enables critical care teams to better meet their needs.

Although people's ethnicities or nationalities may provide a clue to their culture, it is not a reliable indicator and ignores the multiple cultural groups people belong to that extend beyond ethnicity, such as age and gender. Furthermore, with increasing migration globally and inter-ethnic marriages, some people identify with more than one ethnic group. Making assumptions about a person's culture and reliance on universal approaches to direct nursing practice creates risks to nursing practice and potentially compromises the outcomes of interactions and interventions. Even within cultural groups (e.g. indigenous, racial or ethnic underserved groups, immigrant groups, and other marginalised cultural groups such as LGBTQ+ communities), variations and sharing in beliefs and practices can exist. Such differences result from the interactions with the various groups a person belongs to, responses to societal changes and the socialisation of immigrants into a new country or those countries where colonisation has occurred. Acculturation (whereby people acquire aspects of the dominant culture such as food or dress) and assimilation (the integration and adoption of dominant cultural practices by people from ethnic minority groups) are two concepts that are associated with cultural diversity.[121] People are also influenced by the other 'cultural' groups they belong to (e.g. women's or men's groups, belonging to the disabled community, older people's groups), which all have their own particular views of the world, values, beliefs and practices. Therefore, person-centred care of patients and their families is imperative to incorporating specific cultural needs in the planning and delivery of interventions. This section outlines important strategies that critical care nurses can develop for working with patients and their families in order to identify the essential beliefs and practices they need to have incorporated into treatment and intervention plans during a stressful time in an unfamiliar environment. Such actions can optimise their spiritual well-being and lessen stress.

Defining culture

Wepa describes culture as follows:[122]

> Our way of living is our culture. It is our taken-for-grantedness that determines and defines our culture. The way we brush our teeth, the way we bury people, the way we express ourselves through art, religion, eating habits, rituals, humour, science, law and sport; the way we celebrate occasions is our culture. All these actions we carry out consciously and unconsciously (p. 31).

Reid and colleagues[123] describe culture as:

- an intergenerational transmission of patterns of meaning using a variety of modes such as stories, song and cultural symbols
- a social construction that shapes our sense of being and social expectations of behaviour and communication
- a sense of belonging through a system of meaningful actions and behaviours so that we know who we are and how we belong.

Simply, culture refers to the values, beliefs and practices that patients, family members and nurses undertake in their daily lives. It determines how they view the world, and their orientation to health, illness, life and death.[124,125]

Culture involves a shared set of rules and perspectives acquired through the processes of socialisation and internalisation. These provide a frame of reference to guide how members interpret such phenomena as health and illness and death and dying. This, in turn, influences their actions and interactions.[125] Culture is a more-specific way of describing how groups of people function on a daily basis, influenced by their beliefs, relationships and the activities they engage in.

Understanding that culture, ethnicity and race are not the same thing is crucial to meeting the cultural needs of patients and their families. Race is generally determined on the basis of physical characteristics and is often used to socially classify people broadly as Caucasians, Europeans, Polynesians or Asians, for example.[126] However, assigning people to a homogeneous group is problematic, and is the antithesis of cultural diversity,[122] particularly as globally countries are becoming increasingly ethnically diverse. Furthermore, considering everyone as the same does not account for the diversity that exists within many groups in contemporary society, which is increasing with globalisation, marriage between people from different ethnic groups, and the subsequent acculturation and assimilation that occurs. For example, new immigrants may adhere more strongly to traditional cultural values, beliefs and practices than those who have been in a country for two or more generations. Ethnicity extends beyond the physical characteristics associated with race to include such factors as common origins, language, history and dress – it is usually associated with nations,[127] although a number of ethnic groups often exist within a nation.

Culture is internalised and embodied; therefore, it is important for critical care nurses to understand that it is something that is not always visible or identifiable by people's everyday behaviours, especially for those who belong to the dominant culture. It is often implicit, such as our values and beliefs that guide what is important in our lives, and is not something people have had to share until such a time that their cultural values, beliefs and practices become challenged[106] – for instance, when a person and their family are in the foreign environment of a critical care unit, or they are facing the end of life of one of their family members. At this time, what is important for many patients and their families seems to become secondary to the illness or trauma that led to their being in a critical care setting and can cause distress and conflict if left unresolved. At this point it may be helpful to ask the simple question, 'If you were home (in your home country) is there anything different that you would be doing to honor your customs or traditions?' Then, 'Is there anything we can do differently to help support you in fulfilling those customs?'

Differing world views

Culture influences how people view the world, what they believe in and how they do things, particularly with regard to practices around health, dying and death. The critical care environment is unfamiliar for patients and families, especially as health professionals' beliefs, practices and world views may not align with their own. What is important for critical care nurses may not be important for the patient or the family, and may lead to tension and dissatisfaction when patients' and families' views are at variance. This does not mean that one world view is necessarily more right or wrong – they are different. The term for this in biomedical ethics is 'accepting the dynamic of difference'. As nurses we need the insight to be open to the fact that family needs of your patient may be different than what yours might be if you were in the same situation.

The biomedical model influences the way healthcare services are structured and delivered.[77] As a dominant model it heavily influences the necessary focus on the physical well-being of patients within critical care environments. Focusing on the management of disease and illness, and using processes that lead to health issues being fragmented and reduced to presenting signs and symptoms and diagnoses, risks excluding what is important for the patient and family.[128] This contrasts with Indigenous and minority group cultures, for example, which tend to have a holistic eco-spiritual world view, with a strong spiritual dimension that extends beyond a disease and illness focus.[129] As will be discussed later in this chapter, spiritual well-being has greater value and importance for some people – it can be just as significant, and for some, more important than their physical well-being. The world view of critical care nurses is influenced by the cultural beliefs, practices and life circumstances of each nurse, and the 'world view' of the critical care service that drives its service delivery. The result is that, consequently, patients and their families become sandwiched between differing world views. Culturally responsive practice is contingent on nurses having respectful relationships and being willing to let the person and family lead in terms of what they need (all the while balancing the critically ill patient's physical needs).[130,131] Research highlights the lack of alignment that can occur between the needs of consumers of health services and the intentions of healthcare providers such as nurses.[129] It is the potential for the non-alignment between patients and families and healthcare providers that critical care nurses need to be aware of, as dissatisfaction with the care being delivered can arise when the patient's and family's needs are not recognised or attended to,[132] leading to unnecessary tensions and conflicts between patients, families and nurses. A nurse's willingness to acknowledge and respect patients' world views and the things that are important to them minimises the likelihood of any dissatisfaction occurring,[129] as it values their specific needs during their critical care experience. The tension caused by conflict between clinicians and family, or even family-witnessed conflict between clinicians and other clinicians, can erode the family's ability to cope during the crisis of critical illness.[133]

Practice tip

Being able to deliver culturally responsive nursing care requires nurses to undergo a process of education and critical self-reflection of culture, their own cultural beliefs and practices, and the possible influences these may have on practice.[134]

Where the world views of patients and families are considerably different from that of the nurse, nurses should identify the beliefs they hold about the patient and family, the impact of these interactions on the patient and family, and the power the nurse can utilise during such interactions.[135] Sometimes a nurse's personal beliefs will be in conflict with professional nursing beliefs, which necessitates choosing between personal and professional beliefs in the practice setting. For example, a nurse's personal beliefs about life, death and body tissues may be compromised by the duty to care for a patient with brain death awaiting the removal of organs for transplant. This may also be compounded by nursing staff shortages, less-than-desirable skill mixes, and the acuity and complexity that critical care nurses are faced with daily. Therefore, it is vital, not only for the individual nurse, but also for the team of critical care nurses to develop strategies, such as processes and procedures, that can improve the development of working relationships with patients from different cultural backgrounds.[135]

Cultural responsiveness

Cultural responsiveness refers to strategies for responding to a patient's and their family's cultural backgrounds, and depends on the cultural competence of nurses so that they feel culturally safe.[128] An important factor to consider regarding culturally responsive care is recognising the individualistic culture on which many health services are based. That is, the focus is only on patients and their presenting illness or trauma. This is mostly because health systems and services are designed on western biomedical approaches to healthcare. However, for many people belonging to minority cultural groups, their focus is on the collective family – that is, all members and the family as a whole. This collective concept is similar to the notion of holism whereby the whole is greater than the sum of its parts. From a cultural perspective, embedded in families that function collectively is the notion that the family is an integral part of a person and likewise each of its members is critical to the family as a whole. Therefore, the focus of the family is on the responsibilities and obligations that each of its members has to other members as well as to the family as a whole. These families have extended family networks that extend in composition beyond that of nuclear family constructions, which are more constrained in size and make-up.

Different models exist to assist in the integration of the cultural beliefs and practices of patients and their family in critical care nursing practice. For example, Leininger's cultural care diversity and universality theory[136] requires nurses to deliver culturally congruent nursing care for people of varying or similar cultures. Ramsden's work on cultural safety[137,138] focuses on the delivery of nursing care to patients (whose cultural beliefs and practices differ from that of the nurse) that is determined appropriate and effective by the patients and families who are the recipients of that care. These models have been used to guide nursing practice in Australia, New Zealand and North America. Such models require that critical care nurses recognise patients' and families' views of their health experience and any that subsequently have discordant priorities.

Practice tip

Culturally responsive care leading to a patient and their family feeling culturally safe is not a destination or an endpoint. It is a career-long endeavour aided by being humble and critically self-reflective, and drawing on past experiences that were both optimal and less than optimal – the outcome should be improving the quality of care for future patients and families.[139]

Wood and Schwass have described three levels at which a nurse may practise with respect to cultural issues (Table 7.2).[140] These levels, ranging from cultural awareness to cultural safety, describe the differing characteristics of nurses' cultural care. For example, a nurse practising in an organisation where cultural safety is required would need not only to recognise differences between groups of people, but also to deliver differing cultural care to patients and their families after undergoing appropriate education. It is insufficient for nurses to be simply culturally aware or culturally sensitive because, to a large extent, these are relatively passive activities. Critical care nurses need to demonstrate to patients and their families that they have a genuine desire to incorporate important cultural practices into the patient and family care. Therefore, this requires critical care nurses to demonstrate actions and undertake practices so that patients and their families feel culturally safe.

From a transcultural nursing perspective, culturally responsive nursing care requires the nurse to incorporate cultural knowledge, the nurse's own cultural perspective and the patient's cultural perspective into intervention plans.[128] However, it is not possible to collate cultural knowledge specific to various groups owing to the diversity that exists both among and within groups.[141] This difficulty in 'knowing' a culture relates to the diversity not only between different groups of people, but

TABLE 7.2
Levels of cultural practice

LEVEL OF CULTURAL PRACTICE	INDICATORS
1 Awareness	Recognition that differences between groups of people extend beyond socioeconomic differences
2 Sensitivity	Recognition that difference is valid, which initiates a critical exploration of personal cultural beliefs and practices as a 'bearer' of culture that may affect others
3 Safety	Delivery of a safe service as a result of undergoing education about culture and nursing practice, and reflecting on their own and others' practice

Source: Adapted from Wood PJ, Schwass M. Cultural safety: a framework for changing attitudes. Nurs Prax NZ 1993;8(1): 4–15.

also the differences that exist within their 'group', and, despite education in cultural competence, inequities in quality of care continue to exist.[132] Moreover, the reliance on 'evidence' without inclusion of people's sociocultural contexts can result in an incongruence in the health belief systems of patients and their family and nurses.[139] Therefore, critical care nurses are advised to critically examine theories and models to guide their practice, to ensure they deliver appropriate and effective care for the patients and families they work with.

Practice tip

It is important to be mindful of the diversity that exists within 'cultural' groups, and therefore, avoid acting on stereotypes and assumptions.

Competence is an important dimension of nursing practice, as it provides users of nursing services with confidence in nurses' knowledge, skills and attitudes necessary to undertake their practice. Given the importance of culture in the delivery of nursing care, the measurement of cultural competence is also important. There is evidence of numerous variations on the concept of cultural competence.[141-144] The attributes of cultural competence include cultural awareness, cultural knowledge, cultural understanding, cultural sensitivity, cultural interaction and cultural skill.[142-144] However, the inherent need for the acquisition and use of culturally specific information limits the application of these attributes; the collation of culturally specific information is increasingly problematic, particularly as our communities become more diverse in their composition. Therefore, the acquisition of specific knowledge based on a person's racial, ethnic or cultural background is inadequate with increasing cultural diversity. Cultural competence has evolved to be more grounded in person-centred care, aided by a range of skills including compassion, empathy, active listening and attending to the patient's and the family's needs.[145]

Practice tip

The ability to deliver culturally responsive nursing practice involves critical self-reflection to become self-aware, culminating in nurses taking action to improve the patient's and family's health experience and integrating their important beliefs and practices into treatment and intervention plans.

Fundamental to providing culturally responsive nursing care is cultural humility. Minkler[146] maintains '... *cultural humility is the notion that while we can't be competent in another's culture, we can engage in self-reflection, learning our own biases, being open to other's cultures, and committing ourselves to authentic partnership and redressing power imbalances'* (p. 256). Cultural responsiveness is about aiming to practise in a sound manner rather than merely behaving correctly.[128] Durie encouraged the development of cultural safety (which focuses on the patient's and their family's experience and determination of the appropriateness of care received) to a construct that can measure the capability of the health worker, such as the critical care nurse.[147] Culturally competent nursing practice is about:

- the nurses' knowledge about their own cultural beliefs and practices and the impact these may have on others
- the actions and capability of the nurse to improve the patient's health experience, and the integration of culture in clinical practice
- the delivering of culturally competent and safe care.[128]

Cultural competence provides a framework to objectively measure the nurse's performance, although there is variation in frameworks.[135] Fundamental for the critical care nurse to deliver culturally responsive care, which is competent and safe, is determining the cultural needs of patients and families, and the provision of patient-centred care that focuses on their individual needs and expectations.

Working with culturally and linguistically diverse patients and families

Globalisation has resulted in increasing immigration and migration among countries; hence populations are increasing in their cultural and linguistic diversity.

Thirty-four percent of Australians,[148] 27.4% of New Zealanders,[149] 21.9% of Canadians,[150] 13.5% of Americans[151] and 14.3% of those from the UK[152] were born overseas. Immigrants arrive from various countries globally, but especially the European, Asian and African continents. Labels assigned to groups of 'immigrants', such as Asians or Indians, are misleading as the groups are far from the homogeneity they infer. Added to the complexity of trying to determine ways of working with culturally and linguistically diverse patients and families is the variation in their degree of acculturation – for example, some may be second- or third-generation born into another country and highly acculturated into the respective culture of their country of current residence, or they may be new immigrants with traditional cultural beliefs and practices. Therefore, given the diversity that exists, it is difficult to provide specific guidelines on working with culturally and linguistically diverse patients and their families, although some common principles can apply. Ruston and Smith[153] argue that we categorise people according to what we know. When we encounter groups of people that are seen as different or 'outsiders' who disrupt this categorisation, we then tend to classify people using a non-rational approach that lends itself to negative stereotyping, discrimination and stigmatisation. Such approaches are generally based on misinformation that is reinforced by negative societal and media portrayal of such groups.[154]

A fundamental starting point for working with culturally and linguistically diverse patients is to establish their capacity to communicate in the dominant cultural language, for example English. Determining the language a patient uses on a daily basis, and whether they can speak and write in the dominant language, will indicate whether an interpreter is needed. Family members or friends can be used as interpreters when care is being undertaken on a daily basis, although a professional or accredited interpreter should be used when important information is to be shared or when decisions need to be made. This avoids the potential for family members or friends 'censoring' the information conveyed during discussions. How the patient wishes to be addressed, cultural values and beliefs related to communication (e.g. eye contact, personal space or social taboos), preferences related to healthcare providers (that is culture, gender or age), the nature of family support and usual food and nutrition are other areas that should be explored with the patient or family, whichever is appropriate (Table 7.3).

Campinha-Bacote's[155] mnemonic, ASKED, provides a process for self-reflection to make explicit your knowledge and skills and desires to work with people who are culturally and linguistically diverse. The following questions can be asked:

- Awareness: what awareness do you have of the stereotypes, prejudices and racism that you hold about those in cultural groups that are different from your own?

TABLE 7.3

Considerations for working with those from other cultures

ISSUE	CONSIDERATIONS
Holistic, spiritual world view	For some people, health and well-being are not just physical well-being but the social, spiritual, emotional and cultural well-being of the whole family and community. The family and extended family may be more important than individuals on their own.
Beliefs around hospitalisation and places to die	Identify previous healthcare experiences and talk to the family about concerns they may have about the care they will be receiving and the cultural practices they would like observed. Be clear, consistent and honest in responses to questions about a patient's condition – avoid communication that expects people to 'read between the lines'. Avoid doing things that are culturally offensive, so enquire respectfully about what is needed to avoid this.
Traditional healing	Explore traditional healing remedies and 'medicines' that can complement western medicine. Facilitate access for traditional healers when requested.
Connections	In many minority cultural groups, extended families are important and these members should be included. Connections to the environment are important – this means enquiring whether there are cultural processes that need to be undertaken with regard to body tissues/fluids/parts.
Elders	In many minority cultural groups, elders are respected members and hold an important status. An unwell elder may have a lot of visitors because of his/her respected status. An elder may be a spokesperson for the family, making identification of a spokesperson important.
Establishing relationships	Showing attitudes and actions that are genuine, and a willingness to listen and to share where you have come from and who you are, are helpful in establishing relationships. Establish and maintain a positive partnership relationship that promotes participation and that protects people's values and beliefs. Community health workers may provide vital links with cultural minority communities.
Diversity	Often people belonging to minority groups are grouped under one label but are diverse in their values, beliefs and practices. Have conversations with the family and community elders about important cultural information.
Language	Facilitate use of interpreters. Always check out understanding of the information shared. Avoid using healthcare jargon when explaining things. Have culturally appropriate resources developed.

Source: Adapted from Eckermann A-K, Dowd T, Chong E, et al. Binan Goonj: bridging cultures in Aboriginal health. 3rd ed. Sydney, NSW: Churchill Livingstone; 2010, with permission.

- Skill: what skills do you have to undertake a cultural assessment in an appropriate and safe manner?
- Knowledge: how knowledgeable are you about the world views of the various cultural and ethnic groups within your community?
- Encounters: what face-to-face interactions have you initiated with people from different cultural groups than yourself?
- Desire: what is the extent of your desire to be culturally safe or competent in your nursing practice?

When critical care nurses understand their position on nursing people from other cultures, strategies can be adopted to improve their responsiveness and the quality of care delivered. Working with culturally and linguistically diverse people should be based on the following framework:

1 *Relationship:* aim to work in a meaningful relationship with the patient and family. Prior negative experiences may influence the development of a productive relationship. A respectful, genuine, non-judgemental attitude is necessary to develop a productive relationship with the patient and family, and providing time for responses is important.

2 *Participation:* where possible, involve the patient and family in their care, if this is appropriate. This will involve the critical care nurse explaining the treatment and intervention routines.

3 *Protection:* determine specific cultural and spiritual values, beliefs and practices, and enable these to be practised during the patient's time in the critical care unit. Where possible, these should be accommodated, although there may be instances when this is not possible. In such situations, the patient and family should be fully informed of the rationale for this.

4 *Equity:* aim to tailor nursing practice to accommodate patients' and families' life circumstances and beliefs and practices, where possible, to achieve equity in health outcomes.

Determining and inclusion of the cultural needs of patient and family

Given the great diversity that occurs within contemporary cultural groups, it is crucial to develop a relationship so important cultural values, beliefs and practices can be identified and incorporated into the patient's plan of care. Critical care nurses can then better understand a patient's or family's behaviours when the patient is critically unwell. Discovering the values and beliefs a patient and their family have about health, illness, death and dying, and what they believe may make their health worse, is a good starting point and will provide insight into the type of support and caring behaviours that may be observed. In addition to this, identifying how health and illnesses are managed in the person's daily life will provide an indication of whether traditional healers are used, along with healing remedies such as herbs and prayer, for example. Understanding the patient's locus of control can also provide an indication of whether they will play an active role in the outcome of an illness, or whether there is a fundamental belief that illnesses are caused by some external force.

Promoting a genuine, welcoming atmosphere and the use of effective communication (i.e. compassionate and consistent) invites the family to be involved early on in the patient's critical care experience, and are essential to determine the cultural needs of the patient and family (Table 7.4).[156] While communication has been mentioned earlier, interpreting cultural needs requires the critical care nurse to be attentive to communication. Nurses are advised to talk less, attend to details that may arise and simply listen. The need to intervene and to dominate discussions and 'interviews' with the family[156] from the nurse's perspective needs to be curbed, so time is made available for cultural beliefs and practices to be shared.[131,157] Understanding and supporting the patient and family can be improved by the nurse's empowering them through the processes of listening carefully, use of silence (to provide space to process information and questions) and validating what they have to say. The process of involving patients and their family in assessment, decision making and care planning enabling a greater 'client orientation' (versus management orientation) is more likely to be nurses who engage in and facilitate patient/family-centred care that focuses on the individual needs of patients and

their family.[131] Research has found a transformational patient care style that actively involves patients and their family predicts greater satisfaction and is more likely to result in their expectations and needs being met.[158]

Working in partnership with a family can bridge the cultural 'gap', and give families the opportunity to be well informed, which can assist with their stress and coping.[159] However, this is not always easy to achieve in challenging situations, such as when various members of a large family come and go, compounded by changing nurses with shift changes. Receiving clear and consistent information about the patient, including his/her progress, from all members of the healthcare team can reduce cross-cultural confusion and misunderstanding, especially as messages are prone to distortion and change when many are involved. A strategy to manage this may involve discussing the management of information dissemination with the family, and the identification of one or two family members who become the point of contact through which staff discuss and communicate information about the patient.[129,160] Often, apparent 'cultural conflicts' will arise as a result of communication problems with the family; communicating information in a clear and understandable manner helps prevent these problems from occurring.

Practice tip

The EPICS bundle[159] is a mnemonic that helps to plan and provide family-centred care:

- **E**valuate the patient's and family's cultural beliefs, and their needs and expectations and decide what adaptations are needed to their plan of care.
- **P**lan care with the patient and family and validate this with the patient.
- **I**nvolve the family in nursing care decisions.
- **C**ommunicate compassionately and consistently the patient's progress and rationale for any changes in care.
- **S**upport families with compassion and empathy.

For many cultural groups the presence of family is vital to both the patient's and the family's spiritual well-being. Therefore, facilitating a family presence at the patient's bedside and possibly including them in the care of the patient is important. For some cultures, there is a belief that family members should shoulder the burden of information and decision making so the patient can expend their energy and focus on getting better. In some cases to burden the patient with information about their condition, especially its gravity, or having to make decisions, is believed to contribute to a negative outcome. Therefore, positively engaging families and, where practical, patients in collaborative relationships, involving them in the care and decision making and ensuring their cultural values, beliefs and practices are protected are ways

TABLE 7.4

Communication cues and principles

PRINCIPLE	CONSIDERATIONS
Establish a relationship	The first few minutes of your initial interaction with a person from another culture are critical for effective communication. Avoid perpetuating people's experiences with western systems where language has reinforced dominant and submissive power relationships. Obtaining information from patients and family members is regarded as a privilege, not a right. To prove they are worthy and can be trusted with the receipt of knowledge, a nurse may have to spend time building rapport and establishing common ground before exploring the 'business at hand'. Be prepared to share information about yourself. As family and where people are geographically from can be important to people; positioning yourself within your family context and your 'place' is important. For example, sharing where you are from, relationships you are comfortable talking about (children, brothers, sisters, grandparents), the sports team you support and food you like is culturally appropriate.
Consider kinship relationships	Certain people will have rights to access particular knowledge and make specific decisions within family and community. The passing of information often depends on a person's position in the family/community or relationship with the holder of information Identify the relationships between the patient, and his/her attending family and friends and the relationships between family and friends. Establish spokespersons – remembering that there might be different spokespersons for different elements of the person's life. Identify who can make decisions on behalf of the patient (e.g. in the capacity of next of kin). Consider what might constitute gendered or generational considerations in conversations.
Body language	Become familiar with non-verbal forms of communication where possible, e.g. hand signs and facial gestures. Do not assume people from other cultures make direct eye contact. If the person is avoiding eye contact, they will be listening and is not being rude. Body language may also extend into close proximity within the client's personal space; this is particularly evident when the opposite sex is conducting the consultation; ask for permission to conduct any physical examinations.
Use of silence	Use of silence is a key feature of communication with and between people belonging to some cultures. Pauses or silence during an interaction may mean that a person is thinking carefully before speaking or divulging information. The use of silence may also be a time for translation between languages. Pauses may be quite pronounced and time should be allowed for responses before seeking to fill in the silence by repeating the question. Active listening requires that you consider the importance of the use of silence, especially when people are from a different culture, in considering the information shared in the conversation. Cultural protocols may also mean there are times when it is culturally inappropriate to respond. Try reframing the question in a different way, or ask if the person may like someone else to respond.
Shame	Shame is a term often used in some cultures, and will be named accordingly. 'Shame' describes a person's feeling of utmost embarrassment about something. It can be used in both serious and humorous terms.
Providing information and asking questions	'Reading between the lines' is a concept that is difficult to understand if English is not your first language and western culture is unfamiliar. Be direct in your communication – carefully consider how to describe clinical progression, while at the same time not diminishing the severity of a situation because family may need to be informed and travel long distances to join the patient. Do not assume nodding or saying yes means that a message is understood – it is often easier to say yes – this is known as gratuitous concurrence. Perceived/actual power relationships between the health professional and the person and their family may prompt the person not to contradict or disappoint and may lead to the person providing what they think is an agreeable response.
Improve communication outcomes	Provide opportunities for more than one person to ask questions. Follow up on individual messages in different ways to ensure full understanding has been gained. Use open rather than closed questions. Avoid using compound questions (e.g. 'Is it this way, that way or the other way?'). Avoid asking questions in a way that is framed in expectation of a positive response. Ask only one question at a time, and give the person time to consider the question and formulate a response.

critical care nurses can respect the cultural traditions of those patients who are from different cultural and linguistic backgrounds.

A culturally diverse health workforce

Increasing the representation of the workforce to match that of the community and the people served has been recognised internationally as an important mechanism for improving cultural safety within healthcare facilities.[161,162] Research has demonstrated that indigenous people, for instance, are more likely to access mainstream health services if there are indigenous people within the workforce.[163]

Key to culturally responsive care in the critical care setting is a culturally diverse nursing workforce that is reflective of the population the health service serves. Increasing the ethnic and racial diversity among the health workforce is seen as a way to advance the healthcare workforce that is culturally competent and improving the quality of care people receive.[164,165] The under-representation of groups served within the healthcare facility is associated with the lack of culturally competent evidence-based nursing care.[166] Cohen and colleagues maintain,[164] '... *health care providers must have a firm understanding of how and why different belief systems, cultural biases, ethnic origins, family structures, and a host of other culturally determined factors influence the manner in which people experience illness, adhere to medical advice, and respond to treatment. Such differences are real and translate into real differences in the outcomes of care*' (p. 92). Furthermore, they contend that cultural competence cannot be simply learned from textbooks and didactic learning, but instead needs to have people who have 'insider' insights into the way cultural beliefs impact outcomes, and the contribution these can make to the access and quality of care delivered by relatively monocultural healthcare services. To further assure that care is equitably delivered and received, nurses who engage in quality improvement and research efforts are encouraged to stratify outcomes according to demographic variables which would highlight whether one subgroup were inadvertently subject to disparate outcomes. Examples of these variables include gender identity, preferred language, postal code and race/ethnicity.

Cultural responsiveness and patient-centred, individualised care

'*Individualised care requires the patient and nurse to work together to identify a path towards health that maintains the integrity of the patient's sense of self and is compatible with their personal circumstances.*'[167] This means the critical care nurse ideally working in collaboration with the family to identify important cultural needs and the inclusion of beliefs and practices that need to be observed during the patient's critical care experience – in other words, eliciting a patient's view to ensure person-centred care.[168] It is recognised that 'the work' of the nurse involves responding, anticipating, interpreting and enabling, all of which are crucial for individualised care.[169] Indeed, partnership

requires the nurse not only to work with the patient and family but also to identify the power that the nurse possesses and the potential for its inadvertent misuse.[160] Patient- and family-centred care requires critical care nurses to observe each of the following:

- interacting respectfully with the patient and their family, and treating them with dignity
- communicating clearly, without jargon
- sharing information fully and honestly
- using the strengths of the family to enhance their sense of control and independence
- working with patients and their family collaboratively.[170]

Facilitating the inclusion of cultural beliefs and practices requires identification and then incorporation into the patient's plan of care. However, given the resource constraints and the culture of some health services, universal approaches to planning care may be adopted for convenience. The critical care nurse is discouraged from adopting a 'one-size-fits-all' approach to nursing practice, as this disregards the cultural systems of the patient and family.[129] Patient-centred care is optimised by nurses having sufficient information about the patient and family in order to identify their needs and plan interventions. Incorporating each family's cultural beliefs and practices provides a 'bigger picture' of the patient[129] than would have been gained by simply focusing on the presenting disease or illness and its management. Such an approach to patient-centred care enables the critical care nurse to become familiar with the context of the patient's life circumstances and how they interpret illness, and also improves the quality of care and interactions they have with patients and families.[170,171]

Critical care nurses are potentially influential and can advocate for family-centred care,[172] although sometimes the nurse will want to have a full understanding of a cultural belief or practice before being willing to incorporate it. This is an example of where the identification and acceptance of cultural beliefs and practices of the family (to the extent that they will not deliberately harm the patient), and working with the family on how these are incorporated in an intervention plan, can be beneficial to all parties. Once this has occurred, it is crucial this information is documented, thereby making visible the patient's individualised care.[173]

Practice tip

Determining cultural needs means the critical care nurse must:

- identify a spokesperson to communicate information to so the messages the family receives are consistent
- engage in genuine communication and partnership with the patient and family
- be willing to listen, understand and validate information received.

Closely related to cultural aspects of care is spirituality, which for some people is based in religion. Aspects to consider when patients have religious needs are reviewed next.

Spiritual and religious considerations

Spiritual care and being with a patient and family are important in providing quality care, especially near the end of a person's life.[174,175] Despite spirituality being viewed as an important component of holistic nursing care, it is an area that is not always well attended to within the critical care environment.[176-178] While for some people spirituality is embedded within religion, for others it is a metaphysical or existential experience.[176] Therefore, it is important for critical care nurses to avoid assuming that spirituality and religion are the same entity. Spirituality is grounded with a person's culture, the two aligning with their fundamental values and beliefs. It is highly subjective, unique and person or family centred, transcending scientific and objective explanations. When not attended to it can be the source of spiritual distress.[174]

Spiritual and religious beliefs and practices contribute to a person's spiritual well-being,[174,176] on one hand, while on the other a critical care nurse's religion may influence how care is delivered.[179] Spiritual and religious beliefs can be closely aligned with a person's culture and vary in how life, dying and death are viewed, and may dictate how life is conducted.[176,180-182] Any breaches can have profound effects on a patient's well-being and, in some cases, how a family member may consequently interact with the patient. This has important implications for critical care nurses undertaking everyday practices and common procedures where religious beliefs dictate a different approach. A common example is blood transfusions for those belonging to the Jehovah's Witness religion. Having a standardised list of religions and procedural considerations is flawed because of the variations that exist, and in some instances the variations are great. Therefore, as part of the initial assessment the critical care nurse should determine whether the patient has religious beliefs and practices that must be observed or not, and incorporate these into the care plan.

When a family member becomes critically ill, spiritual and religious beliefs and practices become an important coping mechanism in terms of making sense of the experience, as well as being a source of faith and hope. While it can be helpful to the critical care nurse to have an overview of the main religious beliefs and practices (Table 7.5), caution must be used and should not preclude working with the patient's family to ascertain exactly what their beliefs and preferences are. Having said this, a patient may have adopted a religion that is separate from their family. In such circumstances, family cannot be relied upon as informants and, in some situations, there may be a conflict between the religious values and practices of the patient and those of the family. Religious beliefs and practices, like cultural beliefs and practices, will vary between orthodox or traditional and contemporary interpretations.

Patients generally fall into three groups with regard to their religious practices.[180] There are those who:

1 practise their religious beliefs regularly
2 practise their religious beliefs on an irregular basis, often in times of need and stress
3 have no religious interests.

All patients should have access to religious support where they indicate a need. Therefore, it is beneficial for critical care nurses to have knowledge of how to access the relevant religious resources if needed. The focus of the critical care setting often involves going to extreme lengths to keep patients alive, which may well be in direct opposition to some religious beliefs. Spiritual and religious beliefs can either facilitate or disrupt the process of living or dying.[183-185] There are several useful principles underpinning practice when nursing patients with specific religious needs (Table 7.6).

In addition to these principles, contact and communication between the patient, the family and the critical care nurse are important,[176] and can enable a person's spiritual or religious needs to be determined. The critical care nurse should ascertain whether the patient and family have any spiritual or religious beliefs and

TABLE 7.5

Overview of key religious beliefs and practices

RELIGION	PRACTICES TO BE AWARE OF	BELIEFS ABOUT ILLNESS, LIFE AND DEATH
Protestantism	Prayer and the Bible are important for support. A minister, vicar or pastor may visit the sick person and the family.	Illness is an accepted part of life, although euthanasia is not allowed. There is a belief in the afterlife, with the dead being buried or cremated.
Roman Catholicism	Prayer and the Bible are important. Some may have restrictions on eating meat on Fridays of Lent, Ash Wednesday and Good Friday. Priest may undertake communion with and anoint the sick person.	Illness is an accepted part of life, although euthanasia is forbidden. There is a belief in the afterlife, with the dead being buried or cremated.
Judaism	There are orthodox and non-orthodox forms of Judaism. Procedures should be avoided on the Sabbath (from sundown on Friday to sundown on Saturday). Dietary restrictions around pork, shellfish and the combination of meat and dairy products extend to the use of dishes and utensils. Gelatin is a product that is used for medication capsules, for example. Frequent praying, especially for the sick person, who should not be left alone. The Rabbi will attend the sick person.	Illness is an accepted part of life, with euthanasia being forbidden, hence saving or prolonging life is important and those on life support stay on it until death. The Sabbath is a time that is considered sacred and when restrictions on activities are observed. There is a belief that the human spirit is immortal. There are special processes for managing the dead person, who should be buried as soon as possible after death. Therefore, consultation with the Rabbi is important. Postmortem examination is allowed only if necessary.
Buddhism	Prayer and meditation are important, using prayer books and scriptures, supported by teacher and Buddhist monks. Buddhists are generally vegetarian. Patients may refuse treatments (e.g. narcotic medications) that alter consciousness.	Illness originates from a sin in a previous life. There is a belief in afterlife, and the dead are buried or cremated. Living things should not be killed; this belief extends to euthanasia.
Hinduism	Prayer and meditation are important, and are supported by a Guru. Some Hindus are vegetarian. The dying patient may have threads tied around the neck or wrist and be sprinkled with water; these threads are sacred and are not removed after death. The body is not washed after death.	Illness is usually a punishment and must be endured. Some Hindus have healing practices based on their faith. There is a belief that the dead are reincarnated; they are usually cremated.
Sikhism	Morning and evening prayer are important and should not be interrupted for routine care. Some Sikh have undergone initiation and carry on their bodies the 5 Ks (kesh (uncut hair), kengha (wooden comb), kach/kachera (cotton shorts), kara (steel bracelet) and kirpan (strapped sword)) at all times. Hair should not be cut unless urgent for lifesaving treatment. Sikhs may or may not be vegetarians – those who eat meat eat only meat that is not ritually prepared. Gelatin capsules or fish oil may be unacceptable.	Illness and death are believed to be the will of God, and the artificial extension of life over extended periods of time may not be encouraged. Sikhs believe in life after death and in rebirth and, therefore, that the soul's existence is eternal.
Islam (Muslims)	Private prayer, facing Mecca several times a day, requires a private space. The patient may like to be positioned towards Mecca. Guided by the Qur'an (Koran), which outlines the will of Allah (the creator of all) as given through Muhammad (the prophet). Muslims fast during Ramadan, and eating pork and drinking alcohol are forbidden. Stopping treatment goes against Allah. Talking about death should be avoided; designated male relatives will decide what information the patient and family should receive.	Life and death are predetermined by Allah, and any suffering must be endured in order to be rewarded in death. It is believed that dying the death of a martyr will be rewarded in death by going to paradise. Hence, staying true to the Qur'an is crucial. There is a belief in the afterlife, and the dead are buried as soon as possible after death, on the side facing Mecca.

Source: Adapted from Blockley C. Meeting patients' religious needs. Kai Tiaki Nurs NZ 2001/2002;7(11):15–7. Other sources: Hoffman L. A focus on: Judaism. Community Practitioner 2018;91(2):31–3; Nesbitt E. A focus on: Sikhism. Community Practitioner 2018;91(3):33–6.

TABLE 7.6
Principles for recognising religious needs

PRINCIPLE	AREAS FOR CONSIDERATION
Diversity exists between and within the various religions.	Determine values and beliefs related to health, illness, dying, death and any specific requirements for undertaking everyday nursing cares and procedures.
Spirituality is an essential part of care planning and the delivery of quality care.	Spiritual and religious needs should be documented in the care plan to ensure continuity and quality of care.
Interpersonal skills and therapeutic use of self are essential to engaging and being present with the patient and family.	Approach the patient with a genuine, non-judgemental attitude. Avoid imposing own religious or spiritual beliefs on the patient and family.
Being knowledgeable about a patient's religious values about life, health, illness, death and dying enables the critical care nurse to be respectful and accommodating in their care.	Consult family, if they share the same religion, and/or consult appropriate representative of the patient's religion. Areas to explore should include the following to determine: • religious values regarding life, health, illness, dying and death • nature of the ideal environment • processes surrounding dying, if appropriate to the patient • beliefs regarding nutrition and hydration • use of touch • gender-specific care • family presence, involvement and support • care after death.
Philosophies and policies should raise awareness of the cultural and religious diversity within the critical care patient population.	Policies should raise awareness of cultural and religious diversity, and include management of the following: • visiting • modesty • gender-specific care • communication • language and the use of interpreters.

practices to be observed during their time in the critical care setting.[176,180] Once the spiritual or religious beliefs and practices have been determined, the critical care nurse can facilitate opportunities for the patient and/or family to carry out their beliefs and practices, and avoid any insensitive actions and pay attention to any spiritual distress evident in the patient and family members.[180]

> **Practice tip**
>
> Spiritual intelligence enables nurses to be more resilient and adaptable when faced with challenges and stresses often arising within critical care contexts, and is essential for quality of care that includes spiritual care.[186]

A person's spirituality, whether informed by religion or some other basis, manifests in a variety of relationships with self, others, nature and 'divine' beings. It is the essence of who a person is, or who groups of people are. While assessing spiritual or religious needs is one aspect, presence and being with, empathetic listening, determining the reality orientation of the family and enabling visiting

and contact are all important nursing activities that can support the spiritual and religious needs of patients and their families.[179,187,188] When families are confronted with the possibility of death, the documentation of a death plan that outlines the preferred care during the process of dying and death is recommended.[180] Death plans are about what a patient and family want and empowerment, differing from advance directives, which outline what is not wanted (e.g. cardiopulmonary resuscitation). Through formal discussion with the patient and/or family, religious and end-of-life needs can be determined, and a management plan developed for implementation.

> **Practice tip**
>
> Research shows that many critical care nurses feel unprepared and unsupported to deliver spiritual care, making this challenging for them psychologically and emotionally. Make developing spiritual care as part of critical care nursing practice an ongoing professional development activity.

End-of-life care and bereavement

Internationally, mortality rates in ICUs vary considerably and are a feature of the models of care including admission criteria and discharge destinations.[189] Specifically, within Australia and New Zealand the Intensive Care Society Centre for Resource and Evaluation reported on data from 188 (of 221) Australasian ICUs that after-hours discharge from 39 tertiary ICUs varied from 1.4% to 36.8% (mean 16.6%). The ICU mortality rates from New Zealand and Australia across tertiary, metropolitan, rural, paediatric and private ICUs ranged from 7.7% to 9.5%. The impact is that somewhere around 16,300 families in these two countries alone were bereaved during the reporting year of 2019–20.[190] End-of-life and bereavement care therefore constitutes a core component of the comprehensive care provided to patients, families and staff. Death can occur as a result of sudden decline in the patient's condition, or as a result of ceasing active treatment to palliation. Patient death in critical care areas is found to have a significantly different effect on family members from a death in another in-hospital area as the critical illness is often sudden and unexpected. Family may be unprepared for their relative's death in the highly medicalised critical care environment. Where possible, patient, family-centred decision making, together with effective communication and attention to symptom management, is optimal. Practical and emotional support for family and patients is important and scrutiny of the way we manage these important areas provides quality indicators for critical care areas.[45,191] Nurses have crucial influence at end of life. As essential advocates, educators and facilitators, they can initiate conversations and bring patient wishes to the forefront of care ensuring every effort is made to guide care that is patient and family centred.[185]

Patient comfort and palliative care

Maintaining patient comfort and support for families and staff are primary requirements of nursing patients during the end stages of life. Avoiding distress and suffering for patients and their families is a fundamental component to providing a 'good death', together with individualising care by enacting the patient and family's wishes.[192] Advance directives and 'not for resuscitation' orders should be in place to prevent mismanagement and misunderstanding of patient wishes (see Chapter 4).[45] Key elements of palliative care incorporate management of physical, psychological and spiritual symptoms which is a shared responsibility of the healthcare team. Maintenance of patient comfort through protocols or guidelines to reduce symptom distress with non-pharmacological strategies, analgesics and sedatives is extremely important from the patient's, family's and nurses' perspective.[99,193–195] Although this may seem fundamental, there is evidence to suggest that this is still not achieved. Major recommendations from a USA study of 322 critical care nurses indicated end-of-life care needed to be improved in a number of ways including the provision of a private, peaceful environment, timely and truthful communication with patient and family members, the need for 1:1 nurse-to-patient-ratio, and early recognition of futile treatments.[193]

Collaboration and early involvement by palliative care teams is one way to integrate end-of-life care for patients who either remain in critical care areas or are transferred from the unit to other areas. Withholding or withdrawing treatment requires careful consideration and preparation for symptom management for the patient, their family and staff. Choices of bolus or infusion administration of medications need to be based on patient comfort issues. Oxygen therapy is continued in the most appropriate form, and an oral airway may improve patient comfort and aid secretion clearance. Medications may be administered to reduce copious oral secretions and enhance comfort.

The attainment of humane nursing care must include heightened efforts in achieving quality indicators, such as mentioned above – adequate management of pain and nausea, agitation and restlessness. Both critical care staff and families should continue to communicate with the patient by speaking and touching as this can have a calming influence. Comfort measures to enhance holistic care delivery should continue, together with emotional support and environmental modifications promoting a quiet, private and respectful setting.[196]

Patient dignity should be a priority, with gowns or personal attire essential elements of care. The management of symptoms further allows patients to maintain their dignity. Privacy for patients and their families allows an opportunity for them to communicate as they so wish. As indicated in previous sections of this chapter, patient and family culture, beliefs and spiritual values are important considerations that underpin care.[195,197] Caring for patients and their families can be quite challenging and supporting each other in these situations will share the burden and provide direction to novice critical care nurses on ways to alleviate suffering and care for oneself.

Practice tip

Discuss end-of-life care processes in your unit with a colleague. Do you have a current guideline or policy document to provide direction? Are family conferences held regularly to ensure family are kept well informed, or do you use a different method of communicating updates? What would you like to see implemented in your unit to improve end-of-life care?

Family care

Care of the family is supported by proactive palliative care interventions that include empathic, informative communication with interdisciplinary team meetings and family conferences that are not rushed where families are integral to decision making and goal planning.[45,75,198] The desire to participate in decision making varies from family to family, and families' choices cannot be assumed. Decision-making support for family members is complex and to date there is little evidence of effective support mechanisms; however, those that have a patient, family-centred focus are more likely to meet the unique needs of the families.[199] An example of how we should not assume we know best and how to individualise care was reported in a study from The Netherlands where family members were interviewed 2 months following the death of their relative in ICU. Some families wanted the monitoring systems turned off whereas others wanted to be able to see the patient's decline visually.[200] Something that was universal to all family members was the need to have their questions answered and their recognition that nurses did this very well.

Structured communication between the healthcare team and families can assist with timely decisions, goal formation about care and preparation for the process of palliation. Although there are a number of family meeting tools available, they predominantly focus on supporting staff in the process.[201] Ideally, such tools should also support family participation with the preparation of questions, identification of topics for discussion or clarification and sharing concerns and fears, together with overall goals for the meeting. Emotional and practical support can be given to families by providing written material about the critical care area, local facilities and specific information on bereavement.[75] Privacy is not always possible in the busy, sometimes open-plan critical care environment, but maximising efforts in this regard for dying patients and their families provides a more-conducive environment for strengthening patient–family relationships, communication and dignity. Communication is enhanced with family conferences, which provide a structured process where family members and patients' healthcare teams can share goals and understanding of end-of-life care.

Family conferences are a way to meet family needs and enhance communication and understanding of the patient situation. These become an essential element of care when end-of-life discussions are needed. Privacy, away from the direct clinical environment, is important to allow uninterrupted time for families to meet with their relative's healthcare team.[202] When family conferences have been instituted early in the admission, a family/staff relationship will be established that supports ongoing communication about end-of-life care.[73,203]

It is important to have the interprofessional team (e.g. intensivist, social worker, case manager, direct care nurse, chaplain) meeting with the patient's family at this time to ensure a comprehensive approach to the coordination of patient care and family support.[72] This approach helps in both the understanding and the provision of consistent information. Where possible, involving all significant family members in the family conference allows them to hear the same information, ask individual questions and discuss options. These collectively reduce family and/or family/staff conflict[204] and support those families that prefer to make decisions as a collective.

Family members of ICU patients are at a high risk of anxiety and depression. In a large ICU multicentre French study, 73% of family members experienced anxiety and 35% were diagnosed with depression around the time of discharge or death of their relative.[205] This mental health morbidity is likely to be related to the burden of the critical illness and potential or imminent demise of a loved one. Family member's depression, grief and anxiety can be manifested by physiological, behavioural, psychological/cognitive and social indicators. The physiological stress response with increased cortisol excretion and poor sleep patterns[51] can affect family interactions with each other and with staff. At times of end-of-life discussions, family members may exhibit confusion, anger and/or threatening behaviour, making it difficult for everyone involved. Importantly, these emotions make it challenging for family to grasp and understand the often-complex patient situation. Strategies such as family conferences are important as they potentially improve communication channels and promote understanding, thereby reducing conflict situations.

Planning for the family conference around end-of-life issues involves ensuring a common time for significant family members and the critical care team to meet. If a key family member is away or overseas, a conversation over the internet may be the best option as video facilities will allow better communication than with a telephone call. Where there are complex family situations with extended families or previous partners, care must be taken to try to avoid a poorly functioning group. There may also be an estranged partner who wants to be included, which may add to the dynamics of the situation. The critical care team will need to exhibit great diplomacy in such complex situations to keep the group and meeting meaningful and productive. There is no rule as to how to manage these situations but the foremost consideration is how to serve the best interests of the patient. Family members unable to attend the family conferences should be relayed information in a timely way by a self-designated family spokesperson. This person is generally one who is more resilient and coping better than others with the end-of-life discussions who can take the responsibility for communicating the situation to other family members. Reassurance that the patient will not be abandoned and care will remain of the highest quality is important to families and fundamental to the care we provide.

A well-organised critical care team will meet prior to the family conference and ensure all relevant information is gathered and that there is a shared understanding. Curtis and colleagues[206] suggest the use of a five-point approach during the family conference, which may be useful around end-of-life meetings. This approach is termed 'VALUE': (1) **v**aluing family statements, (2) **a**cknowledging emotion, (3) **l**istening, (4) **u**nderstanding the patient as a person and (5) **e**liciting questions. The critical care team's ability to listen to the family is a key element and has been found to significantly increase a family's satisfaction with end-of-life care.[198]

The healthcare team that provides information and discusses palliation and end-of-life care needs to clearly indicate to families that, although they are involved in much of the decision making,[71] the decision to withdraw treatment is a medical one in Australia but may be quite different elsewhere. This notwithstanding, consensus and shared decision making remain the aim as careful consideration of the patient's wishes, the family perspective and the futility or otherwise of further treatment are considered within an ethical framework.[71,202] Importantly, the differences between withdrawal of life-sustaining treatment and the provision of end-of-life care processes need to be distinguished for families.[207] How best to meet the needs of families at these times is not well understood, partly due to the sensitive nature of researching this area of care as we strive to do no harm, and partly due to individual responses to the circumstances that restrict generalisability of findings. Maintaining a patient, family-centred approach seeking feedback on their needs helps us to individualise the care we provide and remains the best available approach in these circumstances where one size does not fit all.

While the family grapple with the process of grieving,[208] we do know that nurses need to provide physical and psychological care for patients and families. This can be achieved when there is patient, family-centred decision making, good communication, continuity of care and emotional and practical support, and spiritual support can assist with this.[209] Individualising the care to the family is essential, and support measures should be instituted based on their needs, which can change rapidly as the situation changes. Importantly, grief manifests in different ways, and grieving is a complex process. Bereaved families in intensive care demonstrate complex bereavement processes and, without support, prolonged grief reactions can occur. In a longitudinal study nearly half (46%) of bereaved family members had complicated grief 1 year later when measured by the Inventory of Complicated Grief Scale.[210] Complicated grief patterns are detrimental as they decrease the family's ability to cope with everyday needs, increase the need for health services and may progress to unresolved grief.[211]

The detrimental effects of long-term unresolved grief after the death of a loved one are well documented.[211] The preferred term is 'prolonged grief disorder' (previously called complicated grief), which has clinically disabling grief symptoms including, amongst others, a preoccupation with thoughts of the loss, avoidance of reminders of the loss, disbelief over the person's death, feeling lonely since the loss, feeling that the future holds no purpose and feeling stunned or shocked by the loss.[212] These symptoms can result in elevated morbidity and mortality levels associated with depression, cardiac events (including a higher risk of sudden cardiac death), hypertension, neoplasms, ulcerative colitis, suicidal tendencies and social dysfunction (including alcohol abuse and violence).[51,211] These potentially harmful outcomes provide strong motivation for critical care clinicians to initiate family support mechanisms such as bereavement services.[213] Bereavement care aims to reduce the immediate physical and emotional distress for those grieving, while improving the long-term morbidity associated with unresolved grief.

Although critical care clinicians in the UK,[214] USA,[213] Europe and Canada[215] are developing guidelines for bereavement care in critical care, little evidence-based research has been conducted on bereavement care strategies.[213] One study, however, conducted a broader evaluation of 113 ICUs in the UK and summarised bereavement care from the perspective of senior nursing clinicians. The senior nurses considered that they were proficient in providing written information to families but lacking in their provision of a respectful and quiet physical environment.[182] Others suggest that our care needs to incorporate key elements including physical and psychosocial comfort and culturally sensitive communication and family care.[216] Bereavement services in 153 Australasian ICUs were reported to also incorporate distribution of information to families in the majority of ICUs; fewer, however, had bereavement follow-up services (50% of ICUs in New Zealand and 23% in Australia).[81] Follow-up services were more common in Denmark, where 72% of the reporting 46 ICUs offered these services to ICU families following the death of a relative in ICU.[217] It is imperative to rigorously assess new and existing bereavement interventions as to how well they meet the needs of families. Legitimising research on this vulnerable group is required to improve end-of-life care for families and patients.

Care of the critical care nurse

The two previous sections have focused on care for the dying patient and their family. Critical care nurses who care for both patients and families also require care in end-of-life situations.[172,218] Caring for dying patients is emotionally draining and highly demanding of the critical care nurse, who may not have the knowledge and understanding of palliative care and death in the critical care environment. Peer support and unit guidelines on palliative care may provide support and reduce caregiver burden.[195,213,219,220]

Dealing with the death of patients may be exacerbated in some critical care environments, particularly in the rural setting, where the nurse may know the patient outside the work environment. Effective palliation is more likely to occur when the interdisciplinary team collectively develops their unit's palliative care and bereavement services with care and attention to staff's needs together with those of patients and their families.[209,213]

In the main, nurses depend on colleagues and friends for support when patients die, and they may value the opportunity to discuss the patient and family situation by way of debriefing sessions. 'Debriefing' sessions can have a number of interpretations. For example, debriefing in critical care often takes the form of an opportunity to share feelings. Alternatively, it may involve a procedural clinical review of events where the objective is to understand and learn from the situation.[221] Both forms of debriefing are important, together with the opportunity for peer discussion to provide mutual support within the interdisciplinary team.[222] Accessing experts from outside the unit's usual resources may also be helpful in particularly challenging situations.[221]

Dealing with death is never easy; however, an awareness of colleagues' needs is a key to providing support as mental and physical exhaustion can develop.[223] The term compassion fatigue is defined as,[224] *'a state of tension and preoccupation with the traumatised patients by re-experiencing the traumatic event … associated with the patient'* (p. 1435). Nurses' experiences of caring for critically ill or dying patients and their families have the potential to gradually lead to compassion fatigue.[223,225] This is detrimental not only to the nurse, but also to patients and families as the nurse endeavours to protect and distance themselves from further emotional situations. A workplace culture that includes positive inter- and intradisciplinary relationships influences the ability of nurses to provide compassionate care. Shared understanding of the plan of care for the patient is an important factor as is having your experiences validated by your team. Influences from outside the workplace also impact on our ability to provide compassionate care. Our values about patient care and lifestyle factors including family demands influence our caring capacity.[226]

One way to explore compassion amongst critical care nurses is to structure 'compassion cafes' into regular education sessions.[227] Compassion cafes are described as a way to provide a safe, supportive space away from the ICU where nurses can share their experiences within a collegial environment. Importantly, they focus on recognition of compassion fatigue and strategies to reduce its occurrence.[228] Sharing experiences and knowledge around end-of-life care[211] helps protect against compassion fatigue[226] and, not unexpectedly, compassion fatigue has been linked to reduced job satisfaction and an intention to leave the profession.[229] A number of strategies are important to enhance the care we are able to provide during end-of-life care. Caring for ourselves and our colleagues is fundamental to being able to care for patients and their families.

Practice tip

Think back to the last time you were involved with a patient who was being palliated. What were the things that worked well for you? Did you feel supported, or provide support to your colleagues? Were you able to care for the patient and their family as you would have liked? Did you have the resources to be able to provide a peaceful and dignified place to be? Having read this chapter, is there feedback you can provide to your colleagues and leadership team on ways to improve palliative care in your unit?

Summary

The psychosocial, cultural and religious needs of critically ill patients and their families are just as important as their physical needs, and care needs to be taken not to overlook these. In this chapter a holistic and patient, family-centred approach to practice is presented, which enables individualised plans of care that include specific psychosocial, cultural and religious needs of critically ill patients and their families. Health, illness, death and dying are sociocultural constructions, and can have different meanings for critically ill patients and their families. Cultural and spiritual care are an important aspect of people's well-being, and essential for critical nurses to be mindful of. Hence, culturally and linguistically diverse patients and families have specific cultural values, beliefs and practices that critical care nurses need to determine, which may involve the assistance of an interpreter. These patients require the critical care nurse to interact with them in a manner that facilitates the identification of their needs on an individual basis. The old adage 'actions speak louder than words' is worthy of consideration when working with these patients in the critical care setting. It is important that individual patient and family plans of care are developed that include their participation and reflect their important beliefs and practices that need to be included in their critical care experience. In order to meet the needs of the critically ill patient and family, the critical care nurse is advised to identify personal beliefs, practices and expectations that may influence professional decision making and interactions with the patient and family.

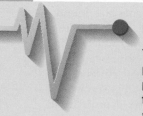

Case study

Your ICU has had a significant number of deaths in a short period of time. The deaths include young people in their 30s, with young children; nearly all of them had declined vaccination for the virus causing a pandemic. Recently a 28-year-old woman, Sheila, was admitted in the active phase of dying from respiratory failure. She is now on the ventilator and sedated. It is likely she will not survive. Her husband had not been able to visit for several days because of the distance he lived from the hospital and his work obligations.

His employer could not release him from duty. He comes to the hospital and on seeing his wife becomes violent with his anger at the situation, hitting his head against the wall and throwing objects in the room. He is shouting at staff, demanding that they save her. He is taken out of the hospital by security. Staff are conflicted about this because he will probably miss the death of his own wife if something is not done to help him cope with the situation. The increase in deaths and anger directed towards staff is taking a toll on everyone in the department. There has been an increase in staff turnover.

CASE STUDY QUESTIONS

1 What would you suggest as a strategy to learn how to meet the needs of Sheila's husband Tom? What actions can be taken to help him de-escalate and cope with the situation?

2 What actions can be taken to support the staff through their grief? What rituals might they perform to help process their grief over the increase in deaths?

3 What actions can be taken to protect staff from violence while providing holistic care to Sheila's family? What is the role of departmental leaders in this situation?

RESEARCH VIGNETTE

Fernández-Martínez E, Mapango EA, Martínez-Fernández MC, et al. Family-centred care of patients admitted to the intensive care unit in times of COVID-19: a systematic review. Intensive Crit Care Nurs 2022;70:103223.

Abstract

Objectives: To describe clinical practice interventions aimed at providing family-centred care in intensive care units during the COVID-19 pandemic.

Research methodology: A systematic review was carried out following the PRISMA recommendations in various databases: PubMed, Cinahl, Web of Science, Scopus, and Google Scholar were consulted, as well as within the grey literature found on the web pages of official organisations related to intensive care medicine and nursing.

Setting: Adult intensive care unit.

Results: The search yielded 209 documents, of which 24 were included in this review: eight qualitative studies, seven protocols and recommendations from official bodies, one mixed-method study, five descriptive studies, one cross-sectional study, one pilot program and one literature review. A thematic analysis revealed four major themes: the use of communication systems, multidisciplinary interventions, the promotion of family engagement and family support. The results show different strategies that can be implemented in clinical practice to solve the difficulties encountered in family-centred care in critical care units during the COVID-19 pandemic.

Conclusions: There is a great variety in the nature of the interventions developed, with the use of telecommunication systems in daily practice being the most repeated aspect. Future research should aim to assess whether the interventions implemented increase the quality of patient and family care by meeting their needs.

Critique

The authors conducted a systematic review adhering to the PRISMA guidelines.[230] A PICO question was crafted to include: Population: Adult ICU Intervention: Strategies to deploy FCC during the pandemic, Outcome: Impact of interventions on family, patients or staff. Because of the relatively small number of studies available 2.5 years after the start of the pandemic (March 2019), both research and non-research reports were considered for inclusion. In addition to the standard method of database retrieval, the grey literature was also queried by searching the websites of intensive care professional societies. Duplicates and reports that were off-topic were removed. There were studies that authors attempted to acquire but were unsuccessful in doing so. Reports were included in multiple languages: English, Spanish, Portuguese or Italian and English translation.

The final 24 reports were critiqued using Joanna Briggs Institute (JBI) tools for systematic reviews, qualitative studies, descriptive studies and opinion pieces to assess the reliability and relevance of each article.[231] As is required when conducting a systematic review, two investigators reviewed each report independently and then compared notes, solving any discrepancies in the review by discussion. Roughly half of the reports came from the United States, while the rest were from the United Kingdom, European Union and Canada.

Communication: Communicating with families electronically was the most frequently used intervention, through either telephone or video calls. Applications such as Facetime or Skype on mobile devices were also used for families to communicate with patients and to engage in daily rounds through video with audio. Videos were advocated because of the ability to read non-verbal language, to see the patient and to develop a stronger relationship with the staff. Pre-existing technology within virtual ICUs were adapted so that the audio or visual recorders were used for the family as well as the staff. Written communication by email was also used. A standardised checklist to guide communication was advocated so that all families received the same contextual information was also advocated. Communication training was recommended especially for those cross-training to the ICU to meet crisis staffing needs. Lastly, the mental health needs of those tasked with communicating with families needed to be addressed because of the relative frequency of imparting bad news and exposure to raw emotion. Readers were cautioned that communicating with families can be psychologically exhausting, necessitating rotation out of this task when communicating as a family liaison was a full-time duty.

Multidisciplinary: Increased referrals to social work and palliative care were recommended. Clinicians from outside the ICU were often relocated to serve the ICU to deal with staffing shortages. These people provided support and consultation, augmented staffing and provided break relief so that FCC could continue in addition to patient care.

Engagement of families: Families were engaged through virtual rounds and decision making via virtual conferencing. An exception to the restrictions on family presence was noted for end-of-life situations, where at least one person was allowed to be present despite the risks. These moments of family presence required education and monitoring regarding use of protective equipment and emotional preparation for what they were likely to see when they entered the room.

Family support: Routine assessment of family needs and early recognition of mental health issues were recommended, as well as the availability of consultation for family psychological support by the ICU team or psychologists.

Harm: Regarding harm, looking back retrospectively it was noted that mortality was higher in patients whose families had less communication, and that goals of care discussions were less frequent with video conferencing than when conducted face to face. There was a psychological burden to staff assigned to communicating with families. Likewise, being the family-designated spokesperson was also psychologically burdensome despite the need for communication.

Discussion: The level of evidence for all of these recommendations is low given that the studies were largely non-experimental in nature and none were controlled studies. However, it would have been nearly impossible and possibly unethical to provide supportive interventions to some but not other families in the name of science. Further, for those studies reporting outcomes, the outcomes were largely satisfaction with the intervention. No attempts were made to measure whether an intervention reduced incidence of PICS-F. The benefit of the tested and proposed interventions appear to outweigh the harm, though training and psychological support for both healthcare professionals and families are indicated.

One would wonder whether any of these changes will endure past the pandemic situation. For instance, in the future will families be allowed to watch patients from home using the adapted tele-ICU technology? Will families continue to benefit from virtual visits when visiting policies return to normal?

This systematic review, by nature of design (publication years 2020–2021) did not capture the previous white paper issued by the Society of Critical Care Medicine on considerations needed to retain FCC during a pandemic. Notably, all of the recommendations outlined above had been advocated prior to the COVID pandemic based upon experiences with previous pandemics.[226] Given this, we have increased confidence that the proposed interventions will not cause harm and could be of benefit to families during a pandemic.

Conclusion: In normal times FCC is difficult to execute uniformly. Pandemics complicate the process of allowing open liberal family presence and/or engagement in decision making and care. The most promising strategies appear to be assigning dedicated staff to communicate with families, followed by daily use of video technology accompanied with structured worktools and staff education. Barriers to operationalising these strategies include the availability of human and technological resources. Pandemics provide an opportunity, though, for innovation, some of which may result in enduring change.

Learning activities

1 In the critical care setting, the focus is on individuals and the physical health status. In this chapter the importance of patient- and family-centred nursing care is discussed, which requires critical care nurses to focus not only on a very unwell patient's physical status but also on their wider health and well-being needs and those of their family. This requires not only consideration of the people before you but also an understanding of the contextual factors that can enhance or impede patient- and family-centred nursing care. Identify the contextual factors in your critical care setting that might influence your practice by completing the following activities:

   a List those organisational policies and practices you can identify in the clinical practice setting that might influence nursing practice.

   b Identify the characteristics of a clinician who practises patient- and family-centred nursing practice and how these promote exemplary nursing care.

   c Imagine you were a patient in the critical care unit in which you work. What would be important to you about the nursing care you received?

   d Think about what you would expect if your immediate family were critically ill during a time when visitors were not allowed in the hospital. How would you suggest that you receive communication from the nurses and clinical team? What would you do to fulfill the need to participate in care?

   e Reflecting on the four activities above, write down how you can improve your patient- and family-centred care practice and identify those factors that would impede this practice and what strategies you could undertake to minimise their effects.

2 When considering culturally responsive care as a career-long endeavour, it is useful for critical care nurses to identify where on that journey they may be and what might be the need to undertake to progress further. Think about two situations involving patients and their families from another culture than your own – one where the interactions went well, the patient's and family's needs were respected and met, and the outcomes were positive, and another where the situation was challenging and marred by conflict and family dissatisfaction. How might you need to develop your knowledge, skills and strategies to optimise your cultural responsiveness? To assist you answer this question, consider the following:

   a Identify the factors that facilitated a positive outcome, and then the challenges and barriers that made reaching a positive outcome problematic.

   b Identify the cultural factors related to your personal and professional expectations, and those of the patient and family. How might these be sources of potential conflict?

   c What knowledge, skills and strategies might be needed for working in a culturally responsive way with patients and families from different cultures?

3 Spiritual intelligence, according to Moradnezhad and colleagues,[186] involves the following activities: creating existential thinking, creating personal meaning, transcendental awareness and consciousness state expansion. In what ways would these activities assist critical care nurses to develop their ability to respond better to

patients' and their families' spiritual needs? To help you assist with this activity, the following questions can guide self-reflection and/or discussion with your peers:

a Why would critical care nurses need to develop their spiritual intelligence?

b What benefits would emerge from having a higher level of spiritual intelligence derived from the activities that Moradnezhad and colleagues[186] suggest within the critical care setting?

c How would critical care nurses having a higher level of spiritual intelligence assist them to respond better to patients' and their families' spiritual needs?

4 You are to attend a family conference for the patient you are caring for. In preparation for this family conference, consider the following:

a What approach you would adopt if this is the first time participating in a family conference.

b The information you would need to gather to prepare in readiness for the family conference.

c The key people you would approach to get additional information, if today is the first time you have cared for the patient.

d What considerations will be needed if children are going to be present.

e The documentation required in the patient's clinical file following the family conference.

f Discussion: what adaptations to the process of FCC do you believe should be maintained as 'enduring change'?

Online resources

Arctic University of Norway's Centre for Sami Studies, https://en.uit.no/enhet/forsiden?p_dimension_id=88182.

Australian Commission on Safety and Quality in Healthcare, Patient-centred care: improving quality and safety by focusing care on patients and consumers: 2010 report, https://www.safetyandquality.gov.au/sites/default/files/migrated/PCCC-DiscussPaper.pdf

Australian Indigenous Health InfoNet, https://healthinfonet.ecu.edu.au

Guide to Māori Culture and Customs https://www.englishnewzealand.co.nz/news/guide-to-maori-culture-and-customs/

Institute for Patient- and Family-Centered Care: this website provides resources and exemplars of best practices: https://www.ipfcc.org/

Lowitja Institute: Cooperative Research Centre for Aboriginal and Torres Strait Islander Health, https://www.lowitja.org.au/page/about-us/our-history/cooperative-research-centre-for-aboriginal-and-torres-strait-islander-health

Māori, https://www.newzealandnow.govt.nz/live-in-new-zealand/tips-for-settling-in/maori-culture

Medical Journal of Australia: articles on Aboriginal health, https://www.mja.com.au/ search?search=Aboriginal+health

New Zealand Ministry of Health website (access to Māori health-related publications and resources), https://www.health.govt.nz/our-work/populations/maori-health

Nursology.net blog, https://nursology.net

WA Health, office of Aboriginal Health, https://www.health.wa.gov.au/Improving-WA-Health/About-Aboriginal-Health

Society of Critical Care Medicine ICU Liberation Bundle (A–F): the 'F' portion of this bundle includes information on how to support family engagement and empowerment: https://www.sccm.org/Clinical-Resources/ICULiberation-Home/ABCDEF-Bundles

Society of Critical Care Medicine, Patient and Family Awards: these annual awards are provided to exemplars providing outstanding and/or creative approaches to family-centered care, https://www.sccm.org/Member-Center/Professional-Development/Awards

YouTube: discrimination of Romani, https://www.youtube.com/watch?v=N8MZz3Ehuil

Further reading

Azoulay É, Curtis JR, Kentish-Barnes N. Ten reasons for focusing on the care we provide for family members of critically ill patients with COVID-19. Intensive Care Med 2021;47(2):230–3.

Best O, Fredericks B, editors. Yatdjuligin: Aboriginal and Torres Strait Islander nursing and midwifery care. 2nd ed. Melbourne, VIC: Cambridge University Press; 2018.

Cormack D, Stanley J, Harris R. Multiple forms of discrimination and relationships with health and wellbeing: findings from national cross-sectional surveys in Aotearoa/New Zealand. Int J Equity Health 2018;17:26.

Creswell JW, Plano Clark VL. Designing and conducting mixed methods research. 3rd ed. Thousand Oaks, CA: SAGE; 2018.

Davey RX. Health disparities among Australia's remote-dwelling Aboriginal people: a report from 2020. J Appl Lab Med 2021;6(1):125–41.

Goldschmidt K, Mele C. 2021 Disruption of patient and family centered care through the COVID-19 pandemic. J Ped Nurs 2021;58:102.

McFadden A, Siebelt L, Gavine A, et al. Gypsy, Roma and traveller access to and engagement with health services: a systematic review. Eur J Pub Health 2018;28(1):74–81.

Nana-Sinkam P, Kraschnewski J, Sacco R, et al. Health disparities and equity in the era of COVID-19. J Clin Transl Sci 2021;5(1):e99.

Papadimos TJ, Marcolini EG, Hadian M, et al. Ethics of outbreaks position statement. Part 2: Family-centered care. Crit Care Med 2018;46(11):1856–60.

Slim MAM, Lala HM, Barnes N, Martynoga RA. Māori health outcomes in an intensive care unit in Aotearoa New Zealand. Anaesth Intensive Care 2021;49(4):292–300.

Stojanovski K, Holla A, Hoxha I, et al. The influence of ethnicity and displacement on quality of antenatal care: the case of Roma, Ashkali, and Balkan Egyptian communities in Kosovo. Health Hum Rights 2017;19(2):35–48.

Strathdee SA, Hellyar M, Montesa C, et al. The power of family engagement in rounds: an exemplar with global outcomes. Crit Care Nurse 2019;39(5):14–20.

Tipa Z, Wilson D, Neville S, et al. Cultural responsiveness and the family partnership model. Nurs Prax N Z 2015;31(2):35–49.

Yi X, Feng X. Study on the current status and influencing factors of workplace violence to medical staff in intensive care units. Emerg Med Int 2022;2022:1792035. doi: 10.1155/2022/1792035.

References

1. Australian Commission on Safety and Quality in Health Care (ACSQHC). The NSQHS standards. Sydney, NSW: ACSQHC; 2017. Available from: https://www.safetyandquality.gov.au/standards/nsqhs-standards. [Accessed 10 February 2023].

2. World Health Organization (WHO). WHO patients for patient safety programme. Geneva: WHO; 2013. Available from: https://www.who.int/initiatives/patients-for-patients-safety. [Accessed 10 February 2023].

3. Mitchell M, Gill F, Grealy B, et al. ACCCN position statement – partnering with families in critical care. Surrey Hills, VIC: ACCCN; 2015. Available from: https://www.acccn.com.au/wp-content/uploads/Partnering-with-Families-in-Critical-Care.pdf. [Accessed 10 February 2023].

4. Jost SG, Bonnell M, Chacko SJ, et al. Integrated primary nursing: a care delivery model for the 21st-century knowledge worker. Nurs Admin Q 2010;34(3):208–16.

5. Jakimowicz S, Perry L, Lewis J. An integrative review of supports, facilitators and barriers to patient-centred nursing in the intensive care unit. J Clin Nurs 2017;26(23-24):4153–71.

6. Jakimowicz S, Perry L. A concept analysis of patient-centred nursing in the intensive care unit. J Adv Nurs 2015;71(7):1499–517.

7. Delaney LJ. Patient-centred care as an approach to improving health care in Australia. Collegian 2018;25(1):119–23.

8. Davidson JE, Aslakson RA, Long AC, et al. Guidelines for family-centered care in the neonatal, pediatric, and adult ICU. Crit Care Med 2017;45(1):103–28.

9. Australian Commission on Safety and Quality in Health Care (ACSQHC). Discussion paper: patient-centred care: improving quality and safety by focusing care on patients and consumers. Sydney, NSW: ACSQHC; 2010. Available from: https://www.safetyandquality.gov.au/wp-content/uploads/2012/01/PCCC-DiscussPaper.pdf. [Accessed 10 February 2023].

10. Epstein RM, Fiscella K, Lesser CS, et al. Why the nation needs a policy push on patient-centered health care. Health Aff 2010;29(8):1489–95.

11. Slatore CG, Hansen L, Ganzini L, et al. Communication by nurses in the intensive care unit: qualitative analysis of domains of patient-centered care. Am J Crit Care 2012;21(6):410–18.

12. Oxford University Press. Oxford English dictionary. Oxford: OUP; 2022. Available from: https://languages.oup.com/research/oxford-english-dictionary/. [Accessed 10 February 2023].

13. Ekman I, Swedberg K, Taft C, et al. Person-centered care: ready for prime time. Eur J Cardiovasc Nurs 2011;10(4):248–51.

14. University of Gothenburg Centre for Person-Centred Care (GPCC). Research. Available from: https://www.gu.se/en/gpcc/about-our-research. [Accessed 10 February 2023].

15. Fumagalli S. Reduced cardiocirculatory complications with unrestrictive visiting policy in an intensive care unit: results from a pilot, randomized trial. Circulation 2006;113(7):946–52.

16. Friedman M. Family nursing: research, theory and practice. 5th ed. Stamford: Appleton & Lange; 2003.

17. Wright LM. Nurses and families: a guide to family assessment and intervention. 6th ed. Philadelphia: F A Davis & Company; 2013.

18. Plaintree International. Resources 2018. Available from: https://planetree.org/certification-resources/. [Accessed 10 February 2023].

19. Espezel HJE, Canam CJ. Parent–nurse interactions: care of hospitalized children. J Adv Nurs 2003;44(1):34–41.

20. Institute for Patient- and Family-Centered Care. Patient- and Family-Centered Care 2012. Available from: https://www.ipfcc.org/about/pfcc.html. [Accessed 10 February 2023].

21. de Beer J, Brysiewicz P. The conceptualization of family care during critical illness in KwaZulu-Natal, South Africa. Health SA Gesondheid 2017;22:20–7.

22. Olding M, McMillan SE, Reeves S, et al. Patient and family involvement in adult critical and intensive care settings: a scoping review. Health Expect 2016;19(6):1183–202.

23. Raiskila S, Lehtonen L, Tandberg BS, et al. Parent and nurse perceptions on the quality of family-centred care in 11 European NICUs. Aust Crit Care 2016;29(4):201–19.

24. Engström B, Uusitalo A, Engström Å. Relatives' involvement in nursing care: a qualitative study describing critical care nurses' experiences. Intensive Crit Care Nurs 2011;27(1):1–9.

25. Garrouste-Orgeas M, Willems V, Timsit JF, et al. Opinions of families, staff, and patients about family participation in care in intensive care units. J Crit Care 2010;25(4):634–40.

26. Mitchell M, Chaboyer W, Burmeister E, et al. Positive effects of a nursing intervention on family-centered care in adult critical care. Am J Crit Care 2009;18(6):543–52.

27. Mitchell M. Family-centred care – are we ready for it? An Australian perspective. Nurs Crit Care 2005;10(2):54–5.

28. Goldfarb MJ, Bibas L, Bartlett V. Outcomes of patient- and family-centered care interventions in the ICU: a systematic review and meta-analysis. Crit Care Med 2017;45(10):1751–61.

29. Mitchell ML. Patient, family centred care. Aust Crit Care 2016;29(4):176–7.

30. Eggenberger SK, Sanders M. A family nursing educational intervention supports nurses and families in an adult intensive care unit. Aust Crit Care 2016;29(4):217–23.

31. de Silva D. Helping measure person-centred care. London: The Health Foundation; 2014. Available from: https://www.health.org.uk/sites/health/files/HelpingMeasurePersonCentredCare.pdf. [Accessed 10 February 2023].

32. Scottish Government. The healthcare quality strategy for NHS Scotland. Edinburgh: The Scottish Government; 2010. Available from: https://www.gov.scot/binaries/content/documents/govscot/publications/strategy-plan/2010/05/healthcare-quality-strategy-nhsscotland/documents/0098354-pdf/0098354-pdf/govscot%3Adocument/0098354.pdf. [Accessed 10 February 2023].

33. Kean S. Children and young people visiting an adult intensive care unit. J Adv Nurs 2010;66(4):868–77.

34. Milner KA, Goncalves S, Marmo S, et al. Is open visitation really "open" in adult intensive care units in the United States? Am J Crit Care 2020;29(3):221–5.

35. Hamilton R, Kleinpell R, Lipman J, et al. International facilitators and barriers to family engagement in the ICU: results of a qualitative analysis. J Crit Care 2020;58:72–7.

36. Papadimos TJ, Marcolini EG, Hadian M, et al. Ethics of outbreaks position statement. Part 2: family-centered care. Crit Care Med 2018;46(11):1856–60.

37. Heesakkers H, van der Hoeven JG, Corsten S, et al. Mental health symptoms in family members of COVID-19 ICU survivors 3 and 12 months after ICU admission: a multicentre prospective cohort study. Intensive Care Med 2022;48(3):322–31.

38. van Veenendaal N, van der Meulen IC, Onrust M, et al. Six-month outcomes in COVID-19 ICU patients and their family members: a prospective cohort study. Healthcare (Basel). 2021;9(7):865.

39. Azoulay E, Resche-Rigon M, Megarbane B, et al. Association of COVID-19 acute respiratory distress syndrome with symptoms of posttraumatic stress disorder in family members after ICU discharge. JAMA 2022;327(11):1042–50.

40. Lopez-Soto C, Bates E, Anderson C, et al. The role of a liaison team in ICU family communication during the COVID 19 pandemic. J Pain Symptom Manage 2021;62(3):e112–19.

41. Rose L, Yu L, Casey J, et al. Communication and virtual visiting for families of patients in intensive care during the COVID-19 pandemic: a UK national survey. Ann Am Thorac Soc 2021;18(10):1685–92.

42. Sasangohar F, Dhala A, Zheng F, et al. Use of telecritical care for family visitation to ICU during the COVID-19 pandemic: an interview study and sentiment analysis. BMJ Qual Saf 2021;30(9):715.

43. Wilson ME, Kaur S, Gallo De Moraes A, et al. Important clinician information needs about family members in the intensive care unit. J Crit Care 2015;30(6):1317–23.

44. Al-Mutair AS, Plummer V, O'Brien A, et al. Family needs and involvement in the intensive care unit: a literature review. J Clin Nurs 2013;22(13-14):1805–17.

45. Nelson JE. Improving comfort and communication in the ICU: a practical new tool for palliative care performance measurement and feedback. Qual Saf Health Care 2006;15(4):264–71.

46. Ekwall A, Gerdtz M, Manias E. The influence of patient acuity on satisfaction with emergency care: perspectives of family, friends and carers. J Clin Nurs 2008;17(6):800–9.

47. Szalados JE. Legal issues in the practice of critical care medicine: a practical approach. Crit Care Med 2007;35(Suppl.):S44–58.

48. Aiken LJ, Bibeau PD, Cilento BJ, et al. A personal reflection: a case study in family-centered care at the National Naval Medical Center in Bethesda, Maryland. Dimens Crit Care Nurs 2010;29(1):13–19.

49. Hwang DY, Yagoda D, Perrey HM, et al. Anxiety and depression symptoms among families of adult intensive care unit survivors immediately following brief length of stay. J Crit Care 2014;29(2):278–82.

50. Bandari R, Heravi-Karimooi M, Rejeh N, et al. Information and support needs of adult family members of patients in intensive care units: an Iranian perspective. J Res Nurs 2015;20(5):401–22.

51. Buckley T, Sunari D, Marshall A, et al. Physiological correlates of bereavement and the impact of bereavement interventions. Dialogues Clin Neurosci 2012;14(2):129–39.

52. Needham DM, Davidson J, Cohen H, et al. Improving long-term outcomes after discharge from intensive care unit: report from a stakeholders' conference. Crit Care Med 2012;40(2):502–9.

53. Lee LYK, Lau YL. Immediate needs of adult family members of adult intensive care patients in Hong Kong. J Clin Nurs 2003;12(4):490–500.

54. Azoulay E, Pochard F, Kentish-Barnes N, et al. Risk of post-traumatic stress symptoms in family members of intensive care unit patients. Am J Respir Crit Care Med 2005;171(9):987–94.

55. McAdam JL, Fontaine DK, White DB, et al. Psychological symptoms of family members of high-risk intensive care unit patients. Am J Crit Care 2012;21(6):386–94.

56. Petrinec AB, Mazanec PM, Burant CJ, et al. Coping strategies and posttraumatic stress symptoms in post-ICU family decision makers. Crit Care Med 2015;43(6):1205–12.

57. de Beer J, Brysiewicz P. The needs of family members of intensive care unit patients: a grounded theory study. S Afr Medcal J 2017;32(2):44–9.

58. Leske J. Protocols for practice: applying research at the bedside, interventions to decrease family anxiety. Crit Care Nurse 2002;22(6):61–5.

59. Jones C, Backman C, Griffiths RD. Intensive care diaries and relatives' symptoms of posttraumatic stress disorder after critical illness: a pilot study. Am J Crit Care 2012;21(3):172–6.

60. Jones C, Skirrow P, Griffiths RD, et al. Post-traumatic stress disorder-related symptoms in relatives of patients following intensive care. Intensive Care Med 2004;30(3):456–60.

61. Davidson JE. Family centered care. In: Goldsworthy S, Kleinpell R, Williams G, editors. International best practices in critical care. 2nd ed. Dayboro, QLD: World Federation of Critical Care Nurses; 2019, p. 96–112.

62. Kinrade T, Jackson AC, Tomnay JE. The psychosocial needs of families during critical illness comparison of nurses' and family members' perspectives. Aust J Adv Nurs 2009;27(1):82–8.

63. Molter NC. Needs of relatives of critically ill patients: a descriptive study. Heart Lung 1979;8(2):332–9.

64. Hickman RL, Douglas SL. Impact of chronic critical Illness on the psychological outcomes of family members. AACN Adv Crit Care 2010;21(1):80–91.

65. Kentish-Barnes N, Lemiale V, Chaize M, et al. Assessing burden in families of critical care patients. Crit Care Med 2009;37:S448–56.

66. Mitchell ML, Courtney M, Coyer F. Understanding uncertainty and minimizing families' anxiety at the time of transfer from intensive care. Nurs Health Sci 2003;5(3):207–17.

67. Nelson DP, Polst G. An interdisciplinary team approach to evidence-based improvement in family-centered care. Crit Care Nurs Q 2008;31(2):110–18.

68. Beck K, Albert E, Johnsen A, et al. Pediatric intensive care unit rounding improvements. BMJ Qual Improv Rep 2016;5(1):u208902.w3600.

69. Santiago C, Lazar L, Jiang D, et al. A survey of the attitudes and perceptions of multidisciplinary team members towards family presence at bedside rounds in the intensive care unit. Intensive Crit Care Nurs 2014;30(1):13–21.

70. Abraham M, Moretz JG. Implementing patient- and family-centered care: part I – understanding the challenges. Pediatr Nurs 2012;38(1):44–7.

71. Cypress BS. Family conference in the intensive care unit: a systematic review. Dimens Crit Care Nurs 2011;30(5):246–55.

72. Moore CD, Bernardini GL, Hinerman R, et al. The effect of a family support intervention on physician, nurse, and family perceptions of care in the surgical, neurological, and medical intensive care units. Crit Care Nurs Q 2012;35(4):378–87.

73. Soltner C, Lassalle V, Galienne-Bouygues S, et al. Written information that relatives of adult intensive care unit patients would like to receive – a comparison to published recommendations and opinion of staff members. Crit Care Med 2009;37(7):2197–202.

74. Nelson JE, Walker AS, Luhrs CA, et al. Family meetings made simpler: A toolkit for the intensive care unit. J Crit Care 2009;24(4):626.e7–14.

75. Lautrette A, Darmon M, Megarbane B, et al. A communication strategy and brochure for relatives of patients dying in the ICU. N Engl J Med 2007;356(5):469–78.

76. Mitchell M, Courtney M. An intervention study to improve the transfer of ICU patients to the ward – evaluation by ICU nurses. Aust Crit Care 2005;18(3):123–8.

77. Kon AA, Davidson JE, Morrison W, et al. Shared decision making in ICUs: an American College of Critical Care Medicine and American Thoracic Society policy statement. Crit Care Med 2016;44(1):188–201.

78. Davidson JE, Daly BJ, Agan D, et al. Facilitated sensemaking: a feasibility study for the provision of a family support program in the intensive care unit. Crit Care Nurs Q 2010;33(2):177–89.

79. Davidson JE. Facilitated sensemaking: a strategy and new middle-range theory to support families of intensive care unit patients. Crit Care Nurse 2010;30(6):28–39.

80. Davidson JE, Zisook S. Implementing family-centered care through facilitated sensemaking. AACN Adv Crit Care 2017;28(2):200–9.

81. Mitchell ML, Coyer F, Kean S, et al. Patient, family-centred care interventions within the adult ICU setting: an integrative review. Aust Crit Care 2016;29(4):179–93.

82. Schwarzkopf D, Behrend S, Skupin H, et al. Family satisfaction in the intensive care unit: a quantitative and qualitative analysis. Intensive Care Med 2013;39(6):1071–9.

83. McGowan C. Patients' confidentiality. Crit Care Nurse 2012;32(5):61–4.

84. Hunter JD, Goddard C, Rothwell M, et al. A survey of intensive care unit visiting policies in the United Kingdom. Anaesthesia 2010;65(11):1101–5.

85. Liu V, Read J, Scruth E, et al. Visitation policies and practices in US ICUs. Crit Care 2013;17(2):R71.

86. Molter NC. Families are not visitors in the critical care unit. Dimens Crit Care Nurs 1994;13(1):2–3.

87. Mitchell ML, Chaboyer W. Family centred care – a way to connect patients, families and nurses in critical care: a qualitative study using telephone interviews. Intensive Crit Care Nurs 2010;26(3):154–60.

88. Guttormson JL, Calkins K, McAndrew N, et al. Critical care nurses' experiences during the COVID-19 pandemic: a US national survey. Am J Crit Care 2022;31(2):96–103.

89. Wendlandt B, Kime M, Carson S. The impact of family visitor restrictions on healthcare workers in the ICU during the COVID-19 pandemic. Intensive Crit Care Nurs 2022;68:103123.

90. Adams A, Mannix T, Harrington A. Nurses' communication with families in the intensive care unit – a literature review. Nurs Crit Care 2017;22(2):70–80.

91. Garrouste-Orgeas M, Philippart F, Timsit JF, et al. Perceptions of a 24-hour visiting policy in the intensive care unit. Crit Care Med 2008;36(1):30–5.

92. Mitchell ML, Aitken LM. Flexible visiting positively impacted on patients, families and staff in an Australian intensive care unit: a before-after mixed method study. Aust Crit Care 2017;30(2):91–7.

93. Van Horn ER, Kautz D. Promotion of family integrity in the acute care setting: a review of the literature. Dimens Crit Care Nurs 2007;26(3):101–7.

94. Maxwell KE, Stuenkel D, Saylor C. Needs of family members of critically ill patients: a comparison of nurse and family perceptions. Heart Lung 2007;36(5):367–76.

95. Skoog M, Milner KA, Gatti-Petito J, et al. The impact of family engagement on anxiety levels in a cardiothoracic intensive care unit. Crit Care Nurse 2016;36(2):84–9.

96. Arockiasamy V, Holsti L, Albersheim S. Fathers' experiences in the neonatal intensive care unit: a search for control. Pediatrics 2008;121(2):e215–22.

97. Davidson JE. Family-centered care: meeting the needs of patients' families and helping families adapt to critical illness. Crit Care Nurse 2009;29(3):28–34; quiz 5.

98. National Institutes of Health (NIH). Health literacy. Bethesda, MD: NIH; 2021. Available from: https://www.nih.gov/institutes-nih/nih-office-director/office-communications-public-liaison/clear-communication/health-literacy. [Accessed 10 February 2023].

99. Beckstrand RL, Lamoreaux N, Luthy KE, et al. Critical care nurses' perceptions of end-of-life care obstacles: comparative 17-year data. Dimens Crit Care Nurs 2017;36(2):94–105.

100. Baumgarten M, Poulsen I. Patients' experiences of being mechanically ventilated in an ICU: a qualitative metasynthesis. Scand J Caring Sci 2015;29(2):205–14.

101. Green A. An exploratory study of patients' memory recall of their stay in an adult intensive therapy unit. Intensive Crit Care Nurs 1996;12(3):131–7.

102. Lawrence M. The unconscious experience. Am J Crit Care 1995;4(3):227–32.

103. Shin JW, Tate JA, Happ MB. The facilitated sensemaking model as a framework for family-patient communication during mechanical ventilation in the intensive care unit. Crit Care Nurs Clin North Am 2020;32(2):335–48.

104. Shin JW, Happ MB, Tate JA. VidaTalk™ patient communication application "opened up" communication between nonvocal ICU patients and their family. Intensive Crit Care Nurs 2021;66:103075.

105. Lorie A, Reinero DA, Phillips M, et al. Culture and nonverbal expressions of empathy in clinical settings: a systematic review. Patient Educ Couns 2017;100(3):411–24.

106. ten Hoorn S, Elbers PW, Girbes AR, et al. Communicating with conscious and mechanically ventilated critically ill patients: a systematic review. Crit Care 2016;20(1):333.

107. McNaughton D, Light J. The iPad and mobile technology revolution: benefits and challenges for individuals who require augmentative and alternative communication. Augment Altern Commun 2013;29(2):107–16.

108. Ahmed S, Lee S, Shommu N, et al. Experiences of communication barriers between physicians and immigrant patients: a systematic review and thematic synthesis. Patient Exp J 2017;4(1):122–40.

109. Travaline J. Communication in the ICU: an essential component of patient care. J Crit Illn 2002;14:451–6.

110. Hupcey JE. Feeling safe: the psychosocial needs of ICU patients. J Nurs Schol 2000;32(4):361–7.

111. Misiak B, Samochowiec J, Bhui K, et al. A systematic review on the relationship between mental health, radicalization and mass violence. Eur Psychiatry 2019;56:51–9.

112. National Council on Interpreting in Health Care (NCIHC). National standards of practice for interpreters in health care. Washington DC: NCIHC; 2005. Available from: https://www.ncihc.org/assets/z2021Images/NCIHC%20National%20Standards%20of%20Practice.pdf. [Accessed 10 February 2023].

113. Dithole K, Sibanda S, Moleki MM, et al. Exploring communication challenges between nurses and mechanically ventilated patients in the intensive care unit: a structured review. Worldviews 2016;13(3):197–206.

114. Dithole KS, Thupayagale-Tshweneagae G, Akpor OA, et al. Communication skills intervention: promoting effective communication between nurses and mechanically ventilated patients. BMC Nurs 2017;16:74.

115. Zaga CJ, Berney S, Vogel AP. The feasibility, utility, and safety of communication interventions with mechanically ventilated intensive care unit patients: a systematic review. Am J Speech Lang Pathol 2019;28(3):1335–55.

116. Hart JT. The inverse care law. Lancet. 971;297:405–12.

117. Buettner-Schmidt K, Lobo ML. Social justice: a concept analysis. J Adv Nurs 2012;68(4):948–58.

118. Faden RR, Powers M. Health inequities and social justice: the moral foundations in public health. Bundesgesundheitsblatt Gesundheitsforschung Gesundheitsschutz 2008;51(2):151–7.

119. Ministry of Health. Achieving equity in health outcomes: summary of a discovery process. 2019. Available from: https://www.health.govt.nz/publication/achieving-equity-health-outcomes-summary-discovery-process. [Accessed 10 February 2023].

120. Francis-Oliviero F, Cambon L, Wittwer J, et al. Theoretical and practical challenges of proportionate universalism: a review. Pan Am J Public Health 2020;44:e110.

121. Lara M, Gamboa C, Kahramanian MI, et al. Acculturation and Latino health in the United States. In: LaVeist TA, Isaac LA, editors. Race, ethnicity and health: a public health reader. 2nd ed. San Francisco, CA: Jossey-Bass; 2013. p. 215–52.

122. Wepa D. Cultural safety in Aotearoa New Zealand. 2nd ed. Melbourne, VIC: Cambridge University Press; 2015.

123. Reid J, Varona G, Fisher M, Smith C. Understanding Māori 'lived' culture to determine cultural connectedness and wellbeing. J Population Res 2016;33(1):31–49.

124. Dempsey J, Hillege S, Hill R, editors. Fundamentals of nursing and midwifery: a person-centred approach to care. 2nd Australian & New Zealand ed. Sydney, NSW: Lippincott, Williams & Wilkins; 2013.

125. Charon JM. Symbolic interactionism: an introduction, an interpretation, an integration. 10th ed. Upper Saddle River, NJ: Prentice-Hall; 2009.

126. Gushue GV, Mejia-Smith BX, Fisher LD, et al. Differentiation of self and racial identity. Counselling Psychol Q 2013;26(3-4):343–61.

127. Wepa D. Cultural safety in Aotearoa New Zealand. Auckland, NZ: Pearson Education New Zealand; 2005.

128. Wilson D, Hickey H. Māori health: Māori- and whānau-centred practice. In: Wepa D, editor. Cultural safety in Aotearoa New Zealand. Melbourne, VIC: Cambridge University Press; 2015. p. 235–51.

129. Wilson D, Heaslip V, Jackson D. Improving equity and cultural responsiveness with marginalised communities: understanding competing worldviews. J Clin Nurs 2018;27(19–20):3810–19.

130. Heyland DK, Davidson J, Skrobik Y, et al. Improving partnerships with family members of ICU patients: study protocol for a randomized controlled trial. Trials 2018;19:1–11.

131. Mol MMC, Boeter TGW, Verharen L, et al. Patient- and family-centred care in the intensive care unit: a challenge in the daily practice of healthcare professionals. J Clin Nurs 2017;26(19-20):3212–23.

132. McKinnon J. The case for concordance: value and application in nursing practice. Br J Nurs 2013;22(13):766–71.

133. Kayser JB, Kaplan LJ. Conflict management in the ICU. Crit Care Med 2020;48(9):1349–57.

134. Almutairi AF, Adlan AA, Nasim M. Perceptions of the critical cultural competence of registered nurses in Canada. BMC Nurs 2017;16:1–9.

135. Gill GK, Babacan H. Developing a cultural responsiveness framework in healthcare systems: an Australian example. Divers Equal Health Care 2012;9(1):45–55.

136. Leininger MM. Cultural care diversity and universality: a theory of nursing. New York: National League for Nursing Press; 2001.

137. Ramsden I. Cultural safety and nursing education in Aotearoa and Te Waipounamu [Doctoral thesis]. Wellington: Victoria University of Wellington; 2002.

138. Ramsden I. Kawa Whakaruruhau: cultural safety in nursing education. Wellington: Ministry of Education; 1990.

139. Lee H, Fitzpatrick JJ, Baik SY. Why isn't evidence based practice improving health care for minorities in the United States? Appl Nurs Res 2013;26(4):263–8.

140. Wood PJ, Schwass M. Cultural safety: a framework for changing attitudes. Nurs Prax N Z 1993;8(1):4–15.

141. McDonagh JR, Elliott TB, Engelberg RA, et al. Family satisfaction with family conferences about end-of-life care in the intensive care unit: increased proportion of family speech is associated with increased satisfaction. Crit Care Med 2004;32(7):1484–8.

142. Perng SJ, Watson R. Construct validation of the Nurse Cultural Competence Scale: a hierarchy of abilities. J Clin Nurs 2012;21(11/12):1678–84.

143. Ingram RR. Using Campinha-Bacote's process of cultural competence model to examine the relationship between health literacy and cultural competence: health literacy and cultural competence. J Adv Nurs 2012;68(3):695–704.

144. Dudas KI. Cultural competence: an evolutionary concept analysis. Nurs Educ Perspect 2012;33(5):317–21.

145. Betancourt JR, Corbett J, Bondaryk MR. Addressing disparities and achieving equity: Cultural competence, ethics, and health-care transformation. Chest 2014;145(1):143–8.

146. Minkler M. Community organizing and community building for health and welfare. 3rd ed. New Brunswick, NJ: Rutgers University Press; 2012.

147. Durie M. Cultural competence and medical practice in New Zealand. Australian and New Zealand Boards and Council Conference; November 21. Wellington, New Zealand; 2001.

148. Australian Bureau of Statistics. Characteristics of recent migrants, Australia, November 2019. June 2020. Available from: https://www.abs.gov.au/statistics/people/people-and-communities/characteristics-recent-migrants/latest-release. [Accessed 10 February 2023].

149. Statistics New Zealand. New Zealand's population reflects growing diversity. September 2019. Available from: https://www.stats.govt.nz/news/new-zealands-population-reflects-growing-diversity. [Accessed 10 February 2023].

150. Statistics Canada. Immigration and ethnocultural diversity in Canada. 2016. Available from: https://www150.statcan.gc.ca/n1/en/subjects/immigration_and_ethnocultural_diversity. [Accessed 10 February 2023].

151. United States Census Bureau. Quick facts United States 2017. Available from: https://www.census.gov/quickfacts/fact/table/US/RH1125220. [Accessed 10 February 2023].

152. UK Office for National Statistics. Census 2021. Overview of the UK population: 2020. February 2022. Available from: https://www.ons.gov.uk/peoplepopulationandcommunity/populationandmigration/populationestimates/articles/overviewoftheukpopulation/2020. [Accessed 10 February 2023].

153. Ruston A, Smith D. Gypsies/travellers and health: risk categorisation versus being 'at risk'. Health Risk Soc 2013;15(2):176–93.

154. Smith D, Ruston A. 'If you feel that nobody wants you you'll withdraw into your own': gypsies/travellers, networks and healthcare utilisation. Sociol Health Illn 2013;35(8):1196–210.

155. Campinha-Bacote J. The process of cultural competence in the delivery of healthcare services: a model of care. J Transcult Nurs 2002;13(3):181–4.

156. Ellis L, Gergen J, Wohlgemuth L, et al. Empowering the "cheerers": role of surgical intensive care unit nurses in enhancing family resilience. Am J Crit Care 2016;25(1):39–45.

157. Boles J. Bearing bad news: supporting patients and families through difficult conversations. Pediatr Nurs 2015;41(6):306–8.

158. Huynh HP, Sweeny K, Miller T. Transformational leadership in primary care: Clinicians' patterned approaches to care predict patient satisfaction and health expectations. J Health Psychol 2018;23(5):743–53.

159. Knapp SJ, Sole ML, Byers JF. The EPICS family bundle and its effects on stress and coping of families of critically Ill trauma patients. Appl Nurs Res 2013;26(2):51–7.

160. Wilson D, Barton P. Indigenous hospital experiences: a New Zealand case study. J Clin Nurs 2011;21(15–16):2316–26.

161. Boucher NA. Direct engagement with communities and interprofessional learning to factor culture into end-of-life health care delivery. Am J Pub Health 2016;106(6):996–1001.

162. Cometto G, Witter S, Boerma T, et al. Tackling health workforce challenges to universal health coverage: setting targets and measuring progress. Bull World Health Organ 2013;91(11):881–9.

163. Mbuzi V, Fulbrook P, Jessup M. Indigenous peoples experiences and perceptions of hospitalisation for acute care: a metasynthesis of qualitative studies. Int J Nurs Stud 2017;71:39–49.

164. Cohen JJ, Gabriel BA, Terrell C. The case for diversity in the health care workforce. Health Aff (Millwood) 2002;21(5):90–102.

165. American Association of Colleges of Nursing (AACN). Diversity, equity and inclusion in academic nursing: AACN position statement. Washington DC: AACN; 2017. Available from: http://www.aacnnursing.org/Portals/42/News/Position-Statements/Diversity-Inclusion.pdf. [Accessed 10 February 2023].

166. Doolen J, York NL. Cultural differences with end-of-life care in the critical care unit. Dimens Crit Care Nurs 2007;26(5):194–8.

167. Procter S. Whose evidence? Agenda setting in multi-professional research: observations from a case study. Health Risk Soc 2002;4(1):45–59.

168. Petroz U, Kennedy D, Webster F, et al. Patients' perceptions of individualized care: evaluating psychometric properties and results of the individualized care scale. Can J Nurs Res 2011;43(2):80–100.

169. Shaw J, Pemberton S, Pratt C, et al. Shadowing: a central component of patient and family-centred care: Joanne Shaw and colleagues explain how an NHS trust incorporates the use of shadowing to improve the care experiences of patients and their families. Nurs Manage 2014;21(3):20–3.

170. Bredemeyer S, Reid S, Polverino J, et al. Implementation and evaluation of an individualized developmental care program in a neonatal intensive care unit. J Spec Pediatr Nurs 2008;13(4):281–91.

171. Suhonen R, Valimaki M, Leino-Kilpi H. Individualized care, quality of life and satisfaction with nursing care. J Adv Nurs 2005;50(3):283–92.

172. Coombs M, Mitchell M, James S, et al. Intensive care bereavement practices across New Zealand and Australian intensive care units: a qualitative content analysis. J Clin Nurs 2017;26(19-20):2944–52.

173. Jansson I, Pilhamar E, Forsberg A. Factors and conditions that have an impact in relation to the successful implementation and maintenance of individual care plans. Worldviews Evid Based Nurs 2011;8(2):66–75.

174. Bone N, Swinton M, Hoad N. Critical care nurses' experiences with spiritual care: the Spirit study. Am J Crit Care 2018;27(3):212–19.

175. Coombs M. A scoping review of family experience and need during end of life care in intensive care. Nurs Open 2015;2(1):24–35.

176. Canfield C. Critical care nurses' perceived need for guidance in addressing spirituality in critically ill patients. Am J Crit Care 2016;25(3):206–11.

177. Abu-El-Noor N. ICU nurses' perceptions and practice of spiritual care at the end of life: Implications for policy change. Online J Issues Nurs 2016;21(1):6.
178. Ramezani M, Ahmadi F, Mohammadi E, et al. Spiritual care in nursing: a concept analysis. Int Nurs Rev 2014;61(2):211–19.
179. Kisorio LC, Langley GC. Intensive care nurses' experiences of end-of-life care. Intensive Crit Care Nurs 2016;33:30–8.
180. Blockley C. Meeting patients' religious needs. Kai Tiaki N Z Nurs J 2001;7(11):15–17.
181. Cook D, Rocker G. Dying with dignity in the intensive care unit. New Engl J Med 2014;370(26):2506–14.
182. Berry M, Brink E, Metaxa V. Time for change? A national audit on bereavement care in intensive care units. J Intensive Care Soc 2017;18(1):11–6.
183. Halligan P. Caring for patients of Islamic denomination: critical care nurses' experiences in Saudi Arabia. J Clin Nurs 2006;15(12):1565–73.
184. Kongsuwan W, Locsin RC. Promoting peaceful death in the intensive care unit in Thailand. Int Nurs Rev 2009;56(1):116–22.
185. Banjar AK. Till death do us part: the evolution of end of life and death attitudes. Can J Crit Care 2017;28(3):34–40.
186. Moradnezhad M, Seylani K, Navab E, et al. Spiritual intelligence of nurses working at the intensive care units of hospitals affiliated with Tehran University of Medical Sciences. Nurs Pract Today 2017;4(4):170–9.
187. Kisorio LC, Langley GC. End-of-life care in intensive care unit: family experiences. Intensive Crit Care Nurs 2016;35:57–65.
188. Sprung CL, Maia P, Bulow HH, et al. The importance of religious affiliation and culture on end-of-life decisions in European intensive care units. Intensiv Care Med 2007;33(10):1732–9.
189. Murthy S, Wunsch H. Clinical review: international comparisons in critical care – lessons learned. Crit Care 2012;16(2):218.
190. Australian and New Zealand Intensive Care Society (ANZICS). ANZICS Centre for Outcome and Resource Evaluation 2020 report. Melbourne, VIC: ANZICS; 2020. Available from: https://www.anzics.com.au/wp-content/uploads/2021/09/2020-ANZICS-CORE-Report.pdf. [Accessed 10 February 2023].
191. Gries CJ, Curtis JR, Wall RJ, et al. Family member satisfaction with end-of-life decision making in the ICU. Chest 2008;133(3):704–12.
192. Kehl KA. Moving toward peace: an analysis of the concept of a good death. Am J Hosp Palliat Care 2006;23(4):277–86.
193. Beckstrand RL, Hadley KH, Luthy KE, et al. Critical care nurses' suggestions to improve end-of-life care obstacles: minimal change over 17 years. Dimens Crit Care Nurs 2017;36(4):264–70.
194. Edwards J, Voigt L, Nelson J, et al. Ten key points about ICU palliative care. Intensive Care Med 2017;43(1):83–5.
195. Gaeta S, Price KJ. End-of-life issues in critically ill cancer patients. Crit Care Clin 2010;26(1):219–27.
196. Ranse K, Yates P, Coyer F. End-of-life care practices of critical care nurses: a national cross-sectional survey. Aust Crit Care 2016;29(2):83–9.
197. Myburgh J, Abillama F, Chiumello D, et al. End-of-life care in the intensive care unit: report from the Task Force of World Federation of Societies of Intensive and Critical Care Medicine. J Crit Care 2016;34:125–30.
198. Schaefer KG, Block SD. Physician communication with families in the ICU: evidence-based strategies for improvement. Curr Opin Crit Care 2009;15(6):569–77.
199. Pignatiello G, Hickman RL Jr, Hetland B. End-of-life decision support in the ICU: Where are we now? West J Nurs Res 2018;40(1):84–120.
200. Noome M, Dijkstra BM, Leeuwen EV, et al. Exploring family experiences of nursing aspects of end-of-life care in the ICU: a qualitative study. Intensive Crit Care Nurs 2016;33:56–64.
201. Singer AE, Ash T, Ochotorena C, et al. A systematic review of family meeting tools in palliative and intensive care settings. Am J Hosp Palliat Care 2016;33(8):797–806.
202. Siegel MD. End-of-life decision making in the ICU. Clin Chest Med 2009;30(1):181–94.
203. Seaman JB. Improving care at end of life in the ICU: a proposal for early discussion of goals of care. J Gerontol Nurs 2013;39(8):52–8.
204. Davis P, Lay-Yee R, Dyall L, et al. Quality of hospital care for Māori patients in New Zealand: retrospective cross-sectional assessment. Lancet 2006;367(9526):1920–5.
205. Pochard F, Darmon M, Fassier T, et al. Symptoms of anxiety and depression in family members of intensive care unit patients before discharge or death. A prospective multicenter study. J Crit Care 2005;20(1):90–6.
206. Curtis JR, Ciechanowski PS, Downey L, et al. Development and evaluation of an interprofessional communication intervention to improve family outcomes in the ICU. Contemp Clin Trials 2012;33(6):1245–54.
207. Coombs MA, Parker R, Ranse K, et al. An integrative review of how families are prepared for, and supported during withdrawal of life-sustaining treatment in intensive care. J Adv Nurs 2017;73(1):39–55.
208. Krueger G. Meaning-making in the aftermath of sudden infant death syndrome. Nurs Inq 2006;13(3):163–71.
209. Nelson JE, Angus DC, Weissfeld LA, et al. End-of-life care for the critically ill: a national intensive care unit survey. Crit Care Med 2006;34(10):2547–53.
210. Anderson WG, Arnold RM, Angus DC, et al. Posttraumatic stress and complicated grief in family members of patients in the intensive care unit. J Gen Int Med 2008;23(11):1871–6.
211. Stroebe M, Schut H, Stroebe W. Health outcomes of bereavement. Lancet 2007;370(9603):1960–73.
212. Golden AM, Dalgleish T. Is prolonged grief distinct from bereavement-related posttraumatic stress? Psychiatry Res 2010;178(2):336–41.
213. Kuschner WG, Gruenewald DA, Clum N, et al. Implementation of ICU palliative care guidelines and procedures. Chest 2009;135(1):26–32.
214. UK Department of Health (DOH). Bereavement care services: a synthesis of the literature. London: DOH; 2011.
215. Cook D, Rocker G, Heyland D. Dying in the ICU: strategies that may improve end-of-life care. Can J Anaesth 2004;51(3):266–72.

216. Preciado A, Vachhani A, Gilbert A, et al. Innovative solutions: the C.O.R.E. to sociocultural care in nursing. Dimens Crit Care Nurs 2012;31(5):283–6.

217. Egerod I, Kaldan G, Coombs M, et al. Family-centered bereavement practices in Danish intensive care units: a cross-sectional national survey. Intensive Crit Care Nurs 2018;45:52–7.

218. Mitchell M, Coombs M, Wetzig K. The provision of family-centred intensive care bereavement support in Australia and New Zealand: results of a cross sectional explorative descriptive survey. Aust Crit Care 2017;30(3):139–44.

219. Quenot JP, Rigaud JP, Prin S, et al. Suffering among carers working in critical care can be reduced by an intensive communication strategy on end-of-life practices. Intensive Care Med 2012;38(1):55–61.

220. Shaw DJ, Davidson JE, Smilde RI, et al. Multidisciplinary team training to enhance family communication in the ICU. Crit Care Med 2014;42(2):265–71.

221. Rogers S, Babgi A, Gomez C. Educational interventions in end-of-life care: part I. Adv Neonatal Care 2008;8(1):56–65.

222. Simpson N, Knott CI. Stress and burnout in intensive care medicine: an Australian perspective. Med J Aust 2017;206(3):107–8.

223. Sacco TL, Ciurzynski SM, Harvey ME, et al. Compassion satisfaction and compassion fatigue among critical care nurses. Crit Care Nurse 2015;35(4):32–43; quiz 1p following.

224. Figley CR. Compassion fatigue: psychotherapists' chronic lack of self care. J Clin Psychol 2002;58(11):1433–41.

225. Alharbi J, Jackson D, Usher K. Compassion fatigue in critical care nurses. An integrative review of the literature. Saudi Med J 2019;40(11):1087–97.

226. Jones J, Winch S, Strube P, et al. Delivering compassionate care in intensive care units: nurses' perceptions of enablers and barriers. J Adv Nurs 2016;72(12):3137–46.

227. Strube P, Henderson A, Mitchell ML, et al. The role of the nurse educator in sustaining compassion in the workplace: a case study from an intensive care unit. J Contin Educ Nurs 2018;49(5):221–4.

228. Winch S, Henderson AJ, Kay M, et al. Understanding compassion literacy in nursing through a clinical compassion cafe. J Contin Educ Nurs 2014;45(11):484–6.

229. Jakimowicz S, Perry L, Lewis J. Compassion satisfaction and fatigue: a cross-sectional survey of Australian intensive care nurses. Aust Crit Care 2018;31(6):396–405.

230. Page MJ, McKenzie JE, Bossuyt PM, et al. Updating guidance for reporting systematic reviews: development of the PRISMA 2020 statement. J Clin Epidemiol 2021;134:103–12.

231. The University of South Australia. Critical appraisal tools. 2022. Available from: https://www.unisa.edu.au/research/allied-health-evidence/resources/cat/. [Accessed 10 February 2023].

Chapter 8

Recovery and rehabilitation

Janice Rattray, Leanne Aitken, Marc Nickels

Learning objectives

After reading this chapter, you should be able to:

- discuss the physical, psychological and cognitive sequelae some survivors experience after critical illness
- identify the risk factors associated with poor physical, psychological and cognitive sequelae
- outline the common functional, psychological, cognitive and health-related quality of life (HRQOL) instruments used to assess patient outcomes after a critical illness
- identify a range of potential interventions that may prevent or reduce the short- and long-term consequences of critical illness.
- examine the benefits and challenges for implementing interventions in the ICU, in hospital after ICU discharge and after hospital discharge to improve recovery and rehabilitation.

Introduction

Millions of people each year experience a critical illness requiring admission to an ICU. Although overall survival rates are generally above 80% at hospital discharge, recovery for individuals is often delayed beyond 6 months post discharge.[1] Physical deconditioning and neuromuscular dysfunction[2] as well as psychological[3–5] and cognitive sequelae[6] are common, adding to the burden of illness for survivors, carers, the healthcare system and broader society.

Although ICU clinicians have traditionally focused on survival as the principal indicator of patient outcome and unit performance, physical, psychological and cognitive functioning and health-related quality of life (HRQOL) have now emerged as legitimate patient outcomes from both practice and research perspectives.[1,7] With this shifting focus towards long–term health and well-being has also come a reconsideration and reconceptualisation of critical care as only one component in the continuum of care for a critically ill patient. An episode of critical illness is now viewed as a continuum that begins with the onset of acute clinical deterioration, includes the ICU admission and continues until the patient's risk of late sequelae has returned to the baseline risk of a similar individual who has not incurred a critical illness.[1,8]

FIGURE 8.1 Prototypical trajectories of recovery. The upper grey line extending past critical illness is the counterfactual trajectory of functioning that would have occurred had the patient not developed critical illness.

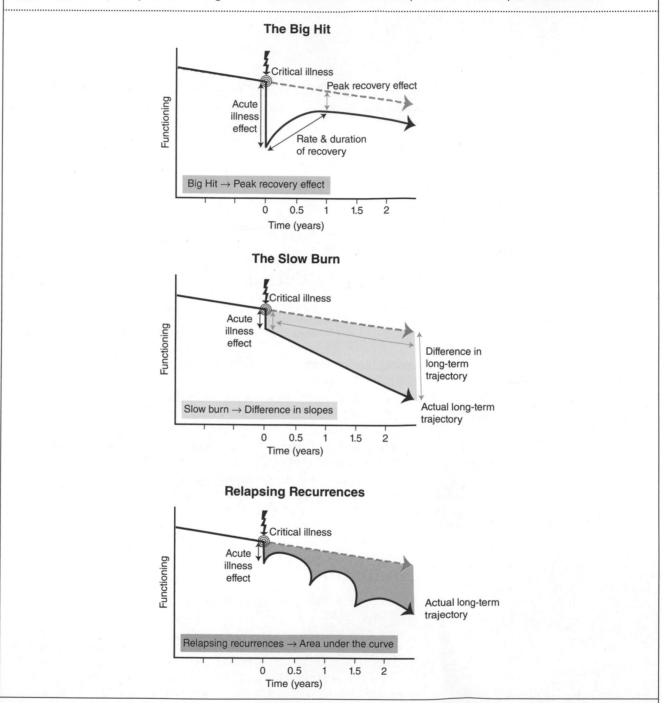

The Big Hit

The Slow Burn

Relapsing Recurrences

Source: Iwashyna, TJ. Trajectories of recovery and dysfunction after acute illness, with implications for clinical trial design. Am J Respir Crit Care Med, 2012;186(4):302–4.

Additionally, a patient's functional recovery is likely to be influenced by their health status prior to an episode of critical illness[9] (Fig. 8.1). As is suggested in Fig. 8.1, patients may not all recover at the same rate or in the same pattern. While we assume that many patients recover as outlined in the 'big hit', i.e. experience an acute loss of function with critical illness and then gradually recover to reach maximum status 1–2 years after critical illness, other patients will recover differently. Various factors are thought to influence this pathway, with pre-existing conditions such as diabetes, cardiac or respiratory disease thought to influence progress. Interventions need to be delivered in a manner that takes into account this recovery trajectory and related factors and incorporates the expertise of all members of the multidisciplinary team.

Reviews of numerous studies confirm delayed recovery in HRQOL[10,11] with physical, psychological and cognitive symptoms prevalent:

- weakness: approximately 40%[2,12,13]
- delirium: up to 81% with average of 32%[14]
- anxiety: up to 45%[3,15]
- depression: approximately 30%[5]
- post-traumatic stress symptoms (PTSS): approximately 20%[4]
- cognitive dysfunction: 36–62%.[6]

Recognition of the frequency, and co-occurrence, of these elements of compromise has led to the development of the term 'post-intensive care syndrome' (PICS) to *'describe new or worsening impairments in physical, cognitive, or mental health status arising after critical illness and persisting beyond acute care hospitalisation'*.[1] It is important to recognise that PICS can affect the family as well as the patient (Fig. 8.2).[1]

While significant sequelae therefore exist for a substantial proportion of critical illness survivors, limited evidence is currently available to support specific interventions for improving their recovery. To help plan support, it is worth recognising that ICU-acquired weakness has been associated with persistent deficits in function and HRQOL at 3 and 6 months post-hospital discharge,[16] although these relationships have not been consistently identified across all cohorts that have been studied.[17] In other groups the best predictors for good

HRQOL 1 year after ICU discharge were identified as time to regain walking ability and mean Montreal Cognitive Assessment (MoCA) at admission to post-acute ICU and rehabilitation units.[18]

In further chapters of this book, patient comfort and psychological issues are discussed including comfort and sedation management and delirium monitoring while in ICU (Chapter 6) and breathing trials and weaning from mechanical ventilation (Chapter 15). Common physical and psychological sequelae associated with a critical illness, and how these impact on a survivor's HRQOL, are discussed in this chapter. Common instruments measuring physical, psychological, cognitive and HRQOL are described. Rehabilitation strategies, commencing in-ICU and extending both post-ICU and post-hospital that can be delivered by the multidisciplinary team are also discussed.

Compromise following a critical illness

Examination of patient outcomes beyond survival is an important contemporary topic for critical care practice and research. Patient outcomes after a critical illness or injury were traditionally measured using a number of objective parameters (e.g. number of organ failure-free days, 28-day status or 1-year mortality). Other measures that examined patient-centred concepts such as functional status, HRQOL, psychological health and cognitive function have become more prevalent in the past 10 years.[1] The notion of 'survivorship' in this patient group is receiving increasing interest,[19,20] recognising that the

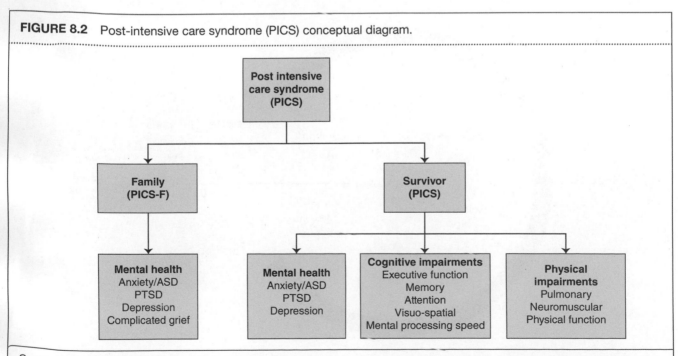

FIGURE 8.2 Post-intensive care syndrome (PICS) conceptual diagram.

Source: Needham DM, Davidson J, Cohen H, et al. Improving long-term outcomes after discharge from intensive care unit: report from a stakeholders' conference. Crit Care Med 2012;40(2):502–9.

recovery trajectory from a critical illness may be long and incomplete, and mapping this path is a complex process.

Disability and health-related quality of life

The World Health Organization (WHO) defines disability as the outcome of the interaction between individuals with a health condition and personal and environmental factors (WHO Policy on Disability, 2021).[21] Survivors of critical illness or trauma experience significant disability.[22,23] Approximately 25% of ICU survivors report moderate to severe disability at 6 months.[23] Mechanically ventilated patients with non-COVID acute respiratory distress syndrome (ARDS) and COVID-19 experienced similar levels of mortality and new disability at 6 months.[24]

The relationship between HRQOL and disability is poorly described.[22,23] The conceptual model presented in Fig. 8.3[24] demonstrates the complex interaction between the effects of critical illness that impact on an individual's function and roles, and limitations in function and roles can be measured and defined as disability. An individual's HRQOL is in turn influenced by factors including resilience, adaptation and environment.[23] Within this chapter, we guide the reader to the commonly used measures but present the physical and psychological issues separately. Ongoing physical and psychological problems tend to impact negatively on social, environmental and economic elements in life.[25] Up to 60% of ICU survivors

are unable to return to work or study following a period of critical illness.[23] Consequently, many patients and families experience a significant economic challenge during the recovery process. A substantial proportion of survivors of critical illness that were employed prior to critical illness were unable to return to employment following hospital discharge, with approximately two-thirds of survivors jobless at 3 months and a third of survivors remaining unemployed 5 years after hospital discharge.[26] These high levels of unemployment are associated with a negative impact on survivors' HRQOL.[26]

Although some patients recover quickly and do not report ongoing issues, others report significant and protracted compromise in their quality of life.[27] It is clear that survivors of critical illness have markedly lower HRQOL than other members in the community when matched for age and gender[11] and, although there is convincing evidence of this widespread compromise, we also know that recovery patterns vary for individual patients, with some recovering rapidly. Factors that have been shown to influence components of quality of life include age, frailty,[28,29] comorbidities,[30] lower socioeconomic status, social integration,[31] gender, severity of illness, primary diagnosis[10] and length of ICU stay, although few of these factors appear to affect people in a consistent manner. Individual characteristics will also influence recovery although this is an area where there is limited research. For example, those with an emotion-focused coping style may have better mental HRQOL.[32]

FIGURE 8.3 Conceptual model of the factors that are included in the WHO International Classification of Functioning after critical illness.

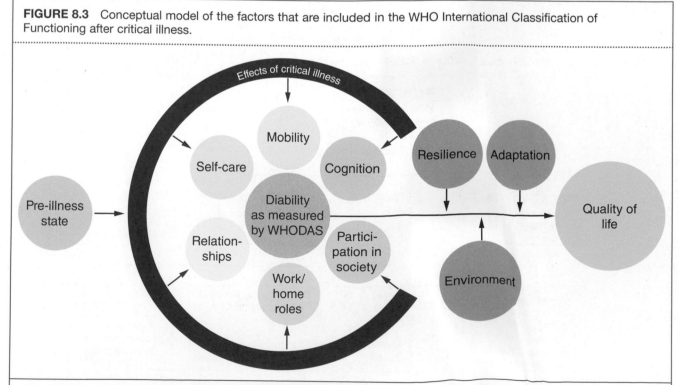

Source: Hodgson CL, Higgins AM, Bailey MJ, et al. The impact of COVID-19 critical illness on new disability, functional outcomes and return to work at 6 months: a prospective cohort study. Crit Care 2021;25(1):382. doi: 10.1186/s13054-021-03794-0.

ICU-acquired weakness

Critical illness myopathy (CIM), polyneuropathy (CIP) and neuromyopathy (CINM) syndromes occur in 50–100% of ICU survivors.[2,12] ICU-acquired weakness (ICU-AW) has come into use as a term that encompasses these syndromes of muscle wasting and functional weakness in patients with a critical illness who have no other plausible aetiology.[33,34] The three syndromes above form the subcategories of ICU-AW, with CINM used when both myopathy and axonal polyneuropathy are evident. Development of ICU-AW is associated with a number of risk factors that occur during intensive care treatment:[35,36]

- *critical illness:* sepsis, systemic inflammatory response syndrome (SIRS), multi-organ system failure, catabolic state
- *treatments:* mechanical ventilation, hyperglycaemia, hypoalbuminaemia, parenteral nutrition, glucocorticoids, sedatives, neuromuscular-blocking agents, immobility.

Local and systemic inflammation acts synergistically with bed rest and immobility to alter metabolic and structural function of muscles,[37] resulting in muscle atrophy and contractile dysfunction, loss of flexibility, CIP, heterotopic ossification and entrapment neuropathy.[34] Muscle wasting can occur rapidly, with patients losing up to 30% of their muscle mass within 10 days of being admitted to the ICU.[38] This muscle loss contributes to weakness, disability and a prolonged recovery period. These neuromuscular dysfunctions are diagnosed by clinical assessment, diagnostic studies (electrophysiology, ultrasound) or histology of muscle or nerve tissue.

The syndrome of ICU-AW manifests as prolonged weaning time, inability to mobilise and reduced functional capacity. Patients with ICU-AW also experience increased mortality.[39] ICU-AW has also been linked with reductions in both functional ability and HRQOL that may persist for months or years after discharge, although effects appear to be inconsistent across different groups of critical illness survivors.[40–42]

Clinical assessment

Clinical assessment includes identification of generalised weakness following the onset of a critical illness, exclusion of other diagnoses (e.g. Guillain–Barré syndrome) and measurement of muscle strength. Instruments are available to assess both volitional and non-volitional muscle strength.[43] Manual muscle testing is commonly assessed using the Medical Research Council (MRC) Scale,[44] a 0–5-point ordinal scale:

0 = no contraction

1 = flicker or trace of muscle contraction

2 = full range of active movement with gravity eliminated

3 = reduced power but active movement against gravity

4 = reduced power but active movement against gravity and resistance

5 = normal power against gravity and full resistance.

For patients who are awake and cooperative, each muscle group is assessed sequentially for strength and symmetry:

- *upper limb:* deltoid, biceps, wrist extensors
- *lower limb:* quadriceps, gluteus maximus, ankle dorsiflexion.

Weakness is evident in patients with an MRC sum score of <48 (<4 in all testable muscle groups); this should be retested after 24 hours. Weakness (<4 MRC Scale) is associated with worse survival up to 5 years after critical illness.[45]

Hand-held dynamometry and handgrip dynamometry can also be used to measure volitional muscle strength using a calibrated device for patients who are conscious and cooperative. The benefit of these measures is increased objectivity to obtain continuous data.[43] The sex-specific thresholds that are indicative of ICU-AW are males <11 kg force and females <7 kg force.[46] All volitional strength measurements may be affected by the level of awareness and cooperation of patients, as well as their motivation, although inter-rater reliability of the MRC sum score as well as hand-held dynamometry and handgrip dynamometry has been shown to be good to very good.[43,44]

Diagnostic testing

Electrophysiological testing (nerve conduction studies, needle electromyography) may be useful to differentiate between CIM and CIP, although this distinction is difficult and often not required in the clinical setting.[36,44] Histology for CIP is primarily noted as distal axonal degeneration in both sensory and motor fibres, while the characteristic findings in CIM are patchy loss of myosin (thick filaments), necrosis and fast-twitch fibre atrophy.[34]

Practice tip

Current clinical recommendations to limit muscle wasting in ICU include:

- minimising patient exposure to corticosteroids and neuromuscular-blocking agents
- limiting depth of sedation
- moderate glycaemic control
- early mobilisation and rehabilitation.

Psychological health

Psychological responses to a critical illness and patients' memories of experiences during an ICU admission have been extensively studied over the past two decades. Some survivors reported increased anxiety, including transfer anxiety (discharge from ICU),[3] depression,[47] post-traumatic stress,[4,48] hallucinations[49] and continuing cognitive dysfunction.[50,51]

Around 50% of survivors will demonstrate significant symptoms of anxiety, depression or post-traumatic stress,[52] and for many these endure for months or years.[52,53] These potentially result in additional health problems, reduced HRQOL,[10,54] reduction in social activities and functioning and failure to engage with rehabilitation programs.[55] Our understanding and awareness of these sequelae and their consequences has improved over the past two decades in part due to increased research activity and the implementation of follow-up services and programs.

Anxiety and depression

One of the challenges of determining prevalence rates is the variability of different measures, the timing of the assessment and the 'cut-off' scores used to determine 'caseness'. The most commonly used measure to assess anxiety and depression in this patient population is the Hospital Anxiety and Depression Scale (HADS),[56] and this was recommended as a core mental health outcome measure in recent consensus discussions.[57] This measure has two 'cut-off' scores to indicate possible (8–10) or probable (≥11) presence of either an anxiety or depressive disorder. Rates of anxiety and depression symptoms have been reported consistently at around 33% for anxiety and 39% for depression at around 12 months after discharge, when applying the lower 'cut-off' score. When the higher 'cut-off' score is applied, these rates reduce to 20% for a potential anxiety disorder at 6 months, reducing to 17% at 12–14 months,[3] and for a potential depressive disorder around 17% at 6 months, reducing to 13% at 12–14 months.[47] Although these latter figures do not represent a clinical disorder, it is clear that for many patients they have ongoing issues.[52] The impact of COVID-19 on critical care survivors' mental health outcomes has yet to be established, but parallels may be drawn from other similar events such as severe acute respiratory syndrome (SARS) and Middle East respiratory syndrome (MERS). A recent systematic review demonstrated that, more than 6 months after discharge, 30% of survivors had significant anxiety symptoms and 33% symptoms of depression.[58] This will have significant implications for care delivery after critical care discharge.

Patients often exhibit high levels of distress at the time of hospital discharge, and these tend to reduce over the first year.[59,60] However, the episodic timing of assessments may not fully capture the potentially varied trajectory of anxiety and depression symptoms, and establish whether full resolution is achieved, or identify a later onset problem. This is an under-researched area. One example is the work of Boede and colleagues,[61] who identified three trajectories of depression in sepsis survivors. These were severe and recovered, mild and recovered, and severe and persistent.[61] This highlights a number of important points; many patients will recover over time but there is a group of patients where this will not occur, symptoms do not reduce and this emphasises the need for ongoing assessment. Our lack of understanding of symptom trajectory has implications for both symptom monitoring and care delivery after ICU discharge.

Patients who have or have had psychological problems prior to intensive care are likely to continue to have or will develop these again after discharge,[47,52,62,63] and this has emerged as one of the main risk factors for subsequent problems. This highlights the importance of ascertaining a patient's pre-ICU mental health.

Although assessment of pre-ICU status is difficult, in some cases this information can be obtained from relatives or caregivers (e.g. if a patient is receiving antidepressant or anxiolytic medication or has seen a psychiatrist or psychologist). It is becoming increasingly clear that anxiety, depression and post-traumatic stress tend to coexist.[52,64] While these may be related, they have important distinct differences and treatments.

Few risk factors for anxiety and depressive symptoms have been consistently identified, but where they are, a useful way to categorise these is: (a) patient-related factors (age, gender, prior mental health problems, illicit drug use and alcohol consumption, educational level and employment status), (b) critical care factors (duration of mechanical ventilation, length of stay and pharmacological treatment) and (c) experience factors (traumatic memories and delirium).[65]

Increased risk of anxiety and depression symptoms is associated with being female (anxiety),[52,66] younger age (anxiety),[66] increased alcohol intake[66] and illicit drug use (mainly depression).[52] Although in a general population, younger age and being female is associated with increased stress symptoms, this is not always the case for ICU survivors, with Milton and colleagues finding that the peak age for psychological problems is between 49 and 65.[67] This is difficult to explain. Other patient-related factors include fewer years of education (mainly depression)[52] and lack of social support.[67] Indeed, Milton and colleagues[67] reported an odds ratio of 3.28 of developing anxiety when social support was low, and Bienvenu and colleagues[52] reported that survivors with some of these characteristics were two times more likely to have prolonged psychological problems. Critical care factors are associated with increased use of pharmacological regimens of opioid (anxiety and depression), benzodiazepines (mainly anxiety) and neuromuscular blockade (anxiety),[63,66] longer duration of mechanical ventilation[63] and a longer ICU stay in some studies, but this is not a consistent finding.[3,47,63,66] The latter finding has implications for subsequent follow-up services, which are often offered to patients based on length of stay. What has been consistent in the literature is the lack of predictive power of illness severity.[52,66] This may be a consequence of how illness severity is measured.[48]

The critical care experience is represented by delirium, delusional and/or traumatic memories. Patients who experience distressing memories that are often described as nightmares or hallucinations or extreme fear are more likely to have ongoing psychological problems.[47,63,67] These will be discussed further in this chapter.

Acute stress disorder/post-traumatic stress

Being critically ill is now a recognised risk factor to developing acute stress disorder and/or significant symptoms of post-traumatic stress.[68,69] PTSD occurs when someone has been exposed to a major life threat and having an episode of critical illness. Given the potential threat to life, a critical care environment that is noisy, with patients experiencing pain, sleep disturbances, invasive procedures and receiving high levels of sedative medications,[68] it is not surprising that these symptoms may develop. In the United Kingdom the prevalence of PTSD is 3.7% for men and 5.1% for women[69] and for intensive care survivors it is around 19.83%.[70] Signs of post-traumatic stress include four main symptom areas: intrusive thoughts, avoidant behaviours, negative alterations in cognitions and mood and hyperarousal symptoms (American Psychiatric Association). Individuals can re-experience a traumatic event through involuntary unwanted thoughts, often in the form of 'flashbacks' and/or 'nightmares'. Individuals experiencing these thoughts often develop avoidant behaviours in the belief this action will reduce the intrusive thoughts. Avoidant behaviours for intensive care patients can range from simply avoiding television programs about hospitals, not talking about their ICU experience to, more seriously, non-attendance at a follow-up clinic or other hospital outpatient appointments. The latter also compounds the issue of accurate prevalence. It is these two symptom clusters (avoidant behaviours and intrusive thoughts) that appear more prevalent in ICU survivors.[69] Negative alterations in cognitions and mood may include continuing self-blame or blaming others about the cause or consequences of the critical illness (American Psychiatric Association). Hyperarousal behaviours include difficulties in concentrating or falling asleep. ICU survivors may be preoccupied with these intrusive thoughts, concerns about future health issues, and may engage in negative health behaviours.[71] To be diagnosed with PTSD, symptoms must last longer than 1 month after the traumatic event, cause significant disruption to an individual's life and be distressing. Individuals are required to meet a number of criteria before a diagnosis of PTSD is considered, and in 2013 the American Psychiatric Association presented the DSM-V criteria for PTSD (see Box 8.1 for these criteria).[72]

What has been difficult to establish is whether it is being critically ill per se or the environment and treatments within critical care, or the experience itself that predispose survivors to develop PTSS.[48] Many symptoms of post-traumatic stress that patients experience in the initial days after intensive care discharge may be considered a normal reaction or an indication of an acute stress response, and it is important that practitioners clearly separate the normal from the abnormal response.[48] This is achieved by assessing the severity and duration of symptoms, and their effect on an individual's life.

Current research has concentrated on prevalence of symptoms at one point in time or group changes over time. Few have considered different trajectories. A number of these have been proposed within the wider PTSS/PTSD literature and include resilience, recovery, delayed reaction and chronic distress.[73] The first trajectory, as the name suggests, consists of those with few symptoms at any time point; a recovery trajectory represents those patients who may exhibit initial distress, but this reduces over time; a delayed reaction will result in symptoms worsening over time and those with chronic distress will have consistently high levels of symptoms.[73] In a study of trauma survivors over a period of 6 years, Bryant and colleagues described these four trajectories but included a fifth – worsening/recovery, where symptoms worsened over time and then recovered. The majority of patients were in the resilient group (73%) with 10% worsening, 8% worsening/recovery, 6% recovery and 5% chronic. An independent predictor of a poorer trajectory was admission to an ICU.[73] We do not know whether ICU patients experience similar trajectories, and this is an important gap. Recognising such trajectories has implications for what and how we deliver short- and long-term psychological therapies.

As with other psychological symptoms such as anxiety and depression, it has been difficult to establish the prevalence of PTSD after intensive care because of the use of self-report measures, different research designs, varied patient case mix and international variations in the delivery of intensive care. These variations have resulted in overestimation of the prevalence of PTSS and PTSD.[74] Patients may have significant PTSS without developing PTSD and it is mainly these symptoms that are assessed using the self-report measures. Reported prevalence of significant PTSS or PTSD varies, with an average of around 20% experiencing significant issues[70,71] during the first year after discharge. This is comparable to civilian war survivors[75] but higher than those exposed to other traumatic events.[70] In a recent systematic review, Righy and colleagues reported an overall prevalence of symptoms of 19.3%, but this ranged from 15.95% at 3 months to 20.25% over 12 months.[70] What is important is that, once PTSS or PTSD is established, it is enduring and without treatment may last for several years.

Similar to symptoms of anxiety and depression, there are certain risk factors that have been associated with PTSS, although also not consistently.[4,48] The literature is equivocal in relation to younger age,[48] female gender, length of stay and duration of mechanical ventilation[63] and sedation regimens,[4,48,66,76] with some studies identifying these as predictors and others not. The lack of consistency of age and gender is difficult to explain as these are cited as risk factors for PTSD in general.[69]

More consistent predictors include previous psychiatric history,[52,55] previous stressful events,[77] lack of social support,[67] educational level,[52] unemployment,[52,66] delirium and frightening and traumatic memories of intensive care,[48,52] care experience, use of restraints[78] and benzodiazepine use.[4,48]

Early signs of acute stress or depression are strong predictors of ongoing problems,[79] and this supports the

---

BOX 8.1

Post-traumatic stress disorder diagnostic criteria[72]

To diagnose PTSD, the person must have been exposed to death, threatened death or life-threatening injuries such as that experienced by intensive care patients and their families. Further, symptoms must be present for more than 1 month, must be distressing for the individual and interfere with different life areas, and must not be due to a medical condition or substance abuse.

1. **One or more: Reliving the event (also called re-experiencing symptoms).** Memories of the traumatic event can come back at any time. They can feel very real and scary. For example:
   - You may have nightmares.
   - You may feel like you are going through the event again. This is called a flashback.
   - You may see, hear, or smell something that causes you to relive the event. This is called a trigger. News reports, seeing an accident or hearing fireworks are examples of triggers.

2. **One or more: Avoiding things that remind you of the event.** You may try to avoid situations or people that remind you of the trauma event. You may even avoid talking or thinking about the event. For example:
   - You may avoid crowds, because they feel dangerous.
   - You may avoid driving if you were in a car accident or if your military convoy was bombed.
   - If you were in an earthquake, you may avoid watching movies about earthquakes.
   - You may keep very busy or avoid getting help so you don't have to think or talk about the event.

3. **Two (or more): Having more negative thoughts and feelings than before the event.** The way you think about yourself and others may become more negative because of the trauma. For example:
   - You may feel numb – unable to have positive or loving feelings towards other people – and lost interest in things you used to enjoy.
   - You may forget about parts of the traumatic event or not be able to talk about them.
   - You may think the world is completely dangerous, and no one can be trusted.
   - You may feel guilt or shame about the event, wishing you had done more to keep it from happening.

4. **Two (or more): Feeling on edge or keyed up (also called hyperarousal).** You may be jittery, or always alert and on the lookout for danger. You might suddenly become angry or irritable. For example:
   - You may have a hard time sleeping.
   - You may find it hard to concentrate.
   - You may be startled by a loud noise or surprise.
   - You might act in unhealthy ways, like smoking, abusing drugs or alcohol, or driving aggressively.

Source: US Department of Veterans Affairs. PTSD: National Center for PTSD. Available from: https://www.ptsd.va. gov/understand/what/ptsd_basics.asp. [Accessed 12 February 2023].

---

importance of early assessment. Ongoing sleep problems, which can be prevalent after intensive care, have been associated with PTSS in one study.[79] However, it is unclear whether poor sleep quality mediates PTSS or PTSS causes sleep problems. This is an area for further study.

We have limited understanding of factors that protect against the development of psychological problems. One significant gap in the literature is the role of personality traits and resources. There is little research in this patient group exploring the role of coping strategies, self-efficacy, resilience, optimism and social support.[48] Given the inconsistencies about risk factors in the literature, understanding these will likely assist us to better predict those at risk.

What is evident in the literature is the effect of patients' subjective intensive care experiences[4,79,80] and traumatic memories.[67] These experiences, reported as unpleasant memories of being in ICU, consistently predict subsequent poorer psychological outcomes.[48,67,81] They are discussed later in this chapter. While this evidence appears strong, that related to delirium is contradictory. No consistent relationship between delirium and subsequent emotional outcome has been identified.[64,82]

Memories and perceptions

An interesting finding in the literature is the lack of support for both length of stay and illness severity as consistent risk factors for subsequent post-traumatic stress reactions.[48,66] If being in intensive care is an independent risk factor, it would be expected that both of these would be key factors with one related to the 'threat to life' and the other increased exposure to the environment. But this is not the case. However, patient-reported memories or lack of memories both consistently emerge as significant factors. This is one of the unique features of being in intensive care: patients have limited recall for factual events and often report large gaps where they remember very little about their critical illness. Some patients will report upsetting or traumatic factual memories such as pain, oxygen masks on their face and difficulty breathing.[83] However, frequently, patients' accounts include disturbing recollections with memories of 'odd perceptual experiences',[81,84,85] 'nightmares' or 'hallucinations'.[83] While not all patients experience these, those who do so tend to report memories that are persecutory in nature,[83] are often associated with feelings of being elsewhere,[86] or fighting for survival.[84] These memories often seemed 'real' and were distressing to patients at the time and may be recalled with the same detail years afterwards.[86] For some, real and unreal memories become blurred, which leads to fear and a feeling of being out of control.[84] For some time it was thought that having factual memories was a protective mechanism[48] to reduce negative psychological outcomes and early work was promising. However, findings have not been replicated consistently,[48] and further work is needed to understand the consequences of these experiences. A range of information-giving interventions has been tested to address these 'memory gaps' and will be discussed later in this chapter.

Cognitive dysfunction

Cognitive impairment in survivors of critical illness has been recognised and measured only in the past decade. Although there is some variation in prevalence and severity, in general more than 50% of survivors report cognitive impairment at the time of hospital discharge and approximately one-quarter continue to have problems 12 months later. Cognitive problems include memory, attention and executive function, which in turn includes reasoning and decision making. These can have significant impact upon the daily life of not just patients but also families and have been linked to other aspects of recovery such as psychological health,[87,88] as well as longer-term dementia.

Various factors have been linked to cognitive impairment including premorbid cognitive function, delirium, hypoxaemia, hypotension, glucose dysregulation, use of sedatives, sepsis and inflammation and sleep efficiency (Table 8.1).[50,89–91] Although many of these relationships appear inconsistent, and may be more problematic in specific subgroups of the critical care population, delirium has repeatedly been shown to be highly predictive of cognitive impairment, particularly in regard to duration of delirium. Characteristics such as age and previous health have not been found to be related to the development of cognitive impairment, with young, previously healthy patients just as likely as older patients to develop problems.

> **Practice tip**
>
> When conducting discharge education for patients and their families, don't forget to tell them that problems with memory, decision making and reasoning are common after critical illness. These will resolve over time for many but, because they persist for some, you may want to suggest where patients and carers may access information about critical illness, recovery and seeking help. (See Online resources at end of this chapter.)

TABLE 8.1

Summary of reviews of cognitive impairment

AUTHORS	NUMBER OF STUDIES	DURATION OF FOLLOW-UP	INCIDENCE OF COGNITIVE IMPAIRMENT	OTHER FINDINGS OF NOTE
Wilcox et al 2013[50]	31 studies: ARDS pts – 11 studies Mixed ICU pts – 20 studies	ARDS pts: 1–241 months Mixed pts: 2 weeks–8.3 years	ARDS pts hosp discharge: 70–100% 1 yr: 46–78% 2 yrs: 25–47% Mixed pts hosp discharge: 39–51% 3–6 mths: 13–79% 12 mths: 10–71%	Mixed findings in relation to the potential predictors of CI including hypoxaemia, pre-existing depression. Some evidence that CI may be more severe or more frequent following sepsis, hypoglycaemia and longer duration of delirium.
Wolters et al 2013[89]	19 studies: ARDS pts – 7 studies mixed ICU pts – 12 studies	2–156 months	ARDS pts: 4–56% Mixed pts: 4–62%	Studies that used only screening test data reported lower rates of CI than studies using neuropsychological testing. No identified higher risk of CI in studies of elderly patients.
Kohler et al 2019[90]	14 studies: non-surgical ICU patients	26–468 weeks (9 years)	17–78%	Rates of cognitive impairment tended to improve over time. Delirium was only risk factor identified.

ARDS = acute respiratory distress syndrome; CI = cognitive impairment
NB: many individual studies are included in multiple reviews

Measuring patient outcomes following a critical illness

The measurement of health outcomes after critical illness is vital – both to determine patient recovery and to inform decisions about ongoing care. Measures related to hospital utilisation, disability, HRQOL and physical, psychological and cognitive function are discussed.

It is unclear how long patient outcomes following critical illness should be measured, but given that ongoing compromise exists for months to years post-hospital discharge, such measurement should continue for a similar time, for example 6–12 months. In the research setting there is a need to extend follow-up of patients beyond 2 years to determine the long-term morbidities associated with critical illness and care.[1]

Hospital utilisation after critical illness

A relatively new measure that incorporates mortality and all hospitalisations into a single measure is days alive and out of hospital (DAOH).[92] This patient-centred outcome measures a patient's ability to survive, return home, and remain free from hospital re-admission.[93] A systematic review and meta-analysis found that participants allocated to rehabilitation groups spent a mean difference of over 9 days alive and out of hospital over 6 months.[94] The Treatment of Invasively Ventilated Adults with Early Activity and Mobilisation (TEAM III) trial is the largest critical care rehabilitation study to be undertaken, and identified DAOH to be the primary outcome.[95] As information for this outcome is relatively easy to obtain and has patient-centred and economic implications, it is likely that this will become commonly incorporated into future research studies. Additionally, it is an outcome measure that could be used by intensive care units to evaluate patient outcomes over time or compare patient outcomes between similar ICUs.

Measures of disability after critical illness

The World Health Organization Disability Assessment Scale 2.0 (WHODAS 2.0) is a 12-level assessment instrument that provides a standardised method for measuring health and disability. The WHODAS 2.0 was developed from a comprehensive set of International Classification of Functioning, Disability and Health (ICF) domains that are sufficiently reliable and sensitive to measure the difference made by a given intervention. The six domains listed were selected to be applicable across cultures in all adult populations:

1 *cognition* – understanding and communicating
2 *mobility* – moving and getting around
3 *self-care* – attending to one's hygiene, dressing, eating and staying alone
4 *getting along* – interacting with other people
5 *life activities* – domestic responsibilities, leisure, work and school
6 *participation* – joining in community activities, participating in society.

The full version has 36 questions and the short version 12 questions. The questions relate to difficulties experienced by the respondent in the above six domains during the previous 30 days. The versions can be administered by a lay interviewer, by the patient or by a proxy (i.e. family, friend or carer). For both versions, general population norms are available.[96]

Measures of HRQOL after a critical illness

The range of instruments available to measure both disability and HRQOL is large. A generic instrument is appropriate for the heterogeneous critical care population and should contain certain attributes: measures baseline HRQOL, is responsive to change over time in a recovering critically ill patient and has demonstrated reliability and validity. Two instruments have been recommended by stakeholder consultations as part of a core outcome set for use after acute respiratory failure.[57] The Short Form Health Survey has been widely used and validated in this population (Fig. 8.4)[1] and includes shorter and longer versions. It measures eight health concepts (physical functioning, physical role limitations, vitality, bodily pain, general health perception, social functioning, emotional role limitations, and mental health) each of which can be scored separately or condensed to two component scores (physical and mental).[97] The EuroQual Five dimension (EQ-5D) is the second instrument. It is also a self-report measure of problems experienced across five domains (mobility, self-care, usual activities, pain/discomfort, anxiety/depression). Two versions are available: one with a three-point response format and one with five (increases the options and sensitivity of the instrument).[98] Following the recommendations from the stakeholder consensus, use of the core outcome measures (Fig. 8.4) is recommended.[99] Table 8.2 summarises the main disability and HRQOL instruments used for patients following a critical illness.[100–109]

Measures of physical function following a critical illness

Numerous instruments have been developed to examine the physical capacity of individuals, usually focusing on functional status ranging from independent to dependent.[110,111] The range of instruments available to measure various aspects of physical function has evolved in the past decade, particularly in regard to the availability of measures useful within the intensive care environment.

The MRC-Sum Score is a manual muscle test and handgrip dynamometry comprises muscle strength tests (described earlier) that can be performed both during a patient's stay in ICU and after a period of critical illness. Additionally, previously available measures such as the Six

FIGURE 8.4 Core outcome measurement set for clinical research in acute respiratory failure survivors. EQ-5D = EuroQual Five dimension; HADS = Hospital Anxiety and Depression Scale; IESR = Impact of Event Scale Revised; MoCA = Montreal Cognitive Assessment; 6MWT = Six Minute Walk Test; SF-36 = Short Form 36.

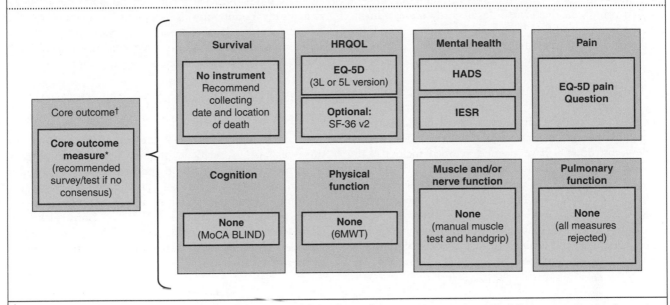

Source: Dinglas VD, Faraone LN, Needham DM. Understanding patient-important outcomes after critical illness: a synthesis of recent qualitative, empirical, and consensus-related studies. Curr Opin Crit Care 2018;24(5):401–9. doi: 10.1097/MCC.0000000000000533.

TABLE 8.2

Disability and HRQOL instruments used for patients following a critical illness

INSTRUMENT	ITEMS	CONCEPTS/DOMAINS
World Health Organization Disability Assessment Scale 2.0 (WHODAS 2.0)[96]	36 (full version) and 12 (short version)	International Classification of Functioning, Disability and Health (ICF) six domains: cognition, mobility, self-care, getting along (interacting with other people), life activities (domestic responsibilities, leisure, work and school), participation
Medical outcomes study (SF-36)[100,101]	36	Physical: functioning, role limitations, pain, general health Mental: vitality, social, role limitations, mental health; health transition; variable response levels (2–5)
Euro–Qol-5 dimensions (EQ-5D)[102,103]	5	Mobility, self-care, usual activities, pain/discomfort, anxiety/depression; 3 or 5 response levels; cost-utility index
15D[103,108]	15	Mobility, vision, hearing, breathing, sleeping, eating, speech, elimination, usual activities, mental function, discomfort, distress, depression, vitality and sexual activity; 5-point ordinal scale (1 = full function; 5 = minimal/no function)
Quality of Life–Italian (QOL–IT)[109]	5	Physical activity; social life; perceived quality of life; oral communication; functional limitation; varied response levels (4–7)
Assessment of Quality of Life (AQOL)[105]	15	Illness (3 items); independent living (3 items); physical senses (3 items); social relationships (3 items); psychological well-being (3 items); 4 response levels; enables cost–utility analysis
Quality of Life–Spanish (QOL–SP)[106]	15	Basic physiological activities (4 items); normal daily activities (8 items); emotional state (3 items)
Nottingham Health Profile (NHP)[107]	45	Experience: energy, pain, emotional reactions, sleep, social isolation, physical mobility Daily life: employment, household work, relationships, home life, sex, hobbies, holidays

Minute Walk Test (6MWT), the Barthel Index and the Functional Independence Measure (FIM) are valuable to assess patients after critical illness. Physical activity associated with cardiac or pulmonary dysfunction may be assessed using perceived breathlessness (dyspnoea) during exercise by the modified Borg scale,[112] ranging from 0 (no dyspnoea) to 10+ (maximal). The Borg scale is commonly used with other physical activity instruments, such as the 6MWT.[113]

The limitation of many of these measures is that they require alert, cooperative patients able to participate in functional activities, whereas critically ill patients are not always able to participate to this level. In response, a range of new instruments have been developed including the Chelsea critical care physical assessment tool (CPAx),[114] the Physical Function ICU Test (PFIT-s),[115] the ICU Mobility Scale (IMS)[116] and the Functional Status Score – ICU (FSS-ICU).[117] Each of these measures has been designed to measure a slightly different aspect of function and they have different benefits and limitations that mean they should be used for different purposes, as outlined in Fig. 8.4. The

Physical Function in Critical Care (PaciFIC) is a new 10-item outcome measure that has been developed incorporating aspects of the PFIT-s and the De Morton Mobility Index (DEMMI) that is intended for use across the acute care continuum.[118] Rigorous evaluation of the robustness of the PaciFIC tool is required in future studies across multiple settings/countries to substantiate the reliability, responsiveness, validity and predictive utility of this tool.[118]

Measures of psychological function after a critical illness

The psychological recovery process and trajectory for survivors of a critical illness remains important. Instruments that assess mood and mental well-being after a critical illness focus on psychological constructs, including anxiety, depression, fear and post-traumatic stress symptoms (Table 8.3).[57,119–124] Constructs that relate to an individual during a critical illness episode also include agitation and confusion/delirium (discussed further in Chapter 6).

TABLE 8.3

Examples of common measures of psychological function after critical illness

INSTRUMENT	MEASUREMENT	SCORE RANGE
Impact of Event Scale (IES);[119] IES-R[120]	15-item; assesses levels of post-traumatic distress; two subscales: intrusive thoughts, avoidance behaviours; revised form (IES-R) adds hyperarousal subscale (7 items).	Frequency of thoughts over past 7 days; 0 = no thoughts; 5 = often; higher scores indicate greater distress: scores ≥11 on either subscale indicates a clinical disorder.
Hospital Anxiety and Depression Scale (HADS)[56]	14-item (4-point scale); measures mood disorders in non-psychiatric patients; focuses on psychological rather than physical symptoms of anxiety and depression.	Score ≥11 on either subscale indicates a clinical disorder.
Center for Epidemiologic Studies – Depression Scale (CES–D)[121]	20-item self-report scale assesses frequency and severity of depressive symptoms experienced in the previous week.	Score range 0–60; higher scores reflect increased symptoms and severity.
Kessler 10 (K-10)[122]	10-item (5-point scale) self-report measure of non-specific psychological distress over the past 4 weeks.	Score range 10–50; higher scores reflect greater distress.
Post-traumatic stress disorder (PTSD) Check List (PCL)[123]	20-item (5-point scale) self-report assessment of symptoms of PTSD corresponding to DSM-V criteria.	Score range 20–100; higher scores reflect increased symptoms of PTSD.
Post-Traumatic Stress Symptoms 14 (PTSS 14)[124]	14-item extended version of the PTSS 10 to cover all aspects of PTSD consistent with Diagnostic and Statistical Manual of Mental Disorders (DSM-IV) symptom categories.	2 parts: Part A – Assessment of traumatic memories from ICU; Part B – Post-traumatic stress disorder symptoms; score range 14–98.
Intensive Care Psychological Assessment Tool (IPAT)[83]	14-item scale covering hopelessness, tension, panic, delusions, intrusive memories, sadness, sleeplessness, communication difficulties, hallucinations and disorientation.	Non-parametric factor analysis reduces this scale to 10 and awaiting further psychometric testing. 3 response formats: no; yes a bit; yes a lot. Trigger scores still require to be confirmed.

Assessment of psychological outcomes has relied mainly on self-report questionnaires administered via either a postal or telephone survey or a structured interview format. Few studies have included clinical assessments such as the Clinical Administered PTSD Scale, the 'gold standard' for diagnosing PTSD.[125] This means, therefore, that such questionnaires are screening tools that can be used to identify individuals at risk of developing a significant clinical problem. They are not diagnostic, and this is an important point when considering designing, implementing and evaluating any intervention. A number of standardised questionnaires have demonstrated reliability and validity in this patient group, but the use of different questionnaires makes it difficult to generalise findings. The Intensive Care Psychological Assessment Tool (IPAT)[83] is slightly different in that it has been designed specifically for the purpose of identifying which ICU patients are at risk of subsequent distress.

These instruments often include 'cut-off' or 'threshold' scores that enable screening for the presence or severity of a disorder. For example, a score of 8–10 on either subscale of the HADS indicates the possible presence of a disorder, while a score of 11 or above indicates probable presence of such a condition.[56] One limitation of these self-report measures is that, while sensitivity (the ability to correctly identify all patients with the condition) can be high, specificity (the ability to correctly identify all patients without the condition) is less easy to determine, and therefore the incidence of psychological distress may be overstated. This makes estimation difficult and is one of the challenges in establishing the actual magnitude of psychological distress after a critical illness. Other challenges include the recruitment of different cohorts or subgroups of patients (e.g. patients with adult respiratory distress syndrome or acute lung injury). Variations in the international provision of ICU services also mean that differences may exist in case mix in the areas of illness severity, planned or unplanned admissions, ages and reasons for admission. The recommendations of core outcome measures will go some way to reducing these variations.

Measures of cognitive function after a critical illness

Cognitive or neuropsychological assessment of critical illness survivors has only become more common in the past 10–15 years. Comprehensive and lengthy testing batteries exist, although those used in studies examining recovery after critical illness have tended to favour slightly shorter testing (Table 8.4).[126–135] Most of these tests require more than 30 minutes for this assessment, which may tire some people, particularly early in their recovery phase after critical illness. In addition, some of the tests need to be administered by qualified psychology or psychiatry personnel, although some instruments that can be administered by research personnel, both in person and over the telephone, have recently been developed. Neuropsychological instruments are non-invasive. Repeated testing with the same instrument on multiple

occasions may lead to practice effects; in other words, the critical illness survivor learns how to perform better on the test. Hence, instruments with multiple versions prove beneficial in some circumstances. Where neuropsychological testing can be carried out, it enables assessment of the nature, severity, prevalence and incidence of cognitive impairment.[126] Cross-cultural differences do exist in some of the domains measured in neuropsychological assessment, so where comparison with normative data is required for analysis and interpretation, for example in the Repeatable Battery for the Assessment of Neuropsychological Status (RBANS), country-specific data are required.[127]

Scales such as the Montreal Cognitive Assessment (MoCA)[129] or the Telephone Interview of Cognitive Status – Modified version (TICS-M)[131] are now frequently used to measure cognitive function after critical illness, as these provide a balance between length and detail, and have versions that can be administered over the telephone. The MoCA is available for use in more than 80 languages and dialects and has received increasing support for use after critical illness.[57]

Improving recovery following a critical illness

Survivors of critical illness experience multidimensional and protracted compromise over weeks to months and often extending to years.[22,23] Interventions to improve recovery following critical illness can be delivered at multiple time points in the critical illness continuum. Some of these interventions are the primary responsibility of the multidisciplinary critical care team, are delivered while the patient remains in ICU and are directed towards limiting the detrimental effects of intensive care or promoting recovery as early as possible. Other interventions to improve recovery may be delivered after the patient has left the ICU but remains in the hospital, or after discharge from hospital. These later strategies are often delivered in collaboration with other members of the healthcare team. Although there is only limited evidence of specific strategies that are effective in improving recovery, the body of evidence unpinning these strategies is starting to build.

Interventions delivered in the ICU

Interventions to improve long-term recovery that are delivered in the ICU focus on strategies to minimise the detrimental effects of critical illness and the associated care. These interventions might focus on one aspect of care (e.g. sedation minimisation or early mobilisation) or might be multidimensional (e.g. targeting sedation minimisation, optimisation of sleep and limitation of the use of restraints as a combined intervention). The majority of interventions delivered within the ICU are targeted at improving physical function. Consensus recommendations have been made to guide clinicians to perform rehabilitation interventions with patients that minimise the risk of exercise-related adverse events.[136] A systematic review and meta-analysis has confirmed that exercise

TABLE 8.4

Neuropsychological instruments to assess cognitive function in patients following a critical illness

INSTRUMENT	MEASUREMENT	SCORE RANGE / COMMENTS
Mini-Mental State Examination (MMSE)[128]	11 items in 5 domains including orientation, memory, attention and concentration, delayed recall, language.	Score of ≤23, or 2 points below maximum in any domain, indicates the presence of moderate-to-severe cognitive impairment; 5–10 minutes to administer.
Montreal Cognitive Assessment (MoCA)[129]	8 cognitive domains including attention and concentration, executive functions, memory, language, visuoconstructional skills, conceptual thinking, calculations, orientation.	Requires 10 minutes to administer; total possible score is 30 with scores ≥26 indicating normal cognition; alternative versions and a version that can be conducted over the phone (referred to as MoCA – Blind) are available.
Repeatable Battery for the Assessment of Neuropsychological Status (RBANS)[130]	Measurement of multiple areas of cognitive functioning across 5 indices covering the domains of immediate memory, visuospatial/constructional, language, attention, delayed memory.	Must be administered by a qualified psychologist; designed as a paper-and-pencil screening battery; has multiple versions to allow for multiple testing without problems of practice effect.
The Telephone Interview of Cognitive Status – Modified (TICS-M)[131,132]	Abbreviated 13-item measure that includes 4 domains: orientation; registration, recent memory and delayed recall (memory); attention/calculation; semantic memory, comprehension and repetition (language).	Maximum score of 39; requires approximately 10 minutes to administer.
Trail Making Test[133]	Part A requires the rapid connection of 25 sequential numbers; part B measures visual scanning, visuospatial sequencing and cognitive set shifting by requiring connection of 25 alternate numbers and letters in ascending sequence.	Score is obtained as the number of seconds required to complete each part (the examiner points out errors as they occur, so correction time is included); this is then converted to a 10-point scale, with 10 as the best possible score in each part; Total score ≤12 indicates impairment.
Wechsler Memory Scale – Revised (WMS-R)[134]	Measures different memory functions in adults; 7 subtests including spatial addition, symbol span, design memory, general cognitive screener, logical memory, verbal paired associates, visual reproducing.	Performance reported as 5 index scores including auditory memory, visual memory, visual working memory, immediate memory, delayed memory.
Wechsler Adult Intelligence Scale – Revised (WAIS-R)[135]	Measures intelligence in adults and older adolescents; although it is used to measure intelligence rather than cognition, it is often used in combination with WMS-R.	10 core subtests and 5 supplemental subtests; 4 index scores (verbal comprehension and working memory that combine to provide Verbal IQ Index; perceptual organisation and processing speed that combine to provide Performance IQ Index) as well as the overall full-scale IQ.

interventions with critically ill patients are safe, with less than 3% potential safety events. Most of these events were minor and transient, with only rare events having any consequence for patient management.[137]

Interventions to minimise ICU-AW, particularly in relation to muscle deconditioning from disuse (e.g. sedation, bed rest), have recently focused on active exercises and mobility, including while patients are intubated and ventilated.[138] Multiple studies and quality improvement projects have demonstrated the safety and feasibility of ICU-based early mobilisation interventions, often with short-term benefits for patients when interventions are delivered early in ICU,[139] although few interventions have

yet had sufficient testing to show sustained improvement in patient outcomes. A systematic review and meta-analysis have shown that physical rehabilitation interventions that commenced in ICU improved physical function at hospital discharge and reduced ICU and hospital length of stay. However, physical rehabilitation does not appear to affect mechanical ventilation duration, muscle strength, HRQOL and mortality.[140] Interventions that have shown initial benefit in small studies include in-bed cycling using an ergometer,[141] a combination of functional electrical stimulation and cycling,[142] early exercise and mobilisation,[143] and studies that focus on multidisciplinary or team-based activities to promote mobilisation[144] (Table 8.5).[145–155] This

TABLE 8.5

Studies of in-ICU mobility over the past 10 years

FIRST AUTHOR/ COUNTRY	DESIGN	N/AGE	COHORT	INTERVENTION	MAIN FINDINGS
Denehy et al 2013,[145] Australia	Single-centre RCT	150/61	>5 days in ICU.	Exercise rehabilitation in ICU, ward and outpatients.	No major adverse events. No significant differences at hospital discharge, 3, 6 or 12 months in 6MWD, TUG, AQOL, SF-36.
Kayambu et al,[146] Australia	Single-centre RCT	50/64	Adult sepsis patients MV >48 h.	Individualised early targeted physical rehabilitation prescribed by ICU physiotherapist for 30 min 1–2/day until ICU discharge.	No differences in physical function measured by Acute Care Index of function, and quality of life (SF-36) at 6-months post-hospital discharge.
Schaller et al 2016,[144] multinational (Austria/ Germany/USA)	Multi-centre RCT	200/65	Surgical ICU patients, MV <48 h and expected to require at least another 24 hours MV.	Goal-directed mobilisation using interprofessional approach incorporating closed loop communication and an algorithm to drive mobilisation.	Improved level of mobilisation. Reduced SICU LOS in intervention group (7 (5–12) vs 10 (6–15) days, $P = 0.0054$). Increased functional mobility at hospital discharge. More adverse events in intervention group compared with control group (25 (2.8%) vs 10 (0.8%)) but no serious adverse event.
Morris et al 2016,[147] USA	Single-centre RCT	300/56	Ventilated (via ETT or NIV) adults, and (PaO_2/FiO_2) ratio less than 300.	Standardised rehabilitation therapy (SRT) passive range of motion, physical therapy, and progressive resistance exercises, and administered by a rehabilitation team; 3 separate sessions every day of hospitalisation for 7 days per week.	No difference in hospital LOS between groups. Similarly, SRT did not affect ventilator-free days or ICU-free days. Functional related and HRQOL outcomes were similar for participants' hospital discharge.
Moss et al 2016,[148] USA	Multi-centre RCT	120/53	Adult who required MV for at least 5 days (modified to MV for at least 4 days after 78 patients had been recruited).	Intensive PT program therapy 7 days/week for up to 28 days after randomisation or until the patient successfully completed 5 stages of the progressive rehabilitation program.	No differences in long-term physical functioning and ICU and hospital free days. Intervention did not commence until ICU Day 8.
Fossat et al 2018,[149] France	Single-centre RCT	314/66	Adults admitted to a medical/surgical ICU.	Cycle ergometry + FES (separate session)	No between group differences in MRC-SS at ICU discharge or HRQOL at 6 months
Eggmann et al 2018,[150] Switzerland	Single-centre RCT	115/64	Adults expected to stay on MV for at least 72 hours and were independent prior to ICU admission.	Progressive early rehabilitation program, including in-bec cycling, resistance training and functional activities.	No differences between group for 6MWD distance and ability to perform ADLs at hospital discharge.

Continued

TABLE 8.5

Studies of in-ICU mobility over the past 10 years—cont'd

FIRST AUTHOR/ COUNTRY	DESIGN	N/AGE	COHORT	INTERVENTION	MAIN FINDINGS
Sarfati et al. 2018,[151] France	Single-centre RCT	125/64	Adults MV for 3 or more days.	Daily passive tilting in addition to standardised rehabilitation therapy.	Did not improve muscle strength measured by the MRC-SS at ICU discharge.
Wright et al 2018,[152] United Kingdom	Multi-centre RCT	308/62	Adults receiving at least 48 hours of mechanical ventilation (including NIV).	90 minutes of targeted physical rehabilitation per day, compared with the control group target of 30 min/day (both Monday to Friday).	No between groups difference in the physical outcomes measured by the Physical component Summary (PcS) measure of SF-36 at 6 months.
Schujmann et al. 2020,[153] Brazil	Single-centre RCT	135/53	Adult ICU patients who were independent prior to hospital admission with an ICU of greater than 4 days.	Progressive early rehabilitation program including functional electric stimulation, in-bed cycling, resisted exercise and functional exercise.	Improved Barthel Index Score after ICU discharge. Control group 76 ± 20, Intervention group 97 ± 5.
Nickels et al 2020,[154] Australia	Single-centre RCT	72/ 56	Adults MV more than 48 hours and recruited within 96 hours of admission.	Progressive in-bed cycling daily for 30 min 6 days per week.	No difference between groups in rectus femoris cross-sectional area and other strength and functional outcomes.
Nakamura et al 2021,[155] Japan	Single-centre RCT	117/68	Adult medical and surgical ICU patients.	Electrical stimulation combined with high-protein or medium-protein nutritional intake.	High-protein delivery provided better muscle volume maintenance, but only with active early rehabilitation.
Hodgson et al 2022,[156] Australia, New Zealand, UK, Ireland, Germany, Brazil	Multi-centre RCT	750/60	Adult MV medical and surgical patients.	Increased early mobilisation compared with usual care	No difference in primary outcome Days Alive and Out of Hospital at Day 180. The intervention was associated with increased adverse events.

6MWD = 6-minute walk distance; ADLs = Activities of Daily Living; AQOL = Assessment of Quality of Life instrument; ETT = Endo tracheal Tube; FES = Functional Electrical Stimulation; HRQOL = Health related Quality of Life; ICU = Intensive Care Unit; LOS = Length of stay; MRC-SS = Medical Research Council Sum Score; MV = mechanical ventilation; NIV = non-invasive ventilation; n.s. = not significant; OT = occupational therapy; PT = physiotherapy; SF-36 = Short Form 36 Health Survey; SICU = Surgical ICU; RCT = randomised controlled trial; TUG = Timed Up and Go test.

is an area where there is increased interest and research activity, with the potential to have an improved evidence base in the near future.

In addition, strategies primarily directed towards minimising sedation, and therefore facilitating more patient movement, have demonstrated effectiveness (see Chapter 6 for further details).

Effective implementation of any of these interventions requires a change in how critical care clinicians care for their patients and this requires a cultural shift with a multidisciplinary team approach and changes in care processes.[157-160] Strong leadership in the process, beliefs about capability and the benefits of the activity, as well as a culture of safety and improvement within the ICU, are perceived as important factors to aid implementation of interventions such as early mobilisation. Involving the family in interventions to support recovery, including early mobilisation, has also been proposed[161] and, although this has not yet been confirmed in research as an effective strategy, it has great potential and few disadvantages if appropriate preparation is provided.

Implementation of 'early' activity for ICU patients relates to after clinical stabilisation is evident, and includes those still intubated. Exercise interventions that can commence early (within 3 days) with critically ill patients may be more effective at improving patient outcomes (function, mobility and quality of life) compared with exercise interventions commencing later (more than 5 days) following ICU admission[162]

Factors to ensure patient safety during mobilisation have been identified, including confirming that a patient has sufficient cardiovascular and respiratory reserve and cognitive function.[136,163] Potential barriers to mobilisation during mechanical ventilation (e.g. acute lung injury, vasoactive infusions) have also been examined and include clinical instability, excessive staff turnover, morale issues and a lack of respect among disciplines.[157,160] Physiotherapy recommendations for physical deconditioning include development of 'exercise prescriptions' and 'mobilising plans'.[164] Activities range from passive stretching and range of motion exercises for limbs and joints to positioning, resistive muscle training to electrical stimulation, aerobic training and muscle strengthening and ambulation.[165,166] Specific mobility activities include:

- in-bed (range of motion, roll, bridge, sitting on the edge of the bed)
- standing at the side of the bed
- standing on the tilt-table
- transfer to and from bed to chair
- marching on the spot
- walking
- neuromuscular electrical stimulation (NMES)
- in-bed cycle ergometry (with and without NMES)
- whole-body vibration.

Patient support for each activity ranges from assistance with 1–2 staff members through to independence under supervision. Inspiratory muscle training (IMT) has been used for weakness associated with prolonged mechanical ventilation, using electronic resistance and mechanical threshold training devices. Results from a systematic review demonstrate that IMT is effective at increasing inspiratory muscle strength and reducing the duration of mechanical ventilation.[167]

Mobilisation practices have been explored in multicentre point prevalence and observational assessments in various countries, with widespread reports of limited mobilisation, especially while patients are mechanically ventilated, despite widespread recognition of the benefits of such mobilisation.[168-172] As noted earlier, a culture of patient wakefulness and early in-ICU activity and mobility is advocated but challenged by the status quo of work practices and health professional role delineations.[160,173] A re-engineering of work processes and practices to promote patient activity is therefore required to ensure optimal outcomes for survivors of a critical illness. Few reports of achieving this change are available, but initial evidence in single centres suggests it is possible to change practice in the local environment using various interventions such as those based on effective teamwork to increase the number of patients mobilising.[174-176]

Interventions to improve psychological recovery

Although there is now strong empirical evidence that some patients experience significant psychological dysfunctions after a critical illness, it is less clear how and when to treat these symptoms. Ongoing psychological problems can impact significantly upon daily life, and this impact should not be underestimated. Increased anxiety and post-traumatic stress symptoms may result in individual ruminating and worrying about subsequent physical health issues, and potentially adopting negative health behaviours such as non-attendance at hospital appointments,[68] and may contribute to an acute re-admission to hospital.[177] This supports the importance of identifying and addressing these issues.

A key role for critical care services is in early detection and identification of patients at risk.[169] Routine and regular monitoring of psychological recovery are included as a quality standard in recent UK National Institute for Health and Care Excellence (NICE) guidelines.[69] Monitoring should be through systematic and standardised screening activities, closely monitoring identified patients and referring to appropriate specialties where appropriate, to optimise their recovery trajectory while not introducing any further harm. Once a patient has a diagnosis of anxiety, depression or post-traumatic stress, treatment should be delivered by an appropriately trained health professional and follow national guidelines, for example NICE guidelines (NICE CG113, NICE CG90, NICE CG116). Recognising the impact of ongoing psychological problems for both patient and families, the UK Intensive Care Society support the inclusion of a clinical psychologist as part of a critical care team. However, in a recent UK survey, 43.3% of services reported that a clinical psychologist was not part of the team and in follow-up services this number reduced to 28%.[178]

Psychological interventions include the importance of developing a trusting relationship between patient and therapist, provision of pragmatic and practical support,[179] 'watchful waiting' incorporating routine and regular monitoring, and psychoeducation to assist patients understand and normalise their experiences and recurring memories. The last item is where information giving is useful.[68] Other therapies include cognitive behavioural therapy (CBT) – trauma focused, eye movement desensitisation and reprocessing (EMDR).[69] It is important that decisions to implement therapies are taken by appropriately trained healthcare professionals.

There may be scope for some specific interventions to be administered when the patient is in intensive care, prior to hospital discharge or when they are at home. There is some evidence to support the minimisation of sedation, particularly with benzodiazepines, while the patient is in ICU, and strategies to achieve this that are relevant to each ICU context should be implemented (see Chapter 6 for more details).[180,181]

The evidence on interventions specifically for critical care patients is limited and a systematic review highlighted the paucity of high-quality studies.[182] In a large multicentre study a nurse-led preventative psychological intervention delivered in intensive care was evaluated; however, improved psychological health for patients was not demonstrated.[183] The role of information giving has been explored also, with varying results (this will be discussed later in the chapter), with some studies indicating benefit and others not. Systematic follow-up services may offer appropriate assessment and support during recovery for individuals identified with psychological disturbances. Intensive care follow-up clinics where patients have the opportunity to discuss their intensive care experiences and receive information about what had happened to them could be a useful intervention, although there are currently no empirical data to support this,[184] and further research work is required. In a recent quasi-experimental study evaluating a nurse-led follow-up program, more severe PTSS in the experimental group receiving the follow-up were reported.[185] This is both an interesting and a concerning finding. Differences between groups go some way in explaining this finding, with the experimental group being younger and having a shorter stay in intensive care, but the authors themselves highlight the need to be cautious about timing interventions and the importance of 'watchful waiting'. We must be mindful also of the premise of 'doing no harm' when developing, delivering and evaluating interventions.

Interventions that include provision of information

Giving information is thought to be important in 'bridging' a perceived memory gap that might help a patient make sense of their critical illness experience, and so improve psychological outcome. This may involve a structured discharge planning process, provision of information through ICU follow-up clinics (see below) or return visits to the ICU, or the use of diaries for intensive care patients. A diary approach has been adopted in a number of European ICUs.[186,187] However, there has been a great deal of variation in how the diaries are compiled and viewed by a patient, as well as how much support is offered to them to explain diary content.[188] To this point in time the use of such diaries tends to be atheoretical,[189] with limited long-term exploration of the effect of the diary intervention on patient outcomes. Evidence of the benefit of diaries remains inconsistent, with some multicentre studies finding benefit[190] while others show no benefit.[191] Inconsistency across outcomes is also reported, with some benefits shown for depression and quality of life, but not for PTSD or anxiety.[192]

The provision of a personalised discharge summary as a component of discharge planning is another approach. This has been shown to be both desired by some survivors[193] and feasible to produce, with an average time to completion of 15 minutes.[194] However, the effectiveness of this as an intervention to reduce negative psychological outcomes has not yet been tested and further research is required.

One further study focusing on psychological rehabilitation after discharge home was conducted to examine the effect of consultations that focused on provision of information and constructing an illness narrative.[195] In this multicentre, non-blinded, randomised controlled trial (RCT), patients received a nurse-led intervention delivered at the ICU follow-up clinic about 3 months after hospital discharge, with further telephone-based consultations 5 and 10 months after discharge. No differences in quality of life were identified between the two groups of patients, although when anxiety was categorised as low or high there were fewer anxious patients in the intervention group, suggesting there may be some benefit in some patients.[195]

It is important to note, however, that not all patients wish to be reminded of their ICU experience; this is especially the case for patients who demonstrate avoidant behaviours. Two studies have reported that approximately 50% of patients do not wish to know what has happened to them during intensive care via receiving a diary,[196,197] or alternatively prefer to receive a simplified version of information in a discharge summary.[198] Others may wish not to be reminded of being critically ill but instead wish to concentrate on recovery.[199] We have to be mindful of not doing harm and that interventions may not be appropriate for all patients at the same point in time.

Interventions to improve cognitive recovery

Although general aspects of critical care such as sedation, delirium prevention and sleep management might affect cognitive function during recovery,[200] strategies that specifically target cognitive function have only recently been developed and tested. Given the nature of critical illness, it is rare that these interventions will be delivered while the patient is still in the ICU but might be delivered in the acute care ward or after discharge home. Interventions frequently rely on computer- or app-based training to provide cognitive training. Despite some initial promising results, more studies are required to determine whether these types of interventions are effective in widespread groups of patients.[201]

Ward-based post-ICU recovery

Follow-up services for survivors of a critical illness have occurred sporadically in individual units with interested clinician teams, but there is currently no widespread systematic approach to recovery and rehabilitation and the management of physical, psychological or cognitive dysfunction.[1]

Commencement or continuation of rehabilitation activities in the general wards after discharge from ICU highlights a potentially different set of challenges, particularly in terms of physiotherapy resources, involvement of other medical teams and compliance to a prescribed plan. Although some cohorts of critically ill patients (e.g. pulmonary, cardiac, stroke, brain injury) have defined rehabilitation pathways, patients with other clinical presentations may not be routinely prescribed a rehabilitation plan or be able to access relevant services.

For patients who survive to ICU discharge, up to 10% will die prior to hospital discharge.[202,203] Some work in Europe on prognosis post-ICU discharge using the 4-point Sabadell Score (0 = good prognosis, 1 = long-term poor prognosis, 2 = short-term poor prognosis, 3 = expected hospital death) demonstrated that subjective intensivist assessment was able to predict the risk of patient mortality and, conversely, those patients potentially suitable for rehabilitation.[204]

Specific ward-based rehabilitation interventions following ICU discharge are beginning to be investigated. Designing and implementing such an intervention is challenging because of the heterogeneous nature of intensive care patients, who have increasing complexity and ill-defined recovery trajectories. Furthermore, these patients tend to be 'scattered' throughout the hospital, making coordination of care post-ICU difficult. Some exploratory work in the UK implemented a generic rehabilitation assistant to support enhanced physiotherapy and nutritional rehabilitation in collaboration with ward-based staff.[205,206] Following the MRC framework for complex interventions, the intervention focused primarily on physical recovery from ICU discharge to 3 months. The generic rehabilitation assistant was able to provide information and explanation of the patient's time in intensive care, facilitate discussions with the multidisciplinary team, assist in goal setting and provide enhanced ward-based rehabilitation.[207] Results demonstrated no significant improvement in primary outcomes (Rivermead Mobility Index) but patients were significantly more satisfied with physiotherapy, nutritional support, coordination of care and information provision.[208] In contrast, in one small Austrian study a ward-based early rehabilitation study was effective in reducing hospital length of stay and improving functional recovery, while also being safe and cost effective.[209] Given the dearth of evidence, and inconsistent results, in this area, further research is required to test specific interventions during the post-ICU hospital period aimed at improving the recovery trajectory and health outcomes for patients with limited physical function. As noted with in-ICU rehabilitation, the optimal duration, intensity and frequency of interventions is not yet clear. A potential shortfall of evaluated post-ICU rehabilitation programs is that a generic approach to rehabilitation has been applied. An individualised rehabilitation program that is tailored to the patients' unique requirements may be more beneficial. For example, if the patient presents with psychological issues following ICU discharge, but not physical issues, a physical rehabilitation program is unlikely to be of additional benefit.

Recovery after hospital discharge

Of patients who survive their critical illness to hospital discharge, up to 20% will die within 12 months, and their risk of death is three times higher than for the general population.[202,210] Functional recovery can be delayed in some individuals for 6–12 months or longer. In an Australian study, 60% of survivors who were working or studying prior to ICU had not returned to work or study at 6 months. Further, 50% of survivors presented with a mild disability and 25% presented with a moderate–severe disability.[23] There were similar findings in a Norwegian study, where only half of 194 patients had returned to work or study 1 year after surviving their critical illness.[211] An Australian multicentre prospective cohort study reported that the independent predictors of death or developing a new disability were higher severity of illness and admission diagnosis. In comparison with surgical admissions patients with diagnosis of cardiac arrest, sepsis or trauma had higher odds of death or new disability.[212] A longitudinal study in the USA reported that pre-ICU frailty status was associated with increased post-ICU disability and new nursing home admission among ICU survivors, and death among all admissions.[28]

There is, however, only limited research and mixed study findings identifying specific interventions during the post-hospital period that may improve a patient's recovery trajectory and health outcomes. Most work has involved practice evaluations or studies of outpatient 'ICU follow-up' clinics, while there is some work exploring home-based programs that predominantly focus on physical recovery.

ICU follow-up programs

Systematic follow-up for survivors of a critical illness after hospital discharge emerged in the UK in the early 1990s, after a number of government reviews on the cost and effectiveness of critical care services highlighted the need to evaluate longer-term patient outcomes, in particular quality of life.[213] These reviews recognised that patients had sequelae that were best understood and managed by ICU clinicians, but importantly also provided support to those relatives supporting the patient's recovery. Globally, over the last decade there have been a range of follow-up rehabilitation programs including attendance at a follow-up clinic, peer support and information giving; however, despite the many imperatives of the need for some form of follow-up, there is limited evidence of their benefits.[214,215] When patients are discharged from hospital after an episode of critical illness, they and their relatives face an uncertain future. As described earlier in this chapter, patients can face a prolonged recovery period with significant physical and psychological problems and their caregivers have to negotiate what is often complex healthcare systems in order to ensure that the correct services and care are provided to their loved ones.[216] This is likely to be even more crucial with the impact of the COVID-19 pandemic.[217]

Follow-up clinics

Intensive care follow-up clinics were established in the UK in the early 1990s,[218] driven by a few interested and committed intensive care clinicians, and are now common in a number of countries. While much of follow-up care is community centred, patients and caregivers find this continued contact with critical care practitioners helpful and reassuring.[215] A recent UK survey indicated that approximately 74% of UK ICUs offered a follow-up service, a rapid rise from the 27% that existed in 2014.[178] There is no one uniform model of a follow-up clinic and many UK clinics are delivered by a multidisciplinary team consisting mainly of nurses, intensivists, physiotherapists and in a number of cases a clinical psychologist, dietitian, pharmacist and speech therapist. Many clinics restrict patients invited to return to those with an ICU length of stay of at least 3 or 4 days. This decision is often based upon resources rather than evidence; patients who have a shorter stay may also have subsequent physical and psychological problems.[219]

Common practice is to invite patients to attend a first clinic appointment approximately 2–3 months after discharge from intensive care or hospital, although timing has to be flexible given the length of hospital stay for some patients. For many, one appointment is sufficient,[220] but others have continuing problems and may need to return on a number of occasions. Some clinics offer return appointments up to 1 year after discharge, determined on an individual patient basis.

Patients who attend clinical appointments tend to report high levels of satisfaction[220] and an Australian study reported that many patients who had received prolonged ventilation indicated that a follow-up clinic would have been beneficial.[221] Despite the evidence of ongoing problems for patients, follow-up services still tend to be underfunded[222] and lack resources in terms of clinic space and administrative support. These can act as barriers to implementation. When there is good interprofessional collaboration, adequate funding and clear and defined operational processes, clinics are more likely to be implemented successfully.[222] Patients and caregivers will have additional attendance challenges and these include ongoing physical problems, financial issues especially if they live a distance from the clinic, work commitments, or importantly because of significant PTSS including avoidant behaviours.[219,223]

Clinic activities

It is undeniable, though, that much of our understanding of the longer-term consequences of critical illness has emerged as a consequence of patients attending follow-up clinics. Patient progress is reviewed for identification of subsequent problems and, crucially, timely referral to appropriate services for further treatment and support. One of the benefits of follow-up is to support patients and caregivers navigate the social and healthcare systems and referral to third-sector or community services can be crucial. Box 8.2 provides examples of areas to be addressed during a clinic visit.

Coordination of care for these patients with complex needs often includes multiple outpatient appointments and investigations at a time when they are least able to cope with this complexity. An additional patient benefit of returning to a follow-up clinic is in supporting them to negotiate their way through this complex care, to coordinate outpatient appointments and to have someone who knows them and understands critical care help them understand and interpret the entire critical illness and recovery experience.[177,224] The benefits of having an opportunity to discuss their experiences with intensive care staff should not be underestimated and, as such, effective communication skills are vital for those delivering ICU clinic services.[225] Patients value being able to speak to 'experts' about their experience, being given information about what happened to them in ICU and also receiving reassurances about the length of time that recovery will take and that their distressing memories are common.

BOX 8.2

Considerations to be addressed at an ICU follow-up clinic[178]

- Assessment of physical, psychological, cognitive and social function using appropriate tools.
- Refer to appropriate specialties when necessary (e.g. psychology, ENT), including third sector and community support.
- Review of medications.
- Consider rehabilitation prescription and plan according to patient recovery trajectory.

Clinics also offer patients and relatives the opportunity to comment on their care both during and after intensive care.[177,220] This is important not just for the patient but also to inform care delivery.

Peer support groups

As with many interventions, a 'one-size fits all' approach will exclude those for whom the intervention is not perceived as appropriate or sufficiently flexible. Recent years have seen an increase in peer support groups.[226] Their premise is to offer support from other intensive care survivors and strategies to improve recovery, and to share experiences.[227] The latter is particularly beneficial for both patients and caregivers in helping to 'normalise' the experience. A range of models have been developed including professional- or patient-led community-based groups such as the ICU Steps group in Dundee, Scotland. This is probably the most common model and tends to be held away from the hospital (e.g. churches). Other models include psychology-led groups, which will be led by a professional with mental health expertise, or the support is embedded with a routine follow-up clinic and supported by both patients and the multidisciplinary team. An online approach can be offered also, which can have different formats, and can be accessed by those with group accessibility issues. Aimed at caregivers, groups based within ICU which tend to be run by ICU staff can be delivered, and one approach that is developing is one-to-one peer mentoring where individual patients are linked to someone further on in their recovery journey.[227] As with follow-up clinics there is limited empirical supporting evidence, but patients and caregivers value these, staff find them beneficial and for this group they particularly value engaging with recovering patients.[225] Similar enablers and barriers exist in the setting up and implementation of these groups. Accessing participants and staffing, along with funding to ensure sustainability, are key issues.[227] A more unique challenge given that many groups and/or individuals meet outside the clinical environment is that of risk management both for the organisation and for staff and volunteers. These involve training, support and, for staff, key governance issues. It is important for both groups that they are adequately prepared to undertake these roles and offered continuing support.

Web-based resources

Telephone contact in the initial weeks after discharge can offer some reassurance to patients and also identify early problems. There may be an opportunity to incorporate technological solutions such as web-based resources, which can provide information about the recovery process and incorporate feedback. One such site is http://edinburghroyalinfirmary.criticalcarerecovery.com/, where patients can access a range of information about the recovery process, be directed to other sites and importantly how to access help.

Summary

In summary we now have increasing evidence of the significant burden of health issues faced by critical illness survivors. We know that many face a prolonged and difficult recovery period that will include physical and psychological problems and that these affect not just the patient themselves but also family members and other carers. Patients' lives may be significantly altered after critical illness, placing a social and economic burden on the patient and family, but also on the healthcare system. Quality of life is often viewed as diminished and we now need to look to focusing on two main areas by identifying (a) effective interventions that can be delivered by the multidisciplinary team that will reduce these burdens and improve overall life quality and (b) the patients most likely to benefit from these interventions. Currently health systems are not organised in such a way as to recognise these problems and, therefore, care after ICU discharge tends to be ad hoc and does not follow a recognised rehabilitation pathway. There is a need to look at and learn from other long-term conditions and to adopt approaches that recognise the concept of survivorship after critical illness[20,228] and develop the appropriate systems and processes that will improve life after critical care.

Case study

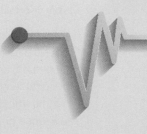

Mr Shaw was a 38-year-old man previously active, independent, and employed full time in an office role. He is married with two young primary school aged children. He was admitted to ICU with acute pancreatitis. He required 25 days of mechanical ventilation, 10 days renal support and a tracheostomy, which was inserted after 12 days. He was in ICU for a total of 30 days. He was sedated through much of the time that he was mechanically ventilated, though in keeping with local policy his sedation was light and titrated according to his Richmond Agitation Sedation Scale (RASS) score. Mr Shaw's wife and young children visited him each day while he was in the ICU. Midway through his stay in ICU, Mr Shaw frequently appeared to be agitated and occasionally aggressive. Mrs. Shaw appeared upset by her husband's behaviour and reported that it was out of character for him. At times, Mr Shaw appeared to recognise his wife and children but they were unsure. After 2 weeks, the physiotherapist assessed Mr Shaw's strength and calculated an MRC Sum Score of 38/60. He remained globally weak when he was discharged from ICU with an MRC Sum Score of 45/60. Mr Shaw was transferred to the high-dependency unit for 3 days and then to a surgical ward for a further 10 days. He was then admitted to an inpatient rehabilitation facility as his level of physical and cognitive function remained well below his pre-illness capabilities. He was discharged home once he was able to manage a flight of stairs independently. An ICU liaison nurse saw him on one occasion prior to him being transferred from the acute ward to rehabilitation. He reported he had some confusion, appeared fatigued and was suffering from hallucinations. He was sent an outpatient appointment to attend the nurse-led ICU follow-up clinic around 3 months after hospital discharge.

Mr Shaw and his wife both attended the clinic. He was progressing slowly and struggling with everyday activities. He was easily tired, and still having some hallucinations from his time in ICU although he was not distressed by these. He indicated to the clinic nurse that he could not understand why he was so tired, and found it hard to concentrate. He was unable to return to his office work. This was causing him and his wife some financial worries and concerns about his progress, and making Mr Shaw irritable and short-tempered with his children. Mrs Shaw was tearful and appeared to be struggling to cope. Mr Shaw had visited his general practitioner (GP) and described these problems, but was told it was quite common to experience these after a lengthy hospitalisation and time in the ICU.

CASE STUDY QUESTIONS

1 What is ICU-acquired weakness? Discuss strategies that can be initiated within the ICU to reduce the development of ICU-acquired weakness.

2 With the exception of the ICU follow-up clinic, Mr Shaw was discharged from rehabilitation without any planned follow-up services. What follow-up services could be suitable to refer Mr Shaw for further follow-up? Are these services available in your local area?

RESEARCH VIGNETTE

Wang YT, Lang JK, Haines KJ et al. Physical rehabilitation in the ICU: a systematic review and meta-analysis. Crit Care Med 2022;50(3):375–88.

Abstract

Objectives: Significant variability exists in physical rehabilitation modalities and dosage used in the ICU. Our objective was to investigate the effect of physical rehabilitation in ICU on patient outcomes, the impact of task-specific training and the dose–response profile.

Methods: A systematic review and meta-analysis by two independent reviewers of randomised controlled trials and controlled clinical trails investigating physical rehabilitation commencing in the ICU in adults was completed. Outcomes included muscle strength, physical function, duration of mechanical ventilation, ICU and hospital length of stay, mortality and health-related quality of life.

Results: Sixty trials were included, with a total of 5352 participants. Random-effects pooled analysis showed that physical rehabilitation improved physical function at hospital discharge (standardised mean difference, 0.22; 95% CI, 0.00–0.44) and reduced ICU length of stay by 0.8 days (mean difference, −0.80 d; 95% CI, −1.37 to −0.23 d), and hospital length of stay by 1.75 days (mean difference, −1.75 d; 95% CI, −3.03 to −0.48 d). Physical rehabilitation had no impact on the other outcomes. The intervention was more effective in trials where the control group received low-dose physical rehabilitation and in trials that investigated functional exercises.

Conclusions: Physical rehabilitation in the ICU improves physical function and reduces ICU and hospital length of stay. However, it does not appear to impact other outcomes.

Critique

This systematic review and meta-analysis synthesised results from 60 trials. Key findings were that physical rehabilitation was more effective in trials where the usual care group received low-dose physical rehabilitation, and interventions that included functional exercises were more effective than trials that compared non-functional experimental interventions such as in-bed cycling and electrical stimulation of muscles.

These results indicate that, for critical care studies to demonstrate a difference between the intervention group and the usual care group, the differences between the physical rehabilitation received need to be substantial. This is often difficult to achieve; sites that complete physical intervention studies are often highly active intensive care units where the culture of early rehabilitation may already be established. Results suggest that the dose–response relationship of physical rehabilitation in the critically ill patient is not linear, with a diminishing benefit at higher doses.

Non-functional experimental interventions often may show benefits such as improved maintenance of muscle mass.[149,154,155] However, these physiological gains may not translate to functional gains.

Overall, the meta-analysis found no differences between the groups for mortality, muscle strength, mechanical-ventilation-free days and HRQOL. However, physical rehabilitation begun in the ICU improved physical function at hospital discharge and reduced ICU and hospital length of stay compared with usual care.

In conclusion, ICUs should have physical rehabilitation services available for up to 5 days per week, as this dosage led to improved physical function and health service outcomes. Wherever possible, functional exercises should be used.

Learning activities

1 Identify the changes in patient care in your ICU that could be introduced to facilitate improved long-term recovery and rehabilitation of your patients. Discuss the potential barriers and facilitators to implementing these changes.

2 Develop an educational plan for delivery in your ICU to help staff understand the physical, psychological and cognitive challenges that patients experience after critical illness.

3 Patients transferred from ICU to the ward may have complex care needs. In your hospital, if a follow-up service was planned how do you think this should be developed?

4 Review the evidence for psychological assessment and management of patients after a critical illness and intensive care admission.

Online resources

ICU Steps, https://icusteps.com

Johns Hopkins Outcomes After Critical Illness and Surgery, https://www.hopkinsmedicine.org/pulmonary/research/outcomes_after_critical_illness_surgery/index.html

Patient-Centered Outcomes Research Institute, https://www.pcori.org/

Patient-reported Outcome and Quality of Life Instruments Database (PROQOLID), https://eprovide.mapi-trust.org/about/about-proqolid

PTSD NICE guidelines, https://www.nice.org.uk/guidance/NG116

Rehabilitation after critical illness in adults, https://www.nice.org.uk/Guidance/CG83, Mobilisation-network.org, http://www.mobilisation-network.org/Network/Welcome.html

Further reading

Azoulay E, Vincent JL, Angus DC, et al. Recovery after critical illness: putting the puzzle together – a consensus of 29. Crit Care 2017;21(1):296. Available from: https://ccforum.biomedcentral.com/articles/10.1186/s13054-017-1887-7. [Accessed 12 February 2023].

Berry A, Beattie K, Bennett J, et al. Physical activity and movement: a guideline for critically ill adults. St Leonards, NSW: Agency for Clinical Innovation, NSW Government; 2017. Available from: https://www.aci.health.nsw.gov.au/__data/assets/pdf_file/0005/239783/ACI17131_PAM_Guideline.pdf. [Accessed 12 February 2023].

National Institute for Health and Care Excellence (NICE). Rehabilitation after critical illness. NICE CG83. London: NICE; 2009. Available from: https://www.nice.org.uk/CG83; 2009 [Accessed 12 February 2023].

References

1. Needham DM, Davidson J, Cohen H, et al. Improving long-term outcomes after discharge from intensive care unit: report from a stakeholders' conference. Crit Care Med 2012;40:502–9. doi: 10.1097/CCM.0b013e318232da75.

2. Jolley SE, Bunnell AE, Hough CL. ICU-Acquired weakness. Chest 2016;150:1129–40. doi: 10.1016/j.chest.2016.03.045.

3. Nikayin S, Rabiee A, Hashem MD, et al. Anxiety symptoms in survivors of critical illness: a systematic review and meta-analysis. Gen Hosp Psychiatry 2016;43:23–9. doi: 10.1016/j.genhosppsych.2016.08.005.

4. Parker AM, Sricharoenchai T, Raparla S, et al. Posttraumatic stress disorder in critical illness survivors: a metaanalysis. Crit Care Med 2015;43:1121–9. doi: 10.1097/ccm.0000000000000882.

5. Rabiee A, Nikayin S, Hashem MD, et al. Depressive symptoms after critical illness: a systematic review and meta-analysis. Crit Care Med 2016;44:1744–53. doi: 10.1097/CCM.0000000000001811.

6. Wilcox ME, Brummel NE, Archer K, et al. Cognitive dysfunction in ICU patients: risk factors, predictors, and rehabilitation interventions. Crit Care Med 2013;41:S81–98. doi: 10.1097/CCM.0b013e3182a16946.

7. Reay H, Arulkumaran N, Brett SJ. Priorities for future intensive care research in the UK: results of a James Lind Alliance priority setting partnership. J Intensive Care Soc 2014;15:288–96. doi: 10.1177/175114371401500405.

8. Angus DC, Carlet J. Surviving intensive care: a report from the 2002 Brussels Roundtable. Intensive Care Med 2003;29:368–77. doi: 10.1007/s00134-002-1624-8.

9. Iwashyna TJ. Trajectories of recovery and dysfunction after acute illness, with implications for clinical trial design. Am J Respir Crit Care Med 2012;186:302–4. doi: 10.1164/rccm.201206-1138ED.

10. Oeyen SG, Vandijck DM, Benoit DD, et al. Quality of life after intensive care: a systematic review of the literature. Crit Care Med 2010;38:2386–400. doi: 10.1097/CCM.0b013e3181f3dec5.

11. Gerth AMJ, Hatch RA, Young JD, et al. Changes in health-related quality of life after discharge from an intensive care unit: a systematic review. Anaesthesia 2019;74:100–8. doi: 10.1111/anae.14444.

12. Appleton RT, Kinsella J, Quasim T. The incidence of intensive care unit-acquired weakness syndromes: a systematic review. J Intensive Care Soc 2015;16:126–36. doi: 10.1177/1751143714563016.

13. Fan E, Dowdy DW, Colantuoni E, et al. Physical complications in acute lung injury survivors: a two-year longitudinal prospective study. Crit Care Med 2014;42:849–59. doi: 10.1097/ccm.0000000000000040.

14. Salluh JI, Wang H, Schneider EB, et al. Outcome of delirium in critically ill patients: systematic review and meta-analysis. BMJ 2015;350:h2538. doi: 10.1136/bmj.h2538.

15. Castillo MI, Cooke M, Macfarlane B, et al. Factors associated with anxiety in critically ill patients: a prospective observational cohort study. Int J Nurs Stud 2016;60:225–33. doi: 10.1016/j.ijnurstu.2016.05.007.

16. Sidiras G, Patsaki I, Karatzanos E, et al. Long term follow-up of quality of life and functional ability in patients with ICU acquired weakness – a post hoc analysis. J Crit Care 2019;53:223–30. doi: 10.1016/j.jcrc.2019.06.022.

17. Eggmann S, Luder G, Verra ML, et al. Functional ability and quality of life in critical illness survivors with intensive care unit acquired weakness: a secondary analysis of a randomised controlled trial. PLoS One 2020;15:e0229725. doi: 10.1371/journal.pone.0229725.

18. Thomas S, Mehrholz J. Health-related quality of life, participation, and physical and cognitive function of patients with intensive care unit-acquired muscle weakness 1 year after rehabilitation in Germany: the GymNAST cohort study. BMJ Open 2018;8(7):e020163. doi: 10.1136/bmjopen-2017-020163.

19. Iwashyna TJ, Netzer G, Langa KM, et al. Spurious inferences about long-term outcomes: the case of severe sepsis and geriatric conditions. Am J Respir Crit Care Med 2012;185:835–41. doi: 10.1164/rccm.201109-1660OC.

20. Kean S, Salisbury LG, Rattray J, et al. 'Intensive care unit survivorship' – a constructivist grounded theory of surviving critical illness. J Clin Nurs 2017;26:3111–24. doi: 10.1111/jocn.13659.

21. World Health Organization (WHO). WHO policy on disability. Geneva: WHO; 2021. Available from: https://www.who.int/about/policies/disability. [Accessed 12 February 2023].

22. Herridge MS, Tansey CM, Matte A, et al. Functional disability 5 years after acute respiratory distress syndrome. N Engl J Med 2011;364:1293–304. doi: 10.1056/NEJMoa1011802.

23. Hodgson CL, Udy AA, Bailey M, et al. The impact of disability in survivors of critical illness. Intensive Care Med 2017;43:992–1001. doi: 10.1007/s00134-017-4830-0.

24. Hodgson CL, Higgins AM, Bailey MJ, et al. The impact of COVID-19 critical illness on new disability, functional outcomes and return to work at 6 months: a prospective cohort study. Critical Care 2021;25:382. doi: 10.1186/s13054-021-03794-0.

25. Griffiths J, Hatch RA, Bishop J, et al. An exploration of social and economic outcome and associated health-related quality of life after critical illness in general intensive care unit survivors: a 12-month follow-up study. Crit Care 2013;17:R100. doi: 10.1186/cc12745.

26. Kamdar BB, Suri R, Suchyta MR, et al. Return to work after critical illness: a systematic review and meta-analysis. Thorax 2020;75:17–27. doi: 10.1136/thoraxjnl-2019-213803.

27. Dowdy DW, Eid MP, Sedrakyan A, et al. Quality of life in adult survivors of critical illness: a systematic review of the literature. Intensive Care Med 2005;31:611–20. doi: 10.1007/s00134-005-2592-6.

28. Ferrante LE, Pisani MA, Murphy TE, et al. The association of frailty with post-ICU disability, nursing home admission, and mortality: a longitudinal study. Chest 2018;153:1378–86. doi: 10.1016/j.chest.2018.03.007.

29. Bagshaw SM, Stelfox HT, Johnson JA, et al. Long-term association between frailty and health-related quality of life among survivors of critical illness: a prospective multicenter cohort study. Crit Care Med 2015;43:973–82. doi: 10.1097/ccm.0000000000000860.

30. Orwelius L, Nordlund A, Nordlund P, et al. Pre-existing disease: the most important factor for health related quality of life long-term after critical illness: a prospective, longitudinal, multicentre trial. Crit Care 2010;14:R67. doi: 10.1186/cc8967.

31. Orwelius L, Backman C, Fredrikson M, et al. Social integration: an important factor for health-related quality of life after critical illness. Intensive Care Med 2011;37:831–8. doi: 10.1007/s00134-011-2137-0.

32. Dettling-Ihnenfeldt DS, de Graaff AE, Beelen A, et al. Coping style and quality of life in Dutch intensive care unit survivors. Rehabil Psychol 2016;61:165–72. doi: 10.1037/rep0000084.

33. Barreiro E. Models of disuse muscle atrophy: therapeutic implications in critically ill patients. Ann Transl Med 2018;6:29. doi: 10.21037/atm.2017.12.12.

34. Stevens RD, Marshall SA, Cornblath DR, et al. A framework for diagnosing and classifying intensive care unit-acquired weakness. Crit Care Med 2009;37:S299–308. doi: 10.1097/CCM.0b013e3181b6ef67.

35. de Jonghe B, Lacherade JC, Sharshar T, et al. Intensive care unit-acquired weakness: risk factors and prevention. Crit Care Med 2009;37:S309–15. doi: 10.1097/CCM.0b013e3181b6e64c.

36. Parry SM, Puthucheary ZA. The impact of extended bed rest on the musculoskeletal system in the critical care environment. Extreme Physiol Med 2015;4:16. doi: 10.1186/s13728-015-0036-7.

37. Winkelman C. Mechanisms for muscle health in the critically ill patient. Crit Care Nurs Q 2013;36:5–16. doi: 10.1097/CNQ.0b013e318275071d.

38. Puthucheary ZA, Rawal J, McPhail M, et al. Acute skeletal muscle wasting in critical illness. JAMA 2013;310:1591–600. doi: 10.1001/jama.2013.278481.

39. Hermans G, Van Mechelen H, Clerckx B, et al. Acute outcomes and 1-year mortality of intensive care unit-acquired weakness. A cohort study and propensity-matched analysis. Am J Respir Crit Care Med 2014;190:410–20. doi: 10.1164/rccm.201312-2257OC.

40. Bein T, Weber-Carstens S, Apfelbacher C. Long-term outcome after the acute respiratory distress syndrome: different from general critical illness? Curr Opin Crit Care 2018;24:35–40. doi: 10.1097/MCC.0000000000000476.

41. Dettling-Ihnenfeldt DS, Wieske L, Horn J, et al. Functional recovery in patients with and without intensive care unit-acquired weakness. Am J Phys Med Rehabil 2017;96:236–42. doi: 10.1097/phm.0000000000000586.

42. Villeneuve PM, Clark EG, Sikora L, et al. Health-related quality-of-life among survivors of acute kidney injury in the intensive care unit: a systematic review. Intensive Care Med 2016;42:137–46. doi: 10.1007/s00134-015-4151-0.

43. Vanpee G, Hermans G, Segers J, et al. Assessment of limb muscle strength in critically ill patients: a systematic review. Crit Care Med 2014;42:701–11. doi: 10.1097/CCM.0000000000000030.

44. Fan E, Cheek F, Chlan L, et al. An official American Thoracic Society clinical practice guideline: the diagnosis of intensive care unit-acquired weakness in adults. Am J Respir Crit Care Med 2014;190:1437–46. doi: 10.1164/rccm.201411-2011ST.

45. Dinglas VD, Aronson Friedman L, Colantuoni E, et al. Muscle weakness and 5-year survival in acute respiratory distress syndrome survivors. Crit Care Med 2017;45:446–53. doi: 10.1097/CCM.0000000000002208.

46. Ali NA, O'Brien JM, Jr., Hoffmann SP, et al. Acquired weakness, handgrip strength, and mortality in critically ill patients. Am J Respir Crit Care Med 2008;178:261–8. doi: 10.1164/rccm.200712-1829OC.

47. Rabiee A, Nikayin S, Hashem MD, et al. Depressive symptoms after critical illness: a systematic review and meta-analysis. Crit Care Med 2016;44:1744–53. doi: 10.1097/ccm.0000000000001811.

48. McGiffin JN, Galatzer-Levy IR, Bonanno GA. Is the intensive care unit traumatic? What we know and don't know about the intensive care unit and posttraumatic stress responses. Rehabil Psychol 2016;61:120–31. 2016/05/20. doi: 10.1037/rep0000073.

49. McKinley S, Fien M, Elliott R, et al. Health-related quality of life and associated factors in intensive care unit survivors 6 months after discharge. Am J Crit Care 2016;25:52–8. doi: 10.4037/ajcc2016995.

50. Wilcox ME, Brummel NE, Archer K, et al. Cognitive dysfunction in ICU patients: risk factors, predictors, and rehabilitation interventions. Crit Care Med 2013;41:S81–98. doi: 10.1097/CCM.0b013e3182a16946.

51. Pandharipande PP, Girard TD, Jackson JC, et al. Long-term cognitive impairment after critical illness. N Engl J Med 2013;369:1306–16. doi: 10.1056/NEJMoa1301372.

52. Bienvenu OJ, Friedman LA, Colantuoni E, et al. Psychiatric symptoms after acute respiratory distress syndrome: a 5-year longitudinal study. Intensive Care Med 2018;44:38–47. doi: 10.1007/s00134-017-5009-4.

53. Kapfhammer HP, Rothenhausler HB, Krauseneck T, et al. Posttraumatic stress disorder and health-related quality of life in long-term survivors of acute respiratory distress syndrome. Am J Psychiatry 2004;161:45–52.

54. de Miranda S, Pochard F, Chaize M, et al. Postintensive care unit psychological burden in patients with chronic obstructive pulmonary disease and informal caregivers: a multicenter study. Crit Care Med 2011;39:112–18. doi: 10.1097/CCM.0b013e3181feb824.

55. Davydow DS, Zatzick D, Hough CL, et al. A longitudinal investigation of posttraumatic stress and depressive symptoms over the course of the year following medical–surgical intensive care unit admission. Gen Hosp Psychiatry 2013;35:226–32. doi: 10.1016/j.genhosppsych.2012.12.005.

56. Zigmond A, Snaith R. The Hospital Anxiety and Depression Scale. Acta Psychiatr Scand 1983;67:361–70.

57. Needham DM, Sepulveda KA, Dinglas VD, et al. Core outcome measures for clinical research in acute respiratory failure survivors. An international modified Delphi Consensus study. Am J Respir Crit Care Med 2017;196:1122–30. doi: 10.1164/rccm.201702-0372OC.

58. Ahmed H, Patel K, Greenwood DC, et al. Long-term clinical outcomes in survivors of severe acute respiratory syndrome and Middle East respiratory syndrome coronavirus outbreaks after hospitalisation or ICU admission: a systematic review and meta-analysis. J Rehabil Med 2020;52:jrm00063. doi: 10.2340/16501977-2694.

59. Chan KS, Aronson Friedman L, Bienvenu OJ, et al. Distribution-based estimates of minimal important difference for hospital anxiety and depression scale and impact of event scale-revised in survivors of acute respiratory failure. Gen Hosp Psychiatry 2016;42:32–5. doi: 10.1016/j.genhosppsych.2016.07.004.

60. Miyamoto K, Shibata M, Shima N, et al. Combination of delirium and coma predicts psychiatric symptoms at twelve months in critically ill patients: a longitudinal cohort study. J Crit Care 2021;63:76–82. doi: 10.1016/j.jcrc.2021.01.007.

61. Boede M, Gensichen JS, Jackson JC, et al. Trajectories of depression in sepsis survivors: an observational cohort study. Crit Care 2021;25:161. doi: 10.1186/s13054-021-03577-7.

62. Dijkstra-Kersten SMA, Kok L, Kerckhoffs MC, et al. Neuropsychiatric outcome in subgroups of intensive care unit survivors: implications for after-care. J Crit Care 2020;55:171–6. doi: 10.1016/j.jcrc.2019.11.006.

63. Karnatovskaia LV, Schulte PJ, Philbrick KL, et al. Psychocognitive sequelae of critical illness and correlation with 3 months follow up. J Crit Care 2019;52:166–71. doi: 10.1016/j.jcrc.2019.04.028.

64. Wolters AE, Peelen LM, Welling MC, et al. Long-term mental health problems after delirium in the ICU. Crit Care Med 2016;44:1808–13. doi: 10.1097/ccm.0000000000001861.

65. Morrissey M and Collier E. Literature review of post-traumatic stress disorder in the critical care population. J Clin Nurs 2016;25:1501–14. doi: 10.1111/jocn.13138.

66. Huang M, Parker AM, Bienvenu OJ, et al. Psychiatric symptoms in acute respiratory distress syndrome survivors: a 1-year national multicenter study. Crit Care Med 2016;44:954–65. doi: 10.1097/ccm.0000000000001621.

67. Milton A, Schandl A, Soliman IW, et al. Development of an ICU discharge instrument predicting psychological morbidity: a multinational study. Intensive Care Med 2018;44:2038–47. doi: 10.1007/s00134-018-5467-3.

68. Murray H, Grey N, Wild J, et al. Cognitive therapy for post-traumatic stress disorder following critical illness and intensive care unit admission. Cogn Behav Therap 2020;13:e13. doi: 10.1017/s1754470x2000015x.

69. National Institute for Health and Care Excellence (NICE). Rehabilitation after critical illness overview. CG83. London: NICE; 2018. Available from: https://www.nice.org.uk/Guidance/CG83. [Accessed 12 February 2023].

70. Righy C, Rosa RG, da Silva RTA, et al. Prevalence of post-traumatic stress disorder symptoms in adult critical care survivors: a systematic review and meta-analysis. Crit Care 2019;23:213. doi: 10.1186/s13054-019-2489-3.

71. Jackson JC, Jutte JE, Hunter CH, et al. Posttraumatic stress disorder (PTSD) after critical illness: a conceptual review of distinct clinical issues and their implications. Rehab Psychol 2016;61:132–40. doi: 10.1037/rep0000085.

72. US Department of Veterans Affairs. PTSD. Washington DC: PTSD: National Center for PTSD; 2023. Available from: https://www.ptsd.va.gov. [Accessed 12 February 2023].

73. Bryant RA, Nickerson A, Creamer M, et al. Trajectory of post-traumatic stress following traumatic injury: 6-year follow-up. Br J Psychiatry 2015;206:417–23. doi: 10.1192/bjp.bp.114.145516.

74. Jackson JC, Hart RP, Gordon SM, et al. Post-traumatic stress disorder and post-traumatic stress symptoms following critical illness in medical intensive care unit patients: assessing the magnitude of the problem. Crit Care 2007;11:1–11.

75. Morina N, Stam K, Pollet TV, et al. Prevalence of depression and posttraumatic stress disorder in adult civilian survivors of war who stay in war-afflicted regions. A systematic review and meta-analysis of epidemiological studies. J Affect Disord 2018;239:328–38. doi: 10.1016/j.jad.2018.07.027.

76. Marra A, Pandharipande PP, Patel MB. Intensive care unit delirium and intensive care unit-related posttraumatic stress disorder. Surg Clin North Am 2017;97:1215–35. doi: 10.1016/j.suc.2017.07.008.

77. Paparrigopoulos T, Melissaki A, Tzavellas E, et al. Increased co-morbidity of depression and post-traumatic stress disorder symptoms and common risk factors in intensive care unit survivors: a two-year follow-up study. Int J Psychiatry Clin Pract 2014;18:25–31. doi: 10.3109/13651501.2013.855793.

78. Wade DM, Howell DC, Weinman JA, et al. Investigating risk factors for psychological morbidity three months after intensive care: a prospective cohort study. Crit Care 2012;16:R192.

79. Elliott R, McKinley S, Fien M, et al. Posttraumatic stress symptoms in intensive care patients: an exploration of associated factors. Rehab Psychol 2016;61:141–50. doi: 10.1037/rep0000074.

80. Jonasdottir RJ, Jonsdottir H, Gudmundsdottir B, et al. Psychological recovery after intensive care: outcomes of a long-term quasi-experimental study of structured nurse-led follow-up. Intensive Crit Care Nurs 2018;44:59–66. doi: 10.1016/j.iccn.2017.06.001.

81. Train S, Kydonaki K, Rattray J, et al. Frightening and traumatic memories early after intensive care discharge. Am J Respir Crit Care Med 2019;199:120–3. doi: 10.1164/rccm.201804-0699LE.

82. Battle CE, James K, Bromfield T, et al. Predictors of post-traumatic stress disorder following critical illness: a mixed methods study. J Intensive Care Soc 2017;18:289–93. doi: 10.1177/1751143717713853.

83. Wade DM, Hankins M, Smyth DA, et al. Detecting acute distress and risk of future psychological morbidity in critically ill patients: validation of the intensive care psychological assessment tool. Crit Care 2014;18:519. doi: 10.1186/s13054-014-0519-8.

84. Maartmann-Moe CC, Solberg MT, Larsen MH, et al. Patients' memories from intensive care unit: a qualitative systematic review. Nurs Open 2021;8:2221–34. doi: 10.1002/nop2.804.

85. Orwelius L, Teixeira-Pinto A, Lobo C, et al. The role of memories on health-related quality of life after intensive care unit care: an unforgettable controversy? Patient Relat Outcome Meas 2016;7:63–71. doi: 10.2147/prom.S89555.

86. Meriläinen M, Kyngäs H, Ala-Kokko T. Patients' interactions in an intensive care unit and their memories of intensive care: a mixed method study. Intensive Crit Care Nurs 2013;29(2):78–87. doi: 10.1016/j.iccn.2012.05.003.

87. Duggan MC, Wang L, Wilson JE, et al. The relationship between executive dysfunction, depression, and mental health-related quality of life in survivors of critical illness: results from the BRAIN-ICU investigation. J Crit Care 2017;37:72–9. doi: 10.1016/j.jcrc.2016.08.023.

88. Brück E, Larsson JW, Lasselin J, et al. Lack of clinically relevant correlation between subjective and objective cognitive function in ICU survivors: a prospective 12-month follow-up study. Crit Care 2019;23:253. doi: 10.1186/s13054-019-2527-1.

89. Wolters AE, Slooter AJ, van der Kooi AW, et al. Cognitive impairment after intensive care unit admission: a systematic review. Intensive Care Med 2013;39:376–86. doi: 10.1007/s00134-012-2784-9.

90. Kohler J, Borchers F, Endres M, et al. Cognitive deficits following intensive care. Dtsch Arztebl Int 2019;116:627–34. doi: 10.3238/arztebl.2019.0627.

91. Müller A, von Hofen-Hohloch J, Mende M, et al. Long-term cognitive impairment after ICU treatment: a prospective longitudinal cohort study (Cog-I-CU). Sci Rep 2020;10:15518. doi: 10.1038/s41598-020-72109-0.

92. Ariti CA, Cleland JG, Pocock SJ, et al. Days alive and out of hospital and the patient journey in patients with heart failure: insights from the candesartan in heart failure: assessment of reduction in mortality and morbidity (CHARM) program. Am Heart J 2011;162:900–6. doi: 10.1016/j.ahj.2011.08.003.

93. Jerath A, Austin PC, Wijeysundera DN. Days alive and out of hospital: validation of a patient-centered outcome for perioperative medicine. Anesthesiology 2019;131:84–93. doi: 10.1097/aln.0000000000002701.

94. Tipping CJ, Harrold M, Holland A, et al. The effects of active mobilisation and rehabilitation in ICU on mortality and function: a systematic review. Intensive Care Med 2017;43:171–83. doi: 10.1007/s00134-016-4612-0.

95. Presneill JJ, Bellomo R, Brickell K, et al. Protocol and statistical analysis plan for the phase 3 randomised controlled Treatment of Invasively Ventilated Adults with Early Activity and Mobilisation (TEAM III) trial. Crit Care Resusc 2021;23:262–72. doi: 10.51893/2021.3.OA3.

96. World Health Organization (WHO). Measuring health and disability, manual for WHO Disability Assessment Schedule (WHODAS 2.0). Geneva: WHO; 2012. Available from: https://www.who.int/publications/i/item/measuring-health-and-disability-manual-for-who-disability-assessment-schedule-(-whodas-2.0). [Accessed 12 February 2023].

97. Ware JE Jr, Sherbourne CD. The MOS 36-item short-form health survey (SF-36). I. Conceptual framework and item selection. Med Care 1992;30:473–83.

98. EuroQol Group. EuroQol – a new facility for the measurement of health-related quality of life. Health Policy 1990;16:199–208. doi: 10.1016/0168-8510(90)90421-9.

99. Mikkelsen ME, Still M, Anderson BJ, et al. Society of Critical Care Medicine's international consensus conference on prediction and identification of long-term impairments after critical illness. Crit Care Med 2020;48:1670–9. doi: 10.1097/ccm.0000000000004586.

100. Ware JE Jr. SF-36 health survey update. Spine 2000;25:3130–9.

101. Ware JE, Snow KK, Kosinski M. SF-36 Health survey: manual and interpretation guide. Lincoln: Quality Metric Incorporated; 2000.

102. Brooks R. EuroQol: the current state of play. Health Policy 1996;37:53–72.

103. Vainiola T, Pettila V, Roine RP, et al. Comparison of two utility instruments, the EQ-5D and the 15D, in the critical care setting. Intensive Care Med 2010;36:2090–3. doi: 10.1007/s00134-010-1979-1.

104. Capuzzo M, Grasselli C, Carrer S, et al. Quality of life before intensive care admission: agreement between patient and relative assessment. Intensive Care Med 2000;26:1288–95.

105. Hawthorne G, Richardson J, Osborne R. The assessment of quality of life (AQoL) instrument: a psychometric measure of health-related quality of life. Qual Life Res 1999;8:209–24.

106. Fernandez RR, Sanchez Cruz SJ, Mata GV. Validation of a quality of life questionnaire for critically ill patients. Intensive Care Med 1996;22(10):1034–42.

107. Hunt S, McKenna S, McEwan J, et al. Measuring health status: a new tool for clinicians and epidemiologists. J R Coll Gen Pract 1985;35:185–8.

108. Sintonen H. The 15D instrument of health-related quality of life: properties and applications. Ann Med 2001;33:328–36.

109. Capuzzo M, Grasselli C, Carrer S, et al. Validation of two quality of life questionnaires suitable for intensive care patients. Intensive Care Med 2000;26:1296–303.

110. Elliott D, Denehy L, Berney S, et al. Assessing physical function and activity for survivors of a critical illness: a review of instruments. Aust Crit Care 2011;24:155–66. doi: 10.1016/j.aucc.2011.05.002.

111. Tipping CJ, Young PJ, Romero L, et al. A systematic review of measurements of physical function in critically ill adults. Crit Care Resusc 2012;14:302–11.

112. Borg AVG. Psychophysical bases of perceived exertion. Med Sci Sports Exerc 1982;14:377–81.

113. American Thoracic Society. Guidelines for the six-minute walk test. Am J Respir Crit Care Med 2002;166:111–17.

114. Corner EJ, Soni N, Handy JM, et al. Construct validity of the Chelsea critical care physical assessment tool: an observational study of recovery from critical illness. Crit Care 2014;18(2):R55.

115. Skinner EH, Berney S, Warrillow S, et al. Development of a physical function outcome measure (PFIT) and a pilot exercise training protocol for use in intensive care. Crit Care Resusc 2009;11:110–15.

116. Hodgson C, Needham D, Haines K, et al. Feasibility and inter-rater reliability of the ICU Mobility Scale. Heart Lung 2014;43:19–24. doi: 10.1016/j.hrtlng.2013.11.003.

117. Thrush A, Rozek M, Dekerlegand JL. The clinical utility of the functional status score for the intensive care unit (FSS-ICU) at a long-term acute care hospital: a prospective cohort study. Phys Ther 2012;92:1536–45. doi: 10.2522/ptj.20110412.

118. Parry SM, Knight LD, Baldwin CE, et al. Evaluating physical functioning in survivors of critical illness: development of a new continuum measure for acute care. Crit Care Med 2020;48:1427–35. doi: 10.1097/ccm.0000000000004499.

119. Horowitz MJ, Wilner N, Alvarez W. Impact of Event Scale: a measure of subjective stres. Psychosom Med 1979;41:209–18.

120. Weiss DS. The impact of event scale – revised. In: Wilson JP, Keane TM, editors. Assessing psychollogical trauma and PTSD. 2nd ed. New York: Guilford Press; 2004, p. 168–89.

121. Radloff LS. The CES-D Scale: a self-report depression scale for research in the general population. Appl Psychol Measure 1977;1:385–401.

122. Kessler RC, Barker PR, Colpe LJ, et al. Screening for serious mental illness in the general population. Arch Gen Psychiatry 2003;60:184–9.

123. Weathers FW, Litz BT, Keane TM, et al. The PTSD Checklist for DSM-5 (PCL-5). Washington DC: PTSD: National Center for PTSD; 2013. Available from: https://www.ptsd.va.gov/professional/assessment/adult-sr/ptsd-checklist.asp. [Accessed 12 February 2023].

124. Stoll C, Kapfhammer HP, Rothenhausler HB, et al. Sensitivity and specificity of a screening test to document traumatic experiences and to diagnose post-traumatic stress disorder in ARDS patients after intensive care treatment. Intensive Care Med 1999;25:697–704.

125. Hull AM, Rattray J. Competing interests declared: early interventions and long-term psychological outcomes. Crit Care 2013;17:111. doi: 10.1186/cc11916.

126. Wergin R, Modrykamien A. Cognitive impairment in ICU survivors: assessment and therapy. Cleve Clin J Med 2012;79:705–12. doi: 10.3949/ccjm.79a.12038.

127. Olaithe M, Weinborn M, Lowndes T, et al. Repeatable Battery for the Assessment of Neuropsychological Status (RBANS): normative data for older adults. Arch Clin Neuropsychol 2019;34:1356–66. doi: 10.1093/arclin/acy102.

128. Folstein MF, Folstein SE, McHugh PR. Mini-mental state. A practical method for grading the cognitive state of patients for the clinician. J Psychiatric Res 1975;12:189–98.

129. Nasreddine ZS, Phillips NA, Bedirian V, et al. The Montreal Cognitive Assessment, MoCA: a brief screening tool for mild cognitive impairment. J Am Geriatr Soc 2005;53:695–9. doi: 10.1111/j.1532-5415.2005.53221.x.

130. Randolph C. Repeatable battery for the Assessment of Neuropsychological Status (RBANS). San Antonio, TX: Psychological Corporation, 1998.

131. de Jager CA, Budge MM, Clarke R. Utility of TICS-M for the assessment of cognitive function in older adults. Int J Geriatr Psychiatry 2003;18:318–24. doi: 10.1002/gps.830.

132. Cook SE, Marsiske M, McCoy KJM. The use of the modified Telephone Interview for Cognitive Status (TICS-M) in the detection of amnestic mild cognitive impairment. J Geriatr Psychiatry Neurol 2009;22:103–9. doi: 10.1177/0891988708328214.

133. Reitan RM. The relation of the trail making test to organic brain damage. J Consult Psychol 1955;19:393–4.

134. Wechsler D. Wechsler Memory Scale – revised San Antonio, TX: Psychological Corporation 1997.

135. Wechsler D. Wechsler Adult Intelligence Scale – revised. San Antonio, TX Psychological Corporation, 1997.

136. Hodgson CL, Stiller K, Needham DM, et al. Expert consensus and recommendations on safety criteria for active mobilization of mechanically ventilated critically ill adults. Crit Care 2014;18:658. doi: 10.1186/s13054-014-0658-y.

137. Nydahl P, Sricharoenchai T, Chandra S, et al. Safety of patient mobilization and rehabilitation in the intensive care unit. Systematic review with meta-analysis. Ann Am Thorac Soc 2017;14:766–77. doi: 10.1513/AnnalsATS.201611-843SR.

138. Calvo-Ayala E, Khan BA, Farber MO, et al. Interventions to improve the physical function of ICU survivors: a systematic review. Chest 2013;144(5):1469–80.

139. Connolly B, O'Neill B, Salisbury L, et al. Physical rehabilitation interventions for adult patients during critical illness: an overview of systematic reviews. Thorax 2016;71:881–90. doi: 10.1136/thoraxjnl-2015-208273.

140. Wang YT, Lang JK, Haines KJ, et al. Physical rehabilitation in the ICU: a systematic review and meta-analysis. Crit Care Med 2022;50:375–88. doi: 10.1097/ccm.0000000000005285.

141. Burtin C, Clerckx B, Robbeets C, et al. Early exercise in critically ill patients enhances short-term functional recovery. Crit Care Med 2009;37:2499–505. doi: 10.1097/CCM.0b013e3181a38937.

142. Parry SM, Berney S, Warrillow S, et al. Functional electrical stimulation with cycling in the critically ill: a pilot case-matched control study. J Crit Care 2014;29:695.e1–7. doi: 10.1016/j.jcrc.2014.03.017.

143. Schweickert WD, Pohlman MC, Pohlman AS, et al. Early physical and occupational therapy in mechanically ventilated, critically ill patients: a randomised controlled trial. Lancet 2009;373:1874–82. doi: 10.1016/s0140-6736(09)60658-9.

144. Schaller SJ, Anstey M, Blobner M, et al. Early, goal-directed mobilisation in the surgical intensive care unit: a randomised controlled trial. Lancet 2016;388:1377–88. doi: 10.1016/s0140-6736(16)31637-3.

145. Denehy L, Skinner EH, Edbrooke L, et al. Exercise rehabilitation for patients with critical illness: a randomized controlled trial with 12 months of follow-up. Crit Care 2013;17:R156. doi: 10.1186/cc12835.

146. Kayambu G, Boots R, Paratz J. Early physical rehabilitation in intensive care patients with sepsis syndromes: a pilot randomised controlled trial. Intensive Care Med 2015;41:865–74. doi: 10.1007/s00134-015-3763-8.

147. Morris PE, Berry MJ, Files DC, et al. Standardized rehabilitation and hospital length of stay among patients with acute respiratory failure: a randomized clinical trial. JAMA 2016;315:2694–702. doi: 10.1001/jama.2016.7201.

148. Moss M, Nordon-Craft A, Malone D, et al. A randomized trial of an intensive physical therapy program for patients with acute respiratory failure. Am J Respir Crit Care Med 2016;193:1101–10. doi: 10.1164/rccm.201505-1039OC.

149. Fossat G, Baudin F, Courtes L, et al. Effect of in-bed leg cycling and electrical stimulation of the quadriceps on global muscle strength in critically ill adults: a randomized clinical trial. JAMA 2018;320:368–78. doi: 10.1001/jama.2018.9592.

150. Eggmann S, Verra ML, Luder G, et al. Effects of early, combined endurance and resistance training in mechanically ventilated, critically ill patients: a randomised controlled trial. PLoS One 2018;13:e0207428. doi: 10.1371/journal.pone.0207428.

151. Sarfati C, Moore A, Pilorge C, et al. Efficacy of early passive tilting in minimizing ICU-acquired weakness: a randomized controlled trial. J Crit Care 2018;46:37–43. doi: 10.1016/j.jcrc.2018.03.031.

152. Wright SE, Thomas K, Watson G, et al. Intensive versus standard physical rehabilitation therapy in the critically ill (EPICC): a multicentre, parallel-group, randomised controlled trial. Thorax 2018;73:213–21. doi: 10.1136/thoraxjnl-2016-209858.

153. Schujmann DS, Teixeira Gomes T, Lunardi AC, et al. Impact of a progressive mobility program on the functional status, respiratory, and muscular systems of ICU patients: a randomized and controlled trial. Crit Care Med 2020;48:491–7. doi: 10.1097/CCM.0000000000004181.

154. Nickels MR, Aitken LM, Barnett AG, et al. Effect of in-bed cycling on acute muscle wasting in critically ill adults: a randomised clinical trial. J Crit Care 2020;59:86–93. doi: 10.1016/j.jcrc.2020.05.008.

155. Nakamura K, Nakano H, Naraba H, et al. High protein versus medium protein delivery under equal total energy delivery in critical care: a randomized controlled trial. Clin Nutr 2021;40:796–803. doi: 10.1016/j.clnu.2020.07.036.

156. TEAM Study Investigators and the ANZICS Clinical Trials Group; Hodgson CL, Bailey M, Bellomo R, et al. Early active mobilization during mechanical ventilation in the ICU. N Engl J Med 2022;387(19):1747–58. doi: 10.1056/NEJMoa2209083. Epub 2022 Oct 26. PMID: 36286256.

157. Barber EA, Everard T, Holland AE, et al. Barriers and facilitators to early mobilisation in Intensive Care: a qualitative study. Aust Crit Care 2015;28:177–82; quiz 183. doi: 10.1016/j.aucc.2014.11.001.

158. Goddard SL, Lorencatto F, Koo E, et al. Barriers and facilitators to early rehabilitation in mechanically ventilated patients – a theory-driven interview study. J Intensive Care 2018;6:4. doi: 10.1186/s40560-018-0273-0.

159. Nickels M, Aitken LM, Walsham J, et al. Clinicians' perceptions of rationales for rehabilitative exercise in a critical care setting: a cross-sectional study. Aust Crit Care 2017;30:79–84. doi: 10.1016/j.aucc.2016.03.003.

160. Carrothers KM, Barr J, Spurlock B, et al. Contextual issues influencing implementation and outcomes associated with an integrated approach to managing pain, agitation, and delirium in adult ICUs. Crit Care Med 2013;41:S128–5. doi: 10.1097/CCM.0b013e3182a2c2b1.

161. Rukstele CD, Gagnon MM. Making strides in preventing ICU-acquired weakness: involving family in early progressive mobility. Crit Care Nurs Q 2013;36:141–7. doi: 10.1097/CNQ.0b013e31827539cc.

162. Hodgson CL, Tipping CJ. Physiotherapy management of intensive care unit-acquired weakness. J Physiother 2017;63:4–10. doi: 10.1016/j.jphys.2016.10.011.

163. Conceicao T, Gonzales AI, Figueiredo F, et al. Safety criteria to start early mobilization in intensive care units. Systematic review. Rev Bras Ter Intensiva 2017;29:509–19. doi: 10.5935/0103-507x.20170076.

164. Gosselink R, Bott J, Johnson M, et al. Physiotherapy for adult patients with critical illness: recommendations of the European Respiratory Society and European Society of Intensive Care Medicine Task Force on Physiotherapy for Critically Ill Patients. Intensive Care Med 2008;34:1188–99. doi: 10.1007/s00134-008-1026-7.

165. Rousseau A-F, Prescott HC, Brett SJ, et al. Long-term outcomes after critical illness: recent insights. Crit Care 2021;25:108. doi: 10.1186/s13054-021-03535-3.

166. Kayambu G, Boots R, Paratz J. Physical therapy for the critically ill in the ICU: a systematic review and meta-analysis. Crit Care Med 2013;41:1543–54. doi: 10.1097/CCM.0b013e31827ca637.

167. Vorona S, Sabatini U, Al-Maqbali S, et al. Inspiratory muscle rehabilitation in critically ill adults. a systematic review and meta-analysis. Ann Am Thorac Soc 2018;15:735–44. doi: 10.1513/AnnalsATS.201712-961OC.

168. Berney SC, Harrold M, Webb SA, et al. Intensive care unit mobility practices in Australia and New Zealand: a point prevalence study. Crit Care Resusc 2013;15:260–5.

169. Hodgson C, Bellomo R, Berney S, et al. Early mobilization and recovery in mechanically ventilated patients in the ICU: a bi-national, multi-centre, prospective cohort study. Crit Care 2015;19:81. doi: 10.1186/s13054-015-0765-4.

170. Jolley SE, Moss M, Needham DM, et al. Point prevalence study of mobilization practices for acute respiratory failure patients in the United States. Crit Care Med 2017;45:205–15. doi: 10.1097/CCM.0000000000002058.

171. Nydahl P, Ruhl AP, Bartoszek G, et al. Early mobilization of mechanically ventilated patients: a 1-day point-prevalence study in Germany. Crit Care Med 2014;42:1178–86. doi: 10.1097/ccm.0000000000000149.

172. Sibilla A, Nydahl P, Greco N, et al. Mobilization of mechanically ventilated patients in Switzerland. J Intensive Care Med 2020;35:55–62. doi: 10.1177/0885066617728486.

173. Bailey PP, Miller RR 3rd, Clemmer TP. Culture of early mobility in mechanically ventilated patients. Crit Care Med 2009;37:S429–35. doi: 10.1097/CCM.0b013e3181b6e227.

174. Dinglas VD, Parker AM, Reddy DR, et al. A quality improvement project sustainably decreased time to onset of active physical therapy intervention in patients with acute lung injury. Ann Am Thorac Soc 2014;11:1230–8. doi: 10.1513/AnnalsATS.201406-231OC.

175. Drolet A, DeJuilio P, Harkless S, et al. Move to improve: the feasibility of using an early mobility protocol to increase ambulation in the intensive and intermediate care settings. Phys Ther 2013;93:197–207. doi: 10.2522/ptj.20110400.

176. Hickmann CE, Castanares-Zapatero D, Bialais E, et al. Teamwork enables high level of early mobilization in critically ill patients. Ann Intensive Care 2016;6:80. doi: 10.1186/s13613-016-0184-y.

177. Donaghy E, Salisbury L, Lone NI, et al. Unplanned early hospital readmission among critical care survivors: a mixed methods study of patients and carers. BMJ Qual Saf 2018;27:915–27. doi: 10.1136/bmjqs-2017-007513.

178. Intensive Care Society/Faculty of Intensive Care Medicine (ICS/FICM). Life after critical illness. 2021. Available from: https://www.ficm.ac.uk/sites/ficm/files/documents/2021-12/LACI%20Life%20After%20Critical%20Illness%202021.pdf. [Accessed 12 February 2023].

179. Bisson JI, Wright LA, Jones KA, et al. Preventing the onset of post traumatic stress disorder. Clin Psychol Rev 2021;86:102004. doi: 10.1016/j.cpr.2021.102004.

180. Long AC, Kross EK, Davydow DS, et al. Posttraumatic stress disorder among survivors of critical illness: creation of a conceptual model addressing identification, prevention, and management. Intensive Care Med 2014;40:820–9. doi: 10.1007/s00134-014-3306-8.

181. Wade D, Hardy R, Howell D, et al. Identifying clinical and acute psychological risk factors for PTSD after critical care: a systematic review. Minerva Anestesiol 2013;79:944–63.

182. Roberts MB, Glaspey LJ, Mazzarelli A, et al. Early interventions for the prevention of posttraumatic stress symptoms in survivors of critical illness: a qualitative systematic review. Crit Care Med 2018;46:1328–33. doi: 10.1097/ccm.0000000000003222.

183. Wade DM, Mouncey PR, Richards-Belle A, et al. Effect of a nurse-led preventive psychological intervention on symptoms of posttraumatic stress disorder among critically ill patients: a randomized clinical trial. JAMA 2019;321:665–75. doi: 10.1001/jama.2019.0073.

184. Schofield-Robinson OJ, Lewis SR, Smith AF, et al. Follow-up services for improving long-term outcomes in intensive care unit (ICU) survivors. Cochrane Database Syst Rev 2018;11:CD012701. doi: 10.1002/14651858.CD012701.pub2.

185. Jonasdottir RJ, Jones C, Sigurdsson GH, et al. Structured nurse-led follow-up for patients after discharge from the intensive care unit: prospective quasi-experimental study. J Adv Nurs 2018;74:709–23. doi: 10.1111/jan.13485.

186. Nydahl P, Knuck D, Egerod I. The extent and application of patient diaries in German intensive care units. Connect 2010;7:122–6.

187. Egerod I, Storli SL, Akerman E. Intensive care patient diaries in Scandinavia: a comparative study of emergence and evolution. Nurs Inq 2011;18:235–46.

188. Aitken LM, Rattray J, Hull A, et al. The use of diaries in psychological recovery from intensive care. Crit Care 2013;17:253. doi: 10.1186/cc13164.

189. Ullman AJ, Aitken LM, Rattray J, et al. Intensive care diaries to promote recovery for patients and families after critical illness: a Cochrane systematic review. Int J Nurs Stud 2015;52:1243–53. doi: 10.1016/j.ijnurstu.2015.03.020.

190. Jones C, Backman CG, Capuzzo M, et al. Intensive care diaries reduce new onset post traumatic stress disorder following critical illness: a randomised, controlled trial. Crit Care 2010;14:168–78.

191. Garrouste-Orgeas M, Flahault C, Vinatier I, et al. Effect of an ICU diary on posttraumatic stress disorder symptoms among patients receiving mechanical ventilation: a randomized clinical trial. JAMA 2019;322:229–39. doi: 10.1001/jama.2019.9058.

192. Barreto BB, Luz M, Rios MNO, et al. The impact of intensive care unit diaries on patients' and relatives' outcomes: a systematic review and meta-analysis. Crit Care 2019;23:411. doi: 10.1186/s13054-019-2678-0.

193. Bench SD, Day T, Griffiths P. Involving users in the development of effective critical care discharge information: a focus group study. Am J Crit Care 2011;20:443–52. doi: 10.4037/ajcc2011829.

194. Bench SD, Heelas K, White C, et al. Providing critical care patients with a personalised discharge summary: a questionnaire survey and retrospective analysis exploring feasibility and effectiveness. Intensive Crit Care Nurs 2014;30:69–76. doi: 10.1016/j.iccn.2013.08.007.

195. Jensen JF, Egerod I, Bestle MH, et al. A recovery program to improve quality of life, sense of coherence and psychological health in ICU survivors: a multicenter randomized controlled trial, the RAPIT study. Intensive Care Med 2016;42:1733–43. doi: 10.1007/s00134-016-4522-1.

196. Rattray J, Crocker C, Jones M, et al. Patients' perception of and emotional outcome after intensive care: results from a multicentre study. Nurs Crit Care 2010;15:86–93.

197. Aitken LM, Rattray J, Kenardy J, et al. Perspectives of patients and family members regarding psychological support using intensive care diaries: an exploratory mixed methods study. J Crit Care 2017;38:263–8. doi: 10.1016/j.jcrc.2016.12.003.

198. Castillo MI, Mitchell M, Davis C, et al. Feasibility and acceptability of conducting a partially randomised controlled trial examining interventions to improve psychological health after discharge from the intensive care unit. Aust Crit Care 2020;33:488–96. doi: 10.1016/j.aucc.2020.01.002.

199. Rattray J, Hull A. Emotional outcome after intensive care: literature review. J Adv Nurs 2008;64:2–13.

200. Deemer K, Zjadewicz K, Fiest K, et al. Effect of early cognitive interventions on delirium in critically ill patients: a systematic review. Can J Anaesth 2020;67:1016–34. doi: 10.1007/s12630-020-01670-z.

201. Muradov O, Petrovskaya O, Papathanassoglou E. Effectiveness of cognitive interventions on cognitive outcomes of adult intensive care unit survivors: a scoping review. Aust Crit Care 2021;34:473–85. doi: 10.1016/j.aucc.2020.11.001.

202. Gayat E, Cariou A, Deye N, et al. Determinants of long-term outcome in ICU survivors: results from the FROG-ICU study. Crit Care 2018;22:8. doi: 10.1186/s13054-017-1922-8.

203. Moran JL, Solomon PJ; ANZICS Centre for Outcome and Resource Evaluation (CORE) of the Australian and New Zealand Intensive Care Society (ANZICS). Fixed effects modelling for provider mortality outcomes: analysis of the Australia and New Zealand Intensive Care Society (ANZICS) Adult Patient Data-base. PLoS One 2014;9:e102297. doi: 10.1371/journal.pone.0102297.

204. Fernandez R, Serrano JM, Umaran I, et al. Ward mortality after ICU discharge: a multicenter validation of the Sabadell score. Intensive Care Med 2010;36:1196–201. doi: 10.1007/s00134-010-1825-5.

205. Salisbury LG, Merriweather JL, Walsh TS. Rehabilitation after critical illness: could a ward-based generic rehabilitation assistant promote recovery? Nurs Crit Care 2010;15:57–65. doi: 10.1111/j.1478-5153.2010.00382.x.

206. Salisbury LG, Merriweather JL, Walsh TS. The development and feasibility of a ward-based physiotherapy and nutritional rehabilitation package for people experiencing critical illness. Clin Rehabil 2010;24:489–500. doi: 10.1177/0269215509360639.

207. Ramsay P, Salisbury LG, Merriweather JL, et al. A rehabilitation intervention to promote physical recovery following intensive care: a detailed description of construct development, rationale and content together with proposed taxonomy to capture processes in a randomised controlled trial. Trials 2014;15:38. doi: 10.1186/1745-6215-15-38.

208. Walsh TS, Salisbury LG, Merriweather JL, et al. Increased hospital-based physical rehabilitation and information provision after intensive care unit discharge: the RECOVER randomized clinical trial. JAMA Intern Med 2015;175:901–10. doi: 10.1001/jamainternmed.2015.0822.

209. Gruther W, Pieber K, Steiner I, et al. Can early rehabilitation on the general ward after an intensive care unit stay reduce hospital length of stay in survivors of critical illness?: a randomized controlled trial. Am J Phys Med Rehabil 2017;96(9):607–15. doi: 10.1097/phm.0000000000000718.

210. Williams TA, Dobb G, Finn J, et al. Determinants of long-term survival after intensive care. Crit Care Med 2008;36:1523–30. doi: 10.1097/CCM.0b013e318170a405.

211. Myhren H, Ekeberg O, Stokland O. Health-related quality of life and return to work after critical illness in general intensive care unit patients: a 1-year follow-up study. Crit Care Med 2010;38:1554–61. doi: 10.1097/CCM.0b013e3181e2c8b1.

212. Higgins AM, Neto AS, Bailey M, et al. Predictors of death and new disability after critical illness: a multicentre prospective cohort study. Intensive Care Med 2021;47:772–81. doi: 10.1007/s00134-021-06438-7.

213. UK National Health Service (NHS) Audit Commission. Critical to success. The place of efficient and effective critical care services within the acute hospital. London: NHS; 1999.

214. Lasiter S, Oles SK, Mundell J, et al. Critical care follow-up clinics: a scoping review of interventions and outcomes. Clin Nurse Spec 2016;30:227–37. doi: 10.1097/nur.0000000000000219.

215. Haines KJ, Beesley SJ, Hopkins RO, et al. Peer support in critical care: a systematic review. Crit Care Med 2018;46:1522–31. doi: 10.1097/ccm.0000000000003293.

216. Sevin CM, Boehm LM, Hibbert E, et al. Optimizing critical illness recovery: perspectives and solutions from the caregivers of ICU survivors. Crit Care Explor 2021;3:e0420. doi: 10.1097/cce.0000000000000420.

217. White C, Connolly B, Rowland MJ. Rehabilitation after critical illness. BMJ 2021;373:n910. doi: 10.1136/bmj.n910.

218. Griffiths JA, Barber VS, Cuthbertson BH, et al. A national survey of intensive care follow-up clinics. Anaesthesia 2006;61:950–5. doi: 10.1111/j.1365-2044.2006.04792.x.

219. Cuthbertson BH, Rattray J, Campbell MK, et al. The PRaCTICaL study of nurse led, intensive care follow-up programmes for improving long term outcomes from critical illness: a pragmatic randomised controlled trial. BMJ 2009;339:b3723. doi: 10.1136/bmj.b3723.

220. Prinjha S, Field K, Rowan K. What patients think about ICU follow-up services: a qualitative study. Crit Care 2009;13:R46. doi: 10.1186/cc7769.

221. Farley KJ, Eastwood GM, Bellomo R. A feasibility study of functional status and follow-up clinic preferences of patients at high risk of post intensive care syndrome. Anaesth Intensive Care 2016;44:413–19.

222. Haines KJ, McPeake J, Hibbert E, et al. Enablers and barriers to implementing ICU follow-up clinics and peer support groups following critical illness: the Thrive Collaboratives. Crit Care Med 2019;47:1194–200. doi: 10.1097/ccm.0000000000003818.

223. Cutler L, Brightmore K, Colqhoun V, et al. Developing and evaluating critical care follow-up. Nurs Crit Care 2003;8:116–25. doi: 10.1046/j.1478-5153.2003.00018.x.

224. McPeake J, Boehm LM, Hibbert E, et al. Key components of ICU recovery programs: what did patients report provided benefit? Crit Care Explor 2020;2:e0088. doi: 10.1097/cce.0000000000000088.

225. Haines KJ, Sevin CM, Hibbert E, et al. Key mechanisms by which post-ICU activities can improve in-ICU care: results of the international THRIVE collaboratives. Intensive Care Med 2019;45:939–47. doi: 10.1007/s00134-019-05647-5.

226. Groves J, Cahill J, Sturmey G, et al. Patient support groups: a survey of United Kingdom practice, purpose and performance. J Intensive Care Soc 2021;22:300–4. doi: 10.1177/1751143720952017.

227. McPeake J, Hirshberg EL, Christie LM, et al. Models of peer support to remediate post-intensive care syndrome: a report developed by the Society of Critical Care Medicine Thrive International Peer Support Collaborative. Crit Care Med 2019;47:e21–7. doi: 10.1097/ccm.0000000000003497.

228. Iwashyna TJ. Survivorship will be the defining challenge of critical care in the 21st century. Ann Intern Med 2010;153:204–5. doi: 10.7326/0003-4819-153-3-201008030-00013.

Chapter 9

Cardiovascular assessment and monitoring

Thomas Buckley, Elliott Williams

KEY WORDS
....

cardiac output

cardiac physiology

cardiovascular
  assessment

cardiovascular
  macrostructure

chest X-ray

coronary perfusion

diagnostic imaging

electrocardiography

haemodynamic
  monitoring

heart sounds

Learning objectives

After reading this chapter, you should be able to:

- describe the normal blood flow through the cardiovascular system
- define each stage of the cardiac action potential and its application to electrocardiography
- describe the determinants of cardiac output and their interpretation in cardiovascular assessment and monitoring
- describe the reasons for the assessment and monitoring of critically ill patients
- summarise the key principles underpinning cardiac assessment and monitoring
- identify the recommended anatomical landmarks for cardiac auscultation and identify normal and common abnormal heart sounds
- describe the physiological bases and reasons for different types of haemodynamic monitoring
- critique and evaluate current clinical practice on haemodynamic monitoring and integrate best evidence in clinical practice.

Introduction

This chapter reviews the support of cardiovascular function in the face of many compromises to the system. It is essential for the reader to have a thorough knowledge of both electrical and mechanical functions of the cardiac system. Methods for assessment of cardiovascular elements are discussed, along with best-practice ideas and diagnostic techniques.

Related anatomy and physiology

The cardiovascular system is essentially a transport system for distributing metabolic requirements to, and collecting byproducts from, cells throughout the body. The heart pumps blood continuously through two separate circulatory systems: to the lungs and to all other parts of the body (Fig 9.1). Structures on the right side of the heart pump blood through the lungs (the pulmonary

FIGURE 9.1 The systemic and pulmonic circulations.

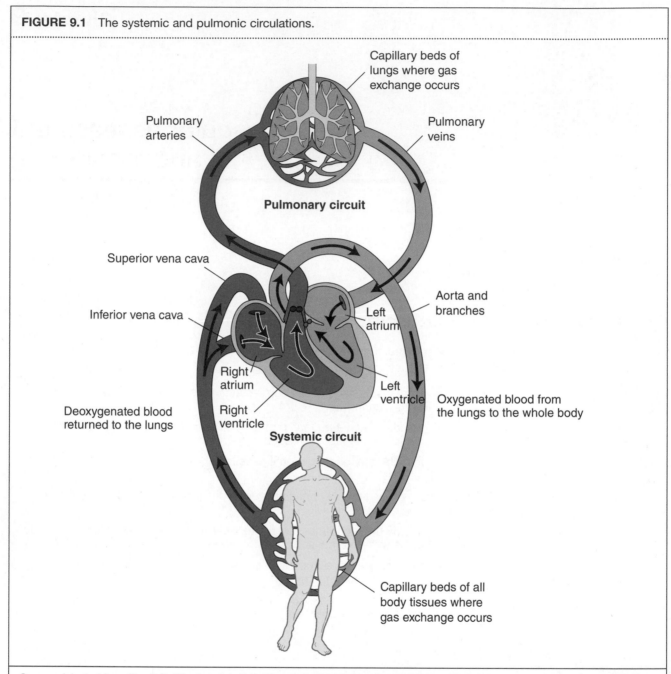

Capillary beds of lungs where gas exchange occurs

Pulmonary arteries

Pulmonary veins

Pulmonary circuit

Superior vena cava

Inferior vena cava

Aorta and branches

Left atrium

Right atrium

Left ventricle

Deoxygenated blood returned to the lungs

Right ventricle

Oxygenated blood from the lungs to the whole body

Systemic circuit

Capillary beds of all body tissues where gas exchange occurs

Source: Adapted from Novak B, Filer L, Latchett R. The applied anatomy and physiology of the cardiovascular system. In: Hatchett R, Thompson D, editors. Cardiac nursing: a comprehensive guide. Philadelphia: Churchill Livingstone Elsevier; 2002, with permission.

circulation) to be oxygenated. The left side of the heart pumps oxygenated blood throughout the remainder of the body (the systemic circulation). The two systems are connected, so the output of one becomes the input of the other.

Cardiac macrostructure

The heart is cone shaped and lies diagonally in the mediastinum towards the left side of the chest. The point of the cone is called the apex and rests just above the diaphragm; the base of the cone lies just behind the mediastinum. The adult heart is about the size of that individual's fist, weighs approximately 300 grams and is composed of chambers and valves that form the two separate pumps. The upper chambers, the atria, collect blood and act as a primer to the main pumping chambers, the ventricles. As the atria are low-pressure chambers, they have relatively thin walls and are relatively compliant. As the ventricles propel blood against either pulmonary or systemic pressure, they have much thicker and more muscular walls than the atria. As pressure is higher in the systemic circulation, the left ventricle (LV) is much thicker than the right ventricle (RV). Dense fibrous connective tissue rings provide a firm anchorage for attachments of atrial and ventricular muscle and valvular tissue.[1]

One-way blood flow in the system is facilitated by valves. Valves between the atria and ventricles are composed of cusps or leaflets sitting in a ring of fibrous tissue and collagen. The cusps are anchored to the papillary muscles by chordae tendineae so that the cusps are pulled together and downwards at the onset of ventricular contraction. The atrioventricular valves are termed the tricuspid valve in the right side of the heart and the mitral or bicuspid valve in the left side of the heart. Semilunar valves prevent backflow from the pulmonary artery (pulmonic valve) and aorta (aortic valve) into the corresponding right and left ventricles. The muscles in the ventricles follow a distinct spiral path so that, during contraction, blood is propelled into the respective outflow tracts of the pulmonary artery and aorta. The aortic valve sits in a tubular area of mostly non-contractile collagenous tissue, which contains the opening of the coronary arteries.

The coronary arteries run through deep grooves that separate the atria and ventricles. The two sides of the heart are divided by a septum, which ensures that two separate but integrated circulations are maintained.[2]

The heart wall has three distinct layers: the outer protective pericardium, a medial muscular layer or myocardium and an inner layer or endocardium that lines the heart. The pericardium is a double-walled, firm fibrous sac that encloses the heart. The two layers of the pericardium are separated by a fluid-filled cavity, enabling the layers to slide over each other smoothly as the heart beats. The pericardium provides physical protection for the heart against mechanical force and forms a barrier to infection and inflammation from the lungs and pleural space. Branches of the vagus nerve, the phrenic nerves and the sympathetic trunk innervate the pericardium.

The myocardium forms the bulk of the heart and is composed primarily of myocytes. Myocytes are the contractile cells and autorhythmic cells which create a conduction pathway for electrical impulses. They are cylindrical in shape (Fig. 9.2) and able to branch to interconnect with each other. The junctions between

FIGURE 9.2   Diagram of an electron micrograph of cardiac muscle showing mitochondria, intercalculated discs, tubules and sarcoplasmic reticulum.

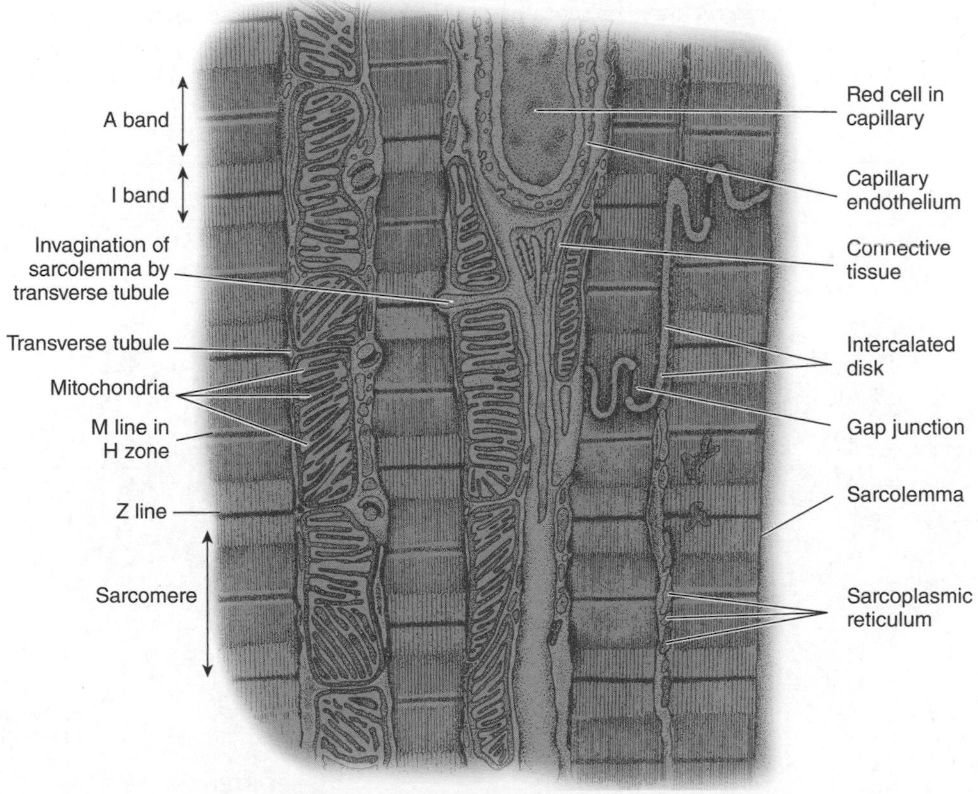

Source: Adapted from Urden L, Stacy KL, Lough ME, editors. Thelan's critical care nursing: diagnosis and management. 6th ed. St Louis: Elsevier; 2010, with permission.

myocytes are termed intercalated discs and contain desmosomes and gap junctions. Desmosomes act as anchors to prevent the myocytes from separating during contraction. Gap junctions contain connexons, which allow ions to move from one myocyte to the next. The movement of ions from cell to cell ensures that the whole myocardium acts as one unit, termed a functional syncytium. When ischaemia occurs, the gap junctions may uncouple, so ions do not move as freely. Uncoupling may also contribute to the poor conduction evidenced on ECG during ischaemia.[3]

The endocardium is composed primarily of squamous epithelium, which forms a continuous sheet with the endothelium that lines all arteries, veins and capillaries. The vascular endothelium is the source of many chemical mediators, including nitric oxide and the endothelin involved in vessel regulation. It has been theorised that the endocardium may also have this function.[1]

Coronary perfusion

The heart is perfused by the right and left coronary arteries, which arise from openings in the aorta called the coronary ostia (Fig. 9.3). The right coronary artery (RCA) branches supply the atrioventricular node, right atrium and right ventricle, and the posterior descending branch supplies the lower aspect of the left ventricle. The left coronary artery divides into the left anterior descending artery (LAD) and the circumflex artery (Cx) shortly after its origin. The LAD supplies the interventricular septum and anterior surface of the left ventricle. The Cx supplies the lateral and posterior aspects of the left ventricle. This is the most common distribution of the coronary arteries, but it is not uncommon for the RCA to be small and the Cx to supply the inferior wall of the left ventricle. The coronary arteries ultimately branch into a dense network of capillaries to support cardiac myocytes. Anastomoses between branches of the coronary arteries often occur in mature individuals when myocardial hypoxia has been present. These anastomoses are termed collateral arteries, but their contribution to normal cardiac perfusion during occlusion of coronary arteries is unclear.

The cardiac veins collect venous blood from the heart. Cardiac venous flow is collected into the great coronary vein and coronary sinus and ultimately flows into the right atrium. Lymph drainage of the heart follows the conduction tissue and flows into nodes and the superior vena cava.

Physiological principles

An understanding of the principles of cardiac physiology is essential for safe management of the critically ill patient. While the primary role of the circulatory system is to provide sufficient blood flow to meet metabolic demands, this requires adequate myocardial contraction, coordinated electrical conduction and adequate intravascular volume.

Mechanical events of contraction

Energy is produced in the myocytes by a large number of mitochondria contained within the cell. The mitochondria produce adenosine triphosphate (ATP), a molecule that is able to store and release chemical energy. Other organelles in the myocyte, called the sarcoplasmic reticulum, are used to store calcium ions. The myocyte cell membrane

---

FIGURE 9.3   Location of the coronary arteries.

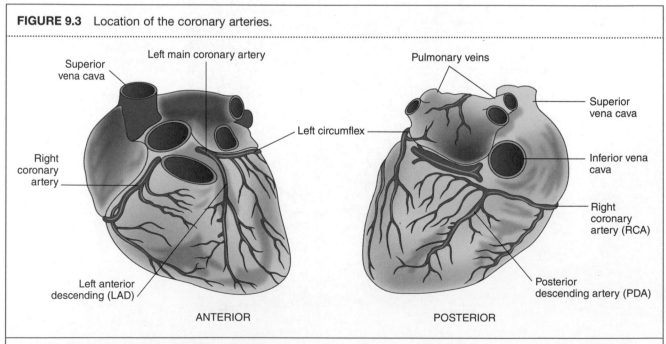

ANTERIOR

POSTERIOR

Source: Adapted from Urden L, Stacy KL, Lough ME, editors. Thelan's critical care nursing: diagnosis and management. 6th ed. St Louis: Elsevier; 2010, with permission.

FIGURE 9.4 Actin and myosin filaments and other cross-bridges responsible for cell contraction.

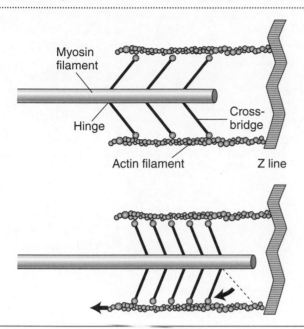

Source: Adapted from Urden L, Stacy KL, Lough ME, editors. Thelan's critical care nursing: diagnosis and management. 6th ed. St Louis: Elsevier; 2010, with permission.

FIGURE 9.5 **(A)** Action potential in a 'fast-response', non-pacemaker myocyte: phases 0–4, resting membrane potential −80 mV, absolute refractory period (ARP) and relative refractory period (RRP). **(B)** Action potential in a 'slow response', pacemaker myocyte. The upward slope of phase 4, on reaching threshold potential, results in an action potential.

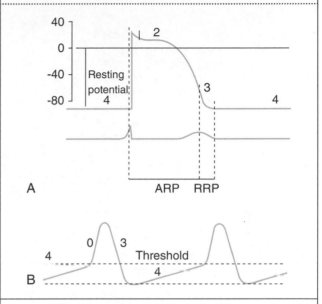

Source: Adapted from Bersten AD, Soni N, Oh TE. Oh's intensive care manual. 7th ed. Oxford: Butterworth-Heinemann; 2013, with permission.

(sarcolemma) extends down into the cell to form a set of transverse tubules (T tubules), which rapidly transmit external electrical stimuli into the cell. Cross-striated muscle fibrils, which contain contractile units, fill up the myocyte. These fibrils are termed sarcomeres.

The sarcomere contains two types of protein myofilaments: one thick contractile protein, myosin, and thin filaments composed of the contractile protein actin and the regulatory proteins troponin and tropomyosin (Fig. 9.4). The myosin molecules of the thick filaments contain active sites that form bridges with sites of the actin molecules on the thin filaments. These filaments are arranged so that, during contraction, bridges form and the thin filaments are pulled into the lattice of the thick filaments. As the filaments are pulled towards the centre of the sarcomere, the degree of contraction is limited by the length of the sarcomere. Starling's law states that, within physiological limits, the greater the degree of stretch, the greater is the force of contraction. The length of the sarcomere is the physiological limit because too great a stretch may disconnect the myosin–actin bridges.[2]

Electrical events of depolarisation, resting potential and action potential

Automaticity and rhythmicity are intrinsic properties of all myocardial cells. However, specialised autorhythmic cells in the myocardium generate and conduct impulses in a specific order to create a conduction pathway. This pathway ensures that contraction is coordinated and rhythmical, so that the heart pumps efficiently and continuously. Electrical impulses termed action potentials are transmitted along this pathway and trigger contraction in myocytes. Action potentials represent the inward and outward flow of negative- and positive-charged ions across the cell membrane (Fig. 9.5).

Cell membrane pumps create concentration gradients across the cell membrane during diastole to create a resting electrical potential of −80 mV. Individual fibres are separated by membranes but depolarisation spreads rapidly because of the presence of gap junctions. There are five key phases to the cardiac action potential:

0 depolarisation

1 early rapid repolarisation

2 plateau phase

3 final rapid repolarisation

4 resting membrane phase.[4]

The contractile response begins just after the start of depolarisation and lasts about 1.5 times as long as the depolarisation and repolarisation (Fig. 9.6).

The action potential is created by ion exchange triggered by an intracellular and extracellular fluid transmembrane imbalance. There are three ions involved: sodium, potassium and calcium. Normally, extracellular

FIGURE 9.6 Action potential.

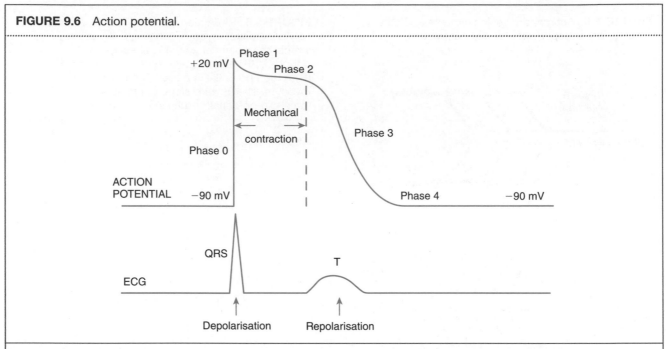

Source: Adapted from Urden L, Stacy KL, Lough ME, editors. Thelan's critical care nursing: diagnosis and management. 6th ed. St Louis: Elsevier; 2010, with permission.

fluid contains approximately 140 mmol/L sodium and 4 mmol/L potassium. In intracellular fluid these concentrations are reversed.[4]

The following is a summary of physiological events during a normal action potential:

- At rest, cell membranes are more permeable to potassium and, consequently, potassium moves slowly and passively from intracellular to extracellular fluid. At this time, fast sodium and slow calcium channels are closed and the resting membrane potential is very negative (−90 mV).

- During depolarisation (phase 0), rapid ion movement caused by sodium flowing into the cell alters the electrical potential from −90 mV to +30 mV. At this time, potassium channels close.

- In phase 1, the sodium channels close and potassium begins to leave the cell. This is followed by a brief influx of calcium via the fast channel and then more via the slower channel to create a plateau (phase 2), the duration of which determines stroke volume due to its influence on the contractile strength of the muscle fibres.

- The third phase occurs when the calcium channels are inactivated allowing potassium to leave the cell more rapidly, restoring the negative charge and causing rapid depolarisation.

- The final resting phase occurs when slow potassium leakage allows the cell to increase its negative potential or charge (phase 4), to ensure that it is more negative than the surrounding fluid, before the next depolarisation occurs and the cycle repeats.[4]

Cardiac muscle is generally slow to respond to stimuli and has relatively low ATPase activity. Its fibres are dependent on oxidative metabolism and require a continuous supply of oxygen. The lengths of fibres and the strength of contraction are determined by the degree of diastolic filling in the heart. The force of contraction is enhanced by catecholamines.

Depolarisation is initiated in the sinoatrial (SA) node and spreads rapidly through the atria, then converges on the atrioventricular (AV) node; atrial depolarisation normally takes 0.1 second. There is a short delay (0.1 s) at the AV node before excitation spreads to the ventricles. This delay is shortened by sympathetic activity and lengthened by vagal stimulation. Ventricular depolarisation takes 0.08–0.1 s, and the last parts of the heart to be depolarised are the posteriobasal portion of the left ventricle, the pulmonary conus and the upper septum.

The electrical activity of the heart can be detected on the body surface because body fluids are good conductors; the fluctuations in potential that represent the algebraic sum of the action potentials of myocardial fibres can be recorded on an electrocardiogram (see later in this chapter).

Cardiac macrostructure and conduction

The electrical and mechanical processes of the heart differ but are connected. The autorhythmic cells of the cardiac conduction pathway ensure that large portions of the heart receive an action potential rapidly and simultaneously. This ensures that the pumping action of the heart is maximised. The conduction pathway is composed of the SA node, the AV node, the bundle of His, right and left

FIGURE 9.7 Cardiac conduction system. AV = atrioventricular; LBB = left bundle branch; RBB = right bundle branch.

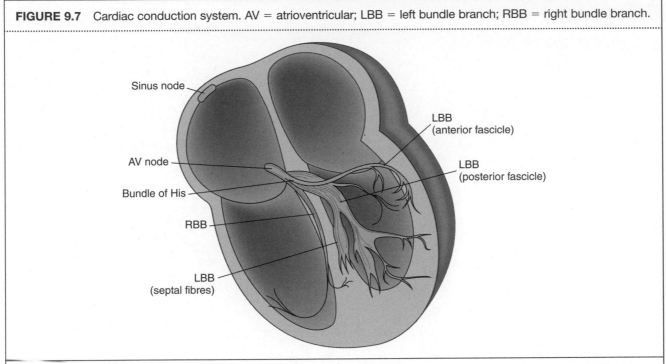

Source: Adapted from Urden L, Stacy KL, Lough MC, editors. Thelan's critical care nursing: diagnosis and management. 6th ed. St Louis: Elsevier; 2010, with permission.

bundle branches and Purkinje fibres (Fig. 9.7). The cells contained in the pathway conduct action potentials extremely rapidly, 3–7 times faster than general myocardial tissue. Pacemaker cells of the SA and AV nodes differ in that they are more permeable to potassium, so that potassium easily 'leaks' back out of the cells triggering influx of sodium and calcium back into cells. This permits the spontaneous automaticity of pacemaker cells.[5]

At the myocyte, the action potential is transmitted to the myofibrils by calcium from the interstitial fluid via channels. During repolarisation (after contraction), the calcium ions are pumped out of the cell into the interstitial space and into the sarcoplasmic reticulum and stored. Troponin releases its bound calcium, enabling the tropomyosin complex to block the active sites on actin, and the muscle relaxes.

The cardiac conduction system and the mechanical efficiency of the heart as a pump are directly connected. Disruption to conduction may not prevent myocardial contraction but may result in poor coordination and lower pump efficiency. Interruption to flow through the coronary arteries may alter depolarisation. Disrupted conduction from the SA to the AV node may allow another area in the conduction system to become the new dominant pacemaker and alter cardiac output. Although the autonomic nervous system influences cardiac function, the heart is able to function without neural control. Rhythmical myocardial contraction will continue because automaticity and rhythmicity are intrinsic to the myocardium.[5]

Cardiac output

Cardiac performance is altered by numerous homeostatic mechanisms. Cardiac output is regulated in response to stress or disease, and changes in any of the factors that determine cardiac output will result in changes to cardiac output (Fig. 9.8). Cardiac output is the product of heart rate and stroke volume; alteration in either of these will increase or decrease cardiac output, as will alteration in preload, afterload or contractility.[1]

Determinants of cardiac output

In the healthy individual, the most immediate change in cardiac output is seen when heart rate rises. However, in the critically ill, the ability to raise the heart rate in response to changing circumstances may be limited, and a rising heart rate may have negative effects on homeostasis because of decreased diastolic filling and increased myocardial oxygen demand.[6]

Preload is the load imposed by the initial fibre length of the cardiac muscle before contraction (i.e. at the end of diastole). The primary determinant of preload is the amount of blood filling the ventricle during diastole and, as indicated in Fig. 9.8, it is important in determining stroke volume. Preload influences the contractility of the ventricles (the strength of contraction) because of the relationship between myocardial fibre length and stretch. However, a threshold is reached when fibres become overstretched, and force of contraction and resultant stroke volume will fall.

Preload reduces as a result of large-volume loss (e.g. haemorrhage), venous dilation (e.g. due to hyperthermia

FIGURE 9.8 Determinants of cardiac function and oxygen delivery.

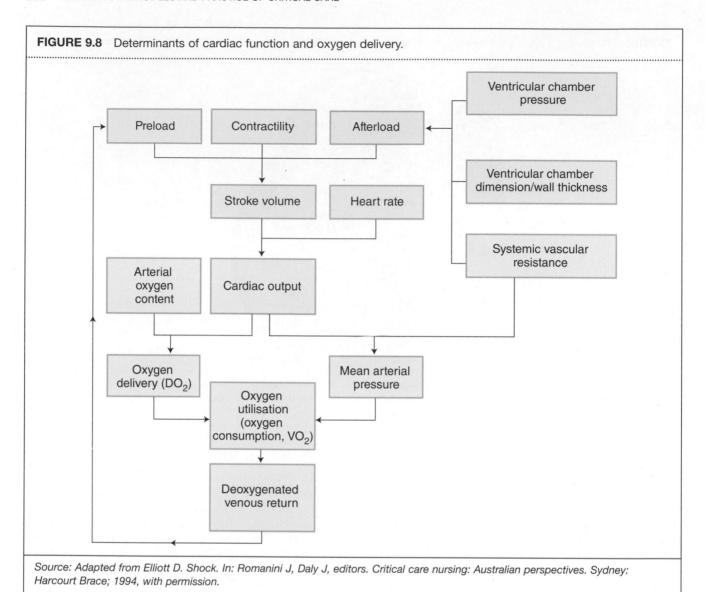

Source: Adapted from Elliott D. Shock. In: Romanini J, Daly J, editors. Critical care nursing: Australian perspectives. Sydney: Harcourt Brace; 1994, with permission.

or drugs), tachycardias (e.g. rapid atrial fibrillation or supraventricular tachycardias), raised intrathoracic pressures (a complication of intermittent positive-pressure ventilation (IPPV)) and raised intracardiac pressures (e.g. cardiac tamponade). Some drugs such as vasodilators can cause a decrease in venous tone and a resulting decrease in preload. Preload increases with fluid overload, hypothermia or other causes of venous constriction, and ventricular failure. Body position will also affect preload through its effect on venous return.

The volume of blood filling the ventricles is also affected by atrial contraction: a reduction in atrial contraction ability, as can occur during atrial fibrillation, will result in a reduction in ventricular volume, and a corresponding fall in stroke volume and cardiac output.[7–9]

Afterload is the load imposed on the muscle during contraction and it translates to systolic myocardial wall tension. It is measured during systole, and is inversely related to stroke volume and therefore cardiac output, but it is not synonymous with systemic vascular resistance (SVR), as this is just one factor determining left ventricular afterload.[10] Factors that increase afterload include:

• increased ventricular radius
• raised intracavity pressure
• increased aortic impedance
• negative intrathoracic pressure
• increased SVR.

As afterload rises, the speed of muscle fibre shortening and external work performed falls, which can cause a decrease in cardiac output in critically ill patients. Afterload of the right side of the heart is assessed during the ejection of blood from the right ventricle into the pulmonary artery. This volume is indirectly assessed by calculating pulmonary vascular resistance. Ventricular afterload can be altered to clinically affect cardiac performance. Reducing afterload will increase the stroke volume and cardiac output, while also reducing myocardial oxygen demand. However, reductions in afterload are associated with lower blood pressure, and this limits the extent to which afterload can be manipulated.[10]

Contractility is the force of ventricular ejection, or the inherent ability of the ventricle to perform external work independently of afterload or preload. It is difficult to measure clinically. It is increased by catecholamines, calcium, relief of ischaemia and digoxin. It is decreased by hypoxia, ischaemia and certain drugs such as thiopentone, beta-adrenergic blockers, calcium channel blockers or sedatives. Such changes affect cardiac performance, with increases in contractility causing increased stroke volume and cardiac output. Increasing contractility will increase myocardial oxygen demand, which could have a detrimental effect on patients with limited perfusion. Stroke volume is the amount of blood ejected from each ventricle with each heartbeat. For an adult, the volume is normally 50–100 mL/beat, and equal amounts are ejected from the right and left ventricle.

Cardiac output is dependent on a series of mechanical events in the cardiac cycle (Fig. 9.9). As a normal average heart rate is maintained at approximately 70 beats per minute (bpm), the average phases of the cardiac cycle are completed in less than a second (0.8 s). Electrical stimulation of myocardial contraction ensures that the four chambers of the heart contract in sequence. This allows the atria to act as primer pumps for the ventricles, while the ventricles are the major pumps that provide the impetus for blood to flow through the pulmonary and systemic vascular systems. The phases of the cardiac cycle are characterised by pressure changes within each of the heart chambers, resulting in blood flow from areas of high pressure to areas of lower pressure.

During late ventricular diastole (rest), pressures are lowest in the heart and blood returns passively to fill the atria. This flow also moves into the ventricle through the open AV valves, producing 70–80% of ventricular filling. The pulmonic and aortic valves are closed, preventing backflow from the pulmonary and systemic systems into the ventricles. Depolarisation of the atria then occurs, sometimes referred to as atrial kick, stimulating atrial contraction and completing the remaining 20–30% of ventricular filling.[1]

During ventricular systole (contraction), the atria relax while the ventricles depolarise, resulting in ventricular contraction. Pressure rises in the ventricles, resulting in the AV valves closing. When this occurs, all four cardiac valves are closed, blood volume is constant and contraction occurs (isovolumetric contraction). When the pressure in the ventricles exceeds the pressure in the major vessels, the semilunar valves open. This occurs when the pressure in the left ventricle reaches approximately 80 mmHg and in the right ventricle approximately 27–30 mmHg. During the peak ejection phase, the pressure in the left ventricle and aorta reaches approximately 120 mmHg and in the right ventricle and pulmonary artery approximately 25–28 mmHg.

During early ventricular diastole, the ventricles repolarise and ventricular relaxation occurs. The pressure in the ventricles falls until the pressures in the aorta and pulmonary artery are higher and blood pushes back against the semilunar valves. Shutting of these valves prevents backflow into the ventricles, and the pressure in the ventricles declines further. During ventricular contraction, the atria have been filling passively, so the pressure in the atria rises to higher than that in the ventricles and the AV valves open, allowing blood flow to the ventricles. Any rise in heart rate will shorten the resting period, which may impair filling time and coronary artery flow as these arteries fill during diastole.[2]

Regulation of cardiac output

The heart is a very effective pump and is able to adapt to meet the metabolic needs of the body. The activities of the heart are regulated by two responsive systems: intrinsic regulation of contraction and the autonomic nervous system.

Intrinsic regulation of contraction responds to the rate of blood flow into the chambers. Blood flow into the heart depends on venous return from systemic and pulmonic veins and varies according to tissue metabolism, total blood volume and vasodilation. Venous return contributes to end-diastolic volume (preload) and pressure, both of which are directly related to the force of contraction in the next ventricular systole. The intrinsic capacity of the heart to respond to changes in end-diastolic pressure can be represented by a number of length–tension curves and the Frank–Starling mechanism (Fig. 9.10). According to this mechanism, within limits, the greater the stretch of the cardiac muscle fibre before contraction, the greater is the strength of contraction. The ability to increase the strength of contraction in response to increased stretch exists because there is an optimal range of cross-bridges that can be created between actin and myosin in the myocyte. Under this range, when venous return is poor, fewer cross-bridges can be created. Above this range, when heart failure is present, the cross-bridges can become partially disengaged, contraction is poor and higher filling pressures are needed to achieve adequate contractile force.[1,2]

Ventricular contraction is also intrinsically influenced by the size of the ventricle and the thickness of the ventricle wall. This mechanism is described by Laplace's law, which states that the amount of tension generated in the wall of the ventricle required to produce intraventricular pressure depends on the size (radius and wall thickness) of the ventricle.[11] As a result, in heart failure, when ventricular thinning and dilation are present, more tension or contractile force is required to create intraventricular pressure and therefore cardiac output.

The heart's ability to pump effectively is also influenced by the pressure that it is required to generate above-end-diastolic pressure to eject blood during systole. This

FIGURE 9.9 The cardiac cycle. AP = action potential.

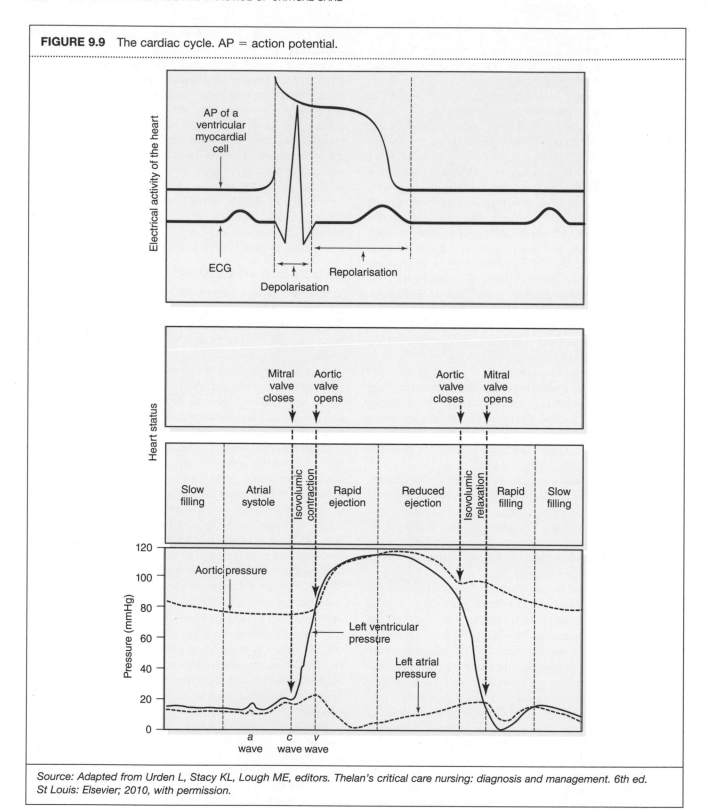

Source: Adapted from Urden L, Stacy KL, Lough ME, editors. Thelan's critical care nursing: diagnosis and management. 6th ed. St Louis: Elsevier; 2010, with permission.

additional pressure is usually determined by how much resistance is present in the pulmonary artery and aorta, and is in turn influenced by the peripheral vasculature. This SVR, known and measured as afterload, causes resistance to flow in relation to the left ventricle and is influenced by vascular tone and disease.[12]

Autonomic nervous system control and regulation of heart rate

Although the pacemaker cells of the heart are capable of intrinsic rhythm generation (automaticity), inputs from the autonomic nervous system regulate heart rate changes in accordance with body needs by stimulating or

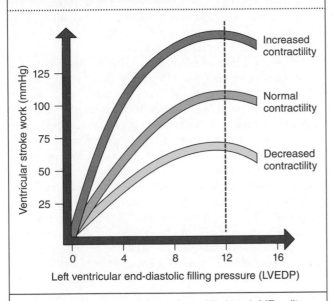

FIGURE 9.10 The Frank–Starling curve. As left ventricular end-diastolic pressure increases, so too does ventricular stroke work.

Source: Adapted from Urden L, Stacy KL, Lough ME, editors. Thelan's critical care nursing: diagnosis and management. 6th ed. St Louis: Elsevier; 2010, with permission.

characteristics are similar. All vessels in the circulatory system are lined by endothelium, including the heart. The endothelium creates a smooth surface, which reduces friction and also secretes substances that promote contraction and relaxation of the vascular smooth muscle. Arteries function to transport blood under high pressure and are characterised by strong elastic walls that allow stretch during systole and high flow. During diastole, the artery walls recoil so that an adequate perfusion pressure is maintained. Arterioles are the final small branches of the arterial system prior to capillaries, and have strong muscular walls that can contract (vasoconstrict) to the point of closure and relax (vasodilate) to change the artery lumen rapidly in response to tissue needs. The lumen created by the arterioles is the most important source of resistance to blood flow in the systemic circulation (just under 50%).

Capillaries function to allow exchange of fluid, nutrients, electrolytes, hormones and other substances through highly permeable walls between the blood plasma and interstitial fluid (Fig. 9.11). Just before the capillary beds are precapillary sphincters, bands of smooth muscle that adjust flow in the capillaries. Venules collect blood from the capillaries to the veins. Excess tissue fluid is collected by the lymphatic system. Lymphatic veins have a similar structure to the cardiovascular system veins

depressing these pacemaker cells. Cardiac innervation includes sympathetic fibres from branches of T1–T5 and parasympathetic input via the vagus nerve. The heart rate at any moment is a product of the respective inputs of sympathetic stimuli (which accelerate) and parasympathetic stimuli (which depress) on heart rate. Rises in heart rate can therefore be achieved by an increase in sympathetic tone or by a reduction in parasympathetic tone (vagal inhibition). Conversely, slowing of the heart rate can be achieved by decreasing sympathetic or increasing parasympathetic activity.[1]

Hormonal, biochemical and pharmacological inputs also exert heart rate influences by their effects on autonomic neural receptors or directly on pacemaker cells. In mimicking the effects of direct nervous inputs, these influences may be described as sympathomimetic or parasympathomimetic. Sympathomimetic stimulation (e.g. through the use of isoprenaline) achieves the same cardiac endpoints as direct sympathetic activity, increasing the heart rate, whereas sympathetic antagonism (e.g. beta-blockade therapy) slows the heart through receptor inhibition.[13] In contrast, parasympathomimetic agonist activity slows the heart rate, whereas parasympathetic antagonism (e.g. via administration of atropine sulfate) raises the heart rate by causing parasympathetic receptor blockade.[1]

The vascular system

The vascular system is specialised according to the different tissues it supplies, but the general functions and

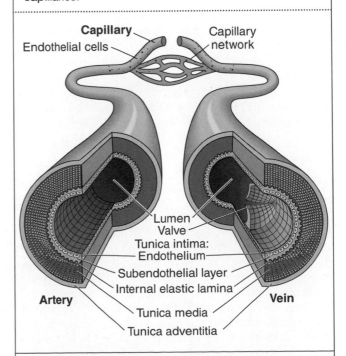

FIGURE 9.11 The structure of arteries, veins and capillaries.

Source: Adapted from Novak B, Filer L, Latchett R. The applied anatomy and physiology of the cardiovascular system. In: Hatchett R, Thompson D, editors. Cardiac nursing: a comprehensive guide. Philadelphia: Churchill Livingstone Elsevier; 2002, with permission.

described below, with lymph returning to this system at the right side of the heart.

Veins collect and transport blood back to the heart at low pressure and serve as a reservoir for blood, with an ability to dilate and constrict as required. Therefore, veins are numerous and have thinner, less muscular walls, which can dilate to store extra blood (up to 70% of total blood volume at any time).[14] Some veins, particularly in the lower limbs, contain valves to prevent backflow and ensure one-way flow to the heart. In addition to intravascular pressure changes, venous return is promoted during standing and moving by the muscles of the legs compressing the deep veins, promoting blood flow towards the heart.

Blood pressure

Blood flow is maintained by pulsatile ejection of blood from the heart and pressure differences between the blood vessels. Traditionally, blood pressure (BP) is measured from the arteries in the general circulation at the maximum value during systole and the minimum value occurring during diastole. The cardiovascular system must supply blood according to varying demands and in a range of circumstances, with at least a minimal blood flow to be maintained to all organs. At a local level, this is achieved by autoregulation of individual arteries, such as the coronary arteries, in response to the metabolic needs of the specific tissue or organ. The exact mechanism is unknown, but it has been proposed that increased vascular muscle stretch and/or metabolites and decreased oxygen levels are detected and cells release substances such as adenosine.[1] These substances result in rapid vasodilation and increased perfusion. The vascular endothelium actively secretes prostacyclin and endothelial-derived relaxing factor (nitric oxide), both of which are vasoactive agents.[15]

There are three main regulatory mechanisms of blood pressure control: (a) short-term autonomic control, (b) medium-term hormonal control and (c) long-term renal system control.

Autonomic control

The cardiovascular control centre connects with the hypothalamus to control temperature, the cerebral cortex and the autonomic system to control cardiac activity and peripheral vascular tone. Information about blood pressure and resistance is sensed by neural receptors (baroreceptors) in the aortic arch and the carotid sinuses, which detect changes in blood supply to the body and the brain. Impulses from these receptors initiate a blood pressure-regulating reflex in the cardiovascular centre, which activates the parasympathetic system and sympathetic system to alter cardiac activity and dilation or constriction of arterioles and veins to lower or raise blood pressure. The cardiovascular system also maintains a constant resting tone of intermediate tension in the arteries.[1]

Hormonal control

Changes in blood pressure are also detected by the adrenal medulla, which secretes catecholamines as cardiac output declines. The two main catecholamines, adrenaline (epinephrine) and noradrenaline (norepinephrine), mimic the action of the sympathetic system by binding to and stimulating adrenergic receptors. Adrenergic receptors are located in smooth muscle cells of vascular beds including the peripheral veins and arterioles supplying the skin, kidneys, skeletal muscles and mucosa.[1]

The main action of adrenaline occurs by binding to the beta-1 adrenoreceptors (located mainly in the heart but also found in platelets and the non-sphincter part of the gastrointestinal tract), causing an increase in the rate and contraction of the heart, aggregation of platelets and relaxation of the non-sphincter part of the gastrointestinal tract. Adrenaline also binds to beta-2 receptors, located on blood vessels, the bronchi, gastrointestinal tract, skeletal muscle, liver and mast cells (inflammatory cells). Activation results in vasodilation of small coronary arteries, bronchodilation, relaxation of the gastrointestinal tract, glycogenolysis (breakdown of glycogen to glucose) in the liver, tremor in skeletal muscle and inhibition of histamine (an inflammatory amine responsible for increased permeability of capillaries).

Noradrenaline binds to both beta and alpha receptors. Alpha-1 and alpha-2 adrenoreceptors are found in the central and peripheral nervous system and are located on vascular and non-vascular smooth muscle. Alpha-1 adrenergic stimulation causes vasoconstriction and is the main mechanism of the vasopressor action of noradrenaline. Presynaptic alpha-2 receptors inhibit the release of noradrenaline and hence serve as an important receptor in the negative-feedback control of noradrenaline release.[16] Postsynaptic alpha-2 receptors are located on liver cells, platelets and the smooth muscle of blood vessels and, when activated, cause platelet aggregation and blood vessel constriction.[17] Noradrenaline results in very little beta-2 activity. Clinically, the positive inotropic and chronotropic effects of noradrenaline from beta-1 simulation are counterbalanced by the increased afterload from elevated SVR (alpha-1 adrenergic agonist effect).[18]

Renal control

Renal control of blood pressure in the long term occurs via control of blood volume. Generally, as blood pressure or volume rises, the kidneys produce more urine; conversely, as blood pressure or volume falls, the kidneys produce less urine.

In addition to longer-term fluid regulation, during acute illness or time of acute hypotension, the renin–angiotensin–aldosterone system (RAAS) plays an important role in maintaining blood pressure. This negative-feedback system both reabsorbs intravascular fluid and increases peripheral resistance in an effort to increase blood pressure.[1] Further details on the RAAS system can be found in Chapter 18.

Assessment

It is essential that the critical care nurse conducts a comprehensive cardiac assessment on a critically ill patient.

The nursing assessment aims to define patient cardiovascular status as well as inform implementation of an appropriate clinical management plan. The focus of the cardiovascular assessment varies according to the setting, clinical presentation and treatments commenced, if any. However, the main priority should be to determine whether the patient is haemodynamically stable or requiring initiation or adjustment of supportive treatments.

A thorough cardiac assessment requires the critical care nurse to be competent in a wide range of interpersonal, observational and technical skills. A cardiac assessment should be performed as part of a comprehensive patient assessment and should consider the following elements.

It is important to create a health history, if not already obtained. This history should aim to elicit a description from the patient or their family of the present illness and chief complaint. A useful guide in taking a specific cardiac history is to use direct questions to seek information regarding symptom onset, course, duration, location and precipitating and alleviating factors. Some common cardiovascular disease-related symptoms to be observed for include: chest discomfort or pain, palpitations, syncope, generalised fatigue, dyspnoea, cough, weight gain or dependent oedema. Chest pain, discomfort or tightness should be initially considered indicative of cardiac ischaemia until proven otherwise by further examination and diagnostic assessment. Additionally, a health history should be inclusive of known cardiovascular risk factors, such as hyperlipidaemia or hypertension, and any medications the patient may be taking including over-the-counter medications.

Prior to inspecting or palpating the patient, the nurse should observe the patient's general appearance, noting whether the patient is restless, able to lie flat, in pain or distress, is pale or has a decreased level of consciousness. Patients with compromised cardiac output will probably have decreased cerebral perfusion and may have mental confusion, memory loss or slowed verbal responses. Additionally, assessment of any pain should be noted.

Specific physical assessment in relation to cardiovascular function should be inclusive of:

- vital signs
- respiratory assessment for signs of pulmonary oedema (shortness of breath or basal crepitations)
- assessment of neck vein distention for signs of right-sided venous congestion
- assessment for signs of peripheral oedema
- capillary refill time with >3 seconds return indicative of sluggish capillary return; indicative of reduced effective circulating volume
- 12-lead ECG for signs of ischaemia or cardiac pathology
- appearance and temperature of the skin for signs of peripheral constriction or dehydration
- core body temperature measurement
- urine output with <0.5 mL/kg/h a potential indicator of decreased renal perfusion.

Assessment of pulse

In the critical care environment, the heart rate can be observed from a cardiac monitor; however, this does not give qualitative information about the arterial pulse. Routinely performed as part of most patient assessments, information gathered from pulse assessment can give useful cues and direct further assessments. Although the radial pulse is distant from the central arteries, it is useful for gathering information on rate, rhythm and strength. A heart rate below 60 bpm is defined as 'bradycardia' (*brady* is Greek for slow, and *kardia* means heart). A heart rate greater than 100 bpm per minute is called 'tachycardia' (*tachy* is Greek for swift). An important aspect of pulse assessment involves assessment for regularity. Detection of an irregular pulse should trigger further investigation and prompt ECG assessment for atrial fibrillation, a condition in which atrial contraction becomes lost because of chaotic electrical activity with variable ventricular response. In addition to rate and rhythm, assessment of the pulse, especially if palpated in the carotid or femoral artery, can reveal a bounding pulse, which may be indicative of hyperdynamic state or aortic regurgitation. An alternating strong and weak pulse, known as *pulsus alternans*, may be observed in advanced heart failure.

Auscultation of heart sounds

Auscultation of the heart involves listening to heart sounds over the pericardial area using a stethoscope. Although challenging to achieve competence in cardiac auscultation, it is an important part of cardiac physical examination and relies on a sound understanding of cardiac anatomy, cardiac cycle and physiologically associated sounds. For accurate auscultation, experience in assessment of normal sounds is critical and can be obtained only through constant practice. When auscultating heart sounds, normally two sounds are readily audible and they are known as the first (S1) and second (S2) sounds. A useful technique when listening to heart sounds is to feel the carotid pulse at the same time as auscultation, which will help identify the heart sound that corresponds with ventricular systole (S1).[19]

> **Practice tip**
>
> When learning to interpret heart sounds, feel the carotid pulse at the same time as auscultation of the heart, which will help identify the heart sound that corresponds with ventricular systole (S1 will be heard simultaneously with the pulse).

The first heart sound S1 occurs at the beginning of ventricular systole, following closure of the intracardiac valves (mitral and tricuspid valves). This heart sound is best heard with the diaphragm of the stethoscope and is loudest directly over the corresponding valves (4th intercostal space (ICS), left of the sternum, for the tricuspid and 5th ICS, left of the mid-clavicular line, for the mitral valve). Following closure of these two valves, ventricular contraction and ejection occur and a carotid pulse may be palpated at the same time that S1 is audible.[19]

The second heart sound S2 occurs at the beginning of diastole, following closure of the aortic and pulmonary valves, and can be best heard over these valves (2nd ICS to the right and left of the sternum, respectively). It is important to remember that both S1 and S2 result from events occurring in *both* left and right sides of the heart. As left-sided heart sounds are normally loudest and occur slightly before right-sided events, careful listening during inspiration and expiration may result in left and right events being heard separately. This is known as physiological splitting of heart sounds, a normal physiological event. A guide to placement of the stethoscope when listening to heart sounds is presented in Table 9.1.

In assessment of the critically ill patient, extra heart sounds, labelled S3 and S4, may be heard during times of extra ventricular filling or fluid overload. Often referred to as 'gallops', these extra heart sounds are accentuated during episodes of tachycardia. S3, ventricular gallop, occurs during diastole in the presence of fluid overload. Considered physiological in children or young people, due to rapid diastolic filling, S3 may be considered pathological when due to reduced ventricular compliance and associated increased atrial pressures. As S3 occurs early in diastole, it will be heard and associated more closely with S2.[19]

S4 is a late diastolic sound and may be heard shortly before S1. S4 occurs when ventricular compliance is reduced secondary to aortic or pulmonary stenosis, mitral regurgitation, systemic hypertension, advanced age or ischaemic heart disease. In patients with severe ventricular dysfunction, both S3 and S4 may be audible, although when coupled with tachycardia these may be difficult to differentiate and will require specialist assessment.[19]

The critical care nurse auscultating the heart should also listen for a potential pericardial rub. This 'rubbing' or 'scratching' sound is secondary to pericardial inflammation and/or fluid accumulation in the pericardial space. To differentiate pericardial rub from pulmonary rub, if possible the patient should be instructed to hold their breath for a short duration as pericardial rub will continue to be audible in the absence of breathing, heard over the 3rd ICS to the left of the mid-sternum. Detection of pericardial rub warrants further investigation by ultrasound.

> **Practice tip**
>
> To differentiate pericardial rub from pulmonary rub, ask the patient to hold their breath for a short duration, as pericardial rub will continue to be audible in the absence of breathing whereas pleural rub will not be audible while the patient is not breathing.

In addition to pericardial rub, murmurs may also be audible. Murmurs are generally classified and characterised by location, with the most common murmurs associated with the mitral or aortic valves, due to either stenosis or regurgitation at these locations. Murmurs are best thought of as turbulent flow or vibrations associated with the corresponding valve and can be of variable pitch. Specialist cardiac referral is indicated upon detection of cardiac murmurs to differentiate pathological murmurs, as seen during valvular dysfunction or myocardial infarction, from innocent systolic 'high-flow' murmurs detected in children or adolescents as a result of vigorous ventricular contraction. Murmurs may be classified using the Levine scale,[20] shown in Table 9.2.

Continuous cardiac monitoring

Internationally, a minimum standard for an ICU requires availability of facilities for cardiovascular monitoring.[21,22]

TABLE 9.1

Guide to placement of the stethoscope when listening to heart sounds

STETHOSCOPE PLACEMENT		AUDITABLE REGION OF HEART
2nd intercostal space	Right of sternum	Aortic valve
2nd intercostal space	Left of sternum	Pulmonary valve
4th intercostal space	Left side of sternum	Tricuspid valve
5th intercostal space	Mid-clavicular line	Mitral valve

TABLE 9.2

Classification of heart murmurs using the Levine scale

Grade 1	Low intensity and difficult to hear.
Grade 2	Low intensity and audible with a stethoscope, but no palpable thrill.
Grade 3	Medium intensity and easily heard with a stethoscope.
Grade 4	Loud and audible and with palpable thrill.
Grade 5	Very loud, but cannot be heard outside the praecordium, and with palpable thrill.
Grade 6	Audible with the stethoscope away from the chest.

Source: Adapted from Olsen K. Oxford handbook of cardiac nursing. 3rd ed. New York: Oxford University Press; 2020.

In the case of the critically ill patient, there are two main forms of cardiac monitoring, both of which are used to generate essential data: continuous cardiac monitoring and the 12-lead ECG. Continuous cardiac monitoring allows for rapid assessment and constant evaluation with, when required, the instantaneous production of paper recordings for more-detailed assessment or documentation into patient records. In addition, practice standards for electrocardiographic monitoring in hospital settings have been established.[23]

It is common practice for five leads to be used for continuous cardiac monitoring, as this allows a choice of seven views. The five electrodes are placed as follows:

- right and left arm electrodes: placed on each shoulder
- right and left leg electrodes: placed on the hips or level with the lowest ribs on the chest
- V-lead views can be monitored: for V1, place the electrode at the 4th ICS, right of the sternum; for V6, place the electrode at the 5th ICS, left mid-axillary line.

The monitoring lead of choice is determined by the patient's clinical situation. Generally, two views are better than one. The V1 lead is best to view ventricular activity and differentiate right and left bundle branch blocks; therefore, one of the channels on the bedside monitor should display a V lead, preferably V1, and the other display lead II or III for optimal detection of arrhythmias. When the primary purpose of monitoring is to detect ischaemic changes, leads III and V3 usually present the optimal combination.[23]

The skin must be carefully prepared before electrodes are attached, as contact is required with the body surface and poor contact will lead to inaccurate or unreadable recordings, causing interference or noise. Patients who are sweaty need particular attention, and it may be necessary to shave the areas where the electrodes are to be placed in very hairy people.

12-lead ECG

The Dutch physiologist Einthoven was one of the first to represent heart electrical conduction as two charged electrodes, one positive and one negative. The body can be likened to a triangle, with the heart at its centre, and this has been called Einthoven's triangle. Cardiac electrical activity can be captured by placing electrodes on both arms and on the left leg. When these electrodes are connected to a common terminal with an indifferent electrode that remains near zero, an electrical potential is obtained. Depolarisation moving towards an active electrode produces positive deflection.

The 12-lead ECG consists of six limb leads and six chest leads. The limb leads examine electrical activity along a vertical plane. The standard bipolar limb leads (I, II, III) record differences in potential between the two limbs by using two limb electrodes as positive and negative poles (Fig. 9.12): leads I, II and III all produce positive deflections on the ECG because the electrical current

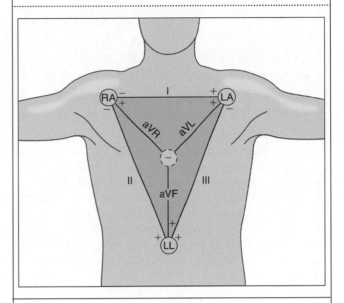

FIGURE 9.12 Einthoven's triangle formed by standard limb leads. aVR, aVL, aVF = unipolar limb leads; LA = left arm; LL = left leg; RA = right arm; I–III = bipolar limb leads.

Source: Adapted from Urden L, Stacy KL, Lough ME, editors. Thelan's critical care nursing: diagnosis and management. 6th ed. St Louis: Elsevier; 2010, with permission.

flows from left to the right and from upwards to downwards. Placement should be:

- I = negative electrode in right arm and positive electrode in left arm
- II = negative electrode in right arm and positive electrode in left leg
- III = negative electrode in left arm and positive electrode in left leg.

The three unipolar limb leads (aVR, aVL and aVF) record activity of the heart's frontal plane. Each of these unipolar leads has only one positive electrode (the limb electrode such as left arm, right arm or left leg), with the centre of Einthoven's triangle acting as the negative electrode. The waveforms of these leads are usually very small; therefore, they are augmented by the ECG machine to increase the size of the potentials on the ECG strip. These three leads view the heart at different angles:

- Lead aVR produces a negative reflection because the electrical activity moves away from the lead. Lead aVR does not provide a specific view of the heart.
- Lead aVL produces a positive deflection because the electrical activity moves towards the lead. Lead aVL views the electrical activity from the lateral wall.
- Lead aVF also produces a positive deflection on the ECG because the electrical activity flows towards this lead. It views the electrical activity from the inferior wall.

The six unipolar chest leads (precordial leads) are designated V1–V6 and examine electrical activity along a horizontal plane from the right ventricle, septum, left ventricle and left atrium. They are positioned in the following way (Fig. 9.13):

- V1 = 4th ICS, to the right of the patient's sternum
- V2 = 4th ICS, to the left of the patient's sternum
- V3 = equidistant between V2 and V4
- V4 = 5th ICS, on the mid-clavicular line
- V5 = 5th ICS, on the anterior axillary line
- V6 = 5th ICS on the mid-axillary line.

Amplitude (voltage) in the ECG is measured by a series of horizontal lines on the ECG trace; lines are 1 mm apart and represent increments of 0.1 mV (Fig. 9.14). Amplitude reflects the wave's electrical force and has no relation to the muscle strength of ventricular contraction. Duration of activity within the ECG is measured by a series of vertical lines also 1 mm apart (see Fig. 9.14). The time interval between each line is 0.04 s. Every fifth line is printed in bold, producing large squares. Each represents 0.5 mV (vertically) and 0.2 s (horizontally).

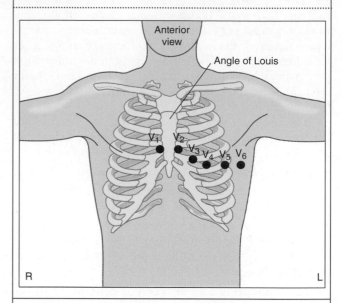

FIGURE 9.13 Position of chest leads. V1–6 = unipolar chest leads.

Source: Adapted from Urden L, Stacy KL, Lough ME, editors. Thelan's critical care nursing: diagnosis and management. 6th ed. St Louis: Elsevier; 2010, with permission.

FIGURE 9.14 ECG graph paper.

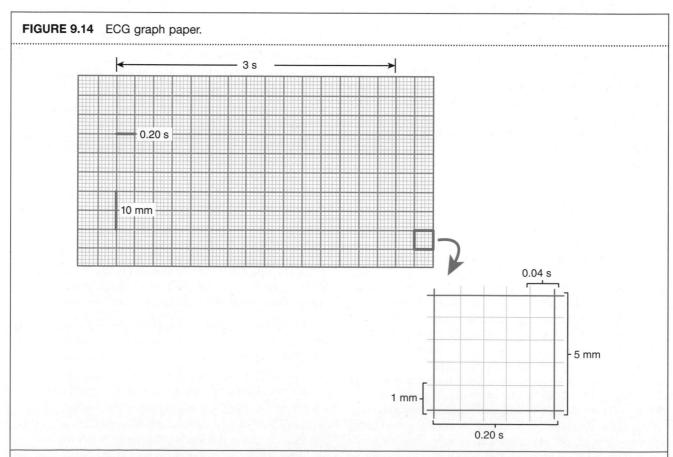

Source: Adapted from Urden L, Stacy KL, Lough ME, editors. Thelan's critical care nursing: diagnosis and management. 6th ed. St Louis: Elsevier; 2010, with permission.

FIGURE 9.15 Normal ECG.

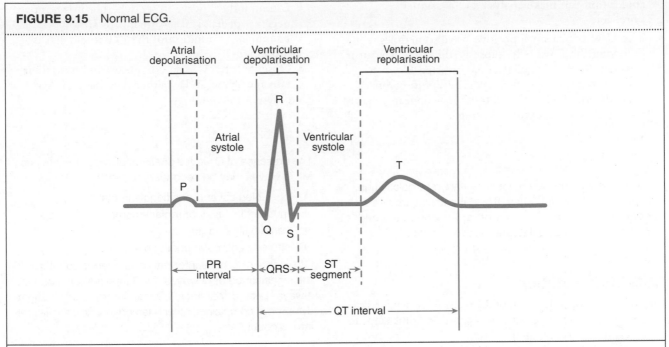

Source: Adapted from Urden L, Stacy KL, Lough ME, editors. Thelan's critical care nursing: diagnosis and management. 6th ed. St Louis: Elsevier; 2010, with permission.

Key components of the ECG

Key components of the cardiac electrical activity are termed P, Q, R, S and T (Fig. 9.15):

- The P wave represents electrical activity caused by spread of impulses from the SA node across the atria and appears upright in lead II. Inverted P waves indicate atrial depolarisation from a site other than the SA node. Normal P-wave duration is considered to be less than 0.12 s.

- The PR interval reflects the total time taken for the atrial impulse to travel through the atria and AV node. It is measured from the start of the P wave to the beginning of the QRS complex, but is lengthened by AV block or some drugs. The normal PR interval is 0.12–0.2 s.

- The QRS complex is measured from the start of the Q wave to the end of the S wave and represents the time taken for ventricular depolarisation. The normal QRS duration is 0.08–0.12 s. Anything longer than 0.12 s is abnormal and may indicate conduction disorders such as bundle branch block.[24] The deflections seen in relation to this complex will vary in size, depending on the lead being viewed. However, small QRS complexes occur when the heart is insulated, as in the presence of pericardial effusion. Conversely, an exaggerated QRS complex is suggestive of ventricular hypertrophy. Normal, non-pathological Q waves are often seen in leads I, aVL, V5 and V6 from septal depolarisation, which are less than 25% of the R height and 0.04 s. A 'pathological'

Q wave (>0.04 s plus >25% of R-wave height) may indicate a previous myocardial infarction; however, not every myocardial infarction will result in a pathological Q wave, and some abnormal Q waves in combination with other ECG changes and patient symptoms may indicate a current myocardial infarction. Pathological Q waves may also be seen in non-ischaemic conditions such as Wolff–Parkinson–White (WPW) syndrome.[25]

- The QT interval is the time taken from ventricular stimulation to recovery. It is measured from the beginning of the QRS to the end of the T wave. Normally, this ranges from 0.35 to 0.45 s, but shortens as heart rate increases. It should be less than 50% of the preceding cycle length.

- The T wave reflects repolarisation of the ventricles. A peaked T wave indicates hyperkalaemia, myocardial infarction (MI) or ischaemia, whereas a flattened T wave usually indicates hypokalaemia. An inverted T wave occurs following an MI or ventricular hypertrophy. A normal T wave is 0.16 s. The height of the T wave should be less than 5 mm in all limb leads, and less than 10 mm in the precordial leads.

- The ST segment is measured from the J point (junction of the S wave and ST segment) to the start of the T wave. It is usually isoelectric in nature, and elevation or depression indicates some abnormality in the onset of recovery of the ventricular muscle, usually due to myocardial injury. Note: it is important that correct filter frequency is applied when recording a 12-lead ECG, as incorrect filter application can make analysis of ST segment unreliable.

- The U wave is a small positive wave sometimes seen following the T wave. Its cause is still unknown but it is exaggerated in hypokalaemia. Inverted U waves may be seen and are often associated with coronary heart disease (CHD),[26] and these may appear transiently during exercise testing.

Practice tip

The 6-second measurement for heart rate calculation is particularly useful when the patient's heart rate is irregular. Count the R waves on a 6-second strip and multiply by 10 to calculate the rate for 1 minute.

ECG interpretation

Interpretation of a 12-lead ECG is an experiential skill, requiring consistent exposure and practice. Some steps to aid interpretation are noted below:

- Calculate heart rate:
  - There are many ways to calculate the heart rate. One way is to count the R waves on a 6-second strip and multiply by 10 to calculate the rate (the top of the ECG paper is usually marked at 3-second intervals).
  - Use an ECG ruler if one is available.
- Check RR intervals (rhythm):
  - Is the rhythm regular?
  - To assess regularity, mark the duration of two neighbouring R waves (RR interval) on a plain piece of paper and move this paper to check other RR intervals on the ECG strip. RR intervals should be uniform in a normal ECG, which indicates that the patient has a regular ECG rhythm.
- Locate P waves (check atrial activity):
  - Observe for the presence or absence of P waves.
  - Check regularity and shape.
  - Is the P wave positive?
  - The relationship between P waves and QRS complexes: is there a P wave preceding every QRS complex?
  - What is the duration of the P wave?
- Measure the PR interval (check AV node activity):
  - What is the duration of the PR interval?
- Measure the QRS duration (check ventricular activity):
  - Is the ventricular electrical activity normal?
  - Is the QRS complex too wide or narrow?
  - Check the presence of a Q wave. If present, is it normal or pathological?
- Note other clues:
  - Observe whether the isoelectric line is present between the S and T waves.

- Examine the T wave to see whether it is positive, negative or flat: is it less than 0.16 s?
- Examine the duration of the QT interval: is it too long?
- Observe for any extra complexes and note their rate and shape, and whether they have the same or different morphology.

Practice tip

The presence of Q waves does not always indicate past MI. Q waves may be secondary to:

- physiological and positional effects
- myocardial injury or replacement
- ventricular enlargement
- altered ventricular conduction.

Other patient clinical information is needed to interpret the significance of Q waves. ECG interpretation should always take a patient's clinical information (patient symptoms, complaints, other haemodynamic information) into account.

Practice tip

Think of the leads I, II, III, aVR, aVL, aVF and V1–V6 as the 'eyes' that are looking at the heart's electrical activity from different angles and view the heart's different areas.

Haemodynamic monitoring

The dynamic movement of the blood in the cardiovascular system is referred to as haemodynamics. Haemodynamic monitoring is performed to provide the clinician with a greater understanding of the pathophysiology of the problem being treated than would be possible with clinical assessment alone. Knowledge of the evidence that underpins the technology and the processes for interpretation is therefore essential to facilitate optimal usage and evidence-based decisions.

This section explores the principles related to haemodynamic monitoring and the different types of monitoring available, and introduces the most recent and appropriate evidence related to haemodynamic monitoring. The reasons for haemodynamic monitoring are generally threefold:

1 to establish a precise health-related diagnosis
2 to determine appropriate therapy
3 to monitor the response to that therapy.

Haemodynamic monitoring can be non-invasive or invasive and may be required on a continuous or intermittent basis, depending on the needs of the patient. In both cases, signals are processed from a variety of physiological variables, and these are then clinically interpreted within the individual patient's context.

Non-invasive monitoring does not require any device to be inserted into the body and therefore does not breach the skin. Directly measured non-invasive variables include body temperature, heart rate, blood pressure, respiratory rate and urine output, while other processed forms can be generated by the ECG, arterial and venous Dopplers, transcutaneous pulse oximetry (using an external probe on a digit such as the finger or on the ear) and expired carbon monoxide monitors.

Invasive monitoring requires the vascular system to be cannulated and pressure or flow within the circulation interpreted. Invasive haemodynamic monitoring technology includes:

- systemic arterial pressure monitoring
- central venous pressure (CVP) monitoring
- pulmonary artery pressure monitoring
- cardiac output monitoring.

Invasive monitoring has also facilitated greater use of blood component analyses, such as arterial and venous blood gases.

The invasive nature of this monitoring allows the pressures that are sensed at the distal ends of the catheters to be transduced, and to continuously display and monitor the corresponding waveforms. The extent of monitoring should reflect how much information is required to optimise the patient's condition, and how precisely the data are to be recorded. It is important to note that these invasive monitoring strategies are not substitutes for careful examination and do not replace the clinicians' clinical decision making. The accuracy of the values obtained and the critical care professionals' ability to interpret the data and choose an appropriate intervention are essential to optimise treatments and patient outcome.

Principles of haemodynamic monitoring

Several key principles need to be understood in relation to invasive haemodynamic monitoring of critically ill patients. These include haemodynamic accuracy, the ability to trend data and the maintenance of minimum standards. These are reviewed below.

Haemodynamic accuracy

Accuracy of the value obtained from haemodynamic monitoring is essential as this information is used to guide patient care. Electronic equipment for this purpose has four components (Fig. 9.16):

1   an invasive catheter attached to high-pressure (non-compliant) tubing
2   a transducer to detect physiological activity
3   a flush system
4   a recording device, incorporating an amplifier to increase the size of the signal, to display information.

High-pressure (non-compliant) tubing reduces distortion of the signal produced between the intravascular device and the transducer, and transmits the hydrostatic pressure to the transducer; the pressure is detected as fluctuations on the diaphragm of the electromanometer within the transducer, and is converted into electrical energy (a waveform). Fluid (0.9% sodium chloride) is routinely used to maintain line patency using a continuous pressure system. No difference in adding heparin in the flush system or using 0.9% sodium chloride alone has been found in maintaining the potency of the pressure system.[27] The pressure of the flush system fluid bag should be maintained at 300 mmHg, which normally delivers a continual flow of 3 mL/h.

Accuracy is dependent on levelling the transducer to the appropriate level (and altering this level with changes in patient position as appropriate), then zeroing the transducer in the pressure-monitoring system to atmospheric pressure, as well as evaluating the response of the system by fast-flush wave testing. The transducer must be levelled to the reference point of the phlebostatic axis, at the intersection of the fourth intercostal space and the mid-thoracic anterior–posterior diameter (not the mid-axillary line). Error in measurement can occur if the transducer is placed above or below the phlebostatic axis. Therefore, when the patient's position changes the transducer must be relevelled in order to maintain the accuracy of the measurement.

Zeroing the transducer system to atmospheric pressure is achieved by turning the three-way stopcock nearest to the transducer open to the air and closing it to the patient and the flush system. The monitor should display zero (0 mmHg), as this equates to current atmospheric pressure (760 mmHg at sea level). With the improved quality of transducers, repeated zeroing is not necessary as, once zeroed, the drift from the baseline is minimal. Some critical care units, however, continue to recalibrate transducer(s) at the beginning of each clinical shift.

Fast-flush square-wave testing, or dynamic response measurement, is a way of checking the dynamic response of the monitor to signals from the blood vessel. It is also a check on the accuracy of the subsequent haemodynamic pressure values. The fast-flush device within the system, when triggered and released, exposes the transducer to the amount of pressure in the flush solution bag (usually 300 mmHg). The pressure waveform on the monitor will show a rapid rise in pressure, which then squares off before the pressure drops back to the baseline (Fig. 9.17).

Interpretation of the square-wave testing is essential; the clinician must observe the speed with which the wave returns to the baseline as well as the pattern produced. One to three rapid oscillations should occur immediately after the square wave, before the monitored waveform resumes. The distance between these rapid oscillations should not exceed 1 mm or 0.04 s. The system is deemed to be adequately damped if these conditions are met. Absence or a reduction of these rapid oscillations, or a square wave with rounded corners, indicates that the

FIGURE 9.16 Haemodynamic monitoring system.

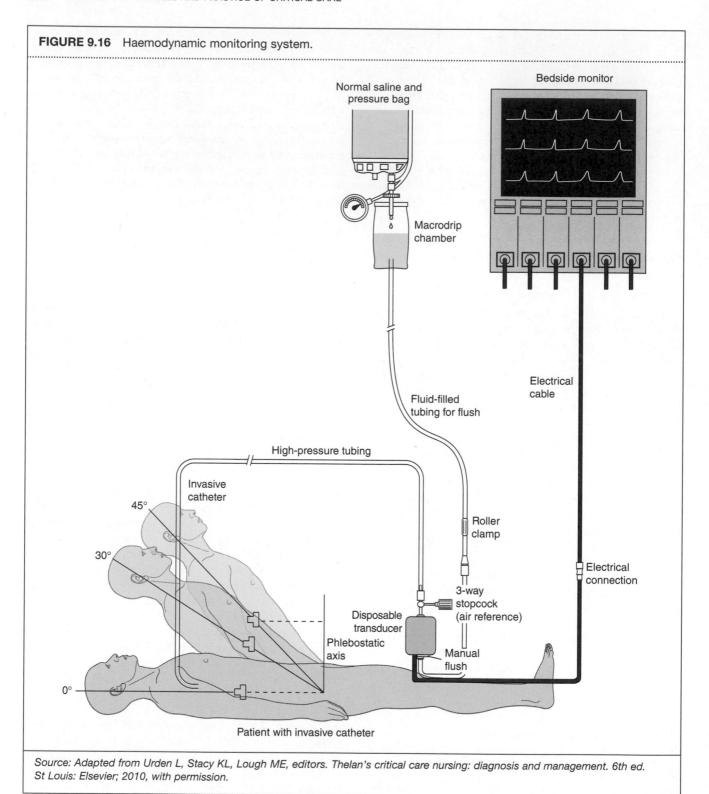

Source: Adapted from Urden L, Stacy KL, Lough ME, editors. Thelan's critical care nursing: diagnosis and management. 6th ed. St Louis: Elsevier; 2010, with permission.

pressure-monitoring system is overdamped; in other words, its responsiveness to monitored pressures and waveforms is reduced (Fig. 9.18). An underdamped monitoring system will produce more-rapid oscillations than usual after the square wave.

Data trends

The ability to read trends in data via a monitor or a clinical information system is essential for critical care practice. Current monitoring systems can retain data for a period of time, produce trend graphs and link to other

FIGURE 9.17 Normal dynamic response test.

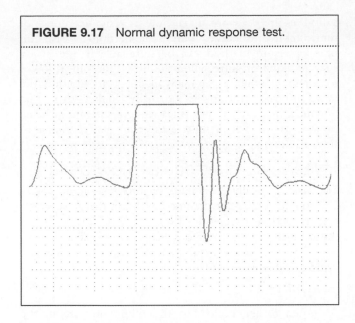

FIGURE 9.18 Overdamped dynamic response test.

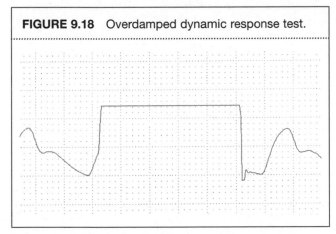

devices to allow review of data from locations other than the immediate bedside. The data trends can be used to assess the progression of a patient's clinical condition and monitor the patient's response to treatment.

Haemodynamic monitoring standards

There are stated minimum standards for critical care units worldwide. The standards require that patient monitoring of the circulation, respiration and oxygenation occurs, with the following essential equipment available for every patient: an ECG that facilitates continual cardiac monitoring, a mechanical ventilator, pulse oximeter and other equipment available where necessary to measure intra-arterial and pulmonary pressures, cardiac output, inspiratory pressure and airway flow, intracranial pressures and expired carbon dioxide.

Blood pressure monitoring

Indirect and direct means of monitoring blood pressure are widely used in critical care units. These are outlined in more detail below.

Non-invasive blood pressure monitoring

Non-invasive blood pressure monitoring requires the use of a manual or electronic sphygmomanometer. Oscillation in the pressure generated by alterations in arterial flow is captured through either auscultation or automatic sensing. On auscultation, several Korotkoff sounds can be heard as the cuff pressure is released:

- a sharp thud that is heard when the patient's systolic pressure is reached
- a soft tapping, intermittent in nature
- a loud tapping, intermittent in nature
- a low, muffled noise that is continuous in nature and is heard when the diastolic pressure is reached; as the cuff pressure diminishes further, the sound disappears.

For critically ill patients, this method of blood pressure monitoring has limitations and is often used when invasive methods cannot be utilised. It is a less-accurate alternative, as results vary with the size of cuff used, equipment malfunction and incorrect placement of the sphygmomanometer (this must be placed at heart level). In addition, the pressures generated by the inflating cuff, particularly those generated by automatic machines, can be high and frequent measurements of blood pressure by this method may become uncomfortable for the patient. It is, therefore, important that skin integrity be checked regularly to prevent ischaemia and that the frequency of automated inflations be minimised.

Invasive intra-arterial pressure monitoring

Arterial pressure recording is indicated when precise and continuous monitoring is required, especially in periods of fluid volume, cardiac output and blood pressure instability. An arterial catheter is commonly placed in the radial artery, although other sites can be accessed, including the brachial, femoral, dorsalis pedis and axillary arteries. Arterial catheter insertion is performed aseptically, and it is important that collateral circulation, patient comfort and risk of infection be assessed before insertion is attempted. The radial artery is the most common site, as the ulnar artery provides collateral supply to the extremity if the radial artery becomes compromised.

Complications of arterial pressure monitoring include:

- infection
- arterial thrombosis
- distal ischaemia
- air embolism
- accidental disconnection leading to rapid blood loss (the insertion sites should be always visible)
- accidental drug administration through the arterial catheter; all arterial lines and connections should be clearly identified as such (e.g. marked with red stickers or have red caps).

Blood pressure is the same at all sites along a vertical level, but when the vertical level is varied the pressure will

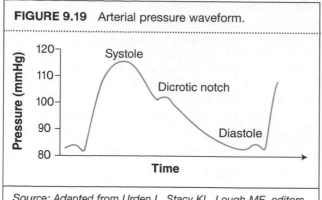

FIGURE 9.19   Arterial pressure waveform.

Source: Adapted from Urden L, Stacy KL, Lough ME, editors. Thelan's critical care nursing: diagnosis and management. 6th ed. St Louis: Elsevier; 2010, with permission.

change. To prevent ventilator-associated pneumonia, ventilated patients are often sat up to 45 degrees. It is important to remember that blood pressures can be measured and recorded at different positions. Consequently, referencing is required to correct for changes in hydrostatic pressure in vessels above and below the heart; if not, the blood pressure will appear to rise when this is not really the case. It is important to zero the monitoring system at the left atrial level.

Arterial waveform

A steep upstroke (corresponding to ventricular systole) is followed by brief, sustained pressure (anacrotic shoulder). At the end of systole, pressure falls in the aorta and left ventricle, causing a downward deflection (Fig. 9.19). A dicrotic notch can be seen in the downward deflection, which represents the closure of the aortic valve when measured directly in the aorta, but is thought to represent peripheral vascular resistance when measured distally. The systolic pressure corresponds to the peak of the waveform. The arterial pressure waveform changes its contours when recorded at different sites. It can become sharper in distal locations.

   Disease process has an effect on waveforms:; for example, atherosclerosis causes an increase in the systolic waveform, as well as a decrease in the size of the diastolic wave and dicrotic notch due to changes in arterial elasticity. Cardiomyopathy causes reduced stroke volume and mean arterial pressure, and there is a late secondary systolic peak seen on the waveform.

Invasive arterial pressure versus cuff pressure

At times, the accuracy of the invasive arterial pressure reading may be checked by comparing the reading with that generated by a non-invasive device using an inflating cuff. However, there is no basis for comparing these values. Invasive blood pressure values are a measure of the actual pressure within the artery whereas those from the cuff depend on flow-induced oscillations in the arterial

wall. Pressure does not equal flow, as resistance does not remain constant. Studies found that the non-invasive cuff blood pressure method can be unreliable in measuring systolic blood pressure when the blood pressure is low – for example, when a patient is in shock. In addition, the radial arterial pressure is normally higher than that obtained by brachial non-invasive pressure monitoring because the smaller vessel size exerts greater resistance to flow, and therefore generates a higher pressure reading.

Invasive cardiovascular monitoring

For many critically ill patients, haemodynamic instability is a potentially life-threatening condition that necessitates urgent action. Accurate assessment of the patient's intracardiac status is therefore essential. Several values can be calculated; the measurements commonly made are listed in Tables 9.3 and 9.4.

Preload

As noted earlier, preload is the filling pressure in the ventricles at the end of diastole. CVP is used clinically as a surrogate estimate of preload in the right ventricle, although this may be an unreliable predictor because CVP is affected by intrathoracic pressure, vascular tone and obstruction. Pulmonary artery occlusion pressure (PAOP), obtained using a pulmonary artery catheter, is sometimes used as a surrogate estimate of left ventricular preload.[28] Other modalities to gain insight into preload are becoming more commonly used in clinical practice, including intrathoracic blood volume measured by transpulmonary thermodilution, left ventricular end-diastolic area measured by echocardiography and, less commonly, right ventricular end-diastolic volume evaluation via fast-response pulmonary artery catheters.

TABLE 9.3

Haemodynamic pressures

PARAMETER	RESTING VALUES
Central venous pressure	0 to +8 mmHg (mean)
Right ventricular pressure	+15 to +30 mmHg systolic; 0 to +8 mmHg diastolic
Pulmonary artery wedge pressure	+5 to +15 mmHg (mean)
Left atrial pressure	+4 to +12 mmHg (mean)
Left ventricular pressure	90–140 mmHg systolic; +4 to +12 mmHg diastolic
Aortic pressure	90–140 mmHg systolic; 60–90 mmHg diastolic; 70–105 mmHg (mean)

TABLE 9.4

Normal haemodynamic values

PARAMETER	DESCRIPTION	NORMAL VALUES
Stroke volume (SV)	Volume of blood ejected from left ventricle/beat: SV = CO/HR	50–100 mL/beat
Stroke volume index (SVI)	Volume of blood ejected/beat indexed to BSA	25–45 mL/beat
Cardiac output (CO)	Volume of blood ejected from left ventricle/min: CO = HR × SV	4–8 L/min
Cardiac index (CI)	A derived value reflecting the volume of blood ejected from left ventricle/min indexed to BSA: CI = CO/BSA	$2.5–4.2$ L/min/m^2 (normal assumes an average weight of 70 kg)
Mean arterial pressure (MAP)	[(2 × diastolic) + systolic] /3	70–105 mmHg
Flow time corrected (FTc)	Systolic flow time corrected for heart rate.	330–360 ms
Systemic vascular resistance (SVR)	Resistance left heart pumps against: SVR = [(MAP − RAP) × 79.9]/CO	900–1300 dyn•s/cm^5
Systemic vascular resistance index (SVRI)	Resistance left heart pumps against indexed to body surface area: SVRI = [(MAP − RAP) × 79.9]/CI	1700–2400 dyn•s/cm^5/m^2
Pulmonary vascular resistance (PVR)	Resistance right heart pumps against: PVR = [(mPAP − LVEDP) × 79.9]/CO	20–120 dyn•s/cm^5
Pulmonary vascular resistance index (PVRI)	Resistance right heart pumps against indexed to body surface area: PVRI = [(mPAP − LVEDP) × 79.9]/CI	255–285 dyn•s/cm^5/m^2
Mixed venous saturation (SvO$_2$)	Shows the balance between arterial O$_2$ supply and oxygen demand at the tissue level.	70%
Left ventricular stroke work index (LVSWI)	Amount of work performed by LV with each heartbeat: (MAP − LVEDP) × SVI × 0.0136	50–62 g-m/m^2
Right ventricular stroke work index (RVSWI)	Amount of work performed by RV with each heartbeat: (mPAP − RAP) × SVI × 0.0136	7.9–9.7 g-m/m^2
Right ventricular end-systolic volume (RVESV)	The volume of blood remaining in the ventricle at the end of the ejection phase of the heartbeat.	50–100 mL/beat
Right ventricular end-systolic volume index (RVESVI)		30–60 mL/m^2
Right ventricular end-diastolic volume (RVEDV)	The amount of blood in the ventricle immediately before a cardiac contraction begins.	100–160 mL/beat
Right ventricular end-diastolic volume index (RVEDVI)		60–100 mL/m^2

BSA = body surface area; HR = heart rate; LVEDP = left ventricular preload; mPAP = mean pulmonary artery pressure; RAP = right atrial pressure.

Source: Adapted from Leeper B. Monitoring right ventricular volumes: a paradigm shift. AACN Clin Issues 2003;14(2):201–19; Schummer W. Central venous pressure. Validity, informative value and correct measurement. Anaesthetist 2009;58(5):499–505.

Central venous pressure monitoring

Centrally inserted central catheters are inserted to facilitate the monitoring of CVP, facilitate the administration of vasoactive medications such as vasopressors or inotropes and large amounts of IV fluid or blood products, and provide short- to intermediate-term access for fluids, drugs, specimen collection and/or the delivery of parenteral nutrition. CVP monitoring has been used for many years to evaluate circulating blood volume, despite discussion as to its validity to do so.[28] However, it is a common monitoring practice and continues to be used. Therefore, clinicians need to be aware of limitations to this form of measurement and interpret the data accordingly. CVP monitoring can produce erroneous results: a low CVP does not always mean low volume and it may reflect other pathology, including peripheral dilation due to sepsis. Hypovolaemic patients may have normal CVP because of sympathetic nervous system activity increasing vascular tone. An increase in CVP can also be seen in patients on mechanical ventilation with application of positive end-expiratory pressure (PEEP).

Central venous catheters used for haemodynamic monitoring are classed as short-term percutaneous (non-tunnelled) devices. Short-term percutaneous catheters are inserted through the skin directly into a central vein, and may remain in situ for up to several weeks. They are easily removed and changed, and are manufactured in single- or multi-lumen configurations. However, they can be easily dislodged, are thrombogenic owing to their material and are associated with a high risk of infection.[29]

Several locations can be used for central venous catheter insertion. The two commonly used sites in critically ill patients are the subclavian and the internal jugular veins. Other less-common sites are the axillary vein, the femoral vein (associated with increased risk of infection) and the external jugular vein (although the high incidence of anomalous anatomy and the severe angle with the subclavian vein make this an unpopular choice).[30]

Internal jugular cannulation has a high success rate for insertion; some complications related to insertion via this route can include carotid artery puncture and laceration of local neck structures arising from needle probing. There are a number of key structures adjacent to the vein, including the vagus nerve (located posteriorly to the internal jugular vein), the sympathetic trunk (located behind the vagus nerve) and the phrenic nerve (located laterally to the internal jugular vein). Damage can also occur to the sympathetic chain, which leads to Horner's syndrome (constricted pupil, ptosis and absence of sweat gland activity on that side of the face). These risks are greatly reduced with the use of ultrasound to aid insertion.[31] Central venous catheters inserted in the internal jugular vein pose several nursing challenges that can cause fixation problems and the need for repeated dressing changes. These include beard growth, diaphoresis and poor control of oral secretions. Recently, these issues have been addressed by cannulating the internal jugular vein low down the neck at the superior margin of the clavicle, with the lower approach allowing for the catheter to be rotated and secured over the supraclavicular region, or even further inferiorly to the chest. This allows for better fixation and dressing integrity and is becoming more frequently used in the Australian context.[30]

The subclavian approach is often used, perhaps because of a reported lower risk of catheter-related bloodstream infection.[32] Despite this, there are several attendant risks which are largely unmodifiable with respect to traditional subclavian vein cannulation. As ultrasound visualisation of the subclavian vein is not possible (because of the clavicle obstructing the transmission of ultrasound waves in the area of interest), and given that the subclavian vein is bounded superiorly by the subclavian artery and inferiorly by the pleura, a 'blind' landmark-only approach is required, which increases iatrogenic complications of arterial puncture, and pneumothorax. Furthermore, bleeding complications are more challenging to manage because of the non-compressible nature of the subclavian vein. Recently, the use of ultrasound and cannulation more laterally into the axillary vein has become a desirable alternative, as the ability to image the pleura and axillary artery, combined with the ability to compress directly over punctured vessels, improves the risk profile during insertion.[33] Complications of any central venous access catheter include air embolism, pneumothorax, hydrothorax and haemorrhage.

Pulmonary artery pressure monitoring

Pulmonary artery pressure (PAP) monitoring began in the 1970s, led by Swan and colleagues,[34] and was subsequently adopted in ICUs worldwide. Pulmonary artery catheterisation facilitates assessment of filling pressure of the left ventricle through the pulmonary artery occlusion pressure (Fig. 9.20). By using a thermodilution pulmonary artery catheter (PAC), cardiac output and other haemodynamic measurements can also be calculated. PAP monitoring is a diagnostic tool that can assist in determining the nature of a haemodynamic problem and improve diagnostic accuracy. In addition to measuring pulmonary artery pressures, PAC may also be used for accessing blood for assessment of mixed venous oxygenation levels (see Chapter 13).

The indications of PAP monitoring are largely based on health professionals' clinical experience and expertise. It has been suggested that PAP monitoring may be indicated for adults in severe hypovolaemic or cardiogenic shock, where there may be diagnostic uncertainty or where the patient is unresponsive to initial therapy. More recently, several systematic reviews and meta-analyses examining the use of PAC in patients with cardiogenic shock found an association with lower short-term mortality rates when a PAC was used to guide treatment.[32,35] The PAP is used to guide administration of fluids, inotropes and vasopressors. PAP monitoring may also be utilised in other cases of haemodynamic instability when the diagnosis is unclear. It may be helpful when clinicians want to differentiate hypovolaemia from cardiogenic shock or, in cases of

FIGURE 9.20 Pulmonary artery catheters.

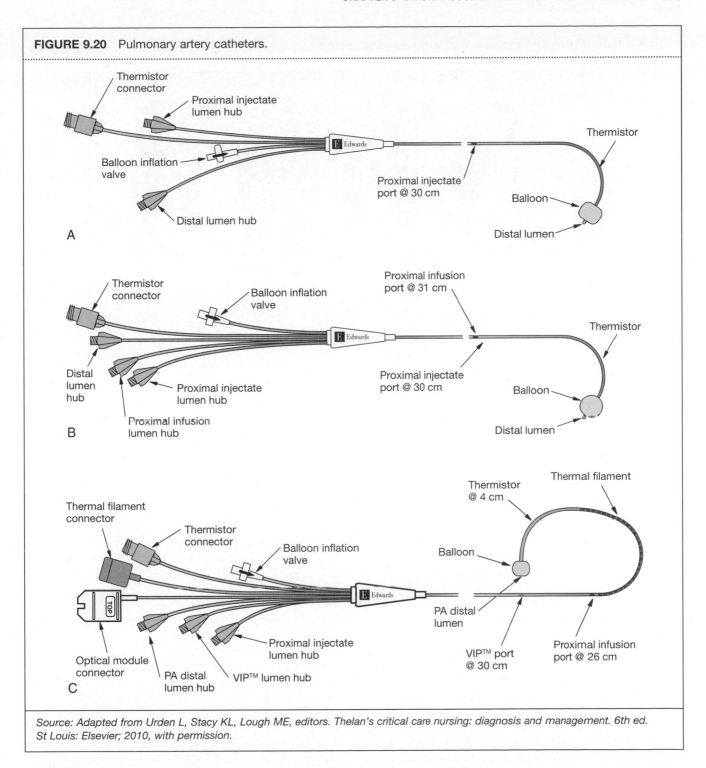

pulmonary oedema, to differentiate cardiogenic from non-cardiogenic origins. Complications do arise from PACs, as these catheters share all the complications of central lines and are additionally associated with a higher incidence of arrhythmia, valve damage, pulmonary vascular occlusion, emboli/infarction (reported incidence of 0.1–5.6%) and, very rarely, knotting of the catheter.[36]

A number of measurements can be taken via the PAC, either by direct measurement, for example using the

pulmonary capillary occlusion pressure (PCOP), which is used as a surrogate estimate of left ventricular preload (LVEDP), or through calculation of derived parameters such as cardiac output (CO) and cardiac index (CI) (see Table 9.4 for descriptors and normal values).

PAOP monitoring

Pulmonary artery occlusion pressure (PAOP), historically referred to as pulmonary capillary wedge pressure (PCWP),

FIGURE 9.21 Pulmonary artery pressure and wedge waveforms.

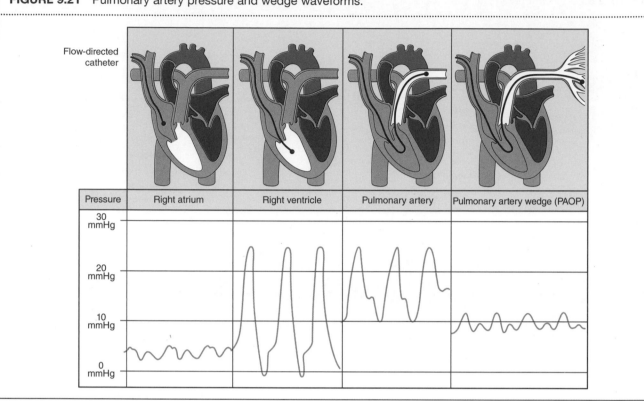

Pressure	Right atrium	Right ventricle	Pulmonary artery	Pulmonary artery wedge (PAOP)

Flow-directed catheter

30 mmHg

20 mmHg

10 mmHg

0 mmHg

Source: Adapted from Urden L, Stacy KL, Lough ME, editors. Thelan's critical care nursing: diagnosis and management. 6th ed. St Louis: Elsevier; 2010, with permission.

is measured when the PAC distal balloon is inflated with no more than 1–1.5 mL air in a branch of the pulmonary artery. The inflated balloon isolates the distal measuring lumen from the pulmonary arterial pressures, and measures pressures in the capillaries of the pulmonary venous system, and indirectly the left atrial pressure. The PAP waveform looks similar to that of the arterial waveform, with the tracing showing a systolic peak, dicrotic notch and a diastolic dip (Fig. 9.21). When the balloon is inflated, the waveform changes shape and becomes much flatter in appearance, providing a similar waveform to the CVP. There are two positive waves on the tracing: the first reflects atrial contraction and the second reflects pressure changes from blood flow when the mitral valve closes and the ventricles contract. The PAOP should be read once the 'wedge' trace stops falling at the end-expiratory phase of the respiratory cycle (see Fig. 9.21).

If balloon occlusion occurs with <1 mL of air, the balloon is wedged in a small capillary and consequently will not accurately reflect left atrial pressure. Conversely, if 1.5 mL air does not cause occlusion, the balloon may have burst (which can result in an air embolus) or it may be floating in a larger vessel. If balloon rupture is suspected, no further attempts to inflate the balloon should be made, and interventions to minimise the risk of air embolism should be initiated.

Note: it is essential that the balloon be deflated as soon as the pressure has been recorded, as continued occlusion will cause distal pulmonary vasculature ischaemia and infarction.

Left atrial pressure monitoring

Left atrial pressure (LAP) monitoring directly estimates left heart preload. It used to require an open thorax to enable direct cannulation of the atrium. It was used only in the postoperative cardiac surgical setting, although such use has been infrequent since the widespread use of PAC. Recent advancement in cardiac implantable devices development enables the patients to self-monitor LAP under their doctors' guidance, which was found to be a valuable tool to improve the management of patients with advanced heart failure. Other modes of monitoring can also be used to achieve comprehensive left atrial assessment, such as Doppler echocardiography.[37]

Afterload

As previously noted, afterload is the pressure that the ventricle produces to overcome the resistance to ejection generated in the systemic or pulmonary circulation by the arteries and arterioles. It is calculated by CO studies: left heart afterload is reflected as SVR, and right heart afterload is reflected as pulmonary vascular resistance (PVR) (see Table 9.4).

Systemic and pulmonary vascular resistance

SVR is a measure of left ventricular afterload and PVR a measure of right ventricular afterload. An elevated SVR can be caused by vasoconstrictors, hypovolaemia or late septic shock. A lowered SVR can be caused by early septic shock, vasodilators, morphine, nitrates or hypercarbia. Afterload is a major determinant of blood pressure, and gross vasodilation causes peripheral pooling and hypotension, reducing SVR. The precise estimation of SVR enables safer use of therapies such as vasodilators and vasoconstrictors. For example, if SVR is elevated, a vasodilator (e.g. hydralazine) may be indicated to lower the blood pressure. If SVR is low, a vasoconstrictor (e.g. noradrenaline) should be considered to treat hypotension.

PVR is a measure of resistance or the impediment of the pulmonary vascular bed to blood flow. An elevated PVR ('pulmonary hypertension') is caused by pulmonary vascular disease, pulmonary embolism, pulmonary vasculitis or hypoxia. A lowered PVR is caused by medications such as calcium channel blockers, aminophylline or isoprenaline, or by the delivery of oxygen.

Contractility

Contractility reflects the force of myocardial contraction, and is related to the extent of myocardial fibre stretch (preload, see above) and wall tension (afterload, see above). It is important because it influences myocardial oxygen consumption. Contractility of the left side of the heart is measured by calculating the left ventricular stroke work index (LVSWI), although the clinical use of this value is not widespread.

The right ventricular stroke work index (RVSWI) can be similarly calculated. Contractility can decrease as a result of excessive preload or afterload, drugs such as negative inotropes, myocardial damage such as that occurring after MI, and changes in the cellular environment arising from acidosis, hypoxia or electrolyte imbalances. Increases in contractility arise from drugs such as positive inotropes.

Cardiac output (CO)

As discussed earlier in the chapter, CO refers to the blood volume ejected by the heart in 1 minute. Stroke volume (SV) is the blood ejected by the heart in one beat. Therefore, CO can be calculated as the heart rate multiplied by SV. The SV is determined by the heart's preload, afterload and the contractility.

The variety of CO measurement techniques has grown over the past decade since the development of thermodilution PACs, pulse-induced contour devices, less-invasive techniques such as Doppler and non-invasive continuous haemodynamic monitoring methods. Vincent and colleagues[38] provide an overview of advantages and disadvantages of these different measurement methods.

As many critically ill patients require mechanical ventilation support, the associated rises in intrathoracic pressure, as well as changing ventricular compliance, make accurate haemodynamic assessment difficult with the older technologies. Therefore, volumetric measurements of preload, such as right ventricular end-systolic volume (RVESV), right ventricular end-diastolic volume (RVEDV) and index (RVESVI/RVEDVI) as well as measurements of right ventricular ejection fraction (RVEF), may be used to determine CO more accurately. The parameters RVEF, CO and/or CI and SV are generated using thermodilution technology, and from these the parameters of RVEDV/RVEDVI and RVESV/RVESVI can be calculated (see Table 9.4 for normal values). The availability of continuous modes of assessment has further improved a clinician's ability to accurately assess, and then effectively treat, these patients.

The Fick principle

Several CO measurement methods use the Fick principle. In 1870, Fick proposed that *'in an organ, the uptake or release of an indicator substance is the product of the arterial–venous concentration of this substance and the blood flow to the organ'*.[39] Using oxygen as the indicator substance, the calculation of CO is as follows:

$$CO = VO_2/(CaO_2 - CvO_2)$$

where VO_2 is oxygen consumption, CaO_2 is arterial oxygen concentration, and CvO_2 is the venous oxygen concentration.

Thermodilution methods

Thermodilution methods calculate CO by using temperature change as the indicator in Fick's method. CO and associated pressures such as global end-diastolic volume can be calculated using a thermodilution PAC. CO can be monitored intermittently or continuously using the PAC. Intermittent measurements obtained every few hours produce a snapshot of the cardiovascular state over that time. By injecting a bolus of 5–10 mL of crystalloid solution and measuring the resulting temperature changes, an estimation of SV is calculated. Cold injectate (run through ice) was initially recommended, but studies now support the use of room temperature injectate, providing there is a difference of 12°C between the injectate and blood temperature. Three readings are taken at the same part of the respiratory cycle (normally end expiration), and any measurements that differ by more than 10% should be disregarded (see Table 9.4 for normal values). Since the 1990s, the value of having continuous measurement of CO has been recognised and this has led to the development of devices that permit the transference of pulses of thermal energy to pulmonary artery blood – the pulse-induced contour method.[40]

Pulse contour cardiac output

Pulse contour cardiac output (PiCCO, note that the lower case 'i' doesn't not stand for anything and is added to make the word pronounceable) provides both intermittent and continuous assessment of CO, and requires a central venous line and an arterial line with a thermistor (not a PAC).[40] A known volume of thermal indicator (usually room temperature saline) is injected into the central vein. The injectate disperses both volumetrically and thermally within the cardiac and pulmonary blood. When the thermal signal is detected by the arterial thermistor, the temperature difference is calculated and a dissipation curve generated. From these data, the CO can be calculated. These continuous CO measurements have been well researched and appear to be equal in accuracy to those produced by intermittent injections required for the earlier catheters.[40] The parameters measured by PiCCO include the following:

- *PiCCO:* is the derived normal value for CI, 2.5–4.2 L/min/m².

- *Global end-diastolic volume (GEDV):* is the volume of blood contained in the four chambers of the heart; it assists in the calculation of intrathoracic blood volume. The derived normal value for global end-diastolic blood volume index is 680–800 mL/m².

- *Intrathoracic blood volume (ITBV):* is the volume of the four chambers of the heart plus the blood volume in the pulmonary vessels; it more accurately reflects circulating blood volumes, particularly when a patient is artificially ventilated. The derived normal value for ITBV index is 850–1000 mL/m².

- *Extravascular lung water (EVLW):* is the amount of water content in the lungs; it allows quantification of the degree of pulmonary oedema (not evident with X-ray or blood gases). The derived normal value for extravascular lung water index is 3–7 mL/kg. EVLW

has been shown to be useful as a guide for fluid management in critically ill patients. An elevated EVLW may be an effective indicator of severity of illness, particularly after acute lung injury or in acute respiratory distress syndrome (ARDS), when EVLW is elevated owing to alterations in hydrostatic pressures. Other patients at risk of high EVLW are those with left heart failure, severe pneumonia and burns. There may be an association between high EVLW and increased mortality, the need for mechanical ventilation and a higher risk of nosocomial infection. A decision tree outlining processes of care guided by information provided by PiCCO is provided in Fig. 9.22.

PiCCO removes the impact of factors that can cause variability in the standard approach of CO measurement, such as injectate volume and temperature, and timing of the injection within the respiratory cycle.[40] The additional fluid volume injected with the standard technique is significant in some patients; with continuous technology, this is eliminated. A further advantage is that virtually real-time responses to treatment can be obtained, removing the time delay that was a potential problem with standard thermodilution techniques.[40]

An arterial catheter is widely used in critical care to enable frequent blood sampling and blood pressure monitoring, and is used to measure beat-by-beat CO, obtained from the shape of the arterial pressure wave. The area under the systolic portion of the arterial pulse wave from the end of diastole to the end of the ejection phase

FIGURE 9.22 PiCCO decision tree. CI = cardiac index; CFI = cardiac function index; ELWI = extravascular lung index; GEDI = global end-diastolic index; GEF = global ejection fraction; ITBI = intrathoracic blood index.

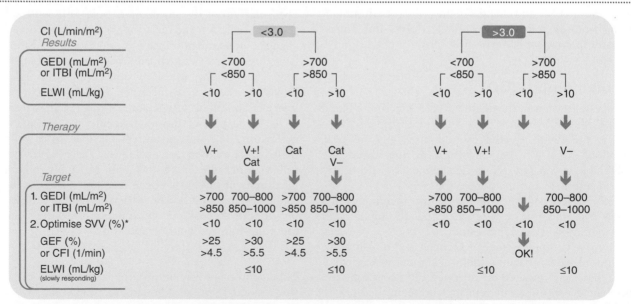

V+ = volume loading (! = cautiously)   V− = volume contraction   Cat = catecholamine / cardiovascular agents
*SVV only applicable in ventilated patients without cardiac arrhythmia

Without guarantee

is measured and combined with an individual calibration factor. The algorithm is capable of computing each single SV after being calibrated by an initial transpulmonary thermodilution.

PiCCO preload indicators of ITBV and GEDV are more sensitive and specific to cardiac preload than the standard cardiac filling pressures of CVP and PAOP, as well as RVEDV. One advantage of ITBV and GEDV is that they are not affected by mechanical ventilation and therefore give correct information on the preload status under almost any condition. EVLW correlates moderately well with severity of ARDS, length of ventilation days, ICU stay and mortality, and appears to be of greater accuracy than the traditional assessment of lung oedema by chest X-ray.[41] Disadvantages of PiCCO include its potential unreliability when heart rate, blood pressure and total vascular resistance change substantially.[40]

Lithium dilution cardiac output (LiDCO)

Lithium can be used as an alternative indicator to estimate CO, which is a method that has been used since its introduction in the 1990s. The LiDCO is calculated using lithium dilution. Isotonic lithium chloride is injected as a bolus (0.002–0.004 mmol/kg) via either a central or a peripheral venous route, then a concentration–time curve is generated by an ex vivo ion-selective electrode attached to the arterial pressure line. The CO is calculated from the lithium dose and the area under the concentration–time curve. It is considered to be a simpler method as it requires only an arterial line. The LiDCO measurement method has been found to be as accurate as the PAC thermodilution technique.[42]

Doppler ultrasound methods

Oesophageal Doppler monitoring enables calculation of CO from assessment of SV and heart rate, but uses a less-invasive technique than those outlined previously.[43] SV is assessed by measuring the flow velocity and the area through which the forward flow travels. Flow velocity is the distance that one red blood cell travels forward in one cardiac cycle, and the measurement provides a time–velocity interval. The area of flow is calculated by measuring the cross-sectional area of the blood vessel or heart chamber at the site of the flow velocity measurement.[43] Oesophageal Doppler monitoring can be performed at the level of the pulmonary artery, mitral valve or aortic valve.

According to Doppler principles, the movement of blood produces a waveform that reflects blood flow velocity, in this case in the descending thoracic aorta (Fig. 9.23), that is captured by the change in frequency of an ultrasound beam as it reflects off a moving object.[44] This measurement is combined with an estimate of the cross-sectional area of the aorta so that the SV, CO and CI can be calculated using the patient's age, height and weight.[44]

Oesophageal Doppler monitoring provides an alternative for patients who would not benefit from PAC insertion,[45] and can be used to provide continuous

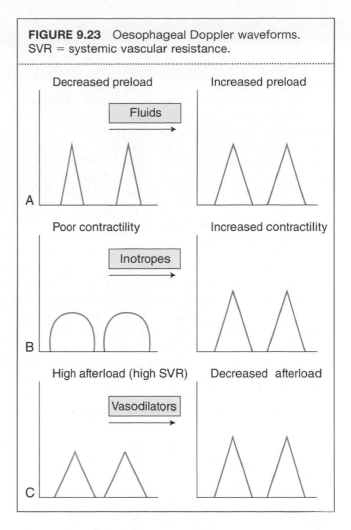

FIGURE 9.23 Oesophageal Doppler waveforms. SVR = systemic vascular resistance.

measurements under certain conditions: the estimate of cross-sectional area must be accurate, the ultrasound beam must be directed parallel to the flow of blood, and there should be minimal variation in the movement of the beam between measurements. This form of monitoring can be used perioperatively and in the critical care unit, on a wide variety of patients.[45] It should not, however, be used in patients with aortic coarctation or dissection, oesophageal malignancy or perforation, severe bleeding problems or with patients on an intra-aortic balloon pump.[45]

The Doppler probe that sits in the oesophagus is approximately the size of a nasogastric tube, is semirigid and is inserted using a similar technique. The patient is usually sedated, but the method has been used in awake patients. In such cases, however, the limitation is that the probe is more likely to require more-frequent repositioning.

The waveform that is displayed on the monitor is triangular in shape (see Fig. 9.23) and captures the systolic portion of the cardiac cycle – an upstroke at the beginning of systole, the peak reflecting maximum systole and the downward slope of the ending of systole. The waveform captures real-time changes in blood flow and can therefore be seen as an indirect reflection of left ventricular function.

Changes to haemodynamic status will be reflected in alterations in the triangular shape (see Fig. 9.23).

Ultrasonic CO monitor

The ultrasonic cardiac output monitor (USCOM) monitors CO non-invasively using continuous Doppler ultrasound waves by placing an ultrasound transducer probe supra- or parasternally. The principles of CO calculation in this method are the same as for oesophageal Doppler monitoring. The use of non-invasive USCOM has been found to provide adequate clinical data in patients in different shock categories, and to be safe and cost effective; however, CO can be difficult to measure in some patients.[46]

Impedance cardiography

Transthoracic bioimpedance (impedance cardiography) is another form of non-invasive monitoring used to estimate CO.[47] It measures the amount of electrical resistance generated by the thorax to high-frequency, low-magnitude currents. This measure is inversely proportional to the content of fluid in the thorax: if the amount of thoracic fluid increases then transthoracic bioimpedance falls. Changes in CO can be reflected as a change in overall bioimpedance. The technique requires six electrodes to be positioned on the patient: two in the upper thorax/neck area and four in the lower thorax. These electrodes also monitor electrical signals from the heart.

Overall, transthoracic bioimpedance is determined by: (1) changes in tissue fluid volume, (2) volumetric changes in pulmonary and venous blood caused by respiration, and (3) volumetric changes in aortic blood flow produced by myocardial contractility. Accurate measurements of changes in aortic blood flow are dependent on the ability to measure the third determinant while filtering out any interference produced by the first two determinants. Any changes to position or to electrode contact will cause alterations to the measurements obtained, and recordings should therefore be undertaken with the electrodes positioned in the same location as previous readings. Caution is required for patients with high levels of perspiration (which reduces electrode contact), atrial fibrillation (irregular RR intervals make estimation of the ventricular ejection time difficult) or pulmonary oedema, pleural effusions or chest wall oedema (which alter bioimpedance readings irrespective of any changes in CO). The use of transthoracic bioimpedance in critically ill patients is less reliable, owing partly to limitations of its usefulness in patients who have pulmonary oedema, and it is not applicable in cardiothoracic surgery.

Practice tip

Current evidence-based literature suggests that haemodynamic measurements such as CVP, PAOP and PAP can be accurately measured with a patient position of supine to head – up to 60 degrees.

Diagnostics

Apart from the haemodynamic monitoring methods to facilitate cardiac assessment of a patient's clinical condition, various diagnostic tests are often used. Echocardiography and blood tests are the most commonly used in critical care. Other tests such as computed tomography (CT) and nuclear medicine cardiac examination are also used when indicated. Exercise stress tests and cardiac angiography are also used and are reviewed in Chapter 10.

Echocardiography

Echocardiography (frequently shortened to ECHO) is often used in critical care to assess cardiovascular conditions such as heart failure, hypertensive heart disease, valve disease and pericardial disease in critically ill patients. It adopts a technique of detecting the echoes produced by a heart from a beam of very-high-frequency sound – ultrasound. Two-dimensional, three-dimensional and contrast ECHO images can be obtained using the non-invasive transthoracic technique or the invasive transoesophageal technique (TOE).[48] The transthoracic ECHO uses a transducer probe externally to the heart to obtain images (the same as a normal ultrasound technique). This method is painless and does not require sedation. The TOE technique involves placing a transducer probe into the oesophageal cavity to assess the function and structure of the heart. This method produces better images of the heart than the normal transthoracic ECHO. However, this method requires sedation during the procedure and the patient needs to fast for a few hours prior to the examination.

Two-dimensional ECHO images are valuable resources for assessment of the function and structure of the heart. Three-dimensional images offer a more-realistic visualisation of its structure and function. Contrast ECHO provides enhanced images of left and right ventricular definition to facilitate the diagnosis of complex cardiac conditions such as congenital heart defects, valve stenosis and regurgitation. The contrast ECHO technique uses gas–air microbubbles, produced by hand-agitating a syringe containing 10 mL of normal saline with a small amount of air, injected into the peripheral vein to produce images of the heart functions.

In the critical care setting, the preparation of critically ill patients for this examination is important. The nurse needs to position the patient to achieve the best results. For TOE preparation, fasting time must be followed so as to avoid complications such as respiratory aspiration. The nurse will also need to assist the anaesthetist and the TOE operator, and continue to monitor the patient's clinical conditions during the procedure.

Blood tests

Several blood tests are often conducted to assist the clinical assessment of critically ill patients in the critical care setting.

Full blood count

The full blood count (FBC) assesses the status of three major cells that are formed in the bone marrow: red blood cells (RBC), white blood cells (WBC) and platelets. Although normal values have been given (see Appendix B), changes will occur in critically ill patients under certain conditions. For example, haemoglobin (Hb) is reduced in the presence of haemorrhage and in acute fluid overload causing haemodilution.

Haemoconcentration can occur during acute dehydration, which would show up as a high Hb. Similar conditions will also affect the haematocrit. WBC levels will be elevated during episodes of infection, tissue damage and inflammation. When infections are severe, the FBC will show a dramatic rise in the number of immature neutrophils. Platelets are easily lost during haemorrhage, and spontaneous bleeding is a danger when the count falls to below 20×10^9/L.[49]

Electrolytes

The assessment of electrolyte levels in critically ill patients is important in diagnosing the patient's condition. Electrolyte imbalances, such as potassium and calcium level changes, can cause cardiovascular abnormalities such as arrhythmias. Electrolyte levels are often checked regularly in critically ill patients.

The functions of electrolytes and their cardiac implications are listed in Table 9.5.

Cardiac enzymes

Cardiac biochemical markers, such as troponin, are proteins released from damaged myocardial cells that are detectable by performing blood tests. Troponin elevation is considered a significant biomarker for patients with MI; however, it can also be elevated in non-MI patients.[50] Therefore, diagnosis for critically ill patients with elevated cardiac troponin levels should be made with support from other data. (See Table 9.6 for cardiac enzyme parameters and normal values. For abnormal cardiac enzymes in MI, please refer to Chapter 10.)

Chest X-ray

Chest X-ray is the oldest non-invasive way to visualise the heart and blood vessels, and is one of the most commonly used diagnostic procedures in critical care. To interpret a chest X-ray for cardiac diagnosis, basic knowledge of the normal anatomical cardiac structure is important to identify abnormality, and a basic understanding of the chest X-ray is essential. Please review the basic concepts, such as what water, air and bone show on X-ray, and the concepts of anteroposterior (AP) and posteroanterior (PA) films, in Chapter 13 before you move on to the next section.

Cardiac chest X-ray interpretation

To interpret the chest X-ray for cardiac assessment, the following steps are recommended to ensure a thorough diagnosis:[51]

1 The heart size needs to be checked first to see whether the size of the heart is appropriate. The cardiac silhouette should be no more than 50% of the diameter of the thorax; this is called the cardiothoracic ratio. The position of the heart should be ⅓ of the heart shadow to the right of the vertebrae and ⅔ of the shadow to the left of the vertebrae. The size of the heart can be determined in a matter of seconds, even by the novice clinician, as this can be simply determined by visualising the cardiothoracic ratio.

2 The shape of the heart should be inspected next. The border of the heart on the X-ray film is determined by the heart anatomy. The border is formed by: the right atrial shadow as the right convex cardiac border, the superior vena cava as the superior border and the left ventricle as the left heart border and cardiac apex. In the frontal chest X-ray, the right ventricle is not a border-forming structure because it is directly superimposed on the cardiac silhouette. Similarly, the normal left atrium should not be visible on a PA film. The border of the heart should be sharp. If the left atrium is enlarged, a convex superior left heart border is seen.

3 On the superior border, the aortic arch and the pulmonary arteries should be identified next. The aortic arch is called the knob. The pulmonary arteries and their branches radiate outwards from the hila (Fig. 9.24). The hilum in the mediastinal region is formed by the pulmonary arteries and the main stem bronchi shadows on the film. The focus of this step is to check for prominence of vessels in this region, as this suggests vascular abnormalities.

Chest X-ray in diagnosing cardiac conditions

For CHD assessment, an initial chest X-ray film is useful to exclude other causes of chest pain, such as pneumonia, pneumothorax and aortic aneurysm, and to assess whether heart failure and/or pulmonary congestion are present. Patients with chronic heart failure show cardiomegaly, Kerley B lines or pulmonary oedema. Cardiomegaly is seen as an enlarged heart on the X-ray film. Kerley B lines on the X-ray film are the result of pulmonary congestion and fluid accumulation in the interstitium. Although cardiomegaly and pulmonary oedema indicate heart failure, the chest X-ray alone cannot diagnose the condition. Other tests are needed to thoroughly assess patients for accurate diagnosis.

> **Practice tip**
>
> Critical care nurses should take a systematic approach to interpreting chest X-rays. The respiratory and cardiac structures, tubes, wires and other devices should all be identified in the chest X-ray film.

A widened mediastinum and abnormal aortic contour may indicate aortic dissection. Similar to heart failure, further tests such as TOE, magnetic resonance imaging (MRI) or

TABLE 9.5
Electrolyte functions and pathophysiology

ELECTROLYTE	FUNCTIONS	COMMON IMBALANCES AND CAUSES	SIGNS AND SYMPTOMS
Potassium	Maintains normal functions of nerve and muscle cells. Acid–base balance.	*Hyperkalaemia* Renal failure, dehydration, diabetes, diuretic medications.	Muscle weakness, ECG changes in cardiac toxicity, severe hyperkalaemia (serum potassium between 6 and 6.5 mEq/L) needs prompt attention because it can cause life-threatening arrhythmia.
		Hypokalaemia Kidney disease, diarrhoea, vomiting, diuretic medications.	Muscle weakness, respiratory failure, ECG changes.
Sodium	Regulates body fluid movement. Maintains cell functions. Acid–base balance.	*Hypernatraemia* Renal failure, dehydration, diarrhoea, vomiting.	Thirst, confusion, hyperreflexia, seizures.
		Hyponatraemia Acute renal failure, heart failure, pancreatitis, peritonitis, burns.	Altered personality, confusion, seizures, coma, death.
Calcium	Bone metabolism. Blood coagulation. Muscle contraction. Nerve conduction.	*Hypercalcaemia* Hyperparathyroidism, vitamin D toxicity, cancer.	Polyuria, constipation, nausea, vomiting, muscle weakness, confusion, coma, ECG changes (shortened QT intervals).
		Hypocalcaemia Hypoparathyroidism, vitamin D deficiency, renal disease.	Paraesthesia, tetany; in severe cases, seizures, encephalopathy, ECG changes (prolonged ST and QT intervals), heart failure.
Magnesium	Activates sodium–potassium pumps. Inactivates calcium channels. Neuromuscular transmission.	*Hypermagnesaemia* Renal failure.	Hypotension, respiratory depression, AV conduction disturbances, which can lead to cardiac arrest (often in renal failure patients).
		Hypomagnesaemia Inadequate intake and absorption, or increased excretion, due to hypercalcaemia or diuretics.	Anorexia, nausea, vomiting, lethargy; it may contribute to hypokalaemia development, therefore cardiac arrhythmias may be present. *Note*: associated hypocalcaemia is common in hypomagnesaemia.
Phosphorus	Intracellular energy production (ATP) and enzyme regulation. Tissue oxygen delivery. Bone metabolism.	*Hyperphosphataemia* Kidney failure, metabolic and respiratory acidosis.	Usually asymptomatic; however, when concurrent hypocalcaemia, symptoms of hypocalcaemia may be present.
		Hypophosphataemia Burns, diuretic medications, respiratory alkalosis, acute alcoholism.	Usually asymptomatic. Severe cases may have muscle weakness, heart failure, coma.

For cardiac implications of electrolytes imbalances, see Chapter 10 and Chapter 11.

Source: Adapted from: Urden LD, Stacey KM, Lough ME, editors. Critical care nursing: diagnosis and management. 7th ed. St Louis: Elsevier; 2014, with permission; Moser DK, Reigel B. Cardiac nursing: a companion to Brauwald's heart disease. St Louis: Elsevier; 2008, with permission.

TABLE 9.6

Cardiac biochemical markers: description and normal values

ENZYME	DESCRIPTION	NORMAL VALUE
Troponin T (cTnT)	Detected within 2–3 h after infarction, and may remain elevated for 7–10 d.	<0.1 ng/mL
Troponin I (cTnI)	Detected within 2–3 h of infarction, and may remain elevated for up to 14 d.	<0.03 ng/mL
Creatine kinase (CK)	Serum CK is elevated following muscle or neurological injury. Creatine kinase myocardial bound (CK–MB) is useful in quantifying the degree of infarction and timing of onset. Levels rise 3–6 h and peak 12–24 h after infarction.	Adult female: 30–135 units U/L; Adult male: 55–170 units U/L CK–MB: 0–5% of total CK
Aspartate aminotransferase (AST)	Detection and monitoring of liver cell damage. No cardiac-specific isoenzymes; today rarely used because it is released after renal, cerebral and hepatic damage.	<40 U/L
Lactate dehydrogenase (LDH)	Of no value in the diagnosis of myocardial infarction. Occasionally useful in the assessment of patients with liver disease or malignancy (especially lymphoma, seminoma, hepatic metastases); anaemia when haemolysis or ineffective erythropoiesis suspected. Although it may be elevated in patients with skeletal muscle damage, it is not useful in this situation. Post-AMI, cardiac-specific isoenzyme LDH peaks between 48 and 72 h.	110–230 U/L
D-dimer	Presence indicates deep vein thrombosis, myocardial infarction, DIC.	<0.25 ng/L

AMI = acute myocardial infarction; DIC = disseminated intravascular coagulation.

Please note different laboratories may use slightly different reference values. Please always check with the values provided by your laboratory.

Source: Adapted from Pragana KD, Pragana TJ. Mosby's diagnostic and laboratory test reference. 13th ed. St Louis: Elsevier; 2016.

FIGURE 9.24 Chest PA radiograph. The convex right cardiac border is formed by the right atrium (thin arrows), and the thick arrows indicate the location of the superior vena cava.

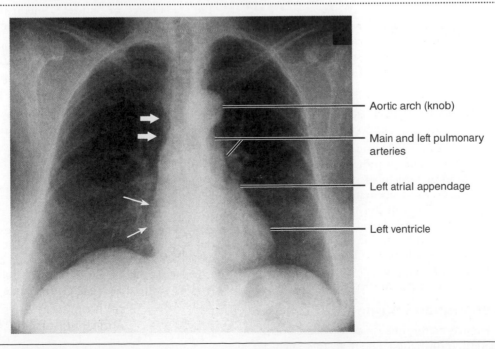

Source: Erkonen WE, Wilbur LS. Radiology 101: the basics and fundamentals of imaging. 3rd ed. Philadelphia, PA: Lippincott Williams and Wilkins; 2009, with permission.

angiography are needed to confirm the diagnosis. Subtle abnormalities in the hilar region may indicate pulmonary arterial hypertension (PAH). A decrease in pulmonary vascular markings and prominent main and hilar pulmonary arterial shadows in the lung fields on the chest film are classic signs of pulmonary hypertension. However, the sensitivity of this for excluding PAH is lacking. In pericardial disease, the chest X-ray often appears normal unless the accumulated fluid in the pericardial space is over 250 mL. Note that accumulation of fluid is indicated in many cardiac conditions; therefore, other tests need to be carried out to confirm the diagnosis.[52]

The positions of a PAC, a central venous catheter and pacing wires can be identified on the chest X-ray. The positions of these catheters need to be checked regularly to ensure the catheters and wires are in appropriate places. More details on how to identify the catheters and pacing wires are given in Chapter 13.

Due to individual variations in shape, size and rotation of the heart, and the complexity of cardiac signs, chest X-rays often play a minor role in cardiac diagnosis. A patient's clinical condition and other diagnostic test results must also be considered when diagnosing a cardiac condition.

> **Practice tip**
>
> Comparison of earlier chest X-ray film(s) with the current film is important to diagnose a patient's clinical progress, response to treatment and any movements of catheter positions.

Other diagnostic tests of cardiac function

Since 2000, more non-invasive diagnostic imaging techniques have been used to aid cardiac assessment. Some of these techniques have shown significant advantages, such as lowered cost, but they also have their limitations.

Cardiac computed tomography

Cardiac CT is a recent development in diagnosing cardiac conditions such as suspected CHD and in the evaluation of coronary artery bypass grafts. It provides a method for visualising the anatomical structures of the heart and coronary arteries reliably and accurately in patients.[53] However, limitations remain with this method including the inability to assess the haemodynamic relevance of a coronary artery lesion. In addition, the most-appropriate radiation and contrast doses have not been determined, though in recent years some progress towards determining a universal approach to these parameters has been made.[54]

Magnetic resonance imaging

MRI is a non-invasive method that can provide cardiac-specific biochemical information about factors such as tissue integrity, cardiac aneurysms, ejection fraction and CO.[55] These techniques are sometimes considered to be superior to radiography and ultrasound examination methods because the MRI is not affected by bone structure. The techniques include perfusion imaging, atherosclerosis imaging and coronary artery imaging. MRI is considered an accurate method for predicting the presence of significant coronary artery disease. However, MRI use in critically ill patients has its limitations. Because of the magnetic field required for this method, the patient cannot be fitted with any pumps or machines that have metal parts in them. Organising appropriate equipment for critically ill patients who are undergoing this test can be a challenge.

Nuclear medicine cardiac studies

There are several types of radionuclide imaging methods available to assess a patient's cardiac status, including radionuclide isotopes, thallium scan and stress test radionuclide scan.[56] The purpose of radionuclide imaging is to assess the perfusion status of cardiac muscle. When lowered perfusion in cardiac muscle is identified, this may indicate heart muscle damage. Radionuclide imaging is often used in patients who have been diagnosed with a MI when further investigation is required to determine whether interventions such as a cardiac stent or coronary artery bypass surgery are likely to benefit the patient.

Nursing care of patients undergoing diagnostic tests

All the above methods have advantages and benefits in assessing the cardiac condition of a patient. For the critical care nurse, preparation of patients for these examinations is important because patients often need to be transported to the radiology or nuclear medicine department. Important considerations include the following:

- A patient's allergy profile in relation to imaging contrast needs to be evaluated before the requests are made.
- These tests all require the patient to lie still for certain periods of time; therefore, explanation is essential and sedation may be required during the procedure.
- Appropriate equipment, such as non-metal equipment, needs to be organised beforehand if the patient is having an MRI study.

> **Practice tip**
>
> Hearing aids and partial dental plates with metal parts must be removed prior to MRI. Additionally, patients with implantable devices such as permanent pacemakers cannot have an MRI. Critical care patients are at increased risk of adverse events during intra-hospital transport; therefore, close monitoring and documenting the patient's clinical condition during transport are imperative.

Summary

The cardiovascular system is essentially a transport system for distributing metabolic requirements to, and collecting byproducts from, cells throughout the body. A thorough understanding of anatomical structures and physiological events is critical to inform a comprehensive assessment of the critically ill patient. Findings from assessment should define patient cardiovascular status as well as inform the implementation of a timely clinical management plan. A thorough cardiac assessment requires the critical care nurse to be competent in a wide range of interpersonal, observational and technical skills.

Current minimum standards for critical care units in many parts of the world require that patient monitoring include circulation, respiration and oxygenation. For many critically ill patients, haemodynamic instability is a potentially life-threatening condition that necessitates urgent action. In the critical care environment, two main forms of cardiac monitoring are commonly employed: continuous cardiac monitoring and the 12-lead ECG. Accurate assessment of the patient's intracardiac status is frequently employed and often considered essential to guide management. Strong research evidence has shown that there is no increased harm or benefit in using pulmonary artery monitoring in critically ill patients; therefore, the decision to use pulmonary artery monitoring as a diagnostic tool depends on the clinical need and clinician expertise. In day-to-day management of critically ill patients, critical care nurses must ensure they are skilled and educated in the techniques of non-invasive and invasive cardiovascular monitoring techniques and technologies, and be able to synthesise all data gathered and base their practice on the best available evidence to date.

Case study

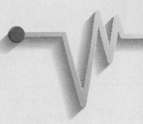

Ms Shirly Wang is a 74-year-old-female who presented to the emergency department (ED) with severe chest pain. On arrival in the ED, her respiratory rate (RR) was 25 breaths/min, heart rate (HR) was 100 bpm, blood pressure (BP) 85/50, peripheral oxygen saturations (SpO_2) 95% on 6 lpm oxygen via face mask, and temperature 36.5°C.

Ms Wang was pale, with cool peripheries, and was speaking in short sentences. She explained that she had been having discomfort in her chest for the past 4 days and that day it had worsened to the point of not being able to stand up from her chair. She has a past medical history of type 2 diabetes mellitus, hypertension, for which she does not take medication, and hypercholesterolaemia.

ED tests included a troponin blood test and a 12-lead ECG. The troponin levels were substantially elevated and the 12-lead ECG showed ST segment elevation in leads V2, V3 and V4. Ms Wang was given a small bolus of IV fluid and was transferred to the cardiac catheter laboratory for emergency percutaneous coronary intervention, where her left anterior descending coronary artery was found to have 90% occlusion. A drug-eluting stent was inserted and Ms Wang's coronary blood flow is restored.

While in the cardiac catheter laboratory, Ms Wang suffered a cardiac arrest, and required two defibrillator shocks. She was intubated and transferred to the ICU for monitoring.

Shortly after arrival in ICU, she remained hypotensive with a BP of 88/60. She had a central venous catheter (centrally inserted central catheter) inserted into the right internal jugular vein, an arterial line inserted in the right radial artery, and was commenced on a milrinone infusion at 0.375 micrograms/kg/min and a noradrenaline infusion at 0.5 micrograms/kg/min.

Ms Wang was ventilated on pressure-regulated volume control, tidal volumes of 400, RR 12, PEEP 8, pressure support of 10, and fraction of inspired oxygen (FiO_2) of 0.4. Her arterial blood gas showed a pH 7.32, partial pressure of oxygen (PaO_2) 90 mmHg, partial pressure of carbon dioxide ($PaCO_2$) 48 mmHg, bicarbonate 22 mmol/L, base excess −3.0 and lactate 3.9 mmol/L.

DISCUSSION

This patient was in cardiogenic shock from an anterioseptal MI, for which she had had symptoms for the preceding 4 days. She showed signs of cardiogenic shock such as pale and cool peripheries, hypotension and a history suspicious of acute coronary syndrome. Myocardial irritability probably contributed to her cardiac arrest and the definitive treatment for her syndrome of revascularisation was undertaken appropriately. Her hypotension on arrival at the ICU was likely to be due to myocardial injury and a potential systemic inflammatory response from having had a cardiac arrest.

CASE STUDY QUESTIONS

1 On admission to ICU, what cardiac and haemodynamic monitoring should be commenced and why?

2 Is CO monitoring needed for Ms Wang? If yes, what monitoring option is appropriate and why?

RESEARCH VIGNETTE

Saugel B, Hoppe P, Nicklas JY, et al. Continuous noninvasive pulse wave analysis using finger cuff technologies for arterial blood pressure and cardiac output monitoring in perioperative and intensive care medicine: a systematic review and meta-analysis. Br J Anaesth 2020;125(1):25–37.

Abstract

Background: Finger cuff technologies allow continuous non-invasive arterial blood pressure (AP) and cardiac output/index (CO/CI) monitoring.

Methods: The authors performed a meta-analysis of studies comparing finger cuff-derived AP and CO/CI measurements with invasive measurements in surgical or critically ill patients. They calculated overall random-effects model-derived pooled estimates of the mean of the differences and of the percentage error (PE; CO/CI studies) with 95% confidence intervals (95% CI), pooled 95% limits of agreement (95% LOA), Cochran's Q and I^2 (for heterogeneity).

Results: The pooled mean of the differences (95% CI) was 4.2 (2.8–5.62) mmHg with pooled 95% LOA of −14.0 to 22.5 mmHg for mean AP ($Q = 230.4$; $P < 0.001$; $I^2 = 91\%$). For mean AP, the mean of the differences between finger cuff technologies and the reference method was ≤5 ± 8 mmHg in 9/27 data sets (33%). The pooled mean of the differences (95% CI) was −0.13 (−0.43–0.18) L/min with pooled 95% LOA of −2.56 to 2.23 L/min for CO ($Q = 66.7$; $P < 0.001$; $I^2 = 90\%$) and 0.07 (0.01–0.13) L/min/m² with pooled 95% LOA of −1.20 to 1.15 L/min/m² for CI ($Q = 5.8$; $P = 0.326$; $I^2 = 0\%$). The overall random effects model-derived pooled estimate of the PE (95% CI) was 43 (37–49)% ($Q = 48.6$; $P < 0.001$; $I^2 = 63\%$). In 4/19 data sets (21%), the PE was ≤30%, and in 10/19 data sets (53%) it was ≤45%.

Conclusions: Study heterogeneity was high. Several studies showed interchangeability between AP and CO/CI measurements using finger cuff technologies and reference methods. However, the pooled results of this meta-analysis indicate that AP and CO/CI measurements using finger cuff technologies and reference methods are not interchangeable in surgical or critically ill patients.

Critique

The aim of this systematic review and meta-analysis of clinical studies was to compare continuous non-invasive finger cuff technology-derived arterial blood pressure (AP) and CO/CI (adjusts its pressure to keep the blood volume in the finger artery constant throughout the cardiac cycle).

The authors identified 24 studies that met predetermined criteria and categorised these studies into three categories for analysis: different software versions of the test device, CO/CI measurements with invasive reference measurements in adult surgical or critically ill patients. Finger cuff technologies continuously record the AP waveform using a finger cuff with an infrared photodiode (device that converts light into an electrical current) and light detector. The finger cuff measurements were taken before and after cardiopulmonary bypass, and during induction and maintenance of general anaesthesia. Studies included had a total number of patients of 1164, with a median of 42 patients included per study (range 10–182 patients). Sixteen of these studies were performed in the operating room and eight in intensive care. Two commercially available systems, the ClearSight and the CNAP system, were included in this meta-analysis.

The authors reported that their meta-analysis showed that there was substantial variability in the AP and CO/CI measurement performance between studies, suggesting that many patient-, clinical setting- and device-related factors may have contributed to this observed heterogeneity. One observation highlighted by authors was the wide variability in reference methods to which finger cuff methods are compared, highlighting the need for standardisation of procedures when using finger cuff technologies.

The authors highlight that, while several studies suggest interchangeability between non-invasive finger cuff technologies and invasive reference methods for AP and CO/CI measurements, overall meta-analyses results suggest that methods are not interchangeable in adult surgical or critically ill patients.

Learning activities

1 Briefly discuss the main ion movement at each of the following phases of the cardiac action potential:

   a depolarisation

   b early rapid repolarisation

   c plateau phase

   d final rapid repolarisation

   e resting membrane phase.

2 Describe the correct placement of the precordial leads when doing a 12-lead ECG.

3 Describe what PQRST represents on an ECG and identify the normal duration for each segment.

4 Describe what systemic vascular resistance (SVR) is and what clinical condition can cause an elevated or lowered SVR.

5 Describe the main determinants of CO.

6 Describe the limitations of CVP monitoring and why.

Online resources

American Heart Association, https://www.heart.org

Australian and New Zealand Intensive Care Society, https://www.anzics.com.au

Australian College of Critical Care Nurses, https://www.acccn.com.au

British Association of Critical Care Nurses, https://www.baccn.org.uk

Critical Care Forum, https://ccforum.biomedcentral.com

European Society of Cardiology, https://www.escardio.org/

National Heart Foundation of Australia, https://www.heartfoundation.org.au

United Kingdom Intensive Care Society, https://www.ics.ac.uk/

World Federation of Critical Care Nurses, https://wfccn.org

Further reading

Mehraeen E, Seyed Alinaghi SA, Nowroozi A, et al. A systematic review of ECG findings in patients with COVID-19. Indian Heart J 2020;72(6):500–7.

Nachman D, Eisenkraft A, Maor Y, et al. Continuous monitoring of advanced hemodynamic parameters shows early cardiovascular changes in a cohort of 492 COVID-19 hospitalized patients. Eur Heart J 2021;42(Suppl 1). doi: 10.1093/eurheartj/ehab724.3090.

Siontis KC, Noseworthy PA, Attia ZI, et al. Artificial intelligence-enhanced electrocardiography in cardiovascular disease management. Nat Rev Cardiol 2021;18,465–78.

Vincent J-L, Joosten A, Saugel B. Hemodynamic monitoring and support. Crit Care Med 2021;49(10):1638–50.

References

1. Hall E, Guyton A. Textbook of medical physiology. 14th ed. Philadelphia: Elsiever Saunders; 2020.

2. Costanzo L. Physiology. 7th ed. Philadelphia: Elsevier; 2021.

3. Chen X, Ashraf S, Ashraf N, et al. UCP3 (uncoupling protein 3) insufficiency exacerbates left ventricular diastolic dysfunction during angiotensin II-induced hypertension. J Am Heart Assoc 2021;10(18):e022556.

4. Varro A, Tomek J, Nagy N, et al. Cardiac transmembrane ion channels and action potentials: cellular physiology and arrhythmogenic behavior. Physiol Rev 2021;101(3):1083–76.

5. Burkhard S, van Eif V, Garric L, et al. On the evolution of the cardiac pacemaker. J Cardiovasc Dev Dis 2017;4(2):4.

6. Billman GE. Homeostasis: the underappreciated and far too often ignored central organizing principle of physiology. Front Physiol 2020;11:200.

7. Denham NC, Pearman CM, Caldwell JL, et al. Calcium in the pathophysiology of atrial fibrillation and heart failure. Front Physiol 2018;9:1380.

8. Reddy YNV, El-Sabbagh A, Nishimura RA. Comparing pulmonary arterial wedge pressure and left ventricular end diastolic pressure for assessment of left-sided filling pressures. JAMA Cardiol 2018:3(6):453–4.

9. Musu M, Guddelmoni L, Murgia F, et al. Prediction of fluid responsiveness in ventilated critically ill patients. J Emerg Crit Care Med 2020;4:26. doi: 10.21037/jeccm.2020.03.03.

10. King J LD. Physiology, cardiac output. Treasure Island, FL: StatPearls Publishing; 2022. Available from: https://www.ncbi.nlm.nih.gov/books/NBK470455/. [Accessed 13 February 2023].

11. Tsuda T. Clinical assessment of ventricular wall stress in understanding compensatory hypertrophic response and maladaptive ventricular remodeling. J Cardiovasc Dev Dis 2021;8(10):122.

12. Centorbi CS, Lazzeroni D, Moderato L, et al. 342 Cardiorespiratory fitness and systemic vascular resistance: oxygen pressure as a novel marker of peripheral vascular response during cardiopulmonary exercise testing. Eur Heart J Suppl 2021;23(Suppl G):suab145.002. doi: 10.1093/eurheartj/suab145.002.

13. Kotecha D, Flather MD, Altman DG, et al. Heart rate and rhythm and the benefit of beta-blockers in patients with heart failure. J Am Coll Cardiol 2017;69(24):2885–96.

14. Thiriet M. Physiology and pathophysiology of venous flow. In: Lanzer P, editor. Panvascular medicine. Berlin, Heidelberg: Springer; 2015, p. 569–89.

15. Nava E, Llorens S. The local regulation of vascular function: from an inside–outside to an outside–inside model. Front Physiol 2019;10:729.

16. Russell JA. Presynaptic alpha-2 receptors inhibit norepinephrine release in tracheal smooth muscle. Respir Physiol 1987;70(1):25–35.

17. Gavras I, Gavras H. Role of alpha2-adrenergic receptors in hypertension. Am J Hypertens 2001;14(6 Pt 2):171S-7S.

18. Foulon P, De Backer D. The hemodynamic effects of norepinephrine: far more than an increase in blood pressure! Ann Transl Med 2018; 6(Suppl 1):S25.

19. Meyer T, Gersh B, Yeon S. Auscultation of heart sounds. UpToDate; 2021. Available from: https://www.uptodate.com/contents/auscultation-of-heart-sounds. [Accessed 13 February 2023].

20. Silverman ME, Wooley CF. Samuel A. Levine and the history of grading systolic murmurs. Am J Cardiol 2008;102(8):1107–10.

21. The Faculty of Intensive Care Medicine (FICM). Guidelines for the provision of intensive care service. Version 2.1. London: FICM; 2022. Available from: https://www.ficm.ac.uk/standardssafetyguidelinesstandards/guidelines-for-the-provision-of-intensive-care-services. [Accessed 13 February 2023].

22. Australian and New Zealand College of Intensive Care Medicine (CICM). Minimum standards for intensive care units. Prahran, VIC: CICM; 2011. Available from: https://www.cicm.org.au/CICM_Media/CICMSite/CICM-Website/Resources/Professional%20Documents/IC-1-Minimum-Standards-for-Intensive-Care-Units.pdf. [Accessed 13 February 2023].

23. Sandau KE, Funk M, Auerbach A, et al. Update to practice standards for electrocardiographic monitoring in hospital settings: a scientific statement from the American Heart Association. Circulation 2017;136(19):e273–344.

24. Tan NY, Witt CM, Oh JK, et al. Left bundle branch block. Circ Arrhythm Electrophysiol 2020;13(4):e008239.

25. Kulig J, Koplan BA. Wolff–Parkinson–White syndrome and accessory pathways. Circulation 2010;122(15):e480–3.

26. Pregerson B. Bradycardia: don't be fooled by U waves. Emerg Med News 2021;43(1):19.

27. Zhong L, Wang HL, Xu B, et al. Normal saline versus heparin for patency of central venous catheters in adult patients – a systematic review and meta-analysis. Crit Care 2017;21(1):5.

28. Su L, Pan P, Li D, et al. Central venous pressure (CVP) reduction associated with higher cardiac output (CO) favors good prognosis of circulatory shock: a single-center, retrospective cohort study. Front Med (Lausanne) 2019;6:216.

29. Rockholt MM, Thorarinsdottir HR, Lazarevic V, et al. Central venous catheter-related complications in hematologic patients: an observational study. Acta Anaesthesiol Scand 2022;66(4):473–82.

30. Cancer Institute NSW. eviQ clinical resource: central venous access devices. In: eviQ cancer treatments. Alexandria, NSW: NSW Government; 2021. Available from: https://www.eviq.org.au/clinical-resources/central-venous-access-devices-cvads. [Accessed 13 February 2023].

31. Hanauer LPT, Comerlato PH, Papke A, et al. Reducing central vein catheterization complications with a focused educational program: a retrospective cohort study. Sci Rep 2020;10(1):17530.

32. Bertaina M, Galluzzo A, Rossello X, et al. Prognostic implications of pulmonary artery catheter monitoring in patients with cardiogenic shock: a systematic review and meta-analysis of observational studies. J Crit Care 2022;69:154024.

33. Sidoti A, Brogi E, Biancofiore G, et al. Ultrasound- versus landmark-guided subclavian vein catheterization: a prospective observational study from a tertiary referral hospital. Sci Rep 2019;9(1):12248.

34. Swan HJC, Ganz W, Forrester J, et al. Catheterization of the heart in man with use of a flow-directed balloon-tipped catheter. New Engl J Med 1970;283(9):447–51.

35. Chow JY, Vadakken ME, Whitlock RP, et al. Pulmonary artery catheterization in patients with cardiogenic shock: a systematic review and meta-analysis. Can J Anesth/J Canadien d'Anesthésie 2021;68(11):1611–29.

36. Rajaram SS, Desai NK, Kalra A, et al. Pulmonary artery catheters for adult patients in intensive care. Cochrane Database Syst Rev 2013; 2:CD003408.

37. Mitchell C, Rahko PS, Blauwet LA, et al. Guidelines for performing a comprehensive transthoracic echocardiographic examination in adults: recommendations from the American Society of Echocardiography. J Am Soc Echocardiogr 2019;32(1):1–64.

38. Vincent JL, Joosten A, Saugel B. Hemodynamic monitoring and support. Crit Care Med 2021;49(10):1638–50.

39. Schmücker G, Burgdorf C, Blohm J-H, et al. Modern gold standard of cardiac output measurement – a simplified bedside measurement of individual oxygen uptake in the cath lab. J Basic Clin Physiol Pharmacol 2022;33(5):639–44.

40. Grensemann J. Cardiac output monitoring by pulse contour analysis, the technical basics of less-invasive techniques. Front Med 2018;5:64.

41. Rasch S, Schmidle P, Sancak S, et al. Increased extravascular lung water index (EVLWI) reflects rapid non-cardiogenic oedema and mortality in COVID-19 associated ARDS. Sci Rep 2021;11(1):11524.

42. Senoner T, Velik-Salchner C, Tauber H. The pulmonary artery catheter in the perioperative setting: should it still be used? Diagnostics 2022;12(177):1–10.

43. Uemura K, Nishikawa T, Kawada T, et al. A novel method of trans-esophageal Doppler cardiac output monitoring utilizing peripheral arterial pulse contour with/without machine learning approach. J Clin Monit Comput 2022;36(2):437–49.

44. Hoskins PR. Principles of Doppler ultrasound. In: Diagnostic ultrasound. 3rd ed. Boca Raton, FL: CRC Press; 2019, p. 143–58.

45. Jasinska-Gniadzik K, Szwed P, Gasecka A, et al. Haemodynamic monitoring in acute heart failure – what you need to know. Adv Intervent Cardiol/Postepy Kardiol Interwencyjnej 2022;18(2):90–100.

46. Zhang Y, Wang Y, Shi J, et al. Cardiac output measurements via echocardiography versus thermodilution: a systematic review and meta-analysis. PLoS One 2019;14(10):e0222105.

47. Li L, Ai Y, Huang L, et al. Can bioimpedance cardiography assess hemodynamic response to passive leg raising in critically ill patients: a STROBE-compliant study. Medicine (Baltimore) 2020;99(51):e23764.

48. Patel AR, Patel AR, Singh S, et al. Cardiac ultrasound in the intensive care unit: a review. Cureus 2019;11(5):e4612.

49. Estcourt LJ, Birchall J, Allard S, et al. Guidelines for the use of platelet transfusions. Br J Haematol 2017;176:65–394.

50. Akwe J, Halford B, Kim E, et al. A review of cardiac and non-cardiac causes of troponin elevation and clinical relevance part II: non cardiac causes. J Cardiol Curr Res 2018;11(1):9–16.

51. Klein JS, Rosado-de-Christenson ML. A systematic approach to chest radiographic analysis. In: Hodler J, Kubik-Huch RA, von Schulthess GK, editors. Diseases of the chest, breast, heart and vessels 2019–2022: diagnostic and interventional imaging. Cham, CH: IDKD Springer; 2019, p. 1–16.

52. Manea M, Bratu OG, Bacalbasa N, et al. Diagnosis and management of pericardial effusion. J Mind Med Sci 2020;7(2):148–55.

53. Nazir MS, Nicol ED. Cardiovascular CT: the role of the cardiologists. Heart BMJ 2019;105(17):1–2.

54. Stocker TJ, Deseive S, Leipsic J, et al. Reduction in radiation exposure in cardiovascular computed tomography imaging: results from the PROspective multicenter registry on radiaTion dose Estimates of cardiac CT anglOgraphy iN daily practice in 2017 (PROTECTION VI). Eur Heart J 2018;39(41):3715–23.

55. Zhang C, Liu J, Qin S. Prognostic value of cardiac magnetic resonance in patients with aortic stenosis: a systematic review and meta-analysis. PLoS One 2022;17(2):e0263378.

56. Ora M, Gambhir S. Myocardial perfusion imaging: a brief review of nuclear and nonnuclear techniques and comparative evaluation of recent advances. Indian J Nucl Med 2019;34(4):263–70.

Chapter 10

Cardiovascular alterations and management

Andrea Driscoll, Lorelle Martin

Learning objectives

After reading this chapter, you should be able to:

- explain the pathophysiology of coronary artery disease, clinical manifestations of acute coronary syndromes and management of events
- discuss the care for a patient with chest pain
- list the diagnostic tests used to assess myocardial ischaemia
- discuss the pathways for reperfusion therapies in STEMI
- outline the clinical manifestations of right and left ventricular failure
- discuss the goals of heart failure treatment
- discuss the pathophysiologies of the four different types of cardiomyopathy and how they affect cardiac function
- outline the actions of angiotensin-converting enzyme inhibitors, angiotensin neprilysin receptor inhibitors, beta-blockers, loop diuretics and spironolactone and how they relate to the pathophysiology of heart failure.

Introduction

The support of cardiovascular function in the face of many compromises is reviewed in this chapter. It focuses on two of the most prevalent and fatal cardiovascular diseases: coronary heart disease (CHD) and heart failure (HF). These diseases are also a common comorbidity in elderly patients admitted to critical care units. The first section on coronary heart disease reviews the pathophysiological concepts of acute coronary syndromes (ACS), associated myocardial ischaemia and complications, with detailed consideration of the clinical implications, assessment and associated management. Heart failure is discussed in terms of the body's compensatory mechanisms and the clinical sequelae and associated clinical features of heart failure. Nursing and medical management is outlined including the management of acute exacerbations of heart failure. Finally, other cardiovascular disorders commonly managed in critical care units are reviewed, ranging from other forms of heart failure to hypertensive emergencies and aortic aneurysms. The case study presented at the end of the chapter highlights the key aspects of the management of heart failure in patients admitted to critical care units.

KEY WORDS

acute coronary syndrome

acute heart failure

aortic aneurysm

arrhythmia

cardiomyopathy

chronic heart failure

endocarditis

hypertensive emergencies

left ventricular failure

myocardial infarction

percutaneous coronary intervention

right ventricular failure

ST-segment elevation

ventricular aneurysm

Cardiovascular disease

Cardiovascular disease (CVD), encompassing diseases of the heart and circulation, retains a key influence on morbidity, mortality and health care expenditure.[1] CVD has been reported to be responsible for an estimated 17.9 million deaths worldwide in 2019, reflecting 32% of all global deaths.[2] Of these approximately 6.8 million have been associated with CHD,[2–4] a condition resulting from a reduction or complete obstruction of blood flow through the coronary arteries due to narrowing from atherosclerosis and/or thrombus formation. Death rates over the last three decades have fallen by about 75%, primarily due to improvements in risk factors and healthcare for those at risk.[4] However, in the most recent decade there has been a plateau in this mortality decline in the 55–69 year olds.[4] Despite improvements, in 2020–2021, 2.9% of the adult population reported living with CHD, and the prevalence of CHD increases rapidly with age, affecting around 1 in 9 (11%) adults aged 75 and over.[4]

Although some patients may be asymptomatic, the most common manifestations of CHD are chest pain due to angina, ACS, which includes unstable angina and myocardial infarction (MI), and sudden death due to cardiac arrest. CHD may also cause arrhythmias and heart failure.

Myocardial ischaemia

When coronary blood supply is insufficient to meet myocardial tissue demand for oxygen, myocardial ischaemia occurs. Critical restriction to blood flow occurs when the diameter of the lumen of the blood vessel is reduced by more than half as a result of either coronary artery narrowing through the build-up of fatty deposits and the development of plaque (atherosclerosis) or the formation of a thrombus or blood clot causing occlusion. Coronary blood flow is also determined by perfusion pressure, which can be adversely affected by abnormalities in blood flow (valvular disease), vessel wall (coronary spasm) and the blood (anaemia, polycythaemia).[5] Myocardial oxygen demand is influenced by heart rate, strength of myocardial contraction and left ventricular wall tension. The myocardium receives most of its blood supply during diastole; therefore, a rise in heart rate that decreases the duration of diastole will also decrease coronary perfusion. Sympathetic stimulation increases the force of contraction and hence oxygen demand. Left ventricular wall tension increases with the changes in preload associated with filling and afterload associated with systemic vascular resistance. During activity, pyrexia and arrhythmias, these effects may compound because of sympathetic stimulation, causing increased oxygen demand and reduced coronary perfusion resulting in symptoms of angina.

Angina

Angina (angina pectoris) is the most common manifestation of CHD and is the term used to describe the symptoms of discomfort that occur during myocardial ischaemia. The classic angina pattern consists of retrosternal constricting chest pain/discomfort, which may radiate to the arms, throat, jaw, teeth, back or epigastrium. Associated symptoms often include shortness of breath, nausea, vomiting, sweating, palpitations and weakness.

A fixed coronary artery lesion, causing limitation of oxygen supply at times of increased demand, results in stable angina. Therefore, symptoms arise during periods of physical and emotional stress and resolve within 2–10 minutes of rest. Symptoms tend to be worse in the morning (coinciding with a peak in blood pressure), after heavy meals and in cold weather. The severity of symptoms has little correlation with the progress of the disease. However, a patient with a typical history of angina has a high probability of CHD and a higher risk of MI and coronary death during the next 5 years.[6]

Acute coronary syndromes

ACS is an umbrella term applied to the spectrum of myocardial injury to categorise and determine treatment strategies. ACS categories range from unstable angina, often related to transient ischaemia at rest, to MI associated with myocardial necrosis. According to electrocardiographic changes, MI is further classified into ST elevation myocardial infarction (STEMI) and non-ST elevation MI (NSTEMI). ACS is associated with the underlying disease process of arthrosclerosis and the development of atheromatous plaque consisting of lipids, fibrin and cell debris which forms over time causing narrowing of the vessel lumen.

ACS, in particular STEMI and NSTEMI, develop due to the fissuring or rupture of the plaque leading to release of vasoconstrictor substances and potentially triggering coagulation activity (Fig. 10.1) causing a reduction in coronary blood flow and subsequent damage to myocardial cells.[5] The diagnosis of ACS will be made based on the combination of clinical history, the presence or absence of ST elevation on a 12-lead electrocardiograph (ECG) and alterations in cardiac biomarkers (commonly troponin), as defined in the fourth universal definition of MI.[5] The presence of ST elevation in the 12-lead ECG will activate well-defined time-sensitive care pathways to achieve rapid revascularisation of the culprit epicardial artery using primary percutaneous coronary intervention (PCI) or thrombolysis. STEMI is considered a medical emergency with the risk of mortality substantial; in-hospital mortality ranges between 4% and 12%, and 1-year mortality reported to be around 10%.[7]

STEMI typically presents as a recent history of angina (within the past 4–6 weeks), a change in symptoms including increased frequency, more easily provoked or occurring in the absence of physical or emotional stress, more severe or prolonged and/or less responsive to nitrate therapy.

STEMI occurs when blood flow to the myocardium is severely impaired for more than 20 minutes as myocardial cell necrosis begins. A coronary artery thrombus arising

FIGURE 10.1 **(A)** Plaque rupture exposes thrombogenic lipid. A white thrombus is formed by activated platelets adhering. This lesion is unstable and may lead to thrombin activation. **(B)** Thrombin activation leads to a mesh of fibrin and red blood cells, leading to a 'red thrombus'.

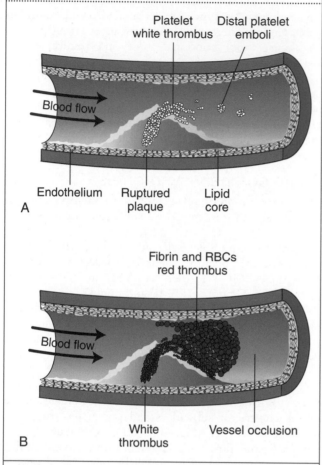

Source: Adapted from Bersten AD, Soni N, Oh TE. Oh's intensive care manual. 5th ed. Oxford: Butterworth–Heinemann; 2003 with permission.

The location and impact of the infarction will depend on which coronary artery has been obstructed:

- Left anterior descending (LAD) affects the function of the left ventricle and interventricular septum, including ventricular conduction tissue. Patients with anteroseptal MI are at high risk of heart failure, cardiogenic shock and mortality due to pump deficits.
- Circumflex (CX) affects the left ventricle lateral and posterior walls and the sinoatrial (SA) node in 40% of people.[5] The impact on pump efficiency of lateral and posterior wall necrosis is not as severe as anteroseptal infarctions, although patients are at more risk of arrhythmias.
- Right coronary artery (RCA) affects the inferior wall of the left ventricle and the right ventricle, as well as the AV node in most patients (90%) and the SA node in 60% of people. There is potentially severe impact on ventricular function if both the inferior wall and the right ventricle are affected, as well as a high risk of arrhythmias due to SA and AV node involvement.

Clinical features

Patients with MI most often present with chest pain. This pain is described as central crushing retrosternal pain which lasts longer than 20 minutes and is not relieved by nitrate therapy. The pain may radiate to the neck, jaw, back and shoulders and is often accompanied by 'feelings of impending doom', sweating and pallor. Nausea is often associated with the pain, due to vagal nerve stimulation. Depending on the size and location of the MI, patients may also present with sudden death or with varying degrees of syncope and heart failure. Women may present with different symptoms from men.[7]

Patient assessment and diagnostic features

A key feature of assessment of the patient with chest pain is the use of protocols and guidelines to promote rapid implementation of revascularisation procedures such as primary PCI and thrombolysis when no contraindications to treatment exist. This process begins at the point of first medical contact, often in the community with 12-lead ECG transmission to the hospital where rapid, early triage models of care are in place. Clinical assessment methods used will depend on the condition of the patient but should occur within 10 minutes of arrival.[7–9] This initial history will focus on the nature of presenting symptoms such as pain and symptoms; assessment can be aided by the use of an acronym such as PQRST or OLDCARTS (Tables 10.1 and 10.2) to incorporate precipitating and palliative factors, qualitative descriptors, onset, location, radiation, severity and duration.[10] Intensity can be rated on a pain scale. Asking patients for descriptive words is useful in assessment as many patients will deny pain and instead use words such as pressure, tightness or constriction. It is essential not to ignore other presentations, as patients with atypical symptoms, such as women, diabetics and the elderly, often have a delayed

from an atherosclerotic plaque is found in the majority of patients affected by STEMI. Cellular death begins in the subendocardial layer and progresses through the full muscle thickness, so that by 2–4 hours with total occlusion a full 'transmural' infarction will result. However, the full extent of tissue death may occur as a single incident or evolve over several days, depending on the degree of obstruction to blood flow. The size and location of the infarction will influence the clinical manifestations and risk of death and determine treatment. The size of the infarction is determined by the extent, severity and duration of the ischaemic event, the amount of collateral circulation and the metabolic demands placed on the myocardium. Usually the ventricle wall is affected, with a small infarction often resulting in a hypokinetic (reduced movement) or dyskinetic wall (altered movement), whereas a large infarction may result in akinesis (no movement).

TABLE 10.1
The PQRST criteria for assessing chest pain

P	Precipitating	Exercise and activity. Stress and anxiety. Cold weather.
	Palliating	Stop activity. Rest. Nitroglycerine.
Q	Quality	Heavy, tight, choking, vice-like, constricting.
R	Region, Radiation	Left side of chest, shoulder, arm and jaw. Retrosternal and radiating to the neck.
S	Severity	Rate pain on scale of 1 (no pain) to 10 (worst pain possible).
T	Time	Pain lasts longer than 10 min despite nitroglycerine. Pain comes and goes but lasts longer than 20 min.

Source: Adapted from Hudak CM, Gallo BM, Morton PG. Critical care nursing, a holistic approach. 7th ed. Philadelphia: Lippincott; 1998.

diagnosis and treatment and a higher mortality.[7,9] Differentiating current pain from any previous pain is also useful in differential diagnosis. Pain relief in the form of narcotics should be a priority not only for comfort but also to reduce associated physiological responses including sympathetic stimulation and vasoconstriction, which are detrimental to an already compromised coronary circulation. Recurrent chest discomfort requires urgent reassessment, including immediate ECG.

The brief history should also include a short cardiovascular risk profile: previous cardiac history such as angina, previous MI, or revascularisation, family history, and past medical history of smoking, hypertension and/or diabetes. A more complete history, which includes detailed information about risk factors, can be acquired when the patient is stabilised. This information will be essential to guide patient education and rehabilitation and to plan discharge.

Practice tip

Due to changes in neuroreceptors, older patients and diabetic patients may not describe the typical anginal pain. Women also may not describe classic angina symptoms and may use different descriptors from men. Be alert for prodromal symptoms, such as increased shortness of breath, weakness and fainting.

TABLE 10.2
OLDCARTS framework for assessing chest pain

DESCRIPTION	QUESTIONS TO ASK TO YIELD THE INFORMATION
Onset	When did the pain begin?
Location	Where is the pain? Can the patient point to the location of the pain?
Duration	How long does the pain last? Is it persistent or intermittent?
Characteristics	Describe the pain: is it crushing, stabbing, indigestion-like, dull, or an ache, for example?
Associating factors	What other symptoms are associated with the pain, such as nausea and/or vomiting, weakness, fatigue, breathlessness, syncope, feeling cold and clammy?
Relieving factors/radiation	Does the pain radiate, such as down the arm or up into the neck, for example? Does the pain stop when activity ceases, or is it relieved by sitting forward or resting?
Treatment/temporal factors	Is pain relieved by rest or a decrease in physical activity? Is it relieved by the use of glyceryl trinitrate? Is pain comparable to previous ischaemic chest pain?
Severity (intensity)	A numerical scale (1 no pain to 10 worse pain experienced) is used to gauge pain severity

Source: Seidel HM, Ball JW, Dains JE, et al. Mosby's guide to physical examination. 6th ed. Mosby, 2003.

Physical examination

Physical manifestations vary and depend on the impact of pain, size and location of the infarction in the individual. Heart rate and blood pressure may be raised because of anxiety. Impaired left ventricular function may result in dyspnoea, tachycardia, hypotension, pallor, sweating, nausea and vomiting. Impaired right ventricular function may be indicated by jugular vein distention and peripheral oedema. Abnormalities in heart sounds may be present, including a muffled and diminished first heart sound due to decreased contractility. A fourth heart sound is common, whereas a third heart sound is uncommon. Many patients develop a pericardial rub after about 48–72 hours owing to an inflammatory response to the damaged myocardium. Additional findings occur with complications, and these are discussed in the related specific sections below.

Electrocardiographic examination

Patients with chest discomfort should be assessed by an appropriately qualified person and have a 12-lead ECG recorded within 10 minutes of first acute clinical contact to determine the presence and extent of myocardial ischaemia and the risk of adverse events, and to provide a baseline for subsequent changes.[7–9] Most importantly, the ECG is essential to determine whether emergency reperfusion is required, and is recommended as the sole test for selecting patients for PCI or thrombolysis. Where ST-segment monitoring is available, this should be continuous. Alternatively, if chest discomfort persists, ECGs should be repeated every 15 minutes. Even when chest pain resolves it is important to record a series of 12-lead ECGs during admission to determine changes over time. (The normal ECG is covered in Chapter 9, whereas this section addresses ischaemic changes in the ECG.)

Myocardial ischaemia, injury or infarction causes cellular alterations and affects depolarisation and repolarisation resulting in T-wave inversion or ST-segment depression in the leads facing the ischaemic area.[11] Ischaemic T waves are usually symmetrical, narrower and more pointed. ST-segment depression of 1 mm for 0.08 seconds is indicative of ischaemia. These changes are reversible with reduction in demand (e.g. rest, nitrates).

MI is associated with a typical pattern of ECG changes over time including evolution of the ST segments, Q-wave development and T-wave inversion as described below, but these changes too are not universal. The distinction between the types of ACS, including ST-elevation acute coronary syndrome (STEACS), ST-elevation MI (STEMI) and non-ST-elevation MI (NSTEMI), is important for ensuring appropriate assessment and protocol-based treatment.

The location and extent of ischaemia or infarction may be evident on the ECG leads overlying the affected area, as follows:

- anteroseptal wall of left ventricle, V1–V4
- anterior wall of the left ventricle, V1–V6, I and aVL
- lateral wall of left ventricle, I, aVL, V5 and V6
- inferior wall of left ventricle, II, III and aVF.

Additional electrodes can be placed on the right chest wall using the same landmarks as the left chest to view the right ventricle (see Chapter 9). Further posterior electrodes, V7–V9, may be placed over the posterior left chest to view the posterior wall. Other indicative signs of posterior wall damage are a dominant r wave in V1 and/or ST depression in V3 and V4, as these may be reciprocal changes. If these signs are present, a left-sided ECG, V7–V9, should be done to confirm or rule out a posterior infarction.

Continuous ECG monitoring is essential for the early detection of arrhythmias, which often accompany myocardial ischaemia or infarction and may be life threatening. The arrhythmia may be due to poor perfusion of the conduction tissue. More often, arrhythmias occur because ischaemic tissue has a lower fibrillatory threshold and ischaemia is not being managed. Arrhythmias also result from left ventricular failure.

Typical ECG evolution pattern

The initial ECG features of MI are ST-segment elevation with tall T waves recorded in leads overlying the area of damaged myocardium. These changes gradually change, or evolve, over time, with ST segments returning to baseline (within hours), while Q waves develop (hours to days) and T waves become inverted (days to weeks). The time course for the evolutionary changes is accelerated by reperfusion – for example, PCI, thrombolysis or surgery. Therefore, an almost fully evolved pattern may be seen within hours if successful reperfusion has been undertaken (see Figs 10.2–10.4 for examples). Given the expected time course for evolution, it is possible to approximate how recently infarction has occurred, which is essential in determining management:

- Acute (or hyperacute): there is ST elevation, but Q waves or T inversion has not yet developed (Fig. 10.5).
- Recent: Q waves have developed. ST-segment elevation may still be present. Evolution is under way. The infarction is more than 24 hours old.
- Old (fully evolved): Q waves and T inversion are present. ST segments are no longer elevated. Infarction occurred anything from a few days to years ago.

Biomarkers

Cardiac troponins T and I are structural proteins, which now are the preferred biomarkers for identification of myocardial necrosis given their sensitivity and specificity. Furthermore, high-sensitivity troponin assays can detect plasma elevation, within 1–3 hours, supporting early diagnosis and subsequent risk stratification of patients with suspected ACS.[7–9] Troponin elevation is defined as at least one value exceeding the 99th percentile of the assay's upper reference limit, and detection of a rise and/or fall of the measurements is essential to support the diagnosis of acute MI.[7–9] Measurement of troponin should occur at hospital presentation and predefined time periods

FIGURE 10.2 Acute inferoposterior infarction: ST elevation in indicative leads II, III and aVF. The ST-segment depression in I and aVL is reciprocal to the inferior infarction. Also, ST depression in anterior leads (V1–V3) is reciprocal to posterior wall infarction. Posterior leads (not shown here) were recorded and revealed ST elevation in V7, V8 and V9. This patient had acute (100%) obstruction at the ostium of the right coronary artery (RCA).

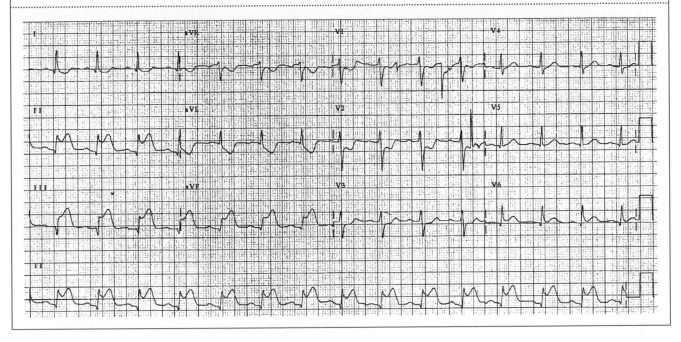

FIGURE 10.3 The same patient as in Fig. 10.2 recorded only 1 hour later, after stenting of the RCA with an evolving inferoposterior infarction. Note the ST segments in II, III and aVF are still elevated but returning to baseline. The reciprocal ST depression is likewise diminishing and can now be seen only in aVL, V1 and V2. Q waves have already developed in inferior leads.

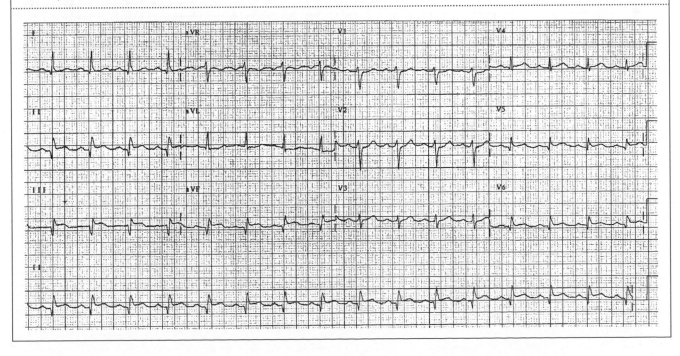

FIGURE 10.4 The same patient again, recorded a further 21 hours later. An almost fully evolved pattern is now present. Note the ST segments inferiorly have almost completely returned to baseline (as have the reciprocal changes). The Q waves remain, and T waves have now inverted inferiorly.

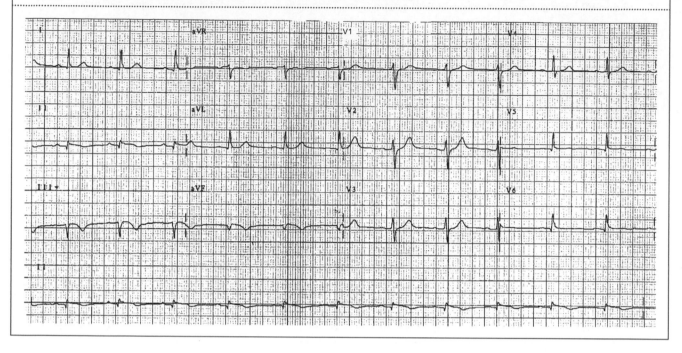

FIGURE 10.5 Acute anterolateral infarction in a patient with anterior descending coronary artery obstruction. Note the ST elevation and tall (hyperacute) T waves across the chest leads V1–V6 recorded on admission.

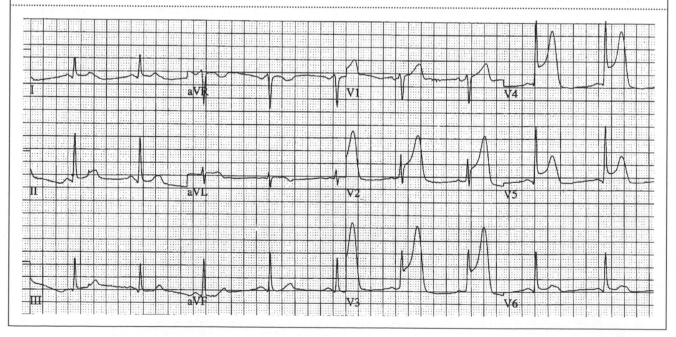

according to unit protocols alongside thorough clinical assessment to allow accurate differential diagnosis of acute MI from other medical conditions associated with elevations in cardiac troponin levels (e.g. including myocarditis, heart failure and renal disease).

Coronary angiography and left heart catheterisation

Coronary angiography gives a detailed picture of coronary artery disease. Specially designed catheters are advanced with the assistance of a guidewire into the ascending aorta via the radial[7] or less frequently the femoral arteries and manoeuvred into the ostium of each coronary artery. Contrast media is then injected and images are taken from several views to provide detailed information on the extent, site and severity of coronary artery lesions and the blood flow into each artery. This flow is graded using the Thrombolysis in Myocardial Infarction (TIMI) studies system (Table 10.3). Typically, a left ventricular angiogram is performed during the same procedure to assess the appearance and function of the left ventricle, mitral and aortic valves. If CHD is visualised on angiography, subsequent treatment is determined according to the severity of the culprit lesions(s) such as percutaneous coronary intervention, coronary artery bypass grafting or medical therapy. In addition to angiography, adjunctive physiological assessment and imaging such as fractional flow reserve (FFR), intravascular ultrasound (IVUS) and optical coherence tomography (OCT) assist in diagnosing the severity and subsequent management of coronary disease.[12-14] FFR is widely used to provide physiological assessment of a suspected culprit coronary lesion(s) and has robust evidence to support the decision to proceed with coronary intervention or medically manage the lesion(s).[14] The nursing care for coronary angiography is similar to PCI and is covered under that section.

Given that conventional angiography provides only information related to the lumen of the artery, the use of alternative imaging techniques is increasing, such as computed tomographic coronary angiography (CTCA) or magnetic resonance imaging (MRI) angiography to visualise the coronary anatomy and provide additional information about the atherosclerotic plaques within the vessel wall.

Non-invasive investigations

A number of investigations may aid the clinical diagnosis for patients with a suspected diagnosis of angina. These investigations which may be either anatomical (e.g. CTCA) or functional (e.g. exercise tolerance testing (ETT) or cardiac imaging) can help confirm the presence of underlying atherosclerotic disease and guide risk stratification related to severity of ischaemia.[15] A baseline 12-lead electrocardiogram (ECG) should be performed in every patient with suspected angina. While an abnormal resting ECG increases the probability that a patient has coronary artery disease (CAD) and may highlight the presence of other conditions such as atrial fibrillation or left ventricular hypertrophy, it is important to remember that a normal 12-lead ECG does not exclude a diagnosis of CAD and further investigation may be required.

Recent guidelines have reduced the emphasis of ETT within the diagnostic screening process; however, practice may be influenced by the availability of local investigative resources.[16] For some time it has recognised that false-positive ETTs are more common in populations with a lower incidence of CHD, including women.[15,16] The main diagnostic ECG abnormality during ECG exercise testing consists of a horizontal or down-sloping ST-segment depression >0.1 mV, persisting for at least 0.06–0.08 seconds after the J-point, in one or more ECG leads. Stress imaging techniques – that is, echocardiography performed in the presence of physical (treadmill or bike) or pharmacological (e.g. dobutamine) stressors, myocardial perfusion scintigraphy (SPECT/PET), or stress MRI – may also detect ischaemic change and wall motion abnormalities. Comparisons of the diagnostic accuracy of various non-invasive tests used in patients with suspected stable angina favour CTCA because of its high sensitivity and specificity (0.96 and 0.79, respectively) in detecting obstructive CAD.[15] Given the high negative predictive value of CTCA in the absence of stenosis, patients and

---

TABLE 10.3

Thrombolysis in myocardial infarction (TIMI) flow grades in coronary arteries

TIMI 0	No perfusion and no antegrade flow beyond the occlusion.
TIMI 1	Penetration with minimal perfusion, and contrast does not opacify the entire bed distal to the stenosis during the picture run.
TIMI 2	Partial perfusion and contrast opacifies the entire coronary bed distal to the stenosis, although entry to this area is slower than with unaffected coronary beds.
TIMI 3	Complete perfusion and filling and clearance of contrast is rapid and comparable to other coronary beds.

Source: Adapted from Belenkie I, Knudtson ML, Roth DL, et al. Relation between flow grade after thrombolytic therapy and the effect of angioplasty on left ventricular function: a prospective randomized trial. Am Heart J 1991;121(2 Pt 1):407–16.

referring physicians can be reassured that initiating medical therapy is sufficient without the need for further testing or invasive therapies.[16] Furthermore, initial trial data suggest that the inclusion of CTCA can clarify diagnosis and aid the implementation of more-appropriate treatment plans with the potential of preventing future coronary events.[16]

Chest radiography

An initial chest X-ray film is useful to exclude other causes of chest pain, such as pneumonia, pneumothorax and aortic aneurysm, and to assess whether heart failure and/or pulmonary congestion are present. If the diagnosis is clearly STEMI, this step can wait until after thrombolysis or PCI.

Patient management

The management of stable angina patients is aimed at: (1) secondary prevention of cardiac events, (2) symptom control with medication, (3) revascularisation and (4) rehabilitation (Fig. 10.6).[9] (Revascularisation by coronary artery bypass graft is reviewed in Chapter 12; revascularisation by percutaneous coronary angioplasty is reviewed in the next section.)

Treatment of patients with ACS aims at rapid diagnosis, identification of the presence or absence of ST elevation and risk stratification. When ST elevation is present, optimal reperfusion strategies are immediately implemented to re-establish flow to the occluded coronary artery, ensure myocardial perfusion and minimise the area of myocardial ischaemia/infarction. In those without ST elevation, the priority is risk stratification using a validated tool such as Global Registry of Acute Events (GRACE) or TIMI to allow early implementation of evidence-based therapies and interventions.[9]

The optimal place to manage ACS or MI patients is in the coronary or cardiac care unit, where continuous, specialised nursing care is available and there is rapid access to treatments. Secondary prevention of cardiac events includes the provision of medications, such as antiplatelet therapy and lipid-lowering therapy.

In addition, treatment aims to:

- stabilise the patient's condition
- decrease myocardial workload
- maximise oxygen delivery to tissues
- control pain and sympathetic stimulation
- prevent and detect complications
- preserve ventricular function
- reduce morbidity and mortality.

Reperfusion therapy

Reperfusion therapy includes coronary angioplasty, ideally with a stent, or thrombolytic therapy (also termed fibrinolysis). Patients fast-tracked for reperfusion therapy have one or more of the following indications: (1) ischaemic or infarction symptoms for longer than 20 minutes, (2) onset of symptoms within 12 hours, and (3) ECG changes (ST elevation of 1 mm in contiguous limb leads, ST elevation of 2 mm in contiguous chest leads, left bundle branch block (LBBB)). Systematic reviews have highlighted the superiority of primary PCI over thrombolysis in relation to short- and long-term mortality, stroke, re-infarction, recurrent ischaemia and the need for coronary artery bypass grafting for STEMI patients. The greatest benefits were noted within the first 12 hours of symptom onset. As such, STEMI guidelines recommend immediate treatment with primary PCI when this can be delivered within 90 minutes of first medical contact.[7-9] However, when primary PCI is not available many will still benefit from immediate thrombolysis and transfer to a facility providing PCI.[7-9]

Thrombolytic therapy

Thrombolytic therapy has been demonstrated to produce a significant reduction in mortality in the high-risk group described above.[7-9] The greatest reduction in mortality occurs if reperfusion occurs within the first 'golden' hour of presentation.[7-9] Thrombolysis can be delivered effectively in many settings where other methods of reperfusion are not available. Clots formed in response to injury normally dissolve using the body's fibrinolytic processes as tissue repair takes place. This requires the presence of the proenzyme plasminogen, which is converted into the enzyme plasmin when activated by macrophages and degrades the clot. Thrombolytic agents, including tissue-type plasminogen activator (tPA), have been developed that trigger conversion of plasminogen to plasmin and therefore break down clots. It is essential to screen patients for contraindications to thrombolysis quickly but thoroughly so that therapy can be commenced as soon as possible. Contraindications are given in the National Health Foundation of Australia (NHFA) Guidelines (see Fig. 10.6).[9]

Tenecteplase is one of the most commonly prescribed thrombolytic agents and is a drug tissue-type plasminogen activator (tPA) that is available as alteplase, tenecteplase and reteplase. These agents are of human origin, made by recombinant DNA techniques.[17] The drug activates only plasminogen present in blood clots, so the risk of haemorrhage is decreased. Unlike streptokinase, tPA can be given repeatedly without risk of anaphylactic reaction. Often patients with anterior ischaemic changes are treated with tPA (alteplase) based on the GUSTO-1 trial that showed improved outcomes in terms of reduction of ischaemia.[18] Alteplase is usually given by infusion, whereas reteplase, which has a longer half-life, can be given in two bolus injections. In the pre-hospital setting, weight-adjusted tenecteplase is the preferred agent for ease of administration through an IV bolus in a pre-hospital setting.[9,17]

Nursing management of the patient post-thrombolysis focuses on monitoring and detection of bleeding complications and/or return of ischaemia. Care is as follows:

- Continuous observations to assess changes in neurological state including orientation, any IV sites

FIGURE 10.6   Management of acute coronary syndromes.

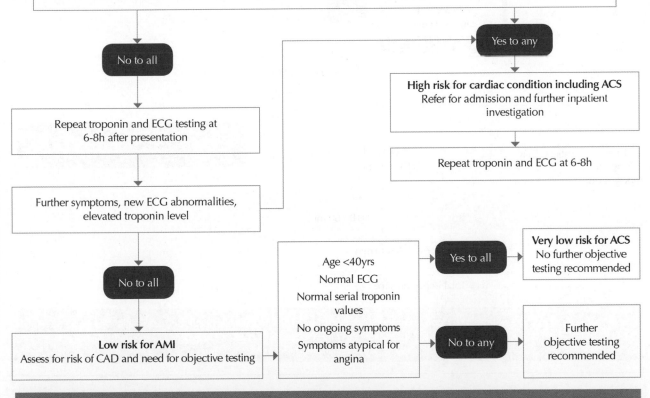

IMPORTANT NOTICE: Management protocols never replace clinical judgement. The care outlined in this protocol must be altered if it is not clinically appropriate for the individual patient.

Troponin and ECG testing on presentation (0h)

High risk features for possible cardiac cause of chest pain (including ACS and other cardiac diagnoses)

- Ongoing or repetitive chest pain despite initial ED treatment
- Elevated level of cardiac troponin*
- Persistent or dynamic electrocardiographic changes of ST-segment depression ≥0.5 mm or new T-wave inversion ≥2 mm in more than two contiguous leads
- Transient ST-segment elevation (≥0.5 mm) in more than two contiguous leads
- Haemodynamic compromise — systolic blood pressure <90 mmHg, cool peripheries, diaphoresis, Killip Class > I, and/or new-onset mitral regurgitation
- Sustained ventricular tachycardia
- Syncope
- Known left ventricular systolic dysfunction (left ventricular ejection fraction <40%)
- Prior AMI, percutaneous coronary intervention or prior coronary artery bypass surgery within 6 months

No to all

Yes to any

High risk for cardiac condition including ACS
Refer for admission and further inpatient investigation

Repeat troponin and ECG testing at 6-8h after presentation

Repeat troponin and ECG at 6-8h

Further symptoms, new ECG abnormalities, elevated troponin level

No to all

Age <40yrs
Normal ECG
Normal serial troponin values
No ongoing symptoms
Symptoms atypical for angina

Yes to all

Very low risk for ACS
No further objective testing recommended

No to any

Further objective testing recommended

Low risk for AMI
Assess for risk of CAD and need for objective testing

Note: It is important to validate the local Suspected ACS assessment protocol (Suspected ACS-AP). We recommend evaluating three components: Routinely monitor and assess patients receiving the local Suspected ACS-AP; continuously evaluate adherence to the Suspected ACS-AP; conduct ongoing assessment of the 30-day outcome associated with the application of the Suspected ACS-AP. *Elevated troponin defined as >99th percentile of a normal reference population.
AMI: acute myocardial infarction; CAD: coronary artery disease; ECG: electrocardiogram; ED: emergency department

Source: Reproduced from National Heart Foundation of Australia and Cardiac Society of Australia and New Zealand (NHFA and CSANZ); Chew DP, Scott IA, Cullen L, et al. NHFA and CSANZ: Australian clinical guidelines for the management of acute coronary syndromes 2016. Heart Lung Circ 2016;25:895–951. © 2016 National Heart Foundation of Australia, ABN 98 008 419 761.

Continued

FIGURE 10.6, cont'd

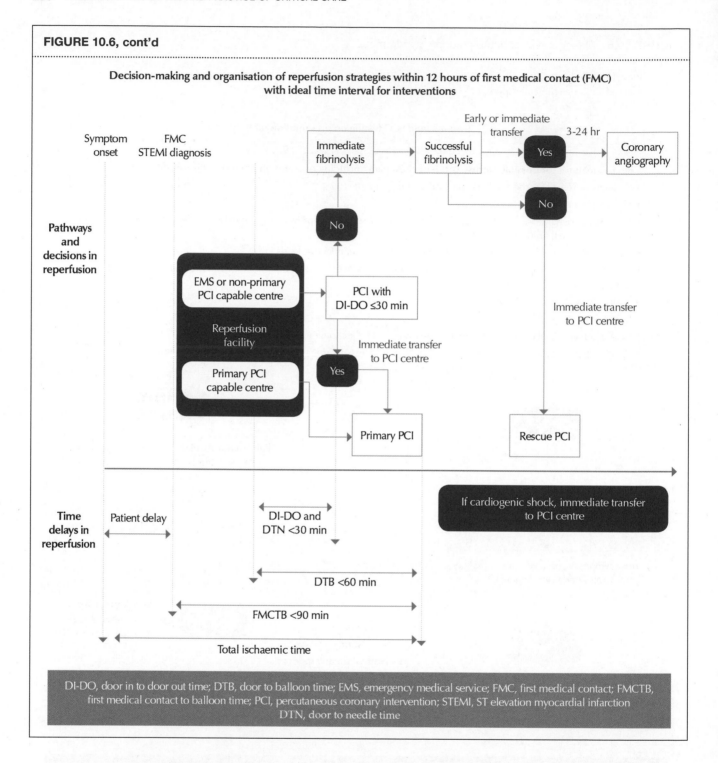

Decision-making and organisation of reperfusion strategies within 12 hours of first medical contact (FMC) with ideal time interval for interventions

DI-DO, door in to door out time; DTB, door to balloon time; EMS, emergency medical service; FMC, first medical contact; FMCTB, first medical contact to balloon time; PCI, percutaneous coronary intervention; STEMI, ST elevation myocardial infarction DTN, door to needle time

and urinalysis for the presence of bleeding. Along with vital signs, these are attended every 15 minutes for the first hour, half-hourly for an hour and then hourly according to the patient's condition; however, patients are advised to report any bleeding post–discharge as well.

- ECG monitoring: includes 12-lead ECG on return and continuous ECG monitoring and chest pain assessment to detect reocclusion and arrhythmias. Some arrhythmias, particularly idioventricular arrhythmias, are associated with reperfusion and tend to be benign. ST-segment monitoring and assessment of pain help evaluate the effectiveness of the thrombolysis. Patients need to be requested to inform nursing staff of any chest pain or discomfort. Should this be present, a repeat 12-lead ECG should be completed.

- IV anticoagulants such as heparin and/or oral antiplatelet drugs, such as ticagrelor or clopidogrel, may be given following thrombolysis to prevent reocclusion in the stent.

Thrombolysis is considered to have failed if the patient is still in pain and the ST segment has not resolved within 60–90 minutes.[7] If thrombolysis fails, patients are at high risk for other interventions, so repeat thrombolysis is often the only treatment option. Salvage or rescue angioplasty may be undertaken if available at the site.

Coronary angioplasty

Following an identified need for coronary revascularisation, clinicians decide whether this should be undertaken non-invasively such as PCI, or invasively such as surgery. Coronary artery bypass grafting was traditionally the first-line option but the role of surgery has been challenged with the evolution of PCI technology, the introduction of drug-eluting stents (DES) and comparable clinical outcomes in specific populations.[15] During PCI a guiding catheter is introduced, commonly through the radial artery, to visualise the affected vessel. A guide wire and balloon are then advanced through the guiding catheter to the area of occlusion or stenosis under the guidance of X-ray imaging. The artery is dilated by inflating a fine balloon to widen the lumen of the artery, and then a coronary artery stent (a fine-lattice scaffold) is inserted to prevent the artery from recoiling (Fig. 10.7). Rapid advances in stent technology and the use of second- and third-generation DESs has helped to prevent or slow down endothelialisation, reducing but not entirely eliminating in-stent restenosis, particularly in small-calibre vessels.[15] The adjunctive intracoronary imaging modalities of OCT and IVUS help visualise the extent of disease, providing vessel lumen dimensions and plaque morphology, along with identification of residual stenosis, giving higher accuracy of stent expansion post dilation, ultimately improving short-term procedural and long-term clinical outcomes.[12]

The choice of revascularisation technique is often complex and will require careful consideration of the individual's medical and surgical suitability for the procedure as well as the patient's individual preferences based on an informed choice associated with risks and benefits. Factors influencing the revascularisation decision may include the extent and severity of underlying CAD – for example, single versus multivessel disease or the presence of left main-stem disease. Associated comorbidities

FIGURE 10.7 PTCA procedure.

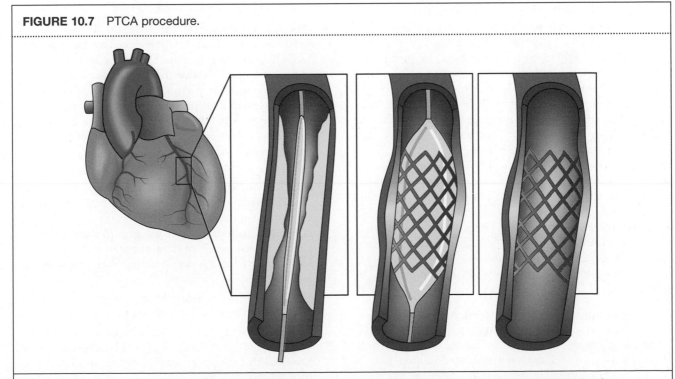

Source: Heart Research Australia, https://www.heartresearch.com.au/living-with-heart-diseases/procedures-and-devices/

(e.g. diabetes mellitus and renal impairment) as well as the patient's age and quality of life may also influence the final decision.[15] Long-term outcomes with PCI for silent ischaemia following MI have demonstrated a significant reduction in cardiac death, recurrent MI, or the need for revascularisation, with less evidence of ischaemia on exercise testing at 4 years despite the PCI patients being on fewer beta-blockers.[19] PCI and CABG now offer comparable outcomes in patients with left main-stem disease in the short to medium term; however, current evidence supports the benefit of CABG over PCI in patients with a greater disease burden and more complex CHD in terms of improved mortality and less need for revascularisation in the longer term.[15]

Primary PCI is the recommended first-line therapy for patients with STEMI as it results in a higher rate of patency of the affected artery (>90%), lower rates of cerebrovascular accident (CVA) and re-infarction and higher short-term survival than thrombolysis.[9,20] Primary PCI is recommended for all patients presenting with chest pain who meet the indications for reperfusion when: (1) facilities are available and it can be achieved within recommended guideline times of 60–90 minutes, (2) there are contraindications to fibrinolytic therapy described above, (3) ischaemia would result in large anterior STEMI within 4 hours, or (4) haemodynamic instability or cardiogenic shock is present.

Following primary PCI, the use of second- and third-generation stents has minimised the incidence of intimal hyperplasia and in-stent restenosis and reduced need for revascularisatrion.[15,19] Research continues to identify optimal strategies for prevention of such complications post-PCI to prevent reduction of blood flow. It is important to complement these procedures, however, with dual antiplatelet therapies and ensure their continuation within agreed timeframes as per unit protocols.

Nursing management of patients post-PCI includes care of the puncture site to prevent bleeding and detect arterial changes (including clot and aneurysm). The increased use of radial access, however, and the use of band-like pressure devices (e.g. TR Bands and Helix) for arterial closure of the radial puncture site has led to fewer issues with haemostasis and vascular complications, and enables earlier mobilisation.[21] Femoral closure is generally done by internal device (e.g. Angio-seal or Perclose). Following closure, oozing may still occur and require the application of additional pressure.

Following PCI, specific care will be determined by access site:

- Observations: observe access site (radial or femoral) for haemorrhage and/or haematoma; assess perfusion to the digits or lower limb, including colour, warmth and pulses. This monitoring is needed frequently in the first few hours, when complications are most likely to occur.
- ECG monitoring: includes 12-lead ECG following completion of the procedure, ongoing ECG

monitoring and chest pain assessment to detect acute reocclusion of the treated vessel. Patients need to be requested to inform nursing staff of any chest pain or discomfort.

- Vital signs: may be recorded every 15 minutes for the first hour, half-hourly for 1 hour and then hourly according to the patient's condition.
- Removal of sheaths: femoral sheaths are usually removed by specially trained nursing staff when the effect of anticoagulation agents are within a recommended range. Removal of the radial sheath is performed at the end of the procedure in the cardiac catheterisation laboratory with a transradial band/ bracelet providing haemostasis.
- Achievement of femoral haemostasis: use either application of pressure for at least 10 minutes or vascular sealing.[10]
  ○ Pressure application can be by a manual compression device (such as Femostop, RADI Medical Systems, Uppsala, Sweden) and less often digital, to maintain a pressure of about 20 mmHg.
  ○ Vascular sealing uses a device such as the Angio-seal vascular closure device (St Jude Medical Inc., St Paul, MN). This includes a collagen plug and a small biodegradable plate inside the artery, which is held in place by a small suture, tamping tube and small spring on the exterior. The tension spring is removed and the suture trimmed half an hour after application. This enables the patient to mobilise and reduces nursing time.
- Assess: international normalised ratio (INR), prothrombin (PT) and partial thromboplastin time (PTT), as bleeding is more likely to occur if anticoagulants are above the therapeutic range. Weight-adjusted heparin (100 units/kg) is usually used during PCI to prevent thrombus formation, and glycoprotein IIb/IIIa inhibitors may be used to prevent platelet aggregation and thrombus formation for patients at high risk of adverse events.
- Bed rest (2–6 h): is used to discourage the patient from moving the joint of the insertion site to prevent clot displacement and haematoma formation. Initially, the patient should lie relatively flat if femoral artery access has been used, then progress to sitting. The period of rest has been demonstrated to be safely reduced to 1 hour in low-risk patients (normotensive and normal platelet count).[10]
- Pain relief: is used primarily to promote comfort for patients who find bed rest causes pain and discomfort.
- Urine output: adequate urine output is essential as radiographic IV contrast is cleared by the kidneys, so it is vital that nurses ensure good hydration and monitor initial urine output.
- Oral antiplatelet drugs, such as ticagrelor or clopidogrel in addition to aspirin: may be given prior to the procedure to prevent later reocclusion in the

stent. Dual antiplatelet therapy should continue for 6 months; however, longer treatment durations may be used where the risks of atherothrombotic events outweigh the risk of bleeding.[20]

Many patients find the PCI procedure and confirmation of CHD diagnosis stressful. It is an important nursing role to provide patients with preparatory information about the procedure and care required during recovery. As family members provide valuable support and reminders about recovery, these people should be included in any information sessions. The patient and family need to be provided with information about the possibility of restenosis, mobility restrictions at home and the lifestyle changes needed to reduce the risk of worsening CHD.

> ### Practice tip
>
> Increased hydration can aggravate problems with urination when on bed rest, particularly in older men with prostate enlargement. If a femoral access site is used in these patients, it is easier for the patient to urinate while turned on their side, using pillow support to maintain the position.

> ### Practice tip
>
> If a femoral access site has been used, bleeding may track between the patient's legs and pool, and this will be invisible to a cursory inspection, particularly if the patient is obese. Always move the patient's thigh during regular inspections.

Nursing management of ACS and MI patients

The nursing role in patients with ACS includes reducing myocardial workload and maximising cardiac output, provision of treatments, careful monitoring to determine the effects of treatment and detect complications, rapid treatment of complications, comfort and pain control, psychosocial support and teaching and discharge planning. Suffering an acute cardiac event results in loss of control over life; the constant presence of nurses and their open and honest communication provides the security and reassurance patients require. A calm, caring manner during nursing care is essential to establish rapport and lower patient and family anxiety. Patients should be given sufficient information to understand their condition and immediate treatment plan but not overloaded with unnecessary facts. Individual evaluation of the patient and the family is necessary to determine the most appropriate management of visiting.

Reduction of myocardial workload includes ensuring the patient has bed rest, providing support with activities and limiting stress. Continuous cardiac monitoring (preferably including ST monitoring) and evaluation of heart rate and rhythm, shortness of breath, chest discomfort and blood pressure are essential to determine ischaemia, treatment effects, myocardial workload and complications. This monitoring should occur within the acute phase, reducing as the patient recovers. Oxygen saturation levels should be routinely assessed and provision of oxygen by mask or nasal cannulae provided only if levels are below 93%.[7–9] A large Swedish registry of 6629 patients with suspected MI found no conclusive evidence to support routine supplementary oxygen therapy in MI.[22] Symptom relief should be provided, including analgesia for pain. Analgesia management should be conducted by nurses because of their continued contact and hence more accurate assessment and treatment of pain.[23,24] It is essential to treat pain, not only for the distress it causes patients but also because pain causes stimulation of the sympathetic nervous system (SNS). SNS responses include elevated heart rate and potential for arrhythmias, peripheral vasoconstriction and increased myocardial contractility and, therefore, an overall increase in myocardial oxygen demand. Effective treatments for pain include IV morphine and nitrates. The IV route is preferable, as absorption is predictable and additional punctures in thrombolysed/anticoagulated patients are not required. Morphine has the additional benefit of reducing anxiety in a distressing situation and should be initially provided at a dose of 2.5–5 mg at 1 mg/min, followed by 2.5-mg doses as indicated. While there is little randomised controlled trial evidence to support this particular practice, it is generally accepted to be appropriate. A standardised method of pain evaluation and charting should be used to ensure consistent assessment and treatment. An antiemetic such as metoclopramide or ondansetron should be given concurrently to lessen and prevent nausea. Other drugs, such as beta-blockers and nitrates, decrease myocardial workload, contributing to pain reduction.

Medications

Provision of medications and assessment of the effectiveness of treatment is a major component of the nurse's role in caring for the cardiac patient. Many of the medications are accompanied by side effects and interactions with other drugs, which the nurse must monitor. An array of medications is used to treat ACS patients, including antiplatelet agents, $P2Y_{12}$ inhibitors, glycoprotein IIB/IIIA inhibitors, anticoagulants, lipid-lowering agents, beta-blockers, ACE inhibitors and organic nitrates (Table 10.4).

Symptom control

Control of anginal symptoms with medication usually includes sublingual glyceryl trinitrate (GTN) for immediate symptom control and one or more antianginal medications for sustained symptom management. These medications are described in the next section. The choice of medication may depend on how acceptable the patient finds the reduction in symptoms and the presence of side effects. Patients need to take antianginal agents continuously, regardless of symptoms. Patients should also be encouraged to take sublingual GTN prophylactically.

TABLE 10.4

Medications used in the treatment of ACS

AGENT	ACTION	SIDE EFFECTS/CAUTION	COMMENTS
ANTIPLATELET Aspirin	Inhibits cyclooxygenase (COX-1) and prevents platelet synthesis of thromboxane A2, a vasoconstrictor and stimulant of platelet aggregation. May provide benefits from anti-inflammatory properties in reducing plaque rupture.	Gastrointestinal (GI) irritation and bleeding; use enteric-coated tablets to minimise gastric irritation.	Noted to reduce the risk of vascular events (cardiovascular death, AMI and non-fatal stroke) by 50%.[15] Lifelong use is recommended for secondary prevention.
$P2Y_{12}$ INHIBITORS Ticagrelor	Reversibly and non-competitively binds the ADP $P2Y_{12}$ receptor on the platelet surface, which prevents ADP-mediated activation of the GP IIb/IIIa receptor complex, thereby reducing platelet aggregation.	Adverse side effects reported for $P2Y_{12}$-receptor antagonists are bleeding, transient bradycardia and dyspnoea. Ticagrelor should be administered with caution or avoided in patients with advanced sinoatrial disease. Caution is advised in patients at risk of increased bleeding owing to trauma, surgery or other pathological conditions and in those with asthma or COPD Care is required when delivering with other drugs and other anticoagulants.	Reversible, direct-acting inhibitor of the ADP receptor $P2Y_{12}$ that has a more rapid onset and more pronounced platelet inhibition than clopidogrel. RCTs have demonstrated reductions in atherothrombotic events (MI or CVA) with no increase in overall rate of major bleeding but had an increase in rate of non-procedural bleeding.
$P2Y_{12}$ INHIBITORS Clopidogrel	ADP receptor agonist; prevents the binding of ADP to its platelet receptor, thus inhibiting platelet aggregation.	Inhibits P450 liver enzyme; care is required when delivering with other drugs and other anticoagulants.	Clopidogrel produces fewer GI effects than aspirin and is more effective in patients with recent stroke, MI and peripheral vascular disease.
GLYCOPROTEIN IIB/IIIA INHIBITORS Tirofiban, eptifibatide, lamifiban, abciximab	Glycoprotein IIb/IIIa receptor antagonists prevent the final step of platelet aggregation and fibrinogen cross-linking. Used most commonly to inhibit thrombus formation in ACS.	Bleeding, thrombocytopenia, nausea, fever and headache; doses need to be reduced in renal failure.	Although much of the evidence for their use precedes the use of the current $P2Y_{12}$ blockers, they are still considered for use in ACS patients at high risk of adverse cardiovascular events or those undergoing complex interventional procedures.
ANTICOAGULANT THERAPY Unfractionated heparin Low-molecular-weight heparin (LMWH) Direct thrombin inhibitors, e.g. hirudin, bivalirudin, Synthetic penta-saccharides, e.g. fondaparinux	Limit further formation of thrombus in the acute phase. The main effect of unfractionated heparin (UH) is on the inhibition of thrombin-induced platelet aggregation. LMWH has been shown to have even greater benefit than UH in reducing subsequent MI and the need for revascularisation, with treatment effects enduring for up to 12 months in NSTEMI. Binds directly to thrombin (factor IIa) and inhibits the conversion of fibrinogen to fibrin. Blocks platelet activation and aggregation. Selectively activated factor X inhibitor.	UH: need for aPTT monitoring. LMWH: convenience in administration, no need for aPTT monitoring. Eliminated even in patients with moderate-to-severe renal function. Require only once a day administration because of long half-life. Caution in impaired liver or renal function where risk of haemorrhage increases. Dose adjustment required for low body weight.	Reduces death and re-infarction. In contrast to UH in STEMI, LMWH prevented 21 deaths or MIs per 1000 patients at the expense of four non-fatal bleeds. Evidence favours progressively LMWHs and treatment durations >48 h. Pentasaccharides appear to have the best safety and efficacy profiles: less adverse bleeding events combined with a reduction in short to medium-term mortality.

TABLE 10.4

Medications used in the treatment of ACS—cont'd

AGENT	ACTION	SIDE EFFECTS/CAUTION	COMMENTS
BETA-BLOCKERS	Reduce cardiac workload (heart rate and force of contraction) and myocardial oxygen demand by blocking beta-adrenergic receptors, preventing sympathetic stimulation of the heart.	Contraindications include significant AV block, bradycardia, hypotension, history of asthma or uncontrolled heart failure.	In the absence of bradycardia or hypotension, immediate IV and oral beta-blockade should be considered in ACS patients.
ACE INHIBITORS e.g. ramipril	Cause dilation of arteries and veins by competitively inhibiting the conversion of angiotensin I to angiotensin II (a potent endogenous vasoconstrictor) and by inhibiting bradykinin metabolism; these actions result in preload and afterload reductions on the heart. ACE inhibitors also promote sodium and water excretion by inhibiting angiotensin II-induced aldosterone secretion; elevation in potassium may also be observed. Can reduce cardiac and vascular remodelling.	Common side effects are dry cough and hypotension. Uncommon but life-threatening effect may be angioedema. Can cause renal impairment – requires monitoring of urea and electrolytes. Exert caution in times of dehydration.	Recommended in high-risk patients with vascular disease (unstable angina) in the absence of documented heart failure. All-cause mortality, MI and stroke are reduced. Observed benefits appear independent of the associated BP reductions particularly marked in patients with diabetes mellitus. Major mortality and morbidity benefits have been reported in patients with HF or LVSD post AMI. Treatment should be initiated within 36 h of the acute event.
NITRATES Glyceryl trinitrate (IV, sublingual and spray) Isosorbide mononitrate	Potent peripheral vasodilators, particularly in venous capacitance vessels, thereby reducing preload and to a lesser extent afterload, to reduce myocardial workload. Dilate normal and atherosclerotic coronary blood vessels to increase myocardial oxygen supply. Used to manage unstable angina and reduce blood pressure in the critical care setting, where there is some evidence for symptomatic relief.	Reflex tachycardia, hypotension, syncope and migraine-like headache; generally occur in first few days of treatment, then subside. Blood pressure should be monitored.	Tolerance to the vasodilator effect occurs, so intermittent treatment is most effective. In the case of transdermal delivery, if treatment is withheld for 8–12 h in every 24 h, therapeutic activity is restored.
LIPID-LOWERING STATINS Atorvastatin, simvastatin, fluvastatin, pravastatin	Inhibit 3-hydroxy-3-methylglutaryl-coenzyme-A (HMG-CoA) reductase, the enzyme that limits the rate of cholesterol synthesis in the liver, thereby reducing plasma cholesterol.	Headache, gastrointestinal upset, inflammation of voluntary muscles and altered liver function; taking statins with food may reduce GI symptoms.	There is strong evidence supporting the secondary prevention benefits of statins; therefore they should be commenced for long-term maintenance before discharge.

ACS = acute coronary syndrome; ADP = adenosine monophosphate; AMI = acute myocardial infarction; aPTT = activated partial thromboplastin time; AV = arteriovenous; BP = blood pressure; COPD = chronic obstructive pulmonary disease; CVA = cerebrovascular accident; HF = heart failure; IV = intravenous; LMWH = low-molecular-weight heparin; LVSD = left ventricular septal defect; MI = myocardial infarction; STEMI = ST-elevation myocardial infarction.

Source: Adapted from Deepak LB, Opie's cardiovascular drugs: a companion to Braunwald's heart disease. 9th ed. Philadelphia: Elsevier; 2020.

Angina may also be managed by treating associated conditions that precipitate angina such as anaemia, thyrotoxicosis and avoiding situations that trigger angina. Education needs to be directed at awareness of symptoms and management of unstable angina and MI symptoms, and the need for emergency care. Although these patients are at low risk of further cardiovascular events in the short term, in the medium to long term the risk may accumulate. Patients with angina may also benefit from comprehensive rehabilitation interventions. While some national guidelines recommend cardiac rehabilitation (CR) for patients with stable angina, a recent Cochrane review focusing on exercise-based interventions highlighted the need for more research in this area.[25]

Angiotensin-converting enzyme (ACE) inhibitors have been recommended for all post-MI patients while in hospital, with review of prescription at 4–6 weeks' post-discharge. Patients with left ventricular failure should be maintained on ACE inhibitors. Similarly, diuretics provide the mainstay of the management of left ventricular failure if it is present. Diabetic patients have a higher mortality after MI in both acute and long-term phases. Guidance supporting the use of insulin for targeted glucose control has become more flexible but still aims to maintain glucose levels below 180 mg/dL or 11 mmol while avoiding hypoglycaemia in ACS patients.[26]

Transfer to a step-down unit or general ward usually occurs when the patient is pain free and is haemodynamically stable. Stability means that patients are not dependent on IV inotropic or vasoactive support and have no arrhythmias. Discharge home after MI varies, but usually occurs at day 2 or 3 for low-risk patients.

Emotional responses and patient and family support

ACS or MI is usually accompanied by feelings of acute anxiety and fear, as most patients are aware of the significant threat posed to their health.[27] For many patients it may also be the first experience of acute illness and associated aspects such as ambulance transport, emergency care and hospitalisation, so they may experience shock and disbelief as well. Fast-track processes such as pre-hospital triage require patients and their families to process a large amount of information and make decisions quickly, and this, added to an alien environment full of unfamiliar technology and personnel, can be quite distressing. However, the environment can also promote a feeling of security for patients and their families.

Anxiety is a common response to the stress of an acute cardiac event and leads to important physiological and psychological changes.[10] The SNS is stimulated, resulting in increased heart rate, respiration and blood pressure. These responses increase the workload of the heart and therefore myocardial oxygen demand. In an acute cardiac event, these demands occur when perfusion is already poor and may lead to worse outcomes, including ventricular arrhythmias and increased myocardial ischaemia. Therefore, staff working in emergency and coronary care should employ strategies to reduce a patient's anxiety. Chapter 6 provides a more detailed description of psychological care.

Increasing a patient's sense of control, calm and confidence in care reduces the patient's sense of vulnerability, whether or not it is realistic. This can be achieved by:

- providing order and predictability in routines, allowing the patient to make choices, providing information and explanations and including the patient in decision making using a calm, confident approach
- open and honest communication with patients and families
- restricting the number and type of visitors in the acute phase, but many patients may feel safer if a family member is present
- provision of comprehensive information to families, with more-concise information in understandable language for patients.

Nurses need to monitor patients for signs of excessive anxiety, including facial expressions and behavioural changes. However, overt behaviours may be controlled by the patient, so careful conversation and/or use of specific assessments may be necessary to detect anxiety. The move to the step-down or general ward may also be stressful to the patient and family. This move needs to be planned and discussed, and promoted as a sign of recovery.

Cardiac rehabilitation

Cardiac rehabilitation (CR) has been defined as *'the coordinated sum of activities required to influence favourably the underlying cause of cardiovascular disease, as well as to provide the best possible physical, mental and social conditions, so that the patients may, by their own efforts, preserve or resume optimal functioning in their community and through improved health behaviour, slow or reverse progression of disease'.*[28] CR is recommended as an integral part of comprehensive care of CHD patients.[9,12,14] Although exercise therapy has consistently been identified as a central element of CR, the British Association for Cardiovascular Prevention and Rehabilitation (BACPR) describes six core components of CR which include: health behaviour change and education; lifestyle risk factor management (including physical activity and exercise, healthy eating and body composition, tobacco cessation and relapse prevention); psychosocial health; medical risk management; long-term strategies; and audit and evaluation (Fig. 10.8).[28]

It is important to identify and address misconceptions and provide information regarding the disease process, prognosis and an optimal approach to recovery. Early mobilisation is encouraged and discharge planning remains a very important element to streamline the transition between hospital and community care. Since discharge may be within 48–72 hours, even from the acute phase, it is important to provide psychological support. Input focusing on health and lifestyle behaviour change, risk

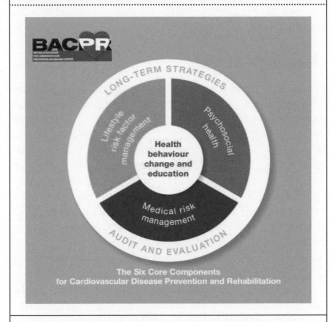

FIGURE 10.8 BACPR core components.

Source: The British Association for Cardiovascular Prevention and Rehabilitation. The BACPR standards and core components for cardiovascular disease prevention and rehabilitation. 3rd ed. British Cardiovascular Society, London: BACPR; 2023. Available from: https://www.bacpr.org/__data/assets/pdf_file/0021/64236/BACPR-Standards-and-Core-Components-2023.pdf.

factor modification and psychosocial well-being can also support self-management of a long-term cardiac condtion.[28 31] There is a strong evidence base supporting the benefits for CR in cardiac conditions, yet many people do not participate in CR following acute events.[31,32] An updated Cochrane review confirmed that exercise-based CR reduces cardiovascular mortality and hospital admissions and improves quality of life.[33] Additional benefits have been shown for improvements in exercise tolerance, symptoms, serum lipids, psychological well-being and cessation of smoking.[33] CR provides adequate and timely assessment of the patients' needs and the provision of a tailored and individualised program to provide support throughout the inpatient, immediate discharge period, and outpatient stages of the patient's recovery focusing on risk modification behaviour. CR incorporates principles of adult learning to optimise learning and behaviour change. These principles include recognition of readiness to learn and change behaviour. Adults are ready to learn most effectively when they are physically and emotionally stable and are aware of the problem or need to learn. Nurses, because of their expertise and continual presence, are best placed to assess and provide education at optimal times.

Complications of myocardial infarction

Despite declines in death rates from MI, many patients will experience complications, most of which occur within the first 24 hours.[34,35]

Cardiogenic shock

Cardiogenic shock occurs as a complication of MI and, although advances in reperfusion therapy have been associated with improvements in survival, in-hospital mortality remains high (27%–51%).[34,35] Results of the CULPRIT-SHOCK trial confirmed that the 30-day risk of a composite of death or severe renal failure leading to renal-replacement therapy was lower among those who initially underwent PCI of the culprit lesion only than among those who underwent immediate multivessel PCI. There were no significant differences in bleeding complications between the two groups.[35]

In addition to revascularisation procedures, efforts to reduce mortality associated with cardiogenic shock have been directed towards improvements in mechanical circulatory support (MCS) therapies. Intra-aortic balloon pumps (IABP) were commonly used to support patients in cardiogenic shock. However, the results of the IABP-SHOCK II trial following acute MI showed no benefit with routine IABP placement in addition to revascularisation.[36] This has resulted in decreased use of IABPs in clinical practice and less prominence of this therapy in guideline recommendations.[7,8] Although other devices and advanced therapies have shown promise in the treatment of cardiogenic shock, more data from randomised clinical trials are needed. Cardiogenic shock and the related management are described in more detail in Chapter 21.

Arrhythmias

Arrhythmias often occur in ACS and are often the cause of death in the pre-hospital phase. Management of the pre-hospital phase focuses on community education and an effective, rapidly responsive ambulance service.[7–9] Arrhythmias may be generated by poorly perfused tissue and electrolyte alterations, and increased sympathetic tone during infarction, but are more often due to a failing left ventricle. Arrhythmias may also be related to revascularisation procedures, although debate exists as to whether this indicates evidence of reperfusion or ongoing ischaemia.[7–9] It is essential to rapidly and effectively treat arrhythmias in the ACS context. The goal of treatment is to maintain hemodynamic stability and cardiac output while reducing workload. Management of arrhythmias is described in Chapter 11.

Pericarditis and pericardial effusion

Pericarditis is inflammation of the visceral and parietal layers of the pericardium that cover the heart. A retrospective analysis of 13,387 ACS patients (2000–13) identified only 90 patients (0.67%) with early post-MI pericarditis, 84.4% of whom had suffered a STEMI. This reflected a 35% reduction in post-MI pericarditis prevalence since 2000.[37]

As pericarditis is associated with chest pain, this is often confused with ischaemic pain, particularly due to the presence of ST-segment elevation on the ECG. However, pericardial pain increases with deep inspiration and a pericardial rub is often present.

Electrocardiographically, the elevated ST segments of pericarditis are typically concave upwards (saddle-shaped) and often widespread, contrasting with convex ST-segment elevation limited to the distribution of a single coronary artery in infarction. In addition, depression of the PR segment is commonly present.[38] Pericarditis normally responds to anti-inflammatory treatment by aspirin, indomethacin and/or corticosteroids. Approximately 1–5% of acute myocardial infarction (AMI) patients develop pericarditis as a late complication, 2 weeks to a few months post-AMI.[12] Usually, this late-onset pericarditis is associated with Dressler's syndrome and may be an autoimmune response to myocardial injury. This is a chronic condition requiring systemic corticosteroid treatment.

Due to the accumulation of excessive pericardial fluid, a pericardial effusion may develop most commonly in anterior STEMI, with large infarcts and when heart failure is present. Patients who develop a pericardial effusion have the potential for rapid deterioration and development of cardiac tamponade and cardiac arrest associated with pulseless electrical activity (PEA). The detection of a moderate-to-severe pericardial effusion ($\geq$10 mm) early after STEMI increases the risk of sudden cardiac death through cardiac tamponade. Although it is often associated with left ventricular free-wall rupture, in 80% of cases it can also be produced by heart failure, and myocardial haemorrhage may result from anticoagulant or antiaggregant therapies. Pericardiocentesis and blood pressure control may also be life saving; however, emergency surgical intervention for tamponade may be required particularly when associated with EMD.

Structural defects

Myocardial tissue death may be catastrophic if it is extensive or results in rupture of ventricular or papillary muscle. These conditions are rare and symptoms develop rapidly. Intraventricular septal rupture is usually associated with anterior MI. The patient develops progressive dyspnoea, tachycardia and pulmonary congestion, as well as a loud systolic murmur associated with a thrill felt in the parasternal area. If a pulmonary artery catheter is present, blood samples from the right atrium and right ventricle will reveal a higher than usual oxygen content. Diagnosis must be confirmed by cardiac catheterisation, and urgent surgery is required.

Papillary muscle rupture most often occurs 2–7 days after MI.[12] Patients experience a sudden onset of pulmonary oedema secondary to pulmonary hypertension and cardiogenic shock. Additional heart sounds and a systolic murmur will be heard. Urgent surgery is required, as the mortality rate for papillary muscle rupture without surgical treatment can reach 80%.[37] Cardiac rupture most often occurs within 5 days of MI and is commonest in older women. The patient experiences continuous chest pain, dyspnoea and hypotension as tamponade develops. Symptoms may worsen rapidly and result in PEA unless surgery is undertaken immediately. Fortunately, with the increasing use of early and effective revasculation therapies,

these complications have become less common, affecting approximately 2.3% of MIs. Clinicians should, however, remain alert to these serious and potentially lethal complications following ACSs.[37]

Heart failure

In normal circumstances, the heart is a very effective, efficient pump with reserve mechanisms available to allow output to meet changing demands. These mechanisms include: (1) increasing heart rate to increase total cardiac output, (2) dilation to create muscle stretch and more-effective contraction, (3) hypertrophy of myocytes over time to generate more force, and (4) increasing stroke volume by increasing venous return and increased contractility. Heart failure is a complex clinical condition characterised by an underlying structural abnormality or dysfunction that results in the inability of the ventricle to fill with or eject blood. The condition is also known as congestive cardiac failure, a term commonly used in the USA but not in Australia. Chronic heart failure (CHF) describes the long-term inability of the heart to meet metabolic demands.

The burden of disease associated with heart failure is on the rise because of our ageing population, the prevalence of CHD and hypertension, the decrease in fatality from ACS and improved methods of diagnosis. Survival rates and prognosis for heart failure patients are extremely poor. Approximately 20% of patients diagnosed with heart failure will die within 1 year of discharge[39,40] and the majority will die within 5 years.[40] The outcomes associated with heart failure are worse than in most common forms of cancer.[41] Heart failure continues to be the most common cause of hospitalisation in the elderly. Over 50% of patients newly diagnosed with heart failure have concurrent ischaemic heart disease, hypertension and diabetes mellitus.[1] The causes of heart failure can be categorised according to: (1) myocardial disease, (2) arrhythmias, (3) valve disease, (4) pericardial disease and (5) congenital heart disease.[42] Myocardial disease may be caused by MI and fibrosis from prolonged ischaemic heart disease, which accounts for approximately two-thirds of heart failure with reduced ejection fraction (HFrEF) causing systolic dysfunction and a reduced ejection fraction.

Arrhythmias, including both brady- and tachyarrhythmias, may cause heart failure due to changes in filling time affecting preload and resultant cardiac output. Myocardial oxygen demand is increased and, if the heart is poorly perfused, muscle contraction will be affected. Frequent premature contractions and atrial fibrillation disturb mechanical coordination so that the ventricles may not be adequately filled for efficient contraction. Heart failure patients are also at high risk of sudden cardiac death due to ventricular fibrillation or tachycardia. Valvular disease-causing heart failure usually involves valves on the left side of the heart (mitral and/or aortic valves). Aortic stenosis results in an increase in afterload and ventricular hypertrophy develops with reduced diastolic compliance resulting in a reduced ejection fraction. Mitral stenosis is usually due to rheumatic heart disease. Valvular incompetence results in a dilated ventricle to accommodate the regurgitant volume. Stroke volume increases in an attempt to empty its contents and ventricular muscle mass increases. However, over time the ventricle is unable to maintain the increased workload and heart failure develops. Valvular heart disease and treatment are described in more detail in Chapter 12.

There are several terms used to describe the pathology and signs and symptoms of heart failure. These include the following:

- *Backward failure:* refers to the systemic and pulmonary congestion that occurs as a result of failure of the ventricle to expel its volume.
- *Forward failure:* is due to an inadequate cardiac output and leads to decrease in vital organ perfusion.
- *Acute heart failure:* includes the initial hospitalisation for the diagnosis of heart failure and exacerbations of CHF.
- *CHF:* develops over time as a result of the inability of compensatory mechanisms to maintain an adequate cardiac output to meet metabolic demands. It refers to a long-term diagnosis of heart failure.
- *HFrEF or systolic heart failure:* refers to the inability of the ventricle to contract adequately during systole resulting in a reduced ejection fraction of <40%[43,44] and an increased end-diastolic volume. In Australia, HFrEF is defined as ejection fraction of <50%.[42] In Europe and USA, an ejection fraction of <40% is defined as HFrEF and an ejection fraction of 41–49% is referred to as mildly reduced heart failure (HFmrEF).[43,44]
- *Heart failure with preserved ejection fraction (HFpEF) or diastolic heart failure:* indicates normal systolic function with a normal ejection fraction (EF ≥50%)[42-44] but impaired relaxation so there is a resistance to filling with increased filling pressures. Diastolic dysfunction usually occurs in conjunction with systolic dysfunction and is more common in the elderly, obesity, diabetes and atrial fibrillation (AF) and females with a history of hypertension.[42–44]
- *Low cardiac output syndrome:* occurs in response to hypovolaemia and/or hypertension. Severe vasoconstriction further reduces the cardiac output.
- *High cardiac output syndrome:* is the result of an increase in metabolic demands causing a decrease in systemic venous return leading to an increase in stroke volume and cardiac output. Burns and sepsis are the main causes.
- *Left-sided heart failure:* occurs when there is a reduced left ventricular stroke volume resulting in accumulation of blood in the pulmonary system.
- *Right-sided heart failure:* is the congestion of blood in the systemic system due to the inability of the right ventricle to expel its blood volume.

Responses to heart failure

When heart failure occurs, several adaptive responses are initiated by the body in an attempt to maintain normal perfusion (Fig. 10.9). These mechanisms are successful in the normal heart but contribute to decreased effectiveness in the failing heart. The compensatory mechanisms include:

- sympathetic nervous system (SNS) response
- renin–angiotensin–aldosterone system (RAAS)
- Frank–Starling response
- neurohormonal response.

The SNS is the first response to be stimulated in heart failure. It occurs within seconds of a reduction in cardiac output and the parasympathetic system becomes inhibited. The baroreceptor reflexes are activated in response to a reduced arterial pressure. The beta-adrenergic receptors located in the heart are activated, resulting in an increase in heart rate and contractility to increase stroke volume and cardiac output. SNS response in the peripheral vascular system results in vasoconstriction, which increases systemic venous return and mean systemic filling pressures. This results in an increase in venous return, preload and afterload (see Fig. 10.9). The consequence of this activation is increased myocardial oxygen demand. Although blood flow to essential organs is maintained, perfusion to the kidneys, gastrointestinal system and skin is reduced and peripheral resistance increased. Chronic activation of vasoconstrictors contributes to the progression of heart failure through increased resistance and effects on cardiac structure, causing hypertrophy and fibrosis and down-regulation of beta-adrenergic receptors and endothelial dysfunction. Chronic poor perfusion to skeletal muscles may contribute to changes in muscle metabolism, resulting in further reductions in exercise tolerance.

The next compensatory mechanism to be activated is the RAAS. This is stimulated within minutes, in response to a decrease in kidney perfusion resulting in a decrease in glomerular filtration rate. Activation of this response results in an increase in systemic venous return and sodium and water reabsorption, which then increases the circulating blood volume, systemic filling pressures and venous return enhancing preload and afterload (see Chapter 9). The Frank–Starling response is also activated. As the end-diastolic volume increases (preload) in response to SNS stimulation, ventricular dilation occurs, stimulating the Frank–Starling response. As the myocardial fibres are stretched during diastole, the force of contractility also increases to expel the increasing preload. This is a major mechanism of the heart to maintain a normal cardiac output. Optimal contractility occurs when the diastolic volume is 12–18 mmHg.[10] However, when the ventricle is damaged, such as in MI, the SNS increases heart rate and contractility, further increasing cardiac workload and exacerbating myocardial dysfunction, which increases end-diastolic volume (preload) and ventricular dilation further, and heart failure progresses. As ventricular dilation

FIGURE 10.9 Flowchart of the pathophysiology of heart failure.

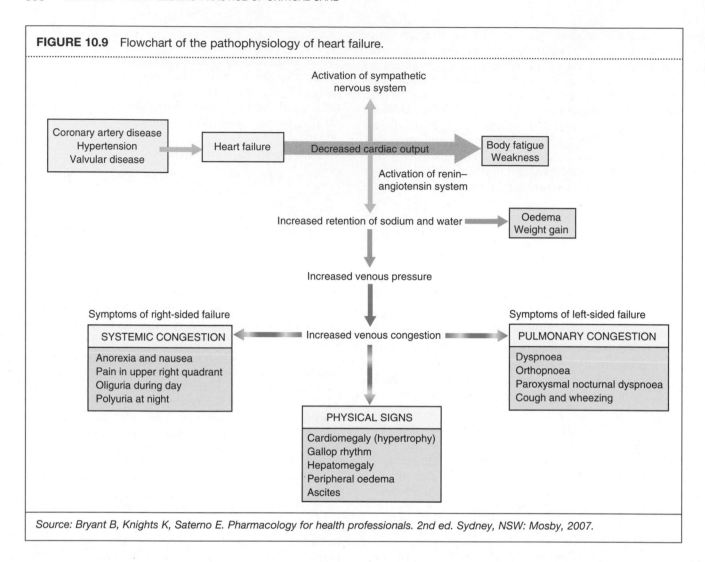

Source: Bryant B, Knights K, Saterno E. Pharmacology for health professionals. 2nd ed. Sydney, NSW: Mosby, 2007.

continues, ventricular hypertrophy results. The myocardium also increases its muscle mass in an attempt to increase contractility, called ventricular remodelling. However, over time ventricular hypertrophy results in changes to end-diastolic compliance and contractility due to the thickened ventricular wall, impaired muscle function and growth of collagen. These result in further impairment of ventricular function (Fig. 10.10). Ventricular hypertrophy also has a depressant effect on ventricular compliance, heart rate and contractility resulting in an increase in end-diastolic pressure with no associated increase in contractility. As the pulmonary artery pressures increase, pulmonary oedema and cardiogenic shock develop.

The final compensatory mechanism to be activated is the neurohormonal response, which takes days to be activated. This response involves the activation of vasopressin and atrial natriuretic peptide (ANP). Vasopressin is a potent vasoconstrictor and also an antidiuretic hormone. ANP is important in the regulation of cardiovascular volume homeostasis. It is released from the atria in response to atrial stretching due to an increased circulating blood volume. ANP blocks the effect of the

SNS, RAAS and vasopressin. It reduces tachycardia via the baroreceptors and reduces circulating blood volume by increasing salt and water excretion in the kidneys. Plasma ANP is increased in acute heart failure (AHF) but depleted in CHF.

While in the healthy heart these compensatory mechanisms would result in an adequate cardiac output, in heart failure they do not, depending on the aetiology. In ischaemic heart failure the damaged myocardium is unable to respond adequately to the Frank–Starling response and ventricular remodelling develops. Heart failure caused by hypertension or valvular heart disease results in persistent pressure or volume overload, which is exacerbated by the Frank–Starling response and SNS compensatory mechanisms. This causes ventricular remodelling and depletion of noradrenaline (norepinephrine) and a reduction of inotropic response to the cardiac SNS. These all exacerbate the reduction in circulating blood volume and kidney perfusion. Many patients with heart failure often have a high plasma renin activity due to the continual activation of the RAAS compensatory mechanism.

In heart failure patients, the inadequate cardiac output results in signs and symptoms of hypoperfusion (oliguria, cognitive impairment and cold peripheries) and congestion of the venous and pulmonary systems (acute pulmonary oedema, dyspnoea, hypoxaemia, peripheral oedema and liver congestion). Classification of signs and symptoms is usually considered in the context of left or right ventricular failure.

Left ventricular failure

Left ventricular failure (LVF), compared with other forms of heart failure, is characterised by breathlessness, orthopnoea and paroxysmal nocturnal dyspnoea, irritating cough and fatigue (Table 10.5). LVF or HFrEF exists when the ventricle has an ejection fraction of less than 50%,[42,44] resulting in increased end-diastolic volume and increased intraventricular pressure. The left atrium is unable to empty into the left ventricle adequately and pressure in the left atrium rises. This pressure is reflected in the pulmonary veins and causes pulmonary congestion. When pulmonary venous congestion exceeds 20 mmHg, fluid moves into the pulmonary interstitium. Raised pulmonary interstitial pressure reduces pulmonary compliance, increases the work of breathing and is experienced by the patient as shortness of breath. Increased blood volume in the lung also initiates shallow, rapid breathing and the sensation of breathlessness. Patients also experience orthopnoea (dyspnoea while lying flat) and paroxysmal nocturnal dyspnoea because, when lying down, blood is redistributed from gravity-dependent areas of the body to the lung. Sitting upright or standing, and sleeping with additional pillows, relieves breathlessness at night.

Acute pulmonary oedema results when pulmonary capillary pressure exceeds approximately 30 mmHg, and then fluid from the vessels begins to leak into the alveoli (Fig. 10.11). This fluid leak decreases the area available for normal gas exchange and severe shortness of breath results, often accompanied by pink, frothy sputum and noisy respirations. This causes patients to experience severe anxiety and decreased oxygen levels. Pulmonary oedema is a medical emergency and requires urgent treatment.

In addition to pulmonary symptoms, patients with LVF experience signs and symptoms related to decreased left ventricular output, including weakness, fatigue, difficulty in concentrating and decreased exercise tolerance. These symptoms may be present for some time before an accurate diagnosis of heart failure is made, because they are non-specific and are consistent with other diagnoses such as depression. Other signs that are

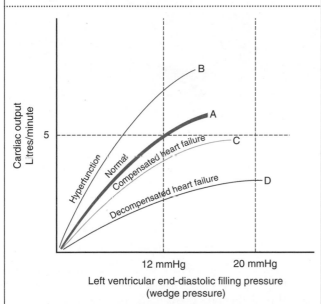

FIGURE 10.10 Function curves of left ventricular pressure during various stages of heart failure.

Source: Michaelson CR. Congestive heart failure. St Louis, MO: Mosby, 1983.

TABLE 10.5

Clinical manifestations of failure of right and left sides of the heart

LEFT VENTRICULAR FAILURE		RIGHT VENTRICULAR FAILURE	
SIGNS	SYMPTOMS	SIGNS	SYMPTOMS
Tachypnoea	Dyspnoea	Peripheral oedema	Fatigue
Tachycardia	Orthopnoea	Raised JVP	Weight gain
Bibasal crackles	PND	Raised central venous pressure	Anorexia
Haemoptysis	Fatigue	Ascites	
Cough	Nocturia	Hepatomegaly	
Pulmonary oedema			
Raised pulmonary artery pressure			
S3 heart sound			

JVP = jugular venous pressure; PND = paroxysmal nocturnal dyspnoea.

FIGURE 10.11   Pathophysiology of pulmonary oedema. As pulmonary oedema progresses, it inhibits oxygen and carbon dioxide exchange at the alveolar–capillary interface. **(A)** Normal relationship. **(B)** Increased pulmonary capillary hydrostatic pressure causes fluid to move from the vascular space into the pulmonary interstitial space. **(C)** Lymphatic flow increases and pulls fluid back into the vascular or lymphatic space. **(D)** Failure of lymphatic flow and worsening of left-sided heart failure causes further movement of fluid into the interstitial space and then into the alveoli.

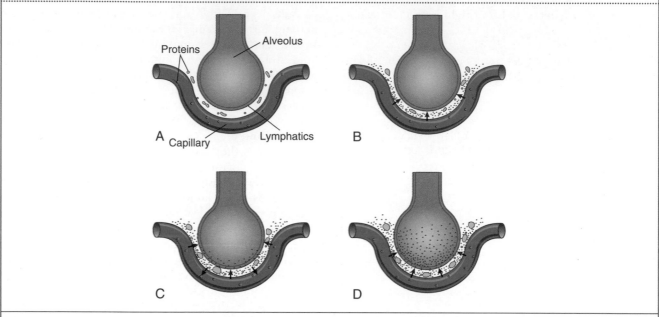

Source: Urden L, Stacy K, Logh M, Thelan's Critical care nursing: diagnosis and management. 5th ed. St Louis, MO: Mosby, 2006.

useful in diagnosis include the presence of S3 (ventricular gallop), crackles over lung fields that do not clear with a cough, cardiomegaly and the presence of pulmonary vessels on chest X-ray.

Right ventricular failure

Right ventricular failure (RVF) does not usually occur in isolation, except in the presence of severe lung disease, such as chronic obstructive pulmonary disease, pulmonary hypertension or a massive pulmonary embolus.[10] In this case, RVF is due to resistance to outflow. The right ventricle can adapt to fairly large changes in volume; however, when cardiac output decreases, end-diastolic volume increases and the right atrium is unable to empty adequately. Right atrial pressure rises and is reflected into the venous system. Jugular vein distention occurs, and the veins are usually visible above the clavicle. Symptoms of right heart failure are not as specific as in LVF and are mostly related to low cardiac output and raised venous pressure (see Table 10.5). Ascites and oedema tend to progress insidiously, and dependent oedema in the feet and ankles is often most prominent. Weight gain is an important sign, as 1 kg of weight gain equals 1 litre of excess fluid. Liver congestion may result in tenderness, ascites and jaundice. Nausea and anorexia may be present and are a result of an increased intra-abdominal pressure. Many signs are not readily distinguishable from LVF, including extra heart sounds.

Patient assessment, diagnostic procedures and classification

Assessment and diagnosis are summarised in a diagnostic algorithm (Fig. 10.12). A full assessment and history are essential to determine the cause(s) of heart failure and to assess the severity of the disease. A careful physical assessment is important for initial diagnosis and to evaluate the effectiveness of treatments and progress of the disease. The depth and time taken to conduct the assessment depend on the severity of symptoms. The physical examination of the patient focuses on cardiovascular and pulmonary assessment.

Cardiovascular assessment includes the following:

- Pulse rate and rhythm: the pulse rate is generally elevated because of a low cardiac output. However, if the patient is prescribed beta-adrenergic blocking agents and/or angiotensin-converting enzyme inhibitors (ACEIs), the pulse rate may be low.

- Palpation of the precordium and apical pulse: these may be displaced laterally and downwards to the left owing to an increased heart size.

- Auscultation of a third heart sound (S3 gallop): occurs because of a low ejection fraction and diastolic dysfunction. A fourth heart sound may also be present owing to a decrease in ventricular compliance.

FIGURE 10.12 Diagnostic algorithm for a patient with suspected heart failure.

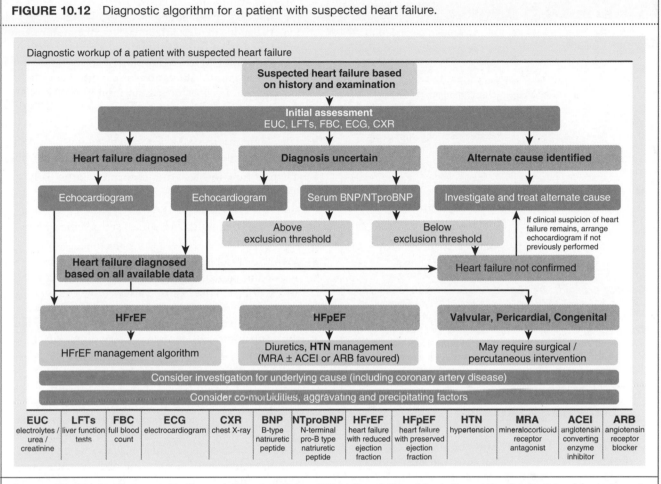

Source: Atherton JJ, Sindone A, De Pasquale CG, et al. National Heart Foundation of Australia and Cardiac Society of Australia and New Zealand: guidelines for the prevention, detection, and management of heart failure in Australia. Heart Lung Circ 2018;27(10): 1123–208, with permission.

- Assessment of jugular venous pressure (JVP): is performed to estimate the degree of venous volume. If raised it reflects hypervolaemia, RVF and reduced right ventricular compliance. It can also be raised in the presence of tricuspid valve disease. The hepatojugular reflex is also assessed by pressing on the liver and observing an increase in JVP. This results in an increase in blood flow to the right atrium.

- Blood pressure: lying and standing blood pressure are measured to assess postural hypotension due to a low cardiac output and also the prescribing of beta-adrenergic blocking agents and ACEIs.

- Peripheries: look for the presence of cyanosis that may be due to vasoconstriction. Assess the fingers for clubbing, which indicates long-term cyanosis usually as a consequence of congenital heart disease. Also, assess the patient for ankle oedema. Peripheral oedema up to the mid-calves indicates a moderate amount of excess fluid and the patient may require a bolus dose of diuretic medication.

Pulmonary assessment includes chest auscultation for inspiratory crepitations that do not clear with coughing. They are initially heard in the bases but as congestion increases they become diffuse. General assessment of the patient includes daily weighing and looking for signs of cachexia (usually associated with severe heart failure), anaemia and dizziness.

Heart failure is usually classified according to the severity of symptoms. In heart failure, the New York Heart Association (NYHA) Functional Classification is commonly used to classify patients based on the activity level that initiates symptoms (Table 10.6).

Diagnostic tests

Tests used to diagnose heart failure include the following:

- Transthoracic echocardiogram (TTE) is the most useful investigation to confirm diagnosis of heart failure. If the TTE visibility is poor, a transoesophageal echocardiogram (TOE) may be done. A TTE is the gold standard diagnostic test for

TABLE 10.6

New York Heart Association functional classification of heart failure

CLASS	DEFINITION
I	Normal daily activity does not initiate symptoms. There are no limitations on activity.
II	Ordinary activities initiate onset of symptoms, but symptoms subside with rest. Slight limitation of daily activities.
III	A small amount of activity initiates symptoms; patients are usually symptom-free at rest. Marked limitation of activity.
IV	Any type of activity initiates symptoms, and symptoms are present at rest.

Source: Adapted from Dolgin M, Association NYH, Fox AC, et al; New York Heart Association. Criteria Committee. Nomenclature and criteria for diagnosis of diseases of the heart and great vessels. 9th ed. Boston, MA: Lippincott Williams & Wilkins; 1994; Criteria Committee, New York Heart Association, Inc. Diseases of the heart and blood vessels. Nomenclature and criteria for diagnosis, 6th ed. Boston, MA: Little, Brown & Co. 1964, p. 114. © 1964 American Heart Association, Inc.

heart failure and should always be undertaken when possible.[42–44] This test is vital, as it can distinguish systolic dysfunction (left ventricular ejection fraction (LVEF) <50%) from diastolic dysfunction, to guide management decisions. Information on left and right ventricular sizes, volumes, left ventricular thrombus and ventricular wall thickness and motion can be provided. Assessment of valve structure and function as well as intracardiac and pulmonary pressures can be determined, without the need for invasive techniques. Pulsed-wave Doppler and tissue Doppler studies can be used to determine diastolic dysfunction.

- Assessment of cardiac function can also be done by invasive techniques (e.g. coronary angiography) and nuclear cardiology tests (e.g. gated radionuclide angiocardiography).
- ECG should be done as an initial investigation. Most common abnormalities include ST-T wave changes, LBBB, left anterior hemiblock, left ventricular hypertrophy, atrial fibrillation and sinus tachycardia.
- Chest X-ray shows cardiomegaly and pulmonary markings, including evidence of interstitial oedema: perihilar pulmonary vessels, small basal pleural effusions obscuring the costophrenic angles, and Kerley B lines (indicating raised left atrial pressure).
- Full blood count checks for anaemia and mild thrombocytopenia. Any signs of anaemia should be further investigated.

- Urea, creatinine and electrolyte tests should be done for dilutional hyponatraemia, hypokalaemia, hyperkalaemia, hypernatraemia, low magnesium and worsening renal function (high urea and creatinine). These should be closely monitored if there are any changes in clinical status and/or drug therapy such as angiotensin receptor neprilysin inhibitors (ARNIs), ACEIs, sodium-glucose co-transporter 2 (SGLT2) inhibitors and diuretics.
- Liver function tests check for elevated levels of AST, ALT, lactate dehydrogenase (LDH) and serum bilirubin.
- Thyroid function tests are performed particularly in patients with no history of coronary artery disease and who develop atrial fibrillation.
- Urinalysis is conducted to measure specific gravity and proteinuria.
- Myocardial ischaemia and viability need to be assessed in patients with heart failure and coronary artery disease. These can be assessed by a stress ECG, stress echocardiography or a myocardial perfusion study. Coronary angiography is useful to determine the contribution of coronary artery disease in these patients.
- Natriuretic peptides include plasma ANP and B-type natriuretic peptide (BNP). BNP or N-terminal proBNP (NTproBNP) is useful when used in conjunction with other diagnostic tests to exclude heart failure. An elevated BNP (>35 pg/mL) or NTproBNP (>125 pg/mL) may also be due to other causes, such as atrial fibrillation, obesity, acute or chronic renal disease or occur in the elderly[42–44] so additional diagnostic tests are warranted to confirm a diagnosis of heart failure. The prescribing of an ARNI will artificially increase BNP levels so NTproBNP should be done on these patients. However, it is useful to use BNP/NTproBNP particularly to differentiate between dyspnoea due to heart failure and dyspnoea due to chronic obstructive pulmonary disease.

Patient management

Treatment of heart failure is lifelong and multifactorial, requiring a well-coordinated, multidisciplinary approach. The goals of heart failure treatment are to identify and eliminate the precipitating cause, promote optimal cardiac function, enhance patient comfort by relieving signs and symptoms and help the patient and family cope with any lifestyle changes. Clinical practice guidelines have been developed to guide the treatment of heart failure on the basis of ventricular dysfunction and grade of symptoms (Figs 10.12 and 10.13).[42–44]

Planning for hospital discharge begins early in the admission and aims to promote quality of life for the patient and prevent unnecessary admissions. Several healthcare services have been implemented to support the transition from hospital to home as it is during the first 30 days post-discharge that a quarter of heart failure

FIGURE 10.13 Management of heart failure with reduced ejection fraction (HFrEF).

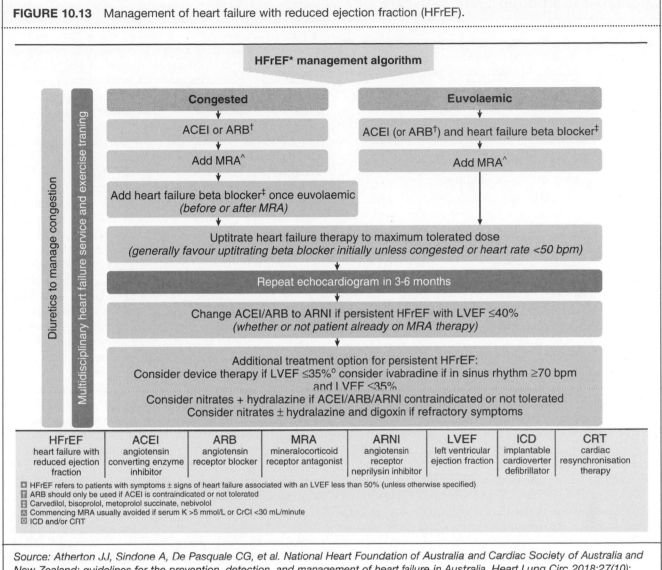

HFrEF	ACEI	ARB	MRA	ARNI	LVEF	ICD	CRT
heart failure with reduced ejection fraction	angiotensin converting enzyme inhibitor	angiotensin receptor blocker	mineralocorticoid receptor antagonist	angiotensin receptor neprilysin inhibitor	left ventricular ejection fraction	implantable cardioverter defibrillator	cardiac resynchronisation therapy

⊞ HFrEF refers to patients with symptoms ± signs of heart failure associated with an LVEF less than 50% (unless otherwise specified)
† ARB should only be used if ACEI is contraindicated or not tolerated
‡ Carvedilol, bisoprolol, metoprolol succinate, nebivolol
∧ Commencing MRA usually avoided if serum K >5 mmol/L or CrCl <30 mL/minute
○ ICD and/or CRT

Source: Atherton JJ, Sindone A, De Pasquale CG, et al. National Heart Foundation of Australia and Cardiac Society of Australia and New Zealand: guidelines for the prevention, detection, and management of heart failure in Australia. Heart Lung Circ 2018;27(10): 1123–208.

patients will be rehospitalised.[45] There are currently over 80 outreach heart failure programs throughout Australia that support heart failure patients post-discharge.[46] The main goals of these programs are to reduce symptom burden, improve functional capacity and minimise hospital readmissions. These programs range from in-hospital visits to facilitate discharge planning to nurse-led heart failure outpatient clinics, home visit programs and heart failure-specific exercise programs. Several meta-analyses of home visit programs have shown a reduction in hospital admissions and mortality[47,48] and these programs are now standard care for heart failure patients.[42–44] Home visit heart failure programs involve a heart failure nurse visiting the patient at home and providing education to the patient and carer, assessing their symptoms and educating the patients and their carers about self-management

strategies. Nurse-led outpatient clinics also reduce hospital admissions and mortality[49,50] and play an important role in the management of heart failure patients post-discharge. These clinics are also recommended as standard care post-discharge.[42]

Management of heart failure after the acute phase is based on three principles: self-care management, long-term lifestyle changes and adherence to pharmacotherapy. Management of self-care is the key to non-pharmacological management of heart failure. Self-care refers to the decision-making process of patients concerning their choice of healthy behaviour and response to worsening symptoms when they occur. It involves cognitive decision making, requiring the recognition of signs and symptoms that indicate a change in condition, which is based on knowledge and prior experiences of deterioration.[51,52]

Lifestyle modification and self-care management

Patient education is the key to self-management and must include family members to be effective. Patient education should include information on the following:

- the disease process – this involves discussing what heart failure is, signs and symptoms and why they occur, and strategies to improve their symptoms
- lifestyle changes
- medications and side effects
- self-monitoring and acute symptoms
- importance of adherence to the medications and management plan.

There are numerous resources available for patient and carer education. The Heart Foundation has an excellent resource titled 'Living well with CHF' and other resources (https://www.heartfoundation.org.au/your-heart/heart-conditions/heart-failure-the-facts). Also 'heart online' (http://www.heartonline.org.au) and 'Heart failure matters' (https://www.heartfailurematters.org/en_GB) are excellent resources for health professionals providing information for patients and carers. Both of these websites also provide resources for health professionals regarding heart failure management and tools such as surveys.

Restriction of fluid to 1.5 L/day is one of the most important strategies that patients can adhere to in order to improve their symptoms. However, it is recommended only in patients with signs and symptoms of fluid overload.[42–44] Patients are encouraged to weigh themselves daily and to identify any increase in weight, as an increase of 1 kg equals 1 litre of excess fluid. International guidelines stipulate that, if their weight increases by 2 kg over 2 days, they need to see their local doctor as soon as possible.[42–44] Patients who adhere to their management plan and closely monitor their daily weight may self-manage their volume status by using a flexible diuretic action plan as developed by their cardiologist. In addition, patients should be advised of early-warning signs of excess fluid volume and decompensation, such as increasing dyspnoea, fatigue and peripheral oedema.

Sleep apnoea also occurs commonly in heart failure patients. There are two types: obstructive sleep apnoea and central sleep apnoea. Obstructive sleep apnoea occurs as a result of airway collapse and is associated with obesity. It can be treated with weight reduction and night-time continuous positive airway pressure (CPAP). The use of CPAP for obstructive sleep apnoea results in an improvement in LVEF due to an increase in left ventricular filling and emptying rates, and a decrease in systolic blood pressure and left ventricular chamber size.[53] Central sleep apnoea (Cheyne–Stokes respiration) occurs as a result of pulmonary congestion and high sympathetic stimulation in patients with severe heart failure and may be treated with CPAP. However, the benefits of oxygen therapy have not been proven. Exercise is equally important, to prevent the deconditioning of skeletal muscle that occurs in heart failure. Exercise training – including walking, exercise bicycle and light resistance – has been shown to improve functional capacity, symptoms, neurohormonal abnormalities, quality of life and mood in heart failure.[54] International heart failure guidelines all recommend that stable heart failure patients, regardless of age, should be considered for referral to a tailored exercise program (preferably a heart failure-specific exercise program) or modified CR program.[42–44] Heart failure exercise programs comprise resistance training and have been shown to improve functional capacity, heart failure symptoms and survival and reduce hospitalisations.[55] In patients with symptomatic heart failure, physical activity should be undertaken under the supervision of trained heart failure specialists (e.g. a physiotherapist or exercise physiologist) who can tailor the level of exercise to the degree of severity of symptoms. Many heart failure patients have comorbidities such as arthritis, which make exercise programs difficult, but maintaining general activity should be encouraged.

Dietary sodium intake should be reduced to 2 g/day for patients with moderate-to-severe heart failure and patients need to eat a healthy diet and maintain a healthy weight.[42–44] Reduction in sodium intake helps reduce fluid retention, diuretic requirements and potassium excretion. A large proportion of an individual's sodium intake can come from processed foods, so patients are encouraged to read nutrition labels and reduce the intake of these foods. Salt intake can also be reduced by avoiding adding salt in cooking or to meals. As heart failure patients who are overweight have an increased demand on their heart, weight loss by lowering dietary fat intake may improve symptoms and quality of life. In patients with moderate-to-severe heart failure, cardiac cachexia and anaemia are common, which further exacerbate weakness and fatigue. These patients will require a referral to a dietitian for nutritional support. Other lifestyle changes are: cease smoking, ideally cease alcohol intake or otherwise limit alcohol to less than two standard drinks/day (alcohol is a myocardial toxin and reduces contractility), limit caffeinated drinks to 1–2 drinks/day (to decrease the risk of arrhythmias), control diabetes and have annual vaccinations for influenza and regular pneumococcal disease vaccinations.[42–44]

Palliative care may be appropriate for patients with end-stage heart failure who are experiencing significant symptoms, prescribed maximal pharmacotherapy and have poor response to treatment. It is important that all patients have an advance care plan in place and that this has been discussed with family members. Advance care plans should be discussed soon after the patient's first hospital admission for treatment of decompensated heart failure.

Pharmacotherapy in patients with heart failure is vital and includes an array of drugs that require careful management. Nurse practitioners are authorised to titrate some heart failure medications, including diuretics, beta-adrenergic blocking agents, ACEIs, angiotension receptor blocking agents (ARBs) and ARNIs. Pharmacists also provide essential patient education and support the management of complex medication schedules. Some major hospitals have a pharmacist outreach program where a pharmacist visits the patient at home.

Practice tip

When considering whether a patient is suitable for palliation, discussion also needs to include deactivation of their pacemaker or implantable cardioverter defibrillator (ICD).

Medications

Pharmacological management relies on the following categories of drugs: ACEIs, ARNI, beta-adrenergic blocking agents, ARBs, SGLT2 inhibitors, mineralocorticoid receptor antagonists (MRA), diuretics, ivabradine, inotropes and antiarrhythmic drugs. Antiarrhythmic drugs are reviewed in Chapter 11. The main actions and adverse effects of these drugs in heart failure are summarised in Table 10.7.

TABLE 10.7

Common medications for the treatment of heart failure

DRUG/EXAMPLE	ACTION	MAJOR ADVERSE EFFECTS
ACEI Captopril Enalapril	Decrease systemic vascular resistance by stopping angiotensin I conversion to II; decreased sodium and water retention.	Symptomatic hypotension Hyperkalaemia Unproductive cough Renal failure Rash
ARNI Entresto	Blocks selective angiotensin I receptor causing a reduction in vasoconstriction, sodium and water retention.	Symptomatic hypotension Hyperkalaemia Risk of angioedema
ARB Candesartan Irbesartan	Block the angiotensin II receptor that responds to angiotensin II stimulation; decreased sodium and water retention. Alternative to ACEI.	Symptomatic hypotension Hyperkalaemia Renal failure
Beta-adrenergic blockers Bisoprolol Carvedilol Metoprolol CR/XL	Reduce systemic vascular resistance and heart rate by blocking adrenoreceptors in arteries and heart.	Hypotension Bronchoconstriction
MRA Spironolactone Eplerenone	Increase urine volume by aldosterone blocking and sodium retention.	Hyperkalaemia Rash Gynaecomastia
SGLT2 inhibitors Empagliflozin Dapagliflozin	Increase diuresis via osmosis through the removal of glucose from the kidneys.	Hypovolaemia Dehyration Genital infections
Ivabradine	Reduces heart rate through inhibition of the sinoatrial node.	Bradycardia Dizziness Ventricular arrhythmias Atrial fibrillation
Loop diuretics Frusemide	Increase urine volume by decreasing reabsorption of chloride and sodium.	Hypokalaemia Ototoxicity Rash
Thiazide diuretics Chlorothiazide Hydrochlorothiazide	Increase urine volume by decreasing reabsorption of sodium.	Hypokalaemia Hyperglycaemia Sensitivity: rash
Cardiac glycosides Digitalis	Increase myocardial contractility and decrease heart rate by inhibiting sodium pump in myocytes.	Tachycardia AV block Nausea and vomiting Disorientation Visual disturbances

ACEI = angiotensin-converting enzyme inhibitors; ARB = angiotension receptor blocking agents; ARNI = angiotensin receptor neprilysin inhibitor; MRA = mineralocorticoid receptor antagonists; SGLT2 inhibitors = sodium–glucose co-transporter 2 inhibitors.

Angiotensin-converting enzyme inhibitors (ACEIs)

ACEIs have been demonstrated to prolong survival, improve patient symptoms and exercise tolerance, prevent hospitalisation and improve ejection fraction in heart failure patients.[56,57] All patients with symptomatic systolic left ventricle (LV) dysfunction should be prescribed either an ACEI, ARNI or ARB.[42–44] ACEIs (such as perindopril, enalapril, lisinopril) act on the renin–angiotensin system by specifically preventing the conversion of angiotensin I to angiotensin II.[26] As a result, systemic vascular resistance (afterload) is decreased. This is particularly important in preventing the progression of heart failure, as blockade of the renin–angiotensin system prevents further development of systolic dysfunction. In addition, because angiotensin II also stimulates the release of aldosterone, sodium and water retention are decreased (preload). This may also be beneficial when ACEIs are prescribed with diuretics, as potassium loss is limited. ACEIs also inhibit the breakdown of bradykinin (a vasodilator), which also contributes to decreasing vascular resistance. The total reduction of systemic vascular resistance reduces the workload of the heart without affecting heart rate or cardiac output.

Common adverse effects of ACEIs primarily result from hypotension, including dizziness and headache. Other side effects include hyperkalaemia, deterioration of renal function and an unproductive cough, which may respond to asthma prophylactic medications. Initial doses of ACEIs should be low, as severe – though transient – symptomatic hypotension can occur, worsening of renal function and hyperkalaemia. The dose of ACEIs needs to be gradually increased to maximum dosage over 2 months to optimise the survival and functional capacity benefits. This group of drugs is contraindicated in patients with bilateral renal artery stenosis because of the danger of developing renal failure. One important adverse effect of ACEIs is that they cannot be taken in conjunction with non-steroidal anti-inflammatory drugs (NSAIDs) as NSAIDs reduce the action of ACEIs.[26]

Practice tip

A dry, non-productive cough is often associated with the introduction of ACEI medication, but is often mistaken for a symptom of other conditions, so patients may not report the symptom as new. The cough usually begins within 1–2 days of commencing therapy and up-titration of dose.

Practice tip

Many heart failure patients have arthritis and take NSAIDs for pain relief. However, heart failure patients must avoid taking NSAID medications when taking ACEIs, as NSAIDs counter the action of ACEIs. In such cases we usually recommend taking long-acting paracetamol or glucosamine for relief from arthritis pain.

Angiotensin receptor neprilysin inhibitor (ARNI)

ARNIs are a class of drugs that act on the RAAS and the neprilysin peptide system. The neprilysin peptide system increases the circulating natriuretic peptides, which reduce the symptoms and progression of heart failure. The first drug in this new class is entresto, a combination of valsartan and sacubitril (neprilysin inhibitor). The valsartan component blocks the AT1 receptor and sacubitril inhibits neprilysin, promoting a higher concentration of circulating natriuretic peptides. In symptomatic patients diagnosed with HFrEF, it is now recommended that patients are prescribed an ARNI to replace ACEI and ARBs.[42–44] ARNIs have demonstrated they reduce hospital re-admissions and improve survival.[58,59] To minimise the risk of angioedema, it is recommended that ACEIs are ceased for at least 36 hours prior to the initiation of an ARNI. There is a contraindication with the combined use of ACEI or ARB and an ARNI. Current clinical guidelines recommend that patients who are eligible to be prescribed an ARNI commence at low dose and then gradually increase 2–4 weekly until optimal dosage is reached. Common adverse effects of ARNIs include: increased risk of angioedema, symptomatic hypotension, hyperkalaemia, renal impairment and a cough.[42,43,58,59]

Angiotensin receptor blocking agents (ARBs)

The primary use of ARBs is in patients who are intolerant of an ARNI or ACEI (e.g. have ACEI-induced cough). They have a similar action as ACEIs; however, ARBs block the angiotensin II receptor that responds to angiotensin II stimulation. ACEIs, on the other hand, act on the enzyme that produces angiotensin II.[26] They have similar benefits to those of ACEIs, such as improving survival, LVEF and heart failure symptoms and reducing hospitalisations.[60] Similar to ACEIs, ARBs are commenced on a low dose and gradually up-titrated to optimal dose over 2 months. Adverse effects are: deterioration in renal function, hyperkalaemia and symptomatic hypotension.[26]

Beta-adrenergic blocking agents

All patients with HFrEF should be prescribed a beta-adrenergic blocking agent. Beta-adrenergic blocking agents (carvedilol, metoprolol CR/XL, bisoprolol, nebivolol) are used in heart failure to inhibit the adverse effects of chronic activation of the SNS and improve ventricular function. In heart failure, beta-2 receptors predominate, with beta-1 receptors being down-regulated. Beta-adrenergic blocking agents reduce this neurohormonal activity. The addition of a beta-adrenergic blocker has been demonstrated to reduce symptoms, reduce hospitalisations and prolong survival in patients.[61] Similar to ARNIs, ACEIs and ARBs, the dose of beta-adrenergic blocking agents is gradually increased. Once the patient is euvolaemic, they should be commenced on a low dose and gradually increased to maximal dose over 2 months.

In patients with chronic obstructive pulmonary disease (COPD), selective beta-1-blockers are prescribed. Patients will require close monitoring for signs of deterioration of their COPD. Other adverse events are: symptomatic hypotension, bradycardia and worsening heart failure. Also, during the up-titration of beta-adrenergic blocking agents, many patients complain of feeling slightly confused in the morning; this usually disappears after 1–2 weeks.

Diuretics

Diuretics are one of the mainstays of management of heart failure, primarily to decrease the sodium and water retention response to the low cardiac output state. A combination of diuretics may be used if oedema persists on one diuretic.

- *Loop diuretics:* (frusemide, ethacrynic acid and bumetanide) act on the ascending limb of the loop of Henle of the nephron. They prevent the reabsorption of chloride and sodium ions from the loop, so that increased concentrations are present in the loop, attracting more water and increasing urine volume. Intravenous administration of frusemide is often used to manage preload in acute exacerbations. In fluid-overloaded patients, the aim is to achieve increased urine output and a weight reduction of 0.5–1 kg daily, until clinical euvolaemia is achieved. Hypokalaemia is a common adverse effect, and patients on long-term diuretics need regular monitoring and may require potassium supplements. Hyponatraemia may also occur at high doses, and needs careful management in heart failure patients. Ototoxicity, presenting as tinnitus, vertigo and deafness, can occur at high doses, so IV delivery of frusemide should be no faster than 4 mg/min.

- *Thiazide and thiazide-like diuretics (chlorothiazide, hydrochlorothiazide, chlorthalidone):* act on the ascending loop of the nephron and decrease sodium reabsorption. As a result, the fluid in the collecting ducts is more concentrated and attracts more water. Thiazides also cause peripheral arteriole vasodilation, which may be beneficial in hypertensive patients. Adverse effects are similar to loop diuretics owing to potassium and sodium loss, and supplementation may be necessary. When ACEIs are prescribed concurrently there is less potassium loss (details below). Hyperglycaemia can occur, so diabetics need monitoring. Impotence may also occur, as well as sensitivity due to the presence of sulfonamide in the drug structure.

- *Mineralocorticoid receptor antagonists (MRAs):* are potassium-sparing diuretics and include spironolactone and eplerenone. Aldosterone acts on the distal convoluted tubule of the nephron to cause sodium retention and hence water retention, although potassium is lost. Antagonists stop this action, so potassium is not lost and not as much sodium retained, so there is minor diuresis. Spironolactone is particularly useful in heart failure because there is excessive aldosterone production,

causing oedema. There is the potential that spironolactone, by blocking aldosterone systemically, may prevent the negative effects of aldosterone on the heart, such as fibrosis, hypertrophy and arrhythmogenesis. Adverse effects include hyperkalaemia, which may occur more readily in heart failure patients because of renal failure, and, because of its potentially lethal effects, spironolactone requires regular monitoring. Other effects include hyponatraemia and feminisation effects such as gynaecomastia. In patients with HFpEF, spironolactone has been shown to reduce heart failure-related hospitalisations; however, there was no reduction in all-cause hospitalisations.[62] MRAs are recommended for use in patients with HFrEF in addition to other pharmacotherapy such as ARNIs, ACEIs or ARBs and beta-adrenergic blockers. MRAs have additional survival benefits and reduce hospital readmission.[63,64]

Sodium–glucose co-transporter 2 (SGLT2) inhibitors

Sodium–glucose co-transporter 2 (SGLT2) inhibitors reduce glucose reabsorption in the kidney and increase its excretion in the urine.[65] SGLT2 inhibitors are a common medication used in diabetes mellitus to lower blood glucose. A meta-analysis of two large international multicentre randomised controlled trials of a total of 8474 HFrEF patients with and without type 2 diabetes mellitus showed that SGLT2 inhibitors reduced the risk of heart failure hospitalisation, cardiovascular rehospitalisations, cardiovascular death and all-cause mortality.[66] SGLT2 inhibitors also reduced the progression of renal disease.[66]

SGLT2 inhibitors have a diuretic effect as glucose is removed via osmosis from the renal tubules. In heart failure patients also prescribed diuretics, SGLT2 inhibitors will increase the diuresis so the dose of loop diuretics may need to be reduced when commencing SGLT2 inhibitors to prevent hypovolaemia. Caution is also required in patients with diabetes and renal impairment as the glucose-lowering effect may be reduced because of impaired renal excretion. Other adverse effects include dehydration, hypotension and genital infections.

Ivabradine

Ivabradine is a sinoatrial node inhibitor resulting in heart rate reduction, which reduces cardiac workload and myocardial oxygen demand. It is recommended for use in patients with HFrEF with EF ≤35%, sinus rhythm >70 beats per minute (bpm) and prescribed optimal dose of medical therapy including beta-adrenergic blocker and ACEI, ARNI or ARB.[42–44] Adverse effects include: bradycardia, dizziness, ventricular arrhythmias and atrial fibrillation (AF). Initially, patients should be prescribed low-dose ivabradine of 2.5–5 mg BD, which is then up-titrated every 2 weeks to a target dose of 7.5 mg BD.

Inotropic agents

This category of drugs increases cardiac contractility. The group includes cardiac glycosides (digoxin) and dopamine agonists (dopamine, dobutamine), sympathomimetics (adrenaline (epinephrine), noradrenaline) and calcium sensitising agents (levosimendan). Inotropes are used as IV infusions in severe heart failure, acute exacerbations of heart failure and for palliative care or bridging to transplant in very severe heart failure. These drugs have both inotropic and chronotropic actions, so that cardiac contractility and heart rate are both increased to improve cardiac output. Continuous ambulatory infusions of inotropic agents such as dobutamine are administered to patients with severe heart failure as a bridge to transplantation, which allows these patients to be discharged home with support from a home visit nurse. A more detailed overview of these medications is in Chapter 21.

Cardiac glycosides

Cardiac glycosides such as digitalis inhibit the sodium pump such that the exchange between sodium and calcium is impaired. This results in calcium stores being released and intracellular calcium levels rising. As more calcium is available for contraction, contractility and cardiac output increase. These changes in ion movement and additional effects, which enhance parasympathetic stimulation, result in decreased impulse generation by the sinoatrial (SA) node. This is known as a negative chronotropic effect. Conduction is also slowed through the atrioventricular (AV) node and ventricles, allowing more filling time, and therefore having a positive effect on cardiac output. The negative chronotropic effects are particularly beneficial in patients with the atrial fibrillation that is so common in heart failure. Digitalis may also affect cardiopulmonary baroreceptors to reduce sympathetic tone, which may be a valuable offset to excessive sympathetic stimulation in heart failure.

The most important adverse effects of digoxin are caused by changes in conduction: tachycardia, fibrillation and AV block. Digoxin may also cause nausea and vomiting due to direct brain effects and gastrointestinal irritation. Digitalis has a narrow margin of safety, a long half-life and side effects that can be fatal, so assay of plasma drug levels must be conducted regularly and at initiation and change of treatment. Excessive digoxin causes disorientation, hallucinations and visual disturbances. Potassium levels directly alter the effect of digoxin, so that low levels enhance effects and high levels reduce effects.

Arrhythmias are common in heart failure. The agent must be carefully selected, as heart failure patients often have complex medication regimens and interactions may occur. Also, some ventricular antiarrhythmics, such as class 1 agents (e.g. flecainide), are associated with sudden death in heart failure. ICD therapy is also effective in treating ventricular arrhythmias. ICDs reduce mortality by 20–30%[67] and are first-line therapy in patients with a history of ventricular fibrillation (VF) or sustained VT. ICDs are also recommended in symptomatic heart failure patients with a LVEF ≤35% with NYHA class II–III, and prescribed optimal pharmacotherapy for at least 3 months.[44] If a patient is to have an ICD implanted, extensive counselling pre- and post-implantation must be undertaken with the patient and carer to ensure they are aware of the painful and unexpected shocks that may be delivered. Cardiac resynchronisation therapy (CRT) (also known as biventricular pacing) is also indicated in patients with symptomatic heart failure to reduce asynchronous pacing of the left ventricle (sinus rhythm, QRS duration 130–149 ms and LBBB despite gold standard pharmacotherapy).[42–44] Systolic function is improved when the left and right ventricles are paced simultaneously. Often patients with a prolonged QRS will have a combination of an ICD with CRT therapy. ICDs and CRT are discussed in more detail in Chapter 11.

In severe heart failure, when patients do not respond to pharmacological treatment, mechanical measures such as cardiopulmonary bypass and left ventricular assist devices may be used. In appropriate candidates, cardiac transplant may also be an option. These procedures are covered under cardiac surgery.

Acute exacerbations of heart failure

Acute exacerbations of heart failure usually occur as episodes of decompensation due to progression of the disease, exacerbation of their comorbidities or non-adherence to their management plan. Acute episodes usually present as congestive heart failure with associated pulmonary oedema, cardiogenic shock (see Chapter 21) or respiratory failure.[42,44] Patients with severe dyspnoea due to pulmonary congestion with an oxygen saturation of less than 94% should be administered oxygen therapy.[42] If their hypoxaemia does not improve and they continue to be tachypnoeic >25 breaths/min despite oxygen therapy, they may benefit from bilevel positive airway pressure (BiPAP) to support ventilation and gas exchange.[42] The use of continuous positive airway pressure ventilation (CPAP) or BiPAP in acute pulmonary oedema will reduce the need for intubation and mechanical ventilation. If their oxygen saturation is greater than 94% then oxygen therapy should not be used as it causes vasoconstriction and reduces cardiac output.[42]

Once the patient has been stabilised in ICU/CCU, it is important to confirm a diagnosis of acute heart failure and to identify and treat potential precipitants. Some of the most common precipitants include: acute myocardial ischaemia or infarction, tachyarrhythmias, sepsis, non-adherence to their heart failure management plan and/or medications, infection, anaemia, hypoxia, acute renal failure, and/or metabolic/hormonal imbalances such as thyroid dysfunction or diabetic ketoacidosis. In addition to a thorough clinical examination, diagnostic tests on admission in the emergency department include: chest X-ray, 12-lead ECG, echocardiography within 48 hours if haemodynamically unstable or suspected cardiac structure dysfunction, natriuretic peptides to exclude acute heart failure (brain natriuretic peptide (BNP) or NTproBNP), cardiac troponins if there is a history of CHD, and other biochemistry and haematology investigations as indicated by their clinical condition.

The mainstay of treatment of an acute exacerbation is pharmacological, so a combination of medications is given, usually comprising diuretics and vasodilators (provided SBP >90 mmHg) such as nitrates. Opiates are to be considered only to relieve anxiety in patients with severe dyspnoea.[42] Opiates are to be used with caution as they reduce the respiratory drive and respiratory workload. Nitrates cause vasodilation and epicardial artery dilation and reduce preload, which also helps to relieve symptoms of pulmonary congestion, particularly at night when filling pressures are increased because of the recumbent position of sleeping. Diuretics should be administered intravenously to optimise the excretion of intra- and extravascular cellular fluid to reduce circulating blood volume to reduce cardiac workload. Thromboembolism prophylaxis with heparin (low molecular weight heparin) or another anticoagulant is recommended. Fluid restriction, usually to 1.5 L in 24 hours, is commenced. Various positive inotropes may be administered at low dose (e.g. IV dobutamine causes vasodilation; IV dopamine improves renal function) to improve contractility and reduce systemic venous return. A higher dose of inotropes should be used only if the patient has symptomatic hypotension or hypoperfusion in order to increase cardiac output and blood pressure. Levosimendan or phosphodiesterase III inhibitors may be used for hypotension or hypoperfusion in order to reverse the effect of beta-blockade to increase cardiac output and blood pressure and improve peripheral perfusion.[10] Vasopressors may also be used in cardiogenic shock (see Chapter 21). Vasopressors should be used only in the short term as they increase afterload, which may further reduce perfusion. If the patient is in rapid atrial fibrillation, digoxin, beta-blockers or amiodarone may be used to control their ventricular rate. A more detailed discussion of these medications is given in Chapter 11.

Various mechanical devices are also available, such as intra-aortic balloon pump, LVAD (discussed in Chapter 12) and pacemakers, particularly ICD or CRT (discussed in Chapter 11). Some patients may also progress to a heart transplant, which is discussed further in Chapter 12.

Most patients in acute heart failure have poor perfusion of the gastrointestinal system and this, combined with dyspnoea, results in a limited appetite. Small, easily ingested meals are best. While the patient is on bed rest, nursing care to prevent problems related to immobility is important. Skin care is particularly important, as poor skin perfusion and oedema place the heart failure patient at higher risk of skin breakdown.

Selected cases

Cardiomyopathy

As the term implies, the cardiomyopathies are primary disorders of the myocardium in which there are systolic, diastolic or combined abnormalities. Classification of the most common forms of cardiomyopathy is made on the basis of the dominant abnormality, which may be dilation, hypertrophy or restricted filling. However, each has different haemodynamic effects and therefore requires different treatment.

Dilated cardiomyopathy

Dilated cardiomyopathy (DCM) is the most common form of cardiomyopathy and is characterised by ventricular and atrial dilation and systolic dysfunction.[68] All four chambers become enlarged, which is not in proportion to the degree of hypertrophy. It presents as heart failure of variable severity, sometimes complicated by thromboembolism at least partly due to atrial fibrillation, which is common. Conduction abnormalities are common in DCM, further exacerbating AV dyssynchrony and left ventricular dysfunction. DCM is the most common cause of sudden cardiac death due to ventricular arrhythmias. Annual mortality from DCM ranges from 10% to 50%.[68] Idiopathic DCM is the most common cause of heart failure in young people. Aetiology of DCM includes CHD, myocarditis, cardiotoxins, genetics and alcohol misuse.

Diagnosis

Many of the features of DCM are non-specific. Heart failure, as mentioned, is present with typical symptoms of dyspnoea, fatigue, peripheral oedema and cardiomegaly. S3 and S4 heart sounds may be present on auscultation. Atrial and ventricular arrhythmias are common, particularly atrial fibrillation, ventricular tachycardia, ventricular fibrillation and torsades de pointes. LBBB is often present, which worsens systolic performance and shortens survival, especially when the QRS interval is markedly prolonged.[68] Echocardiography demonstrates the defining abnormalities and may be useful in revealing atrial thrombus. Occasionally, endocardial biopsy is undertaken to differentiate DCM from myocarditis or rarer causes of cardiomyopathy.

Patient management

Treatment for DCM is similar to that of heart failure and includes beta-adrenergic blocker therapy, ACEIs/ARBs, ARNIs, diuretics and antiarrhythmic therapy where indicated or, if necessary, an ICD for recurrent haemodynamically significant ventricular arrhythmias.[68] The use of CRT has produced significant clinical improvements and is recommended for DCM patients with NYHA functional class II–III, optimal medical therapy, LVEF <35% and sinus rhythm with LBBB with a QRS 130–149 ms.[44] Cardiac transplantation is considered when standard therapies fail to influence clinical progression, and left ventricular assist devices and ICDs may be used as a bridge to transplantation.

Hypertrophic cardiomyopathy

Hypertrophic cardiomyopathy (HCM) is a genetic abnormality that gives rise to inappropriate hypertrophy especially in the intraventricular septum with preserved or hyperdynamic systolic function.[69] The main abnormality with HCM is diastolic rather than systolic as in DCM. The hypertrophy is not a compensatory response to excessive load, such as in aortic stenosis or hypertension. Left ventricular hypertrophy of variable patterns is seen, occasionally with disproportionate septal hypertrophy, which causes left ventricular outflow tract obstruction in which HCM progresses to hypertrophic obstructive cardiomyopathy (HOCM). In HCM the muscle mass is large and hypercontractile, but the left ventricular cavity is small. The increase in left ventricular systolic pressure and the altered relaxation cause diastolic dysfunction and impaired ventricular filling. Mitral regurgitation is common. These abnormalities combine to produce pulmonary congestion and dyspnoea due to raised end-diastolic pressure. Sudden cardiac death, often after exertion or other increases in contractility, is sometimes seen in HCM and is thought to be partly attributable to outflow obstruction.[69] It is the most common cause of death in athletes.[69]

Diagnosis

Echocardiography will confirm the presence and pattern of hypertrophy and the presence (or absence) of an outflow tract gradient. Examination findings include cardiomegaly and pulmonary congestion. An S4 heart sound is common, and the ECG shows left ventricular hypertrophy and often ventricular arrhythmias. When the obstructive form HOCM is present, a systolic murmur, mitral regurgitation murmur and deep narrow Q waves on ECG may be present.[69] The majority of patients are asymptomatic and, when they present to hospital, it will be with severe symptoms of dyspnoea, angina and syncope. In HOCM, angina is the result of an imbalance between oxygen supply and demand due to the increased myocardial mass and not due to atherosclerosis.

Patient management

Treatment for HCM is aimed at the prevention of sudden cardiac death and pharmacotherapy to increase diastolic filling and to reduce the left ventricular outflow tract obstruction. Pharmacotherapy includes beta-adrenergic blocker or calcium channel blocker therapy, as these decrease contractility and lessen outflow tract obstruction. Care is necessary with medication selection, as vasodilation may worsen obstruction, causing haemodynamics to suffer.[69] The impact of atrial fibrillation, by worsening the ventricular filling defect, can be dramatic in HCM patients and will require antiarrhythmics and anticoagulation. If ventricular arrhythmias are present, or there is a family history of sudden cardiac death, treatment with an ICD should be considered.[69] For severely symptomatic patients or those worsening despite maximal drug treatment, surgical myectomy to reduce the size of the septum and lessen obstruction may be necessary and can result in a marked improvement of symptoms.[69] Septal ablation with alcohol injected into the first septal branch of the LAD artery is a less invasive alternative, a procedure that is usually undertaken with pacemaker

insertion as AV block is produced. Although surgical myectomy remains the gold standard, both treatments provide effective symptom relief and improvement in heart failure severity.[69] If the patient with HCM deteriorates and is hospitalised, positive inotropes, chronotropes and nitrates worsen left ventricular outflow tract obstruction and should be avoided. However, beta-adrenergic blockers, amiodarone and calcium antagonists such as verapamil are indicated.[69] Due to the familial nature of HCM, relatives aged 12–18 years also need to be screened for HCM.

Restrictive cardiomyopathy

Restrictive cardiomyopathies (RCMs) limit diastolic distensibility or compliance of the ventricles. The stiff ventricular walls produce diastolic dysfunction and there is impaired ventricular filling. Infiltrates into the interstitium and the replacement of normal myocardium with abnormal tissue hamper this relaxation.[68] Initially, systolic function and wall thickness are normal. However, as the disease progresses, systolic dysfunction occurs. RCM is commonly caused by myocardial infiltration, as in amyloidosis, sarcoidosis, fibrosis or cardiac metastases, or may be idiopathic. Endomyocardial disease is more common in tropical countries, but in the Western world RCMs are the least common form of cardiomyopathy.[68]

Diagnosis

Clinically, heart failure (increase in JVP, dyspnoea, S3 and S4 heart sounds and oedema), particularly right ventricular, and infiltration of the conduction system may cause conduction defects and heart block. Low-voltage ECGs are commonly seen. Patients commonly present with decreased exercise tolerance owing to the impaired ability to increase heart rate and cardiac output because of reduced ventricular filling. RCM must be distinguished from constrictive pericarditis (which it may closely resemble), as pericarditis may be easily managed. If echocardiography demonstrates a restrictive pattern, a myocardial biopsy may be undertaken to determine its aetiology, especially in the case of systemic infiltrative disease.

Patient management

There is no treatment for RCM so the aim of therapy is to relieve symptoms. This includes diuretics, corticosteroids and pacing. The use of nitrates should be initiated with caution as the filling defect can be worsened by decreased venous return or hypovolaemia. Generally, prognosis is poor, with many dying within 1–2 years of diagnosis.[68]

Hypertensive emergencies

Acute, uncontrolled hypertension is often divided into two categories: hypertensive emergencies and hypertensive urgencies. In hypertensive emergencies, blood pressure needs to be reduced within 1 hour to prevent end-organ damage, such as hypertensive encephalopathy, papilloedema or aortic dissection.[70] Immediate blood pressure reduction with IV agents under critical care monitoring is needed. By contrast, hypertensive urgencies are those in which end-organ damage is not occurring and, although prompt management is required, this can be approached more gradually with oral antihypertensive agents under close supervision, without necessarily requiring admission to a critical care unit. Previous hypertension is not always present, but because of chronic adaptive vascular changes it may provide some level of protection against acute tissue injury. Symptoms may not develop until the blood pressure exceeds 220/110 mmHg, whereas hypertensive emergencies in patients without previous hypertension may occur at levels of even 160/100 mmHg.[70] When the diastolic pressure is persistently above 130 mmHg, there is risk of vascular damage and it must be treated.

Diagnosis

A thorough history is taken, including any hypertension management, known renal or cerebrovascular disease, eclampsia in previous pregnancies if gravid or use of stimulants or illicit drugs such as cocaine. Patient assessment should include evidence of: end-organ damage, such as back pain (aortic dissection); neurological damage, such as headache, altered consciousness, confusion, visual loss, stupor or seizure activity (encephalopathy); cardiac damage, such as chest pain, ST-segment changes, cardiac enlargement or the development of heart failure or pulmonary oedema; and renal damage, such as oliguria and azotaemia.[70] Serum urea, creatinine, electrolytes, urinalysis, ECG and chest X-ray should be performed.

Patient management

More severe, or malignant, hypertension may cause retinal haemorrhage or papilloedema, and emergency treatment should immediately be instituted. Other contexts in which there is a need for rapid treatment of severe hypertension include intracranial bleeding, AMI, phaeochromocytoma, recovery from cardiac surgery and bleeding from vascular procedure sites. Hypertensive emergencies in pregnancy threaten both the mother and the fetus.[71]

The aim of treatment is to lower the blood pressure acutely, but neither too quickly nor too dramatically. Recommendations vary, but an initial aim of 150/110–160/100 mmHg within 2–6 hours, or a 25% reduction in mean arterial pressure (MAP) within 2 hours, has been described.[70] Continuous direct arterial pressure monitoring should be in place during treatment. Intravenous sodium nitroprusside, a rapidly acting arterial and venous dilator, is most frequently used, at doses of 0.25–10 micrograms/kg/min.[70] Weaning of nitroprusside is undertaken after the later introduction of oral antihypertensives. Care is required to avoid hypotension during treatment, as well as rebound hypertension as nitroprusside is withdrawn. Rapidly acting beta-adrenergic blocking agents with short half-lives, such as IV esmolol, may be used at doses of 50–100 micrograms/kg/min (or higher) in patients without standard contraindications to beta-adrenergic blockers (e.g. asthma, heart failure).[70] Glyceryl trinitrate infusions at 10–100 micrograms/min or higher are used for combined venous and arterial dilation, especially if there is angina.[7] Intravenous frusemide may be introduced during the acute phase. After intravenous therapies have been established and progress towards target pressures is made, oral agents are introduced. These include oral beta-adrenergic blockers, calcium channel blockers, ACEIs and diuretics.

Infective endocarditis

Infective endocarditis (IE) remains a potentially life-threatening disorder. Despite improvements in the management of IE it is still associated with high mortality and severe complications.[72] Infective endocarditis is no longer isolated to the native valve and may include an infection of any structure within the heart (e.g. prosthetic valves, implanted devices and chordae tendineae). The development of endocarditis has been observed, with factors such as longer life, IV drug use, prosthetic valves, greater rates of cannulation during hospitalisation, cardiac surgery, resistant organisms and increased numbers of immunocompromised patients from immunosuppressant drugs and human immunodeficiency virus/acquired immune deficiency (HIV/AIDS) syndrome.[72]

Infection of the endocardium, often with involvement of the cardiac valves, occurs most commonly as a result of staphylococcal, streptococcal, enterococcal and HAECK (*Haemophilus parainfluenzae*, *H. aphrophilus*, *H. paraphrophilus*, *H. influenzae*, *Actinobacillus actinomycetemcomitans*, *Cardiobacterium hominis*, *Eikenella corrodens*, *Kingella kingae* and *K. denitrificans*) organisms.[72] IE can be acute or subacute. Acute IE progresses over days to weeks with destruction of valves and metastatic infection. Subacute IE occurs over weeks to months and is milder than acute IE. Endothelial damage occurs in the endocardium. Platelet–fibrin deposits form and a lesion develops. Bacterial colonisation then occurs and vegetation adheres to the endocardial lesion. Many of the signs and symptoms of IE are due to the immune response to the microorganism. The patient presents with fever, and general features of febrile illness, which may include septic shock. Joint pain is common and septic arthritis is sometimes seen. Cardiac symptoms develop when there is valvular involvement, which may manifest as erosion through valve leaflets producing regurgitation, fusing of valve leaflets or vegetations (outgrowths from valve structures) producing valvular stenosis or regurgitation.[73] The mitral valve is more commonly affected, but aortic valve involvement carries a worse prognosis.[72,73] Conduction system involvement manifests as arrhythmias and conduction defects. Embolic complications are relatively common and multifactorial. Septic emboli, embolisation of atrial thrombi when atrial fibrillation is present and fragmentation of vegetations may all give rise to pulmonary and systemic emboli. These most often present as splenic infarction, stroke, peripheral vascular occlusion and renal failure.[73]

Diagnosis

Diagnosis of IE is based on the modified Duke criteria, with echocardiography (transthoracic or transoesophageal) alongside clinical judgement.[72,73] These are based on the presence of microorganisms (identified in blood cultures), pathological lesions (vegetation or abscess present) and clinical criteria. The clinical criteria are based on two major criteria, or one major and three minor criteria, or five minor criteria.

Major clinical criteria are:

- positive blood culture
- evidence of endocardial involvement (positive echocardiography, abscess, partial dehiscence of a prosthetic valve or new valvular vegetation).
Minor clinical criteria include:
- fever with body temperature >38°C
- predisposing heart condition or intravenous drug use
- vascular signs: arterial emboli, intracranial haemorrhage, Janeway lesions (erythematous spots on the palms and feet) or conjunctival haemorrhages
- immunological signs: Osler nodes (painful, reddened nodules on the fingers and the feet) or glomerulonephritis.[73]

Echocardiography may reveal vegetations, abscess and valvular abnormalities, but endocarditis is more a clinical diagnosis based on the appearance of febrile illness, positive blood cultures with organisms known to cause endocarditis, new murmur and vascular features. Positive blood cultures remain central to the diagnosis. At least three sets are taken at 30-minute intervals, each containing 10 mL of blood, which should be obtained from a peripheral vein rather than from a central venous catheter (because of the risk of contamination and misleading interpretation) using a meticulous sterile technique. Once the causative microorganism has been identified, blood cultures should be repeated after 48–72 hours to check the effectiveness of treatment.[72]

Patient management

Prosthetic valve endocarditis must be aggressively managed, as mortality may be high.[72] Current guidelines recommend a multidisciplinary team-based approach to improve outcomes.[74] This approach includes standardised medical therapy, recommended surgical interventions and close follow-up for 1 year. Approximately 50% of patients undergo cardiac surgery during hospitalisation.[73]

During hospitalisation, close observation is required to identify and manage any infection-related complications (e.g. perivalvular abscesses, progressive HF, septic emboli and stroke). HF is the most frequent complication of IE (42–60% of cases) and one of the most frequent reasons for surgery. It is associated with new or worsening regurgitation, more often in the aortic rather than the mitral valve, and less commonly due to intracardiac fistulae. Valve obstruction, although more rare, may also lead to HF (see section, Acute exacerbations of heart

failure). Due to the febrile illness, it is important not to overlook hydration and dietary status. Uncontrolled infection is the second commonest indication for surgical intervention, although optimal timing for this remains unclear. The observation that persistently positive blood cultures 48–72 hours after initiation of antibiotics are an independent risk factor for hospital mortality suggests that surgery should be considered at this time after the exclusion of other causes of persistent positive blood cultures.[72] The aim of surgery is the total removal of infected tissues and repair or replacement of the affected valve(s).

Antibiotic therapy is provided empirically until blood culture and sensitivities are established, after which specific therapy will be delivered. The first 2 weeks of inpatient therapy are often considered as the critical phase with the option to consider outpatient antibiotic therapy beyond this point.

Prophylactic antibiotic coverage should be undertaken for at-risk patients 1 hour before dental procedures are to be performed, in particular for those with previous rheumatic fever or endocarditis, or prosthetic valves.[72] Antibiotic prophylaxis for genitourinary and gastrointestinal procedures is no longer recommended.[72]

Patients who have suffered from IE remain at high risk of relapse and reoccurrence risk (2–6%) and therefore they and their families need to be aware of the importance of obtaining blood cultures (×3) if they develop a fever before taking any antibiotics. If bloodstream infection is confirmed as the cause, then re-evaluation for possible IE is required. Regular clinic review within the first year is recommended with blood sampling where infection may be suspected and reinforcement of the principles of IE prevention at each follow-up visit. Echocardiography should be performed at the completion of antimicrobial therapy and repeated at intervals, particularly during the first year of follow-up to monitor the development of secondary HF. Good oral health maintenance, preventive dentistry and advice about skin hygiene, including tattoos and skin piercing, are mandatory.

Aortic aneurysm

The aorta is the major blood vessel leaving the heart. An aneurysm is a local dilation or outpouching of a vessel wall and comes in several forms (Fig. 10.14). Most aortic aneurysms are fusiform and saccular, and occur in the abdominal aorta creating an increase in aortic diameter to 3 cm or more. A fusiform aneurysm is uniform in shape with symmetrical dilation that involves the whole circumference of the aorta.[75] A saccular aneurysm has dilation of part of the aortic wall so the dilation is very localised.[75] A dissecting aneurysm occurs when the layers of the wall of the aorta continue to separate and fill with blood, resulting in obstructed blood flow. The aorta is particularly susceptible to aneurysm formation because of constant stress on the vessel wall and the absence of penetrating vasa vasorum that normally provide perfusion to the adventitia. As the blood flows through the aneurysm

FIGURE 10.14 Major types of aneurysm: (**A**) fusiform aneurysm has an entire section of an artery dilated, occurring most often in the abdominal aorta, due to atherosclerosis; (**B**) sacculated aneurysm affects one side of an artery, usually in the ascending aorta; (**C**) dissecting aneurysm results from a tear in the intima, causing blood to shunt between the intima and media; (**D**) pseudoaneurysm usually results from arterial trauma, such as intra-aortic balloon pump catheter or an arterial introducer; the opening does not heal properly and is covered by a clot that can burst at any time.

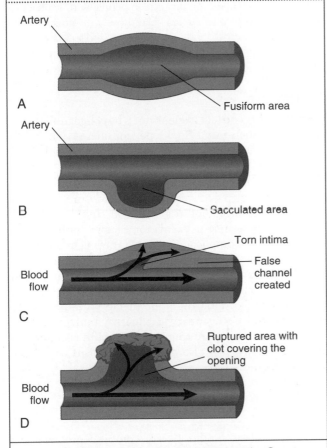

A — Artery / Fusiform area

B — Artery / Sacculated area

C — Torn intima / False channel created / Blood flow

D — Ruptured area with clot covering the opening / Blood flow

Source: Fibrinolytic Therapy Trialists' Collaborative Group. Indications for fibrinolytic therapy in suspected acute myocardial infarction: collaborative overview of early mortality and major morbidity results from all randomised trials of more than 1000 patients. Lancet 1994;343(8893):311–22.

left retroperitoneum, which may contain the rupture. However, the other 20% rupture into the peritoneal cavity and uncontrolled haemorrhage results.[75]

Patients often experience no symptoms until the aneurysm is extensive or ruptures. Clinical presentation varies and depends on the location and expansion rate. Aneurysms of the ascending aorta tend to affect the aortic root and cause valve regurgitation. Expansion of the aneurysm may also compress the vena cava, leading to engorged neck and superficial veins, or compress the large airways, causing respiratory distress. The first symptom most patients experience is pain, which may be steady and continuous from local compression or sudden and severe in the case of dissection or rupture, usually in the lower back. In this case, the pain is usually associated with syncope and is an acute emergency. Depending on the site of the aneurysm, there is usually an absence or decrease in the pulses below the site of the aneurysm, most commonly in the limbs. The renal arteries may be affected, resulting in decreased urine output and renal failure. The spinal blood flow may also be affected, resulting in paraplegia and, if the carotid arteries are affected, there may be altered consciousness. Infrarenal aneurysms are the most common form of aortic aneurysm and are located below the renal arteries. Bruits can also be heard over the aneurysm.

Diagnosis

A chest X-ray is usually the first investigation and may reveal a widened mediastinum or enlarged aortic knob. Some aneurysms will be hidden, so normal chest X-ray does not exclude the diagnosis. If available, a CT scan using contrast dye provides accurate information on the location and size of the aneurysm. Transoesophageal echocardiography (TOE) provides an accurate diagnosis and is the preferred investigation in dissecting aneurysms. A TOE can clearly identify the tear/flap, to enable classification of the aneurysm. There are some limitations in viewing the ascending aorta, and patients with respiratory dysfunction may have difficulty with lying flat for the procedure and having a light anaesthetic.

Patient management

Management of asymptomatic aneurysms is conservative, unless the size of the aneurysm is >1.5 times the normal size of the aortic segment[75] or the situation is acute. The primary aim is to lower hypertension and prevent increases in thrombus size and emboli through the administration of aspirin. Usually, the patient has regular monitoring to assess the aneurysm and to determine the timing and need for surgical repair.

Acute and dissecting aortic aneurysms are life-threatening emergencies, and surgery is often the only option. The development of new or worsening lower back pain may indicate impending rupture and there may be a palpable pulsatile abdominal mass. The faster treatment is initiated, the higher are the chances of survival with optimal recovery. The primary goal is to control blood pressure. If hypertensive, beta–adrenergic blockers or

it becomes turbulent and some blood may stagnate along the walls, allowing a thrombus to form. This thrombus in addition to atherosclerotic debris may embolise into the distal arteries, compromising their circulation. Atherosclerosis is the most common cause of aneurysm, because plaque formation erodes the vessel wall.[75] Other causes include syphilis, infection, inflammatory diseases and trauma. Aneurysms occur most often in men and in people with the risk factors of hypertension or smoking. Approximately 80% of aortic aneurysms rupture into the

sodium nitroprusside are used to reduce further arterial wall stress. If the patient is hypotensive, IV fluid and inotropes may be necessary.

Nursing management of dissecting aortic aneurysm involves the following:

- support during the diagnostic phase
- assessment of pain and provision of analgesia
- stabilising and monitoring of the clinical condition
- provision of psychological support to patient and family
- preparation for surgery and long-term care.

Assessment of the patient's symptoms and effects of the aneurysm is essential. This includes careful assessment and recording of symptoms, including pain level and intensity, peripheral pulses, oxygen saturation levels, blood pressure in both arms and neurological symptoms to assist with diagnosis and detect progression. Intravenous analgesia is essential to control the severe pain, and an antiemetic is useful to prevent opiate side effects. Opiates may also contribute to a sedative effect and slight vasodilation, which are both beneficial. Oxygen therapy via mask should be administered as indicated by oxygen saturation levels. Blood pressure control is vital, and usually IV medications are titrated to a narrow MAP range of 60–75 mmHg. Close observation of fluid balance to detect changes in renal perfusion and maintain appropriate blood volume is also essential. Finally, preparation for surgery is necessary, and must include the patient and family.

Ventricular aneurysm

Less than 5% of patients post-STEMI, particularly a transmural anterior infarction, develop a left ventricular aneurysm.[76] Post-STEMI, dyskinetic or akinetic areas of the left ventricle are common and are known as regional wall motion abnormalities. It is in these areas that there is a risk of an aneurysm developing. Ventricular aneurysms are more likely to develop post-anterior STEMI with a totally occluded LAD with poor collateral circulation.

Aneurysms form when the intraventricular tension stretches the dyskinetic area and a thin, weak layer of necrotic muscle and fibrous tissue develops and bulges with each contraction of the ventricle, resulting in a reduction in stroke volume. Aneurysms range from 1 to 8 cm in diameter and are four times more likely to occur at the apex and anterior wall rather than the inferoposterior wall.[76] Large ventricular aneurysms may result in a reduction in stroke volume, causing an increase in myocardial oxygen demand resulting in angina and heart failure. The mortality rate in people with ventricular aneurysms is four times higher than those with no aneurysm owing to a higher risk of tachyarrhythmias and sudden cardiac death. Unlike aortic aneurysms, these aneurysms rarely rupture so their management is usually conservative.

Diagnosis

Diagnosis of a ventricular aneurysm is by echocardiography. Ventricular aneurysm should be considered when ST-segment elevation persists beyond 1 week after MI.

Patient management

Management of a left ventricular aneurysm consists of aggressive management of STEMI and reperfusion therapy. Long-term anticoagulation therapy with warfarin is required. A complication of a ventricular aneurysm includes the development of an intraventricular thrombus within the aneurysmal pocket, which, if mobilised, becomes an arterial embolus. Also, due to the high risk of tachyarrhythmias, antiarrhythmic therapy is indicated. An ICD may also be necessary if antiarrhythmic therapy is unsuccessful in suppressing tachyarrhythmias. Surgical aneurysmectomy may also be required if heart failure and angina become severe, and is usually successful.

Summary

Compromise of the cardiovascular system, as either a primary or secondary condition, is a common problem that necessitates admission of patients to a critical care area. Prompt and appropriate assessment and treatment are required to ensure adequate oxygen supply to the tissues throughout the body. The most common cardiovascular problems experienced by patients include CHD, arrhythmias and cardiogenic shock; however, heart failure and selected conditions such as cardiomyopathies, hypertensive emergencies, endocarditis and aortic aneurysm also occur. Appropriate assessment and management are essential to prevent secondary complications arising. Important principles covered in this chapter are summarised below.

- CHD:
  - Incorporates myocardial ischaemia, angina and ACS.
  - Early patient assessment and diagnosis are essential to facilitate prompt intervention.
  - Initial diagnosis is based on history, clinical assessment, electrocardiographic and biochemical examination, with coronary angiography, exercise testing and chest radiography available to provide later detail.
  - Early restoration of blood flow – including reperfusion therapy and coronary angioplasty – to reduce myocardial damage is a core component of treatment.
  - Other goals of care include reducing plaque and clot formation in coronary arteries, reducing the workload of the heart, controlling symptoms, providing psychosocial support to the patient and family and educating the patient about the disease process, lifestyle and future responses to illness.

- HF:
  - May affect either the left, right or both ventricles, resulting in different signs and symptoms.
  - Diagnosis is usually made on the basis of echocardiography, ECG and chest X-ray.
  - In AHF, CPAP or BiPAP may be necessary to improve hypoxaemia.
  - Pharmacological therapy of AHF consists of ARNIs/ACEIs/ ARBs, beta-adrenergic blockers, MRAs, SGLT2 inhibitors and diuretics. Inotropes may also be used, such as low-dose dopamine and dobutamine, to improve renal perfusion and contractility.
  - Many patients with HF will also have a pacemaker with CRT and/or a defibrillator to improve cardiac function and reduce the incidence of sudden death.
  - Patient care must be lifelong and coordinated between all members of the healthcare team. Broad interventions, including medications, diet and lifestyle modification, may be appropriate for some patients, while palliative care might be more appropriate for other patients.

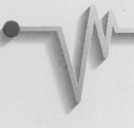

Case study

Mr Smith, a 71-year-old man, presented to his GP with intermittent chest pain. His GP did some urea and electrolytes (U&Es) and noted a troponin rise of 0.08 micrograms/L. Mr Smith decided to go home and experienced no more chest pain. However, he presented to the emergency department (ED) 2 days later with increasing shortness of breath (SOB), paroxysmal nocturnal dyspnoea and orthopnoea but no chest pain. He had been sleeping in a chair at night due to SOB.

He had no past medical history and was previously well. He was not taking any medications. He lived at home with his wife and daughter.

On presentation to ED, his ECG was abnormal (Fig 10.15). His chest X-ray (CXR) in ED showed acute pulmonary oedema with bilateral pleural effusions suggestive of acute pulmonary oedema. In ED, he was afebrile, with pulse 114 bpm and regular, respiratory rate of 26 breaths/min, blood pressure 170/110 and oxygen saturation 98% on room air. NYHA functional class was IV (SOB at rest). His JVP was +2 and he had no peripheral oedema. He had dual heart sounds (S1, S2) and a third heart sound (S3). U&E blood test results included: Na$^+$ 143 mmol/L; K$^+$ 4.5 mmol/L, urea 6.1 mmol/L, creatinine 103 micromols/L and eGFR 58. LFTs were normal. Other pathology included: NTproBNP 3307 ng/L and his troponin T 282 ng/L. He had an elevated D-dimer, which was due to the bilateral pleural effusions.

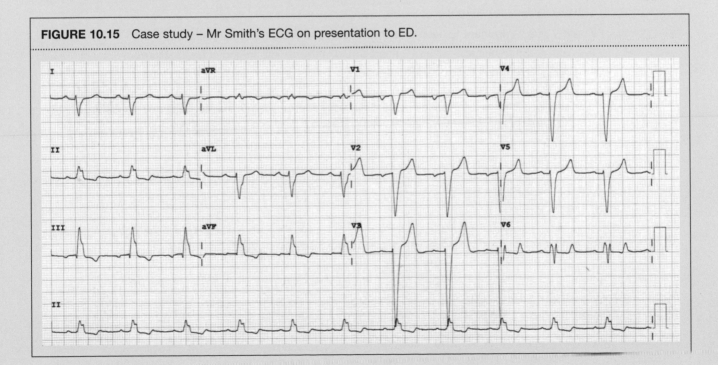

FIGURE 10.15 Case study – Mr Smith's ECG on presentation to ED.

In ED, Mr Smith was prescribed frusemide 80 mg IV and transferred to ward for further diuresis. During his inpatient stay, Mr Smith had an echocardiography which showed a mildly dilated left ventricle with moderate-to-severe left ventricular systolic dysfunction and mild right ventricular systolic dysfunction with a LVEF of 33% and e/e ratio of 13.2%. An e/e >15% is indicative of diastolic dysfunction. He also had a moderately enlarged left atrium, mild aortic and tricuspid regurgitation, and moderate-to-severe mitral regurgitation. His troponin peaked at 1815 2 days later.

Two days post admission, he underwent a coronary angiogram which showed occluded mid left circumflex artery (LCx) with mild LAD. Patient had a drug-eluting stent to his LCx. The LV gram during his coronary angiogram showed severe LV systolic dysfunction with posterior and lateral akinesis. He also had mild RV systolic dysfunction and moderate-to-severe functional mitral regurgitation. During the angiogram, he experienced a PEA arrest and was intubated. CPR commenced and adrenaline given with recovery of blood pressure. Post-arrest he experienced two episodes of monomorphic ventricular tachycardia, which responded to cardioversion. Amiodarone bolus was given and an infusion commenced. Also tirofiban and milrinone infusions were commenced. Mr Smith was transferred to ICU post-PCI. His angiogram showed mild irregularities in the left main coronary artery, mild proximal LAD disease, occluded proximal circumflex and mild right coronary artery stenosis. A drug-eluting stent was implanted in the left circumflex artery with good flow post implantation.

In ICU, he regained consciousness and was slowly weaned off the ventilator and extubated and amiodarone, milrinone and tirofiban infusions ceased. He was discharged from ICU the next day.

During his hospital stay, Mr Smith was gradually commenced on the gold standard pharmacotherapy for heart failure: beta-adrenergic blocker, ACEI, SGLT2I and aldosterone antagonist. During his hospital stay he lost a total of 12 kg of weight. This equates to 12 L of additional fluid in his body. His remaining hospitalisation was uneventful and he was discharged home a few days later. His fluids were restricted to 1.5 L/day, and he was instructed to weigh himself daily. Education was provided to him and his family about the diagnosis of heart failure, prognosis and management of his heart failure at home. On discharge his medications were: aspirin 100 mg mane, atorvastatin 80 mg mane, carvedilol 3.25 mg BD, ramipril 2.5 mg daily, GTN spray SL prn, pantoprazole 40 mg mane, empagliflozin on 10 mg mane, ticagrelor 90 mg BD, spironolactone 12.5 mg daily, and frusemide 40 mg mane. Once he has recovered from his hospitalisation, his ramipril will be changed over to Entresto 24/26 mg BD. He was also referred to a heart failure management program and to be seen in heart failure clinic within 2 weeks of discharge.

CASE STUDY QUESTIONS

1 What is your interpretation of the 12-lead ECG in Fig. 10.15?
2 Why was it important to determine the aetiology of Mr Smith's heart failure?
3 What is the significance of an S3 heart sound in the clinical setting of heart failure?
4 What are common causes of a PEA arrest?
5 When Mr Smith was discharged from hospital, why was he prescribed carvedilol, emapagliflozin, spironolactone and frusemide? Include in your answer the reason for prescribing these medications and their actions and major side effects.

RESEARCH VIGNETTE

Pareek N, Kordis P, Beckley-Hoelscher N, et al. A practical risk score for early prediction of neurological outcome after out-of-hospital cardiac arrest: MIRACLE2. Eur Heart J 2020;41(47):4508–17.

Abstract

Aims: The purpose of this study was to develop a practical risk score to predict poor neurological outcome after out-of-hospital cardiac arrest (OOHCA) for use on arrival to a heart attack centre.

Methods and results: From May 2012 to December 2017, 1055 patients had OOHCA in our region, of whom 373 patients were included in the King's Out of Hospital Cardiac Arrest Registry (KOCAR). We performed prediction modelling with multivariable logistic regression to identify predictors of the primary outcome to derive a risk score. This was externally validated in two independent cohorts comprising 473 patients. The primary endpoint was poor neurological outcome at 6-month follow-up (Cerebral Performance Category 3–5). Seven independent predictors of outcome were identified: missed (unwitnessed) arrest, initial non-shockable rhythm, non-reactivity of pupils, age (60–80 years: 1 point; >80 years: 3 points), changing intra-arrest rhythms, low pH <7.20, and adrenaline administration (2 points). The MIRACLE2 score had an area under the curve (AUC) of 0.90 in the development and 0.84/0.91 in the validation cohorts. Three risk groups were defined: low risk (MIRACLE2 <2: 5.6% risk of poor outcome), intermediate risk (MIRACLE2 of 3–4: 55.4% of poor outcome), and high risk (MIRACLE2 >5: 92.3% risk of poor outcome). The MIRACLE2 score had superior discrimination to the OOHCA (median AUC 0.83 (0.818–0.840); $P < 0.001$) and Cardiac Arrest Hospital Prognosis models (median AUC 0.87 (0.860–0.870; $P = 0.001$), and equivalent performance to the Target Temperature Management score (median AUC 0.88 (0.876–0.887); $P = 0.092$).

Conclusions: The MIRACLE2 is a practical risk score for early accurate prediction of poor neurological outcome after OOHCA which has been developed for simplicity of use on admission.

Critique

The decision to provide ongoing care to patients who have suffered an OOHCA can be perceived as futile when the likelihood of recovery is small. This paper presents a risk score called the MIRACLE2 score to predict neurological recovery, to be used upon presentation to hospital and assist the complex decision-making process clinicians face when treating this patient cohort.

This study used data from a cardiac arrest registry in the United Kingdom to develop a practical risk score to predict poor neurological outcome for patients presenting to hospital following an OOHCA. Data from 1055 patients who were over the age of 18 years who presented to hospital with OOHCA and had return of spontaneous circulation (ROSC) in the community between May 2012 and December 2017 were included. Any patients who had intact conscious state, as determined by Glasgow Coma Score (GCS) of 15/15 on arrival, were excluded.

Multivariate logistic regression identified predictors of poor neurological outcome at 6-month follow-up to derive a risk score. Neurological outcome was classified using the cerebral performance category (CPC), a five-category ordinal scale: CPC-1 represents normal function, CPC-2 represents moderate impairment with independent living, CPC-3 is consciousness with severe impairment, CPC-4 is a persistent coma and CPC-5 represents death. For this study a poor neurological outcome was defined as a CPC score 3–5 as assessed at 6 months.

Seven independent predictors were identified and included in the final derivation of the MIRACLE$_2$ risk score: unwitnessed arrest: 1 point; initial non-shockable rhythm: 1 point; non-reactivity of pupils: 1 point; age (60–80 years: 1 point; >80 years: 3 points); changing intra-arrest rhythms: 1 point; low pH<7.2: 1 point; and adrenaline administration: 2 points – giving a risk score ranging from 0 to 10.

Modelling validated three risk groups:

- low risk (MIRACLE$_2$ score ≤2 = 5.6% chance of poor neurological outcome);
- intermediate risk (MIRACLE$_2$ score 3–4 = 55% chance of poor neurological outcome); and
- high risk (MIRACLE$_2$ score ≥5 = 93% chance of poor neurological outcome).

This study used a development cohort of 1055 patients to derive the risk score and externally validated the results in two independent cohorts comprising of 473 patients. The MIRACLE$_2$ score had an area under the curve (AUC) discrimination of 0.90 in the initial development cohort and an AUC of 0.84 and 0.91 in the two independent cohorts, demonstrating excellent-to-outstanding utility.

Predictive risk scores for the OOHCA patient cohort are useful as decision tools to identify circumstances where limiting care may be more appropriate. Around 90% of patients who suffer cardiac arrest will die, mostly before arriving to hospital. While there are established guidelines that provide some recommendations, namely to continue life support for at least 4–5 days after arrest with targeted temperature management,[2–4] they fail to address the dynamic clinical state of the patient, particularly in the early minutes of arrival to hospital. A score such as the MIRACLE$_2$ score provides some guidance when considering long-term outcomes for patients presenting in cardiac arrest. However, any risk score should not be utilised as the sole factor to decide who should have active and aggressive care withheld, rather than employed as one of several decision tools.

The authors acknowledge there are limitations to this study. The risk score was validated in retrospective cohorts, which may increase the risk of bias. Additionally, the data for the regression models were from Heart Attack Centres or HAC hospitals in London. The authors identify this to potentially affect the transferability of the results to non-HAC hospitals particularly when these institutions lack immediate access to 24-hour specialist cardiology, cardiothoracic and intensive care expertise. The research group associated with this publication are currently validating the risk score in a prospective international cohort.

In summary, the MIRACLE$_2$ predictive risk score offers practical guidance to the often-challenging clinical decision making required when caring for this patient cohort.

Learning activities

1   Follow two ACS patient journeys, one each for patient presenting with either a STEMI or NSTEMI, consider their immediate management and longer-term care needs. Compare and contrast the patient experiences from the two pathways.

2   Examine the 12-lead ECG of a patient with ACS, and identify the key features of this ECG in relation to STEMI or non-STEMI. Compare this with the features of a normal ECG.

3   Discuss the compensatory mechanisms that are activated in heart failure and their effects on the cardiovascular system.

4   Discuss the gold standard pharmacotherapy for patients with HFrEF. Relate the action of each group to their effect on the pathophysiological compensatory mechanisms.

5   Analyse the ECG of a patient with heart failure. What are the electrocardiographical features of left and/or right ventricular hypertrophy? Why do these changes occur in terms of the electrophysiological pathway?

6   Observe an echocardiograph and ask the sonographer to explain what is visualised on the screen, particularly in Doppler mode. Ask them to identify areas of valvular dysfunction and any evidence of dyssynchrony between the ventricles.

Online resources

American Heart Association, www.heart.org/HEARTORG/

Australian Institute of Health and Welfare, www.aihw.gov.au

British Heart Foundation, www.bhf.org.uk

Cardiac Society of Australia and New Zealand, www.csanz.edu.au

European Society of Cardiology, www.escardio.org

Heart Education Assessment and Rehabilitation Toolkit (HEART), www.heartonline.org.au

HEARTe. Chest Heart and Stroke Scotland (CHSS) educational resource, www.heartelearning.org

Heart failure matters, www.heartfailurematters.org

National Heart Foundation of Australia, www.heartfoundation.com.au

National Heart Foundation of New Zealand, www.heartfoundation.org.nz

Patient information on living with heart failure, www.heartfoundation.org.au/SiteCollectionDocuments/Living well with chronic heart failure.pdf

Further reading

Libby P, Bonow RO, Mann DL et al, editors. Braunwald's heart disease: a textbook of cardiovascular medicine. 12th ed. Philadelphia: Elsevier; 2021.

Perpetua EM, Keegan P. Editors. Cardiac nursing. 7th ed. Baltimore: Lippincott, Williams & Wilkins; 2021.

References

1. Benjamin EJ, Virani SS, Callaway CW, et al. Heart disease and stroke statistics – 2018 update: a report from the American Heart Association. Circulation 2018;137:e67–492.

2. World Health Organization Cardiovascular disease fact sheet; deaths from coronary heart disease. Geneva: WHO; 2021. Available from: https://www.who.int/news-room/fact-sheets/detail/cardiovascular-diseases-(cvds). [Accessed 27 February 2023].

3. Lozano R, Naghavi M, Foreman K, et al. Global and regional mortality from 235 causes of death for 20 age groups in 1990 and 2010: a systematic analysis for the Global Burden of Disease Study 2010. Lancet 2012;380(9859):2095–128.

4. Australian Institute of Health and Welfare (AIHW). Australia's health. Canberra, ACT: AIHW; 2022.

5. Hall JE, Hall ME, editors. Guyton and Hall textbook of medical physiology. 14th ed. Philadelphia: Saunders; 2020.

6. Rapsomaniki E, Shah A, Perel P, et al. Prognostic models for stable coronary artery disease based on electronic health record cohort of 102 023 patients. Eur Heart J 2014;35(13):844–52.

7. Ibanez B, James S, Agewall S, et al. 2017 ESC guidelines for the management of acute myocardial infarction in patients presenting with ST-segment elevation. The Task Force for the Management of Acute Myocardial Infarction in Patients Presenting with ST-segment Elevation of the European Society of Cardiology (ESC). Eur Heart J 2018;39(2):119–77.

8. O'Gara PT, Kushner FG, Ascheim DD, et al. 2013 ACCF/AHA guideline for the management of ST-elevation myocardial infarction: a report of the American College of Cardiology Foundation/American Heart Association Task Force on Practice Guidelines. Circulation 2013;127(4): e362–425.

9. Chew DP, Scott IA, Cullen L, et al. National Heart Foundation of Australia and Cardiac Society of Australia and New Zealand Australian clinical guidelines for the management of acute coronary syndromes. Med J Aust 2016;2016:128–33.

10. Perpetua EM, Keegan P, editors. Cardiac nursing. 7th ed. Philadelphia: Lippincott, Williams & Wilkins; 2021.

11. Jacobs AK, Ali MJ, Best PJ, et al. Systems of care for ST-segment–elevation myocardial infarction: a policy statement from the American Heart Association. Circulation 2021;144:e310–27.

12. Chamie D, Costa JR Jr, Damiani LP, et al. Optical coherence tomography versus intravascular ultrasound and angiography to guide percutaneous coronary interventions: the iSIGHT randomized trial. Circ Cardiovasc Interv 2021;14(3):e009452.

13. van Nunen LX, Zimmermann FM, Tonino PAL, et al. Fractional flow reserve versus angiography for guidance of PCI in patients with multivessel coronary artery disease (FAME): 5-year follow-up of a randomised controlled trial. Lancet 2015;386(10006):1853–60.

14. Zimmermann FM, De Bruyne B, Pijls NHJ, et al. A protocol update of the Fractional flow reserve versus Angiography for Multivessel Evaluation (FAME) 3 trial: a comparison of fractional flow reserve-guided percutaneous coronary intervention and coronary artery bypass graft surgery in patients with multivessel coronary artery disease. Am Heart J 2019;214:156–7.

15. Scottish Intercollegiate Guidelines Network (SIGN). Management of stable angina. SIGN publication no. 151. Edinburgh: SIGN; 2018. Available from: https://www.sign.ac.uk. [Accessed 27 February 2023].

16. Williams MC, Hunter A, Shah ASV, et al. Use of coronary computed tomographic angiography to guide management of patients with coronary disease. J Am Coll Cardiol 2016;67(15):1759–68.

17. Guillermin A, Yan DJ, Perrier A, et al. Safety and efficacy of tenecteplase versus alteplase in acute coronary syndrome: a systematic review and meta-analysis of randomized trials. Arch Med Sci 2016;12(6):1181–7.

18. Investigators GUSTO. An international randomized trial comparing four thrombolytic strategies for acute myocardial infarction. N Engl J Med 1993;329(10):673–82.

19. Siontis GCM, Stefanini GG, Mavridis D, et al. Percutaneous coronary interventional strategies for treatment of in-stent restenosis: a network meta-analysis. Lancet 2015;386(9994):655–64.

20. Scottish Intercollegiate Guidelines Network (SIGN). Acute coronary syndrome. SIGN publication no. 148. Edinburgh: SIGN; 2016. Available from: https://www.sign.ac.uk. [Accessed 27 February 2023].

21. Ferrante G, Rao SV, Jüni P, et al. Radial versus femoral access for coronary interventions across the entire spectrum of patients with coronary artery disease. JACC Cardiovasc Interv 2016;9(14):1419–34.

22. Hofman R, James SK, Jernberg T et al. Oxygen therapy in suspected acute myocardial infarction. N Engl J Med 2017; 377:1240–9.

23. Jarvis S. Diagnosis, management and nursing care in acute coronary syndrome. Nurs Times 2017;113(3):31–5.

24. Task Force Members; Montalescot G, Sechtem U, Achenbach S, et al. 2013 ESC guidelines on the management of stable coronary artery disease. The Task Force on the Management of Stable Coronary Artery Disease of the European Society of Cardiology. Eur Heart J 2013; 34(38):2949–3003.

25. Long L, Anderson L, Dewhirst AM, et al. Exercise-based cardiac rehabilitation for adults with stable angina. Cochrane Database Syst Rev 2018;(2):CD012786.

26. Laffin LJ, Bakris GL. Antihypertensive therapies. In Bhatt DL, Opie's cardiovascular drugs: a companion to Braunwald's heart disease. 9th ed. Philadelphia: Elsevier; 2021. p. 97–146.

27. Blumenthal JA, Feger BJ, Smith PJ, et al. Treatment of anxiety in patients with coronary heart disease: rationale and design of the UNderstanding the benefits of exercise and escitalopram in anxious patients WIth coroNary heart Disease (UNWIND) randomized clinical trial. Am Heart J 2016;176:53–62.

28. The British Association for Cardiovascular Prevention and Rehabilitation. The BACPR standards and core components for cardiovascular disease prevention and rehabilitation. 3rd ed. British Cardiovascular Society, London: BACPR; 2017. Available from: https://www.bacpr.org/resources/bacpr-publications. [Accessed 27 February 2023].

29. Long L, Anderson L, Dewhirst AM, et al. Exercise-based cardiac rehabilitation for adults with stable angina. Cochrane Database Syst Rev 2018;(2):CD012786.

30. Marx N, Inzucchi SE, McGuire DK. Diabetes and the cardiovascular system. In: Mann DL, Zipes DP, Libby P, et al, editors. Braunwald's heart disease: a textbook of cardiovascular medicine. 12th ed. Philadelphia: Elsevier Saunders; 2021. p. 1556–78.

31. Dalal HM, Doherty P, Taylor RS. Cardiac rehabilitation. BMJ 2015;351:h5000. doi: 10.1136/bmj.h5000.

32. Herber OR, Smith K, White M, et al. 'Just not for me' – contributing factors to nonattendance/noncompletion at phase III cardiac rehabilitation in acute coronary syndrome patients: a qualitative enquiry. J Clin Nurs 2017;26(21–22):3529–42.

33. Anderson L, Thompson DR, Oldridge N, et al. Exercise-based cardiac rehabilitation for coronary heart disease. Cochrane Database Syst Rev 2016;1:CD001800.

34. Van Diepen S, Katz JN, Albert NM, et al. Contemporary management of cardiogenic shock: a scientific statement from the American Heart Association. Circulation 2017;136(16):E232–68.

35. Thiele H, Akin I, Sandri M, et al. PCI strategies in patients with acute myocardial infarction and cardiogenic shock. N Engl J Med 2017;377(25):2419–32.

36. Thiele H, Zeymer U, Neumann F-J, et al. Intraaortic balloon support for myocardial infarction with cardiogenic shock. N Engl J Med 2012;367(14):1287–96.

37. Lador A, Hasdai D, Porter A, et al. Trends in frequency and prognosis of post myocardial infarction pericarditis: ACSIS 2000–2013. Eur Heart J 2017;38(Suppl 1):ehx504.P3646.

38. Strauss DG, Schocken DD. Marriott's practical electrocardiography. 13th ed. Philadelphia: Lippincott, Williams Williams & Wilkins; 2021.

39. Gerber Y, Weston SA, Redfield MM, et al. A contemporary appraisal of the heart failure epidemic in Olmsted County, Minnesota, 2000 to 2010. JAMA Intern Med 2015;175:996–1004.

40. Tsao CW, Lyass A, Enserro D, et al. Temporal trends in the incidence of and mortality associated with heart failure with preserved and reduced ejection fraction. JACC Heart Fail 2018;6:678–85.

41. Australian Bureau of Statistics. Causes of death Australia 2021. Online. Available from: https://www.abs.gov.au/statistics/health/causes-death/causes-death-australia/latest-release. [Accessed 27 February 2023].

42. Atherton JJ, Sindone A, De Pasquale CG, et al. National Heart Foundation of Australia and Cardiac Society of Australia and New Zealand: guidelines for the prevention, detection, and management of heart failure in Australia. Heart Lung Circ 2018;27(10):1123–208.

43. Yancy CW, Jessup M, Bozkurt B. 2013 ACCF/AHA guideline for the management of heart failure: a report of the American College of Cardiology Foundation/American Heart Association Task Force on practice guidelines. Circulation 2013;128:1810–52.

44. McDonagh TA, Metra M, Adamo M, et al. 2021 ESC Guidelines for the diagnosis and treatment of acute and chronic heart failure. Eur Heart J 2021;42(36):3599–726. doi: 10.1093/eurheartj/ehab368.

45. Driscoll A, Dinh D, Prior D, et al. The effect of transitional care on 30-day outcomes in patients hospitalised with acute heart failure. Heart Lung Circ 2020;29(9):1347–55. doi: 10.1016/j.hlc.2020.03.004.

46. Driscoll A, Worrall-Carter L, Hare DL, et al. Evidence-based chronic heart failure management programs: reality or myth? Qual Saf Health Care 2009;18(6):450–5.

47. McAlister FA, Stewart S, Ferrua S, et al. Multidisciplinary strategies for the management of heart failure patients at high risk for admission. J Am Coll Cardiol 2004;44(4):810–19.

48. Whellan DJ, Hasselblad V, Peterson E, et al. Meta-analysis and review of heart failure disease management randomized controlled clinical trials. Am Heart J 2005;149(4):722–9.

49. Phillips CO, Singa RM, Rubin HR, et al. Complexity of program and clinical outcomes of heart failure disease management incorporating specialist nurse-led heart failure clinics. A meta-regression analysis. Eur J Heart Fail 2005;7(3):333–41.

50. Driscoll A, Currey J, Tonkin A, et al. Nurse-led titration of angiotensin converting enzyme inhibitors, beta-adrenergic blocking agents, and angiotensin receptor blockers for people with heart failure with reduced ejection fraction. Cochrane Database Syst Rev 2015;(12):CD009889.

51. Driscoll A, Davidson P, Clark R, et al. Tailoring consumer resources to enhance self-care in chronic heart failure. Aust Crit Care 2009;22(3):133–40.

52. Riegel B, Dickson VV. A situation-specific theory of heart failure self-care. J Cardiovasc Nurs 2008;23(3):190–6.

53. Kaneko Y, Floras JS, Usui K, et al. Obstructive sleep apnea in heart failure: review of prevalence, treatment with continuous positive airway pressure, and prognosis. Texas Heart Inst J 2018;45(3):151–61.

54. Jewiss D, Ostman C, Smart NA. The effect of resistance training on clinical outcomes in heart failure: a systematic review and meta-analysis. Int J Cardiol 2016;221:674–81.

55. Ellingsen Ø, Halle M, Conraads V, Støylen A, Dalen H, Delagardelle C, et al. High-intensity interval training in patients with heart failure with reduced ejection fraction. Circulation 2017;135:839–49.

56. Group CTS. Effects of enalapril on mortality in severe congestive heart failure. N Engl J Med 1987;316(23):1429–35.

57. Investigators SOLVD. Effect of enalapril on survival in patients with reduced left ventricular ejection fractions and congestive heart failure. N Engl J Med 1991;325(5):293–302.

58. McMurray JJV, Packer M, Desai AS, et al. Angiotensin-neprilysin inhibition versus enalapril in heart failure. N Engl J Med 2014;371(11):993–1004.

59. Packer MMJ, Desai AS, et al; on behalf of the PARADIGM-HF Investigators and Committees. Angiotensin receptor neprilysin inhibition compared with enalapril on the risk of clinical progression in surviving patients with heart failure. Circulation 2015;131(1):54–61.

60. McMurray JJV, Östergren J, Swedberg K, et al. Effects of candesartan in patients with chronic heart failure and reduced left-ventricular systolic function taking angiotensin-converting-enzyme inhibitors: the CHARM-Added trial. Lancet 2003;362(9386):767–71.

61. Hjalmarson Å, Goldstein S, Fagerberg B, et al. Effects of controlled-release metoprolol on total mortality, hospitalizations, and well-being in patients with heart failure: the metoprolol CR/XL randomized intervention trial in congestive heart failure (MERIT-HF). JAMA 2000;283(10):1295–302.

62. Pitt B, Pfeffer MA, Assmann SF, et al. Spironolactone for heart failure with preserved ejection fraction. N Engl J Med 2014;370(15):1383–92.

63. Pitt B, Remme W, Zannad F, et al. Eplerenone, a selective aldosterone blocker, in patients with left ventricular dysfunction after myocardial infarction. N Engl J Med 2003;348(14):1309–21.

64. Pitt B, Zannad F, Remme WJ, et al. The effect of spironolactone on morbidity and mortality in patients with severe heart failure. N Engl J Med 1999;341(10):709–17.

65. Thomson S, Vallon V. Renal effects of sodium–glucose co-transporter inhibitors. Am J Med 2019:132(10):S30–8.

66. Zannad F, Ferreira JP, Pocock SJ, et al. SGLT2 inhibitors in patients with heart failure with reduced ejection fraction: a meta-analysis of the EMPEROR-Reduced and DAPA-HF trials. Lancet 2020;396(10254):819–29. doi: 10.1016/S0140-6736(20)31824-9.

67. Lambiase PD, Theuns DA, Murgatroyd F, et al. Subcutaneous implantable cardioverter–defibrillators: long-term results of the EFFORTLESS study. Eur Heart J 2022;43(21):2037–50.

68. Hershberger RE. The dilated, restrictive and infiltrative cardiomyopathies. In: Libby P, Bonow RO, Mann DL et al, editors. Braunwald's heart disease: a textbook of cardiovascular medicine. 12th ed. Philadelphia: Elsevier; 2021, p. 1031–51.

69. Ho CY, Ommen ST. Hypertrophic cardiomyopathy. In: Libby P, Bonow RO, Mann DL et al, editors. Braunwald's heart disease: a textbook of cardiovascular medicine. 12th ed. Philadelphia: Elsevier; 2021, p. 1062–76.

70. Bakris GL, Sorrentino MI. Systemic hypertension: mechanisms, diagnosis and treatment. In: Libby P, Bonow RO, Mann DL et al, editors. Braunwald's heart disease: a textbook of cardiovascular medicine. 12th ed. Philadelphia: Elsevier; 2021, p. 471–501.

71. Vidaeff A, Carroll MA, Ramin S. Acute hypertensive emergencies in pregnancy. Crit Care Med 2005;33(10):S307–12.

72. Habib G, Lancellotti P, Antunes MJ, et al. 2015 ESC guidelines for the management of infective endocarditis. The Task Force for the Management of Infective Endocarditis of the European Society of Cardiology (ESC) endorsed by: European Association for Cardio-Thoracic Surgery (EACTS), the European Association of Nuclear Medicine (EANM). Eur Heart J 2015;36(44):3075–128.

73. Baddour LMFW, Anavekar NS, Crestanello JA, et al. Infectious endocarditis and infections of indwelling devices. In: Libby P, Bonow RO, Mann DL et al, editors. Braunwald's heart disease: a textbook of cardiovascular medicine. 12th ed. Philadelphia: Elsevier; 2021, p. 1505–30.

74. Baddour LMFW, Wilson WR, Bayer AS, et al. Infective endocarditis in adults: diagnosis, antimicrobial therapy, and management of complications. A scientific statement for healthcare professionals from the American Heart Association. Circulation 2015;132:1435–86.

75. Braverman AC, Schermerhorn M. Diseases of the aorta. In: Libby P, Bonow RO, Mann DL et al, editors. Braunwald's heart disease: a textbook of cardiovascular medicine. 12th ed. Philadelphia: Elsevier; 2021, p. 806–36.

76. Bohula EA, Morrow DA. ST-elevation myocardial infarction management. In: Libby P, Bonow RO, Mann DL et al, editors. Braunwald's heart disease: a textbook of cardiovascular medicine. 12th ed. Philadelphia: Elsevier; 2021, p. 662–713.

Chapter 11

Cardiac rhythm assessment and management

Malcolm Dennis, Michael Sampson

Learning objectives

After reading this chapter, you should be able to:

- describe the mechanisms implicated in the development and propagation of cardiac arrhythmias
- recognise commonly observed arrhythmias and discuss the factors that lead to their development
- understand the haemodynamic consequences of each arrhythmia, and their prognostic implications
- identify assessment and treatment strategies that ensure that specific arrhythmias are managed safely and effectively
- discuss the principles and indications for pacemaker therapy
- recognise abnormal pacemaker activity on the ECG and discuss the causes and corrective actions for complications during temporary pacing
- describe the principles and benefits of cardiac resynchronisation therapy (CRT), including the factors that limit the effectiveness of the therapy
- discuss the principles and indications for treatment of arrhythmias including permanent pacing, cardioverter defibrillators, cardioversion and defibrillation.

Introduction

Normal cardiac function relies on electrical excitation of the myocardium under control of the intrinsic conduction system. A tightly controlled sequence of excitation and conduction through the atria, atrioventricular (AV) node and ventricles results in optimum contraction patterns, with heart rates matched to metabolic demands by the sinus node.[1] Cardiac arrhythmias are disturbances in this normal electrical activity, with variable effect on the individual. Symptoms may be absent or mild, or may result in rapid decline in cardiac output. In addition, they may progressively worsen in severity after initially being tolerated. When severe and sustained, the patient may become shocked or suffer cardiac arrest.[2] Certain arrhythmias increase the risk of heart failure and stroke.[3]

The haemodynamic impact of arrhythmias depends on the type of arrhythmia, the resultant ventricular rate, current health, left ventricular (LV) function and comorbidities.[4] The likelihood of severe compromise is greater in arrhythmias developing during critical illness, where metabolic demand is already high or unmet. Cardiac rhythm assessment and management demands an understanding of why arrhythmias develop and their anticipated effects, as well as a systematic assessment of the patient and ECG. A good grasp of this topic is important, given the frequency of arrhythmia in critically ill people. Atrial fibrillation (AF), for example, affects between 1% and 4% of the population of high-income countries; studies have demonstrated an incidence of new-onset AF exceeding 40% in some critical care populations.[5,6]

This chapter covers the mechanisms of arrhythmia formation, their causes and prognostic features, ECG recognition and treatment in the acute setting. Cardiac rhythm management devices (pacemakers and defibrillators) are covered later in the chapter.

The cardiac conduction system

The contraction of cardiac myocytes is initiated and coordinated by electrical activity created by the depolarisation and repolarisation of the cardiac cell membrane.[7] This is discussed in more detail in Chapter 9. Key points to bear in mind during cardiac rhythm assessment and management are as follows:

- Cardiac electrical activity is the product of ion movement through ion channels in the cell membrane and can be disturbed by ion (electrolyte) concentrations or factors which alter the cell membrane permeability and ion channel function.
- Although the sinus node acts as the pacemaker in normal health, all parts of the conduction system have automaticity and are therefore capable of generating electrical impulses and rhythms.
- In the normal heart, the AV node and bundle of His are the only electrical connection between the atria and ventricles.
- Slow conduction in the AV node prevents it conducting rapid atrial rates to the ventricles. As a result, physiological block occurs in arrhythmias such as atrial fibrillation and flutter.

Sinus rhythm

The normal rhythm of the heart originates in the sinus node and is referred to as sinus rhythm. The sinus rate is varied constantly to closely match the cardiac output to changes in metabolic demand and is influenced predominantly by nervous and endocrine inputs. In normal health, the heart rate during sinus rhythm is between 60 and 100 beats per minute (bpm), varying with activity and other influences.[8] Sinus rates less than 60 are termed sinus bradycardia, and rates greater than 100 as sinus tachycardia.[9] The key features of normal sinus rhythm are as follows:

- Regular P waves have a normal and consistent morphology; P waves are upright in most leads (always inverted in aVR, usually biphasic in V1) (Fig. 11.1).
- One P wave precedes each QRS complex.
- A P-wave rate between 60 and 100 bpm.

The QRS complex is usually narrow during sinus rhythm (less than 0.12 seconds) unless there is bundle branch block. A number of variations of sinus rhythm occur, and these are discussed below. The ECG criteria for rhythms arising in the sinus node are summarised in Table 11.1.

Sinus bradycardia

The sinus rate is primarily regulated by autonomic innervation, with parasympathetic stimulation slowing the rate and sympathetic stimulation increasing it. Sinus bradycardia can therefore result from increased parasympathetic tone (e.g. during sleep or from vagal stimulation such as nausea, vomiting or painful procedures[7]) or from decreased sympathetic stimulation (e.g. from beta-blockers, spinal trauma or spinal anaesthesia). Other causes of sinus bradycardia include hypoxaemia, myocardial ischaemia, hypothyroidism, athletic training, impaired adrenal function, and drugs, notably antiarrhythmics.[1] Sinus bradycardia also features among the rhythm disturbances of sick sinus syndrome, which increases in prevalence with age.[10]

In sinus bradycardia the P-wave appearance is the same as in sinus rhythm, but at a rate less than 60/min (Fig. 11.2). Patients may be asymptomatic, but when marked bradycardia occurs or in the presence of limited cardiovascular reserve there may be symptoms of low cardiac output such as

---

FIGURE 11.1 Sinus rhythm 78 bpm. Every P wave is identical, and is followed by a narrow QRS. The rhythm is regular and the PR interval is normal (0.12 s).

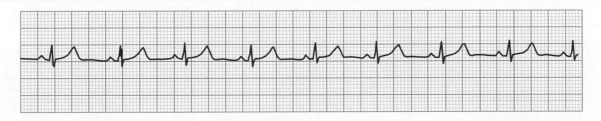

TABLE 11.1

ECG criteria for rhythms arising in the sinus node

RHYTHM	ECG CRITERIA
Sinus rhythm (SR)	Regular rhythm. Heart rate between 60 and 100 bpm. QRS complex usually narrow. Upright P waves precede the QRS complex (inverted in aVR, may be inverted in III, V1). PR interval is consistent, and between 120 and 200 ms (3–5 small squares).
Sinus bradycardia (SB)	As SR, but heart rate less than 60 bpm.
Sinus tachycardia (ST)	As SR, but heart rate greater than 100 bpm.
Sinus arrhythmia	As SR, but PP interval increases with inspiration and decreases with expiration.
Sinus exit block	SR with a sudden missed beat. Pause is a multiple of the usual PP interval.
Sinus arrest	SR with a sudden missed beat. Pause is not a multiple of the usual PP interval.

dopamine. Glucagon can be useful in beta-blocker or calcium channel blocker overdose.[12] Temporary cardiac pacing may be used until acute reversible factors are overcome;[13] for persistent bradycardia, permanent pacemaker implantation may be necessary.

Sinus tachycardia

Sinus tachycardia (>100 bpm[9]) is rarely a manifestation of sinus node disease or dysfunction. Instead, it is most commonly part of normal sympathetic (compensatory) responses to physical or psychological stressors (e.g. exertion, blood loss, pain, any acute illness, hypoxaemia), or unmet metabolic demand (e.g. shock states, anaemia, hypoglycaemia).[8] As such, identification and management of the underlying trigger for sinus tachycardia is the real focus, rather than attempting to slow the heart rate directly. Sinus tachycardia is common in critically ill patients, and may be due not just to the illness, but also to their treatments as well such as bronchodilators, inotropic agents and sympathomimetics.

In sinus tachycardia the P-wave rate is greater than 100/min. Sinus rates of 160–180/min may occasionally be seen. At such rates the P waves are difficult to identify, as they merge with the preceding T wave. (See Fig. 11.3 for sinus tachycardia.)

Practice tip

The severity of sinus tachycardia usually has some relationship to the severity of the trigger – changes in the tachycardia rate can be useful for detecting any worsening of the underlying cause.

In the critically ill patient, it is not uncommon to have more than one trigger for sinus tachycardia. Be alert to additional contributors (including psychological factors) beyond any already identified.

---

lightheadedness or dizziness, fatigue, exercise intolerance, and syncope if bradycardia is marked.[11] If treatment is necessary, heart rate-slowing drugs (negative chronotropes) should be discontinued if possible, and positive chronotropes given to increase the heart rate. Intravenous atropine increases heart rate by blocking parasympathetic activity, and is given in increments of 500 micrograms, up to a maximum of 3 micrograms.[2] Alternative drugs include glycopyrrolate, adrenaline (epinephrine), isoprenaline and

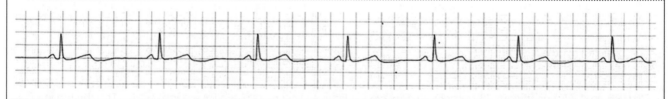

FIGURE 11.2 Sinus bradycardia. There is minor irregularity but the rate is slow throughout at 37–42 bpm. The P waves have normal appearance.

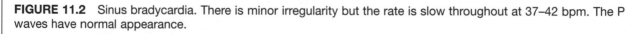

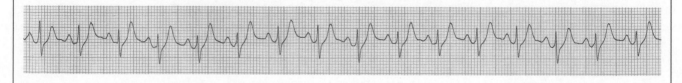

FIGURE 11.3 Sinus tachycardia. The heart rate is 114 bpm and regular.

FIGURE 11.4 Sinus arrhythmia. All P waves are identical but their rhythm is irregular, accelerating gradually at each end of the strip, and slowing in the middle.

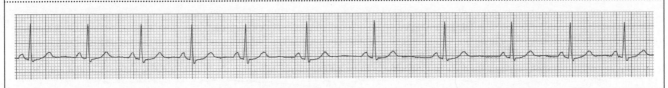

FIGURE 11.5 Sinus exit block. An abrupt rate drop follows the first three sinus beats. The PP interval spanning the pause is exactly twice the PP interval of the preceding beats, consistent with sinus exit block.

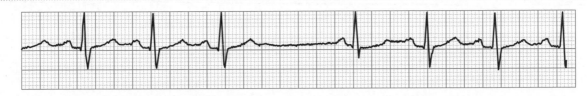

It is very uncommon to see sinus tachycardia without an underlying trigger. A rare exception is 'inappropriate sinus tachycardia', a condition in which unexplained sinus tachycardia is seen at rest.[14] Such patients may need chronic treatment to directly slow the sinus rate, such as beta-blockers, calcium channel blockers, or the selective sinus node inhibitor ivabradine.[15,16] Slowing the heart rate during sinus rhythm also has therapeutic benefit in the long-term management of coronary heart disease and chronic heart failure.

Sinus arrhythmia

Rhythmic variation in the sinus rate can often be seen, resulting in irregularity of sinus rhythm. This is referred to as sinus arrhythmia, most commonly caused by variations in vagal tone during breathing.[1] During inspiration, vagal tone declines and heart rate increases. During expiration, the opposite occurs, and heart rate slows (Fig. 11.4). As with normal sinus rhythm, P waves are of a single morphology, and the PR interval is constant. The variation in rate is usually gradual rather than sudden, and more marked with increased respiratory effort (e.g. snoring, sleep apnoea or dyspnoea). Sudden changes in sinus rate do not characterise sinus arrhythmia and may instead be due to sinus pauses or atrial ectopics.[1] Sinus arrhythmia is usually a normal finding but may also accompany sinus node dysfunction. It does not require treatment.

Sinus pause, arrest and exit block

Sinus pause, arrest and exit block appear as abrupt interruptions to the regular discharge of the sinus node, resulting in delayed appearance of sinus P waves. Sinus pauses are momentary delays in sinus node discharge and P waves fail to appear at the expected time.[8] By convention, the term sinus pause is usually used for shorter rather than longer pauses (e.g. less than 3 seconds), while sinus arrest

is used for longer pauses (greater than 3 seconds) with greater likelihood of symptoms or syncope. In contrast, in sinus exit block the sinus node does discharge but impulses fail to exit the sinus node and excite atrial tissue.[17] The resultant pause duration may be (though not always) a multiple of the previous PP interval, suggesting regular sinus node discharge without exciting the atria (Fig. 11.5). Differentiation of sinus pause, arrest and exit block is imperfect and the emphasis should be on detecting and treating extended periods of sinus node failure/P-wave absence (Fig. 11.6). Permanent pacing is often necessary if syncope has occurred.[17]

Practice tip

Very early atrial ectopic beats may not conduct through the AV node, and the resultant compensatory pause may be misinterpreted as a sinus pause. Observe the T wave prior to the pause for evidence of partially concealed P waves distorting the T wave. Causes (and treatment) of atrial ectopics are quite different to those of sinus pauses.

Arrhythmia mechanisms

Arrhythmias arise from disorders of electrical impulse formation or conduction.[1] They may emerge from locations other than the sinus node (ectopic foci), from continued re-excitation by impulses circulating around distinct pathways (reentry), 'triggered' by repolarisation abnormalities, or in the case of bradyarrhythmias from failure of impulse formation or conduction throughout the heart.

FIGURE 11.6 Sinus pause and sinus arrest. Terminology is a little arbitrary but the first of the pauses in the top strip (duration 2 s) is termed sinus pause and the second, at greater than 3 s, could be termed sinus arrest. In practice, however, the term sinus arrest is usually used to convey longer 'pauses', as in the lower strip where sinus activity convincingly ceases, reappearing spontaneously in this case some 20 s later.

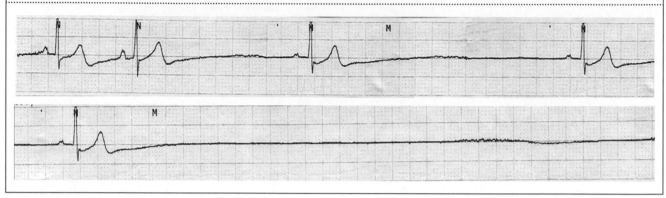

Arrhythmias may occur from cardiac disease or may complicate any acute (non-cardiac) illness. Myocardial infarction or ischaemia, and electrolyte or metabolic disturbances are common acute causes,[8] and scar formation from myocardial injury increases the risk of chronic arrhythmias. Idiopathic degeneration and fibrosis of conduction tissue is also a common cause, especially in the elderly.[18] Pre-existing arrhythmic tendencies may be exacerbated during acute illness or when sympathomimetics or antiarrhythmic drugs are administered.[1]

The mechanisms underpinning abnormal impulse generation and tachyarrhythmias include abnormal automaticity, triggered activity and reentry.[19]

Abnormal automaticity

Automaticity describes the ability of cardiac electrical cells to spontaneously depolarise, and thereby give rise to cardiac rhythms.[7] All cells within the cardiac conduction system have automaticity; under normal circumstances the sinus node has the highest rate of spontaneous depolarisation, and therefore acts as the primary pacemaker.

Under abnormal conditions, such as ischaemia or autonomic changes, automaticity may be depressed or enhanced. When tissues other than the sinus node have enhanced automaticity, they may discharge more rapidly and take control of the cardiac rhythm as ectopic atrial, junctional or ventricular rhythms. These may be as accelerated ectopic rhythms or tachycardias. Abnormalities which enhance such ectopic automaticity are frequently present in critical care patients and include sympathetic responses to illness (or sympathomimetic treatment), hypoxaemia, shock states, hypokalaemia and acidaemia.[20] Depressed automaticity results in bradycardia.

Triggered activity

Triggered activity describes abnormal electrical impulses arising during the repolarisation phase of the action potential. During the return towards resting membrane potential, membrane voltages can be disturbed, especially by abnormal calcium loading of myocytes.[19] These voltage changes may be sufficient for cells to prematurely return to the threshold potential for re-excitation, giving rise to ectopic beats or sustained ventricular arrhythmias. When occurring during phase 2 or 3 of the action potential, these voltage changes are termed 'early after-depolarisations', and when in phase 4, 'late after-depolarisations'.[20]

The major culprit for triggered activity is increased intracellular calcium, seen in digitalis toxicity and during catecholamine administration. It also occurs with muscle fibre stretch as in ventricular hypertrophy or heart failure, partly explaining the increased arrhythmic risk of heart failure patients. Other causes of triggered activity include structural heart disease, myocardial infarction, repolarisation (QT interval)-lengthening drugs and abnormal cardiac ion channel function.[21,22] Common critical care drugs which alter ion channel function include amiodarone, sotalol, erythromycin and propofol.[23] Triggered arrhythmias, especially torsades de pointes (TdP), occurs more readily when there is bradycardia, electrolyte disturbance or ischaemia.[1]

Reentry

Reentry is the most common mechanism responsible for tachyarrhythmias and describes the phenomenon in which cardiac electrical activity continuously conducts around a circuit within the heart (a reentry circuit), generating another P wave or QRS with each transit around the circuit.[20] Reentry permits the atria, AV node or ventricles (or combinations) to continuously re-excite themselves at rapid rates. Underlying reentry is the need for a circuit around which abnormal impulse propagation can occur. This is commonly a pathway around an area of scar from previous myocardial injury (e.g. infarction, infection, fibrosis). To utilise this pathway, however, requires additional conditions, primarily a region of myocardium where conduction block momentarily occurs, with a neighbouring region of slow conduction properties. With these two properties, reentry may occur as follows: a premature beat conducting through the myocardium encounters the area of conduction block because that tissue is still refractory from the preceding beat. If conduction is sufficiently slow through adjacent tissue, it may find a route back to the 'blocked' area and depolarise it if it has by now recovered excitability. Conduction through this area will largely be in the reverse direction to its usual direction (retrograde). Impulses can thus arrive back at the slow conduction area and recommence the same route repetitively. A continuing wave of depolarisation may thus continue to spread around the established circuit, repeatedly exciting the heart at rapid rates.

The so-called 'circuit' used for reentry is often an anatomical obstacle such as scarred myocardium following myocardial infarction, infection, inflammation or fibrosis.[21] Such obstacles create an unusual path for conduction to allow it to return to areas of initially blocked conduction.

Apart from myocardial scars, some normal cardiac structures favour reentry on a larger scale (macro reentry). Atrial flutter, for example, is a continuously propagating wavefront of conduction usually around the tricuspid valve annulus within the right atrium. Reentry may also involve both atria and ventricles together in patients who have accessory pathways linking them. This enables impulses which have conducted from atria to ventricles via the AV node to return to the atria via the accessory pathway and re-excite the atria. A continuing wavefront can thus be established involving the atria, the AV node, the ventricles and the accessory pathway.[24] Continuous reentry around the circuit produces a fast, regular rhythm.[25]

Practice tip

Antiarrhythmic drugs such as flecainide, sotalol and amiodarone alter conduction velocity and refractory period duration. These actions may terminate and prevent cardiac arrhythmias but may also affect conduction system properties in ways which favour the development of other arrhythmias (proarrhythmic effect). Proarrhythmia is a major factor limiting the safety of antiarrhythmic drugs.[26]

Arrhythmia recognition and management

Arrhythmia recognition requires familiarity with P–QRS–T morphologies and their relationships to each other. This is discussed in detail in Chapter 9. To ensure that important information is not overlooked requires an organised method for working through arrhythmia ECGs. Fig. 11.7 provides a systematic, step-wise approach to rhythm

interpretation, which can help guide the ECG reader to a diagnosis. Such approaches are useful for general interpretation, but condensed approaches for use in emergencies and cardiac arrest are also very valuable for rapid decision making.[27,28] Note also that going back through telemetry records permits you to see how the arrhythmia began. This can be extremely helpful, as the onset of arrhythmias may provide greater clarity regarding the diagnosis and mechanism.

Atrial arrhythmias

Atrial arrhythmias are commonly encountered in clinical practice.[1] While they rarely result in death, they frequently cause symptoms such as palpitations, shortness of breath, fatigue, dizziness and syncope. They also increase the risk of thromboembolic events such as stroke, particularly atrial fibrillation. Atrial arrhythmias present as persistent rhythms, or in paroxysmal episodes that terminate spontaneously within minutes, hours or days. In critically ill people, they often cause haemodynamic instability, prolong hospital stay and increase morbidity.[3,25] Atrial arrhythmias include ectopic beats, atrial fibrillation, atrial flutter and atrial tachycardia. The ECG rhythm criteria for these arrhythmias are summarised in Table 11.2.

Atrial ectopic beats

Atrial ectopics, or premature atrial contractions (PACs), are beats occurring singly or in groups, and arising from atrial tissue.[1] On the ECG, atrial ectopics appear as early beats usually with the same QRS morphology as preceding sinus beats (Fig. 11.8). The P wave typically has a different morphology to the sinus P wave because of a different point of origin within the atria. Ectopics can arise in either atrium and are common and usually benign; they rarely require treatment on their own account, but the underlying cause (e.g. heart failure) should be assessed and managed.[3] If atrial ectopics are very premature they may fail to conduct through the AV node (blocked or non-conducted atrial ectopics). If sufficiently premature, the P wave may be less than clear and appear as distortions of the ST segment or T wave and be followed by an apparent pause in the sinus rate.

Atrial fibrillation

Atrial fibrillation (AF) is the most common cardiac arrhythmia; as noted above, it affects up to 4% of the general population and is a common complication of critical illness.[4,6] The arrhythmia occurs most frequently because of atrial fibre stretch as in hypertension or heart failure; it is also common in individuals with chronic pulmonary or other cardiac disease.[3] Other conditions associated with AF include systemic infection, hyperthyroidism, hypokalaemia and alcohol abuse. In a minority of individuals, no underlying cause is found, in which case a genetic predisposition may be present.[29] In some, the trigger for AF initiation is rapid ectopy arising from the pulmonary veins at their junction with the atria, an abnormality which is amenable to ablation therapy.[30]

FIGURE 11.7 Stepwise, systematic approach to rhythm interpretation.

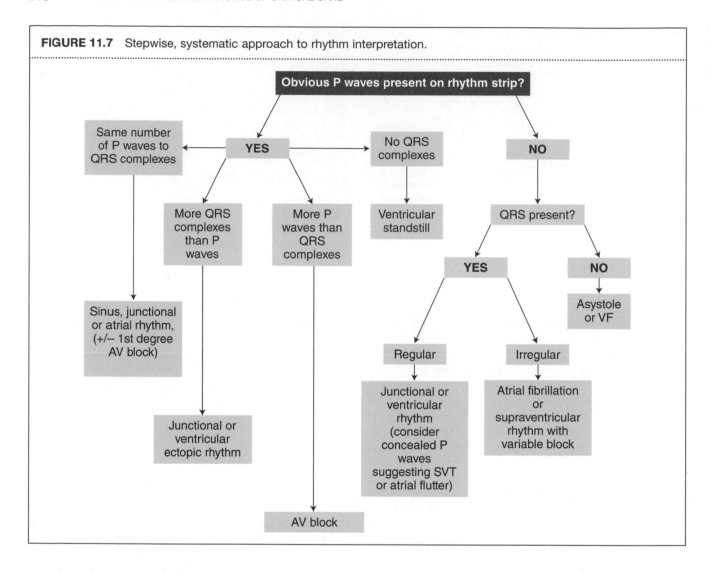

These pulmonary vein ectopics initiate multiple reentry circuits which collide, extinguish and reform, leading to uncoordinated atrial depolarisation.

The term fibrillation refers to a visible quivering motion of the atria resulting from the uncoordinated contraction of groups of muscle segments rather than an organised contraction of the atria as a whole. This accounts for the tendency towards thrombus formation within the atria, due to relative stasis of blood in areas of the chambers, and to decreased emptying of the atria and loss of effective atrial kick.

On the ECG, AF is characterised by an irregularly irregular rhythm (Fig. 11.9).[8] The QRS is narrow, unless there is conduction delay in the ventricles (e.g. bundle branch block). P waves are replaced by fibrillatory waves, which appear as irregular undulations of the electrical baseline at rates of 400–600/min. These conduct irregularly through the AV node so that the ventricular rate is irregular, and usually rapid. The rate may be as high as 160–180/min, and occasionally higher. If there is AV node disease, or the patient is taking drugs that slow AV node conduction, the heart rate may be normal or slow.[3] ST

segment depression may occur even in the absence of chest pain.

> **Practice tip**
>
> AF and heart failure go hand in hand, and each can cause the other. It may not be clear which came first, but be sure to check for both when assessing one of either heart failure or AF.

Acute management

Loss of effective atrial contraction during AF has two important consequences. Firstly, cardiac output and blood pressure may fall due to reduced preload.[7] Secondly, altered flow and stasis of blood within the left atrium can result in thrombus formation and increased risk of thromboembolic events including stroke, limb ischaemia and bowel infarction.[31]

The management of AF in the acute setting is largely based on ensuring adequate haemodynamics and

TABLE 11.2
ECG criteria for rhythms arising in the atria

RHYTHM	ECG CRITERIA
Atrial ectopics (AE) Also known as premature atrial contraction (PAC).	Premature beats with a normal QRS morphology. P waves have a different morphology to sinus P waves. Compensatory pause may occur after the premature beat.
Atrial fibrillation (AF)	Irregularly irregular rhythm. Narrow QRS complex (usually). Discrete P waves not seen – irregular fibrillatory baseline. Rate depends on atrioventricular (AV) node conduction, rarely >180 bpm.
Atrial flutter (AFl)	Regular or regularly irregular rhythm. Narrow QRS complex (usually). Sawtooth flutter waves in inferior leads, atrial rate 200–430/min, commonly around 300/min. 2:1 conduction is common (heart rate around 150 bpm), 1:1 rare unless atrial rate less rapid. Higher degree of AV block in diseased AV nodes, or when rate control drugs given.
Atrial tachycardia (AT)	Regular or regularly irregular rhythm. Narrow QRS complex (usually). P-wave morphology different morphology to sinus rhythm. P waves may be hidden in T waves. Rate depends on AV conduction; may be rapid if 1:1, 2:1. May show 'warm up' in rate or sudden onset, depending on mechanism.

FIGURE 11.8 Sinus rhythm with two atrial ectopic beats (*). The first is premature and has a subtly different P-wave morphology. It conducts normally to the ventricles after a slightly prolonged PR interval. The second ectopic P wave can be seen distorting the ST segment/T wave but is much more premature and is blocked by the AV node – a non-conducted atrial ectopic.

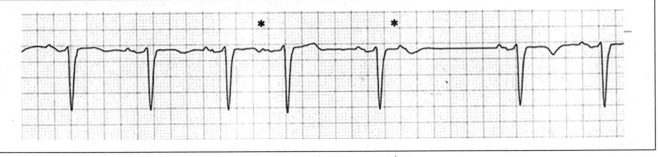

FIGURE 11.9 Atrial fibrillation with a rapid (uncontrolled) ventricular response. The rate is around 170/min and the rhythm irregularly irregular.

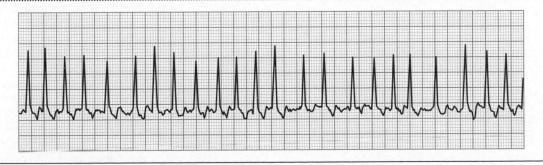

anticoagulation, along with management of the rate and the arrhythmia itself.[32] In patients without adverse features (shock, syncope, myocardial ischaemia or severe heart failure), slowing the ventricular rate (rate control) may be sufficient to stabilise cardiovascular function and manage symptoms.[2] Beta-blockers are commonly used although their negative inotropic properties make them problematic for patients with poor LV function; in these individuals, digoxin or amiodarone may be preferred.[3] If beta-blockers are contraindicated (e.g. in asthma or diabetes), diltiazem and verapamil are alternatives; they are also negative inotropes.[33]

If adverse features are present, direct current (DC) cardioversion may be necessary (see discussion below).[2] Although DC cardioversion has a high success rate, recurrence of AF is common; antiarrhythmic drugs (usually amiodarone) may be given to maintain sinus rhythm.[32] Amiodarone has a high success rate in both restoring and maintaining sinus rhythm.[34] In cases where DC cardioversion is unavailable, or restoration of sinus rhythm is not deemed urgent, it can be used to revert the rhythm. Amiodarone is given as an intravenous loading dose of 300 mg over 1 hour, followed by an infusion of up to 900 mg over 24 hours. Hypotension, bradycardia and phlebitis may occur during acute loading with amiodarone.[35] Hypotension is usually due to rapid administration; using a central venous catheter is recommended to avoid phlebitis.

All patients with AF must be assessed for stroke risk, which increases with age, comorbidity, duration of the arrhythmia and the use of cardioversion. Intrinsic patient factors should be assessed using the CHA$_2$DS$_2$-VASC score (Table 11.3).[36] Any patient with a score of two or more should be offered long-term anticoagulation.[3,32] Anticoagulation must be considered in patients undergoing cardioversion (whether electrical or chemical) if AF has been present for 48 hours or more, or if the patient has a significant risk of stroke (CHA$_2$DS$_2$-VASC score of $\geq$2 in men and $\geq$3 in women).[32] Ideally, oral anticoagulation is given for 3 weeks prior to cardioversion.[37] This may not be practical in acute settings; the use of low-molecular-weight or unfractionated heparin given as soon as possible before cardioversion is a reasonable alternative if cardioversion is deemed urgent, as is transoesophageal echocardiogram to exclude left atrial thrombus.[2] Bleeding risk should also be assessed; in some patients, this may outweigh the benefits of anticoagulation – for example, immediately after major surgery or trauma. Where possible, anticoagulation should be continued for 4 weeks after cardioversion in all individuals, and long term in those with a CHA$_2$DS$_2$-VASC score of 2 or more.[3,32]

Long-term management

In the longer term, some individuals with AF will benefit from catheter ablation.[3] In the 'pulmonary vein isolation' procedure, ablation catheters are inserted via the femoral vein and advanced to the right atrium. The left atrium is then entered using a transeptal puncture. Energy sources including radiofrequency (heat) or cryothermal (freezing) are used to create encircling lesions around the pulmonary veins and/or within the atrial myocardium.[38] Success rates are as high as 90% in patients with paroxysmal AF and normal hearts but decline as comorbidity and persistence of the arrhythmia increase.[38]

If ablation and drug therapy are unsuccessful or contraindicated, a 'pace and ablate' strategy offers a treatment of last resort.[39] Ablation of the AV node is used to create complete heart block (CHB) so that rapid responses to AF no longer occur. A permanent pacemaker is necessary for future rate support (usually with rate responsive pacing), and patients are rendered pacemaker dependent for life.[39]

Atrial flutter

Atrial flutter arises from the same causes as AF and has a similar thromboembolic risk; acute management is identical to AF.[32] Unlike AF, the mechanism underlying atrial flutter is a single macro-reentrant circuit, usually occurring in the right atrium. In typical atrial flutter, the most common variant, depolarisation sweeps continuously around the tricuspid valve annulus in a counterclockwise direction.[20] This produces an organised rhythm in which 'sawtooth' flutter waves, without an intervening isoelectric line, are seen at rates between 220 and 400/min. Most commonly the rate is close to 300/min. Flutter waves are best seen in inferior ECG leads (Fig. 11.10). There is commonly 2:1, 3:1 or 4:1 AV block, resulting in a regular, narrow complex rhythm with a ventricular rate of approximately 150, 100 or 75/min respectively (when the flutter rate is 300).[1] If variable AV conduction occurs, the rhythm is regularly irregular. Conduction at 1:1 ratios is rare in adults unless the flutter rate itself is slow.

TABLE 11.3

CHA$_2$DS$_2$-VASC score. Anticoagulation is mandated if the individual scores $\geq$2

RISK FACTORS	POINTS
Congestive heart failure/left ventricular dysfunction	1
Hypertension	1
Age 75 or more	2
Diabetes mellitus	1
Stroke/transient ischaemic attack/thromboembolic event	2
Vascular disease (coronary heart disease, peripheral vascular disease, aortic plaque)	1
Age 65–74	1
Female gender	2
Maximum score	9

FIGURE 11.10 Atrial flutter with variable block. Note the obvious sawtooth baseline. The atrial rate is regular and a little faster than 300/min, while the ventricular rate is irregular because of the variable block. At times the ventricular rate is close to 150/min (when there is 2:1 block) and at other times close to 100/min (when there is 3:1 block).

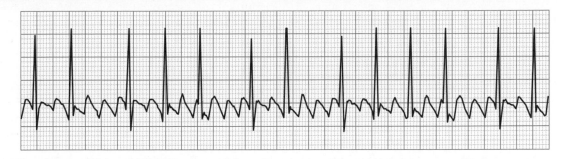

FIGURE 11.11 Atrial tachycardia onset with the often-seen 'warm up'. After three sinus beats at 60/min the first atrial ectopic emerges at a rate of 105/min and the atrial rate then accelerates over four beats before settling at the atrial tachycardia rate of 160/min. The rhythm becomes regular, with a different P-wave morphology and shorter PR interval. Despite merging with the T waves, the abnormal P waves are still easily identified. The QRS during tachycardia is unchanged from that during sinus rhythm.

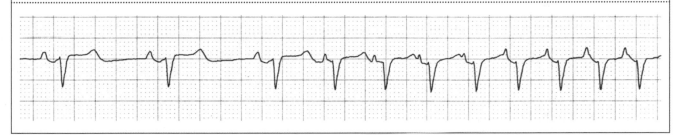

Atrial flutter is highly amenable to catheter ablation, which has a class I indication in clinical guidelines.[25] A lesion is created across the cavotricuspid isthmus (CTI), a narrow part of the reentry circuit bordered by the inferior vena cava and tricuspid valve annulus. CTI ablation can be performed under conscious sedation and has a success rate in excess of 90%; complications are rare.[25]

Atrial tachycardia

Atrial tachycardia describes a rhythm arising in either atrium, usually due to a rapidly firing ectopic focus or a reentry circuit.[20] The atrial rate can be from 100 to 250 bpm and the atrial rhythm is very regular. The ventricular rhythm is regular if there is 1:1 or 2:1 conduction but will be regularly irregular if there is variable AV block; 1:1 conduction is more common than in atrial flutter. P waves may be appreciably different to the sinus P waves, although it is common for them to be concealed in the T wave owing to the rate[9] (Fig. 11.11). When atrial tachycardia is accompanied by high-degree AV block (multiple consecutive non-conducted P waves), digoxin toxicity is the major cause and should be investigated.

Atrial tachycardia is less common than AF or flutter, and variable in its presentation. In younger patients with normal hearts, it often arises from abnormal automaticity in the right atrium and has a benign prognosis with no increase in stroke risk.[1] In older patients, and those with structural heart disease, it more commonly arises from the left atrium or pulmonary veins, in which case it has a similar prognosis to AF. Left atrial tachycardia may occur following AF ablation, and often involves a macro-reentrant circuit around the mitral valve annulus or roof of the left atrium.[38] Atrial tachycardias are treated in the same way as AF and flutter in the acute setting; catheter ablation is often used in long-term management.

Multifocal atrial tachycardia

Multiple rapidly discharging ectopic foci may participate together to form multifocal atrial tachycardia at rates above 100/min. This makes for an irregular tachycardia in which three or more distinct P-wave morphologies can be seen (Fig. 11.12). Multifocal atrial tachycardia may be seen incidentally in the young but is most commonly seen in chronic obstructive pulmonary disease, particularly if the patient is mechanically ventilated because of disease exacerbation. It is also seen in other chronic pulmonary conditions.

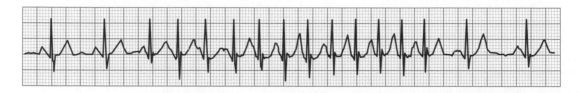

FIGURE 11.12 Multifocal atrial tachycardia at around 100/min. At least three distinct P wave morphologies which are different to the slower sinus P waves are evident, and at different rates creating irregularity. From a patient with chronic obstructive pulmonary disease.

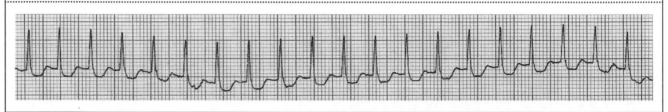

FIGURE 11.13 Supraventricular tachycardia. There are regular, narrow QRS complexes at a rate of 180 bpm. No atrial activity can be seen (the biphasic waveform between the QRS complexes is the T wave).

Supraventricular tachycardia

The term supraventricular tachycardia (SVT) may be used for any tachycardia originating in the atria or AV node. However the distinct diagnosis of atrial fibrillation or flutter can usually be made from the ECG and so the term SVT is generally reserved for atrioventricular nodal reentry tachycardia (AVNRT), atrioventricular reciprocating tachycardia (AVRT) or atrial tachycardia (AT). Typically, these have narrow QRS complexes and P waves are often difficult or impossible to see[40] (Fig. 11.13). In 90% of SVTs the cause is a reentrant circuit that includes the AV node; in the remaining 10% the rhythm is AT.[20] Reentrant SVT results from minor congenital abnormalities in the conduction system and occurs in people of all ages, including children. Unlike AF or flutter, it is not associated with structural heart disease or other chronic disorders.[25] When SVT is associated with a wide QRS (most commonly bundle branch block), the term SVT with aberrancy is used.

SVT is usually paroxysmal in nature, with episodes lasting from seconds to hours. These often terminate spontaneously without intervention. The most common symptom is palpitations; more rarely, breathlessness, chest pain, dizziness or syncope occur.[40] Reentrant SVT falls into two distinct types: AVNRT and AVRT.[20]

Atrioventricular nodal reentrant tachycardia

AVNRT accounts for 60% of SVT, is more common in women, and commonly presents in the middle years of life.[25] Typically the rate is between 140 and 180/minute and the QRS is narrow. It is common for sufferers to seek

medical attention because of palpitations, lightheadedness or shortness of breath. AVNRT requires two distinct pathways connecting the atrium to the AV node ('dual AV node physiology'), described as the 'slow' and 'fast' pathways. The fast pathway conducts quickly but has a long refractory period and the slow pathway conducts slowly but with shorter refractory duration.[20] Normally, the fast pathway accounts for conduction to the AV node, contributing to the normal PR interval of 0.12–0.20 seconds. If the fast pathway is blocked, conduction via the slow pathway would see a longer PR interval of 0.30 seconds or more.

With a longer refractory duration, the fast pathway is more prone to developing block. Premature P waves (ectopics) may be blocked but conduction still occurs down the slow pathway, with an evidently longer PR interval.[41] If the fast pathway has recovered by the time the impulse arrives in the AV node, retrograde conduction back to atria may occur via the fast pathway and re-excite the atria. Conduction may then continue around this reentry circuit of slow pathway–AV node–fast pathway–atria producing tachycardia. There is usually 1:1 conduction to the ventricles. Conduction time from the AV node to the ventricles is generally similar to the time for retrograde conduction to the atria and so P waves are either hidden within the QRS or may be seen just at the end of the QRS or early ST segment.[1] The P wave often distorts the final part of the QRS and gives the impression of a small R wave late in the QRS in V1 (pseudo-R wave in V1) or a small S wave (pseudo-S wave) in lead II. This is a useful feature for diagnosis as the pseudo-R or S waves are present during the tachycardia but not during sinus rhythm before onset.[41] See Fig. 11.14 for this appearance and onset pattern of AVNRT.

FIGURE 11.14 Atrioventricular nodal reentry tachycardia (AVNRT). Lead V1. After two beats of sinus rhythm initially, there is a slightly premature atrial ectopic which conducts with a short PR interval. Another atrial ectopic follows which is more premature and is followed by the characteristic onset of AVNRT: the PR interval increases abruptly to 0.36 s, with onset of tachycardia at 140 bpm. The P waves during the tachycardia can be seen distorting the end of the QRS (the 'pseudo R wave in V1' of AVNRT), which is not present before the tachycardia.

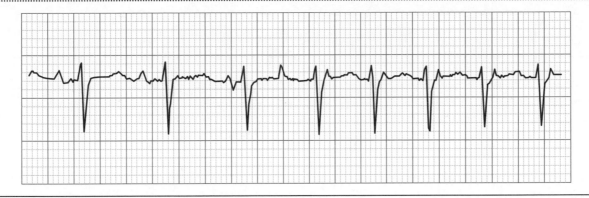

FIGURE 11.15 Antidromic AVRT, recorded using an ambulatory monitor. The patient was a fit young man, who complained of palpitation during exercise. Antidromic AVRT was reproduced during an electrophysiology study, and a left-sided accessory pathway found and ablated. Note the wide QRS, which can be indistinguishable from ventricular tachycardia.

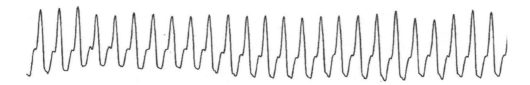

Atrioventricular reentrant tachycardia

Atrioventricular reentrant tachycardia (AVRT) occurs in patients with an accessory pathway, also known as a bypass tract or bundle of Kent.[24] In the normal heart, the bundle of His is the only electrical connection between atria and ventricles.[7] An accessory pathway is a minor congenital abnormality in which strands of myocardium cross the AV fibrous ring, creating an extra conduction pathway between the atria and the ventricles.[20] AVRT is a reentry arrhythmia involving the atria, AV node, ventricles and the accessory pathway. The majority of AVRT is orthodromic, meaning that initial conduction to the ventricle occurs in the normal fashion through the AV node. An atrial ectopic conducts to the ventricles via the AV node and returns to the atria via the accessory pathway, creating a rapid, regular narrow complex tachycardia. Retrograde P waves are sometimes visible in the ST segment or T wave.[40] Less commonly, P waves conduct to the ventricles via the accessory pathway and return to the atria via retrograde conduction through the AV node (antidromic AVRT). In these cases the QRS is wide and resembles monomorphic ventricular tachycardia (VT). P waves are usually difficult to discern, hidden within T waves (Fig. 11.15).

Around 50% of accessory pathways conduct only in a retrograde direction (from ventricles to atria).[24] These pathways are described as 'concealed' because their presence cannot be deduced from the 12-lead ECG during sinus rhythm. They can only support orthodromic AVRT. The remaining 50% conduct in an antegrade fashion across the accessory pathway (atria to ventricles), or in both directions. These pathways are described as 'manifest' because they cause pre-excitation, which can be seen on the 12-lead ECG.[24] Pre-excitation is early electrical activation of the ventricle via the accessory pathway. During sinus rhythm, depolarisation spreads to the ventricles via the accessory pathway and the cardiac conduction system; it arrives earlier via the pathway because this lacks the delay that occurs in the AV node.[7] The main ECG signs of pre-excitation are a short PR interval and a slurring of the first part of the QRS complex, referred to as a delta wave (Fig. 11.16).[9]

FIGURE 11.16   Pre-excitation during sinus rhythm. Note the short PR interval (<120 ms) and slurred upstroke of the QRS complex (delta wave).

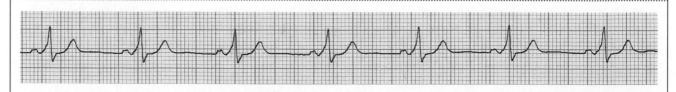

FIGURE 11.17   Pre-excited AF in a young woman. Note the irregular rhythm. Most of the QRS complexes are wide, as the impulses from the atria have conducted down the accessory pathway. Conduction via the AV node rather than the accessory pathway is seen in the middle four beats, the first of which is probably fusion with accessory pathway conduction. The pathway was successfully ablated.

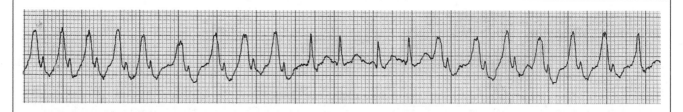

Patients with a pre-excited ECG and symptoms of arrhythmia are said to have Wolff–Parkinson–White (WPW) syndrome, which is associated with a small increased risk of sudden cardiac death (SCD).[25] In patients with WPW syndrome, atrial fibrillation becomes a potentially lethal arrhythmia because conduction via the accessory pathway can occur at rates up to 300/min, producing an irregular broad complex tachycardia at rates which produce syncope.[1] (Fig. 11.17) If sustained at such rapid rates, degeneration into ventricular fibrillation is likely.[42] Pre-excited AF should be terminated with antiarrhythmic drugs or DC cardioversion. Digoxin and other AV conduction-slowing drugs must be avoided as they may accelerate conduction across the accessory pathway.[2]

Practice tip

Narrow complex tachycardias are sometimes difficult to differentiate once they have settled at their tachycardia rate. However, the onset pattern may offer definitive information about the arrhythmia and so it is useful to go back through telemetry records to capture the moment of onset. Many arrhythmias will be clearer with this step.

Treatment of SVT due to AVNRT and AVRT

In both AVNRT and AVRT, the AV node is part of the reentry circuit. Slowing AV node conduction terminates reentry and is the primary approach to acute management.[2]

Vagal manoeuvres (non-invasive techniques that increase parasympathetic tone to the heart) are recommended first-line interventions; they include carotid sinus massage and the Valsalva manoeuvre. They are effective in only 25% of cases, although a UK study demonstrated a 43% success rate using a modified Valsalva in which the patients' legs were raised at the end of the manoeuvre.[2,43] If vagal manoeuvres are unsuccessful or impractical, intravenous adenosine should be given. The initial dose is 6 mg, increased to 12 mg if ineffective, and again to 18 mg if necessary.[2] Adenosine briefly blocks the AV node; it is highly effective but causes unpleasant, albeit transient, symptoms such as chest pain, dizziness and breathlessness. Conscious patients should be warned of these prior to administration.[40] Adenosine is contraindicated in asthma; verapamil 2.5–5 mg intravenously (IV) is a good alternative.[2] SVT rarely causes serious haemodynamic compromise; if this occurs, DC cardioversion should be performed.

Practice tip

Failure to terminate SVT with adenosine suggests that either the drug has been given too slowly (it has a half-life of <10 seconds) or that the rhythm is not reentrant SVT. Adenosine should be given as a rapid bolus in a large, proximal vein followed by an immediate flush. Always record a rhythm strip during drug administration; if the rhythm is not SVT, the underlying atrial activity (P, flutter or fibrillation waves) will be apparent during the pause in ventricular activity.

Although reentrant SVT can be managed using vagal techniques and/or antiarrhythmics drugs over the long term, the most effective treatment is catheter ablation. This has a success rate above 90% and a complication rate below 1% in experienced centres.[25] In WPW syndrome, ablation is a class I recommendation as it reduces the risk of SCD.[44]

Ventricular arrhythmias

Ventricular arrhythmias occur as single ectopic beats or couplets (two consecutive ectopics). Ventricular tachycardia is defined as three or more beats in succession at a rate greater than 100/min.[45] VT may be self limiting, and when lasting less than 30 seconds is termed non-sustained. Self-limiting runs of ventricular arrhythmia are sometimes asymptomatic, but more frequently cause palpitations, dizziness and even loss of consciousness. Symptoms depend on rate, underlying ventricular status and duration.[1] Sustained ventricular arrhythmias (>30 s duration) more commonly cause haemodynamic compromise, and may cause cardiac arrest; immediate assessment and treatment are therefore required.[45] The ECG rhythm criteria for ventricular arrhythmias are summarised in Table 11.4.

Ventricular ectopic beats

Ventricular ectopic beats are also known as premature ventricular contractions (PVCs).[9] On the ECG, they appear as premature beats with a broad QRS complex (Fig. 11.18). There is no preceding P wave, and the ST segment and T waves are discordant (in the opposite direction to the QRS complex). The QRS complex is often tall and bizarre in appearance; it may be notched.[8]

Single PVCs are common and relatively benign, especially in structurally normal hearts.[1] They frequently arise from a single ventricular focus producing a single, uniform QRS shape (monomorphic). Increasing frequency of PVCs may precede more sustained arrhythmias, especially if they are polymorphic or occur in couplets. In critically ill patients, an increasing PVC frequency suggests a heightened risk of sustained ventricular arrhythmia and should prompt patient assessment and optimisation. Electrolytes should be checked and replaced if necessary, especially potassium and magnesium.[46] Oxygenation, tissue perfusion and acid–base status should be optimised. When ventricular ectopics alternate with sinus beats, the resulting rhythm is referred to as ventricular bigeminy (Fig. 11.19) and, if every third beat, ventricular trigeminy. Box 11.1 lists

TABLE 11.4

ECG rhythm criteria for ventricular and cardiac arrest arrhythmias

RHYTHM	ECG CRITERIA
Ventricular ectopics (VE) Also known as premature ventricular contraction (PVC)	Premature beats with a broad QRS complex (≥0.12 s) Discordant T wave No preceding P wave Compensatory pause may occur after beat Occur in single beats, couplets and triplets
Monomorphic ventricular tachycardia (VT)	Three or more consecutive broad QRS beats (≥0.12 s). Every QRS has the same morphology Regular rhythm with heart rate >100/min P waves do not precede the QRS but dissociated P waves may be seen in the T-waves and ST segments
Torsades de pointes (TdP)	Three or more consecutive broad QRS beats (≥0.12 s). Obvious polymorphism of QRS with 'sinusoidal twisting' around the baseline and transitions between polarity of QRS complexes – first positive then negative. Slightly irregular rhythm with a heart rate 220–330 bpm. No P waves seen. ECG during sinus rhythm shows QT prolongation
Ventricular fibrillation (VF)	No recognisable/organised QRS. Irregular baseline deflections of variable amplitude at 300–500/min. P waves not discernible
Asystole	Absence of QRS complexes. ECG baseline commonly shows slow undulation.
Ventricular standstill	Regular P waves but no QRS complexes or T waves
Agonal rhythm	Extremely slow ventricular rate (<20 bpm). QRS complexes usually very wide. Merging of QRS and T wave produces a 'sine wave' rhythm.

FIGURE 11.18 Monomorphic ventricular ectopics. The second and fifth beats are PVCs. Note their prematurity, broad QRS complex, discordant T wave and lack of preceding P waves.

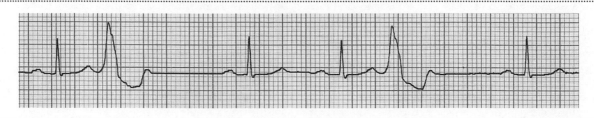

FIGURE 11.19 Ventricular bigeminy. Sinus beats alternate with broad complex QRS complexes (PVCs) which are not preceded by P waves.

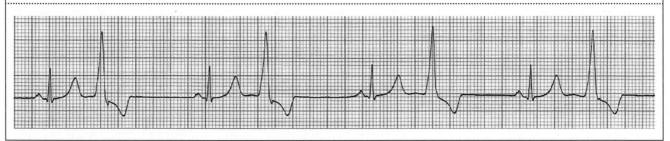

BOX 11.1

Patterns of ventricular ectopy suggestive of a higher risk of arrhythmia

- Increasing frequency of ectopy
- Polymorphic ectopics
- Couplets or triplets
- Bigeminy or trigeminy
- Three or more ectopics in a row (non-sustained ventricular tachycardia)
- R-on-T ectopics
- Bradycardia-dependent ectopics when the QT interval is long

---

patterns of ectopy suggesting increased risk of sustained arrhythmia.

Monomorphic ventricular tachycardia

Ventricular tachycardia describes a run of three or more consecutive beats of ventricular origin, at a rate greater than 100/min.[47] Most VT is monomorphic (all beats of a single shape); on the ECG, it appears as a rapid, regular rhythm with broad QRS complexes that are often bizarre and notched (Fig. 11.20).[8] There may be minor irregularity at the onset of VT and prior to self termination. P waves do not precede the QRS complex, although dissociated P waves (P waves that have no causal relationship with the QRS) may be visible at a slower rate than the VT.

Dissociated P waves are a useful diagnostic feature as they rule out non-VT causes of broad complex tachycardia. These include supraventricular arrhythmia with aberrant conduction and antidromic AVRT.[48] Other features that are diagnostic of VT include capture and fusion beats, seen more in slower VTs. Capture beats are sinus impulses which conduct to the ventricles as single beats amongst the broad VT beats. Fusion beats too are conducted beats but which coincide with VT beats, also as single beats. They are slightly narrower than the VT beats and with some variation in morphology to the VT beats. Both capture and fusion beats are slightly premature compared with the VT rhythm. Very fast VT is sometimes described as ventricular flutter (Fig. 11.21).

The most common cause of monomorphic VT is structural heart disease, especially coronary artery disease.[1] The rhythm is common during acute myocardial infarction (MI) and is a common cause of SCD in this setting.[47] The usual mechanism of monomorphic VT is reentry; in critical illness the rhythm also arises owing to abnormal automaticity or triggered activity, secondary to metabolic derangement, increased sympathetic drive and medication use.[20] In 10% of patients evaluated in the outpatient setting, monomorphic VT occurs in the context of a normal heart and has a relatively benign prognosis.[49]

In critically ill people, monomorphic VT frequently causes haemodynamic compromise, and may result in cardiac arrest. Immediate assessment is necessary. If the patient is pulseless, immediate defibrillation and cardiopulmonary resuscitation (CPR) are indicated.[2] If a cardiac output is present, the patient should be assessed for

FIGURE 11.20 The onset of ventricular tachycardia. There are three sinus beats, followed by a ventricular ectopic which emerges from the T wave of the final sinus beat, precipitating VT. The resulting rhythm is fast and regular, with a wide QRS, discordant T waves and no obvious P waves.

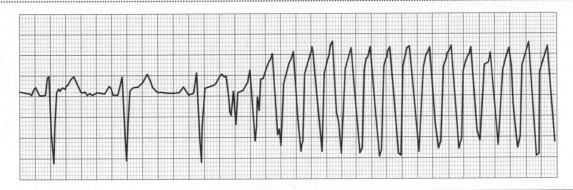

FIGURE 11.21 Ventricular flutter in a 16-year-old female recovering from tricyclic antidepressant overdose. The heart rate is an astonishing 350 bpm, with broad QRS complexes. It is very regular and monomorphic, though it is almost impossible to say which is QRS and which is T wave.

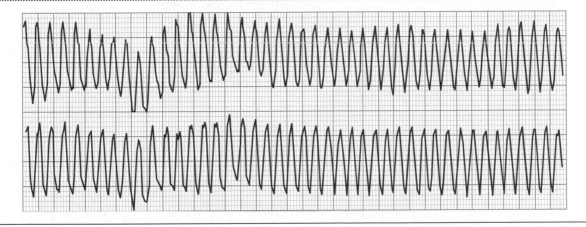

haemodynamic instability, shock, myocardial ischaemia, severe heart failure and syncope.[2] If any of these are present, DC cardioversion is recommended in clinical guidelines.[2] Intravenous amiodarone may be given post-cardioversion to prevent recurrence. In stable patients without adverse features, drug therapy alone is sufficient (typically using amiodarone); careful monitoring for clinical deterioration is necessary. As with ventricular ectopics, patient optimisation is essential. Overdrive pacing may terminate VT if available; the ventricles are briefly paced at a higher rate than the VT, and then the pacing abruptly terminated, hopefully interrupting the reentrant circuit and allowing sinus rhythm to resume. There is a small risk of converting the rhythm to ventricular fibrillation (VF), so this treatment is usually reserved for situations where drugs are ineffective.[1] Cardioversion equipment should be on hand.

> **Practice tip**
>
> Although amiodarone is currently the drug of choice for ventricular arrhythmias, lignocaine (lidocaine) was widely used in the past and remains an effective alternative, especially in the context of myocardial ischaemia. Like amiodarone, it may cause hypotension. Overdose can cause central nervous system dysfunction including slurred speech, dizziness, numbness and seizures.[50]

Polymorphic ventricular tachycardia

In polymorphic VT, the shape and orientation of the QRS complex is variable. The QRS may undergo transitions between upright and inverted (negative) QRS complexes, or may alternate between two discrete morphologies on a beat-to-beat basis (bidirectional VT, seen most commonly in digitalis intoxication) or switch between groups of beats, with first one morphology and then another.[47]

Torsades de pointes is the most common polymorphic VT.[1] In TdP, the QRS undergoes a gradual transition from a negative QRS complex to a positive one, and then back again. There is usually an ill-defined transition between the two, and the amplitude of the QRS complex tends to rise and fall, producing an overall appearance that is sometimes described as 'sinusoidal twisting around the baseline'.[51] The key ECG features of TdP are a rapid, broad complex tachycardia with a varying QRS morphology (Fig. 11.22). The rate is often around 300 bpm and somewhat regular, although irregularity may be more apparent during the transitions between QRS directions. No atrial activity can be seen.

TdP is caused by triggered activity and is associated with delayed repolarisation, seen as QT interval prolongation on the ECG during sinus rhythm (a corrected QT (QTc) of more than 450 ms in men, or 460 ms in women).[52] Bradycardia or pauses increase the risk of TdP in susceptible patients, as does electrolyte depletion.[53] The rhythm often occurs in short, self-terminating bursts which are recurrent, or it may be sustained and eventually degrade to ventricular fibrillation. First-line treatment is intravenous magnesium sulfate 2 g (8 mmol), given over 1–2 minutes and repeated if necessary.[45] Of equal importance is cessation of any agents which are known to prolong the QT interval; the list of such agents is impressive and includes amiodarone and sotalol. Increasing the heart rate with pacing, if available, or isoprenaline is effective at preventing recurrence, but not for interrupting actual episodes of TdP.[53] Other aspects of management include replacement of electrolytes, and correction of ischaemia and acid–base status.[53] Many antiarrhythmics have the potential to prolong the QT interval. The exception is lignocaine, although evidence of efficacy in TdP is limited to animal studies and clinical case reports.[54]

If TdP is sustained, syncope usually occurs and degradation to ventricular fibrillation is likely. Immediate DC cardioversion is indicated.[53]

Ventricular fibrillation

During VF there are no recognisable QRS complexes; the rhythm is fast, chaotic and disorganised. On ECG there is rapid fluctuation of the baseline at rates of 400–600/min, which may be fine or coarse (Fig. 11.23).[51] The ventricles fibrillate (quiver), causing loss of effective ventricular contraction and cardiac arrest. Immediate defibrillation and CPR are required; if unsuccessful, intravenous adrenaline is used to facilitate CPR, and amiodarone may be given before consideration of second-line antiarrhythmics.[2] VF is a common cause of sudden cardiac death, and may accompany myocardial ischaemia or infarction, although like VT it also occurs in the context of non-cardiac critical illness. VF may be a primary arrhythmia or may be the end point of deterioration of other sustained tachyarrhythmias (secondary). VF is the mechanism of sudden death in some inherited cardiac conditions, for example the Brugada syndrome.[45]

Long-term management of ventricular arrhythmias

Any patient surviving a cardiac arrest due to VT or VF should be offered an implantable cardioverter defibrillator (ICD), unless there is a clear and reversible cause.[45] ICD

FIGURE 11.22 Torsades de pointes (TdP) polymorphic ventricular tachycardia. After three beats of sinus tachycardia, a ventricular ectopic beat emerging from the T wave triggers the onset of TdP. Note the characteristic sinusoidal twisting around the baseline, with the QRS increasing and decreasing in amplitude, along with transitions between directions of the QRS. The rate is extremely rapid, exceeding 300/min at times. It is much more common to see TdP emerging from bradycardia or pauses rather than sinus tachycardia as here.

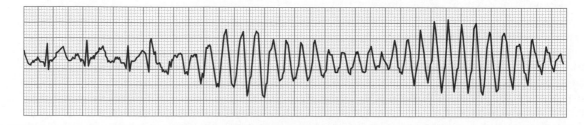

FIGURE 11.23   Ventricular fibrillation. The rhythm is rapid, irregular and wholly disorganised. Variations in rate, amplitude and morphology sometimes conspire to approximate the appearance of VT-like beats but are not convincing and sporadic. No clear-cut QRS complexes are present. The early part of the strip is sometimes termed 'coarse' VF and the later a little more 'fine' based on amplitude.

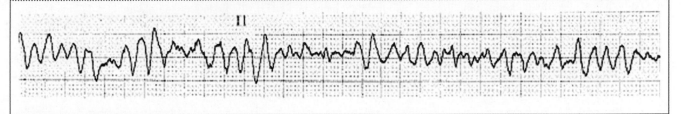

FIGURE 11.24   Asystole. No electrical activity can be seen. Note the often-seen fluctuation of the baseline.

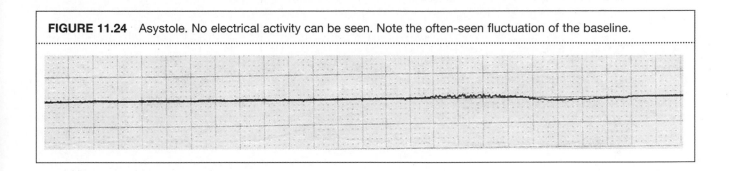

implantation may also be indicated in patients with sustained VT without cardiac arrest, and in individuals with significant LV systolic dysfunction in whom VT risk is greater.[56] Most patients benefit from beta-blockade, and some will need additional antiarrhythmic drug therapy. The choice of antiarrhythmics is influenced by known efficacy, contraindications and any identifiable mechanisms or behaviours. Ablation of VT is now commonplace, with success rates exceeding 80% in patients without structural heart disease.[57] When heart disease is present, outcomes are less certain; success approaches 80% in patients with an ischaemic substrate but is lower in non-ischaemic patients.[57] The aim of ablation may be to prevent recurrent VT, VT storms and ICD shocks rather than complete freedom from arrhythmia. Catheter ablation of VF is less commonly attempted and is limited by an incomplete understanding of the mechanisms that trigger and sustain the arrhythmia; despite this, some success has been demonstrated in certain subgroups, for example those with Brugada syndrome.[58,59]

Asystole, ventricular standstill and agonal rhythm

In a significant proportion of cardiac arrests, asystole, ventricular standstill or agonal rhythm are the primary arrhythmia, or they may develop during attempted resuscitation.[60] Ischaemia, hyperkalaemia and acidosis should be considered when asystole, ventricular standstill or agonal rhythms occur. The ECG rhythm criteria for these arrhythmias are summarised in Table 11.4.

Asystole

Asystole is the complete absence of cardiac electrical activity (Fig. 11.24).[8] The heart does not contract, and cardiac arrest occurs. Commonly, the ECG baseline has a slight wander; if it is completely flat, ECG leads may not be properly connected and should be checked. The treatment of asystole is CPR, intravenous adrenaline and reversal of underlying causes.[2] Additional sympathomimetics may be attempted, and atropine is sometimes used although unsupported by resuscitation guidelines. Temporary cardiac pacing should be attempted if available, particularly in the post-cardiac surgical patient. Major haemorrhage is a common cause of asystole, although the rhythm is also seen late in cardiac arrest when defibrillation has been unsuccessful. The outcomes in asystolic arrest are poor; national audit data from the UK revealed that only 1 in 10 patients with asystole survived to hospital discharge.[61]

Ventricular standstill

In ventricular standstill, the sinus node continues to discharge but without a ventricular response, and no escape rhythm emerges; cardiac arrest occurs.[8] The ECG appearance is similar to asystole, except that regular P waves are seen (Fig. 11.25). There are no QRS complexes or T waves. Ventricular standstill may develop from CHB, which is discussed below.[2] Emergency pacing is the first-line treatment if available.[8] If this is unsuccessful, CPR, adrenaline and a search for reversible causes must be commenced.

FIGURE 11.25   Ventricular standstill. P waves at a rate of 80/min can be seen, but there are no QRS complexes. The patient may respond to emergency pacing.

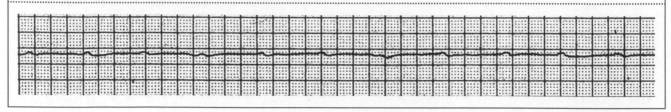

FIGURE 11.26   Agonal rhythm. Note the extremely wide QRS complexes with uncertain, but long, T-wave duration, slow rate (45/min) and low amplitude. Terminal rhythm in a palliative patient.

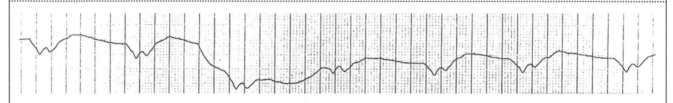

Agonal rhythm

Agonal rhythm may be seen as the final rhythm in terminal illness before progression to asystole, in which case it is largely due to metabolic failure of the heart and inability to sustain the normal electrochemical membrane concentrations necessary for conduction. In critical care it may also be seen in the late stages of unsuccessful resuscitation attempts.[2] It rarely produces a palpable pulse. On the ECG, slow, often irregular and increasingly wide QRS complexes of varying amplitude are seen, with no P waves (Fig. 11.26). As time elapses, the rhythm slows further and the QRS complexes broaden until asystole occurs.[1] At times the very wide QRS and the T wave blend and come to resemble a sine wave. This appearance may also accompany extremes of hyperkalaemia, and if appearing unexpectedly may be due to inadvertent rapid potassium administration. Acute causes of agonal rhythm include tricyclic antidepressant or flecainide overdose. Paced rhythm QRS complexes develop these same agonal patterns of widening/sine wave appearance before eventual loss of capture for the same reasons as above.

Escape rhythms

In sinus node failure or AV block, the inherent automaticity of distal tissues can provide a cardiac rhythm.[8] This phenomenon is described as 'escape'.[1] Escape beats may arise from the AV junction, in which case the QRS complex is narrow, or from the distal (ventricular) conduction system, in which case it is broad. Escape occurs in single beats following a pause, or as sustained rhythms during bradycardia. Table 11.5 summarises the ECG features of the escape rhythms.

Junctional rhythm

Junctional rhythm is an escape rhythm arising from the AV junction, which comprises the AV node and bundle of His.[20] The rhythm is regular, with a narrow QRS complex and a rate typically between 40 and 60 bpm.[51] P waves may be present or absent. Depending on the site of origin of the impulse within the AV junction, inverted P waves are seen before the QRS (with a short PR interval) within the ST segment or are hidden within the QRS complex (Fig. 11.27).[1] If there is abnormal enhancement of automaticity, an accelerated junctional rhythm may be seen; this has the same ECG features, but the heart rate is between 60 and 100 bpm. Junctional tachycardia may also occur, at rates above 100/min. Junctional rhythm is often well tolerated, but the slow heart rate and loss of atrial contribution to ventricular filling can compromise patients who are acutely unwell or who have limited haemodynamic reserve. If treatment is necessary, it follows the same format as sinus bradycardia.

Idioventricular rhythm

If both the sinus and AV nodes fail, an idioventricular escape rhythm may arise from the distal conduction system. These distal pacemakers are slow (20–40/min) and unreliable; there is a small risk of asystole or ventricular standstill.[1] The heart rate may be too slow to generate an adequate cardiac output, so acute rate restoration is often necessary. Positive chronotropes and/or pacing may be necessary.[2] On the ECG, the QRS complex is wide and bizarre, with discordant T waves. If P waves are present, they are dissociated from the QRS complex.

TABLE 11.5

ECG rhythm criteria for escape rhythms

RHYTHM	ECG CRITERIA
Junctional escape beat	Beat following a pause in SR; escape rate 40–60 bpm. Narrow QRS complex. Inverted P waves may precede the QRS with short PR interval, be concealed by the QRS, or occur in ST segment.
Junctional rhythm	Regular rhythm with a heart rate of 40–60 bpm. Narrow QRS complex. Inverted P waves may precede the QRS with short PR interval, be concealed by the QRS, or occur in ST segment.
Accelerated junctional rhythm	As per junctional rhythm, but heart rate 60–100 bpm.
Junctional tachycardia	As per junctional rhythm, but rate >100 bpm.
Idioventricular rhythm	Regular rhythm with a rate 20–40 bpm. Broad QRS complex. P waves may be absent, retrogradely conducted, or dissociated from ventricular rhythm.
Accelerated idioventricular rhythm (AIVR)	As idioventricular rhythm, but heart rate >60 bpm.

FIGURE 11.27 Sinus bradycardia followed by onset of junctional escape rhythm. The sinus rate is initially 37 bpm, but then slows further, allowing the junctional escape to emerge at 35/min. The junctional beats are not preceded by P waves; instead, P waves can be seen distorting the ST segment of the last 2 beats.

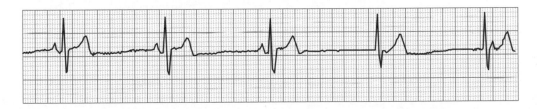

Accelerated idioventricular rhythm

Accelerated idioventricular rhythm (AIVR) is a regular ventricular ectopic rhythm occurring faster than the normal escape rate (between 40 and 100/min). Causes include digitalis toxicity, hyperkalaemia, myocarditis and following successful reperfusion via percutaneous coronary intervention or thrombolytic therapy (Fig. 11.28).[62] AIVR is caused by increased automaticity and like other automatic rhythms may display 'warm-up' behaviour – gradually accelerating rather than displaying the sudden jump in heart rate typical of reentrant arrhythmias.[20] In most cases, it produces a stable cardiac output and requires no treatment; termination usually occurs spontaneously.[62]

Atrioventricular block

AV block is impairment of conduction from the atria to ventricles. It may appear as slowing of AV conduction (long PR interval) or failure to conduct some or all beats.[1] The block may be intermittent or persistent, and the severity of block may change because of changes in the AV node or with changes in the atrial rate. The site of block may be within the AV node itself or in distal conduction tissue

(bundle of His or bilateral bundle branches). The clinical impact depends on the degree of block, the resulting heart rate, metabolic demand at the time, the width of the QRS complex and cardiac reserves. Careful evaluation of the ECG and the patient are therefore required.[2]

AV block occurring within the AV node may be benign and result from changes in autonomic tone, as during sleep.[1] AV node ischaemia may induce block, especially during MI resulting from right coronary artery occlusion.[63] Rate-limiting medications such as digoxin, beta-blockers and calcium channel blockers may also cause or worsen AV block.

AV block occurring below the AV node itself (within the bundle of His or bilateral bundle branches) results from a number of acute and chronic cardiovascular diseases including anterior MI, myocarditis, hypertension and cardiomyopathy.[8] Idiopathic fibrosis of conduction tissues is also common, especially in the elderly. In some cases, the underlying problem relates to a systemic condition; examples include Lyme disease, sarcoidosis and rheumatoid arthritis.[64] Haemodynamic compromise or cardiac arrest are more likely when block arises below the

FIGURE 11.28 Accelerated idioventricular rhythm (AIVR) following reperfusion in myocardial infarction. An accelerated ventricular focus emerges at 65/min, taking over from the slower sinus rate of 60/min. It then accelerates gradually until settling at a rate of 85/min by the end of the second strip. This display of rate 'warm up' at onset is a characteristic of arrhythmias due to increased automaticity. The distortion of the ST segment from the third beat of AIVR onwards is due to retrograde conduction to the atria, creating an inverted P wave.

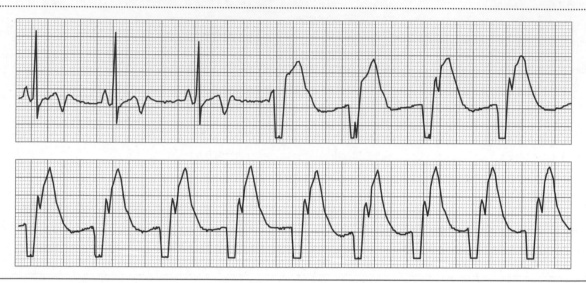

TABLE 11.6
ECG rhythm criteria for atrioventricular (AV) block

RHYTHM	ECG CRITERIA
First-degree AV block (1° AVB)	Regular rhythm. Every P wave followed by a QRS complex. PR interval >0.20 s. QRS usually narrow.
Second-degree AV block Mobitz type I (Wenckebach)	Regularly irregular rhythm. Intermittent non-conducted P waves. PR intervals show progressive PR interval prolongation until 'dropped' beat. QRS usually narrow.
Second-degree AV block Mobitz type II	Regularly irregular, or regular rhythm. Intermittent non-conducted P waves. PR intervals of conducted beats is consistent. QRS often broad.
Third-degree AV block (3° AVB) Also known as complete heart block (CHB)	Slow, regular rhythm (usually <60/min). No causal relationship between P waves and QRS complexes. P waves may be buried in QRS complex and T wave. QRS is usually narrow if there is junctional escape or wide if ventricular.

AV node, and patients often need permanent pacing.[65] The ECG rhythm criteria for atrioventricular block are summarised in Table 11.6.

First-degree AV block

In first-degree AV block, conduction is slow, but every impulse from the sinus node is conducted to the ventricles.[8]

The rhythm may therefore be more accurately defined as AV conduction delay, as no impulses are blocked.[63] On the ECG, the PR interval is greater than 0.20 seconds, but every P wave is followed by a QRS, which is usually narrow (Fig. 11.29).

Conduction delay in first-degree AV block is usually within the AV node; it is a common and benign finding

FIGURE 11.29   First-degree AV block. The PR interval is prolonged at 250 ms, but every P wave is followed by a normal QRS complex (no dropped beats).

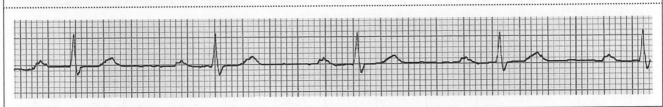

in athletes and during sleep.[1] It rarely causes significant haemodynamic change unless the PR is very long and does not usually require treatment.[8] Monitoring for progression of first-degree block to higher degrees of block is required if it develops during an acute event such as ACS, or upon commencement of conduction-slowing drugs.[63] In the long term, first-degree AV block is associated with an increased risk of atrial fibrillation but does not progress to higher degrees of block in healthy individuals.[65]

Second-degree AV block

In second-degree AV block, conduction failure is intermittent; some impulses are conducted from the atria to the ventricles, while others are blocked.[8] It can be further divided into several categories according to ECG appearance:

- Mobitz type I, also referred to as Wenckebach
- Mobitz type II
- 2:1 AV block.

Mobitz type I (Wenckebach)

Mobitz type I block is usually caused by conduction delay within the AV node. It can be a normal finding during sleep and in athletes, reflecting high vagal tone.[63] Like first-degree heart block, it may complicate acute MI, in which case vigilance for clinical deterioration or progression to higher degrees of block is necessary. The heart rate is often preserved, and treatment is rarely required.

On the ECG, the key feature of Mobitz type I is progressive prolongation of the PR interval over several

beats, followed by conduction failure.[51] The PR interval lengthens, until a P wave is not followed by a QRS complex, commonly referred to as the 'dropped beat' (Fig. 11.30). After the dropped beat, the PR interval returns to baseline and the cycle recurs. The frequency of dropped beats determines the clinical impact and dropped beats become more frequent with worsening of AV node dysfunction, but also with increases in the sinus rate. If every fifth P wave is not conducted then a ratio of 5 P waves to 4 QRSs is present and the 'Wenckebach cycle' can be described as 5 to 4 (5:4). Improvement would see fewer beats dropped and the Wenckebach cycle lengthened to 6:5, 7:6, etc. Worsening of AV conduction sees cycles or ratios shorten to 4:3 or 3:2. Such notation is useful for understanding and documentation of severity or progression. An eye-catching feature of Wenckebach is 'grouped beating' – for example, a group of 4 beats of reasonably regular QRSs, followed by a pause, then another group of 4 and so on. QRS complexes are typically narrow. Symptoms are generally proportional to the frequency of dropped beats and the resultant ventricular rate.[64]

Mobitz type II

Mobitz type II is regarded as more serious AV block and typically pathological rather than benign. The block may be within the AV node or the distal conduction system, and commonly reflects cardiovascular disease.[63] There is a greater risk of progression to CHB, so assessment and monitoring are required.[1] If the heart rate is slow, significant haemodynamic impairment may occur, necessitating drug therapy or pacing.[2] High-grade AV

FIGURE 11.30   Second-degree AV block, Mobitz type I. Every third P wave is not conducted (3:2 conduction). The PR interval can be seen to lengthen before the dropped beats (*). After the dropped beats the cycle starts with a PR interval of 0.18 s. It then extends to 0.25 s before again dropping a beat.

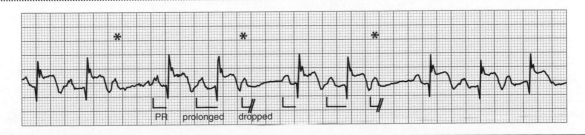

FIGURE 11.31 Second-degree AV block Mobitz type II. There is atrial pacing which does not interfere with any categorisation of the AV block. Initially every fourth paced P wave is blocked before 2:1 block develops midway through the strip. Note the constant PR interval on the conducted beats rather than the progressive PR prolongation typical of type I.

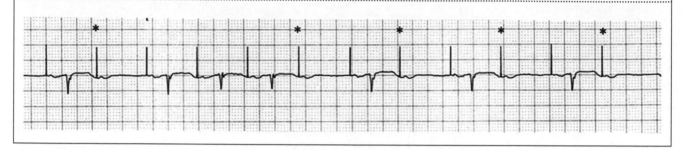

FIGURE 11.32 2:1 AV block. Every second P wave is blocked, with a ventricular rate of 37/min being half the atrial rate. The non-conducted P waves are readily seen just after the T wave of each beat. The PR intervals of conducted beats are uniform in duration (0.20 s).

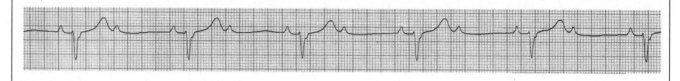

block occurs in some cases, defined as two or more consecutive non-conducted P waves.[63]

On the ECG, some P waves will be followed by QRS complexes, while others will not.[8] Unlike Mobitz type I, the PR interval of the conducted beats is uniform, not lengthening (Fig. 11.31). The rhythm may be regularly irregular; regular for the conducted beats and with the dropped beats providing the irregularity. The same description of dropped beat cycling (4:3, 5:4, etc.) used above can be applied to documenting severity. The QRS is often wide, reflecting distal conduction system disease.[1]

2:1 AV block

Second-degree AV block sometimes occurs in a pattern where every other P wave is blocked, resulting in 2:1 conduction to the ventricles (Fig. 11.32).[51] Using ECG criteria, it is impossible to classify this as either Mobitz I or Mobitz II, because only one PR interval is seen before each dropped beat. The presence or absence of progressive lengthening of the PR is therefore not available to distinguish type I from type II. It should simply be documented, therefore, as 2:1 AV block. In 2:1 AV block with a broad QRS complex, there is greater likelihood that the block is Mobitz type II; an electrophysiological study can be performed if there is doubt about the level of the block.[64]

Third-degree AV block (complete heart block)

In CHB, there is no conduction between the atria and the ventricles.[8] An escape rhythm usually arises below the

level of the block; however, if this fails then ventricular standstill or asystole occurs. Urgent intervention and close monitoring are required; continuous ECG with appropriate alarms is essential.[2] Depending on the site of block within the AV node, there may be junctional escape (narrow QRS, 40–60/min) or ventricular (wide QRS, 20–40/min).[63] Emergency treatment is recommended for CHB with the slower ventricular escape, even when patients appear well.[2]

On the ECG, CHB appears as non-conducted P waves, which are dissociated from the ventricular rhythm.[51] Escape rhythms are usually quite regular and it is usually possible to identify the distinctly unrelated rates of the atria and ventricles (Fig. 11.33).

Practice tip

In atrial fibrillation these degrees of AV block do not apply, with the exception of CHB. Poor AV conduction during AF results in a slow rate but it will be irregular. If CHB develops then the ventricular rate becomes regular, under the control of an escape focus.

Management of AV block

Emergency treatment should be given if adverse features are identified during patient assessment (shock, syncope, myocardial ischaemia or heart failure) or if there is a risk of asystole (recent asystole, Mobitz II AV block, CHB with a

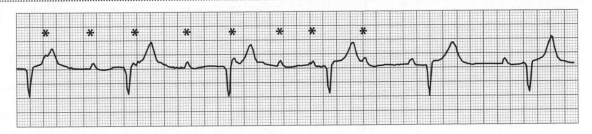

FIGURE 11.33 Complete heart block. The P waves (*) at 90–100/min are regular and at times partially concealed in the QRS or ST segments. A narrow complex escape rhythm is present at 40/min which has no relationship to the P waves (dissociated). The seventh P wave is premature and different in morphology, suggesting it is an (also non-conducted) atrial ectopic beat.

broad QRS, ventricular pauses >3 seconds).[2] As with sinus bradycardia, atropine 500 micrograms IV, repeated up to 3 milligrams, is the first-line recommendation.[63] Atropine reduces the effect of parasympathetic nerves on the heart; the ventricles are poorly supplied with parasympathetic fibres, so atropine may be ineffective in Mobitz II and CHB.[7] If atropine is ineffective, pacing is usually required; other drugs can be used in the interim, as discussed in the management of sinus bradycardia above. Rate-slowing drugs should be stopped or withheld if appropriate.[61]

In the longer term, patients with Mobitz II or complete AV block need permanent pacing unless a reversible cause is identified.[63] AV blocks are often transient and reversible during inferior MI, but permanent and irreversible in anterior MI.[51] When recovery is not expected, a permanent pacemaker should be implanted as soon as possible, as temporary systems are less reliable and more prone to complication.[13] In all forms of AV block, the 12-lead ECG should be carefully evaluated for evidence of underlying conduction system disease, in particular bundle branch blocks and axis deviation.[64]

Antiarrhythmic drugs

Most antiarrhythmic drugs block selective ion channels in the cell membrane, or alter autonomic tone. Their effects include changes in automaticity, conduction velocity, action potential duration and repolarisation.[20] The Vaughan Williams classification organises these drugs into five groups (I–V) based on the principal effect of the drug at the cell membrane. However, the system is imperfect; many drugs have effects from several classes, and classification does not necessarily predict clinical utility (Table 11.7).[66]

The drugs most commonly used in critical care, including notes on their uses and limitations in the acute setting, are listed in Table 11.8. Common (but not universal) problems include negative inotropy, hypotension, depressed sinus and AV node function, and proarrhythmia, along with drug-specific systemic complications.[33] During IV drug administration, the ECG should be continuously monitored for the development of new arrhythmias, bradycardia or AV block, and resuscitation facilities should be immediately available.[67] Of all the drugs, amiodarone

is probably the safest in the acute setting, and the most effective.[66] When used as chronic therapy, however, amiodarone is associated with a worrying range of potentially serious adverse effects.[1]

Cardiac pacing

Cardiac pacing was initially developed to overcome bradycardia and/or AV block.[68] However, applications have expanded, and pacing is also now used to treat tachyarrhythmias (antitachycardia pacing) and to improve left ventricular performance in patients with severe heart failure (cardiac resynchronisation therapy).[69]

Standard antibradycardia pacing allows the heart to be stimulated at a desired rate whenever the heart rate falls below a programmed value, e.g. 50–80 bpm, and for pacing to be withheld when the intrinsic rate is above this rate. Temporary pacing may be provided in an emergency, providing rhythm protection while reversible factors are overcome (e.g. myocardial ischaemia, biochemical or drug influence) or as a bridge to permanent pacemaker implantation.[70]

Principles of pacing

A paced rhythm can be achieved by delivering electrical stimuli through pacing leads attached to the myocardium. Pacing lead systems require two electrodes: a negative electrode via which impulses are delivered to the myocardium, and a positive electrode via which the electrical circuit is completed. Electrical impulses of sufficient strength stimulate the myocardium surrounding the electrode to depolarise and then propagate through the entire myocardium to initiate contraction.[68,71]

Pacing leads (electrodes) may be advanced transvenously to the right ventricular endocardial surface or attached to the epicardium at the time of cardiac surgery.[72]

For epicardial pacing, two separate leads are usually attached to each chamber paced (atrial/ventricular), with one lead connected to each of the negative and positive terminals of the pacemaker (pulse generator).[72] For transvenous pacing, a single lead is used which incorporates both the negative electrode (at the lead tip) and the positive

TABLE 11.7
Vaughan Williams classification system

CLASS	ACTION	DRUGS
IA	Block sodium channels. Prolong the action potential and decrease conduction velocity, increase refractory period. Atrial and ventricular arrhythmias.	Ajmaline Cibenzoline Disopyramide Pilsicainide Procainamide Quinidine
IB	Block sodium channels. Shorten action potential duration and decrease refractory period. Ventricular site of action.	Lignocaine (lidocaine) Mexiletine Phenytoin
IC	Block sodium channels. Marked slowing of conduction velocity with little effect on duration of action potential or refractory period. Atrial and ventricular arrhythmias.	Flecainide Propafenone
II	Block beta-adrenoceptors on the heart (and elsewhere). Decrease sympathetic tone to the heart. Decrease SA and AV node automaticity and conduction velocity.	Atenolol Carvedilol Esmolol Metoprolol Nadolol Propranolol Sotalol
III	Block potassium channels. Increase duration of action potential by prolonging repolarisation.	Amiodarone Dronedarone Dofetilide Ibutilide Sotalol
IV	Block calcium channels. Decrease SA and AV node automaticity and conduction velocity.	Diltiazem Verapamil
V	Other: various mechanisms that do not fit into original classification.	Adenosine Atropine Digoxin Ivabradine Ranolazine Vernakalant

Sources: Fogoros RN, Mandrola JM. Fogoros' electrophysiologic testing. 6th ed. Oxford: Wiley Blackwell; 201;[20] and Dan GA, Martinez-Rubio A, Agewall S, et al Antiarrhythmic drugs – clinical use and clinical decision making: a consensus document from the European Heart Rhythm Association (EHRA) and European Society of Cardiology (ESC) Working Group on Cardiovascular Pharmacology, endorsed by the Heart Rhythm Society (HRS), Asia-Pacific Heart Rhythm Society (APHRS) and International Society of Cardiovascular Pharmacotherapy (ISCP). Europace 2018; Feb 9.[66]

electrode slightly proximal to the tip. In an emergency, these transvenous ventricular pacing wires can be inserted promptly and establish a supportive ventricular rate.[73] Temporary transvenous pacing is almost always undertaken as ventricular pacing only. In the cardiac surgical patient, where direct lead attachment to the epicardium can be performed, pacing may be undertaken as single chamber (atrial or ventricular) or dual chamber (atrial and ventricular).[74]

A major change to placement of ventricular leads has developed more recently. Instead of pacing into the myocardium as described above, leads are increasingly being implanted directly into parts of the conduction system (see section Conduction system pacing below).[75] The two sites currently used are the bundle of His and the left bundle branch. Both are used for standard bradycardia support and as alternatives to cardiac resynchronisation, and both have distinct advantages and disadvantages.[75] These approaches are rapidly growing.

Temporary transvenous wires are vulnerable to movement. Unlike permanent pacing leads, which are 'fixed' in some manner to the myocardium so as to prevent dislodgement,[76] temporary leads are not fixed in place. Loss of contact with the endocardium, with loss of capture, may occur with lead movement. Activity limitation and strict rest in bed are therefore recommended for the patient with temporary transvenous pacing who is pacemaker dependent.[77]

The details and descriptions of pacing in this section apply equally to temporary and permanent pacing. However, strategies for the correction of problems are oriented more towards temporary pacing, where clinicians can perform corrective actions.

Bipolar vs unipolar pacing: achieving capture and sensing

Most commonly, both negative and positive electrodes (also termed poles) are positioned on or within the chamber being paced, a configuration labelled bipolar pacing. Alternatively, unipolar pacing is sometimes necessary, in which only one (the negative) electrode is in contact with the heart, while the positive pole/electrode is positioned elsewhere on the body. Conversion of the usual bipolar configuration to unipolar is a relatively simple but important emergency management option for failure to pace and failure to capture or sense. A discussion of applications and video demonstration of conversion can be seen in the free online lectures 'Temporary ventricular pacing' (detailed in 'Online resources' at the end of this chapter). Both pacing and sensing of the intrinsic rhythm require continued function of both electrodes and leads. Interrupting the integrity or the connections of either the positive or the negative lead will interrupt both sensing and pacing, as neither is possible with/out a complete electrical circuit.[78]

The term 'capture' is used to denote successful stimulation of the atria or ventricles. As the spread of excitation through the myocardium occurs in patterns which differ from intrinsic conduction, the resultant P waves and QRS complexes differ from normal. Atrial-paced P waves may be of relatively low amplitude, whereas the paced QRS is

TABLE 11.8

Antiarrhythmic drugs commonly used in critical care[2,20,33,66]

DRUG	INTRAVENOUS DOSE	INDICATION	CONSIDERATIONS	POSSIBLE ADVERSE EFFECTS
Adenosine	6 mg by rapid bolus into central or large peripheral vein. Increase to 12 mg if second dose required, 18 mg if third dose needed.	Termination of AVNRT or AVRT Diagnostic application to induce AV block and reveal atrial activity.	Avoid in asthma, heart failure or second-/third-degree AV block unless pacemaker fitted. Warn patient of unpleasant but transient effects (e.g. chest pain).	AVB/ventricular standstill; transient chest pain/ nausea/ dizziness/ breathlessness.
Amiodarone	Loading dose of 300 mg IV over 20–60 min, followed by maintenance infusion of 900 mg over 23–24 hours.	Atrial and ventricular arrhythmias.	Potentiates digoxin and warfarin. Causes phlebitis so CVC administration recommended Hypotension linked to speed of administration. Little negative inotropy.	Hypotension; bradycardia; AVB; QT prolongation; with long-term use – thyroid and hepatic dysfunction, pulmonary fibrosis, photosensitivity.
Atropine	500 micrograms IV, repeated every 3–5 min to a max of 3 mg.	Bradycardia.	Blocks vagal tone and therefore less effective in ventricular escape rhythms.	Tachycardia, blurred vision; dry mouth; urinary retention; confusion.
Digoxin	0.75–1 mg IV over at least 2 h then oral/NGT if necessary (usual daily dose 125–250 micrograms).	Rate control of narrow complex arrhythmias, especially AF and flutter.	Narrow therapeutic index and renal excretion – toxicity more likely in renal impairment, hypokalaemia and older patients. Mild positive inotropic effect.	Bradycardia; AVB; nausea/ vomiting; dizziness; blurred or yellow vision (suggests toxicity). At toxic levels, causes atrial or ventricular arrhythmia.
Flecainide	2 mg/kg over 10–30 min (150 mg max), followed if necessary by infusion of 1.5 mg/kg/h for 1 h, then 100–250 micrograms/kg/h for up to 24 h. Max dose in 24 h 600 mg.	Supraventricular and ventricular arrhythmias, pre-excited AF.	Avoid in structural heart disease (increased risk of proarrhythmia). Negative inotrope.	Hypotension; bradycardia; AVB; proarrhythmia; QRS prolongation.
Lignocaine (lidocaine)	Loading bolus of 50–100 mg over a few minutes, immediately followed by a reducing infusion of 4 mg/min for 30 min, 2 mg/min for 2 h, then 1 mg/min.	Ventricular tachycardia, especially after acute MI.	If hepatic/renal dysfunction: dose modification necessary to avoid toxicity. Avoid hypokalaemia.	Dizziness, paraesthesia or drowsiness; confusion; respiratory depression; convulsions; hypotension; bradycardia; AVB.
Metoprolol	Up to 5 mg at 1–2 mg/min. Repeat after 5 min if necessary, max dose 10–15 mg.	Rate control of narrow complex arrhythmias. Termination of SVT.	Contraindicated in asthma, high-grade AV block. Negative inotrope.	Hypotension; bradycardia; AVB; symptom provocation in asthma, COPD, diabetes and peripheral vascular disease.
Sotalol	75–150 mg over 5 h. Usual maintenance dose 75–150 mg once or twice daily (equivalent to 80–160 mg oral).	Supraventricular and ventricular arrhythmias.	Highest risk drug for QT prolongation and torsades de pointes – QTc monitoring recommended. Negative inotrope. Avoid in significant renal impairment.	As for metoprolol; QT prolongation.
Verapamil	5–10 mg over 2–3 min, a further 5 mg after 5 min if required.	Rate control of narrow complex arrhythmias. Termination of SVT and some normal heart VT.	Potentiates digoxin, negative inotrope.	Hypotension; bradycardia; AVB; constipation; flushing/ headache.

AVB = atrioventricular block; COPD = chronic obstructive pulmonary disease; CVC = central venous catheter; GI = gastrointestinal; NGT = nasogastric tube.

Sources: Resuscitation Council UK. Advanced Life Support. 8th edition. London; Resuscitation Council UK. 2021.[2] Fogoros RN, Mandrola JM. Fogoros' electrophysiologic testing. 6th ed. Oxford: Wiley Blackwell; 2018.[20] Joint Formulary Committee (2022) British National formulary (online), London: BMJ Group and Pharmaceutical Press.[33] Dan GA, Martinez-Rubio A, Agewall S, et al Antiarrhythmic drugs – clinical use and clinical decision making: a consensus document from the European Heart Rhythm Association (EHRA) and European Society of Cardiology (ESC) Working Group on Cardiovascular Pharmacology, endorsed by the Heart Rhythm Society (HRS), Asia-Pacific Heart Rhythm Society (APHRS) and International Society of Cardiovascular Pharmacotherapy (ISCP). Europace 2018; Feb 9.[66]

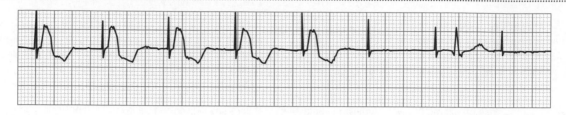

FIGURE 11.34   Ventricular pacing at 86/min. There is capture on the first five beats but none of the remaining pacing spikes is followed by the expected wide QRS of capture. Note that, while there is capture, the patient's own rhythm is suppressed. When capture is lost, the patient's slower rate emerges. Note also that the narrow QRS is not sensed by the pacemaker and does not disturb the regular, fixed rate pacing at 86/min.

recognisably wide (>0.12 seconds) and often notched. ST segments and T waves are typically in opposite direction to the QRS direction (depressed ST, inverted T wave in leads where the QRS is upright, and ST elevation with upright T waves in leads with negative QRS complexes). Together the QRS and ST/T patterns are those of a ventricular ectopic rhythm with an overall morphology resembling left bundle branch block (LBBB)[79] (Fig. 11.34). Note that newer practices of pacing directly into the conduction system are now in use and can result in very different appearances of the paced QRS to those described above. It is now possible for pacing to create normal, narrow QRS complexes with these approaches (discussed further below).

Typically, capture can be achieved with electrical currents of less than 10 milliamps (mA). However, myocardial disease may decrease the responsiveness (increase the capture threshold) of the tissue surrounding the electrode and interfere with successful capture.[80] This may be overcome by increasing the pacemaker output but may require repositioning of the lead to contact more responsive tissue. Where repositioning of the lead is not practical, configuring the system as unipolar may restore capture.[81] To do this a 'skin electrode' is necessary. This is in the form of a commercially available 'skin suture': an electrode which is positioned subcutaneously and connected to the positive terminal of the pacemaker. The anterior torso is a practical location for insertion. This alters the current path of the pacemaker stimulus and the new current path may encounter responsive tissue, restoring capture. This unipolar adaptation is also useful for correcting failure to sense and failure to pace.

Pacing terminology

To aid in communication when discussing pacing functions, international agreement on terminology has been reached (Table 11.9). A 5-letter code[82] describes the pacing (and/or defibrillation) capabilities of any given device in terms of chambers involved in pacing, sensing or other functions such as rate-responsive pacing capabilities. A pacemaker programmed as VVIR, for example, is capable of **V**entricular pacing, sensing of **V**entricular activity, **I**nhibiting pacing in response to sensing of ventricular activity, as well as possessing **R**ate responsiveness. When programmed to VOO there is **V**entricular pacing, but no **(O)** sensing capability, or capability to respond to sensing **(O)**. While the first three letters of this code relate to all pacing, the fourth and fifth letters relate only to permanent pacing and have not been used further in this chapter.

Major pacemaker controls

All temporary pacemakers give the operator control over the pacing mode, rate, output (strength of the applied

TABLE 11.9

Pacemaker terminology[56]

CHAMBER PACED	CHAMBER SENSED	RESPONSE TO SENSING	PROGRAMMABLE FUNCTIONS	ANTITACHYARRHYTHMIA FUNCTIONS
O, none	O, none	O, none	O, none	O, none
A, atrium	A, atrium	T, triggered	P, simple programmable	P, pacing
V, ventricle	V, ventricle	I, inhibited	M, multi-programmable	S, shock
D, dual (A & V)	D, dual (A & V)	D, dual (T & I)	C, communicating R, rate responsive	D, dual (P & S)

Source: Al-Khatib SM, Stevenson WG, Ackerman MJ, et al. 2017 AHA/ACC/HRS guideline for management of patients with ventricular arrhythmias and the prevention of sudden cardiac death: a report of the American College of Cardiology/American Heart Association Task Force on Clinical Practice Guidelines and the Heart Rhythm Society. J Am Coll Cardiol 2017;24390.56

stimulus), sensitivity (for detection of intrinsic rhythm) and (in dual-chamber modes) the AV interval. Additional controls such as output pulse width, upper tracking rate and the post-ventricular atrial refractory period (for DDD mode; see section 'DDD pacing: the 'universal' pacing mode') are available on some temporary and all permanent devices. Table 11.10 describes the major parameters that can be directly controlled on temporary devices.

Mode selection

Emergency transvenous pacing is usually applied as ventricular pacing only. Almost always, this will be in VVI (**V**entricular pacing, **V**entricular sensing, **I**nhibiting pacing; demand) mode. VOO may also be used (rarely) when oversensing is causing unwanted inhibition in pacemaker-dependent patients. In the post-cardiac surgical patient where atrial and ventricular leads can readily be inserted, DDD is the preferred mode (see section 'DDD pacing: the 'universal' pacing mode'). DDD use is also almost universal in permanent pacing, with the exception being when there is atrial fibrillation. Atrial capture is not possible during AF and remaining in DDD during AF may result in undesirable rapid ventricular pacing or may precipitate ventricular arrhythmias. Dual-chamber pacemakers may still be implanted if AF is paroxysmal or where future reversion of AF is thought possible. In these cases, DDD is usually programmed but with a feature which allows automatic mode switching (AMS) to VVI during AF episodes, and back to DDD upon reversion to sinus rhythm.[83]

Atrial modes (AAI and AOO) are used less commonly as they provide no protection against AV block. They are used when there is pure sinus node dysfunction without AV block (see Fig. 11.34).

Output and threshold

The strength of the pacing stimulus applied is termed the pacing 'output' and is adjustable by the operator. For temporary pacing this is more often an adjustable current (from 0.1 to 25 mA), and with permanent pacing an adjustable voltage (0.1–7.5 volts). The minimum output required to achieve capture is termed the output threshold. This pacing threshold may vary significantly with changes in biochemistry, arterial pH, myocardial perfusion, drugs and other factors.[80,84,85] Output settings on the pulse generator are set at double the threshold value to ensure a safety margin to accommodate potential threshold changes.[80]

In addition to the strength of the applied stimulus, some temporary pacemakers feature an adjustable pulse width. This is the duration over which the stimulus is applied and typical ranges are 0.1–2.0 milliseconds. Capture is a product of pulse amplitude and pulse

TABLE 11.10
Pacemaker controls and settings

CONTROL	FUNCTION
Base rate	Sets the rate at which the pacemaker will discharge: pacing occurs at this rate unless the patient's own rate is faster and is sensed by the pacemaker. Typically set at 60–100/min.
Maximum tracking rate (also upper tracking rate)	Sets the upper limit for which atrial tracking will be permitted – i.e. the fastest rate which ventricular pacing will occur in response to atrial rhythms. Usually 130–140 per min. Provides protection against tracking atrial tachyarrhythmias.
Ventricular output	The size, or strength, of the stimulus delivered to the ventricles. In temporary devices this is an adjustable current (measured in milliamperes (mA)). Output is increased until capture (successful stimulation) is achieved. The minimum current required to achieve capture is termed the output threshold. Impulses delivered below the threshold value will not capture the myocardium. Temporary pacemakers have an adjustable output range of 0.1–25 mA.
Atrial output	The size or strength of the stimulus delivered to the atria. Range 0.1–20 mA.
Atrial and ventricular pulse width	Adjustable on only some devices. Allows adjustment of the duration for which the pacemaker output is applied to the myocardium. Selectable range typically 1.0–2.0 ms in 0.25-ms increments. Increasing the pulse width enhances ability to gain capture.
Atrioventricular delay	The interval between the delivery of the atrial and ventricular pacing stimuli. Normally this is set in the same range as normal PR intervals (between 0.12 and 0.20 s).
Sensitivity	Affects the ability of the pacemaker to detect the presence of spontaneous cardiac activity. Sensitivity settings can be adjusted between 1.0 and 20 millivolts (mV). Set at 1.0 mV the device is very sensitive (able to sense small electrical signals from the heart). Set at higher values, the device becomes less sensitive (higher voltage signals required to be detected), with the risk that QRS complexes or P waves will not be sensed.

duration,[69] and so increasing pulse width, if available, is valuable for restoring capture even when maximum output has been unable to capture.

Practice tip

Thresholds for stimulation are more volatile in the temporary pacemaker patient in whom ischaemia or postoperative biochemical, pH and haemodynamic changes are common. Monitoring should be focused on confirming capture and low heart rate limits on monitors should be set to 5 or 10 beats below the base pacing rate. Even single-beat loss of capture should be addressed, as it may be the first emergence in progressive loss of capture.

Sensitivity

QRS complexes recorded by pacemakers typically vary between 1 and 10 mV in amplitude, occasionally higher, and sensitivity is programmed according to the individual's measured QRS (the sensing threshold). Programmable sensitivity values are 0.5–20 mV, with 0.5 mV being *the most* sensitive (smaller voltages can be sensed) and 20 mV being *the least* sensitive (only very large QRS signals would be sensed).[86] If there is failure to sense the intrinsic rhythm,

the pacemaker is made more sensitive by decreasing the sensitivity value, and to correct oversensing the pacemaker is made less sensitive by increasing the sensitivity value. Sensitivity can also be turned off (asynchronous pacing). Sensitivity is typically set to half the numerical value of the measured QRS (see pacemaker testing below).[86]

Demand versus asynchronous pacing

Demand pacing

The so-called 'demand' modes (AAI, VVI, DDD) predominate in pacing, sometimes termed synchronous pacing. In these modes, pacing is provided only on demand – that is, when the heart rate falls below a nominated level (the demand rate) (Fig. 11.35). Demand pacing requires pacemaker detection, or 'sensing' of the patient's intrinsic cardiac rhythm. If an intrinsic rhythm is sensed, it 'inhibits' the pacemaker from delivering a pacing stimulus (pacing is not delivered and a timer for delivery of the next stimulus is reset). The demand modes ensure that pacing is provided only when needed, and also protect against pacing during arrhythmically vulnerable moments in the cardiac cycle. Ventricular pacing delivered at the time of the T wave may induce ventricular tachyarrhythmias[87] (Fig. 11.36), while atrial pacing during atrial repolarisation (shortly after the P wave) may precipitate atrial tachyarrhythmias.

FIGURE 11.35 Atrial fibrillation with demand ventricular pacing at a rate of 60/min. The patient's rate increases after the first two paced beats and inhibits the pacemaker. It then slows to below 60/min and the pacemaker recommences 'on demand'.

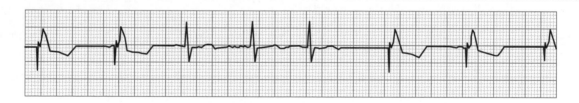

FIGURE 11.36 Intermittent asynchronous pacing due to incomplete failure to sense. Set pacing rate 65/min. The first, third and fourth beats are sensed and appropriately inhibit pacing. However, a pacing spike can be seen at the apex of the T wave of the second beat because of failure to sense that beat. The next pacing spike, just after the apex of the T wave of the fifth beat, arrives during the period of increased excitability in the action potential and precipitates ventricular tachycardia.

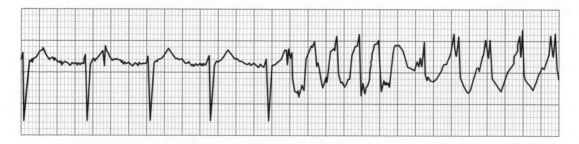

FIGURE 11.37 Commencement of ventricular pacing. The sinus rate is around 70/min. The pacemaker is then turned on with the rate set at 80/min. Capture is achieved immediately and, because the pacing rate is faster, there is suppression of the patient's own rhythm. Note the wide QRS, with ST segments and T waves in an opposite direction to the QRS deflection as expected.

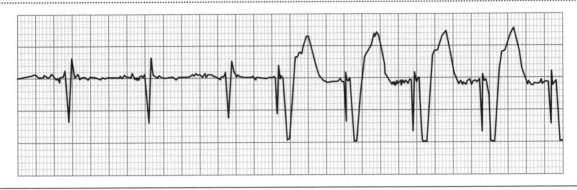

Asynchronous pacing

Pacing may be delivered in an asynchronous mode – that is, without the capability of sensing and synchronising with the heart's inherent rhythm. This is sometimes referred to as 'fixed-rate pacing'. When in an asynchronous mode, the pulse generator will pace perpetually at the set rate, continuing even if an intrinsic rhythm is present. The main application of non-sensing modes is to protect against false inhibition of pacing such as when: (1) there is oversensing, or risk of oversensing, such as in environments with strong electromagnetic fields, and (2) when patients would otherwise be asystolic or critically bradycardic if pacing were inhibited (pacemaker dependent).[80,88] Temporary reprogramming to non-sensing modes (AOO, VOO, DOO) is commonly undertaken during surgery to prevent false pacemaker inhibition by electrocautery.[89] The appropriateness of continuing in an asynchronous mode should always be reconsidered if the patient's rate re-emerges in competition with the pacing because of the risk of precipitating arrhythmias.

Single-chamber pacing: ventricular pacing

Pacing of just the ventricles results in the generation of a ventricular ectopic rhythm (see Fig. 11.34). Functionally, this will be no different from an intrinsic idioventricular rhythm. There will be loss of atrioventricular synchrony, and the loss of atrial kick may cause low cardiac output and hypotension.[90,91] Patients with symptoms of low cardiac output due to just ventricular pacing are said to have pacemaker syndrome. To offset the loss of atrial kick, ventricular pacing is sometimes undertaken at slightly higher rates than normally seen in the resting patient (e.g. 70–80/min rather than 50–60/min).

Ventricular pacing protects against bradycardia or AV block by stimulating the ventricles at a set rate (Fig. 11.37). Temporary ventricular pacing may also be undertaken to

prevent bradycardia-dependent tachyarrhythmias such as TdP.[92] In that context, pacing at faster rates provides protection by reducing the QT interval, as well as preventing pauses which commonly give rise to ectopy and onset of TdP.[92]

> **Practice tip**
>
> If haemodynamics are poor during ventricular pacing (low blood pressure and/or cardiac output), consider changing the pacing rate. A faster pacing rate may offset the loss of atrial kick and so restore cardiac output despite low stroke volume. Alternatively, turning down the pacing rate may reveal an underlying (slower) sinus rhythm that produces improved cardiac output due to the inclusion of atrial kick.

Single-chamber pacing: atrial pacing

Atrial pacing alone (AAI) may be used when there is sinus node dysfunction in the presence of reliable AV conduction.[93] Typically there is sinus bradycardia, pauses or sinus arrest, or there may chronotropic incompetence where the sinus node does not accelerate sufficiently during activity. There needs to be confidence that AV conduction is intact, and that it will remain intact in the future as the annual incidence of progression to AV block is 1% in these patients.[94] If in doubt, dual-chamber pacing is provided. An advantage of atrial pacing over ventricular pacing is that atrial kick is maintained, benefiting cardiac output and blood pressure.[91,95] Atrial-only pacing is uncommon.

Atrial pacing tends to produce low-amplitude P waves, which vary from the typical P waves of sinus rhythm (Fig. 11.38). They may at times be difficult to identify on the ECG. Appropriate lead selection is important to reveal the atrial depolarisation and confirm atrial capture. It is common for the AV interval (PR interval) to extend

FIGURE 11.38 Commencement of atrial pacing. The patient's own sinus rhythm is around 65/min at the start of the strip. Pacing is turned on at 70/min, and capture is immediately evident with altered P waves of low amplitude and very slight extension of the PR interval.

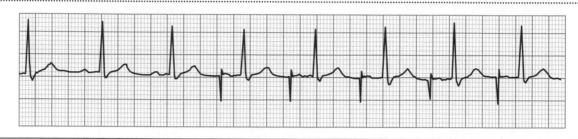

slightly (e.g. to 0.20–0.22 seconds) during atrial pacing compared with sinus rhythm, as the time taken for atrial impulses to traverse the atria from the pacing focus is longer than the sinus-to-AV node conduction interval.

Atrial pacing and AV block

Any degree of AV block is possible during atrial pacing and it must be remembered that AV block is rate dependent. Thus, the severity of AV block may be worsened not only by AV node deterioration but also by changes in the atrial pacing rate. Thus, a patient with first-degree block may develop second-degree block if the atrial pacing rate is increased, without this implying worsening AV node function. Conversely, AV block developing during atrial pacing may be lessened or overcome by reducing the atrial pacing rate. An example of such rate-dependent AV block behaviour is demonstrated in Figs 11.39–11.41.

Practice tip

If AV block is encountered during atrial pacing and is causing significant bradycardia, consideration should be given to reducing the atrial pacing rate to see whether the severity of the AV block can be reduced.

Dual-chamber pacing

Pacing of both the atria and ventricles offers the benefit of atrial kick as well as a guarantee of a ventricular rhythm. Therefore, it provides protection against both sinus bradycardia and AV block. As with either atrial or ventricular pacing, demand modes have been preferred in dual-chamber pacing, unless oversensing and pacemaker dependence warrant asynchronous pacing. Particular features of the DDD pacing mode have made it the predominant mode in both permanent and postsurgical temporary pacing.

Pacing stimuli are delivered to the atria and ventricles at a selected rate. After delivery of the atrial stimulus there is a programmed delay of usually 0.16–0.24 seconds (equivalent to a PR interval) before delivery of the ventricular pacing stimulus (Fig. 11.42). If the patient is able to conduct the atrial depolarisation to the ventricles themselves before the ventricular pacing is due, then the pacemaker senses the resultant QRS and inhibits ventricular pacing. Promoting intrinsic conduction has become an emphasis in modern pacing as ventricular pacing may contribute to the development of heart failure.[96]

A dual-chamber pacemaker may demonstrate atrial and ventricular pacing at the set rate and at the set AV delay as described above, or may operate as simply atrial pacing if normal AV node conduction occurs before the programmed AV delay has elapsed. Deliberately prolonging the programmed AV delay provides greater opportunity for patients to conduct to the ventricles by themselves. In permanent pacing, there is emphasis on avoiding ventricular pacing, but increasing the AV delay beyond the range of a normal PR interval carries an arrhythmic risk[97] (Fig. 11.43).

FIGURE 11.39 Atrial pacing at 70/min with first-degree AV block (and left bundle branch block). Note the long PR interval (0.34 s); particular caution is warranted in increasing the rate as, although AV conduction is 1:1, it is already very slow. See Figs 11.40 and 11.41 for worsening of the AV block as the atrial rate is increased.

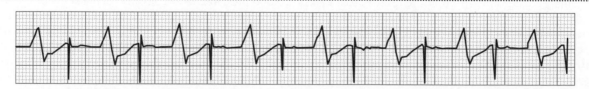

FIGURE 11.40 Second-degree AV block type I with 3:2 conduction. The same patient as above, with worsening AV block after increasing the atrial pacing rate from 70 to 80/min. Note 1:1 conduction has been lost and every third P wave is blocked (non-conducted). The PR interval can be seen to gradually prolong – from 0.34 to 0.46 s before the dropped beat of each cycle.

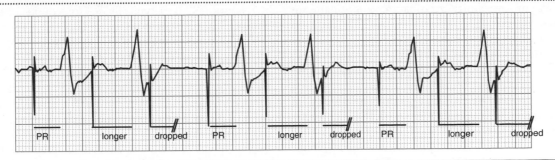

FIGURE 11.41 The same patient again, now with the atrial pacing at 86/min. At the faster atrial rate, AV conduction has worsened further. There is now a 2:1 block yielding a ventricular rate of 43/min.

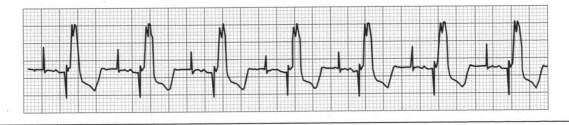

FIGURE 11.42 Dual-chamber pacing at a rate of 72/min. The atrial spikes capture (with low-amplitude P waves) and then, after the AV interval of 0.20 s, ventricular pacing, with capture, is seen.

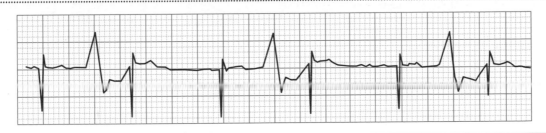

FIGURE 11.43 Extending the AV delay to promote intrinsic conduction. There is initially AV pacing at a rate of 75/min, with an AV delay of 0.16 s. The AV delay is then increased to 0.40 s, permitting the patient to conduct spontaneously with a PR interval of 0.26 s and narrow QRS. The intrinsic QRS complexes are sensed and ventricular pacing is inhibited.

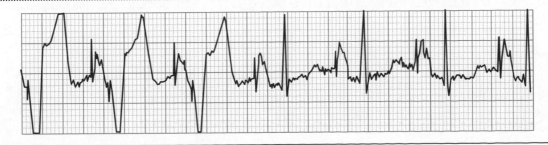

DDD pacing: the 'universal' pacing mode

The introduction of the DDD mode (**D**ual-chamber pacing, **D**ual-chamber sensing and **D**ual responses (inhibition and triggered ventricular pacing)) added an important dimension to dual-chamber pacing: the ability to synchronise ventricular pacing to spontaneous atrial activity in patients with AV block.[84] In addition to the normal demand mode behaviours, the DDD mode features a 'triggered' function. If the pacemaker detects a P wave but a QRS does not follow within the preset AV interval (AV block), the pacemaker will be triggered to provide ventricular pacing at the end of the programmed AV interval.[98] In short, the pacemaker triggers pacing of the ventricles after any P wave, a very physiological approach if the patient has normal sinus node function but pure AV block. In DDD, ventricular pacing will be seen at a range of rates above the programmed base rate as it follows changes in the sinus rate. This triggered behaviour of the DDD device is sometimes called 'P-synchronous ventricular pacing',[98] although 'atrial tracking' is a more practical term as the ventricular pacing 'tracks' the atrial rate (Figs 11.44 and 11.45).

The potential downside of atrial tracking lies in the fact that pacemakers cannot discriminate between the P waves of sinus rhythm and other atrial activity such as atrial tachycardia, flutter or fibrillation. One-to-one tracking of sinus rhythm is appropriate, but 1:1 tracking of very rapid atrial arrhythmias would produce intolerable ventricular rates. For this reason, an 'upper rate' for atrial tracking is programmed in the DDD pacemaker. The upper rate controls the maximal rate at which ventricular pacing can be provided (how fast it may track the atria at a 1:1 ratio). This is typically set to around 120–130 per minute. In younger patients it may be set higher (e.g. 140–170/min). If the atrial rate exceeds the upper rate for tracking, then it is no longer possible for all of the atrial beats to be tracked. DDD pacemakers will start 'dropping' beats when the atrial rate exceeds the upper tracking rate, analogous to the behaviour of the AV node. An additional layer of protection is automatic mode switching, in which permanent pacemakers switch to non-tracking mode (VVI) if the atrial rate exceeds a programmed value (usually >170/min). Temporary pacemakers do not have mode-switching capabilities and so it is the responsibility of clinicians to manually change from DDD to VVI during atrial arrhythmias.

Documentation of paced rhythm

It will be apparent from the descriptions above that at different times the DDD pacemaker may be pacing either the atria *or* the ventricles, pacing both the atria *and* the ventricles, or pacing neither, depending on the patient's sinus and AV node capabilities. Merely documenting 'DDD' does not convey anything about pacemaker dependence or reveal recovery of sinus or AV

FIGURE 11.44 ECG excerpt from a patient with sinus rhythm and 2:1 AV block. The non-conducted P waves are partially concealed but can be seen distorting the T waves (arrows). Although the sinus node can generate a rate of 75/min, the patient is rendered bradycardic (37/min) by the AV block.

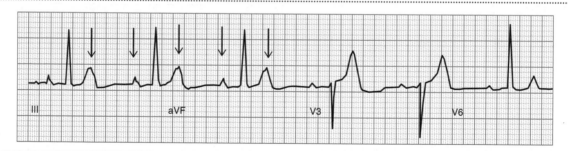

FIGURE 11.45 The same patient as above, 2 h later. A DDD pacemaker has been inserted and, although some of the pacing spikes are difficult to see, all QRSs are paced beats. The sinus rate is again close to 75/min, and atrial tracking ensures that a paced QRS follows each P wave. The ventricular rate has been brought back under control of the sinus node. The tracking of the sinus rate permits pacing (at 75/min) to be faster than the programmed base rate of 60/min.

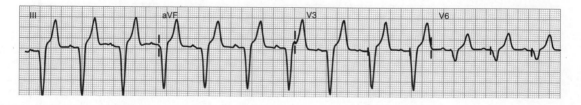

TABLE 11.11

Representative documentation of current rhythm during dual-chamber pacing

SUGGESTED DOCUMENTATION	INFORMATION CONVEYED
AP-VP Atrial paced, ventricular paced	Sinus rate is less than base rate. AV conduction has not occurred before the AV delay times out.
AP-VS Atrial paced, ventricular sensed	Sinus rate is less than base rate. AV conduction is occurring normally (recovered).
AS-VP Atrial sensed, ventricular paced	Sinus rate is greater than base rate. AV block is first degree or worse.
AS-VS Atrial sensed, ventricular sensed	Sinus rate is greater than base rate. Normal AV conduction is present.

nodal capabilities. A representation which conveys atrial and ventricular activity is more useful and is shown in Table 11.11. Note that the information contained may be obtained from either cardiac monitoring or from the pace indicators on the pacemaker.

External (transcutaneous) pacing

Emergency pacing may be undertaken non-invasively via external pacing electrodes, and is termed 'external' or 'transcutaneous' pacing. Adhesive defibrillation pads are applied in either the anteroposterior (preferred) or standard apicobasal positions as per defibrillation. These are connected to a defibrillator with additional pacing capability. Large pacing stimuli (10–200 mA) are necessary to achieve myocardial capture; this frequently causes stimulation of skeletal muscles, which can be uncomfortable or painful. It is also less reliable than transvenous or epicardial pacing.[99] For these reasons its use is reserved for the emergency management of life-threatening bradyarrhythmias, and only as a short-term bridge to invasive pacing. Sedation is usually required.

Transcutaneous pacing provides ventricular pacing only, and the patient should be assessed not only for reliable capture, but also for an adequate pulse and blood pressure during pacing.[100]

Pacing may be in either demand or asynchronous mode, usually at rates of 40–80 bpm.

Practice tip

The high-current pacing spikes of transthoracic pacing may conceal the resultant QRS on bedside monitors. Filters on the monitors of the pacer/defibrillator unit make them a more reliable source of capture confirmation than bedside monitors.

Complications of pacing

Effective pacing may be disturbed by problems related to pacing leads, changes in myocardial responsiveness, programmed values, external electromagnetic fields, the pulse generator itself (including power sources) and interactions between these factors. Four major disturbances to pacing are described below. These provide the bulk of pacing problems encountered and, because they may either interrupt pacing or precipitate serious arrhythmias, critical care nurses need to be competent in their recognition and management.

Failure to capture

Failure to capture is said to be present when pacing stimuli (pacing 'spikes') are present but do not successfully stimulate the heart – that is, pacing spikes are not followed by either QRS complexes (in ventricular pacing) or P waves (in atrial) (Figs 11.46 and 11.47). Failure to capture may occur when the myocardial responsiveness (threshold) worsens, or when impulses do not reach responsive myocardium. Note that dislodgement of a lead from the myocardium will still usually show pacing spikes on the ECG as long as the lead is in contact with body fluids or tissue. This is a critical distinction when troubleshooting failure to capture (spikes are present) from failure to pace (no spikes are present), as management of the two is distinctly different. A chest X-ray

FIGURE 11.46 Intermittent failure to capture. The first, second, sixth and seventh spikes gain ventricular capture but the rest do not. Note the significant pause during failure to capture, in which there is atrial but not ventricular activity. No escape rhythm emerges.

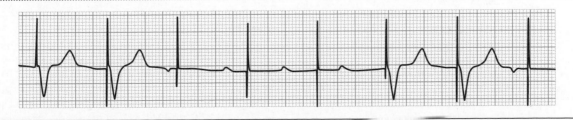

FIGURE 11.47 Atrial pacing with intermittent failure to capture (output set at 14 mA). Note that capture is evident following the first, third, fifth, seventh and eighth pacing spikes, but not the others. Fortunately, here the patient has an underlying sinus rate of 54/min, so that the impact of failure to capture is of no great consequence.

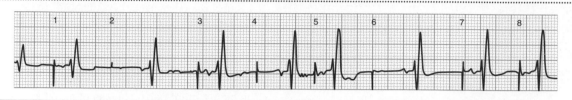

may confirm lead migration. Repositioning of leads must therefore be included in considerations during management of failure to capture.

Failure to capture may present as a clinical emergency and requires immediate attention. With failure to capture, patients are left to generate their own rhythm, which may be unacceptably slow. Failure to capture may be complete (no spikes capturing) or intermittent (with only some spikes achieving capture). Even occasional spikes with failure to capture require immediate attention, as complete failure to capture may ensue. Causes and management of failure to capture[73,85,95,101] are listed in Table 11.12. Patient factors which cause failure to capture are the same as causes of bradycardia and/or AV block, and are essentially causes of conduction system depression. This is useful in guiding investigation of clinical reasons for failure to capture. Likewise, treatment includes the same measures used to treat

bradycardia and AV block. Positive chronotropes are useful both for managing the resultant bradycardia and for potentially restoring capture.

Failure to sense

Sensing of the intrinsic cardiac rhythm is necessary to achieve demand pacing.[78,80,86] If rhythms are not sensed, pacing will proceed at a fixed rate and in competition with the intrinsic rhythm (Figs 11.48 and 11.49). Functionally, inadvertent failure to sense is the same as deliberate asynchronous pacing (as AOO, VOO, DOO) discussed earlier. Normal inhibition cannot occur and competitive pacing may be proaarhythmic[87] (see Fig. 11.36). Arrhythmic risk increases when there is myocardial ischaemia or infarction, hypokalaemia or hypomagnesaemia. Immediate restoration of appropriate sensing needs to be undertaken. Causes and management of failure to sense[80,86,88] are detailed in Box 11.2. Remember, however, that sensing controls are inverse: lowering numerical settings (e.g. from 5 to 2 mV) increases the sensitivity (as does unipolar configuration), while increasing the sensitivity value (from 1 to 4 mV) makes the pacemaker less sensitive.

Failure to pace

Failure to pace is an imperfect term but is used when the pacemaker indicators show that pacing is occurring but spikes do not appear on the ECG. It is also sometimes termed 'failure to output'. Most commonly, this is because of disconnection, or a loose connection between the pacing lead and the bridging cable, or between the bridging cable and the pacemaker. In such instances, the electrical circuit is interrupted and pacing impulses do not reach the patient.[80] If connections have been confirmed and the problem persists then there is fault with the lead itself, the bridging cable or (rarely) the pacemaker. Note that the fault (or connection) could be of either the negative or positive leads, as both must be intact for a complete circuit.

Electrocardiographically, failure to pace appears as failure of the pacing spikes to appear when expected, despite pacing indicators flashing. As with failure to capture, bradycardia may ensue. Failure to pace may present as complete loss of pacing, or just pacing at a slower rate than set (Figs 11.50 and 11.51). Causes and management of failure to pace[74,80,81] are detailed in Box 11.3.

TABLE 11.12

Failure to capture: causes and management

CAUSES	MANAGEMENT
Output too low	Increase output. Increase pulse width if feature is available.
Changing capture threshold	Check for and treat ischaemia, hyperkalaemia, acidosis or alkalosis. Lead maturation.
Antiarrhythmic drugs	Consider cessation, dose reduction or alternative drug.
Lead migration/ dislodgement	Reposition lead if able. Reverse polarity of leads (for epicardial wires). Position patient on left side (if transvenous lead). Consider unipolar pacing via application of a skin suture (or electrode). Treat the resultant rhythm (e.g. atropine, isoprenaline). Place another lead. Consider transcutaneous pacing.

FIGURE 11.48   Ventricular pacing with failure to sense. At the start of the strip there is ventricular pacing with capture. A junctional rhythm emerges at a slightly faster rate than the ventricular pacing, but despite this the pacemaker continues to discharge at a fixed rate. Pacing is not inhibited by the intrinsic rhythm and spikes are delivered into the ST segment and T waves. Note also that the pacing spikes delivered into the QRS and ST segment do not capture because of normal tissue refractoriness at those moments.

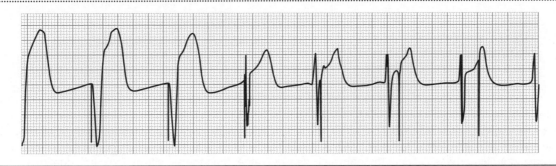

FIGURE 11.49   Atrial failure to sense. The first three beats show atrial pacing. Then there are two spontaneous (faster) P waves (fourth and fifth beats). These P waves should have inhibited the atrial pacing, but pacing spikes can be seen at the start of the QRS of the fourth beat and in the ST segment of the fifth beat. (Note also, the third pacing spike is strictly a fusion beat as the intrinsic P wave and the pacing spike have occurred simultaneously.)

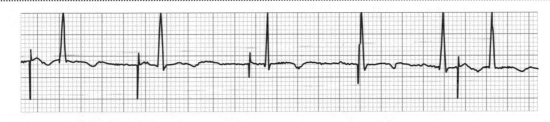

BOX 11.2

Failure to sense: causes and management

Causes:

- Sensitivity set too low (too high a number).
- Programmed to asynchronous mode (AOO, VOO or DOO).
- Altered sensing threshold (lead maturation).
- Decreased myocardial voltages.
- Lead movement/dislodgement.

Management:

- Increase sensitivity (to a lower number).
- Check/tighten connections.
- If epicardial leads, reverse the polarity of the electrodes (reverse connections of positive and negative electrodes).
- Increase the pacing rate to overdrive the competing rhythm.
- If underlying rhythm satisfactory, consider turning pacemaker off.
- Consider placement of an alternative sensing electrode (skin suture) to create unipolar pacing.

Practice tip

If during pacing there is abrupt loss of a paced rhythm with resultant bradycardia, observe the pacing indicators. If indicator lights show that pacing is occurring then look further for the presence or absence of pacing spikes on the ECG. If spikes are present, the problem is failure to capture, corrected by increasing output or treating causes of an increase in threshold. If spikes are absent, the problem is failure to pace and attention is directed to restoring the integrity of the electrical circuit/connections.

Oversensing

Oversensing is the false detection of electrical signals other than genuine cardiac signals (P waves or QRS complexes). Such sensing inhibits pacing and, as in failure to pace, appears as loss of pacing spikes on the ECG.[69,78,89] Sources of electrical interference may originate from the patient (muscle movement, shivering, convulsions), from the heart itself (T-wave oversensing) or from external sources (e.g. diathermy, other electrical stimulation therapies or electrical equipment).

FIGURE 11.50 Ventricular failure to pace. The regular ventricular pacing at 90 bpm is interrupted after three beats. Pacing spikes abruptly cease and, despite reappearing, do so at a slower rate than expected. Both cessation and pacing slower than the programmed rate could be due to either failure to pace or oversensing. Examination of pacing indicators revealed repeated flashing of the 'pace' indicator despite the absence of pacing spikes. This was a case of ventricular failure to pace due to a loose connection of the pacing leads to the bridging cable.

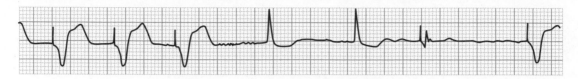

FIGURE 11.51 Atrial pacing with failure to pace. There is sudden disappearance of the pacing spikes after the first three beats. From this strip alone, the distinction between failure to pace and oversensing cannot be made. However, the atrial pacing indicator was flashing through such pauses, rather than the sensitivity indicator, confirming failure to pace. Atrial capture is present but the P waves are not visible on this strip. Capture is instead confirmed by the fact that AV conduction occurs with an unvarying PR interval of 0.26 s after each pacing spike. A single junctional escape beat eventually emerges.

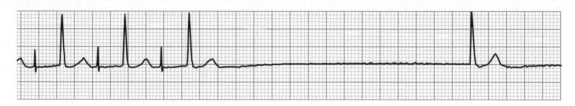

BOX 11.3

Failure to pace: causes and management

Causes:

- Disconnected lead/loose connections – commonest cause.

- Pacemaker turned off or dysfunctional.

- Output turned off.

- Battery depleted.

- Fractured lead (may be internally fractured but outwardly intact).

Management:

- Check that pacemaker is turned on.

- Check all connections and leads, and tighten/replace if necessary.

- Change battery.

- Replace the bridging cable between the pacemaker and the pacing leads.

- Ensure output is turned on.

- Complete circuit with skin suture to positive terminal of the pacemaker, and try each of the existing wires in the negative terminal.

- Differentiate from oversensing.

- Assess and support rhythm and haemodynamics.

Differentiation of oversensing from failure to pace requires observing the pacemaker flashing indicators. Both complications result in loss of pacing spikes, but of course during oversensing the 'sense' indicator will be flashing as opposed to the 'pacing' indicator illuminating during failure to pace.

Oversensing may result in momentary interruptions to pacing (pauses) or complete cessation of pacing. The clinical impact depends on the duration of oversensing, and on the patient's ability to generate an underlying rhythm. The sources of oversensing[69,78] may be difficult to establish clinically but, whether identified or not, treatment is the same: the pacemaker should be made less sensitive. If necessary, sensitivity may be disabled completely by choosing an asynchronous mode (AOO, VOO or DOO) until the source has been confidently addressed. Causes and management of oversensing are detailed in Box 11.4.

For a permanent pacemaker, oversensing can be overcome by positioning a ring magnet over the pacemaker. This will cause it to operate in an asynchronous mode (VOO or DOO), at an increased rate of 90–100/min to reduce the risk of competing with any emerging intrinsic rhythm. A magnet is commonly used when diathermy is in use intraoperatively to prevent oversensing and inappropriate inhibition. If the surgical site precludes magnet placement then intraoperative programming to VOO or DOO mode is undertaken.

BOX 11.4

Oversensing: causes and management

Causes:

- Muscle potentials other than QRS complexes:
  - Cardiac: T waves, U waves, P waves
  - Non-cardiac: shivering, fasciculations, seizure activity, any skeletal muscle movement.
- External electrical interference:
  - Electrocautery, TENS machines
  - Electrical devices (rare)
  - Movement of the connecting pins at the connection to the pulse generator (common).

Management:

- Reduce sensitivity (turn sensitivity to higher number).
- Consider disabling the sensitivity altogether (i.e. asynchronous, VOO, AOO, DOO mode).
- Consider reversing the polarity of the wires (positive to negative).
- Remove the source of interference where it can be identified.

Practice tip

Perhaps a useful guide for rapid differentiation of bradycardia or asystole while pacing is in use is to ask:

- Are pacing spikes present?
  - Yes (but no QRS) – failure to capture.
  - No – failure to pace or oversensing. Ask:
- Which pacing indicator is flashing?
  - Pacing – failure to pace (a loose connection or broken lead or bridging cable).
  - Sensing (but no QRSs) – oversensing.

Care of the patient with temporary pacing

Monitoring and management of the patient and pacing largely fall to the nursing staff. Nurses monitor pacing performance and the detection of pacing abnormalities, the integrity of the pacing system, the avoidance of clinical situations, or physical changes that may alter pacing effectiveness, and troubleshooting complications.

Nursing responsibilities in the care of the patient with a pacemaker include:

- ensuring the integrity of the pacing circuit; physically check/tighten all connections each shift
- pacemaker site inspection for inflammation/swelling/haematoma

- avoidance of hip flexion and rest in bed if femoral insertion
- avoidance of traction on leads and/or bridging cables which may cause lead dislodgement
- vital signs, circulatory observations, etc., at intervals appropriate to the overall patient context
- rhythm monitoring:
  - return of intrinsic rhythm or progression to pacemaker dependence
  - detection of pacing-associated arrhythmias
- confirmation of capture and sensing
- assessment of haemodynamic adequacy during both paced and spontaneous rhythms (BP, CO, perfusion, symptoms)
- strip documentation of rhythm 6-hourly and daily 12-lead ECG
- chest X-ray to confirm the position of the wire/absence of complications
- confirmation of battery status on each shift
- performance of pacemaker threshold assessment on each shift or daily.

Protection against microshock

Even very small electrical currents (termed microshock) can induce VT or VF if they reach the myocardium.[102] Such currents applied to the body surface normally dissipate in body fluids and do not reach sufficient current density at the heart to cause arrhythmias. But pacing leads are a direct route to the heart and so even tiny voltages such as the static electricity generated from bed making or walking on carpet may be sufficient if they reach pacing leads. For this reason, insulating gloves are necessary when handling pacing leads.[102] Patients with temporary pacemakers should be nursed in cardiac-protected areas, but such areas do not protect against the type of current transmission described above. If leads have been disconnected, pending later removal, the connector pins should be insulated.

Battery depletion in a temporary pacemaker

Standard batteries power temporary pacemakers for about a week, and it is good practice to commence treatment with a fresh battery to avoid unexpected power failure during use. Various 'low-battery' indicators exist: some digital devices display a low-battery icon on screen; others will sacrifice power to the flashing pacing indicators (while still pacing) as a marker that there is less than 24 hours remaining power.

Many devices hold a small stored charge, which permits batteries to be replaced without interrupting pacing or powering down. Pacing can be sustained for around 10 seconds, which is enough to replace the battery if a planned, well-rehearsed procedure is undertaken. It is clearly necessary to know the behaviour upon battery removal for the devices in your department.

Pacemaker function testing

Routine pacemaker checks should be undertaken regularly in the patient with a temporary pacemaker. Pacemaker tests are performed to look for return of an underlying rhythm, which may be being concealed by pacing, and to measure thresholds for capture and sensing, as these values may change with time and in response to changing myocardial responsiveness.[103,104] Regular checking allows detection of threshold changes, and the setting of safety margins for output and sensing, in order to avert unexpected failure to capture or sense.

Practices employed to test temporary pacemakers vary widely, as do attitudes to whether this may or may not be undertaken by nurses. The sample protocol shown in Box 11.5 provides an organised approach to testing in which safety has been emphasised. Because of the varying attitudes to nursing responsibilities, the use of this approach should be ratified at individual institutions before use. Many departments stipulate competency certification and may further stipulate that these procedures apply to routine testing only in patients without haemodynamic compromise. An alternative approach to the compromised or unstable patient is also provided below.

Testing pacemaker thresholds is performed daily or on each shift using the steps described in Box 11.5. The test should be carried out promptly, with attention to avoiding undue bradycardia or periods of asynchronous pacing. The patient should be advised to report any sensations/symptoms during testing.

Pacemaker testing in the unstable or pacemaker-dependent patient

Greater caution must be applied in the testing of pacemaker functions if the patient has marked haemodynamic instability or has little or no underlying rhythm. Routine testing of pacemaker function as described in Box 11.5 may not be suitable, but testing for underlying rhythm and some level of confirmation of an output safety margin are of value.

For such patients, testing can be useful to reveal sinus node capability, which may be concealed during ventricular pacing. Figure 11.52 shows that briefly reducing the pacing rate may reveal a useful sinus rate, which because of atrial kick may improve haemodynamics substantially. It is advisable to have additional cardiology or intensive care personnel present during such non-routine testing.

Instead of creating loss of capture to determine capture threshold, a safety margin may still be revealed by reducing the output, but not to values below a previously measured threshold. For example, if the pacemaker is

---

BOX 11.5

Routine temporary pacemaker testing protocol: underlying rhythm, output and sensitivity threshold test

1 Store current values in memory (for devices with memory). If rhythm difficulty is encountered during testing, these original settings can be immediately re-established by depressing the stored values mode selector.

2 Test for underlying rhythm. Gradually decrease rate in 10 bpm steps until evidence of underlying rhythm (ULR) emerges:

   a. If ULR present, observe whether sensing is now occurring.

   b. If still pacing at 50/min (no emergence of ULR), return to initial settings; do not continue to test sensitivity or output thresholds.

   c. Document attempt and ULR less than 50/min.

If ULR is haemodynamically acceptable, continue.

3 Test sensitivity threshold. Having confirmed haemodynamically adequate ULR:

   a. Turn pacing rate to half the patient's rate.

   b. Turn output to minimum (not off).

(NB: Sensitivity testing requires that failure to sense is created for a brief period, so steps 3a and 3b are designed to minimise danger of arrhythmias.)

While observing the sense indicator on the pacemaker:

   a. Decrease sensitivity (increasing the number) until failure to sense (the sense indicator stops flashing – pacing indicator will now be flashing).

   b. Increase sensitivity (decreasing the number) until sensing resumes.

   c. Note the value at which sensing returns – this is the threshold value for sensing.

   d. Set sensitivity to half this value.

4 Test output threshold (continuing from step 3 above the pacing will now be set at a low rate, and at minimum output):

   ○ Increase the pacing rate to 10 greater than ULR.

While watching the monitor:

   a. Gradually increase the output until capture is achieved.

   b. Note the value at which capture occurs – this is the threshold value.

   c. Set output to double this value as a safety margin (minimum 5 mA).

5 Store new values in memory and document settings.

FIGURE 11.52 Revealing concealed sinus capability to improve haemodynamics (ECG and arterial pressure waveform, continuous strip). Initially there is ventricular pacing at a rate of 68/min with no evidence of atrial activity. Blood pressure 85/50 mmHg with noradrenaline (norepinephrine) support at 8 micrograms/min. Across the top strip the pacing rate is reduced and P waves emerge at a rate of 60/min (arrow) before gradual acceleration to 70/min across the lower strip. With restoration of atrial kick the BP increases impressively to 125/65 mmHg, with cardiac index improvement from 1.7 L/min/m^2 to 2.3 L/min/m^2, allowing discontinuation of noradrenaline infusion. Importantly, there was no suggestion of sinus capability until cautiously sought via rate reduction, and the final sinus rate (but with atrial kick) was the same as the initial pacing rate.

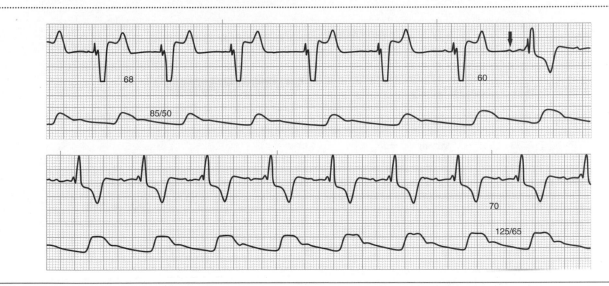

capable of delivering 20 mA, then demonstrating that capture is still present at 10 mA confirms an adequate safety margin without losing capture.

Permanent pacing

For bradyarrhythmias that are not due to temporary reversible factors or that are likely to be sustained or recurrent, permanent pacemaker implantation may be undertaken. A dual-chamber device is usually implanted to allow DDD pacing unless there is permanent atrial fibrillation[83] or an indication for cardiac resynchronisation therapy, discussed below. Rate-responsive pacing is commonly employed in permanent pacing, permitting the pacing rate to be varied during exercise and activity. Virtually all permanent pacing leads are steroid tipped to limit any lead contact-induced inflammatory changes, which can increase threshold.[105]

Pacemaker parameters: programming and status reports

Knowledge of current pacemaker programming is crucial in interpreting pacemaker behaviour to enable determination of whether a change in pacing behaviour represents a pacing problem or is simply an automated behaviour. Device printouts should be available whenever a device is interrogated or reprogrammed, and the summary pages outline the operating parameters, active automated features,

results from recent tests and battery status (see Fig. 11.53 for an example). Important elements include:

- patient/device details: patient name, type of device, date and time of the printout
- predicted battery longevity (assuming 100% pacing), and magnet rate (the asynchronous rate which will apply upon magnet placement)
- current parameters: base rate, maximum atrial tracking rate, AV delay, output settings and pulse widths for both chambers
- episodes: summary of any arrhythmia episodes that have been recorded since the last interrogation and any automatic mode switching events that have occurred
- test results: the results of capture and sensing tests, including graphic trends over time for each parameter.
- lead impedance measurements (high impedance suggests damage to lead conductors while low impedance indicates degradation of the lead insulation).

Cardiac resynchronisation therapy

Cardiac resynchronisation therapy (CRT) involves the use of pacing to improve the performance of the left ventricle in patients with symptomatic heart failure despite optimal

FIGURE 11.53 FastPath Summary from a St Jude Medical Assurity MRI™ dual-chamber pacemaker (St Jude Medical Sylmar CA), highlighting remaining battery longevity, basic parameters, events and test results recorded during pacemaker interrogation. The report shows current mode, rate and AV delay, along with output and sensitivity settings and results of testing in clinic. Test results followed by 'A' in black circles indicate automatic measurements which are performed 8–24-hourly and which allow automatic adjustment of outputs and sensitivity at home according to test results. Lead impedance measurements are shown for testing the integrity of pacing leads. Diagnostics include percentage of pacing, frequency and burden of atrial fibrillation and any episodes of high ventricular rates (usually >175 bpm). Arrhythmia recordings and details of duration/date and time are available in separate sections of device printouts.

ST. JUDE MEDICAL

DEMO PATIENT
Assurity MRI™ 2272 Pacemaker DEMO

12 Jul 2022
10:02 am
In-Clinic

FastPath™ Summary

⚠ 2 Alerts

Page 1 of 1

Battery
Longevity: 10.3–11.2 yrs

~ERI   >5 yrs

Implant Date:	7 Jul 2021
Voltage	3.07 V
Magnet Rate	100.0 ppm
Battery Current	9 uA
Remaining Capacity to ERI	>95%

Test Results   12 Jul 2022   Ⓐ Automatic

	Capture	Sense	Lead Impedance
A	0.625V @ 0.5ms (Bi) Ⓐ 0.5V @ 0.4ms (Bi) 14 Mar 2022	4.0mV (Bi) Ⓐ 4.1mV (Bi) 14 Mar 2022	600 Ω (Bi) Ⓐ 600 Ω (Bi) 14 Mar 2022
V	1.25V @ 0.5ms (Bi) Ⓐ 1.5V @ 0.4ms (Bi) 14 Mar 2022	>12.0mV (Bi) Ⓐ >12.0mV (Bi) 14 Mar 2022	580 Ω (Bi) Ⓐ 580 Ω (Bi) 14 Mar 2022

Parameters

Mode	DDDR
Base Rate	60 bpm
Max Track Rate	130 bpm
Paced AV Delay	200 ms
Sensed AV Delay	150 ms

Capture & Sense	**A**	**V**
ACap™ Confirm/V. AutoCapture	On	On
Pulse Amplitude	1.625 V Ⓐ	1.625 V Ⓐ
Pulse Width	0.4 ms	0.4 ms
AutoSense	Off	Off
Sensitivity (Safety Margin)	0.5 mV (7.8:1)	2.0 mV (6:1)

Diagnostics Summary   Since 7 Jul 2021

AP	11 %
VP	24 %
AMS Episodes	6
Mode Switch	<1%
AT/AF Burden	<1%

Episodes Summary   Since 7 Jul 2021

	Counts	EGMs
AMS Entry	6	6
High Ventricular Rate	2	2
Magnet Response	0	0

Note
This is a demo application.

Alerts
⚠ Device cybersecurity upgrade is available
High Ventricular Rate detected (1)

medical therapy. Patients do not need bradycardia to qualify for this form of pacing. Originally CRT was undertaken only in patients with severe heart failure (New York Heart Association class III–IV with ejection fraction <30%) due to dilated cardiomyopathy and with wide LBBB.[106,107] However, its proven efficacy in all major randomised controlled studies[108–112] has seen the range of indications expand to include patients with less severe heart failure (New York Heart Association classes I and II). Ischaemic cardiomyopathies with LBBB are also amenable to CRT. In the absence of LBBB, CRT is less successful and carries only class IIa/b recommendations in international guidelines.[113] Tailoring new approaches to resynchronisation for non-LBBB patients may improve effectiveness.[114]

Optimum systolic performance requires all segments of the ventricles to contract synchronously, and more or less simultaeously. However, this synchrony is disturbed in LBBB, in which septal depolarisation occurs first, followed by delayed conduction to the posterolateral walls of the left ventricle. The pattern of contraction is similarly disturbed, termed 'mechanical dyssynchrony'. The septum contracts early, followed by contraction of the posterolateral walls, resulting in reduced pumping efficacy, and contributing to low ejection fraction and heart failure.[115,116] Generally, the degree of dyssynchrony and impact on heart failure is worse at longer QRS duration,[117,118] and in dilated cardiomyopathy the QRS may reach 200 ms (0.20 seconds) duration.

CRT overcomes this dyssynchrony by pacing both the right and left ventricles simultaneously, or near-simultaneously, which restores synchronous contraction of the septum and the posterolateral left ventricular wall. This has also been termed biventricular pacing. This abolishes the slow conduction of LBBB, and the QRS duration can be seen to shorten, often to normal durations. Restoration of contractile synchrony improves the ejection fraction, and heart failure features and symptoms improve in at least 80% of patients.[117] Left ventricular dilation may be reversed and at times normal cardiac function is completely restored. The major determinant of CRT success is the degree of reduction in QRS duration.[117,118]

Possible outcomes of CRT include:[115–121]

- reduction in QRS duration, increased ejection fraction
- reduction in size of the left ventricle (reverse remodelling)
- reversal or limitation of the progression of heart failure
- improvement in New York Heart Association functional class
- improvement in quality of life
- improvement in physical function
- reduced hospitalisations for heart failure
- cardiovascular mortality reduction.

The right ventricular lead is implanted in standard fashion, positioned at either the RV apex or the ventricular septum. Most commonly, the left ventricular lead is also positioned transvenously, with the lead advanced to the right atrium and then via the coronary sinus into a coronary vein on the lateral or posterolateral LV wall. In a minority of cases when access is poor or a suitable target vein is unavailable, a separate mini-thoracotomy may be necessary for positioning of an epicardial LV lead.

CRT may be provided by a specialised pacemaker (CRTP (pacemaker)), or as CRTD (defibrillator) if ventricular arrhythmias are occurring.

Clinical response to CRT

CRT may result in immediate improvement, as well as further incremental improvement over the next 3–12 months as the left ventricle adapts to the new pattern of contraction, and to its own improved performance. It is important to stress to patients that they should not be discouraged by absence of obvious early improvement. A significant additional benefit can be anticipated for most patients as they undergo ventricular alterations to the new pattern of LV contraction under biventricular pacing.[119, 120]

Rehospitalisation for worsening of heart failure in patients already implanted with a CRT device may be due to clinical factors but may also be due to correctable CRT problems. The most easily identified of these are AF and loss of capture by either of the ventricular leads such that resynchronisation is not occurring.

In AF, spontaneous conduction at faster rates than the programmed pacing rate will inhibit the pacing, reducing how much biventricular pacing is being provided. In addition, the loss of atrial kick has a significant impact in heart failure patients.[122] Early identification of AF in hospital is therefore important. If there is loss of capture by either the RV or the LV lead (but not both) then the QRS becomes wider than on previous ECGs. Left ventricular leads have a higher incidence of failure to capture.[105] Device interrogation should be undertaken during admission in order to confirm and correct loss of capture or to optimise programming for better resynchronisation.[123]

Recognising failure to capture in a CRT device

Recognising failure to capture in CRT is made difficult by the fact that both ventricles are paced, and a paced-QRS will still be produced when only one lead is capturing.[124] Failure of one lead results in loss of synchronisation and can lead to deterioration of heart failure. Usually it can be recognised by the QRS becoming wider than on previous ECGs and from the appearance of lead V1 on ECG. If only the RV is capturing, ventricular conduction occurs from right to left (left axis deviation) and V1 appears as a negative QRS complex which is also wider than previously (>0.12 s). If only the LV lead is capturing, conduction occurs from left to right (right axis

FIGURE 11.54 Comparative appearance of lead V1 during biventricular pacing, and alternately with loss of capture by the left ventricular, then right ventricular lead. In the top strip, there is Bi-V pacing with a narrow QRS, which is negative in V1. In the same strip, loss of LV capture results in RV-only pacing. The QRS widens to beyond 0.12 s and becomes more deeply negative in V1. In the second strip, RV-only becomes Bi-V pacing after re-establishing LV capture. The QRS narrows and returns to its initial morphology as in strip 1. In the third strip, Bi-V pacing is present initially followed by loss of RV capture, resulting in LV-only pacing. Note that the QRS becomes upright in V1 and again widens to well beyond 0.12 s. In the lower strip, LV-only pacing precedes the return to the previous Bi-V morphology as RV capture is restored.

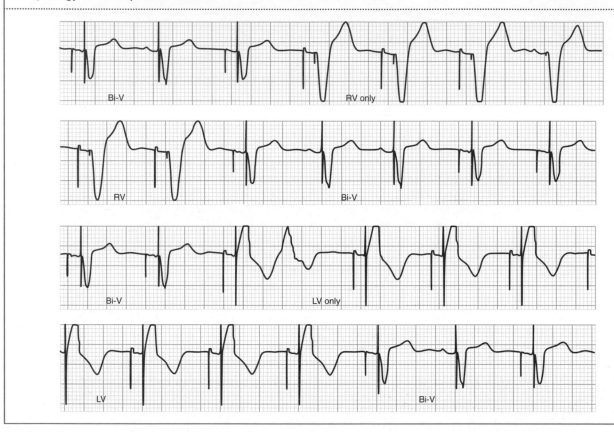

deviation) and V1 usually displays an entirely upright QRS which is wide (>0.12 s). Specific changes include:

- Loss of LV capture (= RV capture only): the QRS widens, V1 is usually entirely negative, left (or leftward) axis[125] (Fig. 11.54).

- Loss of RV capture (= LV capture only): the QRS widens, often markedly, V1 becomes upright complexes (R wave, RsR), right axis deviation, occasionally axis in no man's land[125] (see Fig. 11.54).

- Biventricular capture: the QRS may be entirely negative (but narrow) in V1, or biphasic (RS or rS pattern),[125] with the axis deviated most commonly to the right.

Conduction system pacing

There is currently a rapidly growing shift away from the traditional implantation of ventricular pacing leads into the myocardium of the right ventricular septum or apex. As discussed earlier, the wide QRS of right ventricular pacing results in dyssynchrony of left ventricular contraction and is associated with the development of dilated cardiomyopathy. Two main approaches, collectively termed conduction system pacing, involve implanting leads directly into the bundle of His[126] or the left bundle branch.[127] Both can be used for standard bradycardia support, and because they may restore normal intraventricular conduction (even correcting an existing LBBB) they can be used for cardiac resynchronisation.[128,129]

Conduction system pacing presents a new challenge for ECG interpretation – recognising capture and failure to capture.[130] Historically, recognising ventricular capture was largely straightforward and based on seeing a wide QRS immediately following the pacing stimulus on ECG, and narrow QRS complexes were used to suggest that capture was not occurring. Now with conduction system pacing able to produce narrow QRS complexes, confirmation of capture becomes uncertain unless it is known that conduction system pacing is in use. This uncertainty is compounded by the fact that often a brief

FIGURE 11.55 His bundle pacing. DDD mode with AV pacing at 70/min. The ventricular spikes capture the His bundle and take 40 ms to conduct through the bundle branches before the onset of the QRS. As ventricular excitation occurs via normal ventricular conduction pathways the resultant QRS is narrow, and because the QRS is not wide the strip could easily be interpreted as sinus rhythm with intrinsic conduction to the ventricles, and failure to capture by the pacing stimuli.

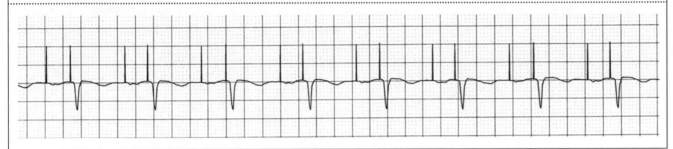

(40 ms) isoelectric interval can follow the pacing stimulus while conduction down the bundle branches occurs before the QRS begins.[130] In Fig. 11.55 this 40-ms isoelectric period can be seen following the ventricular pacing spikes, and the paced QRS is narrow and of normal appearance. This could be mistaken for ventricular failure to capture if it is not known that it is a His bundle pacing system.

Cardioversion and defibrillation

The aim of cardioversion for reversion of tachyarrhythmias is to depolarise all myocardial cells at the same time, with the result that all of the heart will also be refractory at the same time. If this is achieved, the circulating wavefronts of reentry die out for lack of non-refractory tissue to conduct through. If the applied shock does not depolarise the greater bulk of myocardium, then non-depolarised cells are still available for conduction and the arrhythmia may persist. External shocks of 100–200 joules (biphasic) are required for sufficient current density to reach the myocardium and depolarise the greater bulk of cells, extinguishing available pathways.[131] Shocks delivered directly to the heart via an ICD need only be of 20–40 joules strength for the same effect. Drugs or biochemical correction may be necessary to prevent recurrence. Success rates from cardioversion range from 70% to 95% depending on the rhythm.[131] Arrhythmias due to increased automaticity are less amenable to cardioversion, as there is a higher chance of early arrhythmia recurrence; for arrhythmias occurring as a complication of digitalis toxicity, cardioversion (but not defibrillation) is contraindicated.

Early defibrillation increases survival from VF. The success of public-access defibrillator schemes has warranted their increased availability.[132,133] Automatic external defibrillators (AEDs) in the home or community simplify the task of applying defibrillation by non-healthcare responders and increase access to definitive electrical management for patients suffering ventricular arrhythmias.[134]

For patients at increased risk for arrhythmia development, or for those who have survived previous arrhythmic cardiac arrest, an ICD may be necessary. Emergency defibrillation is discussed more completely in Chapter 25.

Elective cardioversion

Elective direct current reversion (DCR, or cardioversion) applied under short-acting sedation or anaesthesia is undertaken for non-cardiac arrest arrhythmias.[135] These include AF, atrial tachycardia or flutter, conscious VT, AV nodal reentry tachycardia, and conscious tachyarrhythmias complicating WPW syndrome. The time available for preparation is variable and depends on haemodynamic status. Patients admitted for reversion of AF or flutter may be stable throughout their hospitalisation, whereas patients with conscious VT may initially demonstrate stability only to decompensate later without warning.

Unlike emergency defibrillation, cardioversion shocks are synchronised to the cardiac cycle so that they are delivered into the QRS complex.[135] Unsynchronised shocks, if delivered into the T wave, may precipitate VF. Confirmation of synchronisation should be sought via markers inscribed over the QRS (and not the T wave) on the debrillator screen.

When time permits the patient should be thoroughly investigated, including physical examination, neurological assessment, palpation of peripheral pulses, electrocardiograph, biochemistry, and serum drug levels where necessary.[133,135] Fasting should be ensured. If not already anticoagulated, transoesophageal echocardiography may be necessary to exclude left atrial thrombus. The patient should be fully informed of the rationale for and nature of the procedure and have all necessary preparatory tasks explained to them.

The cardioversion team should include a minimum of one medical officer, skilled in emergency rhythm management and airway management including intubation, and two critical care nurses, who prepare the patient and equipment, assist in sedation, perform the cardioversion, document events and manage aftercare. All team members should confirm readiness, confirm synchronisation and correct defibrillator energy settings (in joules). The patient is sedated (e.g. midazolam) or anaesthetised (e.g. propofol), preoxygenated and cardioverted under ECG and oximetry monitoring. Electrical safety, and ensuring that all personnel are clear of the bed, is the responsibility of the nurse delivering cardioversion, whether via paddles or hands-free electrodes.

After the procedure the patient should be closely monitored for return to wakefulness, airway protection capability, effective respiration and gas exchange, rhythm stability, blood pressure, and any changes in neurological status or peripheral pulses. Energy requirements for reversion of atrial tachycardia or flutter may be as little as to 50 joules (J).[136] Shock strength escalation following unsuccessful shocks is recommended, with initial shocks at 70–120 J (biphasic) for atrial flutter and 120–150 J for VT cardioversion.[133] These guidelines also suggest commencing at maximum joules for reverting AF.

Implantable cardioverter defibrillators

ICDs were initially implanted for survivors of sudden cardiac death (SCD) or haemodynamically significant, potentially lethal, ventricular arrhythmias.[132,137] They have been repeatedly demonstrated in large clinical trials to provide significantly improved survival compared with pharmacological treatment.[138–142] This 'secondary prevention' application dominated the early indications for ICD devices, with a 31% mortality reduction at 3 years post implant compared with antiarrhythmics in the AVID study.[138] ICD indications have expanded to 'primary prevention' in patients without prior cardiac arrest, as it has become clear that heart failure patients with ejection fractions <30%,[141] inherited arrhythmic disorders[143] and congenital heart diseases[144] have greater risk of sudden cardiac death due to ventricular arrhythmias.

ICDs features both antibradycardia and antitachycardia capabilities. As antibradycardia devices they possess all the capabilities of standard pacemakers, increasingly in the DDD mode. However, if there is no history of bradycardia, they may be programmed at low base pacing rates (e.g. 40/min). If there is significant heart failure the antibradycardia arm may be provided as biventricular pacing (to achieve cardiac resynchronisation). Antitachycardia features are those therapies provided to treat ventricular tachyarrhythmias and include antitachycardia pacing (ATP), also termed overdrive pacing, as well as cardioversion (for VT) and defibrillation (for very fast VT or VF). Refer to Fig. 11.56 for an example of antitachycardia pacing.

ICDs are most commonly positioned in the left pectoral region, leaving the right side of the chest available for conventional placement of external defibrillator pads should they ever become necessary. Atrial leads are normal atrial pacing leads, but the ventricular ICD leads are slightly larger than pacing leads and carry the normal ventricular pacing circuitry, as well as coils encircling the lead that emit the high-energy shock discharges. Single-coil systems have one coil positioned on the lead at the level of the RV cavity, and shocks conduct from this coil to the metal casing of the ICD. Dual-coil leads feature this same RV coil as well as a second coil in the superior vena cava. In these systems, shocks can be configured to conduct from the RV coil to the superior vena cava coil, from the RV coil to the ICD, or from the RV coil to both the superior vena cava coil and the ICD. Configurations can impact significantly on the defibrillation threshold, and changes to the shock vector may be undertaken for patients with high defibrillation thresholds.

All modern ICDs provide biphasic shock waveforms only. Arrhythmia detection and classification usually require only a few seconds. Charge times to maximum joules in a new device are up to 10 seconds. As the battery declines, charge time may increase to 15–20 seconds or longer. Maximum energy delivery capabilities vary between manufacturers but are all in the range of 30–40 J.

Typically, shocks for VF and very fast VT are provided at the maximum available capability of the device, but for less-rapid ventricular tachycardia, lower 'cardioversion' shocks may be attempted first (e.g. 15–25 J). If initial shocks are unsuccessful, progressive shock strength escalation occurs.[145]

Defibrillation thresholds may be measured at the time of implantation of the ICD; however, this practice has decreased significantly because of inherent risks in inducing VF, and because it is recognised that clinical VF may behave differently to induced VF.[146]

ICDs are usually programmed to deliver up to six 'therapies' during a tachyarrhythmia episode. For VF, this usually means six attempts at defibrillation at maximum joules, after which further antitachycardia therapies are aborted. No more shocks will be delivered. Antibradycardia pacing operation will continue. If the tachyarrhythmia is interrupted at any point and then recurs, this six-therapy counter will recommence.

For VT, attempts may first be made to overdrive pace. So-called ATP aims to interrupt VT by pacing the ventricles slightly faster than the VT rate so as to interrupt reentry, the major cause of VT (see Fig. 11.56 for an example of reversion). A number of attempts at ATP may be programmed, often with slightly faster rates at each successive attempt. This is especially true if the patient is known to tolerate their VT reasonably well. If ATP is unsuccessful, devices progress to shocks of increasing strength.

Tachyarrhythmia detection and classification

ICDs are configured to classify and treat arrhythmias first on the basis of rate. Defibrillation algorithms using high-energy settings (30–40 J) are followed when the rate is very fast (e.g. >200/min), as syncope is likely even if the rhythm is not VF (e.g. very fast VT). At slower rates, other antitachycardia options may first be attempted. Additionally, at rates where the rhythm could be either

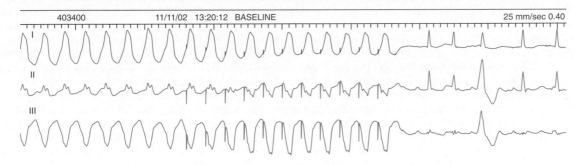

FIGURE 11.56 Successful antitachycardia pacing (ATP) delivered by an implantable cardioverter defibrillator. Three simultaneous strips show the presence of sustained ventricular tachycardia (VT). After the first eight beats, pacing is applied at a rate slightly faster than the tachycardia. Entrainment, or capture, by the pacemaker is best seen in lead II, where the QRS morphology clearly changes. After 11 paced beats, ATP is ceased, revealing interruption of the VT.

ventricular or supraventricular, attempts are made to discriminate between ventricular and supraventricular tachycardias (SVTs) using a variety of criteria. SVT discrimination by a device uses similar criteria to those by which a clinician would differentiate between VT and SVT and include regularity or irregularity of the rhythm, sudden or gradual onset, similar or different morphology to the previous sinus rhythm and atrioventricular relationships. If these discriminators indicate that a tachyarrhythmia is supraventricular, therapy can be withheld, avoiding inappropriate therapy. The major device capabilities and programming options of an ICD are shown in Fig. 11.57.

Patients receiving ICDs require particular education and support, as the experience of shocks can be painful and disturbing. Anticipation of shocks can cause anxiety and/or depression,[147,148] especially in patients who have experienced shocks while conscious. Inappropriate therapy delivery remains a significant problem, and as many as 25% of ICD therapies were reported as inappropriate shocks during early experience, delivered due either to supraventricular arrhythmias or to oversensing of electromagnetic interference.[149,150] Refinement of rhythm discrimination has seen the incidence of inappropriate shocks reduced significantly with time. The avoidance of strong electrical fields (welding, generators) should be stressed, as well as direct contact with devices such as transcutaneous electrical nerve stimulation (TENS) machines or electrocautery devices.[150] If surgery requiring diathermy becomes necessary, antitachycardia therapies are usually programmed to 'OFF' to avoid inappropriate detection and treatment. The ability to undergo magnetic resonance imaging (MRI) should be determined on an individual basis, as some but not all ICDs are approved for use in the MRI environment.

Patients should be encouraged to rest after receiving ICD shocks and report to a healthcare facility for assessment.[151] If inappropriate shocks are being delivered (shocks delivered despite the patient not being in VT or VF), further shocks may be suspended by the placement

of a ring magnet over the device.[152] No VT or VF treatment will be delivered while the magnet is in place over the device. Cardiac monitoring is imperative in case genuine ventricular arrhythmias subsequently develop. Removal of the magnet will immediately reactivate antitachycardia therapies. Backup (antibradycardia) pacing functions remain active and unaffected during magnet application.

In the event of unsuccessful reversion of a ventricular arrhythmia by ICD therapy, standard advanced life support protocols should be applied. External defibrillation can be undertaken with pads in the normal apicobasal or anteroposterior positions, taking care to avoid positioning paddles over the ICD.[153]

Practice tip

If cardiac arrest occurs in a patient with an ICD in place, all standard therapies should be undertaken, including CPR, drug administration and immediate preparation for external defibrillation. If device shocks are unsuccessful, proceed to external defibrillation.

End-of-life care in the patient with an ICD

ICDs often create uncertainty among healthcare workers as to how death may occur. In the end-of-life patient, where active resuscitation is not to be pursued, the decision to disable antitachycardia therapies is often taken. This can be achieved by reprogramming the ICD, and there is often sufficient time to incorporate this step into palliative planning. If time does not permit this, tachyarrhythmia treatment can be suspended by securing a ring magnet over the ICD (tape it in place). Therefore, if the terminal rhythm is VT or VF, shocks and ATP will not be delivered.

FIGURE 11.57 Implantable cardioverter defibrillator (ICD) programmed parameter summary report from St Jude Medical Gallant HF™ ICD with CRT capabilities. (St Jude Medical, Sylmar CA). Similar to the report shown earlier for a pacemaker, the report includes battery status and test results for lead impedances, sensing and capture thresholds for the atrial and ventricular lead. The battery status section also displays the most recent time (in seconds) taken for the device to charge to a maximum joule shock. In the parameters section are the programmed settings for pacing and defibrillation behaviours. The tachyarrhythmia treatments are shown at the right of the parameters section and show the device therapies available for tachycardias occurring at different rates. In the designated 'VF zone', the ICD will respond to any arrhythmia faster than 214 bpm (whether it is VF or fast VT). Immediate high shock strengths are typical for this rate range, though a single attempt at ATP may be attempted while the device is charging for the first shock. In the VT-2 zone, a different strategy has been programmed for VT between 181 and 214/min. Three attempts at delivering ATP have been programmed and, if unsuccessful, the ICD will progress to increasing energy levels (20, 30, 36 J) if reversion is not achieved. A third treatment zone can be programmed for slower VTs, often in the range of 150–180/min. As these rates may be better tolerated, programming is often less aggressive, with a greater number of attempts at ATP before progressing to shocks. Details of how the device is set to discriminate between VT and SVT, as well as the set-up of the pacing strategies, are given in separate sections of these reports. VT/VF episodes since last device check are shown; in this case there has been a single VF episode for which three shocks were delivered. Recordings of these arrhythmias and treatments are recorded elsewhere in the report.

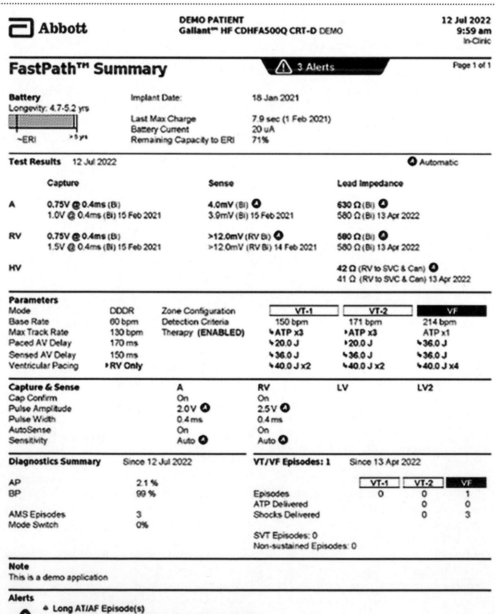

Other than by disabling therapy, cardiac death may occur by normal mechanisms. What would otherwise be a bradyarrhythmic death will instead become eventual failure to capture by the pacemaker. The paced QRS may be seen to significantly widen, similar to an agonal-type rhythm (described earlier) prior to the loss of capture. Similarly, if the cardiac impact of acute or terminal illness produces tachyarrhythmias, these same influences will increase the defibrillation threshold and shocks would become unsuccessful if they are still turned on. Devices offer no protection against pulseless electrical activity.

Note that, although tachyarrhythmia therapies may be disabled for end of life care, the same is not true of basic bradycardia pacing functions. These are left active (ON) and the patient is allowed to eventually lose capture.

Summary

Alteration to the electrophysiological function of the heart is very common in patients admitted to critical care settings. Arrhythmia detection is largely the responsibility of the critical care nurse, who must maintain accurate monitoring, constantly observe for the development of arrhythmias, assess their clinical impact and assist in identifying causative factors. The critical care nurse must also deliver the care and management of arrhythmias, including pharmacological and electrical therapies, being aware of complications and management of complications of these treatments.

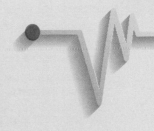

Case study

UNEXPLAINED RAPID PACING IN THE CORONARY CARE UNIT

A 69-year-old male with known ischaemic heart disease and a history of pacemaker implantation had been admitted to CCU with recent gastrointestinal bleeding. Telemetry records showed multiple instances of pacing at 100 bpm instead of the programmed base rate of 65 bpm. These began as abrupt rate increases (rather than gradual accelerations) and abrupt terminations. Many were sustained for long periods (Fig. 11.58).

In a dual-chamber pacemaker, pacing at faster than the programmed base rate may be appropriate under certain conditions but may also be unintended and therefore in need of identification and correction. To interpret such strips, first determine whether there is *dual-chamber* pacing at the elevated rate, or just *ventricular* pacing. If it is only ventricular, then atrial tracking is occurring. It, too, may be appropriate or inappropriate. Tracking sinus rhythm at a rate of 100/min is entirely appropriate but still requires

FIGURE 11.58 DDD pacemaker programmed to base rate 60/min. There is initially dual-chamber pacing at 100/min before the rate abruptly drops to 60/min (as atrial pacing with intrinsic conduction). After eight beats it abruptly returns to the elevated rate of 100/min.

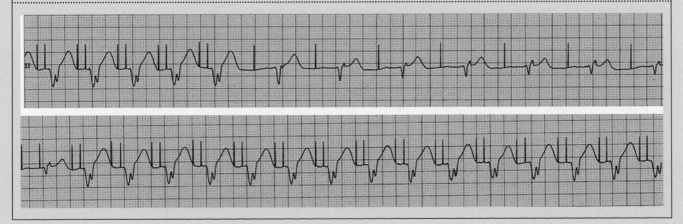

investigation into why the sinus rate is high. Against the known history of this patient, the elevated rate could be due to further bleeding, myocardial ischaemia, or other causes.

Inappropriate tracking may occur when there is sensing of atrial activity which is not sinus in origin and include the following:

- Tracking of an intermittent atrial arrhythmia – depending on the rhythm, the ventricular pacing could be regular or irregular and likely to be faster than seen here.

- Recurrent pacemaker-mediated tachycardia (PMT) – ultimately this is a form of tracking but in PMT the P waves are a result of ventricular pacing conducting retrogradely to the atria – again, it appears as only ventricular pacing and is often brief (e.g. 12 beats) because of automated correction algorithms in pacemakers.

- Electrical interference being sensed in the atrial channel. False signals may occur in the atrial channel because of environmental electrical interference. Oversensing of such 'noise' may be tracked by the pacemaker.

The example here is not atrial tracking because there is dual-chamber pacing, not just ventricular.

Dual-chamber pacing at rates above the programmed base rate can occur as a result of rate-responsive pacing, in which the rate is accelerated in response to activity or an increase in minute ventilation (respiratory rate and depth). Rate-responsive pacing can look like the appearance here but the changes in rate are gradual (for both increasing and decreasing the rate) rather than the abrupt, sudden changes seen here. For this patient who is at rest, and without tachypnoea, rate response does not explain the appearance.

Pacemaker interrogation revealed frequent 'magnet responses' in event logs limited to the period of the patient's hospital stay. This explained the behaviour, but not the source, of the magnetic field which was influencing the pacemaker.

Magnet responses feature in all permanent pacemakers and have important considerations. When a ring-shaped magnet is placed over a pacemaker it will revert to asynchronous pacing (DOO for a dual-chamber device) at the 'magnet rate' (here 100/min). Its main therapeutic application is to protect against pacing inhibition by actual or potential oversensing. With sensing turned off (DOO), false inhibition of pacing cannot occur. Diathermy is a common cause of oversensing, so ring magnets are often positioned over pacemakers intraoperatively for protection. The elevated rate usually ensures overdrive of the intrinsic rhythm to prevent competitive pacing and risk of inadvertent pacing into T waves. Asynchronous pacing carries the very real risk of precipitating VT or VF if the patient's rate overlaps with the asynchronous pacing rate.

The source of magnetic field exposure could not be determined, even with magnetic field testing of the patient's room. After troubleshooting, however, the patient returned to watching television and the asynchronous pacing at 100/min promptly recurred, revealing the source. In consideration to the other patients in the room, he had positioned his television speaker (in the nurse-call handset) on his left shoulder for quiet listening (Fig. 11.59). The magnet in the speaker was the source. Asynchronous pacing was repeatedly reproduced with repositioning of the handset, and interestingly was sometimes volume related, only occurring at higher volumes when the speaker magnetic field increased.

With awareness, it is now apparent that using handsets/speakers in this manner is ubiquitous throughout the hospital. Awareness of this risk to pacemaker patients appears very limited, and, even in CCU, pacemaker patients are not warned about the risk it poses to them. In every case of magnet exposure subsequently investigated in CCU, the source has been confirmed as the handset/speaker placed over the pacemaker for quiet listening.

A more concerning risk occurs when ICDs are exposed to magnets in this way. Unlike pacemakers, magnets do not cause asynchronous pacing in ICDs. Instead, they disable (turn OFF) tachyarrhythmia therapies while the magnet is over the ICD. Therefore, the patient would remain untreated if VT or VF occurred. At the same hospital, one patient with previous recurrent VF was encountered on an (unmonitored) general medical ward using the speaker/handset as above. A routine check of the ICD showed it had undergone frequent magnet reversions. The patient confirmed using the handset in the manner above and triggering of the magnet response was reproducible. As cardiac monitoring was not present, the patient would simply not have received VF treatment, and even had he been in CCU significant delays in defibrillation were conceivable as staff waited for the ICD to operate.

FIGURE 11.59 Nurse-call handset with speaker positioned directly over the patient's pacemaker, evoking frequent magnet responses/asynchronous (DOO) pacing.

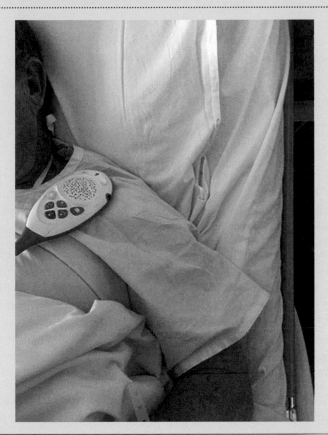

For ICD patients, deliberate magnet application is used in certain contexts:

- To prevent ICD shocks during diathermy, as diathermy currents could be detected and interpreted as VF.

- To suspend ICD therapies when inappropriate shocks are being delivered owing to misdiagnosis of atrial tachyarrhythmias (until device reprogramming is undertaken).

- In end-of-life care, until ICD therapies can be disabled.

The seemingly benign but widespread use of speakers/nurse call handsets in the manner outlined carries significant risks to patients with cardiac devices. These risks should be highlighted and shared with staff and patients in departments where pacemaker patients are accommodated.

CASE STUDY QUESTIONS

1 Under what circumstances can a pacemaker pace faster than the programmed base rate?

2 Outline how to differentiate the various possible causes of more-rapid pacing than expected, including the ECG features which help to discriminate between them.

3 Describe the distinct responses of pacemakers and ICDs to exposure to magnetic fields.

4 Describe the clinical contexts in which a ring magnet may be deliberately placed over a pacemaker or defibrillator.

RESEARCH VIGNETTE

Marcus GM, Vittinghoff E, Whitman IR, et al. Acute consumption of alcohol and discrete atrial fibrillation events. Ann Intern Med 2021;174(11):1503–9.

Abstract

Background: Patients' self-reports suggest that acute alcohol consumption may trigger a discrete atrial fibrillation event.[154]

Design: A prospective, case-crossover analysis.

Setting: Ambulatory persons in their natural environments.

Participants: Consenting patients with paroxysmal AF.

Measurements: Participants were fitted with a continuous electrocardiogram (ECG) monitor and an ankle-worn transdermal ethanol sensor for 4 weeks. Real-time documentation of each alcoholic drink consumed was self-recorded using a button on the ECG recording device. Fingerstick blood tests for phosphatidylethanol (PEth) were used to corroborate ascertainments of drinking events.

Results: Of 100 participants (mean age, 64 years (standard deviation (SD), 15); 79% male; 85% white), 56 had at least 1 episode of AF. Results of PEth testing correlated with the number of real-time recorded drinks and with events detected by the transdermal alcohol sensor. An AF episode was associated with twofold higher odds of 1 alcoholic drink (odds ratio (OR), 2.02; 95% confidence interval (CI), 1.38–3.17) and greater than threefold higher odds of at least 2 drinks (OR, 3.58; 95% CI, 1.63–7.89) in the preceding 4 hours. Episodes of AF were also associated with higher odds of peak blood alcohol concentration (OR, 1.38; 95% CI, 1.04–1.83) per 0.1% increase in blood alcohol concentration) and the total area under the curve of alcohol exposure (OR, 1.14; 95% CI, 1.06–1.22) per 4.7% increase in alcohol exposure, inferred from the transdermal ethanol sensor in the preceding 12 hours.

Limitation: Confounding by other time-varying exposures that may accompany alcohol consumption cannot be excluded, and the findings from the current study of patients with AF consuming alcohol may not apply to the general population.

Conclusion: Individual AF episodes were associated with higher odds of recent alcohol consumption, providing objective evidence that a modifiable behaviour may influence the probability that a discrete AF event will occur.

Primary funding source: National Institute on Alcohol Abuse and Alcoholism.

Critique

AF is the most common arrhythmia in developed countries, with an estimated prevalence of between 1% and 4% in Australia, Europe and the USA, making it a significant burden on individual health and healthcare systems.[5] Although AF is common, its causes remain poorly understood, making it difficult to predict who will be affected by the arrhythmia. Known risk factors for AF include hypertension, chronic diseases of the heart and lungs, systemic infection and thyrotoxicosis.[3] In terms of lifestyle, chronic alcohol use has been identified as a significant risk factor, with studies demonstrating an increased incidence of AF with even a modest, regular alcohol intake.[154,155]

Although the link between alcohol and AF is well established, several major limitations have been identified in the evidence base. Firstly, studies correlating alcohol consumption with AF incidence have previously used questionnaires to assess alcohol intake, rather than objective data. Self-report is prone to external bias, as individuals may report what they feel researchers want to hear, or what they perceive as being socially acceptable, rather than their true behaviour.[156] Secondly, although previous studies have shown that AF risk increases with regular alcohol intake, they have not demonstrated a temporal relationship between alcohol consumption and individual episodes of AF. In other words, they have not shown that discrete episodes of AF have been triggered by drinking alcohol.

In the study by Marcus and colleagues, objective evidence of alcohol consumption was compared with AF occurrence over a 4-week period. A Zio monitor was used to continuously measure heart rhythm and detect episodes of AF.

This device has a button that patients press to record the presence of symptoms, allowing correlation with rhythm changes when the recording is analysed. In the study, patients were asked to press the button every time they had an alcoholic drink, rather than symptoms, allowing accurate timing of when alcohol was consumed. To provide further objective evidence, patients wore a transdermal alcohol monitor, allowing changes in body alcohol to be tracked. As an additional check, PEth testing was performed. This measures serum phosphatidylethanol, a biomarker that reflects alcohol consumption in the previous 4 weeks.

The study showed that patients with paroxysmal AF were twice as likely to experience an episode of the arrhythmia after drinking a single glass of wine, beer or other alcoholic beverage. The increase in risk was threefold after two or more drinks.

There are some limitations to the study; 85% of the participants were white and 79% were male, so it may not be possible to apply these findings to a wider population. Confounding from other factors cannot be excluded, for example other foods or behaviours that might have accompanied alcohol consumption. Nonetheless, the study's great strength is that it objectively demonstrates for the first time that consuming alcohol triggers episodes of AF in some people, a phenomenon which has been widely reported by AF patients but never previously proven. The study gives clinicians stronger evidence on which to base lifestyle advice, and in particular avoidance strategies for AF.

The study also adds to the growing evidence base on the relationship between alcohol and cardiovascular disease. Although the harmful effects of heavy alcohol consumption on the heart and circulation have long been appreciated, light-to-moderate alcohol consumption has previously been associated with a reduced risk of cardiovascular disease.[157] This view was based on the findings of observational studies, which are prone to confounding by uncontrolled variables. Recent research suggests that the lower risk of cardiovascular disease seen in light-to-moderate drinkers may be due to other lifestyle factors such as diet and exercise, which offset the harmful effects of alcohol on cardiovascular health.[158] Emerging evidence suggests that even small amounts of alcohol may increase the risk of cardiovascular disease when compared with abstinence, even when individuals are drinking within government guidelines on 'safe' drinking.[158]

Although clinicians should continue to use government guidelines when delivering health education, they should also be aware that drinking alcohol probably has no cardiovascular health benefits. In people with established cardiovascular disease, especially AF, it is likely to be harmful. This message may be at odds with public perceptions, which are often based on outdated information provided by the mainstream media, rather than a health professional.[159]

Learning activities

1   Review the current national recommendations for alcohol consumption. These can be found on government websites and should form the starting point for health promotion activities with patients.

2   Consider how you assess alcohol consumption during patient assessment. Are you up to date with the current systems for measuring units of alcohol? Is there a standard tool used in your organisation? How would you approach a conversation about alcohol consumption?

3   Think about how alcohol fits into the wider debate on lifestyle, diet and obesity. Do you know how many calories a unit of alcohol contains? How about mixers that may be added, for example cola or tonic water? What effect does alcohol have on other health-related behaviours such as diet and exercise?

4   Our understanding of the factors that contribute to AF, and the way that we classify the disease, have undergone considerable change in recent years. Update your knowledge by reading the introductory sections of the most recent clinical guidelines on the topic – see references 3 and 32, which are both free to download from the internet.

Online resources

ECG quizzes and teaching materials: https://library.med.utah.edu/kw/ecg/, https://ekgreview.com/, https://quizizz.com/admin/quiz/5e68decd2452f2001c742dc6/biotel-systems-review, https://www.ecglibrary.com/ecghome.html, https://en.ecgpedia.org, https://www.healio.com/cardiology/learn-the-heart/quizzes-and-cases, https://www.ecri.org/forms/pages/Alarm_Safety_Resource.aspx

'Life in the fast lane' is an excellent online resource for concise information on arrhythmias and 12-lead ECG abnormalities. It is to the point, up to date and discusses features, clinical considerations and management.

Online manuals and education resources for pacemakers/defibrillators (manufacturer-specific):

Abbott (formerly St Jude Medical), https://www.abbott.com

Boston Scientific (including Guidant devices), https://www.bostonscientific.com

Medtronic, https://www.medtronic.com

'Temporary ventricular pacing Parts 1 and 2'. Lectures by Malcolm Dennis 2022. Appears in the free global Critical Care Nursing Education platform 'Continulus'. The lectures include useful discussions and video demonstration of techniques and methods in pacing management, https://www.continulus.com

To check whether a device is approved for MRI testing, https://www.MRIsafety.com

Further reading

Conover MB. Understanding electrocardiography. 8th ed. St Louis, MO: Mosby; 2002.

Drew B, Ackerman M, Funk M, et al. Prevention of torsades de pointes in hospital settings: a scientific statement from The American Heart Association and The American College of Cardiology Foundation. J Am Coll Cardiol 2010;55(9):934–47.

Epstein A, DiMarco J, Ellenbogen K, et al. American College of Cardiology Foundation; American Heart Association Task Force on Practice Guidelines; Heart Rhythm Society. 2012 ACCF/AHA/HRS focused update incorporated into the ACCF/AHA/HRS 2008 guidelines for device-based therapy of cardiac rhythm abnormalities: a report of the American College of Cardiology Foundation/American Heart Association Task Force on Practice Guidelines and the Heart Rhythm Society. J Am Coll Cardiol 2013;61(3):e6–75.

For down-to-earth discussion of pacemakers and ICDs, the 3-part series by Tom Kenny is valuable; the new editions are imminent:
- The nuts and bolts of cardiac pacing. 2nd edn. Hoboken, NJ: Wiley-Blackwell; 2008.
- The nuts and bolts of ICD therapy. Malden, MA: Blackwell-Futura; 2005.
- The nuts and bolts of cardiac resynchronization therapy. Malden, MA: Blackwell-Futura; 2007.

Glikson M, Nielsen JC, Kronborg MB, et al. 2021 ESC Guidelines on cardiac pacing and cardiac resynchronization therapy: developed by the Task Force on cardiac pacing and cardiac resynchronization therapy of the European Society of Cardiology (ESC) With the special contribution of the European Heart Rhythm Association (EHRA). Eur Heart J 2021;42(35):3427–520.

References

1. Prystowski EN, Klein GJ, Daubert JP. Cardiac arrhythmias: interpretation, diagnosis and treatment. 2nd ed. New York: McGraw Hill; 2020.
2. Resuscitation Council UK. Advanced life support. 8th ed. London; Resuscitation Council UK; 2021.
3. Hindricks G, Potaro T, Dagres N, et al. 2020 ESC Guidelines for the diagnosis and management of atrial fibrillation developed in collaboration with the European Association for Cardio-Thoracic Surgery (EACTS) The Task Force for the diagnosis and management of atrial fibrillation of the European Society of Cardiology (ESC) developed with the special contribution of the European Heart Rhythm Association (EHRA) of the ESC. Eur Heart J 2021;42(5):373–498.
4. Bosch NA, Cimini J, Walkey AJ. Atrial fibrillation in the ICU. Chest 2018;154(6):1424–34.
5. Zulkifly H, Lip GY, Lane DA. Epidemiology of atrial fibrillation. Int J Clin Pract 2018 Mar;72(3):e13070.
6. Wetterslev M, Haase N, Hassager C, et al. New-onset atrial fibrillation in adult critically ill patients: a scoping review. Intensive Care Med 2019;45(7):928–38.
7. Mohrman DE, Heller LJ. Cardiovascular physiology. 9th ed. New York: McGraw Hill; 2018.
8. Houghton, AR. Making sense of the ECG: a hands-on guide, fifth edition, Boca Raton, FL: CRC Press; 2019.

9. Hampton JR. The ECG made easy. 9th ed. London: Churchill Livingstone; 2019.

10. Chang W, Li G. Clinical review of sick sinus syndrome and atrial fibrillation. Herz 2022;47(3):244–50.

11. Hafeez Y, Grossman SA. Sinus bradycardia. StatPearls. Treasure Island, FL: StatPearls Publishing; 2021. Available from: https://www.ncbi. nlm.nih.gov/books/NBK493201/. [Accessed 27 February 2023].

12. Palatnick W, Jelic T. Calcium channel blocker and beta blocker overdose, and digoxin toxicity management. Emerg Med Pract 2020;22 (Suppl. 9):1–42.

13. Suarez K, Banchs JE. A review of temporary permanent pacemakers and a comparison with conventional temporary pacemakers. J Innov Card Rhythm Manag 2019;10(5):3652.

14. Ahmed A, Pothineni NV, Charate R, et al. Inappropriate sinus tachycardia: etiology, pathophysiology, and management: JACC review topic of the week. J Am Coll Cardiol 2022;79(24):2450–62.

15. Knuuti J, Wijns W, Saraste A, et al. 2019 ESC Guidelines for the diagnosis and management of chronic coronary syndromes: the Task Force for the diagnosis and management of chronic coronary syndromes of the European Society of Cardiology (ESC). Eur Heart J 2020;41(3): 407–77.

16. Heidenreich PA, Bozkurt B, Aguilar D, et al. 2022 AHA/ACC/HFSA guideline for the management of heart failure: a report of the American College of Cardiology/American Heart Association Joint Committee on Clinical Practice Guidelines. J Am Coll Cardiol 2022; 79(17):e263–421.

17. Hawks MK, Paul ML, Malu OO. Sinus node dysfunction. Am Fam Physician 2021;104(2):179–85.

18. Kerola T, Eranti A, Aro AL, et al. Risk factors associated with atrioventricular block. JAMA Netw Open 2019;2(5):e194176.

19. Clauss S, Bleyer C, Schuettler D, et al. Animal models of arrhythmia: classic electrophysiology to genetically modified large animals. Nature Rev Cardiol 2019;16(8):457–75.

20. Fogoros RN, Mandrola JM. Fogoros' electrophysiologic testing. 6th ed. Oxford: Wiley Blackwell; 2018.

21. Kistamas K, Veress R, Horvath B, et al. Calcium handling defects and cardiac arrhythmia syndromes. Front Pharmacol 2020;11:72.

22. Mellor GJ, Behr ER. Cardiac channelopathies: diagnosis and contemporary management. Heart 2021;107(13):1092–9.

23. Hickey KT, Elzomor A. Cardiac channelopathies: recognition, treatment, management. AACN Adv Crit Care 2018;29(1):43–57.

24. Leung LW, Gallagher MM. Review paper on WPW and athletes: let sleeping dogs lie? Clin Cardiol 2020;43(8):897–905.

25. Brugada J, Katritsis DG, Arbelo E, et al. 2019 ESC guidelines for the management of patients with supraventricular tachycardia the task force for the management of patients with supraventricular tachycardia of the European Society of Cardiology (ESC) developed in collaboration with the Association for European Paediatric and Congenital cardiology (AEPC). Eur Heart J 2020;41(5):655–720.

26. Klotzbaugh RJ, Martin A, Turner JR. Drug-induced proarrhythmia: discussion and considerations for clinical practice. JAAPA 2020;32(2): 128–35.

27. Resuscitation Council UK. Adult tachycardia. London: Resuscitation Council UK; 2021. Available from: https://www.resus.org.uk/sites/ default/files/2021-04/Tachycardia%20Algorithm%202021.pdf. [Accessed 27 February 2023].

28. Resuscitation Council UK. Adult bradycardia. London: Resuscitation Council UK; 2021. Available from: https://www.resus.org.uk/sites/ default/files/2021-04/Bradycardia%20Algorithm%202021.pdf. [Accessed 27 February 2023].

29. Feghaly J, Zakka P, London B, et al. Genetics of atrial fibrillation. J Am Heart Assoc 2018;7(20):e009884.

30. Haisseguerre M, Jais P, Shah DC, et al. Spontaneous initiation of atrial fibrillation by ectopic beats originating in the pulmonary veins. N Engl J Med 1998;339:659–66.

31. Li YG, Lip GY. Stroke prevention in atrial fibrillation: state of the art. Int J Cardiol 2019;287:201–9.

32. January CT, Wann LS, Calkins H, et al. 2019 AHA/ACC/HRS focused update of the 2014 AHA/ACC/HRS guideline for the management of patients with atrial fibrillation: a report of the American College of Cardiology/American Heart Association Task Force on Clinical Practice Guidelines and the Heart Rhythm Society. J Am Coll Cardiol 2019;74(1):104–32.

33. Joint Formulary Committee. British national formulary (online), London: BMJ Group and Pharmaceutical Press; 2022. Available from: https:// about.medicinescomplete.com/publication/british-national-formulary/. [Accessed 27 February 2023].

34. Mujović N, Dobrev D, Marinković M, et al. The role of amiodarone in contemporary management of complex cardiac arrhythmias. Pharmacol Res 2020;151:104521.

35. Oragano CA, Patton D, Moore Z. Phlebitis in intravenous amiodarone administration: Incidence and contributing factors. Crit Care Nurse 2019;39(1):e1–2.

36. Lip GY, Nieuwlaat R, Pisters R, et al. Refining clinical risk stratification for predicting stroke and thromboembolism in atrial fibrillation using a novel risk factor-based approach: the Euro Heart Survey on atrial fibrillation. Chest 2010;137:263–72.

37. Warden BA, MacKay J, Jafari M, et al. Use of direct oral anticoagulants among patients undergoing cardioversion: the importance of timing before cardioversion. J Am Heart Assoc 2018;7(22):e010854.

38. Calkins H, Hindricks G, Cappato R, et al. 2017 HRS/EHRA/ECAS/APHRS/SOLAECE expert consensus statement on catheter and surgical ablation of atrial fibrillation. Heart Rhythm 2017;14(10):e275–444.

39. Gupta D, Ding WY. Contemporary management of persistent atrial fibrillation. Heart 2022;108(2):145–51.

40. Kotadia ID, Williams SE, O'Neill M. Supraventricular tachycardia: an overview of diagnosis and management. Clin Med 2020;20(1):43.

41. Do DH, Boyle NG, Glover BM, et al. AV nodal re-entry tachycardia (AVNRT). In: Glover BM, Brugada P, editors. Clinical handbook of cardiac electrophysiology. Champaign, IL: Springer; 2021, p. 91–104.

42. Timme N, Opgen-Rhein B, Weber-Bärenbrinker S, et al. Aborted sudden cardiac death and ventricular fibrillation in patients with Wolff–Parkinson–White syndrome. Thorac Cardiovasc Surg 2022;70(S 02):DGPK-V57.

43. Appelboam A, Reuben A, Mann C, et al. Postural modification to the standard Valsalva manoeuvre for emergency treatment of supraventricular tachycardias (REVERT): a randomised controlled trial. Lancet 2015;386(10005):1747–53.

44. Brado J, Hochadel M, Senges J, et al. Outcomes of ablation in Wolff-Parkinson-White-syndrome: data from the German ablation registry. Int J Cardiol 2021;323:106–12.

45. Priori SG, Blomström-Lundqvist C, Mazzanti A, et al. 2015 ESC Guidelines for the management of patients with ventricular arrhythmias and the prevention of sudden cardiac death: the Task Force for the Management of Patients with Ventricular Arrhythmias and the Prevention of Sudden Cardiac Death of the European Society of Cardiology (ESC) endorsed by: Association for European Paediatric and Congenital Cardiology (AEPC). Europace 2015;17(11):1601–87.

46. Tongyoo S, Viarasilpa T, Permpikul C. Serum potassium levels and outcomes in critically ill patients in the medical intensive care unit. J Int Med Res 2018;46(3):1254–62.

47. Foth C, Gangwani MK, Alvey H. Ventricular tachycardia. StatPearls. Treasure Island, FL: StatPearls Publishing; 2021. Available from: https://www.ncbi.nlm.nih.gov/books/NBK532954/. [Accessed 27 February 2023].

48. Ding WY, Mahida S. Wide complex tachycardia: differentiating ventricular tachycardia from supraventricular tachycardia. Heart 2021;107(24):1995–2003.

49. Pathak RK, Ariyarathna N, Garcia FC, et al. Catheter ablation of idiopathic ventricular arrhythmias. Heart Lung Circ 2019;28(1):102–9.

50. Chia KK, Kanagaratnam L, Hellestrand K, et al. Pharmacological therapy for ventricular arrhythmias: a state-of-the art review. Heart Lung Circ 2019;28(1):49–56.

51. Strauss DG, Schocken DD. Marriott's practical electrocardiography. 13th ed. Philadelphia: Lippincott, Williams & Wilkins; 2021.

52. Rautaharju PM, Surawicz B, Gettes LS. AHA/ACCF/HRS recommendations for the standardization and interpretation of the electrocardiogram. Part IV: the ST segment, T and U waves, and the QT interval. A scientific statement from the American Heart Association Electrocardiography and Arrhythmias Committee, Council on Clinical Cardiology; the American College of Cardiology Foundation; and the Heart Rhythm Society. Circulation 2009;119:e241–50.

53. El-Sherif N, Turitto G, Boutjdir M. Acquired long QT syndrome and torsade de pointes. Pacing Clin Electrophysiol 2018;41(4):414–21.

54. Thomas SH, Behr ER. Pharmacological treatment of acquired QT prolongation and torsades de pointes. Br J Clin Pharmacol 2016;81(3):420–7.

55. Sandau KE, Funk M, Auerbach A, et al. Update to practice standards for electrocardiographic monitoring in hospital settings: a scientific statement from the American Heart Association. Circulation 2017;136:e273–344.

56. Al-Khatib SM, Stevenson WG, Ackerman MJ, et al. 2017 AHA/ACC/HRS guideline for management of patients with ventricular arrhythmias and the prevention of sudden cardiac death: a report of the American College of Cardiology/American Heart Association Task Force on Clinical Practice Guidelines and the Heart Rhythm Society. J Am Coll Cardiol 2018;72(14):e91–220.

57. Shivkumar K. Catheter ablation of ventricular arrhythmias. N Engl J Med 2019;380(16):1555–64.

58. Anderson RD, Kumar S, Kalman JM, et al. Catheter ablation of ventricular fibrillation. Heart Lung Circul 2019;28(1):110–22.

59. Brugada J, Pappone C, Berruezo A, et al. Brugada syndrome phenotype elimination by epicardial substrate ablation. Circ Arrhythm Electrophysiol 2015;8(6):1373–81.

60. Oving I, de Graaf C, Karlsson L, et al. Occurrence of shockable rhythm in out-of-hospital cardiac arrest over time: a report from the COSTA group. Resuscitation 2020;151:67–74.

61. Nolan JP, Soar J, Smith GB, et al. Incidence and outcome of in-hospital cardiac arrest in the United Kingdom National Cardiac Arrest Audit. Resuscitation 2014;85(8):987–92.

62. Wang L, Liu H, Zhu C, et al. Clinical characteristics and therapeutic strategy of frequent accelerated idioventricular rhythm. BMC Cardiovasc Disord 2021;21(1):1–9.

63. Nikolaidou T, Ghosh JM, Clark AL. Outcomes related to first-degree atrioventricular block and therapeutic implications in patients with heart failure. JACC Clin Electrophysiol 2016;2(2):181–92.

64. Kusumoto FM, Schoenfeld MH, Barrett C, et al. 2018 ACC/AHA/HRS guideline on the evaluation and management of patients with bradycardia and cardiac conduction delay: executive summary: a report of the American College of Cardiology/American Heart Association Task Force on Clinical Practice Guidelines, and the Heart Rhythm Society. J Am Coll Cardiol 2019;74(7):932–87.

65. Sidhu S, Marine JE. Evaluating and managing bradycardia. Trends Cardiovasc Med 2020;30(5):265–72.

66. Dan GA, Martinez-Rubio A, Agewall S, et al. Antiarrhythmic drugs – clinical use and clinical decision making: a consensus document from the European Heart Rhythm Association (EHRA) and European Society of Cardiology (ESC) Working Group on Cardiovascular Pharmacology, endorsed by the Heart Rhythm Society (HRS), Asia-Pacific Heart Rhythm Society (APHRS) and International Society of Cardiovascular Pharmacotherapy (ISCP). Europace 2018;20(5):731–2an.

67. Sandau KE, Funk M, Auerbach A, et al. Update to practice standards for electrocardiographic monitoring in hospital settings: a scientific statement from the American Heart Association. Circulation 2017;136(19):e273–344.

68. Mond HG, Wickham GG, Sloman JG. The Australian history of cardiac pacing: memories from a bygone era. Heart Lung Circ 2012;21(6-7): 311–19. doi: 10.1016/j.hlc.2011.09.004.

69. Mulpuru S, Madhavan M, McLeod C, et al. Cardiac pacemakers: function, troubleshooting, and management. J Am Coll Cardiol 2017;69(2):189–210. doi: 10.1016/j.jacc.2016.10.061.

70. Epstein AE, DiMarco JP, Ellenbogen KA. 2012 ACCF/AHA/HRS focused update incorporated into the ACCF/AHA/HRS 2008 guidelines for device-based therapy of cardiac rhythm abnormalities. Circulation 2012;127(3):e283–352. doi: 10.1161/CIR/)b)13e31827ce9b.

71. Kusumoto F, Schoenfeld MH, Barrett C, et al. 2018 ACC/AHA/HRS guideline on the evaluation and management of patients with bradycardia and cardiac conduction delay: a report of the American College of Cardiology/American Heart Association Task Force on Clinical Practice Guidelines and the Heart Rhythm Society. Circulation 2019;140:e382–482. doi: 10.1161/CIR.0000000000000628.

72. Rajappan K. Permanent pacemaker implantation technique: part 1. Heart 2009;95:259–64.

73. Sullivan BL, Bartels K, Hamilton N. Insertion and management of temporary pacemakers. Semin Cardiothorac Vasc Anesth 2016;20(1):52–62. doi: 10.1177/1089253215584923.

74. Lazarescu C, Mertes PM, Longrois D. Temporary epicardial pacing following cardiac surgery: practical aspects. Ann Fr Anaesth Reanim 2013;32(9):592–601. doi: 10.1016/j.annfar.2013.07.805.

75. Arnold AD, Whinnett ZI, Vijayaram P. His-Purkinje conduction system pacing: state of the art in 2020. Arrhythm Electrophysiol Rev 2020;9(3): 136–45. doi: 10.1540/aer.2020.14.

76. Overbay D, Criddle L. Mastering temporary invasive cardiac pacing. Crit Care Nurse 2004;24(3):25–32.

77. Laczika K, Thalhammer F, Locker G, et al. Safe and efficient emergency transvenous ventricular pacing via the right supraclavicular route. Anesth Analg 2000;90(4):784–9.

78. Swerdlow CD, Gillberg JM, Olson WH. Sensing and detection with cardiac implatable detection devices. In: Ellenbogen KA, Wilkoff BL, Kay GN, et al, editors. Clinical cardiac pacing, defibrillation, and resynchronization therapy. 5th ed. Philadelphia: Elsevier Saunders; 2017, p. 114–67.

79. Gutiérrez O. Different QRS morphologies in a dual-chamber pacemaker: what is the mechanism? J Thorac Dis 2017;9(11):4674–5. doi: 10.21037/jtd.2017.10.90.

80. Safavi-Naeini P, Saeed M. Pacing troubleshooting: common clinical scenarios. Tex Heart Inst J 2016;43(5):415–18. doi: 10.14503?THIJ-16-5918.

81. Loy SJ, Koulaoic D. Temporary pacing after cardiac surgery. AACN Adv Crit Care 2015;26(3):275–80.

82. Bernstein AD, Camm AJ, Fletcher RD, et al. The NASPE/BPEG generic pacemaker code for antibradyarrhythmic and adaptive rate pacing and antitachyarrhythmic devices. PACE 1987;10:794–9.

83. Stabile G, Simone A, Romano, E. Automatic mode switching in atrial fibrillation. Indian Pacing Electrophysiol J 2005;5:186–96.

84. Kay GN, Shepard RB. Stimulation and excitation of cardiac tissues. In: Ellenbogen KA, Wilkoff BL, Kay GN, Lau CP, et al, editors. Clinical cardiac pacing, defibrillation, and resynchronization therapy. 5th ed. Philadelphia: Elsevier Saunders; 2017, p. 61–113.

85. Schuchert A, Frese J, Stammwitz E, et al. Low settings of the ventricular pacing output in patients dependent on a pacemaker: are they really safe? Am Heart J 2002;143(6):1009–11.

86. Coombes D. Pacemaker therapy 2: pacing functions and their role in patient care. Nurs Times 2021;117(12):29–32. Available from: https://www.nursingtimes.net/clinical-archive/cardiovascular-clinical-archive/pacemaker-therapy-2-pacing-functions-and-their-role-in-patient-care-15-11-2021/. [Accessed 27 February 2023].

87. Tommaso C, Belic N, Brandfonbrener M. Asynchronous ventricular pacing: a rare cause of ventricular tachycardia. PACE 1982;5(4):561–3.

88. Mond HG. Unipolar versus bipolar pacing – poles apart. Pacing Clin Electrophysiol 1991;14(9):1411–24.

89. Bryant HC, Roberts PR, Diprose P. Perioperative management of patients with cardiac electronic devices. BJA Educ 2016;16(11):388–96. doi: 10.1093/bjaed/mkw020.

90. Farmer DM, Mark Estes NA 3rd, Link MS. New concepts in pacemaker syndrome. Indian Pacing Electrophysiol J 2004;4;195–200.

91. Slink M, Hellkamp A, Estes M, et al. High incidence of pacemaker syndrome in patients with sinus node dysfunction treated with ventricular-based pacing in the Mode Selection Trial (MOST). J Am Coll Cardiol 2004;43(11):2066–71.

92. Viskin S, Glikson M, Fish R, et al. Rate smoothing with cardiac pacing for preventing torsade de pointes. Am J Cardiol 2000;86(9):111K-15K.

93. Brandt J, Anderson H, Fahraeus T, et al. Natural history of sinus node disease treated with atrial pacing in 213 patients: implications for selection of stimulation mode. J Am Coll Cardiol 1992;20(3):633–9.

94. Kristensen L, Nielsen JC, Pedersen AK, et al. AV block and changes in pacing mode during long-term follow-up of 399 consecutive patients with sick sinus syndrome treated with an AAI/AAIR pacemaker. Pacing Clin Electrophysiol 2001;24(3):358–65.

95. Reade MC. Temporary epicardial pacing after cardiac surgery: a practical review. Part 2: selection of epicardial pacing modes and troubleshooting. Anaesthesia 2007;62:364–73. doi: 10.1111/j.1365–2044.2007.04951.x.

96. Wilkoff BL, Cook JR, Epstein AE, et al. Dual chamber pacing or ventricular backup pacing in patients with an implantable defibrillator: the Dual Chamber and VVI Implantable Defibrillator (DAVID) trial. JAMA 2002;288:3115–23.

97. Dennis MJ, Sparks PB. Pacemaker mediated tachycardia as a complication of the autointrinsic conduction search function. Pacing Clin Electrophysiol 2004;27(6Pt1):824–6.

98. Lamas GA, Ellenbogen KA. Evidence base for pacemaker mode selection. Circulation 2004;109:443–51. doi: 10.1161/01.CIR.0000115642. 05037.OE.

99. Sherbino J, Verbeek R, Russell D, et al. Prehospital transcutaneous cardiac pacing for symptomatic bradycardia or bradyasystolic cardiac arrest: a systematic review. Resuscitation 2006;70(2):193–200. doi: 10.1016/j.resuscitation.2005.11.019.

100. Bektas F, Soyuncu S. The efficacy of transcutaneous cardiac pacing in ED. Am J Emerg Med 2016;34(11):2090–3. doi: 10.1016/j.ajem.2016.07.022.

101. Chan T, Brady W, Harrigan R. Diagnosis: pacemaker failure to capture. Emerg Med News 2007;29(1):11.

102. Boumphrey S, Langton JA. Electrical safety in the operating theatre. Br J Anaesth 2003;3(1):10–14.

103. Martinez JC, Khiatah B, Jazayeri S, et al. Increased device thresholds with subsequent improvement status post-systemic therapy in a patient with multiple myeloma. Heart Rhythm Case Rep 2021;7(11):717–21. doi: 10.1016/jhcr.2021.06.005.

104. Edafe EA, Okoro TEO, Akpa MR, et al. Effects of cardiac drugs on pacemaker therapy: a review article. J Med-Clin Res Rev 2019;3(6):1–3.

105. Yang Z, Kirchhof N, Li S, et al. Effect of steroid elution on electrical performance and tissue responses in quadripolar left ventricular cardiac vein leads. Pacing Clin Electrophysiol 2015;38(8):966–72. doi: 10.1111/pace.12624.

106. Bakker P, Meijburg H, De Vries JW, et al. Biventricular pacing in end-stage heart failure improves functional capacity and left ventricular function. J Interv Card Electrophysiol 2000;4(2):395–404.

107. Hawkins NM, Petrie MC, MacDonald MR, et al. Selecting patients for cardiac resynchronization therapy: electrical or mechanical dyssynchrony? Eur Heart J 2006;27:1270–81.

108. Linde C, Leclerq C, Rex S, et al. Long-term benefits of biventricular pacing in congestive heart failure: results from the MUSTIC study. J Am Coll Cardiol 2002;40:433–40.

109. Cleland JGF, Subert JC, Erdmann E, et al. Longer-term effects of cardiac resynchronization therapy on mortality in heart failure [The Cardiac Resynchronisation-Heart Failure (CARE-HF) trial extension phase]. Eur Heart J 2006;27:1928–32.

110. Auricchio A, Stellbrink C, Sack S, et al. Pacing Therapies in Congestive Heart Failure (PATH-CHF) Study Group. Long-term clinical effect of hemodynamically optimized cardiac resynchronisation therapy in patients with heart failure and ventricular conduction delay. J Am Coll Cardiol 2002;39:2026–33.

111. Young JB, Abraham WT, Smithe AL, et al. Combined cardiac resynchronization and implantable cardioverter defibrillation in advanced chronic heart failure: the MIRACLE ICD trial. JAMA 2003;289:2685–94.

112. Bristow MR, Saxon LA, Boehmer J, et al. Comparison of Medical Therapy, Pacing, Defibrillation in Heart Failure (COMPANION) Investigators. Cardiac resynchronization therapy with or without an implantable defibrillator in advanced chronic heart failure. N Engl J Med 2004;350:2140–50.

113. Aurichio A, Lumens J, Prinzen FW. Does cardiac resynchronization therapy benefit patients with right bundle branch block: Cardiac resynchronization has a role in patients with right bundle branch block. Circ Arrhythm Electrophysiol 2014;7:532–42. doi: 10.1161/CIRCEP.113.000628.

114. Dennis MJ, Sparks PB, Capitani G. Tailoring cardiac resynchronization therapy to non-left bundle branch block: successful cardiac resynchronization for right bundle branch block with left posterior fascicular block without implantation of a left ventricular lead. Indian Pacing Electrophysiol J 2022;22(4):207–11.

115. Ghi S, Constantin C, Klersy C, et al. Interventricular and intraventricular dyssynchrony are common in heart failure patients, regardless of QRS duration. Eur Heart J 2004;25:571–8.

116. Littmann L, Symanski JD. Hemodynamic implications of left bundle branch block. J Electrocardiol 2000;33(Suppl. 1):115–21.

117. Varma N, O'Donnell D, Bassiouny M, et al. Programming cardiac resynchronization therapy for electrical synchrony: reaching beyond left bundle branch block and left ventricular activation delay. J Am Heart Assoc 2018;7(3):e007489. doi: 10.1161/JAHA.117.007489.

118. Alonso C, Leclercq C, Victor F, et al. Electrocardiographic predictive factors of long-term clinical improvement with multisite biventricular pacing in advanced heart failure. Am J Cardiol 1998;84:1417–21.

119. Verrnooy K, Verbeek XA, Peschar M, et al. Left bundle branch block induces ventricular remodelling and functional septal hypoperfusion. Eur Heart J 2005;26:91–8.

120. Sundell J, Engblom E, Koistinen J, et al. The effects of cardiac resynchronization therapy on left ventricular function, myocardial energetics and metabolic reserve in patients with dilated cardiomyopathy and heart failure. J Am Coll Cardiol 2004;43:1027–33.

121. Peichl P, Kautzner J, Cihak R, et al. The spectrum of inter- and intraventricular conduction abnormalities in patients eligible for cardiac resynchronization therapy. Pacing Clin Electrophysiol 2004;27(8):1105–12.

122. Daubert JC. Atrial fibrillation and heart failure: a mutually noxious association. Europace 2004;5:S1–4.

123. Pujol-Lopez M, San Antonio R, Mont L, et al. Electrocardiographic optimization technique in resynchronization therapy. Europace 2019;21:1286–96. doi: 10.1093/europace/euz126.

124. Sweeney MO, Hellkamp AS, van Bommel RJ, et al. QRS fusion complex analysis using wave interference to predict reverse remodeling during cardiac resynchronization therapy. Heart Rhythm 2014;11(5):806–13. doi: 10.1016/j.hrthm.2014.01.021.

125. Barrold SS, Herweg B. Usefulness of the 12 lead electrocardiograph in the follow-up of patients with cardiac resynchronization devices. Part 1. Cardiology J 2011;18(5):476–86. doi: 10.5603/CJ.2011.0002.

126. Ali N, Keene D, Arnold A, et al. His bundle pacing: a new frontier in the treatment of heart failure. Arrhythm Electrophysiol Rev 2018;7(2):103–10. doi: 10.15420/aer.2018.6.2.

127. Huang W, Chen Z, Su Lan, et al. A beginner's guide to permanent left bundle branch pacing. Heart Rhythm 2019;16(12):1791–6. doi: 10.1016/hrthm.2019.06.016.

128. Teng AE, Massoud L, Ajijola OA. Physiological mechanism of QRS narrowing in bundle branch block patients undergoing permanent His bundle pacing. J Electrocardiol 2016;49(5):644–8. doi: 10.1016/j.electrocard.2016.07.013.

129. Sharma PS, Vijayaraman P. Conduction system pacing for cardiac resynchronisation. Arrhythm Electrophysiol Rev 2021;10(1):51–8. doi: 10.15420/aer.2020.45.

130. Jastrzebski M. ECG and pacing criteria for differentiating conduction system pacing from myocardial pacing. Arrhythm Electrophysiol Rev 2021;10(3):172–80. doi: 10.15420/aer.2021.26.

131. Dosdall DJ, Fast VG, Ideker RE. Mechanisms of tailoring cardiac resynchronization therapy to non-left bundle branch block: successful cardiac resynchronization for right bundle branch block with left posterior fascicular block without implantation of a left ventricular lead. Annu Review Biomedic Eng 2010;12:233–58. doi: 10.1146/annurev-bioeng-070909-105305.

132. The Public Access Defibrillation Trial Investigators. Public-access defibrillation and survival after out-of-hospital cardiac arrest. N Engl J Med 2004;351:637–46.

133. Perkins G, Graesner J-T, Semeraro F. European Resuscitation Council guidelines 2021: executive summary, Resuscitation 2021;161:1–60. doi: 10.1016/j.resuscitation.2021.02.003.

134. Valenzuela TD, Bjerke HS, Clark LL, et al. Rapid defibrillation by nontraditional responders: the Casino Project. Acad Emerg Med 1998;5: 414–15.

135. Sucu M, Davutoglu V, Ozer O. Electrical cardioversion. Ann Saudi Med 2009;29(3):201–6. doi: 10.4103/0256-4947.51775.

136. Pinski SL, Sgarbossa EB, Ching E, et al. A comparison of 50-J versus 100-J shock for direct current cardioversion of atrial flutter. Am Heart J 1999;137:439–42.

137. Pinski KL, Fahy GJ. Implantable cardioverter defibrillators. Am J Med 1999;106:446–58.

138. The Antiarrhythmics versus Implantable Defibrillators (AVID) Investigators. A comparison of antiarrhythmic-drug therapy with implantable defibrillators in patients resuscitated from near-fatal ventricular arrhythmias. N Engl J Med 1997;337:1576–83.

139. Conolly SJ, Gent M, Roberts RS, et al. Canadian Implantable Defibrillator Study (CIDS): a randomized trial of the implantable cardioverter defibrillator against amiodarone. Circulation 2000;101:1297–302.

140. Kuck KH, Cappato R, Siebels J, et al. Randomized comparison of antiarrhythmic drug therapy with implantable defibrillators in patients resuscitated from cardiac arrest. The Cardiac Arrest Study Hamburg (CASH). Circulation 2000;102;748–54.

141. Moss AJ, Hall WJ, Cannom D, et al. Improved survival with an implanted defibrillator in patients with coronary artery disease at high risk for ventricular arrhythmias. Multicentre Automatic Defibrillator Implantation Trial Investigators. N Engl J Med 1996;335(26):1933–40.

142. Mark DB, Nelson CL, Anstrom KJ, et al. Cost-effectiveness of ICD therapy in the sudden cardiac death in heart failure trial (SCD-HeFT). Circulation 2006;114(2):135–42.

143. Schwartz PJ, Spazzolini C, Priori SG, et al. Who are the long-QT syndrome patients who receive an implantable cardioverter-defibrillator and what happens to them? Circulation 2010;122(13):1272–82. doi: 10.1161/CIRCULATIONAHA.110.950147.

144. Khairy P, Silka MJ, Moore JP, et al. Sudden cardiac death in congenital heart disease. Eur Heart J 2022;43(22):2103–15. doi: 10.1093/eurheartj/ehac104.

145. Swerdlow C, Shivkumar K, Zhang J. Determination of the upper limit of vulnerability using implantable cardioverter defibrillator electrograms. Circulation 2003;107:3028–33.

146. Viskin S, Rosso R. The top 10 reasons to avoid defibrillation threshold testing during ICD implantation. Heart Rhythm 2008;5(3):391–3.

147. Sola CL, Bostwick JM. Implantable cardioverter-defibrillators, induced anxiety, and quality of life. Mayo Clinic Proc 2005;80(2):232–7.

148. Qintar M, George JJ, Panko M, et al. A prospective study of anxiety in ICD patients with a pilot randomized controlled trial of cognitive behaviour with moderate to severe anxiety. J Interv Card Electrophysiol 2015;43(1):65–75. doi: 10.1007/s10840-015-9990-7.

149. Daubert JP, Zareba W, Cannom DS, et al; MADIT II Investigators. Inappropriate implantable cardioverter-defibrillator shocks in MADIT II: frequency, mechanisms, predictors and survival impact. J Am Coll Cardiol 2008;51(14):1357–65.

150. Karnik AA, Helm RH, Monahan KM. Mechanisms and management of inappropriate therapy in subcutaneous implantable defibrillators. J Cardiovasc Electrophysiol 2019;30(3):402–9. doi: 10.1111/jce.13831.

151. Braunschweig F, Boriani G, Bauer A, et al. Management of patients receiving implantable cardiac defibrillator shocks: recommendations for acute and long-term patient management. Europace 2010:12(12):1673–90. doi: 10.1093/europace/euq316.

152. Jacob S, Panaich SS, Maheshwari R, et al. Clinical applications of magnets on cardiac rhythm management devices. Europace 2011:13(9); 1222–30. doi: 10/1093/europace/eur137.

153. Luker J, Sultan A, Plenge T, et al. Electrical cardioversion of patients with implanted pacemakers or cardioverter-defibrillator: results of a survey of German centers and systematic review of the literature. Clin Res Cardiol 2018;107:249–58. doi: 10.1007/s00392-017-1178-y.

154. Johansson C, Lind MM, Eriksson M, et al. Alcohol consumption and risk of incident atrial fibrillation: a population-based cohort study. Eur J Intern Med 2020;76:50–7.

155. Csengeri D, Sprünker NA, Di Castelnuovo A, et al. Alcohol consumption, cardiac biomarkers, and risk of atrial fibrillation and adverse outcomes. Eur Heart J 2021;42(12):1170–7.

156. Althubaiti A. Information bias in health research: definition, pitfalls, and adjustment methods. J Multidiscip Healthc 2016;9:211.

157. Hansel B, Thomas F, Pannier B, et al. Relationship between alcohol intake, health and social status and cardiovascular risk factors in the urban Paris-Ile-de-France cohort: is the cardioprotective action of alcohol a myth? Eur J Clin Nutr 2010;64(6):561–8.

158. Biddinger KJ, Emdin CA, Haas ME, et al. Association of habitual alcohol intake with risk of cardiovascular disease. JAMA Netw Open 2022; 5(3):e223849.

159. Whitman IR, Pletcher MJ, Vittinghoff E, et al. Perceptions, information sources, and behavior regarding alcohol and heart health. Am J Cardiol 2015;116(4):642–6.

Chapter 12

Cardiac surgery and transplantation

Sher Michael Graan, Janelle McLean

Learning objectives

After reading this chapter, you should be able to:

- explain cardiac surgical procedures including coronary artery bypass graft surgery and valve repair and replacement
- describe the indications, advantages and disadvantages of using cardiopulmonary bypass
- outline methods of myocardial preservation during cardiac surgery
- discuss immediate postoperative management of cardiac surgical patients
- describe the principles of counterpulsation in the intra-aortic balloon pump (IABP)
- explore the benefits and timing methods of balloon inflation and deflation, including assessment of timing and timing errors
- describe the nursing management of IABP complications, including limb perfusion, bleeding and immobility-related complications
- discuss methods of weaning IABP and management of intra-aortic balloon catheter removal
- discuss the immediate postoperative care of heart transplant recipients
- describe the clinical manifestations of postoperative complications in heart transplant recipients
- identify signs and symptoms of rejection in heart transplant recipients
- evaluate the effectiveness of nursing interventions in the postoperative management of heart transplant recipients.

Introduction

Many critically ill patients experience compromised cardiac function, as either a primary or secondary condition. This chapter follows on from those situations examined in Chapter 10, and reviews care of patients with cardiac conditions that lead to admission to specialised critical care units. The burden of cardiovascular disease (CVD) is the highest globally; the World Health Organization (WHO) reported that CVD was the number one cause of death in 2019, with 17.9 million deaths, which is 32% of all global deaths (16%, i.e. 8.9 million of total global deaths, an increase from 2 million in 2000, were due to ischaemic heart diseases (IHD) alone) and 38% of death caused by CVD were premature deaths (under the age of 70).[1] In Europe, cardiovascular diseases accounted for 45% of all deaths (229 million) in females and 39% (1.9 million) in males; coronary heart diseases were the most common cause of CVD death both in females (38%) and males (44%) in 2021. In 2019, 113 million people were living in Europe with CVD.[2] Cardiovascular diseases in Australia affect one in six (16.6%) Australians and accounted for 25% of all deaths in 2019, with acute coronary events affecting an estimated 58,700 Australians and contributing to 13% of all deaths in 2019.[3] The rate of CHD is more than twice in Indigenous than in non-Indigenous adults (7.4% and 2.7%) and even higher in Indigenous women (3.3 times).[3] Coronary heart diseases still is the leading cause of burden in Australia, despite the rate having fallen by 50% between 2003 and 2018.[4] In 2018–19 there were 161,000 hospitalisations (1.4% of all hospitalisation) due to CHD, which caused 11% of all deaths.[3]

In this chapter, three topics will be discussed. First, the management of a patient who requires cardiac surgery for coronary artery disease or valvular disease, including the use of cardiopulmonary bypass, will be described. Second, the use and management of intra-aortic balloon counterpulsation in cardiac surgical and medical patients will be explored. Finally, the management of patients following heart transplantation, including the prevention and management of immediate postoperative complications, will be reviewed.

Cardiac surgery

The focus of this section is on cardiac surgery for repair of structural abnormalities and repair or replacement of stenotic or regurgitant valves, as well as bypass grafting of coronary artery lesions. The structural abnormalities resulting from myocardial infarction (MI) have been described in Chapter 10. In this chapter, structural and functional abnormalities that are causing valvular disease (mitral, aortic, tricuspid or pulmonic valves) and ventricular defects will be discussed.

Valvular disease

The incidence and types of valvular disease have changed over the past 50 years.[5] Valvular disorders, such as mitral stenosis and aortic regurgitation, often arising from infectious diseases – for example, rheumatic fever (β-haemolytic streptococcal pharyngitis) and syphilis – are much less common today. Conversely, there has been a rise in the rate of degenerative valvular diseases including leaflet degeneration and/or annulus calcification, due to longer life expectancy of populations. In contrast to these trends, the prevalence of rheumatic fever and rheumatic valvular disorders among Aboriginal people (one of the highest in the world) and Pacific Islanders living in

New Zealand is five times higher than the general population.[6] Globally, rheumatic heart diseases are the most common cause of acquired cardiac disease affecting 41 million people mainly in developing countries, with 470,000 new cases annually,[7,8] causing 288,438 deaths per year.[9] Other causes of valvular diseases are congenital valve diseases (common in the younger population, with bicuspid aortic valves) and endocarditis.

Two valvular abnormalities that alter the blood flow across the valve are common. Stenotic valves have a tightened, restricted orifice causing the valve to not fully open. There is a restriction to forward flow of blood, which must be forced through the valve at higher pressure (Fig. 12.1). The high pressure combined with incomplete emptying of the chamber may increase the end-systolic volume, which will result in hypertrophy and dilation of the affected chamber(s) as a compensatory mechanism. The second valvular abnormality is valve regurgitation, which is also called incompetence or insufficiency. In this condition the incomplete closure of the valve leaflets results in backflow of blood into the chamber increasing its end diastolic volume, which may cause chamber hypertrophy and dilation.

Valvular stenosis and/or regurgitation may lead to heart failure as the pressure in the ventricles and atria grows and this pressure is reflected back into the pulmonary (left heart failure) or venous system (right heart failure). Although the heart contains four valves (aortic, pulmonic, mitral and tricuspid), the mitral and aortic valves in the left side of the heart are most commonly affected.

Aortic valve disease

The aortic valve is located between the left ventricle and the aorta, with a normal surface area of 2–3 cm. Mild aortic stenosis is a narrowing of the opening of the valve area to less than 1.5 cm² and a pressure gradient between the left ventricle and aorta of more than 25 mmHg; severe aortic stenosis is defined as a valve area of less than 1.0 cm² and a pressure gradient of more than 55 mmHg (see Fig. 12.1). Aortic stenosis often results from degenerative changes or congenital abnormalities such as a bicuspid aortic valve (with a prevalence of 0.5% in the general population), which may also cause regurgitation. Aortic stenosis increases left ventricle afterload, causing impedance to left ventricle ejection. This increases the left ventricle end-systolic volume and left ventricle systolic pressure, resulting in left ventricle hypertrophy and dilation. Increased myocardial oxygen demands from the hypertrophied muscle also mean that angina is common.

Clinical manifestations of aortic stenosis include low cardiac output, increased left ventricle workload, angina, dyspnoea, syncope and fatigue. On auscultation, additional heart sounds are heard as a systolic ejection murmur and a loud S4. Left heart failure with pulmonary congestion is usually a late sign. The ECG may show left ventricular hypertrophy with strain patterns.

Aortic regurgitation may occur acutely when the aortic valve is damaged by endocarditis, trauma or aortic

FIGURE 12.1   Valvular stenosis and regurgitation: (**A**) normal position of valve leaflets (cusps) when the valve is open and closed; (**B**) open position of a stenosed valve (left) and closed position of a regurgitant valve (right); (**C**) haemodynamic effect of mitral stenosis shows the mitral valve is unable to open completely during left atrial systole, limiting left ventricular filling; (**D**) haemodynamic effect of mitral regurgitation shows the mitral valve does not close completely during left ventricular systole, allowing blood to re-enter the left atrium.

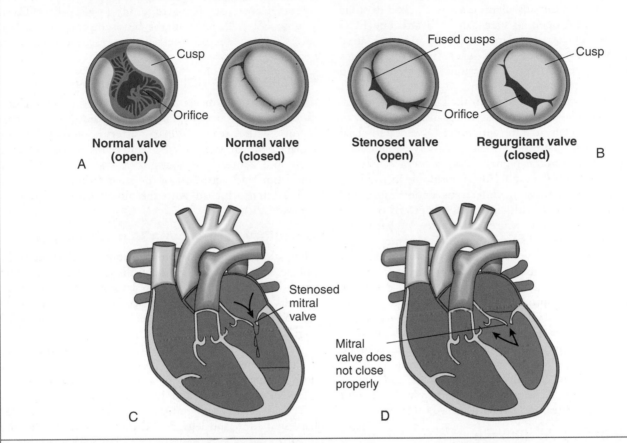

Source: Adapted from Badhwar V, Esper S, Brooks M, et al. Extubating in the operating room following adult cardiac surgery safely improves outcomes and lowers costs. J Thorac Cardiovasc Surg 2014;148(6):3101–9.e1, with permission.

dissection, and presents as a life-threatening emergency. Chronic aortic regurgitation usually results from rheumatic heart disease, syphilis or congenital conditions. In aortic regurgitation the reflux of blood to the left ventricle during diastole, due to incomplete closure of the valve, increases left ventricle end-diastolic pressure and volume. This results in left ventricle dilation and hypertrophy and left heart failure. When left heart failure occurs, left atrial pressure rises and may cause pulmonary congestion and pulmonary hypertension.

In acute aortic regurgitation, the patient presents with signs and symptoms of acute left ventricle failure, cardiogenic shock and acute pulmonary oedema.[10,11] Patients with chronic aortic regurgitation may remain asymptomatic for years, finally presenting with signs of left heart failure including fatigue, palpitation, syncope, angina and dyspnoea. On auscultation, a diastolic murmur can be heard. The ECG may show left ventricular hypertrophy due to volume overload and a chest X-ray may reveal cardiomegaly and features of acute pulmonary oedema.

Mitral valve disease

Mitral stenosis is a chronic and progressive narrowing of the mitral valve orifice (normally 4–6 cm^2), restricting blood flow from the left atrium to the left ventricle. Patients may exhibit symptoms when the valve area is <2 cm^2 and they will have symptoms at rest when the valve area is <1 cm^2.

Mitral valve stenosis often occurs as a result of rheumatic heart disease, degenerative valve diseases and, less often, from systemic lupus erythematosus. These diseases cause damage to the leaflets and chordae tendineae, so that during healing the scars contract and seal, restricting the aperture. The incomplete emptying of the left atrium causes increased left atrial pressure and left atrial enlargement, and results in pulmonary congestion and pulmonary hypertension. In chronic conditions this pressure may also affect the right ventricle, causing right ventricular failure, but left ventricular function is usually intact. Lung compliance is reduced, causing dyspnoea, orthopnoea and nocturnal paroxysmal dyspnoea. Patients may complain of fatigue, low exercise tolerance, cough and haemoptysis. On auscultation a low-pitched diastolic murmur and an opening snap can be heard. The ECG may show left atrial enlargement and possibly atrial fibrillation (AF), and a chest X-ray may reveal right ventricular hypertrophy, left atrium enlargement and features of pulmonary congestion.

In mitral valve regurgitation, the mitral valve is not closing during left ventricular systole, causing backflow of blood into the left atrium, which creates elevated atrial and pulmonary pressures and possibly pulmonary oedema.[11] Acute mitral regurgitation is often caused by acute myocardial infarction (AMI), resulting in papillary muscle rupture, trauma or infectious endocarditis, and patients may present with signs and symptoms of acute left ventricular failure, acute pulmonary oedema and cardiogenic shock. The causes of chronic mitral regurgitation include rheumatic diseases, congenital mitral valve prolapse and degenerative changes. The patient may complain of weakness, fatigue, exertional dyspnoea, palpitation and symptoms of pulmonary congestion and right ventricular failure such as cough, dyspnoea, orthopnoea and lower extremity oedema. On auscultation, a third heart sound and a pansystolic murmur can be heard. ECG may show left atrial enlargement, P mitrale, left ventricular hypertrophy and possibly AF, and a chest X-ray may reveal left ventricular hypertrophy, left atrium enlargement and features of pulmonary congestion.

Tricuspid valve disease

Tricuspid stenosis (normal area is 7 cm^2) is often seen with aortic or mitral valve diseases, and rarely in isolation. The restriction of blood flow from the right atrium to the right ventricle causes systemic venous congestion. On auscultation, a diastolic murmur can be heard. Tricuspid regurgitation is most commonly a functional disorder due to annulus dilation as a result of increased right ventricle pressure and hypertrophy, mitral stenosis, pulmonary embolism, cor pulmonale or right ventricle AMI. The backflow of blood from the right ventricle to the right atrium causes systemic venous congestion. On auscultation, a pansystolic murmur can be heard. In both stenosis and regurgitation of the tricuspid valve patients present with a high central venous pressure (CVP) and jugular venous pressure (JVP), hepatomegaly, ascites and peripheral oedema, and their ECG may show right atrium enlargement, P pulmonale and possibly AF, and a chest X-ray may reveal a prominent right heart border.

Pulmonic valve disease

Pulmonic valve stenosis is rare in isolation and is often due to a congenital defect. The restriction to blood flow

from the right ventricle to the pulmonary arteries causes right ventricular hypertrophy and dilation, and the patient presents with exertional dyspnoea, syncope, cyanosis, a systolic murmur and a split S2 heart sound. The ECG may show right ventricular hypertrophy.

Pulmonic valve regurgitation is also a rare condition that is usually caused by a congenital defect or pulmonary hypertension or is iatrogenic (e.g. post-balloon valvuloplasty). Patients might be asymptomatic, but in severe cases they present with signs and symptoms of right ventricular failure.

Cardiac surgical interventions

The most common cardiac surgical procedures include coronary artery bypass graft (CABG) surgery, to bypass lesions within the coronary arteries, and repair or replacement of stenotic or regurgitant valves. During these procedures, preservation of systemic circulation, ventilation and perfusion of the myocardium is required and is often achieved with the aid of cardiopulmonary bypass (CPB).

Coronary artery bypass graft surgery

The pathophysiology and implications of ischaemic heart disease are explained in detail in Chapter 10. Single lesions can be treated by angioplasty and stent; however, patients with a left main coronary artery lesion, multiple (double- or triple-vessel) disease, longer lesions and failed angioplasty may need CABG surgery.[12]

In CABG a section of vein or artery is used to bypass a blockage in the patient's coronary artery. The vessels used for grafting arise from arteries (internal mammary artery or radial artery and, less commonly, gastroepiploic artery) or veins (saphenous vein). Saphenous veins are harvested from the legs, and the radial artery from the forearm, and each is used as a free graft with anastomoses at the ascending aorta and distal to lesions to one or more coronary arteries. When saphenous veins are used as grafts, they often develop diffuse intimal hyperplasia, which ultimately contributes to restenosis. Patency rates are lowest in saphenous vein grafts (SVGs) attached to small coronary arteries or coronary arteries supplying myocardial scars. Consequently, arterial grafts are used more often, as they are more resistant to intimal hyperplasia. Internal mammary arteries (IMAs) and radial artery grafts may be used.[10,13] The IMA remains attached to the subclavian artery and is mobilised from the chest wall and anastomosed to the coronary artery distal to the occlusion (Fig. 12.2). If the radial artery is being harvested for grafting, the collateral circulation in the forearm is assessed. Echo colour Doppler provides the best accuracy in assessing forearm circulation, although the clinical Allen test is quite commonly used. The disadvantage of the Allen test is that it gives false patency results around 5% of the time.[14] A selection of IMA, SVG and radial artery grafts may be necessary over time as repeat procedures are needed or in patients with extensive disease requiring multiple grafts.

FIGURE 12.2 Coronary artery bypass grafts.
CX = circumflex artery; LAD = left anterior descending;
LIMA = left internal mammary artery; LM = left main;
RCA = right coronary artery; SVG = saphenous vein graft.

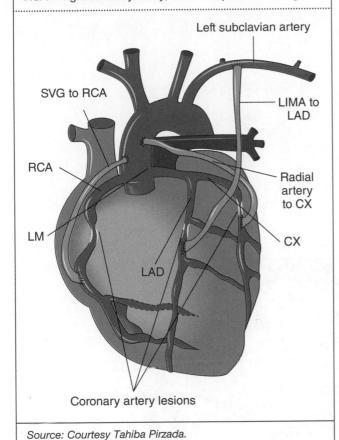

Left subclavian artery

SVG to RCA

LIMA to LAD

RCA

Radial artery to CX

LM

CX

LAD

Coronary artery lesions

Source: Courtesy Tahiba Pirzada.

For single-vessel disease, particularly of the left anterior descending (LAD) artery, a new approach to CABG – minimally invasive direct coronary artery bypass grafting (MIDCABG) – has been used.[15] This procedure uses intercostal incisions and a thoracoscope instead of a sternotomy to access the heart and coronary arteries. MIDCABG is also often performed without CPB (off-pump coronary artery bypass, OPCAB); instead, the heart is slowed with beta-blockers to allow the surgery to be performed on a beating heart.[16,17] OPCAB procedures may also be performed using full or partial sternotomy to provide access for multiple vessel grafting. Both procedures have been successful responses to the drive to reduce the need for transfusion; recovery times, length of stay in hospital, costs and long-term outcomes are comparable with conventional methods.[16,17]

In the last decade, robotically assisted cardiac surgery has evolved in America and Europe and has been introduced at a small number of Australian hospitals for CABG and mitral valve surgery. This technique has further reduced the invasiveness of cardiac surgery, as little more than stab wounds are required in the right chest for

thoracoscopy and the robotic instruments. Avoiding true thoracotomy or sternotomy improves postoperative pain experience, and is associated with quicker recovery time and shorter length of stay.[18,19]

Although CABG is the most common cardiac surgical procedure undertaken in Australia, the incidence of hospitalisation for CABG has declined since 2000/01 from 1.41 to 0.72 procedures/1000 population in 2018–19,[3] but the rate of CABG has not changed in major European countries from 2006 to 2014.[20] The decline in surgery rates is due to changes in the treatment of CHD, including the advent of percutaneous coronary intervention (PCI). More procedures are now being performed in older patients, with 83% of current patients aged over 55 years. CABG is used to relieve the symptoms of angina by increasing coronary blood flow distal to occlusive coronary lesions. It is a palliative, not curative, treatment as the underlying disease process continues. CABG is more effective than percutaneous transluminal coronary angioplasty (PTCA) in patients with extensive, multivessel disease, with improved survival over a 3–5-year period by 5%, and a 4–7-fold reduction in the need for re-intervention.[21] CABG is also used in left main vessel lesions owing to the high risk of extensive infarction associated with PTCA in this area. CABG surgery is commonplace, and many cardiothoracic centres have highly efficient, effective systems in place, with mortality rates as low as 2%.

Valve repair and replacement

Valve surgery is usually undertaken to repair the patient's valve or, more often, to replace the valve with a mechanical or tissue prosthesis. The clinical decision for valve surgery is primarily based on the clinical state of the patient using the New York Heart Association (NYHA) classification system and echocardiographic findings.[10] The type of surgery used will depend on the valves involved, the valvular pathology, the severity of the condition and the patient's clinical condition. Often, valve surgery is not a single procedure, and it may involve multiple valves, CABG, pacemaker and an implantable cardioverter defibrillator (ICD). Valve surgery is palliative, not curative, and patients will require lifelong healthcare.

Valve repair may involve resecting and/or suturing prolapsed or torn leaflets (valvuloplasty) and repairing the ring of collagen the valve sits in (annuloplasty) and is commonly used for mitral and tricuspid regurgitation. Commissurotomy (incising valve leaflets and debriding calcification) is the treatment of choice for mitral stenosis. Both repair processes have demonstrated lower operative mortality than replacement, although complete valve competence may not be achievable. Open procedures are preferred because thrombi and calcification can thereby be removed.

In some instances, valve replacement is necessary but could be associated with higher risks due to the long-term disease process and poor underlying left ventricular function. The most common indication for valve

FIGURE 12.3 Prosthetic valves: **(A)** the Bjork–Shiley valve, with a pyrolyte–carbon disc that opens to 60 degrees; **(B)** the Starr–Edwards caged-ball valve model 6320, with satellite ball; **(C)** the St Jude Medical mechanical heart valve, with a mechano-central flow disc; **(D)** the Hancock II porcine aortic valve, with stent and sewing ring covered in Dacron® cloth 5.

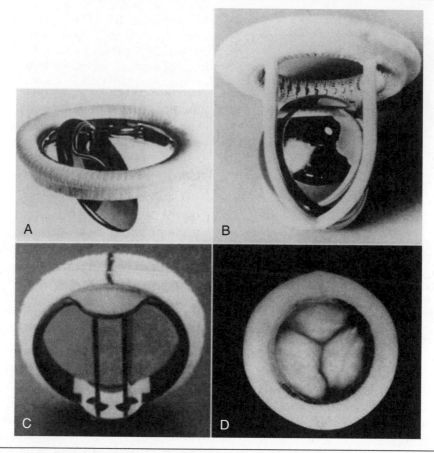

Source: Urden L, Stacy K, Lough M. Critical care nursing: diagnosis and management. 9th ed. St Louis: Elsevier; 2022.

replacement is aortic stenosis, which accounts for around 60% of valve surgery.[10] Prosthetic valves may be mechanical or biological. Mechanical valves are made of metal alloys, pyrolite carbon and Dacron® (Fig. 12.3). Biological valves are constructed from porcine, bovine or human cardiac tissue. Mechanical valves are more durable but have an increased risk of thromboembolism, so lifelong anticoagulation is required. Biological valves suffer from the same problems as the patient's valve (i.e. calcification and degeneration). The choice of valve depends on the age of the patient and potential difficulties and risks with taking anticoagulants.

For elderly patients with high risk of open-heart surgery and higher comorbidity, transcatheter aortic valve implantation (TAVI) of commercial artificial valves (for example Medtronic CORE Valve® or Edwards Sapien®) has been used. This procedure is usually performed in a catheter laboratory, via femoral artery approach, similar to angiography procedure (with larger catheter size) and light anaesthesia. The custom-made artificial valve is deployed precisely over the patient's current diseased valve as a palliative measure to improve the quality of patient life. This procedure carries higher risks of all-cause 1-year mortality of 13.9–16.3%, major vascular complications of 9.3–12.3% and a 2.6% incidence of stroke.[22,23] However in low-risk patients at 3 years follow-up, surgical aortic valve replacement has significantly better survival rate (83.4% vs 72%), and freedom from major cardiac and cerebrovascular events (80.9% vs 67.3%) compared with TAVI.[24]

Mortality is higher for valvular surgery than for CABG, reflecting the underlying loss of ventricular function and additional procedures that are common during valvular surgery. Risk stratification models have been developed to help determine the patients who are most likely to have poor recovery and outcomes.[25] The major factors that contribute to poor outcomes are worse left ventricular function and age over 70 years.[21]

Cardiopulmonary bypass

CPB was developed to enable surgery to be performed on a still, relatively bloodless heart, while preserving the patient's circulation. CPB temporarily performs the functions of the heart in circulating blood and of the lungs by enabling gas exchange. Silicone cannulae are inserted into the venae cavae or right atrium, and venous blood is circulated through a circuit outside the body. In this circuit the blood is oxygenated, carbon dioxide removed and blood temperature controlled. Drugs and anaesthetics may be added. A roller pump is generally used to provide the pressure to create blood flow in the circuit and back to the patient's aorta.

Adverse effects of CPB are diverse, and include the following (Table 12.1):[10,17,26]

- Haematological effects due to exposure of the blood to tubing and gas exchange surfaces, which initiates surface activation of the clotting cascade; also blood component damage due to shear stress from the roller action of the pump, which may reduce haematocrit, leukocyte and platelet count.

- Pulmonary effects due to activation of systemic inflammatory response syndrome (SIRS), which increases capillary leakage, and lung deflation during surgery leading to postoperative atelectasis.

- Cardiovascular effects due to volume changes, fluid shifts and decreased myocardial contractility, which decreases cardiac output; this is most severe during the first 6 hours, but usually resolves within 48–72 hours.

- Neurological effects due to poor cerebral perfusion and generation of thromboemboli from aortic cannulation, which can lead to cerebrovascular accidents.

- Renal effects due to decreases in cardiac output during initiation of CPB, which decreases renal perfusion.

- Post-pump delirium or psychosis, which occurs in 32% of CPB patients, although the cause has not been identified; symptoms include short-term memory deficit, decreased attention and inability to respond to and integrate sensory information.

- Activation of a systemic inflammatory response, which may cause vasodilation and increased cardiac output.

These effects are well documented, and routine CPB management and postoperative care are designed to minimise and treat the complications. Heparin is added at the commencement of CPB and is reversed with protamine (1 mg of protamine for every 100 U of heparin) when CPB ceases; activated clotting times are monitored throughout and after CPB. Blood returning to the circulation is filtered, and surgical procedures proceed carefully to reduce microemboli. Monitoring and maintenance of adequate arterial flow rates are used to prevent low perfusion. Temperature gradients and a rewarming process are instituted slowly so that cardiac output can meet metabolic demands.

Myocardial preservation

One of the processes involved in CPB is that the aorta is clamped where a cannula is inserted to return blood to the circulation. This clamp prevents blood flow into the coronary arteries; therefore, the myocardium must be protected from ischaemia during the cardiac surgical procedure. This protection is achieved through several mechanisms directed towards reducing oxygen demand: first, oxygen demand is reduced by mild-to-moderate hypothermia (28–32°C); second, myocardial temperature is reduced (0–4°C) by infusing cold fluids directly into the coronary arteries; third, normal conduction is prevented by arresting the heart during diastole, by infusing a concentrated potassium solution into the coronary arteries. Return to normal rhythm is usually achieved by circulation of warm blood, though defibrillation may be necessary.

TABLE 12.1

Summary of the impact and side effects of CPB

BODY SYSTEM	CPB IMPACT	SIDE EFFECTS
Haematology	Surface activation of clotting cascade	↓ WBC, ↓ HcT, ↓ platelets Thromboembolism formation
Pulmonary	SIRS activation (CPB circuit) Lung deflation (during surgery)	↑ Capillary permeability and leakage Pulmonary congestion ↓ Surfactant production Atelectasis Impaired gas exchange
Cardiovascular	Volume changes SIRS activation	Fluid shift ↓ Myocardial contractility and CO Vasodilation and ↓ SVR
Neurological	Poor cerebral perfusion Thromboembolism Post-pump delirium or psychosis	↑ Risk of CVA Short-term memory deficit ↓ Attention Sensory deficit
Renal	↓ CO and renal perfusion	↓ Urine output, and ↑ risk of AKI

AKI = acute kidney injury; CO = cardiac output; CPB = cardiopulmonary bypass; CVA = cardiovascular accident; HcT = haematocrit; SIRS = systemic inflammatory response syndrome; SVR = systemic vascular resistance; WBC = white blood cells.

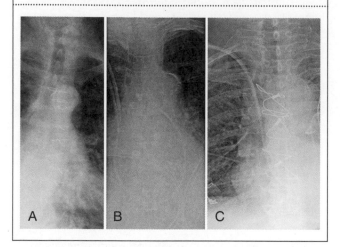

FIGURE 12.4 Sternal closing options: (**A**) use of sternal wire; (**B**) use of sternal clip; and (**C**) use of sternal wires 'figure of 8' method.

Sternal-closing options

The traditional wire closure of the sternum has been used for decades but, due to high risk of infection and postoperative sternal wound dehiscence, other techniques have developed.[27] One method is the use of a biological bone adhesive, such as Kryptonite®, when combined with a standard sternal wire has shown enhancement of mechanical strength, prevention of sternal dehiscence, reduction in postoperative pain and improvement in quality of life, but further research is needed.[28,29] Other techniques such as the use of sternal clips or rigid fixation (e.g. using the SternaLock® system) have been developed, although they still require further evaluation to determine effectiveness and confirm the lack of complications.[30] Use of these methods of sternal closure necessitates having the correct equipment available to enable rapid reopening of the sternum in case of emergency (Fig. 12.4).

Patient management

The often-rapid turnaround of patients from complete dependence in intensive care to discharge in post-cardiothoracic surgery can provide particularly rewarding nursing experiences. However, this rapid progression is also often marked by haemodynamic instability, arrhythmias and biochemical and haematological changes. The increased emphasis on rapid weaning and extubation, often occurring during turbulent anaesthetic recovery, presents one of the more volatile periods in ventilatory support, requiring knowledgeable and skilled nursing and medical management. In addition to the management of ventilation, temporary pacemaker therapies and mechanical circulatory-assist devices (IABP and ventricular assist), effective pain management and rapid mobilisation provide an opportunity for the development of broad and detailed expertise.

Patients are usually admitted to the intensive care unit for 1–2 days although, when early extubation is undertaken, they may spend only hours in a recovery unit before progressing to a cardiothoracic high-dependency area, where nurse-to-patient ratios may be 1:2 to 1:3.

The immediate postoperative period

Patients should be transported to intensive care accompanied by at least an anaesthetist, an appropriately qualified nurse and transport personnel under continuous cardiac monitoring and assisted ventilation. It is a requirement to include capnography during patient transport to detect ventilator disconnection, dysfunction or endotracheal tube migration. Intensive care or theatre nursing staff may be a component of the transport team. The admission to intensive care requires a team approach, with the participation of intensive care nursing and medical staff and/or technician input.[31] The immediate postoperative decision making on patient management is influenced by handover from anaesthetists and the surgical team, settling-in procedures and collegial assistance.[10,32] Admission activities are commonly divided between nurses, with one nurse taking responsibility for the patient and establishing monitoring and haemodynamic assessment and management, and a second nurse managing ventilation and endotracheal tube security, as well as managing chest drains, gastric tube and urinary catheter. If staffing permits, additional nurses may take responsibility for documentation, performing arterial blood gases and 12-lead ECG, and providing assistance as required.

The objectives of immediate postoperative management of cardiac surgical patients may include:

- optimisation of cardiovascular performance
- re-establishment and/or maintenance of normothermia
- promotion of haemostasis
- ventilatory support and management
- prevention and management of arrhythmias
- optimisation of organ perfusion.

Haemodynamic monitoring and support

Typical haemodynamic monitoring includes an intraarterial catheter for continuous blood pressure monitoring and arterial blood sampling. Cardiac output and preload measurement are achieved most commonly with either a pulmonary artery or central venous catheter configured for pulse contour cardiac output (PiCCO) monitoring (see Chapter 9).

Preload measures provided by the pulmonary artery catheter include right atrial pressure (RAP) to approximate right ventricular filling and pulmonary artery pressure (PAP) to approximate right ventricular systole and provide insight into pulmonary vascular resistance and left heart function. The pulmonary capillary wedge pressure (PCWP) is available to approximate left ventricular filling and left heart function. Alternatively, the PiCCO monitoring system represents preload by the intrathoracic blood volume index (ITBVI) and global end-diastolic volume index (GEDVI). In addition, the extravascular lung water index (EVLWI) can demonstrate the accumulation of interstitial lung water.[33]

Cardiac output is measured by either intermittent or continuous thermodilution via pulmonary artery catheters, or measured intermittently and then approximated continuously on a beat-to-beat interpretation of pulse contour by the PiCCO monitoring system. Cardiac output measurement can be combined with other pressure variables to calculate systemic and pulmonary vascular resistance, stroke volume and measures of ventricular work.

Certain common haemodynamic patterns are seen in the early postoperative phase. These must be detected through thorough monitoring and interpretation of variables, and managed according to specific needs. During the initial 2 hours of recovery period, 95% of patients will experience haemodynamic instability.[34,35]

Practice tip

The choice of inotropes and vasoactive drugs should be based on the haemodynamic findings. For example,: a patient with low systemic vascular resistance (SVR) and low contractility (low cardiac output (CO) and blood pressure (BP)) will need an ino-constrictor such as adrenaline (epinephrine) or dopamine; a patient with high SVR and low contractility will need an ino-dilator such as milrinone or dobutamine.

Hypertension

Hypertension is present in up to 30% of patients initially,[36] as hypothermia, stress responses, pain and hypovolaemia contribute to vasoconstriction. When the SVR is excessive, the high afterload may contribute to low CO. Rewarming to normothermia with space blankets or heated air blankets, fluid administration, administration of sedation or analgesics and infusion of intravenous (IV) vasodilators (glyceryl trinitrate or sodium nitroprusside) are all commonly used to overcome vasoconstriction when contributing to hypertension.[37] Occasionally, beta-blockers are used. Hypertension increases myocardial workload and contributes to bleeding.

Hypotension

Transient hypotension requiring treatment is common at some stage during the postoperative period. Contributing factors to hypotension include hypovolaemia and decreased venous return (from polyuria, bleeding, ventilation and positive end-expiratory pressure and excess vasodilation), contractile impairment (from ischaemia or infarction, hypothermia and negative inotropic influences), pericardial tamponade and vasodilation (from excess vasodilator therapy, or as part of an inflammatory response to CPB).[34,36]

Hypotension may present with reduced or elevated preload, reduced or elevated cardiac output and reduced or elevated SVR. When hypovolaemia is present, cardiac output will be low and SVR usually high. Hypovolaemia is diagnosed by measuring preload indicators, as pressure (RAP, PAP, PCWP) or volume (ITBVI, GEDVI).[38,39] Choice of colloids or crystalloid fluids for volume restoration in the postoperative period has no effect on mortality,[40–42] but colloids affect clot formation and strength and also produce greater haemodilution, which is associated with more blood product transfusion.[43] Blood returned from the CPB circuit ('pump blood') usually accompanies the patient to ICU, and this should be re-administered at a rate suitable to filling indices and blood pressure.

Hypotension accompanied by elevated preload and low cardiac output usually represents cardiac dysfunction or pericardial tamponade, and the distinction should be quickly sought.[44,45] When such left ventricular dysfunction is present, there is usually compensatory vasoconstriction and tachycardia, although heart rate responses may be unreliable because of cardioplegia, cold, conduction disease[10] and preoperative beta-blocking agents. Inotropic agents, including milrinone hydrochloride, adrenaline, dopamine or dobutamine, may become necessary (these are covered more completely in Table 21.7 and its accompanying text). When the profile of severe left ventricular dysfunction is persistent (either at the time of coming off bypass or later in intensive care), IABP may be instituted. ECG assessment for new ischaemia or infarction should be made, which, if of significant size, may warrant surgical re-exploration or angiographic investigation. Pericardial tamponade is also a cause of hypotension (covered later in this chapter).

A fourth common postoperative profile is hypotension with normal or elevated cardiac output in the presence of low SVR. This may occur with excess vasodilator administration, the use of postoperative epidural infusions and vasodilation from a systemic inflammatory response to CPB and other factors such as re-infusion of collected operative site blood. The inotrope milrinone hydrochloride is popular in the postoperative phase because of its dilating effect on radial artery grafts,[46] but often contributes to hypotension through its systemic vasodilator properties. When hypotension is attributable to vasodilation, metaraminol or noradrenaline (norepinephrine) may be used.[34,46] Arginine vasopressin, by infusion, could be used as an effective alternative vasoconstrictor for cardiac surgical patients, but early introduction of vasopressin demonstrated improved haemodynamic response.[34]

A mean arterial pressure of 70–80 mmHg is generally targeted in the postoperative period.[36,47] This can sometimes be reduced if there has been ventriculotomy or if there is concern about the status of the aorta. The cardiac index should be maintained above 2.2 L/min/m^2, as hypoperfusion develops below these values. When at these levels, additional assessments are often undertaken, such as mixed venous oxygen saturation measurement (to assess oxygen delivery deficits) and arterial pH and lactate measurements (to detect metabolic acidosis from anaerobic metabolism).

In addition to assessment of preload, contractility and afterload, heart rate and rhythm should be assessed for their input to cardiac output and blood pressure. Extremes of rate and arrhythmias alter ventricular filling and may need correction. If temporary pacing wires are present, pacing strategies for haemodynamic improvement include rate rises (even if already in the normal range)[48] and the provision of dual-chamber or atrial pacing as alternatives to ventricular pacing only, in order to maximise atrioventricular synchrony and the contribution of atrial kick to blood pressure. Alternatively, if ventricular pacing is present, reducing the rate to permit expression of a slower sinus rhythm may, with the provision of atrial kick, improve cardiac output and blood pressure (refer to Chapter 11 for more information on pacing).

> **Practice tip**
>
> Be aware of an apparent paradox: hypertension may occur even if there is hypovolaemia. The intense vasoconstriction often seen postoperatively not only raises blood pressure but also aids venous return so that RAP is normal. It may not be until the patient has warmed and dilated that the true filling status is revealed. When the patient is cold and has normal filling pressures, be prepared for possible hypotension, and the need for significant fluid resuscitation on rewarming.

Rhythm monitoring and postoperative arrhythmias

Continuous rhythm monitoring is necessary while the patient is in intensive care, and telemetry monitoring is usually continued until discharge from hospital. Lead selection is often haphazard, but a chest lead in the V1 position (or lead MCL1) generally provides the best information on atrial and ventricular activity.[49] Unlike many leads, these two leads reliably demonstrate normal rhythms, bundle branch block and ventricular rhythms,[49] and may be useful in confirming pulmonary artery catheter irritation as the cause of ventricular arrhythmias.

A 12-lead ECG is performed on admission to the ICU and should be compared with the preoperative ECG. It should be assessed for signs of new ischaemia or infarction, new bundle branch block and arrhythmias or conduction disturbances. Pericarditis, a frequent complication of surgery, appears as ST-segment elevation (often, but not always, in many leads), and may mask or mimic myocardial infarction. The nurse should look for the classic concave upward or 'saddle-shaped' ST segment, to distinguish pericardial changes from the more convex upward ST segment of infarction. Worsening of pain on inspiration and a pericardial rub help to confirm pericarditis.[50]

Atrial fibrillation is the most common postoperative arrhythmia and contributes significantly to postoperative morbidity and hospital length of stay.[51] It occurs in up to 30–50% of patients, most often on days 2–3 postoperatively.[52] Many patients revert without treatment, but, when treatment becomes necessary, beta-blockers and amiodarone appear to be the most successful agents for correction.[53]

Digitalis is effective for rate control and IV magnesium is often used, although further evidence for its use is needed. Atrial pacing to prevent AF is being increasingly explored but a clear recommendation on pacing sites and protocols has yet to emerge. In contrast, atrial overdrive pacing can be an effective means to immediately and safely interrupt atrial flutter.[52]

Ventricular ectopic beats are common and by themselves do not require treatment unless they accompany ischaemia or biochemical disturbance,[54] in which case they may progress to more complex arrhythmias. Consideration should always be given to the pulmonary artery catheter as the cause (including both correctly and incorrectly positioned catheters), as this is an easily corrected influence. Ventricular tachycardia and fibrillation are uncommon and usually denote myocardial disturbance such as ischaemia or infarction, shock, electrolyte disturbance, hypoxia or increased excitation due to high circulating catecholamine levels.[54] Standard approaches to resuscitation according to protocols in Chapter 24 apply, including standard cardiopulmonary resuscitation (CPR) over the recent sternotomy. However, cardiac advanced life support (CALS) has been introduced in many cardiothoracic centres aiming to avoid CPR and its complications over the recent sternotomy and utilise defibrillation (three consecutive shocks) for shockable rhythms and pacing for non-shockable rhythm and prepare to open the chest as soon as possible. Cardiothoracic ICU and wards have been equipped with a special CALS trolley to accommodate chest opening and appropriate training for medical and nursing staff has been provided. The number of sternal wires has been included in handover and patient journey board for ease of access in case of patient deterioration, and most centres will follow CALS protocol up to day ten of operation. In centres without CALS, when ventricular fibrillation cannot be corrected, consideration is often given to re-exploration of the chest to examine graft patency and/or provide internal cardiac massage. These cardiac surgical intensive care units should be equipped to enable emergency re-exploration for such purposes.[55]

> **Practice tip**
>
> Appropriate patient management should be based on frequent assessment and evaluation of their condition, especially during the immediate postoperative period, to achieve:
> - optimal preload
> - optimal contractility
> - optimal afterload.

Ventilatory support

Ventilation should be approached according to the general principles described in Chapter 15. As anaesthesia is not typically reversed at the end of the operation, patients are generally admitted apnoeic, and within 1–3 hours return to wakefulness and spontaneous breathing.

Ensuring a secure airway is an initial priority; the following should be undertaken:

- Confirmation of endotracheal tube (ETT) position and its security immediately on admission:
  - auscultation for equal bilateral air entry to rule out right main bronchus intubation
  - recording of the ETT insertion length to detect ETT migration
  - postoperative chest X-ray, taken within 30 minutes, to examine for ETT positioning.
- Continuous end-tidal CO_2 monitoring to ascertain ETT placement and detect tube migration.
- Initial ETT care:
  - assessment for air leak around the cuff (via performance of minimal occlusive volume or pressure tests) and auscultation of the neck
  - ensure ETT is adequately secured and positioned so as not to apply undue pressure against soft tissues of the mouth and lips.

There has been a general trend to more-rapid ventilatory weaning in recent years, and in some centres 'fast-track' cardiac surgical recovery includes extubation at the end of the operation before transfer to a recovery unit for suitable patients. Indices of respiration show no improvement when intubation is maintained for longer compared with early extubation,[56,57] and pooled results from randomised early extubation trials show earlier ICU discharge and shorter lengths of stay (by 1 day) when early extubation is undertaken.[56,58]

Apart from these fast-track approaches, ventilation is commonly employed for 2–6 hours in the uncomplicated patient. Reasons for continuing ventilation beyond this time frame may include:

- intraoperative neurological event
- gas exchange deficit with unresolved hypoxaemia
- ventilatory inadequacy
- significant haemodynamic insufficiency or instability
- patients returning from theatre late in the evening may sometimes continue ventilation overnight to optimise postextubation breathing ability.

For many patients, ventilation is provided purely for initial airway and apnoea protection rather than for treatment of pulmonary deficits. In the absence of pulmonary disease, many centres provide fairly uniform approaches to parameter settings that aim at sustaining ventilation and oxygenation, while limiting traumatic risk to the lungs (Table 12.2). However, approaches to ventilation will need to be tailored in the presence of operative complications or coexisting lung disease.

Ventilation challenges specific to the postoperative cardiac setting include:

- atelectasis due to operative access and lungs collapse/deflation

- pneumothorax (pleural opening for grafts, or ventilation-induced trauma)
- pulmonary hypertension from cardiac failure or valve disease
- cardiogenic shock/post-pump failure
- SIRS due to CPB
- early or rapid weaning that is undertaken before complete readiness, leading to failure at weaning attempt
- surgical pain limiting spontaneous effort and potentially leading to atelectasis or sputum retention.

Approaches to weaning

As patients often have no underlying pulmonary pathology, and have been ventilated for brief periods only, rapid weaning phases have become the norm in most centres. In many instances, as soon as the patient wakes and begins spontaneous breathing activity, they may be suitable for at least a trial of spontaneous breathing in continuous positive airway pressure (CPAP) mode, usually with some modest level of pressure support (e.g. 5–10 cmH_2O). If tolerated and the patient maintains an adequate minute volume, SpO_2 and $PaCO_2$, extubation may be considered within as little as another 30 minutes. Normal demonstrations of airway protection capability (e.g. neuromuscular control, gag, swallow, cough and patient strength) should be sought before extubation (see Chapter 15 for details).

These short ventilation times and rapid weaning carry a greater risk of weaning failure. Patients may initially wake and appear to sustain spontaneous ventilation well for some time, only to lapse back under anaesthetic influence. A return to greater ventilatory support may be necessary. Failure to wean carries greater significance in the cardiac surgical patient with existing pulmonary hypertension, as respiratory acidosis causes pulmonary vasoconstriction, abruptly worsening pulmonary hypertension and the risk of pulmonary oedema and/or right ventricular failure.

When ventilation has been more prolonged because of postoperative pulmonary problems, weaning may be approached more cautiously, as might be applied to the general longer-term ventilated patient. Gradual mandatory rate reduction or increasing periods of spontaneous ventilation interspersed with periods of greater assistance have been employed.[56,59]

Postoperative bleeding

The harvest sites for radial arteries or saphenous veins are uncommon sources of significant blood loss and are generally easily managed with dressings or compression. Intrathoracic bleeding, however, may be torrential and threaten life. Occasionally, surgical bleeding from the aorta, arterial grafts or myomectomy sites may exceed replacement capabilities, and at times patients succumb to overwhelming haemorrhage. Maintenance of drain patency and strict recording of losses and total fluid balance are paramount, and fluid balance assessments over shorter intervals, even every 5–10 minutes, become

TABLE 12.2

Postoperative ventilation settings

NOMINAL OR GENERALLY ACCEPTABLE SETTINGS	ALTERNATIVES TO NOMINAL SETTINGS AND REASONS FOR VARIATION
SIMV with volume control ventilation.	Pressure control suitable. Generally used only if there is significant hypoxaemia or the need to exert greater control on pulmonary pressure. Hybrid modes such as autoflow, pressure-regulated volume control (PRVC) or volume control plus (VC+) are also suitable, generally for the same indications as pressure control.
Tidal volume 8–10 mL/kg.	Lower tidal volumes (6–8 mL/kg) when there is known compliance disorder (atelectasis, pulmonary oedema, fibrosis) or unexplained high plateau pressures.
Mandatory rate 10 breaths/min.	Faster rates may be necessary if low tidal volume strategies become necessary. Lower rates if gas-trapping risk due to airways disease. Also adjusted according to $PaCO_2$ level.
Inspiratory flow 30–50 L/min to provide I:E ratio of 1:2 to 1:4 acceptable.	Slower flows to prolong the inspiratory time may be necessary if there is atelectasis and hypoxaemia, or if there is a desire to lessen inspiratory pressures. Faster flows to enhance expiratory time necessary only if gas-trapping risk.
PEEP minimum levels of 5 cmH$_2$O.	Higher levels of PEEP according to severity of hypoxaemia.
Pressure support 5–10 cmH$_2$O.	Automated pressure support modes such as automatic tube compensation (auto-adjusted pressure support to overcome flow resistance of tracheal tubes) or volume support (auto-adjusted pressure support to achieve target tidal volume on spontaneous breaths) exist. There is no pressing indication for their use in uncomplicated cardiac surgical patients.
Permissive hypercapnoea rarely necessary.	Particularly important to avoid if existing pulmonary hypertension, as may worsen acutely with respiratory acidosis.
FiO$_2$ initially 0.8–1.0 then wean down according to PaO$_2$/SaO$_2$. Aiming to reduce to <0.5 as soon as possible.	According to PaO$_2$/SaO$_2$.

FiO$_2$ = fraction of inspired oxygen; PEEP = positive end expiratory pressure; SIMV = synchronised intermittent mandatory ventilation mode.

necessary during active bleeding. Because of the potential rates of bleeding, the cardiac surgical unit must be equipped to institute rapid volume replacement, and have access to adequate blood and blood product stores, blood warmers and all necessary procoagulant therapies. In addition, dedicated equipment should be available to facilitate emergency resternotomy to control haemorrhage.

One or more chest drains are inserted to remove and monitor blood loss, but the positioning of drains is variable, depending in part on the procedure performed, the surgical route taken and surgeon preference. Regardless of these considerations, there will always be a retrosternal/anterior mediastinal drain, as the sternum is generally the major source of bleeding in the absence of complications. Additional drains may be inserted in the pericardial or pleural spaces. Pericardial drains are more likely to be inserted following aortic valve surgery, whereas pleural drains become necessary following mammary artery harvesting or when the pleura is opened for any other

reason. Pleural drains may be anterior, posterior or 'wrap-around' configurations in which they project over the anterior lung, following the pleural space first from midline to lateral and then, finally, the posterior pleural space.

Reportable postoperative blood losses vary, but greater than 100 mL/h, or greater than 400 mL in the first 4 hours, would generally be regarded as excessive and worthy of surgeon notification. Importantly, excessive bleeding does not always represent a surgical defect that reoperation might correct, as there are many contributors to impaired haemostatic capability in the cardiac surgical patient (see below).

Chest drainage should be monitored closely and, while bleeding is active, volumes should be assessed every 5 minutes and patency of drains ensured to avert tamponade. Sudden cessation of drainage should always raise the possibility of the loss of tube patency and risk of tamponade, but tamponade may also occur while drainage continues, as collections and compressions may occur at sites isolated from drains, or losses may simply be occurring faster than that able to be removed by patent drains.

Chest drains should also be observed for bubbling, to assess for air leaks originating from either system faults or patient leaks. When bubbling can be attributed to the patient, the patency of tubes becomes additionally important to avert tension pneumothorax, which may accumulate rapidly, even over the course of a few breaths in the ventilated patient.

Blood transfusions are not aimed at restoring haemoglobin to normal levels and, despite variations in acceptable levels, relative anaemia is almost universally tolerated. Haemoglobin levels are therefore not routinely treated unless below 80 g/L, except in the elderly or when there are significant comorbidities.[60–62] From these levels, patients return to normal haemoglobin status within 1 month postoperatively.

Contributors to impaired haemostatic capability

Many factors may contribute to postoperative bleeding by their influence on coagulation and haemostatic ability. CPB is used in the majority of cardiac surgical cases and exerts many influences on coagulation, as do additional factors such as preoperative medications, anaemia or coagulopathies. Contributing factors include:

- CPB influences:
  - heparinisation, haemodilution, platelet damage and altered function
  - disseminated intravascular coagulation (DIC) following activation of the SIRS post CPB
- preoperative anticoagulant/antiplatelet medications commonly encountered
- aspirin, warfarin, clopidogrel and other NOACs (novel oral anticoagulants)
- preoperative anaemia due to aortic valve disease, autologous blood donation or the various chronic anaemias
- clotting factor deficiency
- hypothermia
- coexisting coagulopathies
- increased fibrinolytic activity
- surgical defects such as failure of access site closure, or vascular anastomosis defects.

Bedside assessment of bleeding

The activated clotting time (ACT) is the most commonly used assessment of coagulation and heparin activity during cardiac surgery and subsequently in intensive care. It measures the time to onset of fibrin formation (initial clot development). The ACT has been valuable because it can be inexpensively and efficiently performed at the bedside, providing prompt results and requiring only modest personnel training. Bleeding patients with a prolonged ACT come under consideration for administration of protamine or other agents.[63] Treatable levels vary from greater than 120 seconds to greater than 150 seconds among different centres.

A limitation of ACT measurements is that they provide no information about clotting processes beyond initial fibrin formation, so clotting deficits such as impaired clot strength or the presence of significant fibrinolysis as contributors to bleeding are not revealed by this test.[64,65] In contrast, the thromboelastograph (TEG) measures the clotting process as it proceeds over time. TEG monitoring reveals not only abnormalities early in the clot process (time to fibrin formation, as would be demonstrated by the ACT) but also the subsequent development of clot strength, clot retraction and, finally, fibrinolytic activity for each of their contributions in the bleeding patient.[64,65] TEG monitoring, although considerably more expensive than the ACT, is now available as a bedside or operating room technology and offers better insight into bleeding causes. In addition, because TEG monitoring identifies deficiencies at the various stages of clot formation, development of clot strength and the presence of undue fibrinolytic activity, it may permit better matching of procoagulant, blood product or antifibrinolytic therapy to needs.[63,65]

No matter which of the above technologies is used at the bedside, the patient with significant bleeding should be evaluated more fully as soon as bleeding develops. Blood should be drawn and sent for laboratory assessment, including full blood examination, clotting profile and measures of fibrinolytic activity.

Heparin reversal

CPB requires full heparinisation (initially 300 IU/kg), which is reversed at end-operation.[66,67] The specific antidote, protamine sulfate, is administered as bypass is ceased, at a dose of 1 mg per 100 IU heparin used (i.e. 3 mg/kg).[67] If reversal is less than complete, as evidenced by a prolonged ACT, further protamine sulfate (at doses of 25–50 mg over 5–10 minutes) may be necessary.

Management of bleeding

Treatment approaches to bleeding once the patient is in intensive care include further protamine administration if the ACT remains prolonged, blood and blood product administration (platelets, clotting factors, fresh frozen plasma), procoagulants (desmopressin acetate (DDAVP)) and anti-fibrinolytic agents (see Table 12.3 for more details). Other general measures such as rewarming the patient and preventing or treating hypertension should be undertaken.

Autotransfusion

Chest drain systems used in cardiothoracic surgery can be configured for retransfusion of collected blood during rapid blood loss. If losses are fresh, and are collected with reliable sterility, they can be transfused back into the patient. Blood that has been collected and left standing in the drain receptacle rapidly becomes unsuitable for

TABLE 12.3

Management of the bleeding patient post-cardiac surgery[60,61,64,67,68]

THERAPY	DOSE	COMMENTS/ISSUES
Protamine sulfate	25–50 mg slow IV (<10 mg/min); may be repeated if ACT is prolonged.	Specific antidote to heparin. May cause hypotension. Contraindicated in patient with seafood allergy.
Aprotinin (Trasylol)	Continuous infusion of 2 million units over 30 min, then 500,000 units per hour.	Antifibrinolytic. Proteinaceous. Anaphylaxis risk on re-exposure. Alert should be posted on history.
Desmopressin acetate (DDAVP)	0.4 micrograms/kg IV.	Promotes factor VIII release; limited evidence for use.
'Pump blood' (blood retrieved from bypass circuit at end-operation)	Often 400–800 mL.	This is the remaining blood in bypass circuit; usually centrifuged before returning to patient. Note: this blood contains heparin from CPB.
Whole blood/packed cells	As necessary to achieve Hb >80 g/L or more, according to needs.	Autologous blood sometimes available when patients have donated blood preoperatively.
Fresh frozen plasma	As necessary.	'Broad-spectrum' factor replacement; contains most factors. Useful adjunct to massive blood transfusion.
Platelet concentrates	As necessary.	Generally ABO and Rh compatible preferred.
Epsilon-aminocaproic acid (Amicar)	100 mg/kg IV followed by 1–2 g/h.	Antifibrinolytic. Inhibits plasminogen activation.
Cryoprecipitate	10 units IV.	Contains factor VIII and fibrinogen (factor I).
Calcium chloride or gluconate	10 mL 10% solution.	Used to offset citrate binding of calcium in stored blood.
Prothrombinex	20–50 IU/kg IV.	Contains factors II, IX and X.

ACT = activated clotting time; CPB = cardiopulmonary bypass.

Sources: Boxma RPJ, Garnier RP, Bulte CSE, et al. The effect of non-point-of-care haemostasis management protocol implementation in cardiac surgery: a systematic review. Transfus Med 2021;31(5):328–38; Fischer M-O, Guinot P-G, Debroczi S, et al. Individualised or liberal red blood cell transfusion after cardiac surgery: a randomised controlled trial. Br J Anaesth 2022;128(1):37–44; Kheiri B, Abdalla A, Osman M, et al. Restrictive versus liberal red blood cell transfusion for cardiac surgery: a systematic review and meta-analysis of randomized controlled trials. J Thromb Tthrombolysis 2019;47(2):179–85; Miles LF, Burt C, Arrowsmith J, et al. Optimal protamine dosing after cardiopulmonary bypass: the PRODOSE adaptive randomised controlled trial. PLoS Med 2021;18(6):e1003658; Ranucci M, Baryshnikova E, Pistuddi V, et al. The effectiveness of 10 years of interventions to control postoperative bleeding in adult cardiac surgery. Interact Cardiovasc Thorac Surg 2017;24(2):196–202.

retransfusion, and so autotransfusion is generally limited to blood that has collected over 1–2 hours, rarely longer. Blood filters should always be used for protection against clots that may have developed in the drain receptacle. A small proportion of centres are using intraoperative cell salvage (e.g. Cell Saver® autologous blood recovery system) to recover blood loss from the chest drain system, wash the red blood cells and re-infuse to the patient in case of postoperative massive bleeding.[68,69]

Pericardial tamponade

Postoperative pericardial tamponade results from the accumulation of blood or effusion fluid within the pericardium. An increasing volume within the pericardial space eventually compresses cardiac chambers, impeding venous return and therefore causing low cardiac output and hypotension. Pericardial tamponade is an emergency and varies in severity from shock to pulseless electrical activity.[45,70] Described as one of the extracardiac obstructive shocks, pericardial tamponade often resembles cardiogenic shock. The low cardiac output and hypotension result in oliguria, altered mentation, peripheral hypoperfusion and development of lactic acidosis. Compensation includes tachycardia and marked vasoconstriction, elevating the SVR. As in cardiogenic shock, there is usually elevation of the filling pressures (right atrial, pulmonary artery and PCWPs), sometimes with a particularly suggestive merging of the pulmonary artery diastolic, right atrial and pulmonary artery wedge pressures.[45,70] Additional features that may be present include muffled heart sounds, decreased QRS voltage, electrical alternans, narrowing pulse pressure and pulsus paradoxus, along with features of increasing anxiety and/or dyspnoea in the awake patient.

Echocardiography is the definitive assessment tool to reveal the presence of pericardial collections as well as identifying the impact on relaxation, filling and contraction of each cardiac chamber. The chest X-ray is of limited use and may show little, even with significant pericardial collections.

Importantly, the 'classic' or typical haemodynamic profile described above is not uniformly seen in tamponade, and tamponade should never be excluded because the haemodynamic status does not match this profile. This may be because classic tamponade implies uniform compression of the entire heart, which may not be the case with haemorrhagic tamponade. A clot may develop over just one chamber rather than occupying the entire pericardium, and so there may be compromise to only a single chamber rather than the whole heart.[45,70]

Management of pericardial tamponade

The management of pericardial tamponade includes limiting further losses into the pericardium, relief of pericardial pressure through evacuation of blood or clots and management of the haemodynamic impact of tamponade.

Steps to control bleeding and blood pressure as described above may limit further losses into the pericardium. All steps should be taken to maintain or re-establish chest tube patency (crushing clots within tubing – often referred to as 'milking' the tubes – is not recommended but continues to be used as a last resort) and to ensure free flow of blood from the chest by avoiding dependent tubing loops or by instigating side-to-side rolling of the patient to possibly bring collections into proximity of drain tubes. When tube patency is in doubt, the surgeon may even pass a suction catheter or a balloon-tipped catheter (such as Fogarty catheter) through the chest drain under aseptic conditions in an attempt to remove clots at the drain tip.[45,70] If the above measures do not relieve tamponade, consideration is given to re-exploring the pericardium, either by returning to the operating theatre or, in an emergency, to the ICU or cardiothoracic ward and activation of a CALS protocol if available, although this is less preferable.

Emergency opening of the sternotomy and mediastinal re-exploration requires a coordinated team response and, where possible, operating room staff should be included to manage the sterile field and assist the surgeon. Equipment and disposable materials should be counted and documented in the manner normally applied in theatre. When the situation has been stabilised, consideration should be given to returning to theatre for final assessment and chest closure.[45,70]

Assessment and management of postoperative pain

As much an art as a science, pain control in the cardiac surgical patient remains a major challenge and continues to provide uncertainty and opportunities for nursing clinicians and researchers. Principles are similar to those outlined in Chapter 6. Surgical pain is often complicated by pericardial inflammation and pain management must be balanced against the promotion of spontaneous breathing, chest physiotherapy, mobilisation and participation in education and lifestyle modification programs.

Analgesic options for pain control include intravenous, oral or rectal analgesics, non-steroidal anti-inflammatory medications and, less commonly, epidural therapies and nerve blocks. Intravenous opiates and codeine/paracetamol preparations provide the mainstay of postoperative analgesia. In recent years, postoperative pain has been well managed by a combination of regular oral slow-release narcotic analgesics such as tapentadol, Targin (oxycodone with naloxone) and oxycodone and paracetamol in addition to the immediate release of those narcotics for breakthrough severe pain. When insufficient, or when clinical and electrocardiographic features suggest pericarditis, non-steroidal anti-inflammatory drugs (NSAIDs) such as rectal indomethacin are appropriate, except in patients with renal impairment owing to their renal side effects of reducing glomerular filtration rate and acute deterioration of renal function.[71,72] The place of intravenous (IV) cyclo-oxygenase-2 inhibitors such as parecoxib appears uncertain, as analgesic efficacy now must be weighed against emerging data suggesting increased thrombotic complications.[71,72] Chronic postsurgical pain could persist in up to 10% of patients especially those of female gender, younger ages and/or overweight. Although the main mechanism of this chronic pain is not yet established, well-controlled perioperative pain management regardless of the methods has shown to be a convincing preventative strategy.[73,74]

Fluid and electrolyte management

Fluid therapy in the postoperative period is aimed at maintaining blood volume, replacing recorded and insensible losses and providing adequate preload to sustain haemodynamic status. Isotonic dextrose solutions (5%) or dextrose 4% plus saline 0.18% are commonly used at approximately 1.5 L/day as maintenance fluids.[75] Fluid boluses, crystalloids and/or colloids (as per unit protocol and clinician's preference) are administered as required, based on patient haemodynamic profiles.

Potassium replenishment is generally necessary according to measured serum potassium. Polyuria is usually evident in the early postoperative period owing to

---

Practice tip

Given the variability of presentation of cardiogenic shock, and the importance of accurate identification, clinicians should search for tamponade whenever there is haemodynamic instability postoperatively, especially when the haemodynamic status does not match classic patterns for the major shock states. The management of postoperative cardiac arrest accompanying any arrhythmia, as well as pulseless electrical activity, should include consideration of tamponade.

deliberate haemodilution while on CPB. With polyuria comes potassium loss, which must be treated to avert atrial or ventricular ectopy and tachyarrhythmias. Because of these predictable potassium losses, protocols for potassium replacement may be instituted, with standing orders for potassium replacement (e.g. 10 mmol over 1 hour if the serum potassium is <4.5 mmol/L, or 20 mmol over 2 hours if <4.0 mmol/L). Main-line hydration infusions may also have added potassium to avoid hypokalaemia. Hypomagnesaemia may also develop as a result of polyuria, and is likewise proarrhythmic. Supplementation (magnesium chloride) is often used for arrhythmia management postoperatively, but its effectiveness has been questioned in many trials.[76,77]

Hyperkalaemia occurs less often but is seen particularly when there is impaired renal function. Additional contributors to a rising potassium level include acidosis, administration of stored blood, haemolysis, inotrope use and any postoperative use of depolarising muscle relaxants such as suxamethonium.

Emotional responses and family support

The experience of being diagnosed with a cardiac disorder, waiting for surgery, the surgical experience and recovery is an emotional journey for patients and their families. Regardless of low mortality rates, the possibility of death and painful wounds can concern patients. Consequently, patients undergoing cardiac surgery often experience anxiety and depression,[78] and women appear to be more vulnerable to these emotions in relation to cardiac surgery than men.[79] In addition, the same levels of anxiety, depression and stress have been experienced by patients' spouses but significantly reduce over time in both patients and their families. It has been suggested that providing appropriate information about the procedures to both patients and their spouses will assist them to deal better with their psychological state in the recovery period.[80] The use of a 30-minute preoperative education session on psychosocial well-being has been shown to significantly reduce the rate of pre- and postoperative anxiety in cardiac surgical patients; therefore, training provided to nurses and physicians on emotional support of these patients is essential.[80,81]

Similarly, adequate preparation of the patient and their family in the preoperative period will assist them with their stress and anxiety coping strategies as well as reduce their work stress after their return to work.[80,81] The preoperative preparation is usually provided by nurses and should incorporate information and support about the procedures and recovery period, so that patients and their families are better equipped during their recovery. Emphasis should be on identifying the intrapersonal stressors, such as pain and discomfort, invasive lines and surgical procedures, for individual patients to assist them to cope with their perioperative and rehabilitation period.[81,82] However, patients who have had their surgery postponed or who have been operated on in an emergency setting may need additional support. Also, critical pathways for cardiac surgery do not include assessing the patient's psychological state, so nurses must take care to consider this aspect. Printed information regarding the surgery, recovery and emotions will be useful for the patient and family (for further information refer to Chapter 6 and Chapter 7).

Intra-aortic balloon pumping

Intra-aortic balloon pumping is a widely used circulatory assist therapy that has become straightforward in application and relatively free of complications.[83,84] The primary aim of IABP is to assist in repairing an existing imbalance between myocardial oxygen supply and demand. The main indications are cardiogenic shock, myocardial infarction or ischaemia, and as haemodynamic support for PCI and weaning from CPB. The combined effects of increasing cardiac output and mean arterial pressure (increasing oxygen supply) and decreasing myocardial workload (reducing oxygen demand) make IABP therapy ideal for the management of infarct-related cardiogenic shock,[84,85] for which it should be regarded as standard management.

IABP therapy involves placement of a balloon catheter in the descending thoracic aorta. This catheter is most commonly advanced from a percutaneous femoral artery access until the tip of the catheter is situated just below the left subclavian artery (Fig. 12.5). A chest X-ray or fluoroscopy should reveal the catheter tip just below the aortic arch, or at the level of the second anterior intercostal space or fifth posterior intercostal space (Fig. 12.6). The conventional catheter has two lumens: a monitoring lumen, which opens at the catheter tip from which the aortic pressure waveform is monitored, and a helium drive lumen, through which the helium is shuttled from the pumping console to the catheter balloon. The newer fibreoptic catheter has an additional lumen for electrical signal acquisition and transmission from the tip of catheter; together with the automation mode this has improved IABP timing through enabling faster adjustment to patient rate and rhythm changes. Balloon volumes range from 25 mL (paediatric use) to 34–50 mL in adults (most commonly used is a 40-mL balloon) and are selected according to patient height (e.g. a 40-mL balloon is used for a patient height of 162–183 cm).

Principles of counterpulsation

When IABP is initiated, the balloon will be inflated rapidly at the onset of diastole of each cardiac cycle and then deflated immediately just before the onset of the next systole; this sequence is referred to as counterpulsation (Fig. 12.7).

Balloon inflation

At the onset of diastole, the balloon is rapidly inflated with (most commonly) 40 mL of helium. This inflation causes a sudden rise in pressure in the aortic root during diastole, raising mean arterial pressure and, importantly,

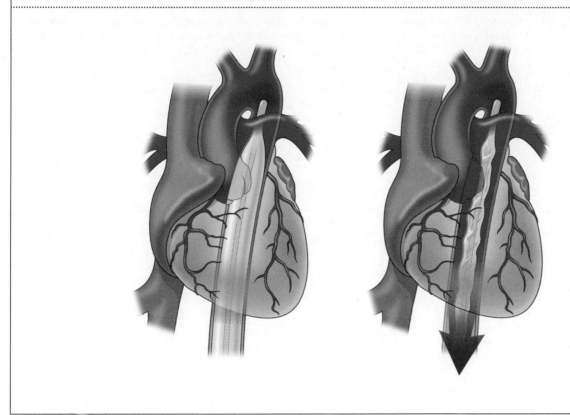

FIGURE 12.5 Intra-aortic balloon catheter. On the left the inflated catheter can be seen behind the heart, with its tip below the arch of the aorta and the left subclavian artery. The balloon cycles between inflated (during diastole) and deflated (during systole), as on the right. Blood fills the aorta while the balloon is deflated, and with inflation the balloon almost fills the descending aorta, displacing 40 mL blood from the aorta to the coronary and systemic circulation.

FIGURE 12.6 IABP catheter position in chest X-ray; the tip is located in the second intercostal space anterior ribs or fifth intercostal space posterior ribs.

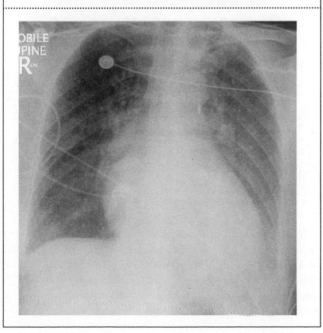

coronary perfusion pressure. The blood displaced by the balloon expansion improves blood flow into the coronary circulation (which fills largely during diastole), as well as to the brain and systemic circulation. Hence, there is improved myocardial oxygen supply and increased mean arterial pressure, as well as improved systemic perfusion.[10,86] The balloon remains inflated for the duration of diastole. The arterial pressure wave should reveal a sharp rise in pressure at the dicrotic notch, with a second pressure peak now appearing on the waveform, described as the 'augmented diastolic' or 'balloon-assisted peak diastolic' pressure. This peak is usually at least 10 mmHg higher than the systolic pressure (see Fig. 12.7).

Balloon deflation

As the inflated balloon largely obstructs the aorta, it must be deflated to permit systolic emptying of the left ventricle. Two separate approaches to the timing of balloon deflation have emerged: 'conventional timing' and 'real timing'.

Conventional timing

In conventional timing, the balloon is deflated immediately prior to systole and deflation timing is predicted from an average of last R–R interval (up to eight) and commonly

FIGURE 12.7 Intra-aortic balloon pump (IABP) during 1:1 assist (counterpulsation on every beat). Balloon inflation at the start of diastole and deflation just before the next systole. IABP during 1:2 assist (counterpulsation on every second beat). Inflation of the balloon rapidly at the inflation point (IP) raises diastolic pressure, producing a peak diastolic pressure (PDP) that exceeds the peak systolic pressure (PSP). The balloon remains inflated during diastole. With balloon deflation just prior to the next systole, there is a rapid decline in pressure to the balloon-assisted end-diastolic pressure (BAEDP), which is lower than normal non-assisted end-diastolic pressure (EDP), reducing afterload. The ensuing systole is achieved with a reduced systolic pressure (the assisted peak systolic pressure, APSP).

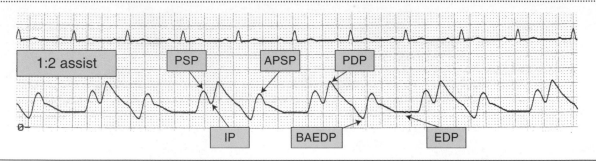

selected for regular rhythms. Rapid deflation induces a precipitous drop in aortic pressure at the end of diastole (a reduced aortic end-diastolic pressure). This reduces the duration of the left ventricle isovolumetric contraction phase of the cardiac cycle (the most oxygen-consuming phase of the cardiac cycle), reduces the left ventricular afterload and improves left ventricular emptying, improving stroke volume and cardiac output. In addition, less pressure is required for left ventricular emptying, so systolic work and oxygen demands on the myocardium are reduced.[10,86] Therefore, deflation during conventional timing should see the aortic pressure drop to below normal at end-diastole, just in advance of the subsequent systole. Systolic pressure should also be lower than during a non–assisted beat. In case of premature cardiac contraction such as atrial or ventricular ectopics, R-wave deflate is active during conventional timing to deflate the balloon and empty the aorta for those beats.

Real timing

In contrast to conventional timing, during real timing (also referred to as R-wave deflate) the balloon remains inflated for slightly longer and is deflated not before but at the same time as systole and is commonly selected for irregular rhythms. The reduction in aortic end-diastolic pressure is therefore not seen, but deflating simultaneously with left ventricular contraction still favourably affects left ventricular emptying.[10,86] Thus, there is improved stroke volume, systolic pressure reduction and decreased ventricular work and oxygen demand as seen during conventional timing.[10,87] Box 12.1 summarises the impact of balloon inflation and deflation on haemodynamic status and the oxygen supply/demand balance.

The arterial pressure wave reveals the impact of IABP therapy on haemodynamic status. Placing the pump into 1:2 assist (balloon pumping on only every second beat) is

---

BOX 12.1

Effects of intra-aortic balloon counterpulsation

- Balloon inflation:
  - increased aortic diastolic pressure (augmented, or balloon-assisted peak diastolic pressure, or balloon aortic end-diastolic pressure (BAEDP))
  - increased mean arterial pressure
  - increased coronary and myocardial perfusion and oxygen supply
  - increased cerebral and systemic perfusion
- Balloon deflation:
  - decreased afterload
  - increased stroke volume and cardiac output
  - decreased LV congestion, decreased PCWP, decreased pulmonary congestion
  - decreased duration of isovolumetric contraction
  - decreased left ventricular workload
  - decreased systolic pressure
  - decreased myocardial oxygen demand

LV = left ventricle; PCWP = pulmonary capillary wedge pressure.

---

useful to highlight balloon pump impact and how assisted beats vary from the normal pressure cycle during systole and diastole. Clinician should be mindful that placing the pump into 1:2 assist will reduce the support by 50%, therefore it should be avoided or minimised to shortest time possible. Fig. 12.7 depicts the impact of IABP on haemodynamic status and the arterial pressure waveform.

Complications of intra-aortic balloon pumping

Serious complications are uncommon during IABP treatment and have continued to decrease in frequency during the past decade with advances in pump technology and the advent of smaller catheter sizes.[88,89] Limb ischaemia remains the most common serious complication, especially in patients with existing vasculopathy,[88,90] providing impetus to the development of smaller catheters, which have now reached 7.0 French gauge. Additional complications, such as bleeding, catheter migration, thromboembolism, insertion site vascular damage, thrombocytopenia and device-related problems such as timing inaccuracy, device failure and gas leaks, also occur but are less common. These are described below.

Patient management

Prevention of complications, as well as optimisation of the impact of counterpulsation, form the major components of nursing care of a patient being treated with IABP. Thorough understanding of the impact of the presence of the balloon, as well as the beneficial and detrimental effects of counterpulsation, is essential.

Maintenance of limb perfusion

The use of smaller-gauge catheters has reduced the potential for obstruction of arterial flow past the catheter to the lower limbs, as has the trend to sheath-less insertion. Nevertheless, the threat of limb ischaemia remains an important issue in patient care, as IABP is most commonly undertaken in patients with atherosclerosis, potentially involving the lower limbs, even in the absence of overt peripheral vascular deficits. Identification of patients at risk (known claudication, chronically cold feet and peripheral vascular diseases) may be useful to ensure appropriate vigilance and prompt intervention where necessary. Peripheral perfusion may also be compromised by arterial embolisation should thrombi develop on the catheter. Although catheter materials are non-thrombogenic, the risk of thrombus formation remains and is heightened if periods of catheter stasis (interrupted pumping) are encountered. Systemic heparinisation is not recommended routinely for thromboembolic prevention except for specific indications as it increases the risk of bleeding.[91]

Hourly assessments of peripheral perfusion (colour, warmth, movement, sensation) should be performed to identify potential deficits. The dorsalis pedis and posterior tibialis pulses should be palpated and may sometimes require examination with a Doppler probe. Deficits should be promptly reported, and consideration given to catheter removal or re-insertion on the contralateral limb. When pulses cannot be demonstrated, the limb should be assessed for the development of compartment syndrome. At times, the viability of a limb must be weighed against the potential survival benefit of IABP to the patient.

Prevention and treatment of bleeding

Significant bleeding is uncommon,[92] but blood loss may occur from the femoral arterial access site. In addition to physical factors at the insertion site, contributors to bleeding include heparinisation, thrombocytopenia from the physical effect of the pump on platelets and/or other anticoagulants or antiplatelet agents used for the primary disease. Regular observation should be made of the insertion site for bruising or external bleeding, as well as other possible sites of bleeding due to heparinisation. Treatment includes manual pressure at the insertion site or use of compression devices such as FemoStop®, reinforcement of dressings and/or topical procoagulant agents. Monitoring of coagulation status and haemoglobin should be undertaken and blood or blood products may (uncommonly) be required.

Prevention of immobility-related complications

The need for immobilisation of the patient, and in particular the leg, is often overemphasised, and may heighten the risk of atelectasis, pressure area development and venous stasis and thrombosis. Sensible limitation of leg movement is advised, but patients can generally still move in bed, and should still be turned 2-hourly for pressure relief as long as the insertion site is adequately protected and supported. The femoral access limits flexion at the hip beyond 30 degrees, which may also hamper effective chest physiotherapy and increase the risk of atelectasis and pneumonia. As the catheter is fixed with sutures at the femoral insertion site, flexion of the hip by more than 30 degrees may cause its migration towards the aortic arch and possible left subclavian or left carotid artery occlusion.

Migration of the balloon catheter towards the aortic arch or towards the abdominal aorta may cause compromised perfusion to the left arm (occlusion of left subclavian artery), kidneys (renal arteries) or abdominal viscera (superior mesenteric artery). Therefore, neurovascular observation of the upper limbs, urine output and bowel sounds are part of nursing management of the patient with IABP in situ.

Weaning of IABP

Weaning of IABP therapy is generally undertaken once the patient has stabilised, is free of ischaemic signs and symptoms and is on minimum or no inotropic support. Algorithms have been offered for approaches to weaning therapy, with no haemodynamic or mortality benefit.[93,94] Weaning is carried out by either gradual reductions in balloon inflation volume (volume weaning) or gradual reductions in assist frequency from 1:1 through 1:2 and 1:4 (ratio weaning). Hybrids of the two approaches are sometimes used. Support is reduced at intervals while the patient is observed for haemodynamic deterioration, pulmonary congestion and the return of ischaemic signs and symptoms.

Assessment of timing and timing errors

Accurate timing of inflation and deflation in relation to the cardiac cycle is required to maximise IABP benefit. Errors in timing may lessen the potential benefit, or in some cases may worsen cardiac performance and increase demands on the myocardium. Nurses are required to continually assess the haemodynamic impact of balloon pumping and the accuracy of timing via inspection of the arterial pressure waveform, and to adjust timing to optimise the impact of balloon pumping. The development of automated IABP counterpulsation has reduced timing errors by automatic trigger signal recognition and selection, accuracy of automatic setting for optimal inflation and deflation timing and automatic adjustment to changing patient conditions. Therefore, the automated mode of counterpulsation is recommended.[95,96] In addition to automated mode, the use of a fibreoptic catheter has reduced timing errors owing to its accurate and faster signals acquisition.[96]

Early inflation

Early inflation will at times be difficult to differentiate from correct inflation timing but is recognised by the onset of inflation soon after the peak systolic pressure, before the pressure has declined to the level of the dicrotic notch (Fig. 12.8). Early inflation may limit the stroke volume and cardiac output, as terminal systole is impeded, and may result in increased myocardial oxygen demands, increased left ventricle workload and premature valve closure. The inflation point should be adjusted (to later) until the inflation upstroke emerges smoothly out of the dicrotic notch.

Late inflation

The arterial pressure waveform reveals the onset of diastole (the dicrotic notch) before balloon inflation commences (Fig. 12.9). This generally results in a lower augmented diastolic pressure than could otherwise be achieved. As the duration of balloon inflation is lessened,

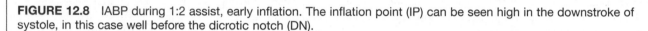

FIGURE 12.8 IABP during 1:2 assist, early inflation. The inflation point (IP) can be seen high in the downstroke of systole, in this case well before the dicrotic notch (DN).

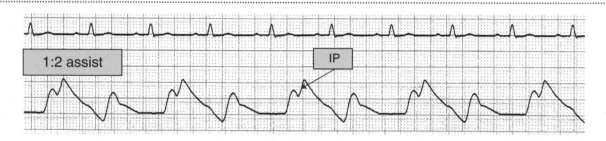

FIGURE 12.9 IABP during 1:2 assist, late inflation. Note that the inflation point (IP) occurs well after the dicrotic notch (DN). Late inflation is also obvious in 1:1 assist with balloon inflation well after the dicrotic notch.

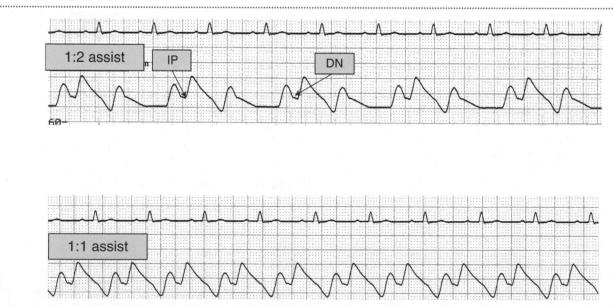

the desired rise in mean arterial pressure and coronary perfusion will not be achieved. The inflation marker should be set to 'earlier' until the inflation upstroke emerges smoothly out of the dicrotic notch.

Early deflation

Deflating the balloon earlier than necessary shortens the duration for which the balloon remains inflated and therefore limits the benefit of IABP. When deflation is very early, it may cause harm. Deflation sees the aortic pressure drop markedly but there is now time for blood to fill the space left by the balloon before systole commences. Aortic end-diastolic pressure increases and may even exceed the normal end-diastolic pressure, increasing the duration of the isovolumetric phase, worsening left ventricular afterload and increasing myocardial oxygen demand. One other potential problem with early deflation is backflow of blood from the coronary and carotid arteries (coronary and carotid 'steal') due to reduction of pressure in the aorta well ahead of ventricular systole and ejection (Fig. 12.10). Correction is achieved by setting deflation to later until the pressure drop of deflation occurs just in advance of the succeeding systole.

Late deflation

When deflation begins too late, systole commences before complete emptying of the intra-aortic balloon. The typical reduction of aortic end-diastolic pressure is not seen. When significantly late, the end-diastolic pressure may even be increased, prolonging the duration of the isovolumetric contraction phase and worsening afterload. As systole occurs against an incompletely deflated balloon,

the stroke volume and cardiac output suffer and ventricular work and oxygen demand increase (Fig. 12.11). Deflation should be set to earlier until the systolic upstroke emerges out of the reduced end-diastolic pressure dip.

Alarm states

Alarm functions vary according to manufacturer and model. The main alarm states common to most devices, and their causes and significance, are shown in Table 12.4. Importantly, in most alarm states the pump consoles will revert to standby, suspending pumping. The balloon is at risk of developing thrombi within the folds of the balloon while deflated, and these can be liberated as arterial emboli on recommencement of pumping. Therefore, it is important to treat alarm states promptly, to limit the duration of balloon stasis. If interruption to pumping is prolonged, intermittent manual inflation of the balloon with a syringe is recommended (e.g. once every 5–10 minutes).

Gas loss alarms

Most devices will determine the severity of gas losses and classify them as slow, rapid or disconnect. In all gas loss states it is imperative that assessments be made to exclude balloon rupture and helium leak into the arterial circulation. Small gas losses of helium may or may not be of clinical significance, but the delivery of sizeable helium volumes may behave as gas emboli and, if delivered into the coronary circulation, may result in lethal arrhythmias or neurological complications if delivered into the cerebral circulation.[97,98] In all gas loss alarm states, the helium drive line should be inspected for the presence of blood to

---

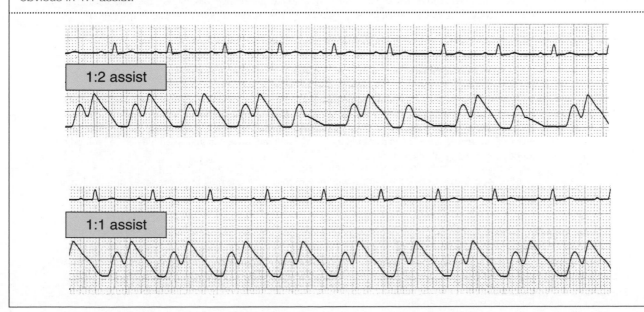

FIGURE 12.10 IABP during 1:2 assist, early deflation. The balloon has been deflated well in advance of the subsequent systole. The aortic pressure does drop off (not much from non-assisted diastole) but then begins to rise again before the next systole gets underway and may even exceed the normal end-diastolic pressure. Early deflation is also obvious in 1:1 assist.

1:2 assist

1:1 assist

FIGURE 12.11   IABP during 1:2 assist, late deflation. The late deflation is seen here as the sharp drop-off before systole and a balloon-assisted end-diastole that does not fall to below the normal patient end-diastolic pressure.

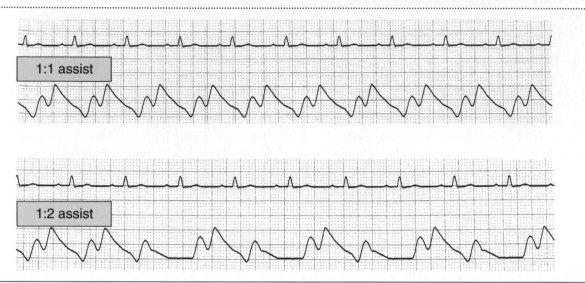

TABLE 12.4

Intra-aortic balloon pump alarm states

ALARM STATE	CAUSES/SIGNIFICANCE
Catheter alarm	Obstruction (complete or subtotal) of the catheter, drive line or balloon. Device reverts to standby (non-assist); commonly due to catheter flexion at insertion site due to limb position or excessive surface-to-vessel depth.
Loss of trigger	ECG trigger: signal disrupted or low in amplitude, or asystole. Pressure trigger: pulse pressure below threshold for detection. Pacer trigger: pacing spikes not detected or absent (including demand pacing). Device reverts to standby until restoration of trigger; alternative trigger selection may be necessary. Automatic mode will search for the best available trigger (different leads or pressure), but ECG trigger is always selected once re-established.
Gas loss alarms	Leak in circuit/drive line or balloon; gas leak may be to the environment or into the patient as a helium embolus. Pump reverts to standby; always check helium drive line for blood before refilling of the circuit.
Low augmentation	Augmented diastolic pressure is lower than operator-selected alarm level. Possible causes: low balloon volume selection, IABC is positioned lower in aorta, vasodilation or late inflation of the balloon. Pumping is not interrupted.
Pneumatic drive	Functional problem with the pump inflation/deflation pneumatic system. Device reverts to standby; alarm may sometimes be activated during tachycardia; 1:2 assist or assist at reduced augmentation may be possible until a replacement device is accessed (newer generation devices function well with higher heart rate).
Autofill failure	Routine 2-hourly refilling of the system with helium may fail if gas tank is incompletely open or if circuit leaks cause volume loss during the filling attempt. Device reverts to standby.
System failure	Console self-testing has identified component malfunction. Device reverts to standby; restarting may be possible, but a replacement device should be accessed.
Low helium supply	Helium tank empty or incompletely opened.
Low battery	Reconnect to power and recharge.

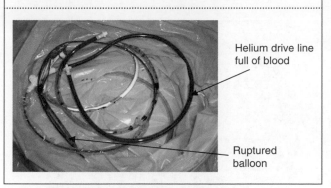

FIGURE 12.12   Intra-aortic balloon rupture and presence of blood in the helium drive line.

Helium drive line full of blood

Ruptured balloon

indicate loss of integrity of the balloon. If blood is present in the drive line (Fig. 12.12), pumping should be suspended and no attempts at recommencing balloon pumping should be made. Prompt removal and/or replacement, along with thorough patient assessment and support, is essential.

Heart transplantation

The ultimate goal of organ transplantation is to provide an improved quality of life and long-term survival for patients with end-stage heart disease. To optimise patient outcomes, the early postoperative management of these patients requires critical care clinicians with specific expertise to collaborate with a multidisciplinary team of health professionals. In the following sections, the important management issues in the early postoperative period for heart transplant recipients are discussed. The major long-term complications of heart transplantation are also discussed briefly as recipients may be re-admitted to critical care with life-threatening complications years after their transplant.

Patients with certain chronic and less commonly acute heart diseases may be referred for organ transplantation assessment when their disease state is such that their life expectancy is less than 2 years and their quality of life intolerable. Patients who receive organ transplants are commonly debilitated and may have an acute-on-chronic presentation at the time of surgery. The surgical procedure is lengthy, up to 12 hours, and involves CPB. The duration and nature of the surgery in patients with severely compromised health status serve to compound the often-critical condition of such patients in the early postoperative period.

The immediate period following surgery is commonly the first contact that critical care clinicians have with transplant recipients and their families. The exception may be patients in the ICU with acute heart failure awaiting heart transplantation who are on temporary or durable mechanical support. Durable mechanical circulatory support, also known as a ventricular assist device (VAD), is used as a 'bridge to transplantation' (Fig. 12.13). Patients

can also be supported by a temporary support device; an intra-aortic balloon pump, Impella® or extracorporeal membrane oxygenation (ECMO) (these are far less common). Ideally, patients with mechanical circulatory support are returned to a sound physical, mental and nutritional state prior to receiving a transplant and, as part of their recovery, await transplantation in the ward or most commonly in the home setting. For specific management of patients on mechanical circulatory support, readers are referred to specific resources (e.g. websites and operating manuals for individual mechanical circulatory support devices: Abbott (Thoratec® HeartMate 3 and HeartMate II), Medtronic (HeartWare® HVAD) and SynCardia.

Heart transplantation is a life-saving and cost-effective form of treatment that enhances the quality of life for many people with severe heart failure. Legislation that defined brain death and enabled beating-heart retrieval was enacted in Australia in 1982. This legislation heralded the establishment of formal transplant programs. In Australia, the first heart program commenced in 1983.[99,100] With worsening shortage of donor hearts, the growing interest of using DCD (donation after cardiac death) hearts has emerged, especially as the use of DCD livers, kidneys and lungs has significantly contributed to transplant numbers. St Vincent's in Sydney performed the world's first DCD heart using the TransMedics Organ Care System (OCS) in 2014. This allows for ongoing assessment of function of the donor heart. Published data on 5-year experience with early-to-medium-term outcomes have been excellent in terms of survival and no difference in rejection rates when compared with heart recipients from donation after brain death (DBD). The experience to date suggests that DCD donors do contribute significantly (~30%) to transplant numbers.[101–104] The non-ischaemic heart preservation (NIHP) XVIVO Heart Box System is another emerging technology to reduce donor injury from long ischaemic times (time from donor explant to recipient implant) by perfusion of the donor heart during transport. This will hopefully increase the use of donor hearts by enabling the procurement of donors a long distance from the implanting centre.[105] At time of writing, within Australia and New Zealand there is a trial of the XVIVO Heart Box System for donor heart procurement and transportation to the recipient hospital in long-ischaemic-time donors.

Another new advance is the utilisation of hepatitis-C-positive heart donors. Over the last 10 years in the United States the opioid epidemic has led to an increase in hepatitis C transmission due to use of shared needles. Nucleic acid testing (NAT) is now standard practice for detecting hepatitis C. The application of direct-acting antiviral treatments in transplant recipients with hepatitis-C-positive donors shows great efficacy and safety. So the increase in utilisation of hepatitis-C-positive heart donors should contribute to addressing donor organ shortages.[106–108] For more information see the International Society for Heart Lung Transplantation (ISHLT) expert consensus statement on the utilisation of hepatitis-C-infected organ donors in cardiothoracic transplantation.[100]

FIGURE 12.13 Pump, monitor and controller. **(A)** HeartMate 3 Controller, Batteries and Battery Clips. **(B)** HeartMate 3.

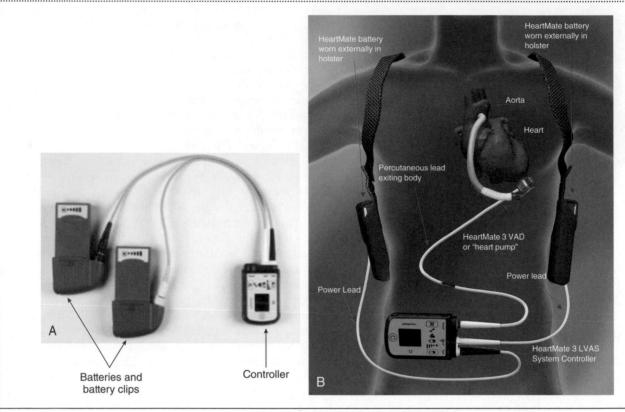

Source: HeartMate 3TM Left Ventricular Assist System Instructions For Use with HeartMate Touch © 2022 Abbott.

The success of transplantation in the current era as a viable option for end-stage organ failure is primarily due to the discovery of the immunosuppressive agent cyclosporine A. In this section, heart transplantation as a component of critical care nursing is discussed, with reference to evidence-based practices.

History

Heart transplant surgery for refractory heart failure was first performed in Australia in 1968, only months after the first heart transplant was performed by Christiaan Barnard at Groote Schur Hospital in Cape Town, South Africa in December 1967.[110] However, high mortality rates associated with severe acute rejection and infection within months of surgery led to a reduction in the number of heart transplants performed worldwide, and in effect a moratorium occurred with the procedure. Heart transplantation was finally established in the modern era as a viable treatment option for end-stage heart failure during the early 1980s when cyclosporine A, a then-novel immunosuppressive agent, dramatically improved patients' survival rates by reducing episodes of acute rejection and lowering attendant infectious complications.[111]

Incidence

Heart transplants in the modern era have been performed in Australia since 1986 and in New Zealand since 1987. In 2018, 141 heart transplants were performed in Australia and New Zealand (the last-published data from the Australia and New Zealand Cardiothoracic Organ Transplant Registry (ANZCOTR)).[112] In Europe in 2020, 587 heart transplants were performed,[113] an annual figure that has been relatively static for the past 5 years. As the annual number of transplants globally is likely to remain relatively stable because of limited organ availability, future management of end-stage heart failure may involve the insertion of a left ventricular assist device (LVAD) designed for long-term permanent mechanical circulatory support, so-called 'destination therapy'. In the early years, the VADs available were primarily used as 'bridge to transplantation' therapy (i.e. support for a failing native heart until a suitable heart became available), not 'destination therapy', although both purposes were shown to be viable options in the REMATCH study.[114] Although this is still the case in Australia and New Zealand, recent global reports show about 56% of VADs are now used as 'destination therapy'.[115] This change has been facilitated by improvements in device technologies and the experiences of clinicians in managing this unique cohort. Survival with current-technology continuous-flow VADs is now at 82% to the first year and 73% at 2 years,[115] with approximately 45% of patients supported on a VAD at time of transplant.[116] The notion of patients with VADs permanently owing to advances in device design and capability (e.g. fully implantable with internal batteries) may not be as futuristic as once thought.

Outcomes from heart transplantation

Currently, the centres around the world that submit data to the ISHLT indicate a 1-year survival at 86%[117] and a 5-year survival at 72.5%, with a 21% survival at 20 years.[118] In Australia and New Zealand, approximately 90% of heart transplant patients survive to 1 year, and 85.4% survive to 5 years.[119]

Survival after heart transplant is improving over time. The median survival of heart transplant recipients who survive beyond 12 months is 14.8 years.[116]

Indications

The vast majority of patients referred for heart transplantation have persistent NYHA functional class IV symptoms (see Chapter 10), secondary to ischaemic heart disease or some form of dilated cardiomyopathy.[116] In ICUs and cardiac units, patients with end-stage cardiomyopathy requiring either continuous intravenous inotropic support or cardiovascular support with an intra-aortic balloon pump, VAD or other mechanical circulatory support device may be referred for transplant consideration.[116] Commonly, patients listed for transplantation have a life expectancy of less than 2 years without transplantation. Accepted contraindications for heart transplantation include active malignancy, complicated diabetes, morbid obesity, uncontrolled infection, active substance abuse and an inability to comply with complex medical regimens.[120] The median recipient age for adult heart recipients is 55 years; however, the percentage of recipients greater than 60 years of age continues to rise.[116] Age has become a relative contraindication. However, higher recipient age is linked with lower long-term survival.[116] The presence of multiple comorbidities in patients over 70 years of age would be expected to exclude the majority of such patients from consideration.[120,121] Other relative contraindications include renal failure and an irreversible high transpulmonary gradient (mean PAP minus pulmonary artery wedge pressure) of greater than 15 mmHg (see following section on Early allograft dysfunction and failure). In the context of a rigorous postoperative regimen of polypharmacy, frequent follow-up medical appointments and routine cardiac biopsies, a strong social support network, absence of psychiatric illnesses and a willingness to participate actively in the recovery process are highly desirable characteristics of prospective recipients.[122]

Patients referred for heart transplant assessment must have exhausted all other accepted pharmacological and surgical treatment options for end-stage heart failure, such as optimal therapeutic doses of common heart failure medications, revascularisation via CABG surgery or PTCA, continuous IV infusions of dobutamine or milrinone in the community/home setting, IV levosimendan (a calcium sensitiser), antiarrhythmic drugs to suppress or an internal cardiac defibrillator to treat potentially lethal arrhythmias, and insertion of a biventricular pacemaker (i.e. chronic resynchronisation therapy) to re-establish atrioventricular synchrony (see Chapter 11).

The median costs associated with heart transplantation are high, at approximately AUD$146,000 for the index admission and approximately AUD$33,000 for subsequent admissions over the first 12 months after heart transplantation, depending on the drug regimen and episodes of rejection or infection.[123] As some immunosuppressant drugs have come off patent, these costs have been reduced. However, the high incidence of chronic heart failure and associated hospitalisation costs are also considerable. The number of Australians aged >65 years developing any form of heart failure is estimated to be more than 68,500 per annum.[124] The prevalence of Australians with heart failure is estimated to be 480,000. The number of hospitalisations reported as heart failure or cardiomyopathy (principal and/or additional diagnosis) was 179,000 between 2020 and 2021; this equates to 1.5% of all hospitalisations in Australia during that time period.[124] The annual direct cost of managing heart failure in the community is close to $900 million and as part of an acute hospitalisation $1.8 billion (total direct cost = $2.7 billion). Transplantation for end-stage heart failure is a viable and economical treatment option for individuals and society; it is, however, a limited resource available to only a few recipients.[125,126]

Forms of heart transplant surgery

The most common heart transplant surgery is orthotopic transplantation, with two surgical techniques used: the standard or bicaval approaches. The standard technique has been used since the 1960s and involves anastomoses of the donor and native atria.[127] Complications associated with the standard technique can include abnormal atrial contribution to ventricular filling and tricuspid and mitral valve insufficiency.[128,129] Since the mid 1990s, the bicaval technique as described by Dreyfus and colleagues[130] is now used almost uniformly. The main advantage of the bicaval approach is the maintenance of atrial-conducting pathways and the likelihood of promoting sinus rhythm and its associated superior atrial haemodynamics[130] (Fig. 12.14). Reported potential disadvantages include stenoses in the inferior and superior vena cava at the anastomosis sites.[130]

The second form of heart transplant surgery, which is rarely utilised now, is heterotopic transplantation. These account for only a handful of heart transplants globally. In this procedure, the donor heart is implanted in the right side of the chest next to the native heart[131] to augment native systolic function. Heterotopic heart transplantation is primarily indicated in patients with pulmonary

FIGURE 12.14 **Left**: Completion of bicaval transplant technique, showing the inferior vena caval, superior vena caval, aortic and pulmonary artery anastomoses. **Right**: Commencement of the left atrial anastomosis.

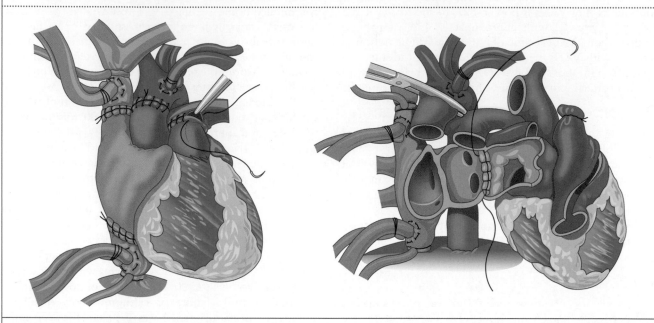

Source: Adapted from Kirklin JK, Young JB, McGiffin DC. Heart transplantation. Philadelphia: Churchill Livingstone; 2002, with permission.

FIGURE 12.15 Chest X-ray showing heterotopic heart transplant.

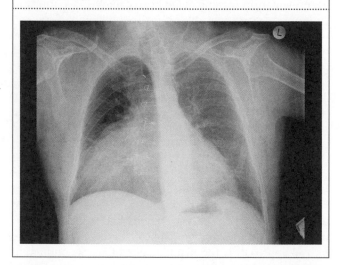

FIGURE 12.16 Heterotopic heart transplant (LVAD configuration).

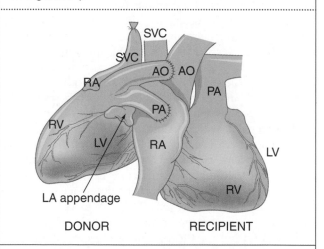

Source: Adapted from Newcomb AE, Esmore DS, Rosenfeldt FL et al. Heterotopic heart transplantation: an expanding role in the twenty-first century? Ann Thorac Surg 2004;78(4):1345–50, with permission.

hypertension refractory to pulmonary vasodilator therapies. It may also be considered in patients with a large body surface area who are unlikely to receive a suitably large-sized donor heart to enable an orthotopic procedure to take place.[127,132] Heterotopic transplantation is usually performed to support the left ventricle (LVAD configuration), but can be configured to support biventricular function (biventricular ventricular assisted device configuration). Fig. 12.15 shows a chest X-ray of the donor heart next to the native heart, and the LVAD

configuration for heterotopic heart transplantation is illustrated in Fig. 12.16.

Patient management

Postoperative nursing and collaborative management of orthotopic heart transplant recipients involve full haemodynamic monitoring with a pulmonary artery

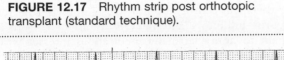

FIGURE 12.17 Rhythm strip post orthotopic transplant (standard technique).

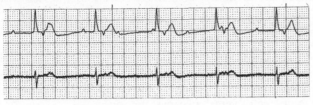

catheter (PAC), a triple- or quad-lumen central venous catheter (CVC), arterial line, indwelling urinary catheter and 5-lead cardiac monitoring to assist in arrhythmia discrimination. A 12-lead ECG is also recorded. If the orthotopic transplant is performed with the standard technique, a remnant P wave from the native heart may be visible on the ECG or cardiac monitor (Fig. 12.17). As the native sinus node cannot conduct across the right atrial suture line, the recipient's heart rate is determined by the conduction system of the donor heart, not the native heart. Of interest, it is possible for the native heart to generate a P wave while the donor heart is in AF or other arrhythmia. (More-detailed discussion of cardiac monitoring and haemodynamic management of patients with a heterotopic heart transplant is available.[133])

Monitoring data are combined with physical assessment information from all body systems to determine nursing and collaborative interventions. Intensive continuous monitoring and assessment of haemodynamic parameters according to evidence-based practices and overall clinical status allow nurses to detect and subsequently respond to emergent postoperative complications. Comprehensive guidelines for the care of heart transplant recipients, supported by the level of evidence for relevant practices, are detailed in a paper published by the ISHLT.[134] The role of nurses in cardiothoracic transplantation continues to evolve. In order to support nurses working at the fullest extent of their education and licensure, a consensus document from ISHLT provides recommendations and areas for future research.[135]

Full ventilatory support is required until the patient's haemodynamic status is stable. Respiratory status is monitored via clinical, radiological and laboratory-derived data (see Chapter 13). Enteral feeding is usually commenced on the day of admission. Renal and neurological function are closely monitored, as tacrolimus and cyclosporine can have a deleterious effect on renal function and can lead to failure as well as neurotoxicity.[136–138] For the small number of patients who develop allograft dysfunction requiring mechanical circulatory support (i.e. ECMO (most common), LVAD or IABP (rare)), or acute renal failure requiring haemofiltration, hospitalisation in the critical care unit tends to last for weeks rather than for days. Each centre will have a clear escalation pathway for initiating mechanical circulatory support.

The immediate period after transplantation can be a time of great hope and joy for recipients and their family and friends; however, complications and setbacks can make the path to recovery prolonged, unpredictable and difficult. The provision of psychosocial support by all members of the transplant/critical care team to family members and friends is an important part of patients' recovery from organ transplantation. Meetings with family that convey honest and open information about a patient's progress need to be conducted regularly. Supporting and managing patients and families following transplant is consistent with support provided to other critically ill patients (see Chapter 8). In addition, there is the issue of dealing with lost hope if the transplant fails: a very distressing time for all involved. In the immediate postoperative period, transplant recipients are at risk of developing complications that include hyperacute rejection, acute rejection, infection, haemorrhage and renal failure. In the immediate postoperative period, heart transplant recipients may experience morbidity specific to the heart transplant procedure, such as early allograft dysfunction (i.e. organ failure due to preservation injury), bleeding, right ventricular failure and acute rejection. Long-term complications include chronic renal failure, hypertension, malignancy, infection, diabetes mellitus and cardiac allograft vasculopathy. The common immediate potential complications and associated clinical management for heart recipients are discussed in the following sections.

All patients receive immunosuppression after transplant. Initially this is high dose, gradually reducing over time. The highest-risk period for rejection is the first 6–9 months post transplant. Standard immunosuppressant agents include prednisolone, calcineurin inhibitor (tacrolimus, cyclosporine), an antiproliferative agent (mycophenolate mofetil or azathioprine) and in some cases, an mTOR inhibitor (everolimus, sirolimus).[139]

Hyperacute rejection

Hyperacute rejection is now a rare form of humoral rejection that occurs minutes to hours after transplantation and results from ABO blood group incompatibility or the recipient having preformed, donor-specific antibodies. ABO blood group and panel reactive screening of anti-human lymphocyte antigen (anti-HLA) antibodies preoperatively minimises the possibility of hyperacute rejection, particularly in healthcare systems where blood that has been prospectively cross-matched is routinely used.[140] If it occurs, hyperacute rejection leads to organ failure and rapid activation of the complement cascade, producing severe damage to endothelial cells, platelet activation, initiation of the clotting cascade and extensive microvascular thrombosis.[141] Plasmapheresis and an intense immunosuppression regimen to eliminate preformed antibodies can be used while the patient is supported on mechanical circulatory support.[139] However, retransplantation may be the most effective treatment for hyperacute rejection.[142]

Acute rejection

Acute rejection can be classified as either cellular or humoral rejection, otherwise known as antibody-mediated rejection (AMR).[140,143] Cellular rejection involves T-cell infiltration of the allograft. Cellular rejection occurs much more commonly than AMR,[140,143] but both may occur simultaneously.[142,143] AMR is a B-cell-mediated release of antibodies.[140] A review in 2013 by key stakeholders has resulted in the publication of standardised nomenclature for antibody-mediated rejection.[143] A further update on AMR in cardiac transplantation has emerged in 2015, in a scientific statement from the American Heart Association.[142] Risk factors for AMR include: presence of a positive donor-specific cross-match, in a sensitised recipient with preformed anti-HLA antibodies, recipient cytomegalovirus seropositivity and patients with previous mechanical circulatory support.[142] Percutaneous transvenous endomyocardial biopsy is considered the gold standard for detecting cardiac rejection. Grading of cardiac rejection has a standardised nomenclature globally.[142,144] In AMR, endomyocardial biopsy reveals increased vascular permeability, microvascular thrombosis, interstitial oedema and haemorrhage, and endothelial cell swelling and necrosis.[143,145] An echocardiogram is also performed regularly to evaluate systolic and diastolic cardiac function.[142] Cardiac MRI also has a role in identifying cardiac rejection[146] by identifying myocardial oedema, signs of inflammation and increased left ventricular wall thickness.[142,146]

Therapeutic interventions for rejection vary between centres and are based on the grade of rejection, degree of haemodynamic compromise, clinical findings and time elapsed since transplantation. Asymptomatic mild rejection (grade 1R) is not usually treated specifically but may involve augmentation of baseline immunosuppression.[147] Moderate rejection (grade 2R) with myocyte necrosis requires treatment.[147] Rejection grade 1R and 2R can progress to a higher grade of rejection in 15–20% of cases.[144] Grade 3R rejection is often associated with haemodynamic compromise and is always treated aggressively. Standard first-line treatment for grade 2 or grade 3 cellular rejection is with high-dose corticosteroids. This is usually given as 1–3 g of IV methylprednisolone over 3 days, known as a 'steroid pulse'. In advanced cases with haemodynamic compromise, antilymphocyte antibody agents (ATG(rabbit), ATGAM(equine)) are used. First-line treatment for significant AMR includes high-dose corticosteroids, antilymphocyte antibodies (ATG, ATGAM), plasmapheresis and IV immunoglobulin (IVIg). Treatment measures (rare) for refractory AMR include monoclonal antibodies (rituximab, alemtuzumab), bortezomib, complement inhibitor (eculizumab) and photopheresis.[142]

For both forms of rejection, other immunosuppressant agents such as a calcineurin inhibitor (tacrolimus, cyclosporine) and an antiproliferative agent (mycophenolate mofetil, azathioprine), sometimes in combination with an mTOR inhibitor (everolimus, sirolimus), are continued.[148] The presence of rejection requires assessment of baseline immunosuppression and doses, with target aims increased where therapeutic drug monitoring is utilised (e.g. for calcineurin inhibitors and mTOR inhibitors).[142] It is important to note that many medications interact with calcineurin inhibitors and mTOR inhibitors through induction or inhibition of the CYP450 enzyme system, which may therefore provoke rejection. In addition to augmentation of immunosuppression therapy, fluid, pharmacological and mechanical therapeutic interventions are instituted to support cardiac function, depending on the degree of ventricular dysfunction.

Nurses have an important role in detecting acute rejection. While rejection may be asymptomatic, it is often diagnosed by clinical signs and supported by histological findings from an endomyocardial biopsy. Low-grade rejection can be suspected when non-specific signs such as malaise, lethargy, low-grade fever and mood changes are present. Acute rejection causing cardiac inflammation is revealed by a sinus tachycardia greater than 120 beats per minute (bpm), a pericardial friction rub, or new-onset atrial arrhythmias such as premature atrial contractions, atrial flutter or fibrillation.[147] More severe forms of acute rejection are suspected when signs and symptoms of varying degrees of heart failure emerge. If patients are awake and alert, they may complain of severe fatigue, sudden onset of dyspnoea during minimal physical effort, syncope or orthopnoea. Physical assessment and haemodynamic monitoring will reveal clinical signs of left and right cardiac failure (see Chapter 9).

Immunosuppression therapy

In this section, a brief discussion of immunosuppression therapies and associated nursing implications is provided. To prevent rejection of the transplanted organ, recipients receive a combination of 2–4 immunosuppression agents, with most patients being discharged from hospital on a triple therapy combination. Triple therapy usually consists of corticosteroids (prednisolone), a calcineurin inhibitor (CNI) (tacrolimus, cyclosporine, with a preference for tacrolimus) and an antiproliferative agent (mycophenolate mofetil or azathioprine, with a preference for mycophenolate mofetil). mTOR inhibitors (everolimus, sirolimus) may also be added to the triple therapy combination as CNI-sparing agents or used instead of CNIs where renal dysfunction is present.[140,148,149] For some heart transplant recipients, everolimus may be favoured because of a lower incidence of cardiac allograft vasculopathy and reduced renal dysfunction compared with calcineurin inhibitors.[150] Everolimus is often added after 3–6 months. Earlier use is limited because of adverse effects on wound healing and higher rate of mortality due to infections.[151]

Trough or predose levels are used to titrate drug dosing for calcineurin inhibitors and mTOR inhibitors but not for mycophenolate or prednisolone. Desired therapeutic drug levels must be balanced against risk of side effects and infection. For example, renal dysfunction commonly limits calcineurin inhibitor dosing and gastrointestinal side effects similarly with mycophenolate. For calcineurin inhibitors, tacrolimus is now considered first line because of the lower rates of rejection and a more favourable adverse effect profile compared with cyclosporine.[149,152] In terms of a preferred antiproliferative, mycophenolate mofetil has now replaced the use of azathioprine in most settings, as it has shown improved survival and reduced rates of rejection.[149,153]

Immunosuppression therapy is commenced preoperatively or in the operating theatre. A maintenance immunosuppression regimen is usually instituted within hours of admission to ICU, with each patient's immunosuppressive needs individually assessed and titrated. For instance, the administration time for introduction of the selected immuno-suppressive agent(s) may be delayed in patients with pre-existing renal dysfunction.[149] When the administration of the usual regimen of immunosuppression is delayed, induction therapy with antilymphocyte agents (antithymocyte globulin (ATG(rabbit)), ATGAM(equine)) or interleukin-2 receptor antagonist (basiliximab) may be used in the immediate post-operative period and calcineurin inhibitor withheld.[140,149] Induction therapy may also be used in circumstances of primary allograft failure perioperatively – HLA mismatch (rare) or early AMR – or to allow for a delay in initiating tacrolimus in patients at risk of renal failure.[149] The common drugs used to suppress the immune system and the nursing implications are illustrated in Table 12.5. As highlighted in Table 12.5, some immunosuppressive agents are hazardous

---

TABLE 12.5

Immunosuppression medications[a]

DRUG NAME	STANDARD DOSE	SIDE EFFECTS	NURSING CONSIDERATIONS
Calcineurin inhibitors (maintenance)			
Tacrolimus (1st line)	Starting dose: 0.01–0.02 mg/kg/day IV 24-hour continuous infusion, followed by titration of dose to levels. Maintenance dose: 0.5–15 mg BD titrated to target level. When switching from IV to oral administration approximately 4× the total daily dose is required. Typical trough level range targeting 10–15 in the first 6 months and 5–10 thereafter.	Infection Renal impairment Tremor Abnormal LFTs Hypercholesterolaemia Headaches Hypomagnesaemia Diabetes (tacrolimus only) Gingival hypertrophy (cyclosporine only) Hirsutism (cyclosporine only)	Monitor renal function. Trough levels should be taken approximately 12 hours after last dose for BD dosing (time sampling of serum drug levels with dosage times). Do not crush tablets/capsules.
Cyclosporine (2nd line)	Starting dose: 3–5 mg/kg/day in two divided doses When switching from IV to oral administration approximately 3× the total daily dose is required. Typical trough level range targeting 250–375 mg in the first 6 months and 150–250 mg thereafter.		
Antiproliferative agents (maintenance)			
Mycophenolate mofetil (1st line)	Starting dose: 2–3 g/day in divided doses. Maintenance dose: 250 mg BD – 1.5 g BD.	Infection Bone marrow suppression Gastrointestinal tract irritation, i.e. nausea, vomiting, diarrhoea (more with mycophenolate)	IV dose same as oral dose. TPMT level must be checked prior to initiating azathioprine. Reduces antibody response to vaccines.
Azathioprine (2nd line)	1–2 mg/kg/day		
mTOR inhibitors (maintenance)			
Everolimus Sirolimus	Dose should be titrated to target trough levels, typically 4–12 ng/mL. Targets trough levels will depend on indication (i.e. additional immunosuppression vs CNI sparing vs CAV prophylaxis).	Bone marrow suppression Hypercholesterolaemia Hypokalaemia Mouth ulcers Pleural and pericardial effusions	Only available as oral formulation.

Continued

TABLE 12.5

Immunosuppression medications—cont'd

....

Corticosteroids (maintenance or rejection)

Prednisolone	Starting dose: 1 mg/kg/day in 2 divided doses, followed by a slow wean as per local protocols. Normally weaned to off within 1 year post transplant. Dose for rejection: 'pulse' 2–2.5 g over 3 days.	Mood change Weight gain Steroid-induced diabetes Osteopenia/osteoporosis Muscle weakness Face swelling 'moon face' Hyperlipidaemia Opportunistic infections	Monitor blood glucose levels.

Interleukin-2 receptor antagonist (induction)

Basiliximab	20 mg IV at time of operation (day 0) and day 4.	Few and infrequent Hypersensitivity reaction	Often used in patients with pre-existing renal dysfunction when tacrolimus initiation may be delayed.

Antilymphocyte preparations (induction or treatment of rejection)

ATG/ATGAM	Refer to local protocols – dosing dependent on indication and CD 2/3 T-lymphocyte levels.	Anaphylaxis Thrombocytopenia Pulmonary oedema Serum sickness	Pre-medication with paracetamol, an antihistamine and steroid may be required. Monitor T-cell markers.

aAll doses and drug combinations are individualised and depend on multiple factors including rejection history, presence of organ dysfunction, side effects, infective issues and time since transplantation. Medications and doses can be broadly categorised into induction immunosuppression and maintenance immunosuppression. Always refer to centre-specific administration protocols and resources with current product information such as MIMS and the Australian Medicines Handbook.

ATG/ATGAM = anti-thymocyte globulin; CAV = cardiac allograft vasculopathy; CD = cluster of differentiation; CNI = calcineurin inhibitor; IV = intravenous; LFT = liver function test; TPMT = thiopurine S-methyltransferase.

non-cytotoxic agents (e.g. mycophenolate mofetil) and require safety measures during preparation, delivery and disposal. In addition, some immunosuppressive agents will be given IV (e.g. tacrolimus, mycophenolate mofetil) until patients can eat and drink as they cannot be crushed for nasogastric administration. Specifically, for azathioprine, thiopurine S-methyltransferase (TPMT) must be checked prior to initiation to ensure the drug does not accumulate and cause bone marrow toxicity. Furthermore, as blood levels of some immunosuppression agents (e.g. tacrolimus, everolimus) are taken regularly to assess efficacy, nurses need to be aware of timing blood sampling to dosage times in order to obtain accurate data to inform doses.

Infection

Infection is a major risk factor for transplant recipients because of their immunosuppressed state. The periods of greatest risk for patients are the first 3 months after transplantation, and after episodes of acute rejection when immunosuppression agents are increased.[154] In addition to the nosocomial bacterial infections that all surgical patients are exposed to in critical care (see Chapter 5), immunosuppressed transplant recipients are at risk of acquiring opportunistic bacterial, viral or fungal infections; latent infections acquired from the donor organ such as cytomegalovirus (CMV); or reactivation of their own latent infections (e.g. CMV or *Pneumocystis jiroveci (formerly carinii)*.[154] To combat *P. jiroveci*, patients receive trimethoprim with sulfamethoxazole,[154] the standard dosing being 800/160 mg three times a week. Despite preoperative screening for CMV, the shortage of donor organs often necessitates CMV mismatching, which is donor CMV-positive serostatus with recipient CMV-negative serostatus. Mismatched patients are at highest risk of CMV infection; however, CMV recipients who are seropositive are also at risk. Effective gold standard prophylaxis for CMV infection is provided by administering oral valganciclovir or intravenous ganciclovir for 3–6 months. Some centres may add CMV hyperimmune globulin to CMV-mismatched patients.[154–156] To prevent infection, standard precautions and meticulous handwashing (see Chapter 5) are performed, rather than isolation procedures.[157] Mandatory measures to prevent overwhelming sepsis are a high level of vigilance by clinicians for signs of infection; obtaining empirical evidence from blood, sputum, urine, wound and catheter-tip cultures; and aggressive and prompt treatment for specific organisms. Although typical signs and symptoms of infection are blunted in transplant recipients, clinicians should suspect infections when patients have a low-grade fever, hypotension, tachycardia, a high cardiac output/ index, a decrease in SVR, changes in mentation, a new cough or dyspnoea.[158,159] Elevated white cell count, the presence of dysuria, purulent discharge from wounds, infiltrates on chest X-ray, sputum production or pain also indicate infection.

Prior to administering blood products, nurses may be required to ascertain the CMV status of the patient and donor. Recipients who are seronegative for CMV and who receive a heart from a seronegative donor must receive whole blood, packed/red cells or platelets that are CMV negative, leuko depleted or both in order to avoid development of a primary CMV infection.[127,134,156] In Australia, any cellular products (red cells and platelets) are leuko reduced, which is considered CMV safe. Please refer to the institution's policy in regards to administration of blood products and CMV infection risk to heart transplant recipients.

Coronavirus 2 (SARS-CoV-2) caused the COVID-19 pandemic. Since early 2020 to the current time, it has had a significant impact on morbidity and mortality in solid organ transplant recipients. Additionally, it has impacted donors, waiting-list patients and healthcare personnel. During the pandemic, donor numbers reduced and there has been increased demand on healthcare resources.[160,161]

To date, the Transplantation Society of Australia and New Zealand (TSANZ) outlines that non-lung donation can be considered when donors are no longer classified as infectious.[162]

The key TSANZ recommendations are:

1   Transplant patients greater than 18 years of age are advised to have three COVID vaccinations, with a booster 4 months after the third dose.

2   Transplant patients should be advised that COVID vaccination acts to prevent infection, decrease the severity and mortality of infection, and also to limit the transmission of disease.

3   If a transplant recipient becomes infected with COVID, they should contact their transplant team as they have an increased risk of morbidity and mortality. Recipients may be suitable for other treatment options, including monoclonal antibodies.[163]

The use of monoclonal antibodies is in place at ANZ transplant centres to treat heart transplant recipients with COVID-19 and is utilised for post-exposure prophylaxis (see local centre guidelines, as recommendations continue to evolve).

Haemorrhage/cardiac tamponade

The risk of haemorrhage or cardiac tamponade is greater for heart transplant recipients than for patients undergoing CABG or valvular surgery. There are many precipitating factors which contribute to this risk, including perioperative use of anticoagulation for LVAD or AF, impairment of hepatic function secondary to right heart failure, redo surgery, surgical suture lines connecting major vessels and atria, and a larger-than-usual pericardium. As the promotion of haemostasis is a major therapeutic goal postoperatively, blood products, procoagulants and antifibrinolytics are commonly administered according to laboratory and clinical data.

Early detection of haemorrhage is achieved by close monitoring of the following: haematological status; chest tube patency, drainage volume and drainage consistency; and trends in haemodynamic data that suggest cardiac tamponade (see earlier in this chapter). Our clinical experience suggests that, if patients are hypotensive sporadically for no apparent reason, efforts should be made to urgently evaluate them for presence of cardiac tamponade. Suspicion of cardiac tamponade may be confirmed by chest X-ray or echocardiogram if the patient's haemodynamic status is stable. Sudden cardiac arrest or haemodynamic collapse secondary to cardiac tamponade warrants an immediate return to theatre or a sternotomy in critical care.

Acute kidney injury

Acute kidney injury or varying degrees of renal dysfunction can occur in the initial postoperative period owing to pre-existing renal dysfunction, tacrolimus therapy, other nephrotoxic agents or sustained periods of hypotension secondary to CPB or allograft dysfunction. Diuretic therapy is invariably needed in the initial postoperative period because of hypervolaemia, which may be caused by fluid retention effects of corticosteroids and raised filling pressures secondary to a transient loss of right and/ or left ventricular compliance.[164] High doses or continuous infusions of diuretics may be required in patients who were on diuretic therapy preoperatively owing to frusemide resistance. Close monitoring of serum electrolyte levels are required, with hypokalaemia often associated with diuretic therapy. Nurses play a crucial role in the prevention, detection and support for renal dysfunction/failure in patients following cardiac surgery on CPB (see earlier in this chapter and Chapter 18). In addition to this, the type and dose of immunosuppressive agents in the postoperative period are carefully selected and initiated according to individual risk factors and clinical status. Experience suggests that early intervention with haemofiltration to support renal function is preferable to continued use of high-dose diuretics and deferred haemofiltration. This is because there is little scope to maintain low doses of renal toxic immunosuppressants for weeks given the imminent risk of rejection and resultant allograft failure.

Early allograft dysfunction and failure

Primary allograft failure is the leading cause of death in the first month and year after surgery.[141] In the immediate postoperative period, myocardial performance may be depressed because of the clinical sequelae of CPB and ischaemic injury associated with surgical retrieval, hypothermic storage, prolonged ischaemic times and reperfusion.[141] A prolonged ischaemic time increases the risk of primary graft failure and 1-month mortality after cardiac transplantation.[165,166] Despite an optimal time period between organ retrieval and reimplantation of less than 4 hours, the vast distances between capital cities in Australia (up to 3000 km) over which donor hearts may be transported, and a decision to accept marginal, suboptimal organs, led Australian researchers and transplant teams to pioneer techniques for use of prolonged-ischaemic-time organs of up to 8 hours (New Zealand, 7 hours).

To better address challenges at donor procurement, which have been limited by the cold storage and heart preservation method, the TransMedics OCS and NIHP XVIVO Heart Box system have been developed. These portable, perfusion systems are designed to increase transplant volumes, improve patient outcomes and reduce transplant costs.[101–105] Refer to TransMedics OCS and XVIVO Heart Box instructions for use; also, using the TransMedics OCS is the standard of care for DCD donors.[101–104,167]

Primary graft dysfunction is diagnosed within 24 hours after surgery, and clinicians must rule out secondary graft dysfunction from causes of hyperacute rejection, pulmonary hypertension and surgical complications such as bleeding. Early allograft dysfunction can present as left, right or biventricular dysfunction. Left ventricular failure is classified as mild, moderate and severe.[141] The severity classification for primary graft dysfunction is described in Table 12.6. The RADIAL risk score is a validated tool that can be utilised to categorise recipients as low, intermediate or high risk for obtaining primary graft failure post heart transplantation.[168–170]

Management of cardiac dysfunction is dependent on clinical signs and underlying aetiologies that include pulmonary hypertension, acute rejection and ischaemic injury. Right ventricular dysfunction is usually secondary to pulmonary hypertension, whereas left ventricular or biventricular dysfunction results from acute rejection and ischaemic injury.

Left ventricular dysfunction cannot always be anticipated preoperatively, so when signs first emerge peri- or postoperatively, fluid management strategies (filling or diuresis as deemed appropriate) and inotropic agents are commenced immediately.[134] In patients with prolonged ischaemic times, mechanical assistance may be required perioperatively.

TABLE 12.6
Severity scale for primary graft dysfunction[141]

DEFINITION OF SEVERITY SCALE FOR PRIMARY GRAFT DYSFUNCTION (PGD)

1. PGD-left ventricle (PGD-LV)	Mild PGD-LV One of the following criteria must be met.	LVEF ≤40% by echocardiography or haemodymanics with RAP >15 mmHg, PCWP >20 mmHg, CI <2.0 L/min/m² (lasting more than 1 hour) requiring low-dose inotropes.
	Moderate PGD-LV. Must meet one criterion from I and another criterion from II.	I. One criteria from the following: LVEF ≤40% or haemodymanic compromise with RAP >15 mmHg, PCWP >20 mmHg, CI <2.0 L/min/m², hypotension with MAP <70 mmHg (lasting more than 1 hour). II. One criteria from the following: i. High-dose inotropes – inotrope score >10, or ii. Newly placed IABP (regardless of inotropes).
	Severe PGD-LV.	Dependence on left or biventricular mechanical support including ECMO, LVAD, BiVAD or percutaneous LVAD. Excludes requirement for IABP.
2. PGD-right ventricle (PGD-RV)	Diagnosis requires either both i and ii, or iii alone.	i. Haemodymanics with RAP >15 mmHg, PCWP <15 mmHg, CI <2.0 L/min/m² ii. TPG <15 mmHg and/or pulmonary artery systolic pressure < 50 mmHg, or iii. Need for RVAD.

BiVAD = biventricular assist device; CI = cardiac index; ECMO = extracorporeal membrane oxygenation; IABP = intra-balloon pump; LVAD = left ventricular assist device; LVEF = left ventricular ejection fraction; PCWP = pulmonary capillary wedge pressure; RAP = right atrial pressure; RVAD = right ventricular assist device; TPG = transpulmonary pressure gradient.

Inotrope score = dopamine (×1) + dobutamine (×1) + amrinone (×1) + milrinone (×15) + adrenaline (×100) + noradrenaline (×100) with each drug dosed in micrograms/kg/min.

Source: Kobashigawa J, Zuckermann A, Macdonald P, et al. Report from a consensus conference on primary graft dysfunction after cardiac transplantation. J Heart Lung Transplant. 2014;33(4):327–40, table 6 on p. 337.

In the initial postoperative period, cardiac dysfunction can also occur as a result of a low-SVR syndrome, characterised by a calculated SVR of less than 750 dynes/s/cm^{-5} in the presence of an unsustainable high cardiac output.[171,172] The cause of low-SVR syndrome is not fully understood, although it has been linked with SIRS associated with CPB (see Chapter 21), the chronic use of angiotensin-converting enzyme inhibitors for end-stage heart failure (see Chapter 10) and a deficiency of vasopressin.[172,173] Noradrenaline is titrated to achieve a calculated SVR within normal parameters and to lower the unsustainably high cardiac index. In severe cases, vasopressin may be infused at doses of 0.04–0.1 units/min concurrently with noradrenaline.[174] Experience suggests that the dose of adrenaline should be minimised in the presence of metabolic acidosis, and the noradrenaline infusion increased to achieve normotension, a calculated SVR higher than 900 dynes/s/cm^{-5} and a sustainable cardiac index.

Patients with depressed left ventricular compliance and contractility due to cardiac dysfunction present clinically with reduced cardiac index, bradycardia, reduced tissue and end-organ perfusion (decreased mental status, oliguria, poor peripheral perfusion, slow capillary refill and raised serum lactate), low systemic venous oxygenation and dyspnoea. Bradycardia may not be evident due to chronotropic support of the denervated heart with atrial pacing and/or isoprenaline.

The immediate haemodynamic management of left ventricular dysfunction/failure secondary to acute rejection or ischaemic injury often involves fluid resuscitation to a pulmonary artery diastolic pressure of 16–20 mmHg, high-dose inotropes, vasodilator agents and possibly the insertion of an IABP to achieve a cardiac index greater than 2.2 L/min/m^2 and adequate end-organ perfusion. The insertion of an LVAD (e.g. Rotoflow®, Rotoflow II®, CardioHelp® or CentriMag® centrifugal pump) or full mechanical circulatory support with extracorporeal membrane oxygenation (ECMO) is indicated when other therapeutic regimens fail to produce a cardiac output that provides adequate end-organ perfusion.[134,141,175–178] VA ECMO being the most common method to treat severe early graft failure compared with temporary VAD support because of favourable outcomes.[175–178] As noted earlier, augmentation of the immunosuppression regimen may also be necessary to manage the acute rejection.

To prevent right ventricular dysfunction and failure secondary to raised pulmonary pressures, prospective heart transplant recipients are screened preoperatively for the degree and reversibility of pulmonary hypertension. Reversible pulmonary hypertension is a transpulmonary gradient less than 15 mmHg that responds to pulmonary vasodilator therapies, such as prostaglandin E1, prostacyclin or inhaled nitric oxide (NO).[179] Right ventricular dysfunction or failure can also occur in the postoperative context as a result of ischaemic injury, an undersized heart (greater than 20% difference in body surface area between donor and recipient) or hypoxic pulmonary vasoconstriction.[127] Isoprenaline or milrinone, dobutamine and adrenaline are administered in this situation.[134]

Right heart dysfunction/failure should be suspected in patients with pre-existing pulmonary hypertension or a haemodynamic profile in the intra- or postoperative context that includes a rising CVP, low-to-normal pulmonary artery diastolic/pulmonary artery wedge pressure (PAWP), high calculated pulmonary vascular resistance, raised PAPs, systemic hypotension and oliguria. The haemodynamic management of patients with right ventricular dysfunction/failure involves optimising right ventricular preload and afterload by titrating fluid and pharmacological therapies to achieve adequate tissue and end-organ perfusion. Fluid resuscitation to a CVP between 14 and 20 mmHg and inotropic therapy are necessary to ensure that the failing right ventricle continues to act as a conduit for the left ventricle. NO by inhalation is the therapy of choice, as it provides selective pulmonary vasodilation at doses of 20–40 ppm, thereby reducing right ventricular afterload without producing systemic hypotension.[179] A secondary benefit of inhaled NO is improved oxygenation due to reduced mismatching of ventilation/perfusion.[180] If inhaled NO is not available, IV prostaglandin E1 or prostacyclin may be used to reduce right ventricular afterload when pulmonary pressures exceed 50 mmHg.[181]

Mild right ventricular dysfunction may be treated with milrinone at doses of 0.375–0.750 micrograms/kg/min or drug combinations that provide afterload reduction and inotropic support (e.g. sodium nitroprusside and adrenaline). Appropriate respiratory management is essential, as hypoxaemia and metabolic or respiratory acidosis can exacerbate right ventricular failure. If pharmacological, fluid and inhaled NO therapies do not produce sustained improvement in right ventricular performance, a right VAD (e.g. Rotoflow®, Rotoflow II®, CardioHelp® or CentriMag® centrifugal pump) is indicated to provide temporary support for the failing right ventricle.[141] For further information on management of right heart dysfunction/failure and left heart dysfunction/failure, see Chapter 10.

Denervation

Donor heart implantation severs both afferent and efferent nervous system connections to the heart. Hence, the transplanted heart has no direct autonomic nervous system innervation but is responsive to circulating catecholamines. The normal heart is under predominant parasympathetic control. Denervation therefore allows the heart to beat faster: typically 90–110 beats per min.[182] Denervation impairs circulatory system homeostasis, as evidenced by: a volume-expanded state, a tendency to hypertension, no sensation of angina pectoris, a high resting heart rate, a slow or absent baroreceptor reflex (to increase heart rate/cardiac output in response to hypotension) and no rises in heart rate and contractility owing to hypovolaemia or vasodilation.[127] As the cardiac allograft is dependent on an adequate preload, the effects of postural changes in recipients are important. (A detailed discussion of physiology of the transplanted heart is provided elsewhere.[127])

There are four important clinical manifestations of denervation in the early postoperative period. First, drugs that act directly on the autonomic nervous system to modify heart rate (e.g. atropine, digoxin) and vagal manoeuvres (carotid sinus massage) are ineffective. Amiodarone and adenosine are effective antiarrhythmic agents. Neither amiodarone nor sotalol interact with immunosuppressive agents.[134] However, as the denervated donor sinus node is more sensitive to exogenous adenosine than a sinus node innervated in the normal way,[183] it has been suggested that adenosine be avoided.[127] That is, a usual adenosine dose may produce toxic-like effects in the context of a denervated heart. Overdrive atrial pacing is a viable alternative to drug therapy to treat a tachyarrhythmia such as atrial flutter.[184]

Second, although a high resting heart rate is possible from efferent cardiac denervation, sinus or junctional bradycardias may occur in the early postoperative period because of transient sinus node dysfunction or preoperative amiodarone. Studies suggest that sinus node dysfunction occurs in about 20% of cases,[185] although anecdotal experience suggests a higher percentage. To prevent low cardiac output secondary to bradycardias, atrial and ventricular epicardial pacing wires are inserted and atrial pacing of >90 bpm,[134] and often 110 bpm, is commenced. Atrial pacing at 110 bpm appears to 'train' the sinus node to conduct at rates of 70–100 bpm in the long term. A resting sinus or junctional heart rate below 70 bpm prior to hospital discharge is predictive of long-term sinus node dysfunction.[127] Insertion of a permanent pacemaker for long-term heart rate control is rarely required. Isoprenaline infusions at doses of 0.5–2 micrograms/min may be used for chronotropy in combination with atrial pacing. As noted earlier, atrial arrhythmias such as atrial flutter may be an early indication of acute rejection. Ventricular arrhythmias are rare and often lethal in spite of aggressive resuscitation attempts. Persistent arrhythmias should always prompt investigation of the patient's rejection level.[134]

Third, as patients rely on circulating catecholamines, orthostatic hypotension is common. Patients are educated to sit up slowly from a lying position. Fourth, patients rarely feel anginal pain for the first 5 years or so after surgery; however, there are certainly reports of patients regaining feelings of angina pectoris due to re-innervation.[186] The inability of patients to feel angina pectoris is important, because all heart transplant recipients are at risk of developing accelerated allograft coronary artery disease.[187] As part of discharge education, patients are taught to identify clinical signs of angina other than chest pain, such as shortness of breath and sweating. A summary of the main clinical manifestations and nursing practice issues for patients following heart transplantation is included in Table 12.7.

> ### Practice tip
>
> Heart transplant patients have a denervated heart, so carotid sinus massage will not slow a tachyarrhythmia and atropine will not increase sinus node firing or atrioventricular conduction.

Medium- to long-term complications

There are six major long-term complications associated with heart transplantation: (1) infection, (2) cardiac allograft vasculopathy, (3) malignancy, (4) renal dysfunction, (5) hypertension and (6) diabetes mellitus.[149,188] Infections are a common complication following transplantation owing to immunosuppressive therapy that is required for the remainder of the recipient's life.[189] Infection is one of the leading causes for long-term mortality in heart transplant recipients.[116] Opportunistic infections are common within the first year post transplantation; however, after this time the most common infections are from community-based pathogens and the incidence of opportunistic infections is reduced. Latent viral infections such as CMV and herpes virus may reactivate or may be acquired from the donor organ. As time post transplant progresses and patients who are low risk for rejection, immunosuppression medications can be altered to reduce the chance of infections occurring.[151] A more detailed overview on infection was discussed earlier in this chapter.

Cardiac allograft vasculopathy (CAV) is a diffuse, proliferative form of obliterative coronary arteriosclerosis[190] that has experienced some improvement in survival, probably due to modalities to prevent progression of the disease.[116] At 5 years after heart transplant, 30% of recipients have developed CAV,[191] whereas almost 50% have CAV at 10 years after transplant.[116]

Notably, CAV is a leading cause of long-term morbidity and mortality, beyond a year post transplant.[192,193] Sudden death, ventricular arrhythmias and symptoms of congestive heart failure may be the first signs of significant CAV. The aetiology of CAV is multifactorial, including immunological factors (e.g. episodes of acute rejection and anti-HLA antibodies), non-immunological cardiovascular risk factors (e.g. hypertension, hyperlipidaemia, pre-existing diabetes and new-onset diabetes), surgical factors (e.g. donor age, ischaemic time and reperfusion injury) and side effects of immunosuppressive drugs such as tacrolimus and corticosteroids (e.g. CMV. infection and nephrotoxicity).[134,149,190,192,193] Statins have been shown to reduce the incidence of CAV.[192,194,195] Statins at doses less than that prescribed for hyperlipidaemia are commenced within 2 weeks of surgery irrespective of cholesterol levels to reduce episodes of rejection and CAV.[134] Use of everolimus or sirolimus, and subsequent dose reduction or cessation of tacrolimus, has been shown to reduce the onset and progression of CAV.[134,192,196,197] In addition, early commencement of low-dose aspirin may delay the progression of CAV.[198,199] Combination therapy of an

TABLE 12.7

Nursing care of patients after heart transplantation

CLINICAL MANIFESTATION	NURSING PRACTICE CONSIDERATIONS
Acute rejection	Detect acute rejection by clinical signs and endomyocardial biopsy. Suspect low-grade rejection when malaise, lethargy, low-grade fever and mood changes are present. Acute rejection is manifested by a sinus tachycardia >120 bpm, a pericardial friction rub or new-onset atrial arrhythmias. Suspect severe acute rejection with manifestations of left and right heart failure; awake patients may complain of severe fatigue, sudden onset of dyspnoea during minimal physical effort, syncope or orthopnoea.
Infection	Standard infection control precautions and meticulous handwashing is required. Observe for signs of infection: low-grade fever, hypotension, tachycardia, a high cardiac output/index, a decrease in SVR, changes in mentation, a new cough, dyspnoea, dysuria, sputum production or pain. Monitor blood, sputum, urine, wound and catheter-tip cultures, infiltrates on chest X-ray and institute aggressive and prompt treatment for specific infective organisms. Check CMV status and institution's protocol before administering blood products.
Haemorrhage/ cardiac tamponade	Monitor: haematological status; chest tube patency, drainage volume and drainage consistency; and trends in haemodynamic data that suggest cardiac tamponade. Patients who are hypotensive sporadically should be assessed to eliminate cardiac tamponade as a cause.
Acute renal failure	Support renal function, including titration of immunosuppressive agents to individual risk factors and clinical status, and early haemofiltration.
Early allograft dysfunction	Augment the immunosuppression regimen to manage the acute rejection.
Left heart failure	Observe for depressed left ventricular compliance and contractility: reduced cardiac index, possible bradycardia (may not be evident due to atrial pacing and/or isoprenaline), decreased mental status, oliguria, poor peripheral perfusion, slow capillary refill and raised serum lactate, low systemic venous oxygenation and dyspnoea. Fluid resuscitate to a PAWP of 14–18 mmHg, high-dose inotropes, vasodilator agents, IABP to achieve a cardiac index >2.2 L/min/m^2 with adequate end-organ perfusion. Insertion of full mechanical circulatory support (ECMO or LVAD) is indicated when other interventions do not provide adequate end-organ perfusion.
Right heart failure	Observe for right heart dysfunction/failure: rising CVP, low-to-normal PAD/PAWP, high calculated pulmonary vascular resistance, raised PAPs, systemic hypotension and oliguria. Optimise right ventricular preload and afterload: titrate fluid and medications to achieve adequate end-organ perfusion; fluid resuscitate to a CVP of 14–20 mmHg; consider inhaled NO (selective pulmonary vasodilation and improved oxygenation from reduced ventilation/perfusion mismatch), prostaglandin E1 or prostacyclin, milrinone or drug combinations with afterload reduction and inotropic support (e.g. sodium nitroprusside and adrenaline). Institute appropriate respiratory management to minimise hypoxaemia and metabolic or respiratory acidosis. If no sustained improvement in right ventricular performance, a right VAD is indicated for temporary support.
Denervation	Drugs with direct autonomic nervous system actions on heart rate (e.g. atropine, digoxin) and vagal manoeuvres (carotid sinus massage) are ineffective. Use overdrive atrial pacing to treat tachyarrhythmias. Sinus or junctional bradycardias may occur, and atrial/ventricular epicardial pacing is used to 'train' the sinus node. Orthostatic hypotension is common: patients should sit up slowly from a lying position. Patients rarely feel anginal pain after surgery: they need to identify other clinical signs of angina, such as shortness of breath and sweating.

CMV = cytomegalovirus; CVP = central venous pressure; ECMO = extracorporeal membrane oxygenation; IABP = intra-aortic balloon pump; LVAD = left ventricular assist device; PAD = pulmonary artery diastolic; PAP = pulmonary artery pressure; PAWP = pulmonary artery wedge pressure; SVR = systemic vascular resistance.

angiotensin-converting enzyme inhibitor with a calcium channel blocker has been shown not only to reduce hypertension but also the microvascular and antiproliferative effects may ameliorate the progression and development of CAV.[190,192,200]

Diagnosis of CAV is difficult, because of allograft denervation, and because a coronary angiogram underestimates the extent of the disease and is insensitive to early lesions.[149,201]

Intravascular ultrasound (which occurs at the same time as a coronary angiogram) provides the most reliable quantitative information about the degree of CAV.[190,201–203] Even so, coronary angiography is the universal assessment utilised as it is readily available in transplant units.[190,201,204] Some non-invasive methods for assessment of CAV and its effects include dobutamine stress echocardiography, positron emission tomography, computer tomography, angiography and cardiac magnetic resonance.[192] Although PCI and CABG can be done, the definitive treatment for severe CAV is retransplantation. Ongoing research into the prevention of CAV[192] will be the most important factor in reducing the incidence and associated mortality.

All heart transplant recipients are at a greater risk of developing malignancies than the general population,[189,205,206] particularly carcinoma of the skin[116,206–208] and lymphoproliferative disorders,[116,209,210] as a consequence of long-term immunosuppression therapy.[140,189,205] Morbidity related to malignancy (primarily skin cancers) is 28% at 10 years after transplant.[116] Nurses play an important role in educating patients about how to avoid and reduce the risks of sun exposure, monitoring for skin changes and having regular skin check-ups. Treatment options in transplant recipients are the same as for the general population (e.g. chemotherapy, radiation therapy and surgical excision), in addition to a reduction in immunosuppression therapy; however, outcomes remain poor.[189,208,211]

Long-term renal dysfunction occurs primarily post transplantation owing to tacrolimus nephrotoxicity. Careful monitoring of tacrolimus levels and avoidance of hypovolaemia and other nephrotoxic drugs are important measures in reducing progression to renal failure. Importantly, research indicates that CNI nephrotoxicity can be reversed by eliminating CNIs from immunosuppression regimens,[212,213] although the benefit needs to be balanced against the risk of rejection.

Progression to end-stage renal failure requiring dialysis or renal transplantation may be required after prolonged exposure to CNIs.[214]

Systemic hypertension following transplantation has been linked with CNI-induced tubular nephrotoxicity, peripheral vasoconstriction and fluid retention.[215] Tacrolimus has been shown to exert a lower incidence of hypertension compared with cyclosporine,[216,217] and is the preferred first-line CNI in most centres. Blood pressure control can be achieved by addressing lifestyle factors plus modification to medication regimens. Lifestyle modifications such as weight loss, exercise programs, low-sodium diet and control of diabetes and hyperlipidaemia should be instituted.[134] Calcium channel blockers and angiotensin-converting enzyme inhibitors may be commenced and adjustment of tacrolimus dosing should be considered to achieve blood pressure control.[134,218]

Post-transplant diabetes mellitus (PTDM) is a common comorbidity after heart transplantation.[188,219] Corticosteroid use, which is initiated in all post-transplant immunosuppressive regimens, causes hyperglycaemia and impaired glucose metabolism.[219] PTDM is seen in 23–39% of recipients within the first 2 years.[188] Risk factors for PTDM are age >50 years, higher BMI, prior ischaemic heart disease, recipient CMV seropositivity, smoking, and use of tacrolimus and steroids.[188] Steroid wean and cessation by 12 months after heart transplant can result in reduced PTDM.[188,220] Due to the microvascular effects of PTDM recipients can be at increased risk of CAV, stroke, renal impairment and infection.[188] In the long term, lifestyle modification, oral hypoglycaemic medication and insulin therapy are recommended as the staged approach to manage PTDM.[221] Multi-disciplinary team approach, including a diabetes educator, nutritionist and endocrinologist, is key to enhancing long-term outcomes.[221]

Lifestyle issues

Following heart transplant surgery, patients require sound advice regarding returning to driving, work, exercise and sexual activity. Cardiac rehabilitation with aerobic and resistance exercise is recommended to prevent short-term weight gain and glucose intolerance, as well as adverse effects of immunosuppressive therapy on skeletal muscle.[134] Return to work or education is expected and encouraged after surgery. Driving a vehicle can be considered once medical issues are stabilised, and bradycardia managed appropriately.[134] In Australia, following heart transplant surgery, patients must not drive a car for at least 6 weeks for private use and 3 months for commercial use.[222] While pregnancy is possible after transplantation, careful planning and explanation of risks to mother and fetus need to be very carefully discussed. Changes to medications are often required to avoid teratogenicity and risks of rejection may be increased as a result of changes to treatment regimens. Pregnancy should be contraindicated for at least 1 year following transplantation and appropriate contraceptive advice is essential. If pregnancy is to be considered, it must be done only under the management of the multidisciplinary team.[134,223,224]

Summary

Primary compromise of the cardiovascular system causes patients to require admission to a critical care area and the need for specialised care including IABP and post-cardiac surgery management. Appropriate assessment and management are essential to prevent secondary complications arising. Important principles of care are summarised below.

Surgical procedures may be performed as treatment for structural abnormalities, ischaemic lesions within coronary arteries and repair or replacement of cardiac valves. Haemodynamic stability constitutes the most common challenge in the postoperative period and may be managed with fluids, cardiovascular medications, cardiac pacing and IABP. Bleeding in the postoperative period may be due to inadequate reversal or heparin, coagulopathy or surgical bleeding; therefore, appropriate diagnosis must occur before relevant treatment is instigated.

IABP is one therapy that is used to provide support in the period after cardiac surgery. Major benefits of IABP include increasing cardiac output, increasing myocardial oxygen supply and decreasing myocardial oxygen demand. Appropriate timing is essential to obtain maximum benefits, so correction of timing errors forms a central component of care. In addition, assessment of limb perfusion, with timely intervention when perfusion is inadequate, is essential to prevent limb ischaemia.

Cardiac transplantation is the gold standard of care used to provide support to patients with end-stage heart failure. Cardiac transplant centres face significant challenges with donor numbers remaining static. Despite this, advancing technology and the increasing use of perfusion systems for organ retrieval has the potential to increase transplant numbers by allowing the use of marginal and DCD donors, as well as donors a long distance from the transplanting centre, without relying on an increase in donor rates. Indications for heart transplantation include end-stage heart failure secondary to ischaemic heart disease and cardiomyopathy. Possible complications in the early postoperative period include acute rejection, infection, haemorrhage, renal failure, right ventricular failure and allograft dysfunction (left ventricular dysfunction/failure). Combination therapy consisting of corticosteroids, a calcineurin inhibitor and an antiproliferative agent are the most common immunosuppressive regimens used to prevent rejection after heart transplantation. An mTOR inhibitor may be added to this combination, or used instead of CNIs where renal dysfunction, or CAV is present. Although early signs of low-grade rejection can be non-specific, signs of moderate rejection usually present as organ dysfunction or failure. Nursing practices for managing patients with heart transplantation focus on prevention and management of complications, maintenance of comfort and promotion of long-term survival with a favourable quality of life.

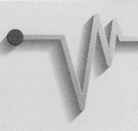

Case study

Ms Ali, a 56-year-old patient, presented by ambulance to the emergency department (ED) in early hours of the morning with chest pain and shortness of breath. The catheter laboratory (cath lab) team was activated by the hospital once they had received the ambulance call of inferior STEMI. Her past history was high cholesterol and hypertension (non-compliant with treatment). She was transferred to the cath lab for angiography that showed subtotal occlusion of proximal right coronary artery (RCA) that the wire could not cross, 60% occlusion mid left circumflex artery and 50% mid anterior descending (LAD) artery. Ms Ali was prepared for emergency CABGs and had three grafts performed for her triple vessels disease. Her ICU stay was uneventful and discharged to cardiothoracic ward on day one. Ms Ali was recovering well from her STEMI and CABGs until day 5, when she complained of severe shortness of breath, cough and pink frothy sputum. On examination, she appeared very anxious and severely dyspnoeic with use of accessory respiratory muscle. Her oxygen saturation was 82%, ST, low blood pressure. Medical emergency team was activated and oxygen via mask applied. At the same time, the CALS preparation was underway. The team initiated non-invasive ventilation for suspected acute pulmonary oedema and cardiogenic shock. An urgent echocardiogram showed acute severe mitral regurgitation with flail leaflet and rupture chordae tendineae. Due to COVID 19 restriction, and unavailability of cardiac surgical team in hospital, Ms Ali was transferred to the cath lab and an IABP was inserted via her left femoral artery to manage her cardiogenic shock state. In a few hours, Ms Ali was admitted back to ICU after surgery and repair of chordae tendineae with minor valve regurgitation that did not require repair or replacement.

Ms Ali's ventilation was weaned and extubated the next morning, and her IABP ratio reduced in the afternoon and the intra-aortic balloon catheter was removed that afternoon as she was on minimal vasopressor support for her blood pressure. Despite the high mortality rate of a combination of the emergency CABGs, cardiogenic shock status, resternotomy and emergency IABP insertion, Ms Ali's cardiac recovery progressed well and she was discharged from hospital on day 16 of her admission and referred to her local cardiac rehabilitation program.

CASE STUDY QUESTIONS

1 Discuss the causes, pathophysiology, treatment (medical and surgical) and prognosis of acute mitral regurgitation.

2 Outline the risks and outcomes of emergency cardiac surgery and same-admission resternotomy for adult cardiac surgical patients.

RESEARCH VIGNETTE

Guertin L, Earle M, Dardas T, et al. Post-heart transplant care pathway's impact on reducing length of stay. J Nurs Care Qual 2021;36(4):350–4.

Abstract

Background: Prolonged length of stay (LOS) has undesirable consequences including increased cost, resource consumption and morbidity and disruptions in hospital flow.

Local problem: A high-volume heart transplant centre in the Pacific Northwest (United States) had a mean index hospital LOS of 23 days, with a goal of 10 days according to the institutional heart transplant care pathway.

Methods: A retrospective, regression analysis was used to identify the factors contributing to LOS of 41 post-heart transplant patients.

Interventions: The post-heart transplant care pathway and order set were modified accordingly and reintroduced to the healthcare team.

Results: Factors contributing to LOS included number of days (1) until the first therapeutic calcineurin inhibitor level, (2) until intravenous diuretics were no longer required, and (3) outside of a therapeutic calcineurin inhibitor range. The interventions reduced the mean LOS by 8 days.

Conclusions: Increased awareness of LOS, education and consistent use of care pathways can significantly reduce length of stay.

Critique

For heart transplant patients there are many factors that contribute to the hospital LOS, some of which are modifiable. A prolonged LOS leads to increased costs, resources and morbidity. Interventions to aid certain factors can then reduce LOS and aim to improve patient satisfaction and hospital flow. Clinical pathways have been shown to improve patient flow and reduce LOS.

This single-centre study identified a local problem that their LOS following heart transplant had increased to 23 days, from an expected care pathway LOS of 10 days. The centre benchmarked mean LOS against similar-sized heart transplant programs, which ranged from 15.1 to 18.1 days. The centre also found that hospital costs had increased by $23,000 because of the increased LOS.

The centre implemented a quality improvement project. Three modifiable factors that could contribute to LOS were identified, and the heart transplant care pathway was modified and reimplemented into the program. The study used a retrospective analysis over a 9-month period, of a small cohort of 41 post-heart-transplant patients.

The three modifiable factors contributing to LOS included number of days: (1) until the first therapeutic calcineurin inhibitor level, (2) until intravenous diuretics were no longer required, and (3) outside of a therapeutic calcineurin inhibitor range. Factors 2 and 3 met statistical significance. The number of days intravenous diuretics was required reduced from 15 to 8, by change to the care pathway reviewing haemodynamic parameters and diuretics at postoperative days (POD) 0 and 1, compared with POD 4. The number of days outside of a therapeutic calcineurin inhibitor range reduced from 8 to 3; the new recommendation assisting this outcome was initiation of calcineurin inhibitor on POD 1 based on serum creatine level 1.8 mg/dL, instead of postextubation and a serum creatinine less than 1.6 mg/dL.

The quality improvement project had clear measurable interventions to reduce LOS. Staff obtained increased awareness of LOS and changes made to the care pathway through education, in addition to changes in the care set orders and standardised guidelines. The education provided was ultimately aimed at changing the culture to drive measurable interventions to improve patient outcomes and reduce LOS on an ongoing basis. The study achieved their outcomes by reducing LOS from 23 to 15 days, aligning them with other benchmarked centres. Furthermore, cost savings were made from the reduced LOS.

The study had strength in the quality improvement design, definitions of the modifiable factors, clear intervention to change the care pathway and measure outcomes. The study had support and collaboration of multiple stakeholders within the hospital and used a statistician to analyse the data. Clear documentation and education to increase multidisciplinary team awareness to the change in care pathway was a key factor to achieve a change in culture: a strong outcome with 8-day reduction in LOS and cost savings. Limitations to the study are: single centre, retrospective study, small volume of patients, short time frame and certain exclusion criteria for heart transplant patients. Furthermore, the data do not consider other factors that influence LOS such as patient adverse events, clinical decision making and change in care providers.

This article outlines the importance of quality improvement within an institution to improve patient care and outcomes, improve culture and hospital flow and reduce LOS and expenses. Nurses play a key role in quality improvement projects across institutions and can be at the forefront in leading such projects: as seen in this article, the first and second authors are registered nurses.

Learning activities

1 Outline the principles of caring for a postoperative cardiac surgical patient during the first 4 hours of ICU admission. Provide a rationale for why these aspects of care are a priority.

2 Discuss the options available in your unit if a patient fails extubation post-cardiac surgery.

3 What haemodynamic values could assist you in deciding the choice of inotropes and vasopressors? Provide rationales.

4 Discuss the management of a patient with cardiac arrest due to pericardial tamponade after minimally invasive cardiac surgery.

5 Compare and contrast the automated and semi-automated modes of intra-aortic balloon counterpulsation.

6 Discuss with a senior colleague the main complications of IABP therapy and what strategies should be included in your care of a patient receiving IABP therapy to minimise the likelihood or impact of these complications.

7 Discuss how you would identify an intra-aortic balloon catheter rupture and immediate management.

Online resources

Abbott, https://www.cardiovascular.abbott/us/en/hcp/products/heart-failure/left-ventricular-assist-devices/heartmate-3/about.html

American Heart Association, http://www.heart.org/HEARTORG

Asian Pacific Society of Cardiology, http://www.apscardio.org

Australian and New Zealand Intensive Care Society (ANZICS), www.anzics.com.au

Australian Institute of Health and Welfare, www.aihw.gov.au

Australian Organ Donor Register (AODR), www.medicareaustralia.gov.au/public/services/aodr/index.jsp

Cardiac Society of Australia and New Zealand, www.csanz.edu.au

Donate Life, www.donatelife.gov.au

European Heart Association, www.heartassociation.eu

European Society of cardiology www.escardio.org

National Health Priorities and Quality, https://www.health.gov.au/ The International Society for Heart and Lung Transplantation (ISHLT), www.ishlt.org

National Heart Foundation of Australia, www.heartfoundation.org.au

National Heart Foundation of New Zealand, www.heartfoundation.org.nz

Transplant Nurses' Association (TNA), https://transplantnurses.org.au/

Transplantation Society of Australia and New Zealand (TSANZ), www.tsanz.com.au

Further reading

Aslam S, Grossi P, Schlendorf KH, et al. Utilization of hepatitis C virus-infected organ donors in cardiothoracic transplantation: an ISHLT expert consensus statement. J Heart Lung Transplant 2020;39(5):418–32.

Coleman B, Blumenthal N, Currey J, et al. Adult cardiothoracic transplant nursing: an ISHLT consensus document on the current adult nursing practice in heart and lung transplantation. J Heart Lung Transplant 2015;34:139–48.

Fishman JA. Infection in organ transplantation. Am J Transplant 2017;17:856–79.

Kobashigawa J, Zuckermann A, Macdonald P, et al. Report from a consensus conference on primary graft dysfunction after cardiac transplantation. J Heart Lung Transplant 2014;33(4):327–40.

McGiffin D, Kure C, McLean J, et al The results of a single-centre experience with HeartMate 3 in a biventricular configuration. J Heart Lung Transplant 2020;40(3):193–200.

Mehra M, Uriel N, Naka Y, et al. A Fully Magnetically Levitated Left Ventricular Assist Device-Final Report. N Engl J Med 2019;380:1618–27.

Pellegrino V, Hockings LE, Davies A. Veno-arterial extracorporeal membrane oxygenation for adult cardiovascular failure. Curr Opin Crit Care 2014;20:484–92.

Razonable RR, Humar, A. Cytomegalovirus in solid organ transplant recipients – guidelines of the American society of transplantation infectious diseases community of practice. ClinTransplant 2019;33(9):e13512.

Scheuer S, Jansz, PC, Macdonald, PS. Heart transplantation following donation after circulatory death: expanding the donor pool. J Heart Lung Transplant 2021;40(9):882–9.

References

1. World Health Organization (WHO). The top 10 causes of death. Geneva: WHO; 2-2-. Available from: https://www.who.int/news-room/fact-sheets/detail/the-top-10-causes-of-death. [Accessed March 2023].
2. Timmis A, Vardas P, Townsend N, et al. European Society of Cardiology: cardiovascular disease statistics 2021. Eur Heart J 2022;43(8):716–99.
3. Australian Institute of Health and Welfare (AIHW). Heart, stroke and vascular disease – Australian facts. Canberra, ACT: AIHW; 2021.
4. Australian Institute of Health and Welfare (AIHW). Australian Burden of Disease Study 2018: key findings. Canberra, ACT: AIHW; 2021.
5. Baker Heart and Diabetes Institute. About heart valve disease. Melbourne, VIC: Baker Heart and Diabetes Institute; 2021.
6. Australian Institute of Health and Welfare (AIHW). Acute rheumatic fever and rheumatic heart disease in Australia, 2016–2020. Canberra, ACT: AIHW; 2022.

7. Menzies School of Health Research. Global and tropical health: rheumatic heart disease. Darwin, NT: Menzies School of Health Research; 2022.

8. Coffey S, Roberts-Thomson R, Brown A, et al. Global epidemiology of valvular heart disease. Nature Rev Cardiol 2021;18(12):853–64.

9. World Health Organization (WHO). Fact sheet: rheumatic heart disease. Geneva: WHO; 2022.

10. Urden L, Stacy K, Lough M. Critical care nursing: diagnosis and management. 9th ed. St Louis, MO: Elsevier; 2022.

11. Talukdar M, Gogoi PC, Konwar R. Clinical assessment of mitral valvular diseases requiring its prosthetic replacement. Indian J Forensic Med Toxicol 2021;15(3):5365–71.

12. Lisko J, Kamioka N, Grubb KJ. The eternal debate: CABG vs PCI. Current status of the literature. Semin Thorac Cardiovasc Surg 2019;31(4):734–9.

13. Jannati M, Navaei M, Ronizi L. A comparative review of the outcomes of using arterial versus venous conduits in coronary artery bypass graft (CABG). J Family Med Prim Care 2019;8(9):2768–73.

14. Di Santo P, Harnett DT, Simard T, et al. Photoplethysmography using a smartphone application for assessment of ulnar artery patency: a randomized clinical trial. CMAJ 2018;190(13):E380–8.

15. Kofidis T, editor. Minimally invasive cardiac surgery: a practical guide. Boca Raton, FL: CRC Press; 2021.

16. Torregrossa G, Sá MP, Van den Eynde J, et al. Hybrid robotic off-pump versus conventional on-pump and off-pump coronary artery bypass graft surgery in women. J Card Surg 2022;37(4):895–905.

17. Taggart DP, Altman DG, Gray AM, et al. Effects of on-pump and off-pump surgery in the Arterial Revascularization Trial. Eur J Cardiothorac Surg 2015;47(6):1059–65.

18. Ravikumar N, George V, Shirke MM, et al. Robotic coronary artery surgery: outcomes and pitfalls. J Card Surg 2020;35(11):3108–15.

19. Stepan C, Wouter O, Burak O, et al. Robotic cardiac surgery in Europe: status 2020. Front Cardiovasc Med 2022;8:827515.

20. Wilkins E, Wilson L, Wickramasinghe K, et al. European cardiovascular disease statistics 2017. Brussels: European Heart Network 2017.

21. Sousa-Uva M, Neumann F-J, Ahlsson A, et al. 2018 ESC/EACTS guidelines on myocardial revascularization. Eur J Cardiothorac Surg 2018;55(1):4–90.

22. Chieffo A, Buchanan GL, Van Mieghem NM, et al. Transcatheter aortic valve implantation with the Edwards SAPIEN versus the Medtronic CoreValve revaling system devices: a multicenter collaborative study: The PRAGMATIC Plus Initiative (Pooled-RotterdAm-Milano-Toulouse in collaboration). J Am Coll Cardiol 2013;61(8):830–6.

23. Popma JJ, Adams DH, Reardon MJ, et al. Transcatheter aortic valve replacement using a self-expanding bioprosthesis in patients with severe aortic stenosis at extreme risk for surgery. J Am Coll Cardiol 2014;63(19):1972–81.

24. Rogato S, Santini F, Barbanti M, et al. Transcatheter aortic valve implantation compared with surgical aortic valve replacement in low-risk patients. Circ Cardiovasc Interv 2016;9(5):e003326.

25. Sun LY, Chu A, Tam DY, et al. Derivation and validation of predictive indices for 30-day mortality after coronary and valvular surgery in Ontario, Canada. CMAJ 2021;193(46):E1757–65.

26. Belov A, Katkov K, Vinokurov IA, et al. [Cardiopulmonary bypass duration as predictor of immediate results after cardiac surgery]. Khirurgiia 2015(5):4–13.

27. Shafi AMA, Abuelgasim E, Abuelgasim B, et al. Sternal closure with single compared with double or figure of 8 wires in obese patients following cardiac surgery: a systematic review and meta-analysis. J Card Surg 2021;36(3):1072–82.

28. Spooner A, Mewhort H, DiFrancesco L, et al. Adhesive-enhanced sternal closure: feasibility and safety of late sternal reentry. Case Rep Surg 2017:2017:8605313.

29. Nenna A, Nappi F, Dougal J, et al. Sternal wound closure in the current era: the need of a tailored approach. Gen Thorac Cardiovasc Surg 2019;67(11):907–16.

30. Royse AG, El-Ansary D, Hoang W, et al. A randomized trial comparing the effects of sternal band and plate fixation of the sternum with that of figure-of-8 wires on sternal edge motion and quality of recovery after cardiac surgery. Interact Cardiovasc Thorac Surg 2020;30(6):863–70.

31. Leonardi S, Capodanno D, Sousa-Uva M, et al. Composition, structure, and function of heart teams: a joint position paper of the ACVC, EAPCI, EACTS, and EACTA focused on the management of patients with complex coronary artery disease requiring myocardial revascularization. Eur J Cardiothorac Surg 2021;59(3):522–31.

32. de Carvalho IM, Soares Ferreira DK, Cortês Nelson AR, et al. Systematization of nursing care in mediate post-operative of cardiac surgery. Revista de Pesquisa: Cuidado e Fundamental 2016;8(4):5062–7.

33. Broch O, Bein B, Gruenewald M, et al. Accuracy of cardiac output by nine different pulse contour algorithms in cardiac surgery patients: a comparison with transpulmonary thermodilution. Biomed Res Int 2016;2016:3468015.

34. Guarracino F, Habicher M, Treskatsch S, et al. Vasopressor therapy in cardiac surgery – an experts' consensus statement. J Cardiothorac Vasc Anesth 2021;35(4):1018–29.

35. Epting CL, McBride ME, Wald EL, et al. Pathophysiology of post-operative low cardiac output syndrome. Curr Vasc Pharmacol 2016;14(1):14–23.

36. Demirci C, Zeman F, Schmid C, et al. Early postoperative blood pressure and blood loss after cardiac surgery: a retrospective analysis. Intensive Crit Care Nurs 2017;42:122–6.

37. Balzer F, Aronson S, Campagna JA, et al. High postoperative blood pressure after cardiac surgery is associated with acute kidney injury and death. J Cardiothorac Vasc Anesth 2016;30(6):1562–70.

38. Fot EV, Izotova NN, Smetkin AA, et al. Invasive and non-invasive dynamic parameters to predict fluid responsiveness after off-pump coronary surgery. Turk J Anesth Reanim 2022;50(1):59–64.

39. Habicher M, Zajonz T, Heringlake M, et al. et al. [S3 guidelines on intensive medical care of cardiac surgery patients: hemodynamic monitoring and cardiovascular system – an update]. Anaesthesist 2018;67(5):375–9.

40. Pfortmueller CA, Kindler M, Schenk N, et al. Hypertonic saline for fluid resuscitation in ICU patients post-cardiac surgery (HERACLES): a double-blind randomized controlled clinical trial. Intensive Care Med 2020;46(9):1683–95.

41. Otero TMN, Aljure OD, Yu S. Postoperative resuscitation with hypertonic saline or hyperoncotic albumin in patients following cardiac surgery: a review of the literature. J Card Surg 2021;36(3):1040–9.

42. Wei L, Li D, Sun L. The comparison of albumin and 6% hydroxyethyl starches (130/0.4) in cardiac surgery: a meta-analysis of randomized controlled clinical trials. BMC Surg 2021;21(1):342.

43. Skhirtladze K, Base EM, Lassnigg A, et al. Comparison of the effects of albumin 5%, hydroxyethyl starch 130/0.4 6%, and Ringer's lactate on blood loss and coagulation after cardiac surgery. Br J Anaesth 2014;112(2):255–64.

44. Foroughi M, Conte AH. Cardiovascular complications and management after cardiac surgery. In: Dabbagh A, Esmailian F, Aranki SF, editors. Postoperative critical care for cardiac surgical patients. Berlin: Springer; 2014, p. 197–211.

45. Ristic AD, Imazio M, Adler Y, et al. Triage strategy for urgent management of cardiac tamponade: a position statement of the European Society of Cardiology Working Group on Myocardial and Pericardial Diseases. Eur Heart J 2014:35(34):2279–84.

46. Mai Mohsen A, Hadil Magdi A. Terlipressin versus norepinephrine to prevent milrinone-induced systemic vascular hypotension in cardiac surgery patient with pulmonary hypertension. Ann Card Anaesth 2019;22(2):136–42.

47. Schub TB, Balderrama DRM. Pulmonary artery catheter: measuring cardiac output. Ipswich, MA: EBSCO Publishing; 2017.

48. Francis J, Prothasis S, Hegde R, et al. Management of temporary epicardial pacing wires in the cardiac surgical patient. Br J Hosp Med 2021;82(6):1–7.

49. Wagner GS, Strauss DG. Marriott's practical electrocardiography. 12th ed. Baltimore, MD: Lippincott, Williams & Wilkins; 2014.

50. Schub TB, Oji ODAF-B. Pericarditis. Ipswich, MA: EBSCO Publishing; 2018.

51. Greenberg JW, Lancaster TS, Schuessler RB, et al. Postoperative atrial fibrillation following cardiac surgery: a persistent complication. Eur J Cardiothorac Surg 2017;52(4):665–72.

52. Raiten J, Patel PA, Gutsche J. Management of postoperative atrial fibrillation in cardiac surgery patients. Semin Cardiothorac Vasc Anesth 2015;19(2):122–9.

53. White CM, Caron MF, Kalus JS, et al. Intravenous plus oral amiodarone, atrial septal pacing, or both strategies to prevent post-cardiothoracic surgery atrial fibrillation: the Atrial Fibrillation Suppression Trial II (AFIST II). Circulation 2003;108(10 Suppl 1):II-200-II-6.

54. Peretto G, Durante A, Limite LR, et al. Postoperative arrhythmias after cardiac surgery: incidence, risk factors, and therapeutic management. Cardiol Res Pract 2014;2014:615987.

55. Society of Thoracic Surgeons Task Force on Resuscitation After Cardiac Surgery. The Society of Thoracic Surgeons expert consensus for the resuscitation of patients who arrest after cardiac surgery. Ann Thorac Surg 2017;103(3):1005–20.

56. Bignami E, Di Lullo A, Saglietti F, et al. Routine practice in mechanical ventilation in cardiac surgery in Italy. J Thorac Dis 2019;11(4):1571–9.

57. Badenes R, Lozano A, Belda FJ. Postoperative pulmonary dysfunction and mechanical ventilation in cardiac surgery. Crit Care Res Pract 2015;2015:420513.

58. Bignami E, Saglietti F, Di Lullo A. Mechanical ventilation management during cardiothoracic surgery: an open challenge. Ann Transl Med 2018;6(19):380.

59. Bansal S, Thai HM, Hsu CH, et al. Fast track extubation post coronary artery bypass graft: a retrospective review of predictors of clinical outcomes. World J Cardiovasc Surg 2013;3:81–6.

60. Kheiri B, Abdalla A, Osman M, et al. Restrictive versus liberal red blood cell transfusion for cardiac surgery: a systematic review and meta-analysis of randomized controlled trials. J Thromb Thrombolysis 2019;47(2):179–85.

61. Fischer M-O, Guinot P-G, Debroczi S, et al. Individualised or liberal red blood cell transfusion after cardiac surgery: a randomised controlled trial. Br J Anaesth 2022;128(1):37–44.

62. Joshi RV, Wilkey AL, Blackwell JM, et al. Blood conservation and hemostasis in cardiac surgery: a survey of practice variation and adoption of evidence-based guidelines. Anesth Analg 2021;133(1):104–14.

63. Bolliger D, Tanaka KA. Point-of-care coagulation testing in cardiac surgery. Semin Thromb Hemost 2017;43(4):386–96.

64. Ranucci M, Baryshnikova E, Pistuddi V, et al. The effectiveness of 10 years of interventions to control postoperative bleeding in adult cardiac surgery. Interact Cardiovasc Thorac Surg 2017;24(2):196–202.

65. Sharma S, Kumar S, Tewari P, et al. Utility of thromboelastography versus routine coagulation tests for assessment of hypocoagulable state in patients undergoing cardiac bypass surgery. Ann Card Anaesth 2018;21(2):151–7.

66. Hällgren O, Svenmarker S, Appelblad M. Implementing a statistical model for protamine titration: effects on coagulation in cardiac surgical patients. J Cardiothorac Vasc Anesth 2017;31(2):516–21.

67. Miles LF, Burt C, Arrowsmith J, et al. Optimal protamine dosing after cardiopulmonary bypass: the PRODOSE adaptive randomised controlled trial. PLoS Med 2021;18(6):e1003658.

68. Boxma RPJ, Garnier RP, Bulte CSE, et al. The effect of non-point-of-care haemostasis management protocol implementation in cardiac surgery: a systematic review. Transfus Med 2021;31(5):328–38.

69. Yousuf MS, Samad K, Ahmed SS, et al. Cardiac surgery and blood-saving techniques: an update. Cureus 2022;14(1):e21222.

70. You SC, Shim CY, Hong G-R, et al. Incidence, predictors, and clinical outcomes of postoperative cardiac tamponade in patients undergoing heart valve surgery. PLoS One 2016;11(11):e0165754-e.

71. Marshall K, McLaughlin K. Pain management in thoracic surgery. Thorac Surg Clin 2020;30(3):339–46.

72. Gunter BR, Butler KA, Wallace RL, et al. Non-steroidal anti-inflammatory drug-induced cardiovascular adverse events: a meta-analysis. J Clin Pharm Ther 2017;42(1):27–38.

73. Bjørnnes A K, Parry M, Lie I, et al. Pain experiences of men and women after cardiac surgery. J Clin Nurs 2016;25(19-20):3058–68.

74. Williams JB, McConnell G, Allender JE, et al. One-year results from the first US-based enhanced recovery after cardiac surgery (ERAS Cardiac) program. J Thorac Cardiovasc Surg 2019;157(5):1881–8.

75. Menger J, Edlinger-Stanger M, Dworschak M, et al. Postoperative management of patients undergoing cardiac surgery in Austria. Wiener Klin Wochensch 2018;130(23):716–21.

76. Ronsoni RM, Souza AZM, Leiria TLL, et al. Update on management of postoperative atrial fibrillation after cardiac surgery. Braz J Cardiovasc Surg 2020;35(2):206–10.

77. Muehlschlegel JD, Burrage PS, Ngai JY, et al. Society of Cardiovascular Anesthesiologists/European Association of Cardiothoracic Anaesthetists practice advisory for the management of perioperative atrial fibrillation in patients undergoing cardiac surgery. Anesth Analg 2019;128(1):33–42.

78. Prado-Olivares J, Chover-Sierra E. Preoperatory anxiety in patients undergoing cardiac surgery. Diseases 2019;7(2):46.

79. Tavares Gomes E, Muniz da Silva Bezerra SM. Anxiety and depression in the preoperative period of cardiac surgery. Revista da Rede de Enfermagem do Nordeste 2017;18(3):420–7.

80. Lai VKW, Ho KM, Wong WT, et al. Effect of preoperative education and ICU tour on patient and family satisfaction and anxiety in the intensive care unit after elective cardiac surgery: a randomised controlled trial. BMJ Qual Saf 2021;30(3):228–35.

81. Koyuncu A, Yava A, Yamak B, et al. Effect of family presence on stress response after bypass surgery. Heart Lung 2021;50(2):193–201.

82. Mendonça KMB, Andrade TMD. Patient's perception about coronary artery bypass grafting. Braz J Cardiovasc Surg 2015;30(5):544–51.

83. Shah M, Patnaik S, Patel B, et al. Trends in mechanical circulatory support use and hospital mortality among patients with acute myocardial infarction and non-infarction related cardiogenic shock in the United States. Clin Res Cardiol 2018;107(4):287–303.

84. Deppe A-C, Weber C, Liakopoulos OJ, et al. Preoperative intra-aortic balloon pump use in high-risk patients prior to coronary artery bypass graft surgery decreases the risk for morbidity and mortality-A meta-analysis of 9,212 patients. J Card Surg 2017;32(3):177–85.

85. Hou D, Yang F, Hou X. Clinical application of intra-aortic balloon counterpulsation in high-risk patients undergoing cardiac surgery. Perfusion 2018;33(3):178–84.

86. Gajanan G, Brilakis ES, Siller-Matula JM, et al. The intra-aortic balloon pump. J Vis Exp 2021 Feb 5;(168).

87. De Lazzari C, De Lazzari B, Iacovoni A, et al. Intra-aortic balloon counterpulsation timing: A new numerical model for programming and training in the clinical environment. Comput Methods Programs Biomed 2020;194:105537.

88. Vallabhajosyula S, Subramaniam AV, Murphree DH Jr, et al. Complications from percutaneous-left ventricular assist devices versus intra-aortic balloon pump in acute myocardial infarction-cardiogenic shock. PLoS One 2020;15(8):e0238046.

89. Rustum S, Schrimpf C, Haverich A, et al. Intra-aortic balloon pump associated vascular complications in cardiac surgical patients: the past and the future. Indian J Thorac Cardiovasc Surg 2017;33(3):200–4.

90. Özen Y, Aksut M, Cekmecelioglu D, et al. Intra-aortic balloon pump experience: a single center study comparing with and without sheath insertion. J Cardiovasc Thorac Res 2018;10(3):144–8.

91. Allender JE, Reed BN, Foster JL, et al. Pharmacologic considerations in the management of patients receiving left ventricular percutaneous mechanical circulatory support. Pharmacotherapy 2017;37(10):1272–83.

92. de Jong MM, Lorusso R, Al Awami F, et al. Vascular complications following intra-aortic balloon pump implantation: an updated review. Perfusion 2018;33(2):96–104.

93. Woten MRB, Caple CRBM. Intra-aortic balloon pump: weaning from and removing. Ipswich, MA: EBSCO Publishing; 2019.

94. Rogers L, Cochrane E, Blundell D, et al. What is the optimum method of weaning intra-aortic balloon pumps? Interact Cardiovasc Thorac Surg 2016;23(2):310–3.

95. Telukuntla KS, Estep JD. Acute mechanical circulatory support for cardiogenic shock. Methodist DeBakey Cardiovasc J 2020;16(1):27–35.

96. Yarham G, Clements A, Morris C, et al. Fiber-optic intra-aortic balloon therapy and its role within cardiac surgery. Perfusion 2013;28(2):97–102.

97. Sebastián CG, Sanz AP, Gómez JLZ. Non-sustained ventricular tachycardia induced by helium leak due to intra-aortic balloon pump rupture. Eur Heart J Cardiovasc Imaging 2021;22(12):e167–e6.

98. Mihatov N, Dudzinski DM. Intraaortic balloon pump rupture. J Invasive Cardiol 2015;27(9):E203.

99. Chapman JR. Transplantation in Australia – 50 years of progress. Med J Aust 1992;157(1):46–50.

100. McBride M, Chapman JR. An overview of transplantation in Australia. Anaesth Intensive Care 1995;23(1):60–4.

101. Chew HC, Iyer A, Connellan M, et al. Outcomes of donation after circulatory death heart transplantation in Australia. J Am Coll Cardiol 2019;73(12):1447–59.

102. Dhital K, Ludhani P, Scheuer S, et al. DCD donations and outcomes of heart transplantation: the Australian experience. Indian J Thorac Cardiovasc Surg 2020;36(Suppl 2):224–32.

103. Scheuer SE, Jansz PC, Macdonald PS. Heart transplantation following donation after circulatory death: expanding the donor pool. J Heart Lung Transplant 2021;40(9):882–9.

104. Messer S, Cernic S, Page A, et al. A 5-year single-center early experience of heart transplantation from donation after circulatory-determined death donors. J Heart Lung Transplant 2020;39(12):1463–75.

105. Nilsson J, Jernryd V, Qin G, et al. A nonrandomized open-label phase 2 trial of nonischemic heart preservation for human heart transplantation. Nat Commun 2020;11(1):2976.

106. Rochlani Y, Diab K, Jorde UP. Hepatitis C-positive donors in cardiac transplantation: problems and opportunities. Curr Heart Fail Rep 2020;17(4):106–15.

107. Siddiqi HK, Schlendorf KH. Hepatitis C positive organ donation in heart transplantation. Curr Transplant Rep 2021;8(4):359–67.

108. Kilic A, Hickey G, Mathier M, et al. Outcomes of adult heart transplantation using hepatitis c-positive donors. J Am Heart Assoc 2020;9(2):e014495.

109. Aslam S, Grossi P, Schlendorf KH, et al. Utilization of hepatitis C virus-infected organ donors in cardiothoracic transplantation: an ISHLT expert consensus statement. J Heart Lung Transplant 2020;39(5):418–32.

110. Barnard CN. The operation. A human cardiac transplant: an interim report of a successful operation performed at Groote Schuur Hospital, Cape Town. S Afr Med J 1967;41(48):1271–4.

111. Excell LWP, Russ, GR. Australia and New Zealand organ donation registry 2010. Adelaide, SA: ANZDATA Registry; 2010.

112. The Australian and New Zealand Cardiothoracic Organ Transplant Registry (ANZCOTR). Twenty-third annual report 1984–2018. Sydney, NSW: ANZCOTR; 2018.

113. Eurotransplant International Foundation. Annual report 2020. Leiden, Eurotransplant International Foundation; 2020. Available from: https://www.eurotransplant.org/wp-content/uploads/2022/03/ET_AR2020_LR_def.pdf. [Accessed March 2023].

114. Rose EA, Moskowitz AJ, Packer M, et al. The REMATCH trial: rationale, design, and end points. Randomized evaluation of mechanical assistance for the treatment of congestive heart failure. Ann Thorac Surg 1999;67(3):723–30.

115. Molina EJ, Shah P, Kiernan MS, et al. The Society of Thoracic Surgeons Intermacs 2020 annual report. Ann Thorac Surg 2021;111(3):778–92.

116. Khush KK, Cherikh WS, Chambers DC, et al. The International Thoracic Organ Transplant Registry of the International Society for Heart and Lung Transplantation: Thirty-sixth adult heart transplantation report – 2019; focus theme: donor and recipient size match. J Heart Lung Transplant 2019;38(10):1056–66.

117. Hayes D Jr, Harhay MO, Cherikh WS et al; International Society for Heart and Lung Transplantation. Heart transplantation, adult recipients. Focus theme: trends in recipient characteristics and impact on outcomes. J Heart Lung Transplant 2021;40(10):1023–72.

118. Wilhelm MJ. Long-term outcome following heart transplantation: current perspective. J Thorac Dis 2015;7(3):549–51.

119. ANZOD Registry. 2019 annual report. Section 12: Deceased organ transplant outcome data; section 12. Adelaide, SA: ANZDATA Registry; 2019. Available from: https://www.anzdata.org.au/wp-content/uploads/2019/07/s12_tx-outcome_2018_v1.0_20190807.pdf. [Accessed March 2023].

120. Mehra MR, Canter CE, Hannan MM, et al. The 2016 International Society for Heart Lung Transplantation listing criteria for heart transplantation: a 10-year update. J Heart Lung Transplant 2016;35(1):1–23.

121. Goldstein DJ, Bello R, Shin JJ, et al. Outcomes of cardiac transplantation in septuagenarians. J Heart Lung Transplant 2012;31(7):679–85.

122. Transplantation Society of Australia and New Zealand (TSANZ). Clinical guidelines for organ transplantation from deceased donors. Canberra, ACT: Australian Government Organ and Tissue Authority; 2021. Available from: https://tsanz.com.au/storage/documents/TSANZ_Clinical_Guidelines_Version-18_Final.pdf. [Accessed March 2023].

123. Marasco SF, Summerhayes R, Quayle M, et al. Cost comparison of heart transplant vs. left ventricular assist device therapy at one year. Clin Transplant 2016;30(5):598–605.

124. Australian Institute of Health and Welfare (AIHW). Heart, stroke and vascular disease: Australian facts. Canberra, ACT: AIHW; 2023. Available from: https://www.aihw.gov.au/reports/heart-stroke-vascular-diseases/hsvd-facts/contents/about. [Accessed March 2023].

125. Chan YK, Tuttle C, Ball J, et al. Current and projected burden of heart failure in the Australian adult population: a substantive but still ill-defined major health issue. BMC Health Serv Res 2016;16(1):501.

126. Chan YK, Gerber T, Tuttle C, et al. Rediscovering heart failure: the contemporary burden and profile of heart failure in Australia. Melbourne, VIC: Mary MacKillip Institute for Health Research; 2015. Contract No.: Key findings 9 and 12.

127. Kirklin JK, Young, JB, McGiffin DC. Heart transplantation. Philadelphia: Churchill Livingstone; 2002.

128. Angermann CE, Spes CH, Tammen A, et al. Anatomic characteristics and valvular function of the transplanted heart: transthoracic versus transesophageal echocardiographic findings. J Heart Transplant 1990;9(4):331–8.

129. Kendall SW, Ciulli F, Mullins PA, et al. Total orthotopic heart transplantation: an alternative to the standard technique. Ann Thorac Surg 1992;54(1):187–8.

130. Dreyfus G, Jebara V, Mihaileanu S, et al. Total orthotopic heart transplantation: an alternative to the standard technique. Ann Thorac Surg 1991;52(5):1181–4.

131. Nakatani T, Frazier OH, Lammermeier DE, et al. Heterotopic heart transplantation: a reliable option for a select group of high-risk patients. J Heart Transplant 1989;8(1):40–7.

132. Newcomb AE, Esmore DS, Rosenfeldt FL, et al. Heterotopic heart transplantation: an expanding role in the twenty-first century? Ann Thorac Surg 2004;78(4):1345-50; discussion 50–1.

133. Neerukonda SK, Schoonmaker FW, Nampalli VK, et al. Ventricular dysrhythmia and heterotopic heart transplantation. J Heart Lung Transplant 1992;11(4 Pt 1):793–6.

134. Costanzo MR, Dipchand A, Starling R, et al. The International Society of Heart and Lung Transplantation guidelines for the care of heart transplant recipients. J Heart Lung Transplant 2010;29(8):914–56.

135. Coleman B, Blumenthal N, Currey J, et al. Adult cardiothoracic transplant nursing: an ISHLT consensus document on the current adult nursing practice in heart and lung transplantation. J Heart Lung Transplant 2015;34(2):139–48.

136. Wu Q, Marescaux C, Wolff V, et al. Tacrolimus-associated posterior reversible encephalopathy syndrome after solid organ transplantation. Eur Neurol 2010;64(3):169–77.

137. Bechstein WO. Neurotoxicity of calcineurin inhibitors: impact and clinical management. Transpl Int 2000;13(5):313–26.

138. Naesens M, Kuypers DR, Sarwal M. Calcineurin inhibitor nephrotoxicity. Clin J Am Soc Nephrol 2009;4(2):481–508.

139. Westerdahl DE, Kobashigawa JA. Heart transplantation for advanced heart failure. In: Brown DL, editor. Cardiac intensive care, 3rd ed. Philadelphia: Elsevier; 2019, p. 504–24.

140. Awad MA, Shah A, Griffith BP. Current status and outcomes in heart transplantation: a narrative review. Rev Cardiovasc Med 2022;23(1):11.

141. Kobashigawa J, Zuckermann A, Macdonald P, et al. Report from a consensus conference on primary graft dysfunction after cardiac transplantation. J Heart Lung Transplant 2014;33(4):327–40.

142. Colvin MM, Cook JL, Chang P, et al. Antibody-mediated rejection in cardiac transplantation: emerging knowledge in diagnosis and management: a scientific statement from the American Heart Association. Circulation 2015;131(18):1608–39.

143. Berry GJ, Burke MM, Andersen C, et al. The 2013 International Society for Heart and Lung Transplantation working formulation for the standardization of nomenclature in the pathologic diagnosis of antibody-mediated rejection in heart transplantation. J Heart Lung Transplant 2013;32(12):1147–62.

144. Stewart S, Winters GL, Fishbein MC, et al. Revision of the 1990 working formulation for the standardization of nomenclature in the diagnosis of heart rejection. J Heart Lung Transplant 2005;24(11):1710–20.

145. Berry GJ, Angelini A, Burke MM, et al. The ISHLT working formulation for pathologic diagnosis of antibody-mediated rejection in heart transplantation: evolution and current status (2005–2011). J Heart Lung Transplant 2011;30(6):601–11.

146. Taylor AJ, Vaddadi G, Pfluger H, et al. Diagnostic performance of multisequential cardiac magnetic resonance imaging in acute cardiac allograft rejection. Eur J Heart Fail 2010;12(1):45–51.

147. Lloveras JJ, Escourrou G, Delisle MB, et al. Evolution of untreated mild rejection in heart transplant recipients. J Heart Lung Transplant 1992;11(4 Pt 1):751–6.

148. Maravic-Stojkovic V, Stojkovic B, Peric M. Modern immunosuppressive agents after heart transplantation. Curr Trends Cardiol 2017;1(2):41–8.

149. Stehlik J, Kobashigawa J, Hunt SA, et al. Honoring 50 years of clinical heart transplantation in circulation: in-depth state-of-the-art review. Circulation 2018;137(1):71–87.

150. Andreassen AK, Andersson B, Gustafsson F, et al. Everolimus initiation and early calcineurin inhibitor withdrawal in heart transplant recipients: a randomized trial. Am J Transplant 2014;14(8):1828–38.

151. Eisen HJ, Kobashigawa J, Starling RC, et al. Everolimus versus mycophenolate mofetil in heart transplantation: a randomized, multicenter trial. Am J Transplant 2013;13(5):1203–16.

152. Taylor DO, Barr ML, Radovancevic B, et al. A randomized, multicenter comparison of tacrolimus and cyclosporine immunosuppressive regimens in cardiac transplantation: decreased hyperlipidemia and hypertension with tacrolimus. J Heart Lung Transplant 1999;18(4):336–45.

153. Kobashigawa J, Miller L, Renlund D, et al. A randomized active-controlled trial of mycophenolate mofetil in heart transplant recipients. Mycophenolate Mofetil Investigators. Transplantation 1998;66(4):507–15.

154. Fishman JA. Infection in organ transplantation. Am J Transplant 2017;17(4):856–79.

155. Razonable RR, Humar A. Cytomegalovirus in solid organ transplant recipients – guidelines of the American Society of Transplantation Infectious Diseases Community of Practice. Clin Transplant 2019;33(9):e13512.

156. Kotton CN, Kumar D, Caliendo AM, et al. The third international consensus guidelines on the management of cytomegalovirus in solid-organ transplantation. Transplantation 2018;102(6):900–31.

157. Walsh TR, Guttendorf J, Dummer S, et al. The value of protective isolation procedures in cardiac allograft recipients. Ann Thorac Surg 1989;47(4):539–44; discussion 544-5.

158. Husain S, Mooney ML, Danziger-Isakov L, et al. A 2010 working formulation for the standardization of definitions of infections in cardiothoracic transplant recipients. J Heart Lung Transplant 2011;30(4):361–74.

159. Luckraz H, Goddard M, Charman SC, et al. Early mortality after cardiac transplantation: should we do better? J Heart Lung Transplant 2005;24(4):401–5.

160. Danziger-Isakov L, Blumberg EA, Manuel O, et al. Impact of COVID-19 in solid organ transplant recipients. Am J Transplant 2021;21(3):925–37.

161. Azzi Y, Bartash R, Scalea J, et al. COVID-19 and solid organ transplantation: a review article. Transplantation 2021;105(1):37–55.

162. Boan P, Marinelli T, Opdam H. Solid organ transplantation from donors with COVID-19 infection. Transplantation 2022;106(4):693–5.

163. Transplantation Society of Australia and New Zealand (TSANZ). Updated TSANZ COVID-19 Vaccination recommendations for transplant recipients. Canberra, ACT: Australian Government Organ and Tissue Authority; 2022. Available from: https://tsanz.com.au/storage/COVID_Communiques/TSANZ-COVID-19-Vaccination-udpate—-17-Jan-2022_Final.pdf. [Accessed March 2023].

164. Cooper DKC, Lidsky NM. Immediate postoperative care and potential complications. In: Cooper DKC, Miller LW, Patterson, GA, editors. The transplantation and replacement of thoracic organs. Boston, MA: Kluwer; 1996. p. 221–7.

165. Marasco SF, Kras A, Schulberg E, et al. Impact of warm ischemia time on survival after heart transplantation. Transplant Proc 2012;44(5):1385–9.

166. Squiers JJ, Saracino G, Chamogeorgakis T, et al. Application of the International Society for Heart and Lung Transplantation (ISHLT) criteria for primary graft dysfunction after cardiac transplantation: outcomes from a high-volume centre. Eur J Cardiothorac Surg 2017;51(2):263–70.

167. Messer S, Page A, Colah S, Axell R, et al. Human heart transplantation from donation after circulatory-determined death donors using normothermic regional perfusion and cold storage. J Heart Lung Transplant 2018;37(7):865–9.

168. Segovia J, Cosio MD, Barcelo JM, et al. RADIAL: a novel primary graft failure risk score in heart transplantation. J Heart Lung Transplant 2011;30(6):644–51.

169. Foroutan F, Alba AC, Stein M, et al. Validation of the International Society for Heart and Lung Transplantation primary graft dysfunction instrument in heart transplantation. J Heart Lung Transplant 2019;38(3):260–6.

170. Subramani S, Aldrich A, Dwarakanath S, et al. Early graft dysfunction following heart transplant: prevention and management. Semin Cardiothorac Vasc Anesth 2020;24(1):24–33.

171. Myles PS, Leong CK, Currey J. Endogenous nitric oxide and low systemic vascular resistance after cardiopulmonary bypass. J Cardiothorac Vasc Anesth 1997;11(5):571–4.

172. Kristof AS, Magder S. Low systemic vascular resistance state in patients undergoing cardiopulmonary bypass. Crit Care Med 1999;27(6):1121–7.

173. Landry DW, Levin HR, Gallant EM, et al. Vasopressin deficiency contributes to the vasodilation of septic shock. Circulation 1997;95(5):1122–5.

174. Argenziano M, Choudhri AF, Oz MC, et al. A prospective randomized trial of arginine vasopressin in the treatment of vasodilatory shock after left ventricular assist device placement. Circulation 1997;96(9 Suppl):II-286–90.

175. Karamlou T, Gelow J, Diggs BS, et al. Mechanical circulatory support pathways that maximize post-heart transplant survival. Ann Thorac Surg 2013;95(2):480–5; discussion 485.

176. Phan K, Luc JGY, Xu J, et al. Utilization and outcomes of temporary mechanical circulatory support for graft dysfunction after heart transplantation. ASAIO J 2017;63(6):695–703.

177. Loforte A, Fiorentino M, Murana G, et al. Mechanically supported early graft failure after heart transplantation. Transplant Proc 2021;53(1):311–7.

178. Takeda K, Li B, Garan AR, et al. Improved outcomes from extracorporeal membrane oxygenation versus ventricular assist device temporary support of primary graft dysfunction in heart transplant. J Heart Lung Transplant 2017;36(6):650–6.

179. Pons J, Leblanc MH, Bernier M, et al. Effects of chronic sildenafil use on pulmonary hemodynamics and clinical outcomes in heart transplantation. J Heart Lung Transplant 2012;31(12):1281–7.

180. Rossaint R, Falke KJ, Lopez F, et al. Inhaled nitric oxide for the adult respiratory distress syndrome. N Engl J Med 1993;328(6):399–405.

181. Armitage JM, Hardesty RL, Griffith BP. Prostaglandin E1: an effective treatment of right heart failure after orthotopic heart transplantation. J Heart Transplant 1987;6(6):348–51.

182. Kansara P, Kobashigawa JA. Management of heart transplant recipients: reference for primary care physicians. Postgrad Med 2012;124(4):215–24.

183. Ellenbogen KA, Thames MD, DiMarco JP, et al. Electrophysiological effects of adenosine in the transplanted human heart. Evidence of supersensitivity. Circulation 1990;81(3):821–8.

184. Macdonald P, Hackworthy R, Keogh A, et al. Atrial overdrive pacing for reversion of atrial flutter after heart transplantation. J Heart Lung Transplant 1991;10(5 Pt 1):731–7.

185. Mackintosh AF, Carmichael DJ, Wren C, et al. Sinus node function in first three weeks after cardiac transplantation. Br Heart J 1982;48(6):584–8.

186. Awad M, Czer LS, Hou M, et al. Early denervation and later reinnervation of the heart following cardiac transplantation: a review. J Am Heart Assoc 2016;5(11):e0004070.

187. Parry A, Roberts M, Parameshwar J, et al. The management of post-cardiac transplantation coronary artery disease. Eur J Cardiothorac Surg 1996;10(7):528–32; discussion 553.

188. McCartney SL, Patel C, Del Rio JM. Long-term outcomes and management of the heart transplant recipient. Best Pract Res Clin Anaesthesiol 2017;31(2):237–48.

189. Potena L, Zuckermann A, Barberini F, et al. Complications of cardiac transplantation. Curr Cardiol Rep 2018;20(9):73.

190. Spartalis M, Spartalis E, Tzatzaki E, et al. Cardiac allograft vasculopathy after heart transplantation: current prevention and treatment strategies. Eur Rev Med Pharmacol Sci 2019;23(1):303–11.

191. Hayes D Jr, Harhay MO, Cherikh WS et al; International Society for Heart and Lung Transplantation. Heart Transplantation, adult recipients. Focus theme: trends in recipient characteristics and impact on outcomes. J Heart Lung Transplant 2021;40(10):1023–72: slide deck, slide 35.

192. Lee MS, Tadwalkar RV, Fearon WF, et al. Cardiac allograft vasculopathy: a review. Catheter Cardiovasc Interv 2018;92(7):E527–E36.

193. Chih S, Chong AY, Mielniczuk LM, et al. Allograft vasculopathy: the Achilles' heel of heart transplantation. J Am Coll Cardiol 2016;68(1):80–91.

194. Kobashigawa JA, Moriguchi JD, Laks H, et al. Ten-year follow-up of a randomized trial of pravastatin in heart transplant patients. J Heart Lung Transplant 2005;24(11):1736–40.

195. Wenke K, Meiser B, Thiery J, et al. Simvastatin initiated early after heart transplantation: 8-year prospective experience. Circulation 2003;107(1):93–7.

196. Keogh A, Richardson M, Ruygrok P, et al. Sirolimus in de novo heart transplant recipients reduces acute rejection and prevents coronary artery disease at 2 years: a randomized clinical trial. Circulation 2004;110(17):2694–700.

197. Eisen H. Long-term cardiovascular risk in transplantation – insights from the use of everolimus in heart transplantation. Nephrol Dial Transplant 2006;21(Suppl 3):iii9–13.

198. Asleh R, Briasoulis A, Smith B, et al. Association of aspirin treatment with cardiac allograft vasculopathy progression and adverse outcomes after heart transplantation. J Card Fail 2021;27(5):542–51.

199. Kim M, Bergmark BA, Zelniker TA, et al. Early aspirin use and the development of cardiac allograft vasculopathy. J Heart Lung Transplant 2017;36(12):1344–9.

200. Erinc K, Yamani MH, Starling RC, et al. The effect of combined angiotensin-converting enzyme inhibition and calcium antagonism on allograft coronary vasculopathy validated by intravascular ultrasound. J Heart Lung Transplant 2005;24(8):1033–8.

201. Kittleson MM. The role of intravascular ultrasound in heart transplant recipients in the modern era. J Card Fail 2021;27(4):473–6.

202. Kobashigawa JA, Tobis JM, Starling RC, et al. Multicenter intravascular ultrasound validation study among heart transplant recipients: outcomes after five years. J Am Coll Cardiol 2005;45(9):1532–7.

203. Tuzcu EM, Kapadia SR, Sachar R, et al. Intravascular ultrasound evidence of angiographically silent progression in coronary atherosclerosis predicts long-term morbidity and mortality after cardiac transplantation. J Am Coll Cardiol 2005;45(9):1538–42.

204. Mehra MR, Crespo-Leiro MG, Dipchand A, et al. International Society for Heart and Lung Transplantation working formulation of a standardized nomenclature for cardiac allograft vasculopathy – 2010. J Heart Lung Transplant 2010;29(7):717–27.

205. Jaamaa-Holmberg S, Salmela B, Lemstrom K, et al. Cancer incidence and mortality after heart transplantation – a population-based national cohort study. Acta Oncol 2019;58(6):859–63.

206. Na R, Grulich AE, Meagher NS, et al. De novo cancer-related death in Australian liver and cardiothoracic transplant recipients. Am J Transplant 2013;13(5):1296–304.

207. De Rosa N, Paddon V, Glanville A, et al. Dermatological disease in Australian heart and lung transplant recipients. Dermatology 2021;237(4):629–34.

208. Veness MJ, Quinn DI, Ong CS, et al. Aggressive cutaneous malignancies following cardiothoracic transplantation: the Australian experience. Cancer 1999;85(8):1758–64.

209. Aversa SM, Stragliotto S, Marino D, et al. Post-transplant lymphoproliferative disorders after heart or kidney transplantation at a single centre: presentation and response to treatment. Acta Haematol 2008;120(1):36–46.

210. Sica A, Rimini MLDE, Sagnelli C, Casale B, et al. Post-heart transplantation lymphoproliferative diseases (PTLDs) and the diagnostic role of [18f] FDG-PET/CT. Minerva Med 2021;112(3):338–45.

211. Alba AC, Bain E, Ng N, et al. Complications after heart transplantation: hope for the best, but prepare for the worst. Int J Transplant Res Med 2016;2(2):1–11.

212. Andreassen AK, Andersson B, Gustafsson F, et al. Everolimus initiation with early calcineurin inhibitor withdrawal in de novo heart transplant recipients: three-year results from the randomized SCHEDULE study. Am J Transplant 2016;16(4):1238–47.

213. Ahmed SB, Waikar SS, Rennke HG, et al. Cardiac transplantation and cyclosporine nephrotoxicity. Kidney Int 2007;72(8):1029–33.

214. Grupper A, Grupper A, Daly RC, et al. Kidney transplantation as a therapeutic option for end-stage renal disease developing after heart transplantation. J Heart Lung Transplant 2017;36(3):297–304.

215. Eisen HJ. Hypertension in heart transplant recipients: more than just cyclosporine. J Am Coll Cardiol 2003;41(3):433–4.

216. McCormack PL, Keating GM. Tacrolimus: in heart transplant recipients. Drugs 2006;66(17):2269–79; discussion 2280–2.

217. Penninga L, Moller CH, Gustafsson F, et al. Tacrolimus versus cyclosporine as primary immunosuppression after heart transplantation: systematic review with meta-analyses and trial sequential analyses of randomised trials. Eur J Clin Pharmacol 2010;66(12):1177–87.

218. Przybylowski P, Malyszko J, Malyszko JS, et al. Blood pressure control in orthotopic heart transplant and kidney allograft recipients is far from satisfactory. Transplant Proc 2010;42(10):4263–6.

219. Heegaard B, Nelson LM, Gustafsson F. Steroid withdrawal after heart transplantation in adults. Transpl Int 2021;34(12):2469–82.

220. Feng KY, Henricksen EJ, Wayda B, et al. Impact of diabetes mellitus on clinical outcomes after heart transplantation. Clin Transplant 2021;35(11):e14460.

221. Shivaswamy V, Boerner B, Larsen J. Post-transplant diabetes mellitus: causes, treatment, and impact on outcomes. Endocr Rev 2016; 37(1):37–61.

222. Austroads. Assessing fitness to drive; conditional licences and periodic review; medical standards for licensing – cardiovascular conditions – heart transplant. Sydney, NSW: Austroads; 2022. Available from: https://austroads.com.au/publications/assessing-fitness-to-drive/ap-g56/cardiovascular-conditions/medical-standards-for-licensing-1/conditional-licences-and-periodic-review#Standards_cardio. [Accessed March 2023].

223. Defilippis EM, Kittleson MM. Pregnancy after heart transplantation. J Card Fail 2021;27(2):176–84.

224. Boyle S, Sung-Him Mew T, et al. Pregnancy following heart transplantation: a single centre case series and review of the literature. Heart Lung Circ 2021;30(1):144–53.

Chapter 13

Respiratory assessment and monitoring

Kalliopi Kydonaki, Rachael Parke

Learning objectives

After reading this chapter, you should be able to:

- understand respiratory anatomy and normal physiology
- understand mechanisms contributing to altered respiratory function
- identify key principles underpinning assessment and monitoring of respiratory function
- describe nursing assessment and monitoring activities for critically ill patients with respiratory dysfunction
- discuss the importance of patient assessment skills, and the contribution of diagnostic and laboratory findings to ongoing clinical management
- outline the physiological basis for different types of monitoring
- describe common diagnostic procedures used in critical care.

Introduction

The respiratory system ensures adequate tissue and cellular oxygenation for the body. It is responsible for gas exchange through the uptake of oxygen (O_2) and excretion of carbon dioxide (CO_2), assists in optimal organ function, contributes to acid–base balance and plays a large role in maintaining homeostasis. As respiratory conditions account for large numbers of admissions to ICUs, a thorough understanding of the anatomy, physiology and pathophysiology of this complex system is required to accurately assess critically ill patients and monitor response to treatment or early signs of deterioration. Recent studies have reported that the prevalence of respiratory viral illnesses was as high as 16–41% in critically ill patients with community-acquired pneumonia and 17–29% in patients admitted with hospital-acquired pneumonia.[1-3]

In this chapter a comprehensive description of the principles and practice of respiratory assessment, monitoring and diagnostics is provided. These are foundational concepts underpinning timely and effective interventions for critically ill patients. Management of respiratory alterations, oxygenation and ventilation is discussed in Chapters 14 and 15.

Related anatomy and physiology

The thoracic cavity contains the trachea and bronchial tree, the two lungs, the pleura and the diaphragm. The mediastinum, located between the lungs, houses and protects the heart, great vessels and the oesophagus. Twelve pairs of ribs cover the lungs. Ten are connected to the spine posteriorly and to the sternum or to the cartilage of the above rib anteriorly (ribs 8–10). The 11th and 12th ribs have no anterior attachment (Fig. 13.1).[4]

The respiratory system is divided into the upper and lower respiratory tracts: the upper airways consist of the nose, nasal conchae, sinus and pharynx; the lower respiratory tract includes the larynx, trachea, bronchi and lungs.[5] Larger airways are lined with stratified epithelial tissue, which has a relatively high cellular turnover rate; these cells protect and clear these large airways. Additional specialised features of this tissue include an extensive distribution of mucous/goblet cells and cilia, which facilitate the mucociliary clearance system of the airway.

Upper respiratory tract

The nasal cavities contain an extremely vascular and mucoid environment for warming and humidifying inhaled gases. To maximise exposure to this surface area, the nasal conchae create turbulent gas flow. Mucus is moved by the cilia at the top of the epithelial cells lining the conducting airways. Mucus moves towards the pharynx at a rate of 1–2 cm per minute, providing filtration and cleaning of the inhaled air. One litre of mucus is produced every day, with only a small part not reabsorbed by the body.[6]

The pharynx is a muscular tube that transports food to the oesophagus and air to the larynx. Inferior to the pharynx, the larynx consists mostly of cartilage attached to other surrounding structures and houses the vestibular (false) vocal folds, which do not produce any sounds but help to close the larynx during swallowing. The lower true vocal cords create the vocal sounds (Fig. 13.2).[7] The pyramid-shaped arytenoids, an important pair of cartilages within the larynx, act as attachment points for the vocal cords. This area is easily damaged, causing arytenoid subluxation. Protrusion of an endotracheal tube stylet, an unanticipated difficult airway leading to prolonged or traumatic intubations, the use of a gum elastic bougie, blind intubation techniques (e.g. utilisation of a lighted stylet or light-wand) and insertion of bulky double-lumen tubes have all been implicated in injury of the arytenoids.[8] The thyroid cartilage ('Adam's apple') and the cricoid cartilage protect the glottis and entrance to the trachea. Another cartilage in the larynx is the leaf-shaped elastic epiglottis, which protects the lower airways from aspiration of food and fluids into the lungs. The epiglottis usually occludes the inlet to the larynx during swallowing. The primitive cough, swallow and gag reflexes further protect the airway.[6] Laryngospasm is a dangerous complication

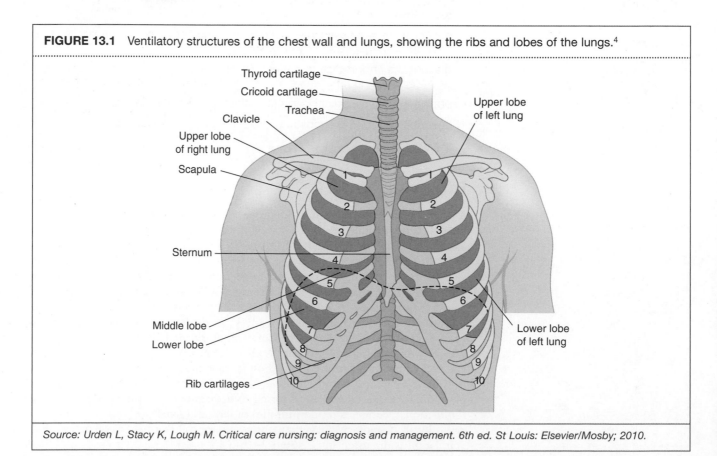

FIGURE 13.1   Ventilatory structures of the chest wall and lungs, showing the ribs and lobes of the lungs.[4]

Source: Urden L, Stacy K, Lough M. Critical care nursing: diagnosis and management. 6th ed. St Louis: Elsevier/Mosby; 2010.

FIGURE 13.2 Larynx. **(A)** Cartilages and ligaments. **(B)** Neck muscles.[7]

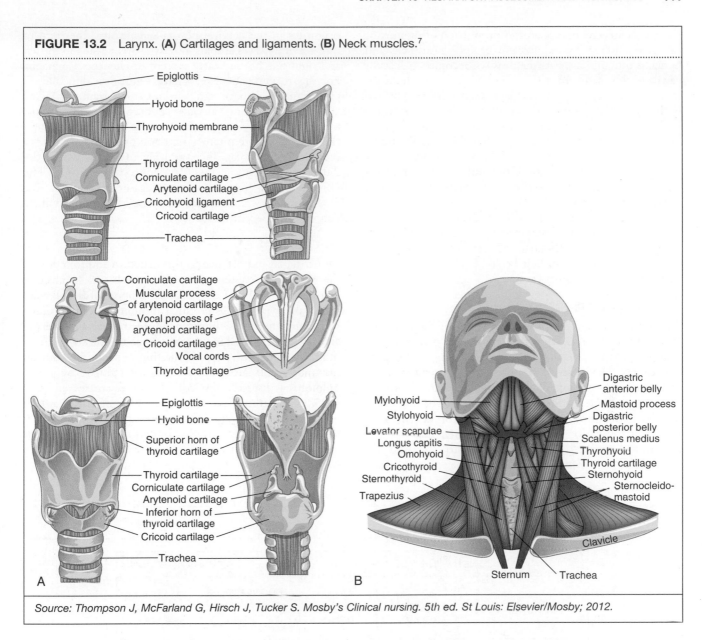

Source: Thompson J, McFarland G, Hirsch J, Tucker S. Mosby's Clinical nursing. 5th ed. St Louis: Elsevier/Mosby; 2012.

caused by irritation of the vocal cords. When the muscles of the vocal cords spasm, the flow of air into the lungs is restricted, leading to airway obstruction. Laryngospasm can be triggered by suctioning of the airways in non-intubated patients or when intubation is performed.[9]

Lower respiratory tract

The trachea is a hollow tube approximately 11 cm long and 2.5 cm in diameter that marks the beginning of the lower respiratory tract. The trachea is supported by 16–20 C-shaped cartilages and is another area at risk of pressure damage from artificial airways. The trachea divides at the carina into the left and right main bronchi. The bronchial tree has two main-stem bronchi that are structurally different. The right bronchus is wider and angles slightly, where it divides further into the three lobes of the right lung. The most common site of aspiration of foreign objects is the right bronchus because of its anatomical position. The acutely angled left main bronchus divides further into the two lobes of the left lung.

The airways within each lung branch further into secondary (or lobar) bronchi, then tertiary (or segmental) bronchi. Further divisions within these conducting airways end with the terminal bronchioles, the smallest airways without alveoli. These conducting airways do not participate in gas exchange but rather form the anatomical dead space (approximately 150 mL).[10] This anatomical dead space provides the important function of humidifying and warming inspired air. It is important to remember that, when a patient is mechanically ventilated, the ventilator tubing extends the dead space and may reduce the volume of fresh air that reaches the patient; this may be similar to the experience of breathing through a snorkel.

Larger airways have a greater proportion of supporting cartilage, ciliated epithelium, goblet and serous cells and, hence, a mucous layer. As the airways become smaller, the cartilage transition from C-shaped rings, which hold the trachea open, to strips of cartilage, then finally to airways with no cartilage but with smooth muscle that forms the walls of the bronchioles. The importance of this is that the diameter of the bronchioles is, therefore, totally under autonomic nervous system control. Smooth muscle surrounds and supports the bronchioles, enabling airway diameter change and subsequent changes in airway resistance to gas flow.[11]

The number of goblet cells and amount of mucus decrease until, at the alveolar level, there is only a single layer of squamous epithelial cells. Alveolar macrophages present among these epithelial cells phagocytose any small particles that enter the alveoli.

Thorax/lungs

The lungs and heart are protected within the thoracic cage. When inspiration is triggered, expansion of the thorax creates a negative pressure, causing air to flow into the lungs. The thorax then passively compresses to expel air from the lungs during expiration. The diaphragm separates the thorax from the abdomen and is the most important inspiratory muscle, performing approximately 80% of the work of breathing. Inspiration is initiated from the medulla, sending impulses through the phrenic nerve to stimulate the diaphragm to contract and flatten. The phrenic nerve originates in the cervical plexus and involves the third to fifth cervical nerves. It splits into two parts, passing to the left and right side of the heart before it reaches the diaphragm. For this reason, patients can have ventilation difficulties if phrenic nerve damage results from C3–C5 trauma.[12]

The conducting airways, ending in the terminal bronchioles, move inspired air towards the respiratory unit (Fig. 13.3).[7] The respiratory unit comprises the respiratory bronchioles, alveolar ducts and alveolar sacs, where the diffusion of gas molecules, or gas exchange, occurs. The pores of Kohn help to distribute gases between alveoli. The respiratory unit makes up most of the lung with a volume of 2.5–3 litres during rest.[11]

Surfactant

Of particular importance to the structure and function of the respiratory system are the types I and II alveolar epithelial cells. Type I cells provide support of the alveolar unit walls. Type II cells produce an important lipoprotein, surfactant, that lines the inner alveolar surface, lowering alveolar surface tension, stabilising the alveoli to optimise lung compliance and facilitating expansion during inspiration.[11] If surfactant synthesis is reduced owing to pulmonary disease, lung compliance decreases and the work of breathing increases. The role of surfactant in managing the respiratory function of premature infants is well described and inactivation or dysfunction of surfactant in adults can contribute to lung disease such as acute respiratory distress syndrome (ARDS).[13]

FIGURE 13.3 Lower airway branches.[7]

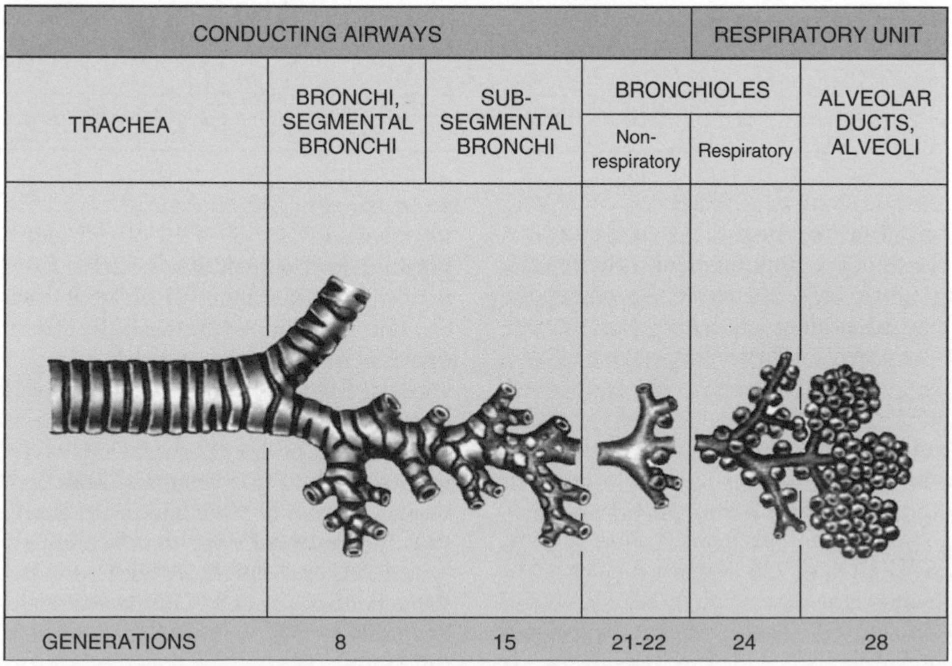

CONDUCTING AIRWAYS					RESPIRATORY UNIT
TRACHEA	BRONCHI, SEGMENTAL BRONCHI	SUB-SEGMENTAL BRONCHI	BRONCHIOLES		ALVEOLAR DUCTS, ALVEOLI
			Non-respiratory	Respiratory	
GENERATIONS	8	15	21-22	24	28

Source: Thompson J, McFarland G, Hirsch J, Tucker S. Mosby's Clinical nursing. 5th ed. St Louis: Elsevier/Mosby; 2012.

Pleura

Each lung is contained within a continuous thin membrane called the pleura, creating the pleural sac that surrounds each lung. The two pleural sacs, one on each side of the midline, are separate from each other. The parietal pleura lines the inner surface of the chest wall and is in close contact with the visceral pleura, which covers the lungs. The pleural space, between these two layers, contains a small amount of serous fluid, which limits friction during lung expansion.[14]

The intrapleural pressure in the pleural space under normal circumstances is always negative with a range of −4 to −10 cmH$_2$O; this negative pressure keeps the lungs inflated. During inhalation the pressure becomes more negative as both the lungs and the chest wall are elastic structures. These elastic fibres of the lung pull the visceral pleura inwards while the chest wall pulls the parietal pleura outwards. The pressure difference between the alveolar pressure (0 cmH$_2$O pressure in the lungs) and the intrapleural pressure (−4 cmH$_2$O) across the lung wall is termed the transpulmonary pressure (+4 cmH$_2$O[0 − (−4) = +4]), and is the force that holds the lungs open[14] (Fig. 13.4).[15]

Pulmonary circulation

The circulatory system of the lungs receives the entire cardiac output but operates as a low-pressure system; it directs blood only back to the left side of the heart (unlike the systemic circulation, which pumps blood to different regions of the entire body). Within the pulmonary circulation, the right ventricle pumps oxygen-depleted blood to the lungs via the pulmonary artery, with oxygen-rich blood returning to the left atrium via the pulmonary veins. Pulmonary blood vessels follow the path of the bronchioles, with capillaries forming a dense network in the walls of the alveoli. As illustrated in Fig. 13.5,[16,17] the entire surface area of the alveolar wall is covered by capillaries, just large enough for a red blood cell to pass through, allowing gas exchange.

Pulmonary vessels are short and thin and have relatively little smooth muscle. The pressure inside the vessels is remarkably low (normal pulmonary artery pressure is only 25/8 mmHg; mean 15 mmHg).[11] This low-pressure system ensures that right heart workload is minimised, while promoting efficient gas exchange in the lungs (Fig. 13.6).[10]

Bronchial circulation

The bronchial circulation, part of the systemic circulation, supplies oxygenated blood, nutrients and heat to the conducting airways (to the level of the terminal bronchioles) and to the pleura. Drainage of this deoxygenated blood is predominantly through the bronchial network, although some capillaries drain into the pulmonary arterial circulation, contributing to venous admixture or right-to-left shunt[11] (see Pathophysiology section for further discussion).

Control of ventilation

Normal breathing occurs automatically and is a complex function not fully understood. It is coordinated by the

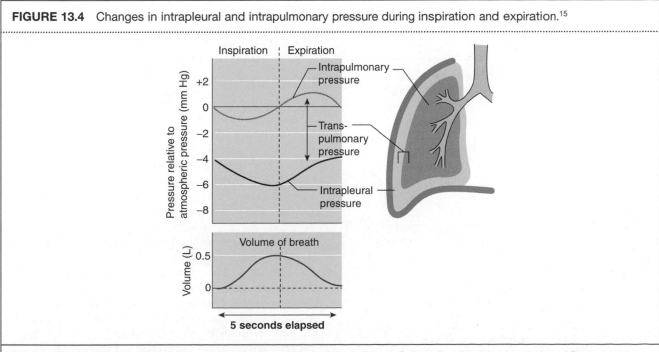

FIGURE 13.4 Changes in intrapleural and intrapulmonary pressure during inspiration and expiration.[15]

FIGURE 13.5 Terminal ventilation and perfusion units of the lung.[17]

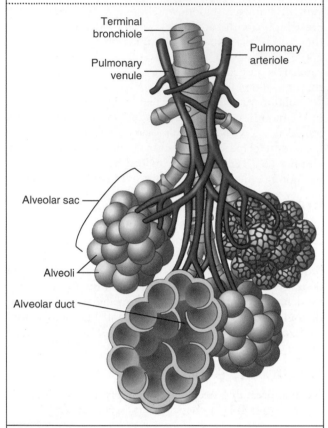

Source: Urden LD, Stacy KM, Lough ME. Critical care nursing: diagnosis and management. 7th ed. St Louis: Elsevier/Mosby; 2014.

FIGURE 13.6 Comparison of pressure in the pulmonary and systematic circulations (mmHg).[10]

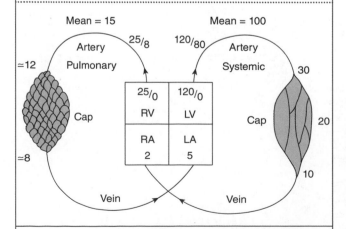

Source: West J, Luks A. Respiratory physiology: the essentials. 10th ed. Philadelphia: Wolters Kluwer; 2016.

respiratory centre, regulated by controllers in the brain, effectors in the muscles and sensors including chemoreceptors and mechanoreceptors. There are also protective reflexes such as sneezing and coughing that respond to respiratory tract irritation by mechanical or chemical stimuli. Sneezing clears the upper respiratory tract and coughing clears the lower respiratory tract. The larynx and carina are particularly sensitive to mechanical stimuli, requiring only minor irritants to stimulate a cough. The terminal bronchioles and alveoli are responsive to chemical stimuli such as chlorine or sulphur dioxide gas.[18]

Controller

In the brainstem, the medulla oblongata and the pons regulate automatic ventilation while the cerebral cortex regulates voluntary ventilation (Fig. 13.7).[15] The respiratory rhythmic centre in the medulla can be divided into inspiratory and expiratory centres, with the following functions:[11]

- The inspiratory centre (or dorsal respiratory group) triggers inspiration.

- The expiratory centre (or ventral respiratory group) functions only during forced respiration and active expiration.

- The pneumotaxic and apneustic centres in the pons adjust the rate and pattern of breathing.

- The cerebral cortex provides conscious voluntary control over the respiratory muscles. This voluntary control cannot be maintained when the partial pressure of carbon dioxide in the arterial blood ($PaCO_2$) and the hydrogen ion (H^+) concentration become markedly elevated; an example is the inability to hold your breath for very long. Emotional and autonomic activities also affect the pace and depth of breathing.

Effectors

The diaphragm is the major muscle of inspiration, although the external intercostal muscles also contribute. The accessory muscles of inspiration (the scalenes, sternocleidomastoid muscles and pectoralis minor) are active only during exercise or strenuous breathing. Expiration is a passive act and only the internal intercostal muscles are involved at rest. During exercise, the abdominal muscles also contribute to expiration. Inspiration is triggered by a stimulus from the medulla, causing downward contraction of the diaphragm, and contraction of external intercostal muscles, lifting the thorax up and out. This action lowers pressure within the alveoli (intra-alveolar pressure) relative to atmospheric pressure. Air rushes into the lungs to equalise the pressure gradient. After contraction has ceased, the ribs and diaphragm relax, the pressure gradient reverses and air is passively expelled from the lungs, which return to their resting state because of elastic recoil.

FIGURE 13.7 Respiratory centres and reflex.[15]

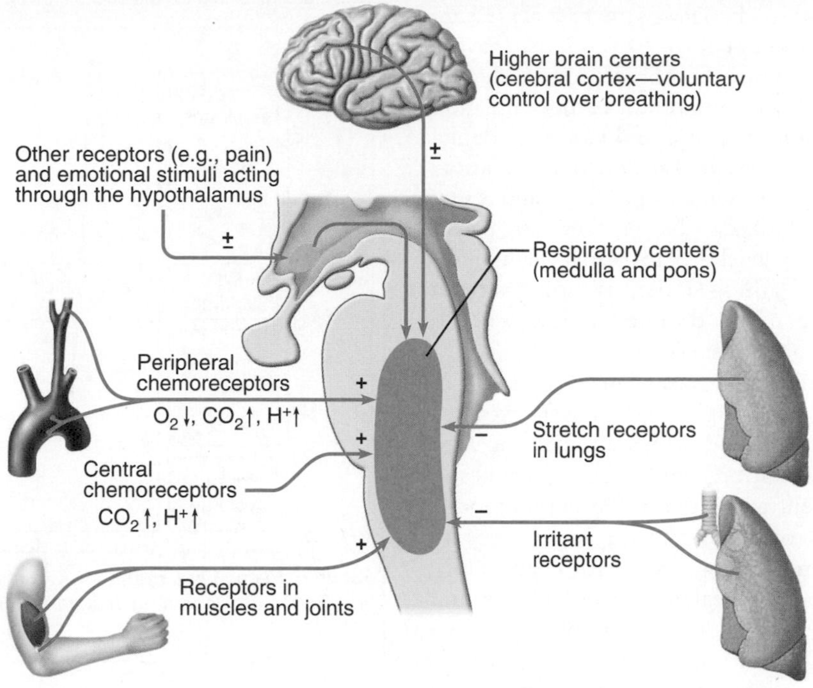

Source: Elaine N. Marieb, Katja Hoehn. Human anatomy and physiology. 8th ed. © 2010 Reprinted by permission of Pearson Education, Inc., New York.

BOX 13.1

Oxygen delivery in COPD

Patients with chronic respiratory conditions including COPD often exhibit signs of hypoxia and hypercarbia, particularly during an acute exacerbation of a chronic condition. There is a strongly held belief that patients who chronically retain CO_2 no longer have a central chemoreceptor response to increased $PaCO_2$ and their drive to breathe is in relation to peripheral chemoreceptor response which detects hypoxia. However, the control of ventilation in such patients is highly complex and involves adaptations of the respiratory control system including changes to respiratory muscles, chemoreceptor signalling and central respiratory drive.[19] While it is true that an uncontrolled administration of oxygen to patients who chronically retain CO_2 results in hypercarbia, this is mainly because of reversal of hypoxic vasoconstriction and changes to ventilation and perfusion matching. To a lesser extent, arterial CO_2 increases because of a rightward shift in the CO_2 dissociation curve (the Haldane effect).[20]

Those patients most likely to develop hypercarbia associated with oxygen administration are also those with significant hypoxaemia. For patients who chronically retain CO_2 and are hypoxic, the hypoxia must be treated and should be tailored to the patient's clinical condition. Evidence suggests that aiming for oxygen saturation between 88% and 92% results in improved patient outcome.[20] For more in-depth description of the physiological changes associated with COPD, please refer to Further reading at the end of this chapter.

Sensors

A chemoreceptor is a sensor that responds to a change in the chemical composition of the blood; there are two types: central and peripheral. Central chemoreceptors account for 70% of the feedback controlling ventilation and respond quickly to changes in the pH of cerebrospinal fluid and increases in $PaCO_2$.[14] If the $PaCO_2$ remains high for a prolonged period, as in chronic obstructive pulmonary disease (COPD), a compensatory change in bicarbonate (HCO_3^-) occurs and the pH in cerebrospinal fluid returns to its near-normal value (Box 13.1).[19,20]

Central chemoreceptors located in the medulla respond to changes in H^+ concentration in the surrounding cerebrospinal fluid. A change in the $PaCO_2$ causes movement of CO_2 across the blood–brain barrier into the cerebrospinal fluid and alters the H^+ concentration. This increase in H^+ stimulates ventilation. Central chemoreceptors do not, however, respond to changes in the partial pressure of oxygen in arterial blood (PaO_2). Opiates also have a negative influence on these chemoreceptors, reducing sensitivity to changing H^+ concentration.[11] Hyperventilation may reduce $PaCO_2$ to a level that could cause accidental unconsciousness if the breath is held after hyperventilation. This phenomenon is well known among divers and is due to increasing levels of CO_2 as the primary trigger of breathing. If the CO_2 level is too low owing to hyperventilation, the breathing reflex is not triggered until the level of oxygen has dropped below what is necessary to maintain consciousness.

Peripheral chemoreceptors also play a role in controlling ventilation, although to a lesser extent.[21] Located in the common carotid arteries and in the arch of the aorta, peripheral chemoreceptors detect changes in $PaCO_2$ and H^+ concentration/pH in arterial blood.[11] Peripheral chemoreceptors are sensitive to changes in PaO_2 and are the primary responders to hypoxaemia, stimulating the glossopharyngeal and vagus nerves and providing feedback to the medulla. In response to low PaO_2, such as below 70 mmHg (8 kilopascals (kPa)),[11] they are stimulated and contribute to maintaining ventilation. Other receptors include stretch receptors located in the lungs, which inhibit inspiration and protect the lungs from overinflation (Hering–Breuer reflex), and in the muscles and joints (see Fig. 13.7).

Pulmonary volumes and capacities

In healthy individuals, the lungs are readily distensible or compliant; when exposed to high, expanding pressures or in disease states, compliance is increased or decreased. Ranges of lung volumes and capacities are illustrated in Fig. 13.8.[22] Tidal volume is the volume of air entering the lungs during a single inspiration and is normally equal to the volume leaving the lungs on expiration (around 500 mL). During inspiration, the tidal volume of inspired air is added to the 2400 mL of air already in the lungs. This remaining volume of air in the lungs after normal expiration is the functional residual capacity,[14] which:

- has an important role in keeping small alveoli open and avoiding atelectasis
- can be reduced during anaesthesia or neuromuscular blockade, most likely due to supine positioning, loss of muscle tone and resulting atelectasis[23]
- if reduced, results in the smallest alveoli closing at the end of the expiration (the 'closing volume').

The closing volume plus the residual volume is called the 'closing capacity'. The closure of the smallest airways may occur because dependent areas of the lungs are compressed, although this is not the only mechanism as these airways also close in the weightlessness of space. The closing volume is dependent on patient age: in a young healthy person it is 10% of vital capacity while for an

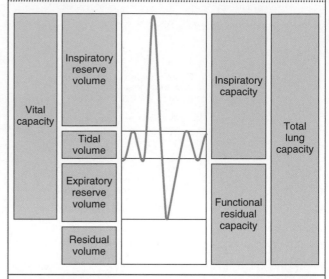

FIGURE 13.8 For lung volume measurements, all values are approximately 25% lower in women.[22]

Source: Pagana KD, Pagana TJ, Pagana TN. (2017). Mosby's diagnostic and laboratory test reference. 13th ed. Philadelphia: Elsevier.

individual aged 65 years it increases to 40%, approximating total functional residual capacity.[11]

Alveolar ventilation

Minute volume represents the volume of gas inhaled or exhaled in 1 minute and is calculated by multiplying the tidal volume by the respiratory frequency (e.g. 500 mL × 12 breaths per min = 6000 mL).[24] In this example only the first 350 mL of inhaled air in each breath reaches the alveolar exchange surface, with 150 mL remaining in the conducting airways, referred to as the 'anatomical dead space'. Alveolar ventilation is the amount of inhaled air that reaches the alveoli each minute (e.g. 350 mL × 12 = 4200 mL of alveolar ventilation).[11]

Work of breathing

At rest, the energy required to breathe is minimal (less than 5% of total oxygen consumption).[11] However, changes in airway resistance and lung compliance affect the work of breathing, resulting in increased oxygen consumption.[24] Airway resistance is determined by the diameter of the airways and the air flow: laminar air flow creates lower resistance whereas turbulent air flow creates higher resistance. Airway resistance is not constant. Certain disease states impact airway resistance – for example, during an exacerbation of asthma, where the constricted airways increase resistance.[11] As noted earlier, the lungs are very distensible, expanding during inspiration. This expansion is called the elastic or compliance work and it refers to the ease with which lungs expand under pressure. Lung compliance is often monitored when patients are mechanically ventilated, and is calculated by dividing the change in lung volume by the change in transpulmonary pressure (i.e. the difference between the alveolar pressure and pleural pressure).[23] For the lung to expand, it must overcome lung viscosity and chest wall tissue (called tissue resistance work). Finally, there is airway resistance work – the movement of air into the lungs via the airways. The work associated with resistance and compliance is easily overcome in healthy individuals, but in pulmonary disease both resistance work and compliance work are increased.[23] During exertion, when increased muscle function heightens metabolic rate, oxygen demand rises to match consumption and avoid anaerobic metabolism, and the work of breathing is increased. The term 'work of breathing' is often used in critical illness, when basic respiratory processes are challenged and breathing consumes a far greater proportion of total energy.

Principles of gas transport and exchange in alveoli and tissues

Oxygen and CO_2 are transported in the bloodstream between alveoli and the tissue cells. Delivery of oxygen to tissues and transfer of CO_2 from the tissues to the capillaries occurs by diffusion and is therefore dependent on the pressure gradient between the capillary and the cell. Diffusion involves molecules moving from areas of high concentration to those of low concentration. Other determinants of the rate of diffusion include the thickness of the alveolar membrane, the surface area of the membrane available for gas transfer and the inherent solubility of the gas. Carbon dioxide diffuses about 20 times more rapidly than oxygen, being much more soluble in blood.[25] At the most distal ends of the conducting airways lies an extensive network of approximately 300 million alveoli. The surface area of the lungs, if spread out flat, would be about 90 m^2 – about 40 times greater than the surface area of the skin.[14] Gas exchange occurs through the exceptionally thin alveolar membranes. Oxygen uptake takes place from the external environment via the lungs through to the blood in the adjacent alveolar capillary networks. Similarly, CO_2 diffuses from the capillaries to the alveoli and is then expired.

Oxygen transport

In oxygenated blood transported by the pulmonary capillaries, there are 20 mL of oxygen in each 100 mL of blood. Oxygen is transported in two ways: dissolved in plasma (about 0.3 mL; 1.5%) with the remainder bound to haemoglobin.[11] Measured by arterial blood gases (ABGs), the 1.5% of oxygen dissolved in blood constitutes the PaO_2.[6] One gram of haemoglobin carries 1.34 mL of oxygen. The level of saturation within the total circulating haemoglobin can be measured clinically, by pulse oximetry. The amount of oxygen actually bound to haemoglobin compared with the amount of oxygen the haemoglobin can carry is commonly reported as arterial oxygen saturation (SaO_2). Oxygen is attached to the haemoglobin molecule at four haem sites. As the majority of oxygen

transport is via haemoglobin, if all four sites are occupied by oxygen molecules the blood is determined to be 'fully saturated' ($SaO_2 = 100\%$).[23]

A large reserve of oxygen is available if required, without the need for any increase in respiratory or cardiac workload. Oxygen extraction is the percentage of oxygen extracted and utilised by the tissues. At rest, just 25% of the total oxygen delivered to the tissue is extracted, although this amount does vary throughout the body, with some tissue beds extracting more and others taking less. Normally, the oxygen saturation of venous blood is 60–75%; values below this indicate that more oxygen than normal is being extracted by tissues. This can be due to a reduction in oxygen delivery to the tissues or to an increase in the tissue consumption of oxygen.[11]

Oxygen delivery and oxygen consumption are important considerations in the management of critically ill patients. Normal oxygen delivery in a healthy person at rest is approximately 1000 mL/min. Normal oxygen consumption is 200–250 mL/min,[11] but this can increase significantly during episodes of sepsis, fever, hypercatabolism and shivering.[23] The difference between normal delivery and normal consumption highlights the large degree of oxygen reserve available to the body.

Oxygen–haemoglobin dissociation curve

As blood is transported to the tissues and end-organs, the tendency of haemoglobin and oxygen to combine decreases relative to the surrounding arterial oxygen tension. This relationship is illustrated by the oxygen–haemoglobin dissociation curve (Fig. 13.9).[26] As oxygen is offloaded at the tissue level, CO_2 binds more readily with haemoglobin, to be transported back to the lungs for removal.[6]

The oxygen–haemoglobin dissociation curve relates the partial pressure of oxygen (PaO_2) to the haemoglobin saturation in blood. While the initial part of the curve rises steeply, the latter part of the curve flattens, representing the binding of oxygen to haemoglobin in the lungs. In the upper part of the curve (within the lungs), relatively large changes in the PaO_2 cause only small changes in haemoglobin saturation. Therefore, if the PaO_2 drops from 100 to 60 mmHg (14–8 kPa), the saturation of haemoglobin changes by only 7% (from a normal 97% to 90%). As long as PaO_2 remains above 60 mmHg (7.8 kPa), haemoglobin will be more than 90% saturated. The minimal changes in oxygen binding within this substantial PO_2 range allow survival at high altitudes.[11] The lower portion (steep component) of the oxygen–haemoglobin dissociation curve, between 40 and 60 mmHg (5–8 kPa), represents the release of oxygen from haemoglobin in tissue capillaries. At this point, a small drop in PaO_2 will cause a large increase in oxygen unloading. As haemoglobin is further desaturated, larger amounts of oxygen are released for tissue use, ensuring an adequate oxygen supply to peripheral tissues even when oxygen delivery is reduced. Oxygen saturation remains at 70–75%, leaving a significant amount of oxygen in reserve. Normally only 25% of

FIGURE 13.9 Shift of the oxygen–haemoglobin dissociation curve: (**A**) to the right and (**B**) to the left.[26]

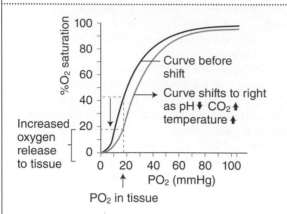

In the tissues, the oxygen–haemoglobin dissociation curve shifts to the right. As pH decreases, PCO_2 increases, or as temperature rises, the curve (black) shifts to the right (blue), resulting in an increased release of oxygen.

A

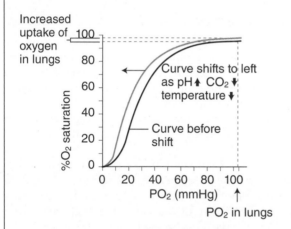

In the lungs, the oxygen–haemoglobin dissociation curve shifts to the left. As pH increases, PCO_2 decreases, or as temperature falls, the curve (black) shifts to the left (blue), resulting in an increased ability of haemoglobin to pick up oxygen.

B

Source: Seely R, Stephens T, Tate P. Anatomy and physiology. 7th ed. Boston: McGraw Hill; 2006.

bound oxygen is unloaded during one systemic circuit. However, during exercise, when the muscles need more oxygen, the PaO_2 drops and more oxygen dissociates from haemoglobin for use by muscle cells without any complementary increase in respiratory rate or cardiac output.[11]

The relationship between the two axes of this curve assumes that values for haemoglobin, pH, temperature,

$PaCO_2$ and 2,3-bisphosphoglycerate, a product of the breakdown of red blood cells that binds reversibly with haemoglobin, are normal. Changes to any of these values will shift the curve to the right or left and therefore reflect different values for PaO_2 and SaO_2[11] (see Fig. 13.9).

Both the binding and the dissociation of oxygen to haemoglobin are reversible reactions depending on the surrounding tissue. When the curve shifts to the right there is a reduced capacity for oxygen binding to haemoglobin in the lungs, but oxygen is more readily released to the tissues. At a local level, in active tissue such as working muscle that generates lactic acid, acid release lowers the pH, resulting in release of oxygen from haemoglobin molecules to the surrounding tissue. The same process occurs when active skeletal muscle generates heat. The increase in local temperature leads to oxygen release for use by the surrounding muscle.[11]

As blood is transported to the tissues and end-organs, the binding affinity of haemoglobin and oxygen decreases relative to the surrounding arterial oxygen tension. As oxygen is offloaded at the tissue level, CO_2 binds more readily with haemoglobin, to be transported to the lungs for removal.[6]

Carbon dioxide transport

Carbon dioxide is transported by blood in three forms: combined with water as carbonic acid (80–90%), dissolved (5%) or attached to plasma proteins (5–10%) including haemoglobin. The dissolved CO_2 constitutes $PaCO_2$ and is measured by ABGs. The greater solubility of CO_2 compared with oxygen results in its rapid diffusion across the capillary membranes and its easy removal.[6] As a byproduct of cellular respiration, CO_2 is produced at a rate of 200 mL/min, with only minor differences in normal concentrations in arterial (480 mL/L) and venous (520 mL/L) blood.[27]

Relationship between ventilation and perfusion

Gas exchange is the key function of the lungs, and the unique anatomy of capillaries and alveoli facilitates this process. However, because of a number of physiological factors, the ventilation to perfusion ratio (V/Q) is not matched in a 1:1 relationship. As normal alveolar ventilation is about 4 L/min and pulmonary capillary perfusion is about 5 L/min, the normal V/Q is 0.8.[11] In addition, pressure in the pulmonary circulation is low relative to systemic pressure and is influenced much more by gravity and hydrostatic pressure. In the upright position, lung apices receive less perfusion compared with the bases.[11] In the supine position, apical and basal perfusions are almost equal, but the posterior (dependent) portion of the lungs receives greater perfusion than the anterior lung area. Ventilation is also uneven throughout the lung, with the bases receiving more ventilation per unit volume than the apices.[11]

Pressure within the surrounding alveoli also influences blood flow through the pulmonary capillary network. The pressure gradients between the arterial and venous ends of a capillary network normally determine blood flow.

However, alveolar pressure (P_A) can be greater than venous (P_v) and/or arterial (P_a) pressure, and this therefore influences blood flow and gas exchange.

For a patient in an upright position, perfusion and ventilation vary as follows:

- *Zone 1 (upper area of the lungs):* alveolar pressure is generally greater than both arterial and venous capillary pressure ($P_A > P_a > P_v$), and blood flow is reduced, leading to alveolar dead space (alveoli ventilated but not adequately perfused).
- *Zone 2 (middle portion of the lungs):* perfusion and gas exchange are influenced more by pressure differences between arterial and alveolar pressures than by the usual difference between arterial and venous pressures ($P_a > P_A > P_v$), with a normal V/Q ratio.
- *Zone 3 (lung bases):* alveolar pressure is lower than both arterial and venous pressures ($P_a > P_v > P_A$), and ventilation is reduced, leading to intrapulmonary shunting (alveoli perfused but not adequately ventilated)[11] (Fig. 13.10).[17]

These physiological relationships are more complex in a critically ill patient when ventilation and/or lung perfusion is further compromised by disease processes and positive pressure ventilation, and the patient is in a supine or semirecumbent position.[11,24]

Acid–base control: respiratory mechanisms

The respiratory system plays a vital role in acid–base balance. Changes in respiratory rate and depth can produce changes in body pH by altering the amount of carbonic acid (H_2CO_3) in the blood. The body has substantial control over acid–base balance by altering alveolar ventilation and the elimination of CO_2 through the lungs. The elimination of acid through the lungs is more than 100 times more efficient than the elimination of acid through the kidneys. If the level of CO_2 in body water increases because of low alveolar ventilation, more H^+ will be produced because CO_2 combines with H_2O to form H_2CO_3. This breaks down to HCO_3^- and H^+ resulting in a decrease in pH:

$$CO_2 + H_2O \leftrightarrow H_2CO_3 \leftrightarrow HCO_3^- + H^+$$

The strength of the dissociation is defined by the Henderson–Hasselbalch equation, which describes the relationship between HCO_3^-, CO_2 and pH, and explains why an increase in dissolved CO_2 causes an increase in the acidity of the plasma, while an increase in HCO_3^- causes the pH to rise, resulting in more alkaline plasma:

$$pH = 6.1 + log\,(HCO_3^-)(CO_2)$$

where 6.1 = the negative logarithm of the acid dissociation constant in plasma for carbonic acid.[11]

Respiratory acidosis is caused by CO_2 retention and it increases the denominator in the Henderson–Hasselbalch equation, resulting in a decreased pH level. In a spontaneously breathing patient, this condition is caused by hypoventilation from either shallow breaths and/or a low respiratory rate. In the acute state the body cannot compensate. If the patient develops chronic CO_2 retention over a long period, there will be a renal response to the increase in CO_2. The renal system retains HCO_3^- to

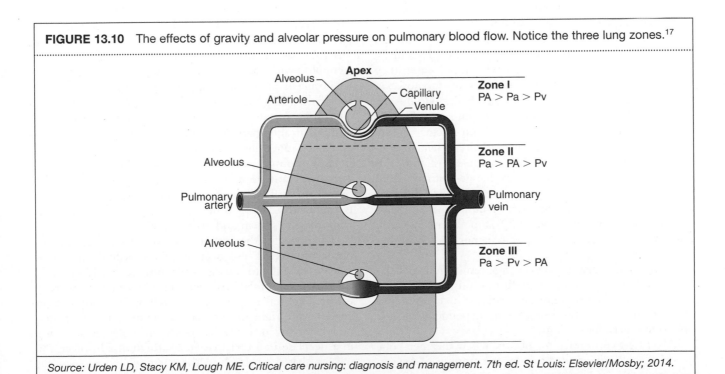

FIGURE 13.10   The effects of gravity and alveolar pressure on pulmonary blood flow. Notice the three lung zones.[17]

Source: Urden LD, Stacy KM, Lough ME. Critical care nursing: diagnosis and management. 7th ed. St Louis: Elsevier/Mosby; 2014.

return the pH to normal (i.e. respiratory acidosis is compensated).

Respiratory alkalosis occurs when a patient hyperventilates and alveolar ventilation is increased as a result of large, frequent breaths; CO_2 decreases in arterial blood and the pH rises. If this condition is maintained (e.g. walking at high altitude), the kidneys excrete HCO_3^- and the pH returns to normal (i.e. the respiratory alkalosis is compensated).[11]

Pathophysiology

Three common pathophysiological concepts that influence respiratory function in critically ill patients are hypoxaemia, inflammation and oedema. Related disease states including respiratory failure, pneumonia, ARDS, asthma and COPD are described in Chapter 14.

Hypoxaemia

Hypoxaemia describes a PaO_2 of less than 60 mmHg (7.99 kPa).[6] This leads to less-efficient anaerobic metabolism at the tissue and end-organ level and compromised cellular function. Hypoxia is abnormally low PO_2 in the tissues, and can be due to:

- 'hypoxic' hypoxia – low PaO_2 in arterial blood due to pulmonary disease
- 'circulatory' hypoxia – reduction of tissue blood flow due to shock or local obstruction
- 'anaemic' hypoxia – reduced ability of the blood to carry oxygen due to anaemia or carbon monoxide poisoning
- 'histotoxic' hypoxia – a cellular environment that does not support oxygen utilisation due to tissue poisoning (e.g. cyanide poisoning).[11]

A hypoxic patient can show symptoms of fatigue and shortness of breath if the hypoxia has developed gradually. If the patient has severe hypoxia with rapid onset, they will have ashen skin and blue discoloration (cyanosis) of the oral mucosa, lips and nail beds. Confusion, disorientation and anxiety are other symptoms. In later stages, unconsciousness, coma and death occur.[28] Acute respiratory failure is a common patient presentation in ICU, occurring in 10% of ICU admissions, and it is characterised by decreased gas exchange with resultant hypoxaemia. ARDS is one such example.[29] Two different mechanisms cause acute respiratory failure: type 1 presents with low PaO_2 and normal $PaCO_2$; type 2 presents with low PaO_2 and high $PaCO_2$ (see Chapter 14 for further discussion).

In general, impaired gas exchange results from alveolar hypoventilation, ventilation/perfusion mismatching and intrapulmonary shunting, each resulting in hypoxaemia. Hypercapnia may also be present, depending on the underlying pathophysiology.[30]

Alveolar hypoventilation occurs when the metabolic needs of the body are not met by the amount of oxygen delivered and CO_2 removed from the alveoli. Alveolar hypoventilation causing hypoxaemia is usually extrapulmonary (e.g. altered metabolism, interruption to neuromuscular control of breathing/ventilation) and is associated with hypercapnia.[31]

V/Q mismatch results when areas of lung that are perfused are not ventilated (no participation in gas exchange) because alveoli are collapsed or infiltrated with fluid from inflammation or infection (e.g. pulmonary oedema, pneumonia). This results in an overall reduction in blood oxygen levels, which is usually countered by compensatory mechanisms.[31]

Intrapulmonary shunting is an extreme case of V/Q mismatch. Shunting occurs when blood passes alveoli that are not ventilated. If there is significant intrapulmonary shunting, there may be overwhelming reductions in PaO_2.[32] Carbon dioxide levels may still be normal but, depending on the onset and progression of respiratory pathophysiology, compensatory mechanisms may not be able to maintain homeostasis[6] (Fig. 13.11).[33]

Tissue hypoxia

There are few physiological changes with mild hypoxaemia (when oxygen saturation remains at 90% despite a PaO_2 of 60 mmHg (8 kPa)), with only a slight impairment in mental state. If hypoxaemia worsens and the PaO_2 drops to 40–50 mmHg (5.3–6.7 kPa), severe tissue hypoxia ensues. Hypoxia at the central nervous system level manifests with headaches and somnolence. Compensatory mechanisms include catecholamine release, and a decrease in renal function results in sodium retention and proteinuria.[11]

Different tissues vary in their vulnerability to hypoxia, with the central nervous system and myocardium at most risk. Hypoxia in the cerebral cortex results in a loss of function within 4–6 seconds, loss of consciousness in 10–20 seconds and irreversible damage in 3–5 minutes. In an environment that lacks oxygen, cells function by anaerobic metabolism and produce much less energy. For example, with aerobic metabolism 38 molecules of adenosine triphosphate are generated compared with 2 molecules of adenosine triphosphate generated in anaerobic metabolism. During anaerobic metabolism, lactic acid also increases. With less energy available, the efficiency of cellular functions such as the sodium–potassium pump, nerve conduction, enzyme activity and transmembrane receptor function is diminished.[11] The overall effect of interruption to these vital cellular activities is a reduction in organ or tissue function, which in turn compromises system and body functions.

Changes to the oxygen–haemoglobin association–dissociation curve also occur in states related to hypoxia. The curve shifts to the right when there is acidosis and/or raised levels of $PaCO_2$, as commonly seen in respiratory failure. The shift in the oxygen–haemoglobin dissociation curve to the right means that, in the lung, fewer oxygen molecules attach to the haemoglobin molecule, resulting in a decrease in arterial oxygen saturation. However, the oxygen that does attach to the haemoglobin molecule is more readily released at the tissue level.[11]

FIGURE 13.11 Ventilation/perfusion mismatch.[33]

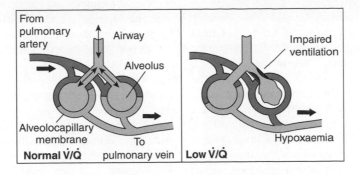

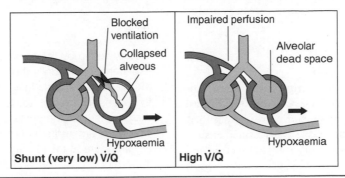

Source: Carlson K. Advanced critical care nursing. St Louis: Saunders Elsevier; 2009.

Compensatory mechanisms to optimise oxygenation

When PO_2 in the alveoli is reduced, regional hypoxic pulmonary vasoconstriction occurs, with contraction of smooth muscles in the small arterioles, directing blood flow away from the hypoxic area of the lung.[11] Peripheral chemoreceptors also detect hypoxaemia and initiate compensatory mechanisms to optimise cellular oxygen delivery. Initial responses are increased respiratory rate and depth, resulting in increased minute ventilation, and a raised heart rate with possible vasoconstriction as the body attempts to maintain oxygen delivery and uptake. An increased respiratory rate is the first 'best' sign that a patient is compensating for an underlying condition. This overall up-regulation cannot be sustained indefinitely, however, particularly in a person who is critically ill, and compensatory mechanisms begin to fail, with worsening hypoxaemia and cellular and organ dysfunction. Unless the hypoxaemia is reversed and/or respiratory and cardiovascular support is provided, irreversible hypoxia and death will ensue.

Inflammation

Inflammatory processes can occur at a local level (e.g. as a result of inhalation injuries, aspiration or respiratory infections) or are secondary to systemic events (e.g. sepsis, trauma). Damage to the pulmonary endothelium and type I alveolar cells appears to play a key role in the inflammatory processes associated with ARDS.[34] Once triggered, inflammation results in platelet aggregation and complement release. Platelet aggregation attracts neutrophils, which release inflammatory mediators (e.g. proteolytic enzymes, oxygen free radicals, leukotrienes, prostaglandins and platelet-activating factor). Neutrophils also appear to play a key role in the perpetuation of ARDS.[31] As well as altering pulmonary capillary permeability, resulting in haemorrhage and leaking of fluid into the pulmonary interstitium and alveoli, mediators released by neutrophils and some macrophages precipitate pulmonary vasoconstriction. Resulting pulmonary hypertension leads to diminished perfusion to some lung areas, with dramatic alterations to both perfusion and ventilation leading to significant V/Q mismatch, and the subsequent signs and symptoms typically seen in patients with pulmonary inflammation/oedema.

Oedema

Pulmonary oedema also alters gas exchange, and results from abnormal accumulation of extravascular fluid in the lung. Two main reasons for this are an increase in hydrostatic or osmotic forces, as seen in left ventricular dysfunction or volume overload, and increased membrane permeability of the lung epithelium or endothelium, allowing accumulation of fluid. This is referred to as non-cardiogenic pulmonary oedema. ARDS may result from increased permeability of the epithelium. A more-detailed discussion of ARDS is provided in Chapter 14.

Changes to respiratory function

During the early exudative phase of ARDS, tachypnoea, signs of hypoxaemia (apprehension, restlessness) and an increase in the use of accessory muscles are usually evident. These symptoms result from infiltration of fluid into the alveoli. With impaired production of surfactant during the proliferative phase, respiratory function deteriorates, and dyspnoea, agitation, fatigue and the emergence of fine crackles on auscultation are common.[31] Airway resistance is increased when oedema affects larger airways. Lung compliance is reduced as interstitial oedema interferes with the elastic properties of the lungs, and it may become challenging to adequately ventilate patients. Infiltration of type II alveolar cells into the epithelium may lead to interstitial fibrosis on healing, causing chronic lung dysfunction.[35]

Respiratory dysfunction: changes to the work of breathing

Without reversal of respiratory compromise, significant increases to the work of breathing will result. Clinical manifestations include tachypnoea, tachycardia, dyspnoea, low tidal volumes and diaphoresis. Hypercapnia ensues, which further compromises respiratory muscle function and precipitates diaphragmatic fatigue. Oxygen consumption during breathing can be so great that reserve capacity is reduced. If patients with pre-existing COPD (who may breathe close to the fatigue work level) experience an acute exacerbation, this can easily tip them into a fatigued state. Early identification and management of respiratory compromise before these stages improve patient outcomes.[11]

Assessment

Respiratory insufficiency is a common reason for admission to ICU, for either a potential or an actual problem, so comprehensive and frequent respiratory assessments are an essential practice role. This section outlines history taking, physical examination, bedside monitoring and diagnostic testing focused on a critically ill patient with respiratory dysfunction.

Assessment is a systematic process comprising history taking of a patient's present and previous illnesses and physical examination of their thorax, lungs and related systems. History taking and physical examination can occur simultaneously if the patient is very ill. Related diagnostic findings inform an accurate and comprehensive assessment. A thorough assessment, followed by accurate ongoing monitoring, enables early detection of changes in condition and the impact of treatment. Depending on a patient's situation, assessment can be either brief or detailed.

Patient history

History taking determines a patient's baseline respiratory status on ICU admission. If the patient is distressed, the nurse should ask only a few questions, but if the patient is able then a more comprehensive interview can be performed, focusing on four areas: the current problem, previous problems, symptoms and personal and family history. Question a family member or close friend if a patient is unable to provide their own history.

When introducing yourself, ask the patient's name, seek eye contact and create a rapport with the patient and the family. Ensure that the patient is in a comfortable position, ideally sitting up in bed. Provide privacy so that the interview is confidential. The physical examination should maintain the patient's dignity and modesty. To minimise distress for a patient who is acutely breathless, the use of short, closed questions is preferable.

Practice tip

History taking by the nurse should be an interactive experience, especially the initial interview where both the patient and nurse learn a lot about each other. If the patient is too sick to be interviewed, as often is the case in ICU, the nurse can instead invite a person who is considered a 'significant other' to the patient to contribute to the patient history. This may capture important information and can contribute to patient and family participation in care through the meaningful bringing together of patient, family and nurse.

Current respiratory problems

Begin by asking the patient about their difficulty breathing. If possible, let the patient describe the respiratory problem in his or her own words. Be focused and listen actively. Ask for location, onset and duration of the respiratory symptoms.

Previous respiratory problems

Many respiratory disorders can be chronic and pulmonary diseases may recur (e.g. asthma). New diseases can complicate existing ones.[36] Problems with breathing and chest problems, and the number of hospitalisations, treatments and childhood respiratory diseases should be discussed with the patient.

Symptoms

Assess the onset and duration, pattern, severity and episodic or continuous nature of presenting symptoms. Also ask about the patient's perception of their respiratory problem, their opinion about its cause and whether the symptoms cause fatigue, anxiety or stress. Ask specifically about dyspnoea, cough, sputum production, haemoptysis, wheezing, chest pain or other pain, sleep disturbances and snoring.

Dyspnoea (shortness of breath) is subjective and therefore difficult to grade. The mechanism that underlies the sensation of dyspnoea is poorly understood, but it is extremely uncomfortable and frightening.[36]

Assess the severity of dyspnoea by asking about breathing in relation to activities (e.g. breathlessness when dressing, walking across a room or even talking). Ask the patient how many pillows they need to sleep as this may indicate the severity of any *orthopnoea* (shortness of breath when lying flat). Orthopnoea can be a symptom of increased blood in the pulmonary circulation due to left ventricular failure, pulmonary oedema, bronchitis, asthma or obstructive sleep apnoea.

A cough can be dry or productive, episodic or continuous and, if exacerbated when the patient is lying flat, can imply heart failure. A cough can also be related to viral infections and allergies, or may indicate intrathoracic disease. Ask the patient if they wake at night due to the cough, how long the cough has been present and if it is getting better or worse.

Sputum production should be considered for amount, colour or the presence of blood. Yellow or green sputum is typical in bacterial infection. Haemoptysis or sputum mixed with blood is a significant finding and can indicate tuberculosis or lung cancer. Wheezing can indicate vocal cord disorder or asthma.[36]

Chest pain can result from multiple causes; therefore, appropriate assessment is essential. Chest pain that occurs during inspiration can be due to irritation or inflammation of the pleural surface. Pleural pain is experienced mostly on one side of the chest, is knifelike in character and occurs in pneumonia, pleurisy and pneumothorax. Chest pain also occurs with fractured ribs.

The most ominous chest pain occurs as a result of myocardial ischaemia due to poor oxygen delivery to the coronary vessels. This pain is termed angina pectoris and can arise from chronic stable angina or acute coronary syndrome[36] (see Chapter 10 for further discussion).

Sleep disturbance and snoring may be related to obstructive sleep apnoea. If the patient complains about drowsiness in the daytime, ask how many hours of continuous sleep they have at night, and whether they take a nap during the day.

Personal and family history

Family history and environment can influence pulmonary presentations. The focus of this questioning is on: tobacco use, medication, recreational drugs, allergies, recent travel, occupational risk, home situation and family history. Use of tobacco, current or past, is important in evaluating pulmonary symptoms. Ask the patient to quantify the amount of cigarette packs per week and how many years they have smoked. The majority of smokers have reduced lung function. Tobacco smoking is responsible for 80% of the risk of developing COPD. Exposure to second-hand smoke may also be of interest, with evidence that extended exposure is a major cause of chronic bronchitis.[37] A history of recent travel increases possible exposure to infectious respiratory diseases.[38] Recent long flights increase the possibility of deep venous thrombosis, which can lead to pulmonary embolism.[39] An occupation with exposure to allergens and toxins is important to document, as this can be associated with declining lung function.[40]

Ask about the patient's home situation and whether they live with someone with an illness such as influenza or tuberculosis. Ask about children who are close to the patient, as innocuous viral infections in small children may account for severe disease in adults.[36] Also check for a family history of cancer and heart or respiratory diseases.

Physical examination

The four activities of physical examination are inspection, palpation, percussion and auscultation. Prior to commencing the examination, prepare the patient as well as possible by providing privacy, warmth, good light and quiet surroundings. Explain that the examination is a standard procedure and you will use your eyes, hands and a stethoscope. Help the patient into a comfortable sitting position in the bed if possible and have all necessary equipment easily accessible.

Inspection

Inspection involves carefully observing the patient from head to toe for signs of respiratory problems. Focus on patient position, chest wall inspection, respiratory rate and rhythm, respiratory effort, central or peripheral cyanosis and clubbing. Note what position appears preferable for the patient, and whether they look comfortable in bed, have trouble breathing or appear anxious. Observe chest wall symmetry during the respiratory cycle, anatomical structures and the presence of scars. The most important sign of respiratory distress is respiratory rate and rhythm. The respiratory rate should be assessed over a 1-minute period so that an accurate measurement is obtained. The normal respiratory rate for adults is 12–20 per minute.[6] Abnormal breathing patterns are noted in Table 13.1.[41] Observe respiratory effort, in particular the use of accessory muscles, abdominal muscles, nasal flaring, body position and mouth breathing.

Inspect the lips, tongue and sublingual area for central cyanosis (a late sign of hypoxia that is almost impossible to detect in a patient with anaemia).[31] Observe the extremities for oedema (which can be a sign of heart failure), fingers and toes for peripheral cyanosis and clubbing of the nail beds. Peripheral cyanosis may indicate low blood flow to peripheral areas. Clubbing of finger or toenail beds can be idiopathic or more commonly due to respiratory or circulatory diseases (e.g. chronic hypoxia in congenital heart disease).[36] Note whether the patient requires oxygen and if so record the dose and method of delivery. If the patient is intubated and mechanically ventilated (monitoring is explained later in this chapter), ensure that the airway is adequately secured. If the patient is orally intubated, observe the mouth for the presence of lesions or pressure on the oral mucosa and lips, and observe the size of the tube, the length at the lips or teeth margin and how it is secured. If the patient has a tracheostomy, observe the stoma for signs of infection or pressure areas, the type and size of tracheostomy tube, the length at the hub if it is a tracheostomy with an adjustable flange and the manner of securement.

TABLE 13.1

Description of different respiratory patterns[41]

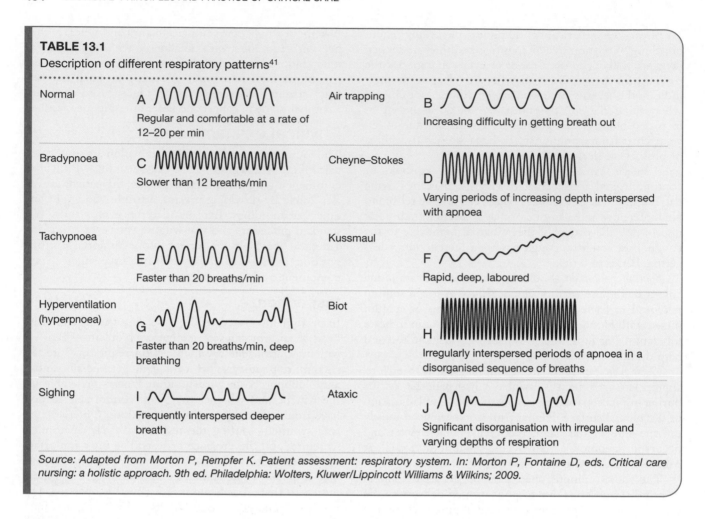

Normal	A — Regular and comfortable at a rate of 12–20 per min	Air trapping	B — Increasing difficulty in getting breath out
Bradypnoea	C — Slower than 12 breaths/min	Cheyne–Stokes	D — Varying periods of increasing depth interspersed with apnoea
Tachypnoea	E — Faster than 20 breaths/min	Kussmaul	F — Rapid, deep, laboured
Hyperventilation (hyperpnoea)	G — Faster than 20 breaths/min, deep breathing	Biot	H — Irregularly interspersed periods of apnoea in a disorganised sequence of breaths
Sighing	I — Frequently interspersed deeper breath	Ataxic	J — Significant disorganisation with irregular and varying depths of respiration

Source: Adapted from Morton P, Rempfer K. Patient assessment: respiratory system. In: Morton P, Fontaine D, eds. Critical care nursing: a holistic approach. 9th ed. Philadelphia: Wolters, Kluwer/Lippincott Williams & Wilkins; 2009.

Palpation

Palpate the patient's chest with warm hands, focusing on areas of tenderness, the tracheal position, and the presence of subcutaneous emphysema and tactile fremitus (vibration intensity felt on the chest wall). Assess for symmetry (left compared with right) and follow a systematic sequence of palpation over the anterior and posterior surfaces (Fig. 13.12).[42] Check the thorax for areas of tenderness or bony deformities and note the symmetry of chest movement during breathing. Use the palm of your hand to assess skin temperature, noting clammy, hot or cold skin. To test for chest wall symmetry on inspiration, place both hands with thumbs together on the patient's posterior thorax and ask them to take a deep breath. Your thumbs should separate equally 3–5 cm during normal deep inspiration[31] (Fig. 13.13).[4] Asymmetry can occur in pneumothorax, pneumonia or other lung disorders where inspiration is affected.

Palpation of the tracheal position is useful to detect a mediastinal shift; deviation of the trachea from midline may indicate a pulmonary problem such as large pneumothorax or previous pneumonectomy.[43] The presence of subcutaneous emphysema indicates air in the subcutaneous tissue and feels like crackling under your fingers due to air pockets in the tissue.[44] This most commonly occurs in the face, neck and chest after blunt or penetrating trauma to the chest (e.g. stabbing, gun shot, fractured ribs), and in facial fractures, tracheostomy, respiratory tract surgery and patients who are mechanically ventilated.

Palpation is also used to assess for tactile (vocal) fremitus, a normal palpable vibration. Place your hands on the patient's chest and ask them to vocalise repeatedly the term 'ninety-nine'. Fremitus is decreased (i.e. impaired transmission of sounds) in pleural effusion and pneumothorax. Fremitus is increased over regions of lung where transmission is increased (e.g. in pneumonia, consolidation).[36] In mechanically ventilated patients, fremitus can be detected when there are secretions in the airways.

Percussion

By tapping the chest with the bony structures of the hands, percussion can help to determine if the lung spaces are filled with air, fluid or sputum consolidation. Place your non-dominant hand with your middle finger extended over the area of chest to be examined. Using the middle finger of your dominant hand, tap on the distal knuckle of the finger resting on the chest wall. Starting from the upper chest wall and moving from side to

FIGURE 13.12 Sequence of systematic movements for palpation, percussion and auscultation of the posterior (**A**) and anterior (**B**) chest. Comparison of the right and left sides of the chest should be performed by moving from side to side, beginning proximally and moving distally down the chest wall.[42]

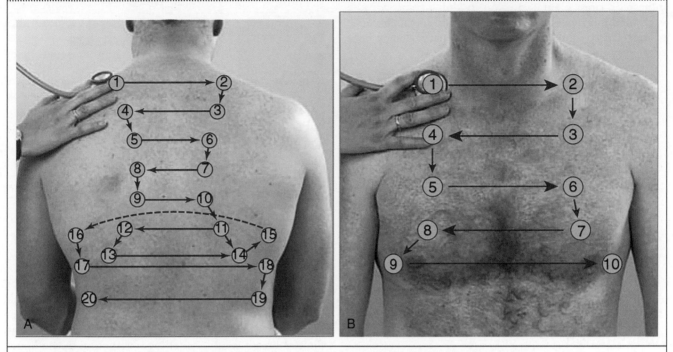

Source: Weber J, Kelly J. Health assessment in nursing. Philadelphia: Lippincott, Williams & Wilkins; 2010.

FIGURE 13.13 Assessment of thoracic expansion. (**A**) Exhalation. (**B**) Inhalation.[4]

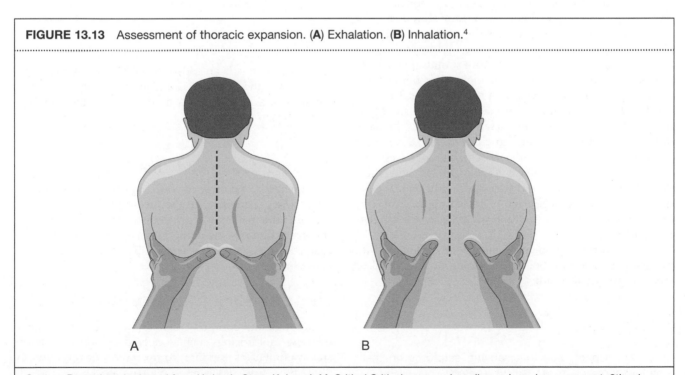

Source: Reproduced adapted from Urden L, Stacy K, Lough M. Critical Critical care nursing: diagnosis and management. 6th ed. St Louis: Elsevier/Mosby; 2010, with permission.

side, following the same sequence as for palpation (see Fig. 13.12), compare one side with the other for variation in sound. Normally, the chest has a resonant percussion tone. A flat percussive note, soft and high-pitched, may indicate a large pleural effusion. A dull percussive note with medium intensity and pitch is heard in the presence of atelectasis, pulmonary oedema, pulmonary haemorrhage or pneumonia.[23]

> **Practice tip**
>
> When performing palpation or percussion of the chest with your hand and auscultation of the chest with a stethoscope, the patient will appreciate the hand and stethoscope being warmed prior to placing them on the skin.

> **Practice tip**
>
> When performing chest inspection, percussion and auscultation, always compare one side of the body with the other.

Auscultation

Careful interpretation of breath sounds and integration of this assessment data with other findings can provide important information about lung disorders.[45–48] Use the diaphragm of the stethoscope and ensure full contact with the skin for optimal listening. For a spontaneously breathing patient, ask them to breathe through their mouth (nose breathing may alter the pitch of the breath sounds). Auscultation is performed in a systematic way so as to compare the symmetry of breath sounds (Fig. 13.12). Normal breath sounds reflect air movement through the bronchi, and sounds change as air moves from larger to smaller airways. Sounds also change when air passes though fluid or narrowed airways. Breath sounds therefore differ depending on the area auscultated. The three types of normal breath sounds are bronchial, bronchovesicular and vesicular breath sounds (Table 13.2),[4] and these should be heard only in the areas specific to their region. If heard in the wrong place – for example, bronchial breath sounds heard in the lung peripheries – it suggests consolidation.

It is important to identify and become familiar with normal breath sounds before beginning to listen for and identify abnormal breath sounds.

> **Practice tip**
>
> Use an alcohol wipe to clean the earpieces on the stethoscope prior to use to protect yourself from infection.

TABLE 13.2

Characteristics of normal breath sounds[4]

SOUND	CHARACTERISTICS
Vesicular	Heard over most of the lung field; low pitch; soft and short exhalation and long inhalation.
Bronchovesicular	Heard over main bronchus area and over right posterior lung field; medium pitch; exhalation equals inhalation.
Bronchial	Heard only over trachea; high pitch; loud and long exhalation.

Source: Adapted from Urden L, Stacy K, Lough M. Critical care nursing: diagnosis and management. 6th ed. St Louis: Elsevier/Mosby; 2010.

Abnormal breath sounds are either continuous or discontinuous. Continuous sounds include wheezes and rhonchi, while discontinuous sounds include crackles (Table 13.3).[4,48] Stridor is an abnormal, loud, high-pitched breath sound caused by obstruction in the upper airways as a result of a foreign body, tissue or vocal cord swelling; this emergent condition requires immediate attention.[45,46] Absent or diminished breath sounds also require immediate treatment, indicating no air flow through that area of the lung.[45]

> **Practice tip**
>
> Respiratory rate is an early warning sign for respiratory distress. If the patient has a high respiratory rate, this can be a sign of hypoxia as the patient attempts to compensate for low PaO_2.

Documentation and charting

Document the findings of your respiratory assessment in the patient's chart; if this is the first respiratory assessment, describe the patient's respiratory history carefully. Any abnormal findings including abnormal sounds and their characteristics should be described to enable subsequent reassessment.

Respiratory monitoring

A thorough and comprehensive assessment, with accurate ongoing monitoring, enables early detection of changes and assessment of responses to treatment for the critically ill. This section describes the main aspects of bedside respiratory monitoring and the instruments used to assess the efficiency of a patient's gas transfer mechanisms,

TABLE 13.3
Description of abnormal breath sounds[4,48]

ABNORMAL SOUND	DESCRIPTION	CONDITION
Absent breath sounds	No air flow to particular portion of lung	Pneumothorax Pneumonectomy Emphysematous blebs Pleural effusion Lung mass Massive atelectasis Complete airway obstruction
Diminished breath sounds	Little air flow to particular portion of lung	Emphysema Pleural effusion Pleurisy Atelectasis Pulmonary fibrosis
Displaced bronchial sounds	Bronchial sounds heard in peripheral lung fields	Atelectasis with secretions Lung mass with exudates Pneumonia Pleural effusion Pulmonary oedema
Crackles (rales)	Short, discrete popping or crackling sounds	Pulmonary oedema Pneumonia Pulmonary fibrosis Atelectasis Bronchiectasis
Rhonchi	Coarse, rumbling, low-pitched sounds	Pneumonia Asthma Bronchitis Bronchospasm
Wheezes	High-pitched, squeaking, whistling sounds	Asthma Bronchospasm
Pleural friction rub	Creaking, leathery, loud, dry, coarse sounds	Pleural effusion Pleurisy

Source: Adapted from Urden L, Stacey K, Lough M. Critical care nursing: diagnosis and management. 6th ed. St Louis: Elsevier/Mosby; 2010.

provide information on the patient's ventilatory state but may determine oxygen saturation and detect hypoxaemia. This prompt, non-invasive detection of hypoxaemia enables detection of clinical deterioration and more-rapid treatment to avoid associated complications.[49]

Pulse oximetry works by emitting two wavelengths of light, red and infrared, that pass through a pulsatile flow of blood from a diode (positioned on one side of the probe) to a photodetector (positioned on the opposite side). The signal emitted is measured over five pulses, causing a slight delay when monitoring. Oxygenated blood absorbs light differently from deoxygenated blood; the oximeter measures the amount of light absorbed by the vascular bed and calculates the percentage of haemoglobin saturation in the capillaries.

Indirect measurement of arterial oxygen saturation via the peripheral circulation using pulse oximetry is referred to as SpO_2 (the symbol 'p' denotes peripheral) and is displayed digitally on the monitor as a percentage, along with heart rate and a plethysmographic waveform. Interpreting this waveform is essential in distinguishing a true oximetry signal from one displaying dampening or artefact (Fig. 13.14). The probe is commonly placed on a finger, but can also be placed on the toe, earlobe or forehead, with forehead probes having the highest accuracy.[50] Change the probe position frequently to maintain adequate perfusion of the site and skin integrity.

Practice tip
In cool environments, wrap the hand or foot that has the sensor attached. This may improve saturation readings.

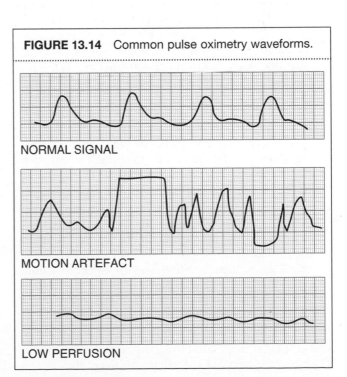

FIGURE 13.14 Common pulse oximetry waveforms.

NORMAL SIGNAL

MOTION ARTEFACT

LOW PERFUSION

including pulse oximetry, capnography, airway pressures and ventilator waveforms and loops.

Pulse oximetry
Pulse oximetry is a non-invasive device that measures the oxygen saturation of haemoglobin in a patient's arterial blood. The technology is common in critical and acute care areas. It is important to note that the device does not

It is important to understand that pulse oximetry measures the saturation of haemoglobin as an estimate of peripheral arterial oxygen saturation (SpO_2). SpO_2 differs from PaO_2 but they are physiologically related, and this relationship is illustrated by the two axes of the oxygen–haemoglobin dissociation curve (for more discussion see Fig. 13.9 and the section Principles of gas transport and exchange in alveoli and tissues). A fit healthy adult, at sea level, with a normal haemoglobin level breathing room air would usually have a SpO_2 of 97–99%. Normal values decline with age, with lower limits of normal being 96% for an 18-year-old and 94% for a 70-year-old person.[50]

Practice tip

Try to place the pulse oximeter on the finger of the opposite arm to where blood pressure is taken, particularly if you have no arterial line and are doing frequent non-invasive blood pressure measurements.

Limitations of pulse oximetry

- Pulse oximetry in isolation does not provide all the necessary information to evaluate oxygenation, ventilation status or acid–base balance. ABG testing is required to assess other parameters.

- Pulse oximetry readings are reasonably reliable when the SaO_2 is 90% or above; accuracy deteriorates when the SaO_2 falls below 90%.[51] When low SpO_2 readings occur and you are confident that the device is not influenced by artefact, formal ABG analysis should be conducted.

- Satisfactory arterial perfusion of the monitored tissue is required; low cardiac output states, vasoconstriction, peripheral vascular disease and hypothermia can cause inaccurate pulse signals and falsely low oxygen saturation readings. Low perfusion will result in a flattened oximetry waveform (see Fig. 13.14). In such cases, confirm oxygen saturation with intermittent ABG testing. In these cases, moving the probe to another location, such as the earlobe or forehead, can improve signal quality. Forehead probes provide higher accuracy and also respond more quickly to changes in saturation. If using an earlobe probe, application of a vasodilator cream can improve both perfusion and signal quality.[50]

- Motion artefact (see Fig. 13.14), caused by patient movement or shivering, is a significant cause of erroneously low readings and false alarms.[51] Keeping the patient warm (if not contraindicated) and encouraging them to minimise movement may limit this problem. Using an earlobe or forehead probe may also reduce motion artefact.[50] The pulse oximetry waveform is useful to distinguish a true reading from a reading influenced by artefact.[51]

- Dark blue, green and black nail varnishes have been shown to affect SpO_2 accuracy, although the differences may not be clinically significant. There is conflicting advice on whether placing the sensor probe sideways on the finger eliminates this effect.[50,51] To ensure accuracy, it is recommended that nail varnish and acrylic nails be removed if possible.

- Modern pulse oximeters are relatively unaffected by light sources, the thickness of tissue or skin pigmentation. In patients with very dark skin, hypoxaemia has been detected less frequently and oxygen saturation may be overestimated when readings are below 90%.[52] Conventional pulse oximetry sensors cannot differentiate between oxyhaemoglobin, carboxyhaemoglobin and methaemoglobin, and therefore provide a false estimation of oxygen saturation. An example of high levels of non-functioning haemoglobin is that of carbon monoxide poisoning; high carboxyhaemoglobin levels give a falsely high SpO_2 reading, leading to an overestimation of oxygenation. New multi-wavelength oximeters that can estimate carboxyhaemoglobin and methaemoglobin are now available but are not accurate in the presence of low SaO_2 readings and, for carboxyhaemoglobin, are not necessarily interchangeable with standard laboratory tests.[51]

- In the presence of anaemia it is possible to have good oxygen saturation of available haemoglobin but poor tissue oxygenation, owing to a deficiency in the ability of the blood to transport oxygen.[51] In anaemia, the pulse oximetry readings may be accurate, but it is the clinician's interpretation of these readings that is important. If we are looking at SpO_2 as a marker of oxygenation, a reduced amount of functioning haemoglobin may be well saturated with oxygen but is a poor reflection of tissue oxygenation. Correction of anaemia is required to improve tissue oxygenation.

- Injection of intravenous dyes[51] (e.g. methylene blue, indocyanine green, indigo carmine) may lead to a false underestimation of SpO_2 for up to 20 minutes after their administration.

Practice tip

Assess the agreement between the heart rate reading displayed in the pulse oximetry section of the monitor and the heart rate calculated by the ECG. Lack of agreement may indicate that not all pulsations are being detected and the pulse oximetry reading may not be accurate.

Practice tip

Patients with COPD who are hypoxic (SpO_2 <88%) should receive supplemental oxygen. The SpO_2 targets for patients with COPD are lower, with SpO_2 generally maintained at 88–92% during an exacerbation if the patient is at risk of hypercapnia.[53] It is important to frequently assess these patients receiving oxygen so that any compromise in breathing is noted and acted upon.

Capnography

Capnography, using infrared spectrometry, monitors expired CO_2 during the respiratory cycle and is referred to as end-tidal CO_2 (PetCO$_2$). The percentage of exhaled CO_2 at end-expiration is displayed on the monitor.

A waveform called a capnogram is produced (Fig. 13.15),[54] and it is important that ICU staff receive training in interpretation of capnography waveforms.[55] Continuous capnography detects subtle changes in patients' lung dynamics (i.e. changes to physiological shunting or alveolar recruitment) and can be measured in both intubated and non-intubated patients. It can be used to estimate $PaCO_2$ levels in patients with a normal ventilation/perfusion ratio (usually 1–5 mmHg less than $PaCO_2$). Levels are, however, affected by conditions common in the critically ill (e.g. low cardiac output states, elevated alveolar pressures, sepsis, hypo/hyperthermia, pulmonary embolism, alterations in tidal volume and respiratory rate), so use PetCO$_2$ to estimate $PaCO_2$ levels in these patients with caution. The amount of dead space in the circuit will also change the correlation between PetCO$_2$ and $PaCO_2$, and the use of filters between the patient airway and the capnography sampling line can cause an artificially low reading.[55] Investigate any sudden changes in PetCO$_2$ levels with ABG analysis. PetCO$_2$ monitoring has many uses in the critical care unit including:

- indicating correct endotracheal tube placement while awaiting chest X-ray (CXR), assessing tube patency and detecting leaks or disconnection of the circuit

- monitoring ventilation status during and after weaning from mechanical ventilation
- assessing the effectiveness of cardiopulmonary resuscitation compressions and detecting the return of spontaneous circulation
- monitoring ventilation continuously during sedation and anaesthesia
- assessing ventilation/perfusion status.[55]

> **Practice tip**
>
> The capnography monitoring line can fill with condensation, particularly if the patient has a humidified ventilator circuit. Regularly check for this and drain or replace the line as necessary. Condensation can interfere with the reading.

Capnography is recommended as a standard component of respiratory monitoring in mechanically ventilated patients in the ICU, during transport of critically ill patients, during anaesthesia and conscious sedation, and during cardiopulmonary resuscitation.[55]

Ventilation monitoring

Mechanical ventilation is a common intervention for patients who require respiratory support in the ICU. Advances in ventilation technology have enhanced our ability to monitor many ventilator parameters. A detailed understanding of mechanical ventilation principles and functions enables patient data to be interpreted accurately and managed appropriately. Chapter 15 provides a detailed discussion of mechanical ventilation, including ventilation monitoring, airway pressures (peak airway pressure, plateau pressure and positive end-expiratory pressure), and waveforms and loop displays.

Bedside and laboratory investigations

Bedside and laboratory investigations add to available information about a patient's respiratory status and assist in diagnosis and treatment. This section focuses on common investigations used to assess a patient's respiratory status and their response to treatment: ABG analysis, blood testing, and sputum and tracheal aspirates. Given the unfamiliar nature of the ICU environment for patients and families, explanation of the purpose of respiratory monitoring procedures and devices may reduce fear and uncertainty.

Blood gas analysis

ABGs are one of the most commonly performed laboratory tests in critical care. Therefore, accurate ABG interpretation is an important clinical skill. ABG measurements enable rapid assessment of oxygenation and

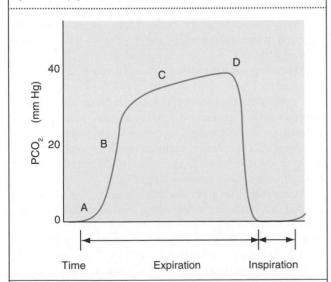

FIGURE 13.15 Normal capnogram.[54] **(A)** end inspiration; **(B)** expiratory upstroke; **(C)** expiratory plateau; **(D)** end-tidal carbon dioxide tension (PetCO$_2$).

Source: Reproduced from Miller-Keane M, O'Toole M. Miller-Keane encyclopedia and dictionary of medicine, nursing, and allied health. 7th ed. Philadelphia: Saunders, 2003.

ventilation, and all ICUs are recommended to have a blood gas analyser as a minimum standard.[56]

Blood for ABG analysis is sampled by arterial puncture or, more commonly in critically ill patients, from an arterial catheter usually sited in the radial or femoral artery. Both techniques are invasive and allow for only intermittent analysis. The advantage of the arterial catheter is that it facilitates ABG sampling without repeated arterial punctures. Continuous blood gas monitoring is possible using an in-line fibreoptic sensor as part of the arterial line, but this practice is yet to have wide application because of technological limitations.[57] Questions also remain regarding the possibility for arteriovenous shunting, blood loss and infection risk with continuous systems.[58]

Sampling technique

A correct sampling technique is essential for accurate results. Prior to arterial sampling from the radial artery, a modified Allen's test should be performed. The patient should initially hold their hand high and clench their fist tightly. Occlusive pressure is then applied by the clinician's thumbs to both the ulnar and radial arteries, to obstruct blood flow to the hand. While maintaining this pressure, the patient is asked to relax their hand, and check whether the palm and fingers have blanched. Occlusive pressure is then released on the ulnar artery only. The modified Allen's test is positive if the hand flushes within 5–15 seconds, indicating that the ulnar artery has good blood flow and radial sampling is safe.[59]

Approximately 2 mL of arterial blood is collected anaerobically and aseptically using a premixed syringe containing dry heparin.[60] If drawing the sample from an intra-arterial line, a portion of blood is discarded to prevent dilution and contamination of the sample from the saline in the flush line. The discard amount is twice the dead space volume in order to ensure clinically accurate ABG and electrolyte measurement, and to prevent unnecessary blood loss.[61] Dead space is defined as the priming volume from the sampling port to the catheter tip; this differs depending on the arterial line setup used. Arterial blood exerts its own pressure, which is sufficient to fill the syringe to the required level; active negative pressure is to be avoided, as this causes frothing. Any excess air will cause inaccurate readings and is expelled before the syringe is capped with a hub, preventing further air contamination. The sample is analysed within 10 minutes if not packed in ice, or within 60 minutes if iced; delays cause degradation of the sample.[60] The use of ice is controversial: while it was appropriate for older-style glass syringes, it is now recognised that plastic syringes become more permeable to gas at lower temperatures, allowing oxygen (but less so carbon dioxide) to escape. For this reason, using ice to preserve samples in plastic syringes is not recommended, and this increases the importance of prompt ABG analysis.[62] Degradation also occurs if the sample is shaken; therefore, gently roll the syringe/collection tube between your fingers to mix the sample with the heparin and

prevent clotting. The frequency of ABG sampling should be carefully considered and based on patient need. ABG sampling may lead to losses of up to 70 mL per day and the cumulative effect may worsen anaemia and increase the need for transfusion. Evidence-based blood conservation strategies should be included in local unit guidelines. This is particularly important in the paediatric population, where the use of small-volume collection tubes have reduced iatrogenic blood loss.[63]

The question of whether or not to adjust the ABG analysis according to the patient's body temperature (by inputting the actual patient temperature result into the blood gas analyser) remains controversial. Hypothermia and hyperthermia can affect gas solubility, and so impact on pCO_2, pO_2 and pH. Body temperature can also shift the oxyhaemoglobin dissociation curve, as well as altering oxygen consumption and production of carbon dioxide. If local unit protocol is to adjust for temperature, it is recommended that both corrected and uncorrected ABG results are reported so as to avoid potentially unsafe decisions based on erroneous assumptions.[64]

There is a difference in the way bicarbonate is determined between an ICU-based ABG machine (which derives its value based on the pCO_2 and the pH) and a biochemistry laboratory that directly measures bicarbonate using an enzymatic assay. The true bicarbonate value is best determined by the Henderson–Hasselbalch equation. Any differences between an ABG machine value and that reported by a laboratory are usually within 3 mmol and are most likely explained by preanalytical errors or how quickly the sample was analysed, rather than one device being superior.[65]

Arterial blood gas analysis

ABG analysis includes measurement of the PaO_2, the $PaCO_2$, the H^+ concentration (pH) and the concentration of chemical buffer, HCO_3^-. Normal values for ABG parameters are listed in Table 13.4. Use a systematic approach when interpreting the results of ABG analysis (Table 13.5).

Assessing oxygenation: when assessing oxygenation, hypoxaemia (PaO_2 <60 mmHg or <7.8 kPa) will be the most common abnormality and may indicate the need for supplemental oxygen to maintain adequate arterial oxygenation.[66] Conversely, hyperoxia rarely occurs unless a patient is receiving supplemental oxygen therapy. Oxygen can be toxic to cells if delivered at high concentrations for a prolonged period.

Assessing the pH: the body's acid–base balance is affected by both the respiratory and metabolic systems and is evaluated by measuring the pH of arterial blood. On the pH scale of 1 to 14 (where 1 = the strongest acid and 14 = the strongest alkali), a pH of 7.4 is the middle of the normal range. Acidaemia is present with a pH of <7.35; alkalaemia is present with a pH of >7.45. The pH changes depending on the amount of H^+ or HCO_3^- in the blood, with H^+ reflecting the acidic component and HCO_3^- the base or buffer component.[66]

TABLE 13.4

Arterial blood gas normal values[a]

BLOOD GAS MEASUREMENT	DESCRIPTION	NORMAL VALUE
Temperature	Patient's body temperature. Analyser defaults to 37°C if not entered.	37°C
Haemoglobin	Samples should be fully mixed so should be constantly agitated until analysed.	Females: 115–165 g/L Males: 130–180 g/L
Acid–base status	Overall acidity or alkalinity of blood.	7.35–7.45 (36–44 nmol/L)
Carbon dioxide (CO_2)	Partial pressure of arterial CO_2. A potential acid.	35–45 mmHg (4.7–6.0 kPa)
Oxygen (O_2)	Partial pressure of O_2. Varies with age.	80–100 mmHg (10.7–13.3 kPa)
Bicarbonate (HCO_3^-)	Standardised HCO_3^- (actual HCO_3^- minus the HCO_3^- produced by respiratory dysfunction) estimates true metabolic function. An alkali or base.	22–26 mmol/L
Base excess	Measures acid–base balance. The number of molecules of acid or base required to return 1 L of blood to the normal pH (7.4).	−2 to +2 mmol/L
Oxygen saturation	Haemoglobin saturation by oxygen in arterial blood.	94.5–98.2%

[a] Institutional norms may vary slightly.

TABLE 13.5

Steps for arterial blood gas (ABG) interpretation

STEP	INTERPRETATION
1	Assess oxygenation: PaO_2 <60 mmHg (<8 kPa) indicates hypoxaemia.
2	Assess the pH level: <7.35 indicates acidosis; >7.45 indicates alkalosis.
3	Assess $PaCO_2$ level: <35 mmHg (<4.7 kPa) indicates respiratory alkalosis; >45 mmHg (>6.0 kPa) indicates respiratory acidosis.
4	Assess HCO_3^- level: <22 indicates metabolic acidosis; >26 indicates metabolic alkalosis.
5	Assess pH, CO_2 and HCO_3^-: is there an acid–base disturbance and is it fully compensated, partially compensated or uncompensated?.
6	Assess other ABG results: are they within normal limits for the patient?

indicates alveolar hypoventilation, due to COPD, pulmonary oedema, airway obstruction, oversedation, narcosis, drug overdose, pain, neurological deficit or permissive hypercapnia in mechanically ventilated patients. Conversely, a $PaCO_2$ of <35 mmHg (4.7 kPa) reflects alveolar hyperventilation, and can be due to hypoxia, pain, anxiety, pregnancy, liver failure, sepsis, early stages of asthma, permissive hypocapnia in mechanically ventilated patients or as a compensatory mechanism for metabolic acidosis.[66]

Assessing for metabolic mechanisms: when there is a metabolic cause to a change in pH, the primary alteration will be to the HCO_3^- level. This may be due to a change in alkaline substances (such as excessive intake of an antacid) or a change in acid substances (such as an excess of lactic acid in the blood).[66] The level of HCO_3^- is regulated by the renal system. A HCO_3^- concentration of <22 mmol/L can lead to metabolic acidosis, caused by renal failure, ketoacidosis, lactic acidosis, diarrhoea, salicylate overdose, a large volume of intravenous saline or cardiac arrest. A HCO_3^- of >26 mmol/L can lead to metabolic alkalosis, caused by severe vomiting, continuous nasogastric suction, diuretics, corticosteroids or excessive citrate administration from stored blood or renal replacement therapy.[66]

The base excess (BE) is an additional value included in the ABG report and it reflects the excess (or deficit) of base to acid in the blood. Normal BE ranges from −2 to +2. If the BE is +2 mmol/L, removal of 2 mmol of base per litre of blood is required to return the pH to 7.4. If the BE is −2 mmol/L (i.e. a base deficit), 2 mmol of base per litre of blood needs to be added to achieve a pH of 7.4. A BE greater than +3 indicates that there is more

Assessing for respiratory mechanisms: $PaCO_2$ indicates the effectiveness of ventilation and rises when ventilation is suboptimal; CO_2 combines with water to form carbonic acid (H_2CO_3), so can alter the pH of blood.

Retention of CO_2 through hypoventilation or air trapping leads to an increased number of H^+ ions, resulting in a lower pH and development of respiratory acidosis. Alternatively, a loss of CO_2 through hyperventilation results in a higher pH and development of respiratory alkalosis. A $PaCO_2$ of >45 mmHg (6 kPa)

base than acid present and therefore alkalosis. A BE below −3 indicates that there is more acid than base.[66] Understanding this concept is useful as it can determine how much treatment is necessary to restore a patient's pH to normal.

Mixed disorders: sometimes there will be both a respiratory and a metabolic cause for a disturbance in pH and this is referred to as a mixed disorder. For example, a cardiac arrest may result in a period of poor perfusion causing metabolic acidosis, and poor ventilation causing a concomitant respiratory acidosis.[66]

Assessing for compensation: the final step of interpretation is to examine the pH, CO_2 and HCO_3^- levels collectively, to determine whether the patient has either fully or partially compensated the primary dysfunction or is in an uncompensated state. With the respiratory system regulating CO_2 and the metabolic system regulating HCO_3^-, restoration of normal acid–base balance and homeostasis is possible. The ability of the body to achieve homeostasis and acid–base balance depends on the ability of the respiratory and renal systems to adjust to the underlying imbalance. The degree of compensation depends on whether the pH returns to normal; full compensation results in a normal pH, whereas in partial compensation the pH remains outside normal limits. In an uncompensated acid–base imbalance, there has been no attempt by the body to correct the acid–base imbalance, and the pH, as well as either the CO_2 or the HCO_3^-, is abnormal.[66]

To assess compensation, the pH, CO_2 and HCO_3^- are examined in the context of a patient's clinical presentation:

- In a fully compensated state, the pH is returned to within normal limits, but the other two parameters will be outside normal limits as the body has successfully manipulated CO_2 and HCO_3^- levels to restore the pH.

- In a partially compensated state, the pH is not within normal limits, and the other parameters will also be outside of normal limits but not enough to bring the pH back to normal.

- In a non-compensated state, the pH will be outside normal limits, and the primary disruption (either CO_2 or HCO_3^-) will also be outside normal limits while the remaining parameter has not compensated for this derangement and has stayed within normal limits.

It can be difficult to differentiate the patient's primary problem from their compensatory response. As a quick guide, if the CO_2 is moving in the opposite direction to the pH, then the primary disruption is respiratory; if the HCO_3^- is moving in the same direction as pH, the disruption is metabolic.[66] Table 13.6 provides a guide to ABG findings for each acid–base disorder.

Other parameters measured on the ABG sample, such as lactate, electrolytes, haemoglobin and glucose, are also considered in determining patient status. Lactate is a useful indicator of anaerobic metabolism due to poor tissue oxygenation. In healthy people, a normal lactate is 0.5–1 mmol/L, while in critically ill patients a normal lactate is considered less than 2 mmol/L. Hyperlactataemia exists where there is a persistent lactate level of 2–4 mmol/L without metabolic acidosis, and this can occur with adequate tissue perfusion. Lactic acidosis is present where a hyperlactataemia and metabolic acidosis coexist. Hypoxic causes of lactic acidosis include respiratory failure, ischaemia, severe anaemia and shock, while non-hypoxic causes include renal or hepatic dysfunction, ketoacidosis, an excess of catecholamines and sepsis. Improved lactate levels are a useful indicator of successful therapy for these derangements.[67]

The Stewart approach

As an adjunct to traditional ABG interpretation, Peter Stewart's seminal concepts on acid–base assessment[68] suggest that, in our body's fluids, pH and HCO_3^- are merely dependent variables that cannot be directly manipulated. Stewart was particularly interested in considering the influence of resuscitation fluid management on acid–base balance. He developed six equations to assist clinicians to analyse the physiological basis of acid–base shifts, considering the impacts of strong cations, the total concentration of weak acids and CO_2.[69] Stewart's intention was not to replace traditional methods of determining acid–base balance, but rather to extend their usefulness and to further explain the physiological basis of complex disorders.[70] An example of the utility of Stewart's work is evident in a study of 300 patients with abdominal sepsis.[71] This report demonstrated that a modification of the Stewart approach was able to identify mixed acid–base disorders which would otherwise remain undetected.[71]

Stewart's complex equations have been made more user friendly with the development of online calculators[72] where the clinician can enter patient chemistry data online to receive an online decision support related to complex acid–base disorders (see Online resources). Once patient data are entered, the site offers clinicians a breakup of the relative contributions to the overall disturbance in pH by its main controlling elements. When displayed graphically, this gives the user a sense of the severity of each contributing factor and allows input of these individual factors into virtual scenarios to predict the possible impact of specific interventions.[69]

Venous blood gas analysis

Where an arterial blood sample is difficult to collect, an alternative is to perform the same measurements on a venous blood sample. Venous blood collection may involve a peripheral venous sample using venipuncture, a central venous sample from a central line, or a mixed venous sample from the distal port of a pulmonary artery catheter. Central venous sampling has the highest evidence for correlation with ABGs. If taking a peripheral sample using venipuncture, release the tourniquet at least 1 minute before the blood is drawn so as to reduce the impact of local ischaemia.[73]

TABLE 13.6

Arterial blood gas findings for acid–base disturbances

	PH	PACO₂, MMHG (KPA)	HCO₃⁻, MMOL/L
RESPIRATORY ACIDOSIS			
Uncompensated	<7.35	>45 (6.0)	Within normal limits
Partially compensated	<7.35	>45 (6.0)	>26
Fully compensated	Within normal limits	>45 (6.0)	>26
RESPIRATORY ALKALOSIS			
Uncompensated	>7.45	<35 (4.7)	Within normal limits
Partially compensated	>7.45	<35 (4.7)	<22
Fully compensated	Within normal limits	<35 (4.7)	<22
METABOLIC ACIDOSIS			
Uncompensated	<7.35	Within normal limits	<22
Partially compensated	<7.35	<35 (4.7)	<22
Fully compensated	Within normal limits	<35 (4.7)	<22
METABOLIC ALKALOSIS			
Uncompensated	>7.45	Within normal limits	>26
Partially compensated	>7.45	>45 (6.0)	>26
Fully compensated	Within normal limits	>45 (6.0)	>26

The partial pressure of venous oxygenation is not useful for measuring oxygenation, as oxygen has already been extracted at tissue level. However, ventilation and acid–base balance can be analysed using the partial pressure of carbon dioxide in venous blood ($PvCO_2$), venous pH and venous serum HCO_3^-. Venous oxygen saturation (SvO_2) can be used in goal-directed therapy for severe sepsis and septic shock.[74]

The minor corrections when converting venous blood gas to ABG equivalents vary slightly according to sampling site. For central sampling, add 0.03–0.05 to the pH and subtract 4–5 mmHg from the $PvCO_2$. For peripheral samples add 0.02–0.04 to the pH and subtract 3–8 mmHg from the $PvCO_2$. Caution should be used in patients with shock where there is poor correlation between venous and arterial samples, particularly for PCO_2 where the differences may increase by a factor of three.[73]

Continuous central venous oxygenation monitoring

$SvO_2/ScvO_2$ (mixed or central venous oxygen saturation) has been a useful assessment of oxygen delivery and consumption, particularly for patients following cardiac surgery and those with sepsis. Continuous $SvO_2/ScvO_2$ is measured using various wavelengths of light via a pulmonary artery catheter to measure SvO_2 or via a central line in the superior vena cava to measure SvO_2, or via a peripherally inserted central line. Normal venous oxygenation is around 70–80%, meaning that healthy people consume around 25% of the oxygen available to them. When oxygen demand is higher, healthy people are able to compensate by increasing their respiratory rate and heart rate. Critically ill patients may have difficulty compensating for increased oxygen demand, and so extract more oxygen from the tissues, leading to a lower venous oxygen saturation. Causes of decreased $ScvO_2$ include increased oxygen consumption, decreased cardiac output, decreased oxygen supply and nursing interventions such as positioning. These may indicate a need to respond through decreasing metabolic demand, increasing inspired oxygen, correcting haemoglobin or increasing cardiac output.[75]

There are slight differences in venous oxygenation values according to the measure used. $ScvO_2$, which measures oxygen saturation from the upper part of the body, will have a value 5–10% higher than the saturation measured using SvO_2, which uses blood returning from both the upper and lower body circulation, and from the coronary circulation. These differences correlate consistently, meaning that the less-invasive $ScvO_2$

monitoring, requiring only a central line, is a satisfactory surrogate.[75]

Oxygen tension-derived indices

The alveolar–arterial gradient is a marker of intrapulmonary shunting (i.e. blood flowing past collapsed areas of alveoli not involved in gas exchange). The index is calculated as $PAO_2 - PaO_2$ (where PAO_2 is the partial pressure of oxygen in the alveoli). PAO_2 is determined by a complex equation, the alveolar gas equation. PAO_2 and PaO_2 are equal when perfusion and ventilation are perfectly matched. The gradient increases with age, but a value of 5–15 mmHg is normal up until approximately middle age. Despite questions about its clinical usefulness, particularly in the critically ill, it is used in clinical practice as a trending tool to track intrapulmonary shunting. Simply put, the larger the gradient between PAO_2 and PaO_2, the larger is the degree of intrapulmonary shunting.[76]

The ratio of PaO_2 to the fraction of inspired oxygen (FiO_2), commonly referred to as the PaO_2/FiO_2 (or P/F) ratio, was introduced as a simple way of estimating pulmonary shunting, even though it does not formally measure alveolar partial pressure. A consensus paper outlines criteria known as the Berlin Definition[77] to define stages of ARDS. According to this definition, a PaO_2/FiO_2 ratio of 200–300 mmHg (≤ 39.9 kPa) indicates mild ARDS, a ratio of 100–200 mmHg (≤ 26.6 kPa) indicates moderate ARDS, while a ratio of less than or equal to 100 mmHg (< 13.3 kPa) indicates severe ARDS. For example, in a patient receiving a FiO_2 of 0.65 who has a PaO_2 of 90 mmHg (12 kPa), their PaO_2/FiO_2 ratio would be 138.5 mmHg, indicating a moderate ARDS state. A diagnosis of ARDS also requires the above reductions in the PaO_2/FiO_2 ratio to be present with the patient receiving at least 5 cmH_2O of positive end-expiratory pressure or continuous positive airway pressure. It requires this state to have developed within 1 week of a known clinical insult or worsening respiratory symptoms. A CXR should show bilateral opacities not fully explained by other causes and respiratory failure not fully explained by cardiac failure or fluid overload.[77]

Blood tests

Haematology and biochemistry investigations should inform treatment for patients with respiratory dysfunction. Full blood count, including a leukocyte differential count, can monitor white cell activity for patients with a confirmed or suspected infective process. When infections are severe, the full blood count will show a dramatic rise in the number of immature neutrophils. Blood cultures can also assist in diagnosis of bacterial or yeast infections and isolation of the causative organism. Viral studies may aid diagnosis for respiratory infections of unknown origin. Where pulmonary embolism is suspected, a D-dimer test can assist diagnosis of a thrombus. Routine measurement of urea and electrolytes can track renal function and acid–base status.[78]

> ### Practice tip
>
> Monitoring lactate levels is important as the levels can be used to assess the effectiveness and efficiency of resuscitative therapies. A persistently elevated lactate level is associated with higher morbidity and poorer patient outcomes. Caution should be used in interpreting lactate levels in patients with liver dysfunction; lactate clearance and normalisation are impaired for these patients during early resuscitation management.[79]

Sputum, tracheal aspirates and nasopharyngeal aspirates

Colour, consistency and volume of sputum provide useful information in determining changes in a patient's respiratory status and progress. Regular cultures of tracheal sputum reveal colonisation by opportunistic organisms and can identify the cause of an acute chest infection or sepsis. Some ICUs have routine (weekly or twice-weekly) surveillance monitoring of tracheal aspirates in long-term mechanically ventilated patients. In spontaneously breathing patients, sputum specimens can be collected in a sterile specimen receptacle. Specimens should be collected prior to commencement of antibiotic therapy and are best collected early in the morning.[80] In intubated patients, using a sputum trap between the suction catheter and suction tubing assists sputum collection. A sterile technique should be maintained to reduce sample contamination.[80]

If obtaining an adequate sputum specimen in non-intubated patients is difficult, there is evidence that administration of nebulised saline (isotonic or hypertonic) may assist sputum collection. There is no evidence to support this among mechanically ventilated patients but, anecdotally, nebulised normal saline may assist sputum production by moistening the airways and thinning secretions. Physiotherapy in the form of manual hyperinflation and head-down tilt during therapy has been shown to increase sputum production for sample collection.[80]

Instilling normal saline in an endotracheal tube to facilitate clearance and/or collection of tenacious sputum remains a controversial issue. There is no evidence that instillation facilitates secretion clearance, while there is some evidence that it increases both patient discomfort and the risk of bacterial contamination of the lower airway. Therefore, this practice is not recommended.[81]

Nasopharyngeal aspirate or swabs may be necessary to diagnose viral respiratory infections. The nasopharyngeal aspirate is collected by inserting a fine, sterile suction catheter (8 or 10 F) attached to a sputum trap through the nares and back to the nasopharynx. Suction is applied while withdrawing and slowly rotating the catheter. The catheter is flushed through to the sputum trap with sterile normal saline or transport medium if available. A nasopharyngeal swab is collected by inserting a specially designed swab to the back of the nasopharynx and rotating for 5–10 seconds. The swab is then withdrawn slowly and placed in the plastic vial containing transport medium.[82] As close contact with the patient is necessary, and the procedure can generate aerosols and droplets, personal protective equipment should be worn.

Diagnostic procedures

Assessment and monitoring of the respiratory status of a critically ill patient may rely on various medical imaging tests and bronchoscopy to determine the cause and severity of the illness episode, relevant comorbidities and the patient's response to treatment.

Medical imaging

A range of imaging techniques may be available for supporting care of a critically ill patient with a respiratory dysfunction, depending on the level of broader health service resources available. This subsection describes X-ray, ultrasound, computerised tomography (CT), magnetic resonance imaging (MRI) and ventilation/perfusion scan techniques.

Chest X-ray

Chest radiography is a common diagnostic tool used for respiratory examination of critically ill patients. CXR allows basic information regarding abnormalities in the chest to be obtained relatively quickly. The image provides information about lung fields and other thoracic structures as well as the placement of invasive lines and tubes. In the ventilated patient, serial CXRs also enable sequential assessment of lung status in relation to therapy,[83] although the value-add of routine CXRs should be considered to maximise benefit and minimise cost.[84]

In-unit X-rays of patients using portable equipment are inferior to those taken using a fixed camera in the radiology department. Patient preparation is therefore important to optimise the quality of the film.[85] Patients should ideally be positioned sitting or semi-erect; CXRs using a supine position are less effective at revealing gravity-related abnormalities such as haemothorax. Lateral view CXRs may assist identification of lesions in the thorax. Film plate location against the patient's thorax determines the view: for posteroanterior (PA) the plate is positioned against the anterior thorax (Fig. 13.16), while the anteroposterior (AP) view has the plate against the patient's back. For mobile CXRs, the AP view is used. The AP view can magnify thoracic structures and can be less

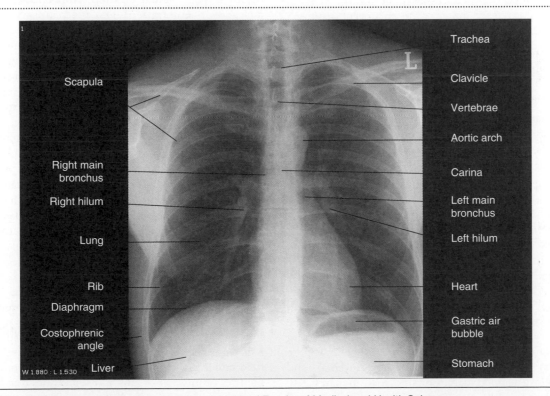

FIGURE 13.16   Chest X-ray, PA view.

Source: Published with permission from University of Auckland Faculty of Medical and Health Sciences.

distinct or even distorted, so interpret findings with caution, particularly if comparing them with previous PA images.[86]

Practice tip

When preparing your patient for a CXR, minimise the number of monitoring leads and unnecessary equipment in the CXR field to optimise the image. Note all lines and tubes present on the CXR request form to aid interpretation.

CXR interpretation follows a systematic process designed to identify common pathophysiological processes and the locations of lines and other items. Table 13.7[87] provides a comprehensive guideline for viewing and interpreting a CXR. Common abnormalities that can be detected by CXR include the following:

- Lobar collapse or atelectasis: loss of lung volume, displacement of fissures and vascular markings and/or diaphragmatic elevation on the affected side.
- Pneumothorax: lack of pulmonary vascular markings on the affected side so the lung field appears black. There will be mediastinal and possible tracheal shift away from the affected side in tension pneumothorax.
- Pleural effusion: in the dependent areas of the pleural spaces, costophrenic angles are blunted by fluid and there may be a mediastinal shift away from a large effusion. Effusions are best visualised with the patient upright and will be evident only on an AP image with 200–400 mL of fluid in the pleural space.
- Pulmonary oedema: lung fields, particularly central and perihilar areas, appear white. Kerley B lines (small horizontal lines <2 cm long) may be present in the lung periphery near the costophrenic angles.
- Pulmonary embolism: although not the optimal diagnostic tool, areas of infarction may be visualised on CXR and may be mistaken for collapse or consolidation.
- Pneumoperitoneum: free air under the diaphragm elevates the diaphragm.[86]

Ultrasound

Ultrasound imaging (sonography) is a useful bedside diagnostic tool for a select group of critically ill patients and can add to the diagnostic information provided by CXR and CT scanning. Ultrasound uses high-frequency sound waves which, when probed on the body, reflect and scatter. The advantages are that the procedure can take place within the ICU and it is radiation free.[88] Ultrasound is most useful for patients with fluid in the pleural space (i.e. pleural effusion, haemothorax or empyema), and provides more-detailed diagnostic information than CXR alone. Ultrasound allows an estimate of the volume and exact location of the fluid present and reduces the

potential for serious complications during aspiration of fluid or chest tube insertion. Newer applications of lung ultrasound technology include assessment of lung recruitment arising from positive end-expiratory pressure, and of reaeration of the alveoli following therapy for ventilator-associated pneumonia.[89] Useful, simplified diagnostic ultrasound protocols are the Bedside Lung Ultrasound in Emergency (BLUE) protocol that guides users through signs of abnormal lung surfaces, pleural effusions, consolidation, interstitial syndrome and pneumothorax for rapid diagnosis of acute respiratory failure, and the Fluid Administration Limited by Lung Sonography (FALLS) protocol that directs scanning activities towards identifying or ruling out causes of shock (i.e. obstructive, cardiogenic, hypovolaemic or distributive), thereby identifying which patients are most likely to benefit from fluid resuscitation.[90]

Computed tomography (CT)

CT is a diagnostic investigation that provides greater specificity in chest anatomy and pathophysiology than a plain CXR, using multiple beams in a circle around the body. These beams are directed to a specific body area and provide detailed, consecutive cross-sectional slices of the scanned regions. CT scans can be performed with or without intravenous contrast. Contrast improves diagnostic precision but is used with caution in patients with renal impairment, as renal failure may preclude a patient from receiving contrast. CT scanning is useful in the detection and diagnosis of pulmonary, pleural and mediastinal disorders (e.g. pleural effusion, empyema, haemothorax, atelectasis, pneumonia, ARDS). CT scans are useful where there are discrepancies between clinical and radiographic findings, or where the patient is not responding as expected to therapy.[91] CT pulmonary angiography produces a detailed view of blood vessels and is, therefore, the most definitive method for diagnosing pulmonary embolism, particularly in the presence of an abnormal CXR.[92]

A significant limitation of CT scanning is that the patient is transported away from the ICU. Transport increases the risks for critically ill patients and usually requires at least two appropriately trained staff to accompany the patient. Detailed planning by the healthcare team (including imaging staff) includes ventilator support, monitoring requirements and maintenance of infusions during scanning. Portable CT scanners are available in some centres and may reduce the risks associated with transportation of critically ill patients to fixed CT scanners.[93] (See Chapter 6 for discussion of in-hospital transfers, and Chapter 23 for inter-hospital transport.)

Magnetic resonance imaging (MRI)

MRI uses radiofrequency waves and a strong magnetic field rather than X-rays to provide high-contrast, detailed pictures of internal organs and soft tissues that are clearer than those generated by X-ray or CT scans. It is not the imaging of choice for respiratory assessment in the

TABLE 13.7

Guide to normal chest X-ray interpretation[87]

Technical issues	• Check X-ray belongs to correct patient; note date and time of film. • Ensure you are viewing X-ray correctly (i.e. right and left markings correspond to thoracic structures). • Determine whether X-ray was taken supine or erect, and whether PA or AP. • Check X-ray was taken at full inspiration (posterior aspects of 9th/10th ribs and anterior aspects of 5th/6th ribs should be visible above diaphragm). • Note the penetration of the film: dark films are overpenetrated and may require a strong light to view; white films are underpenetrated; good penetration will allow visualisation of the vertebrae behind the heart.
Bones	• Check along each rib from vertebral origin, looking for fractures. • Ensure clavicles and scapulas are intact.
Mediastinum	• Check for presence of trachea and identify carina (approximately level of 5th–6th vertebrae). • Check width of mediastinum: should not be more than 8 cm.
Apex	• Ensure blood vessels are visible in both apices, particularly looking to rule out pneumothoraces that present as clear black shading on the X-ray. Erect X-rays are essential to facilitate visibility of pneumothoraces.
Hilum	• Check for prominence of vessels in this region: it generally indicates vascular abnormalities such as pulmonary oedema or pulmonary hypertension, or congestive heart failure.
Heart	• Cardiac silhouette should be not more than 50% of the diameter of the thorax, with 1/3 of heart shadow to the right of the vertebrae and 1/3 of shadow to the left of the vertebrae; this positioning helps to rule out a tension pneumothorax. It should be noted that, post-cardiac surgery, if the mediastinum is left open the heart may appear wider than this; also in AP films this may be the case due to the plate being further away from the heart.

Lung	• Identify the lobes of the lungs and determine if infiltrate or collapse is present in one or more of them. Lobes are approximately located as follows:
	  ○ left upper lobe occupies upper half of lung
	  ○ left lower lobe occupies lower half of lung
	  ○ right lower lobe occupies costophrenic portion of lung
	  ○ right middle lobe occupies cardiophrenic portion of lung
	  ○ right upper lobe occupies upper portion of lung.

Diaphragm	• Check levels of diaphragm: right diaphragm will normally be 1–2 cm above the left diaphragm to accommodate the liver.
Gastric	• Check for pneumoperitoneum and dilated loops of bowel.
Catheters and lines	• Identify distal end of endotracheal tube and ensure it is placed above the carina (i.e. not in the right main bronchus). • Trace nasogastric tube along length and ensure tip is in stomach, or below stomach if a nasoenteric tube. • Check position of intra-aortic balloon pump and ensure it is in the descending thoracic aorta. • Trace all central catheters and ensure distal tip is in correct location. • Identify other lines (e.g. intercostal catheters, pacing wires) and note location.

PA = posteroanterior; AP = anteroposterior.

Source: Adapted from Lareau C, Wootton J. The 'frequently' normal chest x-ray. Can J Rural Med 2004;9(3):183–6.

critically ill, being most useful for detecting neurological or spinal cord injury and congenital heart disease. The strong magnetic field around the scanner means that ferromagnetic objects containing material that can be attracted by magnets, such as iron or steel, can become potentially fatal projectiles. MRI scans may, therefore, be unsuitable for some patients.[94] While the use of MRI is discouraged where permanent pacemakers and implantable defibrillators are in situ, recent research suggests MRIs may be safe if certain precautions are taken: MRI should be conducted only where it is absolutely necessary, and implantable devices should be checked immediately afterwards.[95] Some types of neurostimulation devices and intracranial aneurysm clips[96] have been designed for safe use in MRI, but careful screening should precede MRI to determine patient- and device-specific risks. Dental fillings, braces and retainers are usually safe but may distort images of the face or brain.[94] MRI in people with such devices should be used only where the potential benefit clearly outweighs the risks. The strong magnetic fields also have the potential to interfere with ventilators, infusion pumps and monitoring equipment.

Ventilation/perfusion (V/Q) scan

A V/Q scan is indicated when a mismatch of lung ventilation and perfusion is suspected, most commonly for pulmonary embolism. The scan is performed with the patient inhaling a radioisotopic gas, while the perfusion scan is performed using an intravenous radioisotope that reveals the distribution of blood flow in the pulmonary vessels. These two scans are then compared, seeking mismatches between perfusion and ventilation.

Bronchoscopy

Bronchoscopy is a bedside technique used for both diagnostic and therapeutic purposes. The bronchoscope can be either rigid or flexible, with the flexible fibreoptic bronchoscope most widely used in critical care. A flexible fibreoptic bronchoscope allows direct visualisation of respiratory mucosa and thorough examination of the upper airways and tracheobronchial tree. The scope is passed into the trachea via the oropharynx or nares. In mechanically ventilated patients, the scope can be passed quickly and easily down the endotracheal or tracheostomy tube using a specially adapted valve that allows passage of the scope without disconnection of mechanical ventilation. During bronchoscopy, supplemental oxygen can be administered in non-intubated patients and the FiO_2 can be increased in intubated patients. Accurate continuous monitoring during the procedure includes continuous pulse oximetry, electrocardiography, and monitoring of respiratory rate, heart rate and blood pressure. Equipment for advanced airway management, suctioning, cardiac defibrillation and advanced life support medications is immediately available. In intubated patients, one person is responsible for security of the airway in order to reduce the risk of displacement during the procedure.

When performed by an experienced operator, fibreoptic bronchoscopy is a relatively safe procedure in critically ill patients. In mechanically ventilated patients, the correct diameter of bronchoscope relative to the endotracheal tube diameter is important in order to avoid decreases in tidal and minute volumes, decreased PaO_2 and increased $PaCO_2$. Serious complications such as bleeding, bronchospasm, arrhythmia, pneumothorax and pneumonia occur rarely.[97] Patient preparation may include CXR, haemoglobin and coagulation profile particularly if a biopsy is to be performed, baseline ABGs and fasting or cessation of feeds for 4–6 hours prior.

Diagnostic indications for bronchoscopy include further investigation of poor gas exchange; evaluation of haemoptysis; collection of specimens (e.g. bronchoalveolar lavage, bronchial washings, bronchial brushings, lung biopsy); diagnosis of infection, interstitial lung disease, rejection post lung transplantation or malignancy; and diagnosis of airway injury due to burns, aspiration or chest trauma. Therapeutic indications include removal of mucous plugs, removal of foreign bodies, treatment of atelectasis, assistance during tracheostomy, airway dilation and stenting for tracheobronchomalacia and tracheobronchial stenosis, and lung volume reduction for emphysema.[97]

Summary

In this chapter a comprehensive overview is provided of assessment and monitoring of a patient with respiratory dysfunction to aid clinical decision making. Acute respiratory dysfunction is a major cause for admission to a critical care unit. Whether due to a primary or a secondary condition, compromise of the respiratory system can be a life-threatening situation. The related respiratory physiology, pathophysiology, assessment and respiratory monitoring, bedside laboratory investigations and medical imaging are outlined:

- Critical care nurses are in a prime position to provide systematic and dynamic bedside assessments of a patient's respiratory status, including past and presenting respiratory history, and physical examination of the thorax and lungs using inspection, palpation and auscultation techniques.

- Monitoring of a patient's respiratory function includes pulse oximetry and capnography. Bedside and laboratory investigations including ABG analysis, blood tests and sputum and tracheal aspirates add to available information and assist in both diagnosis and treatment. ABG testing is common and ABG interpretation is an important clinical skill for critical care nurses.

- CXR is the most common diagnostic imaging tool in the ICU. CXR interpretation follows a systematic process to identify common pathologies and to locate lines and other items. Bronchoscopy is a useful bedside diagnostic and therapeutic device. CT provides greater specificity than CXR. Ultrasound imaging is useful to diagnose fluid in the pleural space. MRI and V/Q scans are more-sophisticated diagnostic tools.

Careful patient assessment is essential, as respiratory dysfunction can be immediately life threatening. Contemporary critical care practice involves comprehensive clinical assessment skills and use of a range of monitoring devices and diagnostic procedures. This challenges critical care nurses to be adaptable and willing to embrace new skills and knowledge.

Case study

You are working as a staff nurse on a day shift in the emergency department when Ruairi Moran, a 41-year-old man with breathlessness, arrives by ambulance from his general practitioner's office. He presented with a 10-day history of cough, and a 3-day history of expectorating tenacious yellow-green sputum, fever and shakes, decreased appetite and mild right-sided chest pain with increasing dyspnoea and a hoarse voice. The paramedics reported that his respiratory rate was 35 bpm and shallow. He maintained SpO_2 at 93% while receiving oxygen 6 L/min via Hudson Mask.

During your history taking, it is revealed that Ruairi has no past medical history. He is normally fit and well and enjoys running regularly. He does not smoke, and occasionally drinks a glass of wine when out with friends. He reported that, 2 weeks ago, he was on a holiday in the South of France. He is an office manager in a large solicitor company. He reported that he is married and has two children, 2 and 5 years old. He lives in a semi-detached house.

CLINICAL ASSESSMENT

A clinical assessment is undertaken following the ABCDE Framework as follows:

ABCDE FRAMEWORK ELEMENTS	CLINICAL SIGNS	RATIONALE
Airway	Check for patency	To assess the risk of obstruction (partial or full). If the patient speaks in full sentences, the airway is patent. If they cannot speak in full sentences, there is a risk of partial or full obstruction.
Breathing	RR, SpO_2, use of accessory muscles, nasal flare, skin colour for signs of hypoxaemia	The RR is the first sign of patient deterioration. Increased RR is a compensatory mechanism to hypoxaemia, when the central nervous system is activated with the stimulation of low levels of PaO_2 that are detected by the central and peripheral chemoreceptors.
	Auscultation	Normal SpO_2 is 94–98% and measures % of oxygen saturation.
	Palpation	The use of accessory muscles (trapezius, abdominal muscles) is activated when the diaphragm and intercostal muscles can no longer be used for breathing owing to increased work of breathing. Skin colour is assessed for signs of cyanosis.
	Percussion	
	ABG	
	CXR	Auscultation to assess for bronchial sounds.
		Palpation to assess for deformities of the chest and equal chest expansion.
		Percussion to assess for presence or absence of fluid in the lungs.
		ABG will provide information on the gas exchange and severity of hypoxaemia.
		CXR will demonstrate changes in the lung tissue and help with diagnosis.
Circulation	HR, BP, CRT, temperature	Increased HR is a sign of compensation of the body to the low levels of PaO_2 that are detected by the chemoreceptors. Adrenaline (epinephrine) is excreted to increase the HR and BP in order to improve blood supply and oxygenation.
		Prolonged CRT (>2 s) means peripheral vasoconstriction and it is also a compensatory mechanism that is activated in order to improve the blood supply.
		Temperature to assess for signs of infection.
Disability	AVPU or GCS	To assess the consciousness level of the patient.
	Blood glucose levels	Blood glucose levels can alter consciousness level.

ABCDE FRAMEWORK ELEMENTS	CLINICAL SIGNS	RATIONALE
Exposure	Full body assessment for drains, wounds, skin condition, rash, etc.	To fully assess the body of the patient for signs of haemorrhage, allergic reaction, etc.
		Use AMPLE to assess factors that relate to the episode.
	Allergies	
	Medication	
	Past medical history	
	Last meal	
	Events leading to the episode	
Investigations	Order laboratory tests	CURB65 is a tool to measure risk and severity of CAP and is used in emergency departments.
	CURB65	

ABG = arterial blood gas; AMPLE = allergies, medications, past medical history, last meal eaten, events leading; AVPU = alert, voice, pain, unresponsive; BP = blood pressure; CAP = community-acquired pneumonia; CRT = capillary refill time; CURB65 = confusion, urea, respiratory rate, blood pressure, age 65 or older; CXR = chest X-ray; GCS = Glasgow Coma Score; HR = heart rate; PaO_2 = partial pressure of arterial oxygen; RR = respiratory rate, SpO_2 = peripheral oxygen saturation.

The medical staff members order laboratory and radiological investigations to assist with the diagnosis:

Sodium 132 mmol/L

Potassium 3.7 mmol/L

Creatinine 112 micromol/L

Estimated glomerular filtration rate >90

Urea 14.0 mmol/L

Blood glucose level 8.5 mmol/L

bHCG <0.5

Haemoglobin 130 g/L

White cell count 15.89 $\times$ 10^9/L

Neutrophils 174 $\times$ 10^9/L, PLT 38 $\times10^9$/L

Alanine aminotransferase 55 units/L

Gamma-glutamyl transferase 11 units/L

International normalised ratio 1.8

C-reactive protein 13.5 mg/dL

The chest X-ray shows right lower lobe consolidation

PROGRESS

The patient is transferred from the emergency department to a respiratory medicine ward for close monitoring and management. Four hours later, the nurse looking after him in the ward made a further assessment of his clinical condition, identifying the following:

Unable to speak in full sentences, confused

Respiratory rate 40 breaths/min, rapid and shallow

Use of accessory muscles and nasal flaring

Coarse crackles and bronchial breathing in the right lower lobe on auscultation

SpO_2 93% on 8 L/minute oxygen

Arterial blood gas:

pH: 7.32

PaO_2 8.6 kpa (64.5 mmHg)

$PaCO_2$ 4.7 kpa (35.2 mmHg)

HCO_3^- 18

Lactate 3.5

Heart rate 140 beats/min regular, sinus rhythm

Blood pressure 95/55 mmHg

Capillary refill 4 s, peripheries cool

Temperature 39°C

Blood glucose level 8.5 mmol/L.

He was transferred to the ICU for intubation and mechanical ventilation. He remained ventilated in the ICU for 5 days and was then successfully extubated. He remained in hospital for another 4 days before being discharged.

CASE STUDY QUESTIONS

1 Using the systematic assessment framework ABCDE, explain how you would assess Ruairi and provide a rationale for what you are assessing (use the ABCDE Framework table above to guide you). Remember to make the assessment relevant to this patient.
2 Describe how the underlying physiological changes will affect the patient's tissue oxygenation.
3 Explain how the physiological changes that occur in pneumonia are contributing to the clinical signs exhibited in the patient.
4 As the nurse looking after this patient, what are your priorities of care in the first 24 hours in ICU?
5 Interpret the following blood gas values:
   pH: 7.32 (usual range: 7.36–7.44)
   H^+: 47.4
   PaO_2: 8.6 kPa (usual range 10.5–14 kPa)
   $PaCO_2$: 4.7 kPa (usual range 4.7–6.0 kPa)
   HCO_3^-: 18 (usual range 22–32 mmol/L)
   Lactate: 3.5

RESEARCH VIGNETTE

Holm A, Viftrup A, Karlsson V, et al. Nurses' communication with mechanically ventilated patients in the intensive care unit: Umbrella review. J Adv Nurs 2020;76(11):2909–20.

Abstract

Aim: To conduct a review summarising evidence concerning communication with mechanically ventilated patients in the ICU.

Background: ICU patients undergoing mechanical ventilation are unable to communicate verbally, causing many negative emotions. Due to changes in sedation practice, a growing number of patients are conscious and experience communication difficulties.

Design: The umbrella review method guided by the Joanna Briggs Institute was applied.

Data sources: A systematic search was done in the Cochrane Library, the Joanna Briggs Institute database, Cinahl, Pubmed, PsycINFO and Scopus between January and April 2019. Search terms were 'nurse–patient communication', 'mechanical ventilation', 'intensive care', and 'reviews as publication type'. Literature from 2009–19 was included.

Review methods: Following recommendations by the Joanna Briggs Institute, a quality appraisal, data extraction and synthesis were done.

Results: Seven research syntheses were included. There were two main themes and six subthemes: (1) characterisation of the nurse–patient communication: (a) patients' communication, (b) nurses' communication; (2) nursing interventions that facilitate communication: (a) communication assessment and documentation, (b) communication methods and approaches, (c) education and training of nurses, and (d) augmentative and alternative communication.

Conclusion: Nurse–patient communication was characterised by an unequal power relationship with a common experience – frustration. Four key interventions were identified and an integration of these may be key to designing and implementing future communication packages in the ICU. Findings are transferable to ICU practices where patients are conscious and experience communication difficulties.

Critique

This umbrella review provides an overview of seven research syntheses, all of which concern communication with patients who are mechanically ventilated in the ICU. The objective was to explore nurse–patient communication and to determine which nurse-led interventions may facilitate communication.

As we know, patients who are receiving mechanical ventilation are voiceless for a period of time. Nowadays, we are moving to targeting lighter levels of sedation wherever possible. Because of this, patients are conscious and able to interact more. As nurses, we have the most contact with patients during this time and effective nurse–patient communication is of paramount importance to promote a therapeutic relationship.

While intubated, patients may struggle to express their needs, thoughts and wishes promoting negative thoughts such as frustration, fear, anger and loss of control. However, nursing care characterised by patience, calmness and empathy can alleviate negative experiences. Nurses may also experience negative emotions while caring for patients who are mechanically ventilated if they are unable to alleviate a conscious patient's suffering or understand their wishes.

Communication is a basic right and skill and a key element of patient-centred care. Good nurse–patient communication in the ICU is vital to ensure good care and safety.

Aim of the review: The authors had two review questions:

1. What characterises nurse–patient communication?
2. Which nursing interventions can facilitate communication?

What is an umbrella review?

This umbrella review provides an overall synthesis of existing reviews addressing nurse–patient communication in the ICU. The authors used guidelines developed by the Joanna Briggs Institute to guide the review. A comprehensive search was undertaken using key terms 'nurse–patient communication', 'mechanical ventilation', 'intensive care', and 'reviews as publication type'. Synonyms and Boolean operators (AND/OR) were used. Language bias was limited, with the authors including articles published between 2009 and 2019, in either English or Nordic languages.

Two authors systematically searched five electronic databases with the assistance of a librarian, adding rigour to the search process. A total of 272 articles were identified and 7 were included in the umbrella review. The processes described are clear and transparent, and able to be reproduced.

Two of the researchers independently used an 11-question appraisal tool developed by the Joanna Briggs Institute then pooled their results for an overall appraisal. Use of two reviewers in the quality appraisal and search is recommended and increases the rigour of the process.

A total of 229 findings were compared and contrasted in this review. Two main themes (characterisation of the nurse–patient communication and nursing interventions that facilitate communication) and six subthemes (patients' communication, nurses' communication, communication assessment and documentation, communication methods and approaches, education and training of nurses and augmentative and alternative communication) were identified. The findings show that nurse–patient communication is often burdened with negative experiences and a joint experience of frustration for both nurses and patients. This review also described that while nurses hold the control of communication contents and duration, they also play a vital role in facilitating positive communication experiences. This review suggests that a systematic approach to communication assessment and documentation be implemented, that methods of communication employed by nurses are of great importance, that education and training of nurses in communication is a significant factor in its success or not, and that different approaches to communication aids may be useful in the ICU.

One possible limitation of using an umbrella review approach is that previous errors in the previous reviews may be amplified in this review, leading to incorrect findings. Another limitation may be that of including only reviews that analysed nurses' perspectives of communication. As we know, the ICU is a very multidisciplinary environment and patients, and other allied health professionals, may see communication differently to nurses.

This review suggests that time and effort should be spent on the development and use of a communication package involving communication assessment tool, communication method or approach, a training and education program and the use of both aided and unaided tools and techniques, available in multiple languages, to support effective nurse–patient communication.

Learning activities

1   What are some limitations of using pulse oximetry?
2   When might you decide to use $PetCO_2$ monitoring in clinical practice?
3   When might you use a venous blood gas analysis in critical care practice?
4   Is lactate a good measure of oxygenation in critical illness?

Online resources

Acidbase.org, https://www.acidbase.org

American Association for Respiratory Care, https://www.aarc.org

American Thoracic Society, https://www.thoracic.org

ARDS Network, www.ardsnet.org

Asian Pacific Society of Respirology, https://www.apsresp.org

Australian & New Zealand Society of Respiratory Science, https://www.anzsrs.org.au

Australian Lung Foundation, https://www.lungfoundation.com.au

Australian Resuscitation Council. Arterial blood gas analysis workshop, https://resus.org.au/download/als2_instructor/clinical/skill_stations/arterial_blood_gas_analysis/abg-workshop-guidance-jun-2016.pdf

Basic Lung Sounds Tutorial, https://www.littmann.com.au/3M/en_AU/littmann-stethoscopes-au/education-center/training/

Capnography: a comprehensive educational website, https://www.capnography.com

Chest X-rays, https://www.learningradiology.com

European Respiratory Journal, https://erj.ersjournals.com

Lung Health Promotion Centre, The Alfred Hospital, Victoria, https://www.lunghealth.org

Respiratory Care online, https://rc.rcjournal.com

Thoracic Society of Australia and New Zealand, https://www.thoracic.org.au

Thorax: an international journal of respiratory medicine, http://thorax.bmj.com

Further reading

Bansal T, Beese R. Interpreting a chest X-ray. Br J Hosp Med 2019;80(5):C75–9.

Brochard L, Martin GS, Blanch L, et al. Clinical review: respiratory monitoring in the ICU – a consensus of 16. Crit Care 2012;16(2):219. doi: 10.1186/cc11146.

de Haro C, Ochagavia A, López-Aguilar J, et al. Patient–ventilator asynchronies during mechanical ventilation: current knowledge and research priorities. Intensive Care Med Exp 2019;7(Suppl. 1):43.

Demoule A, Hajage D, Messika J, et al. Prevalence, intensity, and clinical impact of dyspnea in critically ill patients receiving invasive ventilation. Am J Resp Crit Care Med 2022;205(8):917–26.

Duckworth R. How to read and interpret end-tidal capnography waveforms. J Emerg Med Services 2017;42(8). Epub 1 August 2017. Available from: https://www.jems.com/patient-care/how-to-read-and-interpret-end-tidal-capnography-waveforms/. [Accessed 12 February 2023].

Metkus TS, Kim BS. Bedside diagnosis in the intensive care unit. Is looking overlooked? Ann Am Thorac Soc 2015;12(10):1447–50.

Mowery NT. Ventilator strategies for chronic obstructive pulmonary disease and acute respiratory distress syndrome. Surg Clin North Am 2017;97(6):1381–97.

Singer M, Young PJ, Laffey JG, et al. Dangers of hyperoxia. Crit Care 2021;25(1):440.

References

1. Kim JY, Yang KS, Chung Y, et al. Epidemiologic characteristics and clinical significance of respiratory viral infections among adult patients admitted to the intensive care unit. Front Med (Lausanne) 2022;9:829624.

2. Celik I, Saatci E, Eyuboglu AF. Emerging and reemerging respiratory viral infections up to Covid-19. Turk J Med Sci 2020;50(SI-1):557–62.

3. Wiemken T, Peyrani P, Bryant K, et al. Incidence of respiratory viruses in patients with community-acquired pneumonia admitted to the intensive care unit: results from the Severe Influenza Pneumonia Surveillance (SIPS) project. Eur J Clin Microbiol Infect Dis 2013;32(5):705–10.

4. Urden L, Stacy K, Lough M. Critical care nursing: diagnosis and management. 6th ed. St Louis: Elsevier/Mosby; 2010.

5. Stanfield C. Principles of human physiology. 6th ed. London: Pearson Education; 2016.

6. Marieb E, Wilhelm P, Mallatt J. Human physiology. 8th ed. London: Pearson Education; 2017.

7. Thompson J, McFarland G, Hirsch J, et al. Mosby's clinical nursing. 5th ed. St Louis: Elsevier/Mosby; 2012.

8. Lombardi RA, Arthur ME. Arytenoid subluxation. StatPearls Publishing; 2021. Available from: https://www.ncbi.nlm.nih.gov/books/NBK544264/. [Accessed 12 February 2023].

9. Sibert KS, Long JL, Haddy SM. Extubation and the risks of coughing and laryngospasm in the era of coronavirus disease-19 (COVID-19). Cureus 2020;12(5):e8196.

10. West J, Luks A. Respiratory physiology: the essentials. 10th ed. Philadelphia: Wolters Kluwer; 2016.

11. Martini F, Cober W, Nath J, et al. Visual anatomy and physiology. 3rd ed. Harlow, Essex: Pearson Education; 2017.

12. Mandoorah S, Mead T. Phrenic nerve injury. Treasure Island, FL: StatPearls Publishing; 2022. Available from: https://pubmed.ncbi.nlm.nih.gov/29489218/. [Accessed 12 February 2023].

13. Aly H, Mohamed MA, Wung JT. Surfactant and continuous positive airway pressure for the prevention of chronic lung disease: history, reality, and new challenges. Semin Fetal Neonatal Med 2017;22(5):348–53.

14. Marieb E, Wilhelm PB, Mallatt JB. Human anatomy. 8th ed. New York: Pearson; 2016.

15. Marieb EN, Hoehn K. Human anatomy and physiology. 8th ed. New York: Pearson Education, Inc; 2010.

16. Stacy K. Pulmonary anatomy and physiology. In: Urden L, Stacy K, Lough M, editors. Critical care nursing: diagnosis and management. 8th ed. St Louis: Elsevier/Mosby; 2018, p. 411–30.

17. Urden L, Stacy K, Lough M. Critical care nursing: diagnosis and management. 7th ed. St Louis: Elsevier/Mosby; 2014.

18. Barrett KE, Barman SM, Yuan J, et al. Ganong's review of medical physiology. New York: McGraw-Hill Education; 2018.

19. Jonkman AH, de Vries HJ, Heunks LMA. Physiology of the respiratory drive in ICU patients: implications for diagnosis and treatment. Crit Care 2020;24(1):104.

20. Csoma B, Vulpi MR, Dragonieri S, et al. Hypercapnia in COPD: causes, consequences, and therapy. J Clin Med 2022;11(11):3180.

21. Shier D, Butler J, Lewis R. Hole's human anatomy and physiology. 14th ed New York: McGraw-Hill; 2016.

22. Pagana KD, Pagana TJ, Pagana TN. Mosby's diagnostic and laboratory test reference. 13th ed. Philadelphia: Elsevier; 2017.

23. Lumb AB. Why do patients need extra oxygen during a general anaesthetic? BJA Educ 2019;19(2):37–9.

24. McIntyre NR. Physiologic effects of non-invasive ventilation. Resp Care 2019;64(6):617–28.

25. Castro D, Patil SM, Keenaghan M. Arterial blood gas. Treasure Island, FL: StatPearls Publishing; 2022. Available from: https://pubmed.ncbi.nlm.nih.gov/30725604/. [Accessed 12 February 2023].

26. Seely R, Stephens T, Tate P. Anatomy and physiology. 7th ed. Boston: McGraw-Hill; 2006.

27. Vasileiadis I, Alevrakis E, Ampelioti S, et al. Acid–base disturbances in patients with asthma: a literature review and comments on their pathophysiology. J Clin Med 2019;8(4):563.

28. Luks A, Schoene R, Swenson E. High altitude. In: Broaddus VC, Mason R, Ernst J, et al., editors. Murray and Nadel's textbook of respiratory medicine. 6th ed. Philadelphia: Elsevier; 2016, p. 1367–84.

29. Hendrickson KW, Peltan ID, Brown SM. The epidemiology of acute respiratory distress syndrome before and after coronavirus disease 2019. Crit Care Clin 2021;37(4):703–16.

30. Hill NS. Acute ventilator failure. In: Broaddus VC, Mason R, Ernst J, et al., editors. Murray and Nadel's textbook of respiratory medicine. 6th ed. Philadelphia: Elsevier; 2016, p. 1723–39.

31. Urden L, Stacy K, Lough M. Critical care nursing: diagnosis and management. 8th ed. St Louis: Elsevier/Mosby; 2018.

32. Powell F, Wanger P, West J. Ventilation, blood flow and gas exchange. In: Broaddus VC, Mason R, Ernst J, et al, editors. Murray and Nadel's Textbook of respiratory medicine. 6th ed. Philadelphia: Elsevier; 2016, p. 45–75.

33. Carson K. Advanced critical care nursing. St Louis: Elsevier; 2009.

34. Shi R, Lai C, Teboul JL, et al. COVID-19 ARDS is characterized by higher extravascular lung water than non-COVID-19 ARDS: the PiCCOVID study. Crit Care 2021;25(1):186.

35. Cottin V, Price LC, Valenzuela C. The unmet medical need of pulmonary hypertension in idiopathic pulmonary fibrosis. Eur Respir J 2018; 51(1):1702596.

36. Harper N. Respiratory assessment and examination. Practice Nurse 2021;51(10):26–32.

37. Miao JL, Cai JJ, Qin XF, et al. Analysis of the clinicopathological characteristics and risk factors in patients with lung cancer and chronic obstructive pulmonary disease. Biomed Res Int 2018;2018:8398156.

38. Trimble A, Moffat V, Collins AM. Pulmonary infections in the returned traveller. Pneumonia (Nathan) 2017;9:1.

39. Krasinski Z, Chou A, Stepak H. COVID-19, long flights, and deep vein thrombosis: what we know so far. Cardiol J 2021;28(6):941–53.

40. Perlman DM, Maier LA. Occupational lung disease. Med Clin North Am 2019;103(3):535–48.

41. Morton P, Rempfer K. Patient assessment: respiratory assessment. In: Morton P, Fontaine D, editors. Critical care nursing: a holistic approach. 9th ed. Philadelphia: Kluwer/Lippincott Williams & Wilkins; 2009.

42. Weber J, Kelly J. Health assessment in nursing. Philadelphia: Lippincott, Williams & Wilkins; 2010.

43. Light R. Pneumothorax, chylothorax, hemothorax and fibrothorax. In: Broaddus VC, Mason R, Ernst J, et al., editors. Murray and Nadel's Textbook of respiratory medicine. 6th ed. Philadelphia: Elsevier; 2016, p. 1439–60

44. Cheng G, Vergheso T, Park D. Pneumomediastinum and mediastinitis. In: Broaddus VC, Mason R, Ernst J, et al., editors. Murray and Nadel's textbook of respiratory medicine. 6th ed. Philadelphia: Elsevier; 2016, p. 1496–510.

45. Bidkar P, Prabhakar H. Stridor. In: Prabhakar H, editor. Complications of neuroanesthesia. Cambridge, MA: Academic Press; 2016, p. 237–47.

46. Sicari V, Zabbo CP. Stridor. Treasure Island, FL: StatPearls Publishing; 2022. Available from: https://pubmed.ncbi.nlm.nih.gov/30252251/. [Accessed 12 February 2023].

47. Holm A, Viftrup A, Karlsson V, et al. Nurses' communication with mechanically ventilated patients in the intensive care unit: umbrella review. J Adv Nurs 2020;76(11):2909–20.

48. Talley N. Correlation of physical signs and respiratory disease. In: Talley N, O'Connor S, editors. Talley & O'Connor's Clinical examination. 9th ed. Elsevier; 2022, p. 39–58.

49. Torp KD, Modi P, Simon LV. Pulse oximetry. StatPearls. Treasure Island, FL: StatPearls Publishing; 2022. Available from: https://pubmed.ncbi.nlm.nih.gov/29262014/. [Accessed 12 February 2023].

50. Pretto J, Roebuck T, Beckert L, et al. Clinical use of pulse oximetry: official guidelines from the Thoracic Society of Australia and New Zealand. Respirology 2014;19:38–46.

51. Jubran A. Pulse oximetry. Crit Care 2015;19:272.

52. Sjoding MW, Dickson RP, Iwashyna TJ, et al. Racial bias in pulse oximetry measurement. N Engl J Med 2020;383(25):2477–8.

53. Barnett A, Beasley R, Buchan C, et al. Thoracic Society of Australia and New Zealand position statement on acute oxygen use in adults: 'swimming between the flags'. Respirology 2022;27(4):262–76.

54. Miller-Keane M, O'Toole M. Miller-Keane encyclopedia and dictionary of medicine, nursing and allied health. 7th ed. Philadelphia: Saunders; 2003.

55. Kremeier P, Bohm SH, Tusman G. Clinical use of volumetric capnography in mechanically ventilated patients. J Clin Monit Comput 2020; 34(1):7–16.

56. College of Intensive Care Medicine of Australia and New Zealand (CICM). Minimum standards for intensive care units. Melbourne, VIC: CICM; 2016.

57. Bockholt R, Paschke S, Heubner L, et al. Real-time monitoring of blood parameters in the intensive care unit: state-of-the-art and perspectives. J Clin Med 2022;11(9):2408.

58. Gelsomino S, Lorusso R, Livi U, et al. Assessment of a continuous blood gas monitoring system in animals during circulatory stress. BMC Anesthesiol 2011;11:1.

59. Zisquit J, Velasquez J, Nedeff N. Allen test. StatPearls. Treasure Island, FL: StatPearls Publishing; 2022. Available from: https://pubmed.ncbi.nlm.nih.gov/29939593/. [Accessed 12 February 2023].

60. Danckers M, Fried ED. Arterial blood gas sampling: MedScape; 2022. Available from: https://emedicine.medscape.com/article/1902703-overview. [Accessed 12 February 2023].

61. Wiegand D. AACN procedure manual for high acuity, progressive and critical care. 7th ed. Philadelphia: Elsevier; 2017.

62. Baird G. Preanalytical considerations in blood gas analysis. Biochem Med (Zagreb) 2013;23(1):19–27.

63. Ullman AJ, Keogh S, Coyer F, et al. 'True blood' the critical care story: an audit of blood sampling practice across three adult, paediatric and neonatal intensive care settings. Aust Crit Care 2016;29(2):90–5.

64. Chaney B, Emmady PD. Blood gas temperature correction. Treasure Island, FL: StatPearls Publishing; 2022. Available from: https://pubmed.ncbi.nlm.nih.gov/32491701/. [Accessed 12 February 2023].

65. Krzych L, Wojnarowicz O, Ignacy P, et al. Be cautious during the interpretation of arterial blood gas analysis performed outside the intensive care unit. Acta Biochim Pol 2020;67(3):353–8.

66. McLeod A. Arterial blood gas analysis – making it easy: M&K Publishing; 2016.

67. Foucher CD, Tubben RE. Lactic acidosis. Treasure Island, FL: StatPearls Publishing; 2022. Available from: https://pubmed.ncbi.nlm.nih.gov/29262026/. [Accessed 12 February 2023].

68. Stewart P. How to understand acid–base: a quantitative acid-base primer for biology and medicine. New York: Elsevier; 1981.

69. Morgan TJ. The Stewart approach – one clinician's perspective. Clin Biochem Rev 2009;30(2):41–54.

70. Magder S, Emami A. Practical approach to physical–chemical acid–base management. Stewart at the bedside. Ann Am Thorac Soc 2015;12(1):111–17.

71. Ahmed SM, Maheshwari P, Agarwal S, et al. Evaluation of the efficacy of simplified Fencl–Stewart equation in analyzing the changes in acid base status following resuscitation with two different fluids. Int J Crit Illn Inj Sci 2013;3(3):206–10.

72. Elbers P, Gatz R. acidbase.org: Bringing Stewart to the bedside. Available from: https://www.acidbase.org/. [Accessed 12 February 2023].

73. Theodore AC. Venous blood gases and other alternative to arterial blood gases 2022. Available from: https://www.uptodate.com/contents/venous-blood-gases-and-other-alternatives-to-arterial-blood-gases. [Accessed 12 February 2023].

74. Evans L, Rhodes A, Alhazzani W, et al. Surviving sepsis campaign: international guidelines for management of sepsis and septic shock 2021. Intensive Care Med 2021;47(11):1181–247.

75. Chetana Shanmukhappa S, Lokeshwaran S. Venous oxygen saturation. Treasure Island, FL: StatPearls Publishing; 2022. Available from: https://www.ncbi.nlm.nih.gov/books/NBK564395/. [Accessed 12 February 2023].

76. Hantzidiamantis PJ, Amaro E. Physiology, alveolar to arterial oxygen gradient. Treasure Island, FL: StatPearls Publishing; 2022. Available from: https://pubmed.ncbi.nlm.nih.gov/31424737/. [Accessed 12 February 2023].

77. Force ADT, Ranieri VM, Rubenfeld GD, et al. Acute respiratory distress syndrome: the Berlin Definition. JAMA 2012;307(23):2526–33.

78. Royal College of Pathologists of Australia (RCPA). RCPA manual: manual of use and interpretation of pathology tests. Surry Hills, NSW: RCPA; 2022. Available from: https://www.rcpa.edu.au/Manuals/RCPA-Manual/. [Accessed 12 February 2023].

79. Shadvar K, Nader-Djalal N, Vahed N, et al. Comparison of lactate/albumin ratio to lactate and lactate clearance for predicting outcomes in patients with septic shock admitted to intensive care unit: an observational study. Sci Rep 2022;12(1):13047.

80. Shepherd E. Specimen collection 4: procedure for obtaining a sputum specimen. Nurs Times 2017;113(10):49–51.

81. Wang CH, Tsai JC, Chen SF, et al. Normal saline instillation before suctioning: a meta-analysis of randomized controlled trials. Aust Crit Care 2017;30(5):260–5.

82. Marty FM, Chen K, Verrill KA. How to obtain a nasopharyngeal swab specimen. N Engl J Med 2020;382(22):e76.

83. Ganapathy A, Adhikari NK, Spiegelman J, et al. Routine chest x-rays in intensive care units: a systematic review and meta-analysis. Crit Care 2012;16(2):R68.

84. Trumbo SP, Iams WT, Limper HM, et al. Deimplementation of routine chest x-rays in adult intensive care units. J Hosp Med 2019;14(2):83–9.

85. Canadian Agency for Drugs and Technologies in Health (CADTH). Portable versus fixed x-ray equipment: a review of the clinical effectiveness, cost-effectiveness and guidelines. Ottawa: CADTH 2016.

86. Raoof S, Feigin D, Sung A, et al. Interpretation of plain chest roentgenogram. Chest 2012;141(2):545–58.

87. Lareau C, Wootton J. The "frequently" normal chest x-ray. Can J Rural Med 2004;9(3):183–6.

88. Guevarra K, Greenstein Y. Ultrasonography in the critical care unit. Curr Cardiol Rep 2020;22(11):145.

89. Volpicelli G, Mayo P, Rovida S. Focus on ultrasound in intensive care. Intensive Care Med 2020;46(6):1258–60.

90. Lichtenstein DA. BLUE-protocol and FALLS-protocol: two applications of lung ultrasound in the critically ill. Chest 2015;147(6):1659–70.

91. Bentz MR, Primack SL. Intensive care unit imaging. Clin Chest Med 2015;36(2):219–34, viii.

92. Zantonelli G, Cozzi D, Bindi A, et al. Acute pulmonary embolism: prognostic role of computed tomography pulmonary angiography (CTPA). Tomography 2022;8(1):529–39.

93. Xie Z, Liao X, Kang Y, et al. Radiation exposure to staff in intensive care unit with portable CT scanner. Biomed Res Int 2016;2016:5656480.

94. Mittendorff L, Young A, Sim J. A narrative review of current and emerging MRI safety issues: what every MRI technologist (radiographer) needs to know. J Med Radiat Sci 2022;69(2):250–60.

95. Maass AH, Hemels MEW, Allaart CP. Magnetic resonance imaging in patients with cardiac implantable electronic devices. Neth Heart J 2018;26(12):584–90.

96. De Andres J, Martinez-Sanjuan V, Fabregat-Cid G, et al. MRI-compatible spinal cord stimulator device and related changes in patient safety and imaging artifacts. Pain Med 2014;15(10):1815–19.

97. Patolia S, Farhat R, Subramaniyam R. Bronchoscopy in intubated and non-intubated intensive care unit patients with respiratory failure. J Thorac Dis 2021;13(8):5125–34.

Chapter 14

Respiratory alterations and management

Jennifer McGaughey, Amanda Corley

Learning objectives

After reading this chapter, you should be able to:

- discuss the underlying pathophysiology and evidenced-based management of acute respiratory failure and acute respiratory distress syndrome
- differentiate between hypoxaemic and hypercapnoeic respiratory failure
- critically review the incidence of respiratory alterations in the critical care context
- discuss the aetiology, pathophysiology, clinical manifestations and management of common respiratory disorders managed in intensive care, specifically pneumonia, pandemic respiratory infections, asthma, chronic obstructive pulmonary disease, pneumothorax and pulmonary embolism
- describe the evidence base for key components of nursing and collaborative practice involved in the management of patients with acute respiratory failure in the intensive care unit
- outline the principles and immediate postoperative management for lung transplant recipients.

Introduction

A common reason for admission to an ICU is for support of the respiratory system. The proportion of adult patients admitted to ICU in Australia and New Zealand in 2019/20 receiving invasive mechanical ventilation was 33.6%, slightly down from 35.4% the previous reporting year. Non-invasive ventilation was used in 10.8% of patients during the 2019/20 reporting period, compared with 12.2% in the 2018/19 period.[1,2] Failure or inadequate function of the respiratory system occurs as a result of direct or indirect pathophysiological conditions. The process of mechanical ventilation may also injure a patient's lungs, further impacting functioning of the respiratory system. Preventing or minimising ventilator-associated lung injury is therefore also a primary goal of patient care.

In Chapter 13 the relevant assessment and monitoring practices for a patient with life-threatening respiratory dysfunction are described. In this chapter the incidence, pathophysiology, clinical manifestations and management of common respiratory disorders that result in acute respiratory failure are described. Specific conditions of pneumonia, pandemic respiratory infections, asthma, chronic obstructive pulmonary disease (COPD), respiratory failure, acute respiratory distress syndrome (ARDS), pulmonary embolism, pneumothorax and lung transplantation are discussed. Respiratory support strategies including oxygenation and ventilation to support respiratory function during a critical illness are presented in Chapter 15.

Incidence of respiratory alterations

In 2017, chronic respiratory diseases were the third leading cause of death and the leading cause of mortality worldwide, with a global increase in the total cases between 1990 and 2017.[3,4] The Global Burden of Diseases, Injuries and Risk Factors study (2017) estimated that 544.9 million people worldwide had a chronic respiratory disease, representing an increase of 39.8% compared with 1990, with the highest prevalence in high-income regions (10% of the population).[5] In 2015, the United Kingdom and Ireland had the highest age-standardised death rates from respiratory diseases among European Union countries.[6] The main causes of death from respiratory diseases are COPD, pneumonia, asthma, lung cancer and influenza.[6,7] Of these, COPD remained the most prevalent chronic respiratory disease (55%) worldwide in 2017[4,5] and accounted for over 40% of all respiratory mortality across European Union countries (40%) in 2015.[6] Asthma is the second most leading cause of death among chronic respiratory diseases worldwide and smoking remains the main risk factor for chronic respiratory disease-related disability.[5,6] Common respiratory alterations managed in ICU are discussed in the following sections.

Respiratory failure

Respiratory failure occurs when there is a reduction in the body's ability to maintain either oxygenation or ventilation, or both. It is defined as hypoxaemia with or without hypercapnia,[8] which may occur acutely, as observed in pneumonia, or may persist in chronic form, as observed in asthma and COPD.

Aetiology of respiratory failure

For the respiratory system to function effectively, the rate and depth of breathing has to be controlled appropriately by the brain, the chest wall must expand adequately, air needs to flow easily through the airways and effective exchange of gases needs to occur at the alveolar level. Conditions that impact one or more aspects of normal physiological functioning of the respiratory system can cause respiratory failure. Acute hypoxaemic respiratory failure is a leading cause of admission and need for mechanical ventilation in ICU.[9] A prospective, multicentred observational study across 50 countries (LUNG SAFE) found that more than one-third of ICU patients requiring mechanical ventilation have hypoxaemic respiratory failure, with a hospital mortality rate of 39%.[9]

Respiratory failure is classified on the basis of onset (acute, chronic or acute on chronic) or blood gas (hypoxaemic, hypercarbic or combined oxygen and ventilatory failure).[8]

Acute respiratory failure is characterised by life-threatening alterations in function, the manifestations of chronic respiratory failure are more subtle and potentially more difficult to diagnose. Patients with chronic respiratory failure often experience acute exacerbations of their disease, also resulting in the need for intensive respiratory support.[10]

Classification and pathophysiology

Respiratory failure occurs when the respiratory system fails to achieve one or both of its essential gas exchange functions – oxygenation or elimination of carbon dioxide – and can be described as hypoxaemic respiratory failure, which is primarily a failure of oxygenation, or hypercapnoeic respiratory failure, which is primarily a failure of ventilation.[8]

Hypoxaemic respiratory failure: failure to oxygenate

A patient with hypoxaemic respiratory failure presents with a low partial pressure of oxygen (PaO_2) and a normal partial pressure of carbon dioxide ($PaCO_2$).[8,11] It is defined as hypoxaemia that is refractory to supplemental oxygen (PaO_2 <8 kPa/<60 mmHg).[12]

Hypoxaemic respiratory failure may be caused by a reduction in inspired oxygen pressure as might occur at extreme altitude, alveolar hypoventilation, impaired oxygen diffusion or ventilation/perfusion (V/Q) mismatch.[8,11,13] Most major respiratory alterations can cause hypoxaemic respiratory failure, usually as a result of alveolar collapse or consolidation as occurs in severe pneumonia, sepsis[8] or excess fluid in the lungs (decompensated chronic heart failure, renal failure or ARDS).[12] These alterations disrupt the ability of lung tissue to transfer oxygen across the alveolar membrane and hypoxaemia ensues. Abnormal V/Q matching is a prominent feature in ARDS associated with coronavirus disease 2019 (COVID-19).[14] A severe form of mismatch known as intrapulmonary shunting occurs when adequate perfusion exists but there are sections of lung tissue that are not ventilated. In these alveoli, the oxygen content is similar to that of the mixed venous blood and the carbon dioxide is elevated. In other instances, ventilation may be adequate, but perfusion is impaired (e.g. pulmonary embolus). In its severe form, this is known as dead space ventilation as the lungs continue to be ventilated but there is limited or no perfusion, and therefore no gas exchange. In this situation, the alveolar oxygen content is similar to that of the inspired gas mixture and the carbon dioxide is minimal (see Chapter 13 for further discussion).[8,12]

Hypercapnoeic respiratory failure: failure to ventilate

A patient with hypercapnoeic respiratory failure is characterised by high carbon dioxide levels, defined as a pH <7.35 and a $PaCO_2$ <6.7kPa (50 mmHg).[12,15] This failure is caused by alveolar hypoventilation, where the respiratory effort or minute ventilation is insufficient to allow adequate exchange of oxygen and carbon dioxide. This may be caused by conditions that reduce respiratory drive (sedation, head injury, central nervous system infection), abnormalities of the spinal cord, neuromuscular diseases (Guillain–Barré syndrome, muscular dystrophies), chest wall abnormalities (flail chest, kyphoscoliosis), severe air-flow obstruction/V/Q mismatch (exacerbations of asthma or COPD) or increased carbon dioxide production (sepsis, burns).[8,11] COPD is one of the most common causes of hypercapnoeic acute respiratory failure, with 44% of patients admitted with acute exacerbations showing a degree of hypercapnia.[10]

Clinical manifestations

Patient presentations in acute respiratory failure can be quite diverse and are dependent on the underlying pathophysiological mechanism, the specific aetiology and any comorbidities that may exist. Specific clinical manifestations for the disorders discussed in this chapter are provided in each section. Dyspnoea is the most common symptom associated with acute respiratory failure.[16] Changes to breathing patterns result in hyperventilation due to high respiratory drive and inspiratory effort leading to high tidal volumes, increased respiratory rates and, finally, to hypocapnia.[17] Patients may also present with fever, cough, cyanosis, anxiety, confusion and/or sleepiness.[10,15]

A systematic approach to clinical assessment and management of patients with acute respiratory failure is crucial, given the large number of possible causes. Clinical investigations to assess the cause of respiratory failure vary depending on the suspected underlying aetiology and the progression of disease. Arterial blood gas (ABG) analysis, the measurement of PaO_2, $PaCO_2$, alveolar–arterial PO_2 difference and patient response to supplemental oxygen are key elements in determining the cause of acute respiratory failure. Continuous monitoring of oxygen saturation using pulse oximetry, ABG analysis and analysis of chest X-rays (CXR) is used in almost all cases of respiratory failure. Other more-specialised tests such as computed tomography (CT), magnetic resonance imaging (MRI), pulmonary angiography and other specialised investigations may be used in specific circumstances (see Chapter 13).[12]

Patient management

The primary survey (airway, breathing and circulation) and immediate management form initial routine practice.[10]

Supplemental oxygen is always indicated in acute respiratory failure,[15] which requires frequent assessment and monitoring of respiratory function, including a patient's response to supplemental oxygen and/or the need for further ventilatory support. Additional ventilatory support can be achieved through a variety of interfaces and ventilatory modes (see Chapter 15). Patient comfort and compliance with the ventilation mode, ABG analysis and pulse oximetry guide any titration of ventilatory support. The key goals of management are to treat the primary cause of respiratory failure, maintain adequate gas exchange and prevent or minimise the potential complications of positive pressure mechanical ventilation.[18] Comorbidities add to the complexity of managing a patient's primary condition and increase the risk of additional organ dysfunction or failure.

Maintaining oxygenation

The therapeutic aim is to titrate the fraction of inspired oxygen (FiO_2) to achieve a PaO_2 of 9.3 kPa/70 mmHg and to maintain minute ventilation to achieve $PaCO_2$ within normal limits where possible.[15] In acute hypoxaemic respiratory failure the use of high-flow nasal cannula appears to be superior to conventional oxygen therapy and non-invasive ventilation (NIV) in improving oxygenation and lung mechanics, reducing all-cause mortality and intubation rates.[19–21] The use of high-flow nasal oxygen therapy should be considered in patients who do not achieve target oxygen levels with traditional supplemental oxygen delivery devices. Systematic review evidence on the use of high-flow nasal cannulae (HFNC) versus NIV in hypercapnic respiratory failure found no differences between their intubation or mortality rates.[20,22] The American College of Physicians recommends the use of HFNC versus NIV for the management of hospitalised adults with ARF.[19]

Oxygen administration targets should be adjusted for patients with chronic hypercapnia, and the administration of controlled oxygen therapy should be used to achieve a target saturation of 88–92% in all causes of acute hypercapnoeic respiratory failure.[15] Trials of non-invasive ventilation should be started when pH<7.35 and $PaCO_2$ >6.5 kPa/50 mmHg persist or develop despite optimal medical therapy.[15] The use of NIV for the management of patients with an acute exacerbation of COPD and acute hypercapnoeic respiratory failure is now considered to be standard care[23,24] and has been demonstrated to reduce endotracheal intubation and patient mortality.[25,26] It is recommended that NIV be attempted prior to invasive ventilation using portable bilevel ventilators or specifically designed ICU ventilators with non-invasive mode in critically ill patients.[27] A management plan should provide measures to be taken in the event of NIV failure and ceilings of therapy agreed (see Chapter 15 for further detail on assessment and management of oxygenation).[23]

Supporting ventilation

Ventilator-associated lung injury is also a concern when managing patients with acute respiratory failure. A lung can be injured when it is stretched excessively as a result of tidal volume settings that generate high pressures, often referred to as barotrauma. The most common injury is that of alveolar rupture and/or air in the pleural space, resulting in pneumothorax. An approach known as 'lung protective ventilation' aims to minimise overdistention of the alveoli through careful monitoring of tidal volumes and airway pressures. This method of ventilation recommends targeted tidal volumes of 4–8 mL/kg per breath, based on predicated body weight, and plateau pressures <30 cmH_2O for all ventilated patients (see Chapter 15 for further discussion).[28]

Development of ventilator-induced diaphragm dysfunction has been reported as a significant issue when the respiratory muscles are rendered inactive by long-term mechanical ventilation and administration of pharmacotherapy.[29] A higher rate of weaning failure and mortality is associated with diaphragm dysfunction.[30] The introduction of early, graduated rehabilitation exercises was found to improve diaphragm dysfunction and reduce duration of ventilation and intubation in patients with prolonged mechanical ventilation in a single-centre, prospective randomised controlled trial (RCT).[31] The use of prone positioning (>16 h) in patients with moderate to severe respiratory failure (PROSEVA study) reduced mortality in intubated patients by improving the ventilation perfusion ratio mismatching, without increasing the rate of complications,[32] and is recommended management for ARDS.[33]

Prevention or minimisation of complications associated with positive pressure mechanical ventilation remains a major focus of nursing practice.[34] These complications may relate to the patient–ventilator interface (artificial airway and ventilator circuitry), infectious complications or complications associated with sedation and/or immobility. The implementation of an early mobilisation protocol can improve PaO_2, oxygen saturation, PaO_2/FiO_2 ratio and pulmonary compliance in patients with respiratory failure receiving mechanical ventilation.[35] Some common complications and the appropriate management strategies are briefly outlined in Table 14.1[36,37] and are discussed further in Chapter 15.

Chest physiotherapy is a routine activity for managing patients with acute respiratory failure. This involves positioning, manual hyperinflation, percussion and vibration, and suctioning. A single-centre study in Brazil found physiotherapy care provided 24 h/day in ICU reduced length of hospital stay, mechanical ventilation, mortality and lowered incidence of respiratory infections.[38] In patients with COPD pulmonary rehabilitation which focuses on individualised assessment to improve disease control through education and self-management is recommended to reduce hospitalisations and improve dyspnoea, health status and exercise intolerance.[39] Table 14.2 provides an outline of management interventions for patients with respiratory failure,[40–45] particularly those who may require prolonged mechanical ventilation.

Medications

Medications commonly prescribed in respiratory failure include inhalation/intravenous steroids and bronchodilators, antibiotic therapy, analgesia and sedation to maintain patient–ventilator synchrony. Stress ulcer and venous thromboembolism prophylaxis should also be given.[46] A patient's condition, comorbidities and the above-mentioned pharmacological therapy may also be supported with inotropic and other resuscitation therapies (see Chapters 11 and 21). As the use of medications will vary depending on the underlying cause of respiratory failure, these are discussed separately in the sections below.

Practice tip

Obesity hypoventilation syndrome

Obesity hypoventilation syndrome is a specific form of chronic respiratory failure defined as a combination of obesity, hypercapnia when awake and features of obstructive sleep apnoea and/or hypoventilation.[27] NICE guidance recommends use of continuous positive airway pressure as first-line treatment and NIV as an alternative if symptoms do not improve or hypercapnia persists in patients who do not have acute respiratory failure.[47] When patients with obesity hypoventilation syndrome present with acute hypercapnic or acute on chronic respiratory failure, guidance recommends the use of NIV.[27] As the risk of acute respiratory failure is high it is recommended that these patients are managed in a high-dependency area with expertise in the use of continuous positive airway pressure, bilevel positive airway pressure and NIV.[15]

Practice tip

Respiratory failure in the elderly

Older adults have ageing organs and systems and other comorbidities that may exacerbate respiratory dysfunction. Frail hospitalised patients with acute respiratory failure requiring mechanical ventilation were found to be at greater risk of mortality and prolonged length of hospital stay compared with those without frailty.[48] Identification of prehospital frailty using a diagnosis-based approach is suggested to risk stratify acutely ill patients and to focus on innovative approaches to improve long-term outcomes.[48]

Pneumonia

Pneumonia is an infection of the lung. Depending on the type and severity of the infection and the overall health of the person, it may result in acute respiratory failure. Pneumonia can be caused by most types of microorganisms

TABLE 14.1

Complications of mechanical ventilation and associated management strategies[36,37]

PATIENT–VENTILATOR INTERFACE COMPLICATION	MANAGEMENT STRATEGIES
Airway dislodgement/disconnection	Endotracheal tube or tracheostomy tube is secured to optimise ventilation and prevent airway dislodgement or accidental extubation.
Circuit leaks	Cuff pressure assessment. Circuit checks. Exhaled tidal volume measurement.
Airway injury from inadequate heat/humidity	Maintain humidification of the airway using either a heat–moisture exchanger or a water-bath humidifier.
Obstructions from secretions	Assess the need for suctioning regularly and suction as required.
Tracheal injury from the artificial airway	Assessment of airway placement and cuff pressure (minimal occlusion method).
INFECTIOUS COMPLICATION	**MANAGEMENT STRATEGIES**
Ventilator-associated pneumonia (VAP)	Alcohol-based hand hygiene. Appropriate antibiotic therapy. Oral decontamination. Semirecumbent positioning, 30–45 degrees. Daily sedation holds. Peptic ulcer disease prophylaxis. Minimising interruptions to ventilator circuit (e.g. closed suctioning technique). Use of oropharyngeal vs nasopharyngeal feeding tubes. Drainage of subglottic secretions. Small bowel feeding rather than gastric feeding. Aerosolised antibiotics for patients who are colonised. Early discontinuation mechanical ventilation using nurse-led weaning protocols. Early tracheostomy. Prophylactic probiotics.
COMPLICATION ASSOCIATED WITH IMMOBILITY/SEDATION	**MANAGEMENT STRATEGIES**
Gastrointestinal dysfunction	Prokinetic medication. Constipation – bowel therapy regimen.
Muscle atrophy	Passive limb movements, foot splints (see Chapter 5) and early activity/mobility (see Chapter 5).
Pressure injuries	Pressure-relieving mattresses, regular repositioning. Assessment of risks and management of pressure injuries by wound care specialists, nutrition advice.

Sources: Elliot ZJ, Elliot SC. An overview of mechanical ventilation in the intensive care unit. Nursing standard. 2018;32(28):41–9; Bhandary R. Practical ventilator management. Surgery. 2021;39(10):665–70.

but is most commonly a result of bacterial or viral infection. In critical care the key distinctions in assessing and managing a patient with pneumonia relate to the specific aetiology or causative organism.[49] In this section the pathophysiology of pneumonia, as well as the clinical presentation and management of two classifications of pneumonia often seen in the ICU are reviewed:

1 community-acquired pneumonia (CAP)
2 ventilator-associated pneumonia (VAP) and ventilator-associated events.

TABLE 14.2

Long-term patient management in respiratory failure[40–45]

MANAGEMENT	BEST PRACTICE
Tracheostomy	The need for tracheostomy should be individualised and performed early where prolonged ventilation is anticipated. Tracheal stenosis occurs in 30% of patients.
Weaning protocols	Nurse-led individualised weaning protocols have a positive impact on weaning outcomes and patient safety.
Nutrition	ESPEN guidelines on clinical nutrition in ICU recommend assessment of malnutrition in patients >48 h in ICU, oral diet preferred over enteral nutrition or parenteral nutrition, measuring glucose and preventing refeeding syndrome, physical activity to improve beneficial effects of nutritional therapy and in non-intubated patients consider nutritional supplementation and texture-adapted food for patients with dysphagia.
Swallow assessment	Assess for dysphagia to improve oral intake and reduce aspiration due to trauma caused by prolonged intubation.
Mobilisation	Early mobilisation and daily exercise programs to minimise loss of muscle mass and ICU-acquired weakness (passive and active range of motion).
Communication	Encourage use of glasses/hearing aids, communication aids, speaking valves.
Delirum prevention	Assess and screen for delirium (CAM-ICU). Manage pain, agitation and delirium (PAD) using spontaneous breathing trials and minimising sedation. Prevent sleep deprivation by using eye masks, ear plugs and bundled care to minimise external stimuli. Multicomponent interventions to include early mobility and exercise.
Family support	Importance of providing physical, emotional and/or spiritual support to family members.
End-of-life decisions in acute respiratory failure	When clinically appropriate, the withholding and withdrawal of life-sustaining therapy is supported by ethical and legal principles. Advance care planning and palliative care pathways.
Rehabilitation	Multidisciplinary rehabilitation after critical illness to include individualised plan using national post-intensive care rehabilitation collaborative framework to assess needs.
Discharge	Recommend ICU follow up program 2–3 months post-discharge.

Sources: Morgan A. Long-term outcomes from critical care. Surgery. 2020;39(1):53–7; Lai CC, Tseng KL, Ho CH, et al. Prognosis of patients with acute respiratory failure and prolonged intensive care unit stay. J Thorac Dis. 2019;11(5):2051–7; Singer P, Blaser AR, Berger MM, et al. ESPEN guideline on clinical nutrition in the intensive care unit. Clin Nutr. 2019;38(1):48–79; Hirzallah FM, Alkaissi A, Do M, et al. A systematic review of nurse-led weaning protocol for mechanically ventilated adult patients. Nurs Crit Care. 2019;24(2):89–96; Duncan S, McAuley DF, Walshe M, et al. Interventions for oropharyngeal dysphagia in acute and critical care: a systematic review and meta-analysis. Intensive Care Med. 2020;46(7):1326–38; van de Boogaard M, Slooter AJC. Delirium in critically ill patients: current knowledge and future perspectives. BJA Education. 2019;19(12):398–404.

Pathophysiology

The normal human lung was previously considered to be sterile; however, recent developments in microbiological diagnostics using molecular gene-sequencing techniques have demonstrated that the healthy lung is colonised with microorganisms.[50] The term 'lung microbiome' refers to every organism (not only bacteria, but also archaea, fungi and viruses) that is present in the lower respiratory tract and lung tissues. Understanding how the lung microbiome affects human health and disease is an emerging area of research.[51] Current research has established that healthy lungs have characteristic flora that is not observed in individuals with chronic respiratory conditions such as asthma and COPD. A range of predominantly non-pathogenic bacteria are present at low levels in the lungs of healthy individuals, in contrast to diseased states, where colonies of potentially pathogenic bacteria become more dominant.[50,52–54]

FIGURE 14.1 Environmental, microbial, structural and immunological factors influencing the lung microbiome during health and disease.[55]

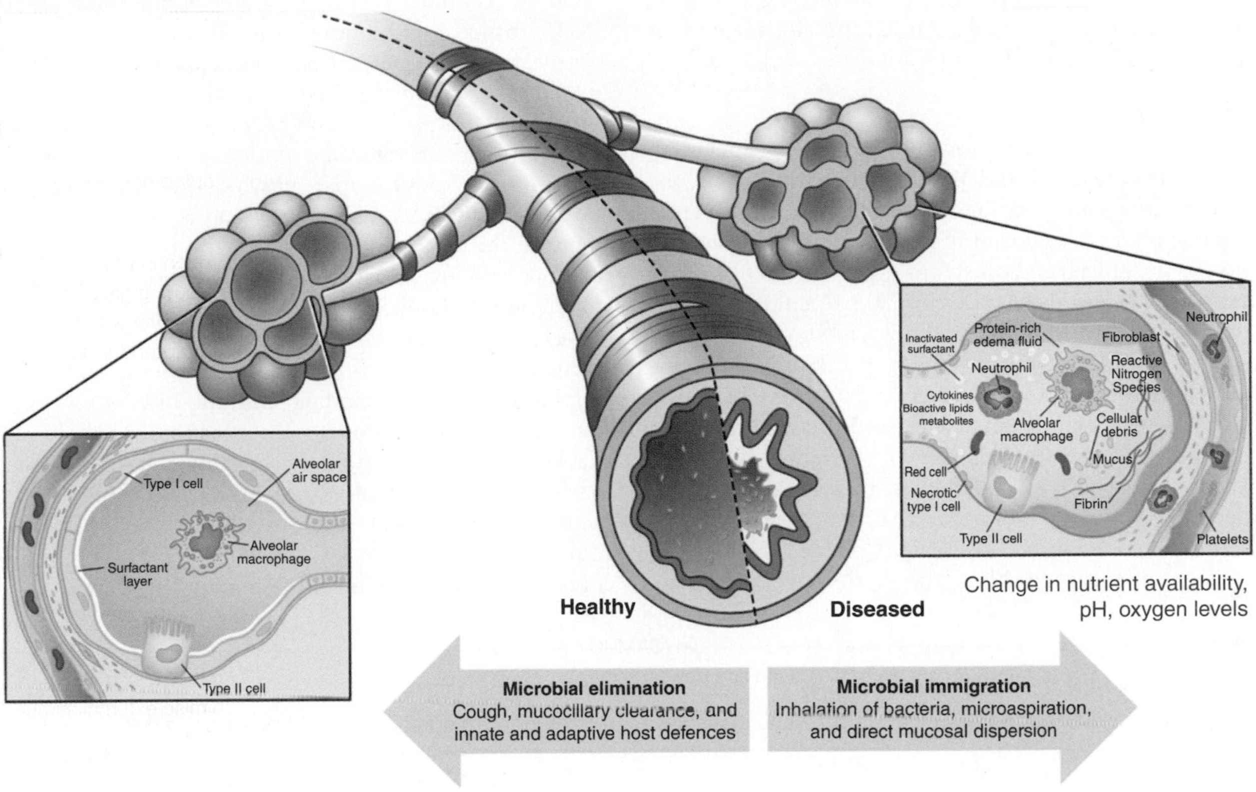

Healthy   Diseased

Change in nutrient availability, pH, oxygen levels

Microbial elimination
Cough, mucociliary clearance, and innate and adaptive host defences

Microbial immigration
Inhalation of bacteria, microaspiration, and direct mucosal dispersion

Source: Huffnagle GB, Dickson RP, Lukacs NW. The respiratory tract microbiome and lung inflammation: a two-way street. Mucosal Immunol. 2017;10(2):299–306.

A number of defence mechanisms exist to prevent microorganisms entering the lungs, such as particle filtration in the nostrils, sneezing and coughing to expel irritants, and mucus production to trap dust and infectious organisms and move particles out of the respiratory system. Infection occurs when one or more of these defences are not functioning adequately or when an individual encounters a large number of microorganisms and the defences are overwhelmed.[55] The lung microbiome during health and disease is depicted in Fig 14.1. An invading pathogen provokes an immune response in the lungs, resulting in the following pathophysiological processes:

- alteration in alveolar–capillary permeability that leads to an increase in protein-rich fluid in the alveoli; this impacts on gas exchange and causes the patient to breathe faster in an effort to increase oxygen uptake and remove carbon dioxide
- mucus production increases and mucous plugs may develop that block off areas of the lung, further reducing capacity for gas exchange
- consolidation occurs in the alveoli, which fill with fluid and debris; this occurs particularly with

bacterial pneumonia, where debris accumulates from the large number of white blood cells involved in the immune response.[51,55]

> **Practice tip**
>
> **Pneumonia in the elderly**
> Pneumonia disproportionately affects older adults and they are at higher risk of hospitalisation, complications and death. One-year mortality has been estimated at 33% in hospitalised adults ≥65 years. Risk factors to be aware of in older adults include: frailty index, swallowing deficits, ethnicity and comorbidities. *Streptococcus pneumoniae* is the most common causative organism for CAP (65–74 years: 48%; >74 years: 66%); however, the incidence of viral infection also increases with increasing age. Immunisation with pneumococcal and influenza vaccines reduces the risk of older adults developing pneumonia.[56,57]

Community-acquired pneumonia

CAP is an acute infection of the pulmonary parenchyma which was contracted by the patient while in the community. CAP has a high hospitalisation rate, with between 22% and 42% of adults presenting with lower respiratory tract infection requiring hospitaliation, and between 1.2% and 10% of those people needing admission to ICU. For adults admitted to ICU, the risk of dying is approximately 30%, a risk which increases with age.[58]

Aetiology

CAP is caused by a variety of microorganisms, including bacteria, viruses, fungi and parasites. In many cases, the causative organism may not be known and current practice in many cases is to initiate antimicrobial treatment as soon as possible, based on symptoms and patient history, rather than waiting for microorganism culture results. Antibiotic stewardship guidelines recommend early review of antibiotic therapy and adjustment of therapy based on microbiological results. As the causative organism for CAP is frequently unidentified and there are regional differences in the prevalence of different causative organisms, use of local guidelines is recommended to guide the selection of antibiotic treatment.[59]

Clinical assessment, especially patient history, is important in distinguishing the aetiology and likely causative organism in patients with CAP. Different ages and characteristics of patients are often associated with different causative organisms. Viral pneumonias, especially influenza, are most common in young children, while adults are more likely to have pneumonia caused by bacteria such as *Streptococcus pneumoniae*, *Haemophilus influenzae*, *Mycoplasma pneumoniae*, *Chlamydophila pneumoniae* or other respiratory viruses. Specific information regarding exposure to animals, travel history, nursing home residency and any occupational or unusual exposure may provide the key to diagnosis. Personal habits such as smoking and alcohol consumption increase the risk of developing pneumonia and should be explored. Many patients admitted to hospital with CAP have comorbidities, suggesting those who are chronically ill have an increased risk of developing acute respiratory failure. The most common chronic illnesses involved are respiratory disease, including smoking history, COPD and asthma, congestive cardiac failure and diabetes mellitus. Table 14.3 outlines aspects of the clinical history associated with particular causative organisms in CAP.[59-63] CAP caused by the novel severe acute respiratory syndrome coronavirus-2 (SARS-CoV-2; COVID-19) will be discussed in the section on Respiratory pandemics.

TABLE 14.3

Clinical history/comorbidities associated with causative organisms of community-acquired pneumonia[59-63]

CONDITION	CAUSATIVE ORGANISMS
Individual factors	
Alcoholism	*S. pneumoniae* (including penicillin-resistant), anaerobes, gram-negative bacilli (possibly *K. pneumoniae*), tuberculosis
Poor dental hygiene	Anaerobes
Elderly	Group B streptococci, *M. catarrhalis*, *H. influenzae*, *L. pneumophila*, gram-negative bacilli, *C. pneumoniae* and polymicrobial infections
COPD or smoking (past or present)	*S. pneumoniae*, *L. pneumophila*, *H. influenzae*, *M. catarrhalis*, *C. pneumoniae*, *Legionella* spp., *Aspergillus* spp.
IV drug use	*S. aureus*, anaerobes, CA-MRSA, *M. tuberculosis*, *S. pneumoniae*
Comorbidities	
Post-influenza pneumonia	*S. pneumoniae*, *S. aureus*, *H. influenzae*
Structural disease of lung (e.g. bronchiectasis, cystic fibrosis)	*P. aeruginosa*, *B. cepacia*, *S. aureus*
Sickle cell disease, asplenia	Pneumococcus, *H. influenzae*
Previous antibiotic treatment and severe pulmonary comorbidity (e.g. bronchiectasis, cystic fibrosis and severe COPD)	*P. aeruginosa*
Malnutrition-related diseases	*S. pneumonia*, *M. tuberculosis*, *M. catarrhalis*
Environmental exposure	
Air conditioning	*L. pneumophila*
Residents in nursing home	*S. pneumoniae*, gram-negative bacilli, *H. influenzae*, *S. aureus*, *C. pneumoniae*; consider *M. tuberculosis*; consider anaerobes, but less common

TABLE 14.3

Clinical history/comorbidities associated with causative organisms of community-acquired pneumonia—cont'd

CONDITION	CAUSATIVE ORGANISMS
Homeless population	*S. pneumoniae, S. aureus, H. influenzae, C. gattii*: caused by inhalation of spores while sleeping, associated with red gum trees (Australia, Southeast Asia, South America)
Suspected bioterrorism	*B. anthracis, F. tularensis, Y. pestis*
Animal exposure	
Bat exposure	*H. capsulatum*
Bird exposure	*C. psittaci, C. neoformans, H. capsulatum*
Rabbit exposure	*F. tularensis*
Exposure to farm animals or parturient cats	*C. burnetii* (Q fever)
Travel history	
Travel to southwestern USA	Coccidioidomycosis; hantavirus in selected areas
Travel to Asia	Severe acute respiratory syndrome (coronavirus), *M. tuberculosis, B. pseudomallei*
Residence or travel to rural tropics	*B. pseudomallei*
Travel to area of known epidemic	Avian influenza (H5N1), swine influenza (H1N1), severe acute respiratory syndrome (coronavirus)

B. anthracis = Bacillus anthracis, B. pseudomallei = Burkholderia pseudomallei; CA-MRSA = community-associated methicillin-resistant *Staphylococcus aureus; C. burnetii = Coxiella burnetii; C. gattii = Cryptococcus gattii; C. neoformans = Cryptococcus neoformans;* COPD = chronic obstructive pulmonary disease; *C. pneumoniae = Chlamydophila pneumoniae; C. psittaci = Chlamydia psittaci; F. tularensis = Francisella tularensis; H. capsulatum = Histoplasma capsulatum; H. influenzae = Haemophilus influenzae;* IV = intravenous; *K. pneumoniae = Klebsiella pneumoniae; L. pneumophila = Legionella pneumophila; M. catarrhalis = Moraxella catarrhalis; M. tuberculosis = Mycobacterium tuberculosis; P. aeruginosa = Pseudomonas aeruginosa; P. cepacia = Pseudomonas cepacia; S. aureus = Staphylococcus aureus; S. pneumoniae – Streptococcus pneumoniae; Y. pestis = Yersinia pestis.*

Sources: Dockrell DH, Ho A, Gordon SB. Community acquired pneumonia. In: Broaddus VC, Ernst JD, King TE, et al, editors. Murray & Nadel's textbook of respiratory medicine. 7th ed. Philadelphia: Elsevier; 2022, p. 600–21; Lanks CW, Musani AI, Hsia DW. Community-acquired pneumonia and hospital-acquired pneumonia. Med Clin North Am. 2019;103(3):487–501; Chan KM, Gomersall CD. Pneumonia. In: Bersten AD, Handy JM, editors. Oh's intensive care manual. 8th ed. Philadelphia: Elsevier; 2019; p. 467–82; Nair G, Niederman P. Community acquired pneumonia. In: Vincent J, Abraham E, Moore F, et al, editors. Textbook of critical care. 7th ed. Philadelphia: Elsevier; 2017; King J, Chandrasekar PH. Cryptococcosis. 2021. Available from: https://emedicine.medscape.com/article/215354-overview. [Accessed 18 February 2023].

Clinical manifestations

Symptoms for pneumonia are both respiratory and systemic. Common characteristics include fever, sweats, rigours, cough, sputum production, pleuritic chest pain, dyspnoea, tachypnoea, pleural rub and inspiratory crackles on auscultation, plus radiological evidence of infiltrates or consolidation. Some people present with atypical symptoms such as malaise, myalgia, confusion and diarrhoea, with atypical symptoms experienced more often in older adults.[60]

Diagnosis

To aid diagnosis of severe presentations of CAP requiring admission to critical care, the following specimens are recommended to be collected: culture and gram stain of lower respiratory tract specimens, pretreatment blood cultures, urine for pneumococcal and legionella antigens, and rapid molecular testing for influenza virus. Routine screening of patients with suspected pneumonia continues to rely on microscopy and blood cultures, detection of antigens in urine and serology. Methods for detection of antigens are now widely available for several pneumonia pathogens, particularly *S. pneumoniae*, *Legionella* and some respiratory viruses. Culture of respiratory secretions may be limited owing to difficulty in obtaining sputum samples. For this reason, nasopharyngeal aspirates or swabs for respiratory virus detection using polymerase chain reaction techniques may be taken as part of the routine screening for CAP. The use of serum procalcitonin to distinguish bacterial from viral aetiology of pneumonia and guide the need for initial antibiotic therapy has been debated in the literature; however, current clinical practice guidelines do not recommend using procalcitonin alone to justify withholding antibiotics.[64]

Severity assessment scoring

To streamline decision making around where and how to treat patients presenting with CAP, severity scores indices have been developed. International guidelines recommend a severity-based approach to management of CAP, in relation to the initial site of treatment (e.g. home, hospital ward, ICU) and appropriate level of intervention, including antibiotic therapy.[64] Several severity scores have been developed and validated; however, to date there is no agreement on the optimal tool or an agreed definition of the term 'severe pneumonia'. CURB-65 and the Pneumonia Severity Index are the most widely recommended systems that produce scores and assess severity based on patient demographics, risk factors, comorbidities, clinical presentation and laboratory results (Box 14.1).[65,66] Clinical practice guidelines from the American Thoracic Society recommend the use of the PSI tool over the CURB-65 tool.[64] The Australian CAP Collaboration team devised and validated the SMART-COP scoring system for predicting the need for intensive respiratory or vasopressor support in patients with CAP. The acronym relates to the factors: low systolic blood pressure, multilobar involvement, low albumin level, high respiratory rate, tachycardia, confusion, poor oxygenation, and low arterial pH.[67]

BOX 14.1

Severity scoring in CAP

CURB-65[65]

The score is an acronym for each of the risk factors measured. One point is allocated for each risk factor present (maximum of 5):

- C – **c**onfusion: a new onset of confusion, defined as an abbreviated mental test score of 8 or less
- U – **u**rea: blood urea nitrogen level >19 mg/dL
- R – **r**espiratory rate: ≥30 breaths/min
- B – **b**lood pressure: ≤90 mmHg systolic or ≤60 mmHg diastolic
- 65 – age: ≥**65** years

Score of 0 or 1: low mortality. Likely suitable for home treatment.

Score of 2: intermediate mortality. Consider hospital supervised treatment.

Score of ≥3: high mortality. Manage in a hospital as severe pneumonia. Assess for ICU admission if score = 4–5.

Pneumonia severity index[66]

The pneumonia severity index (PSI) considers a range of patient characteristics, comorbid diseases, signs and symptoms, and laboratory findings with the intent of classifying the severity of a patient's pneumonia at a risk level ranging from I to V, with V being the most severe. An online PSI calculator (see Online resources for link) is available to assist clinicians in applying the scoring system.

- PSI risk class I – patient can be sent home on oral antibiotics
- PSI risk class II–III – patient should be treated with IV antibiotics and may need to be monitored in hospital for 24 h
- PSI risk class IV–V – patient should be hospitalised for treatment

SMART-COP[67]

Systolic BP <90 mmHg (2 points)

Multilobe infiltrate (1 point)

Albumin <35g/L

RR (age adjusted <50 yrs >25/min, >50 yrs >30/min) (1 point)

Tachycardia >125 bpm (1 point)

Confusion (acute onset) (1 point)

Oxygenation (age adjusted: SpO_2 <93%, PaO_2 <9.3 kPa/70 mmHg, PaO_2/FiO_2 ratio <333) (2 points)

pH <7.35 (2 points)

Scoring:

0–2 points: low risk (<2% 30-day mortality)

3–4 points: moderate risk (5–13% 30-day mortality)

5–6 points: high risk (11–18% 30-day mortality)

7 or more points: very high risk (33% 30-day mortality)

Sources: Adapted from CURB-65: Lim WS, van der Eerden MM, Laing R, et al. Defining community acquired pneumonia severity on presentation to hospital: an international derivation and validation study. Thorax 2003;58:377–82.
Pneumonia severity index (PSI): Fine MJ, Auble TE, Yealy DM, et al. A prediction rule to identify low risk patients with community-acquired pneumonia. N Engl J Med 1997;336:243–50.
SMART-COP: Charles P, Wolfe R, Whitby M, et al. SMART-COP: a tool for predicting the need for intensive respiratory or vasopressor support in community-acquired pneumonia. Clin Infect Dis 2008;47(3):375–84.

Medications

Antibiotic administration is fundamental to a patient's clinical progress. The importance of accurate and timely administration of antibiotics directly impacts on patient outcome. In particular, in critically ill patients the first dose of antibiotics should be administered within an hour of the diagnosis of pneumonia being made.[68] Antibiotic cover depends on the causative organism and sensitivity to drugs (Table 14.4); however, empirical therapy should be commenced in patients with clinically suspected and radiologically confirmed CAP. The need for ongoing antibiotic therapy should be reviewed on a regular basis and de-escalation of antibiotic treatment considered once the clinical signs of infection have resolved.[69]

Hospital-acquired and ventilator-associated pneumonia

Hospital-acquired pneumonia is defined as pneumonia occurring more than 48 hours after hospital admission. It is the second most common nosocomial infection and the leading cause of death from infection acquired in hospital in critically ill patients. VAP is a form of hospital-acquired pneumonia that occurs in patients who have been mechanically ventilated for at least 48 hours.[49] The incidence of VAP is reported at 5–40% among patients requiring mechanical ventilation for more than 48 hours, and is associated with higher mortality, longer mechanical ventilation times, extended lengths of stay, overprescribing of antibiotics and higher healthcare costs. Rates vary widely depending on the country (e.g. North American hospitals report less VAP than European centres, and lower income countries report higher rates than high income countries) and the study population (patients with cancer, trauma, neurological compromise and COPD have higher rates of VAP, as do male patients and those with ARDS or receiving extra-corporeal membrane oxygenation (ECMO)).[70]

Aetiology

Invasively ventilated patients lack the normal defence mechanisms protecting the respiratory tract from infection. Protective mechanisms in the upper and lower airways which are altered by the insertion of an endotracheal tube (ETT) include the anatomical barriers of the glottis and larynx, cough reflexes, normal mucociliary clearance functions, and epithelial lining fluid and surfactant. Due to the loss of these and other functions, bacterial translocation occurs from the oropharynx to the lower airway as a result of microaspiration of secretions around the ETT or via

---

TABLE 14.4

Preferred antimicrobial agents in community-acquired pneumonia and influenza[59]

TYPE OF INFECTION	PREFERRED AGENT(S)
Community-acquired pneumonia	
Streptococcus pneumoniae	Penicillin-susceptible organisms: penicillin G (benzylpenicillin), amoxicillin, doxycycline Penicillin-resistant organisms: cefotaxime, ceftriaxone, vancomycin
Mycoplasma pneumonia	Doxycycline, macrolide
Chlamydophila pneumoniae	Doxycycline, macrolide
Legionella	Azithromycin, fluoroquinolone (levofloxacin or moxifloxacin)
Haemophilus influenzae	cephalosporin, beta-lactam/beta-lactamase inhibitor
Moraxella catarrhalis	Third-generation cephalosporin, beta-lactam/beta-lactamase inhibitor
Streptococci (other than *S. pneumoniae*)	Penicillin, cephalosporin
Anaerobes	Beta-lactam/beta-lactamase inhibitor, beta-lactam plus metronidazole
Staphylococcus aureus	Methicillin-susceptible: oxacillin, nafcillin Methicillin-resistant: vancomycin, linezolid
Klebsiella pneumoniae and other Enterobacteriaceae (excluding *Enterobacter* spp.)	Sensitive organism: third-generation cephalosporin, beta-lactam/beta-lactamase inhibitor, carbapenem (all + aminoglycoside) Carbapenemase-producing *Klebsiella*: ceftazidime–avibactam
Influenza	Oseltamivir, zanamivir, peramivir, baloxavir marboxil

Source: Dockrell DH, Ho A, Gordon SB. Community-acquired pneumonia. In: Broaddus VC, Ernst JD, King TE, et al, editors. Murray & Nadel's textbook of respiratory medicine. 7th ed. Philadelphia: Elsevier; 2022, p. 600–21.

contamination of the ventilator circuit. The patient's severity of disease, physiological reserve and comorbidities influence the development of infection and the likely causative organisms. The likely causative organisms also differ between early (<5 days after intubation) and later (≥5 days)-onset VAP. In early-onset VAP, *S. pneumoniae*, *H. influenzae* and methicillin-sensitive *S. aureus* are frequent. In contrast, in late-onset VAP multi-drug resistant pathogens are more common including *Pseudomonas aeruginosa*, *Acinetobacter baumannii*, methicillin-resistant *S. aureus* and other gram-negative bacilli.[49]

Diagnosis

VAP can be difficult to diagnose, as clinical features can be non-specific and other conditions may cause infiltrates on CXR. Additionally, ambiguity in the definition of VAP has led to inconsistencies in interpretation and application of the definition; therefore, meaningful comparison of incidence and/or treatment effects has been difficult. The current consensus definition developed by a joint international consortium of experts focuses on more-objective data.[49] VAP is suspected when additional support is required to maintain oxygenation, such as increased FiO_2 or higher positive end-expiratory pressure (PEEP); when clinical signs of infection begin to develop, including new onset of pyrexia or raised white blood cell counts; or when indicated by microbiological culture.[71]

Specific risk factors associated with increased mortality in VAP have been identified over the past decade. The most widely recognised risk minimisation factor is the provision of appropriate antibiotic treatment, which has reduced mortality and the rate of complications. Timeliness of antibiotic administration is an independent risk factor for mortality – mortality was increased where administration of antibiotics was delayed for more than 24 hours after diagnosis.[49,68]

When VAP is suspected, two diagnostic strategies are commonly used to guide antibiotic prescribing:

1 *Clinical strategy:* this involves treatment of patients with antibiotics which they have not recently received, based on patient risk factors and local microbiological and resistance patterns. Antibiotic therapy is adjusted based on culture results and the patient's response to treatment.

2 *Invasive strategy:* this involves collection and quantitative analysis of respiratory secretions from samples obtained by fibreoptic bronchoscopy or mini-bronchoalveolar lavage to confirm the diagnosis and causative organism. Antibiotic therapy is then guided by specific protocols based on the quantitative analysis of the specimens.[72,73]

Findings from a systematic review of these strategies did not demonstrate any differences in patient outcome measures including mortality, length of ICU stay or length of ventilation period.[74] Current guidelines recommend that, where possible, invasive strategies are used to collect samples from the distal lower airways, as this decreases

contamination with upper airway secretions and may help to minimise inappropriate antibiotic use.[49]

Patient management

VAP prevention strategies

Prevention of VAP is a key emphasis in the care of all mechanically ventilated patients and involves a number of interventions. VAP prevention has a focus on decreasing the risk of aspiration of upper airway secretions, decreasing microorganism load in the oropharynx and decreasing the introduction of microorganisms into the lower airways from the use of contaminated equipment.

A ventilator care bundle is a strategy which has been used to target VAP prevention and is a combination of evidence-based individual interventions that when used together can improve patient outcomes. Individual components that may be included in a ventilator care bundle can be found in Box 14.2.[71,75,76]

There is strong evidence that successful implementation of a care bundle decreases VAP rates,[71,74,75,77] with a recent meta-analysis also finding a reduction in mortality.[78] However, further research is required to determine what

---

BOX 14.2

Possible ventilator care bundle components[71,75,76]

- Semirecumbent positioning
- Daily sedation holds and assessment for extubation
- Stress ulcer disease prophylaxis
- Avoidance of elective changes of ventilator circuits
- Minimising duration of mechanical ventilation
- Regular oropharyngeal/subglottal suctioning
- Provision of regular mouth care including tooth brushing
- Maintenance of endotracheal tube cuff pressure at 20–30 mmHg
- Selective oropharyngeal decontamination
- Closed in-line suctioning equipment to decrease contamination of the ventilator circuit

Sources: Okgun Alcan A, Demir Korkmaz F, Uyar M. Prevention of ventilator-associated pneumonia: use of the care bundle approach. Am J Infect Control 2016; 44(10):e173–6; Álvarez-Lerma F, Palomar-Martínez M, Sánchez-García M, et al. Prevention of ventilator-associated pneumonia: the multimodal approach of the Spanish ICU "Pneumonia Zero" program. Crit Care Med 2018;46(2):181-8; Khan R, Al-Dorzi HM, Al-Attas K, et al. The impact of implementing multifaceted interventions on the prevention of ventilator-associated pneumonia. Am J Infect Control 2016;44(3):320–6.

individual strategies work together for the maximum effect, and additionally are sustainable and cost effective.

Regular oral hygiene and frequent removal of oropharyngeal secretions can reduce the risk of microaspiration around the ETT cuff.[79,80] Despite the reported benefits, there is currently a debate about the safety of using chlorhexidine mouthwash in intubated patients,[49] as two recent systematic reviews found non-statistically significant upward trends in patient mortality associated with the use of chlorhexidine for oral mouthcares.[81,82] In response, the joint international guidelines issued no recommendation about its general use until more evidence becomes available; however, evidence did determine that it was safe to use in settings of low antibiotic resistance and consumption.

Tooth brushing is essential to maintaining the basic hygiene needs of the patient and current evidence supports the role of tooth brushing in the improvement of oral health and subsequent removal of dental plaques. While there is no identified evidence of harm, there is no definitive evidence that tooth brushing decreases the occurrence of VAP.[83]

Selective oral or digestive decontamination involves prevention of colonisation by potentially pathogenic microorganisms, such as gram-negative aerobic microorganisms and methicillin-sensitive *S. aureus* and yeasts, from the oropharyngeal and intestinal tracts.[49,84] Current guidelines recommend that, in ICUs with low levels of antibiotic resistance, selective oral decontamination with non-absorbable antibiotics may be beneficial.[50] Although this strategy has been shown to be effective in reducing morbidity and mortality, it is yet to be widely adopted in clinical practice, in part due to concerns regarding antimicrobial resistance.[82] Selective digestive decontamination to reduce the incidence of VAP is not currently recommended as it has not been shown to reduce hospital mortality in critically ill patients receiving mechanical ventilation.[85]

Several other novel strategies have been suggested and evaluated for their effectiveness in reducing VAP rates. Specialised ETT tubes that allow for aspiration of subglottic secretions[86,87] and ETT tubes with silver antimicrobial coating may reduce VAP rates but need further evaluation before practice recommendations can be made.[88] ETT tubes with modified cuff shapes and devices to continuously maintain ETT cuff pressure more effectively maintain cuff pressures but there is no evidence of change in VAP rates.[89–91]

Management

Early recognition of pneumonia, timely administration of appropriate antibiotic therapy and supportive care are key aspects in pneumonia management. Supportive ventilation is a key focus for managing patients with pneumonia. In some instances, this may include increased oxygen delivery and PEEP to maintain oxygenation and prevent alveolar collapse. Chest physiotherapy remains a key component of management of all ventilated patients.[38] However, its

contribution towards reducing VAP, duration of mechanical ventilation and length of ICU stay is unclear.[92] Semirecumbent positioning (≥30 degrees)[93] and early mobilisation[94] are important elements of both prevention and management of pneumonia. The evidence supporting use of additional strategies, such as beds with a continuous lateral rotation or a vibration function, is limited and has been associated with complications, so recommendations for their use cannot be made.[95] See Chapter 15 for further discussion.

Practice tip

Pneumonia during pregnancy
Pneumonia is a leading cause of maternal and fetal morbidity and mortality. It also increases the likelihood of complications from pneumonia, including requirement for mechanical ventilation. Bacterial pneumonia is the most common type experienced in pregnancy, although diagnosis is often delayed as a result of the reluctance to obtain a CXR. Management is similar to that in a non-pregnant patient, with antibiotic therapy adjusted to consider the impact on the fetus.

Respiratory pandemics

Serious outbreaks of respiratory infections that spread rapidly on a global scale are termed pandemics. Their spread is rapid because the infection is usually associated with the emergence of a new virus where the majority of the population has no immunity. These infections are characterised by extremely rapid transmission with concurrent outbreaks throughout the globe; the occurrence of disease outside the usual seasonality, including during the summer months; high attack rates in all age groups, with high levels of mortality particularly in healthy young adults; and multiple waves of disease immediately before and after the main outbreak.[96]

Several severe respiratory infections have progressed to become pandemics in recent years. These have been associated with the coronavirus and influenza viruses. Most notable is the current COVID-19 pandemic, which continues to spread via the development of new variants.[97] Prediction of the interval between pandemics is difficult, but occurrence is likely to continue and this therefore requires that the healthcare community be well prepared. The InFACT H1N1 Research Collaborative is an example of a global public health initiative aimed at reducing the mortality associated with the H1N1 influenza virus through clinical research groups and professional organisations working together to gain a rapid understanding of the epidemiology and clinical presentation of the disease, and the identification of effective management strategies.[98] The public health response to the current COVID-19 global pandemic has built on lessons learned from previous global collaborations and has been the most rapid of any pandemic, particularly around epidemiological data sharing to quickly characterise the novel disease (https://isaric.org/).

Influenza epidemics

Epidemics of influenza occur regularly and are associated with high morbidity and mortality.[98] A feature of the influenza virus that explains why it continues to be associated with epidemic and pandemic disease is its high frequency of antigenic variation. This occurs in two of the external glycoproteins and is referred to as antigenic drift or antigenic shift, depending on the extent of the variation. The result of this is that new viruses are introduced into the population and, due to the absence of immunity to the virus, a pandemic of influenza results.[96]

Pandemics of influenza were observed a number of times in the 20th century and were believed to have involved viruses circulating in humans that originated from influenza A viruses in birds. The most recent influenza pandemic was declared by the World Health Organization (WHO) in 2009 when a novel H1N1 influenza A virus emerged in Mexico and the United States of America. The disease spread globally, with millions of cases reported, and resulted in over 16,000 deaths by March 2010.[99] Australian and New Zealand communities had a high proportion of cases of H1N1 influenza A infection, with 856 patients being admitted to ICU, 15 times the incidence of influenza A in other recent years.[100,101]

Priorities for prevention and management of future influenza pandemics involve development of an international surveillance and response network for early detection and containment of the disease, local preparation for controlling the spread of the infection and further development of vaccines and antiviral agents.[96,98]

Patient management

Vaccination

Influenza vaccines are formulated annually based on current and recent viral strains. Success in protecting an individual against influenza requires that the virus strains included in the vaccine are the same as those currently circulating in the community. Vaccines are commonly effective in preventing influenza in 70–90% of healthy adults younger than 65 years of age. Efficacy appears lower in elderly people. Healthcare workers are a key target group for the influenza vaccine, at the very least to reduce absenteeism over what is often the busiest period for most health services and to reduce the risk of nosocomial influenza infections in hospitalised patients.[102,103]

Isolation precautions and personal protective equipment

Key aspects of infection control in an epidemic or pandemic situation focus on limiting opportunities for nosocomial spread and the protection of healthcare workers. Guidelines for institutional management of these infections involve designing and implementing appropriate isolation procedures and recommending appropriate personal protective equipment (PPE).[104] Specific infection control guidelines are usually developed for individual institutions, based on government recommendations for management of staff, appropriate PPE and isolation procedures. This topic is covered in detail in Chapter 5.

COVID-19 coronavirus pandemic

COVID-19 was named by the World Health Organization in February 2020 as the human disease caused by SARS-CoV-2, the most recent in the family of coronaviruses. Its emergence was first detected in the city of Wuhan, China in early December 2019 and these cases were associated with the Wuhan Huanan Seafood Wholesale Market. The intermediate host of the SARS-CoV-2 virus has not been definitively established; however, bats and subsequently pangolins may have played a role in transmission of the virus to humans.[105] According to the WHO online dashboard (https://covid19.who.int/), as of 14 February 2023 there have been 756,135,075 confirmed cases of COVID-19, including 6,841,152 deaths, reported to WHO. As of 13 February 2023, a total of over 13.18 billion vaccine doses have been administered. It is the largest global pandemic since the Spanish influenza (H1N1) of 1918.

COVID-19 has put significant strains on critical care resources worldwide, and public health measures, such as prolonged periods of lockdown, have been put in place to mitigate hospital and ICU overload. Despite these measures, some countries have had insufficient resources to meet demand and availability of ICU beds. Equipment such as ventilators and ECMO machines were rationed, resulting in extreme moral dilemmas for frontline physicians involved in such decision making and ICU triage protocols have been developed to assist in triage decision making.[106]

COVID-19 appears not only to be an acute disease but also results in chronic ill health and disability after acute symptoms subside, and this condition is known as long COVID.[107] Long COVID has been reported in significant numbers of people, with a reported incidence at 6 months of 37% in a cohort of 273,618 people aged 10 years and over.[108] A recent systematic review including 8591 adults reported the most commonly reported symptoms at least 1 year after COVID-19 infection were fatigue/weakness (28%), dyspnoea (18%), arthromyalgia (26%), depression (23%), concentration difficulties (18%) and memory loss (19%). Risk factors for long-COVID symptoms at 1 year were having more-severe disease and being female.[109] However, as this is an emerging and ever-changing field, more high-quality research is needed before definitive conclusions regarding incidence, risk factors and best management of long COVID can be determined with any certainty. These data are crucial for future planning of healthcare services.

Patient management

Vaccine

Rapid and expedited development of an effective vaccine against COVID-19 led to the first vaccination being delivered outside a clinical trial on 8th December 2020. Vaccination is the most effective strategy to reduce serious illness and death from COVID-19 and it has been estimated that nearly 20 million deaths have been avoided in the first year of vaccine availability owing to uptake of COVID-19 vaccination.[110] However, vaccine rollout has been slower in low-income countries than in high-income countries, and this inequitable access to vaccines is likely to extend the end of the pandemic globally.[111]

ICU care

COVID-19 presents in the ICU as a complex disease which may compromise the lung, heart, kidney, brain, liver and coagulation system. Estimates suggest that around 14% of cases will require hospitalisation and 5% will be admitted to a critical care unit (https://ourworldindata.org/covid-hospitalizations). The consensus recommendations of COVID-19 disease severity from the National COVID-19 Clinical Evidence Taskforce (https://covid19evidence.net.au/) is contained in Table 14.5[112] and, using these criteria, patients with severe or critical disease severity would require admission to an ICU.

In a setting of rapidly emerging evidence of varying quality, contemporaneous clinical practice guidelines from peak healthcare bodies, whether professional societies or government departments, has become very important in ensuring that the most robust and up-to-date evidence is available for clinicians to guide patient care. Table 14.6[112,113] details current ICU management practices for adults with COVID-19, and more information on respiratory pathophysiology can be found in the Further reading section.

Acute respiratory distress syndrome (ARDS)

ARDS is an acute, diffuse inflammatory lung injury that causes acute respiratory failure, characterised by hypoxaemia, bilateral infiltrates and decreased lung compliance due to increased alveolar capillary permeability leading to non-hydrostatic pulmonary oedema.[114,115] ARDS should be suspected if hypoxia does not resolve with supplemental oxygen.[39]

Aetiology

ARDS is a characteristic inflammatory response of the lung to a wide variety of insults. Epidemiological studies show a variable incidence of ARDS. A multicentre prospective cohort study (LUNG SAFE) involving 29,144 patients from 50 countries showed that 10% of all patients admitted to the ICU had ARDS, with a 46% mortality for those with severe ARDS.[116] Evidence from individual studies among COVID-19 patients transferred to ICU found an increased prevalence of ARDS (75%), with an associated mortality rate of 45%.[117] Clinical disorders that are commonly associated with ARDS can be separated into those that directly or indirectly injure the lung

TABLE 14.5

Definition for COVID-19 disease severity in adults[112]

Mild illness	An individual with no clinical features suggestive of moderate or more severe disease: • no *or* mild symptoms and signs (fever, cough, sore throat, malaise, headache, muscle pain, nausea, vomiting, diarrhoea, loss of taste and smell) • no new shortness of breath or breathing difficulty on exertion • no evidence of lower respiratory tract disease during clinical assessment or on imaging (if performed)

Moderate illness	A stable patient with evidence of lower respiratory tract disease:
	• during clinical assessment, such as
	  ○ oxygen saturation 92–94% on room air at rest
	  ○ desaturation or breathlessness with mild exertion
	• *or* on imaging

Severe illness	A patient with signs of moderate disease who is deteriorating *or* A patient meeting any of the following criteria: • respiratory rate ≥30 breaths/min • oxygen saturation <92% on room air at rest or requiring oxygen • lung infiltrates >50%

Critical illness	A patient meeting any of the following criteria:
	• respiratory failure (defined as any of)
	  ○ severe respiratory failure (PaO_2/FiO_2 <200)
	  ○ respiratory distress or acute respiratory distress syndrome (ARDS)
	  ○ deteriorating despite non-invasive forms of respiratory support (i.e. non-invasive ventilation (NIV), or high-flow nasal oxygen (HFNO))
	  ○ requiring mechanical ventilation
	• hypotension or shock
	• impairment of consciousness
	• other organ failure

Source: Adapted from National COVID-19 Clinical Evidence Taskforce. Australian guidelines on the clinical care of people with COVID-19 (version 57). 2022. Available from: https://covid19evidence.net.au/. [Accessed 18 February 2023].

TABLE 14.6

Current recommendations for ICU management of adult patients with COVID-19[112,113]

Respiratory support	*Managing risk of infection:*
	• All patients receiving respiratory support should be in a negative-pressure room where possible. If this is not possible, single room or cohorting with other COVID-19 positive patients are alternatives.
	• Contact, droplet and airborne precautions should be in place.
	Oxygenation and ventilation:
	• Target oxygen saturation:
	  ○ 92–96% in most patients
	  ○ 88–92% in those at risk of hypercapnia.
	• For patients with acute hypoxaemic respiratory failure not responding to low-flow oxygen therapy, consider a trial of HFNO. If no response, do not delay non-invasive ventilation or invasive mechanical ventilation.
	• CPAP is the preferred non-invasive positive pressure ventilation therapy for patients with ongoing hypoxaemia (i.e. $FiO_2 \geq 0.4$ to maintain target oxygen saturation). CPAP of 10–12 cmH_2O is recommended.
	• Prone positioning (face-down):
	  ○ Non-mechanically ventilated patients: consider prone positioning for at least 3 hours per day as tolerated.
	  ○ Mechanically ventilated patients: consider prone positioning for at least 12 hours per day.
	• For mechanically ventilated patients with ARDS, recommendations are:
	  ○ Lung-protective ventilation (VT 4–8 mL/kg PBW)
	  ○ Plateau pressures of <30 cmH_2O
	  ○ Conservative fluid strategy rather than liberal
	  ○ No routine use of inhaled nitric oxide (or other pulmonary vasodilator) unless refractory hypoxaemia develops
	  ○ Higher PEEP (>10 cmH_2O) for moderate to severe ARDS
	  ○ Neuromuscular-blocking agents only if lung protective ventilation strategies cannot be achieved.

Haemodynamic support	*Fluid resuscitation:* • In severe or critical COVID-19, restrictive fluid management is recommended. • For acute resuscitation, use buffered/balanced rather than unbalanced crystalloids, and avoid synthetic colloids. *Vasoactive agents:* • Use noradrenaline as the first-line vasoactive agent. If unavailable, use vasopressin or adrenaline. • Target a mean arterial pressure of 60–65 mmHg. If this is not reached with a single vasoactive agent, add a second.
ECMO	• Early referral for consideration of ECMO is recommended. • Select patients may benefit; however, no firm recommendations can be made.
Pharmacological interventions	• Empirical broad-spectrum antibiotics are not recommended unless there is a proven or suspected bacterial infection. • Daily reassessment of the need for antibiotics is recommended. • Prophylactic doses of anticoagulants (preferably low-molecular-weight heparin) are recommended unless contraindicated. • Dexamethasone plus remdesivir should be considered for patients with deteriorating oxygenation and systemic inflammation. • Interleukin-6 inhibitors (e.g. tocilizumab, sarilumab), or Janus kinase inhibitors (e.g. baricitinib, tofacitinib) may reduce the risk of death. • Hydroxychloroquine, ivermectin, aspirin, azithromycin and convalescent plasma are not recommended for use.

ARDS = acute respiratory distress syndrome; CPAP = continuous positive airway pressure; ECMO = extracorporeal membrane oxygenation; FiO_2 = fraction of inspired oxygen; HFNO = high-flow nasal oxygen; PEEP = positive end expiratory pressure; PBW = predicted body weight.

Sources: National COVID-19 Clinical Evidence Taskforce. Australian guidelines for the clinical care of people with COVID-19. 2022 [version 57]. Available at: https://covid19evidence.net.au/; COVID-19 Treatment Guidelines Panel. Coronavirus disease 2019 (COVID-19) treatment guidelines. National Institutes of Health. Available at https://www.covid19treatmentguidelines.nih.gov/.

TABLE 14.7

Direct and indirect causes of acute lung injury[118]

DIRECT LUNG INJURY	INDIRECT LUNG INJURY
Pneumonia (COVID-19)	Sepsis
Aspiration of gastric contents	Multiple trauma
Pulmonary contusion	Cardiopulmonary bypass
Fat, amniotic fluid or air embolus	Drug overdose
Near drowning	Acute pancreatitis
Inhalational injury (chemical or smoke)	Transfusion of blood products
Reperfusion pulmonary oedema	

Source: Adapted from Thompson BT, Chambers RC, Liu KD. Acute respiratory distress syndrome. N Engl J Med 2017; 377(19):1904–5.

(Table 14.7).[118] The most common causes are pneumonia arising from direct injury (30–50%) and sepsis due to indirect injury (30%).[119,120] The risk of developing ARDS increases significantly when more than one predisposing factor is present.

Pathophysiology

Inflammatory damage to alveoli from locally or systemically released inflammatory mediators causes a change in pulmonary capillary permeability, with resulting fluid and protein leakage into the lung extravascular spaces and activation of the extrinsic coagulation cascade.[121] Dilution and loss of surfactant causes diffuse alveolar collapse and a reduction in pulmonary compliance and may also impair the defence mechanisms of the lungs. Intrapulmonary shunt is confirmed when hypoxaemia does not improve despite supplemental oxygen administration.[118,122] The characteristic course of ARDS is described as having three phases:[38,120]

1 *Exudative phase:* injury to the alveolar–capillary membrane results in the migration of neutrophils and secretion of mediators by alveolar microphages into the alveolar compartment causing increased vascular permeability and tissue injury. In response, proinflammatory cytokines and mediators are released that amplify the inflammatory response in the lung. Significant ventilation/perfusion (intrapulmonary shunt) mismatch evolves, causing hypoxaemia and reduced lung compliance within the first 6 days of the disease.

2 *Proliferative phase:* this begins after 2–3 weeks as pulmonary infiltrates resolve and fibrosis and

remodelling occur to re-establish epithelial integrity or may progress to the fibroproliferation phase. This phase is characterised by reduced alveolar ventilation and pulmonary compliance and ventilation/perfusion mismatch. Reduced compliance causes further atelectasis in the mechanically ventilated patient as alveoli are damaged by increased volume and/or pressure on inspiration.

3 *Fibrotic phase:* this occurs after 14 days or may not occur in all patients. It is characterised by ongoing inflammation and microvascular damage where alveoli become fibrotic and the lung is left with emphysema-like alterations, and is linked to prolonged mechanical ventilation and increased mortality.

Diagnosis

Diagnosis of ARDS is based on the Berlin definition (2012)[123] developed by the European Society of Intensive Care Medicine. This definition established three mutually exclusive categories (mild, moderate, severe) that are based on the degree of hypoxaemia (PaO_2/FiO_2 ratio) measured with at least 5 cmH_2O of applied PEEP (Table 14.8).[116,123] These categories correspond to prognosis, with higher severity associated with increased mortality rates.[124] The criteria include onset within 1 week of a known clinical insult or new or worsening symptoms, bilateral opacities on chest imaging, hypoxaemia and unexplained pulmonary oedema. To date, no diagnostic biomarkers are available and definitions rely on clinical presentation and chest imaging. Chest radiograph, lung ultrasound or computed tomography to confirm the presence of bilateral opacities of non-cardiogenic origin on imaging is diagnostic of ARDS.[125,126]

Clinical manifestations

ARDS should be considered in any patient with a predisposing risk factor who develops severe hypoxaemia, reduced compliance and diffuse pulmonary infiltrates on CXR.[118,122,123,127] Clinical manifestations usually occur 72 hours following onset of a presenting condition (e.g. sepsis, pneumonia, trauma, COVID-19) and is characterised by rapid clinical deterioration. Common symptoms include severe dyspnoea, cough, fever, fatigue, pleuritic chest pain, tachypnoea, oedema, hypoxaemia requiring rapidly escalating amounts of supplemental oxygen and persistent coarse crackles on auscultation.[46,128]

Assessment

A patient with ARDS requires ongoing monitoring of oxygenation and ventilation through pulse oximetry, serum lactate and ABG analysis, especially $PaCO_2$ to monitor permissive hypercapnia.[127,128] Monitoring of ventilatory pressures and volumes ensures that additional lung injury is prevented.[129] As many patients with ARDS require cardiovascular support, assessment of haemodynamics and peripheral perfusion is important to ensure that oxygen delivery to cells is achieved.

TABLE 14.8

Acute respiratory distress syndrome: the Berlin definition[123]

....

Timing	Within 1 week of a known clinical insult or new or worsening respiratory symptoms.
Chest imaging[a]	Bilateral opacities – not fully explained by effusions, lobar/lung collapse, or nodules.
Origin of oedema	Respiratory failure not fully explained by cardiac failure or fluid overload.
	Need objective assessment (e.g. echocardiography) to exclude hydrostatic oedema if no risk factor present.
Oxygenation[b]	
Mild	200 mmHg $<PaO_2/FiO_2$ ratio $\leq$300 with PEEP or CPAP $\geq$5 cmH_2O^c
Moderate	100 mmHg $<PaO_2/FiO_2$ ratio $\leq$200 with PEEP or CPAP $\geq$5 cmH_2O
Severe	PaO_2/FiO_2 ratio $\leq$100 with PEEP $\geq$5 cmH_2O

CPAP = Continuous positive airway pressure; FiO_2 = fraction of inspired oxygen; PaO_2 = partial pressure arterial oxygen; PEEP = positive end-expiratory pressure.

[a] Chest radiograph or computed tomography scan.

[b] If altitude is higher than 1000 m, the correction factor should be calculated as follows: PaO_2/FiO_2 × (barometric pressure/760).

[c] This may be delivered non-invasively in the mild acute respiratory distress syndrome group.

Source: Adapted from ARDS Definition Task Force; Ranieri VM, Rubenfeld GD, Thompson BT, et al. Acute respiratory distress syndrome: the Berlin definition. JAMA 2012;307(23):2526–33.

Patient management

Despite decades of research, treatment options for ARDS are limited.[130] The key principles of management are treatment of the precipitating cause and provision of supportive care to minimise iatrogenic injury during the period of respiratory failure.[46,131] The most significant advances in the supportive care of ARDS patients have been associated with improved ventilator management using a protective lung ventilation strategy targeting a tidal volume <6 mL/kg predicted body weight and plateau pressure <30 cmH_2O as standard in ARDS management.[33,131,132] However, protective lung ventilation alone may be insufficient and other adjunctive therapies may be required.[130] In patients with increasing severity of ARDS, the most frequently used adjunctive measures are continuous neuromuscular-blocking agents, high-dose steroids and recruitment maneouvres (i.e. transient elevations in applied airway pressures).[116] Other supportive strategies include cautious fluid management, nutritional support, prevention of VAP, prophylaxis for deep vein thrombosis and gastric ulcers, weaning of sedation, prone positioning, physiotherapy, ECMO and rehabilitation.[46]

Ventilation strategies

The goals of mechanical ventilation for ARDS are to prevent ventilator-associated lung injury[114] and refractory hypoxaemia. Lung-protective strategies that use lower tidal volumes (4–8 mL/kg predicted body weight)[133] and inspiratory pressures (plateau pressure <30 cmH_2O) with higher levels of PEEP (>12 cmH_2O)[33,46,114,134] are associated with decreased mortality[135] and are recommended guidance in moderate to severe ARDS.[33,131,132] However, a large international trial found that less than two-thirds of ARDS patients received a tidal volume of 8 mL/kg or less, 40% measured plateau pressure and 83% received PEEP less than 12 cmH_2O,[116] highlighting the difficulty of achieving lung protective ventilation in practice. A conservative oxygenation (PaO_2 9.3 kPa/70 mmHg, SaO_2 88–95%) is recommended, along with a higher inspiratory/expiratory ratio and respiratory rate, prone positioning and neuromuscular blockade, inhaled vasodilator therapies and conservative fluid therapy.[127,131] The evidence to support the use of lung recruitment manoeuvres to improve patient outcomes remains unclear. American guidance recommends that adult patients with ARDS receive recruitment manoeuvres based on low-to-moderate confidence of the evidence,[33] whereas French formal guidelines do not recommend routine use.[132] High-frequency oscillatory ventilation is currently not recommended in patients with ARDS.[33,130–132]

Some therapies have demonstrated improved oxygenation, which may be an important goal in many patients who experience severe hypoxaemia. ECMO is considered a viable treatment option for severe ARDS, given the increased evidence of its effectiveness beyond a rescue therapy for refractory ARDS.[114,136] Guidelines recommended its use with protective lung ventilation in selected patients with severe ARDS.[33,131,132] Systematic review evidence showed a reduced 60-day mortality in patients with severe ARDS following use of ECMO compared with conventional mechanical ventilation.[137] Further systematic reviews found a significantly higher PaO_2/FiO_2 ratio and probability of surviving without major complications (cumulative survival of 57%)[138,139] or reduced 28-day mortality[130] in patients that underwent prone positioning during venovenous ECMO. Early use of prone positioning and ECMO should therefore be considered.[130] This strategy is described in more detail in Chapter 15.

The use of prone position ventilation results in better oxygenation than supine ventilation; this is largely due to the prevention of ventilator-associated lung injury and should be first-line therapy for patients with moderate to severe ARDS.[33] The result is a more homogeneous ventilation of the lungs and improved ventilation/perfusion matching via recruitment of the alveoli in dependent lung regions.[114] Systematic review evidence[130,140] and findings from the PROSEVA study[32] suggest that use of early prone positioning compared with supine position reduced mortality in patients with severe ARDS who underwent a longer duration of prone ventilation and lung-protective ventilation strategy. A network meta-analysis of RCTs to compare a range of ventilation strategies in patients with moderate to severe ARDS showed that prone positioning with low tidal volume was associated with the greatest reduction in mortality.[141] As a result, guidelines recommend prone positioning for at least >12–16 hours per day in patients with moderate to severe ARDS[33,115,127,132] and implementation of a weaning protocol[142] for patients who have been on mechanical ventilation for more than 24 hours. See Chapter 15 for further information regarding mechanical ventilation strategies.

Medications

Pharmacological interventions are limited in the management of ARDS. It is recommended that neuromuscular-blocking agents are administered early by continuous infusion in ARDS patients, with a PaO_2/FiO_2 ratio <150 for no more than 48 hours with daily evaluation to reduce mortality.[132] Limited evidence suggests that the use of neuromuscular-blocking agents may improve oxygenation and perhaps a reduction in inflammatory mediators in the critically ill. Further research is required to illicit further information on this area.[128,143] Their use should be based on individual assessment, given concerns related to critical illness polyneuromyopathy[120,121] and systematic review evidence suggesting the use of neuromuscular-blocking agents did not improve mortality in moderate to severe ARDS.[130]

The role of corticosteroids in ARDS remains uncertain. A multicentre trial of patients with ARDS due to COVID-19 showed no significant difference in ventilator-free days between high- and low-dose dexamethasone.[144] The use of corticosteroids is not recommended as further evidence of potential benefits and harms is required.[131,145]

The use of inhaled nitric oxide to improve oxygen is controversial, with conflicting guidance on its use as a result of limited evidence to support improved patient outcomes. Guidelines reviewed and endorsed by La Société de Réanimation de Langue Française in France[132] suggest that nitric oxide can be used for patients with severe hypoxaemic ARDS, despite implementation of a protective lung strategy and prone positioning and before venovenous ECMO, based on expert opinion. However, the Faculty of Intensive Care Medicine and Intensive Care Society guidance supported by the British Thoracic Society recommends that inhaled nitric oxide is not used, given the lack of mortality benefit and association with renal dysfunction.[131] A number of drug therapies continue to be investigated to treat ARDS in acute and subacute exudative phases. These include agents that target neutrophil recruitment and activation (neutrophil elastase inhibitors), activation of the coagulation cascade (heparin, aspirin and statins), microvascular injury and leak (beta$_2$-agonists,

angiotensin-converting-enzyme inhibitors; low-dose corticosteroids) and tissue regeneration (growth factors, stem cell therapy).[145,146] The evidence on the role of these pharmacological agents remains unclear; although an improvement in oxygenation has been reported, improvements in other outcomes such as duration of mechanical ventilation, length of ICU stay or improved survival have not been shown.[147] The use of antiplatelet therapy has been associated with a moderately improved survival, reduced incidence of ARDS and need for mechanical ventilation in a recent systematic review, although there is a need for further robust research in this area.[148]

Asthma and chronic obstructive pulmonary disease (COPD)

Asthma is primarily a chronic inflammatory disease that varies over time and intensity, which is defined by the history of respiratory symptoms, wheeze, cough, shortness of breath, with variable expiratory air-flow limitation.[149] COPD is a chronic respiratory condition where air-flow limitation is progressive and not fully reversible, although there may be some reversibility of air-flow limitation with bronchodilators.[23,150] The partial air-flow responsiveness to therapy in COPD results in a clinical overlap between COPD and asthma, as well as chronic bronchitis and emphysema (Fig. 14.2). Each disease is increasingly recognised as a complex of multiple phenotypes with different pathogenic mechanisms (type 2 inflammation, viral infection, bacterial colonisation or impaired lung growth) requiring specific treatment.[151] Increasingly, the coexistence of asthma and COPD is recognised as asthma–COPD overlap, which describes chronic air-flow limitation in adults over 40 years with different forms of airways disease and frequent exacerbations.[152] It is, however, important to differentiate between COPD and asthma as they have different management and illness trajectories.

Asthma is the second most prevalent chronic respiratory disease worldwide, affecting 334 million people.[3] It is a cause of substantial burden of disease, including both premature death and reduced quality of life in people of all ages.[153] In 2017, asthma accounted for 69% of the total incidence of chronic respiratory disease, although, in aggregate, its prevalence had decreased since 1990,[3] with large reductions in the number of hospital admissions over the past decade in several countries.[153] The global incidence rate in males and females were similar, with a decreased rate in those under 10 years of age and an increased rate in people aged 65–74.[4] Asthma is a rare cause of mortality, contributing less than 1% of all deaths in most countries.[153]

Worldwide COPD remained the most prevalent disease-specific chronic respiratory disease in 2017[3] and a leading cause of mortality and morbidity associated with

FIGURE 14.2 Obstructive lung diseases: overlap between asthma, chronic bronchitis and emphysema.

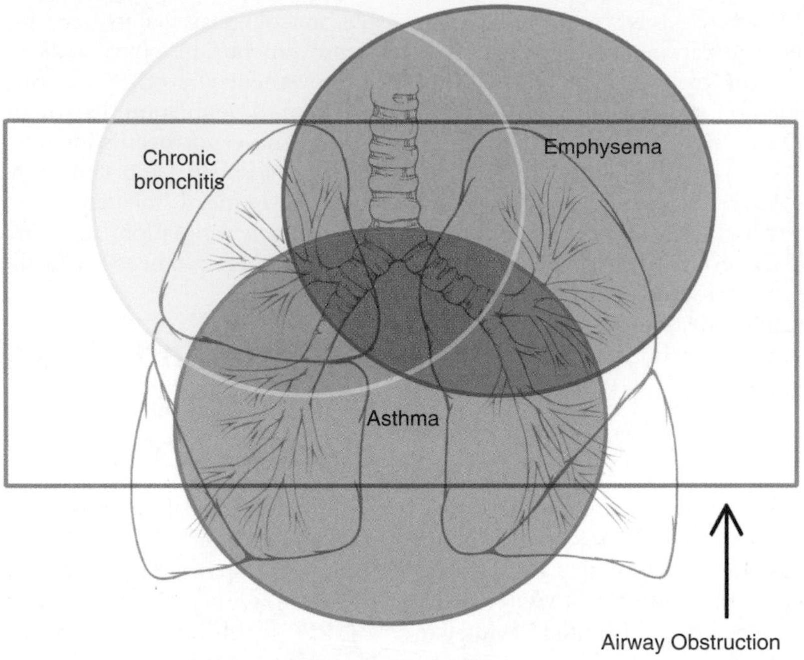

Chronic bronchitis

Emphysema

Asthma

Airway Obstruction

Source: Reproduced from Des Jardins T, Burton GG. Clinical manifestations and assessment of respiratory disease. 8th ed. St Louis, MO: Elsevier; 2020.

substantial economic burden.[39] It is the most common cause of chronic respiratory disease-attributable deaths, at 41.9 deaths per 100,000 individuals[3] with the bulk of the burden occurring in the low-sociodemographic countries.[4] In 2017, COPD was most prevalent in central and eastern Europe and central Asia.[3] The incidence rate of COPD increased with age in both sexes and decreased in all age groups from 1990 to 2017, except for patients older than 80 years.[4] Given the increasing ageing population and continued exposure to risk factors, the prevalence and burden of COPD will continue to increase.[154] Analysis of patients admitted to an ICU with acute exacerbations of COPD in Australia and New Zealand between 2005 and 2017 found that 8.7% died in ICU and 15.4% died in hospital, with an increasing rate of ICU admissions and decreasing rate of mortality.[155] Deaths from COPD were eight times more common than deaths from asthma.[5]

Pathophysiology

Asthma is a complex syndrome of unknown aetiology. However, it is known to be influenced by genetic, immunological and environmental factors, and epidemiological studies show strong associations with respiratory pathogens.[151] Analysis of 2019 global burden of disease data found that high body–mass index (BMI), smoking and occupational factors were the main attributable risk factors across 204 countries.[156] These factors lead to

infection and allergic responses, airway inflammation, airway hyperresponsiveness, bronchoconstriction and oedema that result in wheezing, breathlessness and coughing. The pathophysiology of life-threatening asthma involves constriction of the bronchioles and subsequent air trapping in the alveoli beyond the constriction, leading to hyperinflation, expiratory air-flow limitation and generation of intrinsic PEEP. This is exacerbated by increased resistance in expiratory gas flow due to a loss of elastic recoil and rapid respiratory rates. The patient increases the work of breathing, becomes rapidly fatigued and anxious and there is diminished gas exchange. These factors reduce carbon dioxide elimination while increasing its production and eventually will progress to muscle fatigue and respiratory failure.[157]

In contrast to asthma, COPD is a preventable and treatable disease associated with an inflammatory response due to airway/alveolar abnormalities caused by significant exposure to noxious gases or particles.[39] This causes respiratory symptoms and significant air-flow narrowing that result in a permanent and progressive condition.[23] Smoking (both active and passive) is the most prevalent risk factor for chronic respiratory diseases worldwide and continuation is the most significant determinant for disease progression.[3] Other environmental risk factors include occupational exposure to dusts, fumes and chemicals, air pollution, age, genetic factors and socioeconomic status.[6,39] Disease progression in susceptible individuals is most likely to be dependent on the synergistic effects of these factors. COPD is characterised by persistent air-flow limitation[158] and air-flow obstruction caused by an immune response to long-term inhaled noxious gases.[159] The acute inflammation releases several cytokines and chemotactic factors which cause bronchoconstriction, oedema and mucus hypersecretion[159] as a result of three different pathological mechanisms. First, chronic inflammation leads to remodelling and narrowing of the small airways. Second, loss of elastic support and lung recoil leads to airway collapse because the small airways close on expiration. Third, the mucous and plasma exudate from the inflammation obstructs the airway lumen. These mechanisms lead to air trapping and lung hyperinflation due to reduced air flow on expiration, which consequently produces dyspnoea and exercise limitation for the patient.[160] Perfusion abnormalities arise from hypoxaemia-induced vasoconstriction of the capillary beds. Pulmonary ventilation/perfusion abnormalities and hyperinflation contribute to increased pulmonary vascular resistance and respiratory muscle fatigue. Increased pulmonary vascular resistance and hypoxaemia require the right side of the heart to work harder and may lead to right ventricular hypertrophy, dysfunction and failure (cor pulmonale). Chronic hypoxia causes pulmonary artery constriction and pulmonary hypertension is a common complication in COPD linked to increased mortality and morbidity.[159]

Clinical manifestations

With asthma and COPD, a patient may present with symptoms of wheeze, chest tightness, cough and/or dyspnoea which are triggered by exercise, allergens, viral infections or irritants.[149,161,162] History and physical assessment are fundamental to determining the severity of presentation and should be conducted concurrently with prompt initiation of therapy.[150] Acute severe asthma or asthma exacerbations are characterised by a progressive increase in symptoms and decrease in lung function.[151,162]

Respiratory alkalosis is the most common abnormality found during asthma exacerbations due to increased respiratory drive, but, as bronchoconstriction worsens, hypercarbia and respiratory acidosis develop.[163] Presence of diminished or silent breath sounds, sitting hunched forward, agitated, severe breathlessness, an inability to complete sentences, an altered level of consciousness, use of accessory muscles, hyperinflation of the chest, tachypnoea >30/min, tachycardia >120 bpm, SaO_2 on air <90% and diaphoresis indicate a life-threatening case.[149,162,164] Chest pain or tightness may be present.

Patients with COPD present with recurrent history of lower respiratory tract infections or history of exposure to risk factors with dyspnoea, chronic cough and sputum production.[39] An exacerbation of COPD is defined as an acute worsening of respiratory symptoms that results in additional therapy.[23,39] Key symptoms of an exacerbation are increased dyspnoea, cough and wheeze as a result of increased airway inflammation, tachypnoea, mucus production, fatigue, confusion and marked gas trapping.[23,39]

Assessment and diagnostics

Diagnosis is based on clinical history, physical assessment and objective tests[165] which demonstrate evidence of reversible air-flow obstruction, airway hyperresponsiveness or the presence of airway inflammation.[149] The clinical history provides details of variability in expiratory lung function and respiratory symptoms such as wheeze, cough, breathlessness or chest tightness.[149] Physical assessment includes details regarding exacerbation severity, pulse rate, oxygen saturation, respiratory rate, accessory muscle use, ability to complete sentences and equal bilateral air entry,[162,165] the purpose of which is to determine the level of severity (moderate acute, acute severe, life-threatening or near fatal) of acute asthma attacks.[164] In asthma, a positive spirometry test showing a reduced forced expiratory volume in 1 second/forced vital capacity (FEV_1/FVC) ratio of <0.75, or a positive bronchodilator reversibility test with an increase in FEV_1 of >12% and >200 mL from baseline after inhalation of short-acting beta$_2$-agonists, is diagnostic of obstructive airway disease.[149,165,166] In addition to spirometry and peak flow measures for airway obstruction, the Scottish Intercollegiate Guidelines Network/British Thoracic Society, NICE and National Asthma Education and Prevention Program[164,165,167] recommend the use of fractional concentration of exhaled nitric oxide testing to detect type 2 airway inflammation, although the Global Initiative for Asthma 2022 indicates that this diagnostic testing has not been established.[149]

In COPD a history of exposure to risk factors and comprehensive assessment of symptoms/risk of exacerbations using the COPD assessment test or Medical Research Council (MRC) dyspnoea scale[23] and the COPD control questionnaire is recommended.[39] Spirometry is required to determine diagnosis, and a post-bronchodilator FEV_1/FVC ratio <0.7 confirms the presence of persistent air-flow limitation.[23] The level of air-flow limitation is classified as a spirometric grade (mild, moderate, severe or very severe) based on postbronchodilator FEV_1.[39,168,169] This assessment approach emphasises the importance of patient symptoms and exacerbation risks in guiding therapies in COPD.[39] Further diagnostic tests and procedures involve peak flow monitoring, spirometry,[23] exercise testing/assessment of physical activity, oximetry, radiology and ABGs.[150] Forward planning for potential deterioration and constant assessment of respiratory, cardiovascular and neurological systems are fundamental in determining optimal clinical progress for these patients.[23]

Patient management

Contemporary management of asthma follows a stepwise asthma management or action plan to recognise and respond to worsening symptoms in order to minimise acute exacerbations.[149] Many presentations will be managed in the emergency department (see Chapter 23 for further discussion) and do not require inpatient acute admission. Parameters which guide the need for referral to critical care include persistent hypoxia despite supplemental oxygen, hypercapnia, acidosis, exhaustion, reduced level of consciousness, haemodynamic instability, respiratory arrest[164] and presenting with a silent chest.[149]

Hypoxaemic patients with acute severe asthma require administration of supplementary oxygen via nasal cannulae or mask titrated to maintain an SpO_2 level of 94–98%.[149,164] Controlled low-flow oxygen is associated with better physiological outcomes than high-concentration (100%) oxygen therapy. There should be monitoring and review of the response of symptoms, oxygen saturation and lung function 1 hour after administration of medications.[149] Reassessment and ongoing management require monitoring of peak flow, vital signs, SaO_2, ABGs and potassium and blood sugar levels, as hypokalaemia and hyperglycaemia can result from beta$_2$-agonist and corticosteroid use.[162,164] For patients requiring ventilatory support, intubation and positive pressure ventilation is required, as the use of non-invasive ventilation is not recommended in patients with asthma.[164] Reassessment and ongoing management require monitoring of peak flow, SaO_2, ABGs, and potassium and blood sugar levels.[164] Indications for ventilation are decreased conscious level, respiratory arrest and worsening hypoxia/hypercapnia.[162]

The goals of treatment for COPD are to minimise the impact of the current exacerbation as either an outpatient or an inpatient depending on the severity of the underlying disease.[39] Exacerbations should be managed promptly to prevent hospitalisation.[170] Evidence suggests that more than 80% of exacerbations are managed as outpatients with pharmacological intervention.[39] Potential indications for ICU admission include severe dyspnoea that fails to respond to initial emergency treatment, confusion, hypoxaemia (PaO_2 <5.3 kPa/40 mmHg) or respiratory acidosis (pH <7.5) despite supplemental oxygen or NIV, and the need for mechanical ventilation or vasopressors.[39] Oxygen therapy should be administered to keep the SaO_2 within the individualised target range.[23] Systematic review evidence on the efficacy and safety of HFNC therapy in COPD and hypercapnic respiratory failure is conflicting owing to the small number of studies and low to very low certainty of evidence.[20,22,171] NIV is the treatment of choice for persistent hypercapnic respiratory failure.[23] Patients unable to tolerate NIV or those who have diminished consciousness, haemodynamic instability or life-threatening hypoxia require initiation of invasive mechanical ventilation during an exacerbation.[39]

However, as the mortality of COPD patients who develop acute hypercapnic respiratory failure remains high, supportive, palliative and end-of-life care planning prior to exacerbations is crucial.[24,170] Longer-term tackling of the main risk factors along with better primary care management could also help reduce health complications of asthma and COPD.[6]

Medications

First-line management of acute severe or life-threatening asthma exacerbations includes administration of controlled oxygen therapy (94–98% SaO_2) and high doses of short-acting beta$_2$-agonists (salbutamol) via continuous nebulisation or repeated every 15–30 minutes.[149,162,164] Adding anticholinergics (ipratropium bromide) to nebulised beta$_2$-agonists every 4–6 hours produces greater bronchodilation, faster recovery and shorter admissions.[162,164] Nebulisers should be oxygen driven at 6 L/min to prevent desaturation.[172] Systemic oral corticosteroids (prednisolone) are the mainstay of treatment and should be administered within the first hour to reduce mortality, relapse and ICU admission rates of asthma.[149] Treatments are normally administered concurrently to achieve rapid improvement.[150] Patients with acute severe or life-threatening asthma should be given a single dose of intravenous magnesium sulfate when there is a poor response to initial treatment.[149,164]

First-line management of acute exacerbations of COPD includes administration of short-acting beta$_2$-agonists (salbutamol), with or without muscarinic receptor antagonists (ipratropium), controlled oxygen therapy and systemic corticosteroids.[23,39] Bronchodilators can be given by pressurised metered-dose inhaler and spacer, or by air-driven nebulisation to avoid worsening hypercapnia.[23] The dose interval is titrated to the response and can range from hourly to 6-hourly. Prescription of supplemental oxygen to COPD patients with arterial hypoxaemia (IaO_2 7.3 kPa/<55 mmHg) should be titrated to keep IaO_2 >90%.[39] An oral mucolytic for a chronic cough with productive sputum and antibiotic therapy for purulent sputum should be considered[173] to shorten recovery time and hospitalisation duration. Methylxanthines (theophylline) are not recommended.[39]

See Table 14.9 for key medications used in the treatment of asthma and COPD. Once the acute exacerbation of both asthma and COPD has resolved, it is important that the severity of the individual's condition is reassessed, action plans are developed and patients are educated about the importance of maintenance therapy to prevent future severe exacerbations.[39]

Pneumothorax

A pneumothorax occurs when air that has escaped from a defect in the pulmonary tree is trapped in the potential space between the two pleurae. A pneumothorax can be classified as spontaneous, traumatic or iatrogenic and can be life threatening. A spontaneous pneumothorax can be primary (in persons without lung disease) or secondary (in persons with lung disease). A pneumothorax is traumatic if caused by a blunt or penetrating injury, or iatrogenic if caused by complications from diagnostic or therapeutic interventions.[174]

In some cases, the amount of air trapped increases markedly if the defect in the pulmonary tree functions as a one-way valve. In this case, air enters the pleural cavity on inspiration but is unable to exit on expiration, leading to increasing intrapleural pressure. This is termed a tension pneumothorax. A patient with tension pneumothorax presents with acute pleuritic pain, severe dyspnoea,

TABLE 14.9

Key medications in an acute episode of asthma[149,164]

TYPE OF DRUG	GENERIC MEDICATION	ACTION	NURSING CONSIDERATIONS
Controlled oxygen therapy	Oxygen	Increases supply of oxygen for uptake.	Titrate FiO_2 to SaO_2 (aim 94–98%) via nasal cannulae or mask.
Inhaled beta$_2$-agonist	Salbutamol	Produces relaxation of bronchial smooth muscle and air-flow improvement by action at beta$_2$ receptors.	Metered-dose inhaler 4 puffs initially via spacer and then 2 puffs every 2 min up to 10 puffs maximum in moderate asthma. In acute severe asthma give oxygen driven nebulised salbutamol 5 mg every 15–30 min (6 L/min) to prevent desaturation. In life-threatening asthma consider continuous salbutamol nebuliser 5–10 mg/h. Side effects include muscle tremor, tachycardia and palpitations.
Systemic corticosteroids	Hydrocortisone	Rapid onset (5–6 h after administration). Increases beta-responsiveness of airway smooth muscle and suppresses inflammatory cytokines and chemokines.	Intravenous hydrocortisone 400 mg daily (100 mg × 6-hourly) until conversion to oral prednisolone is possible.
	Prednisolone	Decreases inflammatory response and mucus secretion.	Oral dose 40–50 mg daily × 5 days minimum. Oral as effective as intravenous administration. Tapering not required for oral dose less than 2 weeks. Do not stop inhaled steroids when prescribed oral coriticosteriods.
Methylxanthine	Aminophylline	Bronchodilator. Inhibits the inflammatory phase in asthma. Stimulates the medullary respiratory centre.	Intravenous aminophylline/theophylline should be reserved for near-fatal asthma patients who fail to respond or are intolerant of β$_2$-adrenoreceptor agonists. 5 mg/kg loading dose over 20 min, then infusion 0.5–0.7 mg/kg/h. Poor efficacy and safety profile with potentially fatal side effects.
Muscarinic antagonists	Ipratropium bromide	Competitively inhibit the action of acetylcholine at the muscarinic receptors, blocking airway smooth muscle contraction.	Anticholinergics exert an additional bronchodilator effect to that provided by β$_2$-adrenoreceptor agonists alone. Dose 0.5 mg 4–6 hourly via oxygen driven nebuliser.
	Magnesium sulfate	Inhibit calcium influx into airway smooth muscle, causing bronchodilation.	Not recommended for routine use in asthma exacerbations. Single dose of magnesium sulfate (1.2–2 g intravenously over 20 min) in acute severe asthma. Dose should not be repeated, as hypermagnesaemia is associated with muscle weakness and respiratory failure.

Sources: Scottish Intercollegiate Guidelines Network, British Thoracic Society, Healthcare Improvement Scotland. British guideline on the management of asthma: a national clinical guideline. Edinburgh: Healthcare Improvement Scotland. Available from: https://www.sign.ac.uk; Global Initiative for Asthma. Global strategy for asthma management and prevention. Fontana, WI: Global Initiative for Asthma; 2022. Available from: https://ginasthma.org.

tachycardia, hypoxia, decreased air entry on the affected side, hyperexpansion of the chest and agitation. The actual incidence of tension pneumothorax is not accurately established but is associated with significant morbidity and mortality.[175]

Pathophysiology

Tension pneumothorax occurs when a one-way valve forms, allowing air to flow into the pleural space but stopping air from flowing out. The volume of intrapleural air increases with each inspiration. Consequently, pressure rises within the thoracic cavity, the lung collapses and hypoxaemia ensues. Further pressure causes a mediastinal shift towards the unaffected side that subsequently compresses the lung (causing further hypoxaemia) and the superior and inferior vena cava entering the right atrium of the heart (causing compromised venous return). Untreated, the resultant hypoxaemia, metabolic acidosis and decreased cardiac output can lead to cardiac arrest and death.[175]

Clinical manifestations

Severe presentations are identified by history and clinical examination (respiratory distress, cyanosis, tachycardia, tracheal shift towards the unaffected side and unilateral movement of the chest). Point-of-care lung ultrasound by an experienced operator can rapidly and accurately diagnose tension pneumothorax with greater sensitivity than supine CXR.[176] When CXR is used for diagnosis, lung markings will be absent and a translucent appearance of the pleural air will be evident (see Chapter 13 for information on CXR interpretation).[175]

Patient management

It is essential to check airway, breathing and circulation in all patients with chest trauma. Upright positioning may be beneficial if there is no contraindication. Penetrating wounds should be covered immediately with an occlusive or pressure bandage. If a tension pneumothorax leading to haemodynamic instability is suspected, a thin needle can be used to relieve the pressure and allow the lung to re-inflate (needle decompression). Needle decompression is not always successful and it may be difficult to ensure that the needle has reached the thoracic cavity. An alternative method is finger thoracostomy and the method used is often based on clinician preference, as there is little evidence to support one method over another. Insertion of a chest tube attached to a water-seal drain, consisting of interconnected collection chamber, water-seal chamber and suction control chamber, may be necessary to allow the collapsed lung to re-expand. Recent evidence regarding the chest tubes sizing has led to a trend towards the use of smaller-sized tubes or pigtail catheters, even in the setting of haemothorax.[175] If a haemothorax is present or if the pneumothorax is not resolving, suction on the pleural drain (~5–20 mmHg) may expedite drainage and re-expansion of the lung and reduce length of stay.[177] To aid recovery from traumatic pneumothorax, it is important to support the respiratory system with strategies such as oxygen therapy or non-invasive/invasive ventilation, optimal patient positioning to reduce pain and allow lung expansion, and encouragement of deep breathing and coughing. Pain control is important in the management of traumatic pneumothorax and includes epidural analgesia, paravertebral blocks, intercostal nerve blocks, intrapleural analgesia, intravenous opioids, oral or transdermal analgesics, and combinations of these. Epidural analgesia and combination therapy appear the most effective;

however, patient preference must also be considered.[178] Regular monitoring of the chest tube for the presence of air leak and serous or haemoserous drainage should be performed, as should frequent respiratory assessment. Chapter 12 discusses chest tube management in more detail.

Pulmonary embolism

In the United States, venous thromboembolism (VTE) is the third leading cause of cardiovascular death, accounting for an estimated 94,000 new cases annually, with an increasing incidence with age.[179] VTE includes both deep vein thrombosis (DVT) and pulmonary embolism (PE), which occur respectively when a blood clot forms in a deep vein (leg, thigh, pelvis) or when a clot (embolism) travels through the bloodstream to the lungs.[180] Predisposing risk factors for thrombosis are venous stasis, vein wall injury and hypercoagulability (obesity, disseminated intravascular coagulation, hormone therapy) of blood. Clinical risk factors are immobility, surgery, trauma, cancer, pregnancy or genetic conditions (thrombophilia).[181,182] However, in as many as 40% of patients with PE, no provoking factors are detected (see Table 14.10 for a list of risk factors).[183] Critically ill patients are at increased risk of developing DVT and acute PE.[184] Acute PE is the most serious clinical presentation of VTE.[185]

Clinical manifestations

PE interferes with both circulation and gas exchange.[183] Pulmonary artery obstruction causes release of vasoactive agents, with a subsequent increase in pulmonary vascular resistance and right ventricular afterload.[183] Systemic vasoconstriction increases the pressure in the pulmonary artery, resulting in increased contractility and tachycardia as the right ventricle dilates and left ventricle filling is impeded. This reduces coronary blood flow and cardiac output, resulting in systemic hypotension, haemodynamic instability, and hypoxia as a result of V/Q mismatch.[182] Resultant increases in pulmonary hypertension induce right-sided heart failure, which is the main cause of mortality in patients with acute PE.[183,184]

Acute PE presentation can vary widely from asymptomatic to severe haemodynamic collapse or death.[186,187] Early recognition is of utmost importance. Suspect PE if patients develop a sudden onset of dyspnoea, pleuritic/substernal chest pain, haemoptysis, syncope or complete circulatory collapse.[183,187] Physical exam reveals tachypnoea, tachycardia, hypotension and increased jugular venous pressure.[187,188] Dyspnoea may be acute and severe, with hypoxaemia due to the mismatch between ventilation and perfusion.[183,189]

Assessment and diagnostics

Diagnosis includes a detailed clinical history and assessment of risk factors, presenting symptoms and physical examination to determine probability of PE and the need

TABLE 14.10

Risk factors for venous thromboembolism[182,183,185]

Individual	Age >70 years
	Previous venous thromboembolism
	Pregnancy and the puerperium
	Active or occult malignancy
	Varicose veins
	Obesity
	Prolonged severe immobility (bed rest, long-haul flights)
	Oestrogen therapy (hormone replacement therapy or oral contraceptives)
	Inherited or acquired thrombophilia
Medical	Heart failure or atrial fibrillation/flutter
	Myocardial infarction
	Congestive heart failure or respiratory failure
	Spinal cord injury
	Diabetes
	Chemotherapy
	Malignancy
	Acute inflammatory bowel disease
	Hormone replacement therapy
Surgical	All surgical procedures, especially abdominal, pelvic, thoracic, orthopaedic (hip and knee replacement)
	Major trauma
	Fractured lower limb
ICU	Central venous catheters
	Sepsis
	Mechanical ventilation
	Pharmacological sedation
	Vasopressor use
	End-stage renal failure

Sources: Sista AK, Kuo WT, Schiebler M, et al. Stratification, imaging, and management of acute massive and submassive pulmonary embolism. Radiology 2017;284(1):5–24; Konstantinides SV, Meyer G, Bueno H, et al. 2019 ESC guidelines for the diagnosis and management of acute pulmonary embolism developed in collaboration with the European respiratory society (ERS). Eur Heart J 2020;41(4): 543–603; Alhassan S, Pelinescu A, Gandhi V, et al. Clinical presentation and risk factors of venous thromboembolic disease. Crit Care Nurs Q. 2017;40(3):201–9.

for further testing.[185] Assessment and stratification of risk is of paramount importance to guide treatment options given the wide presentation of PE.[186] European Society of Cardiology guidelines (2020) recommend that risk assessment and classification of PE severity should be initiated early as part of the diagnostic assessment in order to identify patients at high risk of mortality based on haemodynamic instability.[183] Patients who are haemodynamically stable undergo a tiered diagnostic strategy based on the

clinical probability of PE. In patients with low suspicion of PE, the PE rule-out criteria can be used to determine whether further investigations are needed. When PE is suspected, the two validated clinical/diagnostic prediction tools – the Wells' Criteria for Pulmonary Embolism and the Geneva Score (Revised) – are widely used to assess pretest probability for the diagnosis of PE in adults.[188,190] These tools assign points to a list of criteria of known risk factors and clinical signs to produce an overall score indicating clinical probability of a PE. A Wells score of 4 points or more requires hospital admission and immediate computed tomography pulmonary angiogram (CTPA).[185,188] Evidence-based literature supports the practice of using these pretest assessment tools before proceeding to diagnostic testing.

The American Heart Association and the European Society of Cardiology use the Pulmonary Embolism Severity Index to classify PE into three categories (massive/high risk, submassive/intermediate risk, low risk).[186,191] This index, or its simplified version, considers risk, clinical status and comorbidities to predict 30-day mortality and determine risk-adjusted management strategies.[192] Risk stratification is based on clinical assessment, objective markers of cardiac injury and assessment of right ventricular dysfunction.[186] Assessment of right ventricular dysfunction radiographically (echocardiography, CT) and/or laboratory (B-type natriuretic peptide, troponin level) is suggested by the European Society of Cardiology guidelines to aid risk stratification.[183] Stratification and scientific guidelines allow for early identification and more-invasive interventions of higher-risk patients.[186]

Diagnostic investigations include: lower limb compression ultrasonography for a suspected DVT, pathology test for elevated levels of d-dimer in plasma and V/Q scan or CT pulmonary angiography for definitive diagnosis of PE.[192,193] CT pulmonary angiography is considered the gold standard for diagnosis of PE.[187] A CXR and electrocardiogram are undertaken for differential diagnosis.[183,188]

Patient management

All patients in ICU are at high risk of venous thromboembolism and policies should be implemented for thromboembolic prophylaxis.[194] Recommended VTE prophylactic pharmacological interventions include administration of low-molecular-weight heparin or, for patients at high risk of bleeding, mechanical prophylaxis (inferior vena cava filter) when anticoagulation is contraindicated in patients with proximal DVT or PE.[188,189]

Early anticoagulation therapy is the main treatment option, and choice of treatment will depend on comorbidities, bleeding risk, concurrent medications and cost.[191] Unstable patients and patients with a high probability of PE require cardiopulmonary support, anticoagulation and reperfusion.[187] Haemodynamic and respiratory support includes administration of oxygen in patients with PE and a SaO_2 <90%, inotropes to support right ventricular failure and modest (500 mL) fluid challenge, and use of HFNC or NIV is preferred. Invasive mechanical ventilation using protective lung strategies should be used with caution for severe hypoxaemia that is refractory to conventional oxygen supplementation, given its haemodynamic adverse effects.[183] Advanced therapeutic intervention options for certain high-risk patients may include catheter-directed thrombolysis, surgical pulmonary embolectomy or mechanical circulatory support (right ventricular assist devices and ECMO), given improved evidence of outcomes.[186,191]

The complex management of patients with intermediate–high-risk PE has led to the development of pulmonary embolism response teams to provide a multidisciplinary approach for individualised advanced treatment strategies. The European Society of Cardiology recommends establishment of such interdisciplinary teams if resources are available.[183,195]

Medications

Medications commonly prescribed for PE include inotropes, analgesics, and thrombolytic and anticoagulant therapy. Supportive treatment of acute right ventricular failure and hypotension is vital. Inotropic drugs such as adrenaline (epinephrine), noradrenaline (norepinephrine) and dobutamine need to be carefully administered because of associated peripheral vasodilation, which may exacerbate the problem. In general, anticoagulation treatment plays the major role in patient therapy. The European Society of Cardiology[183] recommends low-molecular-weight heparin, direct Xa inhibitor (fondaparinux) or direct oral anticoagulants as first-line therapies for high or intermediate clinical probability of PE owing to a lower risk of major bleeding.[191,196] Unfractionated heparin is limited to situations of diminished renal function or haemodynamic instability where primary reperfusion is considered.

In patients at high risk with haemodynamic instability, systemic thrombolysis (e.g. tissue plasminogen activator) should be the first-line treatment as it restores pulmonary perfusion and haemodynamic stability more rapidly than does anticoagulation.[184,191] Table 14.11 outlines some of the key anticoagulant medications recommended and prescribed for patients with PE.[183,188,197]

Lung transplantation

Transplantation is a life-saving and cost-effective form of treatment that enhances the quality of life for people with chronic respiratory disease.[198] Survival rates post-transplant have improved over time, with a median survival rate of 6.7 years for transplantation for any indication occurring between 2010 and 2017 (1-year survival 85%; 5-year survival 59%).[199] Lung transplantation is facilitated by organ donation after neurological death or circulatory death. Donation after circulatory death is a relatively recent practice, with the first successful lung transplant performed in 1995 using this technique, which significantly increases the number of organs available for lung

transplantation. Registry data from the International Society for Heart and Lung Transplantation confirm that early and intermediate patient outcomes for lung transplantation using donation after circulatory death are equivalent to outcomes for donation after neurological death. For lung transplants performed between 2003 and 2017, there was no difference in survival between lung recipients of donors after neurological death versus circulatory death at 1 year or 5 years (88% vs 89% and 61% vs 63%, respectively).[200]

Indications

The main criteria for lung transplantation in Australia are: COPD (including individuals with alpha$_1$-antitrypsin disorder, a genetic abnormality associated with early-onset emphysema), cystic fibrosis, pulmonary fibrosis, pulmonary arterial hypertension and bronchiectasis. Patients with advanced lung disease have poor quality of life, often struggling to perform activities of daily living, are usually oxygen dependent and have symptoms consistent with New York Heart Association functional class III or IV symptoms.[198]

Patient selection

Careful selection of appropriate candidates for lung transplantation is recognised as an important predictor of outcomes and selection is based on who will gain the most benefit in survival and quality of life. Guidance for clinicians regarding timing of referral, evaluation, determination of candidacy and eventual listing is provided by the global heart and lung transplantation body and provides a framework for decision making. Early referral is preferred so that modifiable risk factors for complications can be addressed so as to optimise physical health as well as ensuring adequate psychological and social supports are in place. Risk factors considered by the multidisciplinary transplant team include age, malignancy, renal function, cardiovascular function, functional status, infectious disease status and human leukocyte antigen antibodies. Also critical to optimal patient outcomes are psychosocial factors such as psychological function, cognitive impairment, social support, behavioural adherence to future treatment and substance use.[201]

Surgical technique

The four possible techniques of isolated lung transplantation and indications for each technique are outlined in Table 14.12.[202] The surgery can be performed with or without cardiopulmonary bypass, during which cardiorespiratory support is delivered via an extracorporeal circuit, thereby leaving the surgical field blood free. Currently, lung transplantation takes two main forms: bilateral sequential lung transplantation (BSLTx) and single-lung transplantation (SLTx). BSLTx is the most common form of lung transplantation and has a survival advantage over and above SLTx. However, the advantage of SLTx over BSLTx is that twice as many people receive life-saving surgery. For SLTx recipients with COPD, there

TABLE 14.11
Anticoagulation medications for pulmonary embolism[183,188,197]

TYPE OF DRUG	GENERIC MEDICATION	ACTION	NURSING CONSIDERATIONS
Anticoagulant	Unfractionated heparin	A strongly acidic mucopolysaccharide with rapid anticoagulant effects. Binds to antithrombin III and inhibits factor Xa and thrombin. Standard heparin has a molecular weight of 5000–30,000 daltons.	Restricted use to haemodynamic instability and renal impairment (creatinine clearance CrCL <30 mL/min) or severe obesity. Dosing adjusted based on partial thromboplastin time (aPPT) and patient-related factors. Short half-life (1 h) and reversed by protamine sulfate. Efficacy controlled by monitoring antifactor Xa.
	Low-molecular-weight (LMW) heparin	LMW heparin ranges from 1000 to 10,000 daltons, resulting in distinct properties. Factor Xa inhibitor LMW heparin binds less strongly to protein, has enhanced bioavailability, interacts less with platelets and yields a very predictable dose response, eliminating the need to monitor aPPT.	Initial anticoagulation in PE. Lower risk of inducing major bleeding. Administered subcutaneously. Fondaparinux contraindicated in renal failure (creatinine clearance <30 mL/min) as it accumulates increasing risk of haemorrhage.
	Direct oral anticoagulant/ non-vitamin K antagonist oral anticoagulants	Factor Xa inhibitor.	Apixaban/rivaroxaban no need to monitor INR Avoid use CrCl <15 mL/min. Reduced rates of bleeding.
	Vitamin K antagonists	Inhibits the recycling of Vitamin K.	Continued in parallel with oral anticoagulation for >5 days until INR 2.0–3.0 for 2 consecutive days. Daily dose adjusted to INR over next 5–7 days Reduced risk of bleeding.
Thrombolysis	Recombinant tissue-type plasminogen activator (rt-PA) alteplase, urokinase and streptokinase	Thrombolysis results in restoration of pulmonary arterial blood flow and is urgently required in massive pulmonary embolism to minimise right ventricular failure.	Greatest benefit when initiated within 48 hours of symptoms. The risks of therapy include haemorrhage. Safety and monitoring of the patient's clinical state are paramount.

Sources: Konstantinides SV, Meyer G, Bueno H, et al. 2019 ESC Guidelines for the diagnosis and management of acute pulmonary embolism developed in collaboration with the European Respiratory Society (ERS). Eur Heart J 2020;41(4):543–603; National Institute for Health and Care Excellence (NICE). Venous thromboembolic diseases: diagnosis, management and thrombophilia testing. London: NICE; 2020. Available from: https://www.nice.org.uk/guidance/ng158; Nagraj S, Li W, Zamora C, Barakakis PA, et al. Pharmacological and interventional management of pulmonary embolism: where do we stand? Future Cardiol 2022;18(3):191–206.

is an increase in the complexity of postoperative respiratory management, and for this reason some centres may perform BSLTx for patients with COPD. SLTx is also utilised for patients with idiopathic pulmonary fibrosis and other forms of interstitial lung disease who have a high waiting-list mortality.[198] The majority of lung transplants performed are bilateral lung transplants; however, a single lung may be transplanted, or bilateral lungs may be transplanted with another organ, most commonly the heart then the liver. Of the 167 recipients receiving transplanted lungs in Australia in 2021, 139 received double lungs and 28 received single lungs; there were four heart/double lung transplants and two double lung/liver transplants.[203]

Postoperative management of complications

A multidisciplinary approach by skilled clinicians is important in successfully managing the lung transplant recipient during the complex immediate postoperative period in order to maximise their longer-term outcomes.

TABLE 14.12

Comparison of the four standard lung replacement techniques, including their common indicators [202]

	HEART–LUNG	BILATERAL SEQUENTIAL LUNG	SINGLE LUNG	LIVE DONOR LOBAR
Incision	• Midline sternotomy	• Transverse sternotomy, i.e. horizontal 'clam shell' • Midline sternotomy	• Lateral thoracotomy • Midline sternotomy	• Transverse sternotomy, i.e. horizontal 'clam shell'
Anastomoses	• Tracheal • Right atrial • Aortic	• Left and right bronchial • 'Double' left atrial • Right and left pulmonary artery	• Bronchial • Left atrial • Pulmonary artery	• Lobar bronchus to bronchus • Lobar vein to superior pulmonary vein • Lobar artery to main pulmonary artery
Advantages	• Airway vascularity • All indications	• Access to pleural space • No cardiac allograft • Less cardiopulmonary bypass	• Easiest procedure • Increases recipients	• Increases donors • Can be performed 'electively'
Disadvantages	• Cardiac allograft • Organ 'consumption'	• Airway complications • Severe postoperative pain	• Airway complications • Poor reserve	• Complex procedure • Donor morbidity
Common indications	• Congenital heart disease with pulmonary hypertension • Heart and lung disease • Primary pulmonary hypertension	• Cystic fibrosis • Bullous emphysema • Primary pulmonary hypertension • Bronchiectasis	• Emphysema • COPD • Pulmonary fibrosis • Primary pulmonary hypertension	• Cystic fibrosis • Pulmonary fibrosis • Primary pulmonary hypertension

COPD = chronic obstructive pulmonary disease.

Source: Adapted from McShane PJ, Ruiz, LG, Garrity ER. Lung transplantation. In: Spiro SG, Silvestri GA, Agusti A. editors. Clinical respiratory medicine. St Louis, MO: Mosby; 2012, p. 831–45, with permission.

High-level evidence guiding the management of lung transplant recipients in ICU is surprisingly scarce, and recommendations for practice often come from observational studies and/or clinical expertise and opinion. The following sections outline common postoperative complications and current best-practice patient management.

Respiratory dysfunction

Respiratory dysfunction can develop owing to severe dysfunction of the transplanted lung resulting from ischaemia–reperfusion injury, pulmonary oedema, hyperacute rejection and pulmonary venous or arterial anastomotic obstruction.[204] Other major complications in the early postoperative period affecting respiratory management include severe pain, diaphragmatic dysfunction, acute rejection and infection.

Respiratory dysfunction within the first 72 hours postoperatively is commonly due to primary graft dysfunction (PGD), a form of acute lung injury characterised by non-specific alveolar damage, lung oedema and hypoxaemia. Clinical signs of PGD range from mild hypoxaemia with infiltrates on CXR to severe

ARDS requiring high-level ventilatory support, pharmacological support and ECMO. Early recognition and management of this complication reduces early mortality. PGD may be aggravated by factors associated with the donor (e.g. advanced age, trauma, history of smoking, aspiration, pneumonia and hypotension), the pre- and intraoperative period (e.g. prolonged ischaemic time of the organ while in transit, single-lung transplant, use of cardiopulmonary bypass) or the recipient (e.g. pulmonary hypertension, high BMI, preoperative sarcoidosis). Lung transplant recipients exhibiting signs of PGD should be ventilated using lung-protective strategies similar to those used to manage ARDS.[198] Table 14.13 details the grading system for PGD from the International Society of Heart and Lung Transplantation.[205]

Respiratory dysfunction beyond 72 hours can be due to infection, allograft rejection or hemidiaphragm paralysis secondary to phrenic nerve damage.[206] Long-term respiratory complications include airway anastomotic problems (stricture and dehiscence), suboptimal exercise performance and chronic rejection manifesting as bronchiolitis obliterans syndrome.[207,208]

TABLE 14.13

Primary graft dysfunction definition from the 2016 International Society for Heart and Lung Transplantation[205]

GRADE[a]	PULMONARY OEDEMA ON CHEST X-RAY	PAO$_2$/FIO$_2$ RATIO[b]
PGD grade 0	No	Any
PGD grade 1	Yes	>300
PGD grade 2	Yes	200 to 300
PGD grade 3	Yes	<200

FiO$_2$ = fraction of inspired oxygen; PaO$_2$ = partial pressure of arterial oxygen; PGD = primary graft dysfunction.

[a]PGD is graded at 4 time-points within the first 72 hours post-transplant, with the first grading performed at reperfusion of the second lung (0, 24, 48 and 72 hours).

[b]Take the worst available PaO$_2$/FiO$_2$ ratio in the grading period

Source: Snell GI, Yusen RD, Weill D, et al. Report of the ISHLT Working Group on Primary Lung Graft Dysfunction, part I: definition and grading – a 2016 Consensus Group statement of the International Society for Heart and Lung Transplantation. J Heart Lung Transpl 2017;36(10):1097–103.

Patient management

Mechanical ventilation is essential after lung transplant, and most patients will require it for a duration of 2–3 days, with around 14% of recipients requiring prolonged mechanical ventilation.[198] The goal of mechanical ventilation in the immediate postoperative period is to minimise ventilator-induced lung injury to the allograft, maintain adequate gas exchange and facilitate early ventilator weaning. In BSLTx, lung protective ventilation[209] should be used to protect the transplanted lungs, with tidal volumes based on the donor's predicted body weight (~6 mL/kg) and an inspiratory plateau pressure of <25–30 cmH$_2$O.[210] To prevent disruption to the healing bronchial anastomosis and to prevent alveolar overdistention, high PEEP levels (i.e. >12–14 cmH$_2$O) are not usually used even in the setting of hypoxia. Targets for SpO$_2$ and PaO$_2$ should be around 90% and 8–10.7 kPa/60–80 mmHg respectively, using the minimum FiO$_2$ to achieve this. Commonly, ventilator settings and respiratory weaning are guided by pH rather than PaCO$_2$ levels.[211] A modest degree of hypercarbia is anticipated postoperatively and resolves over time. Lung-protective ventilation has a positive impact on recovery and long-term outcomes in patients with ARDS and it is now recommended that SLTx and BSLTx recipients receive similar ventilator settings.[212] In SLTx recipients, ventilation/perfusion mismatches may be improved by inhaled nitric oxide and by positioning patients regularly with the allograft uppermost. Timely extubation onto high-flow nasal cannulae or low-flow oxygen is very important to encourage early mobilisation and chest physiotherapy as a way of optimising respiratory function.[210]

In recipients who have developed PGD, slower weaning from sedation and mechanical ventilation is required and employing ultraprotective lung ventilation (tidal volumes ≤6 mL/kg) is warranted, provided gas exchange can be maintained. Severity of PGD is assessed by ABG analysis, CXR, bronchoscopy and haemodynamic parameters.[206]

For patients with PGD accompanied by high pulmonary pressures, inhaled nitric oxide may be useful in decreasing high pulmonary pressures and reducing intrapulmonary shunting; however, currently no high-level evidence exists to demonstrate that inhaled nitric oxide prevents PGD. Other therapies used for severe refractory PGD are prone positioning, neuromuscular blockade and venovenous or venoarterial ECMO support.[210] Many diagnostic tests will be performed in the immediate postoperative period and they include CXR, bronchoscopy, ABG analysis and echocardiography. CXR provides vital information about ETT position, lung expansion, lung size, position of the diaphragm and mediastinum and the presence of pneumothorax, oedema and atelectasis. PGD appears on CXR as a rapidly developing diffuse alveolar pattern of infiltration that is greater in the lower regions, and most commonly seen on the first postoperative day but may occur up to 72 hours following surgery. The presence of rapidly worsening pulmonary infiltrates (especially if associated with low cardiac indices) should, however, prompt urgent echocardiography to assess cardiac function and pulmonary venous anastomosis patency.

Beyond 72 hours, alveolar and interstitial infiltration may indicate either acute rejection or an infective process. In critical care, patients with allograft dysfunction are rigorously assessed for the emergence of rejection and pulmonary infection using transbronchial biopsy and bronchoalveolar lavage. Evidence of rejection will be treated with changes in immunosuppression regimen and appropriate ventilatory and haemodynamic supports. Subtle changes in respiratory effort, gas exchange and minute ventilation may be the only signs to alert the nurse to respiratory dysfunction secondary to rejection or infection during mechanical ventilation. Clinical signs of pulmonary infection include a low-grade fever, increasing dyspnoea and sputum production, cough and infiltrates on CXR. Hypotension, a reduced cardiac index and subtle changes in respiratory parameters during mechanical ventilation, noted above, may also be present. Pulmonary infections may be acquired through nosocomial, community or donor means, with recipient-colonised and opportunistic infections prevalent. Regardless of the route of transmission, all infections require prompt antimicrobial therapy.[206] Healthcare workers play an important role in preventing transmission of infection between patients and translocation of bacteria within patients. Meticulous handwashing between patients and between procedures are important measures in reducing infection rates.

Specific considerations regarding postoperative management of SLTx for chronic obstructive pulmonary disease are required, owing to the unique phenomenon of acute native lung hyperinflation (ANLH), which occurs in around 15–30% of recipients (Fig. 14.3). ANLH leads to mediastinal shift and diaphragmatic flattening, ultimately resulting in respiratory failure and haemodynamic instability requiring vasopressors and independent lung ventilation to restore cardiorespiratory function.[213] Nurses need to be aware of the patients who can potentially develop ANLH and to remain hypervigilant, as early signs and opportunities to rapidly stabilise patients' haemodynamic and respiratory status can be easily missed. Early stages of ANLH in a patient with left SLTx for COPD can be seen on the CXR in Fig. 14.4.

If tailoring ventilatory settings to minimise hyperinflation fails, insertion of a dual-lumen ETT is required so that independent protective lung ventilation can be initiated for the allograft. Precise positioning and secure placement of the tube is vital, to avoid slight movement of the position and consequent displacement of correct cuff placement (see Fig. 14.5 for correct positioning of a dual-lumen ETT). Timely extubation is paramount in patients receiving SLTx in order to mitigate the harmful effects of positive pressure ventilation.[198]

Pain

Optimal analgesia post-lung transplant is essential to facilitate extubation, optimise lung mechanics, re-establish cough mechanism and participate in physiotherapy. Recipients of lung transplantation can experience significant postoperative pain, more so than patients undergoing general thoracic procedures. Furthermore, recipients of BSLTx performed via transverse sternotomy (clamshell incision) can experience severe postoperative pain. Thoracic epidural analgesia has been associated with improved acute postoperative pain control, decreased

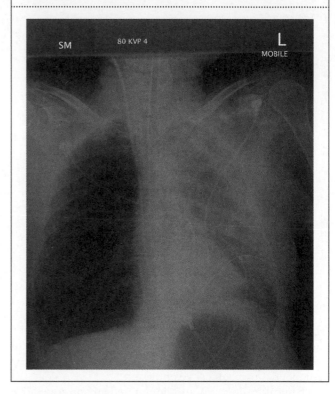

FIGURE 14.4 Chest X-ray of a patient with left single-lung transplant for COPD who has developed acute native lung hyperinflation.

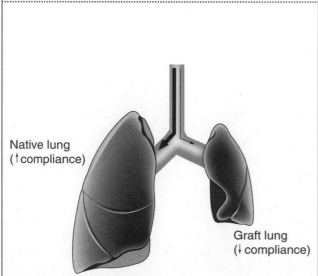

FIGURE 14.3 Mechanism of acute native lung hyperinflation: distribution of inspiratory gas.

Native lung (↑compliance)

Graft lung (↓ compliance)

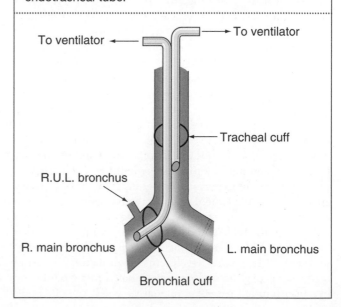

FIGURE 14.5 Correct positioning of a double-lumen endotracheal tube.

To ventilator

To ventilator

Tracheal cuff

R.U.L. bronchus

R. main bronchus

L. main bronchus

Bronchial cuff

duration of mechanical ventilation and reduced ICU length of stay.[214] Ideally, all lung transplant recipients should receive epidural analgesia; however, the insertion of an epidural catheter at the time of surgery may be delayed because of preoperative anticoagulation therapy and/or perioperative coagulopathy. In these circumstances, epidural analgesia should be instituted as soon as appropriate after surgery in suitable patients. Opioids are commonly used for pain control and can be delivered as a continuous intravenous infusion or via a patient-controlled analgesia infusion; however, limiting their use postoperatively is advisable. More recently, multimodal opioid-sparing pain management protocols have been examined as a way to further enhance postoperative recovery.[215] These protocols include preoperative analgesia of paracetamol and gabapentin, intraoperative fentanyl and placement of an intercostal nerve block (around the fifth intercostal space) with bupivacaine, and, postoperatively, sedation with dexmedetomidine, routine paracetamol and gabapentin, and intravenous opioids as needed which are switched to orals as soon as practicable. This approach has been shown to reduce opioid use in the postoperative period and at discharge[215] and is recommended for the management of postoperative pain generally; however, more research is needed to determine whether this approach reduces adverse events and length of hospital stay post-lung transplantation.[216]

Patient management

Consultation with pain services to ensure patients receive optimal analgesic regimens should be an integral component of patients' postoperative management (see Chapters 6 and 26). Paracetamol is beneficial in relieving mild to moderate pain and may be used as an adjunct to centrally acting analgesics for moderate to severe pain. The use of non-steroidal anti-inflammatory drugs should be avoided, owing to their detrimental effects on renal and gastrointestinal function. If patient-controlled analgesia has been prescribed, education on how to use the analgesia is required, as well as close observation of the patient's haemodynamic, respiratory and neurological status. Adjuvant non-pharmacological interventions can also be extremely effective in managing acute postoperative pain, including careful patient positioning, pressure area care, distraction therapies and the presence of family.[216]

Haemodynamic instability

All lung transplant patients can experience haemodynamic compromise postoperatively. Myocardial contractility may be compromised owing to hypoxaemia, electrolyte imbalances and acidosis; therefore, most recipients will require vasopressors for initial cardiac support. Cautious use of fluids is indicated but there is evidence that a central venous pressure greater than 0.9 kPa/7 mmHg leads to increased duration of mechanical ventilation and hospital mortality.[217] Recipients with preoperative pulmonary hypertension and right ventricular dysfunction

may require inhaled pulmonary vasodilators to reduce right ventricular afterload.[198] Arrhythmias are common in the postoperative period, particularly atrial arrhythmias which occur in around 30% of recipients, and is associated with increased perioperative mortality, hospital length of stay and the requirement for tracheostomy.[218] Known risk factors for the development of atrial fibrillation include electrolyte imbalances, pain, fluid overload, poor gas exchange and the use of vasopressors and inotropes.

ECMO may be used for haemodynamic support in the setting of refractory low cardiac output states. The decision to choose venoarterial ECMO over venovenous may be made if both the respiratory and cardiac systems require support, despite the higher risk profile of venoarterial ECMO for complications such as bleeding and cannulation-related adverse events. More details regarding the choice of ECMO mode can be found in Chapter 15.

Patient management

Haemodynamic management goals are to maintain sufficient preload and to deliver adequate cardiac output by balancing stroke volume and heart rate. To closely monitor rapidly changing haemodynamic status post-transplant, invasive cardiac output monitoring may be required (pulmonary artery catheter) in addition to the regular monitoring seen in ICU. Intravenous crystalloid or colloid fluids may be administered judiciously to support blood pressure; however, pulmonary oedema and graft dysfunction can ensue if too much fluid is given.[219] Therefore the patient should be kept 'dry' with a central venous pressure less than 0.9 kPa/7 mmHg. Fluid resuscitation should include products to correct anaemia and preoperative low plasma protein levels.

Vasopressors and inotropes may be used to enhance left ventricular contractility, in addition to vasodilators to offload the left ventricle. In patients requiring intraoperative cardiopulmonary bypass, high doses of inotropes are often needed to overcome transient relative hypovolaemia. Echocardiography is an extremely useful bedside tool which can be used to assess volume status and myocardial function so as to guide the careful titration of fluids and vasopressors necessary to protect the allograft.

Immediately postoperatively, gentle rewarming measures are needed to re-establish normothermia in order to prevent haemodynamic instability and the haematological and peripheral perfusion impairments associated with hypothermia. Regular monitoring of serum electrolytes is important to ensure adequate levels of potassium, magnesium and calcium and to reduce the incidence of postoperative arrhythmias. Intravenous or oral antiarrhythmics may also be required to treat persistent rhythm disturbances, particularly to achieve rate control. Management of the patient receiving ECMO is a complex task requiring skilled input from the multidisciplinary team. Refer to the Further reading section for more information.

Renal and gastrointestinal dysfunction

Renal dysfunction in the early postoperative period is common and has been reported in up to 65% of recipients within 2 weeks of transplant. It is often compounded, often as a result of the present of renal impairment pre-transplant due to factors such as age, diabetes and poorly controlled hypertension.[219] Factors in the early preoperative period which predispose the lung transplant patient to renal injury include restrictive fluid management and aggressive diuresis to prevent pulmonary oedema; commencement of immunosuppressants, particularly calcineurin inhibitors; and hypotension. Patients who require lung transplantation due to cystic fibrosis have long-standing gastrointestinal problems and in the postoperative period are at risk of distal intestinal obstruction syndrome.[198]

Patient management

Early renal replacement therapy to reduce kidney injury should be considered. Management of gut function is an important aspect of nursing practice, including the prevention of constipation with stool softeners and osmotic laxatives (see Chapter 6). For patients receiving transplantation for cystic fibrosis, pancreatic enzyme supplements are required postoperatively. As these patients can be debilitated preoperatively, enteral feeds not requiring pancreatic enzyme supplements should be commenced as soon as possible after surgery, as these enzymes cannot be administered via enteral feeding tubes. To protect the allograft from gastroesophageal reflux, proton-pump inhibitors should be used to prevent gastroesophageal reflux and appropriate patient positioning should be maintained if possible, ideally a reverse Trendelenburg position if tolerated.[198]

Psychosocial care

In the early postoperative period, corticosteroids, sedatives, sleep deprivation and persistent pain contribute to delirium.[220] Rejection episodes can be emotionally demanding, and the requirement for higher doses of corticosteroids can lead to irritability, insomnia, profound depression, mania or psychosis.

Although lung transplantation offers recipients relief from shortness of breath and increased exercise tolerance, many patients have to continue managing other aspects of their underlying disease (e.g. cystic fibrosis). Hence the burden of living with a chronic illness remains. Conversely, some recipients experience wellness for the first time in a long period, and this can alter family and relationship dynamics. Lung transplant recipients often experience persistent symptoms of depression and anxiety. Heightened levels of depression have been associated with decreased survival, highlighting the need for ongoing psychosocial support for lung transplant recipients.[221]

Post-traumatic stress disorder is also experienced in up to 15% of lung recipients by the end of the first year post-transplant, owing to the traumatic events which may occur during their journey to and after transplant, such as life-threatening deteriorations, intractable dyspnoea, failed transplant call-ups, memories of surgery and ICU, and the many post-transplant complications which occur.[222] However, overall, lung transplantation improves health-related quality of life and confers a survival benefit to the majority of recipients.[223] In circumstances where lung function deteriorates after initial success, patients and families experience feelings of devastation and hopelessness. Counselling services are essential in both the preoperative and the postoperative phase.[222]

Long-term sequelae

Survival after lung transplant has improved significantly from earlier years, owing to improvements in donor selection, pre-transplant optimisation of recipients, organ preservation and postoperative management. Global survival rates have improved significantly over the last 20 years, with median survival rates now 6.7 years compared with 4.7 years.[199] Chronic rejection, also termed bronchiolitis obliterans syndrome, is the major complication post-lung transplant, with a quarter of recipients experiencing one or more episodes in the first year.[224] It negatively affects long-term outcomes, with the risk of developing this complication increasing to 60–80% at 5–10 years post-transplant.[198] Long-term sequelae for lung transplant recipients also include renal impairment, with an incidence of 25% at 1 year and 37% at 5 years, infections resulting in increased mortality, and increased risk of malignancies.[198,225] Further information is available about long-term complications specific to lung transplantation, such as bronchiolitis obliterans syndrome and other non-pulmonary complications.

Summary

Respiratory alterations – whether a primary condition or a secondary complication of comorbidity – are a common reason for ICU admission. Vigilant assessment, monitoring and provision of a rapid response to a deteriorating state are central to critical care nursing practice. Contemporary approaches to respiratory support focus on preserving a patient's respiratory function, including use of NIV, using less-controlled ventilation when appropriate and consideration of weaning from mechanical ventilation at the earliest opportunity.

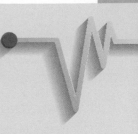

Case study

A 67-year-old female with severe breathlessness is brought into the emergency department by ambulance. The breathlessness has been progressively worsening for 2 days and is accompanied by right-sided chest pain, which she describes as sharp, stabbing and worse on inspiration. She had been discharged from hospital 1 month earlier after a 3-week admission with COVID-19, which included a 9-day ICU stay requiring mechanical ventilation. She has a history of obesity, hypertension and hyperlipidaemia, and has no history of venous thromboembolism. Her regular medications are candesartan and atorvastatin. Low-molecular-weight heparin, which she was receiving during her hospitalisation with COVID-19, was discontinued on discharge.

On examination, she is diaphoretic, agitated and cannot speak in sentences. She is tachypnoeic (respiratory rate 36 breaths/min) receiving oxygen at 15 L/min via a non-rebreather mask; her oxygen saturation is 86%. Her chest is clear with decreased air entry basally. She is tachycardic (heart rate 125 bpm), hypotensive (systolic blood pressure 85 mmHg) and has dual heart sounds with nil added. She reports no pain or swelling of the lower limbs. Abdominal examination is unremarkable.

Investigations ordered include: ABGs (pH 7.28, $PaCO_2$ 7.2 kPa/54 mmHg, and PaO_2 7.7 kPa/58 mmHg), electrocardiograph (sinus tachycardia with signs of right heart strain), chest radiography and urgent CTPA, based on her risk factors. CTPA showed bilateral pulmonary emboli with some saddling across the main pulmonary artery.

The patient continued to be hypotensive, tachypnoeic with increased accessory muscle use and hypoxic (repeat ABG: pH 7.18, $PaCO_2$ 9.2 kPa/69 mmHg, and IaO_2 6.9 kPa/52 mmHg); therefore rapid sequence induction and tracheal intubation was performed. Inotropes were commenced to support her blood pressure. Based on the CTPA results, intravenous thrombolysis was administered (tissue plasminogen activator). She was transferred to ICU for further management.

DISCUSSION

This patient presented with a massive pulmonary embolism post-COVID-19 infection. Although there is still much to understand about COVID-19 as a novel disease, it has emerged that it is an independent risk factor for VTE, a risk which is present both while in hospital and also extending up to 45 days after hospital discharge. This has prompted further examination of VTE prophylaxis in the post-hospital setting. It has been suggested that patients hospitalised with COVID-19 with known VTE risk factors should receive extended VTE prophylaxis up to 45 days after hospital discharge using a subcutaneous low-molecular-weight heparin or oral factor Xa inhibitors, such as rivaroxaban.[226]

CASE STUDY QUESTIONS

1 Review the risk factors this patient presents with using two clinical prediction calculators: the Wells' Criteria for Pulmonary Embolism (https://www.mdcalc.com/wells-criteria-pulmonary-embolism) and the Geneva Score (Revised) for pulmonary embolism (https://www.mdcalc.com/geneva-score-revised-pulmonary-embolism). What is the patient's risk stratification? Was previous COVID-19 infection included within the risk profile of these calculators?
2 Interpret the results from the patient's ABG analysis.
3 Consider the benefits of institutional antithrombotic protocols by reading this article: Cohoon KP, Mahé G, Tafur AJ, et al. Emergence of institutional antithrombotic protocols for coronavirus 2019. Res Pract Thromb Haemost 2020;4:510–17. What treatment regimen would be appropriate for the patient in this case study, given her history of obesity (body mass index 42 kg/m²)?

RESEARCH VIGNETTE

Bloomfield R, Noble DW, Sudlow A. Prone position for acute respiratory failure in adults. Cochrane Database Syst Rev 2015;11:CD008095. doi: 10.1002/14651858.CD008095.pub2.

Abstract

Background: Acute hypoxaemia de novo or on a background of chronic hypoxaemia is a common reason for admission to intensive care and for provision of mechanical ventilation. Various refinements of mechanical ventilation or adjuncts are employed to improve patient outcomes. Mortality from ARDS, one of the main contributors to the need for mechanical ventilation for hypoxaemia, remains approximately 30–40%. Ventilation in the prone position (PP) may improve lung mechanics and gas exchange, and could improve outcomes.

Objectives: The objectives of this review are to ascertain whether prone ventilation offers a mortality advantage when compared with traditional supine or semirecumbent ventilation in adult patients with severe acute respiratory failure requiring conventional invasive artificial ventilation.

Search methods: We searched CENTRAL, MEDLINE, EMBASE, CINAHL and LILACS up to May 2020 for eligible RCTs using an updated version of the search strategy from the earlier version of the review. We added a search in the Cochrane COVID-19 Register. We also searched for studies by hand-searching reference lists and citations of relevant articles, by contacting colleagues and by hand-searching published proceedings of relevant journals. We searched trial registers for ongoing studies in November 2020. We applied no language or publication status constraints.

Selection criteria: We included RCTs that examined the effects of PP versus supine/semirecumbent position during conventional mechanical ventilation in adult participants with acute hypoxaemia.

Data collection and analysis: We used standard methodological procedures expected by Cochrane. We analysed data using Review Manager software and pooled included studies to determine the risk ratio (RR) for mortality and the risk ratio or mean difference (MD) for secondary outcomes; we also performed subgroup analyses and sensitivity analyses.

Main results: We identified nine relevant open-label (unblinded) RCTs (12 publications), which enrolled a total of 2165 participants. All recruited participants suffered from disorders of lung function causing moderate to severe hypoxaemia and requiring mechanical ventilation, so they were fairly comparable within what is the great diversity of specific disease diagnoses in intensive care. Blinding of participants, carers, clinical triallists and other decision makers to treatment allocation was not possible (face-up vs face-down). This predisposes to bias with regards to use of co-interventions and also initiation of withholding or withdrawing life-support, a common practice in intensive care.

Primary analyses of short- and longer-term mortality pooled from six trials demonstrated an RR of 0.84 to 0.86 in favour of PP, but findings were not statistically significant. In the short term, mortality for those ventilated prone was 33.4% (363/1086) and supine 38.3% (395/1031). This resulted in an RR of 0.84 (95% confidence interval (CI) 0.69–1.02). For longer-term mortality, results showed 41.7% (462/1107) for prone and 47.1% (490/1041) for supine positions, with an RR of 0.86 (95% CI 0.72–1.03). The quality of the evidence for both outcomes was rated as low because of important potential bias and serious inconsistency. Subgroup analyses for mortality identified three groups consistently favouring PP: those recruited within 48 hours of meeting entry criteria (five trials; 1024 participants; RR of 0.75 (95% CI 0.59–94)), those treated in the PP for 16 or more hours per day (five trials; 1005 participants; RR of 0.77 (95% CI 0.61–0.99)), and participants with more severe hypoxaemia at trial entry (six trials; 1108 participants; RR of 0.77 (95% CI 0.65–0.92)). The quality of the evidence for these outcomes was rated as moderate as a result of a potentially important risk of bias.

Prone positioning appeared to influence adverse effects: pressure ulcers (four trials; 823 participants), with an RR of 1.25 (95% CI 1.06–1.48), and tracheal tube obstruction, with an RR of 1.78 (95% CI 1.22–2.60), were increased with prone ventilation. Reports of arrhythmias were reduced with PP, with an RR of 0.64 (95% CI 0.47–0.87).

Conclusions: We found no convincing evidence of benefit or harm from universal application of PP in adults with hypoxaemia, mechanically ventilated in ICUs. This is despite the benefits observed in one of the open-label trials restricted to participants with greater disease severity. Three subgroups (early implementation of PP, prolonged adoption of PP and severe hypoxaemia at study entry) suggested that prone positioning may confer a benefit for mortality, but these results should be interpreted with caution. Additional adequately powered studies would be required to definitively confirm or refute these observations of subgroup benefit. This is problematic, given the results of the most recent open-label trial showing a benefit and recommendations derived from several published subgroup analyses. If replication and confirmation of such trial results, which would be desirable, are not realistic then formal meta-analysis of individual patient data and post-trial observational studies (as occur after phase III clinical drug trials) could be utilised to confirm apparent benefit in at-risk populations. Complications such as tracheal tube obstruction and pressure ulcers are increased with the use of prone ventilation. Long-term mortality data (12 months and beyond), as well as functional, neuropsychological and quality-of-life data, are required if future studies are to better inform the role of prone positioning in the management of hypoxaemic respiratory failure in the ICU.

Critique

Patients in ICU with acute respiratory failure present with profound hypoxia, and providing ventilation in the prone position could have beneficial effects on oxygenation and mortality.

Focus: Adult patients in ICU with acute respiratory failure have a high mortality risk. Managing patients with invasive ventilation to improve hypoxia is a cornerstone of treatment. The use of prone positioning, which requires patients to lie face down for up to 16 hours a day, could have beneficial effects on gaseous exchange, hypoxia and mortality in patients who are mechanically ventilated. However, there is limited evidence on whether the intervention of prone positioning compared with conventional modes of mechanical ventilation in the supine or semirecumbent position improves mortality in adult ICU patients with acute respiratory failure. The purpose of this updated systematic review was to evaluate the effectiveness of mechanical ventilation in PP compared with mechanical ventilation in the supine or semirecumbent position in critically ill ICU adult patients with acute respiratory failure to determine mortality (primary 10–30 days or ICU mortality), longer-term mortality (>30 days or hospital mortality), VAP rate, ventilator days, length of ICU stay, length of hospital stay, improvement in oxygenation, adverse events, quality of life and economic outcomes.

Methodological quality: The review used Cochrane methodology, which strengthened the overall methodological quality of the review. The authors reported transparent processes demonstrating robustness in meeting the PRISMA checklist standards. An updated and revised search strategy to include additional terms and filters for RCTs was undertaken across all major healthcare databases (May 2020) and repositories/registries for trials (November 2020) so as to ensure a comprehensive and reproducible search. Additional hand searching of books (critical care and mechanical ventilation), reference lists, review articles and citations, communicating with published triallists, and subject-specific search in the journals, which was undertaken in January 2014, was not updated. Selection, data extraction and quality assessment of studies were undertaken by two authors independently in order to minimise the risk of bias and enhance transparency. A third author checked the data for accuracy and completeness. The quality of each study was assessed using the Cochrane risk-of-bias tool to evaluate the validity of the included studies. Statistical methods were used to combine individual studies in a meta-analysis to allow the results of a number of similar trials to be summarised so as to give an overall picture of the findings. The differences between them includes studies (i.e. heterogeneity was assessed using I^2 statistic) to estimate the proportion of variability in the meta-analysis. Subgroup analyses were undertaken to identify differences in mortality (short and long term) of prone positioning compared with recumbent or semiprone positioning across interventions (duration of prone ventilation (>16 vs <16 hours a day), recruitment timing (<48 vs >48 hours), Simplified Acute Physiology Score II, tidal volume in relation to body weight, and acute lung injury and ARDS (pulmonary and extrapulmonary) versus other causes of acute hypoxaemic respiratory failure. This allows the overall findings from the meta-analysis to be broken down into smaller similar subsets based on a shared characteristic in order to compare differences between them. A sensitivity analysis to determine the effect on the quality of evidence across outcomes excluded studies at high risk of bias. The certainty of the evidence for each outcome study was assessed using the Grades of Recommendation, Assessment, Development and Evaluation system. This allowed authors to make recommendations based on the strength of the evidence evaluated. These practices demonstrate a reliable process and reflect high standards in conducting the Cochrane systematic review.

Study findings and interpretation: The review included nine RCTs including 2165 participants reported in 12 publications. All recruited ICU patients required mechanical ventilation as a result of hypoxaemia due to disorders of lung function. The methods for generating and concealing randomisation were unclear or inadequate for a small number of included studies. As it was impossible to blind participants and personnel to the intervention (face down or face up), all included studies were at high risk of performance and detection bias. This suggests that there may have been systematic differences between baseline characteristics of groups and differences in the care provided or how outcomes were determined as a result of researcher influence on selection or treatment of patients.

Interpretation of results: Results showed low certainty of evidence of mortality benefit (short and long term) for prone positioning compared with traditional supine or semirecumbent ventilation. Secondary outcomes showed prone positioning reduced the mean duration of ventilation, improved PaO_2/FiO_2 ratio and increased length of ICU stay. There was no difference in rate of ventilator-associated pneumonia. Prone positioning increased adverse events (pressure ulcer events, tracheal tube obstruction and tracheal tube displacement). It reduced reports of arrhythmias. When results were divided into subgroups to make comparisons with regards to long-term mortality, those patients who were ventilated in PP <16 hours per day were assessed with severe hypoxaemia at trial entry or were recruited within 48 hours of meeting entry criteria (resulting in limited exposure to supine position over 48 hours) favoured prone positioning. The quality of the evidence for these outcomes was rated as moderate owing to risk of bias. No studies reported on economic outcomes. Sensitivity analysis for risk of bias or confounding showed little effect on most results.

These findings show low certainty of evidence that, for a subgroup of patients with acute respiratory failure, early prone positioning (>16 hours) may provide short- and long-term mortality benefit. However, researchers recommended that further adequately powered research needs to be undertaken to confirm or refute the observations of subgroup benefit and further functional, psychological and quality-of-life outcome data is required to inform management in ICU.

Learning activities

1 A 56-year-old male patient is admitted to your ICU with difficulty breathing. He has a history of diabetes and has recently had the flu. His body mass index is 46. How might you manage this patient, given his clinical condition?

2 The rate of VAP has recently increased in your ICU. What strategies might be implemented to reduce the rate of this hospital-acquired complication?

3 What is the mechanism behind a tension pneumothorax? Why is it regarded as a critical event?

4 What rescue therapies might be implemented for the patient with ARDS and refractory hypoxaemia?

5 When initiating and managing respiratory support, what patient assessment should be considered to optimise this therapy?

6 Chlorhexidine mouthwash (selective oral decontamination) has been commonly used as a strategy to prevent VAP.[227] Why is it currently not recommended, except in certain settings?

Online resources

American Association for Respiratory Care, https://www.aarc.org

Asthma Australia, https://www.asthma.org.au

Asthma UK, https://www.asthma.org.uk

Australian Lung Foundation, https://lungfoundation.com.au

British Thoracic Society, https://www.brit-thoracic.org.uk

Centers for Disease Control and Prevention, https://www.cdc.gov

Lung Health Promotion Centre, https://www.lunghealth.org

National Confidential Enquiry into Patient Outcome and Death. Pulmonary embolism: know the score (2019). https://www.ncepod.org.uk/2019pe.html

National COVID-19 Clinical Evidence Taskforce, https://covid19evidence.net.au/

NHLBI ARDS Network, www.ardsnet.org

NIH COVID-19 treatment guidelines, https://www.covid19treatmentguidelines.nih.gov/management/critical-care-for-adults/

Organ and Tissue Authority: Donate Life Australia, https://www.donatelife.gov.au

PSI/PORT Score: Pneumonia Severity Index for CAP, https://www.mdcalc.com/psi-port-score-pneumonia-severity-index-cap

Respiratory Care online, https://rc.rcjournal.com

Respiratory Research, http://respiratory-research.biomedcentral.com

Thoracic Society of Australia and New Zealand, https://thoracic.org.au

World Health Organization, https://www.who.int

Further reading

Althoff MD, Holguin F, Yang F, et al. Noninvasive ventilation use in critically ill patients with acute asthma exacerbations. Am J Respir Crit Care Med 2020(11);202:1520–30.

Attaway AH, Scheraga RG, Bhimraj A, et al. Severe COVID-19 pneumonia: pathogenesis and clinical management. BMJ 2021;372:n436.

Ball L, Silva PL, Giacobbe DR, et al. Understanding the pathophysiology of typical acute respiratory distress syndrome and severe COVID-19. Expert Rev Respir Med 2022;16(4):437–46.

Combes A, Schmidt M, Hodgson CL, et al. Extracorporeal life support for adults with acute respiratory distress syndrome. Intensive Care Med 2020;46(12):2464–76. doi: 10.1007/s00134-020-06290-1.

Lewis SR, Baker PE, Parker R, et al. High-flow nasal cannulae for respiratory support in adult intensive care patients. Cochrane Database Syst Rev 2021;3:CD010172. doi: 10.1002/14651858.CD010172.pub3.

Mir T, Almas T, Kaur J, et al. Coronavirus disease 2019 (COVID-19): multisystem review of pathophysiology. Ann Med Surg (Lond) 2021;69:102745.

Weinberger J, Rhee C, Klompas, M. Incidence, characteristics, and outcomes of ventilator-associated events during the COVID-19 pandemic. Ann Am Thorac Soc 2022:19(1):82–9. doi: 10.1513/AnnalsATS.202103-364OC.

References

1. Australian and New Zealand Intensive Care Society (ANZICS). Centre for Outcome and Resource Evaluation, 2019 report. Melbourne, VIC: ANZICS; 2019. Available from: https://www.anzics.com.au/annual-reports/. [Accessed 15 February 2023].

2. Australian and New Zealand Intensive Care Society (ANZICS). Centre for Outcome and Resource Evaluation, 2020 report. Melbourne, VIC: ANZICS; 2020. Available from: https://www.anzics.com.au/annual-reports/. [Accessed 15 February 2023].

3. Soriano JB, Kendrick PJ, Paulson KR, et al. Prevalence and attributable health burden of chronic respiratory diseases, 1990–2017: a systematic analysis for the Global Burden of Disease Study 2017. Lancet Respir Med 2020;8(6):585–96.

4. Xie M, Liu X, Cao X, et al. Trends in prevalence and incidence of chronic respiratory diseases from 1990 to 2017. Respir Res 2020;21:49. doi: 10.1186/s12931-020-1291-8.

5. Soriano JB, Abajobir AA, Abate KH, et al. Global, regional, and national deaths, prevalence, disability-adjusted life years, and years lived with disability for chronic obstructive pulmonary disease and asthma, 1990–2015: a systematic analysis for the Global Burden of Disease Study 2015. Lancet Respir Med 2017;5(9):691–706.

6. OECD/European Union. Mortality from respiratory diseases. In: Health at a glance: Europe 2018: state of health in the EU cycle. Brussels: OCED Publishing; 2018, p. 94–5.

7. Forum of International Respiratory Societies. The global impact of respiratory disease. 2nd ed. Sheffield: European Respiratory Society; 2017.

8. Slattery M, Vasques F, Srivastava S, et al. Management of acute respiratory failure. Medicine 2020;48(6):397–403.

9. Pham T, Pesenti A, Bellani G, et al. Outcome of acute hypoxaemic respiratory failure: Insights from the LUNG SAFE Study. Eur Respir J 2021;57:2003317.

10. Gadre SK, Duggal A, Mireles-Cabodevila E, et al. Acute respiratory failure requiring mechanical ventilation in severe chronic obstructive pulmonary disease (COPD). Medicine 2018; 97(17):e0487.

11. Prasad S, O'Neill S. Respiratory failure. Surgery 2021;39(10):654–9.

12. Shebl E, Mirabile VS, Sankari A, et al. Respiratory failure. Treasure Island, FL: StatPearls Publishing; 2022. Available from: https://www.ncbi.nlm.nih.gov/books/NBK526127/. [Accessed 15 February 2023].

13. Summers C, Todd RS, Vercruysse GA, et al. Acute respiratory failure. In: Newman M, Fleisher L, Ko C, et al, editors. Perioperative medicine. 2nd ed. Philadelphia: Elsevier; 2022, p. 576–86

14. Brosnahan SB, Jonkman AH, Kugler MC, et al. Covid-19 and respiratory system disorders. Current knowledge, future clinical and translational research questions. Arterioscler Thromb Vasc Biol 2020 Nov;40:2586–97.

15. Davidson AC, Banham S, Elliott M, et al. British Thoracic Society/Intensive Care Society guideline for the ventilatory management of acute hypercapnic respiratory failure in adults. BMJ Open Resp Res 2016;3:e000133.

16. Dangers L, Montlahuc C, Kouatchet A, et al. Dyspnoea in patients receiving noninvasive ventilation for acute respiratory failure: prevalence, risk factors and prognostic impact. Eur Respir J 2018;52:1702637.

17. Frat JP, Le Pape S, Coudroy R, et al. Noninvasive oxygenation in patients with acute respiratory failure: current perspectives. Int J Gen Med 2022;15:3121–32.

18. Lamba TS, Sharara RS, Leap J, et al. Management of respiratory failure. Crit Care Nurs Q 2016;39(2):94–109.

19. Qaseem A, Etxeandia-Ikobaltzeta I, Fitterman N, et al. Appropriate use of high-flow nasal oxygen in hospitalized patients for initial or postextubation management of acute respiratory failure: a clinical guideline from the American College of Physicians. Ann Intern Med 2021;174(7):977–84.

20. Xu Z, Zhu L, Zhan J, et al. The efficacy and safety of high-flow nasal cannula therapy in patients with COPD and type II respiratory failure: a meta-analysis and systematic review. Eur J Med Res 2021;26(1):122.

21. Yasuda H, Okano H, Mayumi T, et al. Association of noninvasive respiratory support with mortality and intubation rates in acute respiratory failure: a systematic review and network meta-analysis. J Intensive Care 2021;9:32.

22. Alnajada AA, Blackwood B, Mobrad A, et al. High flow nasal oxygen for acute type two respiratory failure: a systematic review [version 2; peer review: 2 approved]. F1000Res 2021;10:482.

23. National Institute for Health and Care Excellence (NICE). Chronic obstructive pulmonary disease in over 16s: diagnosis and management. London: NICE; 2018. Available from: https://www.nice.org.uk/guidance/ng115. [Accessed 15 February 2023].

24. Schreiber A, Fusar Poli B, Bos LD, et al. Noninvasive ventilation in hypercapnic respiratory failure: from rocking beds to fancy masks. Breathe 2018;14(3):235–7.

25. Osadnik CR, Tee VS, Carson-Chahhoud KV, et al. Non-invasive ventilation for the management of acute hypercapnic respiratory failure due to exacerbation of chronic obstructive pulmonary disease. Cochrane Database Syst Rev 2017;7:CD004104.

26. Sakuraya M, Okano H, Masuyama T, et al. Efficacy of non-invasive and invasive respiratory management strategies in adult patients with acute hypoxaemic respiratory failure: a systematic review and network meta-analysis. Crit Care 2021;25:414.

27. Chawla R, Dixit SB, Zirpe KG, et al. ISCCM guidelines for the use of non-invasive ventilation in acute respiratory failure in adult ICUS. Indian J Crit Care Med 2020;24(Suppl. 1):S61–81.

28. Narendra DK, Hess DR, Sessler CN, et al. Update in management of severe hypoxemic respiratory failure. Chest 2017;152(4):867–79.

29. Dres M, Dubé BP, Mayaux J, et al. Coexistence and impact of limb muscle and diaphragm weakness at time of liberation from mechanical ventilation in medical intensive care unit patients. Am J Respir Crit Care Med 2017;195(1):57–66.

30. Dres M, Demoule A. Diaphragm dysfunction during weaning from mechanical ventilation: an underestimated phenomenon with clinical implications. Crit Care 2018;22(1):73.

31. Dong Z, Liu Y, Gai Y, et al. Early rehabilitation relieves diaphragm dysfunction induced by prolonged mechanical ventilation: a randomised control study. BMC Pulm Med 2021;21:106.

32. Guérin C, Reignier J, Richard JC, et al. Prone positioning in severe acute respiratory distress syndrome. N Engl J Med 2013;368(23):2159–68.

33. Fan E, del Sorbo L, Goligher EC, et al. An official American Thoracic Society/European Society of Intensive Care Medicine/Society of Critical Care Medicine clinical practice guideline: mechanical ventilation in adult patients with acute respiratory distress syndrome. Am J Respir Crit Care Med 2017;195(9):1253–63.

34. Tobin MJ. Physiologic basis of mechanical ventilation. Ann Am Thorac Soc 2018;15(Suppl. 1):S49–52.

35. Rezvani H, Esmaeili M, Maroufizadeh S, et al. The effect of early mobilization on respiratory parameters of mechanically ventilated patients with respiratory failure. Crit Care Nurs Q 2022;45(1):74–82.

36. Elliot ZJ, Elliot SC. An overview of mechanical ventilation in the intensive care unit. Nurs Stand 2018;32(28):41–9.

37. Bhandary R. Practical ventilator management. Surgery 2021;39(10):665–70.

38. Castro AAM, Calil SR, Freitas SA, et al. Chest physiotherapy effectiveness to reduce hospitalization and mechanical ventilation length of stay, pulmonary infection rate and mortality in ICU patients. Respir Med 2013;107(1):68–74.

39. Global Initiative for Chronic Lung Disease. Global strategy for the diagnosis, management, and prevention of chronic obstructive pulmonary disease. 2022 report. Global Initiative for Chronic Lung Disease; 2021.

40. Morgan A. Long-term outcomes from critical care. Surgery (Oxf) 2020;39(1):53–7.

41. Lai CC, Tseng KL, Ho CH, et al. Prognosis of patients with acute respiratory failure and prolonged intensive care unit stay. J Thorac Dis 2019;11(5):2051–7.

42. Singer P, Blaser AR, Berger MM, et al. ESPEN guideline on clinical nutrition in the intensive care unit. Clin Nutr 2019;38(1):48–79.

43. Hirzallah FM, Alkaissi A, Do M, et al. A systematic review of nurse-led weaning protocol for mechanically ventilated adult patients. Nurs Crit Care 2019;24(2):89–96.

44. Duncan S, McAuley DF, Walshe M, et al. Interventions for oropharyngeal dysphagia in acute and critical care: a systematic review and meta-analysis. Intensive Care Med 2020;46(7):1326–38.

45. van de Boogaard M, Slooter AJC. Delirium in critically ill patients: current knowledge and future perspectives. BJA Educ 2019;19(12):398–404.

46. Saguil, A. Fargo MV. Acute respiratory distress syndrome: diagnosis and management. Am Fam Physician 2020;101(12):730–8.

47. National Institute for Health and Care Excellence (NICE). Obstructive sleep apnoea/hypopnoea syndrome and obesity hypoventilation syndrome in over 16s. London: NICE; 2021. Available from: https://www.nice.org.uk/guidance/ng202/chapter/2-Obesity-hypoventilation-syndrome. [Accessed 15 February 2023].

48. Hope AA, Adeoye O, Chuang EH, et al. Pre-hospital frailty and hospital outcomes in adults with acute respiratory failure requiring mechanical ventilation. J Crit Care 2018;44:212–16.

49. Torres A, Niederman MS, Chastre J, et al. International ERS/ESICM/ESCMID/ALAT guidelines for the management of hospital-acquired pneumonia and ventilator-associated pneumonia. Eur Respir J 2017;50(3):1700582.

50. Moffatt MF, Cookson WO. The lung microbiome in health and disease. Clin Med 2017;17(6):525–9.

51. Smith AD, Zhang Y, Barber RC, et al. Common lung microbiome identified among mechanically ventilated surgical patients. PLoS One 2016;11(11):e0166313.

52. Dickson RP, Schultz MJ, van der Poll T, et al. Lung microbiota predict clinical outcomes in critically ill patients. Am J Respir Crit Care Med 2020;201(5):555–63.

53. Wang Z, Li F, Liu J, et al. Intestinal microbiota – an unmissable bridge to severe acute pancreatitis-associated acute lung injury. Front Immunol 2022;13:913178.

54. Fromentin M, Ricard JD, Roux D. Respiratory microbiome in mechanically ventilated patients: a narrative review. Intensive Care Med 2021;47(3):292–306.

55. Huffnagle GB, Dickson RP, Lukacs NW. The respiratory tract microbiome and lung inflammation: a two-way street. Mucosal Immunol 2017;10(2):299–306.

56. Arnold FW, Reyes Vega AM, Salunkhe V, et al. Older adults hospitalized for pneumonia in the United States: incidence, epidemiology, and outcomes. J Am Geriatr Soc 2020;68(5):1007–14.

57. Furman CD, Loinonbach A, Usher R, et al. Pneumonia in older adults. Curr Opin Infect Dis 2021;34(2):135–41.

58. National Institute for Health and Care Excellence (NICE). Pneumonia in adults: diagnosis and management. Clinical guideline. London: NICE; 2022. Available from: https://www.nice.org.uk/guidance/cg191. [Accessed 15 February 2023].

59. Dockrell DH, Ho A, Gordon SB. Community acquired pneumonia. In: Broaddus VC, Ernst JD, King TE, et al, editors. Murray & Nadel's textbook of respiratory medicine. 7th ed. Philadelphia: Elsevier; 2022, p. 600–21.

60. Lanks CW, Musani AI, Hsia DW. Community-acquired pneumonia and hospital-acquired pneumonia. Med Clin North Am 2019;103(3):487–501.

61. Chan KM, Gomersall CD. Pneumonia. In: Bersten AD, Handy JM, editors. Oh's intensive care manual. 8th ed. Philadelphia: Elsevier; 2019, p. 467–82.

62. Nair G, Niederman P. Community acquired pneumonia. In: Vincent J, Abraham E, Moore F, et al, editors. Textbook of critical care. 7th ed. Philadelphia: Elsevier; 2017, p. 101–2.

63. King J, Chandrasekar PH. Cryptococcosis. 2021. Available from: https://emedicine.medscape.com/article/215354-overview. [Accessed 15 February 2023].

64. Metlay JP, Waterer GW, Long AC, et al. Diagnosis and treatment of adults with community-acquired pneumonia. An official clinical practice guideline of the American Thoracic Society and Infectious Diseases Society of America. Am J Respir Crit Care Med 2019;200(7):e45–67.

65. Lim WS, van der Eerden MM, Laing R, et al. Defining community acquired pneumonia severity on presentation to hospital: an international derivation and validation study. Thorax 2003;58(5):377–82.

66. Fine MJ, Auble TE, Yealy DM, et al. A prediction rule to identify low-risk patients with community-acquired pneumonia. N Engl J Med 1997;336(4):243–50.

67. Charles PGP, Wolfe R, Whitby M, et al. SMART-COP: a tool for predicting the need for intensive respiratory or vasopressor support in community-acquired pneumonia. Clin Infect Dis 2008;47(3):375–84.

68. Levy MM, Evans LE, Rhodes A. The Surviving Sepsis campaign bundle: 2018 update. Intensive Care Med 2018;44(6):925–8.

69. Tiszai-Szucs T, MacSweeney C, Keaveny J, et al. Feasibility of antimicrobial stewardship (AMS) in critical care settings: a multidisciplinary approach strategy. Med Sci (Basel) 2018;6(2):40.

70. Papazian L, Klompas M, Luyt CE. Ventilator-associated pneumonia in adults: a narrative review. Intensive Care Med 2020;46(5):888–906.

71. Okgün Alcan A, Demir Korkmaz F, Uyar M. Prevention of ventilator-associated pneumonia: Use of the care bundle approach. Am J Infect Control 2016;44(10):e173–6.

72. Chastre J, Luyt CE. Ventilator-associated pneumonia. In: Broaddus VC, Ernst J, King TE, et al, editors. Murray & Nadel's textbook of respiratory medicine. 7th ed. Philadelphia: Elsevier; 2021, p. 583–92.

73. Berton DC, Kalil AC, Teixeira PJZ. Quantitative versus qualitative cultures of respiratory secretions for clinical outcomes in patients with ventilator-associated pneumonia. Cochrane Database Syst Rev 2014;10:CD006482.

74. Parisi M, Gerovasili V, Dimopoulos S, et al. Use of ventilator bundle and staff education to decrease ventilator-associated pneumonia in intensive care patients. Crit Care Nurse 2016;36(5):e1–7.

75. Álvarez-Lerma F, Palomar-Martínez M, Sánchez-García M, et al. Prevention of ventilator-associated pneumonia. Crit Care Med 2018;46(2):181–8.

76. Khan R, Al-Dorzi HM, Al-Attas K, et al. The impact of implementing multifaceted interventions on the prevention of ventilator-associated pneumonia. Am J Infect Control 2016;44(3):320–6.

77. DeLuca LA, Walsh P, Davidson DD, et al. Impact and feasibility of an emergency department-based ventilator-associated pneumonia bundle for patients intubated in an academic emergency department. Am J Infect Control 2017;45(2):151–7.

78. Pileggi C, Mascaro V, Bianco A, et al. Ventilator bundle and its effects on mortality among ICU patients. Crit Care Med 2018;46(7):1167–74.

79. Haghighi A, Shafipour V, Bagheri-Nesami M, et al. The impact of oral care on oral health status and prevention of ventilator-associated pneumonia in critically ill patients. Aust Crit Care 2017;30(2):69–73.

80. Chacko R, Rajan A, Lionel P, et al. Oral decontamination techniques and ventilator-associated pneumonia. Br J Nurs 2017;26(11):594–9.

81. Klompas M, Speck K, Howell MD, et al. Reappraisal of routine oral care with chlorhexidine gluconate for patients receiving mechanical ventilation: systematic review and meta-analysis. JAMA Intern Med 2014;174(5):751–61.

82. Price R, MacLennan G, Glen J. Selective digestive or oropharyngeal decontamination and topical oropharyngeal chlorhexidine for prevention of death in general intensive care: systematic review and network meta-analysis. BMJ 2014;348:g2197.

83. Hua F, Xie H, Worthington HV, et al. Oral hygiene care for critically ill patients to prevent ventilator-associated pneumonia. Cochrane Database Syst Rev 2016;10(10):CD008367

84. Daneman N, Sarwar S, Fowler RA, et al. SuDDICU Canadian Study Group. Effect of selective decontamination on antimicrobial resistance in intensive care units: a systematic review and meta-analysis. Lancet Infect Dis 2013;13(4):328–41.

85. SuDDICU Investigators for the Australian and New Zealand Intensive Care Society Clinical Trials Group; Myburgh JA, Seppelt IM, Goodman F, et al. Effect of selective decontamination of the digestive tract on hospital mortality in critically ill patients receiving mechanical ventilation: a randomized clinical trial. JAMA 2022;328(19):1911–21.

86. Huang XA, Du YP, Fu BB, et al. Influence of subglottic secretion drainage on the microorganisms of ventilator associated pneumonia: a meta-analysis for subglottic secretion drainage. Medicine 2018;97(28):e11223.

87. Hubbard JL, Veneman WL, Dirks RC, et al. Use of endotracheal tubes with subglottic secretion drainage reduces ventilator-associated pneumonia in trauma patients. J Trauma Acute Care Surg 2016;80(2):218–22.

88. Tokmaji G, Vermeulen H, Müller MCA, et al. Silver-coated endotracheal tubes for prevention of ventilator-associated pneumonia in critically ill patients. Cochrane Database Syst Rev 2015; 2015(8):CD009201.

89. Monsel A, le Corre M, Deransy R, et al. Modification of tracheal cuff shape and continuous cuff pressure control to prevent microaspiration in an ex vivo pig tracheal two-lung model. Crit Care Med 2017;45(12):e1262–9.

90. Deem S, Yanez D, Sissons-Ross L, et al. Randomized pilot trial of two modified endotracheal tubes to prevent ventilator-associated pneumonia. Ann Am Thorac Soc 2016;13(1):72–80.

91. Rouzé A, Martin-Loeches I, Nseir S. Improved endotracheal tubes for prevention of ventilator-associated pneumonia: better than silver and gold? Respir Care 2019;64(1):108–9.

92. Wang MY, Pan L, Hu XJ. Chest physiotherapy for the prevention of ventilator-associated pneumonia: a meta-analysis. Am J Infect Control 2019;47(7):755–60.

93. Wang L, Li X, Yang Z, et al. Semi-recumbent position versus supine position for the prevention of ventilator-associated pneumonia in adults requiring mechanical ventilation. Cochrane Database Syst Rev 2016;2016(1):CD009946.

94. Agency for Healthcare Research and Quality (AHRQ). Early mobility guide for reducing ventilator-associated events in mechanically ventilated patients. Rockville, MD: AHRQ; 2017. Available from: https://www.ahrq.gov/sites/default/files/wysiwyg/professionals/quality-patient-safety/hais/tools/mvp/modules/technical/early-mobility-mvpguide.pdf. [Accessed 15 February 2023].

95. Coppadoro A, Bittner E, Berra L. Novel preventive strategies for ventilator-associated pneumonia. Crit Care 2012;16(2):210.

96. McIntosh K, Perlman S. Coronaviruses, including severe acute respiratory syndrome (SARS) and Middle East respiratory syndrome (MERS). In: Bennett JE, Dolin R, Blaser MJ, editors. Mandell, Douglas, and Bennett's principles and practice of infectious diseases. 8th ed. Philadelphia: Churchill Livingstone; 2015, p. 1928–36.e2.

97. Boehm E, Kronig I, Neher RA, et al. Novel SARS-CoV-2 variants: the pandemics within the pandemic. Clin Microbiol and Infect 2021;27(8):1109–17.

98. InFACT Global H1N1 Collaboration. InFACT: a global critical care research response to H1N1. Lancet 2010;375(9708):11–13.

99. Neumann G, Noda T, Kawaoka Y. Emergence and pandemic potential of swine-origin H1N1 influenza virus. Nature 2009;459(7249):931–9.

100. ANZIC Influenza Investigators; Webb SAR, Pettilä V, Seppelt I, et al. Critical care services and 2009 H1N1 influenza in Australia and New Zealand. N Engl J Med 2009;61(20):1925–34.

101. ANZIC Influenza Investigators; Webb SAR, Aubron C, Bailey M, et al. Critical care services and the H1N1 (2009) influenza epidemic in Australia and New Zealand in 2010: the impact of the second winter epidemic. Crit Care 2011;15(3):R143.

102. de Serres G, Skowronski DM, Ward BJ, et al. Influenza vaccination of healthcare workers: critical analysis of the evidence for patient benefit underpinning policies of enforcement. PLoS One 2017;12(1):e0163586.

103. Arghittu A, Dettori M, Azara A, et al. Flu vaccination attitudes, behaviours, and knowledge among health workers. Int J Environ Res Public Health 2020;17(9):3185.

104. National Center for Immunization and Respiratory Diseases (NCIRD). Prevention strategies for seasonal influenza in healthcare settings . Atlanta, GA: NCIRD; 2021. Available from: https://www.cdc.gov/flu/professionals/infectioncontrol/healthcaresettings.htm. [Accessed 15 February 2023].

105. Joint WHO-China Study Team. WHO-convened global study of origins of SARS-CoV-2: China part (text extract). Infect Dis Immun 2021;1(3):125–32.

106. Sprung CL, Joynt GM, Christian MD, et al. Adult ICU triage during the coronavirus disease 2019 pandemic: who will live and who will die? Recommendations to improve survival. Crit Care Med 2020;48(8):1196–202.

107. Ward H, Flower B, Garcia PJ, et al. Global surveillance, research, and collaboration needed to improve understanding and management of long COVID. Lancet 2021;398(10316):2057–9.

108. Taquet M, Dercon Q, Luciano S, et al. Incidence, co-occurrence, and evolution of long-COVID features: a 6-month retrospective cohort study of 273,618 survivors of COVID-19. PLoS Med 2021;18(9):e1003773.

109. Han Q, Zheng B, Daines L, et al. Long-term sequelae of COVID-19: a systematic review and meta-analysis of one-year follow-up studies on post-COVID symptoms. Pathogens 2022;11(2):269.

110. Watson OJ, Barnsley G, Toor J, et al. Global impact of the first year of COVID-19 vaccination: a mathematical modelling study. Lancet Infect Dis 2022;22(9):1293–302.

111. Wouters OJ, Shadlen KC, Salcher-Konrad M, et al. Challenges in ensuring global access to COVID-19 vaccines: production, affordability, allocation, and deployment. The Lancet 2021;397(10278):1023–34.

112. National COVID-19 Clinical Evidence Taskforce. Australian guidelines on the clinical care of people with COVID-19 (version 57). 2022. Available from: https://covid19evidence.net.au/. [Accessed 15 February 2023].

113. COVID-19 Treatment Guidelines Panel. National Institutes of Health. Coronavirus disease 2019 (COVID-19) treatment guidelines. 2022. Available from: https://www.covid19treatmentguidelines.nih.gov/. [Accessed 15 February 2023].

114. Fernando SM, Ferreyro BL, Urner M, et al. Diagnosis and management of acute respiratory distress syndrome. CMAJ 2021;193(2):E761–8.

115. Fan E, Brodie D, Slutsky AS. Acute respiratory distress syndrome: advances in diagnosis and treatment. JAMA 2018;319(7):698–710.

116. Bellani G, Laffey JG, Pham T, et al. Epidemiology, patterns of care, and mortality for patients with acute respiratory distress syndrome in intensive care units in 50 countries. JAMA 2016;315(8):788–800.

117. Tzotzos SJ, Fischer B, Fischer H, et al. Incidence of ARDS and outcomes in hospitalized patients with COVID-19: a global literature survey. Crit Care 2020;24(1):516.

118. Thompson BT, Chambers RC, Liu KD. Acute respiratory distress syndrome. N Engl J Med 2017;377(6):562–72.

119. Pham T, Rubenfeld GD. Fifty years of research in ARDS the epidemiology of acute respiratory distress syndrome: a 50th birthday review. Am J Respir Crit Care Med 2017;195(7):860–70.

120. Powers K. Acute respiratory distress syndrome. J Am Acad Physician Assist 2022;35(4):29–33.

121. Meyer NJ, Gattinoni L, Calfee CS. Acute respiratory distress syndrome. Lancet 2021;398:622–37.

122. Yadav H, Thompson BT, Gajic O. Fifty years of research in ARDS. Is acute respiratory distress syndrome a preventable disease? Am J Respir Crit Care Med 2017;195(6):725–36.

123. ARDS Definition Task Force; Ranieri VM, Rubenfeld GD, Thompson BT, et al. Acute respiratory distress syndrome: the Berlin definition. JAMA 2012;307(23):2526–33.

124. Ferguson ND, Fan E, Camporota L, et al. The Berlin definition of ARDS: an expanded rationale, justification, and supplementary material. Intensive Care Med 2012;38(10):1573–82.

125. Chiumello D, Umbrello M, Sferrazza Papa GF, et al. Global and regional diagnostic accuracy of lung ultrasound compared to CT in patients with acute respiratory distress syndrome. Crit Care Med 2019;47(11):1599–606.

126. Liaqat A, Mason M, Foster BJ, et al. Evidence-based mechanical ventilatory strategies in ARDS. J Clin Med 2022;11(2):319.

127. Howell MD, Davis AM. Management of ARDS in adults. JAMA 2018;319(7):711–12.

128. Yadam S, Bihler E, Balaan M. Acute respiratory distress syndrome. Crit Care Nurs Q 2016;39(2):190–5.

129. Bein T, Grasso S, Moerer O, et al. The standard of care of patients with ARDS: ventilatory settings and rescue therapies for refractory hypoxemia. Intensive Care Med 2016;42(5):699–711.

130. Aoyama H, Uchida K, Aoyama K, et al. Assessment of therapeutic interventions and lung protective ventilation in patients with moderate to severe acute respiratory distress syndrome: a systematic review and network meta-analysis. JAMA Netw Open 2019;2(7):e198116.

131. Griffiths MJD, McAuley DF, Perkins GD, et al. Guidelines on the management of acute respiratory distress syndrome. BMJ Open Respir Res 2019;6:e000420.

132. Papazian L, Aubron C, Brochard L, et al. Formal guidelines: management of acute respiratory distress syndrome. Ann Intensive Care 2019;9(1):69.

133. Walkey AJ, Goligher EC, Del Sorbo L, et al. Low tidal volume versus non–volume-limited strategies for patients with acute respiratory distress syndrome: a systematic review and meta-analysis. Ann Am Thorac Soc 2017;14(Suppl. 4):S271–9.

134. Coleman MH, Aldrich JM. Acute respiratory distress syndrome: ventilator management and rescue therapies. Crit Care Clin 2021;37(4):851–66.

135. Wang C, Wang X, Chi C, et al. Lung ventilation strategies for acute respiratory distress syndrome: A systematic review and network meta-analysis. Sci Rep 2016;6:22855.

136. Brodie D, Slutsky AS, Combes A. Extracorporeal life support for adults with respiratory failure and related indications: a review. JAMA 2019;322(6):557–68.

137. Munshi L, Walkey A, Goligher E, et al. Venovenous extracorporeal membrane oxygenation for acute respiratory distress syndrome: a systematic review and meta-analysis. Lancet Respir Med 2019;7(2):163–72.

138. Poon WH, Ramanathan K, Ling RR, et al. Prone positioning during venovenous extracorporeal membrane oxygenation for acute respiratory distress syndrome: a systematic review and meta-analysis. Crit Care 202;25:292.

139. Petit M, Fetita C, Gaudemer A, et al. Prone-positioning for severe acute respiratory distress syndrome requiring extracorporeal membrane oxygenation. Crit Care Med 2022;50(2):264–74.

140. Munshi L, Del Sorbo L, Adhikari NKJ, et al. Prone position for acute respiratory distress syndrome: a systematic review and meta-analysis. Ann Am Thorac Soc 2017;14(Suppl. 4):S280–8.

141. Sud S, Friedrich JO, Adhikari NKJ, et al. Comparative effectiveness of protective ventilation strategies for moderate and severe acute respiratory distress syndrome a network meta-analysis. Am J Respir Crit Care Med 2021;203(11):1366–77.

142. Girard TD, Alhazzani W, Kress JP, et al. An official American Thoracic Society/American College of Chest Physicians clinical practice guideline: liberation from mechanical ventilation in critically ill adults. Rehabilitation protocols, ventilator liberation protocols, and cuff leak tests. Am J Respir Crit Care Med 2017;195(1):120–33.

143. Guervilly C, Bisbal M, Forel JM, et al. Effects of neuromuscular blockers on transpulmonary pressures in moderate to severe acute respiratory distress syndrome. Intensive Care Med 2017;43(3):408–18.

144. Maskin LP, Bonelli I, Olarte GL, et al. High- versus low-dose dexamethasone for the treatment of COVID-19-related acute respiratory distress syndrome: a multicenter, randomized open-label clinical trial. J Intensive Care Med 2022;37(4):491–9.

145. Jeon K. Pharmacotherapy for acute respiratory distress syndrome: limited success to date. Tuberc Respir Dis (Seoul) 2017;80(3):311–12.

146. Sweeney RM, McAuley DF. Acute respiratory distress syndrome. Lancet 2016;388(10058):2416–30.

147. Tongyoo S, Permpikul C, Mongkolpun W, et al. Hydrocortisone treatment in early sepsis-associated acute respiratory distress syndrome: results of a randomized controlled trial. Crit Care 2016;20(1):329.

148. Mohananey D, Sethi J, Villablanca PA, et al. Effect of antiplatelet therapy on mortality and acute lung injury in critically ill patients: a systematic review and meta-analysis. Ann Card Anaesth 2016;19(4):626–37.

149. Global Initiative for Asthma. Global Strategy for asthma management and prevention. Updated 2022. Fontana, WI: Global Initiative for Asthma; 2022

150. Global Initiative for Chronic Lung Disease. Global strategy for the diagnosis, management and prevention of chronic obstructive pulmonary disease. 2022 report. Global Initiative for Chronic Lung Disease; 2021

151. Global Initiative for Asthma. Pocket guide for asthma management and prevention (for adults and children older than 5 years). A pocket guide for health professionals. Fontana, WI: Global Initiative for Asthma; 2021.

152. Yanagisawa S, Ichinose M. Definition and diagnosis of asthma-COPD overlap (ACO). Allergol Int 2018;67(2):172–8.

153. Global Asthma Network. The global asthma report 2018. Auckland; New Zealand: Global Asthma Network; 2018. Available from: globalasthmareport.org. [Accessed 15 February 2023].

154. Rodrigues S de O, da Cunha CMC, Soares GMV, et al. Mechanisms, pathophysiology and currently proposed treatments of chronic obstructive pulmonary disease. Pharmaceuticals 2021;14:979.

155. Berenyi F, Steinfort DP, Abdelhamid YA, et al. Characteristics and outcomes of critically ill patients with acute exacerbation of chronic obstructive pulmonary disease in Australia and New Zealand. Ann Am Thorac Soc 2020;17(6):736–45.

156. Safiri S, Carson-Chahhoud K, Karamzad N, et al. Prevalence, deaths, and disability-adjusted life-years due to asthma and its attributable risk factors in 204 countries and territories, 1990–2019. Chest 2022;161(2):318–29.

157. Sinyor B, Concepcion Perez L. Pathophysiology of asthma. StatPearls. Treasure Island, FL: StatPearls Publishing; 2022. Available from: https://www.ncbi.nlm.nih.gov/books/NBK551579/. [Accessed 15 February 2023].

158. Singh D, Agusti A, Anzueto A, et al. Global strategy for the diagnosis, management, and prevention of chronic obstructive lung disease: the GOLD science committee report 2019. Eur Respir J 2019;53(5):1900164.

159. Leap J, Arshad O, Cheema T, et al. Pathophysiology of COPD. Crit Care Nurs Q 2021;44(1):2–8.

160. Barnes PJ. Cellular and molecular mechanisms of asthma and COPD. Clin Sci 2017;131(13):1541–58.

161. Booth A. Clinical guidelines: which is the best of three? Pract Nurs 2020;31(8):344–51.

162. Carlsson JA, Bayes HK. Acute severe asthma in adults. Medicine 2020;48(5):297–302.

163. Fergeson JE, Patel SS, Lockey RF. Acute asthma, prognosis, and treatment. J Allergy Clin Immunol 2017;139(2):438–47.

164. Scottish Intercollegiate Guidelines Network (SIGN), British Thoracic Society, Healthcare Improvement Scotland. British guideline on the management of asthma: a national clinical guideline. Edinburgh: Healthcare Improvement Scotland; 2019. Available from: https://www.sign.ac.uk/sign-158-british-guideline-on-the-management-of-asthma. [Accessed 15 February 2023].

165. National Institute for Health and Care Excellence (NICE). Asthma: diagnosis, monitoring and chronic asthma management. London: NICE; 2017. Available from: https://www.nice.org.uk/guidance/ng80. [Accessed 15 February 2023].

166. Tan DJ, Lodge CJ, Lowe AJ, et al. Bronchodilator reversibility as a diagnostic test for adult asthma: findings from the population-based Tasmanian Longitudinal Health Study. ERJ Open Res 2021;7(1):00042–2020.

167. Cloutier MM, Dixon AE, Krishnan JA, et al. Managing asthma in adolescents and adults: 2020 asthma guideline update from the National Asthma Education and Prevention Program. JAMA 2020;324(22):2301–17.

168. Holguin F, Cardet JC, Chung KF, et al. Management of severe asthma: a European Respiratory Society/American Thoracic Society guideline. Eur Respir J 2020;55:1900588

169. Wedzicha JA, Miravitlles M, Hurst JR, et al. Prevention of COPD exacerbations: a European Respiratory Society/American Thoracic Society guideline. Eur Respir J 2017;50(3):1602265

170. Yang IA, Brown JL, George J, et al. COPD-X Australian and New Zealand guidelines for the diagnosis and management of chronic obstructive pulmonary disease: 2017 update. Med J Aust 2017;207(10):436–42.

171. Attaway AH, Faress J, Jacono F, et al. Acute responses to oxygen delivery via high flow nasal cannula in patients with severe chronic obstructive pulmonary disease-HFNC and severe COPD. J Clin Med 2021;10:1814.

172. Lombard E, Gates J, Ruickbie S. Acute asthma exacerbations: tips from the shop floor. Br J Hosp Med (Lond) 2020;81(12):1–10.

173. National Institute for Health and Care Excellence (NICE). Chronic obstructive pulmonary disease (acute exacerbation): antimicrobial prescribing. London: NICE; 2018. Available from: https://www.nice.org.uk/guidance/ng114. [Accessed 15 February 2023].

174. Roberts DJ, Leigh-Smith S, Faris PD, et al. Clinical presentation of patients with tension pneumothorax: a systematic review. Ann Surg 2015;261(6):1068–78.

175. Tran J, Haussner W, Shah K. Traumatic pneumothorax: a review of current diagnostic practices and evolving management. J Emerg Med 2021;61(5):517–28.

176. Chan KK, Joo DA, McRae AD, et al. Chest ultrasonography versus supine chest radiography for diagnosis of pneumothorax in trauma patients in the emergency department. Cochrane Database Syst Rev 2020;7(7):CD013031.

177. Feenstra TM, Dickhoff C, Deunk J. Systematic review and meta-analysis of tube thoracostomy following traumatic chest injury; suction versus water seal. Eur J Trauma Emerg Surg 2018;44(6):819–27.

178. Galvagno SM, Smith CE, Varon AJ, et al. Pain management for blunt thoracic trauma. J Trauma Acute Care Surg 2016;81(5):936–51.

179. Heit JA, Spencer FA, White RH. The epidemiology of venous thromboembolism. J Thromb Thrombolysis 2016;41(1):3–14.

180. Banerjee TP, Mora JC. The management of pulmonary embolism. Anaesth Intensive Care Med 2020;21(3):139–46.

181. Wendelboe AM, Raskob GE. Global burden of thrombosis: epidemiologic aspects. Circ Res 2016;118(9):1340–7.

182. Sista AK, Kuo WT, Schiebler M, et al. Stratification, imaging, and management of acute massive and submassive pulmonary embolism. Radiology 2017;284(1):5–24.

183. Konstantinides SV, Meyer G, Bueno H, et al. 2019 ESC Guidelines for the diagnosis and management of acute pulmonary embolism developed in collaboration with the European Respiratory Society (ERS). Eur Heart J 2020;41(4):543–603.

184. Weinstein T, Deshwal H, Brosnahan SB. Advanced management of intermediate-high risk pulmonary embolism. Crit Care 2021;25(1):311.

185. Alhassan S, Pelinescu A, Gandhi V, et al. Clinical presentation and risk factors of venous thromboembolic disease. Crit Care Nurs Q 2017;40(3):201–9.

186. Tice C, Seigerman M, Fiorilli P, et al. Management of acute pulmonary embolism. Curr Cardiovasc Risk Rep 2020;14(12):24.

187. Licha CRM, McCurdy CM, Maldonado SM, et al. Current management of acute pulmonary embolism. Ann Thorac Cardiovasc Surg 2020;26(2):65–71.

188. National Institute for Health and Care Excellence (NICE). Venous thromboembolic diseases: diagnosis, management and thrombophilia testing. London: NICE; 2020. Available from: https://www.nice.org.uk/guidance/ng158. [Accessed 15 February 2023].

189. Yamamoto T. Management of patients with high-risk pulmonary embolism: a narrative review. J Intensive Care 2018;6:16.

190. Klok FA, Mos ICM, Nijkeuter M, et al. Simplification of the revised Geneva Score for assessing clinical probability of pulmonary embolism. Arch Intern Med 2008;168(19):2131–6.

191. Tan CW, Balla S, Ghanta RK, et al. Contemporary management of acute pulmonary embolism. Semin Thorac Cardiovasc Surg 2020;32(3):396–403.

192. Villgran V Das, Lyons C, Nasrullah A, et al. Acute respiratory failure. Crit Care Nurs Q 2022;45(3):233–47.

193. Tomkiewicz EM, Kline JA. Concise review of the clinical approach to the exclusion and diagnosis of pulmonary embolism in 2020. J Emerg Nurs 2020;46(4):527–38.

194. Duranteau J, Taccone FS, Verhamme P, et al; ESA VTE Guidelines Task Force. European guidelines on perioperative venous thromboembolism prophylaxis: intensive care. Eur J Anaesthesiol 2018;35(2):142–6.

195. Roy PM, Douillet D, Penaloza A. Contemporary management of acute pulmonary embolism. Trends Cardiovasc Med 2021;11:48.

196. Todoran TM, Petkovich B. Aggressive therapy for acute pulmonary embolism: systemic thrombolysis and catheter-directed approaches. Semin Respir Crit Care Med 2021;42(2):250–62.

197. Nagraj S, Li W, Zamora C, Barakakis PA, et al. Pharmacological and interventional management of pulmonary embolism: where do we stand? Future Cardiol 2022;18(3):191–206.

198. Nair P, Jansz P, Plit M. Lung transplantation. In: Bersten A, Handy J, editors. Oh's Intensive Care Manual. 8th ed. Oxford: Elsevier; 2019, p. 1244–55.

199. Bos S, Vos R, van Raemdonck DE, et al. Survival in adult lung transplantation: where are we in 2020? Curr Opin Organ Transplant 2020;25(3):268–73.

200. van Raemdonck D, Keshavjee S, Levvey B, et al. Donation after circulatory death in lung transplantation – five-year follow-up from ISHLT Registry. J Heart Lung Transplant 2019;38(12):1235–45.

201. Leard LE, Holm AM, Valapour M, et al. Consensus document for the selection of lung transplant candidates: an update from the International Society for Heart and Lung Transplantation. J Heart Lung Transplant 2021;40(11):1349–79.

202. McShane P, Ruiz L, Garrity E. Lung transplantation. In: Spiro S, Silvestri G, Agusti A, editors. Clinical respiratory medicine. 4th ed. St Louis, MO: Mosby; 2012, p. 882–902.

203. ANZOD Registry. 2022 Annual report, section 8: deceased donor lung donation. Adelaide, SA: Australia and New Zealand Dialysis and Transplant Registry; 2022. Available from: https://www.anzdata.org.au. [Accessed 15 February 2023].

204. Laubach VE, Sharma AK. Mechanisms of lung ischemia-reperfusion injury. Curr Opin Organ Transplant 2016;21(3):246–52.

205. Snell GI, Yusen RD, Weill D, et al. Report of the ISHLT Working Group on Primary Lung Graft Dysfunction, part I: definition and grading – a 2016 consensus group statement of the International Society for Heart and Lung Transplantation. J Heart Lung Transplant 2017;36(10):1097–103.

206. Potestio C, Jordan D, Kachulis B. Acute postoperative management after lung transplantation. Best Pract Res Clin Anaesthesiol 2017;31(2):273–84.

207. Tabarelli W, Bonatti H, Tabarelli D, et al. Long term complications following 54 consecutive lung transplants. J Thorac Dis 2016;8(6):1234–44.

208. Langer D. Rehabilitation in patients before and after lung transplantation. Respiration 2015;89(5):353–62.

209. The Acute Respiratory Distress Syndrome Network. Ventilation with lower tidal volumes as compared with traditional tidal volumes for acute lung injury and the acute respiratory distress syndrome. New Engl J Med 2000;342(18):1301–8.

210. di Nardo M, Tikkanen J, Husain S, et al. Postoperative management of lung transplant recipients in the intensive care unit. Anesthesiology 2022;136(3):482–99.

211. Batra K, Chamarthy MR, Reddick M, et al. Diagnosis and interventions of vascular complications in lung transplant. Cardiovasc Diagn Ther 2018;8(3):378–86.

212. Barnes L, Reed RM, Parekh KR, et al. Mechanical ventilation for the lung transplant recipient. Curr Pulmonol Rep 2015;4(2):88–96.

213. Shehata IM, Elhassan A, Urits I, et al. Postoperative management of hyperinflated native lung in single-lung transplant recipients with chronic obstructive pulmonary disease: a review article. Pulm Ther 2021;7(1):37–46.

214. Pottecher J, Falcoz PE, Massard G, et al. Does thoracic epidural analgesia improve outcome after lung transplantation? Interact Cardiovasc Thorac Surg 2011;12(1):51–3.

215. Lewis TC, Sureau K, Katz A, et al. Multimodal opioid-sparing pain management after lung transplantation and the impact of liposomal bupivacaine intercostal nerve block. Clin Transplant 2022;36(1):e14512.

216. Schug SA, Palmer GM, Scott DA, et al. Acute pain management: scientific evidence. 5th ed. Melbourne, VIC: Australian and New Zealand College of Anaesthetists; 2020. Available from: https://www.anzca.edu.au/. [Accessed 15 February 2023].

217. Pilcher DV, Scheinkestel CD, Snell GI, et al. High central venous pressure is associated with prolonged mechanical ventilation and increased mortality after lung transplantation. J Thorac Cardiovasc Surg 2005;129(4):912–18.

218. Waldron NH, Klinger RY, Hartwig MG, et al. Adverse outcomes associated with postoperative atrial arrhythmias after lung transplantation: a meta-analysis and systematic review of the literature. Clin Transplant 2017;31(4):e12926.

219. Trinh BN, Brzezinski M, Kukreja J. Early postoperative management of lung transplant recipients. Thorac Surg Clin 2022;32(2):185–95.

220. DeBolt CL, Gao Y, Sutter N, et al. The association of post-operative delirium with patient-reported outcomes and mortality after lung transplantation. Clin Transplant 2021;35(5):e14275.

221. Smith PJ, Blumenthal JA, Trulock EP, et al. Psychosocial predictors of mortality following lung transplantation. Am J Transplant 2016;16(1):271–7.

222. Sher Y. Post-transplant psychosocial and mental health care of the lung recipient. In: Sher Y, Maldonado JR, editors. Psychosocial care of end-stage organ disease and transplant patients. Champaign, IL: Springer International; 2019. p. 289–98.

223. Singer JP, Katz PP, Soong A, et al. Effect of lung transplantation on health-related quality of life in the era of the Lung Allocation Score: a U.S. prospective cohort study. Am J Transplant 2017;17(5):1334–45.

224. Chambers DC, Cherikh WS, Harhay MO, et al. The International Thoracic Organ Transplant Registry of the International Society for Heart and Lung Transplantation: thirty-sixth adult lung and heart–lung transplantation report – 2019; focus theme: donor and recipient size match. J Heart Lung Transplant 2019;38(10):1042–55.

225. Chambers DC, Perch M, Zuckermann A, et al. The International Thoracic Organ Transplant Registry of the International Society for Heart and Lung Transplantation: thirty-eighth adult lung transplantation report – 2021; focus on recipient characteristics. J Heart Lung Transplant 2021;40(10):1060–72.

226. Cohoon KP, Mahé G, Tafur AJ, et al. Emergence of institutional antithrombotic protocols for coronavirus 2019. Res Pract Thromb Haemost 2020;4(4):510–17.

227. Zhao T, Wu X, Zhang Q, et al. Oral hygiene care for critically ill patients to prevent ventilator-associated pneumonia. Cochrane Database Syst Rev 2020;12(12):CD008367.

Chapter 15

Ventilation and oxygenation management

Louise Rose, Frederique Paulus

Learning objectives

After reading this chapter, you should be able to:

- describe oxygen therapy, including low-flow and high-flow devices, complications associated with oxygen therapy, and management priorities
- state nursing priorities for airway management strategies including laryngeal masks, endotracheal tubes and tracheostomy tubes
- summarise current knowledge on the physiological benefits, indications for use, associated monitoring priorities, complications, modes, settings and interfaces for non-invasive ventilation
- state the indications for use, associated monitoring priorities, complications, classification framework, modes and settings for invasive mechanical ventilation
- outline the weaning continuum and current evidence for optimising safe and efficient weaning from mechanical ventilation
- discuss ventilation management strategies for refractory hypoxaemia
- discuss ventilation management strategies for severe airflow limitation

Introduction

Support of oxygenation and ventilation are two of the most common interventions in intensive care; in 2020, there were 190,000 adult ICU admissions, with approximately 34% of adult patients in Australian and New Zealand ICUs receiving invasive mechanical ventilation.[1] Similar numbers of critically ill patients receive ventilation in the United Kingdom,[2] whereas in the United States reported numbers range from 21% to 39%.[3] The technology available for supporting oxygenation and ventilation is complex, ranging from simple interventions, such as nasal cannulae, through to invasive mechanical ventilation and extracorporeal support. Additionally, the meaning of ventilator terminology is often unclear and terms may be used interchangeably. Critical care nurses must have a strong knowledge of the underlying principles of oxygenation and ventilation that will facilitate an understanding of respiratory support devices, associated monitoring priorities and risks.

Oxygen therapy

Oxygen is required for aerobic cellular metabolism and ultimately for human survival, with some cells, such as those in the brain, being more sensitive to hypoxia than others. Refer to Chapter 13 for discussion of oxygen delivery and consumption, the oxyhaemoglobin dissociation curve, hypoxaemia and tissue hypoxia; this material provides rationales for clinical decisions regarding the administration of oxygen therapy or ventilation strategies. Oxygen therapy should be considered for patients with a significant reduction in arterial oxygen levels, irrespective of diagnosis and especially if the patient is drowsy or unconscious.

Indications

Indications for oxygen therapy include:

- cardiac and respiratory arrest
- type I respiratory failure
- type II respiratory failure
- chest pain or acute coronary syndrome with hypoxia (i.e. SpO_2 less than 93%) or evidence of shock[4]
- low blood pressure, cardiac output
- increased metabolic demands
- carbon monoxide poisoning.

Complications

Administration of oxygen, regardless of the delivery device, has potential adverse effects. High concentrations of oxygen cause nitrogen washout, resulting in absorption atelectasis.

Hypoventilation and CO_2 narcosis

High-dose oxygen therapy may lead to hypoventilation, hypercapnia and CO_2 narcosis in a small proportion of patients with chronic obstructive pulmonary disease (COPD). The processes underpinning these physiological changes are described in Chapter 13. These patients require close monitoring of $PaCO_2$ levels when oxygen therapy is instituted or increased. Although COPD patients frequently may have a lower baseline SpO_2 (88–94% compared with 96–100% in patients with no lung pathology), treatment of hypoxia is still essential, and oxygen should not be withheld or withdrawn while hypoxia remains, even if hypercapnia worsens.[5,6]

> **Practice tip**
>
> Oxygen should not be withheld or withdrawn while hypoxia remains, even if hypercapnia worsens.

Oxygen toxicity

Administration of high oxygen concentrations may lead to oxygen toxicity; symptoms include non-productive cough, substernal pain, reduced lung compliance,

---

BOX 15.1

Signs and symptoms of oxygen toxicity

Central nervous system:
- nausea and vomiting
- anxiety
- visual changes
- hallucinations
- tinnitus
- vertigo
- hiccups
- seizures

Pulmonary:
- dry cough
- substernal chest pain
- shortness of breath
- pulmonary oedema
- pulmonary fibrosis

---

interstitial oedema and pulmonary capillary haemorrhage. These symptoms may be mistakenly attributed to the underlying illness, especially in a sedated and ventilated patient. Many of the symptoms abate once the fraction of inspired oxygen (FiO_2) is reduced, although irreversible pulmonary fibrosis may occur (Box 15.1). The concentration and duration of oxygen exposure that induces oxygen toxicity varies between patients.[7] The lowest possible FiO_2 should therefore be used to achieve the target partial pressure of oxygen in arterial blood (PaO_2) or peripheral oxygen saturation (SpO_2).

Oxygen administration devices

Initial management of hypoxia in a spontaneously breathing patient with an intact airway is low- or variable-flow oxygen via nasal cannulae (up to 6 L/min) or face mask (up to 15 L/min). Although oxygen devices have traditionally had FiO_2 ascribed to specific flow rates, the FiO_2 delivered to the alveoli is variable due to the influence of:

- patient factors: inspiratory flow rate, respiratory rate, tidal volume (V_T), respiratory pause
- oxygen device factors: oxygen flow rate, volume of mask/reservoir, air vent size, tightness of fit.

Normal inspiratory flow in a healthy adult ranges between 25 and 35 L/min. Patients with respiratory failure tend to increase their flow demand from 50 up to 300 L/min. Patients in respiratory distress are characterised by high respiratory rates and low V_Ts[7,8] that can significantly decrease the FiO_2 available via an oxygen delivery device, depending on the type in use.

All oxygen delivery devices use some type of reservoir to support oxygen delivery and prevent CO_2 rebreathing. For face masks, the reservoir is the mask; for nasal cannulae it is the patient's pharynx. Patients with high inspiratory flow demand will deplete the reservoir faster than it can be replenished, resulting in air entrainment and dilution of the oxygen concentration.

Variable-flow devices

A range of low- or variable-flow oxygen delivery devices is available. These devices range from nasal cannulae and oxygen masks with different features through to bag–mask ventilation.

Low-flow nasal cannulae

Traditional low-flow nasal cannulae sit at the external nares and deliver 1–4 L/min of oxygen. Higher flows may cause discomfort and damage from the drying effect on respiratory mucosa. Increased flow demand with respiratory distress dilutes the oxygen, reducing the FiO_2 to the alveoli.

High-flow nasal cannulae

High-flow nasal cannulae have slightly larger prongs that facilitate oxygen flow of up to 60 L/min leading to less air entrainment than with other oxygen delivery systems.[8,9] High-flow nasal cannulae generate low levels of positive end-expiratory pressure, though this is dependent on the flow rate, trachea size and mouth closing,[10] and can therefore reduce tachypnoea and work of breathing.[11,12] The high gas flow may flush CO_2 from the anatomical dead space preventing CO_2 rebreathing and thereby decreasing $PaCO_2$, although this is not well supported by the literature.[13,14] These systems are generally well tolerated, but must be used with heated humidification to avoid drying the respiratory mucosa.[12] High-flow nasal cannulae are now used frequently in many areas of clinical practice to avoid, or as an alternative to, more-invasive therapies.[15] High-flow nasal cannulae are better tolerated than NIV, giving the advantages of patient comfort and therefore better tolerance of prolonged device use.[16] Current evidence indicates high-flow nasal cannulae may lead to less treatment failure than conventional oxygen therapy but makes little to no difference compared with NIV.[17]

Oxygen masks

Loose-fitting oxygen masks include simple (Hudson) face masks, aerosol masks used in combination with heated humidification and nebuliser treatments, tracheostomy masks and face tents. All are considered low-flow or variable-flow devices, with the delivered FiO_2 varying with patient demand. Flow rates ≥5 L/min minimise CO_2 rebreathing. The addition of 'tusks' to a Hudson mask may increase the oxygen reservoir,[18] but does not guarantee a consistent FiO_2 and has probably been superseded by high-flow systems.[19]

Partial rebreather and non-rebreather masks have an attached reservoir bag that enables delivery of higher levels of FiO_2. Both mask types have a one-way valve precluding expired gas entering the reservoir bag. A non-rebreather mask has two one-way valves preventing air entrainment.[20] The maximum FiO_2 delivery with non-rebreather masks is 0.85 with low-flow demand, with a steep decline in alveolar oxygen concentration as minute volume increases. Non-rebreather masks may perform worse than a Hudson mask without a reservoir bag.[7]

Venturi systems

Venturi systems use the venturi effect to entrain gas via a narrow aperture via a side port increasing gas speed and gaining kinetic energy. FiO_2 concentration can be altered by widening or narrowing the Venturi device aperture to a maximum FiO_2 of 0.6. The FiO_2 concentration using a Venturi system is less affected by changes in respiratory pattern and demand compared with other low-flow oxygen devices.[7]

Bag–mask ventilation

Bag–mask ventilation with a self-inflating bag (and reservoir), non-return valve and mask delivers assisted ventilation at a FiO_2 of 1.0. Addition of a positive end-expiratory pressure (PEEP) valve will improve oxygenation. Manual ventilation requires a good seal between the patient's face and the mask; this may be difficult to achieve as a single operator. One person should hold the mask and lift the patient's chin, while another squeezes the bag. Effective bag–mask ventilation is confirmed when the chest visibly rises as the bag is squeezed as well as improved oxygen saturations.[21] Bag mask ventilation may cause gastric insufflation, increasing the risk of vomiting and subsequent aspiration.

> **Practice tip**
>
> Transparent face masks are recommended for bag–mask ventilation as they allow immediate recognition if a patient vomits.

Airway support

The most common cause of partial airway obstruction in an unconscious patient is loss of oropharyngeal muscle tone, particularly of the tongue. This may be alleviated by tilting the head slightly back and lifting the chin or thrusting the jaw forward. The head-tilt/chin-lift manoeuvre is not used if cervical spine injury is suspected.[22] The jaw-thrust manoeuvre may require two hands to maintain.[23] If more prolonged support is required, an oro- or nasopharyngeal airway can be used that may also facilitate bag–mask ventilation.

Oro- and nasopharyngeal airways

The Guedel oropharyngeal airway is available in various sizes (a medium-sized adult requires a size 4). The airway is inserted into the patient's mouth past the teeth, with the end

FIGURE 15.1 Nasopharyngeal airways.

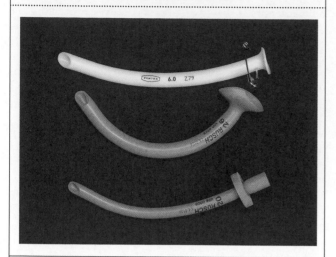

Source: Davey AJ, Diba A. Ward's Anaesthetic equipment. 5th ed. London: Elsevier Saunders; 2005.

FIGURE 15.2 Laryngeal mask airways.

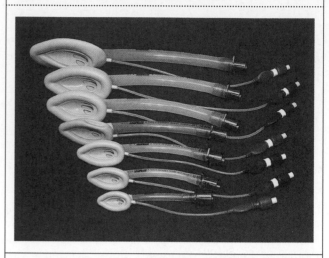

Source: Davey AJ, Diba A. Ward's Anaesthetic equipment. 5th ed. London: Elsevier Saunders; 2005.

facing up into the hard palate, then rotated 180 degrees, taking care to bring the tongue forwards and not push it back. Oropharyngeal airways are poorly tolerated in conscious patients and may cause gagging and vomiting.[21]

A nasopharyngeal airway (Fig. 15.1) is inserted through the nares into the oropharynx; it can be difficult to insert and require generous lubrication to minimise trauma. This type of airway should not be used for patients with a suspected head injury. As well as opening the airway, suction catheters can be passed to facilitate secretion clearance. Once inserted, these airways are better tolerated than an oropharyngeal airway.

Laryngeal mask airway and insertion

The classic laryngeal mask airway (cLMA) (Fig. 15.2) is positioned blindly into the pharynx to form a low-pressure seal against the laryngeal inlet. It is easier and quicker to insert than an endotracheal tube, and is particularly useful for operators with limited airway skills; the cLMA does not carry the same potentially fatal complications such as oesophageal intubation, although the risk of aspiration remains.[24]

Mechanical ventilation can be delivered with low airway pressures (less than 20 cmH$_2$O) via a cLMA. This device is widely used in elective general anaesthesia,[22] and can be used in critical care as an alternative to bag–mask ventilation[24] or endotracheal intubation when initial attempts at intubation have failed.[25] The 'intubating' LMA is most commonly used when a difficult intubation is anticipated or encountered. This device has a handle and is more rigid, wider and curved than the cLMA, enabling passage of a purpose-made endotracheal tube.[26]

Combitube

The combitube is more widely used in North America for emergency situations than in Australia and the UK.[22] It is a

dual-lumen, dual-cuff oesophageal–tracheal airway that enables ventilation if inserted into either the oesophagus or trachea. Inexperienced operators may find a combitube more difficult to insert correctly than a cLMA.[26] Complications may occur in up to 40% of patients and include aspiration pneumonitis, pneumothorax, airway injuries and bleeding, oesophageal laceration and perforation and mediastinitis.[27]

Endotracheal tubes

Endotracheal intubation is the 'gold standard' for airway support, providing airway protection in the presence of airway oedema, absent gag, cough or swallow reflex. Intubation facilitates mechanical ventilation and pulmonary secretion clearance.[23]

Endotracheal tubes (ETT) have common design characteristics, are generally made from polyvinyl chloride, are available with internal diameters ranging from 2 to 10 mm (common adult sizes are 7–9 mm; a size 6 mm should be available for difficult intubations) and are up to 30 cm long. A longitudinal radio-opaque line allows visualisation of tube placement on a chest X-ray. Markings at 1-cm intervals indicate the length from the distal end, a design feature that facilitates the ability to gauge insertion depth and monitor tube movement.[28] Tubes are available with and without a distal cuff, an inflatable balloon that seals the trachea, facilitates positive-pressure ventilation and prevents aspiration of oropharyngeal contents. Cuffs come in a range of profiles and volumes, but are commonly high-volume, low-pressure enabling application of a safe pressure over a larger surface area (Fig. 15.3). A smaller inflatable balloon, attached to the cuff via a pilot line, provides a tactile gauge of cuff pressure and a small air reservoir to prevent minor changes in cuff pressure.[29]

Endotracheal tubes reinforced with a wire coil embedded within the plastic along the entire tube length prevent kinking and occlusion. These tubes are more

FIGURE 15.3 Endotracheal tubes.

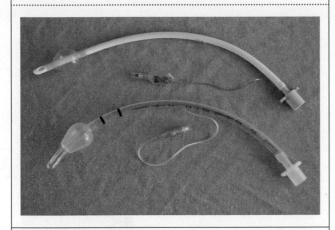

Source: Lewis S, Heitkemper M, Dirksen S, Medical–surgical nursing. 5th ed. St Louis Mosby 2000.

commonly used in the operating room.[30] The wire coils can be irreversibly compressed by a strong bite occluding the airway. Reinforced tubes also increase the risk of tracheal damage and should be replaced with a standard ETT on ICU arrival. Most ETTs have a 'Murphy eye', an oval-shaped hole in the side of the tube between the cuff and the tube end that provides a patent aperture if the distal opening is occluded.[31]

Double-lumen endotracheal tubes (DLT) enable independent lung ventilation (ILV) using two ventilators. ILV was initially developed for thoracic surgical procedures to allow ventilation of one lung while performing surgery on the other. ILV is also used in the critical care setting for isolation of a lung in patients with unilateral lung injury.[32] DLTs have a tracheal and a bronchial lumen; the bronchial lumen can be right or left sided. A left-sided DLT is used most commonly because positioning is easier. Fibreoptic bronchoscopy guidance is required to confirm proper placement. DLTs have a large overall diameter but separate lumens are smaller compared with single-lumen ETT leading to increased airway resistance. Secretion clearance through DLTs can be problematic and special care is needed to prevent tube dislocation and cuff overinflation.[32]

Preparation for intubation

Adequate preparation of the patient, equipment and environment, as well as knowledge of emergency procedures, is important to ensure safe and efficient intubation. Up to 50% of patients undergoing endotracheal intubation in the ICU experience complications; 28% will have a serious complication, including hypoxaemia, circulatory collapse, cardiac arrhythmia, cardiac arrest, oesophageal intubation, aspiration and death.[33] For these reasons, use of a checklist, clear allocation of roles, a time-out procedure, a mitigation plan for any concerns and verbal confirmation between team members are important at the start and during the procedure.

Patient preparation

If appropriate, and time permits, explain the procedure to the patient and family. Prepare the patient with:

- reliable intravenous access established to allow rapid fluid and drug administration
- accurate blood pressure monitoring (preferably intra-arterial)
- continuous oxygen saturation and ECG monitoring
- nasogastric tube (if in situ), which should be aspirated and placed on free drainage
- positioning supine in the 'sniff' position.

Equipment and drugs

All equipment should be available and checked immediately prior to intubation, including:

- oxygen supply
- suction supply, with a range of Yankauer and y-suction catheters/closed suction device
- laryngoscope blades and compatible holder, with a functioning light, including second laryngoscope in case of device failure
- appropriately-sized face mask
- manual ventilation with a bag valve mask (e.g. Ambu® resuscitator) attached to an oxygen supply
- ETT cuff inflated in sterile water to ensure no leaks and even inflation, with additional ETT tubes available if needed
- water-based lubricant of tube and cuff (while maintaining sterility)
- capnography (chemical CO_2 detectors are often used in emergency situations)
- ventilator and circuit
- emergency/resuscitation trolley at bedside
- gloves, eye protection
- drugs (sedative and muscle relaxant; NB: sedatives should be administered before a muscle relaxant so that the patient is unaware of paralysis).

> **Practice tip**
>
> During intubation, know who to call for help, and do not hesitate to do so.

Procedure

The patient is preoxygenated to minimise desaturation during apnoea and laryngoscopy, commonly via bag and mask, although other methods such as NIV,[34] heated and humidified nasal oxygen,[35] and flush rate oxygen by face mask may improve preoxygenation compared with a traditional face mask.[36] The practice of apnoeic oxygenation during endotracheal intubation through the administration of 15 L/min via nasal cannula has become popular in emergency departments. To date there is insufficient evidence to recommend its routine use during endotracheal intubation in the critically ill. Intubation in ICU is usually performed via laryngoscopy with insertion of an oral ETT. Intubation may be performed using a fibreoptic bronchoscope when difficulty is encountered, or for nasal intubation.

Oral vs nasal intubation

Oral intubation is preferred unless there are specific indications for nasal intubation. Oral intubation is easier to perform and allows use of a larger-diameter ETT. While nasal intubation provides better splinting for the ETT and facilitates oral hygiene, it can damage nasal structures, is contraindicated in skull fractures, and due to increased risk of maxillary sinusitis and ventilator-associated pneumonia (VAP) is not recommended for ventilation longer than 24 hours.[37]

Cricoid pressure

The cricoid cartilage, situated below the thyroid prominence, is a closed tracheal ring which, when compressed, closes the oesophagus while the trachea remains open. Cricoid pressure is performed by placing the thumb on one side of the patient's trachea, middle finger on the other side and index finger directly on the cricoid.[38] Although widely used, its efficacy is questionable as technique is frequently poor,[39] and there is wide anatomical variation in the exact orientation of the oesophagus in relation to the trachea.[40]

Backwards, upwards, rightwards pressure manoeuvre

The backwards, upwards, rightwards pressure (BURP) manoeuvre on the thyroid cartilage was introduced in the mid 1990s to improve visualisation during difficult laryngoscopy. The patient's jaw is thrust forward, so the head is in the 'sniffing' position. The thumb and third finger are placed on either side of the thyroid cartilage and the index finger on top. Pressure is applied in the sequence *b*ackwards (towards the spine), *u*pwards (towards the head), *r*ightwards (towards the *p*atient's right side). This is easier to perform following administration of muscle relaxants.

Cuff management

Endotracheal and tracheostomy tube cuffs prevent airway contamination by pharyngeal secretions and gastric contents and loss of V_T during mechanical ventilation. The cuff does not secure the tube in the trachea.

Confirmation of tube position

The correct position of the ETT distal end is 3–5 cm above the carina. A lip level of 20 cm for women and 22 cm for men should prevent endobronchial intubation, with the proximal end fixed at either the centre or the side of the mouth.[41] Confirmation of the ETT position via chest X-ray is required immediately following intubation and at regular intervals thereafter as tube movement can occur.

Chest auscultation and observation of chest expansion to confirm ETT position is unreliable, as the chest may appear to rise with oesophageal intubation. Conversely, the chest may not rise with a correctly positioned tube if the patient is obese or has a rigid chest wall. Patients with left main bronchus intubation may exhibit bilateral breath sounds.[42] End-tidal CO_2 monitoring is the 'gold standard' method to confirm endotracheal placement and exclude oesophageal intubation (see Chapter 13 for further information on end-tidal CO_2 monitoring). Disposable devices that change colour in the presence of CO_2 are inexpensive and easy to use, but may be inaccurate during cardiopulmonary resuscitation, or if contaminated. Capnography is the most reliable technique to identify ETT placement in both arrest and non-arrest situations.[25] Continuous end-tidal CO_2 monitoring during intubation is recommended as a minimum standard by the College of Intensive Care Medicine of Australia and New Zealand.[43]

> **Practice tip**
>
> Always ensure there is someone who is skilled at intubation immediately available when extubating a patient.

Tracheostomy

Tracheostomy may be required for upper airway obstruction, although it is most commonly performed for ICU patients requiring prolonged mechanical ventilation. The advantages of tracheostomy over endotracheal intubation include decreased risk of laryngeal damage and subglottic stenosis, reduced airway resistance and dead space, which decreases the work of breathing and therefore supports weaning[44] and improved patient tolerance, enabling sedation reduction. The optimum time to perform tracheostomy remains contentious, and is often influenced by patient diagnosis.[45]

Procedure

Tracheostomy can be performed using a surgical or percutaneous dilational technique. Percutaneous dilation is contraindicated in patients with anatomical anomalies of the neck and serious bleeding disorders, and should be undertaken with caution in patients who are obese, have a cervical spine injury, coagulopathy, difficult airway or require high levels of ventilatory support.[46] Percutaneous dilation is more commonly performed than the surgical technique in Australian and New Zealand ICUs.[46]

A variety of tracheostomy tubes are available that facilitate secretion clearance, communication and differing patient anatomy. Inner cannulas (reusable or disposable) prevent secretion build up on the tracheostomy tube, while fenestrated and talking tracheostomies facilitate communication, as do one-way valves, such as the Passy–Muir® valve, used with the cuff deflated.

Tracheostomy care

The aim of tracheostomy care is to keep the stoma free of infection and prevent tube blockage or dislodgement. The stoma should be assessed at least every 24 hours for trauma, infection or inflammation and fixation devices are changed with two nurses required to safely perform changes.[47] Velcro tapes are easier to change and more comfortable than cotton tape.[48] Lint-free or superabsorbent foam dressings are used under the flange to absorb secretions. Adequate humidification and suctioning will usually prevent tube obstruction (see later in this chapter). The use of inner cannulae has obviated the need for frequent tracheostomy tube changes. Single-lumen (no inner cannula) tracheostomy tubes should be changed every 7–10 days.[47]

Minitracheostomy

A minitracheostomy, a small-bore tracheal cannula with a diameter of 4 mm, can be inserted percutaneously in patients with an ineffective cough to facilitate respiratory secretion clearance via endotracheal suctioning. A minitracheostomy is generally used after tracheostomy removal but may be used in patients for secretion clearance that have not required tracheostomy such as those with neurological compromise. The minitracheostomy preserves glottic function and maintenance of phonation but does not provide airway protection and therefore cannot be used for invasive ventilation. Complications associated with use of a minitracheostomy occur infrequently; those complications that do occur are associated with difficulty inserting and positioning the tube.[49, 50]

Complications of endotracheal intubation and tracheostomy

Tube blockage, tube dislodgement and aspiration are major complications. Partial ETT or tracheostomy tube dislodgement can cause greater harm than complete removal because of delays in diagnosis and resultant aspiration and worsening gas exchange. Tube dislodgement is most likely to occur when turning the patient, in agitated patients or when nursing staff are busy with other tasks or on breaks.[51] While physical restraint may be considered to prevent tube dislodgement, multiple studies have noted patients were restrained when self-extubation or device removal occurred.[52–55] Appropriate levels of analgesia and sedation are therefore required for minimising self-extubation risk.

Complications during, and immediately after, endotracheal intubation and tracheostomy include cardiovascular compromise, bleeding, tracheal wall injury, vocal cord damage, pneumothorax, pneumomediastinum and subcutaneous emphysema. Late complications of tracheostomy include tracheal stenosis, tracheomalacia and tracheo-oesophageal fistula and infection. As noted

earlier, damage to the trachea is exacerbated by high cuff pressures.[56] Percutaneous tracheostomy results in fewer wound infections, decreased incidence of bleeding and reduced mortality compared with surgical tracheostomy.[57]

Managing endotracheal and tracheostomy tubes

Tracheal suction

Patients with an ETT or tracheostomy tube require tracheal suction to remove pulmonary secretions that can lead to atelectasis or airway obstruction and impair gas exchange.[58] Suction should be performed as clinically indicated, with assessment of visible or audible secretions, rising inspiratory pressure, decreasing V_T or increased work of breathing.[59] A sawtooth pattern on the flow-volume waveform may also indicate the need for suction (discussed later in this chapter).[60]

Preoxygenation using a FiO_2 of 1.0 for approximately 60 seconds prior to suctioning is commonly performed, though not supported by strong evidence unless the patient is experiencing hypoxia or has compromised cerebral circulation.[61] Preoxygenation of patients without hypoxia should be avoided as it may cause harm associated with oxygen toxicity. If a patient's oxygen saturation declines to an unacceptable level during suctioning, the FiO_2 should be increased to 1.0. Manual hyperinflation should be discouraged owing to the risk of haemodynamic compromise, derecruitment, barotrauma and lack of evidence of benefit.[62] Similarly, installation of saline is not supported because of the adverse effect on oxygen saturation.[63]

Methods

The three methods of suctioning are:

- *Open suction:* a suction catheter is passed under aseptic technique directly into the ETT/tracheostomy after disconnection from the ventilator circuit. Disadvantages include loss of PEEP resulting in alveolar derecruitment and increased risk of transmission of infective organisms. A surgical mask and protective eyewear should be worn.[64]

- *Semi-closed suction:* a suction catheter is passed through a swivel connector with a self-sealing rubber flange.

- *Closed suction:* in-line system is attached between the ETT/tracheostomy tube and the ventilator circuit where the suction catheter is contained in an integrated plastic sleeve. Alveolar derecruitment occurs to a lesser degree than with open suction.

There is no difference between techniques in relation to development of VAP and quantity of secretions removed.

The suction catheter diameter should not be greater than half the airway diameter, using the formula: suction catheter size (French) = (ETT size (mm) − 1) × 2. The suction catheter should be inserted to the carina, then withdrawn 2 cm before suction is applied to prevent mucosal damage. Suction should last only 15 seconds, using continuous, rather than intermittent, suction. Suction pressure should be set as low as possible, with <150 mmHg recommended for adults and <100 mmHg for neonates.[59] Use of ETTs or tracheostomy tubes with integrated subglottic suction ports may assist in preventing VAP, especially when performed with other prevention strategies such as semi-recumbent positioning and good cuff seal management.

Adverse effects

Adverse effects of suctioning include hypoxaemia, introduction of infective organisms, tracheal trauma, bradycardia, hypertension and increased intracranial pressure. Tracheal suctioning causes discomfort, and should therefore be performed only when clinically indicated, such as audible presence of secretions, desaturation and when a saw-tooth pattern is observed on the flow time scalar and flow/volume loop.[61,62]

Securing endotracheal and tracheostomy tubes

The purpose of ETT and tracheostomy tube fixation is to maintain the tube in the correct position, prevent unintended extubation or dislodgement and facilitate mechanical ventilation while maintaining skin integrity and oral hygiene.[65] ETT fixation methods include:

- tying cotton tape around the tube, then around the neck
- taping the tube to the face using medical adhesive tape
- commercial tube holders of varying designs.

There is no evidence supporting a preferred method[66] with each having specific strengths and weaknesses. A manikin study comparing cotton tapes with the Thomas Endotracheal Tube Holder demonstrated less ETT movement with the commercial tube holder.[67] Two nurses are required to prevent ETT dislodgement during fixation. Although there is also no evidence recommending a preferred frequency, ETT fixation is generally changed at least daily, to allow assessment of the underlying skin with particular attention to the ears and corners of the mouth and to facilitate oral hygiene.[65] The ETT position in the mouth is alternated at this time. ETT fixation devices including cotton ties, if applied too tightly can compress the internal or external jugular veins, which increases intracranial pressure due to reduced vascular drainage.[68] Avoid compression of internal or external jugular veins with tight cervical collar or tight tape fixation of the endotracheal tube that would impede cerebral venous drainage and result in an increase in the ICP.

> **Practice tip**
>
> Adhesive devices may become dislodged as facial hair grows under them.

Cuff pressure management

Cuff inflation pressures should be maintained at 20–30 cmH$_2$O (15–22 mmHg). Tracheal wall damage may occur if cuff pressure exceeds tracheal capillary perfusion pressure (27–40 cmH$_2$O/20–30 mmHg). Cuff inflation pressures ≤20 cmH$_2$O (15 mmHg) are associated with an increased risk of aspiration and an increase in VAP.[69]

There are four methods for assessing cuff inflation:

1 minimal occluding volume
2 minimal leak test
3 cuff pressure measurement
4 palpation.

Palpation of the pilot balloon is perhaps the most available and easy technique for monitoring cuff inflation but is highly subjective and inaccurate, therefore use of a manometer to measure cuff pressure is recommended.[70] Cuff pressure measurement requires a manometer attached to the pilot balloon. Cuff pressure varies with head and body position, tube position and airway pressures.[71,72] The optimum frequency of cuff pressure monitoring is unclear, with infrequent monitoring probably as safe as frequent monitoring.[73] Continuous cuff pressure measurement may reduce VAP.[74] Even with appropriate cuff inflation micro-aspiration occurs via the longitudinal folds in the cuff.[75]

If performing minimal occluding volume and minimal leak test, aspiration should be prevented by semirecumbent positioning, suctioning the back of the mouth (as far back as tolerated), aspiration of the nasogastric tube and discontinuation of feeds before cuff deflation.

Subglottic secretion management

For the intubated patient, oropharyngeal secretions drain into the subglottic space, pool above the cuff, and gradually leak via the longitudinal cuff folds to the lungs increasing the risk of pneumonia. Subglottic secretion drainage (SSD), a dedicated lumen within the ETT dorsal wall that exits above the cuff, enables removal of subglottic secretions either continuously via low-pressure suction or intermittently via either suction or a syringe. Tracheal mucosa injuries induced by suctioning may occur with both continuous and intermittent suctioning in up to 27% of patients.[76,77] A 2016 systematic review and meta-analysis found SSD to reduce the risk of VAP and the duration of ventilation, though there was no evidence of effect on ICU or hospital mortality or length of stay.[78]

Managing emergencies associated with endotracheal and tracheostomy tubes

Pilot tube

If the pilot tube for the ETT or tracheostomy tube is accidentally cut or a hole is suspected in the tubing or balloon, cannulate the tubing with a 23- or 24-gauge needle to re-inflate the cuff and clamp the tubing. If using a clamp with serrations, place gauze between the tube and the clamps to avoid further damage to the pilot tube.

Cuff herniation

ETT cuff herniation occurs infrequently with low-pressure, high-volume cuffs, may be difficult to diagnose, but can cause life-threatening bronchial obstruction.[79] If cuff herniation is suspected (profound desaturation, loss of breath sounds), deflate and re-inflate the cuff, checking the cuff pressure is within normal range. If the problem persists, the tube will need changing.

Persistent cuff leaks

Cuff leaks may be categorised as leaks around an intact cuff or those due to structural damage to the cuff.[80] Structural damage generally requires replacement of the tube, particularly if leaks are large and ventilation is ineffective.

Practice tip

A persistent cuff leak as indicated by bubbling or other noises suggestive of gas leak and loss of V_T or cuff pressures of ≥ 30 cmH$_2$O (22 mmHg) indicating failure to generate a seal should be reviewed; check ETT position for migration and refer to medical staff.

Extubation

Following successful weaning from mechanical ventilation (see later in this chapter), assessment of the patient prior to extubation should indicate adequate gas exchange, respiratory rate and work of breathing on minimal support, respiratory muscle strength; the ability to cough and clear secretions spontaneously; and a stable haemodynamic and mental status.[81] Serious postextubation complications of laryngospasm and stridor cannot be reliably predicted,[82] so the ease/grade of intubation should be considered prior to extubation and provision made for immediate re-intubation.[83] Methods for extubation are the positive-pressure technique and the more conventional technique, consisting of inserting a suction catheter into the ETT and the trachea, deflating the cuff and removing the ETT while continuously suctioning during the whole procedure. The positive-pressure technique involves applying a pressure level during cuff deflation and extubation. Both strategies aim to minimise leakage of oropharyngeal fluids into the distal airway. There is some evidence that extubation with positive pressure has a lower incidence of complications like upper airway obstruction, desaturation and vomiting.[84]

Mechanical ventilation

Primary goals of mechanical ventilation include ensuring adequate oxygenation, carbon dioxide elimination and respiratory muscle unloading while decreasing the oxygen cost of breathing.[85]

Principles of mechanical ventilation

Mechanical ventilation describes the application of positive- or negative-pressure breaths using non-invasive or invasive techniques. Indications for initiation of mechanical ventilation are discussed below. Table 15.1 lists the patient parameters typically observed in acute and chronic respiratory failure that may influence the decision to ventilate. During positive-pressure ventilation, the type of ventilation used most commonly in critical care, the ventilator delivers a flow of gas into the lungs during inspiration using a pneumatic system. Expiration is passive.

The equation of motion

The equation of motion for the respiratory system is a mathematical model that relates pressure, volume and flow during breath delivery, with the pressure required to deliver a volume of gas determined by the elastic and resistive properties of the respiratory system[86] (Table 15.2).

Compliance and elastance

Compliance refers to the ease with which lung units distend. Elastance is the tendency of the lung units to return to their original form once stretched. Compliance (C) is defined as the change in volume that occurs due to a change in pressure and is expressed as $C = \Delta V/\Delta P$.

Lung tissue and the surrounding thoracic structures contribute to respiratory compliance. Normal compliance for a mechanically ventilated patient ranges from 35 to 50 mL/cmH$_2$O.[87]

Resistance

Resistance refers to the forces that oppose air flow. Resistance in the airways is influenced by large and small airway diameter including the artificial airway, airway length, the gas flow rate and the density and viscosity of the inspired gas. For example, narrowing of airways causes increased resistance, as do higher gas flows owing to turbulent flow. During mechanical ventilation, bronchospasm, airway oedema, endotracheal tube lumen size, increased secretions and inappropriate setting of flow rates can influence airway resistance. Normal resistance for intubated patients is 6 cmH$_2$O/(L/s).[87]

Driving pressure

The driving pressure (ΔP), the pressure that the ventilator applies when delivering a tidal volume, is a measure of the stress that is placed on the lungs with each breath. ΔP can be calculated for patients who are not making inspiratory efforts by subtracting PEEP from the plateau pressure (Pplat). It is advised to minimise the intensity of ventilation by setting the ventilator so that the driving pressure (ΔP) remains below 15 cmH$_2$O.[88]

Mechanical power

Mechanical energy is the energy that is transferred from the ventilator to the lungs. The amount of energy transferred over time that is delivered from the ventilator

TABLE 15.1

Physiological indications suggesting the need for mechanical ventilation

PARAMETER	NORMAL VALUES	ARF	CRF	ASSOCIATED SIGNS AND SYMPTOMS
Respiratory rate	12–20	≥28	≥30	Dyspnoea, increased activation of accessory muscles and active expiration.
pH	7.35–7.45	<7.30 No compensatory changes.	7.35–7.40 May be normal due to metabolic compensation.	Failure to adequately ventilate: elevated $PaCO_2$, acidic pH, headache, confusion or other mental status change, tachypnoea (RR >30), flushed skin.
$PaCO_2$	35–45 mmHg	>50 mmHg and rising.	>50 mmHg and rising.	
PaO_2	80–100 mmHg	<65 mmHg and falling.	<50 mmHg and falling Hb/HCT elevated as compensatory mechanism.	Failure to adequately oxygenate: decreased PaO_2 and SpO_2, tachycardia, hyper- or hypotension, dyspnoea, gasping, nasal flaring, use of accessory muscles, anxiety, agitation and altered mental status, cyanosis.
HCO_3^-	22–26 mmol/L	Within normal Limits.	If chronic hypercapnia, then HCO_3^- >26 mmol/L is a compensatory mechanism. If CRF is primarily failure to oxygenate, then HCO_3^- will be within normal limits.	

ARF = acute respiratory failure; CRF = chronic respiratory failure; HCT = haematocrit; RR = respiratory rate.

TABLE 15.2

Equation of motion

EQUATION:

$P_T (P_{airway} + P_{muscle}) = V_T/C + V_T/T_I \times R + PEEP_T$

Abbreviations:

P_T = total pressure – the sum of the pressure in the proximal airway and the pressure generated by the respiratory muscles
V_T = tidal volume
C = compliance
T_I = inspiratory time
R = resistance
$PEEP_T$ = total positive end-expiratory pressure – alveolar pressure at the end of expiration and is the sum of PEEP applied by the ventilator and any intrinsic (auto) PEEP
Notes: V_T/C: describes the elastic properties of the respiratory system.
V_T/T_I: reflects flow in the system $V_T/T_I \times R$: resistance of the respiratory system.

to the lungs is called mechanical power (MP). It is a summary value; the respiratory rate, tidal volume, peak pressure or maximum pressure and driving pressure are used to calculate the MP.[89]

Ventilator graphics

Analysis of ventilator graphics provides clinicians with the ability to assess patient–ventilator interaction, appropriateness of ventilator settings and lung function.

Scalars: pressure/time, flow/time, volume/time

Many ventilators now offer integrated graphic displays as waveforms that plot one of three parameters – pressure, flow or volume – on the vertical (y) axis against time, measured in seconds, on the horizontal (x) axis, referred to as scalars. Examination of scalars can assist with assessment of patient–ventilator synchrony, patient triggering, appropriateness of inspiratory/expiratory times, presence of gas trapping, appropriateness and adequacy of flow, lung compliance, and airway resistance and circuit leaks.[90–93]

Pressure versus time scalar

The morphology of this waveform depends on the control variable (volume or pressure), breath type (mandatory or spontaneous) and whether the breath is initiated by the ventilator or the patient's inspiratory effort.[92] Pressure–time waveforms reflect airway pressure (P_{aw}) during inspiration and expiration and can be used to evaluate peak and plateau inspiratory pressures and end-expiratory pressures, inspiratory and expiratory times, and appropriateness of flow (Fig. 15.4). The peak pressure represents the maximum pressure achieved during

inspiration. The plateau pressure is measured during an inspiratory hold and represents the pressure applied to the small airways and alveoli. The expiratory pressure is the pressure measured once the patient has expired. Pressure–time scalars vary in appearance depending on the control variable (volume vs pressure). In *volume-control breaths* (see Fig. 15.4) the inspiratory waveform continues to rise until peak inspiratory pressure is achieved according to V_T set. If an inspiratory hold is applied, a plateau pressure will be generated. As the patient expires, airway pressure will drop back to the set PEEP level. *In pressure-control breaths*, the

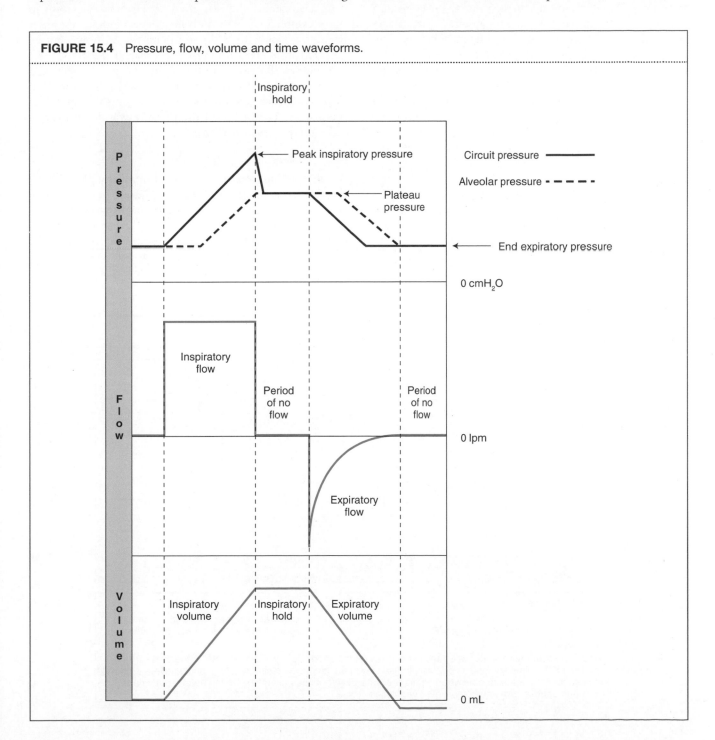

FIGURE 15.4   Pressure, flow, volume and time waveforms.

inspiratory waveform reaches its peak at the beginning of inspiration and remains at this elevation until cycling to expiration.

When interpreting the pressure waveform it is important to recognise that the graphic waveforms display circuit pressure, which does not always represent alveolar pressure. Periods of no flow (inspiratory and expiratory holds/pauses) are required to estimate alveolar pressure. The plateau pressure is a more reliable estimate of inspiratory alveolar pressure than the peak inspiratory pressure. An expiratory hold is required to determine end expiratory alveolar pressure. Estimating alveolar pressure may be useful to assess the patient's respiratory resistance and compliance. Comparing the difference between the peak inspiratory pressure and plateau pressure can give an indication of the patient's inspiratory resistance. Comparing the difference between the plateau pressure and the end-expiratory pressure can provide information about the patient's compliance.

Spontaneous triggering of ventilation can be identified by examination of the pressure–time scalar at the beginning of inspiration. A small negative deflection indicates patient effort. When pressure triggering is used, a breath is triggered when the pressure drops below baseline. The depth of the deflection is proportional to the patient effort required to trigger inspiration (Fig. 15.5). A flow-triggered breath occurs when the flow rises above baseline, although this is frequently accompanied by a small negative deflection in the pressure–time scalar. Patient inspiratory attempts that fail to trigger the ventilator can also be identified as negative deflections in the pressure waveform without corresponding responses from the ventilator.[93] Appropriateness of flow can be detected from the pressure–time scalar. If the flow is set too high or the rise time too short, this can be seen as a sharp peak in the waveform (see Fig. 15.5). Conversely, if flow is inadequate or the rise time too long, the incline of the inspiratory portion of the pressure waveform may be dampened or even negative.[90]

Flow versus time scalar

The flow–time scalar presents the inspiratory phase above the horizontal axis and the expiratory phase below (Fig. 15.6). The shape of the inspiratory flow waveform is influenced by the selection of flow pattern (constant, decelerating, sinusoidal) in volume-control breaths or the variable and decelerating flow waveform associated with

---

Practice tip

- A large difference between peak and plateau pressures indicates high airway resistance.
- An elevated plateau pressure indicates reduced compliance.

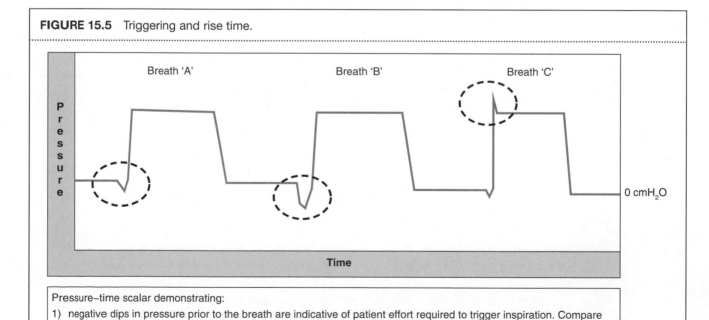

FIGURE 15.5 Triggering and rise time.

Pressure–time scalar demonstrating:

1) negative dips in pressure prior to the breath are indicative of patient effort required to trigger inspiration. Compare the drop in pressure in breath 'A' to breath 'B'. The greater drop in pressure in breath 'B' indicates a greater patient effort to trigger gas flow.

2) the effect on the pressure time scalar when the rise time is set too short. Note the 'overshootx' in the pressure waveform on breath 'C'. This sometimes occurs in patients with a high airway resistance (e.g. acute severe asthma) and a short rise time. It is questionable whether this pressure overshoot has any effect on the patient but it can trigger the high-pressure alarm and compromise ventilation.

FIGURE 15.6 Flow versus time waveform.

Unbel	Flow wave pattern	Description
(Rectangular, square)	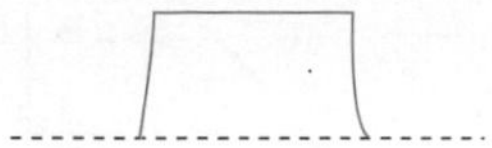	Peak flow rate is delivered immediately at the onset of inspiration, maintained throughout the inspiratory phase, and abruptly terminated at the onset of expiration.
		Common default pattern with volume-targeted modes.
Sinusoidal	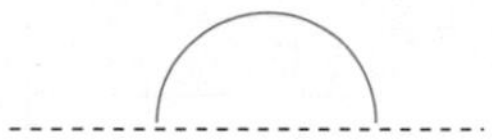	Inspiratory flow rate gradually accelerates to peak flow and then tapers off.
		Believed to mimic spontaneous inspiratory patterns.
		May increase peak inspiratory pressure (PIP).
Accelerating (ascending ramp)	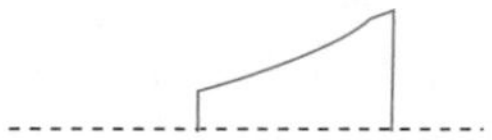	Flow gradually accelerates in a linear fashion to the set peak flow rate.
Decelerating (descending ramp)	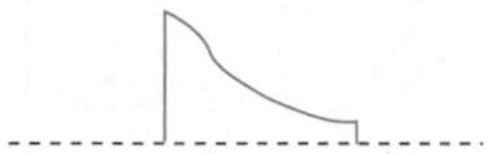	Flow is at peak at onset of inspiration and gradually decelerates throughout inspiratory phase.
		Flow ceases and ventilator cycles to expiratory phase when flow decays to a percentage of peak flow, usually 25% but varies by ventilator model. Terminal flow criteria may be adjustable in some newer ventilators.
		Rapid intial flow raises mean airway pressure and may assist in alveolar recruitment.
		May improve the distribution of gases when there is inhomogeneity of alveolar ventilation.
		Decreases dead space, increases arterial oxygen tension, and reduces PIP.

Source: Reproduced from Pierce LNB. Management of the mechanically ventilated patient. 2nd ed. St Louis, MO: Saunders Elsevier; 2007, Table 6.3, p 195.

pressure-control breaths. The inspiratory flow waveform of spontaneous breaths, those triggered and cycled by the patient, is influenced by the presence or absence of pressure support and the expiratory sensitivity.[90]

Evaluation of the expiratory limb of the flow–time scalar assists with detection of gas trapping and the patient's response to bronchodilators. In the absence of gas trapping, the expiratory limb drops sharply below baseline then gradually returns to zero before the next breath. Failure to return to baseline indicates gas trapping whereby the inspired gas is not totally expired. Gas trapping results in development of intrinsic or 'auto-PEEP'. This can adversely affect a patient's haemodynamic status and cause patient–ventilator asynchrony.[94] Gas trapping may occur in patients with air-flow limitation such as those with COPD and asthma. Consequences of gas trapping include dynamic hyperinflation, reduced respiratory compliance and respiratory muscle fatigue.[95] Evaluation of the expiratory flow waveform also enables evaluation of the effects of bronchodilator therapy as, if efficacious, the expiratory flow waveform will return to baseline (Fig. 15.7).[94] Patient–ventilator asynchrony can be detected in the flow waveform as abrupt decreases in expiratory flow in the expiratory limb and abrupt increases in flow in the inspiratory limb.[93]

Volume versus time scalar

The volume–time waveform originates from the functional residual capacity (baseline), rises as inspiratory flow is delivered to reach the maximum inspiratory V_T, then returns to baseline during expiration. The waveform is useful in troubleshooting circuit leaks (Fig. 15.8) as it will fail to return to baseline if a leak in the circuit–patient interface is present.

Loops: pressure–volume, flow–volume

Most contemporary critical care ventilators allow for monitoring of pressure, flow and volume parameters

FIGURE 15.7 Auto-PEEP and gas trapping.

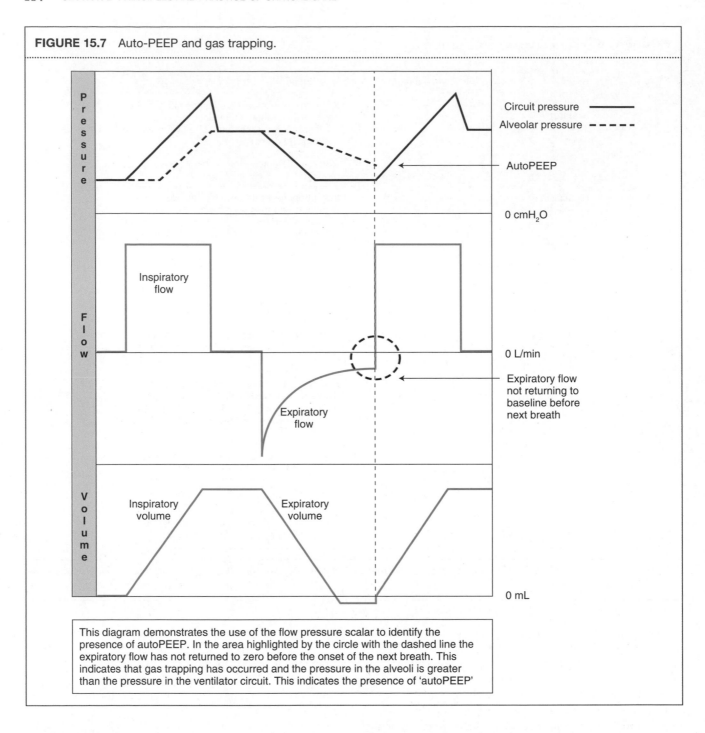

This diagram demonstrates the use of the flow pressure scalar to identify the presence of autoPEEP. In the area highlighted by the circle with the dashed line the expiratory flow has not returned to zero before the onset of the next breath. This indicates that gas trapping has occurred and the pressure in the alveoli is greater than the pressure in the ventilator circuit. This indicates the presence of 'autoPEEP'

FIGURE 15.8 Tidal volume versus time, with and without leak.

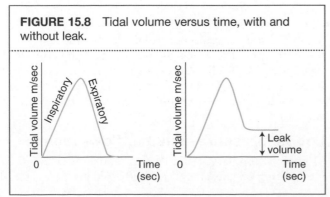

integrated into graphic loops enabling measurement of airway resistance, chest wall and lung compliance.

Pressure–volume loops

The two parameters P_{aw} and V_T are plotted against each other, with P_{aw} on the x axis. For mandatory breaths, the loop is drawn counterclockwise (Fig.15.9). Spontaneous (triggered and cycled) breaths are drawn in a clockwise fashion. When low gas flow is delivered and the patient is unable to initiate ventilation, pressure–volume loops may be used to identify the lower and upper inflection points. The lower inflection point begins near the beginning of inspiration as the P_{aw} starts to rise with little change in V_T. As P_{aw}

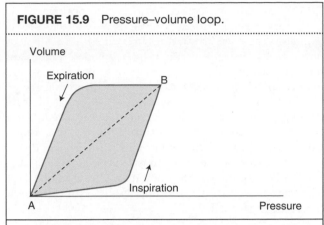

FIGURE 15.9 Pressure–volume loop.

Source: Adapted from: Draegerwerk AG & Co. https://www.draeger.com/sites/assets/Publixhingiages/Products/savina-300/UK/9097421-Figel-Curves_Loops-en.pdf p. 26, with permssion.

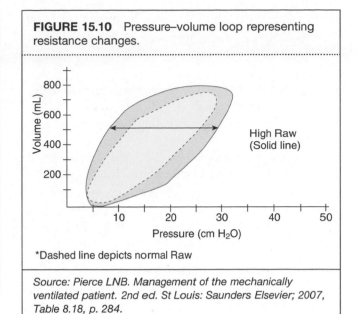

FIGURE 15.10 Pressure–volume loop representing resistance changes.

*Dashed line depicts normal Raw

Source: Pierce LNB. Management of the mechanically ventilated patient. 2nd ed. St Louis: Saunders Elsevier; 2007, Table 8.18, p. 284.

continues to rise, the V_T increases exponentially as alveoli are recruited, resulting in a marked increase in the inspiratory limb slope. This point represents alveolar recruitment and is referred to as the lower inflection point, and may be used to guide PEEP selection.[96,97] The inspiratory limb continues until peak inspiratory pressure and maximal V_T are achieved. The bend in the inspiratory limb towards the end of inspiration is referred to as the upper inflection point, and denotes the point at which small volume increases produce large pressure increases indicating lung overdistention.[96] The expiratory limb represents lung derecruitment and is also useful in guiding PEEP selection.[98,99]

For patient-triggered mandatory breaths, the initial part of the loop occurs to the left of the y axis and flows in a clockwise fashion, reflecting patient effort. The loop then shifts to the right of the y axis and moves in a counterclockwise fashion as the ventilator assumes the work of breathing.[87] Pressure–volume loops reflect dynamic compliance between the lungs and the ventilator circuit. Decreased compliance requires greater pressure to achieve V_T and is reflected in a flattened pressure–volume loop.[100] The area between the loops represents the resistance to inspiration and expiration, known as *hysteresis*. As resistance increases, less V_T is delivered resulting in a shorter and wider loop; conversely, as resistance decreases, a longer, wider loop is generated (Fig. 15.10).[101]

Flow–volume loops

Flow–volume loops recorded during positive-pressure ventilation depict inspiration above the baseline and expiration below it. These loops are useful in determining response to bronchodilators and examining changes in airway resistance.

Ventilator circuits

Delivery of mechanical ventilation requires a ventilator circuit to transport gas flow to the patient. To prevent condensation from cooling of warm humidified gas, inspired gas is heated via a wire inside the circuit wall in either the inspiratory limb alone or both the inspiratory and expiratory limbs.[102] Historically ventilator circuits were changed frequently (48–72 hours) to decrease the risk of VAP.[103] Current guidelines and recommendations for VAP prevention found evidence that the frequency of ventilator circuit changes did not reduce VAP incidence; indeed, frequent changes may increase VAP owing to circuit manipulation. Therefore, routine circuit changes were not necessary and circuits should be changed only when soiled or damaged.[104,105]

Humidification

Humidification warms and moistens gas to facilitate cilia action and mucus removal as well as to prevent drying and irritation of respiratory mucosa and solidification of secretions. During endotracheal intubation and mechanical ventilation, the normal humidification processes of the nasopharynx are bypassed. This, in combination with the use of dry medical gas at high flow rates, means alternative methods of humidification are required. The best conditions for mucosal health and function over prolonged periods are when inspired gas is warmed to core body temperature and is fully saturated with water.[106]

Absolute and relative humidity

Absolute humidity refers to the amount of water vapour in a given volume of gas at a given temperature. Absolute humidity rises with increasing temperature; during mechanical ventilation gas is heated to increase the amount of water vapour it will hold. Relative humidity is expressed as a percentage, and is the actual amount of water vapour in a gas compared with the maximum amount this gas can hold (ratio of absolute to maximal humidity). Ideal humidification is achieved when the:

- inspired gas delivered into the trachea is at 37°C with a water content of 30–43 g/m³ (relative humidity is 100% at 37°C in the bronchi)

- set temperature remains constant without fluctuation
- humidification and temperature are unaffected by large or differing types of gas flow
- device is simple to use
- humidifier can be used with spontaneously breathing and ventilated patients
- safety alarms prevent overheating, overhydration and electrocution
- resistance, compliance and dead-space characteristics do not adversely affect spontaneous breathing modes
- sterility of the inspired gas is not compromised.[107]

Humidification is applied using either a heat–moisture exchanger (HME) or a heated water bath reservoir device in combination with a heated ventilator circuit.

Heat–moisture exchanger

HMEs conserve heat and moisture during expiration, enabling inspired gas to be heated and humidified, and are generally combined with a microbiological filter. Two types of HMEs exist: hygroscopic and hydrophobic. Hygroscopic HMEs absorb moisture onto a chemically impregnated foam or paper material whereas hydrophobic HMEs contain a hydrophobic membrane with small pores. HMEs are placed distally to the circuit Y-piece in line with the ETT and increase dead space by an amount equal to their internal volume.[108] HMEs should be changed every 24 hours or when soiled with secretions and are usually reserved for short-term humidification.

Heated humidification

Heated humidification is often used for patients requiring greater than 24 hours of mechanical ventilation. Various models of heater bases and circuits are on the market and we recommend their use in accordance with manufacturer instructions. However, a recent systematic review and meta-analysis that included 34 trials (2848 participants) reported no difference on artificial airway occlusion, pneumonia or mortality comparing HMEs with heated humidification, although evidence certainty was low.[109] There was some evidence that hydrophobic HMEs may reduce the risk of pneumonia compared with heated humidification.

Non-invasive ventilation

NIV is an umbrella term describing the delivery of mechanical ventilation without the use of an invasive airway, via an interface such as an oronasal, nasal or full-face mask, nasal pillows or helmet. NIV techniques include both negative- and positive-pressure ventilation, although in critical care positive-pressure ventilation is primarily used.

Terminology

NIPPV is the provision of inspiratory pressure support, also referred to as inspiratory positive airway pressure (IPAP) usually in combination with positive end-expiratory pressure (PEEP). PEEP is also referred to as expiratory positive airway pressure (EPAP). CPAP does not actively assist inspiration but provides a constant positive airway pressure throughout inspiration and expiration, which can decrease work of breathing.[110]

The terms biphasic (or bilevel) positive airway pressure (BiPAP®) and non-invasive pressure support ventilation (NIPSV) are also used to refer to NIPPV.[111] The acronym BiPAP® is registered to Respironics (Murrayville, PA), a company that produces non-invasive ventilators including the BiPAP® Vision, which is commonly used in the ICU. The acronym NIPSV is primarily used in European descriptions of NIPPV.

> **Practice tip**
>
> When other members of the ICU team use the term BiPAP/BIPAP, clarify whether they are referring to non-invasive or invasive ventilation.

Physiological benefits

The efficacy of NIV in patients with acute respiratory failure is, at least in part, related to avoidance of inspiratory muscle fatigue through the addition of inspiratory positive pressure hence reducing inspiratory muscle work.[112] Application of positive pressure during inspiration increases transpulmonary pressure, inflates the lungs, augments alveolar ventilation and unloads the inspiratory muscles.[113] Augmentation of alveolar ventilation, demonstrated by an increase in V_T, increases CO_2 elimination and reverses acidaemia. High levels of inspiratory pressure may also relieve dyspnoea.[114]

The main physiological benefit in patients with congestive heart failure (CHF) is attributed to the increase in functional residual capacity associated with the use of PEEP that reopens collapsed alveoli and improves oxygenation.[115] Increased intrathoracic pressure associated with the application of positive pressure also may improve cardiac performance by reducing myocardial work and oxygen consumption through reductions to ventricular preload and left ventricular afterload.[115–117] NIV also preserves the ability to speak, swallow, cough and clear secretions, and decreases risks associated with endotracheal intubation.[118]

Indications for NIV

The success of NIV treatment is dependent on appropriate patient selection.[119] Table 15.3 outlines indications and contraindications to NIV.

Acute respiratory failure

Evidence supporting the role of NIV in patients with de novo acute hypoxaemic respiratory failure (i.e. significant hypoxaemia (an arterial oxygen tension/inspiratory oxygen fraction ratio (PaO_2/FiO_2) ≤ 200), tachypnoea,

TABLE 15.3

Indications and contraindications for non-invasive ventilation

INDICATIONS

Bedside observations	Increased dyspnoea; moderate-to-severe tachypnoea: >24 breaths per min (obstructive) >30 breaths per min (restrictive). Signs of increased work of breathing, accessory muscle use and abdominal paradox.
Gas exchange	Acute or acute-on-chronic ventilatory failure (best indication), $PaCO_2$ >45 mmHg, pH <7.35. Hypoxaemia (use with caution), PaO_2/FiO_2 ratio <200.

CONTRAINDICATIONS

Absolute	Respiratory arrest. Unable to fit mask.
Relative	Medically unstable: hypotensive shock, uncontrolled cardiac ischaemia or arrhythmia, uncontrolled upper gastrointestinal bleeding. Agitated, uncooperative. Unable to protect airway. Swallowing impairment. Excessive secretions not managed by secretion clearance techniques. Multiple (i.e. two or more) organ failure. Recent upper airway or upper gastrointestinal surgery.

$PaCO_2$ = partial pressure of carbon dioxide in arterial blood; PaO_2 = partial pressure of oxygen in arterial blood; PaO_2/FiO_2 = ratio of partial pressure of oxygen in arterial blood to fraction of inspired oxygen.

Source: Reproduced from Nava S, Hill N. Non-invasive ventilation in acute respiratory failure. Lancet 2009;374(9685): 250–9.

and a non-COPD diagnosis) is uncertain, resulting in the inability to make a recommendation for its use in the 2017 European Respiratory Society and American Thoracic Society guidelines on NIV for acute respiratory failure.[120] NIV in these patients may be less effective in reducing the work of breathing compared with patients with hypercapnic respiratory failure.

Acute exacerbation of COPD and CHF

Strong evidence exists to support the use of NIV for patients with acute exacerbation of COPD and CHF. A 2017 systematic review of NIV for patients with hypercapnic respiratory failure due to COPD that included

17 trials enrolling 1264 patients found NIV as a first-line intervention reduced the risk of mortality by 46% and the risk of endotracheal intubation by 65%.[121] COPD patients most likely to respond favourably to NIV include those with an unimpaired level of consciousness, moderate acidaemia, a respiratory rate of <30 breaths/minute and who demonstrate an improvement in respiratory parameters within 2 hours of commencing NIPPV.[112,122]

Early use of NIV in combination with standard therapy for patients with CHF has also been shown to reduce intubation rates and mortality when compared with standard therapy alone.[123–125] The 2019 Cochrane systematic review including 24 trials (2664 participants) with acute cardiogenic pulmonary oedema found NIV reduced hospital mortality and re-intubation rates compared with standard medical care and no increased risk of acute myocardial infarction.[126,127] The authors recommended NIV was a safe option with similar adverse event rates to standard medical care. Practice surveys indicate CPAP may be the preferred method of NIV for patients with CHF in Australia and internationally.

NIV in weaning

NIV provides partial ventilator support without the need for an artificial airway and as such has a role in weaning and avoiding complications associated with invasive ventilation.[128] Patients are extubated directly to NIV and then weaned to standard oxygen therapy. This use of NIV differs from its role in preventing re-intubation in patients that develop, or who are at high risk of, postextubation respiratory failure.[129] Current practice guidelines suggest NIV is used to prevent re-intubation in these high-risk patients.[130] A 2022 systematic review including 36 randomised controlled trials (6806 participants) showed that NIV reduced re-intubation compared with conventional oxygen therapy.[131] There was no difference, however, comparing NIV with HFNC.

A 2021 systematic review and meta-analysis of 28 trials with 2066 participants (45% with COPD) using extubation to NIV as a weaning strategy reported reductions in mortality, weaning failure, VAP, ICU and hospital lengths of stay, and total duration of ventilation.[132,133] Early extubation to NIV restores a patient's ability to communicate using voice, as well as eat and drink. It also affords the opportunity to reduce sedation and enable mobilisation and participation in other rehabilitation activities.

Other indications

Other indications for NIV include:

- asthma[134–136]
- pulmonary infiltrates in immunocompromised patients
- neuromuscular disorders (e.g. muscular dystrophy, amyotrophic lateral sclerosis)
- fractured ribs
- obesity and central hypoventilation syndromes
- palliation.[137,138]

Patient section

Selection of patients to receive NIV depends on the presence of any indications listed above as well as bedside observations and gas exchange parameters found in Table 15.3.

Interfaces and settings

NIV requires an interface that connects the patient to a ventilator, a portable compressor or a flow generator with a CPAP valve. The selection of an appropriate interface can influence NIV success or failure. Oronasal masks cover both the mouth and nose and are the preferred mask type for the management of acute respiratory failure.[139] Nasal masks enable speech, eating and drinking, and therefore are used more frequently for long-term NIV use. An oronasal mask enables delivery of higher ventilation pressures with less leak and greater comfort for the patient.[140] Other interfaces include full-face masks[140] that seal around the perimeter of the face and cover the eyes as well as the nose and mouth, nasal pillows, mouthpieces that are placed between the patient's lips, and helmets that cover the whole head and consist of a transparent plastic hood attached to a soft neck collar. These alternative interfaces have the potential to increase patient tolerance by reducing pressure ulceration, air leaks and patient discomfort.[141,142] In a 2022 systematic review including 16 randomised controlled trials and 8 observational studies (1345 participants), use of helmet NIV was found to reduce mortality and intubation compared with face-mask NIV.[143]

Initiation and monitoring priorities

Successful initiation of NIV is dependent on patient acceptance and tolerance. Patient acceptance may be aided by a brief explanation of the procedure and its benefits. Strategies to enhance patient tolerance include: use of an interface that fits the patient's facial features, commencing with low pressure levels, holding the mask gently in position prior to securing with the straps/headgear, and ensuring straps prevent major leaks but are not so tight they increase discomfort. Once NIV is commenced, the patient should be monitored for respiratory and haemodynamic stability, response to NIV treatment, ongoing tolerance and presence of air leaks (Table 15.4). Arterial blood gas analysis should be performed at baseline and within the first one to two hours of commencement.[144] During the initiation and stabilisation period, patients should be monitored using a nurse-to-patient ratio of 1:1 with ongoing coaching to promote NIV tolerance throughout the early stabilisation period.

Practice tip

NIV tolerance may be promoted with a simple explanation of the therapy, reassurance and constant monitoring for your patient. During initiation, allow them to take short breaks from the mask if they are in discomfort or experiencing claustrophobia.

TABLE 15.4

Monitoring priorities for non-invasive ventilation

PRIORITY	ASSESSMENT
Patient comfort	Restlessness Mask tolerance Anxiety level Dyspnoea score Pain score
Conscious level	Glasgow Coma Scale
Work of breathing	Chest wall motion Accessory muscle activation RR
Gas exchange parameters	Continuous SpO_2 Arterial blood gas analysis (baseline and 1–2-hourly subsequently) Patient colour
Haemodynamic status	Continuous heart rate Intermittent blood pressure
Ventilator parameters	Air leak around mask Adequacy of PS (V_T, pH, $PaCO_2$) Adequacy of peak end-expiratory pressure (SpO_2, PaO_2)

$PaCO_2$ = partial pressure of carbon dioxide in arterial blood; PaO_2 = partial pressure of oxygen in arterial blood; PS = pressure support; RR = respiratory rate; SpO_2 = saturation of peripheral oxygen; V_T = tidal volume.

Source: Adapted from Rose L, Gerdtz M. Use of non-invasive ventilation in Australian emergency departments. Int J Nurs Stud 2009;46(5):617–23, with permission.

Potential complications

Masks need to be tight fitting to reduce air leaks; however, this contributes to pressure ulceration on the bridge of the nose or above the ears (due to mask straps/headgear). Air leaks may cause conjunctival irritation and the high flow of dry medical gas results in nasal congestion, oral or nasal dryness and insufflation of air into the stomach. Claustrophobia associated with the NIV interface may also lead to agitation, reducing the efficacy of NIV treatment due to poor coordination of respiratory cycling between the patient and NIV unit.[112] More serious, yet infrequent, complications include aspiration pneumonia, haemodynamic compromise associated with increased intrathoracic pressures and pneumothorax.[113]

Detecting NIV failure

Failure to respond to NIV within 1–2 hours of commencement is demonstrated by unchanged or worsening gas exchange, as well as ongoing or new onset of rapid shallow breathing and increased haemodynamic instability.[140] Decreased level of consciousness may be indicative of imminent respiratory arrest.

Weaning NIV

Existing guidelines provide little guidance on how to wean NIV.[120,145] In many cases, NIV may be simply withdrawn as opposed to weaned. For those commencing on high levels of IPAP and/or EPAP, these pressures may need weaning based on ongoing assessment of dyspnoea, chest wall movement, as well as ventilation and oxygenation parameters. Another weaning method may be progressive extension of time off NIV, while monitoring tolerance.

Invasive mechanical ventilation

Critically ill patients with persistent respiratory insufficiency (hypoxaemia and/or hypercapnia), due to drugs, disease or other conditions, may require intubation and mechanical ventilation to support oxygenation and ventilatory demands. Clinical criteria for intubation and ventilation should be based on individual patient assessment and patient response to measures aimed at reversing hypoxaemia. Box 15.2 describes some specific considerations for mechanical ventilation of the elderly patient.

Indications

Indications for intubation and mechanical ventilation include:

- apnoea
- inability to protect airway (e.g. loss of gag/cough reflex, decreased Glasgow Coma Scale score)
- clinical signs indicating respiratory distress (e.g. tachypnoea,[146] activation of accessory and expiratory muscles, abnormal chest wall movements,[147] tachycardia and hypertension)
- inability to sustain adequate oxygenation for metabolic demands; e.g. cyanosis, SpO_2 <88%, with supplemental FiO_2 ≥0.5
- respiratory acidosis (e.g. acute decrease in pH <7.25)
- postoperative respiratory failure
- shock.

The goals of mechanical ventilation are to achieve and maintain adequate pulmonary gas exchange, to minimise

---

BOX 15.2

Mechanical ventilation of the elderly patient

1. Elderly survivors of mechanical ventilation may have a greater increase in disability than those hospitalised and not requiring ventilation,[136] information that should be shared with patients and family members when considering treatment options.

2. Frail elderly patients are at increased risk of delirium resulting in prolonged mechanical ventilation.[137]

---

the risk of lung injury, to reduce patient work of breathing and to optimise comfort.

Mechanical ventilators

Contemporary ventilators use sophisticated microprocessor controls with sensitive detection, response and control of pressure and gas-flow characteristics. These ventilators are sensitive to patient ventilatory demands, enabling improved patient–ventilator synchrony during both inspiratory and expiratory breath phases. Parameters commonly manipulated during mechanical ventilation are detailed in Table 15.5. Parameters often observed and documented are discussed below.

Phases of breath delivery

The respiratory cycle comprises both inspiratory and expiratory phases (Fig. 15.11). Pressure, flow, volume and time are parameters used to describe or classify mechanical ventilator breaths during the phases of inspiration. Ventilator breaths are classified by (1) the mechanism (ventilator or patient) that 'triggers' the start of inspiration, (2) the parameter that is 'targeted' (also referred to as 'controlled' or 'limited') during inspiration, and (3) the parameter that 'cycles' the breath from inspiration to expiration.[148]

Pressure versus volume delivery

Volume-control ventilation (VCV) provides the ability to regulate minute ventilation (V_E) and CO_2 elimination with straightforward manipulation of respiratory rate and V_T.[149] This provides consistent V_T delivery, independent of lung mechanics. The set V_T and flow rates used in VCV means that the ventilator is unable to increase volume or flow rates in response to the patient's inspiratory demands during mandatory breaths. This inability to respond to patient's inspiratory flow requirements can lead to dyssynchrony. Another disadvantage of VCV is the lack of control over peak airway pressure that changes in response to altered compliance and resistance. Elevated plateau pressure may cause alveolar overdistention, barotrauma and haemodynamic effects such as reduced venous return and cardiac output, resulting in hypotension and thus decreased organ perfusion.[150] Clinicians need to carefully monitor ventilation to avoid injurious pressures. In VCV the peak airway pressure is achieved towards the end of inspiration, and only for a short duration; therefore distribution of gas may not be optimised and shearing stress can occur.[151] This can be overcome with use of a decelerating waveform and an inspiratory time that produces an inspiratory hold.

Pressure-control ventilation (PCV) allows control over the peak inspiratory pressure and inspiratory time. Clinicians must monitor minute ventilation and gas exchange owing to the lack of a guaranteed V_T and possible changes in respiratory compliance and resistance. The variable flow and V_Ts means that there is the potential for greater interaction between patient efforts and ventilator breaths than is present in volume-controlled ventilation. The variable and decelerating inspiratory gas flow pattern of PCV enables

TABLE 15.5

Set ventilator parameters

PARAMETER	DESCRIPTION
Fraction of inspired oxygen (FiO$_2$)	The fraction of inspired oxygen delivered on inspiration to the patient.
Tidal volume (V_T)	Volume (mL) of each breath.
Set breath rate (f)	The clinician-determined set rate of breaths delivered by the ventilator (bpm).
Inspiratory trigger or sensitivity	Mechanism by which the ventilator senses the patient's inspiratory effort. May be measured in terms of a change in pressure or flow.
Inspiratory pressure (P_{insp}, P_{high})	Clinician-determined pressure that is targeted during inspiration.
Inspiratory time (T_{insp})	The duration of inspiration (s).
Inspiratory:expiratory ratio (I:E)	The ratio of the inspiratory time to expiratory time.
Flow (V)	The speed gas travels during inspiration (L/min).
Pressure support (PS)	The flow of gas that augments a patient's spontaneously initiated breath to a clinician-determined pressure (cmH$_2$O).
Positive end-expiratory pressure (PEEP)	Application of airway pressure above atmospheric pressure at the end of expiration (cmH$_2$O).
Rise time	Time to achieve maximal flow at the onset of inspiration for pressure-targeted breaths.
Expiratory sensitivity	During a spontaneous breath, the ventilator cycles from inspiration to expiration once flow has decelerated to a percentage of initial peak flow.
Minute volume (V_E)	Generally, not set directly but is determined by V_T and f settings. Tidal volume multiplied by the RR over 1 minute (L/min).
Airway pressure (P_{aw})	The pressure measured in cmH$_2$O by the ventilator in the proximal airway.
Plateau pressure (P_{plat})	The pressure, measured in cmH$_2$O, applied to the small airways and alveoli. Pplat is not set but can be measured by performing an inspiratory hold manoeuvre.
Automatic tube compensation	Active during spontaneous breaths to compensate for the work of breathing associated with ETT resistance via closed-loop control of continuously calculated tracheal pressure.
Respiratory rate	The number of breaths measured over 1 minute.

rapid alveolar filling and more even gas distribution compared with the constant flow pattern that may be used with volume control. This decelerating flow pattern also results in improved gas exchange, decreased work of breathing and prevention of overdistention in healthy alveoli.[152–155] During PCV, the set inspiratory pressure is achieved at the beginning of the inspiratory cycle and maintained for the set inspiratory time. This promotes recruitment of alveoli with high opening pressures and long time-constants.

Ventilator parameters

Fraction of inspired oxygen

The FiO$_2$ is expressed as a decimal, between 0.21 and 1.0, when supplemental oxygen is applied. Room air has an oxygen content of 0.21 (21%). Ventilation is commonly commenced on a high FiO$_2$ setting but, as noted earlier, clinicians should consider the risks of oxygen toxicity, which include disruption to the alveolar–capillary membrane and alveolar wall fibrosis.[156]

Tidal volume

V_T is the volume, measured in mL, of each breath. Set or targeted V_T is calculated using the patient's predicted body weight using height and gender-specific tables[157] to achieve 6–8 mL/kg (Table 15.6). Professional society clinical practice guidelines recommend using 4–8 mL/kg predicted body weight[158] or <6 mL/kg ideal body weight[159] targeting lower inspiratory pressures (plateau pressure 30 cmH$_2$O) in patients with acute respiratory distress syndrome (ARDS). A 2017 systematic review including 7 randomised controlled trials and 1481 patients

FIGURE 15.11 Phases of breath delivery.

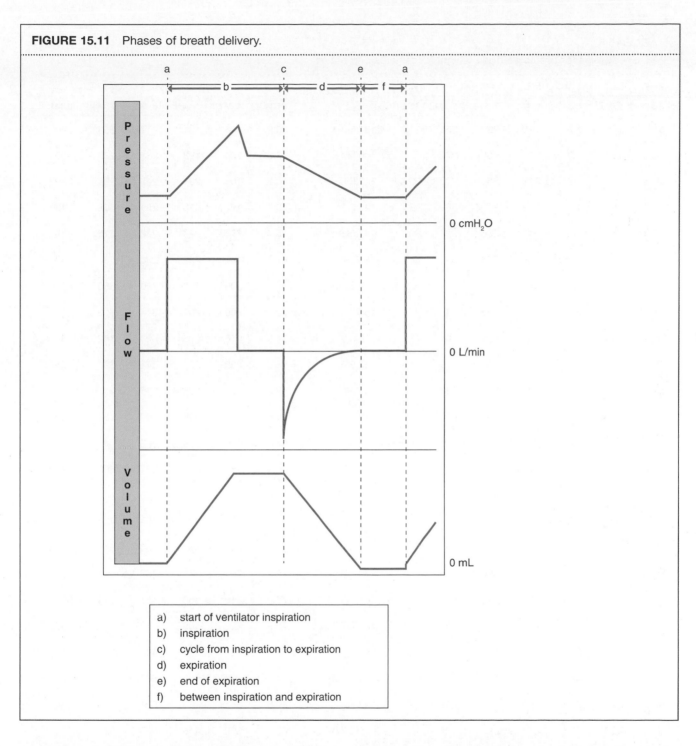

a) start of ventilator inspiration
b) inspiration
c) cycle from inspiration to expiration
d) expiration
e) end of expiration
f) between inspiration and expiration

reported a significant mortality reduction for LTV as compared with conventional ventilation strategies when including trials that also used a high PEEP strategy.[160] No difference was found when excluding studies that also used a high PEEP strategy. As increasing evidence confirms high V_T causes harm,[161] clinicians should consider aiming for 6–8 mL/kg in all ventilated patients.

Respiratory rate

Mandatory frequency (f) or respiratory rate (RR) is set with consideration of the patient's own respiratory effort,

anticipated ventilatory requirements and the effect on the I:E ratio. Use of high doses of sedation with or without neuromuscular blockade requires setting a mandatory rate that facilitates adequate gas exchange and meets oxygenation requirements. A lower frequency can be set for a patient able to breathe spontaneously in modes such as synchronised intermittent mandatory ventilation (SIMV) and assist control (A/C) (see below) to enable spontaneous triggering. Physiologically normal respiratory rates are 12–20 breaths per minute. Patients with hypoxaemic respiratory failure generally breathe 20–30 breaths per minute.[162]

TABLE 15.6

ARDSnet tables for predicted body weight for females and males

PBW	4 ML	5 ML	6 ML	7 ML	8 ML	HEIGHT, CENTIMETRES (INCHES)	PBW	4 ML	5 ML	6 ML	7 ML	8 ML
31.7	127	159	190	222	254	137(54)	36.2	145	181	217	253	290
34	136	170	204	238	272	140(55)	38.5	154	193	231	270	308
36.3	145	182	218	254	290	142(56)	40.8	163	204	245	286	326
38.6	154	193	232	270	309	145(57)	43.1	172	216	259	302	345
40.9	164	205	245	286	327	147.5(58)	45.4	182	227	272	318	363
43.2	173	216	259	302	346	150(59)	47.7	191	239	286	334	382
45.5	182	228	273	319	364	152.5(60)	50	200	250	300	350	400
47.8	191	239	287	335	382	155(61)	52.3	209	262	314	366	418
50.1	200	251	301	351	401	157.5(62)	54.6	218	273	328	382	437
52.4	210	262	314	367	419	160(63)	56.9	228	285	341	398	455
54.7	219	274	328	383	438	162.5(64)	59.2	237	296	355	414	474
57	228	285	342	399	456	165(65)	61.5	246	308	369	431	492
59.3	237	297	356	415	474	167.5(66)	63.8	255	319	383	447	510
61.6	246	308	370	431	493	170(67)	66.1	264	331	397	463	529
63.9	256	320	383	447	511	172.5(68)	68.4	274	342	410	479	547
66.2	265	331	397	463	530	175(69)	70.7	283	354	424	495	566
68.5	274	343	411	480	548	178(70)	73	292	365	438	511	584
70.8	283	354	425	496	566	180(71)	75.3	301	377	452	527	602
73.1	292	366	439	512	585	183(72)	77.6	310	388	466	543	621
75.4	302	377	452	528	603	185.5(73)	79.9	320	400	479	559	639
77.7	311	389	466	544	622	188(74)	82.2	329	411	493	575	658
80	320	400	480	560	640	190.5(75)	84.5	338	423	507	592	676
82.3	329	412	494	576	658	193(76)	86.8	347	434	521	608	694
84.6	338	423	508	592	677	195.5(77)	89.1	356	446	535	624	713
86.9	348	435	521	608	695	198(78)	91.4	366	457	548	640	731

PBW = predicted body weight.

The formulae, when using height in centimetres, are:

• Females = 45.5 + 0.91 × (height in cm − 152.4)

• Males = 50 + 0.91 × (height in cm − 152.3).

Source: Adapted with information from NIH/NHLBI ARDS Network, www.ardsnet.org.

Triggering of inspiration

Depending on the ventilation mode, breaths are triggered by the ventilator or patient in various sequences. A breath may be triggered by the ventilator in response to time elapsed in modes with clinician-determined set frequency such as controlled mandatory ventilation (CMV), and in A/C and SIMV in the absence of spontaneous effort. Patient triggering requires the ventilator to sense the patient's inspiratory effort. Modern generation ventilators use flow triggering, as evidence indicates that flow triggering may be more responsive to patient effort than pressure triggering.[163] Pressure triggering requires the patient to create a negative pressure within the ventilator circuit of sufficient size to enable the ventilator to sense the effort and commence flow of gas. Flow triggering is sometimes used in conjunction with a predetermined flow of gas, usually 5–10 L/min, referred to as the bias (or base) flow, that travels continuously through the ventilator circuit. When the patient makes an inspiratory effort, they divert flow that is sensed by the ventilator. If the flow diversion reaches a clinician-determined set value, a breath is initiated.[164] The flow trigger is usually set at 1–3 L/min (1 L/min represents less patient effort and 3 L/min represents greater patient effort). Despite advances in ventilator technology, various studies continue to identify missed patient triggers that contribute to patient–ventilator asynchrony.[165] Conversely, 'auto-triggering' is ventilator triggering in the absence of spontaneous inspiratory effort. Auto-triggering is sometimes observed in patients with an increased cardiac output, such as those fulfilling brain death criteria.

Rise time

The rise time controls how quickly the ventilator reaches the clinician-determined inspiratory pressure (P_{insp}) for mandatory breaths and pressure support for spontaneous breaths. Reducing the rise time to its lowest value will enable the ventilator to reach target pressure in the shortest time frame resulting in a more rapid delivering of flow in the early phase of inspiration. This reduces work of breathing and improves synchrony. In patients with a high airway resistance (e.g. severe asthma), a short inspiratory time may cause oscillation and overshoot of the pressure waveform. The clinical relevance of this is questionable but it produces an abnormal pressure waveform and results in alarm violations. Increasing the rise time may alleviate this problem. In other patients, an increased rise time may unnecessarily increase their work of breathing.[166]

Inspiratory time and inspiratory: expiratory ratio

The total time available for each mandatory breath is determined by the set inspiratory time and breath frequency. Normal inspiratory time is 0.8–1.2 seconds. Total breath time comprises the inspiratory (I) and expiratory (E) time, which can be expressed as a ratio (I:E). In normal spontaneous breathing, expiratory time is approximately twice the inspiratory time (1:2 ratio). Gas flow also influences inspiratory time, with higher gas flows resulting in decreased time to achieve the target V_T. The I:E ratio can be manipulated to create an inverse relationship (1:1, 2:1, 4:1), with the goal of increased mean airway pressure resulting in alveolar recruitment and improved oxygenation. Prolonging the inspiratory time beyond normal or using inverse ratio ventilation in any mode can result in patient ventilator dyssynchrony and increased risk of barotrauma.[167]

Inspiratory flow and flow pattern

The flow rate refers to the speed of gas, is measured in litres per minute (L/min) and is generally delivered at speeds of 30–60 L/min. Higher flow rates cause turbulent gas flow, resulting in increased peak airway pressures. Lower flow rates result in laminar flow, increased inspiratory time, improved gas distribution and lower peak airway pressures.[168] The flow of inspiratory gas can be delivered in three styles: constant or square wave, decelerating ramp and sinusoidal pattern (see Fig. 15.6). In a constant flow pattern, the peak flow is achieved at the beginning of inspiration and is held constant throughout the inspiratory phase. This may result in higher peak airway pressures. Using a decelerating ramp, the gas flow is highest at the beginning of inspiration and tapers throughout the inspiratory phase. Sinusoidal gas flow resembles spontaneous ventilation.

Peak airway pressure

Airway pressures vary across the respiratory cycle with a number of pressures identifiable (e.g. peak inspiratory, end-expiratory). The airway pressure (P_{aw}) is an important parameter in assessing respiratory compliance and patient–ventilator synchrony, and will vary depending on V_T, RR, ventilator flow pattern, dynamic compliance and airway resistance. In pressure-targeted modes, the peak inspiratory pressure is equivalent to the P_{insp}. In volume-targeted modes, the peak inspiratory pressure is determined by the set V_T and patient compliance and resistance.

Positive end-expiratory pressure

PEEP is the pressure applied at the end of the expiratory cycle to prevent alveolar collapse. PEEP increases residual lung volume thereby recruiting collapsed alveoli, improving ventilation/perfusion match and enhancing movement of fluid out of the alveoli.[169,170] PEEP was originally introduced by Ashbaugh and colleagues[171] in the 1960s as a technique for treating refractory hypoxaemia in patients with ARDS. Ventilator-associated lung injury may be prevented using PEEP by recruiting atelectic alveoli and bronchioles and preventing cyclic opening and closing of alveoli.[172] PEEP may be beneficial, however, only if the lung is recruitable such as in collapsed, as opposed to consolidated, lung.[169] Selection of optimal PEEP remains controversial. A 2021 Cochrane systematic review and meta-analysis including 10 trials (3851 participants) found moderate-certainty evidence that high PEEP levels compared with low PEEP levels do not reduce hospital mortality but do improve oxygenation levels.[173] Current professional society guidelines for ARDS management make a conditional recommendation for use of high PEEP in patients with moderate-to-severe ARDS.[158,159] In patients without ARDS or other causes of significant atelectasis, high PEEP levels should be used with caution.[174]

Pressure support

When triggered by the patient, the ventilator delivers flow to achieve the clinician-determined set pressure support. The flow is variable, depending on the patient demand. The V_T achieved with pressure support is dependent on chest and lung compliance as well as airway and ventilator resistance. Pressure support is generally set at 5–20 cmH$_2$O. Increasing the level of pressure support will result in increased V_T, and improvements in gas exchange if compliance and resistance remain constant.

Expiratory sensitivity

Expiratory sensitivity describes the percentage of decay in peak flow reached during the inspiratory phase that signals the ventilator to cycle to expiration for spontaneous breaths. In some ventilator models this is predetermined at 25%, whereas others allow clinician selection. Premature termination of a breath will increase inspiratory muscle workload whereas delayed breath termination increases expiratory muscle load.[175] Reducing the expiratory sensitivity in patients with COPD may prolong the inspiratory time, thereby increasing the V_T and reducing the respiratory rate and gas trapping.[176]

Practice tip

The P_{insp} setting reflects a different value on different ventilators. P_{insp} equals total pressure including PEEP on some ventilators and P_{insp} above PEEP on others. Use the pressure–time scalar to confirm.

Automatic tube compensation

Automatic tube compensation is active during spontaneous breaths and is designed to compensate for the work of breathing associated with ETT resistance via closed-loop control of continuously calculated tracheal pressure.[177,178] During spontaneous inspiration, a pressure gradient exists between the proximal and distal ends of the ETT owing to resistance created by the tube. A reduced pressure at the proximal end of the tube means a patient needs to produce a greater inspiratory force (greater negative pressure) to generate an adequate V_T.[179] Higher flow rates generate larger pressure gradients and greater resistance. Automatic tube compensation requires the airway type and size to be selected on the ventilator as well as the percentage of automatic tube compensation (ATC) to be applied. Automatic tube compensation may have some

role in assisting with weaning success when used as a spontaneous breathing trial strategy.[180]

Ventilator modes

The mode of ventilation describes inspiratory phase variables; how the ventilator controls pressure, volume and flow during a breath; as well as describing how breaths are sequenced. All breaths have trigger, limit and cycle inspiratory phase variables.[181] Each breath is triggered (started) either by the patient or by the ventilator. During inspiration, the breath is limited to a set target of pressure, volume or flow. This target cannot be exceeded during each breath. The cycling variable determines the end of the inspiratory phase. Again, this variable may be pressure, flow, volume or time. Gas delivery during each breath is described by the control variable. There are five control variables: pressure, volume, flow, time and dual control (such as used in the mode pressure-regulated volume control). Breath sequencing refers to the sequence of mandatory and spontaneous breath. A spontaneous breath is one during which inspiration is both started (triggered) and stopped (cycled) by the patient. Spontaneous breaths may be assisted, as with pressure support, or unassisted. Mandatory breaths are either triggered or cycled by the ventilator.[182] A complete mode description should include: (1) the control variable, (2) the breath sequence and (3) the targeting scheme (limit variable).

Commonly employed ventilation modes

Contemporary ventilators now provide a range of modes to facilitate mechanical ventilation (Table 15.7).

Controlled mandatory ventilation

CMV is a mandatory mode, and is the original and most basic mode of ventilation.[183] CMV delivers all breaths at a clinician-determined set frequency (rate); the patient's spontaneous effort is not acknowledged by the ventilator.[184] VCV requires clinician selection of the frequency, PEEP, FiO$_2$, tidal volume, flow waveform, peak inspiratory flow and either the inspiratory time or I:E ratio. PCV requires clinician selection of rate, PEEP, FiO$_2$, inspiratory pressure, as opposed to tidal volume, and inspiratory time or I:E ratio depending on the ventilator type. Peak inspiratory flow and the flow waveform are manipulated by the ventilator, to achieve the clinician-selected inspiratory pressure within the set inspiratory time. The inability to breathe spontaneously during CMV contributes to diaphragm muscle dysfunction and atrophy, which may result in difficulty weaning from the ventilator.[185]

Assist control

In A/C the patient can trigger the ventilator, however, unlike SIMV, every patient-initiated breath is assisted to the same clinician-determined V_T (volume targeted) or inspiratory pressure (pressure targeted). All breaths are cycled by the ventilator irrespective of being patient- or

TABLE 15.7
Ventilator modes

MODE	DESCRIPTION	CLINICAL IMPLICATIONS
Controlled mandatory ventilation (CMV)	All breaths are mandatory; no patient triggering is enabled. Also called volume-controlled ventilation (volume targeted) (VCV) and pressure-controlled ventilation (pressure targeted) (PCV).	Patients with respiratory effort require sedation and neuromuscular blockade. Potential for respiratory muscle atrophy due to disuse.
Assist control (A/C)	Breaths may be either machine or patient triggered but all are cycled by the ventilator. Assist control may be delivered as volume (AC-VC) or pressure (AC-PC) targeted.	Activation of the diaphragm with patient triggering. Potential for respiratory alkalosis if tachypnoea develops.
Synchronised intermittent mandatory ventilation (SIMV)	Mandatory breaths are delivered using a set rate and volume (SIMV-VC) or pressure (SIMV-PC). Mandatory breaths are synchronised with patient triggers within a timing window. Between mandatory breaths the patient can breathe spontaneously.	Reduced need for sedation. Activation of the diaphragm with patient triggering.
Pressure support ventilation (PSV)	All breaths are patient triggered and cycled. Pressure applied by the ventilator during inspiration (PS) augments patient effort.	Reduced need for sedation. Facilitates ventilator weaning. Level of PS can be adjusted to achieve desired V_T. Sustains respiratory muscle tone and decreases work of breathing.
Variable pressure support ventilation	Mimics variability of breaths in normal spontaneous breathing as opposed to the fixed level of support used in traditional PSV.	May improve patient–ventilator synchrony.
Continuous positive airway pressure (CPAP)	All breaths are patient triggered and cycled. Positive pressure is applied throughout inspiratory and expiratory phases of the respiratory cycle.	Requires intact respiratory drive and patient ability to maintain adequate tidal volumes.
Volume support (VS)	Spontaneous mode with clinician preset target tidal volume delivery achieved with the lowest inspiratory pressure.	Requires intact respiratory drive.
Pressure-regulated volume control (PRVC)	Mandatory rate and target tidal volume are set, and the ventilator then delivers the breaths using the lowest achievable pressure.	Dual control of volume and pressure enables guarantee of volume and pressure.
Airway pressure release ventilation (APRV)	Ventilator cycles between two preset pressure levels for defined time periods. I:E ratio is inverse, often with a prolonged inspiratory time (4 s) and shortened expiratory time (0.8 s). Patient can breathe spontaneously at both pressure levels.	Reduced need for sedation. Activation of the diaphragm with patient triggering. Promotes alveolar recruitment. Considered a rescue mode in ARDS when used with extreme inverse ratio.
Biphasic positive airway pressure (BiPAP/BiLevel/ Bivent)	As with APRV, the ventilator cycles between two preset pressure levels for defined time periods and the patient can breathe spontaneously at both pressure levels. The inspiratory time is generally shorter than, or the same length as, the expiratory time.	Reduced need for sedation. Activation of the diaphragm with patient triggering. Promotes alveolar recruitment.
Adaptive support ventilation (ASV)	Automatic breath-by-breath adaptation of RR and pressure levels based on a clinician-set desired percentage of minute ventilation.[270]	Automatically sets all ventilator settings except PEEP and FiO_2. Potential for use as a weaning mode.

Continued

TABLE 15.7

Ventilator modes—cont'd

MODE	DESCRIPTION	CLINICAL IMPLICATIONS
Intellivent-ASV	Automatically adjusts RR and pressure levels in the same manner as ASV but also aims to achieve a low driving pressure. Automatically adjusts PEEP and FiO_2 comparing the difference between measured SpO_2 and target SpO_2.	Given Intellivent-ASV automates virtually all ventilation it may offer the potential to reduce clinician workload while optimising ventilation and thereby reducing the time mechanical ventilation is needed.
Neurally adjusted ventilatory assist (NAVA®)	Delivers positive pressure proportional to diaphragmatic electrical activity using a clinician-determined proportionality factor set on the ventilator.	Improves patient–ventilator synchrony. Role in weaning, particularly for those patients experiencing difficult or prolonged weaning.
Proportional assist ventilation (PAV)	Delivers positive pressure throughout inspiration in proportion to patient-generated effort, and dependent on the set levels of flow assist (offsets resistance) and volume assist (offsets elastance).	Requires intact respiratory drive. Patients with high respiratory drive as the ventilator may overassist and continue to apply support when the patient has stopped inspiration.
Proportional assist ventilation (PAV+™)	Clinician only sets a percentage of work for the ventilator. The ventilator assesses total work of breathing by randomly measuring compliance and resistance every 4–10 breaths.	Requires intact respiratory drive. Decreases work of breathing and improves patient–ventilator synchrony. Potential for use as a weaning mode.
Volume- assured PS (VAPS)	The ventilator switches from pressure control to volume control, or PS to volume control during inspiration.	Enables maintenance of a preset minimum V_T and reduces work of breathing.

RR = respiratory rate.

ventilator-triggered. In the absence of spontaneous breathing, A/C resembles CMV.

Synchronised intermittent mandatory ventilation (SIMV)

SIMV delivers breaths at a set frequency (rate), and can be either pressure or volume targeted. Setting of the ventilator is similar to setting VCV or PCV. The availability of patient triggering with SIMV facilitates provision of gas flow in recognition of a patient's spontaneous effort. SIMV uses a timing window to deliver mandatory breaths in synchrony with patient inspiratory effort.[186] Additional spontaneous breaths occurring outside of the timing window may be assisted with pressure support to augment the patient's spontaneous effort to a preset pressure level.

Pressure support ventilation (PSV)

PSV is a spontaneous mode in which the patient initiates all breaths, with support of the patient's inspiratory effort by the ventilator using rapid acceleration of flow to achieve a preset (by a clinician) level of inspiratory pressure. Unlike CMV, SIMV or A/C, PSV does not require setting of ventilator (mandatory) breaths. PSV is usually employed with PEEP, which maintains partial inflation of alveoli during the expiratory phase to promote alveolar recruitment and oxygenation. As the support provided in PSV is fixed (i.e. 10 cmH_2O), the ventilator cannot respond to changing patient inspiratory demands.

Continuous positive airway pressure (CPAP)

CPAP applies a set baseline positive pressure throughout the inspiratory and expiratory phase. In this spontaneous breathing mode, unlike PSV, no additional positive pressure is provided to the patient during inspiration. Due to nomenclature used on some ventilator models, PSV is frequently misrepresented as CPAP.

Volume-targeted pressure control breaths

A number of hybrid ventilator modes are commercially available that use an algorithm to target a set V_T by regulating the inspiratory pressure during pressure-controlled breaths based on the patient's resistance, compliance and inspiratory effort. Examples include pressure-regulated volume control, available on the Servo

300 and Servo I (Maquet, Solna, Sweden) and SIMV with autoflow (Dräger, Lübeck, Germany). On initiation of these modes, the ventilator delivers a number of breaths during a 'learning period' to establish an estimate of the pressure required to achieve the targeted V_T. The patient's resistance, compliance and inspiratory effort continue to influence the pressure and flow delivered to attain the targeted V_T. The ventilator constantly regulates inspiratory pressure based on the pressure/volume calculation of the previous breaths and the clinician-determined target tidal volume. Volume control (VC+) on the Puritan Bennett 980 ventilators provides a mandatory, pressure-controlled breath with unrestricted flow during the inspiratory phase. The inspiratory pressure target is again automatically adjusted from breath to breath based on changing lung conditions to achieve the desired tidal volume.

Airway pressure release ventilation (APRV), biphasic positive airway pressure (BiPAP) and BiLevel

APRV, BiPAP and BiLevel are ventilator modes that allow unrestricted spontaneous breathing independent of ventilator cycling, using an active expiratory valve that allows patients to exhale even in the inspiratory phase.[187,188] These modes are pressure limited and time cycled. In the absence of spontaneous breathing, these modes resemble conventional pressure-limited, time-cycled ventilation.[184] In North America the acronym BiPAP® is registered to Respironics non-invasive ventilators (Murrayville, PA). Therefore, ventilator companies have developed brand names such as BiLevel (Puritan Bennett, Pleasanton, CA; GE Healthcare, Madison, WI), Bivent (Maquet, Solna, Sweden), DuoPaP (Hamilton Medical, Rhäzüns, Switzerland), PCV+ (Dräger Medical, Lübeck, Germany) or BiPhasic (Viasys, Conshocken, PA) to describe essentially equivalent modes. BiLevel, available on Puritan Bennett ventilators (Pleasanton, CA, GE Healthcare, Madison, WI), can provide additional pressure support or automatic tube compensation (see below) during spontaneous breaths. Some ambiguity exists in the criteria that distinguish APRV and BiPAP. When applied with the same I:E ratio, no difference exists between the two modes. APRV as opposed to BiPAP, however, is more frequently described with an extreme inverse ratio (i.e. an inspiratory time of 4 seconds and expiratory time of 0.5 seconds). Recent systematic reviews suggest airway pressure release ventilation may confer a mortality benefit and improved oxygenation when compared with conventional ventilation strategies in patients with acute hypoxic respiratory failure.[189]

Proportional modes

Proportional ventilatory modes are designed to optimise patient–ventilator interaction, delivering inspiratory assist in proportion to the patient's inspiratory effort on a breath-by-breath basis. This prevents ventilator under-and-over assistance.[190]

Adaptive support ventilation

Adaptive support ventilation (ASV) is a closed-loop mode that provides automatic adaptation on a breath-by-breath basis of respiratory rate (in patients who require mandatory ventilation) and pressure levels based on a clinician-set-desired percentage of target minute ventilation (MinVol%) aiming to minimise the work and force of breathing.[191] If set at 100%, this is equivalent to 100 mL/kg of ideal body weight/minute. Adaptation of pressure levels provides adaptive pressure control ventilation in patients who require mandatory ventilation and adapts to pressure support ventilation in spontaneously breathing patients.

Intellivent-ASV

Intellivent-ASV is an extension of ASV providing fully automated control of both ventilation and oxygenation settings adjusting tidal volume, respiratory rate and PEEP to achieve a low driving pressure. Minute volume is adjusted according to continuously measured etCO2; PEEP and FiO2 are adjusted according to continuously measured SpO2.[192]

Neurally adjusted ventilatory assist

Neurally adjusted ventilatory assist (NAVA®) is a proportional mode available on the Servo-I® ventilator (Getinge, Sweden). It uses a specialised nasogastric catheter with electrodes to measure the electrical activity of the diaphragm using the electrical activity of the diaphragm (Eadi) signal to control patient–ventilator interaction.[193] This should result in optimal patient–ventilator synchrony as it represents the endpoint of neural output from the respiratory centres and so is the earliest signal of patient inspiratory trigger and expiratory cycling. Pressure delivered to the airways is proportional to inspiratory diaphragmatic electrical activity using a clinician-determined proportionality factor set on the ventilator.[193,194] NAVA® provides breath-by-breath assist in synchrony with, and in proportion to, respiratory demand. NAVA improves patient–ventilator synchrony[195,196] and shows some promise as a weaning adjunct in difficult-to-wean patients.[197]

Proportional assist ventilation (PAV) and proportional assist ventilation plus (PAV+)

PAV is a spontaneous breathing mode that varies pressure support (assist) generated by the ventilator on a breath-by-breath basis based on patient's ventilator demand.[198] PAV+ is an extension of PAV whereby the ventilator measures compliance and resistance every 4–10 breaths to calculate elastance and work of breathing. The ventilator adjusts the level of support based on these measurements to meet a clinician-set level of assistance (e.g. 80%). As with NAVA, both modes may promote patient comfort and ventilator synchrony[196] and may have a role in ventilator weaning though further studies are required.[199]

Variable pressure support ventilation

Variable PSV mimics variability of breaths in normal spontaneous breathing as opposed to the fixed level of support used in traditional PSV. The ventilator generates and applies random variation in pressure support levels causing tidal volume variation. Variable PSV may improve patient–ventilator synchrony though further evidence is needed in this relatively new mode.[200]

Managing the mechanically ventilated patient

Management of refractory hypoxaemia

Refractory hypoxaemia may require strategies in addition to conventional lung-protective mechanical ventilation.[201] These include recruitment manoeuvres (RMs), high-frequency oscillatory ventilation (HFOV), extracorporeal membrane oxygenation (ECMO) and nitric oxide (NO).

Recruitment manoeuvres

RMs refer to brief application of high levels of PEEP to raise the transpulmonary pressure to levels higher than achieved during tidal ventilation, with the goals of opening collapsed alveoli, recruiting slow opening alveoli, preventing alveolar derecruitment and reducing shearing stress.[202] The most common RM is elevation of PEEP to achieve a peak pressure of 40 cmH_2O for a sustained period of 40 seconds, although studies report peak pressure elevations ranging from 25 to 50 cmH_2O for durations ranging from 20 to 40 seconds.[203] Effective recruitment may be difficult to assess with the potential for either alveolar overdistention or failure to recruit.[204] Once the RM is terminated, derecruitment may occur rapidly. Adverse effects, including hypotension, acidosis and desaturation, have been noted during RMs owing to increased intrathoracic and intrapulmonary pressures resulting in reductions in venous return and cardiac output; however, most do not result in serious sequelae.[202] A 2020 systematic review of RMs and high PEEP did not reduce mortality, nor did it increase the risk of barotrauma in patients with ARDS.[205]

High-frequency oscillatory ventilation

HFOV requires a specialised ventilator and manipulation of four variables: mean airway pressure (cmH_2O), frequency (Hz), inspiratory time and amplitude (or power (ΔP)).[206] Alveolar overdistention is limited through the use of sub-dead-space tidal volumes whereas alveolar cyclic collapse is prevented by maintenance of high end-expiratory lung pressures.[207,208] High-frequency (between 3 and 15 Hz) oscillations at extremely fast rates (300–420 breaths/min) create pressure waves enabling CO_2 elimination.[207] Oxygenation is facilitated through application of a constant mean airway pressure via the bias flow (rate of fresh gas).[209] In adults, recommendations for the initiation of HFOV state mean airway pressure should be set 5 cmH_2O above the peak airway pressure achieved with conventional ventilation.[210] The recommended frequency range is 3–10 Hz, with 5 Hz conventionally used to initiate HFOV. Inspiratory time is set at 33% and the amplitude setting is determined by adequate CO_2 elimination.[209] Increased CO_2 elimination is achieved by lowering the frequency and increasing the amplitude.

HFOV is generally considered a rescue mode for adult patients with ARDS experiencing refractory hypoxaemia and failing conventional ventilation.[209] Given evidence indicated HFOV does not improve mortality rates and indeed may be harmful,[211] current guidelines make a strong recommendation to avoid using HFOV.[158,159,212]

Extracorporeal membrane oxygenation

ECMO improves total body oxygenation using an external (extracorporeal) oxygenator, while allowing intrinsic recovery of lung pathophysiology by resting the lung. Indications for ECMO include acute severe cardiac or respiratory failure such as severe ARDS[213,214] and refractory shock or as a bridge to transplantation.[215] There are two types of ECMO. A veno-venous ECMO circuit drains venous blood, oxygenates the blood and pumps the blood back into the same venous compartment.[216] A venoarterial ECMO circuit removes deoxygenated blood from a central vein or the right atrium, oxygenates the blood and returns oxygenated blood to the arterial side of the circulation, typically to the aorta. This form of ECMO partially supports the cardiac output as the flow through the ECMO circuit is in addition to the normal cardiac output. Venoarterial ECMO is required for cardiac support whereas both venoarterial and venovenous ECMO can be used for respiratory support.[215]

ECMO consists of three key components:

1   a blood pump (either a simple roller or centrifugal force pump)

2   a membrane oxygenator (bubble, membrane or hollow fibre)

3   a countercurrent heat exchanger, where the blood is exposed to warmed water circulating within metal tubes.

In addition, essential safety features include bubble detectors that detect gas in the arterial line and shut the pump off; arterial line filters between the heat exchanger and arterial cannula, to trap air thrombi and emboli; pressure monitors placed before and after the oxygenator, which measure the pressure within the circuit and detect rising circuit pressures commonly caused by thrombus or circuit or cannulae occlusion, and continuous venous oxygen saturation and temperature monitoring. On commencement of ECMO, the circuit is primed with fresh blood. The acid–base balance and blood gas of the primer are adjusted to ensure that the pH is within the normal range (7.35–7.45) and PaO_2 is adequate. ECMO can be delivered via venoarterial access, which requires cannulation of an artery. This method bypasses the pulmonary circulation while providing cardiac support to the systemic circulation and achieves a higher PaO_2 with lower perfusion rates. The alternative is venovenous access, used for patients in respiratory failure with adequate cardiac function as there is no support of systemic circulation. Perfusion rates are higher, the mixed venous PO_2 is elevated and the PaO_2 is lower.[217]

Venovenous ECMO in adults with severe ARDS reduces mortality.[218] Bleeding as a complication of anticoagulation is a major risk of ECMO,[219] with cerebral bleeds being the most catastrophic. Another serious complication is limb ischaemia when the femoral artery is used.

Nitric oxide

NO is an endothelial smooth muscle relaxant. Inhaled NO is effective for dilation of pulmonary arteries resulting in reduced pulmonary shunting and reduced right ventricular afterload due to reduced pulmonary artery tone. Pulmonary shunting refers to failure of uptake of alveolar gas by the pulmonary vascular bed owing to vascular constriction or interstitial oedema. Inhaled NO has a role in the management of pulmonary hypertension and was previously thought to have a role in management of refractory hypoxaemia for patients with ARDS. However, the 2016 Cochrane systematic review and meta-analysis of NO in ARDS comprising 14 RCTs and 1275 participants reported no effect on overall mortality despite a statistically significant improvement in oxygenation in the first 24 hours.[220]

Prostacyclin

Prostacyclin, both aerosol and intravenous, is used to treat pulmonary hypertension. Continuously aerosolised prostacyclin is a currently off-label treatment used for pulmonary hypertension and severe hypoxaemic respiratory failure.[221] Although it may offer some advantage by providing the drug directly to the target organ, high doses cannot be administered because of airway irritant effects.[222]

Aerosol therapy

The delivery of inhaled aerosols to invasively ventilated patients via pressurised metered-dose inhalers (pMDIs) and nebulisers is a common practice in the ICU.[223] Inhalation aerosols include bronchodilators, corticosteroids, antibiotics, mucolytics and vasodilators. Jet, ultrasonic and vibrating mesh are the common nebulisers used. Administration during invasive mechanical ventilation is challenging; factors influencing effective aerosol delivery are related to medication type, inhalation device used, type of airway humidification and the placement of the device in the circuit.[224] Deposition of aerosolised drugs in the lungs is as low as 38% with a pMDI and lower than 20% with nebulisers.[223] At present, there are no high-quality trials that prove the effectiveness of aerosol therapy in the different disease conditions.

Positioning

Regular repositioning of critically ill patients is essential for lung recruitment, prevention of atelectasis and maintenance of skin integrity (see Chapter 6).

Head of bed elevation

Supine positioning has been associated with aspiration of abnormally colonised oropharyngeal and gastric contents[225]

and increased incidence of VAP compared with a semirecumbent position, defined as backrest elevation at 45 degrees.[226] Guidelines and care bundles for VAP prevention recommend semirecumbent positioning for all mechanically ventilated patients.[227,228] A more recent trial has, however, questioned the feasibility of 45-degree semirecumbent positioning as this backrest elevation was achieved for only 15% of study observations.[229] A 2022 systematic review of 20 trials on the effect of body positioning concluded that semirecumbent position is the most effective position to reduce VAP incidence, hospital length of stay and the duration of MV.[230]

Contraindications to backrest elevation include:

- suspected or existing spinal injury
- intracranial hypertension (for 45-degree elevation)
- unstable pelvic fractures
- prone positioning
- haemodynamic support devices (intra-aortic balloon pumps, left ventricular assist devices and ECMO)
- femoral catheterisation for continuous renal replacement therapy
- large abdominal wounds
- following femoral sheath removal.

As some degree of semirecumbent positioning is preferable to supine positioning, patients with suspected or existing spinal injury, pelvic fractures, bariatric patients or being managed with prone positioning can have their head elevated by tilting the whole bed. Patients with femoral cannulation and large abdominal wounds can usually achieve 25–30-degree positioning.

Clinical practice audits conducted internationally and in Australia and New Zealand indicate that compliance with a 45-degree semirecumbent position rarely occurs, even when taking contraindications into consideration.[231–234] Similarly, interventions to improve compliance failed to demonstrate adherence to the 45-degree semirecumbent position that can be sustained by the patient over time.[235]

Practice tip

Backrest elevation is difficult to estimate accurately. Use an objective measurement device such as an inclinometer or protractor.

Lateral positioning

Patients with unilateral lung disease experience a mismatch of ventilation to perfusion if the consolidated or atelectic lung is placed in the dependent position.[236] Temporary and early positioning of the affected lung in the dependent position, amongst other strategies such as avoiding manual hyperinflation, for patients with unilateral pneumonia or following aspiration may be beneficial in preventing the movement of bacteria or acidic gastric contents into the non-affected lung.[237] This theory has been coined 'propagation prevention'. While appealing, as yet there have been no adequately powered randomised controlled trials to support its use. Continuous lateral rotational therapy is a positioning therapy advocated for the prevention and management of respiratory complications associated with immobility.[238] The multicentre, randomised, controlled trial found a significant reduction in VAP and shorter durations of ventilation and ICU stay in a mixed ICU population.[239] Some evidence also suggests a role in patients with severe thoracic trauma.[240] Continuous lateral rotation therapy requires a special bed system enabling rotation of the upper part of the body to a maximum angle of 90 degrees.

Prone positioning

Prone positioning has been shown to improve oxygenation and intrapulmonary shunt fraction when compared with rotational turning in invasive ventilated patients with ARDS.[241] Prone positioning may also decrease the risk of VAP owing to improved bronchial secretion drainage, limitation of colonisation of distal lung, decreased atelectasis and increased alveolar recruitment, but may increase spread of pathogens in the lung and the risk of aspiration.[242,243]

Prone positioning results in changes to the distribution of ventilation and pulmonary blood flow. Pleural pressures are lower in non-dependent regions and higher in dependent regions because of gravitational forces, the weight of the overlying lung and mismatch between the local physical structures of the lung and chest wall.[244] The weight of the overlying lung increases in ARDS owing to parenchymal oedema and fluid within the alveoli.[243] This gradient in pleural pressures means transpulmonary pressure is higher in non-dependent lung regions, compared with dependent regions. Perfusion also increases from previously non-dependent to dependent lung regions, resulting in optimal matching of ventilation and perfusion to promote gas exchange.[245]

Increased pleural pressure in the dependent dorsal regions in the supine position can result in airway closure, atelectasis and hypoxaemia.[246] The difference in pleural pressures from non-dependent and dependent lung regions is greater in the supine compared with the prone position. In the supine position, the heart and abdominal contents also compress lung bases and decrease functional residual capacity, whereas in prone positioning the weight of these structures is lifted from the lung.

Prone positioning consistently demonstrated reduced mortality and improved oxygenation for patients with ARDS managed with protective lung ventilation compared with patients who are not proned.[247] Prone positioning is now recommended for adult patients with severe ARDS for more than 12 hours per day.[158,159,212] Adverse events related to prone positioning include increased risk of decubitus ulcer formation, endotracheal obstruction and thoracotomy tube dislodgement, and ocular injury.

Implementing prone positioning requires forward planning to ensure eye care and protection, mouth care, wound dressings and tracheal suction are attended to before positioning the patient prone. Intravenous lines, electrocardiogram leads, urinary catheter drainage, chest drains and ostomy bags need to be secured and repositioned appropriately once the patient is positioned.[248] Prone positioning can be achieved by manual handling of the patient, requiring up to five staff, although commercial devices are available that facilitate the turning and positioning.

Awake prone positioning

The practice of prone position has recently been extended to non-intubated patients with acute hypoxaemic respiratory failure. Best-practice guidelines for prone positioning of non-intubated patients, also referred to as awake prone position, became available after the initial wave of the COVID-19 pandemic.[249] It appears to be a safe and easy to apply strategy, although the optimal timing and duration need to be determined.[250] The effects of this intervention on outcomes including improved oxygenation, reduced intubation rate and mortality are unclear.[251]

Complications of mechanical ventilation

Physiological complications associated with mechanical ventilation include ventilator-induced lung injury (VILI) and nosocomial infection, including VAP and ventilator-associated events (VAE).[252,253] VILI occurs through alveolar overdistention and cyclic opening and closing of alveoli, resulting in diffuse alveolar damage, increased permeability, pulmonary oedema, cell contraction and cytokine production.[254,255] VILI has an important impact on outcome of mechanically ventilated patients.[256] Evidence from randomised controlled trials show that using lung-protective ventilation with low tidal volumes and inspiratory pressures less than 30 cm of water may reduce the risk of VILI and improve outcome.[257] Observational studies have shown that limiting driving pressure and mechanical power to mitigate the risk of VILI have been associated with reduced mortality.[258–260] Currently at bedside, MP is rarely calculated or monitored. VAP substantially increases the duration of ICU stay and is associated with an attributable mortality of 13%.[261] Patients on mechanical ventilation are at risk of developing pulmonary barotrauma. Barotrauma is due to alveolar rupture and causes accumulation of extra-alveolar gas, which could result in pneumothorax or subcutaneous emphysema. Although all mechanically ventilated patients are at risk for barotrauma, inappropriate ventilator settings and underlying lung diseases including COPD, asthma, interstitial lung disease and ARDS may increase the risk of barotrauma.[262] The incidence of barotrauma during mechanical ventilation is less than 3% when high tidal volumes and pressures are limited. The incidence in patients with underlying lung diseases is higher and varies from 3% to 10%.[263] A recent meta-analysis of mechanically ventilated patients with COVID-19 ARDS showed a 14% incidence of barotrauma.[264] Additional complications associated with mechanical ventilation are listed in Table 15.8.

TABLE 15.8

Complications of mechanical ventilation

Barotrauma	Pneumothorax, pneumomediastinum, pneumopericardium, pulmonary interstitial emphysema, subcutaneous emphysema.
Volutrauma	Shearing stress, endothelial and epithelial cell injury, fluid retention and pulmonary oedema, perivascular and alveolar haemorrhage, alveolar rupture.
Biotrauma	Activation of systemic and local inflammatory mechanisms.
Ventilation/perfusion mismatch	Alveolar distention causes compression of the adjacent pulmonary capillaries resulting in dead space ventilation.
↓ Cardiac output	Resulting in hypotension, ↓ cerebral perfusion pressure (CPP), ↓ renal and hepatic blood flow.
↑ Right ventricular afterload	Due to ↑ intrathoracic pressure may result in ↓ left ventricular compliance and preload.
↓ Urine output	Due to ↓ glomerular filtration rate, ↑ sodium reabsorption and activation of the renin–angiotensin–aldosterone system.
Fluid retention	Due to above renal factors as well as ↑ antidiuretic hormone and ↓ atrial natriuretic peptide.
Impaired hepatic function	Due to ↑ pressure in the portal vein, ↓ portal venous blood flow, ↓ hepatic vein blood flow.
↑ Intracranial pressure	Due to ↓ cerebral venous outflow.
Oxygen toxicity	Alterations to lung parenchyma similar to those found in ARDS.
Pulmonary emboli and deep vein thrombosis	Due to immobility.
Ileus, diarrhoea	Due to alterations in gastric motility.
Gastrointestinal haemorrhage	Gastritis and ulceration may occur due to stress, anxiety and critical illness.
ICU-acquired weakness	Neuropathies and myopathies develop in association with critical illness, corticosteroids and neuromuscular blockade.
Psychological issues	Delirium, anxiety, depression, agitation and post-traumatic stress disorder may be experienced by critically ill ventilated patients in the acute and recovery phases.

Weaning from mechanical ventilation

Weaning traditionally occurs via clinician-directed adjustments to the level of support provided by the ventilator, culminating in a spontaneous breathing trial (SBT) comprising either low-level pressure support or a T-piece trial.

Current recommendations

No ventilation strategy is more lung-protective than the timely and appropriate discontinuation of mechanical ventilation. Weaning refers to the transition from ventilatory support to spontaneous breathing.[265] Evidence-based consensus guidelines[266] published for weaning emphasise the importance of preventing unnecessary delays in the weaning process, early recognition of a patient's ability for spontaneous breathing and the use of a systematic method to identify the potential for extubation.

Weaning predictors

Clinician judgement regarding prediction of weaning readiness is known to be imperfect, with unnecessary prolongation of ventilation[267,268] or high rates of re-intubation as resultant consequences, both of which are associated with adverse outcomes.[269] An evidence-based review evaluating over 50 objective physiological measurements for determining readiness for weaning and extubation found most had only a modest relationship with weaning outcome; no single factor or combination of factors demonstrated superior accuracy.[270] The respiratory frequency to tidal volume ratio (f/V_T) (also referred to as the rapid shallow breathing index) is commonly used. However, a recent systematic review and meta-analysis pooling data from 48 studies (10,946 patients) found moderate sensitivity but poor specificity with f/V_T thresholds of <105, 80 to 105 and <80.[271]

Weaning methods

Definitions categorising weaning outcomes group patients into simple or short, difficult and prolonged weaning based on the duration of weaning and number of separation or SBT attempts.[272,273] Prior to separation or SBT attempts, weaning required a switch from a mandatory to a spontaneous breathing mode and generally a reduction of support provided by the ventilator. PSV is the most commonly used weaning mode.[274] Modes such as SIMV and AC may result in delayed weaning.

Spontaneous breathing trials

SBTs incorporate a focused assessment of a patient's capacity to breathe prior to extubation[275,276] and are recommended as the major diagnostic test to determine extubation readiness.[272] Professional society guidelines on liberation from mechanical ventilation recommend use of PSV with 5–8 cmH$_2$O rather than T-piece or CPAP SBTs.[130] As mentioned earlier, ATC may also have a role in the conduct of SBTs. Generally, SBTs should need to last only 30 minutes.[276] Formal daily SBT testing is less common in Australia and New Zealand, in contrast to international findings.[277]

Weaning protocols

Implementation of various organisational strategies such as weaning teams and non-physician-led weaning protocols may assist in the timely recognition of weaning and extubation readiness.[278] Coupling of a sedation and weaning protocol can also reduce the duration of ventilation.[279] Use of protocols to minimise sedation, enabling timely liberation from mechanical ventilation, is another recent professional society recommendation.[130] A Cochrane systematic review and meta-analysis of 17 weaning protocol trials including 2434 patients demonstrated a reduction in the duration of mechanical ventilation with use of a protocol.[278] However, the authors cautioned that the effect of weaning protocols may vary according to the ICU organisational characteristics such as an intensivist-led ICU model, high levels of physician staffing, structured ward rounds, collaborative discussion and more frequent medical review, all characteristics reported for ICUs in Australia and New Zealand.[280-282]

Automated weaning

Automated closed-loop ventilation modes potentially enable more efficient weaning by providing improved adaptation of ventilatory support through continuous monitoring and real-time intervention.[283] Several closed-loop ventilation modes exist including NAVA, PAV or PAV+, adaptive support ventilation (ASV), SmartCare™/PS and Intellivent.

ASV requires clinician-set maximum plateau pressure and desired minute ventilation based on ideal weight. ASV then automatically selects the target ventilatory pattern adjusting respiratory rate, tidal volume and inspiratory time continuously while accounting for respiratory mechanics (resistance, compliance, auto-PEEP). ASV can be used in spontaneously breathing patients as volume-targeted PSV with automatic adjustment of PS based on respiratory rate on a breath-by-breath basis.[284] Intellivent-ASV is an extension of ASV adapting nearly all ventilator settings. Intellivent-ASV enables weaning via gradual reduction in the support provided by the ventilator to sustain minute ventilation.[192] Intellivent-ASV also has a QuickWean setting that comprises reduction, observation and SBT phases of weaning

SmartCare™/PS monitors three respiratory parameters, f, V_T and end-tidal carbon dioxide concentration, every 2 or 5 minutes and periodically adapts PS.[285,286] SmartCare™/PS establishes a respiratory status diagnosis, based on evaluation of the three parameters, and may either decrease or increase PS, or leave it unchanged to maintain the patient in a defined 'respiratory zone of comfort'.[286,287] A 2021 systematic review and network meta-analysis of automated weaning found all automated modes reduced the duration of weaning compared with standard weaning practice, but did not identify a specific automated mode that was more effective in reducing the duration of MV weaning.[288]

The difficult-to-wean patient

International reports indicate patients that require mechanical ventilation for prolonged mechanical ventilation defined as ≥21 days account for approximately 10% of all mechanically ventilated patients, but occupy 40% of ICU bed days and accrue 50% of ICU costs.[289,290] Little evidence defines the optimal method for managing the difficult-to-wean patient. One trial found no difference in weaning duration or success when comparing tracheostomy trials with low-level pressure support in patients with COPD experiencing weaning difficulty.[291] A randomised controlled trial demonstrated increased weaning success with use of a once-daily progressive tracheostomy mask trial compared with pressure support weaning.[292] These patients are most likely to benefit from an individualised and structured approach to weaning using progressive lengthening of tracheostomy trials with supportive ventilation in between, in combination with early physical therapy.

Patients requiring prolonged mechanical ventilation often experience retention of airway secretions due to ineffective cough and reduced mucociliary transport.[293] Retained secretions can lead to atelectasis and may promote ventilator-associated lung injury, which impairs successful weaning. Techniques designed to enhance airway secretion clearance include manually assisted cough and mechanically assisted cough using a mechanical insufflation–exsufflation (MI-E) device. Manually assisted cough consists of a cough timed with an abdominal or lateral costal compression. MI-E devices such as the CoughAssist™ (Philips Respironics Corp, Millersville, PA) or the NIPPY Clear-way (B&D Electromedical, Stratford-Upon-Avon, Warwickshire) alternate positive pressure (insufflation) aimed at expanding the lungs to approximately 90% of capacity[294] and negative pressures (rapid exsufflation) delivered via the ETT, tracheostomy or mask. Although some evidence suggests these techniques reduce re-intubation and are safe in the critically ill, further studies are required.[295]

> **Practice tip**
>
> Tachypnoea and decreased V_T during weaning are indicators that a patient is not ready for extubation.

Summary

Support of oxygenation and ventilation during critical illness are key activities for nurses in ICU. Oxygen therapy promotes aerobic metabolism but has adverse effects that need to be considered. Various oxygen delivery devices provide low or variable flows of oxygen.

Strong evidence supports the use of NIV for COPD and CHF, but caution is required when used for de novo acute respiratory failure. Early extubation to NIV also has a role in promoting weaning success, particularly in COPD patients. NIV success is dependent on patient tolerance, with common complications including pressure ulcers, conjunctival irritations, nasal congestion, insufflation of air into the stomach and claustrophobia.

Airway support can be provided with oro- or nasopharyngeal airways, LMAs and endotracheal intubation; oral intubation is the preferred method. For a patient with an ETT, the key points for practice are:

- ETT placement should be confirmed with end-tidal CO_2 monitoring
- the aim of endotracheal cuff management is to prevent airway contamination and enable positive–pressure ventilation
- closed suctioning reduces alveolar derecruitment compared with open suctioning
- instillation of normal saline is not recommended during routine tracheal suctioning.

The optimal timing of tracheostomy remains uncertain; however, tracheostomy should be considered for patients experiencing weaning difficulty.

The goals of mechanical ventilation are to promote gas exchange, minimise lung injury, reduce work of breathing and promote patient comfort:

- Despite its life-saving potential, mechanical ventilation carries the risk of serious physical and psychological complications.
- Humidification of dry medical gas is required during mechanical ventilation to prevent drying of secretions, mucous plugging and airway occlusion.
- The pressure required to deliver a volume of gas into the lungs is determined by elastic and resistive forces.
- Contemporary ventilators now provide a range of modes to facilitate mechanical ventilation.
- Analysis of ventilator graphics provides clinicians with the ability to assess patient–ventilator interaction, appropriateness of ventilator settings and lung function.
- Semirecumbent positioning at 45 degrees elevation has been shown to reduce VAP but compliance is poor.
- RMs, ECMO and prone positioning are strategies that may facilitate management of refractory hypoxaemia.
- Systematic adoption of strategies such as daily SBTs, weaning protocols and automated closed loop modes may facilitate shorter weaning durations and better rates of weaning success.

Case study

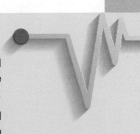

A 67-year-old male (Fred) was admitted to the ICU with acute respiratory failure due to community-acquired pneumonia. Fred was morbidly obese (196 kg) with extensive central obesity and a body mass index of 75.2. He had a history of COPD; however, he was not prescribed steroids and had not been investigated for sleep apnoea.

Fred was commenced on broad-spectrum antibiotic cover in the emergency department. Fred had a trial of NIV with FiO_2 0.65, PEEP 8 cmH_2O (EPAP 7 cmH_2O) and pressure support 5 cmH_2O (IPAP 12 cmH_2O) to reduce his work of breathing and improve gas exchange. The NIV trial was discontinued as Fred's dyspnoea was unrelieved, and hypoxia and hypercapnia persisted. He was intubated with a size 7 oral ETT and a bronchial alveolar lavage was performed to obtain samples for bacterial and viral screening. Nasopharyngeal swabs were also obtained. Ventilator settings following intubation were A/C, FiO_2 1.0, respiratory rate 16 breaths per minute, P_{insp} 30 cmH$_2$O, PEEP 15 cmH$_2$O, and inspiratory time of 1.1 seconds. Initial blood gases were as follows: pH 7.07, PaO_2 71 mmHg, $PaCO_2$ 71 mmHg, HCO$_3$ 16.4 mmol, base excess −9.5, sodium 123 mmol, chloride 94 mmol, lactate 0.7, SpO_2 94%, and PaO_2/FiO_2 (PF) ratio 71. Dynamic compliance was 25.6 mL/cmH$_2$O; resistance was 8.6 cmH$_2$O/(L/s). A chest X-ray showed bilateral pulmonary infiltrates and a lobular pneumonia. Chest auscultation revealed bilateral crackles, late in the inspiratory phase.

Nursing assessment indicated the following issues:
1 Notable audible cuff leak on inspiration despite a cuff pressure of 30 cmH$_2$O.
2 Atelectasis as evidenced by decreased air entry in lung bases, reduced compliance, diminished gas exchange, and obliteration of costophrenic angles on the chest X-ray.

To address the cuff leak, nursing staff connected rigid manometer tubing between the cuff pressure gauge and the ETT pilot tube to enable continuous cuff pressure measurement. Cuff pressure did not decrease over time indicating that the ETT cuff was intact. Therefore, the audible air leak was not caused by a leaking ETT cuff but was due to an air leak around the cuff. On careful examination of the chest X-ray, the ETT cuff was found to be above the level of the vocal cords and therefore needed repositioning.

To address the atelectasis, Fred was repositioned in a high semi-Fowler position (≥45° HOB elevation). This change in positioning resulted in an immediate improvement in compliance from a baseline of 25.6 to 38.4 mL/cmH$_2$O. V_T also increased from 300 mL to 400 mL. These improvements enabled rapid downward titration of FiO_2 to 0.7 while maintaining a SpO_2 >90%. A RM using 40 cmH$_2$O for 40 seconds was performed with further improvement of Fred's oxygenation indicating his lungs were responsive to this strategy. The ventilator mode was changed to APRV with a P_{insp} of 27 cmH$_2$O for 6 seconds and an expiratory pressure of 5 cmH$_2$O for 0.4 seconds. Further improvements in oxygenation were noted (PaO_2 180 mmHg and PF ratio 225).

DISCUSSION

A cuff leak may be assumed to be secondary to a hole in either the cuff or the pilot tube; however, this is relatively rare. Audible cuff leaks are more frequently due to a malpositioned ETT. It is important to note that each time cuff pressure is measured a small volume of gas leaves the cuff to pressurise the pressure gauge. Repeated cuff pressure measurement may cause reduced cuff pressure over time, which may be falsely assumed to indicate the cuff is losing volume due to other causes. Attaching rigid tubing between the cuff and pressure gauge eliminates this problem and facilitates continuous cuff pressure measurement. This is a useful strategy for assessing cuff leak problems. In this case scenario, careful troubleshooting averted the need for ETT replacement and avoided unnecessary risk to the patient.

Patient positioning is extremely important in managing the bariatric patient. Central obesity causes cephalic displacement of the diaphragm resulting in a positive pleural pressure and subsequent alveolar collapse. Box 15.3 describes some specific considerations for mechanical ventilation in the bariatric patient. Inspiratory crackles late in the inspiratory phase indicate late alveolar opening and an increased potential for lung injury due to cyclic alveolar inflation and deflation. Positive pleural pressure decreases transpulmonary pressure and often necessitates the use of higher levels of PEEP to prevent collapse. Positioning in the high semi-Fowler position can have a dramatic and positive effect on lung mechanics for these patients, evidenced by the increase in compliance in this case study. RMs typically have limited period of effectiveness – that is, derecruitment generally occurs following the manoeuvre. APRV maintains the higher level of pressure for a prolonged time so sustaining alveolar recruitment. In this case study, APRV and position changes appeared to promote recruitment and improved oxygenation enabling downwards titration of the FiO_2. When considering extubation for the bariatric patient, maintaining PEEP at a high level prior to extubation and using CPAP following extubation may prevent alveolar de-recruitment.

CASE STUDY QUESTIONS

1 Why should the lowest possible FiO_2 be used to achieve a target partial pressure of oxygen in arterial blood (PaO_2) or peripheral oxygen saturation (SpO_2)?
2 Name three advantages of high-flow nasal cannulae compared with low-flow nasal cannulae.
3 What is the most reliable method for confirming ETT placement after intubation?
4 Volume-control ventilation is a controlled mode of ventilation in which the respirator delivers a preset volume. Name two disadvantages of volume-control ventilation.
5 Mechanical ventilation can cause several serious complications including ventilator-associated pneumonia (VAP) and ventilator-associated lung injury (VALI). What is the best way to prevent these complications?
6 Prone positioning should be maintained for a maximum of 6 hours for patients with severe ARDS: true or false?

BOX 15.3

Mechanical ventilation and the bariatric patient

- Bariatric patients are at increased risk of atelectasis and have decreased chest wall compliance due to the weight of the abdomen.
- Avoid the supine position as this will further decrease lung volumes.
- Bariatric patients may require higher airway pressures to generate adequate tidal volumes.
- Recruitment manoeuvres may improve oxygenation.[230]
- Frail elderly may experience difficult weaning owing to the presence of comorbidities such as CHF, ischaemic heart disease and COPD.

RESEARCH VIGNETTE

Personalised mechanical ventilation tailored to lung morphology versus low positive end-expiratory pressure for patients with acute respiratory distress syndrome in France (the LIVE study): a multicentre, single-blind, randomised controlled trial. *Lancet Respir Med* 2019;7(10):870–80.

Abstract

Background: The effect of personalised mechanical ventilation on clinical outcomes in patients with acute respiratory distress syndrome (ARDS) remains uncertain and needs to be evaluated. We aimed to test whether a mechanical ventilation strategy that was personalised to individual patients' lung morphology would improve the survival of patients with ARDS when compared with standard of care.

Methods: We designed a multicentre, single-blind, stratified, parallel-group, randomised controlled trial enrolling patients with moderate-to-severe ARDS in 20 university or non-university intensive care units in France. Patients older than 18 years with early ARDS for less than 12 hours were randomly assigned (1:1) to either the control group or the personalised group using a minimisation algorithm and stratified according to the study site, lung morphology and duration of mechanical ventilation. Only the patients were masked to allocation. In the control group, patients received a tidal volume of 6 mL/kg per predicted body weight and positive end-expiratory pressure (PEEP) was selected according to a low PEEP and fraction of inspired oxygen table, and early prone position was encouraged. In the personalised group, the treatment approach was based on lung morphology; patients with focal ARDS received a tidal volume of 8 mL/kg, low PEEP and prone position. Patients with non-focal ARDS received a tidal volume of 6 mL/kg along with recruitment manoeuvres and high PEEP. The primary outcome was 90-day mortality as established by intention-to-treat analysis. This study is registered online with ClinicalTrials.gov, NCT02149589.

Findings: From 12 June 2014 to 2 Feb 2017, 420 patients were randomly assigned to treatment; 11 patients were excluded in the personalised group and nine patients were excluded in the control group; 196 patients in the personalised group and 204 in the control group were included in the analysis. In a multivariate analysis, there was no difference in 90-day mortality between the group treated with personalised ventilation and the control group in the intention-to-treat analysis (hazard ratio (HR) 1·01; 95% confidence interval (CI) 0·61–1·66; $P = 0.98$). However, misclassification of patients as having focal or non-focal ARDS by the investigators was observed in 85 (21%) of 400 patients. We found a significant interaction between misclassification and randomised group allocation with respect to the primary outcome ($P < 0.001$). In the subgroup analysis, the 90-day mortality of the misclassified patients was higher in the personalised group (26 (65%) of 40 patients) than in the control group (18 (32%) of 57 patients; HR 2·8; 95% CI 1·5–5·1; $P = 0.012$.

Interpretation: Personalisation of mechanical ventilation did not decrease mortality in patients with ARDS, possibly because of the misclassification of 21% of patients. A ventilator strategy misaligned with lung morphology substantially increases mortality. Whether improvement in ARDS phenotyping can decrease mortality should be assessed in a future clinical trial.

Critique

Not all types of ARDS are the same and should not be treated similarly. The treatment for individual ARDS patients entails adjusting ventilator settings to reduce the risk of VILI. The effect of tailored mechanical ventilation including PEEP settings, recruitment manoeuvres and prone positioning on clinical outcomes in ARDS patients was evaluated in this study. According to the primary analysis, a tailored ventilation strategy based on lung pathology did not reduce 90-day mortality. A major limitation of this study was the low adherence to the study protocol with respect to the assessment of the lung pathology by CT scan, which could have led to the high number of patients whose lung pathology was misclassified. The misclassified patients were excluded in a prespecified subgroup analysis. Correctly classified patients did seem to benefit from the tailored intervention, while misclassified patients had a significantly higher mortality rate. Considerations for translation of this research into practice are as follows.

Personalised medicine aims to deliver a therapy to patients who will benefit and withhold this therapy from patients who will not or even will be harmed. ICU nurses and physicians work hard to offer the best possible care for patients who need mechanical ventilation, but appropriately classifying patients with ARDS at the bedside may be very challenging. The use of a CT scan in critically ill ARDS patients, the gold standard, has its limitations because transporting these patients comes with risks. Furthermore, in critically ill patients the chest radiograph lacks adequate diagnostic accuracy for pulmonary pathology. To avoid misclassification of ARDS patients in daily practice, alternatives for lung imaging are needed. Promising tools are lung ultrasound and electrical impedance tomography, which have become more common in the ICU and can be safely used at the bedside.

Learning activities

1 Describe how the terms IPAP and EPAP used on some NIV ventilators correlate with the more generic terms of PEEP and pressure support (PS).

2 Why is it important to consider the patient's respiratory rate and tidal volume when using a low-flow (variable-flow) oxygen delivery device?

3 How do increasing PEEP and recruitment manoeuvres increase oxygenation?

4 Identify some of the potential risks of recruitment manoeuvres and the nursing observations to detect signs of deterioration.

5 Explain how a reduction in the FiO_2 from 1.0 to 0.8 can increase the SpO_2.

Online resources

American Association for Respiratory Care, https://www.aarc.org/resources/

American Thoracic Society, https://www.thoracic.org/statements/index.php

Anaesthesia UK, https://www.frca.co.uk/default.aspx

ARDS network, www.ardsnet.org/

Australian and New Zealand Intensive Care Society, https://www.anzics.com.au/

Canadian Society of Respiratory Therapists, Respiratory compromise toolkit, https://www.csrt.com/respiratory-compromise-toolkit/

College of Intensive Care Medicine of Australia and New Zealand, https://www.cicm.org.au/

Covidien education resources, https://www.medtronic.com/covidien/en-us/clinical-education.html

Critical Care Medicine Tutorials, https://ccm-tutorials.com

Department of Anaesthesia and Intensive Care, Chinese University of Hong Kong, https://www.cuhk.edu.hk/med/ans/

Intensive Care New South Wales, https://aci.health.nsw.gov.au/networks/icnsw

National Institute for Health and Care Excellence, https://www.nice.org.uk/

Thoracic Society of Australia and New Zealand, https://thoracic.org.au/

VentWorld, ventworld.com/

Further reading

Branson RD, Gomaa D, Rodriquez D Jr. Management of the artificial airway. Respir Care 2014;59(6):974–89.

Canadian Critical Care Trials Group/Canadian Critical Care Society Noninvasive Ventilation Guidelines Group. Clinical practice guidelines for the use of noninvasive positive-pressure ventilation and noninvasive continuous positive airway pressure in the acute care setting. CMAJ 2011;183(3):E195–214.

Chatburn RL, Khatib ME, Mireles-Cabodevila E. A taxonomy for mechanical ventilation: 10 fundamental maxims. Respir Care 2014;59(11):1747–63.

Dhand R. How should aerosols be delivered during invasive mechanical ventilation? Respir Care 2017;62(10):1343–67.

Fan E, Brodie D, Slutsky AS. Acute respiratory distress syndrome: advances in diagnosis and treatment. JAMA 2018;319(7):698–710.

Ferrer M, Sellares J, Torres A. Noninvasive ventilation in withdrawal from mechanical ventilation. Semin Respir Crit Care Med 2014;35(4):507–18.

Jiang JR, Yen SY, Chien JY, et al. Predicting weaning and extubation outcomes in long-term mechanically ventilated patients using the modified Burns Wean Assessment Program scores. Respirology 2014;19(4):576–82.

Suzumura EA, Figueiró M, Normilio-Silva K, et al. Effects of alveolar recruitment maneuvers on clinical outcomes in patients with acute respiratory distress syndrome: a systematic review and meta-analysis. Intensive Care Med 2014;40(9):1227–40.

References

1. Australian and New Zealand Intensive Care Society. Centre for Outcome and Resource Evaluation (ANZICS CORE) annual report 2020. Melbourne, VIC: ANZICS; 2020.

2. Intensive Care National Audit & Research Centre. Key statistics from the Case Mix Programme – adult, general critical care units. 1 January 2019 to 31 December 2021. London: Intensive Care National Audit & Research Centre; 2022.

3. Wunsch H, Wagner J, Herlim M, et al. ICU occupancy and mechanical ventilator use in the United States. Crit Care Med 2013;41:2712–19.

4. Chew D, Aroney C, Aylward P, et al. 2011 Addendum to the National Heart Foundation of Australia/Cardiac Society of Australia and New Zealand Guidelines for the management of acute coronary syndromes (ACS) 2006. Heart Lung Circ 2011;20:487–502.

5. Hoiland RL, Mladinov S, Barak OF, et al. Oxygen therapy improves cerebral oxygen delivery and neurovascular function in hypoxaemic chronic obstructive pulmonary disease patients. Exp Physiol 2018;103(8):1170–7. doi: 10.1113/ep086994.

6. Naughton M, Tuxen D. Acute respiratory failure in chronic obstructive pulmonary disease. In: Bersten A, Soni N, editors. Oh's intensive care manual. 8th ed. Philadelphia: Butterworth-Heinemann Elsevier; 2019; p. 388–401.

7. Wagstaff T, Soni N. Performance of six types of oxygen delivery devices at varying respiratory rates. Anaesthesia 2007;62:492–503.

8. Sampson B, Bihari S. Oxygen therapy. In: Bersten A, Soni N, editors. Oh's intensive care manual. 8th ed. Philadelphia: Butterworth-Heinemann Elsevier; 2019, p. 359–72.

9. Sim M, Dean P, Kinsella J, et al. Performance of oxygen delivery devices when the breathing pattern of respiratory failure is simulated. Anaesthesia 2008;63:938–40.

10. Chanques G, Riboulet F, Molinari N, et al. Comparison of three high flow oxygen therapy delivery devices: a clinical physiological cross-over study. Minerva Anestesiol 2013;79:1344–55.

11. Corley A, Caruana LR, Barnett AG, et al. Oxygen delivery through high-flow nasal cannulae increase end-expiratory lung volume and reduce respiratory rate in post-cardiac surgical patients. Br J Anaesth 2011;107:998–1004. doi: 10.1093/bja/aer265.

12. Kernick J, Magary J. What is the evidence for the use of high flow nasal cannula oxygen in adult patients admitted to critical care units? A systematic review. Aust Crit Care 2010;23:53–70.

13. Fisher and Paykel Healthcare New Zealand. Nasal high flow. https://www.fphcare.com/en-gb/hospital/infant-respiratory/nasal-high-flow/. [Accessed 15 February 2023].

14. Papazian L, Corley A, Hess D, et al. Use of high-flow nasal cannula oxygenation in ICU adults: a narrative review. Intensive Care Med 2016;42:1336–49. doi: 10.1007/s00134-016-4277-8.

15. Peters S, Holets S, Gay P. High-flow nasal cannula therapy in do-not-intubate patients with hypoxemic respiratory distress. Respir Care 2013;58:597–600.

16. Helviz Y, Einav S. A systematic review of the high-flow nasal cannula for adult patients. Crit Care 2018;22:71.

17. Lewis S, Baker P, Parker R, et al. High-flow nasal cannulae for respiratory support in adult intensive care patients. Cochrane Database Syst Rev 2021;3:CD010172.

18. Hnatiuk O, Moores L, Thompson J, et al. Delivery of high concentrations of inspired oxygen via tusk mask. Crit Care Med 1998;26:1032–5.

19. Peruzzi W, Smith B. Oxygen delivery: tusks versus flow. Crit Care Med 1998;26:986.

20. Boumphrey S, Morris E, Kinsella S. 100% Inspired oxygen from a Hudson mask – a realistic goal? Resuscitation 2003;57:69–72.

21. Davies JD, Costa BK, Asciutto AJ. Approaches to manual ventilation. Respir Care 2014;59:810–22; discussion 822–4. doi: 10.4187/respcare.03060.

22. Cook T, Hommers C. New airways for resuscitation? Resuscitation 2006;69:371–87.

23. Choi G, Joynt G. Airway management and acute airway obstruction. In: Bersten A, Soni N, editors. Oh's intensive care manual. 8th ed. Philadelphia: Butterworth-Heinemann Elsevier; 2019, p. 373–87.

24. Donatelli J, Gupta A, Santhosh R, et al. To breathe or not to breathe: a review of artificial airway placement and related complications. Emerg Radiol 2015;22:171–9. doi: 10.1007/s10140-014-1271-8.

25. Nolan J, Hazinski M, Billi J, et al. Part 1: Executive summary: 2010 international consensus on cardiopulmonary resuscitation and emergency cardiovascular care science with treatment recommendations. Resuscitation 2010;81:e1–25.

26. Wahlen B, Roewer N, Lange M, et al. Tracheal intubation and alternative airway management devices used by healthcare professionals with different level of pre-existing skills: a manikin study. Anaesthesia 2009;64:549–54.

27. Vézina M-C, Trépanier C, Nicole P, et al. Complications associated with the Esophageal-Tracheal Combitube® in the pre-hospital setting. Can J Anesth 2007;54:124–8.

28. Haas C, Eakin R, Konkle M, et al. Endotracheal tubes: old and new. Respir Care 2014;59:933–52.

29. Haas C, Branson R, Folk L, et al. Patient-determined inspiratory flow during assisted mechanical ventilation. Respir Care 1995;40:716–21.

30. Ball J, Platt S. Obstruction of a reinforced oral tracheal tube. Brit J Anaesth 2010;105:699–700.

31. Davies R. The importance of a Murphy eye. Anaesthesia 2001;56:906–24.

32. Anantham D, Jagadesan R, Tiew P. Clinical review: independent lung ventilation in critical care. Crit Care 2005;9:594–600.

33. Jaber S, Amraoui J, Lefrant J-Y, et al. Clinical practice and risk factors for immediate complications of endotracheal intubation in the intensive care unit: a prospective, multiple-center study. Crit Care Med 2006;34:2355–61.

34. Weingart S. Preoxygenation, reoxygenation, and delayed sequence intubation in the emergency department. J Emerg Med 2010;40(6):661–7.

35. Vourc'h M, Asfar P, Volteau C, et al. High-flow nasal cannula oxygen during endotracheal intubation in hypoxemic patients: a randomized controlled clinical trial. Intensive Care Med 2015;41:1538–48.

36. Mosier J, Hypes C, Sakles J. Understanding preoxygenation and apneic oxygenation during intubation in the critically ill. Intensive Care Med 2016;43:226–8.

37. Holzapfel L, Chastang C, Demingeon G, et al. A randomized study assessing the systematic search for maxillary sinusitis in nasotracheally mechanically ventilated patients. Influence of nosocomial maxillary sinusitis on the occurrence of ventilator-associated pneumonia. Am J Resp Crit Care Med 1999;159:695–701.

38. Beavers R, Moos D, Cuddeford J. Analysis of the application of cricoid pressure: implications for the clinician. J PeriAnesth Nurs 2009;24:92–102.

39. Brisson P, Brisson M. Variable application and misapplication of cricoid pressure. J Trauma 2010;69:1182–4.

40. Salem MR, Khorasani A, Zeidan A, et al. Cricoid pressure controversies: narrative review. Anesthesiology 2017;126:738–52. doi: 10.1097/aln.0000000000001489.

41. Sitzwohl C, Langheinrich A, Schober A, et al. Endobronchial intubation detected by insertion depth of endotracheal tube, bilateral auscultation, or observation of chest movements: randomised trial. BMJ 2010;341:c5943.

42. Rudraraju P, Eisen L. Confirmation of endotracheal tube position: a narrative review. J Intensive Care Med 2009;24:283–92.

43. College of Intensive Care Medicine of Australia and New Zealand (CICM). Minimum standards for intensive care units. IC-1. Ptahran, VIC: CICM; 1994 (reviewed 2016). Available from: https://www.cicm.org.au/CICM_Media/CICMSite/CICM-Website/Resources/Professional%20Documents/IC-1-Minimum-Standards-for-Intensive-Care-Units_2.pdf.[Accessed 15 February 2023].

44. Mallick A, Bodenham A. Tracheostomy in critically ill patients. Eur J Anaesthesiol 2010;27:676–82.

45. De Leyn P, Bedert L, Delcroix M, et al. Tracheotomy: clinical review and guidelines. Eur J Cardiothorac Surg 2007;2:412–21.

46. Australian and New Zealand Intensive Care Society (ANZICS). Percutaneous dilatational tracheostomy consensus statement. Carlton, VIC: ANZICS; 2014. Available from: https://www.anzics.com.au/wp-content/uploads/2018/08/2014-The-ANZICS-Percutaneous-Dilatational-Tracheostomy-Consensus-Statement.pdf. [Accessed 15 February 2023].

47. Russell C. Providing the nurse with a guide to tracheostomy care and management. B J Nur 2005;14:428–33.

48. Dennis-Rouse M, Davidson J. An evidence-based evaluation of tracheostomy care practices. Crit Care Nurs Q 2008;31:150–60.

49. Beach L, Denehy L, Lee A. The efficacy of minitracheostomy for the management of sputum retention: a systematic review. Physiotherapy 2013;99:271–7.

50. Abdelaziz M, Naidu B, Agostini P. Is prophylactic minitracheostomy beneficial in high-risk patients undergoing thoracotomy and lung resection? Interac Cardiovasc Thorac Surg 2011;12:615–18.

51. Thomas A, McGrath B. Patient safety incidents associated with airway devices in critical care: a review of reports to the UK National Patient Safety Agency. Anaesthesia 2009;64:358–65.

52. Ai ZP, Gao XL, Zhao XL. Factors associated with unplanned extubation in the Intensive Care Unit for adult patients: a systematic review and meta-analysis. Intensive Crit Care Nurs 2018;47:62–8. doi: 10.1016/j.iccn.2018.03.008.

53. Curry K, Cobb S, Kutash M, et al. Characteristics associated with unplanned extubations in a surgical intensive care unit. Am J Crit Care 2008;17:45–51, quiz 52.

54. Chao CM, Lai CC, Chan KS, et al. Multidisciplinary interventions and continuous quality improvement to reduce unplanned extubation in adult intensive care units: A 15-year experience. Medicine 2017;96:e6877. doi: 10.1097/md.0000000000006877.

55. Chuang ML, Lee CY, Chen YF, et al. Revisiting unplanned endotracheal extubation and disease severity in intensive care units. PloS One 2015;10:e0139864. doi: 10.1371/journal.pone.0139864.

56. Engels P, Bagshaw S, Meier M, et al. Tracheostomy: from insertion to decannulation. Can J Surg 2009;52:427–33.

57. Brass P, Hellmich M, Ladra A, et al. Percutaneous techniques versus surgical techniques for tracheostomy. Cochrane Database Syst Rev 2016;7:CD008045. doi: 10.1002/14651858.CD008045.pub2.

58. Fernandez M, Piacentini E, Blanch L, et al. Changes in lung volume with three systems of endotracheal suctioning with and without pre-oxygenation in patients with mild-to-moderate lung failure. Intensive Care Med 2004;30:2210–15.

59. American Association for Respiratory Care. AARC clinical practice guidelines. Endotracheal suctioning of mechanically ventilated patients with artificial airways. Respir Care 2010;55:758–64.

60. Sole ML, Bennett M, Ashworth S. Clinical indicators for endotracheal suctioning in adult patients receiving mechanical ventilation. Am J Crit Care 2015;24:318–24, quiz 325. doi: 10.4037/ajcc2015794.

61. Chaseling W, Bayliss S-L, Rose K, et al. Suctioning an adult ICU patient with an artificial airway, version 2. Chatswood, NSW: Agency for Clinical Innovation NSW Government; 2014.

62. Paulus F, Binnekade J, Vroom M, et al. Benefits and risks of manual hyperinflation in intubated and mechanically ventilated intensive care unit patients: a systematic review. Crit Care 2012;16:R145.

63. Ayhan H, Tastan S, Iyigun E, et al. Normal saline instillation before endotracheal suctioning: "What does the evidence say? What do the nurses think?": multimethod study. J Crit Care 2015;30:762–7. doi: 10.1016/j.jcrc.2015.02.019.

64. National Health and Medical Research Council. Australian guidelines for the prevention and control of infection in healthcare. Canberra, ACT: Commonwealth of Australia; 2010.

65. Intensive Care Coordination and Monitoring Unit. Stabilisation of an endotracheal tube for the adult intensive care patient. NSW Health statewide guidelines for intensive care. Available from: https://aci.health.nsw.gov.au/__data/assets/pdf_file/0003/178554/EOI-ICCMU.pdf. [Accessed 15 February 2023].

66. Gardner A, Hughes D, Cook R, et al. Best practice in stabilisation of oral endotracheal tubes: a systematic review. Aust Crit Care 2005;18:158165.

67. Murdoch E, Holdgate A. A comparison of tape-tying versus a tube-holding device for securing endotracheal tubes in adults. Anaesth Intensive Care 2007;35:730–5.

68. Haddad S, Arabi Y. Critical care management of severe traumatic brain injury in adults. Scand J Trauma Resusc Emerg Med 2012;20:12.

69. Hockey CA, van Zundert AA, Paratz JD. Does objective measurement of tracheal tube cuff pressures minimise adverse effects and maintain accurate cuff pressures? A systematic review and meta-analysis. Anaesth Intensive Care 2016;44:560–70.

70. Bulamba F, Kintu A, Ayupo N, et al. Achieving the recommended endotracheal tube cuff pressure: a randomized control study comparing loss of resistance syringe to pilot balloon palpation. Anesthesiol Res Pract 2017;2017:2032748.

71. Sole M, Penoyer D, Su X, et al. Assessment of endotracheal cuff pressure by continuous monitoring: a pilot study. Am J Crit Care 2009;18:133–43.

72. Lizy C, Swinnen W, Labeau S, et al. Cuff pressure of endotracheal tubes after changes in body position in critically ill patients treated with mechanical ventilation. Am J Crit Care 2014;23:e1–8.

73. Letvin A, Kremer P, Silver P, et al. Frequent versus infrequent monitoring of endotracheal tube cuff pressures. Respir Care 2018;63:495–501.

74. Lorente L, Lecuona M, Jiménez A, et al. Continuous endotracheal tube cuff pressure control system protects against ventilator-associated pneumonia. Crit Care 2014;18:R77.

75. Fernandez J, Levine S, Restrepo M. Technologic advances in endotracheal tubes for prevention of ventilator-associated pneumonia. Chest 2012;142:231–8.

76. Seguin P, Perrichet H, Pabic E, et al. Effect of continuous versus intermittent subglottic suctioning ontracheal mucosa by the Mallinckrodt TaperGuard Evac oral tracheal tube in intensive care unit ventilated patients: a prospective randomized study. Indian J Crit Care Med 2018;22:1–4.

77. Suys E, Nieboer K, Stiers W, et al. Intermittent subglottic secretion drainage may cause tracheal damage in patients with few oropharyngeal secretions. Intensive Crit Care Nurs 2013;29:317–20.

78. Mao Z, Gao L, Wang G, et al. Subglottic secretion suction for preventing ventilator-associated pneumonia: an updated meta-analysis and trial sequential analysis. Crit Care 2016;20:353.

79. Bitgani M, Madineh H. Intraoperative atelectasis due to endotracheal tube cuff herniation: a case report. Acta Medica Iranica 2012;50: 652–4.

80. El-Orbany M, Salem M. Endotracheal tube cuff leaks: causes, consequences, and management. Anesth Analg 2013;117:428–34.

81. AARC. AARC clinical practice guideline: removal of the endotracheal tube. 2007 revision and update. Respir Care 2007;52:81–93.

82. Schnell D, Planquette B, Berger A, et al. Cuff leak test for the diagnosis of post-extubation stridor. J Intensive Care Med 2019;34(5):391–6. doi: 10.1177/0885066617700095.

83. Pluijms WA, van Mook WN, Wittekamp BH, et al. Postextubation laryngeal edema and stridor resulting in respiratory failure in critically ill adult patients: updated review. Crit Care 2015;19:295. doi: 10.1186/s13054-015-1018-2.

84. Andreu MF, Dotta ME, Bezzi MG, et al. Safety of positive pressure extubation technique. Respir Care 2019;64:899–907. doi: 10.4187/respcare.06541.

85. Zhang B, Ratano D, Brochard L, et al. A physiology-based mathematical model for the selection of appropriate ventilator controls for lung and diaphragm protection. J Clin Monit Comput 2021;35:363–78.

86. Hess D. Ventilator waveforms and the physiology of pressure support ventilation. Respir Care 2005;50:166–86.

87. Cairo J. Pilbeam's mechanical ventilation: physiological and clinical applications. 7th ed. St Louis: Mosby Elsevier; 2019.

88. Amato MBP, Meade MO, Slutsky AS, et al. Driving pressure and survival in the acute respiratory distress syndrome. New Engl J Med 2015;372:747–55. doi: 10.1056/NEJMsa1410639.

89. Giosa L, Busana M, Pasticci I, et al. Mechanical power at a glance: a simple surrogate for volume-controlled ventilation. Intensive Care Med Exp 2019;7:61. doi: 10.1186/s40635-019-0276-8.

90. Burns S. Working with respiratory waveforms: how to use bedside graphics. AACN Clin Issues 2003;14:133–44.

91. Rittner F, Doring M. Curves and loops in mechanical ventilation. Hong Kong: Draeger Medical Asia Pacific; n.d.

92. Zanella A, Bellani G, Pesenti A. Airway pressure and flow monitoring. Curr Opin Crit Care 2010;16:255–60. doi: 10.1097/MCC.0b013e328337f209.

93. Nilsestuen J, Hargett K. Using ventilator graphics to identify patient-ventilator asynchrony. Respir Care 2005;50:202–34.

94. Yang S, Yang S. Effects of inspiratory flow waveforms on lung mechanics, gas exchange, and respiratory metabolism in COPD patients during mechanical ventilation. Chest 2002;122:2096–104.

95. Blanch L, Bernabé F, Lucangelo U. Measurement of air trapping, intrinsic positive end-expiratory pressure, and dynamic hyperinflation in mechanically ventilated patients. Respir Care 2005;50:110–23.

96. Lu Q, Rouby J-J. Measurement of pressure-volume curves in patients on mechanical ventilation: methods and significance. Crit Care 2000;4:91–100.

97. Bonetto C, Calo M, Delgado M, et al. Modes of pressure delivery and patient–ventilator interaction. Respir Care Clin N Am 2005;11:247–63.

98. Maggiore S, Jonson B, Richard J, et al. Alveolar derecruitment at decremental positive end-expiratory pressure levels in acute lung injury: comparison with the lower inflection point, oxygenation, and compliance. Am J Respir Crit Care Med 2001;164:795–801.

99. Hickling K. Best compliance during a decremental, but not incremental, positive end-expiratory pressure trial is related to open-lung positive end-expiratory pressure: a mathematical model of acute respiratory distress syndrome lungs. Am J Respir Crit Care Med 2001;163:69–78.

100. Brochard L. What is a pressure–volume curve? Crit Care 2006;10:156. doi: 10.1186/cc5002.

101. Lucangelo U, Bernabé F, Blanch L. Respiratory mechanics derived from signals in the ventilator circuit. Respir Care 2005;50:55–65.

102. Al Ashry HS, Modrykamien AM. Humidification during mechanical ventilation in the adult patient. BioMed Res Int 2014;2014:715434. doi: 10.1155/2014/715434.

103. Branson R. The ventilator circuit and ventilator-associated pneumonia. Respir Care 2005;50:774–85.

104. Muscedere J, Dodek P, Keenan S, et al. Comprehensive evidence-based clinical practice guidelines for ventilator-associated pneumonia: prevention. J Crit Care 2008;23:126–37.

105. Hellyer T, Ewan V, Wilson P, et al. The Intensive Care Society recommended bundle of interventions for the prevention of ventilator-associated pneumonia. J Intensive Care Soc 2016;17:238–43.

106. Kilgour E, Rankin N, Ryan S, et al. Mucociliary function deteriorates in the clinical range of inspired air temperature and humidity. Intensive Care Med 2004;30:1491–4.

107. Gallucio ST, Bersten AD. Humidication and inhalation therapy. In: Bersten A, Soni N, Oh T, editors. Oh's intensive care manual. 8th ed. Oxford: Butterworth-Heinemann; 2019, p. 414–27.

108. Wilkes AR. Heat and moisture exchangers and breathing system filters: their use in anaesthesia and intensive care. Part 1 – history, principles and efficiency. Anaesthesia 2011;66:31–9. doi: 10.1111/j.1365-2044.2010.06563.x.

109. Gillies D, Todd D, Foster J, et al. Heat and moisture exchangers versus heated humidifiers for mechanically ventilated adults and children. Cochrane Database Syst Rev 2017;9:CD004711.

110. Nava S, Hill N. Non-invasive ventilation in acute respiratory failure. Lancet 2009;374:250–9.

111. Rose L, Gerdtz M. Review of non-invasive ventilation in the emergency department: clinical considerations and management priorities. J Clin Nurs 2009;18:3216–24.

112. Mehta S, Hill N. Noninvasive ventilation: state of the art. Am J Respir Crit Care Med 2001;163:540–77.

113. Hill N. Noninvasive positive pressure ventilation. In: Tobin M, editor. Principles and practice of mechanical ventilation. 3rd ed. New York: McGraw-Hill, 2013, p. 435–46.

114. L'Her E, Deye N, Lellouche F, et al. Physiologic effects of noninvasive ventilation during acute lung injury. Am J Respir Crit Care Med 2005;172:1112–18.

115. Hill N, Brennan J, Garpestad E, et al. Noninvasive ventilation in acute respiratory failure. Crit Care Med 2007;35:2402–7.

116. Schulze V, Meyer C, Eickholt C, et al. Impact of continuous positive airway pressure on left ventricular systolic loading and coronary flow reserve in healthy young men. Heart Lung Circ 2018;27:344–9. doi: 10.1016/j.hlc.2017.02.022.

117. Kaye D, Mansfield D, Naughton MT. Continuous positive airway pressure decreases myocardial oxygen consumption in heart failure. Clin Sci 2004;106:599–603.

118. Pladeck T, Hader C, Von Orde A, et al. Non-invasive ventilation: comparison of effectiveness, safety, and management of acute heart failure syndromes and acute exacerbations of chronic obstructive pulmonary disease. J Physiol Pharmacol 2007;58:539–49.

119. Caples S, Gay P. Noninvasive positive pressure ventilation in the intensive care unit: a concise review. Crit Care Med 2005;33:2651–8.

120. Rochwerg B, Brochard L, Elliott M, et al. Official ERS/ATS clinical practice guidelines: noninvasive ventilation for acute respiratory failure. Eur Respir J 2017;50:1602426.

121. Osadnik C, Tee V, Carson-Chahhoud K, et al. Non-invasive ventilation for the management of acute hypercapnic respiratory failure due to exacerbation of chronic obstructive pulmonary disease. Cochrane Database Syst Rev 2017;7(7):CD004104.

122. Confalonieri M, Garuti G, Cattaruzza M, et al. A chart of failure risk for noninvasive ventilation in patients with COPD exacerbation. Eur Respir J 2005;25:348–55.

123. Masip J, Roque M, Sanchez B, et al. Noninvasive ventilation in acute cardiogenic pulmonary edema. JAMA 2005;294:3124–30.

124. Peter JV, Moran JL, Phillips-Hughes J, et al. Effect of non-invasive positive pressure ventilation (NIPPV) on mortality in patients with acute cardiogenic pulmonary oedema: a meta-analysis. Lancet 2006;367:1155–63. doi: 10.1016/S0140-6736(06)68506-1.

125. Winck JC, Azevedo LF, Costa-Pereira A, et al. Efficacy and safety of non-invasive ventilation in the treatment of acute cardiogenic pulmonary edema – a systematic review and meta-analysis. Crit Care 2006;10:R69. doi: 10.1186/cc4905.

126. Berbenetz N, Wang Y, Brown J, et al. Non-invasive positive pressure ventilation (CPAP or bilevel NPPV) for cardiogenic pulmonary oedema. Cochrane Database Syst Rev 2019;4:CD005351.

127. Vital F, Ladeira M, Atallah A. Non-invasive positive pressure ventilation (CPAP or bilevel NPPV) for cardiogenic pulmonary oedema. Cochrane Database Syst Rev 2013;5:CD005351.

128. Juern JS. Removing the critically ill patient from mechanical ventilation. Surg Clin N Am 2012;92:1475–83. doi: 10.1016/j.suc.2012.08.008.

129. Agarwal R, Aggarwal A, Gupta D, et al. Role of noninvasive positive-pressure ventilation in postextubation respiratory failure: a meta-analysis. Respir Care 2007;52:1472–9.

130. Ouellette D, Patel S, Girard T, et al. Liberation from mechanical ventilation in critically ill adults: an official American College of Chest Physicians/American Thoracic Society clinical practice guideline: inspiratory pressure augmentation during spontaneous breathing trials, protocols minimizing sedation, and noninvasive ventilation immediately after extubation. Chest 2017;151:166–80.

131. Fernando S, Tran A, Sadeghirad B, et al. Noninvasive respiratory support following extubation in critically ill adults: a systematic review and network meta-analysis. Intensive Care Med 2022;48:137–47.

132. Burns K, Stevenson J, Laird M, et al. Non-invasive ventilation versus invasive weaning in critically ill adults: a systematic review and meta-analysis. Thorax 2022;77(8):752–61. doi: 10.1136/thoraxjnl-2021-216993.

133. Burns K, Meade M, Premji A, et al. Non-invasive positive pressure ventilation as a weaning strategy for intubated patients with respiratory failure. Cochrane Database Syst Rev 2013:CD004127.

134. Althoff M, Holguin F, Yang F, et al. Noninvasive ventilation use in critically ill patients with acute asthma exacerbations. Am J Respir Crit Care Med 2020;202:1520–30.

135. Lim WJ, Mohammed Akram R, Carson KV, et al. Non-invasive positive pressure ventilation for treatment of respiratory failure due to severe acute exacerbations of asthma. Cochrane Database Syst Rev 2012;12:CD004360. doi: 10.1002/14651858.CD004360.pub4.

136. Pallin M, Naughton M. Noninvasive ventilation in acute asthma. J Crit Care 2014;29:586–93.

137. Diaz de Teran T, Barbagelata E, Cilloniz C, et al. Non-invasive ventilation in palliative care: a systematic review. Minerva Med 2019;110: 555–63.

138. Quill C, Quill T. Palliative use of noninvasive ventilation: navigating murky waters. J Palliat Med 2014;17:657–61.

139. Ozsancak Ugurlu A, Sidhom SS, Khodabandeh A, et al. Use and outcomes of noninvasive positive pressure ventilation in acute care hospitals in Massachusetts. Chest 2014;145:964–71. doi: 10.1378/chest.13-1707.

140. Evans TW. International Consensus Conferences in Intensive Care Medicine: non-invasive positive pressure ventilation in acute respiratory failure. Organised jointly by the American Thoracic Society, the European Respiratory Society, the European Society of Intensive Care Medicine, and the Societe de Reanimation de Langue Francaise, and approved by the ATS Board of Directors, December 2000. Intensive Care Med 2001;27:166–78.

141. Hong S, Wang H, Tian Y, et al. The roles of noninvasive mechanical ventilation with helmet in patients with acute respiratory failure: a systematic review and meta-analysis. PloS One 2021;16:e0250063.

142. Esquinas Rodriguez AM, Papadakos PJ, Carron M, et al. Clinical review: helmet and non-invasive mechanical ventilation in critically ill patients. Crit Care 2013;17:223. doi: 10.1186/cc11875.

143. Chaudhuri D, Jinah R, Burns K, et al. Helmet noninvasive ventilation compared to facemask noninvasive ventilation and high-flow nasal cannula in acute respiratory failure: a systematic review and meta-analysis. Eur Respir J 2022;59:2101269.

144. Davidson AC, Banham S, Elliott M, et al. BTS/ICS guideline for the ventilatory management of acute hypercapnic respiratory failure in adults. Thorax 2016;71(Suppl. 2):ii1–35. doi: 10.1136/thoraxjnl-2015-208209.

145. Keenan S, Sinuff T, Burns K, et al. Clinical practice guidelines for the use of noninvasive positive-pressure ventilation and noninvasive continuous positive airway pressure in the acute care setting. CMAJ 2011;183:E195–214.

146. Laghi F, Tobin M. Indications for mechanical ventilation. In: Tobin M, editor. Principles and practice of mechanical ventilation. 3nd ed. New York: McGraw-Hill, 2013, p. 101–36.

147. Tobin M, Guenther S, Perez W, et al. Konno-Mead analysis of ribcage-abdominal motion during successful and unsuccessful trials of weaning from mechanical ventilation. Am Rev Respir Dis 1987;135:1320–8.

148. Chatburn R, Volsko T, Hazy J, et al. Determining the basis for a taxonomy of mechanical ventilation. Respir Care 2012;57:514–24.

149. Rose L. Advanced modes of mechanical ventilation: implications for practice. AACN Adv Crit Care 2006;17:145–58.

150. Neto AS, Jaber S. What's new in mechanical ventilation in patients without ARDS: lessons from the ARDS literature. Intensive Care Med 2016;42:787–9. doi: 10.1007/s00134-016-4309-4.

151. Habashi N. Other approaches to open-lung ventilation: airway pressure release ventilation. Crit Care Med 2005;33:S228–40.

152. Marik P, Krikorian J. Pressure-controlled ventilation in ARDS: a practical approach. Chest 1997;112:1102–6.

153. Esteban A, Alia I, Gordo F, et al. Prospective randomized trial comparing pressure-controlled ventilation and volume-controlled ventilation in ARDS. Chest 2000;117:1690–6.

154. Campbell R, Davis B. Pressure-controlled versus volume-controlled ventilation: does it matter? Respir Care 2002;47:416–26.

155. Jiang J, Li B, Kang N, et al. Pressure-controlled versus volume-controlled ventilation for surgical patients: a systematic review and meta-analysis. J Cardiothorac Vasc Anesth 2016;30:501–14. doi: 10.1053/j.jvca.2015.05.199.

156. Asfar P, Singer M, Radermacher P. Understanding the benefits and harms of oxygen therapy. Intensive Care Med 2015;41:1118–21.

157. Martin D, Richards G. Predicted body weight relationships for protective ventilation – unisex proposals from pre-term through to adult. BMC Pulm Med 2017;17:85.

158. Fan E, Del Sorbo L, Goligher E, et al. An official American Thoracic Society/European Society of Intensive Care Medicine/Society of Critical Care Medicine clinical practice guideline: mechanical ventilation in adult patients with acute respiratory distress syndrome. Am J Respir Crit Care Med 2017;195:1253–63.

159. Griffiths M, McAuley D, Perkins G, et al. Guidelines on the management of acute respiratory distress syndrome. BMJ Open Respir Res 2019;6:e000420.

160. Walkey A, Goligher E, Del Sorbo L, et al. Low tidal volume versus non-volume-limited strategies for patients with acute respiratory distress syndrome. A systematic review and meta-analysis. Ann Am Thorac Soc 2017;14:S271–79.

161. Neto A, Simonis F, Barbas C, et al. Lung-protective ventilation with low tidal volumes and the occurrence of pulmonary complications in patients without acute respiratory distress syndrome: a systematic review and individual patient data analysis. Crit Care Med 2015;43:2155–63.

162. Holets S, Hubmayr R. Setting the ventilator. In: Tobin M, editor. Principles and practice of mechanical ventilation. 3rd ed. New York: McGraw-Hill, 2013, p. 139–58.

163. Khalil M, Elfattah N, El-Shafey M, et al. Flow versus pressure triggering in mechanically ventilated acute respiratory failure patients. Egypt J Bronchol 2015;9:198–201.

164. Hill L, Pearl R. Flow triggering, pressure triggering, and autotriggering during mechanical ventilation. Crit Care Med 2000;28:579–81.

165. Murias G, Villagra A, Blanch L. Patient--ventilator dyssynchrony during assisted invasive mechanical ventilation. Minerva Anesthesiol 2013;79:434–44.

166. Murata S, Yokoyama K, Sakamoto Y, et al. Effects of inspiratory rise time on triggering work load during pressure-support ventilation: a lung model study. Respir Care 2010;55:878–84.

167. Amato M, Marini J. Pressure-controlled and inverse-ratio ventilation. In: Tobin M (ed) Principles and practice of mechanical ventilation. 3rd ed. New York: McGraw-Hill; 2013, p. 227–52.

168. Pierce L. Management of the mechanically ventilated patient. 2nd ed. St Louis: Saunders: Elsevier; 2007.

169. Gattinoni L, Caironi P, Carlesso E. How to ventilate patients with acute lung injury and acute respiratory distress syndrome. Curr Opin Crit Care 2005;11:69–76.

170. Kallet R. Evidence-based management of acute lung injury and acute respiratory distress syndrome. Respir Care 2004;49:793–809.

171. Ashbaugh D, Bigelow D, Petty T, et al. Acute respiratory distress in adults. Lancet 1967;2:319–23.

172. Vasques F, Duscio E, Cipulli F, et al. Determinants and prevention of ventilator-induced lung injury. Crit Care Clin 2018;34:343–56.

173. Santa Cruz R, Villarejo F, Irrazabal C, et al. High versus low positive end-expiratory pressure (PEEP) levels for mechanically ventilated adult patients with acute lung injury and acute respiratory distress syndrome. Cochrane Database Syst Rev 2021;3:D009098.

174. Serpa Neto A, Schultz M. Optimizing the settings on the ventilator: high PEEP for all? JAMA 2017;317:1413–14.

175. Hess D, Kacmarek R. Essentials of mechanical ventilation. 4th ed. New York: McGraw-Hill, 2018.

176. MacIntyre N. Patient–ventilator interactions: optimizing conventional ventilation modes. Respir Care 2011;56:73–84.

177. Lago A, Goncalves E, Silva E, et al. Comparison of energy expenditure and oxygen consumption of spontaneous breathing trial conducted with and without automatic tube compensation. J Clin Med Res 2015;7:700–5.

178. L'Her E. Automatic tube compensation: is it worthwhile? Respir Care 2012;57:813–14.

179. Unoki T, Serita A, Grap M. Automatic tube compensation during weaning from mechanical ventilation: evidence and clinical implications. Crit Care Nurse 2008;28:34–42.

180. Yi L, Tian X, Chen M, et al. Comparative efficacy and safety of four different spontaneous breathing trials for weaning from mechanical ventilation: a systematic review and network meta-analysis. Front Med 2021;8:731196.

181. Chatburn R. Classification of ventilator modes: update and proposal for implementation. Respir Care 2007;52:301–23.

182. Chatburn R. Understanding mechanical ventilators. Expert Rev Respir Med 2010;4:809–19.

183. Kacmarek R, Branson R. Should intermittent mandatory ventilation be abolished? Respir Care 2016;61:854–66.

184. Chatburn R, El-Khatib M, Mireles-Cabodevila E. A taxonomy for mechanical ventilation: 10 fundamental maxims. Respir Care 2014;59:1747–63.

185. Haitsma J. Diaphragmatic dysfunction in mechanical ventilation. Curr Opin Anaesthesiol 2011;24(2):214–18.

186. MacIntyre NR. Evidence-based guidelines for weaning and discontinuing ventilatory support. Chest 2001;120:375S-95S.

187. Jain S, Kollisch-Singule M, Sadowitz B, et al. The 30-year evolution of airway pressure release ventilation (APRV). Intensive Care Med Exp 2016;4:11.

188. Daoud E, Farag H, Chatburn R. Airway pressure release ventilation: what do we know? Respir Care 2012;57:282–92.

189. Lim J, Litton E. Airway pressure release ventilation in adult patients with acute hypoxemic respiratory failure: a systematic review and meta-analysis. Crit Care Med 2019;47:1794–9.

190. Jonkman A, Rauseo M, Carteaux G, et al. Proportional modes of ventilation: technology to assist physiology. Intensive Care Med 2020;46:2301–13.

191. Boles J-M, Bion J, Connors A, et al. Weaning from mechanical ventilation. Eur Respir J 2007;29:1033–56.

192. Botta M, Wenstedt E, Tsonas A, et al. Effectiveness, safety and efficacy of INTELLiVENT–adaptive support ventilation, a closed-loop ventilation mode for use in ICU patients – a systematic review. Expert Rev Resp Med 2021;15:1403–13.

193. Umbrello M, Antonucci E, Muttini S. Neurally adjusted ventilatory assist in acute respiratory failure-a narrative review. J Clin Med 2022;11:1863.

194. Verbrugghe W, Jorens P. Neurally adjusted ventilatory assist: a ventilation tool or a ventilation toy? Respir Care 2011;56:327–35.

195. Chen C, Wen T, Liao W. Neurally adjusted ventilatory assist versus pressure support ventilation in patient-ventilator interaction and clinical outcomes: A meta-analysis of clinical trials. Ann Transl Med 2019;7:382.

196. Schmidt M, Kindler F, Cecchini J, et al. Neurally adjusted ventilatory assist and proportional assist ventilation both improve patient-ventilator interaction. Crit Care 2015;19:56.

197. Yuan X, Lu X, Chao Y, et al. Neurally adjusted ventilatory assist as a weaning mode for adults with invasive mechanical ventilation: A systematic review and meta-analysis. Crit Care 2021;25:1–11.

198. Kacmarek R. Proportional assist ventilation and neurally adjusted ventilatory assist. Respir Care 2011;56:140–8.

199. Tirupakuzhi Vijayaraghavan B, Hamed S, Jain A, et al. Evidence supporting clinical use of proportional assist ventilation: a systematic review and meta-analysis of clinical trials. J Intensive Care Med 2020;35(7):627–35. doi: 10.1177/0885066618769021.

200. Vargas M, Buonanno P, Sica A, et al. Patient-ventilator synchrony in neurally-adjusted ventilatory assist and variable pressure support ventilation. Respir Care 2022;67:503–9.

201. ARDSnet. Ventilation with lower tidal volumes compared with traditional tidal volumes for acute lung injury and the acute respiratory distress syndrome. N Engl J Med 2000;342:1301–8.

202. Suzumura E, Amato M, Cavalcanti A. Understanding recruitment maneuvers. Intensive Care Med 2016;42:908–11.

203. Hodgson C, Goligher E, Young M, et al. Recruitment manoeuvres for adults with acute respiratory distress syndrome receiving mechanical ventilation. Cochrane Database Syst Rev 2016;11(11):CD006667.

204. Suarez-Sipmann F, Bohm S, Tusman G, et al. Use of dynamic compliance for open lung positive end-expiratory pressure titration in an experimental study. Crit Care Med 2007;35:214–21.

205. Ball L, Serpa Neto A, Trifiletti V, et al. Effects of higher PEEP and recruitment manoeuvres on mortality in patients with ARDS: a systematic review, meta-analysis, meta-regression and trial sequential analysis of randomized controlled trials. Intensive Care Med Exp 2020;8:39.

206. Rose L. Clinical application of ventilation modes: ventilatory strategies for lung protection. Aus Crit Care 2010;23:71–80.

207. Facchin F, Fan E. Airway pressure release ventilation and high-frequency oscillatory ventilation: potential strategies to treat severe hypoxemia and prevent ventilator-induced lung injury. Respir Care 2015;60:1509–21.

208. Goffi A, Ferguson N. High-frequency oscillatory ventilation for early acute respiratory distress syndrome in adults. Curr Opin Crit Care 2014;20:77–85.

209. Hager D. High-frequency oscillatory ventilation in adults with acute respiratory distress syndrome. Curr Opin Anaesthesiol 2012;25:17–23.

210. Ip T, Mehta S. The role of high-frequency oscillatory ventilation in the treatment of acute respiratory failure in adults. Curr Opin Crit Care 2012;18:70–9.

211. Goligher E, Munshi L, Adhikari N, et al. High-frequency oscillation for adult patients with acute respiratory distress syndrome. a systematic review and meta-analysis. Ann Am Thorac Soc 2017;14:S289–96.

212. Papazian L, Aubron C, Brochard L, et al. Formal guidelines: management of acute respiratory distress syndrome. Ann Intensive Care 2019;9:69.

213. Combes A, Hajage D, Capellier G, et al. Extracorporeal membrane oxygenation for severe acute respiratory distress syndrome. N Engl J Med 2018;378:1965–75.

214. Serpa Neto A, Schmidt M, Azevedo L, et al. Associations between ventilator settings during extracorporeal membrane oxygenation for refractory hypoxemia and outcome in patients with acute respiratory distress syndrome: a pooled individual patient data analysis : Mechanical ventilation during ECMO. Intensive Care Med 2016;42:1672–84.

215. Makdisi G, Wang I. Extra corporeal membrane oxygenation (ECMO) review of a lifesaving technology. J Thorac Dis 2015;7:E166–76.

216. Lindholm J. Cannulation for veno-venous extracorporeal membrane oxygenation. J Thorac Dis 2018;10:S606–12.

217. Zangrillo A, Landoni G, Biondi-Zoccai G, et al. A meta-analysis of complications and mortality of extracorporeal membrane oxygenation. Crit Care Resusc 2013;15:172–8.

218. Munshi L, Walkey A, Goligher E, et al. Venovenous extracorporeal membrane oxygenation for acute respiratory distress syndrome: a systematic review and meta-analysis. Lancet Respir Med 2019;7:163–72.

219. Nguyen T, Phan X, Nguyen T, et al. Major bleeding in adults undergoing peripheral extracorporeal membrane oxygenation (ECMO): prognosis and predictors. Crit Care Res Pract 2022;2022:5348835.

220. Gebistorf F, Karam O, Wetterslev J, et al. Inhaled nitric oxide for acute respiratory distress syndrome (ARDS) in children and adults. Cochrane Database Syst Rev 2016;2016(6):CD002787.

221. McPeck M, Ashraf S, Cuccia A, et al. Factors determining continuous infusion aerosol delivery during mechanical ventilation. Respir Care 2021;66:573–81.

222. Hill N, Preston I, Roberts K. Inhaled therapies for pulmonary hypertension. Respir Care 2015;60:794–802.

223. Dugernier J, Ehrmann S, Sottiaux T, et al. Aerosol delivery during invasive mechanical ventilation: a systematic review. Crit Care 2017;21:264.

224. Dhanani J, Fraser J, Chan H, et al. Fundamentals of aerosol therapy in critical care. Crit Care 2016;20:269.

225. Burk R, Grap M. Backrest position in prevention of pressure ulcers and ventilator-associated pneumonia: conflicting recommendations. Heart Lung 2012;41:536–45.

226. Drakulovic M, Torres A, Bauer T, et al. Supine body position as a risk factor for nosocomial pneumonia in mechanically ventilated patients: a randomised trial. Lancet 1999;354:1851–8.

227. Torres A, Niederman M, Chastre J, et al. International ERS/ESICM/ESCMID/ALAT guidelines for the management of hospital-acquired pneumonia and ventilator-associated pneumonia: guidelines for the management of hospital-acquired pneumonia (HAP)/ventilator-associated pneumonia (VAP) of the European Respiratory Society (ERS), European Society of Intensive Care Medicine (ESICM), European Society of Clinical Microbiology and Infectious Diseases (ESCMID) and Asociación Latinoamericana del Tórax (ALAT). Eur Respir J 2017;50(3):1700582.

228. Kalil A, Metersky M, Klompas M, et al. Executive summary: management of adults with hospital-acquired and ventilator-associated pneumonia: 2016 clinical practice guidelines by the Infectious Diseases Society of America and the American Thoracic Society. Clin Infect Dis 2016;63:575–82.

229. van Nieuwenhoven C, Vandenbroucke-Grauls C, van Tiel F, et al. Feasibility and effects of the semirecumbent position to prevent ventilator-associated pneumonia: a randomized study. Crit Care Med 2006;34:396–402.

230. Pozuelo-Carrascosa D, Cobo-Cuenca A, Carmona-Torres J, et al. Body position for preventing ventilator-associated pneumonia for critically ill patients: a systematic review and network meta-analysis. J Intensive Care Med 2022;10:9.

231. Rose L, Baldwin I, Crawford T, et al. A multicenter, observational study of semirecumbent positioning in mechanically ventilated patients. Am J Crit Care 2010;19:e100–8.

232. Wolken R, Woodruff R, Smith J, et al. Observational study of head of bed elevation adherence using a continuous monitoring system in a medical intensive care unit. Respir Care 2012;57:537–43.

233. Liu J, Song H, Wang Y, et al. Factors associated with low adherence to head-of-bed elevation during mechanical ventilation in Chinese intensive care units. Chin Med J 2013;126:834–8.

234. Llaurado-Serra M, Ulldemolins M, Fernandez-Ballart J, et al. Related factors to semi-recumbent position compliance and pressure ulcers in patients with invasive mechanical ventilation: an observational study (CAPCRI study). Int J Nurs Studies 2016;61:198–208.

235. Rose L, Baldwin I, Crawford T. The use of bed-dials to maintain recumbent positioning for critically ill mechanically ventilated patients (the RECUMBENT study): multicentre before and after observational study. Int J Nurs Stud 2010;47:1425–31.

236. Hewitt N, Bucknall T, Faraone N. Lateral positioning for critically ill adult patients. Cochrane Database Syst Rev 2016;12:CD007205.

237. Marini J, Gattinoni L. Propagation prevention: a complementary mechanism for "lung protective" ventilation in acute respiratory distress syndrome. Crit Care Med 2008;36:3252–8.

238. Wanless S, Aldridge M. Continuous lateral rotation therapy – a review. Nurs Crit Care 2012;17:28–35.

239. Staudinger T, Bojic A, Holzinger U, et al. Continuous lateral rotation therapy to prevent ventilator-associated pneumonia. Crit Care Med 2010;38:486–90.

240. Schieren M, Piekarski F, Dusse F, et al. Continuous lateral rotational therapy in trauma – a systematic review and meta-analysis. J Trauma Acute Care Surg 2017;83:926–33.

241. Beitler J, Shaefi S, Montesi S, et al. Prone positioning reduces mortality from acute respiratory distress syndrome in the low tidal volume era: a meta-analysis. Intensive Care Med 2014;40:332–41.

242. Guerin C, Baboi L, Richard J. Mechanisms of the effects of prone positioning in acute respiratory distress syndrome. Intensive Care Med 2014;40:1634–42.

243. Kallet R. A comprehensive review of prone position in ARDS. Respir Care 2015;60(11):1660–87.

244. Gattinoni L, Taccone P, Carlesso E, et al. Prone position in acute respiratory distress syndrome. Rationale, indications, and limits. Am J Respir Crit Care Med 2013;188:1286–93.

245. Jozwiak M, Monnet X, Teboul J. Optimizing the circulation in the prone patient. Curr Opin Crit Care 2016;22:239–45.

246. Fessler H, Talmor D. Should prone positioning be routinely used for lung protection during mechanical ventilation? Respir Care 2010;55: 88–99.

247. Aoyama H, Uchida K, Aoyama K, et al. Assessment of therapeutic interventions and lung protective ventilation in patients with moderate to severe acute respiratory distress syndrome: a systematic review and network meta-analysis. JAMA Netw Open 2019;2:e198116.

248. Dickinson S, Park P, Napolitano L. Prone-positioning therapy in ARDS. Crit Care Clin 2011;27(3):511–23.

249. Stilma W, Åkerman E, Artigas A, et al. Awake proning as an adjunctive therapy for refractory hypoxemia in non-intubated patients with COVID-19 acute respiratory failure: guidance from an international group of healthcare workers. Am J Trop Med Hyg 2021;104:1676–86.

250. Chen L, Zhang Y, Li Y, et al. The application of awake-prone positioning among non-intubated patients with COVID-19-related ARDS: a narrative review. Front Med (Lausanne) 2022;9:817689.

251. Fazzini B, Page A, Pearse R, et al. Prone positioning for non-intubated spontaneously breathing patients with acute hypoxaemic respiratory failure: a systematic review and meta-analysis. Br J Anaesth 2022;128:352–62.

252. Sutherasan Y, D'Antini D, Pelosi P. Advances in ventilator-associated lung injury: prevention is the target. Expert Rev Respir Med 2014;8:233–48.

253. Torres A, Niederman M, Chastre J, et al. Summary of the international clinical guidelines for the management of hospital-acquired and ventilator-acquired pneumonia. ERJ Open Res 2018;4(2):00028–02018.

254. Gattinoni L, Pi A, Caironi P, et al. Ventilator-induced lung injury: the anatomical and physiological framework. Crit Care Med 2010;38:S539–48.

255. Slutsky A, Ranieri V. Ventilator-induced lung injury. N Engl J Med 2013;369:2126–36.

256. Gattinoni L, Marini JJ, Collino F, et al. The future of mechanical ventilation: lessons from the present and the past. Crit Care 2017;21:183. doi: 10.1186/s13054-017-1750-x.

257. Brower RG, Matthay MA, Morris A, et al. Ventilation with lower tidal volumes as compared with traditional tidal volumes for acute lung injury and the acute respiratory distress syndrome. N Engl J Med 2000;342:1301–8. doi: 10.1056/nejm200005043421801.

258. Tonetti T, Vasques F, Rapetti F, et al. Driving pressure and mechanical power: new targets for VILI prevention. Ann Transl Med 2017;5:286. doi: 10.21037/atm.2017.07.08.

259. Costa ELV, Slutsky AS, Brochard LJ, et al. Ventilatory variables and mechanical power in patients with acute respiratory distress syndrome. Am J Respir Crit Care Med 2021;204:303–11. doi: 10.1164/rccm.202009-3467OC.

260. Amato MB, Meade MO, Slutsky AS, et al. Driving pressure and survival in the acute respiratory distress syndrome. N Engl J Med 2015;372:747–55. doi: 10.1056/NEJMsa1410639.

261. Melsen W, Rovers M, Groenwold R, et al. Attributable mortality of ventilator-associated pneumonia: a meta-analysis of individual patient data from randomised prevention studies. Lancet Infect Dis 2013;13:665–71.

262. Kao J, Kao H, Chen Y, et al. Impact and predictors of prolonged chest tube duration in mechanically ventilated patients with acquired pneumothorax. Respir Care 2013;58:2093–100.

263. Anzueto A, Frutos-Vivar F, Esteban A, et al. Incidence, risk factors and outcome of barotrauma in mechanically ventilated patients. Intensive Care Med 2004;30:612–19. doi: 10.1007/s00134-004-2187-7.

264. Umbrello M, Venco R, Antonucci E, et al. Incidence, clinical characteristics and outcome of barotrauma in critically ill patients with COVID-19: a systematic review and meta-analysis. Minerva Anestesiol 2022;88:706–18. doi: 10.23736/s0375-9393.22.16258-9.

265. Thille A, Cortés-Puch I, Esteban A. Weaning from the ventilator and extubation in ICU. Curr Opin Crit Care 2013;19:57–64.

266. Schmidt G, Girard T, Kress J, et al. Liberation from mechanical ventilation in critically ill adults: executive summary of an Official American College of Chest Physicians/American Thoracic Society clinical practice guideline. Chest 2017;151:160–5.

267. Shaikh H, Morales D, Laghi F. Weaning from mechanical ventilation. Semin Respir Crit Care Med 2014;35:451–68.

268. Thille A, Boissier F, Ben Ghezala H, et al. Risk factors for and prediction by caregivers of extubation failure in ICU patients: a prospective study. Crit Care Med 2015;43:613–20.

269. Cavallone L, Vannucci A. Review article: extubation of the difficult airway and extubation failure. Anesth Analg 2013;116:368–83.

270. Meade M, Guyatt G, Cook D, et al. Predicting success in weaning from mechanical ventilation. Chest 2001;120:400S-24S.

271. Trivedi V, Chaudhuri D, Jinah R, et al. The usefulness of the rapid shallow breathing index in predicting successful extubation: a systematic review and meta-analysis. Chest 2022;161:97–111.

272. Béduneau G, Pham T, Schortgen F, et al. Epidemiology of weaning outcome according to a new definition. The WIND study. Am J Respir Crit Care Med 2017;195:772–83.

273. Kampolis C, Mermiri M, 'Mavrovounis G, et al. Comparison of advanced closed-loop ventilation modes with pressure support ventilation for weaning from mechanical ventilation in adults: a systematic review and meta-analysis. J Crit Care 2022;68:1–9.

274. Pellegrini J, Moraes R, Maccari J, et al. Spontaneous breathing trials with T-Piece or pressure support ventilation. Respir Care 2016;61: 1693–703.

275. Rose L. Strategies for weaning from mechanical ventilation: a state of the art review. Intensive Crit Care Nurs 2015;31:189–95.

276. Figueroa-Casas J, Connery S, Montoya R. Changes in breathing variables during a 30-minute spontaneous breathing trial. Respir Care 2015;60:155–61.

277. Burns K, Rizvi L, Cook D, et al. Ventilator weaning and discontinuation practices for critically ill patients. JAMA 2021;325:1173–84.

278. Blackwood B, Burns K, Cardwell C, et al. Protocolized versus non-protocolized weaning for reducing the duration of mechanical ventilation in critically ill adult patients. Cochrane Database Syst Rev 2014;2014(11):CD006904.

279. Girard T, Kress J, Fuchs B, et al. Efficacy and safety of a paired sedation and ventilator weaning protocol for mechanically ventilated patients in intensive care (Awakening and Breathing Controlled trial): a randomised controlled trial. Lancet 2008;371:126–34.

280. Bellomo R, Stow P, Hart G. Why is there such a difference in outcome between Australian intensive care units and others? Curr Opin Anaesthesiol 2007;20:100–5.

281. Rose L, Nelson S, Johnston L, et al. Workforce profile, organisation structure and role responsibility for ventilation and weaning practices in Australia and New Zealand intensive care units. J Clin Nur 2008;17:1035–43.

282. Rose L, Blackwood B, Burns S, et al. International perspectives on the influence of structure and process of weaning from mechanical ventilation. Am J Crit Care 2011;20:e10–18.

283. Branson R. Automation of mechanical ventilation. Crit Care Clin 2018;34:383–94.

284. Fernández J, Miguelena D, Mulett H, et al. Adaptive support ventilation: State of the art review. Indian J Crit Care Med 2013;17:16–22.

285. Rose L, Presneill J and Cade J. Update in computer-driven weaning from mechanical ventilation. Anaesth Intensive Care 2007;35:213–21.

286. Burns K, Lellouche F, Nisenbaum R, et al. Automated weaning and SBT systems versus non-automated weaning strategies for weaning time in invasively ventilated critically ill adults. Cochrane Database Syst Rev 2014;2014(9):CD008638.

287. Rose L, Schultz M, Cardwell C, et al. Automated versus non-automated weaning for reducing the duration of mechanical ventilation for critically ill adults and children. Cochrane Database Syst Rev 2014;2014(6):CD009235.

288. Neuschwander A, Chhor V, Yavchitz A, et al. Automated weaning from mechanical ventilation: results of a Bayesian network meta-analysis. J Crit Care 2021;61:191–8.

289. Rose L, Fowler R, Fan E, et al. Prolonged mechanical ventilation in Canadian intensive care units: a national survey. J Crit Care 2015;30: 25–31.

290. Iwashyna T, Hodgson C, Pilcher D, et al. Timing of onset and burden of persistent critical illness in Australia and New Zealand: a retrospective, population-based, observational study. Lancet Respir Med 2016;4:566–73.

291. Vitacca M, Vianello A, Colombo D, et al. Comparison of two methods for weaning patients with chronic obstructive pulmonary disease requiring mechanical ventilation for more than 15 days. Am J Respir Crit Care Med 2001;164:225–30.

292. Jubran A, Grant B, Duffner L, et al. Effect of pressure support vs unassisted breathing through a tracheostomy collar on weaning duration in patients requiring prolonged mechanical ventilation: a randomized trial. JAMA 2013;309:671–7.

293. Gonçalves M, Honrado T, Winck J, et al. Effects of mechanical insufflation-exsufflation in preventing respiratory failure after extubation: a randomized controlled trial. Crit Care Med 2012;16:R48.

294. Gomez-Merino E, Sancho J, Marin J, et al. Mechanical insufflation-exsufflation: pressure, volume, and flow relationships and the adequacy of the manufacturer's guidelines. Am J Phys Med Rehab 2002;81:579–83.

295. Rose L, Adhikari N, Leasa D, et al. Cough augmentation techniques for extubation or weaning critically ill patients from mechanical ventilation. Cochrane Database Syst Rev 2017;1(1):CD011833.

Chapter 16

Neurological assessment and monitoring

Theresa Green, Kelly Harbour

Learning objectives

After reading this chapter, you should be able to:

- describe the anatomy and physiology of the nervous system
- differentiate between the central and peripheral nervous systems
- describe the techniques used for neurological assessment
- explain the importance and process of serial neurological assessment in the patient with brain injury
- identify the distinction between normal and abnormal neurological responses
- state the determinants of intracranial pressure and describe compensatory mechanisms
- relate the procedures of selected neurodiagnostic tests to nursing implications for patient care.

Introduction

The nervous system, composed of the brain, spinal cord and nerves, is a complex network of neurons that form the major controlling, regulatory and communicating systems in the body. While accounting for a mere 3% of total body weight, it utilises 15–20% of the body's metabolic resources.[1] The brain is the centre of all mental activity, including thought, learning, memory, communication and planning. Because the brain can neither store oxygen nor effectively engage in anaerobic metabolism, any interruption in the blood or oxygen supply to the brain rapidly leads to clinically observable signs and symptoms. Glucose is virtually the sole energy substrate for the brain, and it is entirely oxidised (i.e. consumed to produce energy). Without oxygen and glucose, brain cells continue to function normally for approximately 10 seconds. The brain can be seen as an almost exclusive glucose-processing machine, producing water (H_2O) and carbon dioxide (CO_2).

Together with the endocrine and immune systems, the nervous system is responsible for regulating and maintaining homeostasis for all the organs in the body. Through its receptors, the nervous system responds to the environment, both external and internal. Diseases and disorders of the nervous system are common in the critical care unit, both as primary processes and as complications of multiple organ dysfunction in the critically ill patient. An understanding of basic neuroanatomy and neurophysiology is important if these disorders are to be recognised and treated. This chapter provides an overview of neurological anatomy and physiology and outlines the elements of a comprehensive neurological assessment.

Neurological anatomy and physiology

All the sensory details that incorporate a body's own information systems are related to neurological anatomy and physiology. Composed of central and peripheral components, with the brain as the command centre, the nervous system is responsible for the body's most fundamental activities. Nerves, which are made up of bundles of fibres, deliver impulses to various parts of the body, including the brain. The brain translates the information delivered by the impulses, which then enables the person to react.[2] This section discusses the main components of the nervous system starting from neurons and nervous system transmission. Then the central nervous system (CNS) and the peripheral nervous system (PNS) are examined and aligned with neurological assessments.

Components of the nervous system

The CNS consists of the spinal cord and brain and is responsible for integrating, processing and coordinating sensory data and motor commands (Fig. 16.1).[3] The CNS is linked to all parts of the body by the PNS, which transmits signals to and from the CNS. The PNS is composed of 43 pairs of spinal nerves and 12 pairs of cranial nerves that emerge from the base of the brain. All branch and diversify prolifically as they distribute to the tissues and organs of the body. The peripheral nerves carry input to the CNS via their sensory afferent fibres and deliver output from the CNS via the efferent fibres. Specific physiology of the CNS and PNS is discussed in

FIGURE 16.1 The functional divisions of the nervous system.

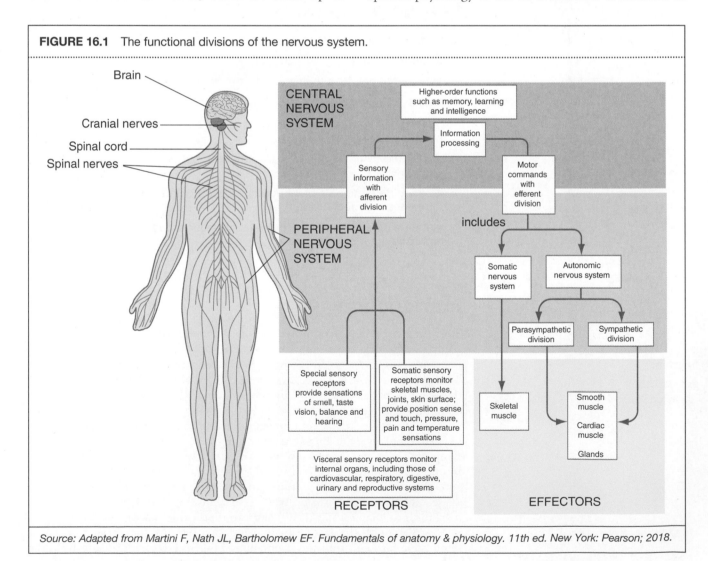

Source: Adapted from Martini F, Nath JL, Bartholomew EF. Fundamentals of anatomy & physiology. 11th ed. New York: Pearson; 2018.

detail later in the chapter. First, however, neuron cell anatomy and physiology are examined.

Neurons

Neurons are specialised cells in the nervous system; each is comprised of a dendrite, cell body (soma) and axon.[3] Each neuron uses biochemical reactions to receive, process and transmit information. Most synaptic contacts between neurons are either axodendritic (excitatory) or axosomatic (inhibitory). A neuron's dendritic tree is connected to many neighbouring neurons and receives positive or negative charges from other neurons. The input is then passed to the soma (cell body).[4] The primary role of the soma and the enclosed nucleus is to perform the continuous maintenance required to keep the neuron

functional. Most neurons lack centrioles, important organelles involved in the organisation of the cytoskeleton and the movement of chromosomes during mitosis. As a result, typical CNS neurons cannot divide and cannot be replaced if lost to injury or disease. The fuel source for the neuron is glucose; insulin is not required for cellular uptake in the CNS.[4]

A myelin sheath, consisting of a lipid–protein casing, covers the neuron.[5] Myelin is not a continuous layer but has gaps called nodes of Ranvier (Fig. 16.2A). The myelin provides protection to the axon and speeds the transmission of impulses along nerve cells from node to node (see Fig. 16.2B). Each synaptic knob contains mitochondria, portions of the endoplasmic reticulum and thousands of vesicles filled with neurotransmitter molecules. Breakdown

FIGURE 16.2 (**A**) Afferent and (**B**) efferent neurons, showing the soma or cell body, dendrites and axon. Arrows indicate the direction for conduction of action potentials.

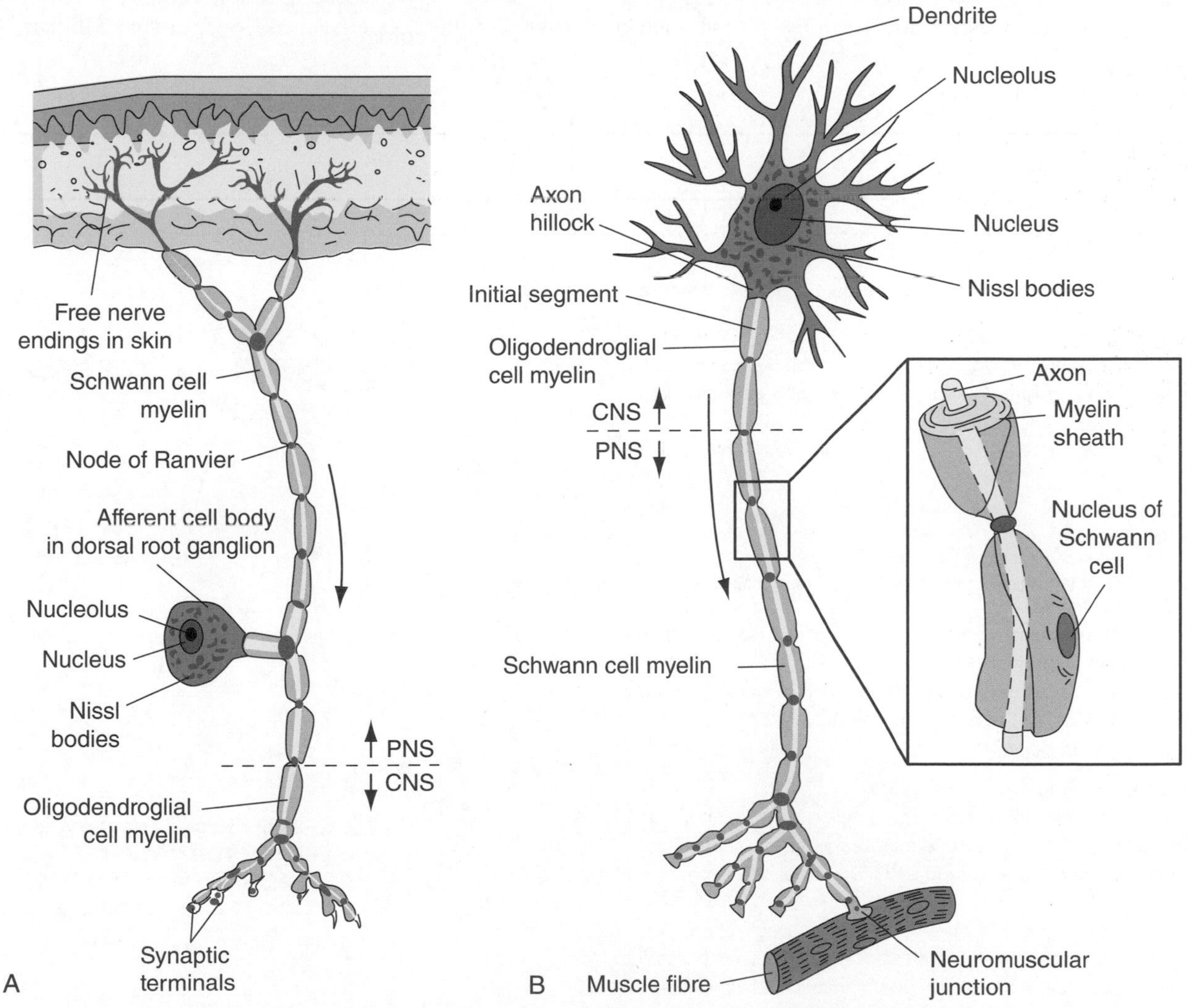

Source: Adapted from Porth C. Pathophysiology concepts of altered health states. 9th ed. Philadelphia: Lippincott, Williams and Wilkins; 2013.

products of neurotransmitter released at the synapse are reabsorbed and reassembled at the synaptic knob. The synaptic knob receives a continuous supply of neurotransmitter synthesised in the cell body, along with enzymes and lysosomes. The movement of materials between the cell body and synaptic knobs is called axoplasmic transport. Some materials travel slowly, at rates of a few millimetres per day. This transport mechanism is known as the 'slow stream'. Vesicles containing neurotransmitter move much more rapidly, travelling in the 'fast stream' at 5–10 millimetres per hour, which increases synaptic activity. Axoplasmic transport occurs in both directions. The flow of materials from the cell body to the synaptic knob is anterograde flow. At the same time, other substances are being transported towards the cell body in retrograde flow ('retro' meaning backward). If debris or unusual chemicals appear in the synaptic knob, retrograde flow soon delivers them to the cell body. The arriving materials may then alter the activity of the cell by turning appropriate genes on or off. Retrograde flow is the means of transport for viruses, pathogenic bacteria, heavy metals and toxins to the CNS, with resulting disease such as

tetanus, viral encephalitis and lead intoxication. Defective anterograde transport seems to be involved in certain neuropathies, including critical illness neuropathies.[6,7]

Synapses

The human brain contains at least 100 billion neurons, each with the ability to influence many other cells. Although there are many kinds of synapses within the brain, they can be divided into two general classes: electrical synapses and chemical synapses. Electrical synapses permit direct, passive flow of electrical current from one neuron to another in the form of an action potential; they are described in Table 16.1. The current flows through gap junctions, which are specialised membrane channels that connect the two cells. Chemical synapses, in contrast, enable cell-to-cell communication via the secretion of neurotransmitters; the chemical agents released by the presynaptic neurons produce secondary current flow in postsynaptic neurons by activating specific receptor molecules (Fig. 16.3).

Myelin increases conduction velocity. Demyelination of peripheral nerves, as occurs in Guillain–Barré

TABLE 16.1

Generation of action potentials (nervous tissue)

STEP 1: Depolarisation
A graded depolarisation brings an area of excitable membrane to threshold (−60 mV).

STEP 2: Activation of sodium channels and rapid depolarisation
The voltage-regulated sodium channels open (sodium channel activation).
Sodium ions, driven by electrical attraction and the chemical gradient, flood into the cell.
The transmembrane potential goes from −60 mV, the threshold level, towards +30 mV.

STEP 3: Repolarisation: inactivation of sodium channels and activation of potassium channels
The voltage-regulated sodium channels close (sodium channel inactivation occurs) at +30 mV.
The voltage-regulated potassium channels are now open, and potassium ions diffuse out of the cell.
Repolarisation begins.

STEP 4: Return to normal permeability
The voltage-regulated sodium channels regain their normal properties in 0.4–1.0 ms. The membrane is now capable of generating another action potential if a larger-than-normal stimulus is provided.
The voltage-regulated potassium channels begin closing at −70 mV. Because they do not all close at the same time, potassium loss continues and a temporary hyperpolarisation to approximately −90 mV occurs.
At the end of the relative refractory period, all voltage-regulated channels have closed, and the membrane is back to its resting state.

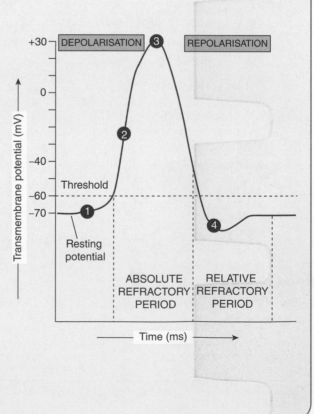

FIGURE 16.3 Sequence of events involved in transmission at a typical chemical synapse.

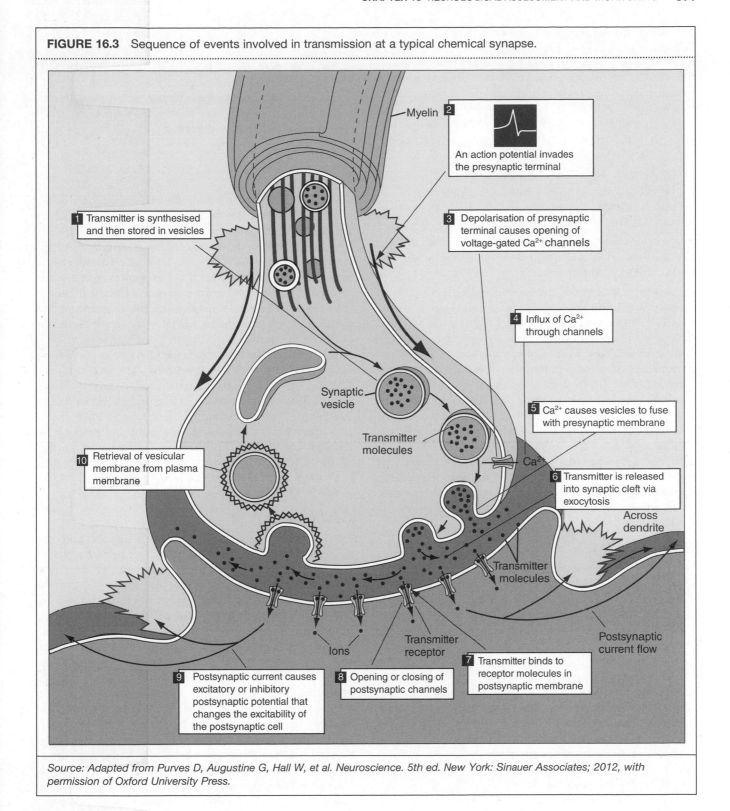

1 Transmitter is synthesised and then stored in vesicles

2 An action potential invades the presynaptic terminal

3 Depolarisation of presynaptic terminal causes opening of voltage-gated Ca^{2+} channels

4 Influx of Ca^{2+} through channels

5 Ca^{2+} causes vesicles to fuse with presynaptic membrane

6 Transmitter is released into synaptic cleft via exocytosis

7 Transmitter binds to receptor molecules in postsynaptic membrane

8 Opening or closing of postsynaptic channels

9 Postsynaptic current causes excitatory or inhibitory postsynaptic potential that changes the excitability of the postsynaptic cell

10 Retrieval of vesicular membrane from plasma membrane

Myelin

Synaptic vesicle

Transmitter molecules

Ca^{2+}

Across dendrite

Transmitter molecules

Postsynaptic current flow

Ions

Transmitter receptor

Source: Adapted from Purves D, Augustine G, Hall W, et al. Neuroscience. 5th ed. New York: Sinauer Associates; 2012, with permission of Oxford University Press.

syndrome, slows conduction and may result in conduction block, which manifests clinically as weakness.[8] Consequently, chronically demyelinated axons become vulnerable, with axon loss being a major cause of disability. In time, remyelination may occur, requiring the generation of myelin-competent oligodendrocytes, but most often it does not fully recapitulate developmental myelination.

Neurotransmitters

Neurotransmitters are chemicals that act as messengers to relay information between neurons.[9] Neurotransmitters are either inhibitory or excitatory.[10] The majority of neurotransmitters are produced in the cell body of neurons in the brain and stored in vesicles. When released, they travel across the synaptic junction and bind to specific neuroreceptor sites on the postsynaptic membrane.[10,11]

Chemically, there are four classes of neurotransmitters:

1 *acetylcholine (ACh):* the dominant neurotransmitter in the PNS, released at neuromuscular junctions and synapses of the parasympathetic division

2 *biogenic amines:* serotonin, histamine and the catecholamines dopamine, adrenaline (epinephrine) and noradrenaline (norepinephrine)

3 *excitatory amino acids:* glutamate and aspartate; and the *inhibitory amino acids*: gamma-aminobutyric acid (GABA), glycine and taurine

4 *neuropeptides:* over 50 are known, amino acid neurotransmitters being the most numerous.

Co-neurotransmitters describe the condition of more than one neurotransmitter per synapse. For example, neuropeptide Y and adenosine triphosphate (ATP) are co-transmitters of noradrenaline; they are released together, mediate their function by activation of α- and β-adrenoceptors and regulate renovascular resistance. Similarly, receptors are an important control point for the effectiveness of synapses. Neurotransmitters are the common denominator between the nervous, endocrine and immune systems. Many neurotransmitters are endocrine analogues and the main parasympathetic neurotransmitter, acetylcholine, interacts with immune cells such as macrophages through the anti-inflammatory cholinergic pathway.[7]

Neuroglia

Neuroglia are the non-neuronal cells of the nervous system and are 10–50 times more prevalent than neurons. They are divided into macroglia (astrocytes, oligodendroglia and Schwann cells) and microglia, and are described in Table 16.2. They not only provide physical support but also respond to injury, regulate the ionic and chemical composition of the extracellular milieu, participate in the blood–brain and blood–retina barriers, form the myelin insulation of nervous pathways, guide neuronal migration during development and exchange metabolites with neurons. The CNS has a greater variety of neuroglia. Unlike neurons, neuroglia continue to multiply throughout life. Because of their capacity to reproduce, most tumours of the nervous system are tumours of neuroglial tissue and not of nervous tissue itself.

Central nervous system

The CNS is composed of the brain and spinal cord (Fig. 16.4). The primary purpose is to acquire, coordinate and disseminate information about the body and its environment. This section describes the anatomy and physiology of the brain and spinal cord.

> ### Practice tip
>
> The brain consists of three major divisions: (1) the massive, paired hemispheres of the cerebrum; (2) the brainstem, consisting of the thalamus, hypothalamus, epithalamus, subthalamus, midbrain, pons and medulla oblongata; and (3) the cerebellum.

Brain

There are different ways of discussing the anatomy of the brain. Commonly, the brain can be divided into three regions: forebrain, midbrain and hindbrain (Table 16.3). The forebrain includes the two large hemispheres of the cerebrum: the basal ganglia and the diencephalon (thalamus and hypothalamus). The outer layer of the cerebrum, the cerebral cortex, contains central masses of grey matter. The midbrain includes the tegmentum and the tectum. The hindbrain includes the cerebellum, the pons and the midbrain.

Functionally, the brain can be divided into the brainstem, the cerebellum and the cerebrum. The parts of the brainstem (midbrain, pons and medulla) are most often visualised including the thalamus (Fig. 16.5). The cerebellum (metencephalon), including two hemispheres and a central zone (vermis), lies below the tentorium and posterior to the pons and medulla. The cerebrum is the largest portion of the CNS and includes the cerebral cortex (frontal, temporal, parietal and occipital lobes) and the basal ganglia, as well as the hippocampus and olfactory bulb.

Cerebral cortex

The forebrain contains the cerebral cortex and the subcortical structures rostral (sideways) to the diencephalon (i.e. thalamus and hypothalamus). The cortex, or outermost surface of the cerebrum, makes up about 80% of the human brain. The cerebral cortex varies in thickness from 2 to 4 millimetres. It contains the cell bodies and dendrites of neurons or grey matter that receive, integrate, store and transmit information.[12] Conscious deliberation and voluntary actions come from the cerebral cortex. White matter lies beneath the cerebral cortex and is composed of myelinated nerve fibres. The cortex is involved in both the processing of sensory information from the body and the delivery of motor commands. These occur in specific areas of the brain and can be mapped. Topographically, the cerebral cortex is divided into areas of specialised functions, including the primary sensory areas for vision (occipital cortex), hearing (temporal cortex) and somatic sensation (postcentral gyrus), and the primary motor area (precentral gyrus). As shown in Fig. 16.6, these well-defined areas comprise only a small fraction of the surface of the cerebral cortex.

Most of the remaining cortical area is known as the association cortex, where the processing of extensive and sophisticated neural information is performed. The association areas are also sites of long-term memory, and

TABLE 16.2

Neuroglia, their location and role as supporting nervous tissue

CELL TYPE	LOCATION	MAIN FUNCTION
Astrocytes 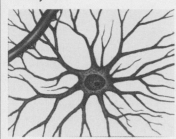	CNS: the largest and most numerous neuroglial cells in the brain and spinal cord.	Astrocytes are considered as important as the neuron in communication and brain regulation. They regulate communication, extracellular ionic and chemical environments between neurons. They respond to injury and have an important role in cerebral oedema.
Ependymal cells 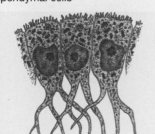	CNS: line the ventricular system of the brain and central cord of the spinal canal.	Transport of CSF and brain homeostasis. Phagocytotic defence against pathogens. Store glycogen for brain tissue.
Microglia 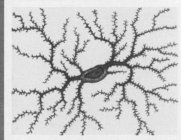	CNS: located within the brain parenchyma behind the blood–brain barrier.	Wander between the peripheral immune system and the CNS as a defence against infection. Displace synaptic input in injured neurons.
Oligodendrocytes 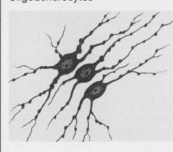	CNS: spiral around an axon to form a multilayered lipoprotein coat in both the white and grey matter in the brain and spinal cord. PNS: Schwann cells are the supporting cells of the PNS.	Responsible for the formation of myelin sheaths surrounding axons. Oligodendrocytes wrap themselves around numerous axons at once. Schwann cells wrap themselves around peripheral nerve axons. Unlike oligodendrocytes, a single Schwann cell makes up a single segment of an axon's myelin sheath.

they are critical to human functions such as language acquisition, speech, musical ability, mathematical ability, complex motor skills, abstract thought, symbolic thought and other cognitive functions. Association areas interconnect and integrate information from the primary sensory and motor areas via intra-hemispheric connections. The parietal–temporal–occipital association cortex integrates neural information contributed by visual, auditory and somatic sensory experiences. The prefrontal association cortex is extremely important as the coordinator of emotionally motivated behaviours, by virtue of its connections with the limbic system.

The prefrontal cortex receives neural input from the other association areas and regulates motivated behaviours

FIGURE 16.4   The subdivisions and components of the central nervous system.

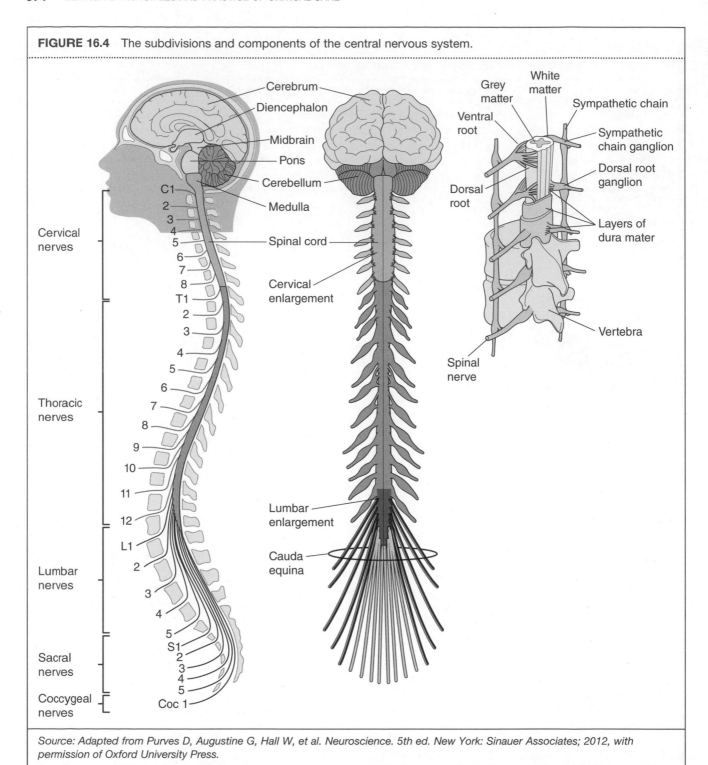

Source: Adapted from Purves D, Augustine G, Hall W, et al. Neuroscience. 5th ed. New York: Sinauer Associates; 2012, with permission of Oxford University Press.

by direct input to the premotor area, which serves as the association area of the motor cortex. Sensory and motor functions are controlled by cortical structures in the contralateral hemisphere. Particular cognitive functions or components of these functions may be lateralised to one side of the brain.

The cerebral cortex receives sensory information, relayed through the thalamus, from many different sensory organs and processes the information. The two hemispheres receive the information from the opposite sides of the body. The parts of the cortex that receive this information are called primary sensory areas and they cross at various points in the sensory pathway, because the cerebral cortex operates on a contralateral basis. The discriminative touch system crosses high, in the medulla. The pain system crosses low, in the spinal cord. The proprioceptive sensory

TABLE 16.3

Organisation of the brain

DIVISION	DESCRIPTION	FUNCTIONS
Forebrain		
Cerebrum	Largest and uppermost portion of the brain. Divided into two hemispheres, each subdivided into the frontal, parietal, temporal and occipital lobes.	Cortex (outer layer) is the site of conscious thought, memory, reasoning and abstract mental functions, all localised within specific lobes.
Diencephalon	Between the cerebrum and the brainstem. Contains the thalamus and hypothalamus.	Thalamus sorts and redirects sensory input; hypothalamus controls visceral, autonomic, endocrine and emotional function, and the pituitary gland. Contains some of the centres for coordinated parasympathetic and sympathetic stimulation, temperature regulation, appetite regulation, regulation of water balance by antidiuretic hormone (ADH) and regulation of certain rhythmic psychobiological activities (e.g. sleep).
Brain stem	Anterior region below the cerebrum: the medulla, pons and midbrain compose the brainstem.	Connects cerebrum and diencephalon with spinal cord.
Midbrain		
Midbrain	Below the centre of the cerebrum.	Has reflex centres concerned with vision and hearing; connects cerebrum with lower portions of the brain. It contains sensory and motor pathways and serves as the centre for auditory and visual reflexes.
Basal ganglia or corpus striatum	The mass of grey matter in the midbrain beneath the cerebral hemispheres. Borders the lateral ventricles and lies in proximity to the internal capsule.	An important role in planning and coordinating motor movements and posture. Complex neural connections link the basal ganglia to the cerebral cortex. The major effect of these structures is to inhibit unwanted muscular activity; disorders of the basal ganglia result in exaggerated, uncontrolled movements.
Pons	Anterior to the cerebellum.	Connects the cerebellum with other portions of the brain; contains motor and sensory pathways; helps to regulate respiration; axons from the cerebellum, basal ganglia, thalamus and hypothalamus; portions of the pons also control the heart, respiration and blood pressure. Cranial nerves V–VIII connect the brain in the pons.
Hindbrain	Contains a portion of the pons, the medulla oblongata and the cerebellum.	
Reticular activation system (RAS)	The reticular formation networks run through the brainstem core, known as the tegmentum.	Activity of the cerebral cortex is dependent on both specific sensory input and non-specific activating impulses from the RAS, and is critical to the existence of the conscious state, states of alertness and arousal.

Continued

TABLE 16.3

Organisation of the brain—cont'd

DIVISION	DESCRIPTION	FUNCTIONS
Medulla oblongata 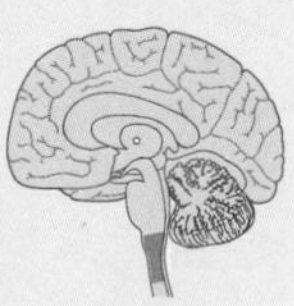	Between the pons and the spinal cord.	The medulla oblongata contains motor fibres from the brain to the spinal cord and sensory fibres from the spinal cord to the brain. Most of these fibres cross at this level. Cranial nerves IX–XII connect to the brain in the medulla, which has centres for control of vital functions such as respiration and the heart rate.
Cerebellum 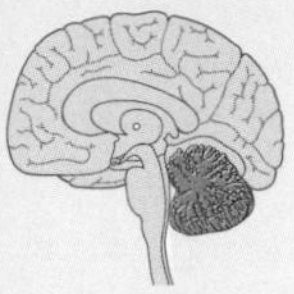	Below the posterior portion of the cerebellum. Divided into two hemispheres.	Coordinates voluntary muscles; maintains balance and muscle tone; has both excitatory and inhibitory actions. It also controls fine movement, balance, position sense and integration of sensory input.

FIGURE 16.5 Lateral view of the brainstem showing the thalamus, midbrain, pons and medulla.

THALAMUS

MIDBRAIN

PONS

MEDULLA

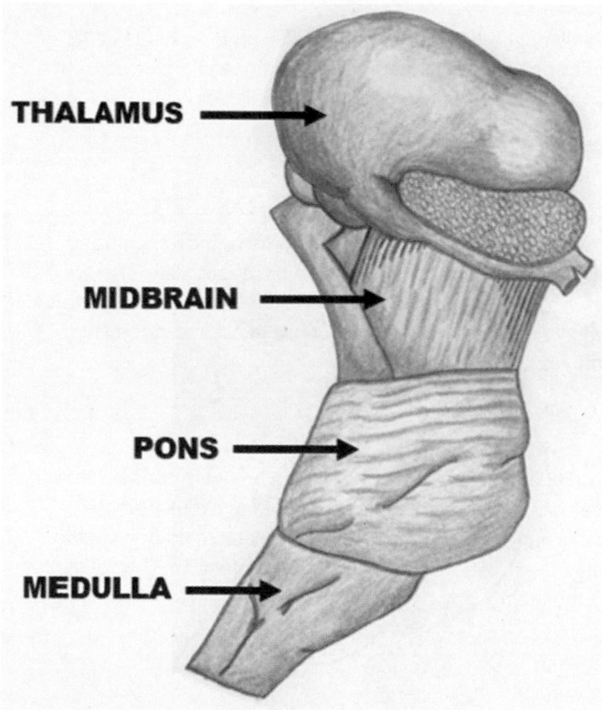

Source: Courtesy Taylore Jansen.

The homunculus (Fig. 16.7) is a visual representation of correlative neuroanatomy. Different areas of the body are shown by the corresponding areas in brain hemispheres. The body on the right side of Fig. 16.7 is the motor homunculus and that on the left the sensory homunculus. Representations of parts of the body that exhibit fine motor control and sensory capabilities occupy a greater amount of space than those that exhibit less precise motor or sensory functions.

Basal ganglia and cerebellum

The olfactory bulb, nucleus accumbens, putamen, globus pallidus, caudate, ventral pallidum, subthalamic nucleus and projections from the substantia nigra are a group of nuclei that collectively make up the basal ganglia. The basal ganglia play an important role in movement, as evidenced by the hypokinetic/rigid and hyperkinetic disorders seen with lesions of related nuclei. Their role in the initiation and control of movement cannot be isolated from the motor activities of the cortex and brainstem centres discussed previously. Procedural memories for motor and other unconscious skills depend on the integrity of the premotor cortex, basal ganglia and cerebellum. The cerebellum plays a more obvious role in coordinating movements by giving feedback to the motor cortex, as well as by providing important influences on eye movements through brainstem connections, and on postural activity through projections down the spinal cord.

Brainstem

The brainstem is composed of the midbrain, pons and medulla oblongata (see Fig. 16.5).[10] These structures connect the cerebrum and diencephalon with the spinal cord. Collectively, they integrate vestibular, visual and somatosensory inputs for the control of eye movements and, through projections to the spinal cord, provide for

system that guards balance and position goes to the cerebellum, which works ipsilaterally and therefore does not cross. Almost every region of the body is represented by a corresponding region in both the primary motor cortex and the somatic sensory cortex.

FIGURE 16.6 (**A**) Major anatomical landmarks on the surface of the left cerebral hemisphere. The lateral sulcus has been pulled apart to expose the insula. (**B**) The left hemisphere usually contains the general interpretive area and the speech centre. The prefrontal cortex of each hemisphere is involved with conscious intellectual functions. (**C**) Regions of the cerebral cortex as determined by histological analysis. Several of the 47 regions described by Brodmann are shown for comparison with the results of functional mapping.

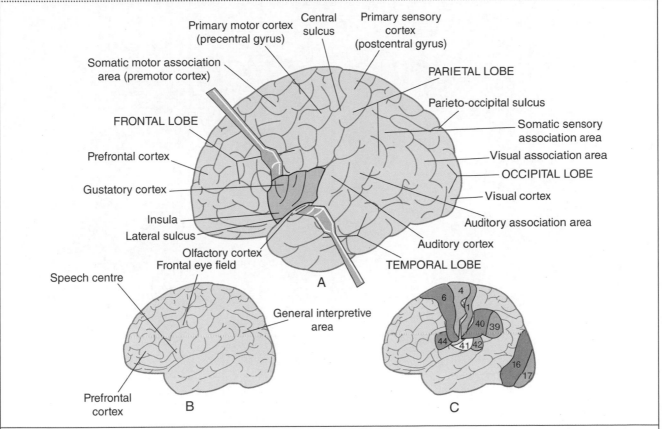

Source: Martini F, Nath JL, Bartholomew EF. Fundamentals of anatomy & physiology. 11th ed. ©2018. Printed and Electronically reproduced by permission of Pearson Education, Inc., New York.

postural adjustments. For example, these centres keep the images on matching regions of the retinas when the head moves by causing conjugate eye movements in the opposite direction to which the head is turned. This is the basis for the oculocephalic reflex test in neurological assessment, in which the head is rapidly turned and the eyes move conjugately in the opposite direction, demonstrating the integrity of much of the brainstem. The sequence of sleep states is governed by a group of brainstem nuclei that project widely throughout the brain and spinal cord.

The midbrain, inferior to the centre of the cerebrum, forms the superior part of the brainstem. It contains the reticular formation (which collects input from higher brain centres and passes it on to motor neurons), the substantia nigra (which regulates body movements – damage to the substantia nigra causes Parkinson's disease) and the ventral tegmental area (which contains dopamine-releasing neurons that are activated by nicotinic acetylcholine receptors). White matter in the anterior

midbrain conducts impulses between the higher centres of the cerebrum and the lower centres of the pons, medulla, cerebellum and spinal cord. The midbrain contains autonomic reflex centres for pupillary accommodations to light (Edinger–Westphal nucleus), which receive stimuli via the optic nerve (cranial nerve (CN-II)) and send signals via the oculomotor nerve (CN-III) to cause pupillary constriction and accommodation of the lens. Hence, damage to CN-III will produce a dilated pupil. It also contains the ventral tegmental area, packed with dopamine-releasing neurons that synapse deep within the forebrain and seem to be involved in pleasure: amphetamines and cocaine bind to the same receptors that it activates, and this may account at least in part for their addictive qualities.

The pons Varolii (pons) lies between the medulla oblongata and the midbrain (mesencephalon). It contains pneumotaxic and apneustic respiratory centres and fibre tracts connecting higher and lower centres, including the cerebellum. The pons seems to serve as a relay station,

FIGURE 16.7 Somatosensory and motor homunculi. Note that the size of each region of the homunculi is related to its importance in sensory or motor function, resulting in a distorted-appearing map.

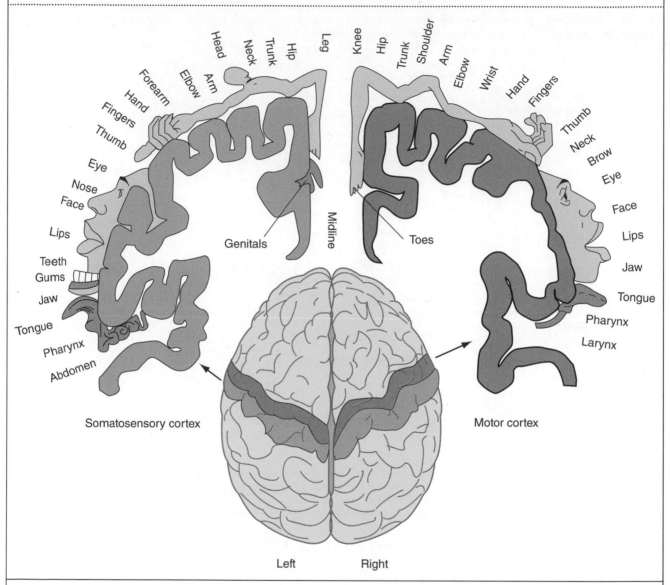

Source: Adapted from Blumenfeld H. Neuroanatomy through clinical cases. New York: Sinauer Associates; 2010, with permission of Oxford University Press.

carrying signals from various parts of the cerebral cortex to the cerebellum. Nerve impulses coming from the eyes, ears and touch receptors are sent on to the cerebellum. The pons also participates in the reflexes that regulate breathing. Table 16.4 contains a description of the cranial nerves including their type of tract, their function and location of origin.

The medulla oblongata lies between the pons and the spinal cord and looks like a swollen tip to the spinal cord. Running down the ventral aspect of the medulla are the pyramids, which contain corticospinal fibres. The medulla oblongata controls automatic functions (e.g. breathing and heart rate) and relays nerve messages from the brain to the

spinal cord. Processing of interaural time differences for sound localisation occurs in the olivary nuclei. The neurons controlling breathing have μ-receptors, the receptors to which opiates bind. This accounts for the suppressive effect of opiates on breathing. Impairment of any of the vital functions or reflexes involving these cranial nerves suggests medullary damage.

Limbic system

The limbic system includes the hypothalamus, the cingulate gyrus of the cortex, the amygdala and hippocampus in the temporal lobes and the septum and interconnecting nerve fibre tracts. The hypothalamus

TABLE 16.4

The cranial nerves, their locations and functions

CRANIAL NERVE	TRACT(S)	FUNCTION	LOCATION OF ORIGIN
I Olfactory	Sensory	Sense of smell	Diencephalon
II Optic	Sensory	Vision	Diencephalon
III Oculomotor	Parasympathetic	Muscles that move the eye and lid, pupillary constriction, lens accommodation.	Midbrain
	Motor	Elevation of upper eyelid and four of six extraocular movements.	
IV Trochlear	Motor	Downward, inward movement of the eye (superior oblique).	Midbrain
V Trigeminal	Motor	Muscles of mastication and opening jaw.	Pons
	Sensory	Tactile sensation to the cornea, nasal and oral mucosa and facial skin.	
VI Abducens	Motor	Lateral deviation of eye (lateral rectus).	Pons
VII Facial	Parasympathetic	Secretory for salivation and tears.	Pons
	Motor	Movement of the forehead, eyelids, cheeks, lips, ears, nose and neck to produce facial expression and close eyes.	
	Sensory	Tactile sensation to parts of the external ear, auditory canal and external tympanic membrane.	
		Taste sensation to the anterior two-thirds of the tongue.	
VIII Vestibulocochlear	Sensory	Vestibular branch: equilibrium. Cochlear branch: hearing.	Pons
IX Glossopharyngeal	Parasympathetic	Salivation.	Medulla
	Motor	Voluntary muscles for swallowing and phonation.	
	Sensory	Sensation to pharynx, soft palate and posterior one-third of tongue.	
		Stimulation elicits gag reflex.	
X Vagus	Parasympathetic	Autonomic activity of viscera of thorax and abdomen.	Medulla
	Motor	Voluntary swallowing and phonation.	
		Involuntary activity of visceral muscles of the heart, lungs and digestive tract.	
	Sensory	Sensation to the auditory canal and viscera of the thorax and abdomen.	
XI Accessory	Motor	Sternocleidomastoid and trapezius muscle movements.	Medulla
XII Hypoglossal	Motor	Tongue movements.	Medulla

and limbic system, which are closely linked to homeostasis, act to regulate endocrine secretion and the autonomic nervous system, and to influence behaviour through emotions and drives. The hypothalamus integrates information from the forebrain, brainstem, spinal cord and various endocrine systems. This area of the brain also contains some of the centres for coordinated parasympathetic and sympathetic stimulation, as well as those for temperature regulation, appetite regulation, regulation of water balance by antidiuretic hormone (ADH) and regulation of certain rhythmic psychobiological activities (e.g. sleep). The release of stored serotonin from axon terminals in the diencephalon suppresses activation of the ascending reticular activating system (ARAS). The ARAS controls sleep, waking and fight-versus-flight responses. Suppression of the ARAS results in increased sleep or sleep-like states. The hypothalamus contains a plethora of neurotransmitters. These are found in the terminals of axons that originate from neurons outside the hypothalamus, but most are synthesised within the hypothalamus itself. The list of chemicals thought to act as neurotransmitters includes the 'classic' transmitters ACh, GABA, glutamate, serotonin, dopamine and noradrenaline, as well as literally dozens of peptides that have been identified in recent years.

Protection and support of the brain

The brain occupies the cranial cavity and is covered by membranes, fluid and the bones of the skull. The delicate tissues of the brain are protected from mechanical forces by (1) the bones of the cranium, (2) the cranial meninges and (3) cerebrospinal fluid. In addition, the neural tissue of the brain is biochemically isolated from the general circulation by the blood–brain barrier.

> **Practice tip**
>
> Openings in the fourth ventricle permit cerebrospinal fluid to enter subarachnoid spaces surrounding both the brain and the spinal cord.

Cerebral spinal fluid

Cerebral spinal fluid (CSF) is an ultrafiltrate of blood plasma composed of 99% water with other constituents, making it close to the composition of the brain extracellular fluid. Approximately 500 mL of CSF are secreted each day, but only approximately 150 mL are in the ventricular system at any one time, meaning that the CSF is continuously being absorbed. The CSF produced in the ventricles must flow through the interventricular foramen, the third ventricle, the cerebral aqueduct and the fourth ventricle to exit from the neural tube.

Three openings, or foramina, allow the CSF to pass into the subarachnoid space (Fig. 16.8). Approximately 30% of the CSF passes down into the subarachnoid space that surrounds the spinal cord, mainly on its dorsal surface, and moves back up to the cranial cavity along its ventral surface. Reabsorption of CSF into the vascular system occurs through a pressure gradient. The normal CSF pressure is approximately 10 mmHg in the lateral recumbent position, although it may be as low as 5 mmHg or as high as 15 mmHg in healthy persons. The microstructure of the arachnoid villi is such that, if the CSF pressure falls below approximately 3 mmHg, the passageways collapse and reverse flow is blocked. Arachnoid villi function as one-way valves, permitting CSF outflow into the blood but not allowing blood to pass into the

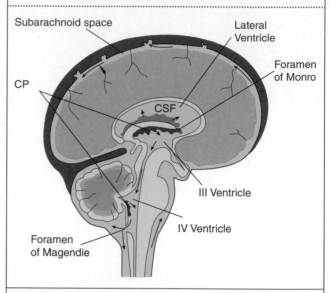

FIGURE 16.8 Circulation of the cerebrospinal fluid (CSF): sagittal section indicating CSF presence (light blue), and routes of circulation of CSF (arrows).

Source: Santos CRA, Duarte AC, Quintela T, et al. The choroid plexus as a sex hormone target: functional implications. Front Neuroendocrinol 2017;44:103–21.

arachnoid spaces. The pressure in the CSF manifests as normal intracranial pressure (ICP).

Blood–brain–CSF barrier

The CNS is richly supplied with blood vessels that bring oxygen and nutrients to its cells. However, many substances cannot easily be exchanged between blood and brain because the endothelial cells of the vessels and the astrocytes of the CNS form extremely tight junctions, collectively referred to as the blood–brain barrier (BBB). In particular, small, non-charged, lipid-soluble molecules can cross the BBB with ease. Evidence suggests that the BBB maintains the chemical environment for neuronal function and protects the brain from harmful substances. Substances in the blood that gain rapid entry to the brain include glucose, the important source of energy, certain ions that maintain a proper medium for electrical activity and oxygen for cellular respiration. Small fat-soluble molecules, like ethanol, pass through the BBB. Some water-soluble molecules pass into the brain carried by special proteins in the plasma membrane of the endothelial cells. Excluded molecules include proteins, toxins, most antibiotics and monoamines (e.g. neurotransmitters). Some of these unwanted molecules are actively transported out of the endothelial cells. When injured (by force, infection or oxidative processes), the permeability of the BBB is disrupted, allowing a proliferation of various chemicals and molecules – even bacteria – into the brain parenchyma, with at times devastating consequences.

Cerebral circulation

The brain must maintain a constant flow of blood for brain activity to occur. The arterial cerebral blood flow (CBF) to the brain consists of approximately 20% of the cardiac output (Fig. 16.9). Normal CBF is 750 mL/min. The brain autoregulates CBF over a wide range of blood pressures by vasodilation or vasoconstriction of the arteries. In response to decreased arterial flow, the arteries that make up the circle of Willis can act as a protective mechanism by shunting blood from one side to the other or from the anterior to posterior portions of the brain. This compensatory mechanism delays neurological deterioration in patients.

The cerebral veins drain into large venous sinuses and then into the right and left internal jugular veins (Fig. 16.10). The venous sinuses are found within the folds of the dura mater. Unlike most veins in the body, the veins and sinuses of the brain do not have valves, so the blood flows freely by gravity. The face and scalp veins can flow into the brain venous sinuses; therefore, infection can

FIGURE 16.9 The major arteries of the brain: (**A**) ventral view: the enlargement of the boxed area showing the circle of Willis; (**B**) lateral and (**C**) mid-sagittal views showing anterior, middle and posterior cerebral arteries; (**D**) idealised frontal section showing the course of middle cerebral artery.

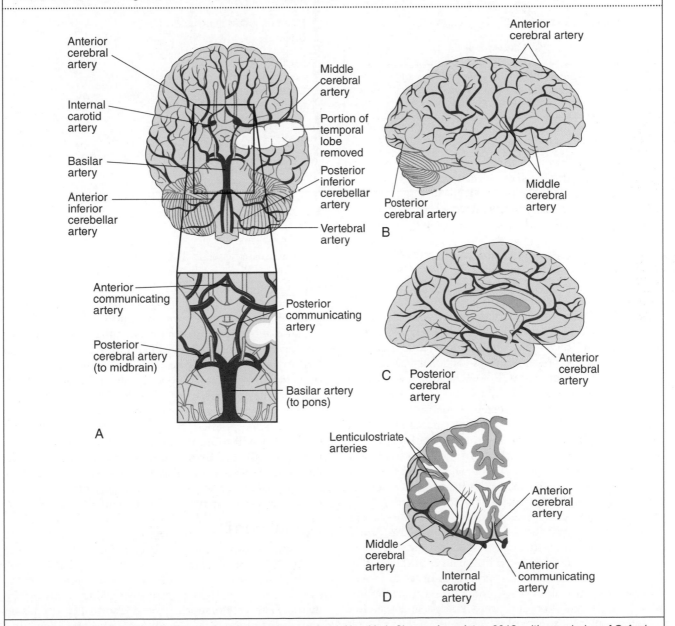

Source: Purves D, Augustine G, Hall W, et al. Neuroscience. 5th ed. New York: Sinauer Associates; 2012, with permission of Oxford University Press.

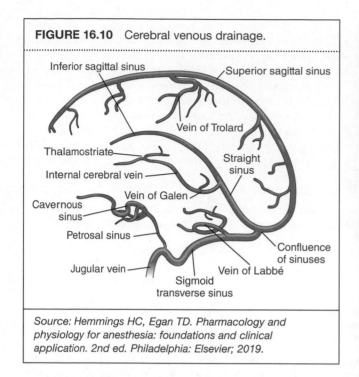

FIGURE 16.10 Cerebral venous drainage.

Source: Hemmings HC, Egan TD. Pharmacology and physiology for anesthesia: foundations and clinical application. 2nd ed. Philadelphia: Elsevier; 2019.

TABLE 16.5

Changes in cerebrovascular and cerebrometabolic parameters when various cerebral variables are reduced with and without intact autoregulation

PRIMARY REDUCTION IN THESE VARIABLES	CBF	CBV (ICP)	AVDO$_2$
CMRO$_2$	↑	↓	—
CPP (autoregulation intact)	—	↑	—
CPP (autoregulation defective)	↓	↓	↑
Blood viscosity (autoregulation intact)	—	↓	—
Blood viscosity (autoregulation defective)	↑	—	↓
PaCO$_2$	↓	↓	↑
Conductive vessel diameter (vasospasm above ischaemic threshold)	↓	↑	↑

AVDO$_2$ = arteriovenous O$_2$ difference; CBF = cerebral blood flow; CBV = cerebral blood volume; CMRO$_2$ = cerebral metabolic rate of oxygen; CPP = cerebral perfusion pressure; ICP = intracranial pressure; PaCO$_2$ = arterial CO$_2$ tension; ↑ = increase; ↓ = decrease; — = no change.

easily be spread into the dural venous sinuses and then enter the brain. Patient position can prevent or promote venous drainage from the brain. Head turning and tilting may kink the jugular vein and decrease or stop venous flow from the brain, which will then raise the pressure inside the cranial vault.

CBF is the cerebral perfusion pressure (CPP) divided by the cerebrovascular resistance (CVR). CVR is the amount of resistance created by the cerebral vessels, and it is controlled by the autoregulatory mechanisms of the brain. Specifically, vasoconstriction (and vasospasm) will increase CVR, and vasodilation will decrease it. It is influenced by the inflow pressure (systole), outflow pressure (venous pressure), cross-sectional diameter of cerebral blood vessels and ICP. CVR is similar to systemic vascular resistance but, due to the lack of valves in the venous system of the brain, cerebral venous pressure also influences the CVR. An important characteristic of the cerebral circulation is its ability to autoregulate – that is, the ability to maintain constant CBF despite variations in perfusion pressure (Table 16.5). This is important in protecting the brain from both ischaemia during hypotension and haemorrhage during hypertension.

CBF is affected by extrinsic and intrinsic factors. Extrinsic factors include systemic blood pressure, cardiac output, blood viscosity and vascular tone. The body responds to these demands with changes in blood flow. Aerobic metabolism requires oxygen in order to process glucose for normal energy production (production of ATP). The brain does not store energy and therefore requires a constant source of oxygen and energy, its supply from CBF can be exhausted within 3 minutes. Intrinsic factors include PaCO$_2$ (pH), PaO$_2$ and ICP. The vessels dilate with increases in PaCO$_2$ (hypercarbia) or low pH (acidosis) and with decreases in PaO$_2$ (hypoxia). This vasodilation increases CBF. The vessels constrict with decreases in PaCO$_2$ or high pH and with increases in local PaO$_2$. This vasoconstriction will decrease the CBF. In addition, intrinsic factors can change the extrinsic factors by altering the metabolic mechanisms. These changes can lead to an alteration in the CBF. For example, there can be a change from aerobic to anaerobic metabolism, which increases the concentrations of other end-products such as lactic acid, pyruvic acid and carbonic acid, which causes a localised acidosis. These end-products result in a decrease in pH that will cause an increase in CBF. Other factors that can affect CBF include pharmacological agents (anaesthetic agents and some antihypertensive agents), rapid-eye-movement sleep, arousal, pain, seizures, elevations in body temperature and cerebral trauma.

Spinal cord

The spinal cord is the link between the PNS and the brain.[5] The spinal cord has a small, irregularly shaped internal section of unmyelinated tissue (grey matter) surrounded by a larger area of myelinated axons (white matter). The grey matter is arranged so that it extends up and down dorsally in a column, one on each side; another column is found in the ventral region on each side (Fig. 16.11).

FIGURE 16.11   The spinal cord and spinal meninges: (**A**) posterior view of the spinal cord, showing the meningeal layers, superficial landmarks and distribution of grey matter and white matter; (**B**) sectional view through the spinal cord and meninges, showing the peripheral distribution of spinal nerves.

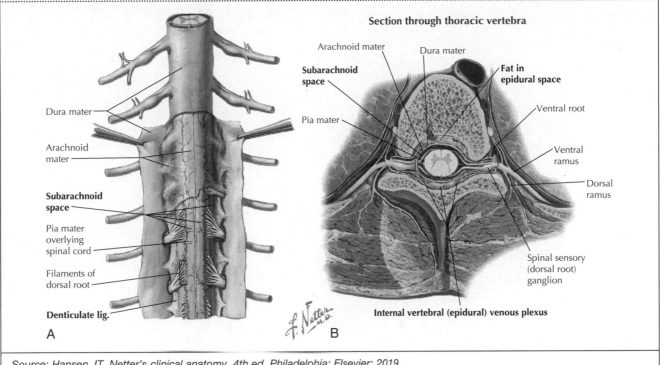

Source: Hansen JT. Netter's clinical anatomy. 4th ed. Philadelphia: Elsevier; 2019.

The spinal cord is an essential component of both the sensory and motor divisions of the nervous system. The first of the primary functions of the spinal cord is to transmit sensory impulses along the ascending tracts to the brain and to transmit motor impulses down the descending tracts away from the brain. The second primary function of the spinal cord is to house and regulate spinal reflexes.[5] Receipt of sensory impulses may cause a reaction anywhere in the body; alternatively, the signal might be stored in the memory to be used at some stage in the future. Within the motor division of the nervous system, the spinal cord helps to control the various bodily activities, including skeletal muscle activity, smooth muscle activity and secretion by both endocrine and exocrine glands.

Sensory neurons from all over the skin, except for the skin of the face and scalp, feed information into the spinal cord through the spinal nerves. As shown in Fig. 16.12, the skin surface can be mapped into distinct regions called dermatomes. Each dermatome corresponds to a single spinal nerve. Sensation from a given dermatome is carried over its corresponding spinal nerve. This information can be used to identify the spinal nerve or spinal segment that is involved in an injury. In some areas, the dermatomes are not absolutely distinct. Some dermatomes may share a nerve supply with neighbouring regions. For this reason, it is often necessary to numb adjacent dermatomes to achieve adequate anaesthesia.

The blood supply to the spinal cord arises from branches of the vertebral arteries and spinal radicular arteries. The mid–thoracic region, at approximately T4–T8, lies between the lumbar and vertebral arterial supplies and is a vulnerable zone of relatively decreased perfusion. This region is most susceptible to infarction during periods of hypotension, thoracic surgery or other conditions, causing decreased aortic pressure and potentially leading to ischaemic spinal injury with devastating consequences.

Peripheral nervous system

The PNS consists of 12 pairs of cranial nerves, 31 pairs of spinal nerves and all neural structures lying outside the spinal cord and brainstem. The cranial nerves have previously been discussed regarding their role in brainstem function (see Table 16.4). The PNS has both motor and sensory components. The former includes the motor neuron cell body in the anterior horn of the spinal cord and its peripheral axonal process travelling through the ventral root and eventually the peripheral nerve. The motor nerve terminal, together with the muscle endplate and the synapse between the two, comprises the neuromuscular junction. The peripheral sensory axon, beginning at receptors in cutaneous and deep structures, as well as muscle and tendon receptors, travels back

FIGURE 16.12 **(A)** Anterior and **(B)** posterior distributions of dermatomes on the surface of the skin.

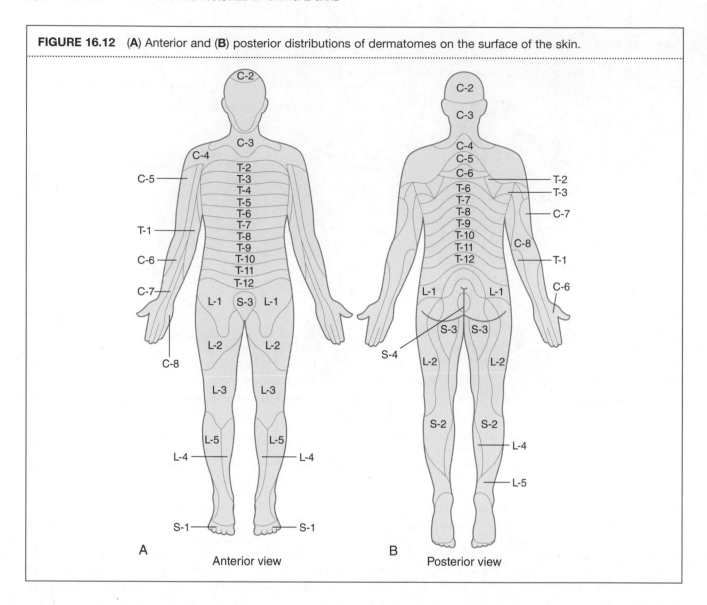

A   Anterior view

B   Posterior view

through peripheral nerves to its cell body located in the dorsal root ganglion. Its central process, travelling through the dorsal root, enters the spinal cord in the region of the dorsal horn. All commands for movement, whether reflexive or voluntary, are ultimately conveyed to the muscles by the activity of the lower motor neurons.

Motor control

Movements can be divided into three main classes: voluntary activity, rhythmic motor patterns and reflex responses. The highest-order activity, voluntary movement, allows for expression of the will and a purposeful response to the environment (e.g. reading, speaking, performing calculations). Such activity is goal directed and largely learned, and improves with practice. In rhythmic motor patterns, the initiation and termination may be voluntary, but the rhythmic activity itself does not require conscious participation (e.g. chewing, walking, running). Reflex responses are simple, stereotyped responses that do not

involve voluntary control (e.g. deep tendon reflexes or withdrawal of a limb from a hot surface). Motor control is carried out in a hierarchical, yet parallel, fashion in the cerebral cortex, the brainstem and the spinal cord. Modulating influences are provided by the basal ganglia and cerebellum through the thalamus.

Sensory control

The sensory control is responsible for detecting, interpreting and transmitting external signals. There are several different types of sensory neurons and these can be either encapsulated or non-encapsulated; both extend to the periphery (i.e. skin) and primarily respond to pressure, vibration or temperature. A very light pressure may be interpreted as light touch, whereas a focalised high pressure may be interpreted as pain. The processing of sensory stimuli begins with a combination of mechanical and chemical signalling that causes ion (sodium) channels to open. The change in polarity becomes an electrical signal that is transmitted along the nerve and processed in the brain as pain, touch, tension, temperature or vibration.

Autonomic nervous system

The autonomic nervous system, with its three major divisions (sympathetic, parasympathetic and enteric), is largely an involuntary system and is part of the efferent division, as shown in Fig. 16.1. The autonomic nervous system allows the body to adjust to rapidly changing external events (the 'flight or fight' response of the sympathetic division) and to regulate internal activities (blood pressure, temperature, airway and breathing, urinary function, and digestion by the parasympathetic and enteric divisions). Whereas the major controlling centres for somatic (i.e. voluntary) motor activity are the primary and secondary motor cortices in the frontal lobes and a variety of related brainstem nuclei, the major locus of central control in the visceral motor system is the hypothalamus and the complex circuitry that it controls in the brainstem tegmentum and spinal cord.[5] The status of both divisions of the visceral motor system is modulated by descending pathways from these centres to preganglionic neurons in the brainstem and spinal cord, which in turn determine the activity of the primary visceral motor neurons in autonomic ganglia.[5]

The postganglionic neurons of the sympathetic system, with few exceptions, act on their effectors by releasing the neurotransmitter adrenaline and the related compound noradrenaline. This system is therefore described as adrenergic, which means 'activated by adrenaline'. The autonomic regulation of various organ systems of particular importance in clinical practice is illustrated in Fig. 16.13.

Neurological assessment and monitoring

This section explores the complex issues surrounding cerebral haemodynamics and assessment. The objective of assessment is to determine the extent of neurological injury, recognise fluctuations in condition and imminent deterioration, and assist in maintaining cerebral perfusion as part of multimodal monitoring.

Physical examination

The neurological exam begins at the onset of patient contact, and the priorities are defined by a primary survey and vital signs. The patient's history and contact with family help to inform the clinical examination. The history should include the patient's normal baseline status and past neurological injury such as previous stroke, and symptoms such as seizures or long-standing weakness. Additional information about medication use and other substance use should be included in the history.[13]

Specific areas tested during the initial neurological exam include the level of consciousness, general behaviour, memory, attention and concentration, abstract thought or

judgement, motor function, sensory function and cranial nerve function. Not every aspect of the examination will be relevant in all critical care situations and so may not be tested. Nevertheless, the clinician should understand how all the components are integrated and how they influence priority decision making for patient care.

While the essential components of the neurological exam are similar, components of the exam should be individualised to the patient's ability. It may be necessary to modify assessment techniques; for example, intubated patients who are otherwise awake and aware may gesture or write answers to questions instead of verbalising them. In addition, when patients are the recipients of very frequent neurological assessment over an extended period (including arousal and awareness, pupil and motor response), sleep and rest deprivation is common.[14,15] Sleep deprivation and sensory overload may confound assessment accuracy. Consideration needs to be given in regard to the priorities of assessment and rest; a plan needs to be implemented to promote rest as neurological injury requires rest and sleep for restoration.[16] See Online resources for links to a full neurological assessment and physical examination protocol.

Conscious state

Consciousness can be defined in terms of an individual's internal awareness of self and external awareness of environment. Hence, awareness, arousal and responsiveness are fundamental constituents of consciousness and should be evaluated and documented repeatedly for trend analysis. Changes in the level of consciousness are often the first sign of neurological deterioration.[17,18]

Arousal or responsiveness assessment

Evaluation of arousal typically scores the patient's response to stimuli. The Alert, Verbal, Pain, Unresponsive (AVPU) scale, the Richmond Agitation Sedation Scale (RASS), the National Institutes of Health Stroke Scale (NIHSS) and the Glasgow Coma Scale (GCS) each have elements that assess the patient's ability to respond to stimuli.[19–23] An initial AVPU assessment during resuscitation is based on the response to stimulation: **A**wake, **V**erbal, **P**ain, or **U**nresponsive. Observe the patient's response (verbal or motor). If there is no response to voice or light touch,

FIGURE 16.13 Sympathetic and parasympathetic divisions of the autonomic nervous system. Sympathetic outputs (**left**) arise from thoracolumbar spinal cord segments and synapses in paravertebral and prevertebral ganglia. Parasympathetic outputs (**right**) arise from craniosacral regions and synapses in ganglia in or near effector organs.

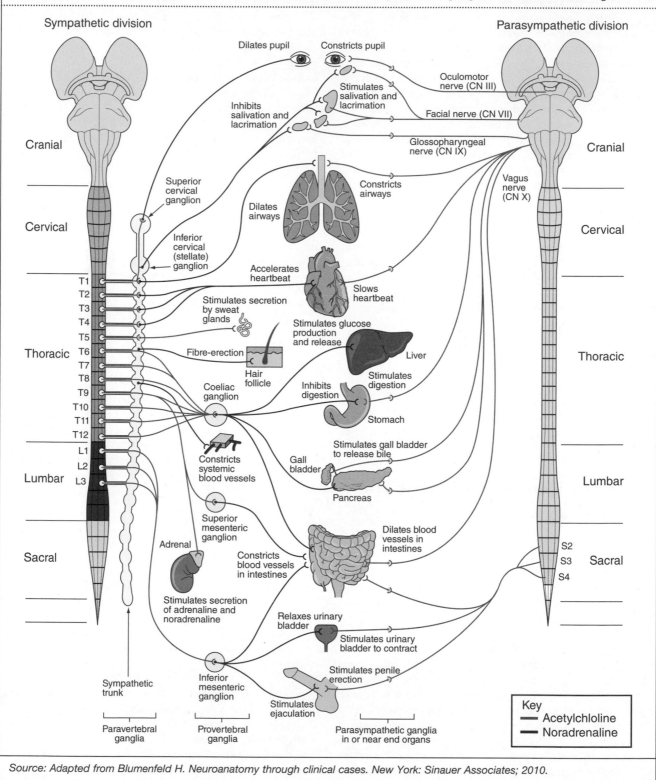

Source: Adapted from Blumenfeld H. Neuroanatomy through clinical cases. New York: Sinauer Associates; 2010.

painful stimulus is needed to assess neurological status. Central pain should be used first and applied with care. Trapezius pinch and supraorbital pressure are methods for introducing central pain. Hand grasp is a reflex and is unreliable to test motor strength or cognitive capacity. If the patient does not respond to verbal stimulus but moves spontaneously in a purposeful manner (picks at linen, pulls at tubes), the patient is localising. Localising is purposeful and intentional movement intended to eliminate a noxious stimulus, whereas withdrawal is a 'smaller' movement used to 'get away from' noxious stimulus. Painful stimulus is not required if spontaneous localisation has been observed. Watch for symmetry. Abnormal flexion differs from withdrawal in that the flexion is rigid and looks abnormal. Abnormal extension is a rigid movement with extension of the limbs.[22,24]

> **Practice tip**
>
> When a patient opens their eyes when you call their name, it is an indication that their reticular activating centre (brainstem) functioning is intact, but it does not tell you if they are awake or aware.[25]

> **Practice tip**
>
> Awareness means that the cerebral cortex is working in conjunction with the reticular activating system (arousal) and that the patient can interact with and interpret their environment.

Assessment of awareness and responsiveness

Awareness and responsiveness in a comatose patient can be assessed using a coma-scoring system such as the GCS or the Full Outline of UnResponsivness (FOUR) score.[26,27] These neurological assessments are used to monitor progression of coma and the patient's response to interventions, and to determine the type of care needed.

The GCS was developed to establish an objective, quantifiable measure to describe the prognosis of a patient with a traumatic brain injury (TBI) and includes scoring of separate subscales related to eye opening, verbal response and motor response (Table 16.6). Originally, the GCS was developed as three separate response areas and reported as such.[21] Contemporary use of the GCS automatically adds the three best response scores, hence limiting the information given from the separate response areas. Reporting the GCS as three numbers and then the total gives a broader assessment interpretation. The advantage of the GCS is that it allows rapid serial comparisons and categorisation of basic neurological function over time.[28] However, it has several recognised weaknesses, including poor prediction of outcome beyond survival, poor inter-rater reliability and inconsistent use in the pre-hospital and

hospital settings. GCS accuracy will be affected if the patient is receiving anaesthetic agents or sedation and noxious stimuli should be avoided. Furthermore, the rare event of a *locked-in syndrome*, where a patient is neurologically aware and awake but not responding, is poorly represented by the GCS. Also, interpretation of response regarding language used or a previous communication disability is important for assessment accuracy.[29] See Online resources for a link to a full GCS procedure.

The FOUR score (Fig. 16.14) is an accurate predictor of outcome in TBI.[30] It is easy to learn, remember and

---

TABLE 16.6
Glasgow Coma Scale

The Glasgow Coma Scale is scored between 3 and 15, 3 being the worst, and 15 the best. It comprises three parameters: best eye response, best verbal response and best motor response. The definition of these parameters is given below

THE GLASGOW COMA SCALE FOR ADULTS	PAEDIATRIC VERSION OF THE GLASGOW COMA SCALE
Best eye response (4)	**Best eye response (4)**
1 No eye opening.	1 No eye opening.
2 Eye opening to pain.	2 Eye opening to pain.
3 Eye opening to verbal command.	3 Eye opening to verbal command.
4 Eyes open spontaneously.	4 Eyes open spontaneously.
Best verbal response (5)	**Best verbal response (5)**
1 No verbal response.	1 No vocal response.
2 Incomprehensible sounds.	2 Occasionally whimpers and/or moans.
3 Inappropriate words.	3 Cries inappropriately.
4 Confused.	4 Less than usual ability and/or spontaneous irritable cry.
5 Orientated.	5 Alert, babbles, coos, words or sentences to usual ability.
Best motor response (6)	**Best motor response (6)**
1 No motor response.	1 No motor response to pain.
2 Extension to pain.	2 Abnormal extension to pain (decerebrate).
3 Flexion to pain.	3 Abnormal flexion to pain (decorticate).
4 Withdrawal from pain.	4 Withdrawal to painful stimuli.
5 Localising pain.	5 Localises to painful stimuli or withdraws to touch.
6 Obeys commands.	6 Obeys commands or performs normal spontaneous movements.

FIGURE 16.14 The Full Outline of UnResponsiveness (FOUR) Score.

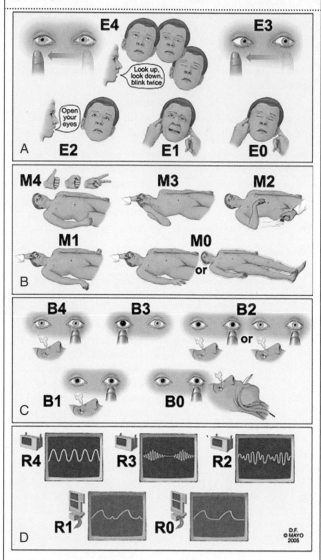

Source: Adapted from Wijdicks EF, Bamlet WR, Maramattom BV, et al. Validation of a new coma scale: the FOUR score. Ann Neurol 2005;58(4):585-593, with permission.

brainstem function. Regular rate of respirations receives a score of 4, irregular a score of 3, Cheyne–Stokes respirations a score of 2, the intubated patient who breathes spontaneously or triggers the ventilator will receive a score of 1 and the patient who fails to trigger the ventilator (no spontaneous breaths) receives a score of 0. If all four components are graded at zero, brain death testing is suggested. The FOUR score may help the examiner to localise lesions and diagnose the patient with locked-in syndrome.

The administration of the FOUR offers a few specific advantages over the GCS.[28] The FOUR adds to the eye opening of the GCS by testing eye tracking, hence incorporating midbrain and pontine functions. It allows for testing of afferent language processing and remains testable regardless of endotracheal intubation, aphasia, aphonia or trauma to the vocal apparatus. It adds to the motor score of the GCS, incorporating hand gestures into the evaluation. The bulk of the motor score is similar to the GCS except that no difference is delineated between flexor posturing and normal flexion to pain. Specific testing of brainstem reflexes via pupillary, corneal and cough reflexes further allows the clinician to localise lesions and track progression of cerebral injury, specifically by addressing unilateral fixed mydriasis, a sign alerting to uncal herniation (a life-threatening situation where raised intracranial pressure causes brain portions to move from one compartment to another).[28–30]

Eye and pupil assessment

Pupillary responses, including pupil size and reaction to light, are important neurological observations and they localise cerebral disease to a specific area of the brain. The immediate constriction of the pupil in response to light is referred to as the direct light reflex or pupillary light reflex (PLR). Removal of the light should result in dilation of the pupil. Introduction of the light into one eye should cause a similar constriction to occur in the other pupil (consensual light reaction).[31]

Other points to consider when conducting pupillary observations include the following:

- Pinpoint non-reactive pupils are associated with opiate use.

- Non-reactive pupils may also be caused by local damage.

- Atropine will cause dilated pupils.

- One dilated or fixed pupil may be indicative of an expanding or developing intracranial lesion, compressing the oculomotor nerve on the same side of the brain as the affected pupil.[32]

- A sluggish pupil may be difficult to distinguish from a fixed pupil and may be an early focal sign of an expanding intracranial lesion and raised ICP. A sluggish response to light in a previously reacting pupil must be reported immediately.[32,33]

Assessment of pupillary function focuses on three areas: (1) estimation of pupil size and shape, (2) evaluation

administer. The four components of the FOUR score are: (1) best eye response, (2) best motor response, (3) best brainstem response, and (4) evaluation of the respiratory pattern. Component subscores range from 0 (worst) to 4 (best), and can be rated in intubated patients, with equal weight given to each component. Best eye response is voluntary eye movement or tracking and worst eye response is no eye opening to painful stimuli. Best motor response is the ability to follow commands and worst is the absence of any motor response to painful stimuli. The best brainstem response is intact pupillary light reflex and corneal reflex; the worst is the absence of pupil, corneal and cough reflexes. Respiratory pattern further evaluates

of pupillary reaction to light and (3) assessment of eye movements. Metabolic disturbances rarely cause pupillary changes; therefore, abnormal pupillary findings are usually due to a nervous system lesion. Irregular-sized pupils are normal for some people and eye prostheses are common; it is important to establish and document these findings so a trend can be established to distinguish normal from altered states. However, subjective observations of pupillary function by human observers are not reliable.[32]

Eye and eyelid movements

Patients who are comatose will exhibit no spontaneous eye opening. In patients with bilateral thalamic damage, there may be normal consciousness, but an eye-opening apraxia (difficulty initiating the act of lid elevation after lid closure) which may mimic coma.[34] If the patient's eyes are closed, the clinician should gently raise and release the eyelids. Brisk opening and closing of the eyes indicates that the pons is grossly intact. If the pons is impaired, one or both eyelids may close slowly or not at all. In the patient with intact frontal lobe and brainstem functioning, the eyes, when opened, should be pointed straight ahead and at equal height. If there is awareness, the patient should look towards stimuli after eye opening. Eye deviation indicates either a unilateral cerebral or a brainstem lesion. If the eyes deviate laterally, gently turn the head to see whether the eyes will cross the midline to the other side. A pattern of spontaneous, slow and random movements (usually laterally) is termed 'roving-eye movements'. This indicates that the brainstem oculomotor control is intact, but awareness is significantly impaired.[35]

Limb movement

Assessment of extremities and body movement (or motor response) provides valuable information about the patient with a decreased level of consciousness. The clinician must observe the patient's spontaneous movements, muscle tone and response to tactile stimuli. Decorticate (flexor) posturing is seen when there is involvement of a cerebral hemisphere and the brain stem. It is characterised by adduction of the shoulder and arm, elbow flexion and pronation and flexion of the wrist while the legs extend.[36] In terms of the GCS motor score, the *withdrawal flexor* scores higher (4/6) than a *spastic flexor* movement (3/6). Decerebrate (extensor) posturing is seen with severe metabolic disturbances or upper brainstem lesions. It is characterised by extension and pronation of the arm(s) and extension of the legs. Patients may have an asymmetrical response and may posture spontaneously or to stimuli.[37]

Motor tone is first assessed by flexing the limbs and noting increased or absent tone. If no tone is present, the hand is lifted approximately 30 cm above the bed and carefully dropped while protecting the limb from injury. The test is repeated with all extremities. Typically, the lower the level of consciousness, the closer to flaccid the limb(s) will be. An asymmetrical examination may indicate a lesion in the contralateral hemisphere or brainstem.

The next assessment, the *peripheral reflex response*, is a response to tactile stimuli peripherally and usually elicits a reflex response rather than a central or brain response. It is important to apply stimuli in a progressive manner, *using the least noxious stimuli necessary to elicit a response*. If there is no response to light or firm pressure, the clinician must use noxious stimuli. Each extremity is assessed individually. The typical technique for peripheral noxious stimuli involves pressure on the nail beds for asserting a peripheral stimulus. The triple-flexion response is a withdrawal of the limb in a straight line with flexion of the wrist–elbow–shoulder or the ankle–knee–hip. This response is considered a spinal reflex and is not an indication of brain involvement in the movement. The triple-flexion response is common in patients with severe neurological impairment and may be seen in patients who progress to brain death. Care must be taken to avoid confusion between brain- and spinal-mediated responses. If the patient has any other motor activity to peripheral extremity noxious stimuli, it is an indication of higher brain function.

If a noxious stimulus is applied *centrally* through a trapezius pinch or supraorbital pressure and the patient moves an extremity, it is an indication of brain involvement in the movement and not a spinal reflex. The movement should be noted as normal, decorticate (flexor: either withdrawal or spastic) or decerebrate (extensor) posturing and documented accordingly. In ventilated patients, endotracheal suction can also be a substitute for a central noxious stimulus, but the choice of stimulus needs to be consistent.

Practice tip

Localising to trapezius pinch requires the patient to cross the midline and purposefully reach towards the clavicle. It is an intentional movement to eliminate a noxious stimulus. Do not apply supraorbital pressure to patients with facial injuries close to the supraorbital region.

Practice tip

The ability to cough with suctioning can be tested in an intubated patient and implies an intact cranial nerve X.

Facial symmetry

Subtle facial symmetry may be difficult to appreciate in patients with oedema, endotracheal tube tape and nasogastric tubes. An asymmetric response is indicative of a lesion of the facial cranial nerve (CN-VII). Complete hemifacial involvement is typically seen in peripheral dysfunction (Bell's palsy), whereas superior division (forehead) sparing weakness indicates a pontine/medullary (central) involvement.

Corneal reflexes

Corneal reflexes are routinely assessed only in the unconscious patient. The corneal reflex is a protective mechanism (protects the eye) and therefore improper testing could result in damage to the eye. This tests the sensory portion of the trigeminal nerve (CN-V) and motor portion of the facial nerve (CN-VII). To test this reflex in the unconscious patient, gently hold the eye open and allow a drop of sterile saline (you may use isotonic eye drops) to land on the cornea. The patient with an intact reflex will blink (also termed 'blink to threat') in response. Due to the risk of corneal abrasion, the practice of touching the cornea with a wisp of cotton should be limited to the outer canthus.

Oropharyngeal reflexes

The oropharyngeal reflex (also called the gag reflex) tests the sensory and motor function of the vagus nerve (CN-X) and glossopharyngeal nerve (CN-IX). The gag reflex is important in providing protection to the airway (to avoid aspiration). Ask the awake patient to open their mouth and then use a soft-tipped applicator or suction catheter to lightly touch the soft palate in the back of their throat. The patient should gag if this reflex is intact. In the less responsive patient, this manoeuvre is often performed when providing oral hygiene, and the patient is assessed for elevation of the uvula when the soft palate is stimulated.

National Institutes of Health Stroke Scale

The National Institutes of Health Stroke Scale, or NIH Stroke Scale (NIHSS), is a validated and universally recognised 15-item neurological assessment for suspected acute ischaemic stroke (Table 16.7). Examination covers levels of consciousness, language, neglect, visual-field loss, extraocular movement, motor strength, ataxia, dysarthria and sensory loss. Point scores range between 0 and 42, where higher scores indicate greater severity. The NIHSS has recently been adopted in an Australian neurocritical care unit for the early detection of delayed cerebral ischaemia in patients with aneurysmal subarachnoid haemorrhage. Training and certification are required by practitioners wishing to use this scale.

See Online resources for a link to the NIHSS procedure.

TABLE 16.7
NIH Stroke Scale

INSTRUCTIONS	SCALE DEFINITION
1a. Level of consciousness	
The investigator must choose a response if a full evaluation is prevented by such obstacles as an endotracheal tube, language barrier, or orotracheal trauma/bandages. A 3 is scored only if the patient makes no movement (other than reflexive posturing) in response to noxious stimulation.	0 = **alert**; keenly responsive. 1 = **not alert**; but arousable by minor stimulation to obey, answer, or respond. 2 = **not alert**; requires repeated stimulation to attend, or is obtunded and requires strong or painful stimulation to make movements (not stereotyped). 3 = Responds only with reflex motor or autonomic effects, or totally unresponsive, flaccid, and areflexic. **Score:**
1b. Level of consciousness questions	
The patient is asked the month and his/her age. The answer must be correct – there is no partial credit for being close. Aphasic and stuporous patients who do not comprehend the questions will score 2. Patients unable to speak because of endotracheal intubation, orotracheal trauma, severe dysarthria from any cause, language barrier or any other problem not secondary to aphasia are given a 1. It is important that only the initial answer be graded and that the examiner not 'help' the patient with verbal or non-verbal cues	0 = **answers** both questions correctly. 1 = **answers** 1 question correctly. 2 = **answers** neither question correctly. **Score:**

TABLE 16.7
NIH Stroke Scale—cont'd

INSTRUCTIONS	SCALE DEFINITION

1c. Level of consciousness commands

The patient is asked to open and close the eyes and then to grip and release the non-paretic hand. Substitute another 1-step command if the hands cannot be used. Credit is given if an unequivocal attempt is made but not completed due to weakness. If the patient does not respond to command, the task should be demonstrated to them (pantomime), and the result scored (i.e. follows none, 1 or 2 commands). Patients with trauma, amputation, or other physical impediments should be given suitable 1-step commands. Only the first attempt is scored.

0 = **performs** both tasks correctly.
1 = **performs** 1 task correctly.
2 = **performs** neither task correctly.
Score:

2. Best gaze

Only horizontal eye movements will be tested. Voluntary or reflexive (oculocephalic) eye movements will be scored, but caloric testing is not done. If the patient has a conjugate deviation of the eyes that can be overcome by voluntary or reflexive activity, the score will be 1. If a patient has an isolated peripheral nerve paresis (CN-III, -IV or -VI), score a 1. Gaze is testable in all aphasic patients. Patients with ocular trauma, bandages, preexisting blindness, or other disorder of visual acuity or fields should be tested with reflexive movements, and a choice made by the investigator. Establishing eye contact and then moving about the patient from side to side will occasionally clarify the presence of a partial gaze palsy.

0 = **normal.**
1 = **partial gaze palsy;** gaze is abnormal in 1 or both eyes, but forced deviation or total gaze paresis is not present.
2 = **forced deviation,** or total gaze paresis is not overcome by the oculocephalic manoeuvre.
Score:

3. Visual

Visual fields (upper and lower quadrants) are tested by confrontation, using finger counting or visual threat, as appropriate. Patients may be encouraged, but if they look at the side of the moving fingers appropriately, this can be scored as normal. If there is unilateral blindness or enucleation, visual fields in the remaining eye are scored. Score 1 only if a clear-cut asymmetry, including quadrantanopia, is found. If patient is blind from any cause, score 3. Double simultaneous stimulation is performed at this point. If there is extinction, patient receives a 1, and the results are used to respond to item 11.

0 = **no visual loss.**
1 = **partial hemianopia.**
2 = **complete hemianopia.**
3 = **bilateral hemianopia** (blind including cortical blindness).
Score:

4. Facial palsy

Ask – or use pantomime to encourage – the patient to show teeth or raise eyebrows and close eyes. Score symmetry of grimace in response to noxious stimuli in the poorly responsive or non-comprehending patient. If facial trauma/bandages, orotracheal tube, tape or other physical barriers obscure the face, these should be removed to the extent possible.

0 = **normal** symmetrical movements.
1 = **minor paralysis** (flattened nasolabial fold, asymmetry on smiling).
2 = **partial paralysis** (total or near-total paralysis of lower face).
3 = **complete paralysis** of 1 or both sides (absence of facial movement in the upper and lower face).
Score:

5. Motor arm

The limb is placed in the appropriate position: extend the arms (palms down) 90° (if sitting) or 45° (if supine). Drift is scored if the arm falls before 10 seconds. The aphasic patient is encouraged using urgency in the voice and pantomime, but not noxious stimulation. Each limb is tested in turn, beginning with the non-paretic arm. Only in the case of amputation or joint fusion at the shoulder should the examiner record the score as untestable (UN) and clearly write the explanation for this choice.

0 = **no drift;** limb holds 90° (or 45°) for full 10 seconds.
1 = **drift;** limb holds 90° (or 45°), but drifts down before full 10 seconds; does not hit bed or other support.
2 = **some effort against gravity;** limb cannot get to or maintain (if cued) 90° (or 45°), drifts down to bed, but has some effort against gravity.
3 = **no effort against gravity;** limb falls.
4 = **no movement.**
UN = **amputation** or joint fusion, explain:
Score 5a (left arm):
Score 5b (right arm):

Continued

TABLE 16.7
NIH Stroke Scale—cont'd

INSTRUCTIONS	SCALE DEFINITION
6. Motor leg	
The limb is placed in the appropriate position: hold the leg at 30° (always tested supine). Drift is scored if the leg falls before 5 seconds. The aphasic patient is encouraged using urgency in the voice and pantomime but not noxious stimulation. Each limb is tested in turn, beginning with the non-paretic leg. Only in the case of amputation or joint fusion at the hip should the examiner record the score as untestable (UN) and clearly write the explanation for this choice.	**0** = **no drift;** leg holds 30° position for full 5 seconds. **1** = **drift;** leg falls by the end of the 5-second period but does not hit the bed. **2** = **some effort against gravity;** leg falls to bed by 5 seconds but has some effort against gravity. **3** = **no effort against gravity;** leg falls to bed immediately. **4** = **no movement.** UN = **amputation** or joint fusion, explain: **Score 6a (left leg):** **Score 6b (right leg):**
7. Limb ataxia	
This item is aimed at finding evidence of a unilateral cerebellar lesion. Test with eyes open. In case of visual defect, ensure testing is done in intact visual field. The finger–nose–finger and heel–shin tests are performed on both sides, and ataxia is scored only if present out of proportion to weakness. Ataxia is absent in the patient who cannot understand or is paralysed. Only in the case of amputation or joint fusion should the examiner record the score as untestable (UN) and clearly write the explanation for this choice. In case of blindness, test by having the patient touch the nose from the extended arm position.	**0** = **absent.** **1** = **present in ONE limb.** **2** = **present in TWO limbs.** UN = **amputation** or joint fusion, explain: **Score:**
8. Sensory	
Sensation or grimace to pinprick when tested, or withdrawal from noxious stimulus in the obtunded or aphasic patient. Only sensory loss attributed to stroke is scored as abnormal and the examiner should test as many body areas [(arms (not hands), legs, trunk, face) as needed to accurately check for hemisensory loss. A score of 2, 'severe or total sensory loss', should be given only when a severe or total loss of sensation can be clearly demonstrated. Stuporous and aphasic patients will, therefore, probably score 1 or 0. The patient with brainstem stroke who has bilateral loss of sensation is scored 2. If the patient does not respond and is quadriplegic, score 2. Patients in a coma (item 1a = 3) are automatically given a 2 on this item.	**0** = **normal;** no sensory loss. **1** = **mild-to-moderate sensory loss;** patient feels pinprick is less sharp or is dull on the affected side; or there is a loss of superficial pain with pinprick, but patient is aware of being touched. **2** = **severe or total sensory loss;** patient is not aware of being touched in the face, arm and leg. **Score:**
9. Best language	
A great deal of information about comprehension will be obtained during the preceding sections of the examination. For this scale item, the patient is asked to describe what is happening in the attached picture, to name the items on the attached naming sheet, and to read from the attached list of sentences. Comprehension is judged from responses here, as well as to all of the commands in the preceding general neurological exam. If visual loss interferes with the tests, ask the patient to identify objects placed in the hand, repeat and produce speech. The intubated patient should be asked to write. The patient in a coma (item 1a = 3) will automatically score 3 on this item. The examiner must choose a score for the patient with stupor or limited cooperation, but a score of 3 should be used only if the patient is mute and follows no 1-step commands.	**0** = **no aphasia;** normal. **1** = **mild-to-moderate aphasia;** some obvious loss of fluency or facility of comprehension, without significant limitation on ideas expressed or form of expression. Reduction of speech and/or comprehension, however, makes conversation about provided materials difficult or impossible. For example, in conversation about provided materials, examiner can identify picture or naming card content from patient's response. **2** = **severe aphasia;** all communication is through fragmentary expression; great need for inference, questioning and guessing by the listener. Range of information that can be exchanged is limited; listener carries burden of communication. Examiner cannot identify materials provided from patient response. **3** = **mute, global aphasia;** no usable speech or auditory comprehension. **Score:**

TABLE 16.7
NIH Stroke Scale—cont'd

INSTRUCTIONS	SCALE DEFINITION
10. Dysarthria	
If patient is thought to be normal, an adequate sample of speech must be obtained by asking patient to read or repeat words from the attached list. If the patient has severe aphasia, the clarity of articulation of spontaneous speech can be rated. Only if the patient is intubated or has other physical barriers to producing speech should the examiner record the score as untestable (UN) and clearly write the explanation for this choice. Do not tell the patient why he/she is being tested.	0 = **normal.** 1 = **mild-to-moderate dysarthria;** patient slurs at least some words and, at worst, can be understood with some difficulty. 2 = **severe dysarthria;** patient's speech is so slurred as to be unintelligible in the absence of or out of proportion to any dysphasia, or is mute/anarthric. UN = **intubated** or other physical barrier, explain. **Score:**
11. Extinction and inattention (formerly Neglect)	
Sufficient information to identify neglect may be obtained during the prior testing. If the patient has a severe visual loss preventing visual double simultaneous stimulation, and the cutaneous stimuli are normal, the score is normal. If the patient has aphasia but does appear to attend to both sides, the score is normal. The presence of visual spatial neglect or anosognosia may also be taken as evidence of abnormality. Since the abnormality is scored only if present, the item is never untestable.	0 = **no abnormality.** 1 = **visual, tactile, auditory, spatial, or personal inattention,** or extinction to bilateral simultaneous stimulation in 1 of the sensory modalities. 2 = **profound hemi-inattention or extinction to more than 1 modality;** does not recognise own hand or orients to only 1 side of space. **Score:**

CATEGORY	SCORE
1a. Level of consciousness	0 = alert 1 = drowsy 2 = stuporous 3 = coma
1b. Orientation questions[a]	0 = answers both correctly 1 = answers one correctly 2 = incorrect
1c. Response to commands[a]	0 = performs both correctly 1 = performs one correctly 2 = incorrect
2. Gaze	0 = normal 1 = partial gaze palsy 2 = forced deviation
3. Visual fields	0 = no visual loss 1 = partial hemianopia 2 = complete hemianopia 3 = bilateral hemianopia
4. Facial paresis	0 = normal 1 = minor 2 = partial 3 = complete
5a. Motor arm – left **5b. Motor arm – right**	0 = no drift 1 = drift 2 = can't resist gravity 3 = no effort against gravity 4 = no movement

Continued

TABLE 16.7

NIH Stroke Scale—cont'd

CATEGORY	SCORE
6a. **Motor leg – left** 6b. **Motor leg – right**	0 = no drift 1 = drift 2 = can't resist gravity 3 = no effort against gravity 4 = no movement
7. **Limb ataxia**	0 = no ataxia 1 = present in one limb 2 = present in two limbs
8. **Sensory**	0 = normal 1 = partial loss 2 = severe loss
9. **Language**	0 = no aphasia 1 = mild-mod aphasia 2 = severe aphasia 3 = mute
10. **Dysarthria**	0 = normal articulation 1 = mild to mod slurring of words 2 = near to unintelligible or worse
11. **Extinction and inattention**	0 = no neglect 1 = partial neglect 2 = complete neglect

Source: Ischemic stroke. Elsevier point of care. Updated December 8, 2021. Copyright Elsevier BV. All rights reserved.

Post-traumatic amnesia scale

Post-traumatic amnesia (PTA) is a disorder after brain injury that is classified as a traumatic delirium and may even be found in patients who rate a GCS of 15.[38] The incidence of delirium after a brain injury event is high, especially with severe injuries and loss of consciousness. Delirium is discussed in detail in Chapter 8; however, traumatic delirium historically has been referred to in the literature as post-traumatic amnesia. Post-traumatic amnesia is defined as the 'time elapsed from injury until recovery of full consciousness and the return of ongoing memory'. It is the initial stage of recovery from brain injury and is characterised by anterograde (formation of new memory) and retrograde (memory before injury) amnesia, disorientation and rapid forgetting. Brief periods of PTA can occur after minor concussion and may be the only clinical sign of any brain injury. This is when PTA is useful for defining the severity of injury and alerting the clinician in regard to greater surveillance and investigation, as described in Table 16.8. Patients often progress directly from coma into delirium without a clearly defined stupor stage, so using a tool to measure PTA can be useful to gauge the actual condition of the patient in the delirium state. Duration of PTA is extremely variable, ranging from

TABLE 16.8

Post-traumatic amnesia (PTA) scale used to determine severity of brain injury

PTA DURATION	SEVERITY
1–4 hours	Mild brain injury
≤1 day	Moderate brain injury
2–7 days	Severe brain injury
1–4 weeks	Very severe brain injury
1–6 months	Extremely severe brain injury
>6 months	Chronic amnesia state

minutes to months. Although the early stages of PTA are easily recognised, identifying the endpoint is difficult and complex.

The duration of PTA is the best indicator of the extent of cognitive and functional deficits after TBI. The two most common means of assessing PTA are the Galveston

Orientation and Amnesia Test (GOAT) and the Westmead PTA scale.[38–40] The GOAT features 10 questions that assess temporal and spatial orientation, biographical recall and memory. The test consists of 10 items that involve the recall of events that occurred right before and after the injury, as well as questions about disorientation. Scores of 75 or more on this scale (out of a total possible score of 100) correspond to the termination of the PTA episode. In the Westmead PTA scale, four pictures, one with the examiner's face and name, are to be recalled by the patient on the next day. Those with severe PTA will have difficulty completing such short-term memory tasks. The duration of PTA correlates well with the extent of diffuse axonal injury and with functional outcomes. A person is said to be absolved of PTA if they can achieve a perfect score for three consecutive days.[39]

Assessment of the injured brain

The primary aims of managing patients with acute brain injury in the critical care unit are to limit the risk of secondary brain injury and maintain cerebral perfusion. There is little that can be done to reverse the primary damage caused by an insult. Secondary insults may be subtle and can remain undetected by routine systemic physiological monitoring. Continuous monitoring of the CNS in the ICU serves three functions:

1 determination of the extent of the primary injury

2 early detection of secondary cerebral insults so that appropriate interventions can be instituted

3 monitoring of therapeutic interventions to provide feedback.

Despite technological advances, computerised tomography (CT), magnetic resonance imaging (MRI) and functional MRI are all limited in that they reflect the brain status at a single moment in time and are not able to provide continuous real-time data.[41] Continuous data can be provided, such as intra-arterial blood pressure, pulse oximetry (SpO_2), end-tidal carbon dioxide ($EtCO_2$) and temperature; however, these data are considered surrogates and may not directly reflect changes in intracranial pathology. Advanced continuous monitoring includes partial pressure of brain tissue oxygen ($PbtO_2$) and CBF, which require invasive technology. Serial neurological evaluation with the GCS or FOUR score can and should be performed routinely. The use of emerging technology through continuous EEG, signal-processed EEG (bispectral index), cerebral oximetry and transcranial Doppler is actively being investigated.

Brain-imaging techniques

Computed tomography

CT is the primary neuroimaging technique in the initial evaluation of the acute brain injury patient; it uses a computer to digitally construct an image based upon the measurement of the absorption of X-rays through the brain.[42] Table 16.9 generally summarises the white-to-black

TABLE 16.9	
The brain and related structures in CT	
STRUCTURE/FLUID/SPACE	GREY SCALE
Bone, acute blood	Very white
Enhanced tumour	Very white
Subacute blood	Light grey
Muscle	Light grey
Grey matter	Light grey
White matter	Medium grey
Cerebrospinal fluid	Medium grey to black
Air, fat	Very black

intensities seen for selected tissues in CT. The advantages of CT are: (1) it is rapidly performed, which is especially important in neurological emergencies, (2) it clearly shows acute and subacute haemorrhages into the meningeal spaces and brain and (3) it is less expensive than an MRI. Disadvantages include: (1) it does not clearly show acute or subacute infarctions or ischaemia, or brain oedema, but shows only injury, (2) it does not differentiate white from grey matter as clearly as an MRI and (3) it exposes the patient to ionising radiation. Despite these limitations, it is still the most prevalent form of neurological imaging.

Practice tip

The mnemonic 'Sometimes Blood Can Be Very Bad' (Symmetry, Blood, Cisterns, Bone, Ventricles, Brain) provides a routine approach when looking at brain CT scans.

Magnetic resonance imaging

The tissues of the body contain large amounts of protons (nuclei of hydrogen atoms) that function like tiny spinning magnets. Normally, these protons are arranged randomly in relation to each other owing to the constantly fluctuating magnetic field produced by the associated electrons. However, when placed in a superconducting magnet, the magnetic moments of the protons will tend to align along the direction of this external field. MRI uses this characteristic of protons to generate images of the brain and body.[42] The advantages of MRI are: (1) it can be manipulated to visualise a wide variety of abnormalities within the brain and (2) it can show much of the detail of the brain in normal and abnormal states. The disadvantages of MRI are: (1) it does not show acute or subacute haemorrhage into the brain in any detail, (2) the time frame and enclosed space required to perform and prepare a patient for the procedure are not advantageous for neurological emergencies, (3) it is relatively more expensive compared with CT, (4) the loud noise of the procedure needs to be considered in patient management, (5) equipment for life support and monitoring needs to be non-magnetic because of the magnetic nature of the procedure and (6) patients with metal objects such as implantable medical devices (pacemakers), shrapnel (e.g. military TBI wounds) or metal shavings (e.g. from welding) may be at increased risk and unable to undergo MRI.

Functional magnetic resonance imaging

Functional magnetic resonance imaging (fMRI) is similar to MRI but uses deoxyhaemoglobin as an endogenous contrast, which serves as the source of the magnetic signal for fMRI.[42] It can determine precisely which part of the brain is handling critical functions such as thought, speech, movement and sensation; help assess the effects of stroke, trauma or degenerative disease on brain function; monitor the growth and function of brain tumours; and guide the planning of surgery or radiation therapy for the brain.

Cerebral angiography

Cerebral angiography involves cannulation of cerebral vessels and the administration of intra-arterial contrast agents and medications for conditions involving the arterial circulation of the brain. This procedure also has the benefit of using non-invasive CT or MRI with or without contrast to guide the accuracy of the procedure. For example, intracranial aneurysms and arteriovenous malformations can be accurately diagnosed and repaired without surgical intervention.

Cerebral perfusion-imaging techniques

Numerous imaging techniques have been developed and applied to evaluate brain haemodynamics, perfusion and blood flow. The main advanced imaging techniques dedicated to brain haemodynamics are positron emission tomography (PET), single photon emission computed tomography (SPECT), xenon-enhanced computed tomography (XeCT), dynamic perfusion computed tomography (PCT), MRI dynamic susceptibility contrast (DSC) and arterial spin labelling (ASL). All of these techniques give similar information about brain haemodynamics in the form of parameters such as CBF or cerebral blood volume (CBV). However, each technique relies upon different technical aspects, contrasts, processing and duration of imaging. Moreover, due to cost, few institutions have invested in providing all of the aforementioned imaging techniques. Hence, the inter-rater reliability for measuring CBF or CBV using one technology versus another is not well defined.

ICP monitoring

Invasive measures for monitoring ICP are commonly used in patients with a severe head injury or after neurological surgery. Normal ICP varies with age, body position and clinical condition. The normal ICP is 7–15 mmHg in a supine adult, 3–7 mmHg in children and 1.5–6 mmHg in term infants. The definition of intracranial hypertension depends on the specific pathology and age, although ICP >20 mmHg is generally considered to be abnormal. Significantly increased ICP may cause a reduction in CPP and CBF; if uncorrected, this may lead to secondary ischaemic cerebral injury. Although studies have shown that high ICP is associated with poor outcome, there is no agreed upon threshold at which treatment should be initiated to reduce ICP and no agreed-upon best intervention. Recent evidence supports that, because ICP varies widely over a short period of time, nurses should observe ICP for at least 5 minutes prior to documenting an ICP value.[43]

ICP varies with arterial pulsation and is not a static pressure. Fluctuations can be seen with breathing and during coughing and straining. Each of the intracranial constituents occupies a certain volume and, being essentially liquid, is incompressible. ICP cannot be reliably estimated from any specific clinical feature or CT finding and must be measured. Different methods of monitoring ICP have been described but two methods are commonly used in clinical practice: intraventricular catheters and intraparenchymal fibreoptic microtransducer systems. The traditional reference point for the transducer is the foramina of Monro (the duct joining the lateral and third ventricle that is in alignment with the middle of the ear) although, in practical terms, the external auditory meatus is often used.[44]

When ICP monitoring is required, the use of ventriculostomy catheters (external ventricular drainage (EVD) catheters) provides similar accuracy to intraparenchymal fibreoptic systems. Fibreoptic systems provide a reflection of ICP in the brain tissue (paren-chyma) and EVD systems provide a reflection of ICP in the ventricular system. The EVD system includes an external drainage system connected to a strain gauge transducer. The drainage system and pressure transducer are primed on insertion with sterile preservative-free saline. The pressure transducer must be calibrated (also termed zero referencing, zero balancing or simply zeroing) to a known value. Commonly, atmospheric pressure is used as a zero-value reference.

Monitoring ICP through an EVD has the advantage of providing a pathway to divert CSF out of the skull to reduce ICP. Alternatively, the EVD catheter may provide a pathway to instill medication into the ventricular system. The primary disadvantage to monitoring ICP through an EVD is the increased risk of infection. When there is a significant amount of blood in the ventricular system, the EVD is also prone to clogging; this loss of patency obliterates the ability to monitor ICP. Ventricular collapse may occur through overdrainage or cerebral oedema. Because the EVD relies upon a continuous column of fluid, this loss of patency affects the accuracy of ICP values. Current evidence supports a higher risk of complications when the EVD is left open to drain for extended periods of time.[45] In addition, limiting ventricular drainage per hour using gravity and three-way taps to 5–10 mL/h has been used to avoid excessively rapid CSF drainage.

Fibreoptic catheter systems are inserted into the intraparenchymal space and provide a continuous record of ICP. Because of the lower complication rate, critical care physicians and advance practice nurses are now placing fibreoptic catheters where previously only neurosurgeons placed invasive ICP monitoring. Many fibreoptic catheter systems are now part of multimodal monitoring systems that provide intracranial temperature, partial pressure of brain tissue oxygen (PbtO$_2$) and CBF.

While Brain Trauma Foundation (BTF) guidelines suggest ICP monitoring for head injury patients with GCS scores <9, there is growing controversy regarding the efficacy of ICP monitoring to improve outcome from severe TBI.[46,47] A review of neurocritical care and outcome from TBI suggested that ICP/CPP-guided therapy may benefit patients with severe head injury, including those presenting with raised ICP in the absence of a mass lesion and those requiring complex interventions.

Practice tip

The fixed volume of brain parenchyma, CSF and intravascular blood contained within the rigid, non-expandable cranium determines ICP. Brain tissue accounts for 80% of this volume, whereas blood and CSF each account for about 10%.

Pulse waveforms

Interpretation of waveforms that are generated by the cerebral monitoring devices is important in the clinical assessment of intracranial adaptive capacity (the ability of the brain to compensate for rises in intracranial volume without raising the ICP). Brain tissue pressure and ICP increase with each cardiac cycle and, therefore, the ICP waveform is a modified arterial pressure wave (Fig. 16.15). The cardiac waves reach the cranial circulation via the choroid plexus and resemble the waveforms transmitted by arterial catheters, although the amplitude is lower.

There are three distinct peaks seen in the ICP waveform:[48]

- P1, the percussion wave, which is sharp and reflects the cardiac pulse as the pressure is transmitted from the choroid plexus to the ventricle
- P2, the tidal wave, which is more variable in nature and reflects cerebral compliance and increases in amplitude as compliance decreases
- P3, which is due to the closure of the aortic valve and is known as the dicrotic notch. Of recent importance is that the elevation of P3 may indicate low global cerebral perfusion.

It is important that the waveform be continuously observed, as changes in mean pressure or in waveform

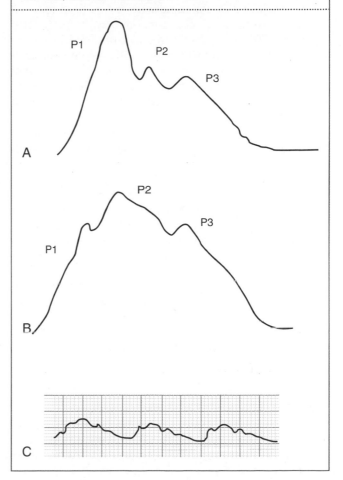

FIGURE 16.15 The intracranial pressure waveforms. **(A)** Depicts the situation of a compliant system; **(B)** a high-pressure wave recorded from a non-compliant system in which P2 exceeds the level of the P1 waveform, due to a marked decrease in cerebral compliance. The lower tracing **(C)** is an example of an ICP waveform from a patient-monitoring system in which the three distinct components, as indicated in the text, can be identified.

shape usually require immediate attention.[48] In acute states such as head injury and subarachnoid haemorrhage, ICP depends greatly on the link between monitoring and therapy, so close inspection of the trend in the ICP and the details derived from the waveform is extremely important. Simple ongoing visual assessment of the ICP waveform for increased amplitude, elevated P2 and rounding of the waveform provides non-specific information suggestive of decreased intracranial adaptive capacity and altered intracranial dynamics.

Assessment of cerebral perfusion

CPP is calculated as the mean arterial pressure (MAP) minus the ICP and represents the pressure gradient across the vessel that drives CBF:

$$CPP = MAP - ICP$$

CPP is a pressure-based surrogate of oxygen and metabolite delivery. There is no evidence for the optimum level of CPP, and it is likely that emerging evidence will support different CPP thresholds based on injury pathology. Higher CPP has been associated with increased lung water and acute respiratory distress syndrome. Furthermore, mortality rises approximately 20% for each 10-mmHg loss of CPP. In those studies where CPP was maintained above 70 mmHg, the reduction in mortality was as much as 35% for those with severe head injury.[49] The BTF provides a level IIB recommendation for CPP goal of 60–70 mmHg despite the lack of definitive data.[50] These guidelines also include a level III recommendation to avoid aggressive attempts to raise CPP >70 mmHg because of the risk for respiratory failure. Despite noting associations between measured decreases in cerebral oxygenation and worse outcomes, the BTF guidelines find inadequate evidence to provide a recommendation for or against intracranial oxygen or jugular bulb oxygen monitoring.[50]

Assessment of cerebral oxygenation

The three main factors determining cerebral oxygenation are CBF, arterial oxygen content and cerebral metabolic rate of oxygen consumption.[51] In clinical practice, monitoring of arterial blood gas tensions is routine in most critically ill patients. Measurement of cerebral metabolic rate of oxygen consumption is, however, not commonplace as it is technically difficult and cumbersome. Therefore, the predominant monitoring strategy in clinical practice has relied on measurements of CBF and its surrogates. This section will outline those modalities.

Jugular venous oximetry

Jugular venous catheterisation is used for deriving oxygen-based variables. It facilitates the assessment of jugular venous oxygenation ($SjvO_2$), cerebral oxygen extraction (CEO_2) and arteriovenous difference in oxygen ($AVDO_2$). All these variables indicate changes in cerebral metabolism and blood flow, and therefore the catheter generates continuous data that reflect the balance between supply and demand of cerebral oxygen.[52] The catheter is inserted in the right jugular vein, as it is slightly larger than the left and provides readings that are more representative of overall brain function. The catheter tip is advanced so that the tip sits in the bulb of the internal jugular vein. The normal requirement for cerebral oxygen delivery is consumption at 35–40% of available oxygen, giving a normal $SjvO_2$ of 60–65%. Changes in $SjvO_2$ reflect changes in cerebral metabolic rate and CBF; however, as it is a global measure, it does not detect regional ischaemia.[53] $SjvO_2$ is also sensitive to operator error, requires frequent recalibration, and patient positioning (e.g. changes in head or neck position) may alter the signal quality and require medical intervention to reposition the catheter. For these reasons, $SjvO_2$ is becoming increasingly less common.

Partial pressure of brain tissue oxygenation monitoring

Changes in ICP values alone may not accurately depict poor CBF or oxygenation deficits to brain tissue and may be late signs, occurring hours later when damage cannot be reversed.[54,55] Consequently, brain tissue hypoxaemia may occur during the first 24 hours after injury despite controlled brain pressures. Monitoring the partial pressure of oxygen in brain tissue ($PbtO_2$) as an adjunct to ICP monitoring may provide more accurate and timelier cerebral oxygen delivery and demand than ICP alone.[55] Normal $PbtO_2$ (20–25 mmHg) emerges as a critical determinant of outcome, with values <20 mmHg associated with higher risk of poor functional outcomes. A $PbtO_2$ value <10 mmHg for more than 10 minutes carries a higher risk of death. Alterations in cerebral metabolic rate can also change tissue oxygen levels. Increased adherence to guidelines and reducing the patient's energy consumption via reduced noise and/or distractions, and increasing their protein caloric intake to complement their increased stress state, may improve tissue oxygenation.[56]

Cerebral microdialysis

Cerebral microdialysis remains primarily a research tool for investigating the metabolic status of one area of brain tissue.[54,57] The microdialysis probe is inserted into the cerebral tissue where substances in the extracellular fluid surround the semipermeable membrane at the tip of the catheter. Following equilibration of the tissue metabolites with the perfusion fluid, the dialysate can be analysed for concentrations of products of energy metabolism (glucose, lactate, pyruvate and glutamate) as indicators of hypoxia and ischaemia. In addition, interstitial glycerol can be determined, which is a parameter of lipolysis and/or cell membrane damage.[58] The products of metabolism are sampled hourly and the trends in values for each metabolite are explored as correlates of changes to cerebral metabolic function. Because of limited outcome data, cerebral microdialysis is primarily used in conjunction with clinical research.

Non-invasive assessment

Invasive methods of measuring ICP, CBF and $PbtO_2$ are associated with complications. Because of this, many patients with low- or moderate-grade TBI do not typically receive invasive monitoring. Non-invasive methods for detecting episodes of cerebral hypoxia and ischaemia are detailed in the following section.

Transcranial Doppler

Transcranial Doppler (TCD) ultrasound has proved to be a safe, reliable and relatively inexpensive technology for measuring cerebrovascular blood velocities and evaluating cerebral circulation and haemodynamics.[59] A handheld transducer is used to direct pulses of ultrasound towards the cerebral arteries at the base of the skull.[60] Velocities from the cerebral arteries, the internal carotids, the basilar and the vertebral arteries can be sampled by altering the transducer location, angle and the instrument's depth setting. The most common windows in the cranium are in the orbit (of the eye) and in the temporal and suboccipital regions. TCD measures systolic, diastolic and mean velocity in middle cerebral artery (MCA) flow; as well as providing the pulsatility index (PI), a derived value. Changes in the PI are sometimes used to identify the threshold of autoregulation. In subarachnoid haemorrhage (SAH) and TBI, this may be due to vasospasm, impaired autoregulation or abnormal intracranial compliance.

Continuous electroencephalography

Electroencephalography (EEG) is used to display and record electrical activity produced by the firing of neurons within the brain. Both scalp (sensors placed on the surface of the scalp) and depth (sensors placed into brain tissue) electrodes are used in EEG monitoring. Continuous EEG (cEEG) has the advantage of being continuous and non-invasive and carries the potential to detect alterations in brain physiology at a reversible stage, which may trigger treatment before permanent brain injury occurs.[61] Currently, the main applications of cEEG are diagnosing and localising seizure, non-convulsive status epilepticus, monitoring and guiding the treatment of status epilepticus and detecting delayed cerebral ischaemia from vasospasm in SAH patients.[62-64] Other applications may include monitoring of reperfusion after interventions for acute stroke patients and detection of intracranial hypertension. Clinically unrecognised electrographic seizures and periodic epileptiform discharges have been shown to be frequent and associated with poor outcome in patients with severe brain injury from different aetiologies, including TBI, ischaemic and haemorrhagic strokes and CNS infection.[65]

The EEG becomes substantially abnormal (suppressed) when CBF declines to 20–30 mL/100 g/min. More-subtle abnormalities accompany lesser degrees of hypoperfusion, including initial loss of beta activity, slowing to the theta range and then to the delta range. Irreversible injury to brain tissue occurs at cerebral flows of about 10–12 mL/100 g/min. Therefore, EEG sensitivity to ischaemia allows its use in situations where cerebral perfusion is at risk. Changes over time in quantitative EEG (qEEG) parameters can trigger remote reading, focused neurological examination, imaging studies and early treatment.[65] Subtle EEG changes may be difficult to interpret in isolation, but may be better understood when interpreted along with other components of a multimodality monitoring (neurological exam, ICP, CBF and $PbtO_2$).

Near-infrared spectroscopy

Near-infrared spectroscopy (NIRS) is a non-invasive method of monitoring continuous trends of cerebral oxygenated and deoxygenated haemoglobin by utilising an infrared light beam transmitted through the skull.[66] Oxygenated and deoxygenated haemoglobin moieties have different absorption spectra, and cerebral oxygenation and haemodynamic status can be determined by their relative absorption of near-infrared light.[67] NIRS allows interrogation of the cerebral cortex using reflectance spectroscopy via optodes, light-transmitting and detecting devices, placed on the scalp. Normal saturation is 70%. Because NIRS interrogates arterial, venous and capillary blood within the field of view, the derived saturation represents regional tissue oxygenation (rSO_2) measured from these three compartments and can be used to identify tissue hypoxia and ischaemia in the brain cortex. Although promising, the clinical and bedside use of NIRS is constrained by sources of error including contamination of the signal by the extracerebral circulation (such as in the scalp), extraneous light and the presence of extravascular blood arising from subarachnoid or subdural haemorrhage.

Bispectral index monitoring

Bispectral index (BIS) monitoring is a neurophysiological monitoring device that continually analyses brain activity non-invasively through the electroencephalogram (EEG).[68] Traditionally used within the operating theatre environment to monitor a patient's level of sedation, it is occasionally used within the intensive care environment to assess brain activity or level of consciousness. Alterations in metabolic activity or metabolic stability within the brain will be reflected on the machine's EEG. The BIS number ranges from 0 to 100.[69] A BIS number of 100 indicates a conscious patient (high metabolic activity), a BIS number of 40–60 indicates a sedation level for general anaesthesia and a BIS number of 0 indicates no brain activity detected (isoelectric/markedly decreased or absent metabolic activity).

Summary

An overview of anatomy and physiology in the context of and as applied to neurological assessment of the critically ill is provided in this chapter. Priorities of clinical assessment are described and include determining the extent of the neurological injury, recognising fluctuations in the patient's condition, and assisting in the maintenance of cerebral perfusion as part of multimodal monitoring. Imaging techniques and assessment incorporate the therapeutics of ICP, CPP, CBF, $PbtO_2$, cEEG, transcranial Doppler and cerebral perfusion imaging. The clinical case demonstrates neurological assessment priorities in an unstable TBI patient and a subarachnoid haemorrhage patient. Clinical, non-invasive and invasive assessment techniques are described within the context of these patients' care.

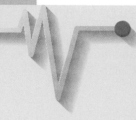

Case study

Mr A was admitted to the emergency department by ambulance after being found by his wife at the bottom of a ladder. He was agitated, confused and not moving his left arm. Mr A had a history of ischaemic heart disease, hypercholesterolaemia and osteoarthritis. His regular medications include aspirin and rosuvastatin. On ambulance arrival to the scene, Mr A's GCS was 11/15 (E3, V3, M5); his pupils were equal and reactive. His blood pressure was 89/76 mmHg and oxygen saturations 93% requiring oxygen administration. A cervical collar was applied. Mr A was taken to the emergency department at a tertiary hospital.

EMERGENCY DEPARTMENT

On arrival, Mr A was taken for a non-contrast CT brain (CTB), which showed multicompartmental intracranial haemorrhage including bilateral frontal contusions, right-sided subdural haemorrhage (SHD) with 5 mm of midline shift, and small intraventricular haemorrhage. While in the CT scanner, Mr A's GCS reduced to 7/15 (E1, V2, M4). He was intubated, platelet infusion was administered, and he was taken then to operating theatre for evacuation of SDH and insertion of an external ventricular drain (EVD).

INTENSIVE CARE UNIT

Day 0:

Mr A was sedated on propofol and fentanyl infusions. On a sedation hold, he localised with his right side and his pupils were equal and reactive. Mr A's blood pressure was maintained between 100 mmHg and 150 mmHg systolic with a noradrenaline infusion. ICP ranged between 4 mmHg and 18 mmHg; his EVD was kept open to drainage 15 cm above the foramen of magnum. The goal was to wean sedation in the next 48 hours and assess for extubation readiness.

Day 2:

Mr A began to experience intracranial hypertension with ICP persistently >22 mmHg, the waveform demonstrating an elevated P2. On neurological assessment with sedation hold, Mr A was no longer localising on application of central stimulus. His ICP spiked intermittently to >30 mmHg,; his pupils were equal and reactive, but sluggish.

Mr A's head of bed was elevated to 30 degrees, and the cervical collar removed with sandbag application. Midazolam and cisatracurium infusions were added, along with the administration of intermittent hypertonic saline (3%) boluses. His ventilation was titrated to target a CO_2 of 35 mmHg and a cooling blanket applied to obtain normothermia. The EVD was lowered to 10 cm above FM for increased CSF shunting. The noradrenaline infusion was titrated to ensure that his CPP was between 60 and 70 mmHg.

Despite these interventions, Mr A continued to experience intracranial hypertension. A repeat CTB demonstrated blossoming of the frontal contusions, significant cerebral oedema and signs of herniation. Mr A was taken urgently to operating theatres for decompressive craniectomy.

Day 3–22:

Mr A made slow neurological improvements over his intensive care journey. On day 14 he underwent an MRI showing possible diffuse axonal injury and bilateral frontal infarcts. His spinal precautions were lifted and the collar removed. Mr A's EEG showed generalised slowing but there were no signs of status epilepticus. On day 18 he was tracheostomised and admitted to the neurosurgical ward on day 26 with a GCS of 10/15 (E4, V3, M5).

DISCHARGE FROM HOSPITAL

Mr A's tracheostomy was removed while on the neurosurgical ward and he was discharged to the brain injury rehabilitation unit.

CASE STUDY QUESTIONS

1 Discuss some of the concerning neurological and hemodynamic findings when Mr A was found by the ambulance, and the implications of these.

2 What are some of the reasons Mr A may have had an external ventricular drain inserted rather than an intraparenchymal monitor?

3   Discuss the role of sedation hold in neurological assessment. How would this have contributed to the recognition of neurological deterioration?

4   How will the use of hypertonic saline play a role in the reduction of ICP?

5   How will the removal of a cervical collar help to reduce ICP?

RESEARCH VIGNETTE

Anestis DM, Tsitsopoulos PP, Tsonidis CA, et al. The current significance of the FOUR score: a systematic review and critical analysis of the literature. J Neurol Sci 2020;409:116600.

Abstract

Background: The Full Outline of Un-Responsiveness Score (FOURs) is a scale for clinical assessment of consciousness that was introduced to overcome disadvantages of the widely accepted Glasgow Coma Score (GCS).

Objective: To carry out a systematic review and critical analysis of the available literature on the clinical application of FOURs and perform a comparison with the GCS, in terms of reliability and predictive value.

Methods: An initial search retrieved a total of 147 papers. After applying strict inclusion criteria and further article selection to overcome data heterogeneity, a statistical comparison of inter-rater reliability, in-hospital mortality and long-term outcome prediction between the two scales in the adult and pediatric populations was done.

Results: Even though FOURs is more complicated than GCS, its application remains quite simple. Its reliability, validity and predictive value have been supported by an increasing number of studies, especially in critical care. A statistically significant difference ($P = 0.034$) in predicting in-hospital mortality in adults, in favour of FOURs when compared with GCS, was found. However, whether it poses a clinically significant advantage in detecting patients' deterioration and outcome prediction compared with other scaling systems remains unclear.

Conclusion: Further studies are needed to discern the FOURs' clinical usefulness, especially in patients in non-critical condition, with milder disorders of consciousness.

Critique

The Full Outline of Un-Responsiveness Score (FOURs) was principally designed to overcome the shortcomings of the widely used and previously considered 'gold standard' GCS. The aim was to provide a tool to test the verbal component of comatose patients, differentiate between patients with low scores, and detect subtle changes in the neurological condition. The FOURs' four components include: eye response, motor response (including gesturing in an attempt to replace verbal response), brainstem reflexes and breathing pattern.

This systematic review aimed to systematically summarise the existing data and provide a critical analysis on the FOURs, emphasising aspects of clinical importance. A strength of the review was the systematic search of the literature from 2005, since the FOURs was first introduced, and the critical analysis of the studies using a predetermined protocol including an assessment of risk of bias using the using the Mixed Methods Appraisal Tool (MMAT).

The authors conclude that the FOURs has been successfully evaluated for its predictive value for various conditions and its close relationship to mortality and poor neurological outcome has been well documented. FOURs' potential superiority to GCS appears to be most evident in studies of intensive care patients, suggesting that the additional neurological elements included in the FOURs are of value especially in critically ill patients. Additionally, the authors reported that mortality was higher in patients with the lowest FOUR score compared with the lowest GCS score, suggesting a potential advantage of the FOURs in patients with severe disorders of consciousness.

Learning activities

1 What are the theoretical advantages to developing nursing practice interventions using a staged approach to research?

2 Discuss the potential implications of observational/feasibility studies on implementation of findings in practice.

3 What are some of the potential threats to validity in this study?

4 What information does the Glasgow Coma Score provide?

5 What information should the nurse convey to staff in the intensive care unit when transferring the patient from the ED?

Online resources

Agency for Clinical Innovation (ACI) Adult neurological observation chart: education package, https://aci.health.nsw.gov.au/__data/assets/pdf_file/0018/201753/AdultChartEdPackage.pdf

American Association of Neuroscience Nurses (AANN), https://aann.org

Australasian Neuroscience Nurses' Association, https://www.anna.asn.au

Brain Explorer, https://brainexplorer.net

Brain Injury Association of America, https://www.biausa.org

Cranial nerves music video, https://www.youtube.com/watch?v=sAFaTaavmO8

FOUR score for Neuro Assessments, https://w3.rn.com/News/clinical_insights_details.aspx?Id=29828

The Glasgow Coma Scale (GCS) Part 1, https://www.youtube.com/watch?v=T93Ah9Zkurl&feature=player_detailpage

The Glasgow Coma Scale (GCS) Part 2, https://www.youtube.com/watch?v=_jTTPjZ_ruE

Neurocritical Care Society, https://www.neurocriticalcare.org

Neurological Foundation of New Zealand, https://neurological.org.nz

Neurotorium, https://neurotorium.org

Official Journal of the American Academy of Neurology (AAN), https://www.neurology.org

Physical Examination and Neurological Assessment, www.neurologyexam.com

Post-traumatic amnesia protocol, https://www.mq.edu.au/about/about-the-university/our-faculties/medicine-and-health-sciences/departments-and-centres/department-of-psychology/the-pta-protocol

Society for Neuroscience, https://www.sfn.org

The Brain Trauma Foundation, www.braintrauma.org

The National Institutes of Health Stroke Scale (NIH Stroke Scale), https://www.youtube.com/watch?v=do2CbY_Nm5c

World Health Organization (WHO), Road traffic injuries, https://www.who.int/news-room/fact-sheets/detail/road-traffic-injuries

Further reading

Blumenfeld H. Neuroanatomy through clinical cases. 3nd ed. Sunderland, MA: Sinauer Associates; 2021.

Carney N, Totten AM, O'Reilly C, et al. Guidelines for the management of severe traumatic brain injury. Neurosurgery 2016;80(1):6–15.

Greenberg MS. General neurocritical care. In: Greenberg MS, editor. Handbook of neurosurgery. 9th ed. New York: Thieme Medical; 2019. p. 126–31.

Hawryluk GWJ, Rubiano AM, Totten AM, et al. Guidelines for the management of severe traumatic brain injury: 2020 update of the decompressive craniectomy recommendations. Neurosurgery 2020;87(3):427–34.

Moini J, Piran P. Functional and clinical neuroanatomy. London; Academic Press; 2020. doi: 10.1016/C2018-0-01786-7.

Wang TY, Park C, Zhang H, et al. Management of acute traumatic spinal cord injury: a review of the literature. Front Surg 2021;8:698736.

Zink EK. Nursing training and management in the neurocritical care Unit. In: Nelson, S, Nyquist, P. (eds). Neurointensive care unit. Current Clinical Neurology series. Champaign, IL: Humana; 2020, p. 381–4. doi: 10.1007/978-3-030-36548-6_30.

References

1. Olsen DM, McNett M, Littejohns LR. AANN core curriculum for neuroscience nursing. 7th ed. Glenview, IL: American Association of Neuroscience Nurses; 2022.

2. Hickey JV. Overview of neuroanatomy and neurophysiology. In: Hickey JV, Staryer AL, editors. The clinical practice of neurological and neurosurgical nursing. 8th ed. Philadelphia: Wolters Kluwer; 2019, p. 47–92.

3. Norris TL. Porth's pathophysiology concepts of altered health states. 10th ed. Philadelphia: Wolters Kluwer; 2019.

4. Hall JE, Hall ME. Transport of substances through cell membranes. In: Guyton and Hall textbook of medical physiology. 14th ed. Philadelphia: Elsevier; 2022, p. 51–62.

5. Wehrwein EA, Orer HS, Barman SM. Overview of the anatomy, physiology, and pharmacology of the autonomic nervous system. Compr Physiol 2016;6(3):1239–78.

6. Armstrong RC, Mierzwa AJ, Marion CM, et al. White matter involvement after TBI: clues to axon and myelin repair capacity. Exp Neurol 2016;275(Pt 3):328–33.

7. Sandring S. Nervous system. In: Sandring S. editor. Grey's anatomy. 42nd ed. Philadelphia: Elsevier; 2021. p. 43–70.

8. Head VA, Wakerley BR. Guillain-Barre syndrome in general practice: clinical features suggestive of early diagnosis. Br J Gen Pract 2016;66(645):218–19.

9. Kandel ER, Koester JD, Mack SH, et al. Principles of neural science. New York: McGraw Hill; 2021.

10. Hickey JV, Strayer, AL. The clinical practice of neurological and neurosurgical nursing. 8th ed. Philadelphia: Wolters Kluwer; 2019.

11. Rudolph LM, Cornil CA, Mittelman-Smith MA, et al. Actions of steroids: new neurotransmitters. J Neurosci 2016;36(45):11449–58.

12. Blumenfeld H. Cerebral hemispheres and vascular supply. In: Blumenfeld H, editor. Neuroanatomy through clinical case. 3rd ed. Sunderland, MA: Sinauer Associates; 2022. p. 389–459.

13. Blumenfeld H. Neuroanatomy through clinical cases. 2nd ed. Sunderland, MA: Sinauer Associates; 2018.

14. Grossman MN, Anderson SL, Worku A, et al. Awakenings? Patient and hospital staff perceptions of nighttime disruptions and their effect on patient sleep. J Clin Sleep Med 2017;13(2):310–15.

15. Medrzycka-Dabrowska W, Lewandowska K, Kwiecień–Jaguś K, et al. Sleep deprivation in intensive care unit – systematic review. Open Med (Wars) 2018;13:384–93.

16. Steaphen A, Olson DM, Stutzman SE. Nurses' perceptions of a novel protocol addressing uniform periods of minimum assessment times. J Neurosci Nurs 2017;49(5):302–6.

17. Whyte J. Disorders of consciousness: the changing landscape of treatment. Neurology 2014;82(13):1106–7.

18. Brogan ME, Provencio JJ. Spectrum of catastrophic brain injury: coma and related disorders of consciousness. J Crit Care 2014;29(4):679–82.

19. Prottengeier J, Moritz A, Heinrich S, et al. Sedation assessment in a mobile intensive care unit: a prospective pilot-study on the relation of clinical sedation scales and the bispectral index. Crit Care 2014;18(6):615.

20. Sessler CN, Gosnell MS, Grap MJ, et al. The Richmond agitation-sedation scale: validity and reliability in adult intensive care unit patients. Am J Respir Crit Care Med 2002;166(10):1338–44.

21. Teasdale G, Jennett B. Assessment of coma and impaired consciousness. A practical scale. Lancet 1974;2(7872):81–4.

22. Mehta R, Chinthapalli K. Glasgow coma scale explained. BMJ 2019;365:l1296.

23. Powers WJ, Rabinstein AA, Ackerson T, et al. Guidelines for the early management of patients with acute ischemic stroke: 2019 update to the 2018 guidelines for the early management of acute ischemic stroke: a guideline for healthcare professionals from the American Heart Association/American Stroke Association. Stroke 2019;50(12):e344–418.

24. Reith FC, Brennan PM, Maas AI, et al. Lack of standardization in the use of the Glasgow Coma Scale: results of international surveys. J Neurotrauma 2016;33(1):89–94.

25. Mattar I, Liaw SY, Chan MF. A study to explore nurses' knowledge in using the Glasgow Coma Scale in an acute care hospital. J Neurosci Nurs 2013;45(5):272–80.

26. Stead LG, Wijdicks EF, Bhagra A, et al. Validation of a new coma scale, the FOUR score, in the emergency department. Neurocrit Care 2009;10(1):50–4.

27. Anestis DM, Tsitsopoulos PP, Tsonidis CA, et al. The current significance of the FOUR score: a systematic review and critical analysis of the literature. J Neurol Sci 2020;409:116600.

28. Wijdicks EF, Kramer AA, Rohs T Jr, et al. Comparison of the Full Outline of UnResponsiveness score and the Glasgow Coma Scale in predicting mortality in critically ill patients. Crit Care Med 2015;43(2):439–44.

29. McNett MM, Amato S, Philippbar SA. A comparative study of Glasgow Coma Scale and Full Outline of Unresponsiveness Scores for predicting long-term outcome after brain injury. J Neurosci Nurs 2016;48(4):207–14.

30. Kasprowicz M, Burzynska M, Melcer T, et al. A comparison of the Full Outline of UnResponsiveness (FOUR) score and Glasgow Coma Score (GCS) in predictive modelling in traumatic brain injury. Br J Neurosurg 2016;30(2):211–20.

31. Greenberg MS. Handbook of neurosurgery. 9th ed. New York: Thieme Medical; 2019.

32. Chen JW, Vakil-Gilani K, Williamson KL, et al. Infrared pupillometry, the Neurological Pupil index and unilateral pupillary dilation after traumatic brain injury: implications for treatment paradigms. Springerplus 2014;3:548.

33. Olson DM, Stutzman S, Saju C, et al. Interrater reliability of pupillary assessments. Neurocrit Care 2016;24(2):251–7.

34. Bledsoe BE, Casey MJ, Feldman J, et al. Glasgow Coma Scale scoring is often inaccurate. Prehosp Disaster Med 2015;30(1):46–53.

35. Spinello IM. Brain death determination. J Intensive Care Med 2015;30(6):326–37.

36. Woischneck D, Skalej M, Firsching R, et al. Decerebrate posturing following traumatic brain injury: MRI findings and their diagnostic value. Clin Radiol 2015;70(3):278–85.

37. Baumann JJ, Blissitt PA, Stewart-Amidei C. Assessment. In: Bader MK, Littlejohns LR, Olson DM, editors. AANN core curriculum for neuroscience nursing. 6th ed. Glenview, NSW: American Association of Neuroscience Nurses; 2016. p. 63–96.

38. Shores EA, Marosszeky JE, Sandanam J, et al. Preliminary validation of a clinical scale for measuring the duration of post-traumatic amnesia. Med J Aust 1986;144(11):569–72.

39. Levin HS, O'Donnell VM, Grossman RG. The Galveston Orientation and Amnesia Test. A practical scale to assess cognition after head injury. J Nerv Ment Dis 1979;167(11):675–84.

40. Davidoff G, Doljanac R, Berent S, et al. Galveston Orientation and Amnesia Test: its utility in the determination of closed head injury in acute spinal cord injury patients. Arch Phys Med Rehabil 1988;69(6):432–4.

41. LeBihan D. Elementary particles. Looking inside the brain: the power of neuroimaging. Princeton: Princeton Univ. Press; 2015. p. 4–21.

42. Ramezani M, Abolmaesumi P, Marble K, et al. Fusion analysis of functional MRI data for classification of individuals based on patterns of activation. Brain Imaging Behav 2015;9(2):149–61.

43. Rogers M, Stutzman SE, Atem FD, et al. Intracranial pressure values are highly variable after cerebral spinal fluid drainage. J Neurosci Nurs 2017;49(2):85–9.

44. Olson DM, Batjer HH, Abdulkadir K, et al. Measuring and monitoring ICP in neurocritical care: results from a national practice survey. Neurocrit Care 2014;20(1):15–20.

45. Chung DY, Leslie-Mazwi TM, Patel AB, et al. Management of external ventricular drains after subarachnoid hemorrhage: a multi-institutional survey. Neurocrit Care 2017;26(3):356–61.

46. O'Phelan K, Shepard SAI, DeJesus-Alvelo I. Controversies in intracranial pressure monitoring. In: Koenig M, editor. Cerebral herniation syndromes and intracranial hypertension. New Brunswick, NJ: Rutgers University Press; 2016. p. 55–77.

47. Chesnut R, Videtta W, Vespa P, et al. Intracranial pressure monitoring: fundamental considerations and rationale for monitoring. Neurocrit Care 2014;21(2):64–84.

48. Hawthorne C, Piper I. Monitoring of intracranial pressure in patients with traumatic brain injury. Front Neurol 2014;5:121.

49. Johnston AJ, Steiner LA, Coles JP, et al. Effect of cerebral perfusion pressure augmentation on regional oxygenation and metabolism after head injury. Crit Care Med 2005;33(1):189–95.

50. Carney N, Totten AM, O'Reilly C, et al. Guidelines for the management of severe traumatic brain injury, fourth edition. Neurosurgery 2017;80(1):6–15.

51. Vos PE, Diaz-Arrastia R. Traumatic brain injury. Chichester: John Wiley; 2015.

52. Wijayatilake DS, Talati C, Panchatsharam S. The monitoring and management of severe traumatic brain injury in the United Kingdom: is there a consensus?: a national survey. J Neurosurg Anesthesiol 2015;27(3):241–5.

53. Korbakis G, Vespa PM. Multimodal neurologic monitoring. Handb Clin Neurol 2017;140:91–105.

54. Le Roux P, Menon DK, Citerio G, et al. Consensus summary statement of the International Multidisciplinary Consensus Conference on Multimodality Monitoring in Neurocritical Care: a statement for healthcare professionals from the Neurocritical Care Society and the European Society of Intensive Care Medicine. Neurocrit Care 2014;21(Suppl. 2):S1–26.

55. Okonkwo DO, Shutter LA, Moore C, et al. Brain oxygen optimization in severe traumatic brain injury phase-II: a phase II randomized trial. Crit Care Med 2017;45(11):1907–14.

56. Saherwala AA, Bader MK, Stutzman SE, et al. Increasing adherence to Brain Trauma Foundation Guidelines for hospital care of patients with traumatic brain injury. Crit Care Nurse 2018;38(1):e11–20.

57. Pinczolits A, Zdunczyk A, Dengler NF, et al. Standard-sampling microdialysis and spreading depolarizations in patients with malignant hemispheric stroke. J Cereb Blood Flow Metab 2017;37(5):1896–905.

58. Carpenter KL, Young AM, Hutchinson PJ. Advanced monitoring in traumatic brain injury: microdialysis. Curr Opin Crit Care 2017;23(2):103–9.

59. Kumar G, Shahripour RB, Harrigan MR. Vasospasm on transcranial Doppler is predictive of delayed cerebral ischemia in aneurysmal subarachnoid hemorrhage: a systematic review and meta-analysis. J Neurosurg 2016;124(5):1257–64.

60. Valdueza JM, Schreiber SJ, Roehl JE, et al. Neurosonology and neuroimaging of stroke: a comprehensive reference. 2nd ed. New York: Thieme; 2017.

61. Herman ST, Abend NS, Bleck TP, et al. Consensus statement on continuous EEG in critically ill adults and children, part II: personnel, technical specifications, and clinical practice. J Clin Neurophysiol 2015;32(2):96–108.

62. Francoeur CL, Mayer SA. Management of delayed cerebral ischemia after subarachnoid hemorrhage. Crit Care 2016;20(1):277.

63. Gollwitzer S, Groemer T, Rampp S, et al. Early prediction of delayed cerebral ischemia in subarachnoid hemorrhage based on quantitative EEG: a prospective study in adults. Clin Neurophysiol 2015;126(8):1514–23.

64. Katyal N, Singh I, Narula N, et al. Continuous electroencephalography (CEEG) in neurological critical care units (NCCU): a review. Clin Neurol Neurosurg 2020;198:106145.

65. Swisher CB, Sinha SR. Utilization of quantitative EEG trends for critical care continuous EEG monitoring: a survey of neurophysiologists. J Clin Neurophysiol 2016;33(6):538–44.

66. Yucel MA, Selb JJ, Huppert TJ, et al. Functional near infrared spectroscopy: enabling routine functional brain imaging. Curr Opin Biomed Eng 2017;4:78–86.

67. Boas DA, Elwell CE, Ferrari M, et al. Twenty years of functional near-infrared spectroscopy: introduction for the special issue. Neuroimage 2014;85(Pt 1):1–5.

68. Mitchell-Hines T, Ellison K, Willis S. Using bispectral index monitoring to gauge depth of sedation/analgesia. Nursing 2016;46(4):60–3.

69. Martini F, Nath JL, Bartholomew EF. Fundamentals of anatomy & physiology. 11th ed. New York: Pearson; 2018.

Chapter 17

Neurological alterations and management

Carolyne Stewart, Elaine McGloin

Learning objectives

After reading this chapter, you should be able to:

- describe alterations in consciousness, and in motor, sensory and autonomic nerve function
- differentiate cerebral hypoxia from cerebral ischaemia, and focal from global ischaemia
- differentiate between primary and secondary brain insults due to brain injury
- describe the characteristics of spinal cord trauma
- explain the characteristics of central nervous system infection and inflammation
- outline neuromuscular disorders that may be present in critically ill patients
- relate the procedures of selected neurodiagnostic tests to nursing implications for patient care
- discuss the rationale for medical and nursing management in the care of the brain-injured patient.

Introduction

Numerous conditions encountered in critical care areas relate to serious neurological dysfunction. While most are associated with critical illness, or are at least well defined, several others occur infrequently and are not addressed extensively in this chapter. The effects of a primary illness frequently obscure the onset of an abrupt neurological complication. For example, a metabolic disorder producing encephalopathy or the use of sedation to allow better synchrony with a mechanical ventilator may delay recognition of an intracerebral haemorrhage. Neurological alterations are generally defined by problems that derive from the acute aspects of diseases such as stroke, brain and spinal cord injury, CNS infections and status epilepticus. This chapter discusses the concepts that underlie neurological abnormalities and addresses current management techniques and modalities.

Neurological dysfunction

This section discusses the concepts of neurological dysfunction including altered levels of consciousness, motor and sensory function, and cerebral metabolism and perfusion.

Alterations in consciousness

Impaired consciousness is often the first sign of a severe pathological process. Consciousness is the recognition of self and the environment, which requires both arousal and awareness. Decreased consciousness can range from mild depression to coma, the most severe form of absolute unconsciousness.

Altered cognition and coma

Coma is a state of unresponsiveness from which the patient, who appears to be asleep, cannot be aroused by verbal and physical stimuli to produce any meaningful response. Therefore, the diagnosis of coma implies the absence of both arousal and consciousness.[1] Coma must be considered a symptom with numerous causes and therefore there are several management strategies to consider. Stupor is a state of unconsciousness from which the patient can be awakened, but produces inadequate responses to verbal and physical stimuli. Somnolence is a state of unconsciousness from which the patient can be fully awakened.

Although there are many specific causes of unconsciousness, the sites of cerebral affection are either the bilateral cerebral cortex or the brainstem reticular activating system. The commonest causes of bilateral cortical disease are deficiencies of oxygen, metabolic disorders, physical injury, toxins, postconvulsive coma and infections.[2] The reticular activating system maintains the state of wakefulness through continuous stimulation of the cortex. Any interruption may lead to unconsciousness. The reticular activating system can be affected in three principal ways: by supratentorial pressure (upper part of the brain), by infratentorial pressure (brainstem or cerebellar) and by intrinsic brainstem lesions. Supratentorial and infratentorial lesions produce impaired consciousness by enlarging and displacing tissue. Lesions that affect the brainstem itself damage the reticular activating system directly.

> **Practice tip**
>
> The first principle of management of a person found unconscious is to maintain their airway.

Recently acquired confusion, severe apathy, stupor or coma implies dysfunction of the cerebral hemispheres, the diencephalon and/or the upper brainstem.[3] Focal lesions in supratentorial structures may damage both hemispheres, or may produce swelling that compresses the diencephalic activating system and midbrain, causing transtentorial

herniation and brainstem damage. Primary infratentorial lesions may compress or directly damage the reticular formation anywhere between the level of the mid-pons and (by upward pressure) the diencephalon. Metabolic or infectious diseases may depress brain functions by a change in blood composition or the presence of a direct toxin. Impaired consciousness may also be due to reduced blood flow (as in syncope or severe heart failure) or a change in the brain's electrical activity (as in epilepsy). Concussion, anxiolytic drugs and anaesthetics impair consciousness without producing detectable structural changes in the brain.

Many of the enzymatic reactions of neurons, glial cells and specialised cerebral capillary endothelium in the brain are catalysed (i.e. accelerated) by the energy-yielding hydrolysis of adenosine triphosphate (ATP) to adenosine diphosphate (ADP) and inorganic phosphate. Without a constant and generous supply of ATP, cellular synthesis slows or stops, neuronal functions decline or cease and cell structures become damaged.[4] The use of lactate for oxidative metabolism becomes prominent when extracellular brain lactate concentration increases to supraphysiological levels, inducing a sparing of cerebral glucose. The brain depends entirely on the process of glycolysis and respiration within its own cells to provide its energy needs. Even short interruptions of blood flow, and thereby of the oxygen and glucose supply, threaten tissue vitality.

Seizures

A seizure is an uninhibited, abrupt discharge of ions from a group of neurons resulting in epileptic activity.[5] The majority of patients experiencing seizures in the ICU do not have pre-existing epilepsy, and their chances of developing epilepsy in the future are usually more dependent on the cause than on the number or intensity of seizures that they experience. However, because of the other deleterious neuronal and systemic effects of seizures, their rapid diagnosis and suppression during a period of critical illness is necessary.

Seizures are classified depending on how they start as: (1) partial or focal seizures, (2) generalised or full-body seizures involving both cerebral hemispheres, or (3) partial seizures with secondary generalisation (for example, the seizure starts focally and ends with bilateral motor activity). Patients may be conscious during a partial seizure, whereas during generalised seizures they are not. As partial seizures may not always progress to tonic–clonic movement or alteration in consciousness, partial seizure represents one of the most elusive diagnoses in neurology and is often misdiagnosed. Patients with partial seizures may describe a pre-epileptic event known as an aura.

Seizures may either prompt the patient's admission to ICU (usually due to status epilepticus) or develop as a complication of another illness.[6] Seizures can be due to vascular, infectious, neoplastic, traumatic, degenerative, metabolic, toxic or idiopathic causes. Factors influencing the development of post-traumatic epilepsy include an early post-traumatic seizure, depressed skull fracture, intracranial haematoma, dural penetration, focal neurological deficit and post-traumatic amnesia over 24 hours with the presence of a skull fracture or haematoma. Seizures in critically ill patients are most commonly due to drug effects; metabolic, infectious or toxic disorders; or intracranial mass lesions, although they may be due to trauma or neoplasm.[7] Conditions producing seizures tend either to increase neuronal excitation or to impair neuronal inhibition. A few generalised disorders (e.g. non-ketotic hyperglycaemia) may produce partial or focal seizures.

Alterations in motor, sensory and autonomic nerve function

Alterations in motor and sensory function include skeletal muscle weakness and paralysis. They result from lesions in the voluntary motor and sensory pathways, including the upper motor and sensory neurons of the corticospinal and corticobulbar tracts, or the lower motor and sensory neurons that leave the central nervous system (CNS) and travel by way of the peripheral nerves to the muscle and sensory receptors.

Muscle tone, which is a necessary component of muscle movement, is a function of the muscle spindle (myotatic) system and the extrapyramidal system, which monitors and buffers input to the lower motor neurons by way of the multisynaptic pathways.[8] Upper motor neuron lesions produce spastic paralysis, and lower motor neuron lesions produce flaccid paralysis. Damage to the upper motor and sensory neurons of the corticospinal, corticobulbar and spinothalamic tracts is a common component of stroke.[9] Polyneuropathies involve multiple peripheral nerves and produce symmetrical sensory, motor and mixed sensorimotor deficits:

- Lesions of the corticospinal and corticobulbar tracts result in weakness or total paralysis of predominantly distal voluntary movement. Babinski's sign (i.e. dorsiflexion of the big toe and fanning of the other toes in response to stroking the outer border of the foot from heel to toe) and spasticity (increased muscle tone and exaggerated deep tendon reflexes) often characterise these lesions.

- Disorders of the basal ganglia (extrapyramidal disorders) do not cause weakness or reflex changes. Their hallmark is involuntary movement (dyskinesia), causing increased movement (hyperkinesias) or decreased movement (hypokinesia) and changes in muscle tone and posture.

- Cerebellar disorders cause abnormalities in the coordination of movement and fine motor skills. Strength is minimally affected.

- Critical illness myopathy and polyneuropathies are the most common causes of neuromuscular weakness in the intensive care setting. Causes include long-term mechanical ventilation, with risks increased by

specific disease processes, female gender and high glucose levels.[10,11] (See Chapter 8 for more information about these conditions.)

Dysfunctions of the autonomic nervous system or autonomic dysreflexia result from failure or imbalance of the sympathetic or parasympathetic components of the autonomic nerve dysfunction, with resultant signs such as: (1) increased (>120/min) or decreased (<50/min) heart rate, (2) increased respiratory rate (>24/min), (3) raised temperature (>38.5°C), (4) increased (>160 mmHg) or decreased (<85 mmHg) systolic blood pressure (BP), (5) increased muscle tone, (6) decerebrate (extensor) or decorticate (flexor) posturing and (7) profuse sweating. For example, in spinal injury the presence of a noxious stimulus can be transmitted from the periphery to the spinal cord and activate a dysfunctional sympathetic response.

Autonomic nervous system dysfunctions reflect the numerous interactions among the CNS, peripheral nervous system (both sympathetic and parasympathetic branches), endocrine system and immune system.[12] Dysfunctions range from alterations in the sympathetic–parasympathetic balance to almost complete cessation of activity, as occurs in spinal cord injury. As the autonomic nervous system controls organ function, dysfunction affects all organs. The immune system is connected to the nervous system through the autonomic nervous system; therefore many patients with infections, systemic inflammatory response and multiorgan failure exhibit autonomic nerve dysfunction. Autonomic nerve dysfunction can be assessed by time and spectral domain heart rate variability.[13]

Alterations in cerebral metabolism and perfusion

Neuronal cell death occurs in both high- and low-oxygenated states during injury. Cerebral metabolism and perfusion are compromised by diverse injury processes and biochemical patterns of ischaemia and mitochondrial dysfunction. These changes commonly occur following a primary brain injury and are therefore termed secondary brain injury processes.[14]

Cerebral ischaemia and mitochondrial dysfunction

Ischaemia results from inadequate delivery of oxygen to and the inadequate removal of carbon dioxide from the cell. This causes an increase in the production of intracellular lactic acid. Ischaemia can be caused by an increase in nutrient utilisation by the brain in a hyperactive state, a decrease in delivery related to either cerebral or systemic complications and/or a mismatch between delivery and demand.[15] The ischaemic cascade is described in Fig. 17.1 and is covered in detail elsewhere.[16] Inflammation together with oxidative stress, excitotoxicity, failure of ionic homeostasis, including disrupted calcium,

FIGURE 17.1 Ischaemic cascade. In cerebral ischaemia, energy failure causes depolarisation of the neuronal membrane, and excitatory neurotransmitters such as glutamate are released together. A marked influx of Ca^{2+} into neurons then occurs, which provokes the enzymatic process leading to irreversible neuronal injury. Inflammation is also a contributing factor in the development of ischaemic damage.

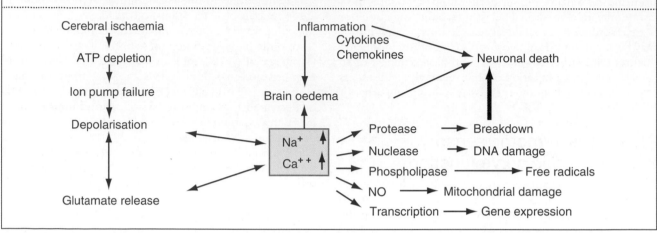

sodium and potassium homeostasis, and energy failure are the key pathological changes in ischaemic brain damage.[17] There is a significant inflammatory response in the ischaemic brain associated with changes in the peripheral immune system. When cerebral blood flow (CBF) falls to about 40% of normal, electroencephalography (EEG) slowing occurs. When CBF falls below 10 mL/100 g/min (i.e. 20%), the function of ionic pumps fails, which leads to membrane depolarisation. Cerebral ischaemia and reperfusion injury contribute to the cascade of physiological events that is termed secondary brain injury.[18]

Mitochondrial dysfunction occurs in the secondary phase of brain injury and is often associated with normal oxygen levels after reperfusion in the brain. Mitochondria are sensitive to the high levels of free glutamate that are the product of injury and reperfusion. Free calcium and nitrous oxide promote excessive production of reactive oxygen species and mitochondrial membrane permeability. Degradation of deoxyribonucleic acid and essential proteins follows and results in neuronal cell death.[18]

Cerebral oedema

Cerebral oedema is defined as increased brain water content. The brain is particularly susceptible to injury from oedema because of its confined space and limitation of expansion. There are no lymphatic pathways within the CNS to carry away the fluid that accumulates. The Monro–Kellie hypothesis states that the contents of the cranium, which is about 80% brain tissue, 10% blood and 10% cerebral spinal fluid (CSF), are incompressible and so an increase in volume in one of the components without a corresponding decrease in another component causes a rise in pressure.[19]

After brain injury, alterations in ionic gradients cause a stepwise progression from cytotoxic to vasogenic oedema.[20] Ischaemia leads to the cessation of primary active transport via the sodium–potassium pump. As a

result, cotransporters (secondary active transport) and passive transporters (via ion channels) attempt to maintain cellular processes.[21] By doing so, neurons and neuroglia accumulate active solutes that cause cellular swelling and eventually passage of fluid into the extracellular space. While the classifications of oedema are useful to define specific treatments, they are somewhat arbitrary, as cytotoxic and vasogenic oedemas often occur concurrently. In fact, each of these processes may cause the other. Ultimately, these changes can lead to raised intracranial pressure (ICP) and herniation.

Cytotoxic oedema, also termed intracellular oedema, is reversible in its early phases. Cellular swelling, usually of astrocytes in the grey matter, generally occurs following a cerebral ischaemia event such as cardiac arrest.[21] The resulting hypoxia or anoxia causes a reduction of the production of ATP, leading to a failure of the sodium–potassium pump and the influx of Na^+ ions into the cell. This in turn increases the intracellular osmolarity, triggering the movement of extracellular water into the cell, so increasing the cell volume. The blood–brain barrier remains intact and capillary permeability is not impaired. However, eventually, endothelial and neuroglial dysfunction impairs the ability to maintain the integrity of the blood–brain barrier and vasogenic oedema ensues.

Vasogenic oedema, sometimes termed extracellular oedema, is caused by increased capillary permeability.[21] Rises in brain water content are often quite dramatic because the fluid that results from increased capillary permeability is usually rich in proteins, resulting in the spread of oedema and brain ischaemia. This can lead to further cytotoxic oedema, and to the progressive breakdown of both astrocytes and neurons.[21]

Interstitial oedema occurs as a result of hydrocephalus, when the pressure within the ventricles is higher than the capacity of the ependymal cells to confine the CSF within the ventricles. The ventricular ependymal lining ruptures, allowing CSF into the extracellular space, most commonly the periventricular white matter. Causes of interstitial oedema include obstructing masses, meningitis, subarachnoid haemorrhage and normal-pressure hydrocephalus.

Hydrocephalus

Hydrocephalus is the result of an imbalance between the formation and drainage and/or reabsorption of CSF. Reduced absorption most often occurs when one or more passages connecting the ventricles become blocked, preventing movement of CSF to its drainage sites in the subarachnoid space just inside the skull. This type of hydrocephalus is called 'non-communicating'. A reduction in the absorption rate called 'communicating hydro-cephalus' can be caused by damage to the arachnoid villi – for example, following a subarachnoid haemorrhage. Both types lead to an elevation of the CSF pressure in the brain. A third type of hydrocephalus, 'normal-pressure hydrocephalus' is marked by ventricle enlargement without an apparent rise in CSF pressure and can be misdiagnosed.[22]

Hydrocephalus may be caused by congenital brain defects, haemorrhage in either the ventricles or the subarachnoid space, CNS infection (syphilis, herpes, meningitis, encephalitis or mumps), cerebral oedema or tumours. Treatment includes ventriculostomy drainage of CSF in the short term or a surgical shunt for those with chronic conditions; either is predisposed to blockage and infection.

> ### Practice tip
>
> The clinical features of idiopathic normal-pressure hydrocephalus are abnormal gait, cognitive impairment and urinary incontinence. In older people, these can be misdiagnosed as dementia.

Intracranial hypertension

The ICP is the pressure exerted by the contents of the brain within the confines of the skull and the blood–brain barrier. It incurs changes to the compensatory reserve and pulse amplitude, as illustrated in Fig. 17.2.[23] Normal ICP

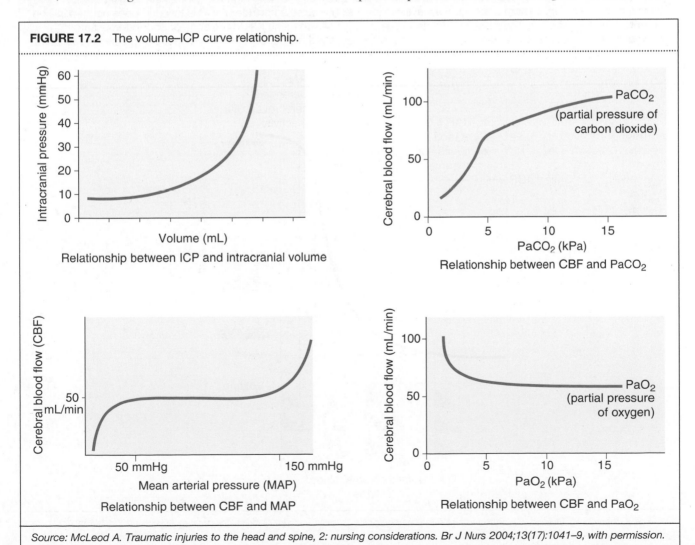

FIGURE 17.2 The volume–ICP curve relationship.

Relationship between ICP and intracranial volume

Relationship between CBF and $PaCO_2$

Relationship between CBF and MAP

Relationship between CBF and PaO_2

Source: McLeod A. Traumatic injuries to the head and spine, 2: nursing considerations. Br J Nurs 2004;13(17):1041–9, with permission.

is 0–10 mmHg. Sustained pressure of >15 mmHg is termed intracranial hypertension, with implications for CBF.[24] Areas of reduced CBF and focal ischaemia appear when the ICP is >20 mmHg, and global ischaemia occurs at >50 mmHg. The ICP waveform contains valuable information about the nature of cerebrospinal pathophysiology. Both autoregulation of CBF and compliance of the cerebrospinal system are reflected in the ICP waveform.[25] Waveform analysis of the ICP is described in Chapter 16.

Initially, intracranial compliance allows compensation for rises in intracranial volume by means of shunting CSF down the thecal sac, increased reabsorption of CSF and vasoconstriction of the cerebral venous vessels reducing the volume of blood within the cranial vault. These mechanisms of autoregulation enable a constant CBF to be maintained over a range of arterial perfusion pressures. During a slow continuous rise in volume, the ICP rises to a plateau level at which the increased level of CSF absorption keeps pace with the rise in volume, with ample compensatory reserve. When these compensatory mechanisms become exhausted, pressure begins to rise and the patient exhibits signs and symptoms of raised ICP. The time taken to overcome these protective processes depends on how quickly the rise of intracranial volume occurs, and is expressed as an index as shown in Fig. 17.3.[26] Intermittent expansion (which in health can be caused by Valsalva manoeuvres such as coughing and straining) causes only a transient rise in ICP at first. When sufficient CSF has been absorbed to accommodate the volume, the ICP returns to normal.

If the ICP rises to the level of arterial pressure, this itself begins to rise, accompanied by bradycardia or other

---

FIGURE 17.3 In a simple model, pulse amplitude of intracranial pressure (ICP) (expressed along the *y*-axis on the right side of the panel) results from pulsatile changes in cerebral blood volume (expressed along the *x*-axis) transformed by the pressure–volume curve. This curve has three zones: a flat zone, expressing good compensatory reserve; an exponential zone, depicting poor compensatory reserve; and a flat zone again, seen at very high ICP (above the 'critical' ICP), depicting derangement of normal cerebrovascular responses. The pulse amplitude of ICP is low and does not depend on mean ICP in the first zone. The pulse amplitude increases linearly with mean ICP in the zone of poor compensatory reserve. In the third zone, the pulse amplitude starts to decrease with rising ICP. RAP = index of compensatory reserve.

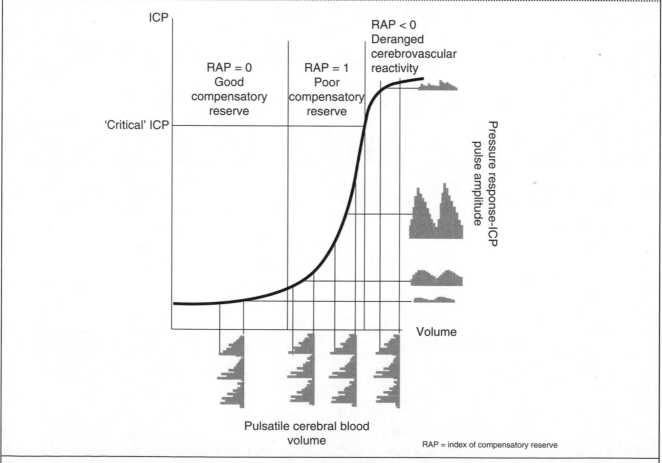

Source: Czosnyka M, Pickard J. Monitoring and interpretation of intracranial pressure. J Neurol Neurosurg Psychiat 2004;75(6):813–21, with permission from BMJ Publishing Group Ltd.

FIGURE 17.4   Injury to the brainstem can result in various abnormal respiratory patterns.

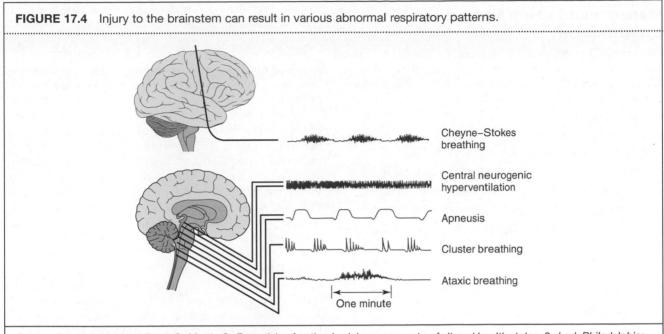

Cheyne–Stokes breathing

Central neurogenic hyperventilation

Apneusis

Cluster breathing

Ataxic breathing

One minute

Source: Reproduced from Porth C, Martin G. Essentials of pathophysiology; concepts of altered health states. 3rd ed. Philadelphia: Lippincott, Williams & Williams 2011 with permission.

disturbances of heart rhythm, termed Cushing's response. Dilation of the small pial arteries and some slowing of venous flow, which is followed by pulsatile venous flow, also occur. The respiratory changes associated with increased ICP depend on the level of brainstem involved. A midbrain involvement results in Cheyne–Stokes respiration. When the midbrain and pons are involved, there is sustained hyperventilation. There are rapid and shallow respirations with upper medulla involvement, with ataxic breathing in the final stages (Fig. 17.4).[27] Neurogenic pulmonary oedema may also occur because of increased sympathetic activity due to the effects of an elevated ICP on the hypothalamus, medulla or cervical spinal cord.

The causes of intracranial hypertension are classified as acute or chronic. Acute causes include brain trauma, ischaemic injury and intracerebral haemorrhage. Infections such as encephalitis or meningitis may also lead to intracranial hypertension. Chronic causes include many intracranial tumours, such as ependymomas, or hydrocephalus that may gradually impinge on CSF pathways and interfere with CSF outflow and circulation. As the ICP continues to increase, the brain tissue becomes distorted, leading to herniation and additional vascular injury.[28]

Neurological therapeutic management

This section explores the management of cerebral perfusion. The objective is to identify deficits in perfusion, allowing the initiation of strategies aimed at preventing secondary insults and further ischaemia. The modalities of

neuroprotection, including the management of intracranial hypertension and cerebral ischaemia, are discussed below and nursing interventions based on published guidelines for the prevention of secondary insults and promotion of cerebral perfusion are considered.

Optimising cerebral perfusion

Intracranial hypertension and cerebral ischaemia are the two most important secondary injury processes that can be anticipated, monitored and treated in the ICU. This applies to all aetiologies of brain injury including trauma. Advanced cerebral-monitoring techniques are described in Chapter 16. Episodes of brain hypoxia are common and may occur even when ICP and cerebral perfusion pressure (CPP) are normal, emphasising the value of multimodal monitoring that integrates data from several physiological monitors.[29] These observations can help clinicians to better understand the complex pathophysiology of the brain after an acute insult, evaluate autoregulation and identify optimal physiological targets and the utility of therapeutic interventions. The selection of oxygenation monitoring focuses on the appropriateness of focal or global monitoring, the location of the monitor in relation to the injury and the intermittent or continuous nature of the monitoring device.

Practice tip

Cerebral perfusion pressure (CPP) = mean arterial pressure (MAP) − ICP. So, if ICP is increased, MAP must also be increased to maintain CPP.

Management of intracranial hypertension

Intracranial hypertension is treated by removing mass lesions and/or increasing the space available for expansion of injured tissue.[30] This may be achieved by reducing one of the other available intracranial fluid volumes such as:

- CSF via ventricular drainage
- cerebral blood volume by osmotic diuretic therapy, hypothermia or hyperventilation
- brain tissue water content by osmotic diuretic therapy
- removing swollen and irreversibly injured brain
- increasing cranial capacity by decompressive craniectomy.

The application of these concepts to the following therapeutic strategies is important in the management of intracranial hypertension.[30]

Practice tip

In brain injury, position the patient at 30 degrees head-up to maximise cerebral perfusion and minimise cerebral oedema.

External ventricular drainage

External ventricular drains allow both the monitoring of ICP levels and the drainage of CSF. The use of continuous versus intermittent drainage systems remains variable, with little evidence to guide practice in the adult population. Open systems where drainage is continuous risk sudden drops in ICP, which can be life threatening, while also allowing only for intermittent ICP monitoring. In contrast, closed systems where ICP is continuously monitored have to be intermittently opened to allow for CSF drainage. The Brain Trauma Foundation guidelines recommend a continuous drainage system zeroed at the level of the midbrain, based on moderate levels of evidence.[31] Both systems carry a high risk of infection.

Ventilation therapies

Hyperventilation reduces $PaCO_2$. It will reduce ICP by vasoconstriction induced by alkalosis, but it also decreases CBF. The fall in ICP parallels the fall in cerebral blood volume. Hyperventilation decreases regional blood flow to hypoperfused areas of the brain. Therefore, generally $PaCO_2$ should be maintained in the low-normal range of about 35–45 mmHg (4.6–6 kPa). Hyperventilation should be utilised only when ICP elevations are refractory to other treatments and when brain tissue oxygenation is in the normal range.[31] The Brain Trauma Foundation Guidelines recommend hyperventilation therapy be used as only a temporary measure to treat a critically elevated ICP, which is refractory to other therapies, and with cerebral oxygen monitoring to allow measurement of oxygen delivery levels. The Brain Trauma Foundation also recommends that it should be avoided during the acute phase (i.e. 24 hours) following initial injury.[31]

Osmotherapy

Acute administration of an osmotic such as mannitol or hypertonic saline produces a potent anti-oedema action, primarily on undamaged brain regions with an intact blood–brain barrier. This treatment causes the movement of water from the interstitial and extracellular space into the intravascular compartment, thereby improving intracranial compliance or elastance. In addition to causing 'dehydration' of the brain, osmotic agents have been shown to exert beneficial non-osmotic cerebral effects, such as augmentation of CBF (by reducing blood viscosity, resulting in enhanced oxygen delivery), free radical scavenging and diminishing CSF formation and enhancing CSF reabsorption.[32]

A 2020 Cochrane review[33] showed there is insufficient evidence available to recommend one type of hyperosmolar agent over another, and the Brain Trauma Foundation acknowledges the increasing use of hypertonic saline.[31] Both intravenous hypertonic saline (3%) and 20% mannitol can help reduce ICP and maintain haemodynamic status. However, mannitol also has a diuretic effect, which is relatively contraindicated in patients with both traumatic brain injury (TBI) and hypovolaemia as it may worsen intravascular volume depletion and decrease cerebral perfusion.[31] A systematic review and meta-analysis found no mortality benefit or effect on controlling ICP with the use of hypertonic saline compared with other solutions.[34]

Targeted temperature management

Targeted temperature management may be used to prevent fever, to maintain normothermia or to reduce core temperature. Hyperthermia is common in brain-injured patients and is independently associated with increased morbidity and mortality, partly because of its effects on ICP. Temperature elevations as small as 1–2°C above normal can aggravate ischaemic neuronal injury and exacerbate cerebral oedema.[35]

ICP falls significantly at brain temperatures below 37°C and CPP peaks at 35–36°C. However, at temperatures below 35°C both oxygen delivery and oxygen consumption decrease. Cardiac output also decreases progressively with hypothermia.[36] Temperatures lower than 34°C substantially increase the volume of intravenous (IV) fluid infusion and inotrope requirements to maintain an adequate mean arterial pressure, and at 31°C the serum potassium, white blood cell count and platelet counts are diminished.[37] Therefore, normothermia should be the standard of care.

In some patients (e.g. those following cardiac arrest or with a TBI), lower target temperatures may be used to reduce intracranial hypertension and maintain sufficient CPP.[38] The target temperature may differ according to the situation. For example, some international guidelines recommend cooling patients post-cardiac arrest to

32–36°C.[39–41] In contrast, the 2017 French guidelines recommend maintaining a target temperature of 35–37°C in severe TBI, lowered to 34–35°C for those with refractory hypertension.[39] They further suggest considering targeted temperature management at 32–35°C in patients with refractory status epilepticus. However, in the trial TTM2 examining optimal temperature for out-of-hospital cardiac arrest patients, targeted hypothermia did not lead to lower mortality rates in comparison with aiming for normothermia.[33]

The optimal length of time or the best method by which to actively cool someone remains unknown, although some studies suggest longer-term cooling for up to 5 days may be most beneficial.[42] Active cooling may be initiated using paracetamol, cooling blankets, evaporative cooling and other innovative cooling technologies. Care should be taken to avoid complications such as hypokalaemia and hyperaemia (increased blood flow), which may occur during rewarming, resulting in dysrhythmias, acute brain swelling and rebound intracranial hypertension.[42] It is also important to avoid shivering, which can be counterproductive. Canadian guidelines recommend a continuous method of temperature assessment, such as oesophageal monitoring.[39]

Corticosteroids

Excessive inflammation has been implicated in the progressive neurodegeneration that occurs in multiple neurological diseases, including cerebral ischaemia. The efficacy of glucocorticoids is well established in ameliorating oedema associated with brain tumours and in improving the outcome in subsets of patients with bacterial meningitis. Despite encouraging experimental results, clinical trials of glucocorticoids in ischaemic stroke, intracerebral haemorrhage, aneurysmal subarachnoid haemorrhage (aSAH) and TBI have not shown a definite therapeutic effect. Furthermore, the CRASH (corticosteroid randomisation after significant head injury) trial reported that risk of death was higher in the treatment group than in the control group.[43] Therefore, high-dose steroids are not indicated for use in TBI. However, anterior pituitary insufficiency is an underrecognised problem in patients with severe TBI, particularly in elderly people or those who have diffuse axonal injury and skull base fracture. In these instances, administration of hydrocortisone in physiological doses and endocrine follow-up are indicated.[44]

Sedatives and analgesics

Appropriate use of sedatives and analgesics can help reduce ICP. They cause a reduction in cerebral blood volume and, therefore, in ICP. They also reduce pain and agitation, which may cause arterial hypertension and an associated increase in ICP. The choice of drug (or combination of drugs) often depends on local protocols and practice. However, for patients with severe intracranial hypertension, the Brain Trauma Foundation guidelines recommend either propofol or barbiturates for first-line management.[31]

Barbiturates exert cerebral protective and ICP-lowering effects through alteration in vascular tone, suppression of metabolism and inhibition of free radical-mediated lipid peroxidation. Barbiturates may effectively lower CBF and regional metabolic demands, which in turn decrease CBF and cerebral volume. This results in beneficial effects on ICP and global cerebral perfusion. However, barbiturates can cause significant hypotension and should be used only to control elevations in ICP which are refractory to other interventions once haemodynamic stability has been achieved.[31]

Propofol has a rapid onset and short duration of action and is commonly used to help lower ICP. At higher doses (>5 mg/kg/h), it can also induce EEG burst suppression, which can effectively treat status epilepticus.[45] However, there is no evidence that it improves mortality or 6-month outcomes and high doses are associated with significant adverse effects, including hypotension. Many other commonly used sedatives, analgesics and anaesthetic agents can also induce hypotension, potentially reducing CPP and increasing ICP. Careful bedside monitoring and titration is therefore required. The use of vasoactive medication may also be required to offset the effects of the sedatives and analgesics.

Surgical interventions

The European TBI guidelines suggest that operative management be considered for large intracerebral lesions within the first 4 hours of injury. The use of unilateral craniectomy after the evacuation of a mass lesion, such as an acute subdural haematoma or traumatic intracerebral haematoma, is accepted practice. Surgery is also recommended for open, compound depressed skull fractures that cause a mass effect.[46] Mass effect on computerised tomography (CT) scan is defined as distortion, compression and/or displacement of intracranial contents, dislocation or obliteration of the fourth ventricle, compression or loss of visualisation of the basal cisterns or the presence of obstructive hydrocephalus.

Decompressive craniectomy (removal of a portion of the skull) for refractory intracranial hypertension has been performed since 1977, with a significant reduction in ICP for both TBI[45] and ischaemic stroke.[47] However, in 2011 a multicentre trial of early decompressive craniectomy in patients with severe TBI (the DECRA trial) reported that, although an early bifrontotemporoparietal decompressive craniectomy in adults with severe diffuse TBI and refractory intracranial hypertension decreased ICP and length of stay in the ICU, it was associated with more-unfavourable outcomes at both 6 and 12 months.[48] The subsequent randomised evaluation of surgery with craniectomy for uncontrollable elevation of ICP (RESCUEicp) trial[49] used a higher threshold for intervention than did the DECRA trial, and included patients with mass lesions and unilateral or bilateral decompressive craniectomy. Nevertheless, conclusions remain the same and indicate that, while decompressive craniectomy lowers mortality, survivors have poorer functional outcomes than those treated conservatively.

Fundamental nursing care considerations

Nurses should consider the impact of the environment and interventions on a patient's ICP and take proactive steps to avoid unnecessary rises, while promptly recognising and treating any increases that do occur, as described in Table 17.1. Clustering of care activities can produce a cumulative and resistant effect on ICP, which can be difficult to return to baseline, resulting in decreased CPP. ICP monitoring allows the clinician to assess the effect of interventions on a patient's ICP and CPP and to individualise care. In the case of uncontrollable ICP rises, non-essential interventions should be terminated and the

---

TABLE 17.1

Nursing interventions for the brain-injured patient with intracranial hypertension

AIM	GOAL	INTERVENTIONS
Maintain adequate oxygenation and ventilation.	PaO_2 100 mmHg (13.3 kPa) $PaCO_2$ 35–40 mmHg (4.6–5.3 kPa) PaO_2/FiO_2 ratio >350 SaO_2 98% SjO_2 50–75% $PbtO_2$ >20 Airway patent Lungs clear on auscultation Prevention of ventilator-associated pneumonia (VAP)	• Maintain airway – will require intubation for Glasgow Coma Scale score <8 or diaphragmatic respiratory insufficiency. • Assess bilateral chest movement: listen for airway obstruction or ET cuff leak; auscultate for air entry. • Assess chest X-ray. • Consider preoxygenation prior to suction/repositioning/other interventions. • Obtain ABG and manipulate set FiO_2 and ventilator settings to meet parameter goals. • Monitor end-tidal CO_2 continuously. • Be aware of the impact of increasing levels of PEEP on ICP levels. Chest physiotherapy and suction patient as needed. • Use frequent subglottal suctioning, and maintain head of bed elevation at 30 degrees or more to prevent aspiration. • In recovery: assess for upper airway weakness and reflex (prevent aspiration), sputum retention and atelectasis.
Maintain haemodynamic stability and CBF.	MAP: ≥90 mmHg Stroke: thrombolytic, embolic and ICH, MAP 90–120 mmHg $PbtO_2$ <20 CVP 5–10 mmHg CPP 60–70 mmHg Haematocrit 33% or haemoglobin content 80–100 g/L	• Maintain euvolaemia. • Give prescribed intravenous fluids (avoiding dextrose solutions) as prescribed to maintain CVP and PCWP within parameters. • Use noradrenaline (norepinephrine) once euvolaemic in order to optimise MAP. • Observe $PbtO_2$ for sedation-induced hypotension. • Transfuse with red blood cells as appropriate. • Monitor BP, CVP and other haemodynamic parameters. • Monitor closely for signs and symptoms of neurogenic pulmonary oedema, especially in patients with cardiac history. • Transcranial Doppler image to check for vasospasm. • Non-traumatic aSAH, administer IV nimodipine infusion to prevent vasospasm as prescribed; consider components of HH therapy. • Ischaemic stroke, administer tPA within 3 h of event. • ICH, prevent rebleeding; administer prescribed haemostatic medications, reduce hypertension.
Maintain ICP and CPP within target range.	ICP <20 mmHg CPP 50–70 mmHg	• Elevate head of bed above the level of the heart to obtain optimal level of ICP and CPP. Monitor ICP, CPP and $PbtO_2$ to ensure optimal level for your patient (15–30 degrees). • Avoid Trendelenburg position, extreme hip flexion and lateral flexion of neck. • Position body with neck straight and no knee elevation in order to maintain venous outflow. • If patient has a ventriculostomy, drain per prescription. • Individualise care to control ICP; terminate non-essential interventions if ICP rises above set parameters. • Administer prescribed hypertonic saline or mannitol infusions. • Consider paralytics if positioning, cooling, sedation and mannitol does not resolve increased ICP. • Prepare for surgical craniotomy if indicated. • Drainage of CSF via EVD.

TABLE 17.1

Nursing interventions for the brain-injured patient with intracranial hypertension—cont'd

AIM	GOAL	INTERVENTIONS
Maintain normothermia.	Core temperature 35–37°C	• Continuous monitoring of temperature, e.g. via oesophageal monitoring or indwelling urinary catheter. • Administration of paracetamol. • Instigate the use of cooling blankets or other devices as necessary. • Avoid shivering of the patient as this can increase ICP.
Maintain environment/ reduce stimulation.	A calm and stress-free environment	• Group necessary interventions in a timely manner to allow adequate rest. • Limit noxious stimuli; minimise noise and lighting. • Avoid overstimulation and limit interventions if ICP is precarious. • Assess the need for and administer analgesia and sedation (e.g. propofol, morphine, fentanyl, lorazepam/midazolam) as prescribed. • Speak to patient using their name and explain procedures even if unconscious. • Sensitively manage visitors remembering the importance of contact with family and friends.
Maintain nutrition.		• Promote early enteric feeding. • Oral enteric feeding tube (nasogastric contradicted in TBI). • Dietitian referral for metabolic requirements.
Essential care.	Patient integument maintained and infection free: skin, mucous membranes, cornea, wounds, invasive lines. Patient safety enabled, preventing nosocomial infection, secondary brain injury, self-harm.	• Head-to-toe assessment of skin integrity, corneas, mucous membranes. • Provide regular eye, oral and hair care. • Instigate a bowel care protocol to avoid constipation. • Deep vein thrombosis prevention as appropriate to patient's condition. • Ensure ETT ties are secure but not too tight, which can impede intracranial venous outflow and lead to raised ICP. • Consider the use of alternative ETT securement, such as taped to the face, when ICP is refractory to treatment. • Regular repositioning for pressure area care and chest management. • Consider a pressure-relieving mattress. • Consider need for kinetic therapy, e.g. rotation/percussion therapy bed (within spinal precautions where necessary). • Maintain infection control interventions and closely monitor for infection related to invasive devices and wounds. • Use of chemical and physical restraint after assessment and prescription, within institutional policy. • Ensure effective verbal and written communication with other health professionals.
Psychological/ family.	Family and significant others informed and supported. Psychological well-being of patient maintained The patient feels safe.	• Refer and coordinate information and service provision from other health professionals. • The provision of quality, informed and inclusive care to the patient provides family and significant others with the confidence that the nurse advocates for the patient in their place. • Ensure psychological assessment and administer prescribed therapy for delirium and post-traumatic stress. • Nursing interventions planned to allow for rest and recovery. • Administer coordinated rehabilitation strategies.

ABG = arterial blood gas; aSAH = aneurysmal subarachnoid haemorrhage; BP = blood pressure; CBF = cerebral blood flow; CPP = cerebral perfusion pressure; CVP = central venous pressure; ET = endotracheal; ETCO$_2$ = end-tidal carbon dioxide; ETT = endotracheal tube; FiO$_2$ = fraction of inspired oxygen; HH = hypervolaemic hypertensive; ICH = intracerebral haemorrhage; ICP = intracranial pressure; IV = intravenous; MAP = mean arterial pressure; PaCO$_2$ = partial pressure of alveolar carbon dioxide; PaO$_2$ = partial pressure of alveolar oxygen; PbtO$_2$ = brain tissue oxygenation; PCWP = pulmonary capillary wedge pressure; PEEP = positive end-expiratory pressure; SaO$_2$ = arterial oxygen saturation; SjO$_2$ = jugular venous oxygen saturation; TBI = traumatic brain injury; tPa = tissue plasminogen activator; VAP = ventilator-associated pneumonia

ICP allowed to return to baseline. Care should be taken to limit noxious stimuli, such as environmental noise and pain, as these can increase ICP and to administer adequate sedation and analgesia to keep the patient calm and pain free. Even though a patient may not be able to respond, nurses should always assume they can hear and understand, addressing them by name and explaining all procedures. Adapting the environment, for example by dimming lights, and giving consideration to family visitation and its effects on a patient's ICP should be made.

Maintaining head position at 30 degrees facilitates cerebral venous drainage while having no adverse effects on CPP, although the results of a trial comparing acute stroke patients nursed flat with those nursed at a minimum of 30 degrees head-up did not show any difference in disability outcomes.[50] Extreme hip flexion, the Trendelenburg position and lateral flexion of the neck should, however, be avoided as these positions increase intrathoracic pressure and hence ICP.[51] Chest physiotherapy and suctioning are important as they improve gas exchange, helping to maintain CPP, but they also increase ICP.[52]

A head-to-toe skin assessment should be carried out every shift. The use of a pressure-relieving mattress should be considered, although, for patients who have either a confirmed or suspected spinal injury, the use of an alternating pressure air mattress is contraindicated as the neutral alignment of the spinal column cannot be guaranteed. Deep vein thrombosis prevention should also be in place, noting that the use of graduated compression stockings may be contraindicated in some patients (e.g. following stroke). Hygiene interventions should include regular oral, eye and hair care and a bowel regimen to avoid constipation, which can increase intra-abdominal pressure and ICP.[51] These essential nursing cares and others are described in Chapter 5. Regular repositioning of nasogastric and endotracheal tubes will help to prevent the development of pressure injury, which could be a source of pain and hence increase ICP. Care should also be taken to avoid overtightening endotracheal tubes, which can restrict venous drainage.

Central nervous system disorders

CNS disorders include brain and/or spinal injury from trauma, infection or immune conditions. The pathophysiology and aetiology of these disorders are discussed here, including management of these conditions.

Traumatic brain injury (TBI)

TBI has replaced the former term 'head injury' and is defined as an alteration in brain function, or other evidence of brain pathology, caused by an external force, which can affect the scalp, skull or brain.[53] The range of severity of TBI is broad, from concussion through to post-coma unresponsiveness. The incidence of TBI is increasing worldwide, though estimates vary considerably between countries.[53,54] Reviewers of the global literature agree that the incidence of TBI is highest in countries of low to middle income; in males and in those aged 15–25 years. Rates in older populations (over 65 years) are also increasing. Outcome data from long-term follow-up of TBI cohorts support that physical and neuropsychological difficulties are common; it is estimated that there are at least 13 million people living with TBI-related disability in the USA and the European Union.[53]

Aetiology

Falls are the leading cause of TBI (35.2%), followed by being struck by/against an object and motor vehicle collisions or traffic accidents.[54,55] However, road traffic accidents and gunshot wounds to the head lead to the most TBI fatalities. In contrast, sporting accidents and falls account for a far greater percentage of mild injuries. Infants and toddlers up to 4 years of age, older adolescents aged 15–19 years and adults older than 65 years of age are the highest-risk age groups for TBI.[56] This trimodal distribution has been demonstrated for most ethnic and racial groups studied, as well as in global studies of TBI. Most studies have found that the highest age-specific incidence is in the young adult years. Injury and debility in this age group also carry significant morbidity, with many more years of potential life lost and lost productivity for injuries incurred in young people. For every age group studied, males are more likely to suffer TBI than females. Among young people, males are up to seven times more likely to suffer a TBI. People of colour and those of lower socioeconomic strata also suffer rates of TBI 30–50% higher than the majority of individuals. Alcohol is involved in 50% of cases of TBI, because of intoxicated drivers or pedestrians, increased risk of falls, suicide attempts or interpersonal violence.[56–58]

The transfer of energy to the brain tissue causes the damage and is a significant determinant in the severity of injury. The introduction of safer car designs, the mandatory use of seatbelts, airbags and other road traffic initiatives (e.g. redesigning hazardous intersections, driver education campaigns, random breath testing and reducing speed limits) has decreased the overall number of road fatalities; improvements in retrieval, neurosurgery and intensive care in the past few decades have enabled many people to survive injuries that would previously have been fatal.

Pathophysiology

TBI is a heterogeneous pathophysiological process (Fig. 17.5). The mechanisms of injury forces inflicted on the head produce a complex mixture of diffuse and focal lesions within the brain.[59] Damage resulting from an injury can be immediate (primary) or secondary in nature. Secondary injury results from disordered autoregulation and other pathophysiological changes within the brain in the days immediately after injury. Urgent neurosurgical intervention for intracerebral, subdural or extradural haemorrhage can mitigate the extent of secondary injury.

FIGURE 17.5 Pathophysiology of traumatic brain injury.

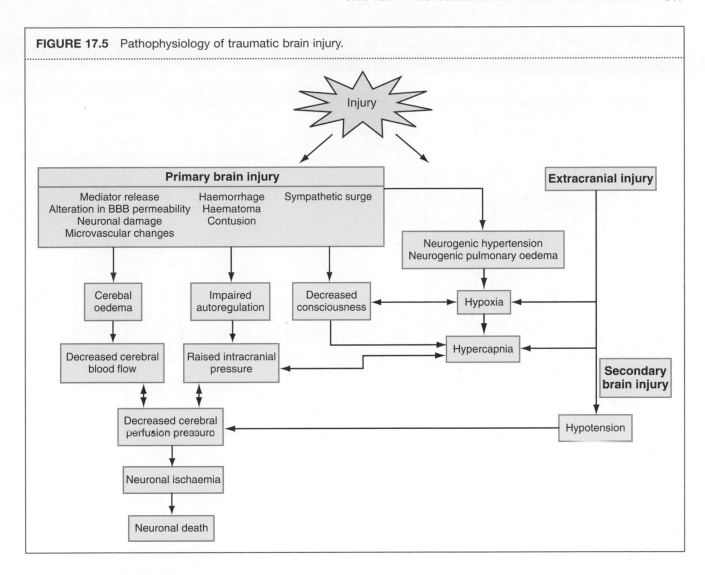

Scalp lesions can bleed profusely and quickly lead to hypovolaemic shock and brain ischaemia. Cerebral oedema, haemorrhage and biochemical response to injury, infection and increased ICP are among the commonest physiological responses that can cause secondary injury. Tissue hypoxia is also of major concern and airway obstruction immediately after injury contributes significantly to secondary injury. Poor CBF, due to direct (primary) vascular changes or damage, can lead to ischaemic brain tissue and eventually neuronal cell death.[60] Systemic changes in temperature, haemodynamics and pulmonary status can also lead to secondary brain injury (Fig. 17.6). In moderate-to-severe and occasionally in mild injury, CBF is altered in the initial 2–3 days, followed by a rebound hyperaemic stage (days 4–7), leading to a precarious state (days 8–14) of cerebral vessel unpredictability and vasospasm.[61] More than 30% of TBI patients have autonomic nerve dysfunction characterised by episodes of increased heart rate, respiratory rate, temperature, BP, muscle tone, decorticate or decerebrate posturing and profuse sweating.[62] Lack of insight into these processes and implementing early weaning of supportive therapies can lead to significant secondary insults.

Classification

Mild TBI is usually defined as when someone has a Glasgow Coma Scale (GCS) score of 13 to 15. It often presents as a component of multitrauma or sports injury and can be overlooked at the expense of other peripheral injuries.[63] Clinical symptoms such as dizziness, confusion, post-traumatic amnesia, nausea and vomiting which persist at 4 hours post-injury require continued observation. Routine head CT is recommended to exclude mass lesions and diffuse axonal injury. Moderate TBI presents with a GCS of 9–12. Patients will require an early CT scan and should be admitted to hospital for at least 24 hours for close observation. A GCS of 8 or less is considered a severe TBI requiring resuscitation, early intubation to prevent hypoxaemia and early CT scan to guide management.

FIGURE 17.6 Conceptual changes in cerebral blood flow (CBF) and intracranial pressure (ICP) over time following traumatic brain injury: (**A**) cytotoxic oedema; (**B**) vasogenic oedema; (**C**) CBF. CPP = cerebral perfusion pressure; MAP = mean arterial pressure.

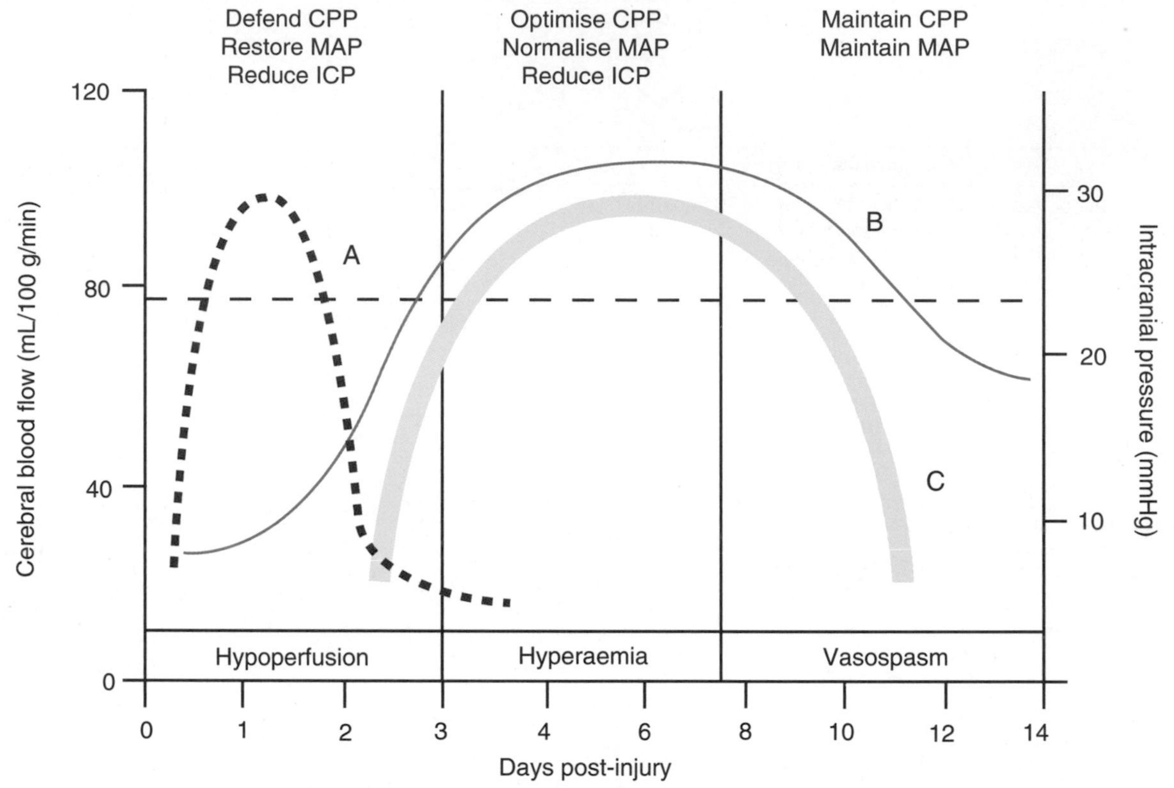

Primary versus secondary injury

Brain injury associated with TBI can be divided into primary and secondary injury. Primary injury is the damage that occurs at the time of the trauma and is a result of mechanical forces being applied to the brain tissue. The mechanisms of injury are contact (coup), acceleration–deceleration (contrecoup) and rotational acceleration–deceleration (diffuse axonal), which result in shearing, compression and stretching (tensile) of the structures of the brain. Secondary injury is the damage occurring after the primary impact and, unlike primary injury, can be prevented and treated. The mechanisms of secondary injury include an inflammatory cascade response, neurotoxicity due to the release of glutamate, and electrolyte imbalances caused by the breakdown of the sodium–potassium pump. Hypoxia, hypotension, intracranial hypertension and changes to CBF will further exacerbate secondary injury. Careful monitoring of the patient is required to reduce or prevent the incidence of secondary injury.

Focal injury

Because of the shape of the inner surface of the skull, focal injuries are most commonly seen in the frontal and temporal lobes, but they can occur anywhere. Contact phenomena or a local blow to the head, or the head coming into contact with another item with force, are commonly superficial and can generate contusional haemorrhages through coup and contrecoup mechanisms.[63] Cerebral contusions are readily identifiable on CT scans, but may become visible on CT only on days 2 or 3. Deep intracerebral haemorrhages can result from either focal or diffuse damage to the arteries.

Diffuse injury

Diffuse (axonal) injury refers to the shearing of axons and supporting neuroglia; it may also traumatise blood vessels and can cause petechial haemorrhages, deep intracerebral haematomas and brain swelling.[63] Diffuse injury results from the shaking, shearing and inertial effects of a traumatic impact, as often seen in high-speed motor vehicle accidents. Mechanical damage to small venules as part of the blood–brain barrier can also trigger formation of haemorrhagic contusions. This vascular damage may increase neuronal vulnerability, causing post-traumatising perfusion deficits and the extravasation of potentially neurotoxic blood-borne substances. The most consistent effect of diffuse brain damage, even when mild, is the presence of altered consciousness. The depth and duration of coma provide the best guide to the severity of the

FIGURE 17.7 Extradural haematoma and a subtle subdural haematoma (**left**), subdural haematoma (**middle left**), diffuse axonal injury (**middle right**) and combination injuries (**right**).

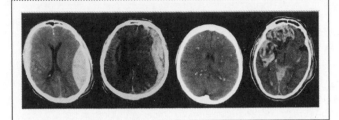

diffuse damage. The majority of patients with diffuse injury will not have any CT evidence to support the diagnosis. Other clinical markers of diffuse injury include the high speed or force strength of injury, absence of a lucid interval, and prolonged retrograde and anterograde amnesia. Fig. 17.7 contrasts CT scans with haematoma formation and diffuse axonal injury.

Skull fractures

Skull fractures are present on CT scans in about two-thirds of patients after TBI. Skull fractures can be linear, depressed or diastatic, and may involve the cranial vault or skull base. In depressed skull fractures the bone fragment may cause a laceration of the dura mater, resulting in a cerebrospinal fluid leak, or become embedded in the parenchyma, requiring surgery to elevate or remove the bone fragment.[63] Basal skull fractures include fractures of the cribriform plate, frontal, sphenoid, temporal and occipital bones. The clinical signs of a basal skull fracture may include: CSF otorrhoea or rhinorrhoea, haemotympanum or presence of blood in the tympanic cavity of the middle ear, postauricular ecchymoses, periorbital ecchymoses and injury to the cranial nerves – VII (weakness of the face), VIII (loss of hearing), I (loss of smell), II (vision loss) and VI (double vision). As it contains glucose, CSF leaks from the nose and ears can also be detected by using a glucometer.

Patient management

The surveillance and prevention of secondary injury is the key to improving morbidity and mortality outcomes in patients with TBI. Interventions are targeted at maintaining adequate CBF and minimising oxygen consumption by the brain in order to prevent ischaemia. The anticipation and prevention of systemic complications are also crucial.

Nursing management of the neurologically impaired, immobilised, mechanically ventilated patient is described in Table 17.1 and is an adaptation of the current guidelines[31] (Table 17.2) to clinical practice (see Online resources for TBI-related protocols). In all TBI multitrauma patients, disability and exposure/environmental control assessment includes further investigations with complete CT scans. Until spinal injury is definitively excluded, TBI management should also include spinal precautions.

Spinal cord trauma

Traumatic spinal cord injury (SCI) is estimated to have a global-incidence rate of 23 cases per million of the population.[64,65] This translates to almost 180,000 cases per year. Traffic-related accidents are the leading cause of traumatic SCI in developed countries, accounting for one-third to one-half of cases.[66] Falls are the next most common cause, with rates increasing in the elderly in particular. In developing countries, traumatic SCI is most often caused by falls at home or in the workplace, with rates as high as 63%.[67] The highest proportion of violence-related traumatic SCI occurs in areas of armed conflict or high availability of weapons. Recreational injuries occur most often with snowboarding, rugby and diving accidents. A systematic review of 13 studies from around the world indicated that in most regions there are peak rates of traumatic SCI in young adults (15–29 years) and that in older age groups the incidence rate increased steadily with increasing age.[68] A predominance of males is also evident.

Of all SCI cases, 51% result in complete tetraplegia (loss of function in the arms, legs, trunk and pelvic organs). The predominant risk factors for SCI include age, gender and alcohol and drug use.[67] The vertebrae most often involved in SCI are the 5th, 6th and 7th cervical (neck), the 12th thoracic and the 1st lumbar. These vertebrae are the most susceptible because there is a greater range of mobility in the vertebral column in these areas. Damage to the spinal cord ranges from transient concussion or stunning (from which the patient fully recovers), through contusion, laceration and compression of the cord substance (either alone or in combination), to complete transection of the cord (which renders the patient paralysed below the level of the injury).[67]

Mechanisms of injury

Cervical injury can occur from both blunt and penetrating trauma but in reality is a combination of different mechanisms of acceleration and deceleration, with or without rotational forces and axial loading.[67] An illustrative example is a diving injury caused by a direct load through the head and cervical spine. Cervical trauma is produced by a combination of the mechanisms listed below:

- *Hyperflexion:* usually results from forceful deceleration and often seen in patients who have sustained trauma from a head–on motor vehicle collision or diving accident. The cervical region is most often involved, especially at the C5–C6 level.

- *Vertical compression or axial loading:* typically occurs when a person lands on the feet or buttocks after falling or jumping from a height. The vertebral column is compressed, causing a fracture resulting in damage to the spinal cord.

- *Hyperextension:* is the most common type of injury. Hyperextension injuries can be caused by a fall, a rear-end motor vehicle collision or hit on the head (e.g. during a boxing match). Hyperextension of the

TABLE 17.2

Summary of Brain Trauma Foundation guidelines of the management of severe traumatic brain injury[29]

ITEM	LEVEL I EVIDENCE	LEVEL II EVIDENCE	LEVEL III EVIDENCE
BP and oxygenation	None.	BP should be monitored and hypotension (SBP <90 mmHg) avoided.	Oxygenation should be monitored and hypoxia (PaO$_2$ <60 mmHg/8 kPa or O$_2$ saturation <90%) avoided.
Hyperosmolar therapy	None.	Mannitol is effective for control of raised ICP at doses of 0.25 g/kg to 1 g/kg body weight. Arterial hypotension (SBP <90 mmHg) should be avoided. Hypertonic saline evidence is limited on the use, concentration and method of administration for the treatment of traumatic intracranial hypertension.	Restrict mannitol use prior to ICP monitoring to patients with signs of transtentorial herniation or progressive neurological deterioration not attributable to extracranial causes.
Prophylactic hypothermia	Insufficient data.	Insufficient data.	Prophylactic hypothermia is not significantly associated with decreased mortality. Prophylactic hypothermia is associated with significant higher Glasgow Outcome Scale scores.
Infection prophylaxis	Insufficient data.	Periprocedural antibiotics for intubation should be administered to reduce the incidence of pneumonia – but does not change length of stay or mortality. Early tracheostomy – reduces mechanical ventilation days.	Routine ventricular catheter or prophylactic antibiotic use for ventricular catheter placement is not recommended to reduce infection. Early extubation in qualified patients, without increased risk of pneumonia.
Deep vein thrombosis prophylaxis	Insufficient data.	Insufficient data.	Graduated compression stockings or intermittent pneumatic compression stockings until ambulatory. Low-molecular-weight heparin or low unfractionated heparin in combination with above. Risk of expansion of intracranial haemorrhage.
Indications for ICP monitoring	Insufficient data.	ICP monitoring recommended for patients with GCS score of 3–8 with abnormal CT.	Normal CT with two or more of the following: • Age 40+ years • Motor posturing • SBP <90 mmHg • GCS score 9–15 with abnormal CT at prescription discretion.
ICP monitoring technology	Insufficient data.	Insufficient data.	Insufficient data. The ventricular catheter with external strain gauge, most accurate low-cost, reliable ICP device. Can also be recalibrated in situ. Parenchymal ICP cannot be recalibrated. Negligible drift.
ICP treatment threshold	Insufficient data.	Treatment initiated ICP above 20 mmHg.	A combination of ICP values, clinical and brain CT should be used to determine the need for treatment.

TABLE 17.2

Summary of Brain Trauma Foundation guidelines of the management of severe traumatic brain injury—cont'd

ITEM	LEVEL I EVIDENCE	LEVEL II EVIDENCE	LEVEL III EVIDENCE
Cerebral perfusion	Insufficient data.	Aggressive attempts to maintain CPP above 70 mmHg with fluids and pressors owing to risk of ARDS.	CPP of <50 mmHg should be avoided. The CPP value to target lies within the range of 50–70 mmHg. Patients with intact pressure autoregulation tolerate higher CPP values. Ancillary monitoring of cerebral parameters that include blood flow, oxygenation or metabolism facilitates CPP management.
Brain oxygen monitoring and thresholds	Insufficient data.	Insufficient data.	Jugular venous oxygenation (<50%) or brain tissue oxygen tension (<15 mmHg) are treatment thresholds and are to be avoided.
Anaesthetics, analgesics and sedatives	Insufficient data.	Manage pain and agitation. High-dose barbiturate may be used in haemodynamically stable patients refractory to other ICP treatments. Propofol for the control of ICP. High-dose propofol can produce significant morbidity.	None advised.
Nutrition	Insufficient data.	Full caloric replacement by day 7 post-injury.	None advised.
Antiseizure prophylaxis	Insufficient data.	Phenytoin or valproate is not recommended for preventing late post-traumatic seizures. Anticonvulsants are indicated to decrease the incidence of early post-traumatic seizures.	None advised.
Hyperventilation	Insufficient data.	Prophylactic hyperventilation ($PaCO_2$ <25 mmHg/3.3 kPa) is not recommended.	Use hyperventilation for temporary reduction of elevated ICP. Hyperventilation should be avoided during the first 24 h after injury when CBF is often critically reduced. If hyperventilation used: SjO_2 or $PbtO_2$ measures recommended to monitor oxygen delivery.
Steroids	Not recommended.	None advised.	None advised.

ARDS = acute respiratory distress syndrome; BP = blood pressure; CBF = cerebral blood flow; CPP = cerebral perfusion pressure; CT = computerised tomography (scan); GCS = Glasgow Coma Scale; ICP = intracranial pressure; $PaCO_2$ = partial pressure of alveolar carbon dioxide; PaO_2 = partial pressure of alveolar oxygen; $PbtO_2$ = brain tissue oxygenation; SBP = systolic blood pressure; SjO_2 = jugular venous oxygen saturation.

Source: Adapted from Brain Trauma Foundation, American Association of Neurological Surgeons, Joint Section on Neurotrauma and Critical Care. Guidelines for management of severe head injury. New York: Brain Trauma Foundation; 2007.

head and neck may cause contusion and ischaemia of the spinal cord without vertebral column damage. Whiplash injuries are the result of hyperextension. Violent hyperextension with fracture of the pedicles of C2 and forward movement of C2 on C3 produces the 'Hangman's fracture'.

- *Extension–rotation:* rotational injuries result from forces that cause extreme twisting or lateral flexion of the head and neck. Fracture or dislocation of vertebrae may also occur. The spinal canal is narrower in the thoracic segment relative to the width of the cord, so when vertebral displacement occurs it is more likely to damage the cord. Until the age of 10, the spine has increased physiological mobility due to lax ligaments, which affords some protection against acute SCI. Elderly patients are at a higher risk owing to the presence of osteophytes and narrowing of the spinal canal.

Classification of spinal cord injuries

SCI can be broadly classified as complete or incomplete.[68] The diagnosis of complete SCI cannot be made until spinal cord shock resolves. There are four incomplete SCI syndromes as follows:

- *Anterior cord syndrome:* injury to the motor and sensory pathways in the anterior parts of the spine. Patients are able to feel crude sensation, but movement and detailed sensation are lost in the posterior part of the spinal cord. Clinically, the patient usually has complete motor paralysis below the level of injury (corticospinal tracts) and loss of pain, temperature and touch sensation (spinothalamic tracts), with preservation of light touch, proprioception and position sense. The prognosis for anterior cord syndrome is the worst of all the incomplete syndrome prognoses.
- *Posterior cord syndrome:* is usually the result of a hyperextension injury at the cervical level and is not commonly seen. Position sense, light touch and vibratory sense are lost below the level of the injury.
- *Central cord syndrome:* this is injury to the centre of the cervical spinal cord, producing weakness, paralysis and sensory deficits in the arms but not the legs. Hyperextension of the cervical spine is often the mechanism of injury, and the damage is greatest to the cervical tracts supplying the arms. Clinically, the patient may present with paralysed arms but with no deficit in the legs or bladder.
- *Brown–Séquard syndrome:* this involves injury to the left or right side of the spinal cord. Movements are lost below the level of injury on the injured side, but pain and temperature sensation are lost on the side opposite to the injury. The clinical presentation is one in which the patient has either increased or decreased cutaneous sensation of pain, temperature and touch on the same side of the spinal cord at the level of the lesion. Below the level of the lesion on the same side,

there is complete motor paralysis. On the patient's opposite side, below the level of the lesion there is loss of pain, temperature and touch because the spinothalamic tracts cross soon after entering the cord.

Pathophysiology

SCIs can be separated into two categories: primary injuries and secondary injuries. Primary injuries are the result of the initial insult or trauma, and are usually permanent. The force of the primary insult produces its initial damage in the central grey matter of the cord. Secondary injuries are usually the result of a contusion or tear injury, in which the nerve fibres begin to swell and disintegrate. Secondary neural injury mechanisms include ischaemia, hypoxia and oedema, cellular and molecular inflammatory injury and cell death. Ischaemia, the most prominent post-SCI event, may occur up to 2 hours post-injury and is intensified by the loss of autoregulation of the spinal cord microcirculation.[69] This will decrease blood flow, which is then dependent on the systemic arterial pressure in the presence of hypotension or vasogenic spinal shock. Oedema develops at the injured site and spreads into adjacent areas. Hypoxia may occur because of inadequate airway maintenance and ventilation. Immune cells, which normally do not enter the spinal cord, engulf the area after a SCI and release regulatory chemicals, some of which are harmful to the spinal cord. Highly reactive oxidising agents (free radicals) are produced, which damage the cell membrane and disrupt the sodium–potassium pump.

Free radical production and the formation of reactive oxygen and nitrogen species or lipid peroxidation lead to vasoconstriction, increased endothelial permeability and increased platelet activation. A secondary chain of events produces ischaemia, hypoxia, oedema and haemorrhagic lesions, which in turn result in the destruction of myelin and axons. Autoregulation of spinal cord blood flow may be impaired in patients with severe lesions or substantial oedema formation. These secondary reactions, believed to be the principal causes of spinal cord degeneration at the level of injury, are thought to be reversible until 4–6 hours after injury. Therefore, if the cord has not suffered irreparable damage, early intervention is needed to prevent partial damage from developing into total and permanent damage.[70,71]

Spinal shock occurs with physiological or anatomical transection or near-transection of the spinal cord. It occurs immediately after or within several hours of a SCI and is caused by the sudden cessation of impulses from the higher brain centres.[72] It is characterised by the loss of motor, sensory, reflex and autonomic function below the level of the injury, with resultant flaccid paralysis. Loss of bowel and bladder function also occurs. In addition, the body's ability to control temperature is lost (i.e. poikilothermia) and the patient's temperature tends to equilibrate with that of the external environment.

Neurogenic spinal shock occurs as a result of mid- to upper-level cervical injuries and is the result of sympathetic vascular denervation and peripheral vasodilation. The loss of spinal cord vasculature autoregulation occurs, causing the blood flow to the spinal cord to be dependent on the systemic BP. Signs and symptoms include hypotension, severe bradycardia and loss of the ability to sweat below the level of injury. The same clinical findings pertaining to disruption of the sympathetic transmissions in spinal shock occur in neurogenic shock (see Chapter 21).[73]

Systemic effects of spinal cord injury

The traumatic insult causing the SCI is associated with an immediate stimulation of central and peripheral sympathetic tone. Initially, the elevated sympathetic activity raises systemic arterial BP and induces cardiac dysrhythmias. At the stage of spinal shock with loss of neuronal conduction, the sympathetic excitation is closely followed by decreases in systemic vascular resistance, arterial hypotension and venous pooling. Lesions above the level of T5 additionally present with severe bradycardia and cardiac dysfunction. The decreases in cardiac output combined with systemic hypotension further aggravate spinal cord ischaemia in tissues with defective autoregulation.[70]

SCI may produce respiratory failure. The extent of respiratory complications is related to the level of the injured segments. Injuries above the level of C4–C5 produce complete paralysis of the diaphragm, with substantial decreases in tidal volume and consecutive hypoxia. With lesions below C6, the function of the diaphragm is maintained and there is incomplete respiratory failure due to paralysed intercostal and abdominal musculature. As a consequence, arterial hypoxia and hypercapnia occur, both of which promote neuronal and glial acidosis, oedema and neuroexcitation.[72]

Patient management

SCI should be suspected in patients with neck pain, sensory and motor deficits, unconsciousness, intoxication, spondylitis or rheumatoid arthritis, all major trauma, distracting injuries, head injury and facial fractures. Where a SCI is suspected, or cannot be excluded, the patient must be placed on a spine board with the head and neck immobilised in a neutral position so as to reduce the risk of neurological deterioration from repeated mechanical insults.[73] Spinal injury patients are susceptible to pressure injuries (see Chapter 5), so time must be considered when hard surfaces are used for immobilisation. Total neck immobilisation should not interfere with maintenance of the airway, and inadequate respiratory function must be avoided.[68]

Practice tip

It is important to appropriately size and fit rigid cervical spine collars, which may be difficult in patients with excess adipose tissue. Collars that are too short or tall can lead to cervical spine flexion or extension. The use of a collar also increases the chances of the patient developing a pressure injury. Care must be taken to assess the skin integrity beneath the collar, particularly on the occiput and chin and across the clavicles.

Resuscitation

Initial treatment aims for decompression of the spinal cord and reversal of neurogenic shock and respiratory failure. Spinal shock is associated with decreases in systemic vascular resistance, arterial hypotension, venous pooling, severe bradycardia and decreased myocardial contractility. Consequently, treatment of neurogenic shock includes fluid replacement to maintain arterial BP, circulatory volume, renal function and tissue oxygenation. Lower-limb compression assists with venous return. Infusion of free water must be avoided, as this decreases plasma osmolarity and promotes spinal cord oedema. Atropine may be administered to reverse bradycardia and increase cardiac output. Administration of vasopressors (e.g. noradrenaline (norepinephrine)) prior to correction of the intravascular volume status may increase systemic vascular resistance (left ventricular afterload) and further impair myocardial contractility. Therefore, careful volume replacement is the first step, and administration of vasopressors the second step, in the treatment of arterial hypotension and low cardiac output after acute cervical SCI.

The major early cause of death in patients with acute cervical SCI is respiratory failure. Tracheal intubation may be indicated in unconscious patients, patients with shock or those with other major associated injuries and during cardiovascular and respiratory distress. It is also indicated in conscious patients presenting with the following criteria: maximum expiratory force below 20 cmH_2O, maximum inspiratory force below 20 cmH_2O, vital capacity below 1000 mL and presence of atelectasis, contusion and infiltrate.[70]

Investigations

Following the initial assessment of the patient, detailed CT diagnostic radiography defines the bone damage and compression of the spinal cord. Cervical spine fractures occur predominantly at two levels: at the level of C2 and at the level of C6 or C7. Unfortunately, 20–30% of these fractures can be missed on plain radiographs. Current recommendations are to consider use of multidetector-row CT as the initial screening examination in suspected cervical trauma instead of radiographs or standard CT. Specific radiological procedures such as cervical myelography, high-resolution CT scan or magnetic resonance imaging (MRI) will identify fractures, dislocation of bony fragments and spinal cord contusion.[73]

Neuroprotective and regenerative strategies

In patients with a dislocated cervical fracture, decompression and anatomical bony realignment may be achieved with traction forces applied manually, or with halo or Gardner–Wells systems under radiological control. If the anatomical bony alignment procedures and traction forces fail to decompress the cord, surgical intervention to remove the lesion is required. The timing of surgical intervention remains controversial. While urgent surgical decompression or internal stabilisation should be performed in all patients with deteriorating neurological status, surgical treatment may be deferred in patients with stable neurological deficits.[74]

The most promising neuroprotective reparative therapeutic strategies undergoing investigation include riluzole, hypothermia, granulocyte colony-stimulating factor, glibenclamide, minocycline, Cethrin (VX-210) and anti-Nogo-A antibody.[74] Apart from hypothermia, most other strategies have not been successful, which has been attributed to attempting to block only one molecular pathway of a complex range of SCI molecular mechanisms. There has been renewed interest in regeneration, which involves stem cell transplantation or similar restorative approaches designed to optimise spontaneous axonal growth and myelination, but human research remains in its infancy owing to limiting legislation in some countries.

Collaborative care interventions

Patients with acute cervical SCI require ICU monitoring, observation and support of ventilation, a nasogastric or orogastric tube to reduce abdominal distention and risk of aspiration (a nasogastric tube should be used only if there is no risk related to TBI and basal skull fracture), a urinary catheter and thermal maintenance. In addition, the following should be noted:[71]

- Tracheostomy is indicated in high cervical spine injury and ischaemia, sometimes temporarily while the early oedema is resolving.

- Spinal alignment and immobilisation require careful positioning with dedicated neck support by experienced clinicians.

- Shoulder and lumbar support pillows are often prescribed. Pressure-relief mattresses must be suitably designed for spine immobilisation and, when prescribed, can be tilted to facilitate ventilation.

- Meticulous integument and bowel care is indicated, with daily protocols for regular stool softeners and peristaltic stimulants essential for the prevention of autonomic dysreflexia (i.e. strong sensory input from the bowel to the spinal cord that evokes a massive reflex sympathetic surge) and autonomic nerve dysfunction.

- Early nutritious feeding is essential, whether oral or enteric; however, aspiration must be prevented. The supplementation of feeding with high-energy protein fluids to match the catabolic state assists with recovery (see Chapter 19).

- Both hyper- and hypoglycaemia must be avoided.[73]

- The concepts of pain relief and sedation in patients with SCI are based on the maintenance of coupling between metabolism and spinal cord blood flow while achieving hypnosis, analgesia and a 'relaxed cord'. These concepts include maintenance of normal to high systemic perfusion pressures, normoxia and normocapnia.

- Psychological and empathetic support is essential and appropriate referral for grieving and stress is

paramount. Rehabilitation counselling and planning starts at the acute stage in order to give the family unit future focus and hope.

See Online resources for specific protocols related to spinal injury.

Cerebrovascular disorders

Cerebral vascular disorders include cerebrovascular disease and cerebral vascular incidents (stroke). A stroke (acute brain injury of vascular origin) is defined as an interruption of the blood supply to any part of the brain, resulting in damaged brain tissue.

According to the World Health Organization (WHO), stroke claims 6.2 million lives each year and globally it is the second most common cause of death, exceeded only by coronary heart disease.[75] The incidence of stroke in the USA is about 7.2 million[76] and in the UK approximately 152,145 people suffer a stroke per annum.[77] Stroke is also the primary cerebrovascular disorder in Australia and New Zealand.[78] The age-adjusted incidence of stroke is higher in men than women in all countries. Those over 65 years are also most at risk.[75]

Stroke is divided into two major categories: ischaemic (85%), in which vascular occlusion and significant hypoperfusion occur; and haemorrhagic (15%), in which there is extravasation of blood into the brain. Although there are some similarities between the two broad types of stroke, the aetiology, pathophysiology, medical management, surgical management and nursing care differ.

Aetiology

Hypertension is the leading risk factor for stroke. Other risk factors include diabetes, cardiac disease, previous cerebrovascular disease (transient ischaemic attack or stroke, or myocardial infarction), age, sex, lipid disorders, excessive ethanol ingestion, elevated haematocrit, elevated fibrinogen and cigarette smoking.[76] Cerebral arteriosclerosis predisposes individuals to both ischaemic and haemorrhagic stroke. Smoking is the strongest risk factor for aSAH. Atrial fibrillation, endocarditis and medications containing supplemental oestrogen are risk factors for embolic stroke. Seizures develop in approximately 10% of cases, usually appearing in the first 24 hours, and more likely to be focal than generalised. Occurrence of seizures within 24 hours of stroke is associated with higher 30-day mortality, which may be a reflection of severe neuronal damage.[78]

Ischaemic stroke

Ischaemic stroke compromises blood flow and energy supply to the brain, which triggers mechanisms that lead to cell death, and are embolic or thrombotic in origin. Infarction occurs rapidly in the region of most severe ischaemia (termed ischaemic penumbra) and expands at the expense of the surrounding hypoxic tissue, from the centre to the periphery. Therapeutic strategies in acute ischaemic stroke are based on the concept of arresting the transition of the penumbral region into infarction, thereby limiting ultimate infarct size and improving neurological and functional outcome. Ischaemic stroke can be further categorised as middle cerebral artery occlusion, acute basilar occlusion and cerebellar infarcts.[79]

Practice tip

For consideration of ischaemic stroke lysis, the timing of the onset of symptoms needs to be very clearly defined. In particular, if a patient wakes from sleep with stroke symptoms, the timing of onset must be assumed to be when they were last well – that is, the time when they went to sleep.

The management of an ischaemic stroke is comprised of four primary goals: restoration of CBF (reperfusion), prevention of recurrent thrombosis, neuroprotection and supportive care.[79] The timing of each element of clinical management needs to be implemented in a decisive manner. For eligible patients, IV tissue plasminogen activator should be administered at a dose of 0.9 mg/kg (maximum of 90 mg), with 10% of the total dose administered as an initial bolus and the remainder infused over 60 minutes, provided that treatment is initiated within 4.5 hours of clearly defined symptom onset.[79] The recommendation assumes a relatively higher value on long-term functional improvement and a relatively lower value on minimising the risk of intracerebral haemorrhage in the immediate peristroke period.

Endovascular clot retrieval is increasingly being used as a reperfusion therapy following ischaemic stroke. This involves the use of a mechanical device to remove the blockage. This therapy can be used in conjunction with IV tissue plasminogen activator. As cardiac dysrhythmias such as atrial fibrillation predispose to embolic events, cardiac monitoring for at least 24 hours should be carried out. Table 17.3 shows the classification and treatment strategies, and the Online resources reflect specific ischaemic stroke protocols.

Haemorrhagic stroke

Haemorrhagic stroke is divided into two main categories: intracerebral haemorrhage and spontaneous subarachnoid haemorrhage.

Intracerebral haemorrhage

Intracerebral haemorrhage (ICH) comprises 10–15% of all strokes, with an incidence of 24.6 per 100,000 person-years, and with a growing incidence associated with the use of anticoagulation, antiplatelet agents and an ageing population.[80] Despite this, ICH remains the last stroke type without a definitive treatment and contributes to significant morbidity and mortality. Up to half of patients die within 30 days, often despite extensive stays in the ICU. Moreover, those who survive have a high degree of long-term disability.[80] Pathogenesis of ICH include hypertension,

TABLE 17.3

Classification and type of ischaemic stroke and treatment options

CLASSIFICATION	TREATMENT OPTIONS
Middle cerebral artery occlusion	Intravenous or intra-arterial tissue plasminogen activator (tPA). Exclusion criteria: >3 h elapsed from stroke onset and widespread early infarct changes on CT scan. Tolerate autoprotective hypertension for perfusion of the ischaemic penumbra.
Acute basilar occlusion	Anticoagulation with intravenous heparin. Thrombolysis up to 12 h after onset.
Cerebellar infarcts	May be difficult to recognise because of the slow evolution of brainstem and cerebellar signs. Aspirin, antihypertensives and conventional cerebral oedema strategies.

vascular malformations, brain tumours, bleeding disorders, or the use of drugs such as cocaine or amphetamines, which elevate BP. Ideally, patients with acute ICH should be admitted to an ICU based on the need for close monitoring of neurological and haemodynamic condition and the risk for early deterioration from haematoma expansion, cerebral oedema, hydrocephalus or airway compromise. Many ICHs continue to grow and expand over several hours after the onset of symptoms.

As with all emergency management, initial assessment of airway, breathing and circulation is critical. Until the diagnosis of ICH is made from neuroimaging, airway and haemodynamic management proceeds in a common pathway with other stroke subtypes. Because many ICH patients are obtunded or comatose, airway management (specifically the need for intubation for airway protection) should be considered throughout the early treatment course. Following the diagnosis of ICH, immediate consideration should be given to the need for (1) acute control of elevated BP, (2) correction of coagulopathy because of medications or underlying medical conditions, and (3) the need for urgent surgical haematoma evacuation.[81] Over 90% of patients have acute hypertension, whether or not there is a history of pre-existing hypertension. It remains unclear whether this response is adaptive (to maintain perfusion to an ischaemic penumbra surrounding the haematoma) or potentially harmful (resulting in rebleeding, perihaematoma oedema expansion, or both).[81] The American Heart Association/American Stroke Association 2019 guidelines recommend that, for patients with hypertension, BP should be carefully lowered to ensure systolic pressure is less than 185 mmHg.[82] Rapid lowering of BP should be considered in patients presenting with a systolic BP >220 mmHg with ICH; it may also be reasonable to consider aggressive reduction of BP with a continuous intravenous infusion and frequent BP monitoring. The aim should be to reach a systolic BP of 140 mmHg or lower while ensuring that the drop is not greater than 60 mmHg in 1 hour.[83]

Use of antithrombotic medications is a risk factor for the occurrence of ICH, as well as for haematoma expansion if an ICH occurs. As there is a broad range of antithrombotic medications, including warfarin, heparin, antiplatelet agents such as aspirin and clopidogrel and agents such as dabigatran and rivaroxaban, the specific risks and interventions to reverse coagulopathy vary. Also, coagulopathies may be due to underlying medical conditions, such as liver disease or haematological malignances.[84] Patients with ICH should have intermittent pneumatic compression for prevention of venous thromboembolism, as compression stockings are not recommended for use in this population.[84] Most of the brain injury and swelling that happens in the days after ICH is the result of inflammation caused by thrombin and other coagulation end-products.[85] Dysautonomia, in the form of central fever, hyperventilation, hyperglycaemia and tachycardia or bradycardia, is common. Hyperglycaemia at the time of hospital admission is associated with early mortality and poor outcome in ICH patients.[86]

Subarachnoid haemorrhage (SAH)

Subarachnoid haemorrhage is defined as a bleed into the subarachnoid space, which can be spontaneous or associated with a TBI. Spontaneous SAH is most commonly due to vascular abnormalities such as cerebral or brain aneurysm. Admission to the ICU is required for grade 4 aneurysmal SAH based on the World Federation of Neurosurgical Societies Scale[87] (Table 17.4). This level

TABLE 17.4

World Federation of Neurosurgical Societies scale for aneurysmal subarachnoid haemorrhage (aSAH)[82]

GRADE	GLASGOW COMA SCALE	MOTOR DEFICIT
I	15	Absent
II	14–13	Absent
III	14–13	Present
IV	12–7	Present or absent
V	6–3	Present or absent

Source: Teasdale GM, Drake CG, Hunt W, et al. A universal subarachnoid hemorrhage scale: report of a committee of the World Federation of Neurosurgical Societies. J Neurol Neurosurg Psychiatry 1988;51(11):1457, with permission from BMJ Publishing Group Ltd.

of severity is at greater risk of systemic complications and clinical deterioration.[88] Resuscitation is directed towards maintaining CPP by ensuring adequate arterial BP (often with the use of inotropes to produce relative hypertension, although reactive hypertension is often present), ensuring euvolaemia and producing relative haemodilution.[89]

Hypovolaemia occurs in 30–50% of patients and hyponatraemia in 30% of patients.[89] In the first 6 days, plasma volume decreases of greater than 10% can occur following aSAH, hence increasing the risk of delayed cerebral ischaemia and vasospasm.[90] Women have been found to have more significant drops in blood volume than men following aSAH. 'Third-space' loss, insensible losses and blood loss account for this drop in fluid volume, as well as electrolyte disturbances.[91]

Practice tip

Fever is the most common medical complication in patients suffering from aSAH and is associated with neurological deterioration.

In the acute stages, other aspects of management include suitable analgesia, seizure control and treatment with nimodipine to prevent delayed cerebral ischaemia and vasospasm.[89] Acute hydrocephalus secondary to aSAH is usually managed by external ventricular drainage and is associated with neurological improvement. ICP monitoring and drainage of CSF via ventriculostomy is also indicated.[90]

Increased sympathetic activation from the presence of haemoglobin in the subarachnoid space results in elevated catecholamine levels. This is characterised by hypothalamically mediated changes including increased sympathetic and parasympathetic activity that causes cardiac and pulmonary complications (neurogenic pulmonary oedema).[92] Manifestations include electrocardiographic changes, dysrhythmias, impaired cardiac contractility, elevated troponin levels and myocardial necrosis. Cardiac and pulmonary complications are associated with delayed cerebral ischaemia and poor outcome after aSAH. As cardiac function is one of the determinants for adequate CBF, it is essential to identify such occurrences early and treat them accordingly.

Hyponatraemia occurs from alterations in atrial natriuretic factor in response to sympathetic nervous system activation. The syndrome of inappropriate secretion of antidiuretic hormone is primarily responsible for hyponatraemia in those with aSAH, as is cerebral salt-wasting syndrome.

Prevention of delayed cerebral ischaemia and cerebral vasospasm

Delayed cerebral ischaemia can occur as a result of aSAH. It is defined as the occurrence of focal neurological impairment (such as hemiparesis, aphasia, apraxia, hemianopia or neglect) or a decrease of at least two points on the GCS (on either the total score or one of its individual components of eye, motor or verbal). This drop in GCS should last for at least 1 hour, is not apparent immediately after aneurysm occlusion and cannot be attributed to other causes by means of clinical assessments, cerebral CT or MRI scanning, and appropriate laboratory studies.[93] Delayed cerebral ischaemia occurs in about 30% of patients surviving the initial haemorrhage, mostly between days 4 and 10 after aSAH. The known clinical symptoms, such as a decrease in the level of consciousness and focal signs (e.g. aphasia and hemiparesis), may be reversible or otherwise progress to cerebral infarction, resulting in an unfavourable outcome or even death. A diagnosis of delayed cerebral ischaemia is made after exclusion of other causes (e.g. infection, hypotension, hyponatraemia and others) and confirmed with angiography, and is especially difficult in patients who are comatose or sedated.[94] The latter are typically patients with a high grade on the World Federation of Neurosurgical Societies scale (grade 4–5), approximately 40–70% of the patient population with ruptured aneurysms.[95] The Fisher scale is also used to classify the amount of subarachnoid blood seen on CT scan and can help predict the likelihood of vasospasm.[96] Early brain injury and cell death, blood–brain barrier disruption and initiation of an inflammatory cascade, microvascular spasm, microthrombosis, cortical-spreading depolarisations and failure of cerebral autoregulation have all been implicated in the pathophysiology of delayed cerebral ischaemia.

Cerebral vasospasm is a self-limited vasculopathy that develops 4–21 days after SAH (see Fig. 17.6). Vasospasm occurs when the clot undergoes lysis (dissolution), increasing the chances of rebleeding. About one-third of aSAH patients develop symptomatic vasospasm, which is associated with neurological signs and symptoms of ischaemia. Post-TBI cerebral vasospasm occurs in approximately 10–15% of patients. Oxyhaemoglobin, a product of haemoglobin (Hb) breakdown, probably initiates vasoconstriction, leading to smooth-muscle proliferation, collagen remodelling and cellular infiltration of the vessel wall. The resulting vessel narrowing can lead to delayed cerebral ischaemia. The initial proinflammatory effect elicited by Hb and Hb-bound cells initiates an inflammatory cascade and cortical-spreading depolarisation involving an increase of cytokines, leukocytes and cell adhesion molecules characterising the inflammatory process. The symptoms are poorly localised and develop gradually over hours, suggesting a progressing, global disease process.

Calcium antagonists have not been effective in TBI SAH with vasospasm. However, nimodipine has demonstrated effectiveness in the treatment of vasospasm in aSAH, reducing the incidence of delayed cerebral ischaemia and poor outcome by 40% without ameliorating vasospasm.[97]

Despite its widespread use as a mainstay therapy for cerebral vasospasm, research evidence does not support the use of 'triple H' therapy (hypervolaemia, hypertension, haemodilution).[97] Clinical studies reveal that hypervolaemia results in pulmonary oedema, as well as haemodilution, and with it a decrease in arterial oxygen and oxygen-carrying capacity. Anaemia has also been associated with a worse outcome after aSAH. Hence, haemodilution has been eliminated from 'triple H' therapy and the target is now euvolaemia rather than hypervolaemia. These changes, along with the established hypertensive therapy, are the mainstays in clinical practice recommended in the Neurocritical Care Society aSAH guidelines.[98]

It is believed that early open surgical clipping or wrapping and endovascular coil embolisation prevent rebleeding and that removal of blood from the basal cisterns around the major cerebral arteries may prevent vasospasm.[99] In aSAH, endovascular therapies should be considered in patients at risk for vasospasm-related ischaemia prior to the development of delayed cerebral ischaemia. Prophylactic angioplasty done without the presence of angiographic arterial narrowing exposes patients to the risk of vessel rupture and death without clear benefit in outcome.[98] Therefore, routine prophylactic cerebral angioplasty is not recommended.[98]

Cerebral venous sinus thrombosis (CVST)

Compared with cerebral infarctions from arterial sources, cerebral venous infarctions are less common, with reported incidences of 0.22 to 1.57 per 100,000.[100,101] Following the SARS-CoV-2 pandemic, cases of vaccine-induced thrombotic thrombocytopenia (VITT) have resulted in patients presenting with CVST.[102] It is particularly important to recognise cerebral venous thrombosis because there is general consensus that early anticoagulation can result in good clinical outcomes. MRI and CT vascular imaging have made it easier to establish the diagnosis, but close monitoring of the patient is essential, as late deterioration can occur.

Patient management

Expected outcomes for patients with acute ischaemic and haemorrhagic stroke include prevention of secondary injury and of airway and respiratory complications, and maintenance of haemodynamic stability. Timely assessment and intervention are paramount in the management of ischaemic stroke, especially regarding interventional pharmacology and prevention of cerebral haemorrhage.[88] See Online resources for specific protocols related to stroke.

Atrial fibrillation and deep vein thrombosis prevention (in ischaemic stroke) both require anticoagulation control. In haemorrhagic stroke, a sequential compression device and stockings are indicated, as anticoagulants are a risk factor for rebleeding. Maintenance of bowel and bladder function and prevention of integumentary complications, malnutrition, seizures and increasing neurological deficits are important goals. Environmental precautions are implemented to provide a non-stimulating environment, preventing rises in ICP and further bleeding.

TABLE 17.5

Typical profiles of cerebrospinal fluid in acute meningitis and encephalitis

		MENINGITIS		ENCEPHALITIS
INVESTIGATION	REFERENCE RANGE	BACTERIAL	VIRAL	BACTERIAL/VIRAL
Opening pressure	<30 mmH$_2$O	Raised	Normal	Raised
White cells:				
Total count	<5 × 10^6/L	Greatly raised	Moderately raised	Moderately raised
Differential	Lymphocytes (60–70%), monocytes (30–50%), no neutrophils or red blood cells	Neutrophils predominate	Lymphocytes predominate	Lymphocytes predominate
Glucose concentration	2.8–4.4 mmol/L	Lowered	Normal	Normal
CSF:serum glucose ratio	>60%	Lowered	Normal	Normal
Protein concentration	<0.45 g/L	Raised	Normal or slightly raised	Normal or slightly raised

Sensory perceptual and motor alterations need to be assessed in regard to effective communication and pain management. Rehabilitation and psychological support for the patient and significant others are integrated into the acute care phase for a smooth transition.

Infection and inflammation

The CNS infections of major interest in the ICU are divided into those that affect the meninges (meningitis) and those that affect the brain parenchyma (encephalitis), which may be viral or bacterial in aetiology. Many medical conditions can mimic viral encephalitis. Particular attention should be given to the possibility of such non-viral infections as cerebral malaria, which may be rapidly fatal if not treated early. Metabolic conditions, such as liver and renal failure and diabetic complications, may also cause confusion due to the manifestation of cerebral oedema. The possible role of alcohol and drug ingestion should also be considered.

Meningitis

Meningitis is inflammation of the pia and arachnoid layers of the meninges. Acute community-acquired meningitis can develop within hours to days and is usually viral or bacterial. Viral meningitis usually has a good prognosis, whereas bacterial meningitis is associated with significant rates of morbidity and death, so it is critical to recognise and differentiate them promptly.[101] The incidence, mortality and morbidity from acute community-acquired meningitis has decreased significantly, especially in high-income countries, probably as a result of vaccination and

better antimicrobial and adjuvant therapy, but the disease still has a high toll.[103,104] Table 17.5 shows the CSF profiles for acute meningitis and encephalitis, and Table 17.6 shows the classification, treatment and clinical presentation of acute meningitis.

Complications of meningitis vary according to the aetiological organism, the duration of symptoms prior to initiation of appropriate therapy, and the age and immune status of the patient. Temporary problems include development of haemodynamic instability and disseminated intravascular coagulopathy, particularly in meningococcal infection, a syndrome of inappropriate secretion of antidiuretic hormone or another dysregulation of the hypothalamic–pituitary axis (e.g. diabetes insipidus) and an acute rise in ICP.

> **Practice tip**
>
> The dose of antimicrobial drug required for treating meningitis is usually higher than normal, as penetration across the blood–CSF barrier is poor.

Focal neurological signs may develop in the early stages of meningitis, but are more common later. The development of subdural empyema, brain abscess and acute hydrocephalus may require surgical intervention. Bacterial meningitis with accompanying bacteraemia can lead to a marked systemic inflammatory response with septic shock and acute respiratory distress syndrome.

TABLE 17.6

Classification of acute meningitis

ACUTE MENINGITIS	BACTERIAL – NOTIFIABLE DISEASE	VIRAL
Aetiology	*Neisseria* meningitis: • Serogroups A, B, C – 90% invasive isolates • Serogroup B – most disease • Serogroup A – epidemic disease and indigenous *Haemophilus influenzae* type B, *Streptococcus pneumoniae*, *Listeria monocytogenes*.	Enteroviruses: 85–95% of cases. Herpes simplex 1 and 2. Varicella zoster. Cytomegalovirus. Epstein–Barr. HIV infection can also present as aseptic meningitis. Postinfectious encephalomyelitis: may occur following a variety of viral infections, usually of the respiratory tract. *Cryptococcus neoformans.* Fungal isolates.
Pathophysiology	Rapid recognition and diagnosis of meningitis is imperative. Quick and insidious progress of disease. Colonisation of mucosal surfaces (nasopharynx). Haematogenous or contiguous spread. Specific antibodies important defence. Bacterial invasion of meninges: inflammatory response, breakdown of the BBB, cerebral oedema, intracranial hypertension. Vasculitis, spasm and thrombosis in cerebral blood vessels.	The physical signs are not so marked and the illness is not as severe and prolonged as bacterial meningitis. Viral infection of mucosal surfaces of respiratory or gastrointestinal tract. Virus replication in tonsillar or gut lymphatics. Viraemia with haematogenous dissemination to the CNS. Meningeal inflammation, BBB breakdown, cerebral oedema, vasculitis and spasm.
Clinical presentation and progression	Presents with sepsis: headache, fever, photophobia, vomiting, neck stiffness, alteration of mental status. Meningococcaemia is characterised by an abrupt onset of fever (with petechial or purpuric rash). Progresses to purpura fulminans, associated with the rapid onset of hypotension, acute adrenal haemorrhage syndrome and multiorgan failure. Kernig's sign. Brudzinski's sign. Cranial nerve palsies (III, IV, VI, VII) uncommon and develop after several days. Focal neurological signs in 10–20% cases. Seizures in 30% of cases. Signs of intracranial hypertension: coma, altered respiratory status. Leads to hypertension and bradycardia before herniation, or brain death, leads to irreversible septic shock.	Presents with non-specific symptoms, viral respiratory illness, diarrhoea, fever, headache, photophobia, vomiting, anorexia, rash, cough and myalgia. Occurs in summer or late autumn Enteroviral, pleurodynia, chest pain, hand–foot–mouth disease. HSV-2: acute genital herpes.
Treatment	If meningococcal infection is suspected, the best way to reduce mortality is to administer empirical IV therapy immediately: ceftriaxone 2 g IV 12-hourly or cefotaxime 2 g IV 6-hourly or immediately. Consequent dose, times and type of antibiotic need to be modified after full investigation and a detailed examination have taken place. Dexamethasone may be prescribed: needs to be at same time as antibiotic as outcome neurologically is reduced if given after antibiotic. Reduces BBB permeability. Supportive treatment and resuscitation. Management of intracranial hypertension/ischaemia.	Administer intravenous aciclovir (acyclovir). Dexamethasone may be prescribed: reduces BBB permeability. Supportive treatment and resuscitation. Management of intracranial hypertension/ischaemia.

BBB = blood–brain barrier; CNS = central nervous system.

Encephalitis

Encephalitis indicates inflammation of the brain substance (parenchyma) and can range from being a mild and self-limiting condition to a serious, life-threatening illness. Inflammation of the meninges (meningoencephalitis) or spinal cord (encephalomyelitis) may also be present.

Herpes simplex virus encephalitis is the most common sporadic viral encephalitis worldwide, with an annual incidence of 1 in 250,000–500,000.[105] Without treatment, herpes simplex virus encephalitis is fatal in up to 80% of cases, and leaves up to 50% of survivors with long-term sequelae.[106] Other common causes include enteroviruses, influenza virus and *Mycoplasma pneumoniae*, with geographical location, history of travel, animal exposure and vaccination determining the likely pathogen. *Mycobacterium tuberculosis*, *Cryptococcus neoformans* and *Treponema pallidum* (syphilis) can also affect the brain parenchyma, but they usually result in chronic or subacute meningitis.

In the majority of encephalitis cases, the offending organism finds access to the brain via the nasopharyngeal epithelium and the olfactory nerve system. Arboviruses are transmitted from infected animals to humans through the bite of infected animals.[107] The cytokine storm results in neural cell damage, as well as the apoptosis of astrocytes. The disruption of the blood–brain barrier progresses to septic shock, disseminated intravascular coagulopathy and multiorgan failure. Encephalitis may present with progressive headache, fever and alterations in cognitive state (confusion, behavioural change, dysphasia) or consciousness. Focal neurological signs (paresis) or seizures (focal or generalised) may also occur. Upper motor signs (hyperreflexia and extensor–plantar responses) are often present, but flaccid paralysis and bladder symptoms may occur if the spinal cord is involved.[107] Associated movement disorders or the inappropriate secretion of antidiuretic hormone may be seen. The most sensitive type of imaging for diagnosis of encephalitis is MRI; in HSV encephalitis, CT scans may initially appear normal, but MRI usually shows involvement of the temporal lobes and thalamus.[107] Examination of CSF can assist in differential diagnosis. Refer to Table 17.6 for CSF profiles. EEG is less sensitive but may be helpful if it shows characteristic features (e.g. lateralising periodic sharp and slow-wave patterns).

Patient management

Neurological derangement often coexists with circulatory insufficiency, impaired respiration, metabolic derangement and seizures. Protecting the patient from injury secondary to raised ICP and seizure activity is essential. Prevention of complications associated with immobility, such as decubitus and pneumonia, is required. It is important to institute droplet infection control precautions in those attending the patient until 24 hours after the initiation of antibiotic therapy (oral and nasal discharge is considered infectious). See Online resources for infection control protocols relating specifically to meningitis.

Support in an ICU is often required in encephalitis to maintain ventilation, protect the airway and manage complications such as cerebral oedema. The management of acute viral encephalitis includes aggressive airway, ventilation, sedation, seizure, haemodynamic, fluid and nutritional support. Clinical deterioration is usually the result of severe cerebral oedema with diencephalic herniation or systemic complications, including generalised sepsis and multiple organ failure. The use of ICP monitoring in acute encephalitis remains controversial but should be considered if there is a rapid deterioration in the level of consciousness, and if imaging suggests raised ICP. Prolonged sedation may be necessary. Decompressive craniotomy may be successful in cases where there is rapid swelling of a non-dominant temporal lobe, as poor outcome is otherwise likely.[108]

Neuromuscular disorders

Generalised muscle weakness can manifest in several disorders that require ICU admission or complicate the clinical course of patients. These may involve motor neuron disease and disorders of the neuromuscular junction, peripheral nerve conduction and muscular contraction. These disorders manifest as Guillain–Barré syndrome, myasthenia gravis and critical illness polyneuropathies and myopathy.

Guillain–Barré syndrome

Guillain–Barré syndrome (GBS) is an immune-mediated disorder resulting from generation of autoimmune antibodies and/or inflammatory cells that cross-react with epitopes on peripheral nerves and roots, leading to demyelination or axonal damage, or both, and autoimmune insult to peripheral nerve myelin. Estimates of GBS incidence range from 0.8 to 1.9 cases per 100,000 person-years, are higher in males and increase with age.[109] Of all patients, 85% recover with minimal residual symptoms; severe residual deficits occur in up to 10%. Residual deficits are most likely in patients with rapid disease progression, those who require mechanical ventilation or those 60 years of age or over. Death occurs in 3–8% of cases, resulting from respiratory failure, autonomic dysfunction, sepsis or pulmonary emboli.[110]

Aetiology

The diagnosis of GBS is confirmed by the findings of cytoalbuminological dissociation (elevation of the CSF protein without concomitant CSF pleocytosis) and by neurophysiological findings suggestive of an acute (usually demyelinating) neuropathy. These abnormalities may not be present in the early stages of the illness.[111] There are two forms of GBS. The demyelinating form, the more common one, is characterised by demyelination and inflammatory infiltrates of the peripheral nerves and roots. In the axonal form the nerves show Wallerian degeneration (the fatty degeneration of a nerve fibre after it has been severed from its cell body) with an absence of inflammation. Discrimination between the axonal and demyelinating forms relies mainly on electrophysiological methods. There is a close association between GBS and a preceding infection, suggesting an immune basis for the syndrome. The commonest infections are due to *Campylobacter jejuni*, cytomegalovirus and Epstein–Barr virus.

Pathophysiology

GBS is the result of a cell-mediated immune attack on peripheral nerve myelin proteins. The Schwann cell is spared, allowing for remyelination in the recovery phase of the disease. With the autoimmune attack there is an influx of macrophages and other immune-mediated agents that attack myelin, cause inflammation and destruction and leave the axon unable to support nerve conduction. This demyelination may be discrete or diffuse, and may affect the peripheral nerves and their roots at any point from their origin in the spinal cord to the neuromuscular junction. The weakness of GBS results from conduction block and concomitant or primary axonal injury in the affected motor nerves. Pain and paraesthesias are the clinical correlates of sensory nerve involvement.

Clinical manifestations

Onset is rapid, and approximately 20% of cases lead to total paralysis, requiring prolonged intensive therapy with mechanical ventilation. The therapeutic window for GBS is short, and the current optimal treatment with whole-plasma exchange or immunoglobulin therapy lacks immunological specificity and only halves the severity of the disease.[112] GBS has three phases – acute, plateau and recovery – each stage lasting from days to weeks and in recovery to months and years. The patient presents with:

- symmetrical weakness, diminished reflexes and upward progression of motor weakness; a history of a viral illness in the previous few weeks suggests the diagnosis
- changes in vital capacity and negative inspiratory force, which are assessed to identify impending neuromuscular respiratory failure.

Indications for ICU admission include the following: ventilatory insufficiency, severe bulbar weakness threatening pulmonary aspiration, autonomic instability or coexisting general medical factors,[110] and often a combination of factors are present. About 30% of patients have respiratory failure that requires mechanical ventilation. Ventilatory failure is primarily caused by inspiratory muscle weakness, although weakness of the abdominal and accessory muscles of respiration, retained airway secretions leading to pulmonary aspiration and atelectasis are all contributory factors. The associated bulbar weakness and autonomic instability reinforce the need for control of the airway and ventilation.

Practice tip

In GBS, vital capacity less than 20 mL/kg is a sign of respiratory fatigue. Early intubation leads to earlier extubation and a better prognosis.

Acute motor and sensory axonal neuropathy, the acute axonal form of GBS, usually presents with a rapidly developing paralysis over hours and a rapid development of respiratory failure requiring tracheal intubation and ventilation. $PaCO_2$ may remain constant until just before intubation, emphasising the importance of not relying purely on arterial blood gas (ABG) analysis to make decisions regarding intubation.

Sensory involvement in relation to pain has been studied, asserting the clinical observation of pain ranging from mild to severe in the acute and rehabilitant phases. Chronic pain is often present in survivors of GBS.[111]

There may be total paralysis of all voluntary muscles of the body, including the cranial musculature, the ocular muscles and the pupils. Prolonged ventilatory support is likely in GBS patients who experience rapid disease progression, bulbar dysfunction, bilateral facial weakness or autonomic nerve dysfunction. Tracheostomy is usually performed within 2 weeks, and mechanical ventilation is delivered in a supportive mode with minimal yet adequate sedation and pain management.[112]

Patient management

Assessment and understanding of neuromuscular weakness through motor and sensory neurological assessment is vital in the acute care and rehabilitation of GBS patients (see Online resources for published guidelines):

- Comprehensive respiratory assessment (level of overall patient comfort, frequency and depth of breathing, forced vital capacity, use of accessory muscles, presence of paradoxical respiration and integrity of upper airway reflexes), ABG data and chest radiography determine levels of fatigue in both the acute stage (for intubation and ventilation) and the rehabilitation (weaning) stage. Long-term ventilation increases the risk of ventilator-associated pneumonia, requiring routine surveillance.
- Cardiovascular assessment is important, as serious tachyarrhythmias and bradyarrhythmias and destabilising fluctuations in BP caused by autonomic impairment are prevalent. This feature is common during fatigue, sleep and states of dehydration. Often, autonomic dysfunction is worst in the early stages of a nosocomial infection.[113]
- Cranial nerve assessment and dermatome (for sensory) and muscle strength assessment assist in mapping the progression, severity and rehabilitation of the disease and determining the risk of aspiration. Pain (especially neuropathic) is particularly common in GBS during changes in myelination, and can be difficult to treat.[114]

A structured care plan involving the patient and family is essential for continuity of care, particularly in the long-term recovery phase. The provision of sleep, good nutrition and prevention of the complications of immobility (nosocomial infections, deep vein thrombosis, integument and muscular weakening, adequate nutrition and constipation) are important.[112] The following points also need consideration:[112,114]

- Endotracheal and pharyngeal suction can be demanding (weakened upper airway reflexes), and sputum plugging and retention requires frequent repositioning and physiotherapy.
- Routine daily gentle exercise as part of a flexible program improves well-being and strength.
- Fatigue must be avoided, as autonomic nerve dysfunction, deafferent pain syndromes, muscle pain and depression can be exacerbated.
- Suctioning, coughing, bladder distention, constipation and the Valsalva manoeuvre can also aggravate autonomic nerve dysfunction instability.
- Therapeutic massage, warm and cold packs and careful positioning contribute to comfort and pain management.
- The patient's surroundings should be pleasant and presentable, especially during long recovery.
- Communication techniques need to be refined to prevent fatigue and frustration.
- Patience, tolerance, empathy, humour and family involvement assist the patient in psychological resilience and recovery.

Intravenous immunoglobulin administration may cause low-grade fever, chills, myalgia, diaphoresis, fluid imbalance, neutropenia, nausea and headaches, and at times acute tubular necrosis. Administration and assessment require adherence to transfusion protocols.[112] Transfusion nurse specialists in collaboration with the patient's nurse perform plasmapheresis.

In the acute phase, accurate diagnosis and timely ventilatory support are provided by effective communication between primary and in-hospital care providers.[112] Multidisciplinary case management is utilised after stabilisation in the acute phase, especially when the level of severity is determined. Recovery and rehabilitation process information is provided to the patient and family so that consultation and communication are effective in recovery.

Myasthenia gravis

Myasthenia gravis is an autoimmune disorder caused by autoantibodies against the nicotinic acetylcholine receptor on the postsynaptic membrane at the neuromuscular junction. It is characterised by weakness and fatiguability of the voluntary muscles. In women, it peaks in the second and third decades of life, while in men it tends to occur in the sixth to eighth decades of life. Although a relatively rare disease, prevalence rates have been rising steadily over time, probably as a result of decreased mortality, longer survival and higher rates of diagnosis.[115] Approximately 20% of patients will experience a myasthenic crisis, typically within 2 years of diagnosis, which can lead to the development of respiratory failure, progressive bulbar weakness, failure of airway protection

and severe limb and truncal weakness causing extensive paralysis, requiring an admission to ICU.[115]

Aetiology

Myasthenic crisis occurs when weakness from acquired myasthenia gravis becomes severe enough to necessitate intubation for ventilatory support or airway protection. Myasthenic crisis is most likely in patients whose history includes previous crisis, oropharyngeal weakness or thymoma. Possible triggers include infections, aspiration, physical and emotional stress and changes in medications.[116] Most antibiotics have a trigger effect and should be carefully prescribed. Median duration of hospitalisation for crisis is 1 month. The patient usually spends half of this time intubated in the ICU. About 25% of patients are extubated on hospital day 7, 50% by hospital day 13, and 75% by hospital day 31. The mortality rate during hospitalisation for crisis has fallen from nearly 50% in the early 1960s to between 3% and 10% today. With the incidence of crisis remaining stable over the past 30 years, this fall in mortality rates probably reflects improvements in the ICU management of these patients.[117]

Pathophysiology

In myasthenia gravis both structural changes in the architecture of the neuromuscular junction and dynamic alterations in the turnover of acetylcholine receptors erode the safety margin and efficiency of neuromuscular transmission. Of all patients with myasthenia gravis, 80–85% have an identifiable and quantifiable antibody found in the immunoglobulin G fraction of plasma, which is responsible for blocking receptors to the action of acetylcholine at the neuromuscular junction.[118] Therefore, successful neuromuscular transmission is markedly affected by small and subtle changes in acetylcholine release and other triggers (as above), and this gives rise to the decrement in transmission with repetitive stimulation and the characteristic fatiguable muscle weakness. Diagnosis is usually by clinical examination and serology testing for antibodies. The 'Tensilon' test, which involves the injection of IV edrophonium and observing the patient for increased eyelid muscle strength, may also be used, although it can cause adverse reactions such as bronchospasm and bradycardia, and false-positive results. Pharmacological management for myasthenia gravis includes the use of anticholinesterases (pyridostigmine), steroids, azathioprine and cyclophosphamide. Thymectomy reduces the antibodies responsible for acetylcholine blockade and is often performed early in the disease.[116,118] Plasmapheresis and IV immunoglobulin are also used in the short term for myasthenic crisis and are especially useful for preventing respiratory collapse or assisting with weaning.

Clinical manifestations

In a myasthenic crisis, vital capacity falls, cough and sigh mechanisms deteriorate, atelectasis develops and hypoxaemia results.[116] Ultimately, fatigue, hypercarbia and ventilatory collapse occur. Commonly, superimposed pulmonary infections lead to increased morbidity and mortality. Assessment for triggers begins with a careful review of systems, with attention to recent fevers, chills, cough, chest pain, dysphagia, nasal regurgitation of liquids and dysuria. Detailed history taking should note any trauma, surgical procedures and medication use. General assessment includes vital signs; ear, nose and throat inspection; chest auscultation; and abdominal check. In addition to supportive care and the removal of triggers, management of myasthenic crisis includes treatment of the underlying myasthenia gravis. An experienced neurologist, who will ultimately provide the patient's care outside the ICU, should be part of the care team. Options for treatment during crisis include: use of acetylcholinesterase inhibitors, plasma exchange, IV immunoglobulins and immunosuppressive drugs, including corticosteroids.[117] Cholinergic crisis and myasthenic crisis are due to two different situations although both cause muscle weakness. Cholinergic activity can increase only if the enzymes that break down acetylcholine are deactivated. This can happen when the patient is taking drugs like neostigmine or pyridostigmine.

Patient management

Careful and accurate assessment in the presenting myasthenic crisis patient determines the triggers of the event and incorporates a history, including infections and prescribed medications. These medications can exacerbate acetylcholine receptor blockade, and respiratory demand proves too much for the patient. Awareness by the nurse of trigger medications ensures advocacy for the patient (see Online resources for published guidelines).

- Respiratory and cardiovascular assessment incorporates upper and lower airway muscle weakness. ABGs are a poor marker for intubation and ventilation because these values change late in the decompensation cycle. Being able to recognise fatigue (inability to speak, poor lung expansion, vital capacity below 1 litre, shoulder and arm weakness) in patients with neuromuscular weakness and air hunger is important.[118]
- Non-invasive ventilation can be difficult to administer safely, with the potential for aspiration due to insidious upper airway weakness; however, the option should be considered with careful assessment of gag, swallow and cough reflexes in order to prevent intubation.[119]
- Neuromuscular blockade should be avoided (because of residual long-term paralysis), with the use of glottal local anaesthetic spray for emergency intubation and ventilation.
- Placement of small-bore duodenal tubes decreases the risk of aspiration and may be more comfortable than regular nasogastric tubes.
- Tracheostomy is generally not needed, as the duration of intubation is often less than 2 weeks.

- Cardiac assessment needs to include assessment for both atrial and ventricular dysrhythmias due to autonomic nerve dysfunction.[117] These can be insidious and can be provoked by subtle changes in electrolytes.
- Nursing care will relate to the needs of long-term immobilised, intubated, ventilated patients with neuromuscular alterations.

Myasthenia gravis patients have similar care needs to those of patients with GBS (refer to Patient management for GBS above). Fatigue and the structure and timing of care are very important. Flexibility of care is important, as energy fluctuates on an hourly basis.[118] Despite having a shorter recovery time than GBS, weaning and recovery in myasthenia gravis is still a slow process and impulsive extubation is discouraged. Therapy should be tailored on an individual basis using best clinical judgement.

Status epilepticus

Status epilepticus is defined as enduring seizure activity that is not likely to stop spontaneously. The traditional definition is 30 minutes of continuous seizure activity (updated to 5 minutes to indicate the point at which treatment should be started) or two or more seizures without full recovery of consciousness between seizures.[119] There are as many types of status epilepticus as there are types of seizures. The distinction between convulsive and non-convulsive status epilepticus depends on clinical observation and on a clear understanding of typology.[120] Estimates of the overall incidence have varied from 9.9 to 41 per 100,000 person-years, depending on the population studied and the definitions used.[121] Over half the cases are acute symptomatic, emphasising the importance of identifying an acute precipitant. In adults, low antiepileptic drug levels, cerebrovascular accident, hypoxia, metabolic causes and alcohol represent the main acute causes. Mortality is about 20%; most patients die of the underlying condition rather than the status epilepticus itself. Status epilepticus can result in permanent neurological and mental deterioration; the risks of morbidity greatly increase with longer duration of the episode. Status epilepticus in the ICU falls into two main groups: those transferred to the ICU because of uncontrolled (refractory) status epilepticus and those who are admitted to the ICU for another reason and have status epilepticus as an additional finding.[122]

Pathophysiology

At a cellular level, status epilepticus results from a failure of normal inhibitory pathways, primarily mediated by gamma-aminobutyric acid acting via gamma-aminobutyric acid A receptors. This loss of inhibitory drive allows the activation of excitatory feedback loops, leading to repetitive, synchronous firing of large groups of neurons. As seizure activity continues, there is a further decline in gamma-aminobutyric inhibitory tone that counterbalances neuronal excitation function. Continued excitatory input mediated primarily by glutamate leads to neuronal cell death.[123]

Clinical manifestations

Convulsive status epilepticus is a medical emergency. The initial consequence of a prolonged convulsion is a massive release of plasma catecholamines, which results in a rise in heart rate, BP and plasma glucose. During this stage, cardiac dysrhythmias are often seen, and may be fatal. CBF is greatly increased, and hence glucose delivery to active cerebral tissue is maintained. As the seizure continues, hyperthermia above 40°C with lactic and respiratory acidosis continues to intensify, especially without adequate resuscitation and control of the seizure.

The status epilepticus may then enter a second, late phase in which cerebral and systemic protective measures progressively fail. The main characteristics of this phase are: a fall in BP, a loss of cerebral autoregulation resulting in the dependence of CBF on systemic BP, and hypoglycaemia due to the exhaustion of glycogen stores and increased neurogenic insulin secretion. ICP can rise precipitously. The combined effects of systemic hypotension and intracranial hypertension may result in a compromised cerebral circulation and cerebral oedema. ICP monitoring is advisable in prolonged cases when raised ICP is suspected. Further complications that can occur include rhabdomyolysis leading to acute tubular necrosis, hyperkalaemia and hyponatraemia.[123]

Patient management

The online resources describe management of seizures in general; however, the following specific status epilepticus aspects of patient management should be considered:

- resuscitation
- specific post-status epilepticus patient assessment
- pharmacological patient management.

Status epilepticus requires control of the seizure and then investigation regarding the cause. Airway protection is often difficult in the seizing patient, so the first line of treatment includes basic life-support measures followed by the administration of IV propofol, midazolam or, in refractory cases, phenytoin. Neuromuscular blockade will be required to facilitate intubation in patients who continue to have tonic–clonic seizure activity despite these pharmacological interventions. A short-acting, non-depolarising muscle relaxant that is devoid of significant haemodynamic effects and does not raise ICP is the preferred agent (e.g. rocuronium). Succinylcholine should be avoided if possible, as the patient may be hyperkalaemic as a consequence of possible rhabdomyolysis. Prolonged neuromuscular blockade should be avoided as it only stops the motor response, hence masking the altered neuronal activity. Once the seizures are controlled, intubation and ventilation can protect the airway and potentially reverse the acidosis.

Practice tip

The three most crucial factors determining the outcome from status epilepticus are the underlying aetiology, the speed of antiseizure treatment and the age of the person. Older-aged individuals with status epilepticus frequently have a symptomatic cause, possess a more limited reserve to recover due to comorbidities and have a higher mortality rate.

Neurological assessment is limited in the sedated patient. Pupillary response is usually sluggish and reflects the medication prescribed. Routine monitoring in an ICU is essential, with CT and MRI to exclude mass lesions. Blood glucose levels should be checked immediately by bedside testing. Blood should be tested for electrolytes, magnesium, phosphate, calcium, liver and renal function, haematocrit, white blood cell count, platelet count, antiepileptic drug levels, toxic drugs and substances (particularly salicylates) and alcohol.

EEG monitoring in the ICU for refractory status epilepticus is essential, as a patient may enter a drug-induced coma with little outward sign of convulsions yet have ongoing electrographic epileptic activity. Furthermore, continuous recording will give an indication of worsening of generalised convulsions regardless of the presence or absence of sedating drugs or paralysing agents. This manifests as bilateral EEG ictal discharges on the monitor. Deeper sedation and anaesthesia are then indicated and can be titrated to EEG results.[124]

The goal of pharmacological therapy is to achieve the rapid and safe termination of the seizure, and to prevent its recurrence without adverse effects on the cardiovascular and respiratory systems or without altering the level of consciousness. Diazepam, lorazepam, midazolam, phenytoin and phenobarbitone have all been used as first-line therapy for the termination of status epilepticus. Sodium valproate may also be used; however, caution should be taken when administering sodium valproate to females of child-bearing age.[125] The best regimen to use will depend on the cause of the seizure and previous antiepileptic drug therapy. A patient who develops status epilepticus during alcohol withdrawal may not need continued medication following the withdrawal process. In contrast, patients with, for example, encephalitis or trauma may require high doses of antiepileptic medication to control seizure activity.

Summary

A description and application of neurological alterations and their management are provided in this chapter, beginning with an overview of neurological dysfunction, specifically pathophysiological alterations of consciousness, alterations in motor and sensory function, and alterations in cerebral perfusion and metabolism. Cerebral oedema is related to ICP preceding the therapeutic management of these conditions. Intracranial hypertension is discussed in association with cerebral perfusion and metabolic events. CNS disorders including traumatic brain and spinal injury, their aetiology, clinical pathophysiology and management are covered. Cerebrovascular disorders that focus on ischaemic stroke, intracerebral haemorrhage and subarachnoid haemorrhage are described. Meningitis and encephalitis are included in the section on infection and inflammation with GBS, myasthenic crisis and status epilepticus in the neuromuscular alterations' component.

Case study

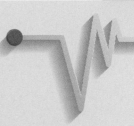

Michael, a 26-year-old male, was holidaying with friends having finished their university course. While out sightseeing, Michael tripped over while crossing a road and fell head first into oncoming traffic. He was struck by a car and was thrown approximately 1.5 metres. An ambulance was called and, when the paramedics arrived, Michael was found to have a decreased level of consciousness. His GCS was initially 10, E 2 V3 and M 5 but as he was being assessed his GCS dropped to 4, E 1 V 1 and M 2. At this time his left pupil was also noted to be unresponsive. The paramedics intubated Michael and administered 100 mL of IV mannitol. Spinal precautions were initiated and Michael was transferred to the emergency department of a large tertiary hospital.

Here a primary trauma survey was carried out and Michael was taken for urgent CT imaging where a CT of head, cervical spine, thorax, abdomen and pelvis was performed. Routine bloods were taken and an ECG was carried out. The results of the CT imaging were:

- comminuted depressed fracture of the left parietal and temporal bones

- extensive contusions of the left parietal and temporal lobes of the brain

- cerebral oedema with 1 cm midline shift

- petechial haemorrhages in the midbrain

- a base of skull fracture

- subarachnoid blood covering the left hemisphere

- all other imaging was clear of injuries.

Michael was taken for emergency surgery where an external ventricular (EVD) drain was inserted and elevation of the depressed skull fracture. On completion of the surgery, Michael remained intubated and was transferred to the ICU. The postoperative orders by the neurosurgeon were to keep the ICP <20 mmHg, place the EVD at 15 cmH$_2$O above the tragus and maintain the cerebral perfusion pressure (CPP) at >65 mmHg.

INITIAL INTENSIVE CARE

In the ICU, Michael remained intubated and ventilated using a mandatory volume-controlled mode with the settings of 12 breaths per minute with tidal volumes of 470 mL, FiO$_2$ 0.3, positive end-expiratory pressure (PEEP) 5 cmH$_2$O and pressure support (PS) 5 cmH$_2$O. End-tidal CO$_2$ (ETCO$_2$) was initiated. Michael was sedated using a propofol infusion and analgesia was a fentanyl infusion. ICP readings fluctuated between 15 and 22 mmHg. An arterial line was inserted with an initial reading of 115/74 mmHg and a MAP of 68 mmHg. A central venous access device (CVAD) was placed and Michael was commenced on a noradrenaline infusion to increase his CPP. Spinal precautions were maintained initially, with Michael positioned using reverse Trendelenburg.

DAYS 1–2

Michael's ICP continued to rise despite optimisation of his ventilation to maintain his PaCO$_2$ on the lower end of normal limits by increasing his respiratory rate to 16/minute. His sedation was increased and a neuromuscular blockade was introduced. The EVD height was reduced to 10 cmH$_2$O. On the 2nd day, Michael had a tonic–clonic seizure lasting approximately 45 seconds, which was treated with clonazepam 1 mg IV. Michael was also loaded with phenytoin 1 g followed by a daily dose of 300 mg. Following this the ICP reading spiked to 36 mmHg and Michael's left pupil dilated and became sluggishly reactive. Hypertonic sodium chloride 3% 100 mL IV was given and Michael was taken for an urgent CT of brain, which showed increased cerebral oedema and midline shift. Based on these results, Michael was taken to theatre for an emergency craniectomy.

DAYS 3–7

Following surgery, Michael's ICP was generally well controlled with his CPP maintained greater than 65 mmHg using a noradrenaline infusion. Michael's pupils had returned to being equal and reactive to light and his spine was radiologically cleared. A progress brain CT showed evolving contusions and a small diffuse axonal injury.

DAYS 8–15

Michael's condition continued to improve with ICP well controlled. The neuromuscular blockade was ceased and sedation lightened. By day 9, Michael obeyed commands for the first time, giving him a GCS score of 10, E 3, V 1, M 6 with a weakness on his right side. Michael was successfully extubated on day 14. His main issue now was confusion and agitation, which was compounded by expressive dysphasia. He was fitted with a helmet to protect the craniectomy site.

DAYS 16–21

On day 16, Michael was considered medically suitable for transfer to the ward setting. While there he progressed with his physio and his confusion and expressive disphasia continued to improve. He was assessed by a rehabilitation specialist and was transferred to a brain injury unit, where he continued to improve. A date was then set for him to return to hospital to have his craniectomy defect repaired with an acrylic cranioplasty.

CASE STUDY QUESTIONS

1 From your reading of the case study, explain the rationale for why pupil dysfunction is ipsilateral while limb movement is contralateral.
2 What is the basis for PaCO$_2$ control in a patient with a traumatic brain injury?
3 Damage to which area of the brain results in Michael having expressive dysphasia? Explain the difference between expressive and receptive dysphasia.
4 Explain the compensatory mechanisms used by the body to help control intracranial pressure.

RESEARCH VIGNETTE

Roberts I, Shakur-Still H, Aeron-Thomas A, et al; CRASH-3 Collaborators. Effects of tranexamic acid on death, disability, vascular occlusive events and other morbidities in patients with acute traumatic brain injury (CRASH-3): a randomized placebo-controlled trial. Lancet 2019;394:1713–23.

Abstract

Background: Tranexamic acid reduces surgical bleeding and decreases mortality in patients with traumatic extracranial bleeding. Intracranial bleeding is common after TBI and can cause brain herniation and death. We aimed to assess the effects of tranexamic acid in patients with TBI.

Methods: This randomised, placebo-controlled trial was done in 175 hospitals in 29 countries. Adults with TBI who were within 3 h of injury, had a GCS score of 12 or lower or any intracranial bleeding on CT scan, and no major extracranial bleeding cases were eligible. The time window for eligibility was originally 8 h, but in 2016 the protocol was changed to limit recruitment to patients within 3 h of injury. This change was made blind to the trial data, in response to external evidence suggesting that delayed treatment is unlikely to be effective. We randomly assigned (1:1) patients to receive tranexamic acid (loading dose 1 g over 10 min then infusion of 1 g over 8 h) or matching placebo. Patients were assigned by selecting a numbered treatment pack from a box containing eight packs that were identical apart from the pack number. Patients, caregivers and those assessing outcomes were masked to allocation. The primary outcome was head injury-related death in hospital within 28 days of injury in patients treated within 3 h of injury. We prespecified a sensitivity analysis that excluded patients with a GCS score of 3 and those with bilateral unreactive pupils at baseline. All analyses were done by intention to treat. This trial was registered with ISRCTN (ISRCTN15088122), ClinicalTrials. gov (NCT01402882), EudraCT (2011-003669-14) and the Pan African Clinical Trial Registry (PACTR20121000441277).

Results: Between 20 July 2012 and 31 Jan 2019, we randomly allocated 12,737 patients with TBI to receive tranexamic acid (6406 (50.3%)) or placebo (6331 (49.7%)), of whom 9202 (72.2%) patients were treated within 3 h of injury. Among patients treated within 3 h of injury, the risk of head injury-related death was 18.5% in the tranexamic acid group versus 19.8% in the placebo group (855 vs 892 events; risk ratio (RR) 0.94 (95% confidence interval (CI) 0.86–1.02)). In the prespecified sensitivity analysis that excluded patients with a GCS score of 3 or bilateral unreactive pupils at baseline, the risk of head injury-related death was 12.5% in the tranexamic acid group versus 14.0% in the placebo group (485 vs 525 events; RR 0.89 (95% CI 0.80–1.00)). The risk of head injury-related death reduced with tranexamic acid in patients with mild-to-moderate head injury (RR 0.78 (95% CI 0.64–0.95)) but not in patients with severe head injury (0.99 (95% CI 0.91–1.07); P value for heterogeneity 0.030). Early treatment was more effective than was later treatment in patients with mild and moderate head injury ($P = 0.005$), but time to treatment had no obvious effect in patients with severe head injury ($P = 0.73$). The risk of vascular occlusive events was similar in the tranexamic acid and placebo groups (RR 0.98 (0.74–1.28)). The risk of seizures was also similar between groups (1.09 (95% CI 0.90–1.33)).

Interpretation: Our results show that tranexamic acid is safe in patients with TBI and that treatment within 3 h of injury reduces head injury-related death. Patients should be treated as soon as possible after injury.

Critique

This study aimed to examine whether early administration of tranexamic acid reduces mortality in patients who have sustained a traumatic brain injury. Previous studies excluded those who sustained a TBI, although it is known that tranexamic acid reduces the risk of bleeding in general trauma patients and is a cost-effective way to reduce risk of death from haemorrhage.

It is well known that those who develop intracranial bleeding following a TBI have an increased risk of death and therefore the CRASH-3 investigators have an excellent rationale for investigating the effect of administration of tranexamic acid on those patients who develop a TBI.

The strengths of this study include the randomised control design. Randomised controlled trials (RCTs) are the gold standard design for establishing cause-and-effect relationships and are ideal for investigating the effect of a drug on a large defined target population such as those patients who develop a TBI. This study was a very large multicentre trial carried out across a range of countries. This increases the external validity as the intervention is examined across different geographical locations and differing economic circumstances. Participating centres were also blinded as to which arm of the trial patients were allocated to. This is a strength, as it prevents detection bias where an intervention may be over- or underestimated according to clinician subjectivity.

There are, however, several limitations which should be considered when applying these results to practice. There was no described standard protocol for management strategies that patients may have received other than the trial intervention. This means that there may be other interventions which contributed to either a lower or higher risk of death, so potentially skewing results.

In the context of critically ill patients who sustain a severe TBI, there was no significant difference in mortality rates between the two arms when all types of TBI (mild, moderate and severe) were grouped together: 18.5% tranexamic acid group vs 19.8% in the placebo group (0.94 (0.86–1.02)). Given that many patients admitted to critical areas are more likely to have sustained a severe TBI, critical care practitioners need to accurately assess severity of TBI so as to avoid futile or even potentially harmful treatments.

Overall, this study suggests that the administration of tranexamic acid reduces mortality in the first 3 hours following a mild-to-moderate TBI. Further investigation examining interventions which may reduce mortality rates for those patients who develop a severe TBI is required.

Learning activities

1 What are the main causes of raised ICP?

2 Describe the management of a patient with raised ICP.

3 Explain the differences between the various types of stroke and briefly outline the management of each.

4 Describe the possible complications associated with a subarachnoid haemorrhage.

5 Explain the treatments available for a patient admitted with an ischaemic stroke.

6 A patient has been admitted following a high-speed motor vehicle accident which resulted in a C4–C5 SCI.

   a Describe the mechanisms of injury to the spinal cord involved with this type of accident.

   b Outline the initial management of this patient.

7 What is the clinical management of a patient who presents in status epilepticus?

8 Define hydrocephalus and the possible causes of the development of this condition.

9 Describe the differences between bacterial and viral meningitis in terms of presentation and treatment.

Online resources

TRAUMATIC BRAIN INJURY

AACN Clinical Practice Guideline series. Care of the patient undergoing intracranial pressure monitoring/external ventricular drainage or lumbar drainage, https://aann.mycrowdwisdom.com/diweb/catalog/item/id/1514646.

Brain Trauma Foundation. Guidelines for the management of severe TBI. 4th ed, https://braintrauma.org/guidelines/guidelines-for-the-management-of-severe-tbi-4th-ed#/

BMJ Best practice. Assessment of traumatic brain injury, acute, https://bestpractice.bmj.com/topics/en-gb/515#referencePop1

Centers for Disease Control and Prevention. Traumatic brain injury and concussion, https://www.cdc.gov/traumaticbraininjury

CSF drainage and ICP monitoring system, https://www.youtube.com/watch?v=MPpH8MnXhb8&list=PLH9gpVKlHL6p09 M1Pz8Upo qggfwLsfxzA

National Resource Centre for Traumatic Brain Injury, https://www.brainlink.org.au

SPINAL CORD INJURY

Academy Spinal Cord Injury Nurses (ASCIP), https://www.academyscipro.org

BMJ Best Practice: acute cervical spine trauma,

Cervical collars, https://www.youtube.com/watch?v=cYxnp6ml8mE

Emergency Neurological Life Support. Traumatic spine injury protocol, 2019, https://higherlogicdownload.s3.amazonaws. com/NEUROCRITICALCARE/fdc4bb32-6722-417b-8839-f68ac1ef3794/UploadedImages/ENLS_Documents/ENLS_V4.0_ protocol%20files/ENLS_V_4_0_Protocol_TSI_FINAL.pdf.

International Spinal Cord Society (ISCoS),

National Institute for Health and Care Excellence (NICE). Guideline NG41. Spinal injury: assessment and initial management, https://www.nice.org.uk/guidance/ng41/evidence/full-guideline-2358425776

STROKE

AHA/ASA GUIDELINE 2012. Guidelines for the management of aneurysmal subarachnoid hemorrhage: a guideline for healthcare professionals from the American Heart Association/American Stroke Association,

AHA/ASA GUIDELINE 2018. Guidelines for the early management of patients with acute ischemic stroke: a guideline for healthcare professionals from the American Heart Association/American Stroke Association, https://stroke.ahajournals. org/content/49/3/e46

AHA/ASA GUIDELINE 2021. 2021 guideline for the prevention of stroke in patients with stroke and transient ischemic attack: a guideline from the American Heart Association/American Stroke Association, https://www.ahajournals.org/doi/10.1161/STR.0000000000000375

AHA/ASA GUIDELINE 2022. Guidelines for the management of patients with spontaneous intracerebral hemorrhage: a guideline for healthcare professionals from the American Heart Association/American Stroke Association, https://www.ahajournals.org/doi/epub/10.1161/STR.0000000000000407

Australian Institute of Health and Welfare. Stroke and its management in Australia: an update, https://www.aihw.gov.au/publication-detail/?id=60129543613

BMJ Best Practice. Ischaemic stroke, https://bestpractice.bmj.com/topics/en-gb/3000114

BMJ Best Practice. Stroke due to spontaneous intracerebral haemorrhage, https://bestpractice.bmj.com/topics/en-gb/3000109

National Institute for Health and Care Excellence (NICE). Stroke and transient ischaemic attack, https://www.nice.org.uk/guidance/conditions-and-diseases/cardiovascular-conditions/stroke-and-transient-ischaemic-attack

National Stroke Foundation of Australia, https://strokefoundation.org.au

INFECTIONS

BMJ Best Practice. Bacterial meningitis in adults, https://bestpractice.bmj.com/topics/en-gb/539

British Infection Association. Published guidelines, https://www.britishinfection.org/guidelines-resources/published-guidelines/

Centers for Disease Control and Prevention. Guideline for isolation precautions: preventing transmission of infectious agents in healthcare settings, https://www.cdc.gov/infectioncontrol/guidelines/isolation/appendix/transmission-precautions.html

GUILLAIN–BARRÉ/MYASTHENIA GRAVIS

BMJ Best Practice. Guillain–Barré syndrome, https://bestpractice.bmj.com/topics/en-gb/176

GBS/CIDP Foundation International, https://www.gbs-cidp.org/

Myasthenia Gravis Foundation America. International consensus guidance for management of myasthenia gravis, https://n.neurology.org/content/neurology/early/2016/06/29/WNL.0000000000002790.full.pdf

STATUS EPILEPTICUS

American Epilepsy Society. Guidelines, https://www.aesnet.org/clinical-care/clinical-guidance/guidelines

BMJ Best Practice. Status epilepticus, https://bestpractice.bmj.com/topics/en-gb/464

Further reading

Hachem LD, Ahuja CS, Fehlings MG. Assessment and management of acute spinal cord injury: from point of injury to rehabilitation. J Spinal Cord Med 2017;40(6):665–75.

Hickey J, Strayer A. The clinical practice of neurological and neurosurgical nursing. 8th ed. Philadelphia: Lippincott Williams & Wilkins; 2019.

Hussein MTEL, Zettel S, Suykens AM. The ABCs of managing increased intracranial pressure. J Nurs Educ Pract 2017;7(4):6–14.

References

1. Cavanna AE, Shah S, Eddy CM, et al. Consciousness: a neurological perspective. Behav Neurol 2011;24(1):107–16.

2. Edlow JA, Rabinstein A, Traub SJ, et al. Diagnosis of reversible causes of coma. Lancet 2014;384(9959):2064–76.

3. Cavanna AE, Cavanna SL, Servo S, et al. The neural correlates of impaired consciousness in coma and unresponsive states. Discov Med 2010;9(48):431–8.

4. Strosznajder RP, Czubowicz K, Jesko H, et al. Poly(ADP-ribose) metabolism in brain and its role in ischemia pathology. Mol Neurobiol 2010;41(2–3):187–96.

5. Huff JS, Fountain NB. Pathophysiology and definitions of seizures and status epilepticus. Emerg Med Clin North Am 2011;29(1):1–13.

6. Varelas PN, Spanaki MV, Mirski MA. Status epilepticus: an update. Curr Neurol Neurosci Rep 2013;13(7):357.

7. Veening JG, Barendregt HP. The regulation of brain states by neuroactive substances distributed via the cerebrospinal fluid; a review. Cerebrospinal Fluid Res 2010;6(7):1.

8. Winhammar J, Rowe D, Henderson R, et al. Assessment of disease progression in motor neuron disease. Lancet Neurol 2005;4(4):229–38.

9. Di Pino G, Pellegrino G, Assenza G, et al. Modulation of brain plasticity in stroke: a novel model for neurorehabilitation. Nat Rev Neurol 2014;10(10):597–608.

10. Shepherd S, Batra A, Lerner DP. Review of critical illness myopathy and neuropathy. Neurohospitalist 2017;7(1):41–8. doi: 10.1177/1941874416663279.

11. Edriss H, Selvan K, Sigler M, et al. Glucose levels in patients with acute respiratory failure requiring mechanical ventilation. J Intensive Care Med 2017;32(10):578–84.

12. Silverman MN, Heim CM, Nater UM, et al. Neuroendocrine and immune contributors to fatigue. PM R 2010;2(5):338–46.

13. Guan L, Collet JP, Mazowita G, et al. Autonomic nervous system and stress to predict secondary ischemic events after transient ischemic attack or minor stroke: possible implications of heart rate variability. Front Neurol 2018;(9):90. doi: 10.3389/fneur.2018.00090.

14. Bulstrode H, Nicoll JAR, Hudson G, et al. Mitochondrial DNA and traumatic brain injury. Ann Neurol 2014;75(2):186–95.

15. Trendelenburg G. Molecular regulation of cell fate in cerebral ischemia: role of the inflammasome and connected pathways. J Cereb Blood Flow Metab 2014;34(12):1857–67.

16. Jhelum P, Karisetty BC, Kumar A, et al. Implications of epigenetic mechanisms and their targets in cerebral ischemia models. Curr Neuropharmacol 2017;15(6):815–30.

17. Kumar VSS, Gopalakrishnan A, Naziroglu M, et al. Calcium ion – the key player in cerebral ischemia. Curr Med Chem 2014;21(18):2065–75.

18. Giacino JT, Fins JJ, Laureys S, et al. Disorders of consciousness after acquired brain injury: the state of the science. Nat Rev Neurol 2014;10(2):99–114.

19. Partington T, Farmery A. Intracranial pressure and cerebral blood flow. Anaesth Intensive Care Med 2014;15(4):189–94.

20. Halstead MR, Geocadin RG. The medical management of cerebral edema: past, present, and future therapies. Neurotherapeutics 2019;16(4):1133–48. doi: 10.1007/s13311-019-00779-4.

21. Stokum JA, Gerzanich V, Simard JM. Molecular pathophysiology of cerebral edema. J Cereb Blood Flow Metab 2016;36(3):513–38.

22. Kiefer M, Unterberg A. The differential diagnosis and treatment of normal-pressure hydrocephalus. Dtsch Arztebl Int 2012;109(1–2):15–26.

23. McLeod A. Traumatic injuries to the head and spine, 2: nursing considerations. Br J Nurs 2004;13(17):1041–9.

24. Cummings BM, Yager PH, Murphy SA, et al. Managing edema and intracranial pressure in the intensive care unit. In: Lo EH, Lok J, Ning MM, et al, editors. Vascular mechanisms in CNS trauma. New York: Springer; 2014. p. 363–78.

25. Di Ieva A, Schmitz EM, Cusimano MD. Analysis of intracranial pressure: past, present, and future. Neuroscientist 2013;19(6):592–603.

26. Czosnyka M, Pickard J. Monitoring and interpretation of intracranial pressure. J Neurol Neurosurg Psychiat 2004;75(6):813–21.

27. Porth C, Gaspard K. Essentials of pathophysiology: concepts of altered health states. 4th ed. Philadelphia: Wolters Kluwer; 2015.

28. Latronico N. The relationship between the intracranial pressure – volume index and cerebral autoregulation. Intensive Care Med 2013;1:153.

29. Kirkman MA, Smith M. Multimodality neuromonitoring. Anesthesiol Clin 2016;34(3):511–23.

30. Stocchetti N, Maas AI. Traumatic intracranial hypertension. N Engl J Med 2014;370(22):2121–30.

31. Brain Trauma Foundation. Guidelines for the management of severe traumatic brain injury. 4th ed. Palo Alto, CA: Brain Trauma Foundation; 2016. Available from: www.braintrauma.org.

32. Kheirbek T, Pascual J. Hypertonic saline for the treatment of intracranial hypertension. Curr Neurol Neurosci Rep 2014;14(9):1–6.

33. Chen H, Song Z, Dennis JA. Hypertonic saline versus other intracranial pressure-lowering agents for people with acute traumatic brain injury. Cochrane Database Syst Rev 2020;1(1):CD010904. doi: 10.1002/14651858.CD010904.pub3.

34. Berger-Pelleiter E, Émond M, Lauzier F, et al. Hypertonic saline in severe traumatic brain injury: a systematic review and meta-analysis of randomized controlled trials. CJEM 2016;18(2):112–20.

35. Yenari MA, Colbourne F, Hemmen TM, et al. Therapeutic hypothermia in stroke. Stroke Res Treat 2011;2011:157969. doi: 10.4061/2011/157969.

36. Akbari Y, Mulder M, Razmara A, et al. Cool down the inflammation: hypothermia as a therapeutic strategy for acute brain injuries. In: Chen J, Hu X, Stenzel-Poore M, et al, editors. Immunological mechanisms and therapies in brain injuries and stroke. Springer Series in Translational Stroke Research 6. New York: Springer; 2014. p. 349–75.

37. Marion DW, Regasa LE. Revisiting therapeutic hypothermia for severe traumatic brain injury … again. Crit Care 2014;18(3):160.

38. Kirkman MA. Targeted temperature management and acute brain injury: an update from recent clinical trials. Curr Anesthesiol Rep 2016;6(3):214–22.

39. Cariou A, Payen JF, Asehnoune K, et al; Société de Réanimation de Langue Française (SRLF) and the Société Française d'Anesthésie et de Réanimation (SFAR) in conjunction with the Association de Neuro Anesthésie Réanimation de Langue Française (ANARLF), the Groupe Francophone de Réanimation et Urgences Pédiatriques (GFRUP), the Société Française de Médecine d'Urgence (SFMU) and the Société Française Neuro-Vasculaire (SFNV). Targeted temperature management in the ICU: guidelines from a French expert panel. Ann Intensive Care 2017;7(70):1–14.

40. Howes D, Gray SH, Brooks SC, et al. Canadian guidelines for the use of targeted temperature management (therapeutic hypothermia) after cardiac arrest: a joint statement from The Canadian Critical Care Society (CCCS), Canadian Neurocritical Care Society (CNCCS), and the Canadian Critical Care Trials Group (CCCTG). Resuscitation 2016;98:48–63.

41. Donnino MW, Andersen LW, Berg KM, et al; the ILCOR ALS Task Force. Temperature management after cardiac arrest. Resuscitation 2016;98:97–104.

42. Povlishock JT, Wei EP. Posthypothermic rewarming considerations following traumatic brain injury. J Neurotrauma 2009;26(3):333–40.

43. Edwards P, Arango M, Balica L, et al. Final results of MRC CRASH, a randomised placebo-controlled trial of intravenous corticosteroid in adults with head injury – outcomes at 6 months. Lancet 2005;365(9475):1957–9.

44. Tritos NA, Yuen KC, Kelly DF, et al. American Association of Clinical Endocrinologists and American College of Endocrinology disease state clinical review: a neuroendocrine approach to patients with traumatic brain injury. Endocr Pract 2015;21:823.

45. Adembri C, Venturi L, Pellegrini-Giampietro DE. Neuroprotective effects of propofol in acute cerebral injury. CNS Drug Rev 2007;13:333–51.

46. Li LM, Timofeev I, Czosnyka M, et al. Review article: the surgical approach to the management of increased intracranial pressure after traumatic brain injury. Anesth Analg 2010;111(3):736–48.

47. Vibbert M, Mayer SA. Early decompressive hemicraniectomy following malignant ischemic stroke: the crucial role of timing. Curr Neurol Neurosci Rep 2010;10(1):1–3.

48. Cooper JD, Rosenfeld JV, Murray L, et al. Decompressive craniectomy in diffuse traumatic brain injury. N Engl J Med 2011;364(16):1493–502.

49. Hutchinson PJ, Kolias AG, Timofeev IS, et al; for the RESCUEicp Trial Collaborators. Trial of decompressive craniectomy for traumatic intracranial hypertension. N Engl J Med 2016;375:1119–30.

50. Anderson CS, Arima H, Lavados P, et al; for the HeadPoST Investigators and Coordinators. Cluster-randomized, crossover trial of head positioning in acute stroke. N Engl J Med 2017;376:2437–47.

51. Haddad SH, Arabi YM. Critical care management of severe traumatic brain injury in adults. Scand J Trauma Resusc Emerg Med 2012;20(12):1–15.

52. Ferreira LL, Valenti VE, Vanderlei LCM. Chest physiotherapy on intracranial pressure of critically ill patients admitted to the intensive care unit: a systematic review. Rev Bras Ter Intensiva 2013;25(4):327–33.

53. Roozenbeek B, Maas AI, Menon DK. Changing patterns in the epidemiology of traumatic brain injury. Nat Rev Neurol 2013;9(4):231–6.

54. Nguyen R, Fiest KM, McChesney J, et al. The international incidence of traumatic brain injury: a systematic review and meta-analysis. Can J Neurol Sci 2016;43(6):774–85.

55. National Center for Injury Prevention and Control. Rates of TBI-related hospitalizations by age group – United States, 2001–2010. Atlanta, GA: Centers for Disease Control and Prevention; 2014. Available from: https://data.cdc.gov/Traumatic-Brain-Injury-/Rates-of-TBI-related-Deaths-by-Age-Group-United-St/nq6q-szvs [Accessed 15 February 2023].

56. Peeters W, van den Brande R, Polinder S, et al. Epidemiology of traumatic brain injury in Europe. Acta Neurochir (Wien) 2015;157(10):1683–96.

57. Myburgh JA, Cooper DJ, Finfer SR, et al. Epidemiology and 12-month outcomes from traumatic brain injury in Australia and New Zealand. J Trauma 2008;64(4):854–62.

58. Iaccarino C, Carretta A, Nicolosi F, et al. Epidemiology of severe traumatic brain injury. J Neurosurg Sci 2018;62(5):535–41. doi: 10.23736/S0390-5616.18.04532-0.

59. Soustiel JF, Sviri GE, Mahamid E, et al. Cerebral blood flow and metabolism following decompressive craniectomy for control of increased intracranial pressure. Neurosurgery 2010;67(1):65–72.

60. Badruddin A, Taqi MA, Abraham MG, et al. Neurocritical care of a reperfused brain. Curr Neurol Neurosci 2011;11(1):104–10.

61. Choi HA, Jeon S-B, Samuel S, et al. Paroxysmal sympathetic hyperactivity after acute brain injury. Curr Neurol Neurosci Rep 2013;13(8):1–10.

62. Zakharova N, Kornienko V, Potapov A, et al. Mapping of cerebral blood flow in focal and diffuse brain injury. In: Zakharova N, Kornienko V, Potapov A, et al, editors. Neuroimaging of traumatic brain injury. Berlin: Springer International Publishing; 2014, p. 107–23.

63. Rabinowitz AR, Li X, Levin HS. Sport and nonsport etiologies of mild traumatic brain injury: similarities and differences. Annu Rev Psychol 2014;65:301–31.

64. Fitzharris M, Cripps RA, Lee BB. Estimating the global incidence of traumatic spinal cord injury. Spinal Cord 2014;52(2):117–22.

65. Singh A, Tetreault L, Kalsi-Ryan S, et al. Global prevalence and incidence of traumatic spinal cord injury. Clin Epidemiol 2014;6:309–31.

66. Jazayeri SB, Beygi S, Shokraneh F, et al. Incidence of traumatic spinal cord injury worldwide: a systematic review. Eur Spine J 2015;24(5):905–18.

67. Wilson JR, Cho N, Fehlings MG. Acute traumatic spinal cord injury: epidemiology, evaluation, and management. In: Patel VV, Patel AP, Harrop JS, et al, editors. Spine surgery basics. Berlin: Springer-Verlag; 2014. p. 399–409.

68. Silva NA, Sousa N, Reis RL, et al. From basics to clinical: a comprehensive review on spinal cord injury. Prog Neurobiol 2014;114:25–57.

69. Evans LT, Lollis SS, Ball PA. Management of acute spinal cord injury in the neurocritical care unit. Neurosurg Clin N Am 2013;24(3):339–47.

70. Lo V, Esquenazi Y, Han MK, et al. Critical care management of patients with acute spinal cord injury. J Neurosurg Sci 2013;57(4):281–92.

71. Eckert MJ, Martin MJ. Trauma: spinal cord injury. Surg Clin North Am 2017;97(5):1031–45.

72. Pimentel L, Diegelmann L. Evaluation and management of acute cervical spine trauma. Emerg Med Clin North Am 2010;28(4):719–38.

73. National Institute for Health and Care Excellence (NICE). Spinal injury: assessment and initial management. NG41. London: NICE; 2016. Available from: https://www.nice.org.uk/guidance/ng41. [Accessed 15 February 2023].

74. Ulndreaj A, Badner A, Fehlings MG. Promising neuroprotective strategies for traumatic spinal cord injury with a focus on the differential effects among anatomical levels of injury. F1000Res 2017;6:1907. doi: 10.12688/f1000research.11633.1.

75. World Health Organization (WHO). The top ten causes of death. Geneva: WHO; 2017. Available from: https://www.who.int/mediacentre/factsheets/fs310/en/. [Accessed 15 February 2023].

76. American Heart Association (AHA). Statistical update. Heart disease and stroke statistics – 2018 update. A report from the American Heart Association. Circulation 2018;137:e67–492.

77. Townsend N, Wickramasinghe K, Bhatnagar P, et al. Coronary heart disease statistics 2012 edition. London: British Heart Foundation; 2012.

78. Chung JM. Seizures in the acute stroke setting. Neurol Res 2014;36(5):403–6.

79. Powers WJ, Rabinstein AA, Ackerson T, et al; on behalf of the American Heart Association Stroke Council. Guidelines for the early management of patients with acute ischemic stroke: a guideline for healthcare professionals from the American Heart Association/American Stroke Association. Stroke 2018;49(3):e46–110. doi: 10.1161/STR.0000000000000158.

80. Van Asch CJ, Luitse MJ, Rinkel GJ, et al. Incidence, case fatality, and functional outcome of intracerebral haemorrhage over time, according to age, sex, and ethnic origin: a systematic review and meta-analysis. Lancet Neurol 2010;9:167–76.

81. Hemphill JC, Greenberg SM, Anderson CS, et al. Guidelines for the management of spontaneous intracerebral hemorrhage: a guideline for healthcare professionals from the American Heart Association/American Stroke Association. Stroke 2015;46(7):2032–60.

82. Powers WJ, Rabinstein AA, Ackerson T, et al. Guidelines for the early management of patients with acute ischemic stroke: 2019 update to the 2018 guidelines for the early management of acute ischemic stroke: a guideline for healthcare professionals from the American Heart Association/American Stroke Association. Stroke 2018;50(12):e344–418. doi: 10.1161/STR.0000000000000211.

83. National Institute for Health and Care Excellence (NICE). Stroke and transient ischaemic attack in over 16s: diagnosis and initial management NG128. London: NICE; 2022. Available from: https://www.nice.org.uk/guidance/ng128/chapter/Recommendations#blood-pressure-control-for-people-with-acute-intracerebral-haemorrhage. [Accessed 15 February 2023].

84. Steiner T, Al-Shahi Salman R, Beer R, et al. European Stroke Organisation guidelines for the management of spontaneous intracerebral hemorrhage. Int J Stroke 2014;9(7):840–55.

85. Zhou Y, Wang Y, Wang J, et al. Inflammation in intracerebral hemorrhage: from mechanisms to clinical translation. Prog Neurobiol 2014;115:25–44.

86. Tan X, He J, Li L, et al. Early hyperglycaemia and the early-term death in patients with spontaneous intracerebral haemorrhage: a meta-analysis. Internal Med J 2014;44(3):254–60.

87. Teasdale GM, Drake CG, Hunt W, et al. A universal subarachnoid hemorrhage scale: report of a committee of the World Federation of Neurosurgical Societies. J Neurol Neurosurg Psychiatry 1988;51(11):1457.

88. Helbok R, Kurtz P, Vibbert M, et al. Early neurological deterioration after subarachnoid haemorrhage: risk factors and impact on outcome. J Neurol Neurosurg Psychiatry 2013;84(3):266–70.

89. Connolly ES, Rabinstein AA, Carhuapoma JR, et al; American Heart Association Stroke Council; Council on Cardiovascular Radiology and Intervention; Council on Cardiovascular Nursing; Council on Cardiovascular Surgery and Anesthesia; Council on Clinical Cardiology. Guidelines for the management of aneurysmal subarachnoid hemorrhage: a guideline for healthcare professionals from the American Heart Association/American Stroke Association. Stroke 2012;43(6):1711–37.

90. Tagami T, Kuwamoto K, Watanabe A, et al. Effect of triple-H prophylaxis on global end-diastolic volume and clinical outcomes in patients with aneurysmal subarachnoid hemorrhage. Neurocrit Care 2014;21(3):462–9.

91. Hamdan A, Barnes J, Mitchell P. Subarachnoid hemorrhage and the female sex: analysis of risk factors, aneurysm characteristics, and outcomes. J Neurosurg 2014;121(6):1367–73.

92. Moussouttas M, Lai EW, Huynh TT, et al. Association between acute sympathetic response, early onset vasospasm, and delayed vasospasm following spontaneous subarachnoid hemorrhage. J Clin Neurosci 2014;21(2):256–62.

93. de Rooij NK, Rinkel GJ, Dankbaar JW, et al. Delayed cerebral ischemia after subarachnoid hemorrhage: a systematic review of clinical, laboratory, and radiological predictors. Stroke 2013;44(1):43–54.

94. Brathwaite S, Macdonald RL. Current management of delayed cerebral ischemia: update from results of recent clinical trials. Transl Stroke Res 2014;5(2):207–26.

95. Sarrafzadeh AS, Vajkoczy P, Bijlenga P, et al. Monitoring in neurointensive care – the challenge to detect delayed cerebral ischemia in high grade aSAH. Front Neurol 2014;5:34.

96. Fisher C, Kistler J, Davis J. Relation of cerebral vasospasm to subarachnoid hemorrhage visualized by computerized tomographic scanning. Neurosurgery 1980;6(1):1–9.

97. Luoma A, Reddy U. Acute management of aneurysmal subarachnoid haemorrhage. Contin Educ Anaesth Crit Care Pain 2013;13(2):52–8.

98. Diringer MN, Bleck TP, Claude Hemphill J 3rd, et al; Neurocritical Care Society. Critical care management of patients following aneurysmal subarachnoid hemorrhage: recommendations from the Neurocritical Care Society's Multidisciplinary Consensus Conference. Neurocrit Care 2011;15:211–40.

99. Sandström N, Yan B, Dowling R, et al. Comparison of microsurgery and endovascular treatment on clinical outcome following poor-grade subarachnoid hemorrhage. J Clin Neurosci 2013;20(9):1213–18.

100. Coutinho JM, Zuurbier SM, Aramideh M, et al. The incidence of cerebral venous thrombosis: a cross-sectional study. Stroke 2012;43:3375.

101. Devasagayam S, Wyatt B, Leyden J, et al. Cerebral venous sinus thrombosis incidence is higher than previously thought: a retrospective population-based study. Stroke 2016;47:2180–2.

102. De Michele M, Kahan J, Berto I, et al. Cerebrovascular complications of COVID-19 and COVID-19 vaccination. Circ Res 2022;130(8):1187–203. doi: 10.1161/CIRCRESAHA.122.319954, 10.1161/CIRCRESAHA.122.319954.

103. World Health Organization (WHO). Meningococcal meningitis. Geneva: WHO; 2021. Available from: http://www.who.int/en/news-room/fact-sheets/detail/meningococcal-meningitis. [Accessed 15 February 2023].

104. Bradshaw M, Venkatesan A. Herpes simplex virus-1 encephalitis in adults: pathophysiology, diagnosis, and management. Neurotherapeutics 2016;13(3):493–508.

105. Hills SL, Rabe IB, Fischer M. Travelers' health. Chapter 4: Infectious diseases related to travel. Japanese encephalitis. Centers for Disease Control and Prevention (CDC). Atlanta, GA: CDC; 2018. Available from: https://wwwnc.cdc.gov/travel/yellowbook/2018/infectious-diseases-related-to-travel/japanese-encephalitis. [Accessed 15 February 2023].

106. Middleton D, Pallister J, Klein R, et al. Hendra virus vaccine, a one health approach to protecting horse, human, and environmental health. Emerg Infect Dis 2014;20(3):372.

107. Rozenberg F. Acute viral encephalitis. Handb Clin Neurol 2013;112:1171–81.

108. Vellozzi C, Iqbal S, Stewart B, et al. Cumulative risk of Guillain–Barré syndrome among vaccinated and unvaccinated populations during the 2009 H1N1 influenza pandemic. Am J Public Health 2014;104(4):696–701.

109. Bhagat H, Dash HH, Chauhan RS, et al. Intensive care management of Guillain–Barré syndrome: a retrospective outcome study and review of literature. J Neuroanaesth Crit Care 2014;1(3):188.

110. Ruts L, Drenthen J, Jongen JLM, et al. Pain in Guillain–Barré syndrome: a long-term follow-up study. Neurology 2010;75(16):1439–47.

111. BMJ Best Practice. Guillain–Barré syndrome. London: BMJ; 2017. Available from: https://bestpractice.bmj.com/topics/en-gb/176. [Accessed 15 February 2023].

112. Yuki N, Hartung H-P. Guillain–Barré syndrome. N Engl J Med 2012;366(24):2294–304.

113. van den Berg B, Walgaard C, Drenthen J, et al. Guillain–Barré syndrome: pathogenesis, diagnosis, treatment and prognosis. Nature Rev Neurol 2014;10(8):469–82.

114. Spilane J, Higham E. Myasthenia gravis. BMJ 2012;345:e8497.

115. Vacca V. Myasthenia gravis and myasthenic crisis. Nurs Crit Care 2017;12(5):38–46.

116. Sakaguchi H, Yamashita S, Hirano T, et al. Myasthenic crisis patients who require intensive care unit management. Muscle Nerve 2012;46(3):440–2.

117. Bhagat H, Grover V, Jangra K. What is optimal in patients with myasthenic crisis: invasive or non-invasive ventilation? J Neuroanaesth Crit Care 2014;1(2):116.

118. Sánchez S, Rincon F. Status epilepticus: epidemiology and public health needs. J Clin Med 2016;5(8):71.

119. Huff JS, Fountain NB. Pathophysiology and definitions of seizures and status epilepticus. Emerg Med Clin North Am 2011;29(1):1–13.

120. Neligan A, Sander JW. Epidemiology of seizures and epilepsy. Epilepsy 2013;28–32.

121. Hocker S, Wijdicks EF, Rabinstein AA. Refractory status epilepticus: new insights in presentation, treatment, and outcome. Neurol Res 2013;35(2):163–8.

122. Fernandez A, Claassen J. Refractory status epilepticus. Curr Opin Crit Care 2012;18(2):127–31.

123. Claassen J, Taccone FS, Horn P, et al. Recommendations on the use of EEG monitoring in critically ill patients: consensus statement from the neurointensive care section of the ESICM. Intensive Care Med 2013;39(8):1337–51.

124. Dankiewicz J, Cronberg T, Lilja G, et al. Hypothermia versus normothermia after out-of-hospital cardiac arrest. N Engl J Med 2021;384:2283–94. doi: 10.1056/NEJMoa2100591

125. National Institute for Clinical Excellence (NICE). Epilepsies in children, young people and adults. NG217. London: NICE; 2022. Available from: https://www.nice.org.uk/guidance/ng217. [Accessed 15 February 2023].

Chapter 18

Support of renal function

Ian Baldwin

Learning objectives

After reading this chapter, you should be able to:

- differentiate between acute and chronic renal failure and describe the most likely causes of kidney injury in the critically ill adult
- outline treatment approaches in managing acute kidney injury (AKI) in critical illness
- describe the indications for renal replacement therapy in critical care
- understand the circuit and key components included for dialysis support and renal replacement therapy in the critically ill
- appreciate the unique and purpose-made fluids used to achieve this along with the importance of fluid balance in the anuric patient with an AKI
- understand the assessment and markers for AKI and the biomarkers for identification of kidney injury
- understand the advanced ICU knowledge and skills for continuous renal replacement therapy in critical care
- consider advanced concepts of blood purification, plasma exchange and kidney support outside the ICU.

Introduction

Deterioration of kidney function as a result of physiological injury to the point where there is retention of nitrogenous wastes is a common manifestation of critical illness and is often associated with failure of other organs.[1] Acute kidney injury (AKI) is a syndrome with susceptibility factors, including age, cardiac disease and diabetes, and then an exposure such as shock and/or sepsis[2,3] leading to a loss of kidney function.[4] Acute tubular necrosis is a collective term commonly used in the past to describe acutely deteriorating renal function, reflecting pathological changes from various renal insults of a nephrotoxic or ischaemic origin. Factors that cause renal function to deteriorate are not always ischaemic or necrotic in origin, and a syndrome with degrees of deterioration prior to an anuric state and failure is often evident. Functional impairment correlates poorly with structural injury; therefore, a consensus definition and classification system has been established that focuses on incremental organ injury and functional loss rather than end-stage organ failure.[5,6]

AKI is defined as a rapid decrease in kidney function, resulting in an inability to maintain acid–base, fluid and electrolyte balance, and to excrete nitrogenous wastes. This new approach describes staging of AKI severity and embraces the concept of organ failure where a dynamic spectrum is found, from small indiscrete changes in function that are immediately reversible through to gross acute signs and irreversible organ failure.[5] With this change of conceptual focus in recent years, new consensus guidelines have been released in an effort to better guide clinical understanding and decision making, the most comprehensive being from the Kidney Disease: Improving Global Outcomes (KDIGO) group.[7] Three stages of AKI are defined and are based on elevation in serum creatinine and/or decline in urinary output, where these data correlate with outcome and prognosis.[8] On average, 5% of hospital admissions and up to 50% of ICU admissions carry a diagnosis of AKI, and it will develop in 10–15% of hospitalised patients.[8] Patients with AKI of any type are at higher risk for all-cause mortality according to prospective cohorts, whether or not there is substantial renal recovery. The rates of AKI in the hospital setting have increased steadily since the 1980s and continue to rise, with older and more-complex people treated in the ICU.[8-10]

Related kidney functions

The renal system has a number of key functions, including regulation and maintenance of fluid and electrolyte balance, clearance of metabolic and other waste products, an indirect role in the maintenance of blood pressure, acid–base balance and endocrine function. A review of key renal functions can be useful additional reading for how the kidneys provide waste and toxin removal, fluid management and balance, blood pressure control and electrolyte and acid–base stability.

This review will assist many aspects of this chapter and AKI pathology; however, it is worth recalling now that the kidneys receive approximately 25% of the cardiac output each minute and excrete approximately 180 L/day of glomerular filtrate. Fortunately, tubular reabsorption accounts for approximately 178.5 L/day of the original filtrate, allowing for a modest daily fluid intake or retention of 1.5 L for fluid homeostasis.[11] During this process of filtration and reabsorption, metabolic byproducts and electrolyte and other wastes (including many drugs) are also excreted and maintained in balance. As with all body organ systems, an adequate blood pressure and supply of oxygen to the kidneys is vital and required for this fluid and electrolyte regulatory role necessary to keep stability across the body and other vital organ function.[12]

The kidneys are vital human body organs essential to sustaining life. An important interrelationship of the kidneys and other body organs exists, known as 'organ cross-talk' with the brain, heart, liver and lungs dependent on receiving 'clean' blood to function. As toxins and fluid rapidly accumulate owing to AKI during critical illness, these changes contribute to other key organ dysfunction.[1] AKI induces remote organ injury in the heart, brain, lungs, liver and gut involving multiple inflammatory pathways, including increased expression of soluble proinflammatory mediators, innate and adaptive immunity, cellular apoptosis, physiological derangements and genomic changes.[13]

Pathophysiology and classification of kidney failure

Diseases of the kidneys affect structure and therefore function of nephrons in some way. Pathology such as this, if untreated, may not cause complete and terminal loss of renal function or end-stage renal disease (ESRD). Depending on the extent of nephron damage or 'injury' occurring at the time, and any previous illness that resulted in undetected or pre-existing kidney damage,[5,6] nephrons may recover or survive an insult.[14,15] This concept of injury with failure and then recovery is more clearly described in the later section on acute tubular damage using current contemporary terminology and diagnostic categories for an AKI. This includes a five-level classification, which has been in place since 2001 and is given the acronym RIFLE (see Fig. 18.1A). For associated guidelines and a more recent and simpler staging at three levels, the KDIGO criteria are also presented (see Fig. 18.1B). AKI has a significant effect on mortality and increased health risks.[10] A systematic review of 25 studies with data from 254,408 adults, of whom 55,150 had AKI,[16] demonstrated that AKI was associated with an 86% increase in cardiovascular mortality and a 38% increased risk of cardiovascular events such as congestive heart failure, acute myocardial infarction and stroke. AKI was also associated independently with a 58% increase in the risk of congestive heart failure and a 40% increase in the risk of acute myocardial infarction.[16]

The conventional classification of AKI is based on the perceived causative mechanisms, which have been a traditional pathway for teaching and link to the clinical state of renal failure:[5,17]

- prerenal
- intrarenal (intrinsic)
- postrenal.

However, more recently AKI in critical illness links to the pathway of susceptibility, exposure and outcome[18] and AKI subtypes such as septic AKI or cardiac failure AKI[19] (see Fig. 18.2), where renal replacement therapies are necessary to support life until recovery may occur.

Prior to considering whether a critically ill patient has suffered acute injury, it has been recommended that the effects of intra-abdominal hypertension be considered.[20] As it is possible that up to half of mechanically ventilated

FIGURE 18.1 (**A**) Criteria for diagnosis of acute kidney injury (AKI): the risk, injury and failure criteria with outcomes of loss and end-stage renal disease (RIFLE). (**B**) Criteria for AKI diagnosis: three stages. ARF = acute real failure; GFR = glomerular filtration rate; s. creat = serum creatinine; UO = urine output.

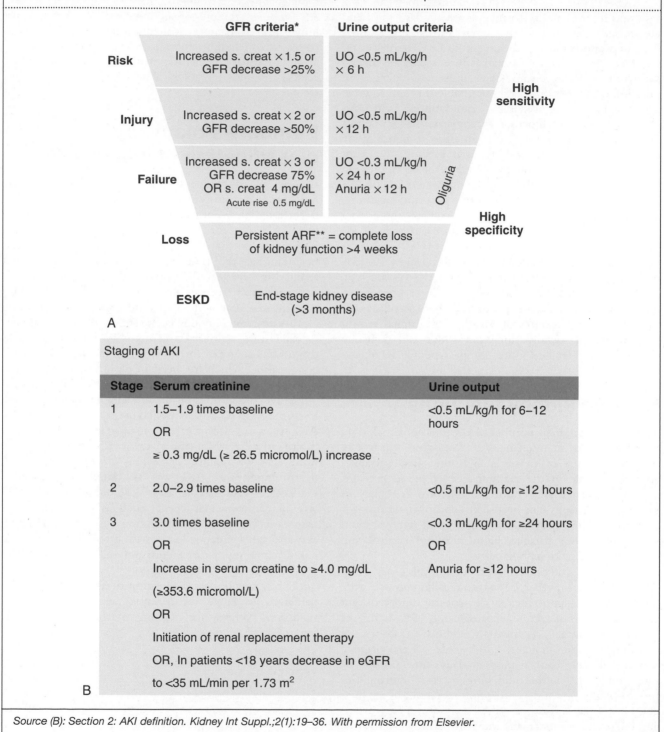

Stage	Serum creatinine	Urine output
1	1.5–1.9 times baseline OR ≥ 0.3 mg/dL (≥ 26.5 micromol/L) increase	<0.5 mL/kg/h for 6–12 hours
2	2.0–2.9 times baseline	<0.5 mL/kg/h for ≥12 hours
3	3.0 times baseline OR Increase in serum creatine to ≥4.0 mg/dL (≥353.6 micromol/L) OR Initiation of renal replacement therapy OR, In patients <18 years decrease in eGFR to <35 mL/min per 1.73 m^2	<0.3 mL/kg/h for ≥24 hours OR Anuria for ≥12 hours

Source (B): Section 2: AKI definition. Kidney Int Suppl.;2(1):19–36. With permission from Elsevier.

patients will have this to some degree, measures to relieve the pressure should be considered, as changes in renal function can be due to either direct pressure on the kidney or drainage system, or to increased pressure within the venous circulation of the kidney. Intra-abdominal hypertension also clouds the assessment of haemodynamic parameters and cardiovascular performance, making it difficult to assess fluid needs and responsiveness to fluid resuscitation.[20,21] For a more detailed discussion of intra-abdominal hypertension, please refer to Chapter 20.

FIGURE 18.2   Neuroendocrine response to shock, resulting in oliguria.

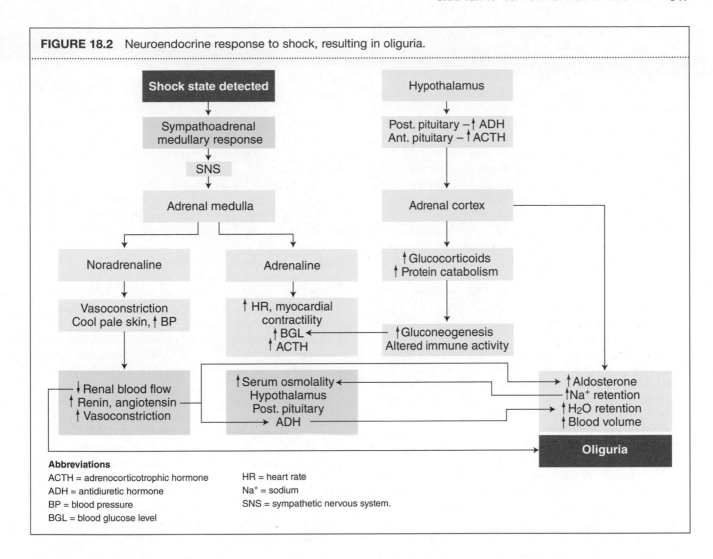

Prerenal causes

Prerenal factors affecting blood supply to the kidneys, such as hypovolaemia, cardiac failure or hypotension and shock, are the most common causes of AKI.[19] The mechanism and outcome are easily related.

Low cardiac output is a state of low or inadequate renal arteriolar blood flow (i.e. nephron afferent vessel). This occurs in states of cardiogenic shock, heart failure, pulmonary embolism and pericardial tamponade. Arrhythmias and valvular disorders can also reduce cardiac output. In the ICU setting, positive-pressure ventilation will decrease venous return, also decreasing cardiac output.

Intrarenal (intrinsic) causes

Intrinsic damage to the nephron structure and function can be due to infective or inflammatory illness, toxic drugs, toxic wastes from inflammation in sepsis, vascular obstructive thrombus or emboli. AKI such as this accounts for approximately 85% of intrinsic kidney failure. The two major causes of acute tubular necrosis (ATN) are ischaemia and nephrotoxin exposure. Ischaemic AKI is characterised not only by inadequate glomerular filtration rate (GFR)

but also by renal blood flow inadequate to maintain parenchymal cellular perfusion. Renal tubular damage with low effective arterial blood flow to the kidney can result in tubular necrosis and cells detaching from the base membrane and cell death or apoptosis.[22] This occurs in the setting of prolonged hypotension or hypoxaemia, such as volume depletion or shock. Underlying sepsis can also be an independent risk factor for ATN. Major surgical procedures can involve prolonged periods of hypoperfusion, which are exacerbated by vasodilating anaesthetic agents.[18,21,23]

ATN describes damage to the tubular portion of the nephron and may range from subtle metabolic changes to total dissolution of cell structure, with tubular cells 'defoliating' or detaching from the tubule basement membrane.[22,24] In critical illness, the most common combination causing AKI is the administration of nephrotoxic agents in association with prolonged hypoperfusion or ischaemia.[15,22] Tubular cells suffer an ischaemic insult, causing a shedding of the cells from the nephron basement membrane. This shedding of cells has an initial loss of cell polarity, and then cell death, with a 'patchy' occurrence along the tubule basement membrane.[24,25] In addition, some cells detach themselves before death in a response known as apoptosis, or cell self-death[26,27] (see Chapter 22). The response is aimed at organ survival, with some individual cells 'sacrificing' themselves during a period of crisis. This protective response reduces oxygen demand by initiating cell death in some tubules, while others differentiate and then proliferate for repair, allowing continuation of some normal function. If the causative process abates, the remaining cells regenerate by epithelial cell differentiation and proliferation, tissue repair occurs with restoration of normal epithelium in some tubules and nephron function returns.

However, with cessation of urine flow, toxicity occurs owing to high serum levels of wastes such as urea, creatinine, potassium and undefined toxins.[22,27] This is the clinical state associated with the pathology of AKI that better describes the total 'picture' of preillness status, immediate causative events and degree of injury determined by patient serum creatinine or urine output.[19,25]

In the past, authors have often employed the term ATN to describe this type of obstructive and ischaemic AKI,[28] using it as a surrogate for AKI in the acute setting, as it focuses on the pathophysiology of tubular damage, recognising this damage as a final outcome of all causative factors. However, more recently, with the development of a consensus definition for AKI describing stages of illness severity, the term AKI is now used, reflecting pathophysiology, the outcome of many causative factors and the clinical context where small derangements may be evident with reversibility of dysfunction and recovery, through to irreversible damage with kidney failure, and cessation of function permanently.[24,29,30] This acronym is associated with stages or levels of kidney dysfunction established by expert and consensus groups in nephrology and critical care.[7,31] This is done with other major organ failures such as heart[32] or liver failure.[33] Importantly, the ability to describe AKI using staging (e.g. 1–3) provides standard clinical reference and language for bedside, research and publications. Other causes of intrinsic AKI are glomerulonephritis, nephrotoxicity and chronic vascular insufficiency and are discussed below.

Glomerulonephritis

This condition is caused by either an infective or a non-infective inflammatory process damaging the glomerular membrane or a systemic autoimmune illness attacking the membrane.[34] Either cause results in a loss of glomerular membrane integrity, allowing larger blood components such as plasma proteins and white blood cells to cross the glomerular basement membrane. This causes a loss of blood protein, tubular congestion and failure of normal nephron activity. Resolution is based on treating the cause, such as an infection or autoimmune inflammatory illness.[17,34]

Nephrotoxicity

Nephrotoxicity occurs as a result of damage to nephron cells from a wide range of agents, including many drugs used in critical care (e.g. antibiotics, anti-inflammatory agents, cancer drugs, radio-opaque dyes). Toxic products of muscle breakdown in severe illness and trauma, commonly called rhabdomyolysis (see Chapter 23),[35,36] blood product administration reactions and blood cell damage associated with major surgery are also causative agents.[36,37] As these agents may often be given concurrently, a cumulative effect, along with intermittent falls in renal perfusion, may result in the development of intrinsic AKI.

Aminoglycosides cause some degree of ATN in up to 25% of hospitalised patients receiving therapeutic levels of the drugs. Non-oliguric kidney injury typically occurs after 5–10 days of exposure. Predisposing factors include underlying kidney damage, volume depletion and advanced age. Aminoglycosides can remain in renal tissues for up to a month, so kidney function may not recover for some time after stopping the medication. Monitoring of peak and trough levels is important, but trough levels are more helpful in predicting renal toxicity. Gentamycin, tobramycin, vancomycin, intravenous acyclovir (aciclovir) and several cephalosporins are nephrotoxic; streptomycin is the least nephrotoxic of the aminoglycosides.[38,39]

Radiographic contrast media may be directly nephrotoxic. Contrast-induced nephropathy is the third leading cause of new-onset AKI in hospitalised patients.[40] It results from a combination of direct renal tubular epithelial cell toxicity and renal medullary ischaemia.[40,41] Predisposing factors include patient comorbidities, amount of contrast administered, concomitant medication use such as non-steroidal anti-inflammatory agents and angiotensin converting enzyme inhibitors.[41] Lower volumes of contrast with lower osmolality agents are recommended in high-risk patients. Toxicity usually occurs within 24–48 hours after the radiocontrast study.[41]

Vascular insufficiency

One-third of patients who develop AKI in the ICU have chronic renal dysfunction.[1,10,19] This chronic dysfunction may be undiagnosed prior to the critical illness, and may be related to diabetes, the ageing process and/or long-term hypertension. These factors create a reduction in both large and microvasculature blood flow into and within the kidney, therefore reducing glomerular filtration activity and affecting the reabsorption and diffusive process of the nephron. This reduction in blood flow is exacerbated by degenerative vessel obstruction with atheromatous plaque, which is particularly pronounced in diabetic patients owing to ineffective glucose metabolism. Diabetic patients are more likely to develop AKI associated with medical care in hospital from what may otherwise seem to be a relatively trivial insult to the kidneys in a younger, healthy patient. The event may be enough to move the patient from kidney injury to ESRD, as they lack any degree of 'renal reserve' or tolerance to events such as low blood pressure or administration of nephrotoxic drugs normally filtered by the kidney.[42]

Postrenal causes

Urinary tract obstruction is the primary postrenal cause of AKI, and is uncommon in the critical care setting as it is rarely associated with acute-onset renal failure.[8] Postrenal causes are the least common reason for AKI, accounting for approximately 5–10% of cases, but are important to detect because of their reversibility. Postrenal azotaemia occurs when urinary flow from both kidneys, or a single functioning kidney, is obstructed. Occasionally, postrenal uropathies can occur when a single kidney is obstructed if the contralateral kidney cannot adjust for the loss in function (e.g. in a patient with advanced chronic kidney disease (CKD)). Obstruction leads to elevated intraluminal pressure, causing kidney parenchymal damage, with marked effects on renal blood flow and tubular function, and a decrease in GFR.

Postrenal causes include urethral obstruction, bladder dysfunction or obstruction, and possibly obstruction within the ureters and renal pelvises. In men, benign prostatic hyperplasia is the most common cause. Patients taking anticholinergic drugs are at risk for urinary retention. Obstruction can also be caused by bladder, prostate and cervical cancers, retroperitoneal fibrosis and neurogenic bladder. Less common causes are blood clots in the urine pathway, bilateral ureteral stones, urethral stones or strictures and bilateral papillary necrosis.[43]

Treatment

Treatment is aimed at hastening recovery and avoiding complications. Preventive measures should be taken to avoid volume overload and hyperkalaemia, both of which occur in the kidney with impaired function. Widespread use of diuretics in critically ill patients with AKI should be encouraged only in states of volume overload and with caution, and close attention paid to responsiveness,[44] where differences may occur for those with low urine output compared with those with elevated creatinine as an indication for use and dosing.[45] Diuretics do not treat or prevent an AKI.[46] Disabling side effects of supranormal diuretic dosing include hearing loss and cerebellar dysfunction. This is mainly due to peak frusemide levels when high bolus doses are used, and this risk can be minimised by using a frusemide infusion.[45]

AKI: clinical and diagnostic criteria for classification

Clinical assessment

Clinical assessment of the patient with impending AKI can involve a limited number of tests and investigations; however, the clinical history is important and part of the susceptibility and exposure pathway with an AKI developing.[7] The patient's age, past medical and surgical history, more-recent illness and management with diabetes are flags or of key importance.[47] After this, key assessments used in monitoring renal function are performed or checked, such as urine output, serum creatinine and urea levels, biochemistry, acid–base measures from arterial blood gas, cardiovascular measures such as heart rate and blood pressure, along with fluid balance status, oxygen requirements and blood gas exchange, chest radiology and current weight. These measures are essential for diagnosis, staging the AKI and management decisions in the critically ill patient.[1,8,48] They also link into the wider assessment of fluid and electrolyte balance, as described in Chapters 9 and 21.

Biomarkers for the detection of AKI

Numerous biomarkers have been identified in the last several years that can indicate whether kidney injury is occurring and when damage has been done. Serum creatinine, a marker of kidney function but not kidney injury,[49] has been a benchmark for decades to determine loss of renal function as a guide to treatment and for renal support techniques, but it has limitations.[50] Normal creatinine is variable and influenced by age, race and sex, and a rise in serum creatinine may not occur until there is a marked decrease in the GFR.[51] Also, creatinine is not adequate for an early identification of reduced GFR and it does not allow differentiation between haemodynamically mediated changes in renal function and intrinsic renal failure or obstructive nephropathy. Most importantly, serum creatinine does not differentiate quickly reversible, volume-sensitive reductions in GFR.[52]

> **Practice tip**
>
> Serum creatinine reflects the real value of GFR under steady-state conditions, but not when renal function is deteriorating. Critically ill patients are not in a steady state so the use of serum creatinine in this patient population as a marker of renal function may be limited.[52,53]

The search for a sensitive and clinically useful biomarker continues, and this is a big difference in early detection and predictive management for AKI compared with the utility of cardiac enzymes and troponin with cardiac ischaemia. Two biomarkers have been investigated for the detection and/or management of AKI, and are available but in limited clinical use.

Neutrophil gelatinase-associated lipocalin (NGAL)

Neutrophil gelatinase-associated lipocalin, a protein of the lipocalin family, is expressed at very low constant levels in different cell types. It is highly expressed after ischaemic or toxic kidney injury in humans and in many animals, and is promoted as useful and a logical step in AKI diagnosis and management.[54] NGAL can be assayed from plasma serum or urine samples, with increasing sensitivity or accuracy as an AKI state progresses (serum). The elevation of NGAL is detectable as early as 3 hours after the injury and peaks approximately 6–12 hours after injury, depending on the severity of injury. The elevation can persist up to 5 days after the initial injury when the injury is severe.[55] NGAL can rise for days before sepsis causing an elevation in serum creatinine and can be influenced by several factors including baseline renal function, sepsis and urinary tract infection.[56,57] Current use of this biomarker is limited and variable in clinical management across different countries.

Kidney injury molecule-1

Kidney injury molecule-1 is a transmembrane glycoprotein which is expressed at low levels in the normal kidney as well as in other organs, but is influenced by comorbidities and therefore may lack specificity.[58] Kidney injury molecule-1 has a protective effect in the kidney in ischaemia/repercussion injury and has been proposed to play an important role in kidney recovery and tubular regeneration because it mediates the phagocytosis of cell debris into cultured renal epithelial cells.[59,60]

Complications of AKI and kidney failure

Uraemic complications

Uraemic complications are influenced by the rate of urea accumulation and vary from patient to patient. As serum urea levels rise rapidly (e.g. over a few days), when above 20 mmol/L the blood coagulation can be affected. A rash and related itchiness can occur. As blood levels continue to rise, neurological function can be affected, and the level of consciousness will deteriorate. In some cases, high levels of urea can result in encephalopathy.[61]

Cardiovascular alterations

Cardiovascular alterations can occur because of AKI[62] as a result of direct effects on the myocardium but also because of fluid accumulation and electrolyte disturbance. The greatest concern is fluid overload as a consequence of failure to excrete the excess quantities of fluid used in resuscitating critically ill patients[63] and the necessity to provide adequate nutrition in the form of parenteral or enteral nutrition.[64] Without appropriate management, heart failure and pulmonary oedema can develop.[65] Refer to Chapter 11 for a more detailed discussion of cardiac arrhythmias associated with electrolyte disturbances.

Respiratory alteration

As noted earlier, with AKI and fluid accumulation, inadequate clearance of the pulmonary interstitial space by the pulmonary lymphatics occurs, resulting firstly in interstitial oedema and moving on to overt pulmonary oedema and serious impairment of pulmonary gas exchange, and then associated oxidative stress with reactive oxygen molecules participating.[66] See Chapter 13 for detailed discussion of ventilation and perfusion matching and pulmonary oedema. Respiratory rate may also

increase as patients develop metabolic acidosis through both renal injury and associated critical illness.

Haematological alterations

The primary haematological concern in AKI is related to the anticoagulatory effects of rapidly increasing serum urea. While the kidney accounts for 90% of circulating erythropoietin production,[67] the acute nature of severe AKI does not influence anaemia to the extent of more-common causes such as haemorrhage related to trauma or surgery, or even iatrogenic blood loss.

Neurological alterations

Changes to central nervous system function can be related to accumulating urea, fluid and disruption of sodium balance.[68] In the most severe form, these can result in loss of consciousness and fits.[66]

AKI diagnosis

The management of AKI begins with the diagnosis, based on the patient's presenting signs and symptoms linked to a patient history. A long-term history of renal disease involving urinary tract infections, diabetes, cardiac failure and systemic inflammatory illnesses is highly relevant.[48] Immediate history of presentation to a hospital involving surgery or any life-threatening illness with associated shock is also highly relevant in association with reduced urine output volumes over time.[8,19]

Nurses in the critical care setting, who measure urine output hourly, readily recognise a key sign of impending renal dysfunction. Oliguria in the absence of catheter obstruction should be responded to quickly, as this suggests inadequate kidney blood flow and, to some extent, is a delayed observation considering the continual moderation of kidney function producing urine output. Persisting oliguria or the onset of anuria with associated rises in blood creatinine fulfils the injury phase of AKI. This sequence of events can be identified in the well-established classification known as the 'RIFLE' criteria: the **r**isk, **i**njury, **f**ailure and outcome criteria of **l**oss and **e**nd-stage disease. This has provided the basis for a widely accepted approach to diagnosing and classifying AKI.[5,6]

Consensus definitions and classification for AKI: the RIFLE criteria and KDIGO staging

The RIFLE criteria are shown in Fig. 18.1A, and use rising creatinine and falling urine output as highly sensitive and specific indicators for a continuum of renal failure.[5,6] This useful classification system, established in the year 2000 by a dialysis quality group, provides grading for loss of kidney function, reflecting stages of injury to the kidney before failure occurs. Without this, the small but important losses of kidney function before the failure state are not adequately considered.[69] This approach provides a consensus definition for loss of kidney function that is useful for clinical practice and research into this area, with clinicians all talking the same 'language' when comparing patients and/or results from clinical trials. The shape of the diagram indicates that more people will develop symptoms of AKI linked to kidney 'injury' and be considered 'at risk' (high sensitivity and a wider shape) than those at the bottom of the definition, who are fewer in number but need to fulfil strict criteria (high specificity and a narrower shape).

Since this time and as a progression in AKI understanding, in 2012 a European consensus group established the KDIGO initiative and combined the work of another expert North American group, the Acute Kidney Injury Network,[31] and published an AKI staging of severity with three stages; it has now become the most used and cited.[70] The Acute Kidney Injury Network and KDIGO expert groups provide many helpful clinical care guidelines[48,71] for identification and care of patients with AKI.

> **Practice tip**
>
> A reduction in urine output is an important sign of impending AKI; however, checking a catheter for blockage is also important. A bladder scanner may also reveal a full bladder where no catheter is in place. The use of newer digital urine output-monitoring systems is helpful to maintain vigilance in urine output monitoring, by using alarms when urine output falls to less than 0.5 mL/kg/h, can function by automatically documenting hourly into the electronic medical record,[72] and may contribute to detecting and managing AKI.[73]

Management of the patient with AKI

Reducing further insults to the kidneys

After diagnosis, the next management principle is to remove or modify any cause that may exacerbate the pathological process associated with AKI. Further interventions and investigations are performed in relation to findings from the history and hospital presentation. These may include:

- further intravenous fluid resuscitation (despite an oligoanuric state) and restoration of blood pressure using inotropic/vasoactive drugs
- physical or diagnostic assessment for renal outflow obstruction and alleviation if present; consider raised abdominal pressure
- avoiding contrast-enhanced radiological investigations
- ceasing or modifying the dose of any nephrotoxic drugs or agents and treating infection with alternative, less toxic antibiotics.[8,74]

Initial management strategies for the early stages of AKI remain conservative, with careful management of fluid (once adequate circulating volume is assured) and haemodynamics, encouraging diuresis if present, monitoring blood profiles for changes in urea and electrolytes and limiting or reformulating administration of agents that may contribute to the accumulation of urea and electrolytes (e.g. enteral or intravenous nutritional supplements). The use of agents such as mannitol, dopamine and frusemide, while popular in practice, have not been shown to be of any value in improving outcome in patients at risk of AKI.[75,76]

Despite these efforts, life-threatening biochemistry may arise in AKI, such as severe acidosis and hyperkalaemia (pH <7.1 and serum potassium >6.5 mmol/L), that requires immediate treatment and is an indication for beginning renal replacement therapy (RRT) without elevation of serum creatinine and oliguria and fluid overload.[77]

Fluid balance

Fluid management has been identified as a key strategy for the management of an AKI.[78,79] As oliguria and anuria are key diagnostic and clinical signs of renal dysfunction, reducing fluid intake is necessary to prevent intravascular overload and tissue oedema until renal recovery begins or a type of RRT is started. Reducing or restricting fluid intake can be a challenge in the critically ill as it is not uncommon for these patients to be administered 3 L of fluid in 24 hours.[80,81] A balance state for this degree of fluid administration suggests a urine output at 3–4 mL/kg/h without considering other insensible losses will rarely cause intravascular volume depletion.[63,65,82] Strategies can be considered to minimise fluid intake such as preparing drug infusions without diluent and in a concentrated version of the usual preparation. Pharmacists may assist with this requirement and offer advice for drug preparation and delivery. Restriction of oral fluids can be implemented and monitored using a fluid chart, with the aim of adhering to the prescribed volume. Nutrition therapy is important for optimising patient outcome but can also contribute to increased fluid intake. Enteral feeding is preferred for most critically ill patients and standard enteral feeding formulas can contribute about 1.5 L of fluid intake per day in an adult.[81] Nutrition is very important in the patient experiencing AKI, where growth and repair is needed with damaged kidney cells and protein depletion is to be avoided. Calorie-dense enteral feeding formulas (2 kcal/mL) can be considered as a strategy to minimise fluid intake associated with enteral feeding (see Chapter 19 for further discussion on nutrition in critical illness). Fluid balance charting and a clear understanding of the maximum fluid intake per day is vital for managing AKI at this stage, and a maximum intake of 1.5 L per day is a common target in the adult patient.[79,83] An inability to prevent a positive fluid balance, largely due to meeting nutritional requirements, is often the reason RRT is initiated.[84] Care should also be taken to prevent fluid overload with AKI at this time. Studies in children show increased morbidity and mortality in fluid-overloaded patients.[85] Fluid volume and overload lead to organ congestion and a resultant decrease in renal blood flow.[82,86]

Electrolyte balance

Managing serum electrolytes, in particular potassium, is essential for patient stability, as low or high levels are more likely to be associated with life-threatening arrhythmias. However, phosphate, calcium and sodium may also be abnormal and require strategies to reduce, supplement or control the serum level away from toxicity.[87] Hyponatraemia, for example, may be associated with altered mental state, impaired consciousness and even seizures.[65,88]

Acid–base balance

Control of the acid–base balance is another essential function of the healthy kidneys and, with failure, metabolic acidosis will develop as a result of decreased buffering and accumulation of many acids not excreted.[89] An increased minute ventilation may be observed in the patient, representing a physiological attempt to control acidaemia. This requires additional energy and caloric consumption and is another indication that RRT should be implemented using bicarbonate fluids to control the acidaemia.[90]

Pharmacotherapy and altered pharmacokinetics

The modification of drug regimens to effect changes to excretion and volume of distribution is a further aspect of clinical management during the onset of AKI. Drugs are excreted from the body after hepatic and other organ metabolism, which converts them to a water-soluble form such that they appear in the urine. Therefore, modification of dose (through reduction or frequency of administration) and monitoring for serum levels helps to prevent further renal insult while ensuring the desired clinical effect.[91,92]

Aminoglycosides are a key group of antibiotics requiring adjustment and monitoring in AKI, if not ceasing and substituting for another appropriate but less nephrotoxic antibiotic.[93] Other drugs administered in the ICU that warrant attention include narcotics, histamine-2 receptor antagonists and beta-blockers. Pharmacy product information attached with packaging and/or local pharmacy information usually provides helpful suggestions and guidelines for relevant drug use in AKI. If RRT is started, and is functioning continuously with efficiency, the clearance and toxicity of drugs is of less concern and dosing may resume to normal for some drugs, with close monitoring continuing.[94]

If conservative measures fail, ongoing management of the patient with AKI requires RRT. This enables control of blood biochemistry, prevents toxin accumulation and allows removal of fluids so that adequate nutrition can be achieved, but importantly this is a support system and not a treatment for AKI.

The criteria and indications for initiating RRT are listed in Box 18.1. One indication is enough to initiate RRT, while two or more make RRT urgent. Combined

---

BOX 18.1

Proposed criteria for the initiation of renal replacement therapy in adult critically ill patients[8,74,77]

- Oliguria (urine output <200 mL/12 h)
- Anuria/extreme oliguria (urine output <50 mL/12 h)
- Hyperkalaemia (K+ >6.5 mmol/L)
- Severe acidaemia (pH <7.1)
- Azotaemia (urea >30 mmol/L)
- Clinically significant organ (esp. lung) oedema
- Uraemic encephalopathy
- Uraemic pericarditis
- Uraemic neuropathy/myopathy
- Severe dysnatraemia (Na+ >160 or <115 mmol/L)
- Hyperthermia
- Drug overdose with dialysable toxin

---

derangements can create the necessity to commence therapy before individually defined limits have been reached. Early initiation of treatment is widely advocated and may confer more-rapid renal recovery, but timing and illness progression and outcomes for best practice is currently of high interest. Evidence from randomised clinical trials using defined 'early' or 'delayed' initiation protocols for starting of RRT with an AKI is variable. However, a meta-analysis of 10 studies[95] suggests that a delayed start does not affect patient survival, and may reduce costs and save resources.

Approaches to renal replacement therapy

A brief review of the historical perspectives associated with the development of modern-day dialysis and RRT provided in the ICU is helpful in understanding key concepts and methods for RRT, and in particular as a continuous (C) method or CRRT (continuous renal replacement therapy).

History

Dialysis is a term describing RRT and refers to the purification of blood through a membrane by diffusion of waste substances.[96–98] Table 18.1 outlines historical events during the development of dialysis in Europe and the USA.

The combination of an extracorporeal circuit (EC), blood pump and filter membrane and the associated nursing management are now commonly known as haemodialysis. With industrial and scientific developments, such as plastics moulding and electronics, current dialysis techniques are safe, effective and a life-sustaining treatment for the millions of people who suffer acute and chronic kidney failure.[96,98]

TABLE 18.1

Historical events in the development of dialysis

TIME PERIOD AND DEVELOPER	DESCRIPTION
1854: Thomas Graham, Scottish chemist	First used the term 'dialysis' to describe the transport of solutes through an ox bladder, which drew attention to the concept of a membrane for solute removal from fluid.
1920s: George Haas, German physician	First human dialysis was carried out, performing six treatments on six patients. Haas failed to make further progress with the treatment but is recognised as an early pioneer of dialysis.
1920–30s	Synthetic polymer chemistry allowed development of cellulose acetate, a membrane integral to the further development of dialysis treatments.
1940s: Willem Kolff, Dutch physician	The discovery of heparin, an anticoagulant, enabled further development of dialysis during World War II, the Kolff rotating drum kidney (see Fig. 18.8)
1940–50s: Kolff and Allis-Chalmers, USA	Further modification of the Kolff dialyser and the development of improved machines.
1950s: Fredrik Kiil, Norway	Developed the parallel plate dialyser made of a new cellulose, cuprophane. This required a pump to push the blood through the membrane and return the blood to the patient.
1950–60s	Dialysis began to be widely used to treat kidney failure.
1960s: Richard Stewart and Dow Chemical, USA	The hollow-fibre membrane dialyser used a membrane design of a cellulose acetate bundle, with 11,000 fibres providing a surface area of 1 m^2.
1970s	Use of the first CAVH circuits for diuretic-resistant oedema by Kramer.
1980s	First continuous therapies using blood pump and intravenous pumps to control fluid removal and substitution; Australia and New Zealand led the way.
1990s	New purpose-built machines used; Gambro Prisma, Baxter BM 11 + 14 to provide pump-controlled therapies with integrated automated fluid balance using scales to measure fluids; cassette circuits, automated priming; new membranes.
2000	Further purpose-built machines using direct measurement for waste and substitution fluids via Kimal Hygieia machine. Introduction of high fluid exchange rates for sepsis treatment. Introduction of dialysis-based machines in the ICU for daily 'hybrid' treatments: SLEDD and SLEDDf.
2010	Multiple CRRT machines; more advanced graphics interface and smart alarms; waste-disposal systems; high flux, porous membranes.
2020	Further advances with CRRT machines enabling mode changes during treatment, increased safety alarms for fluid 'balance', treatment data storage and transmission; automated citrate anticoagulation software.

CAVH = continuous arteriovenous haemofiltration; CRRT = continuous renal replacement therapy; SLEDD = sustained low-efficiency daily dialysis; SLEDDf = sustained low-efficiency daily diafiltration.

Nursing of dialysis patients has developed into a specialist field of knowledge and skill, with nurses combining their holistic view of patient management with the specialist needs of patients with renal failure, from the outpatient setting to the ICU, including a collaborative approach to further adaptations of dialysis best suited to the critically ill.[99–101]

Development of renal replacement therapy in critical care

Historically, AKI was treated in the ICU with the use of peritoneal dialysis (PD), which did not require specialist nurses or doctors. This simple technique removes wastes by infusing a dialysis fluid into the abdomen, allowing diffusion and osmosis to occur between the peritoneum and fluid before draining out again in repeated cycles.[102] This was performed by the ICU nurse and prescribed by ICU doctors, but was inadequate in its clearance of waste and fluid volume, and was associated with infection, limitation of respiratory function and exacerbated glucose intolerance.[103,104] Today, PD is rarely, if ever, used in the management of renal failure in the critical care setting in western and well-funded health care settings; however, it does have a place in low-income areas and those with reduced resources internationally.[103]

In 1977 Peter Kramer, a German ICU doctor, developed a new dialytic technique called continuous arteriovenous haemofiltration (CAVH), which was specifically intended for use in the critically ill patient and required insertion of catheters into an artery and a vein. It was later renamed slow continuous ultrafiltration (SCUF), as it enabled the removal of plasma water in addition to dissolved wastes (convective clearance of solutes) at a flow rate of 200–600 mL/h by passive drainage from the membrane as blood flowed through it.[105] This marked the beginning of continuous RRT in the ICU as an intervention prescribed and managed by ICU nurses and doctors for patients with AKI.[104]

Refinement of renal replacement therapy

Today, CAVH is replaced with a dialysis blood pump mode, and this enables a much more efficient technique for the ICU patient with AKI. Blood pumps generate a reliable flow of blood, eliminating the need for an arterial puncture where the patient's heart was indeed the pump. The insertion of venous access catheters is now used with an external blood pump machine. This is termed continuous venovenous haemofiltration (CVVH), and can reliably pump blood at a constant rate and achieve ultrafiltration volumes of 1000 mL/h. With further modifications to the circuit and filter set-up, a diffusive component was added to the therapy by running a dialysate volume through the haemofilter, flowing between the membrane fibres and counter-current to blood flow. This was termed continuous venovenous haemodiafiltration (CVVHD(f)).[99,106–109]

Principles of extracorporeal CRRT

Both intermittent haemodialysis and CRRT require a machine to pump blood and fluids, pressure and flow devices to monitor treatment, a tubing and filter membrane set that together create an EC (outside the body blood pathway), and a catheter connecting the patient's circulation to the circuit (Fig. 18.3). This catheter enables blood to be drawn from and returned to the patient (known as 'access'). Access can be achieved by three different techniques:

- temporary catheters inserted via a skin puncture into an artery for drawing blood and a vein to return the blood (arteriovenous access)

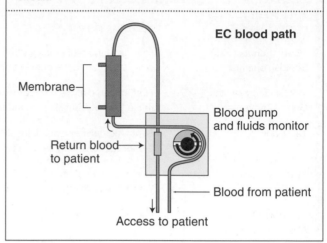

FIGURE 18.3 Renal replacement therapy blood path circuit common to all approaches. EC = extracorporeal circuit.

- a surgical joining of an artery and vein (usually in the forearm), making a large vessel that is punctured with needles to both draw and return the blood (arteriovenous fistula)
- a catheter with two lumens to draw and return blood via a large central vein (a dual venovenous access catheter).

In the AKI setting and where temporary treatment is anticipated, the two-lumen catheter is recommended.[77,110,111]

Haemodialysis, haemofiltration and haemodiafiltration

Haemodialysis, haemofiltration and haemodiafiltration are three common techniques used to achieve artificial kidney support in AKI. The basic blood path or circuit for these therapies is indicated in Fig. 18.3 and is a useful review to understand each therapy and where the RRT fluids are then applied to the circuit, differentiating them as techniques.

The extracorporeal component is a common factor in all these different circuit designs. The difference between treatments is how the solutes such as urea, creatinine and other waste products and the solvent or plasma water are removed from the blood as it passes through the filter membrane (artificial kidney), and the intermittent versus continuous prescription of the therapy. The three physical mechanisms of fluid and solute management are convection, diffusion and ultrafiltration. Fig. 18.4 lists the commonly used abbreviations to describe the timing of treatment, blood access for the therapy and mode of solute removal.

Convection

Convection is the process whereby dissolved solutes are removed along with plasma water as it is filtered through the dialysis membrane. The word is derived from the Latin *convehere*, meaning 'to remove or to carry along with'.[112,113]

FIGURE 18.4 Abbreviations and membrane mechanisms for modes of renal replacement therapy

	Mechanism of solute removal
H (or HF) = haemofiltration – convection CVVH as continuous therapy (CRRT)	**Convection ('solute drag')** 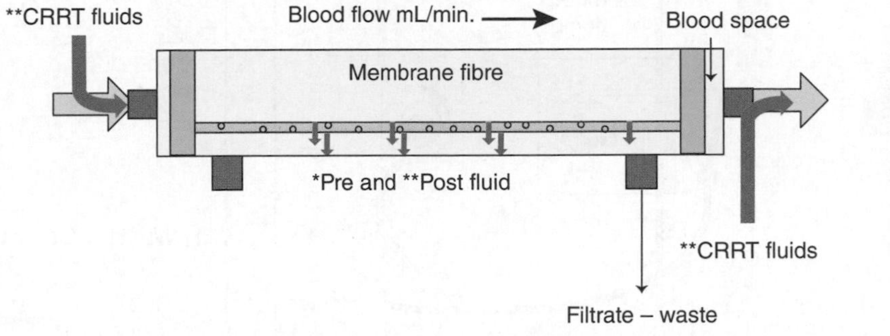
D (or HD) = haemodialysis – diffusion NB: this is slower or of much lower intensity when done as a continuous therapy or CRRT as CVVHD compared with intermittent haemodialysis (IHD).	**Diffusion ('solute exchange')** 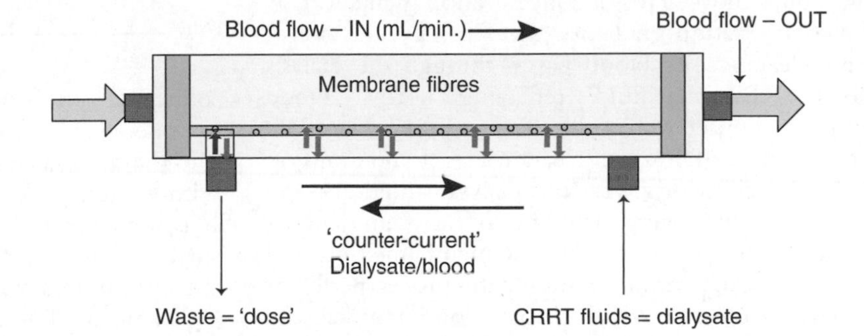
HDF = haemodiafiltration – diffusion and convection CVVHDF as a continuous therapy	**Diffusion & Convection (solute 'drag & exchange')** 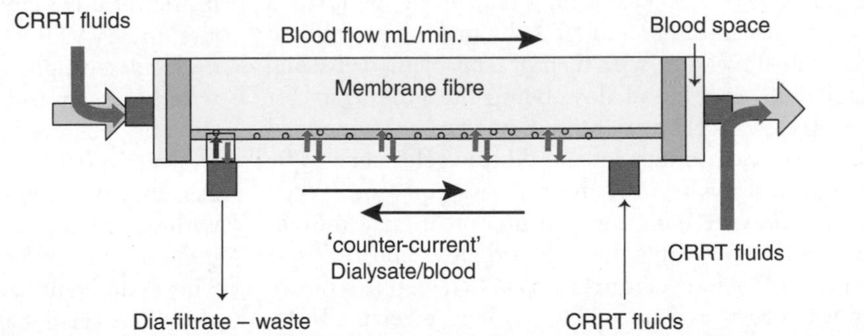

This process is similar to that occurring in the native kidney glomerulus, as plasma water is filtered across the nephron tubule via the Bowman's capsule. In RRT, the plasma water with the dissolved wastes is discarded; the deficit is then replaced with commercially manufactured artificial plasma water in equal or slightly lower amounts to achieve a desired fluid balance. This blood purification process is commonly known as haemofiltration.[107,113,114] When applied on a continuous basis in the ICU,

haemofiltration can adequately replace essential renal functions, and is particularly effective in managing fluid balance.[77,108] Fig. 18.5 illustrates the circuit and set-up for continuous venovenous hemofiltration.

Diffusion

Diffusion refers to the physical movement of solutes across a semipermeable membrane from an area of high concentration to that of a relatively low concentration;

FIGURE 18.5 Continuous venovenous haemofiltration (CVVH) circuit.

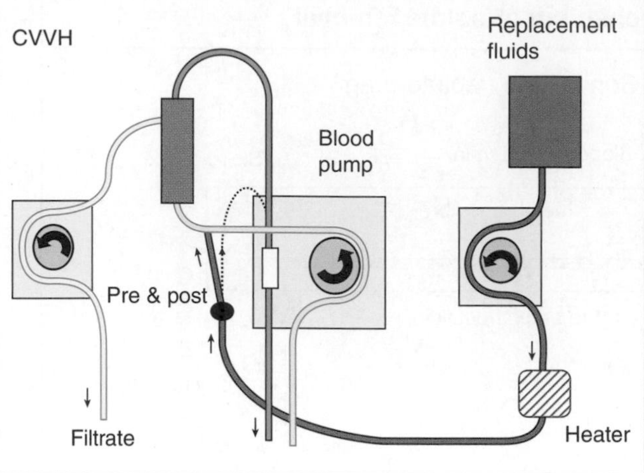

FIGURE 18.6 Intermittent dialysis circuit (IHD). HCO_3^- = bicarbonate; K^+ = potassium; Qdf = flow of dialysis fluid; RO = reverse osmosis; UF = ultrafiltrate.

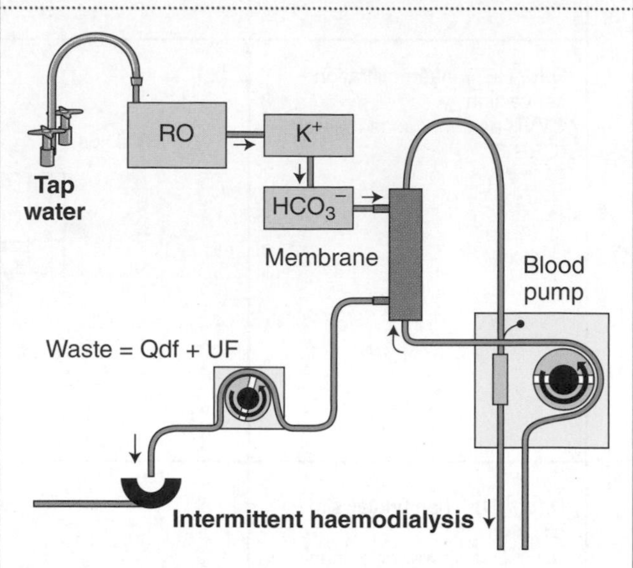

that is, solutes move across a concentration gradient.[113] A higher concentration gradient results in a greater rate of diffusive clearance. As blood passes through the dialysis membrane, dialysate fluid, reflecting normal blood chemistry, is exposed to blood on the opposing side of the membrane fibre. Diffusive clearance is continuous as solute exchange occurs with the dialysate fluid and the blood continually moving in and out of the membrane. As waste-laden blood enters the hollow membrane fibre and fresh dialysate is in continuous supply, this process performs an effective waste-removal function. Blood and dialysate are established in a counter-current or opposing flow to each other to maximise the diffusive process,[115] mimicking the normal nephron function of the kidneys.[116]

A diffusive clearance technique can be performed with increasing intensity and effect by making both blood and dialysate flow faster, with technical problems delivering the high fluid and blood flow being the limiting factor increasing clearance. The two flows need to be maintained in relation to each other; for the diffusive clearance to be efficient, the dialysate flow must always equal or exceed the blood flow. A common setting for an intermittent dialysis treatment would be a blood flow and dialysate fluid flow of 300 mL/min each. When applied on an intermittent basis, as is normal for patients receiving RRT for chronic renal failure, this is called intermittent haemodialysis.[107,117] Fig. 18.6 illustrates the circuit set-up for intermittent haemodialysis.

Ultrafiltration

Ultrafiltration is the process that allows plasma water to leave the blood, achieving body fluid or water loss.[118] Dialysis (or nephrology) nurses measure a fluid loss by weighing the patient before and after a treatment. This process is primarily used to achieve fluid balance, an important function of the kidneys. The only difference between this process and the convective clearance of

solutes is that this fluid is not replaced and is therefore not considered to be an adequate solute management method. Ultrafiltration cannot be undertaken in large amounts without fluid replacement, as it would cause hypovolaemia. It is implemented during a dialysis period by removing small amounts each hour (e.g. 250 mL/h for 4 h) during the intermittent treatment cycle.

There are different therapeutic effects from each form of RRT and different operational prescriptions of blood and fluid flow. Combinations of convection and diffusion can be used, known as CVVHDf.[77,106,114,118] An increase in the diffusive component (i.e. raising the dialysate flow rate in CVVHDf) will increase the removal of small-molecular-weight substances such as potassium and assist with hydrogen ion exchange via buffer solution. This can also be achieved via increasing filtration fluid flow (convective clearance), which will also add an increase in clearance of larger molecules, for example those associated with severe infection and systemic inflammation or sepsis. Fig. 18.7 illustrates the circuit and set-up for CVVHDf. These different modes or methods to achieve solute clearance, acid–base control and fluid balance and supporting the patient with failing kidneys are applied with similar success and outcome. Large randomised controlled trials[81,119] or meta-analysis reviews[120] investigating anticoagulation methods report similar patient demographics, and outcomes for ICU stay, morbidity and mortality. There are some physician preferences for mode choice with CRRT and this is possibly associated with training pathways in medicine.[77,121]

Delivering CRRT

To correctly understand the different variants of RRT, how each achieves waste removal and fluid balance along

FIGURE 18.7 Continuous venovenous haemodiafiltration (CVVHDf) circuit.

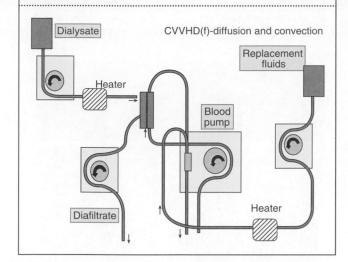

Fluids used for therapy: dialysate, pre- and post-dilution

In diffusive mode such as CVVHDf, fluids are used as a dialysate (i.e. for diffusive molecular exchange). In a convective mode, known as CVVH, fluids are administered into the blood pathway and can be introduced before or after the membrane to provide convection (i.e. plasma water removal and replacement). Fluid administration before the membrane is termed predilution and after the membrane it is referred to as postdilution.[65,79] Any fluid administered predilution changes the blood haematocrit and, unless the blood flow is increased to compensate, subsequent solute clearance within the membrane reduces. This aspect of clearance and the effect of fluids administered and blood flow is known as the filtration fraction.[122,123] However, the dilution does help to prevent clotting within the membrane and is considered clinically beneficial.[124] If the waste-removal rate is increased in either mode for a negative fluid balance, the dose is increased as a result, depending on the amount per hour.[108,123,125]

Membranes

The filter or haemofilter (blood filter) is the primary functional component of the RRT system,[97,126] responsible for separating plasma water from the blood and/or allowing the exchange of solutes across the membrane by diffusion. The filter is made of a plastic casing, containing a synthetic polymer inner structure arranged in longitudinal fibres.[97] A schematic diagram of a haemofilter is shown in Fig. 18.8. The fibres are hollow and have pores along their length with a size of 15,000–30,000 daltons. This allows plasma water to pass through, carrying dissolved wastes out of the blood (most of which have a

with knowledge of how to 'troubleshoot' the machine providing RRT, nurses benefit from a clear understanding of major circuit components, their functions and the blood pathway known as the extracorporeal circuit (EC).[108] For the treatment or therapy, physicians prescribe this as a 'dose'[122] and is the volume of fluid removed as waste in respective modes, as outlined in Figs 18.5 and 18.7. Estimated or actual patient weight can be used, and 25 mL/kg/h is common in adults for the effluent and waste removal. That is, for an 80-kg patient this would be prescribed and set at 2 L/h and automatically controlled by the machine pumps and software.

FIGURE 18.8 Continuous venovenous haemodiafiltration (CVVHDf) haemofilter (dialysis membrane). Cross-sectional view indicating longitudinal synthetic fibres conveying blood into and out of the plastic casing outer structure. Plasma water is removed via the side ultrafiltrate port during CVVH, applying convective clearance. In CVVHDf, the blood is exposed to fluid via the membrane fibres so that diffusive clearance can occur.

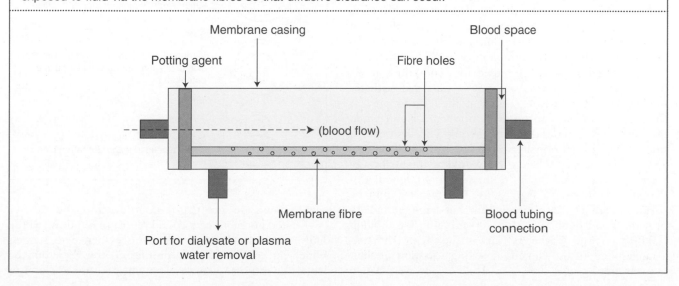

molecular weight <20,000 daltons) while larger plasma proteins and blood cells (at least 60,000–70,000 daltons) are retained.[111] Plasma water separated from the blood in this way is carried away from the filter by a side exit port and a pump, where it is measured and directed into a collection bottle or bag as waste; this convective clearance of solutes is similar to urine produced by the normal kidneys. The plasma water loss is replaced in equal volume with a commercially manufactured plasma water substitute; as previously stated it can be either postdilution, after the 'filtered' blood exits the haemofilter, or predilution, prior to the blood entering the haemofilter, or it can be both at the same time (pre- and postdilution). The plasma water replacement contains no metabolic wastes and achieves blood purification as it is continuously replaced.[113,123]

Filter membrane polymers are made of different materials: AN69 (acrylonitrile/sodium methallyl sulfonate), polyacrylonitrile, polyamide and polysulfone[97] or polyethersulfone.[111] All demonstrate similar artificial kidney effects and are generally chosen according to the supplier circuit provided or, when this is not fixed, by the vendor or prescribing preference.[127] The most important characteristics of filters used in continuous modes of therapy are: (1) a high plasma water clearance rate at low blood flow rates and circuit pressures and (2) high permeability to middle-sized molecular weight substances (500–15,000 daltons, e.g. inflammatory cytokines), which are often encountered in critical illness.[97,128]

More recently, membranes are provided with a heparin coating and charge polarity to promote binding and removal of toxins.[129,130]

Vascular access

As previously noted, to establish CRRT it is necessary to create a blood flow outside the body using the EC.[108] Blood is most commonly accessed from the venous circulation of the critical care patient via a catheter placed in a central vein (e.g. femoral). Blood is both withdrawn from the vein and returned to the same vein – that is, venovenous access by means of a double (dual)-lumen catheter.[111] Venovenous haemofiltration has the advantages of requiring only a single venipuncture, a reliable blood flow delivered from a blood pump and alternative venous access sites if there is site infection or access is difficult.

The dual-lumen catheter used for venovenous access has an internal diameter of 1.5–3 mm and catheter lumens are sufficiently separated at their tip to prevent filtered blood from mixing with unfiltered blood when used in the recommended sequence.[131] This ensures that filtered blood does not simply pass back through the EC and artificial kidney, where there would be minimal waste clearance compared with 'fresh' unfiltered blood; this design is illustrated in Fig. 18.9A. The catheter must be small enough to place into a vein but large enough to provide blood flow of at least 200 mL/min for an adult CRRT circuit. Catheters are made with different arrangements of the lumens revealing variation in their cross-section profile (see Fig. 18.9B); however, design

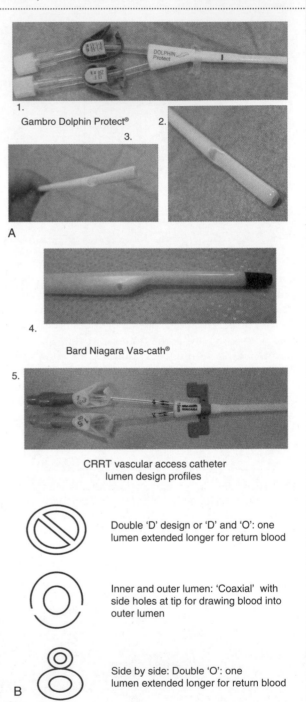

FIGURE 18.9 **(A)** Vascular-access catheters for continuous renal replacement therapy (CRRT). Dual-lumen, Bard® Niagara™ and Gambro Dolphin Protect™ catheters; **(B)** concept diagram of catheter lumen profiles used for dual-lumen CRRT catheters.

1. Gambro Dolphin Protect®
2.
3.
4.
A

Bard Niagara Vas-cath®

5.

CRRT vascular access catheter lumen design profiles

Double 'D' design or 'D' and 'O': one lumen extended longer for return blood

Inner and outer lumen: 'Coaxial' with side holes at tip for drawing blood into outer lumen

Side by side: Double 'O': one lumen extended longer for return blood

B

requirements are such that the outflow from the catheter is via a red end connection, and return blood flow via the blue connection.[110,131] There is no evidence to suggest which internal or distal tip profile is better,[132,133] but the larger the internal diameter, and when advanced closer to the right heart,[134] the less likely it is that flow will be obstructed during patient care with CRRT. After a catheter is threaded into a vein, the blood flow may be adequate, but later during patient care it may be obstructed because of different nursing interventions and patient movement, which may alter blood flows within the low-pressure venous system.[135]

Insertion sites may be affected by nursing care interventions. Placement of the catheter is usually in the femoral or internal jugular vein, and less often the subclavian.[127,136,137] In short-term haemodialysis catheterisation, femoral and internal jugular central venous access routes have similar risks for catheter-related complications, except internal jugular central venous access routes can be associated with a higher risk of mechanical complications.[138] The right internal jugular vein is the vessel of choice for CRRT because it is the shortest, most direct vascular route to the right atrium and therefore provides potentially better blood flow.[137,138] The left internal jugular vein can also be used, but it has a longer and less direct route to the right atrium. Anecdotally, the subclavian position is more easily managed for dressing and securing, continuous observation and patient comfort, but is more problematic in terms of flow reliability. KDIGO practice guidelines[111,131] do not support use of the subclavian vein. Intrathoracic pressure changes associated with physiotherapy or spontaneous patient coughing and breathing, coupled with the upright position of patients, may hinder blood flow from the subclavian-sited access catheter. While these issues are not encountered with a femoral-placed catheter, flow problems can arise due to side lying and flexion at the groin or hip.[99,136,138]

> ### Practice tip
>
> If CRRT circuits clot or fail, remember, if this is associated with failure of the access catheter, restarting a new treatment is also likely to fail unless the catheter is changed or resited. The solution or response is not to prompt an increase in anticoagulant dose.

Blood pump

In venovenous modes, a pump component is essential as part of the patient's blood volume flows externally to the body via the EC. Blood flow is maintained by a rotating wheel with blood-filled tubing inserted, known as a 'roller pump'. This pump allows compression of tubing to move the blood forwards and is designed to avoid causing cell damage when working, provide a reliable flow and be correct for the prescription, as this setting (mL/min) associates with the fluids used (L/h) which together create the clearance or removal of wastes dosage. The tubing in the pump must recoil and fill with new outflow blood for the next compression and stroke volume not unlike the human heart with atrial or ventricular filling. Faster or higher flow rate settings above 300 mL/min. despite the

best vascular access, may not be achieved because of the limitations of roller pumps.[135,139,140]

Venous return line bubble trap chamber

The purpose of using a bubble trap chamber is to prevent any gas bubbles in the EC from entering the patient's circulation by allowing them to rise to the top of a small, vertically positioned collection reservoir (Fig. 18.10). Venous pressure is commonly measured via a tubing connection into the top of this venous chamber, and additional intravenous fluids can be administered into this chamber via a secondary tube connection. The level of blood in the chamber must be below the top, to prevent spillage into the pressure-monitoring line. It is advised that the blood level be adjusted to near full to allow for visual inspection of incoming blood flow and to ensure that any air or gas bubbles are trapped here.[139,141] As this creates a gas–blood interface within the venous chamber, there is a potential source of venous chamber clotting and hence circuit failure.[139,141] Addition of replacement fluids into this chamber when using post-dilution fluid administration can cause a plasma fluid layer to develop above the blood level and may reduce clotting by stopping blood foaming on its surface, and it eliminates air or gas contact with the blood.[141,142] Newer CRRT machine designs either do not have a bubble trap (e.g. NxStage® System[143] (NxStage Medical Inc., Lawrence, MA)), or use a small chamber to remove gas and minimise clotting at this point.

Anticoagulation

There are several different drugs used to prevent blood clotting in the EC; heparin, prostacyclin, thrombin

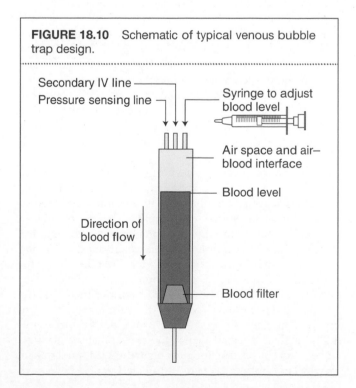

FIGURE 18.10   Schematic of typical venous bubble trap design.

Secondary IV line
Pressure sensing line
Syringe to adjust blood level
Air space and air–blood interface
Blood level
Direction of blood flow
Blood filter

TABLE 18.2

Commonly used anticlotting agents for CRRT

DRUG	BENEFITS	PRECAUTIONS
Heparin	Inexpensive, wide experience, easily reversed, easily monitored, short half-life.	Sensitivity reactions, heparin-induced thrombocytopenia, to be effective means increased risk of bleeding systemically.
Low-molecular-weight heparin (LMWH)	Moderately inexpensive, increasing experience, less likely to result in sensitivity reactions.	Difficult to monitor, not easily reversed, longer half-life, dosing varies between types of LMWH.
Prostacyclin	Very short acting, has a physiological role in inhibiting platelet activity, does not exacerbate other drug reactions.	Expensive, no measure of effectiveness, narrow dose range with associated hypotension, individual patients sensitive to haemodynamic effects, unstable in solution.
Citrate-based solutions or citrate concentrate – as infusion	Limit anticlotting effect to extracorporeal circuit (EC) – 'regional anticoagulation'; results suggest very effective in prolonging circuit life.	Substantial metabolic effect if not adequately managed (serum ionised calcium must be monitored closely); requires additions to EC to administer and reverse and use of specialised replacement/dialysate solutions; not useful when liver failure present, citrate is converted to bicarbonate by the liver providing the necessary buffer for renal replacement therapy (RRT); acidosis may occur in liver failure.
No anticlotting agent (with saline flushes)	No side effects, no exacerbation of unstable haematological status, liver failure.	May encounter very short circuit life that consumes remaining haematological components; risk of fluid overload if saline flushes are not part of fluid balance; no evidence that saline flushes have any benefit.

inhibitors and sodium citrate have been well described in the literature and can be used separately or in various combinations; each has potential complications or side effects (Table 18.2).[131,144–146] As blood comes into contact with the plastic tubing and the polymer fibres of the filter, various clotting systems are activated. This is a normal action of blood when exposed to non-biological surfaces. The aim of anticlotting drugs is to delay clot formation while the blood is outside the body, particularly when within the densely packed fibres of the filter. As calcium, blood platelet cells and thrombin are vital in clot formation, these drugs are targeted to one of these elements. This targeting must not be too pronounced, as the patient may begin to bleed when the blood returns from the EC to the body.

Heparin is the most commonly used agent for the prevention of clotting, as it is inexpensive, widely available and easily reversed by another drug, protamine.[147] Heparin is usually administered into the EC before the blood enters the filter (prefilter or membrane), although the optimal place to administer any anticoagulant drug during CRRT is not agreed upon, before the key area for clotting seems sensible.[148,149] A bolus is often given prior to circuit connection, either in the circuit prime or via the venous access catheter to boost the clotting time before maintenance infusion. A maintenance dose (5–15 units/kg/h) is then adjusted against the relevant laboratory tests and a visual inspection for clotting in the EC is undertaken, particularly noting the venous bubble trap.

Sodium citrate is another popular anticoagulant for CRRT as a first-line agent and method in the critically ill, and replaces the traditional use of heparin.[150] Citrate provides the anticoagulant and the buffer for pH control and chelates calcium, inducing anticoagulation of blood by reducing the serum ionised calcium level.[151] For anticoagulation, the dose and administration rate of citrate are commonly set to achieve a reduction in the CRRT circuit blood ionised calcium level to <0.3 mmol/L.[151,152] As ionised calcium is essential for the progression of the coagulation cascade to form a stable clot, an anticoagulant effect is achieved when the calcium is bound or chelated.[151,152] A continuous infusion of citrate is administered into the CRRT circuit before the membrane, similar to use of heparin. Citrate is provided as an additive to commercially prepared CRRT replacement fluids and this dilute preparation in association with the blood flow rate, as well described in the literature, creates the suitable dose. When circuit blood returns to the patient circulation, it mixes with systemic blood and the calcium concentration is restored to normal; free citrate not binding to calcium is metabolised by the liver to provide carbon dioxide and bicarbonate as a necessary buffer.[153] Citrate-bound calcium is lost in the waste fluid removed with RRT and requires replacement by a separate calcium infusion to maintain serum calcium levels to normal, at 1.0–1.3 mmol/L.[152] Due to the complex nature of the citrate-based anticoagulation approach, a number of different protocols have been proposed and used to optimise dose for the

RRT and the citrate necessary; the fluids used are provided at variable concentrations, and used with variable blood flow rates and, when necessary, calcium free dialysate fluid to prevent excessive loss of citrate, inadequate buffer control and/or toxicity with failed citrate metabolism.[151,153] Not all methods will be applied in the one ICU, and local expertise development of one method and an alternative is common. Recent reviews provide a good synopsis of each method, as they are different depending on the CVVH or CVVHDf mode.[151,154]

Fig 18.8 is a circuit diagram to represent how citrate and bicarbonate fluid are used to provide therapy in CVVHDf mode; this provides anticoagulation and buffer together in association with calcium replacement to the patient.

Thrombin inhibitors are another type of anticoagulant that can be used in CRRT. They inhibit free and clot-bound thrombin and do not react with antibodies to heparin.[155,156] Thrombin inhibitors such as argatroban are useful in patients who have heparin-induced thrombocytopenia associated with heparin anticoagulation.[156,157] These inhibitors are more expensive than heparin but provide effective anticoagulation. The KDIGO guidelines and recent reviews for CRRT[1,7,75,77] provide clinical guidance for the use of thrombin inhibitors and when they are of benefit rather than other anticoagulants or no anticoagulant when heparin-induced thrombocytopenia is suspected or confirmed. Argatroban is cleared by the liver and has a half-life of 31–59 minutes.[156] Dosage includes a loading and a maintenance dose adjusted to keep the activated partial thromboplastin time (aPTT) 1–3 times the reference level.[155,156]

If bleeding occurs during anticoagulation with argatroban, the infusion can be turned off. In an ex vivo study, the effects of argatroban were able to be reversed using recombinant-activated factor VII. In patients with hepatic failure or with multiple organ dysfunction syndrome and sepsis, the clearance of argatroban may be markedly reduced.[157]

When citrate is contraindicated with hepatic failure, and when heparin has either failed or been associated with thrombocytopenia, epoprostenol (prostacyclin PGI2) can be used with effect.[158] The infusion is also administered into the CRRT circuit before the membrane and at an increasing dose for effect but can cause hypotension, limiting dose increases.

Low-molecular-weight heparin drugs such as enoxaparin or danaparoid may also be used with similar context to epoprostenol, and without the concern for vasodilation and reduction in vital blood pressure in the acutely ill. This group of drugs is more expensive and are not easily assayed or monitored and reversed in effect.[159,160]

Fluids and fluid balance

Fluid used during any form of CRRT is a commercially manufactured product with an electrolyte composition similar to blood plasma.[161] This provides a solution useful as a replacement solution for plasma water removed in convective mode such as CVVH, or as a dialysate solution in diffusive mode or CVVHDf.[162] These respective applications allow for plasma water replacement with 'clean' and buffered plasma water following toxin-laden plasma water removal or, during CVVHDf, for plasma water to be exposed to the whole blood across the membrane fibres so that toxins and molecules will diffusively exchange from blood into the fluid. The additives or recipes for three commonly used commercial fluids are listed in Table 18.3 together with saline solution and normal blood plasma chemistry for comparative analysis. The key additives of note in commercial fluids are the elevated level of bicarbonate and a variable concentration of potassium (no potassium option also), providing an effective buffer for the acidaemia and hyperkalaemia associated with AKI.[163]

Throughout the course of a continuous treatment with CRRT, hypokalaemia may occur, and a higher potassium-added solution may be required to correct and maintain normal serum levels. Bicarbonate-added fluid is prepared just prior to use by combining a two-compartment bag (Fig. 18.11) as the two fluids are unstable in long-term storage. The higher cost, problems with reconstituting bicarbonate solution bags and manual handling of large (5 L) fluid bags did increase interest in 'online' fluid production from tap-water at the bedside. This approach can be less expensive and requires no bag changing or reconstituting by nurses,[164] but does require the installation of a complex and expensive reverse osmosis machine, the cost of which would be offset if large volumes of fluid were then consumed from this online manufacture. This approach is used in some centres for these reasons, and is applied as ICU 'daily dialysis' or extended dialysis modes[165] and is the therapy of choice using well-known and understood methods from chronic dialysis methods and technology.[166]

Fluid balance monitoring and adjustment to machine settings is a key nursing responsibility in managing a patient treated with CRRT.[167] This requires an operator of the machine to enter a rate of fluid removal each hour, or for a longer set time period, and the machine is intended to achieve this target for the set time. It is important to remember that this volume of fluid removed is simply the machine-prescribed loss of fluid removed, commonly determined by electronic scales in the machine or the balancing chambers, and does not equate to the overall fluid balance of the patient.[65,79,86,168] A simple fluid balance calculation accounts for addition of all intakes, plus small physician-ordered volume loss, minus outputs each hour. The set volume removal each hour to achieve a desired fluid state must be determined in context for the entire clinical status of a patient where verbal communication and written prescribing orders must be clear to differentiate 'machine loss – setting' from patient net 'loss' or balance per hour.[169] A calculation example is provided in Fig. 18.12. Despite simple software for setting the desired fluid loss or removal per hour during treatment, mistakes and errors occur.[170] In some cases, particularly in

TABLE 18.3
Blood plasma chemistry compared with commonly used commercial CRRT fluids

	BLOOD – PLASMA (A)	SALINE (BAXTER, TOONGABBIE, AUSTRALIA)	BAXTER ACCUSOL	GAMBRO HEMOSOL B0 (GAMBRO, LUND, SWEDEN)	BAXTER HAEMOFILTRATION CITRATE SOLUTION (BAXTER, TOONGABBIE, AUSTRALIA)
Sodium (mmol/L)	136–145	150	140	140	152
Chloride (mmol/L)	98–107	150	113.5	109.5	99
Potassium (mmol/L)	3.5–5.1	0	4.0 or 2.0	4.0 or 2.0	5
Bicarbonate (mmol/L)	22–29	0	35	32	0
Calcium	2.15–2.55	0	1.75	1.75	0
Magnesium	0.66–1.07	0	0.5	0.5	0
Citrate (mmol/L)	0	0	0	0	18
Lactate	0.5–2.2		0	3.0	0.0
pH (range)	7.35–7.45	4.0–7.0	7.4	7.0–8.5	5–6.5
mOsm/kg (listed or estimated)	280–300	300	300.3	287	270

Adult ranges from: https://www.austinpathology.org.au/test-directory.

FIGURE 18.11 Two-compartment bicarbonate bag. CRRT = continuous renal replacement therapy.

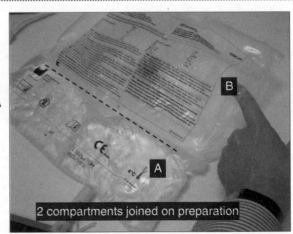

Bicarbonate CRRT fluid
Main bag – bicarbonate – B
Small bag – electrolytes – A

K^+ of 0 or K^+ of 4
No glucose

2 compartments joined on preparation

small children and babies, this can be fatal.[171,172] Most machines now provide limits for the amount of accumulative fluid balance error (+ve or −ve) before an alarm will sound with a display message to advise the nurse. Such errors can occur as a result of fluid bags remaining clamped, or fluid pathway lines kinked or clamped. Logically, the machine is removing or infusing fluid but the machine scales or balancing chambers are not detecting a weight change.[173] The fluids infused as replacement or removed as waste plus additional fluid for a loss are usually all recorded on a fluid balance formula in electronic charting at the bedside. This is presented as inputs and outputs charting, with the difference between these amounts understood as the balance; usually a negative in the context of a patient with AKI, anuric and in the ICU setting is commonly set for a negative balance overall. This fluid balance is achieved easily with recent electronic records included in ICU clinical information

FIGURE 18.12 Continuous renal replacement therapy (CRRT) hourly fluid balance calculation example.

CRRT Typical Fluid Balance Calculation

All intakes (tube feeds, IVs IVBPs, flushes) mL	**A**	110
MD ordered net loss	**B**	(+50 mL)
Total		160 mL
All outputs (nasogastric tube, chest drain(s), urine output or stool)	**C**	−10
	D	(+150 mL)
Actual fluid pumped mL	**E**	142

Actual Fluid Balance = (A − C) − E
Most e-charting will automatically calculate fluid balance

and patient management systems and presented as a spreadsheet, and with similarities to paper charts used many years ago, and accelerated in use during the COVID-19 pandemic.[174]

Irrespective of patient acuity, when CRRT is used, individual patient assessment for fluid status must occur at least twice a day. Subtle temperature changes in the patient, surgical drain losses, diarrhoea and variable fluid intake all contribute to a more precise fluid balance.[79] Regular weighing of patients may assist in assessing overall patient condition,[168,175] in addition to regular physical and clinical assessment of the patient. Electrolyte disturbances may also occur despite use of balanced replacement solutions. Particular attention should focus on regular assessment of fluid and electrolytes, especially potassium, sodium, phosphate and magnesium levels. Fluids and their composition are changing and new additives such as phosphate are being introduced into clinical care: (i) where low phosphate levels are apparent, (ii) with higher volume and treatment dose as phosphate removal is high and (iii) after many weeks of CRRT in the critically ill whose nutrition is poor.[176]

Practice tip

Fluid removal during CRRT is prescribed by doctors and usually to a time frame or target aim for the day. The nurse needs to calculate the rate per hour for the target and perform a recalculation if CRRT is off and there is no treatment for any time.

Patient management

Nursing protocols have previously been focused on machine priming, patient preparation and use of a CRRT system, as this was the essential training pathway for nurses learning the operator–machine–patient interface.[99,177] Current CRRT machines are highly automated and have advanced software with instructional on-screen coloured pictures, circuit diagrams and text prompts providing a sequential step-by-step approach for priming, patient connection and key alarms. Nonetheless, the clinical knowledge, psychomotor skills and the responsibility for managing an EC to efficiently and safely treat a critically ill patient should not be understated.[178] The nurse-to-patient ratio for CRRT is commonly 1:1 worldwide, acknowledging the attention and focus required despite the advances in machine automation.[173,178,179] This is a reasonable approach, as CRRT in the ICU is very different to the use of dialysis for chronic renal failure where a nurse may oversee three or four patients on dialysis under their care and with different start times (overlapping) for a 3–4-hour treatment in each case. In the ICU these patients are usually in a multiorgan failure state, are intubated and require mechanical ventilation, cardiovascular support and/or enteral feeding, need many intravenous drugs and infusions and have reduced neurological function with or without sedation. This is a picture mandating both technical and cognitive tasks in addition to comprehensive nursing care, including full hygiene and all care for the bedridden and often unconscious patient.

Monitoring correct machine function for reliable flow of blood, continuous changing of bags as substitution fluids empty and waste bags fill, adjustment and constant review for stability with anticoagulation agents and the overall monitoring and response to other parameters of patient metabolic stability with electrolyte, acid–base and temperature management represent some of the work associated with the nursing care required.[173,177] Machine and circuit preparation, connection and, when required, stopping and disconnecting a treatment are further skill and knowledge sets for ICU nurses. It is in the key interest of both doctors and nurses in the ICU that the treatment be 'continuous', as frequent stopping and restarting increases nursing workload and may cause instability in the patient.[180,181]

In Table 18.4 a summary of key nursing practice and interventions for bedside use is provided, making this information a suitable reference for nursing knowledge and skills associated with CRRT use in the ICU. Practice recommendations are also included. This information is general to any CRRT machine and does not include a detailed anticoagulation protocol. Anticoagulation technique for CRRT usually dominates any policy and is viewed more frequently in comparison with the psychomotor skills component for machine preparation, connection and fluids bags management. Nursing practice policies can also be supplemented with machine-specific and quick-reference 'one-page' lists for shift check or anticoagulation method. Fig. 18.13 is an example of a shift checklist. Publications for the many aspects of nursing implementation and use of CRRT in the ICU are available and can provide ideas for checklists, teaching

TABLE 18.4

Troubleshooting guide: key nursing practice and interventions for CRRT

	POTENTIAL PROBLEM (NUMBERED LIST)	KEY NURSING INTERVENTIONS REQUIRED, REFERENCED TO LISTED NUMBER
Patient and machine/ system preparation before use	1 Machine alarms and technical failure on starting treatment 2 Air entrainment during prime 3 Fluid setting errors 4 Fluids/electrolytes incorrect 5 Machine and patient too far apart or machine placed out of staff view	1 Machine self-test and/or checklist completed. 2 Double-check all circuit lines around circuit, particularly for clamps ON or OFF as required. 3 Treatment orders cross-checked with settings. 4 Double-check fluids used, e.g. any additives required. 5 Position machine according to access catheter site: at feet for femoral line, at bedside for subclavian and at bed head for jugular with screen faced to staff desk or charts/computer. Recommendation: • Have your own pre-start check routine (paper document list).

Connection to the system and initiation of therapy	1 Access catheter obstruction/failure
	2 Hypotension on start
		1 Prepare access connections with antiseptic, aspirate any instilled drug and test easy flush return (venous) lumen and aspirate outflow (arterial) lumen.
		2 Connect both circuit lines to access catheter administering priming volume to patient:
		  a Increase vasoactive drugs if necessary to increase MAP.
		  b Start blood pump slowly with small increases until blood fills all the circuit.
		Recommendations:
		• Use two nurses for connection routine; start fluid replacement and removal only after blood circuit is full and at prescribed speed; stay with patient until stable ≈ first 15 min.
		• Patient in bed, supine position and MAP >70 mmHg, stable.

In-use troubleshooting alarms and maintenance, fluid balance	1 Excessive negative pressure >−100 mmHg: 'arterial alarm' 2 High pressure >+100 mmHg: 'venous alarm' 3 High TMP alarm 4 Air-detected alarm 5 Hypothermia 6 Fluid balance errors 7 Electrolyte imbalance	1 & 2 Maintain access catheter alignment, preventing kinks in access and circuit lines. 1 & 2 Do not place extra connections or taps between access catheter and circuit lines. 3 Suggests filter clotting or blood flow too slow for fluids settings. 4 Ensure venous chamber is filled with blood, and bubbles are removed regularly with post-dilution fluid into the chamber. 5 Heater set to 37°C or greater to compensate for heat loss from EC. 6 Use fluids charting or similar to account for all fluid inputs including anticoagulant volume. Clarify orders to set machine 'loss' in respect of this. Commonly a net negative. Orders and settings should not be prescribed to administer fluid – no net positive. 7 Potassium additive to CRRT fluid is often required after 24–48 h of treatment; some patients are hypokalaemic despite acute renal failure. Phosphate monitoring and correction are important. Recommendations: • Assess and reset fluid balance settings hourly, particularly in unstable patients and for inexperienced staff. • Fluid gain or positive fluid balance using CRRT should be considered an adverse event or complication of use.

Monitoring and adjustment to anticoagulation	1 Premature clotting in circuit and filter	1 Check and monitor effect of anticoagulant therapy according to local policy. With heparin use this could be after first 6 h and then daily:
		  a Maintain adequate dose to therapeutic range.
		  b Use predilution fluid administration.
		  c Use blood flow greater than 150 mL/min.
		  d Use large-bore access catheter and take care not to obstruct or kink catheter.
		  e Keep blood pump operating: minimise stops >30 s.
		Recommendation:
		• If frequent failure (clotting <4 h), always check for blood-flow obstruction before more, or alternative, anticoagulation; e.g. review to consider change or replacement of access catheter.

TABLE 18.4

Troubleshooting guide: key nursing practice and interventions for CRRT—cont'd

	POTENTIAL PROBLEM (NUMBERED LIST)	KEY NURSING INTERVENTIONS REQUIRED, REFERENCED TO LISTED NUMBER
Access care and dressings	1 Access dislodgement 2 Access catheter infection 3 Access catheter obstruction	1 Ensure catheter sutured in place and well secured with dressing; single or double ('sandwich' technique) biofilm–polyurethane. 2 Use asepsis when flushing or connecting to access catheter; monitor site for infection and patient for suspected line sepsis; use catheter site alcohol patch, e.g. chlorhexidine-impregnated dressing. 3 Use heparin to fill catheter dead space when not in use for >4 h and label accordingly. Recommendation: • Use flexible dressing with application to both sides along catheter allowing movement away off skin surface, preventing obstruction during patient care/ positioning and lifting or tearing off dressing.
Vital sign monitoring	1 Arrhythmias, hypotension, temperature	1 Monitor vital signs hourly; consider any links between changes, and use of RRT; e.g. low CVP and excessive fluid removal, temperature fluctuations when CRRT OFF and ON. Recommendation: • CVP readings should be performed every 2–4 hours during CRRT; CVP can be used as a target for daily fluid loss prescription. Weigh the patient if possible. Do frequent blood gas and electrolytes commonly associated with ICU care.
Assessment of filter function and patency	1 Filter clotting abruptly with inability to return circuit blood to the patient 2 Inadequate solute removal	1 If TMP or pre-filter pressure (P-IN) >250 mmHg is diagnostic of filter clotting, consider electively returning blood by crystalloid infusion into outflow limb of circuit and ceasing treatment – follow local policy. Observe for venous chamber clot development. If excessive and venous pressure >150 mmHg, consider electively returning blood cease treatment. 2 Assess patient's solute levels: urea and creatinine should be reducing or stable. Recommendations: • Predicting circuit or filter clotting can be difficult. TMP and P-IN can rise quickly after being stable or within normal range. If there is a trend upwards reflecting diagnosis of clotting, cease treatment electively to avoid blood flow 'standstill' and a failure to restart and blood loss. • Nurses may document these pressures hourly or check the machine frequently, but they must respond quickly to cease treatment.
Cessation of treatment and disconnection from the extracorporeal circuit	1 Blockage and/or clotting in access catheter 2 Inadvertent blood loss 3 Infectious risk	1 Use concentrated heparin (other anticoagulant) to fill dead space of catheter when not in use >4 h. Use heparin 1000 IU/mL and follow manufacturer's specifications for volume required. 2 Always attempt to cease a circuit before it clots and always return patient blood if possible. 3 Use asepsis for disconnection procedure. Recommendation: • Access catheter should not be used for other purposes/infusions when RRT is not connected.
Temporary disconnection for procedures	1 Maintenance of circuit before reconnection 2 Infection 3 Inadvertent fluid administration	1 Flush out any excess blood residue in circuit; keep blood pump operational with saline (prime) in circuit. 2 For circuits in use for >24 h before disconnection or not restarted after 6 h following temporary disconnection, consider discarding. 3 After restarting circuit, increase fluid loss to remove fluid used to re-establish RRT. Recommendation: • Reuse of circuits in this context is not desirable and with prior planning should be avoidable, e.g. plan for radiology, surgery, etc. when circuit off or restart new circuit around these interventions. If this is done, consider adding heparin 5000 IU to circuit when temporarily disconnected unless contraindicated, but flush this out with 200–300 mL prime solution before reconnection; always use additive label indicating heparin added.

CRRT = continuous renal replacement therapy; CVP = central venous pressure; EC = extracorporeal circuit; MAP = mean arterial pressure; RRT = renal replacement therapy; TMP = transmembrane pressure.

FIGURE 18.13 Shift checklist for continuous renal replacement therapy (CRRT). CVVH = continuous venovenous haemofiltration; UF = ultrafiltrate.

Shift check list CRRT as CVVH: Infomed HF 440

Check	Rationale
Machine position relative to patient with blood lines not too tight – stretched	Patient movement could cause excess drag on vascath site and securing tape
Brakes ON	Machine must have brakes on to prevent inadvertent movement and risk of above
Fluids: correct for K^+ and both bags hanging from same point – height, both line clamps open	Fluids should empty at similar rate, minimise mixing, scales and balance alarms more likely if the bags hanging at different heights
Flush line connected, correct fluid, clamped as close to blood path as possible. Date this bag	Fluid to return patient blood; this may be required any time. Clamp close to blood path to prevent blood tracking back up this line and clotting, only to be flushed in with use
Waste bottle hanging stable and waste pump hose with end plug ready, coiled on machine holder	This bottle will weigh > 16 kg on full. Needs to hang with stability to prevent scales alarms. Hose ready for use with end cap to prevent drips
Venous – bubble chamber full and inspect for clot	Adjust this up slowly, with syringe attached. Keep full to trap gas / air and allow for the level to fall during use with gas entry associated with bicarbonate fluids (CO_2) when heated
Luer syringe (10 mL), 3-way tap and dead end cap (red) in line – for chamber adjustment	Luer syringe will not fall / slip off during use; red cap blocks pathway between venous blood chamber and UF pathway if 3-way tap was accidently opened to both chambers.
Screen settings & alarms	
Blood flow – speed	200 mL/min standard
UF flow	2000 mL/h standard CVVH
Manual Pre-dilution %	50:50 for CVVH (Citrate use 70% pre)
'Weight loss' – Fluid loss rate mL/h	Check orders – fluid loss target
Next intervention (h:min)	Time until fluids bag change or bottle empty
Temperature setting	Default at 37°, maybe ↑↓ to patient need
Venous +10 to + 150 mmHg (influenced by blood flow rate and chamber clotting, access function – blue lumen)	This pressure always positive, measured on the return limb of circuit. ~ +50 to +100 mmHg
Arterial −150 to −10 mmHg (influenced by blood flow rate and access function – red lumen)	This pressure always negative, measured on the outflow limb of circuit. ~ −50 to −100 mmHg
Trans-membrane pressure (TMP) (Pin + Pv)/2 – Puf	Indicative of clotting / clogging in the membrane. Set at 200 mmHg initially. When 250^+ mmHg, usually terminate treatment.
Anticoagulation and prescription orders	Check drug dose and orders correct

tools and policy design for what can be termed a 'CRRT program'. A program representing this support being available and used in an ICU benefits from close links with the vendor or a specific machine supplier, as their 'CRRT package' can include machines, circuit and membrane, vascular access catheters, anticoagulation protocols and CRRT fluids.[173] In ICU, both nursing and medical disciplines have individuals who are expert in CRRT, and doctors will diagnose, prescribe and manage AKI with CRRT independent of nephrologists.[77]

Continuous renal replacement machines

There are many machines available for CRRT in the ICU. How to identify the machine that a particular ICU should use or purchase is a common question from nurses, and there is limited literature available providing comparisons of their technical characteristics,[182,183] and more recent reviews for this decision, their use and the future with further automation are encouraging.[184,185] Table 18.5 outlines the major differences in machines or

TABLE 18.5

Machine design and build approaches

MACHINE TYPE	WASTE COLLECTION	MEMBRANE	CIRCUIT	PRESSURE MEASUREMENT	PRIMING PREPARATION AND SOFTWARE OPTION(S)
A	One 5-L or 10-L bag; empty when full, change bag(s)	AN69, prefitted, not changeable	Cartridge kit-based, multipurpose; all modes	In-line pressure transducers	Fully automated, software for management of citrate anticoagulation
B	One 5-L or two bags; empty when full, change bags	Different membranes possible – polyethersulfone or others	Cartridge kit-based, multipurpose; all modes	In-line pressure transducers	Fully automated, intelligence software for fluid management
C	Drain to bedside outlet; no bag collection required	Company-provided membrane in kit	Cartridge kit-based, multipurpose; all modes	In-line and other pressure transducers	Fully automated, intelligence software for fluid management

system approaches. Three machines adopting common design features from Table 18.5 are shown in Fig. 18.14 (Prismaflex; Hospal, Lyon, France), Fig. 18.15 (Aquarius, Nikkiso, Sydney, Australia) and Fig. 18.16 (NxStage®, Lawrence MA), each highlighting the major technical differences in how CRRT machines are presented and used.

Teaching and training CRRT

Since introduction of CRRT to the ICU in the 1980s and early 1990s, medical companies as machine vendors have developed and expanded their offerings for teaching and training nurses in the use of CRRT machines and the broader aspects of AKI and patient care. More commonly, where CRRT has imbedded in clinical practice for many years, the education focus is with smaller groups teaching new procedures and methods, updates, orientation for new staff and specialist training in association with postgraduate certification. These didactic session topics may be scheduled in the sequence and over several weeks to become more powerful when supplemented with simulation activities linked to live patient care and bedside clinical support.[100,101,106] A recent report suggests that, when simulation is added to didactic CRRT education programs, an improvement in CRRT functional time (filter 'life') is observed – a direct benefit to users, lessening cost and better for patients.[186]

The key to successful CRRT education and training is to develop nurses with clinical experience managing CRRT regularly in the ICU and encourage these experts to teach others around them when they can. Educators may already be in place for broader aspects of ICU education and postgraduate trainees but, for any staffing structure with or without dedicated teaching roles, identifying a small number of nurses as CRRT 'champions' for training and ongoing support when CRRT is in progress is a common and successful approach to provide learning for others over the 24/7 context in the ICU.[99,187]

FIGURE 18.14 Prismax continuous renal replacement therapy machine.

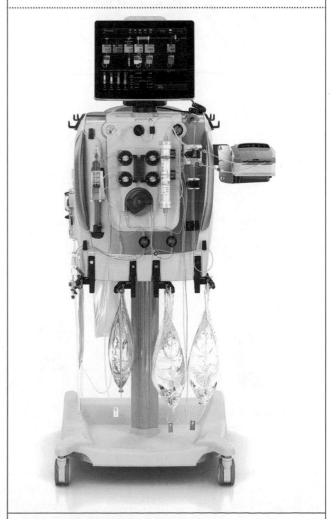

Source: © Baxter Healthcare.

FIGURE 18.15 Aquarius continuous renal replacement therapy machine.

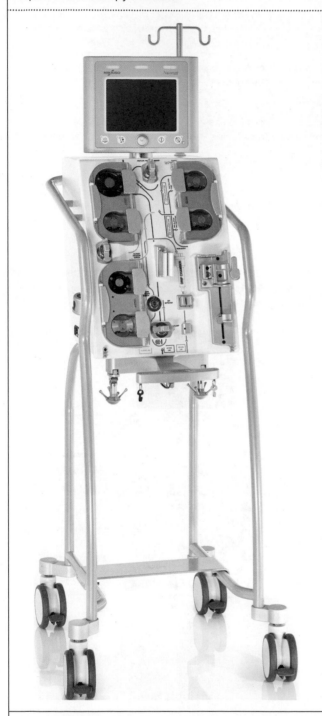

Source: © Nikkiso, Nikkiso ANZ.

FIGURE 18.16 NxStage System One continuous renal replacement therapy machine.

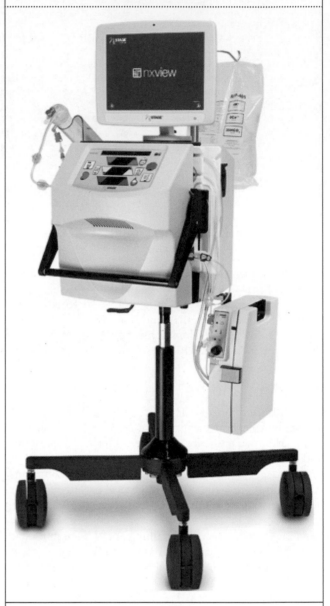

Source: Courtesy NxStage Medical, Lawrence, MA, USA

Quality and measures of success

Maintaining quality and nursing expertise for CRRT in the ICU will be related to the frequency of use and the size of the user group. When there are long periods between CRRT use, and/or when the ICU has a large number of staff members, ensuring competency may be challenging. Regular competency checks and staff assessments can be performed,[177,187] depending upon resource allocation for this task. Shift allocation of the nurse to a patient with AKI and treatment with CRRT care may benefit from predetermined skill sets as a guide to best match the individual nurse's competency with the CRRT-treated patient and ensure safety.[177,179] The most useful measure for quality when using CRRT is the progressive 'life' of the circuit or filter.[187,188] This data point may be recorded on bedside e-charts alongside hourly observations and provides an instant audit for

FIGURE 18.17 Bedside charts concept image with consecutive filter life hours associated with hourly vital signs and charting in the ICU. Time on and off treatment is easily identified, in addition to total hours delivered each day (hours and % of each 24). CRRT = continuous renal replacement therapy.

First entry at 0100 h, beginning a 24-h period of charting or e-recording

Infusion A (mg/h)	30	30	30	30	30	40	40	40	40	40	40	40	40	30	30	30	30	30	30	30	30	30	30	30
Infusion B (mg/h)	5	5	5	5	5	5	5	5	6	6	6	6	6	6	---	---	---	---	---	---	---	---	---	---
CRRT filter 'life' h cumulative	28	29	30	31	32	33	34	35	■	1	2	3	4	5	6	7	8	9	10	11	12	■	■	1

The above charting concepts shows continuity from previous day: filter life(s) of 35, 12 h, 90% delivered time

Infusion A (mg/h)	30	30	30	30	30	40	40	40	40	40	40	40	40	30	30	30	30	30	30	30	30	30	30	30
Infusion B (mg/h)	5	5	5	5	5	5	5	5	6	6	6	6	6	6	---	---	---	---	---	---	---	---	---	---
CRRT filter 'life' h cumulative	---	---	---	1	2	3	4	5	■	1	2	3	4	5	6	7	■	■	1	2	3	■	■	■

The above charting concepts shows CRRT starting day, and filter life(s) of 5, 7, 3 h and 15 h/24 this day. 62%

each circuit used and throughout the patient treatment (see Fig. 18.17, charting filter life or cumulative hours of use for a circuit and filter). This variable is most commonly used to compare efficacy of different anticoagulation techniques, but may also be considered a measure of access catheter and blood flow reliability, machine technical function and staff user competence.[188] Circuit or filter life (these terms are used interchangeably) is reported widely in the literature and, despite lacking a clear bedside definition, published data from large randomised trials indicate that a median life of 21 hours is common.[119,189] Poor circuit life at 4–6 hours reflects clinical problems and an interprofessional review before the next treatment begins is warranted. Machines will usually log this data in the treatment or therapy history along with alarm events, and may also be included in a dashboard view and download.[190] Quality for CRRT programs can include these top ten: (i) dose delivery as set volumes/kg of diffusion and/or convection multiplied by number of hours per day, (ii) filter life or consecutive hours of operation before stopping from clotting, (iii) downtime or the time off treatment after stopping before

restart, (iv) adverse events with blood loss and/or bleeding ranked highly, (v) leadership and prescribing done correctly, (vi) education and teaching completed, (vii) vascular access use and changes needed, along with (viii) machine alarms for this, (ix) AKI and mortality, and (x) cost and wastage tracking.[188]

Special considerations

Paediatrics: babies and small children of 3–30 kg body weight

The use of dialysis and haemofiltration in babies and small children is further developing as a specialty area.[191] However, many aspects of adult CRRT apply, particularly for those patients >15 kg.[192] Key differences, depending on size and weight, for this patient group are: (i) a smaller membrane surface area (size), and smaller circuit tubing to reduce priming and circuit volume, (ii) a smaller access catheter (<7 Fr) depending on body weight and often placed in the femoral vein, (iii) a blood flow rate of 3–5 mL/kg/min, (iv) variable fluids flow (dialysate or substitution) rates depending on mode but 2 L/1.73 m^2/h is common, and (v) increased prevention of hypothermia, as this problem is exacerbated in babies and small infants.[193] Anticoagulation is the same as for adults but with reduced drug doses for the size of the infant or child.[194]

Extracorporeal membrane oxygenation

Increasingly, extracorporeal membrane oxygenation (ECMO) is applied for those with refractory hypoxaemia in association with respiratory failure or used in the context of right heart failure and combined heart–lung failure.[195,196] These critically ill patients frequently have AKI and require CRRT, and useful outcome data is becoming available.[197] It is convenient and often necessary to connect the CRRT circuit into the ECMO circuit, as the patient may have other access sites used for multiple cannulation. In any case, the high blood flow associated with ECMO and the placement of the circuit tubing allow for a connection of the CRRT circuit at many places. The preferred attachment site is preoxygenator.[109,198] The only limiting factor is the positive pressure in the ECMO circuit, which is not compatible with the normally negative access pressure when using venous access with a CRRT machine. Some machines provide a software option to select access pressure positive, allowing this use with ECMO; others do not and may require some alarm override or restrictive device to create negative pressure for the outflow from the ECMO into the CRRT line. Some simple techniques used for insertion of a CRRT circuit into the ECMO circuit can be used to prevent excess pressure alarms.[199]

The anticoagulation provided for the use of ECMO is a convenient state for the successful use of the CRRT and much of this is usually controlled by a perfusionist or a cardiac anaesthetist overseeing the ECMO support in conjunction with the ICU nurse and usually with heparin.[195,196]

Blood purification

This term can be used for all, and any mode or technique associated with an EC and removal of wastes and or toxins by diffusion, convection or both. More advanced in use is removal and discard of whole plasma with equal replacement as plasma exchange,[200] and combined techniques used for isolated cases and/or at some specialist centres where physicians have a dedicated interest and where intermediate hospitals do not have specialist apheresis or nephrology teams available.[201] In some approaches, either whole blood or plasma (after circuit separation from the blood) is pumped through a highly adsorptive membrane to remove toxins or protein-bound drugs, and the clean blood or plasma returned to the EC and patient.[200] In other blood purification methods, different membranes are used to be more selective for larger molecules and target various blood mediators associated with a target illness – sepsis, for example.[202] These are known as high-flux or high-sieving coefficient membranes[97] and are useful when rhabdomyolysis is treated. This condition occurs secondarily to trauma, and particularly crush injury with a high release of myoglobin and myoglobinuria presenting, which is toxic to the kidney and a cause of AKI.[203]

Operating theatre

There are some circumstances when CRRT is useful in the operating theatre. This is in association with any prolonged surgical case where AKI exists in association with a critical illness and specific surgery such as hepatic transplant. Local factors related to ICU staffing, and the surgical and anaesthetic teams' working relationship with the ICU, will influence exactly how this is achieved. The literature in this area is sparse; however, retrospective and small data sets reflect that CRRT in the operating theatre is achievable and safe[204,205] but opinions and data are mixed regarding the benefits.[205–207]

Summary

In this chapter a review of the important physiological functions of the kidney is provided and the context of kidney failure is also defined as an injury, or AKI, and this can be considered in stages of severity and is the basis of classification as for other organ failures. Management of patients with AKI is discussed and includes diagnosis and associated biomarkers, prevention of further injury, fluid and electrolyte balance and aspects of nutrition and pharmacy before consideration of an artificial support or RRT. There are now established criteria for stages of AKI indicating when an artificial kidney support should begin replacing the functions of the kidney. This support is broadly termed dialysis but is provided in the many variants of RRT, and as a continuous therapy in the ICU setting as CRRT. The history of dialysis is relevant as nurses have always played an important role in providing this treatment that, when integrated into the care of the critically ill, requires substantial clinical knowledge and technical skills. The machine and circuit for CRRT are useful to understand and assist in preparation, connection to the patient and then troubleshooting during use. The major failing of CRRT is clotting of the EC, and anticoagulation approaches are the key preventive strategy. When clotting occurs, delays occur and time is lost before restarting, and this is a key communication time with prescribers to prevent a secondary failure of treatment – for example, a positive fluid balance. Teaching CRRT and quality review are very important for a successful program in the ICU. Finally, the concept of blood purification techniques is introduced and the use of CRRT in special considerations is briefly discussed, which includes use in the operating theatre, with small children and with ECMO.

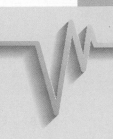

Case study

Mr Kinjury, a 68-year-old male, is a hard-working, active farmer who lives alone after his wife died just over 1 year ago and who presented to the emergency department in a confused and agitated state but also sleepy. He was coughing up fresh-looking blood. His referral letter indicates a history of increased alcohol consumption for many years and recent treatment for a chest infection. He has been provided with some assistance for low mood because of feeling lonely and depressed at times. He is overweight (~115 kg), has diabetes which is normally controlled by diet, but recently has not managed this well. Weight loss and blood sugar monitoring have been encouraged but with his limited attention.

His chest X-ray indicates a lobar pneumonia. His temperature is 38.8°C and he has an elevated white cell count. He is tachycardic and his blood pressure is less than 70 mmHg systolic. His oral intake is uncertain, and his last urine production was approximately 24 hours earlier.

He has a distended abdomen, with ascites, patchy bruising on the chest and legs, oedema of the lower legs and ankles, some scleral icterus and swollen testes. His bowel motions are a dark fluid with spots of black; haemorrhoids are also noted.

His blood work indicates a low sodium, high potassium and significantly elevated creatinine, low haemoglobin and platelet count; liver function tests reflect poor function, with very elevated bilirubin and liver enzymes. His respiratory function and conscious state deteriorate, and he is intubated after ICU admission and mechanically ventilated. Blood cultures, sputum and cardiac echo tests are performed; an abdominal X-ray, gastroscopy before CRRT is prescribed.

DISCUSSION

Mr Kinjury presents with a history of poor attention to his health, and background factors creating susceptibility for any major organ failure if an acute new illness 'episode' arises. The death of his wife has been a factor in changed social and personal interest in his best health, a delayed visit to a doctor with respiratory symptoms and being unwell. This is often considered a 'delayed' or late presentation and makes the illness more difficult to manage and outcomes worse. The AKI will be more acute and rapid in development, with irreversible damage and recovery more in question.

CASE STUDY QUESTIONS

1   Mr Kinjury has developed an AKI. What has caused or triggered this state and what are the key diagnostics features? Consider the staging or level of AKI.
2   CRRT used can be with different modes and anticoagulation strategies. Outline what you would anticipate the physician to prescribe for CRRT to best manage this patient safely.
3   After starting CRRT, what measures, tests or other assessments would reflect a response and success with therapy?
4   List five measures or assessments to check as a quality review of the CRRT used for Mr Kinjury.
5   After 5 days of ICU care, Mr Kinjury has improved, and is extubated with some high-flow nasal oxygen; however, his CRRT continues. What will the prescribing physicians consider when deciding whether CRRT may be stopped?

RESEARCH VIGNETTE

Ruiz EF, Ortiz-Soriano VM, Talbott M, et al. Development, implementation and outcomes of a quality assurance system for the provision of continuous renal replacement therapy in the intensive care unit. Sci Rep 2020;10(1):20616. doi: 10.1038/s41598-020-76785-w.

Abstract

Critically ill patients with requirement of CRRT represent a growing ICU population. Optimal CRRT delivery demands continuous communication between stakeholders, iterative adjustment of therapy, and quality assurance systems. This quality improvement (QI) study reports the development, implementation and outcomes of a quality assurance system to support the provision of CRRT in the ICU. This study was carried out at the University of Kentucky Medical Center between September 2016 and June 2019. We implemented a quality assurance system using a stepwise approach based on the (a) assembly of a multidisciplinary team, (b) standardisation of the CRRT protocol, (c) the creation of electronic CRRT flowsheets, (d) selection, monitoring and reporting of quality metrics of CRRT deliverables and (e) enhancement of education. We examined 34-month data comprising 1185 adult patients on CRRT (~7420 patient-days of CRRT) and tracked selected QI outcomes/metrics of CRRT delivery. As a result of the QI interventions, we increased the number of multidisciplinary experts in the CRRT team and ensured a continuum of education to healthcare professionals. We maximised to 100% the use of continuous venovenous hemodiafiltration and doubled the percentage of patients using regional citrate anticoagulation. The delivered CRRT effluent dose (~30 mL/kg/h) and the delivered/prescribed effluent dose ratio (~0.89) remained stable within the study period. The average filter life increased from 26 to 31 h ($P = 0.020$), reducing the mean utilisation of filters per patient from 3.56 to 2.67 ($P = 0.054$) despite similar CRRT duration and mortality rates. The number of CRRT access alarms per treatment day was reduced by 43%. The improvement in filter utilisation translated into ~20,000 US$ gross savings in filter cost per 100 patients receiving CRRT. We satisfactorily developed and implemented a quality assurance system for the provision of CRRT in the ICU that enabled sustainable tracking of CRRT deliverables and reduced filter resource utilisation at our institution.

Critique

This report provides data for a 3-year before-and-after study in over 1100 adults in ICU managed with CRRT for ~7420 days. The study and project collected data before introducing a stepwise quality assurance list over 10 months for key initiatives and tracked the metrics for these before, during and after the implementation period.

Adult patients were typical and representative; the quality metrics assessed were also useful and well known to all users of CRRT worldwide. The early intervention period also included the implementation of the dedicated teams, education, protocols, prescribing and advanced and super-users.

The outcomes and improvements are listed and described well in the abstract and conclusions, with well-presented graphs and figures.

The report presents the experience of a project to improve CRRT in a single centre in the US and through this report we can learn about strategies for improved care, and that the best and most efficient use of a high-tech intervention in the ICU team, a collaborative approach, standard CRRT protocol, flow and prescribing sheets (electronic), establishing the reporting metrics, education and workforce and clinical experts are common elements in many quality project reports.

The work presented in this report published in 2020 is current and contemporary for CRRT use. The methods and analysis are fitting for a quality process. What is described in this report is applicable to other areas; the initiatives used are practical and could be used in all settings despite the authors' concern that this may not be the case. The analysis and results are open to some interpretation and could be subject to question over which QI intervention has the most association or power for outcome. For example, if filter life as a metric for CRRT is considered, individual and/or grouping of interventions may provide the best outcome and longer filter life. The use of citrate anticoagulation method may not provide the best outcome unless this is grouped with more and new nurse education, establishing

CRRT 'super' users, improved clinical planning to avoid treatment interruptions with unplanned patient imaging, or use of best vascular access siting, with safety and harm minimisation at the forefront. The collection of over 3 years of data in over 1100 patients is to be applauded.

Quality is now a vital aspect of CRRT in the ICU where many people combine to provide this support and can be represented in the concept diagram provided below. CRRT in the Australasian setting has always been with a degree of quality within ICU structure for nursing and medicine. However, as we progress further with the increased demand for CRRT in sicker and older patients, within larger ICUs and nursing teams, quality needs to emerge and be implemented with a clearly identifiable 'champions' group in the ICU. Implementing quality activities and following the list or key metrics is the challenge in an acute and busy ICU.

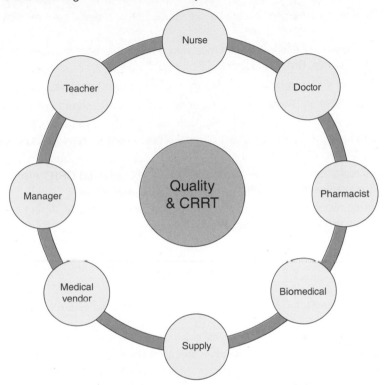

Quality and CRRT concept diagram: the many groups and people needed for effective quality.

Learning activities

1 Review a patient on CRRT and clarify their presentation for how they developed an AKI using the susceptibility, risk and outcome pathway.

2 Think of an area or aspect of CRRT use where the evidence for best practice is unclear and where further research is needed. Start with the idea or question, review any literature, then how you would investigate this, the data needed, how this could be analysed and whether a change of practice or improved care would be an outcome – the research process. Discuss with a more senior or CRRT-experienced colleague.

3 Audit your patient during CRRT and assess the net fluid balance for one day, noting whether the daily targets are achieved. Are the machine, nurse, medical team and others getting this right?

4 Review your key performance and/or clinical data collected in your ICU to evaluate CRRT practice and compare with the list in the Research vignette.

Online resources

Acute Disease Quality Initiative, https://www.adqi.org

Global Health Care Education, https://www.continulus.com/library/fluids-and-fluid-balance-aki-and-crrt

Kidney Diseases Improving Global Outcomes, https://kdigo.org

Pediatric continuous renal replacement therapy, https://www.pcrrt.com

Wolters Kluwer Global Professional Information, https://www.wolterskluwer.com/en/solutions/uptodate

Further reading

Baldwin I:. Is there a need for a nurse emergency team for continuous renal replacement therapy? Contrib Nephrol 2007;156:191–6.

Dunn W, Shyamala S. Filter lifespan in critically ill adults receiving continuous renal replacement therapy: the effect of patient and treatment-related variables. Crit Care Resusc 2014;16(3):225–31.

Karkar A, Ronco C. Prescription of CRRT: a pathway to optimize therapy. Ann Intensive Care 2020;10:32.

Kellum JA, Sileanu FE, Murugan R, et al. Classifying AKI by urine output versus serum creatinine level. J Am Soc Nephrol 2015;26(9):231–8.

Legrand M, Darmon M, Joannidis M, et al. Management of renal replacement therapy in ICU patients: an international survey. Intensive Care Med 2013;39:101–8.

Wilbers TJ, Koning MV. Renal replacement therapy in critically ill patients with COVID-19: A retrospective study investigating mortality, renal recovery and filter lifetime. J Crit Care 2020;60:103–5.

Zhang L, Baldwin I, Zhu G, et al. Automated electronic monitoring of circuit pressures during continuous renal replacement therapy: a technical report. Crit Care Resusc 2015;17(1):1–54.

References

1. Pickkers P, Darmon M, Hoste E, et al. Acute kidney injury in the critically ill: an updated review on pathophysiology and management. Intensive Care Med 2021;47(8):835–50.
2. Leaf DE. Introduction: cross-talk between the kidneys and remote organ systems in AKI. Semin Nephrol 2019;39(1):1–2.
3. Manrique-Caballero CL, Del Rio-Pertuz G, Gomez H. Sepsis-associated acute kidney injury. Crit Care Clin 2021;37(2):279–301.
4. Bellomo R, Kellum JA, Ronco C, et al. Acute kidney injury in sepsis. Intensive Care Med 2017;43(6):816–28.
5. Kellum JA, Bellomo R, Ronco C. The concept of acute kidney injury and the RIFLE criteria. Contrib Nephrol 2007;156:10–16.
6. Kellum JA, Bellomo R, Ronco C. Definition and classification of acute kidney injury. Nephron Clin Pract 2008;109(4):c182–7.
7. Kellum JA, Lameire N, Aspelin P, et al. Kidney disease: improving global outcomes (KDIGO) acute kidney injury work group. KDIGO clinical practice guideline for acute kidney injury. Kidney Int Suppl 2012;2(1):1–138.
8. Ronco C, Bellomo R, Kellum JA. Acute kidney injury. Lancet 2019;394(10212):1949–64.
9. Ng JH, Hirsch JS, Hazzan A, et al. Outcomes among patients hospitalized with COVID-19 and acute kidney injury. Am J Kidney Dis 2021;77(2):204–15.e1.
10. Hoste EAJ, Kellum JA, Selby NM, et al. Global epidemiology and outcomes of acute kidney injury. Nat Rev Nephrol 2018;14(10):607–25.
11. Guyton AC, Hall JE. The body fluids and kidneys. In: Guyton AC, Hall textbook of medical physiology. 13th ed. Philadelphia: WB Saunders; 2016, p. 305–442.
12. Sato R, Luthe SK, Nasu M. Blood pressure and acute kidney injury. Crit Care 2017;21(1):28.
13. White LE, Hassoun HT. Inflammatory mechanisms of organ crosstalk during ischemic acute kidney injury. Int J Nephrol 2012;2012:505197.
14. Forni LG, Darmon M, Ostermann M, et al. Renal recovery after acute kidney injury. Intensive Care Med 2017;43(6):855–66.
15. Basile DP, Anderson MD, Sutton TA. Pathophysiology of acute kidney injury. Compr Physiol 2012;2(2):1303–53.
16. Odutayo A, Wong CX, Farkouh M, et al. AKI and long-term risk for cardiovascular events and mortality. J Am Soc Nephrol 2017;28(1):377–87.
17. Cumming A. Acute renal failure: definitions and diagnosis. In: Ronco C, Bellomo R, editors. Critical care nephrology. Dordrecht: Kluwer Academic; 1998, p. 591–8.
18. Girling BJ, Channon SW, Haines RW, et al. Acute kidney injury and adverse outcomes of critical illness: correlation or causation? Clin Kidney J 2020;13(2):133–41.
19. Kellum JA, Prowle JR. Paradigms of acute kidney injury in the intensive care setting. Nat Rev Nephrol 2018;14(4):217–30.
20. Hedenstierna G, Larsson A. Influence of abdominal pressure on respiratory and abdominal organ function. Curr Opin Crit Care 2012;18(1):80–5.

21. O'Connor ME, Kirwan CJ, Pearse RM, et al. Incidence and associations of acute kidney injury after major abdominal surgery. Intensive Care Med 2016;42(4):521–30.

22. Zuk A, Bonventre JV. Acute kidney injury. Ann Rev Med 2016;67:293–307.

23. Boyer N, Eldridge J, Prowle JR, et al. Postoperative AKI. Clin J Am Soc Nephrol 2022;17(10):1535–45.

24. Sheridan AM, Bonventre JV. Pathophysiology of ischemic acute renal failure. Contrib Nephrol 2001(132):7–21.

25. Gaut JP, Liapis H. Acute kidney injury pathology and pathophysiology: a retrospective review. Clin Kidney J 2021;14(2):526–36.

26. Bonventre JV. Dedifferentiation and proliferation of surviving epithelial cells in acute renal failure. J Am Soc Nephrol 2003;14(Suppl. 1):S55–61.

27. Bonventre JV. Pathophysiology of ischemic acute renal failure. Inflammation, lung-kidney cross-talk, and biomarkers. Contrib Nephrol 2004;144:19–30.

28. Endre ZH. Acute renal failure. In: Whitworth JA, Lawrence JR, editors. Textbook of renal disease. 2nd ed. Edinburgh: Churchill Livingstone; 1994, Chapter 20.

29. Han SS, Kim S, Ahn SY, et al. Duration of acute kidney injury and mortality in critically ill patients: a retrospective observational study. BMC Nephrol 2013;14:133.

30. Uchino S, Bellomo R, Bagshaw SM, et al. Transient azotaemia is associated with a high risk of death in hospitalized patients. Nephrol Dial Transplant 2010;25(6):1833–9.

31. Levey AS, Eckardt KU, Tsukamoto Y, et al. Definition and classification of chronic kidney disease: a position statement from Kidney Disease: Improving Global Outcomes (KDIGO). Kidney Int 2005;67(6):2089–100.

32. Krum H, Abraham WT. Heart failure. Lancet 2009;373(9667):941–55.

33. Kamath PS, Kim WR; Advanced Liver Disease Study Group. The model for end-stage liver disease (MELD). Hepatology 2007;45(3):797–805.

34. Fenoglio R, Sciascia S, Baldovino S, et al. Acute kidney injury associated with glomerular diseases. Curr Opin Crit Care 2019;25(6):573–9.

35. Morales-Alvarez MC. Nephrotoxicity of antimicrobials and antibiotics. Adv Chronic Kidney Dis 2020;27(1):31–7.

36. Petejova N, Martinek A. Acute kidney injury due to rhabdomyolysis and renal replacement therapy: a critical review. Crit Care 2014;18(3):224.

37. Shiba A, Uchino S, Fujii T, et al. Association between intraoperative oliguria and acute kidney injury after major noncardiac surgery. Anesth Analg 2018;127(5):1229–35.

38. Jamal JA, Mueller BA, Choi GY, et al. How can we ensure effective antibiotic dosing in critically ill patients receiving different types of renal replacement therapy? Diagn Microbiol Infect Dis 2015;82(1):92–103.

39. Perazzella MA. Drug-induced acute kidney injury: diverse mechanisms of tubular injury. Curr Opin Crit Care 2019;25(6):550–7.

40. Leisman S. Radiocontrast toxicity. Adv Chronic Kidney Dis 2020;27(1):50–5.

41. Mockel M, Radovic M, Kuhnle Y, et al. Acute renal haemodynamic effects of radiocontrast media in patients undergoing left ventricular and coronary angiography. Nephrol Dial Transplant 2008;23(5):1588–94.

42. Chawla LS, Kimmel PL. Acute kidney injury and chronic kidney disease: an integrated clinical syndrome. Kidney Int 2012;82(5):516–24.

43. Yap E, Salifu M, Ahmad T, et al. Atypical causes of urinary tract obstruction. Case Rep Nephrol 2019;2019:4903693.

44. Patschan D, Patschan S, Buschmann I, et al. Loop diuretics in acute kidney injury prevention, therapy, and risk stratification. Kidney Blood Press Res 2019;44(4):457–64.

45. Zhao GJ, Xu C, Ying JC, et al. Association between furosemide administration and outcomes in critically ill patients with acute kidney injury. Crit Care 2020;24(1):75.

46. McMahon BA, Chawla LS. The furosemide stress test: current use and future potential. Ren Fail 2021;43(1):830–9.

47. Liu KD, Goldstein SL, Vijayan A, et al. AKI!Now initiative: recommendations for awareness, recognition, and management of AKI. Clin J Am Soc Nephrol 2020;15(12):1838–47.

48. Kellum JA, Lameire N. Diagnosis, evaluation, and management of acute kidney injury: a KDIGO summary (Part 1). Crit Care 2013;17(1):204.

49. Waikar SS, Betensky RA, Emerson SC, et al. Imperfect gold standards for biomarker evaluation. Clin Trials 2013;10(5):696–700.

50. Verma S, Kellum JA. Defining acute kidney injury. Critical Care Clin 2021;37(2):251–66.

51. Andreucci M, Faga T, Pisani A, et al. The ischemic/nephrotoxic acute kidney injury and the use of renal biomarkers in clinical practice. Eur J Intern Med 2017;39:1–8.

52. Wang HE, Jain G, Glassock RJ, et al. Comparison of absolute serum creatinine changes versus Kidney Disease: Improving Global Outcomes consensus definitions for characterizing stages of acute kidney injury. Nephrol Dial Transplant 2013;28(6):1447–54.

53. Pakula AM, Skinner RA. Acute kidney injury in the critically ill patient: a current review of the literature. J Intensive Care Med 2016;31(5):319–24.

54. Matsa R, Ashley E, Sharma V, et al. Plasma and urine neutrophil gelatinase-associated lipocalin in the diagnosis of new onset acute kidney injury in critically ill patients. Crit Care 2014;18(4):R137.

55. Mårtensson J, Bellomo R. The rise and fall of NGAL in acute kidney injury. Blood Purif 2014;37(4):304–10.

56. Mishra J, Dent C, Tarabishi R, et al. Neutrophil gelatinase-associated lipocalin (NGAL) as a biomarker for acute renal injury after cardiac surgery. Lancet 2005;365(9466):1231–8.

57. Mishra J, Ma Q, Prada A, et al. Identification of neutrophil gelatinase-associated lipocalin as a novel early urinary biomarker for ischemic renal injury. J Am Soc Nephrol 2003;14(10):2534–43.

58. Ichimura T, Hung CC, Yang SA, et al. Kidney injury molecule-1: a tissue and urinary biomarker for nephrotoxicant-induced renal injury. Am J Physiol Renal Physiol 2004;286(3):F552–63.

59. Alge JL, Arthur JM. Biomarkers of AKI: a review of mechanistic relevance and potential therapeutic implications. Clin J Am Soc Nephrol 2015;10(1):147–55.

60. Meersch M, Schmidt C, Van Aken H, et al. Urinary TIMP-2 and IGFBP7 as early biomarkers of acute kidney injury and renal recovery following cardiac surgery. PLoS One 2014;9(3):e93460.

61. Seifter JL, Samuels MA. Uremic encephalopathy and other brain disorders associated with renal failure. Semin Neurol 2011;31(2):139–43.

62. Grams ME, Rabb H. The distant organ effects of acute kidney injury. Kidney Int 2012;81(10):942–8.

63. Perner A, Prowle J, Joannidis M, et al. Fluid management in acute kidney injury. Intensive Care Med 2017;43(6):807–15.

64. Schrier RW. Fluid administration in critically ill patients with acute kidney injury. Clin J Am Soc Nephrol 2010;5(4):733–9.

65. Ostermann M, Liu K, Kashani K. Fluid management in acute kidney injury. Chest 2019;156(3):594–603.

66. Lee SA, Cozzi M, Bush EL, et al. Distant organ dysfunction in acute kidney injury: a review. Am J Kidney Dis 2018;72(6):846–56.

67. Jelkmann W. Regulation of erythropoietin production. J Physiol 2011;589(Pt 6):1251–8.

68. Tanaka S, Okusa MD. Crosstalk between the nervous system and the kidney. Kidney Int 2020;97(3):466–76.

69. Murugan R, Kellum JA. Acute kidney injury: what's the prognosis? Nat Rev Nephrol 2011;7(4):209–17.

70. Cruz DN, Bagshaw SM, Ronco C, et al. Acute kidney injury: classification and staging. Contrib Nephrol 2010;164:24–32.

71. Ronco C, Levin A, Warnock DG, et al. Improving outcomes from acute kidney injury (AKI): report on an initiative. Int J Artif Organs 2007;30(5):373–6.

72. Otero A, Fernandez R, Apalkov A, et al. An automatic critical care urine meter. Sensors (Basel) 2012;12(10):13109–25.

73. Minor J, Smith A, Deutsch F. Automated versus manual urine output monitoring in the intensive care unit. Sci Rep 2021;11(1):17429.

74. Kellum JA, Bellomo R, Ronco C. Does this patient have acute kidney injury? An AKI checklist. Intensive Care Med 2016;42(1):96–9.

75. Ostermann M, Bellomo R, Burdmann EA, et al. Controversies in acute kidney injury: conclusions from a Kidney Disease: Improving Global Outcomes (KDIGO) conference. Kidney Int 2020;98(2):294–309.

76. Bellomo R, Vaara ST, Kellum JA. How to improve the care of patients with acute kidney injury. Intensive Care Med 2017;43(6):727–9.

77. Bellomo R, Baldwin I, Ronco C, et al. ICU-based renal replacement therapy. Crit Care Med 2021;49(3):406–18.

78. Prowle JR, Bellomo R. Fluid administration and the kidney. Curr Opin Crit Care 2013;19(4):308–14.

79. Murugan R, Hoste E, Mehta RL, et al. Precision fluid management in continuous renal replacement therapy. Blood Purif 2016;42(3):266–78.

80. Finfer S, Norton R, Bellomo R, et al. The SAFE study: saline vs albumin for fluid resuscitation in the critically ill. Vox Sang 2004;87(Suppl. 2):123–31.

81. Investigators RRTS; Bellomo R, Cass A, Cole L, et al. An observational study fluid balance and patient outcomes in the Randomized Evaluation of Normal vs. Augmented Level of Replacement Therapy trial. Crit Care Med 2012;40(6):1753–60.

82. Prowle JR, Echeverri JE, Ligabo EV, Fluid balance and acute kidney injury. Nat Rev Nephrol 2010;6(2):107–15.

83. Peake SL, Chapman MJ, Davies AR, et al. Enteral nutrition in Australian and New Zealand intensive care units: a point-prevalence study of prescription practices. Crit Care Resusc 2012;14(2):148–53.

84. Fiaccadori E, Cremaschi E, Regolisti G. Nutritional assessment and delivery in renal replacement therapy patients. Semin Dial 2011;24(2):169–75.

85. Alobaidi R, Morgan C, Basu RK, et al. Association between fluid balance and outcomes in critically ill children: a systematic review and meta-analysis. JAMA Pediatr 2018;172(3):257–68.

86. O'Connor ME, Prowle JR. Fluid overload. Crit Care Clin 2015;31(4):803–21.

87. Bonavia A, Singbartl K. Kidney injury and electrolyte abnormalities in liver failure. Semin Respir Crit Care Med 2018;39(5):556–65.

88. Ostermann M, Dickie H, Tovey L, et al. Management of sodium disorders during continuous haemofiltration. Crit Care 2010;14(3):418.

89. Ronco C, Ricci Z. Renal replacement therapies: physiological review. Intensive Care Med 2008;34(12):2139–46.

90. Hertzberg D, Rydén L, Pickering JW, et al. Acute kidney injury – an overview of diagnostic methods and clinical management. Clin Kidney J 2017;10(3):323–31.

91. Jang SM, Awdishu L. Drug dosing considerations in continuous renal replacement therapy. Semin Dial 2021;34(6):480–8.

92. Lea-Henry TN, Carland JE, Stocker SL, et al. Clinical pharmacokinetics in kidney disease: fundamental principles. Clin J Am Soc Nephrol 2018;13(7):1085–95.

93. Lewis SJ, Mueller BA. Antibiotic dosing in patients with acute kidney injury: "enough but not too much". J Intensive Care Med 2016;31(3):164–76.

94. Choi G, Gomersall CD, Tian Q, et al. Principles of antibacterial dosing in continuous renal replacement therapy. Crit Care Med 2009;37(7):2268–82.

95. Bouchard J, Mehta RL. Timing of kidney support therapy in acute kidney injury: what are we waiting for? Am J Kidney Dis 2022;79(3):417–26.

96. Cameron JS. Practical haemodialysis began with cellophane and heparin: the crucial role of William Thalhimer (1884–1961). Nephrol Dial Transplant 2000;15(7):1086–91.

97. Ronco C, Clark WR. Haemodialysis membranes. Nat Rev Nephrol 2018;14(6):394–410.

98. Ronco C, La Greca G. The role of technology in hemodialysis. Contrib Nephrol 2002;137:1–12.

99. Baldwin I, Fealy N. Nursing for renal replacement therapies in the intensive care unit: historical, educational, and protocol review. Blood Purif 2009;27(2):174–81.

100. Baldwin IC, Elderkin TD. Continuous hemofiltration: nursing perspectives in critical care. New Horiz 1995;3(4):738–47.

101. Martin RK, Jurschak J, editors. Nursing management of continuous renal replacement therapy. Seminars in dialysis. Chichester, UK: Wiley Online Library; 1996.

102. Wild J. Peritoneal dialysis. In: Thomas N, editor. Renal nursing. 5th ed. Hoboken NJ: Wiley Blackwell; 2019, p. 235–76.

103. Ponce D, Balbi A, Cullis B. Acute PD: evidence, guidelines, and controversies☆. Semin Nephrol 2017;37(1):103–12.

104. Ronco C. Continuous renal replacement therapy: forty-year anniversary. Int J Artif Organs 2017;40(6):257–64.

105. Kramer P, Wigger W, Rieger J, et al. [Arteriovenous haemofiltration: a new and simple method for treatment of over-hydrated patients resistant to diuretics]. Klin Wochenschr 1977;55(22):1121–2.

106. Baldwin I, Fealy N. Clinical nursing for the application of continuous renal replacement therapy in the intensive care unit. Semin Dial 2009;22(2):189–93.

107. Bellomo R, Ronco C, Mehta RL. Nomenclature for continuous renal replacement therapies. Am J Kidney Dis 1996;28(5):S2–7.

108. Boyle M, Baldwin I. Understanding the continuous renal replacement therapy circuit for acute renal failure support: a quality issue in the intensive care unit. AACN Adv Crit Care 2010;21(4):367–75.

109. Seczynska B, Krolikowski W, Nowak I, et al. Continuous renal replacement therapy during extracorporeal membrane oxygenation in patients treated in medical intensive care unit: technical considerations. Ther Apher Dial 2014;18(6):523–34.

110. Davenport A, Mehta S. The Acute Dialysis Quality Initiative – part VI: access and anticoagulation in CRRT. Adv Ren Replace Ther 2002;9(4):273–81.

111. Juncos LA, Chandrashekar K, Karakala N, et al. Vascular access, membranes and circuit for CRRT. Semin Dial 2021;34(6):406–15.

112. Ofsthun NJ, Colton CK, Lysaght MJ. Determinants of fluid and solute removal rates during hemofiltration. In: Henderson LW, Quellhorst G, Baldamus CA, et al, editors. Hemofiltration. Berlin: Springer-Verlag; 1986, p. 17–39.

113. Goldstein SL. Continuous renal replacement therapy: mechanism of clearance, fluid removal, indications and outcomes. Curr Opin Pediatr 2011;23(2):181–5.

114. Neri M, Villa G, Garzotto F, et al. Nomenclature for renal replacement therapy in acute kidney injury: basic principles. Crit Care 2016;20(1):318.

115. Baldwin I, Baldwin M, Fealy N, et al. Con-current versus counter-current dialysate flow during CVVHD. A comparative study for creatinine and urea removal. Blood Purif 2016;41(1-3):171–6.

116. Ronco C, Bellomo R. Basic mechanisms and definitions for continuous renal replacement therapies. Int J Artif Organs 1996;19(2):95–9

117. Fiedling C. Haemodialysis. In: Thomas N, editor. Renal nursing. 5th ed. Hoboken NJ: Wiley Blackwell; 2019, p. 179–234.

118. Villa G, Neri M, Bellomo R, et al. Nomenclature for renal replacement therapy and blood purification techniques in critically ill patients: practical applications. Crit Care 2016;20(1):283.

119. Network VNARFT; Palevsky PM, Zhang JH, O'Connor TZ, et al. Intensity of renal support in critically ill patients with acute kidney injury. N Engl J Med 2008;359(1):7–20.

120. Bai M, Zhou M, He L, et al. Citrate versus heparin anticoagulation for continuous renal replacement therapy: an updated meta-analysis of RCTs. Intensive Care Med 2015;41(12):2098–110.

121. Bellomo R, Cole L, Reeves J, et al. Who should manage CRRT in the ICU? The intensivist's viewpoint. Am J Kidney Dis 1997;30(5 Suppl. 4):S109–11.

122. Neyra JA, Tolwani A. CRRT prescription and delivery of dose. Semin Dial 2021;34(6):432–9.

123. Claure-Del Granado R, Clark WR. Continuous renal replacement therapy principles. Semin Dial 2021;34(6):398–405.

124. Uchino S, Fealy N, Baldwin I, et al. Pre-dilution vs. post-dilution during continuous veno-venous hemofiltration: impact on filter life and azotemic control. Nephron Clin Pract 2003;94(4):c94–8.

125. Murugan R, Hoste E, Mehta RL, et al. Precision fluid management in continuous renal replacement therapy. Blood Purif 2016;42(3):266–78.

126. Vienken J, Diamantoglou M, Henne W, et al. Artificial dialysis membranes: from concept to large scale production. Am J Nephrol 1999;19(2):355–62.

127. Fealy N, Aitken L, Toit E, et al. Continuous renal replacement therapy: current practice in Australian and New Zealand intensive care units. Crit Care Resusc 2015;17(2):83–91.

128. Romagnoli S, Ricci Z, Ronco C. CRRT for sepsis-induced acute kidney injury. Curr Opin Crit Care 2018;24(6):483–92.

129. Honore PM, Jacobs R, Joannes-Boyau O, et al. Newly designed CRRT membranes for sepsis and SIRS – a pragmatic approach for bedside intensivists summarizing the more recent advances: a systematic structured review. ASAIO J 2013;59(2):99–106.

130. Turani F, Barchetta R, Falco M, et al. Continuous renal replacement therapy with the adsorbing filter oXiris in septic patients: a case series. Blood Purif 2019;47(Suppl. 3):1–5.

131. Honore PM, Spapen HD. Evolution of vascular access and anticoagulation. Contrib Nephrol 2018;194:15–24.

132. Fealy N, Kim I, Baldwin I, et al. A comparison of the Niagara and Medcomp catheters for continuous renal replacement therapy. Ren Fail 2013;35(3):308–13.

133. Naka T, Egi M, Bellomo R, et al. Resistance of vascular access catheters for continuous renal replacement therapy: an ex vivo evaluation. Int J Artif Organs 2008;31(10):905–9.

134. Morgan D, Ho K, Murray C, et al. A randomized trial of catheters of different lengths to achieve right atrium versus superior vena cava placement for continuous renal replacement therapy. Am J Kidney Dis 2012;60(2):272–9.

135. Baldwin I, Bellomo R, Koch B. Blood flow reductions during continuous renal replacement therapy and circuit life. Intensive Care Med 2004;30(11):2074–9.

136. Bellomo R, Mårtensson J, Lo S, et al. Femoral access and delivery of continuous renal replacement therapy dose. Blood Purif 2016;41(1–3): 11–17.

137. Schetz M. Vascular access for HD and CRRT. Contrib Nephrol 2007;156:275–86.

138. Crosswell A, Brain MJ, Roodenburg O. Vascular access site influences circuit life in continuous renal replacement therapy. Crit Care Resusc 2014;16(2):127–30.

139. Baldwin I. Factors affecting circuit patency and filter 'life'. Contrib Nephrol 2007;156:178–84.

140. Baldwin I, Bellomo R, Koch B. A technique for the monitoring of blood flow during continuous haemofiltration. Intensive Care Med 2002;28(9):1361–4.

141. Baldwin I, Fealy N, Carty P, et al. Bubble chamber clotting during continuous renal replacement therapy: vertical versus horizontal blood flow entry. Blood Purif 2012;34(3–4):213–18.

142. Davies H, Leslie G. Maintaining the CRRT circuit: non-anticoagulant alternatives. Aust Crit Care 2006;19(4):133–8.

143. Clark WR, Turk JE, Jr. The NxStage System One. Semin Dial 2004;17(2):167–70.

144. Dirkes S, Wonnacott R. Continuous renal replacement therapy and anticoagulation: what are the options? Crit Care Nurse 2016;36(2):34–41.

145. Tolwani AJ, Wille KM. Anticoagulation for continuous renal replacement therapy. Semin Dial 2009;22(2):141–5.

146. Davies H, Leslie G. Anticoagulation in CRRT: agents and strategies in Australian ICUs. Aust Crit Care 2007;20(1):15–26.

147. Karakala N, Tolwani A. We use heparin as the anticoagulant for CRRT. Semin Dial 2016;29(4):272–4.

148. Baldwin I, Tan HK, Bridge N, et al. Possible strategies to prolong circuit life during hemofiltration: three controlled studies. Ren Fail 2002;24(6):839–48.

149. Leslie GD, Jacobs IG, Clarke GM. Proximally delivered dilute heparin does not improve circuit life in continuous venovenous haemodiafiltration. Intensive Care Med 1996;22(11):1261–4.

150. Kindgen-Milles D, Brandenburger T, Dimski T. Regional citrate anticoagulation for continuous renal replacement therapy. Curr Opin Crit Care 2018;24(6):450–4.

151. Tolwani A, Wille KM. Regional citrate anticoagulation for continuous renal replacement therapy: the better alternative? Am J Kidney Dis 2012;59(6):745–7.

152. Davies H, Morgan D, Leslie G. A regional citrate anticoagulation protocol for pre-dilutional CVVHDf: the 'Modified Alabama Protocol'. Aust Crit Care 2008;21(3):154–65.

153. Schneider AG, Journois D, Rimmele T. Complications of regional citrate anticoagulation: accumulation or overload? Crit Care 2017;21(1):281.

154. Morabito S, Pistolesi V, Tritapepe L, et al. Regional citrate anticoagulation for RRTs in critically ill patients with AKI. Clin J Am Soc Nephrol 2014;9(12):2173–88.

155. Grouzi E. Update on argatroban for the prophylaxis and treatment of heparin-induced thrombocytopenia type II. J Blood Med 2014;5:131–41.

156. Link A, Girndt M, Selejan S, et al. Argatroban for anticoagulation in continuous renal replacement therapy. Crit Care Med 2009;37(1):105–10.

157. Saugel B, Phillip V, Moessmer G, et al. Correction: argatroban therapy for heparin-induced thrombocytopenia in ICU patients with multiple organ dysfunction syndrome: a retrospective study. Crit Care 2012;16(2):415.

158. Deep A, Zoha M, Dutta Kukreja P. Prostacyclin as an anticoagulant for continuous renal replacement therapy in children. Blood Purif 2017;43(4):279–89.

159. Tsang DJ, Tuckfield A, Macisaac CM. Audit of safety and quality of the use of enoxaparin for anticoagulation in continuous renal replacement therapy. Crit Care Resusc 2011;13(1):24–7.

160. Davenport A. Management of heparin-induced thrombocytopenia during continuous renal replacement therapy. Am J Kidney Dis 1998;32(4):E3.

161. Godden J, Spexarth F, Dahlgren M. Standardization of continuous renal-replacement therapy fluids using a commercial product. Am J Health Syst Pharm 2012;69(9):786–93.

162. Schetz M, Leblanc M, Murray PT. The Acute Dialysis Quality Initiative – part VII: fluid composition and management in CRRT. Adv Ren Replace Ther 2002;9(4):282–9.

163. Davenport A. Replacement and dialysate fluids for patients with acute renal failure treated by continuous veno-venous haemofiltration and/or haemodiafiltration. Contrib Nephrol 2004;144:317–28.

164. Baldwin I, Bellomo R. Sustained low efficiency dialysis in the ICU. Int J Intensive Care 2002;9(4):177–87.

165. Wang AY, Bellomo R. Renal replacement therapy in the ICU: intermittent hemodialysis, sustained low-efficiency dialysis or continuous renal replacement therapy? Curr Opin Crit Care 2018;24(6):437–42.

166. Zhang L, Yang J, Eastwood GM, et al. Extended daily dialysis versus continuous renal replacement therapy for acute kidney injury: a meta-analysis. Am J Kidney Dis 2015;66(2):322–30.

167. Davies H, Leslie GD, Morgan D. A retrospective review of fluid balance control in CRRT. Aust Crit Care 2017;30(6):314–19.

168. Davies H, Leslie GD, Morgan D, et al. A comparison of compliance in the estimation of body fluid status using daily fluid balance charting and body weight changes during continuous renal replacement therapy. Aust Crit Care 2019;32(2):83–9.

169. Prowle J, Mehta R. Fluid balance management during continuous renal replacement therapy. Semin Dial 2021;34(6):440–8.

170. Bagshaw SM, Baldwin I, Fealy N, et al. Fluid balance error in continuous renal replacement therapy: a technical note. Int J Artif Organs 2007;30(5):434–40.

171. Bouchard J, Soroko SB, Chertow GM, et al. Fluid accumulation, survival and recovery of kidney function in critically ill patients with acute kidney injury. Kidney Int 2009;76(4):422–7.

172. Sutherland SM, Zappitelli M, Alexander SR, et al. Fluid overload and mortality in children receiving continuous renal replacement therapy: the prospective pediatric continuous renal replacement therapy registry. Am J Kidney Dis 2010;55(2):316–25.

173. Baldwin I, Mottes T. Acute kidney injury and continuous renal replacement therapy: a nursing perspective for my shift today in the intensive care unit. Semin Dial 2021;34(6):518–29.

174. Alessandri F, Pistolesi V, Manganelli C, et al. Acute kidney injury and COVID-19: a picture from an intensive care unit. Blood Purif 2021;50(6):767–71.

175. Schneider AG, Baldwin I, Freitag E, et al. Estimation of fluid status changes in critically ill patients: fluid balance chart or electronic bed weight? J Crit Care 2012;27(6):745.e7–12.

176. Chua HR, Schneider AG, Baldwin I, et al. Phoxilium vs Hemosol-B0 for continuous renal replacement therapy in acute kidney injury. J Crit Care 2013;28(5):884.e7–14.

177. Graham P, Lischer E. Nursing issues in renal replacement therapy: organization, manpower assessment, competency evaluation and quality improvement processes. Semin Dial 2011;24(2):183–7.

178. Przybyl H, Evans J, Haley L, et al. Training and maintaining: developing a successful and dynamic continuous renal replacement therapy program. AACN Adv Crit Care 2017;28(1):41–50.

179. Baldwin IC. Training, management, and credentialing for CRRT in the ICU. Am J Kidney Dis 1997;30(5 Suppl. 4):S112–16.

180. Fealy N, Baldwin I, Bellomo R. The effect of circuit "down-time" on uraemic control during continuous veno-venous haemofiltration. Crit Care Resusc 2002;4(4):266–70.

181. Oh HJ, Lee MJ, Kim CH, et al. The benefit of specialized team approaches in patients with acute kidney injury undergoing continuous renal replacement therapy: propensity score matched analysis. Crit Care 2014;18(4):454.

182. Clark WR, Villa G, Neri M, et al. Advances in machine technology. Contrib Nephrol 2018;194:80–9.

183. Ronco C. Machines used for continuous renal replacement therapy. In: Kellum J, Bellomo R, Ronco C, editors. Continuous renal replacement therapy. New York: Oxford University Press; 2010, p. 229–46.

184. Macedo E, Cerdá J. Choosing a CRRT machine and modality. Semin Dial 2021;34(6):423–31.

185. See E, Ronco C, Bellomo R. The future of continuous renal replacement therapy. Semin Dial 2021;34(6):576–85.

186. Mottes T, Owens T, Niedner M, et al. Improving delivery of continuous renal replacement therapy: impact of a simulation-based educational intervention. Pediatr Crit Care Med 2013;14(8):747–54.

187. Rewa OG, Villeneuve PM, Lachance P, et al. Quality indicators of continuous renal replacement therapy (CRRT) care in critically ill patients: a systematic review. Intensive Care Med 2017;43(6):750–63.

188. Ruiz EF, Ortiz-Soriano VM, Talbott M, et al. Development, implementation and outcomes of a quality assurance system for the provision of continuous renal replacement therapy in the intensive care unit. Sci Rep 2020;10(1):20616.

189. Bellomo R, Cass A, Cole L, et al. Intensity of continuous renal-replacement therapy in critically ill patients. N Engl J Med 2009;361(17):1627–38.

190. Broman M, Bell M, Joannes-Boyau O, et al. The novel PrisMax continuous renal replacement therapy system in a multinational, multicentre pilot setting. Blood Purif 2018;46(3):220–7.

191. Lee KH, Sol IS, Park JT, et al. Continuous renal replacement therapy (CRRT) in children and the specialized CRRT team: a 14-year single-center study. J Clin Med 2019;9(1):110.

192. Ricci Z, Goldstein SL. Pediatric continuous renal replacement therapy. Contrib Nephrol 2016;187:121–30.

193. Askenazi DJ, Goldstein SL, Koralkar R, et al. Continuous renal replacement therapy for children ≤10 kg: a report from the prospective pediatric continuous renal replacement therapy registry. J Pediatr 2013;162(3):587–92.e3.

194. John JC, Taha S, Bunchman TE. Basics of continuous renal replacement therapy in pediatrics. Kidney Res Clin Pract 2019;38(4):455–61.

195. Combes A, Bacchetta M, Brodie D, et al. Extracorporeal membrane oxygenation for respiratory failure in adults. Curr Opin Crit Care 2012;18(1):99–104.

196. Combes A, Brodie D, Bartlett R, et al. Position paper for the organization of extracorporeal membrane oxygenation programs for acute respiratory failure in adult patients. Am J Respir Crit Care Med 2014;190(5):488–96.

197. Chen H, Yu RG, Yin NN, et al. Combination of extracorporeal membrane oxygenation and continuous renal replacement therapy in critically ill patients: a systematic review. Crit Care 2014;18(6):675.

198. Seczyńska B, Królikowski W, Nowak I, et al. Continuous renal replacement therapy during extracorporeal membrane oxygenation in patients treated in medical intensive care unit: technical considerations. Ther Apher Dial 2014;18(6):523–34.

199. Garwood C, Sandoval CP, Wonnacott R, et al. Continuous renal replacement therapy: case vignettes. AACN Adv Crit Care 2017;28(1):64–73.

200. Lemaire A, Parquet N, Galicier L, et al. Plasma exchange in the intensive care unit: technical aspects and complications. J Clin Apher 2017;32(6):405–12.

201. Baldwin I, Todd S. Therapeutic plasma exchange in the intensive care unit and with the critically ill, a focus on clinical nursing considerations. J Clin Apher 2022;37(4):397–404.

202. Clark E, Molnar AO, Joannes-Boyau O, et al. High-volume hemofiltration for septic acute kidney injury: a systematic review and meta-analysis. Crit Care 2014;18(1):R7.

203. Esposito P, Estienne L, Serpieri N, et al. Rhabdomyolysis-associated acute kidney injury. Am J Kidney Dis 2018;71(6):A12–14.

204. Douthitt L, Bezinover D, Uemura T, et al. Perioperative use of continuous renal replacement therapy for orthotopic liver transplantation. Transplant Proc 2012;44(5):1314–17.

205. Parmar A, Bigam D, Meeberg G, et al. An evaluation of intraoperative renal support during liver transplantation: a matched cohort study. Blood Purif 2011;32(3):238–48.

206. Safwan M, Gosnell J, Collins K, et al. Effects of intraoperative continuous renal replacement therapy on outcomes in liver transplantation. Transplant Proc 2020;52(1):265–70.

207. Townsend DR, Bagshaw SM, Jacka MJ, et al. Intraoperative renal support during liver transplantation. Liver Transplant 2009;15(1):73–8.

Chapter 19

Nutrition assessment and therapeutic management

Andrea P Marshall, Emma J Ridley

KEY WORDS

anabolism

catabolism

dysphagia

enteral nutrition

glycaemic control

hypermetabolism

indirect calorimetry

parenteral nutrition

Learning objectives

After reading this chapter, you should be able to:

- describe the changes in metabolism associated that occur during critical illness
- describe the consequences of malnutrition and how they influence recovery from critical illness
- identify appropriate nutrition assessment strategies and critique methods of determining nutritional requirements in critical illness
- apply theoretical knowledge to support the optimisation of delivery of prescribed enteral nutrition
- apply theoretical knowledge to support the safe delivery of parenteral nutrition
- rationalise selected nutritional support strategies for specific clinical conditions
- critically analyse the role of glycaemic control in the context of critical illness.

Introduction

Critical illness may be associated with increased catabolism that occurs at a time when oral intake may be difficult or impossible. In patients with severe illness, an accumulated energy and protein deficit may lead to muscle wasting and decreased lean body mass, which are associated with adverse outcomes.[1] Enteral nutrition (EN) is the preferred method of nutrition therapy for the critically ill when mechanically ventilated (MV), although some patients might require parenteral nutrition (PN) or a combination of EN and PN. Oral nutrition is becoming increasingly used during critical illness when appropriate, but specific and important issues exist with regards eating to support recovery with oral nutrition alone. The timing and duration of nutrition provision is also an important consideration when determining the role of nutrition in critical illness.

As part of the interdisciplinary team, nurses play an integral role in the provision of appropriate nutrition and advocacy for patient's nutrition, and are responsible for monitoring achievement of nutrition goals and implementing strategies to optimise nutrition intake. In this chapter an overview of metabolism and the consequences of malnutrition is provided. This is followed by discussion of nutritional assessment and delivery strategies where an emphasis is placed on nutrition therapy through the provision of EN. Tailoring nutrition to specific disease states is also included in this chapter. Lastly, we discuss the importance of glycaemic control in critical illness.

Metabolism

The body requires energy in order to support normal body and cellular function. Energy is derived from the metabolism of macronutrients including carbohydrate, protein and fat. In the normal metabolic process (not in critical illness), carbohydrates are broken down and stored as glycogen in the liver and skeletal muscle, while fat, stored in adipose tissue, is available for long-term energy requirements following food consumption. Proteins and amino acids, however, are not easily stored and so reduced protein intake can result in catabolism of body protein.[2]

The breakdown of food to produce energy is carried out in three phases: (1) the digestion of large macromolecules into simple subunits, (2) intracellular breakdown of subunits to acetyl coenzyme A (CoA) and production of small amounts of adenosine triphosphate (ATP) (2 molecules), and (3) production of ATP through oxidative phosphorylation[3] (Fig. 19.1).

FIGURE 19.1 Three phases of catabolism.[3] ATP = adenosine triphosphate; CoA = coenzyme A; NADH = nicotinamide adenine dinucleotide.

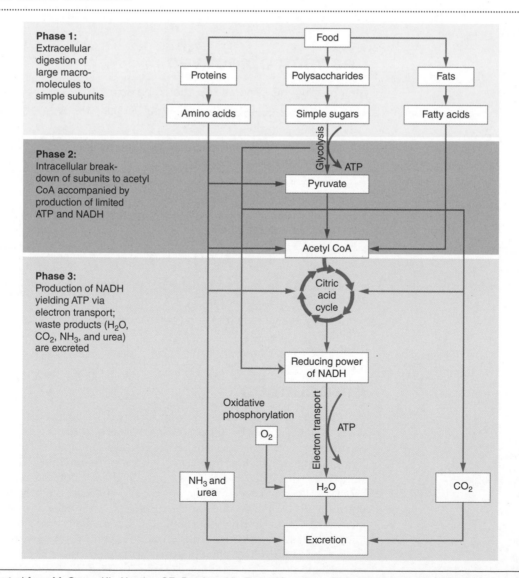

Source: Adapted from McCance KL, Huether SE, Brashers VL, Rote NS, editors. Pathophysiology: the biologic basis for disease in adults and children. 8th ed. St Louis, MO: Elsevier; 2019, Figure 1-26, p. 23, with permission.

Effect of critical illness on metabolism

The stress and injury associated with critical illness triggers the hypothalamus, sympathetic nervous system and adrenal medulla to initiate a response that results in hypercatabolism. Hormones released from the gut and adipose tissue may further trigger the stress response in critically ill patients.[4] Mediators of this response are cytokines including interleukin-1, interleukin-6 and tumour necrosis factor-α, and production of counterregulatory hormones such as catecholamines, cortisol, glucagon and growth hormone induce catabolism (Fig. 19.2) This increased catabolism that occurs in response to these mediators varies across the course of critical illness and can persist well beyond the initial period of critical illness or injury. The ebb phase occurs immediately and can last for 24–48 hours. Haemodynamic instability, reduced cardiac output, reduced oxygen consumption and low body temperature occur alongside increased glucagon, catecholamines and free fatty acid levels. This is followed by a more prolonged phase where oxygen consumption, the metabolic rate and cardiac output are increased and carbohydrates, amino acids and fats are oxidised as fuel sources.[5] The degree of response is associated with the severity of illness or injury. The clinical consequences are outlined in Table 19.1.[6]

Practice tip

Metabolic rate fluctuates throughout an episode of critical illness and can vary significantly between patients. Generally, the sicker a patient is the higher their metabolic rate. These changes in metabolic rate might influence how practitioners decide to prescribe nutrition support.

To maintain normal cellular function, body cells require adequate amounts of the six basic nutrients: carbohydrates, fats and proteins to provide energy, and vitamins, minerals and water to catalyse metabolic processes. How best to provide this nutrition support to critically ill patients remains an area of controversy and

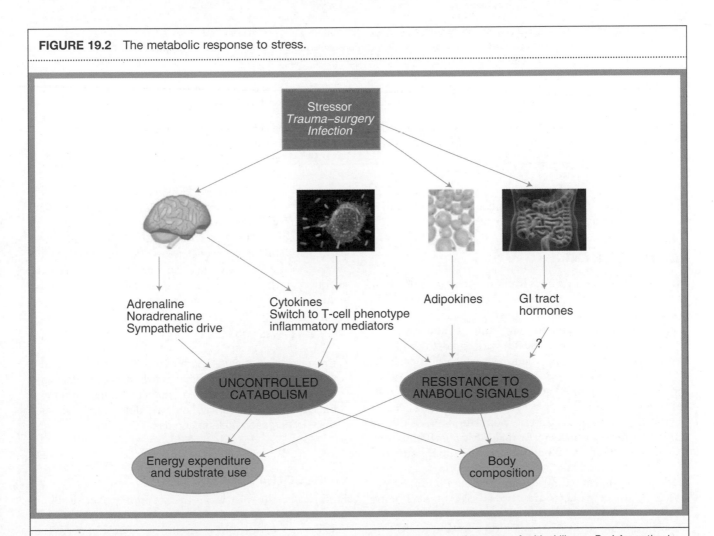

FIGURE 19.2 The metabolic response to stress.

Source: Reproduced from Preiser J-C, Ichai C, Orban J-C, et al. Metabolic response to the stress of critical illness. Br J Anaesthesia 2014;113(6):945–54, with permission.

TABLE 19.1

Clinical consequences of the metabolic response to stress[6]

CONSEQUENCE	DESCRIPTION
Energy expenditure (EE)	In the early phase of critical illness/injury, the EE is usually lower than before the illness/injury; EE increases in the later phases of critical illness/injury. In chronic critical illness the EE is more difficult to predict and is influenced by physiological changes and therapeutic interventions.
Use of energy substrates	The use of proteins, lipids and carbohydrates as energy sources changes during critical illness. Metabolism of macronutrients can be influenced by absorption, intracellular metabolism and substrate oxidation. In the early phases, carbohydrate oxidation is increased. As illness progresses, glucose utilisation decreases and there is increased use of fats and proteins. This can result in loss of muscle which may impact functional recovery.
Stress hyperglycaemia	Metabolism of carbohydrates is changed in critical illness and results in rapid use of glycogen stores as well as increased endogenous glucose production; both result in increased plasma glucose concentrations. Hormone release (catecholamines, growth hormone, cortisol and cytokines) increase glucose production by the liver and contribute to insulin resistance.
Lactate as a substrate	Lactate can be converted to glucose and is possibly a fuel used by organs under conditions of stress. Lactate may be a useful, if not obligatory, substrate used by organs such as the brain and heart during stress conditions.
Lipids	Lipids as an energy source require large amounts of oxygen in order to be converted to ATP by the mitochondria. Metabolism of lipids can be increased but complete oxidation is possible only if the mitochondria are fully functional, although mitochondrial function may be impaired during critical illness.
Proteins	Protein breakdown can exceed synthesis after stress. Stress metabolism can result in increased degradation of protein and contribute to depletion of skeletal muscles and ICU-acquired weakness.
Changes in body composition	Changes include loss of lean body mass and preservation of fat tissue and increased lipid storage. Body cell mass is decreased and extracellular fluid is increased.

requires additional basic and clinical research to inform our understanding of this complex area.

Malnutrition

Malnutrition in critical illness is an important consideration, with a reported prevalence of between 38% and 75%.[7,8] In critical illness, malnutrition can be pre-existing[9] and the result of chronic starvation without inflammation, or associated with chronic disease with mild-to-moderate degrees of inflammation. Malnutrition can also occur as the result of recent and acute disease with marked inflammatory response.[10] Determining the extent of pre-existing malnutrition in critical care is challenging because of the heterogeneous patient populations and use of different criteria to characterise malnutrition.[8] Pre-existing malnutrition in critical illness can increase the absolute risk of 90-day post-discharge mortality and is also a significant predictor of unplanned 30-day hospital re-admission.[9]

Critically ill patients are also at risk of developing iatrogenic or hospital-acquired malnutrition with the prescription and delivery of nutrition contributing factors. The risk of hospital-acquired malnutrition probably increases as length of stay increases and if the patient is receiving oral nutrition alone. Consequently, accurate assessment of nutritional requirements and strategies is vital to ensure the prescribed nutrition is delivered, particularly in longer-stay patients. The patient's clinical presentation can also have an impact on nutritional adequacy with surgical patients receiving less nutrition than medical patients owing to repeated fasting.[11]

> **Practice tip**
>
> Critically ill patients, particularly the elderly, can present to the ICU with existing malnutrition. Obtaining information on pre-admission nutrition status from the patient and/or the family can help determine whether there is increased malnutrition risk.

Consequences of malnutrition

Historically, the provision of nutrition to critically ill patients was considered a supportive strategy which could help provide exogenous macronutrients during periods of critical illness in order to minimise loss of muscle mass. Nutrition is now considered a therapy which can help attenuate stress metabolism, prevent oxidative cellular injury and modulate immune responses.[12]

Patients who experience malnutrition during critical illness often experience unfavourable outcomes including increased infectious morbidity, multiple-organ dysfunction, prolonged hospitalisation and disproportionate mortality.[12] Longer-term malnutrition can contribute to loss of muscle mass and reduced functional recovery. The extent to which the provision of artificial nutrition ameliorates these complications is unclear. The degree of critical illness and hypercatabolism varies between patients and is often difficult to determine. For this reason, it is necessary to assess, as accurately as possible, the nutritional requirements of each individual patient, although there is a lack of consensus on how this is best done.[13]

Nutritional assessment

Not all critically ill patients have the same nutritional needs.[13] Protein and energy requirements are influenced by the underlying disease process and the degree of critical illness. Nutritional assessment guides nutrition therapy for each patient and should incorporate patient history, clinical diagnosis, physical examination, anthropometric data, laboratory tests, dietary assessment and functional outcomes.[14] The degree of acute or chronic inflammation is an important contributing factor to the development of malnutrition.[15]

Not all critically ill patients are alike, with variations in nutrition risk. Energy expenditure varies[4] and is reported to range from 22 to 34 kcal/kg/day, but the difficulty lies in easily knowing where an individual patient sits within this range. Assessing which patients might be at greatest nutritional risk is important so as to identify those likely to benefit most from nutrition therapy. Existing nutrition-screening tools for hospitalised patients have not been validated for use in the critically ill.[16,17] A validated novel scoring tool, the **m**odified **NUT**ritional **Ri**sk in the **C**ritically ill (mNUTRIC) score, which incorporates variables related to acute and chronic starvation, acute and chronic inflammation, age and severity of illness (Table 19.2), has been developed[18–20] with high scores associated with increased ICU length of stay and mortality.[18,21] More-objective approaches to nutritional assessment, such as body composition or assessment of muscle mass using computed tomography (CT),[22] ultrasound[23] or bioelectric impedence,[24] are being explored. A recent study compared ultrasound-derived muscle thickness at five sites to CT muscle area at admission in 50 critically ill patients, with good potential noted for prediction of muscle mass.[25] Further work is needed to refine this or other tools in order to objectively identify nutrition risk in critically ill patients and determine which patients are most likely to benefit from nutrition therapy.

Determining nutritional requirements

Energy expenditure in critical illness is influenced by patient activity, stage of illness, type of injury and previous nutritional status (particularly muscle mass). Resting energy expenditure (REE) is the primary consideration

TABLE 19.2

Conceptual model and variables included in the NUTritional Risk in the Critically ill (NUTRIC) score[18,19,25]

CONCEPTS	PROPOSED VARIABLES	VARIABLES RETAINED IN FINAL SCORE
Acute starvation	Decreased oral intake over the last week	No
	Pre-ICU hospital admission	Yes
Chronic starvation	Weight loss over the last 6 months	No
	BMI <20	No
Acute inflammation	IL-6	Yes
	PCT	No
	CRP	No
Chronic inflammation	Comorbid illness	Yes
Severity of illness	Age	Yes
	APACHE II score	Yes
	SOFA score	Yes

APACHE = Acute physiology and chronic health evaluation; BMI = body mass index; CRP = C-reactive protein; IL-6 = interleukin-6; PCT = procalcitonin; SOFA = sequential organ failure assessment.

when prescribing energy intake because it is the largest component of total energy expenditure for hospitalised patients.[4] REE can be measured using indirect calorimetry or estimated using one of many different predictive equations. Randomised clinical trials have demonstrated that protein and energy intake is increased when indirect calorimetry is used.[26–28] However, evidence quality is limited and further research in this area is needed. Both approaches to determining energy requirements are used in ICUs and both have advantages and limitations.

> ### Practice tip
>
> For severely malnourished patients, introducing nutrition support rapidly can cause refeeding syndrome to occur. In this syndrome, metabolic disturbances occur that are characterised by electrolyte disorders, particularly hypophosphataemia. A slower introduction of nutrition with monitoring and replacement of electrolytes is recommended.

Indirect calorimetry

Indirect calorimetry is the 'gold standard' and most precise way of determining energy expenditure in critical illness,[29,30] but is infrequently used owing to lack of availability and experience.[31] Through indirect calorimetry, energy expenditure is calculated using oxygen consumption and carbon dioxide production.[4] Measurement accuracy can be affected by many factors including instrument performance, user experience, ambient temperature and volume leaks that might occur through the calorimeter, endotracheal tube or chest drains.[4] Patient-related factors also can influence measurement of REE, such as physical activity, food consumption and physiological stress such as pain. To obtain the most accurate measurement of REE, it is recommended that these measurements be taken under steady-state conditions[32] – that is, where there is at least a 5-minute period with ≤10% coefficient of variance in the oxygen consumption and carbon dioxide production.[4] However, metabolic equilibrium is not well defined and variation in how a steady state is determined exists. Comprehensive discussions of practical aspects of indirect calorimetry are published elsewhere.[4]

Predictive equations

Because indirect calorimetry is not available in many ICUs, it is common practice to use predictive equations (Table 19.3) to determine energy requirements.[24,33] The accuracy of predictive equations is poor compared with measurement of REE using indirect calorimetry; however, some predictive equations perform better in critical illness than do others. Some equations use only static variables (such as height, weight, age and sex) to predict REE. Others use more-dynamic variables (such as body temperature, minute ventilation, heart rate) in an attempt to account for the metabolic variation that occurs in critical illness.[34]

Although the accuracy of predictive equations compared with indirect calorimetry has been evaluated in many studies, no single equation is identified as being superior.[35] With over 200 predictive equations described in the literature[12] and variable accuracy of these equations, it makes selection challenging, particularly because of influencing factors such as body mass index (BMI), sex and age.

While most predictive equations are more likely to underestimate measured energy expenditure in the critically ill, wide variations in predicted energy expenditure have been reported and may contribute to both over- and underfeeding.[36] A recent systematic review of 18 studies demonstrated that, at a patient level, predictive equations underestimated energy requirements in 13–90% of patients; overestimation of energy requirements was observed in up to 88% of patients.[36] Despite the variable accuracy of predictive equations, they may provide some guidance for nutrition prescription in the absence of indirect calorimetry, but should be used alongside other assessments of nutritional requirements.

TABLE 19.3

Predictive equations for estimating energy expenditure in critically ill patients[33]

American College of Chest Physicians	25 × weight If BMI 16–25 kg/m² use usual body weight If BMI >25 kg/m² use ideal body weight If BMI <16 kg/m² use existing body weight for the first 7 × 10 days then ideal body weight
Harris–Benedict equation	Men: 66.4730 + (13.7516 × weight) + (5.0033 × height) − (6.7550 × age) Women: 655.0955 + (9.5634 × weight) + (1.8496 × height) − (4.6756 × age)
Ireton–Jones 1992 equation	1.925 − (10 × age) + (5 × weight) + (281 for males) + (292 if trauma present) + (851 if burns present)
Ireton–Jones 1997 equation	(5 × weight) − − (11 × age) + (244 for males) + (239 if trauma present) + (840 if burns present) + 1784
Penn State 1998	(1.1 × value from Harris–Benedict equation) + (140 × T_{max}) + (32 × VE) − 5340
Penn State 2003	(0.85 × value from Harris–Benedict equation) + (175 × T_{max}) + (33 × VE) − 6433
Swinamer 1990	(945 × body surface area) − (6.4 × age) + (108 × temperature) + 24.2 × respiratory rate) + (817 × V_T) − 4349

BMI = body mass index.

Source: Walker RN, Heuberger RA. Predictive equations for energy needs for the critically ill. Respir Care 2009;54(4): 509–21, with permission.

Practice tip

Ongoing patient assessment including regular weighing should be undertaken throughout the critical illness trajectory to ensure the nutrition prescription closely matches patient requirements.

Nutrition support

Prevention, detection and correction of malnutrition are important components of optimal nutritional support in critical illness. Nutrition support is instituted to optimise the patient's metabolic state, reduce morbidity and improve recovery. Additional benefits of nutrition support include attenuation of the metabolic response to stress, restriction of oxidative cellular injury, moderation of the immune response,[37] and decreasing insulin resistance through modulation of metabolism.[38] Most critically ill patients cannot consume food or fluids orally and, in these situations, EN is the preferred method of feeding for patients.[39–41] For some patients, PN alone or combined with EN may also be required to provide optimal nutrition support. Nutrition support is important throughout the trajectory of recovery from critical illness requirements, and nutrition support interventions are likely to vary throughout[42] (Fig. 19.3).

Enteral nutrition

EN has benefits beyond simply the supply of nutrients to the body and any amount is beneficial.[43] EN helps the structural and functional integrity of the gut, increases gastric mucosal blood flow, stimulates brush border enzymes, preserves epithelial tight cell junctions,[37] provides gut-

derived mucosal immunity and prevents rapid change in the gut microbiome.[38] Major effects of EN are: preservation of intestinal epithelium, mucosal mass and microvilli height; prevention of bacterial translocation; and a positive effect on the gut-associated lymphoid tissue, the source of most mucosal immunity in humans.[37] Septic complications may be decreased when EN is provided,[44] although this is not confirmed in all clinical trials.[45,46] Stimulating and improving gastrointestinal immune function is an important goal of early EN,[47] with the gut microbiome maintained in part by luminal nutrient stimulation, which in turn enhances microbial diversity.[48] While there is still much to learn in relation to the nutritional and non-nutritional benefits of EN in critical illness, current research suggests that EN is the preferred strategy of nutritional support for most critically ill patients.

FIGURE 19.3 Nutrition support during recovery from critical illness.

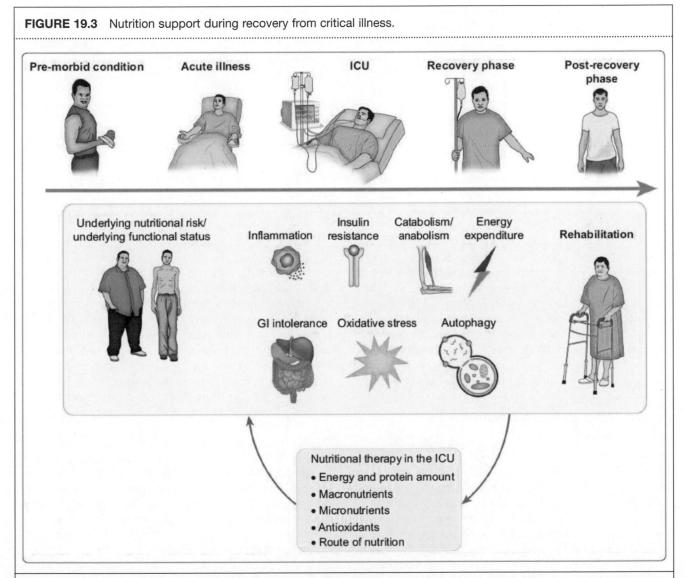

Source: Reprinted by permission of Springer Nature, Arabi YM, Casaer MP, Chapman M, et al. The intensive care medicine research agenda in nutrition and metabolism. Intensive Care Med 2017;43(9):1239–56.

Early or delayed enteral nutrition?

Early EN (within 24–48 hours) is recommended[39,40] and early EN may reduce infectious complications compared with delaying EN beyond 48 hours.[41]

An evidence-based guideline specific to early enteral nutrition in critically ill patients resulted in the formulation of 17 recommendations favouring the initiation of early EN.[40] Early EN was recommended over early parenteral nutrition (PN) and in patients receiving neuromuscular blockade or extracorporeal membrane oxygenation, and those for whom prone positioning is being used. Early EN is also recommended in those patients with traumatic brain injury, stroke, spinal cord injury, severe acute pancreatitis, or who have undergone gastrointestinal or abdominal aortic surgery. Early EN can be used where the patient has an open abdomen or intra-abdominal hypertension, provided that abdominal compartment syndrome is not present. However, EN should be reduced or discontinued if intra-abdominal pressure increases. Bowel sounds are not a reason to delay early EN unless bowel ischaemia or obstruction is expected. Similarly, early EN can be used in patients who have diarrhoea. Low-dose early EN is recommended in the context of therapeutic hypothermia, with the dose being increased after rewarming, and for patients with controlled acute, immediately life-threatening metabolic derangements associated with liver dysfunction, independent on the grade of encephalopathy.[40]

Early EN should be delayed in uncontrolled shock where haemodynamic and tissue perfusion goals have not been reached.[40,49] Once shock is controlled, low-dose EN can be commenced even if vasopressors are in use.[38] Delaying EN should occur in the context of uncontrolled life-threatening hypoxaemia, hypercapnia or acidosis; where overt bowel ischaemia, abdominal compartment syndrome, or active upper gastrointestinal bleeding is present; if a patient has high-output intestinal fistula and feeding access distal to the fistula is not possible; or where the gastric residual volume (GRV) is more than 500 mL in 6 hours.[40] While these recommendations reflect current best evidence, it should be noted that recommendations are based on either low-quality evidence or expert opinion, which highlights the need for further research in these areas.

Energy and protein goals in critical illness

There has been a recent trend towards a more conservative approach to nutrition support for critically ill patients at low nutrition risk because it is believed such patients are unlikely to benefit from aggressive nutrition therapy.[41,50] The potential lack of benefit has resulted in recommendations that specialised nutrition therapy in the first week in ICU is not required for low-risk patients.[50]

There has been much debate recently regarding energy and protein goals in critical illness.[51] The heterogeneity of critical illness means that a one-size-fits-all approach is unlikely to be helpful and the notion of individualising nutrition requirements to need has increasingly been highlighted.[52] Initially, it was thought that aggressive, early nutrition in critical illness could improve outcomes but this has not been substantiated in recent clinical trials.[45,53–55] It is possible that the endogenous production of glucose accompanied by lower energy expenditure in the early, acute phase of critical illness may mean that a beneficial impact of artificial nutrition is limited at this time point. The findings of The Augmented versus Routine approach to Giving Energy Trial (TARGET) support the idea that delivery of energy early in critical illness does not confer more of a benefit than does usual care.[45] However, this study was conducted in a general ICU population and was not focused on patients at highest nutrition risk. Early in critical illness it is also unclear whether low energy/adequate protein or low energy/low protein is more beneficial than usual care, particularly when provided for a short duration.[54,56] Current recommendations suggest that, in the early phase of critical illness, administering up to 70% of measured energy expenditure should be followed,[41] although older clinical practice guidelines do not distinguish energy targets based on the phase of critical illness.[50]

As a patient shifts to that late acute phase (days 3–7), nutrition may be more physiologically available and improved patient outcomes are more likely; however, determining when metabolic effects of critical illness change is difficult to determine in clinical practice. Nevertheless, as patients move into the late acute phase of critical illness, energy delivery can be increased to 80–100% of measured energy expenditure.[41]

In recent years, greater attention has been given to protein prescription in critical illness, as the catabolic response to critical illness can lead to a significant loss of muscle mass, which contributes to ICU-acquired weakness.[57] It is well recognised that protein delivery is well below what is recommended, with patients receiving an average of 0.6 g/kg/day during the 14 days after critical illness or injury.[58,59] In observational studies, higher protein provision is associated with reduced mortality.[15,60] However, prospective clinical trials have shown a limited effect of protein on important clinical outcomes and this continues to be the focus of nutrition research in critical illness. Current recommendations for protein provision vary. The American Society for Parenteral and Enteral nutrition recommends 1.2–2.0 g/kg/day,[50] the European Society of Parenteral and Enteral Nutrition recommends 1.3 g/kg/day[41] and the German Society for Nutritional Medicine recommends 1.0–1.2 g/kg/day.[39] Others have suggested commencing at a lower dose (0.8 g/kg/day) of protein during the early phase, which can be increased to 1.2 g/kg/day later on.[61] Larger clinical trials are needed to inform optimal protein administration in the context of critical illness.

The lack of definite data to inform macronutrient prescription in critical illness is recognised. Nevertheless, underdelivery of prescribed nutrition remains a concern and, in most cases, underdelivery is unnecessary and avoidable.[62,63] Clinician factors that contribute to underdelivery of EN include interruptions and low priorities for feeding,[64] recurrent fasting for clinical investigations and procedures[65] and variability in clinical practice-associated knowledge deficits or clinical uncertainty.[66] Patient factors preventing adequate delivery of prescribed nutrition include perceived intolerance as evidenced by high gastric residual volumes and diarrhoea.[67]

Practice tip

Nurses should regularly assess how well patients are meeting their nutrition goals and identify potential barriers which can be addressed through interdisciplinary collaboration to ensure nutrition intake is optimised.

Management of enteral feeding

Enteral nutrition guidelines and protocols

There are many different evidence-based nutrition clinical practice guidelines (CPGs) specific to critical illness. Comprehensive evidence-based nutrition guidelines are available from professional organisations such as the European Society of Parenteral and Enteral Nutrition,[41] the German Society for Medical Nutrition,[39] the European Society for Intensive Care Medicine,[40] the American Society of Parenteral and Enteral Nutrition,[50] the Malaysian Dietitians' Association[68] and the Metabolism and Nutrition Working Group of the Spanish Society of Intensive Care Medicine and Coronary Units.[69] The Canadian Clinical Practice Guidelines for Nutrition support in mechanically ventilated, critically ill adult patients was first published in 2003,[70] with updates as recently as 2015. While the Canadian CPGs are no longer updated, systematic reviews on the key topic areas continue to be provided.[71] Focused updates to previous guidelines are also available,[72] as are more-specific guidelines relating to critically ill patients with burns[73] and dysglycaemia.[74]

These evidence-based CPGs serve as a strong foundation for the development of local policies, procedures and protocols. Use of protocols to guide EN practice can help improve the delivery of enteral feeds and clinical outcomes.[75,76] However, a positive impact on nutrition intake is not always observed,[77] and can be related to poor adherence to recommendations.[78] Protocol variability exists because of the lack of robust research in the management of EN, as evidenced by the number of guideline recommendations which are based on expert opinion. In the absence of strong research evidence, rituals are embraced and rarely challenged.[79] Furthermore, the implementation and sustainability of guidelines are influenced by multiple factors such as clinician preference, patient population, clinical contexts and content of guidelines.[67,80] Decisions of what to include may be challenged by variations in guideline recommendations.[52]

Routes of enteral feeding

Wide-bore nasogastric or orogastric tubes are most commonly used in the critically ill in the early stages of EN.[61] Should prolonged EN be anticipated (longer than 1 month), or where patients have gastric intolerance, then gastrostomy, duodenostomy or jejunostomy tubes may be used.[41,50] Postpyloric feeding is useful if patients are not tolerating gastric feeding, but has not been shown to be superior to gastric feeding[81] when gastrointestinal function recovery, mortality or hospitalisation expenses are considered.[82] Postpyloric enteral access is also recommended for patients deemed to be at high risk for aspiration.[41] Lower incidence of pulmonary aspiration, gastric reflux and pneumonia ($P < 0.001$, all), and gastrointestinal complications including vomiting, nausea, diarrhoea, abdominal distension, high gastric residual volume and constipation ($P < 0.05$, all), were reported in a systematic review and meta-analysis of gastric versus postpyloric feeding in critically ill patients.[82] However, tube placement of postpyloric tubes can be more challenging and not as simple as placement of a gastric tube.[61,83]

Assessment of enteral feeding tube placement

The correct placement of enteral feeding tubes is crucial to promote adequate nutrition and avoid adverse events. The correct insertion of enteral feeding tubes in the critically ill can be challenging because these patients often have a reduced cough reflex and altered sensorium, and receive sedative and narcotic medications.[84] Misplacement of the feeding tube into the tracheobronchial tree is a potential but infrequent complication of tube insertion in the ICU; however, the consequences can be significant.[85] Complications such as infusion of tube feedings, pneumothorax, pneumonitis, hydropneumothorax, bronchopleural fistula, empyema and pulmonary haemorrhage have been reported.[86] Confirmation of tube placement is routinely done with radiography (Fig. 19.4),[87] which is considered the gold standard.[88] Bedside techniques, such as point-of-care ultrasound,[89] measurement of gastric pH,[90] carbon dioxide monitoring, auscultation and enteral access devices have been identified as alternatives, but all have significant limitations in critically ill patients.[84] For example, in a convenience sample of adult patients, the diagnostic accuracy of pH 5.5 to differentiate gastric from non-gastric samples was low and attributed to limited accuracy of pH measurement and operator interpretation of results.[90] Capnography has a reported sensitivity (100%), specificity (92.5%) and accuracy (95%) for determining gastric placement[91] and is useful in differentiating from inadvertent placement of the tube in the respiratory tract,[92] but does not necessarily indicate that the placement in the alimentary tract is correct.[91] Point-of-care ultrasound may be useful in identifying gastric tube placement.[89] However, in a study of intensive care nurses who were trained to undertake this assessment, the correct placement was verified by ultrasound in 70–78%

FIGURE 19.4   Correct placement of a nasogastric tube.[87]

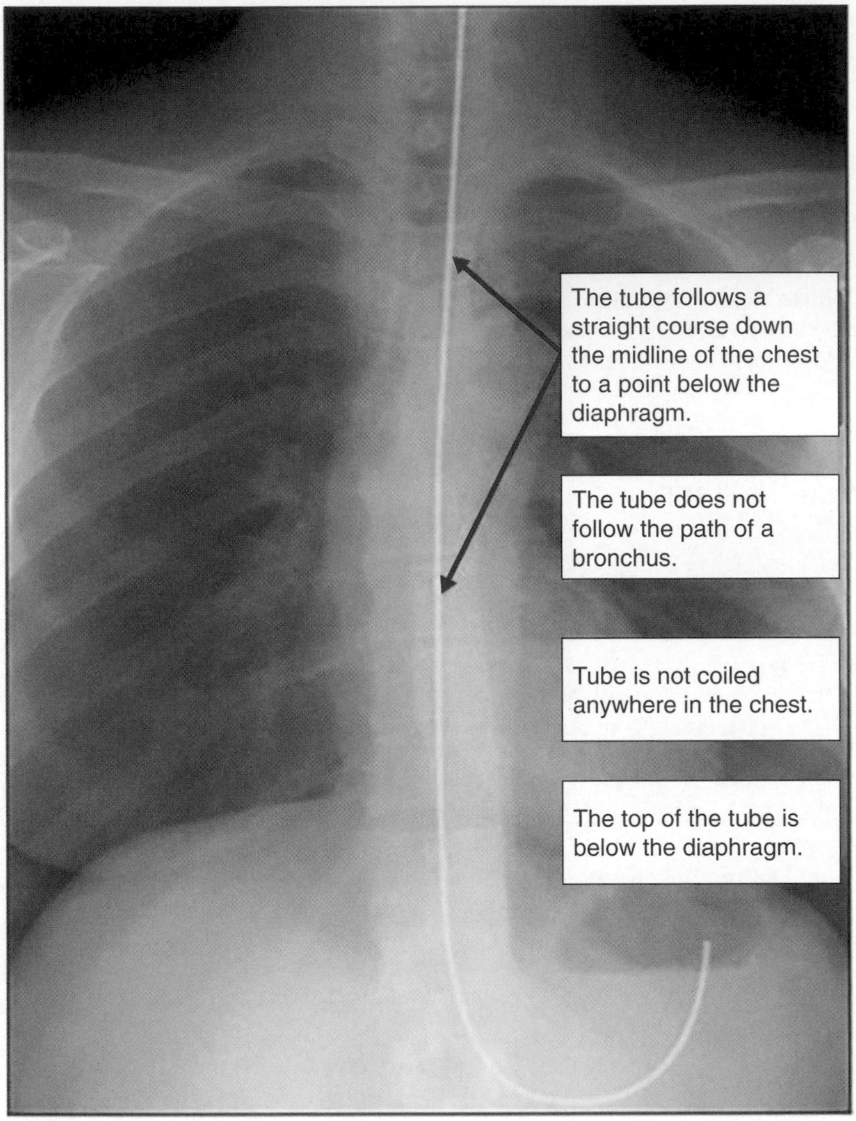

The tube follows a straight course down the midline of the chest to a point below the diaphragm.

The tube does not follow the path of a bronchus.

Tube is not coiled anywhere in the chest.

The top of the tube is below the diaphragm.

Source: © Pennsylvania Patient Safety Authority.

of critically ill patients,[93] much lower than that reported with capnography. Auscultation of the stomach when air is insufflated via the gastric tube is a common and somewhat ritualistic practice that is very unreliable in critically ill patients and no longer recommended,[94,95] yet is difficult to de-implement because the technique is so embedded in clinical practice.[96]

The limitation of these bedside measures means that chest X-ray remains the gold standard when assessing feeding tube placement for critically ill patients[97] and, if unavailable, multiple bedside methods of determining placement should be used so as to improve accuracy of assessment.[84,94]

Newer techniques of assessing gastric tube placement include the use of electromagnetic placement devices, which are most common for small bowel tube placement, where they are reported to be an effective method of feeding tube placement (>94% placement in the desired location).[98] The same technology has been used to evaluate nasogastric tube placement in neuroscience patients, where 32/39 were correctly placed in the stomach (3 results unavailable and 4 tubes placed further than the stomach).[99] This approach shows promise and requires further research. Implementation requires consideration of the training and resource requirements if electromagnetic placement devices are to be widely adopted.

Feeding regimens

Once the enteral feeding tube is successfully placed, administration of the feeding solution can begin using a variety of methods, including bolus, intermittent and continuous enteral feeding (Table 19.4). Bolus enteral feeding is rarely used in the ICU. It is less clear whether intermittent or continuous feeding is the more beneficial. A systematic review of 10 studies (664 patients), most with an overall high risk of bias, showed that the continuous and intermittent routes of enteral feeding of critically ill patients were similar for nutrition intake, gastric residual volume, aspiration pneumonia, diarrhoea, abdominal distention, ICU length of stay and mortality. The only difference was an observed higher incidence of vomiting in patients who were fed continuously (risk ratio (RR), 2.76, 95% confidence interval (CI), 1.23–6.23).[100]

TABLE 19.4

Methods of feed delivery

METHOD	DESCRIPTION
Bolus	• Delivery of a large volume of tube feed into the stomach over a short period of time (>100 mL). • Associated with complications, such as aspiration and vomiting.
Intermittent	• A several-hour infusion a few times a day (e.g. 150 mL/h for 3 hours, three times per day), or delivered over a longer period (12–16 hours) with an 8–12-hour rest period. • Allows gastric acidity and therefore limits bacterial overgrowth. • Requires a higher hourly rate to meet caloric requirements.
Continuous	• The delivery of small amounts of formula per hour over a 24-hour period. • May make caloric requirements more achievable. • Continuous dilution of gastric acid may contribute to bacterial overgrowth.

However, another meta-analysis of 14 randomised controlled trials (1025 critically ill patients) reported that intermittent feeding could significantly increase feeding intolerance, GRV and aspiration. Patients in the intermittent-feeding group received more calories.[101] Like the systematic review of Thong and colleagues,[100] the methodological quality of the studies was low, suggesting that higher-quality evaluative studies are required to determine whether intermittent or continuous feeding in critically ill patients is preferable.[102] Because of inconclusive evidence regarding feeding regimens, decisions are based on individual patient assessment and the clinician's clinical judgement.

Commencing enteral nutrition

For most critically ill patients, EN can be safely commenced. The relatively few reasons for delaying enteral feeding include uncontrolled shock, uncontrolled life-threatening hypoxaemia, hypercapnoea or acidosis, active upper gastrointestinal bleeding, overt bowel ischaemia, high-output intestinal fistula, abdominal compartment syndrome and persistent high GRVs.[41] Where therapeutic hypothermia is being used, or if a patient has increased intra-abdominal hypertension or acute liver failure, it is recommended that EN is commenced at a low rate.[41]

For many years a functioning bowel was considered necessary before EN could be commenced and there were perceptions that bowel rest was necessary. This approach is no longer supported[50] and it is recognised that gastrointestinal dysfunction may occur in up to 70% of critically ill patients.[103] However, gastrointestinal dysfunction (which may include alterations in bowel sounds, gastric emptying, the presence of vomiting and/or diarrhoea) may reflect increased disease severity and reduce the success of EN delivery.[104] While isolated evidence of gastrointestinal dysfunction does not meaningfully inform decisions regarding EN, comprehensive physical assessment of the gastrointestinal system may be useful in informing clinical decision making.[105]

As more is becoming known about metabolism in critical illness[106] and with recognition that the nutrition risk for all critically ill patients differs,[19] the current recommendations suggest that, in the acute early phase of critical illness, energy targets should be <70% of estimated or measured requirements for patients who are well nourished or moderately malnourished. In the context of severe malnutrition, a similar approach can be used provided that serum phosphate levels are normal.[52] Where feeding to goal rate or volume is not possible, trophic feeds can be delivered[107] and may be sufficient to prevent gastric mucosal atrophy and maintain the integrity of the gut.[108] A number of clinical trials have been undertaken to identify whether intentional underfeeding compared with full feeding confers a benefit for critically ill patients. Although many of these clinical trials suggest a benefit with underfeeding, it must be acknowledged that these studies do have methodological limitations, which means

FIGURE 19.5   Recommendations for nutritional management by nutritional status and phase of critical illness.[52] EN = enteral nutrition; IC = intensive care; PN = parenteral nutrition.

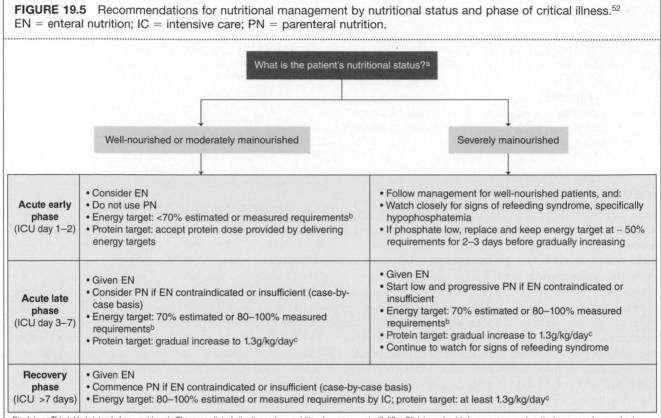

	Well-nourished or moderately mainourished	**Severely mainourished**
Acute early phase (ICU day 1–2)	• Consider EN • Do not use PN • Energy target: <70% estimated or measured requirements[b] • Protein target: accept protein dose provided by delivering energy targets	• Follow management for well-nourished patients, and: • Watch closely for signs of refeeding syndrome, specifically hypophosphatemia • If phosphate low, replace and keep energy target at ~ 50% requirements for 2–3 days before gradually increasing
Acute late phase (ICU day 3–7)	• Given EN • Consider PN if EN contraindicated or insufficient (case-by-case basis) • Energy target: 70% estimated or 80–100% measured requirements[b] • Protein target: gradual increase to 1.3g/kg/day[c]	• Given EN • Start low and progressive PN if EN contraindicated or insufficient • Energy target: 70% estimated or 80–100% measured requirements[b] • Protein target: gradual increase to 1.3g/kg/day[c] • Continue to watch for signs of refeeding syndrome
Recovery phase (ICU >7 days)	• Given EN • Commence PN if EN contraindicated or insufficient (case-by-case basis) • Energy target: 80–100% estimated or measured requirements by IC; protein target: at least 1.3g/kg/day[c]	

Disclaimer: This table is intended as a guide only. There are clinical situations where nutritional management will differ. Clinicians should always assess each patient on a case-by-case basis. [a]Nutrition status should be assessed using local hospital guidelines or Global Leadership Initiative on Malnutrition criteria for diagnosis of malnutrition and clinical judgment (understanding the limitations with malnutrition diagnostic tools in the ICU setting); [b]Measured energy requirements by indirect calorimetry; [c]Adjusted body weight should be used in predictive equations for obese patients (BMI >30kg/m²)

Source: Lambell KJ, Tatucu-Babet OA, Chapple L, et al. Nutrition therapy in critical illness: a review of the literature for clinicians. Crit Care 2020;24:35, Figure 1.

the results should be interpreted cautiously.[51] Nevertheless, current evidence-based recommendations suggest targeting <70% of estimated or measured energy requirements in the first 1–2 days of illness, increasing to 70% of estimated or 80–100% of measured requirements in the late acute phase (days 3–7). In the week following critical illness, the energy target should be 80–100% (Fig. 19.5).[52]

Some patients may develop electrolyte disorders when nutrition therapy is commenced because of a change in fluid status, the electrolyte content in feeding solutions, overfeeding or the development of refeeding syndrome. Refeeding syndrome may occur when the body shifts from the use of fat and protein as energy sources in starvation to the use of carbohydrates for energy; the patient may exhibit abrupt electrolyte shifts and is represented by hypophosphataemia (below 0.65 mmol/L).[109] The prevalence of refeeding syndrome can be difficult to establish because of the variable definitions but can be experienced in up to 40% of critically ill patients. Up to 10% of patients may experience severe hypophosphataemia (<0.32 mmol/L). Identifying which patients are at greater risk of refeeding syndrome is

challenging. Prolonged previous starvation is clearly a risk; however, critical illness with catabolism, hyperglycaemia, fluid shifts and administration of large amounts of insulin can also increase risk.[109] If hypophosphataemia occurs within 72 hours of commencing EN then caloric restriction is warranted.[61]

Managing complications of enteral nutrition

Once EN is established, it is important to assess for potential complications. These can include metabolic changes;[110] feeding intolerance such as increased gastric residual volume,[111,112] gastric distention, vomiting and diarrhoea; pulmonary aspiration;[39] and device-related complications.[113] Ongoing monitoring for these complications should be incorporated into nursing care so that preventative or corrective interventions can be implemented in order to minimise their occurrence or optimise management.

Gastric residual volume

Assessment of feeding tolerance by measuring GRV is a common part of nursing practice despite this representing only upper gastrointestinal intolerance and the fact that evidence is lacking to show GRV measurement positively impacts clinical outcomes including mortality, pneumonia, vomiting and length of hospital stay.[114] The best approach to the measurement of GRV is also unclear. The frequency of assessment can range from every 4 hours to daily, or not at all. There is also variation in what is considered a high GRV.[115] There is a wide range of GRVs that are considered 'high' with volumes ranging from 50 to 500 mL.[116,117] However, current evidence-based nutrition guidelines which have a recommendation specific to the measurement of GRV recommend that it should not be used as part of routine care to monitor ICU patients receiving EN.[50] A recent systematic review of 5 studies involving 998 patients showed no difference in mortality or ventilator-associated pneumonia between patients in whom a GRV was measured and those in whom it was not. Duration of ventilation or ICU length of stay was also similar between the two groups. However, where vomiting was an outcome of interest, there was an increase in vomiting observed when GRV was not measured,[118] with the majority of data being contributed by one study.[119] In three studies which included enteral feeding intolerance as an outcome measure, there was a decrease in the rate of feeding intolerance when GRV was not assessed.[118] For those ICUs where GRVs are still utilised, withholding EN for GRVs <500 mL in the absence of other signs of intolerance should be avoided.[50] Current recommendations are, however, based predominantly on critically ill patients with a medical diagnosis, and surgical patients may need to be managed differently. In a recent multicentre clinical trial evaluating the effectiveness of a promotility drug, surgical patients had a significantly higher incidence of high (>400 mL for one measure, or >250 mL for two consecutive measures) GRV. In this clinical trial, GRV reflected gastric emptying and high GRV was considered an acceptable surrogate marker for delayed gastric emptying.[120]

The most common approach to GRV assessment was using the syringe aspiration methods although the techniques are not well established or described in the literature.[87] Factors such as tube diameter, tube position, type of gastric access and the patient's position can influence GRV measurement accuracy.[121] It is assumed that measuring GRV is accurate and useful, but GRV does not correlate with clinical or radiological abdominal findings.[122] However, in a recent single-centre, prospective cross-sectional study, ultrasound assessment of GRV demonstrated a strong correlation (intraclass correlation coefficient (ICC) 0.814 (0.61–0.92)) with GRV assessment using syringe aspiration, suggesting that this may be an option for assessing GRV, provided adequate training is provided.[123] If gastric contents are aspirated, there is the question about whether to discard or refeed the aspirate. The evidence for discarding gastric aspirate is weak[124] and this continues to be a practice that is inconsistent within and across intensive care units.

Practice tip

In determining feeding intolerance, a single high GRV in the absence of physical examination or radiographic findings should not result in the cessation of enteral feeding. Persisting with enteral feeding has demonstrated benefits.

Prevention or management of gastrointestinal motility that results in increased GRV can include patient position,[125] maintaining electrolyte balance and normoglycaemia, minimising – where possible – the use of catecholamines, analgesic and sedative agents, early enteral feeding and pharmacotherapy.[126] Prokinetic agents are commonly used to promote gastric emptying in critically ill patients and can lead to reduced GRV.[127] Consensus on when prokinetic agents should be commenced is lacking,[128] with the recognition that, in the early phase of critical illness enteral feeding, intolerance may be an adaptive mechanism.[129] Metoclopramide and erythromycin are commonly used as prokinetic agents and one clinical practice guideline recommends that erythromycin be used as a first-line prokinetic therapy,[41] although this is not a consensus recommendation. Metoclopramide alone or in conjunction with erythromycin is also recommended. There is also a range of other agents which have been evaluated in the context of critical illness.[130] A clinical trial of a ghrelin agonist (ulimorelin) and metoclopramide examined the safety and efficacy of these prokinetic agents, demonstrating that both achieve similar rates of feeding success with no safety differences.[131] In both groups, achieving feeding success (≥80% of daily protein prescription) was observed in only 51.6% (ulimorelin) and 55.2% (metoclopramide) of patients. Data were collected over a 5-day period during which enteral feeding intolerance continued to decline, with only 15% of patients exhibiting feeding intolerance at day 5. This suggests that motility disorders for most critically ill patients are transient and highlights the need for further research in this area. Where the use of non-pharmacological strategies (e.g. patient positioning) and prokinetics is unsuccessful in improving gastric emptying, postpyloric feeding could be considered.[108]

Practice tip

When evaluating GRV in relation to the rate of enteral feeding, remember to take into account the production of gastric secretion, which can be as much as 2500 mL/day.

Diarrhoea

Development of diarrhoea in enterally fed patients[61] can occur for a range of different reasons[125] and is not uncommon in critical illness.[132] Unfortunately, defining diarrhoea is problematic, as it is a subjective assessment that relies on nursing interpretation rather than on quantifiable assessment of stool weight.[132] Factors which can influence EN-related diarrhoea include the method of delivery (less likely with continuous infusion), content and composition of the feeds, and bacterial contamination. When causes of diarrhoea are not systematically investigated, EN can often (and incorrectly) be identified as the cause and this may contribute to unnecessary feeding interruptions.[133] Diarrhoea may contribute to fluid and electrolyte disorders, malnutrition, breaches of skin integrity and wound contamination, and consequently effective management needs to be implemented and targeted at the cause.[133,134]

Enteral feeding solutions present an excellent medium for the growth of microorganisms, and bacterial contamination of enteral feeding solutions can occur even when administering prepackaged feeds from a sterile container.[135] Strategies to limit bacterial contamination of enteral feeding solutions include:

- meticulous preparation of feeding solutions and equipment
- using commercially prepared formula in closed systems in preference to decanted feeds
- limiting the time that feeding solution is kept at room temperature once opened
- meticulous attention to handwashing
- limiting manipulation of the EN bags and delivery system at the bedside.[136]

Practice tip

Nurses may be tempted to stop EN in the presence of diarrhoea, but there is no evidence to support withholding enteral feeding in critically ill patients. The only exception may be if there are significant disturbances in fluid and/or electrolyte balance.

Pulmonary aspiration

An important complication of enteral feeding is the development of pulmonary aspiration and nosocomial pneumonia. Determining whether aspiration has occurred is difficult, even for experienced clinicians, and there are no simple, reliable and valid bedside techniques to identify whether a patient has pulmonary aspiration. High GRVs have been linked to the potential for pulmonary aspiration, although this has not been shown in research,[137] and both enteral and parenteral nutrition are associated with high rates of microaspiration.[138] Risk factors for aspiration include an inability to protect the airway, presence of a nasoenteric enteral access device, mechanical ventilation, age ≥70 years, reduced level of consciousness, supine positioning, gastroesophageal reflux and use of bolus intermittent enteral nutrition.[139] Many of the risk factors for aspiration are not directly linked to the provision of EN and current evidence-based guidelines to prevent pulmonary aspiration are appropriately comprehensive.[140]

Recommendations specific to enteral feeding emphasise the need for adequate hand hygiene, a semirecumbent positioning (30–45 degrees), avoidance of gastric overdistention, and removal of the nasogastric tube as soon as possible.[141]

Traditional approaches to assessment of pulmonary aspiration, such as colouring agents and use of glucose oxidase strips, are no longer recommended because they are ineffective.[50] Further, colouring agents such as methylene blue are toxic to the mitochondria and interfere with oxidative phosphorylation.[139]

Practice tip

Nursing patients with the head of the bed elevated is common in ICU; however, more evidence is needed to demonstrate that this practice prevents pulmonary aspiration.

Parenteral nutrition

EN is the preferred method of nutritional support because it is closer to normal volitional eating, leading to physiological advantages, is associated with fewer infectious and metabolic complications and is less expensive than PN. PN bypasses the gastrointestinal system and the crucial role that hormones and nutrients play in regulating gut function, metabolic pathways and hepatic function.

Studies report conflicting results on the benefit of PN for the nutrition support of critically ill patients, with early studies reporting worse clinical outcomes and more-recent studies concluding that there is no difference in clinical outcomes when EN is compared with PN.[46,55,142–144] In a randomised clinical trial (RCT), Harvey and colleagues[143] compared EN with PN and found no significant differences in mortality or infection rate. In a second RCT, the NUTRIREA-2 multicentre study in 44 French ICUs, early isocaloric EN was compared with early isocaloric PN in 2410 critically ill patients with shock. No difference in mortality or risk of secondary infection was observed, but early EN was associated with more digestive complications in the early isocaloric EN group compared with the early isocaloric PN group.[46] Conversely, the EPaNIC trial showed that late (day 8), rather than early (day 3), initiation of PN in a predominantly cardiac surgery population was associated with fewer complications and faster recovery.[55] These conflicting findings are probably due to improvements in management of infection risk and line management, the evolution of PN solutions and careful consideration to the risks of overfeeding patients in applying PN in care.[142,145] Recent guidelines[12] recommend that EN is supplemented with PN in patients who cannot commence early EN or until target nutrition goals are achieved; however, the time period varies between guidelines. McClave and colleagues[12] and the recent update of some recommendations in the previous guideline[72] recommend PN be initiated after

1 week, unless the patient is severely malnourished, largely because of the results of the EPaNIC trial. However, another study[146] found that supplemental PN in the first week of critical illness resulted in a reduction in late infections.

With conflicting evidence, it is necessary for clinicians to carefully assess the patient and apply individual clinical judgement to determine which patients are most likely to benefit from more-aggressive nutrition therapy early in their ICU stay. There can be metabolic, immunological, endocrine and infective complications from infusing solutions of high glucose concentration and fat globules intravenously.[147] PN impairs humoral and cellular immunological defences and the association of PN with increased free radical formation may be important for patients who are critically ill.[121] Attention must be paid to avoid overfeeding, particularly with glucose, when providing PN. This is more likely to occur in those patients who are also receiving pharmacological therapy containing lipids or glucose if these are not also taken into account when determining nutrition prescription.

PN solutions contain carbohydrates, lipids, amino acids, electrolytes, vitamins and trace elements (Table 19.5) and are commonly available as 'all-in-one' admixtures, which simplifies PN use and decreases line infection rates.[148] PN, whether supplementary or complete, provides daily allowances of nutrients and minerals. The addition of vitamins and trace elements to PN solutions is necessary,

TABLE 19.5
Components of PN solutions

COMPONENT	RECOMMENDATION	GRADE[a]
Carbohydrate	The minimal amount of carbohydrate required is about 2 g/kg of glucose per day.	B
	Hyperglycaemia (glucose >10 mmol/L) contributes to death in the critically ill patient and should also be avoided to prevent infectious complications.	B
	Reductions and increases in mortality rates have been reported in ICU patients when blood glucose is maintained between 4.5 and 6.1 mmol/L. No unequivocal recommendation on this is therefore possible at present.	C
	There is a higher incidence of severe hypoglycaemia in patients treated to the tighter limits.	A
Lipids	Lipids should be an integral part of PN for energy and to ensure essential fatty acid provision in long-term ICU patients.	B
	Intravenous lipid emulsions (LCT, MCT or mixed emulsions) can be administered safely at a rate of 0.7 g/kg up to 1.5 g/kg over 12–24 h.	B
	The tolerance of mixed LCT/MCT lipid emulsions in standard use is sufficiently documented. Several studies have shown specific clinical advantages over soybean LCT alone but require confirmation by prospective controlled studies.	C
	Olive oil-based PN is well tolerated in critically ill patients.	B
	Addition of EPA and DHA to lipid emulsions has demonstrable effects on cell membranes and inflammatory processes. Fish oil-enriched lipid emulsions probably decrease length of stay in critically ill patients.	B
Amino acids	When PN is indicated, a balanced amino acid mixture should be infused at approximately 1.3–1.5 g/kg ideal body weight/day in conjunction with an adequate energy supply.	B
	When PN is indicated in ICU patients the amino acid solution should contain 0.2–0.4 g/kg/day of L-glutamine (e.g. 0.3–0.6 g/kg/day alanyl-glutamine dipeptide).	A
Micronutrients	All PN prescriptions should include a daily dose of multivitamins and of trace elements.	C

[a] Grade of recommendation – the grade of recommendation is based on the quality of the evidence where A is high, B is moderate, C is low and D is very low (as quoted in Guyatt GH, Oxman AD, Vist GE, et al. GRADE: an emerging consensus on rating quality of evidence and strength of recommendations. BMJ 2008; 336:924–6).

DHA = docosahexaenoic acid; EPA = eicosapentaenoic acid; LCT = long-chain triglycerides; MCT = medium-chain triglycerides.

Source: Adapted from Singer P, Berger MM, Van den Berghe G, et al. ESPEN guidelines on parenteral nutrition: intensive care. Clin Nutr 2009;28(4):387–400, with permission.

particularly as water-soluble vitamins and trace elements are rapidly depleted (Table 19.6).[149,150] Standardised PN formulations, although as effective as custom-made PN in providing caloric requirements, are less likely to achieve estimated protein requirements and have been noted to be associated with hyponatraemia.[151] Glucose is the primary energy source in PN solutions. Concentrations of 10–70% glucose may be used in PN solutions, although the final concentration of the solution should be no more than 35%. The high concentration of PN solutions can cause thrombosis so PN is normally infused via a central venous catheter. Catheter insertion, ongoing care and replacement are similar to that with any other central venous catheter and, although delivering nutrient-rich solutions, there are insufficient data to suggest whether patients receiving PN are at higher risk of developing a catheter-related bloodstream infection.[152] Although the evidence base is weak, expert recommendations suggest that a dedicated central venous catheter, or lumen of a multilumen catheter, should be used to deliver PN.[153] Manipulation of the catheter and tubing should be avoided in order to minimise infection of the catheter. Peripheral administration can be considered when the final solution concentration is 10–12%,[154] but is not usually used in the context of critical illness because high volumes of PN would be required to meet caloric requirements. Routine monitoring of the patient's fluid balance, glucose, biochemical profile, full blood count, triglycerides, trace elements and vitamins is necessary. The patient is also assessed for signs of complications associated with the administration of PN (Table 19.7).

TABLE 19.6
Trace elements in PN[150]

TRACE ELEMENT	ACTION
Zinc	Wound healing
Iron	Haemoglobin synthesis
Copper	Erythrocyte maturation and lipid metabolism
Manganese	Calcium and phosphorus metabolism
Cobalt	Essential constituent of vitamin B12
Iodine	Thyroxine synthesis
Chromium	Glucose utilisation

TABLE 19.7
Short-term metabolic complications associated with total PN

COMPLICATION	CAUSE	DETECTION AND TREATMENT
Hyperosmolar coma	Occurs acutely if a rapid infusion of hypertonic fluid is administered. Infusion can cause severe osmotic diuresis, resulting in electrolyte abnormalities, dehydration and malfunction of the central nervous system.	Daily blood samples, accurate measurements of fluid balance, routine blood samples. Reduce infusion rate, correct electrolyte imbalances.
Electrolyte imbalance	Disturbances in serum electrolytes, particularly sodium, potassium, urea and creatinine, may occur early in the treatment of TPN. Electrolyte imbalances can be caused by the patient's underlying medical condition; requirements vary with individual patients' needs. Can be caused by inadequate or excessive administration of intravenous fluids.	Daily blood samples taken early in treatment to detect abnormalities. Replacement fluid as required; extra intravenous fluids may be required during the stabilisation period.
Hyperglycaemia	Critically ill patients may be resistant to insulin because of the secretion of ACTH and adrenaline (epinephrine). This promotes the secretion of glycogen, which inhibits the insulin response to hyperglycaemia.	Monitor the patient's blood sugar 4-hourly after commencement of treatment or as required. Monitor daily urinalysis for glucose and ketones. An insulin infusion may be required to keep blood sugar levels within prescribed limits.
Rebound hypoglycaemia	May occur on discontinuation of TPN because hyperinsulinism may occur after prolonged intravenous nutrition. A rise in serum insulin occurs with infusion, and thus sudden cessation of infusion can result in hypoglycaemia.	Glucose infusion rate should be gradually reduced over the final hour of infusion before discontinuing. Some patients may receive a 10% glucose solution after cessation of TPN.

TABLE 19.7

Short-term metabolic complications associated with total PN—cont'd

COMPLICATION	CAUSE	DETECTION AND TREATMENT
Hypophosphataemia	Glucose infusion results in the continuous release of insulin, stimulating anabolism and resulting in rapid influx of phosphorus into muscle cells. The greatest risk is to malnourished patients with overzealous administration of feeding. Patients who are hyperglycaemic, who require insulin therapy during TPN or who have a history of alcoholism or chronic weight loss may require extra phosphate in the early stages of treatment.	Monitor phosphate levels daily. Hypophosphataemia will usually appear after 24–48 h of feeding. Reduce the carbohydrate load and give phosphate supplementation.
Lipid clearance	Lipids are broken down in the bloodstream with the aid of lipoprotein lipase found in the epithelium of capillaries in many tissues. A syndrome known as fat overload syndrome can occur when infusion of lipid is administered that is beyond the patient's clearing capacity, resulting in lipid deposits in the capillaries.	Blood samples should be taken after the first infusion commences (within 6 h) to observe for lipid in the blood.
Side effects of lipid infusion	Some patients suffer symptoms either during or after an infusion of lipid mix PN. The exact cause is unknown. The patient may complain of headache, nausea or vomiting, and generally feels unwell.	Treat mild symptoms. If tolerated, the TPN solution of non-protein calories can be given in the form of glucose. However, it is essential that the regimen includes some fat to prevent the development of fatty acid deficiency.
Anaphylactic shock	This is a rare complication but may occur as a reaction to the administration of a lipid.	It may be necessary to administer adrenaline and/or steroids, and to provide supportive therapy as required.
Glucose intolerance	TPN using glucose as the main source of calories is associated with a rise in oxygen consumption and CO_2 production. The workload imposed by the high CO_2 production may precipitate respiratory distress in susceptible patients, particularly those requiring mechanical ventilation.	Observe patients for signs of respiratory distress. Provide non-protein calories in the form of glucose–lipid mix. Slow initial rate of infusion.
Liver function	Abnormalities with liver function can be associated with TPN. May be attributable to hepatic stenosis with moderate hepatomegaly; patients may also develop jaundice. Liver function tests often return to normal after cessation of therapy; however, TPN can lead to severe hepatic dysfunction in neonates.	Monitor liver function tests twice weekly. There are several factors that may contribute to development of abnormal liver function tests. These most often occur after a period of time and appear to be more of a problem when there is an excess calorie intake or in glucose-based regimens.

ACTH = adrenocorticotrophic hormone; PN = parenteral nutrition; TPN = total parenteral nutrition.

Practice tip

PN solutions are high in glucose and therefore require vigilance in preventing catheter-related infection.

Transition to oral diet and fluids
Dysphagia assessment

The patient's condition, length of stay in ICU and their ability to swallow will influence when and how quickly oral nutrition can commence. Accurate identification of swallowing disorders in critically ill patients is crucial to determine the safety and type of oral nutrition. Dysphagia that occurs in ICU patients following extubation is usually an ICU-acquired disorder,[155] although it is also possible for patients to have an undiagnosed swallowing disease. The prevalence of swallowing disorders in patients with acute respiratory failure who are extubated is unknown. The estimated prevalence of dysphagia ranges between 3% and 62% for patients recovering from critical illnesses.[156] Six potential mechanisms can cause patients in the ICU to develop dysfunctional swallowing. Endotracheal and tracheostomy tubes can cause direct trauma, focal ulceration and inflammation.[157] Neuromyopathy resulting in muscular weakness can also cause postextubation dysphagia. The third mechanism for dysphagia is the development of dysfunctional oropharyngeal and laryngeal sensation. Sensation abnormalities can result from either critical illness polyneuropathy or local oedema.[158] Swallowing dysfunction in critical illness can be related to impaired sensorium as a result of ICU-acquired delirium, underlying critical illness or the effects of sedating medications. Gastro-oesophageal reflux is disordered swallowing in critically ill patients and some of the pathophysiological processes responsible for gastro-oesophageal reflux are likely to continue in the immediate postextubation period.[159]

Swallowing dysfunction can also occur because of dyssynchronous breathing and swallowing in patients with underlying respiratory impairment and tachypnoea. The study of those factors that increase the risk for impaired swallowing in awake, recently extubated patients without strokes or neuromuscular diseases is less advanced. Specific risk factors for this type of postextubation dysphagia have been widely reported, but meaningful analysis is prevented owing to the different approaches to patient populations, assessment methods (including timing) and duration of intubation.[160] Additional research is required to identify risk factors which contribute most to the development of dysphagia after extubation. There are some data to suggest that critically ill patients who have required prolonged intubation may be at increased risk of dysphagia but are also less likely to be referred for screening.[161,162] Comparisons of studies are limited by biased patient selection, heterogeneous study populations and differing diagnostic protocols.

The most common diagnostic test to evaluate for postextubation dysphagia is a bedside swallow evaluation performed by a speech language pathologist. Although the components of this examination are not standardised and can vary by practitioner,[155] patients usually undergo an interview, a structural and functional evaluation of their mouth and their cough response and an assessment of their swallowing function with different food textures and liquid thicknesses. Non-instrumental approaches to dysphagia assessment in critically ill patients have not been widely studied and there is a need for further high-quality research in this area, where assessment approaches are evaluated against a gold standard such as flexible endoscopic evaluation of swallowing (FEES).[159] Additional tests may be ordered to assist in the diagnosis of postextubation dysphagia. A videoendoscopic evaluation of swallowing (VEES), often referred to as a modified barium swallow, is highly sensitive and specific for aspiration. The other gold standard instrumental procedure to evaluate for postextubation dysphagia is a fibreoptic endoscopic swallow study.[155]

Oral nutrition intake

Nutrition intake following ICU admission is important as this is a time where it is recognised that the patient may be at increased nutrition risk and the body more able to process nutrition to facilitate recovery. In an observational study of 50 critically ill patients, oral intake was inadequate in the week following extubation, with no patients consuming more than 50% of daily requirements.[163] Subsequent studies have indicated that oral intake is significantly below predicted energy and protein needs when oral nutrition alone is provided compared with EN or combined enteral and oral nutrition.[164–167] Patients who are being weaned from nutrition support may have oral nutrition slowly introduced. For longer-stay patients, particularly those who have ICU-acquired weakness, weaning from enteral or PN onto oral nutrition may commence with a trial of oral feeding by day supplemented by nutrition support at night.

Many patients resume oral intake after extubation and on discharge from ICU. Strategies to support nutritional intake of patients on an oral diet typically target organisational or patient level factors designed to improve volitional nutritional intake. Use of oral nutrition supplements (ONS) is an additional strategy that can be used to increase protein and calorie intake and may be of benefit to those patients who continue to be at high nutrition risk and who have decreased nutritional intake.[168] A recent systematic review of 94 RCTs (10,284 patients) reported on the evidence for dietary advice with and without the use of ONS in adults with disease-related malnutrition, identifying that in the short-term the use of ONS can improve weight gain in adults although an impact on mortality was not demonstrated.[169] Across the RCTs the size and direction of effect, length of intervention and follow-up was inconsistent, limiting conclusions that can be made. Other novel strategies are being evaluated to address the issue of malnutrition and underfeeding throughout the critical illness recovery trajectory, including complex interventions that incorporate family partnerships.[170,171]

> ### Practice tip
>
> Patients who have been intubated for prolonged periods are at risk for developing dysphagia. Swallowing screening and swallowing assessment might be necessary prior to commencing oral intake. Strategies should be employed to ensure that swallowing assessment is undertaken quickly so nutrition intake is not negatively impacted.

Nutrition in specific clinical conditions

Not all critically ill patients are the same. Age, severity of illness, BMI and specific clinical presentations can each influence nutritional requirements and the nutrition support required. Approaches to nutrition therapy may be similar regardless of clinical presentation, such as the timing and route of feeding and techniques used to monitor nutritional status and tolerance of nutrition. However, every patient should be individually assessed, and nutrition therapy approaches targeted to their specific clinical condition. There are some general recommendations for specific clinical presentations that can serve as a guide for selecting optimal nutrition in some patient groups.

Obesity

As the proportion of the population with obesity increases, so too does the number of obese patients admitted to critical care areas. The key difference for obese patients is the accumulation of body fat. There can also be an increase in muscle mass because of the effort of carrying extra body weight.[172] However, increased muscle mass is not uniformly present in all obese patients and those whose movement is severely restricted, are older or who have chronic illness may have loss of skeletal muscle mass.[173]

Nutrition management for patients with a body mass index ≥ 30 kg/m² is challenging because during critical illness there is a greater risk of insulin resistance and loss of lean body mass, alongside wide variations in macronutrient metabolism.[174] Determining nutrition requirements is also complex. Most predictive equations of energy expenditure are weight based; therefore it is necessary to adjust to ideal body weight to avoid overfeeding, but it should be recognised that most predictive equations underestimate requirements for this patient group.[175] It is important to recognise that, although body weight increases, the energy expenditure does not increase to the same extent.[176] When the BMI is >40 the increase in energy expenditure is only 14%, less than those patients with a BMI <30 or between 30 and 40, where the increase is approximately 25%.

Assessment of the obese critically ill patient should incorporate assessment of central adiposity, metabolic syndrome and sarcopenia.[50] Understanding of how obesity influences energy expenditure can help guide nutrition prescription, though current evidence-based recommendations vary in relation to the composition, energy and protein prescription of nutrition for obese patients[177] and are largely based on expert opinion. Current guidelines recommend the use of indirect calorimetry to guide energy prescription, with one recommending hypocaloric nutrition[50] and another recommending isocaloric nutrition.[41] Predictive equations for determining energy requirements in obese patients is imprecise[178] and nutrition prescriptions should be informed by a comprehensive patient assessment. A high-protein diet is recommended as an important strategy to preserve lean body mass, mobilise adipose stores and minimise metabolic complications of overfeeding,[50] although protein targets differ. Taylor and colleagues[50] recommend 2.0–2.5 g/kg ideal body weight/day whereas Singer and colleagues[41] recommend ⅓ g/kg adjusted body weight/day, but Dickerson[174] highlights that protein prescription should be guided by nitrogen balance where possible. Ongoing assessment of the obese critically ill patient is necessary, with nutrition requirements taking into consideration pre–illness condition, the degree of critical illness and treatment strategies. Monitoring of nutrition therapy is essential in the critically ill obese patient to avoid complications such as hyperglycaemia, dyslipidaemia, hypercapnia, fluid overload and hepatic stenosis.

> ### Practice tip
>
> Obese critically ill patients might have increased GRVs because of increased intra-abdominal pressure, which inhibits gastric emptying.

Sepsis

The incidence of sepsis is on the increase worldwide and, although mortality rates have improved in recent years, these can still be high.[179] Sepsis results in an overwhelming cytokine-mediated, proinflammatory response to the presence of infection and is characterised by widespread inflammation, vasodilation, leukocyte accumulation and increased microvascular permeability.[180]

There is a growing body of literature which specifically addresses the nutritional needs of patients with sepsis; however, evidence is still required to inform clinical decision making regarding nutrition support for these patients. The current Surviving Sepsis guidelines have a nutrition-specific recommendation for the patient with sepsis where early (within 72 hours) initiation of EN is recommended, although this is based on very low quality of evidence.[181] The paucity of research relating to nutrition in sepsis means that current recommendations are based on consensus or low-quality evidence drawn from other clinical trials in which patients with sepsis were included. There are some differences in terms of when EN should commence but agreement that there should be resolution of haemodynamic stability.[40,41,50] In the context of septic shock, intolerance to EN is likely to be high if shock is not controlled, and impaired splanchnic circulation can be aggravated by EN administration because of the increased workload associated with digestion.[41] Where shock is uncontrolled, EN in the first 48 hours after admission has been shown to be less favourable than delayed administration following establishment of haemodynamic stability.[182] Digestive complications were also observed in the early EN group in the NUTRIREA-2 study, suggesting that full feeding during shock be avoided.[46] A clear approach for how nutrition support might be provided is lacking because studies using different methodologies and different patient populations have produced conflicting results. Until further high-quality research is available, decisions on the commencement and progression of nutrition support, particularly EN, should be based on individual patient assessment and clinical judgement.

Renal failure

Critically ill patients with renal failure have widely variable metabolic patterns and nutritional requirements, making decisions about patient-specific nutritional requirements and goals challenging. The optimal nutrition requirements for patients with acute kidney injury are unclear, and assessment of nutritional requirements is complicated not only by fluctuating fluid balance and body weight[183] but also by the underlying disease and type and the intensity of renal replacement therapy.[184] For critically ill patients who require renal replacement therapy, there can be additional loss of glucose, amino acids, proteins, trace elements and vitamins that are water soluble and have a low molecular weight.[184] These losses can be pronounced when highly efficient renal replacement therapy, such as continuous venovenous haemofiltration or prolonged intermittent strategies such as sustained low-efficiency dialysis, is used.

Although each patient requires nutritional assessment and tailored nutritional prescription, it is suggested that a calorie intake of 25–30 kcal/kg/day is required for patients with renal failure, with a protein intake of 1.2–2 g/kg/day[50] or targets similar to other critically ill patients.[185] Protein should not be restricted in patients with renal insufficiency as a means to avoid or delay commencement of dialysis.[50] When patients are receiving haemodialysis or continuous renal replacement therapy, protein can be increased up to 2.5 g/kg/day to achieve a positive nitrogen balance.[186] Using specific formulas for critically ill patients with acute renal failure should be considered on an individual basis.

Pancreatitis

Severe acute pancreatitis is a disease associated with increased morbidity and mortality.[187] It causes both local and systemic complications and results in increased catabolism and hypermetabolism, although the severity of clinical presentations can vary widely.[188]

The European Society of Intensive Care Medicine conditionally recommends early EN in patients with severe acute pancreatitis, while recognising that there is low quality of evidence for this recommendation.[40] The meta-analysis undertaken to support this recommendation identified that early EN reduced infectious complications in patients with severe acute pancreatitis. There was no evidence to support the use of early parenteral nutrition or delayed EN over early EN; however, the evidence quality was recognised as being low.[41] Intragastric delivery of EN is not contraindicated, but there is little evidence comparing the effectiveness of gastric versus jejunal feeding in patients with severe acute pancreatitis, unless there is evidence of gastric outlet obstruction, in which case jejunal feeding should be used.[189] The use of PN in severe acute pancreatitis should be avoided because EN confers greater benefit with a lower mortality rate, shorter duration of hospitalisation, and fewer infectious complications, organ failure or surgical intervention required when EN is used as the nutrition support therapy.[190]

Trauma and surgery

Nutritional recommendations for trauma patients are generally the same as those for all critically ill patients. Guidelines suggest early enteral nutrition can be provided to critically ill adult patients with abdominal trauma, provided that the continuity of the gastrointestinal tract is confirmed/restored,[40] although this recommendation is based on expert opinion and further research in this area is required. Energy and protein targets are similar to that provided for other critically ill patients.[50] Interruptions and underdelivery of prescribed nutrition can be a common problem in patients with traumatic injury. Strategies such as protocolised approaches to nutrition support can help patients reach nutritional adequacy.[11] Nasogastric feeding is suitable for most trauma patients although small bowel feeding might be required for those patients who require longer periods of nutrition support, such as might occur in patients with traumatic brain injury.[11]

Critically ill surgical patients do require special attention because they are at high risk of hospital-acquired malnutrition. Prolonged periods of inadequate oral nutrition are associated with higher mortality and, even for those patients who are well nourished at time of surgery, should they be unable to eat for more than 7 days then nutritional support is indicated.[191]

Postoperative patients may, however, continue to receive little or no nutrition following surgery. Postoperative ileus is often a concern, which means some clinicians do not provide EN. Instead, gastric aspiration is implemented, and the patient is given intravenous fluids. However, studies of gut motility demonstrate that small bowel peristalsis returns within hours following a laparotomy.[121] Therefore, interruption of nutritional intake is not necessary following surgery, even for patients who have undergone gastrointestinal surgery.[50] A meta-analysis of 15 studies that included 1240 patients demonstrated that early postoperative nutrition was associated with significant reductions in complications and there was no evidence of negative outcomes that commonly concern clinicians, including anastomotic dehiscence.[192]

Enteral feeding does not need to be withheld after abdominal or oesophageal surgery, and if the patient is unable to eat orally then EN is the preferred method of feeding unless there is discontinuity or obstruction of the gastrointestinal tract.[41] Parenteral nutrition may be required if there is an unrepaired anastomotic leak, internal or external fistula or if distal feeding accesses cannot be achieved. In the absence of bowel injury, it is also possible to provide EN to the patient with an open abdomen. Additional protein may need to be considered in patients with an open abdomen if there is significant exudate.[50]

Burns

Shortly after injury, severe burns are associated with a high degree of hypermetabolism and hypercatabolism.[193] Burns can also result in destruction of skeletal muscle.[194] The hypermetabolic and hypercatabolic response to severe burn injury can result in significant caloric deficits and weight loss that may lead to immune dysfunction, decreased wound healing, severe infections and death.[195] There are a number of different guidelines to inform nutritional management of the patient with severe burns which differ in content and quality,[196] one of which is specific to burns.[73] As with other nutrition guidelines, there is variability in recommendations, and recommendations are often made on low-quality evidence or expert opinion.

Comprehensive nutritional assessment is important for patients with severe burns[197] and helps to inform nutrition therapy strategies (Table 19.8). Assessing caloric requirements can be challenging and indirect calorimetry is the preferred method of determining REE,[198] but may not be available in all clinical areas. When this equipment is unavailable, there are a range of predictive equations that can be used,[199,200] but each has limitations and some may not be responsive to changes in the patient's clinical condition (Table 19.9).[201]

There are several benefits to early and continuous EN, including a decreased hypermetabolic response; decreased levels of circulating catecholamines, cortisol and glucagon; preservation of gut mucosal blood flow and mucosal integrity; and improved gut motility.[202] Early EN (within 4–6 h of injury) should be provided to patients with burns when oral intake is not possible or is inadequate.[50] PN can be used with EN and/or if oral intake is not possible, as was the case for the majority of patients in a recent

TABLE 19.8

Comprehensive nutrition assessment in the patient with severe burns[197]

HISTORY AND PHYSICAL EXAMINATION	PRE-EXISTING MALNUTRITION
	Malabsorption
	Paralytic ileus
	Severe shock
	Bowel obstruction
	Diffuse peritonitis
Laboratory measurements	Serum albumin and prealbumin
	Nitrogen balance
	Tests for immune function
Clinical examination	Anthropometric measurements
	Fluid intake and output
Metabolic assessment	Indirect calorimetry

TABLE 19.9

Predictive equations for estimating caloric requirements in patients with burns[201]

AGE, YEARS	NAME	FORMULA
0–1	Galveston Infant	2100 kcal/m^2 + 1000 kcal/m^2 burn
1–11	Galveston Revised	1800 kcal/m^2 + 1300 kcal/m^2 burn
12–16	Galveston Adolescent	1500 kcal/m^2 + 1500 kcal/m^2 burn
16–59	Curreri formula	25 kcal/kg body weight + (40) TBSA
	Toronto formula	$-4343 + (10.5 \times TBSA) + (0.23 \times CI) + (0.84 \times HBE) + (114 \times T) - (4.5 \times PBD)$
≥60	Curreri formula	20 kcal/kg body weight + 65 (TBSA)

CI = total calorie intake the previous day; HBE = Harris–Benedict estimates; PBD = number of postburn days to the day preceding the estimation; T = average of core temperatures (°C) the previous day; TBSA = burn size in total body surface area.

Source: Rodriguez NA, Jeschke MG, Williams FN, et al. Nutrition in burns: Galveston contributions. JPEN J Parenter Enteral Nutr 2011;35(6):704–14.

observational study.[203] Protein requirements are similar to that for other critically ill patients and recommendations are for patients with burn injury to receive 1.5–2 g/kg/day of protein.[50]

Coronavirus disease 2019

The ongoing coronavirus disease 2019 (COVID-19) pandemic has stretched hospital systems and ICUs worldwide. While the spectrum of disease is widely variable, approximately 5% of people infected will become critically ill. In such cases, nutrition therapy will often be required. The contagious nature of the severe acute respiratory syndrome coronavirus 2 (SARS-CoV-2) virus means that health professionals need to take extra measures to maintain safety while providing clinical care.[204] The COVID-19 pandemic has resulted in a proliferation of research and discussion papers focusing on clinical management, including in the area of critical care nutrition. This rapid growth in the literature does not necessarily mean that all that is published is of high quality and some basic requirements of good-quality research may have been overlooked, underscoring the need for ongoing quality assessment of research alongside judicial clinical judgement.[205]

There have been several clinical guidelines rapidly developed to guide nutrition practice in patients with COVID-19. Chapple and colleagues[206] in their consensus assessment reviewed 10 ICU nutrition clinical practice guidelines. Similarity between recommendations was noted for the use of high protein, volume-restricted enteral formula delivered gastrically, commenced early and introduced gradually. Specific attention focused on enteral feeding while the patient was in the prone position, and non-intubated patients in the ICU were identified at increased risk of reduced volitional intake. Key areas where differences observed were around the use of indirect calorimetry to guide energy prescription and the use of GRV for monitoring feeding tolerance. Similarities and differences between the various guidelines are summarised in Table 19.10.

> **Practice tip**
>
> Patients being nursed in the prone position can continue to be fed enterally but may experience increased GI intolerance. Ongoing assessment is required so strategies to manage feeding intolerance, such as the use of prokinetics or postpyloric feeding, can be initiated early.

Glycaemic control in critical illness

Hyperglycaemia and increased insulin resistance are characteristics of the body's stress response and activation of the sympathetic, adrenal and hypothalamic–pituitary–adrenal axis responses to critical illness. Hyperglycaemia has been considered a beneficial adaptive response to stress to provide energy substrate to the organs involved in the 'fight or flight' response. In hospitalised patients, hyperglycaemia is associated with increased mortality, although this association is stronger in patients without pre-existing diabetes.[207] Relative hyperglycaemia, which is the acute rise of blood glucose concentration because of stress hyperglycaemia above background levels and assessed by the stress hyperglycaemia ratio, independently predicts in-hospital mortality in critically ill patients across the glycaemic spectrum.[208]

The complexity of the physiological processes associated with hyperglycaemia in critical illness and the sophisticated research required to generate valid information render clinical decision making related to glycaemic control challenging, particularly given that patient response to critical illness and injury will differ. Nevertheless, the concept of glycaemic control is accepted but there are

TABLE 19.10

Summary of content presented in each nutrition guideline for critically ill patients admitted with COVID-19

GUIDELINE OR PRACTICE RECOMMENDATION SOCIETY	NUTRITION RISK SCREENING	NUTRITION REQUIREMENTS/ PRESCRIPTION	TIMING OF INITIATION	ROUTE OF FEEDING	MODE OF FEEDING	FORMULA PRESCRIPTION	MONITORING
ANSISA	✓	✓	✗	✓	✓	✓	✗
ASPEN	✓	✓	✓	✓	✓	✓	✓
AuSPEN	✓	✓	✓	✓	✓	✓	✓
BDA	✗	✗	✗	✓	✓	✓	✓
BRASPEN	✓	✓	✓	✓	✗	✓	✓
ESPEN	✓	✓	✓	✓	✗	✗	✓
IDA	✗	✓	✓	✓	✓	✓	✗
INDI	✓	✗	✓	✓	✓	✓	✓
ATID	✓	✓	✓	✓	✗	✓	✓
TDA	✓	✓	✗	✓	✗	✓	✗

ANSISA = National Association of Specialists in Food Science (Italy); ASPEN = American Society for Parenteral and Enteral Nutrition; ATID = Israeli Dietetic Association; AuSPEN = Australasian Society for Parenteral and Enteral Nutrition; BDA = British Dietetic Association; BRASPEN = Brazilian Society of Parenteral and Enteral Nutrition; ESPEN = European Society for Clinical Nutrition and Metabolism; IDA = Indian Dietetic Association; INDI = Irish Nutrition and Dietetic Institute; TDA = Turkish Dietetic Association.

Source: Chapple LS, Tatucu-Babet OA, Lambell KJ, et al. Nutrition guidelines for critically ill adults with COVID-19: is there consensus? Clin Nutr ESPEN 2021;44:69–77.

variations in the recommended range of acceptable values for glucose levels. The most common recommendation is to target a moderate blood glucose concentration of <180 mg/dL for all critically ill patients, although research to identify targets for specific patient populations continues.[209]

Insulin infusions are used to control high blood glucose levels and nurses have an integral role in the management of these patients. It is recommended that blood glucose values are monitored every 1–2 hours until glucose values and insulin infusion rates are stable, then every 4 hours thereafter.[209] The continuation of insulin infusions in patients who have their EN decreased or ceased requires more-frequent blood glucose monitoring because of the risk of hypoglycaemia.

Strategies to improve glycaemic control in critical illness include the use of protocols and continuous glucose monitoring. In the SPRINT trial, a protocol to support clinicians in achieving tight glycaemic control was evaluated in 371 patients (compared with 413 case-matched controls) and use of the protocol was associated with a mortality reduction.[210]

Validity of blood glucose measurement is also an important consideration. Formal laboratory testing is considered the 'gold standard' for blood glucose measurement but point-of-care testing of blood glucose is common in the critical care setting. Blood glucose may be sampled from arterial, venous and capillary blood. The use of capillary blood in testing blood glucose may be problematic, particularly in those patients for whom hypoperfusion is an issue.[209] It is recommended that point-of-care testing using capillary blood is interpreted with caution because the measurements may not accurately estimate arterial blood or plasma glucose values. Continuous blood glucose monitoring is another alternative that can help reduce hypoglycaemic events.[211] However, their availability in intensive care units worldwide is not widespread.

Further research will be needed to determine the benefit of glycaemic control across a range of specific critical illness presentations and strategies to optimise assessment and management of hyperglycaemia.

Summary

Critically ill patients are at increased risk of malnutrition because of increased metabolic requirements coupled with challenges in delivering prescribed nutrition. Critical care nurses play a pivotal role in ensuring nutritional adequacy and are well positioned to coordinate interdisciplinary collaboration to optimise nutrition therapy. Optimising nutrition in critical illness is assisted by accurate assessment of nutritional requirements and prescribing nutrition that closely matches the patient's individual needs and the various time points throughout their critical illness experience. Delivery of prescribed nutrition is the role of the nurse and attention should be given to minimising interruptions to nutrition therapy and optimising delivery of prescribed nutrition. During recovery from critical illness and when the patient resumes oral intake, nutritional risk can be increased because of factors that impact on the patient's ability to eat. Ongoing nutrition support postextubation and on the ward may be required, through either ongoing EN or use of specialised diets and ONS. Assessment of the ability to safely resume oral intake might be necessary for those patients at risk of dysphagia, and this may require collaboration with a speech language pathologist. Attention to nutritional requirements should commence on admission to the ICU and extend beyond both ICU and hospital discharge.

Case study

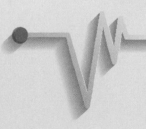

Robert, a 59-year-old builder, was admitted to ICU following a motorbike accident. He sustained multiple injuries including bilateral pneumothoraxes and fracture of the T3 bilateral transverse processes. His admission weight was 88 kg and he was 190 cm tall. His BMI was 24.4.

Robert required intubation and prolonged mechanical ventilation (10 days) and remained in ICU for 2 weeks. Throughout the first week of admission, he was haemodynamically unstable and required noradrenaline (norepinephrine) to support his blood pressure. Glycaemic control with an insulin infusion was required for the first 11 days of his ICU admission.

EN was commenced 10 hours after admission to the ICU with a standard polymeric enteral feeding formula prescribed at 25 kcal/kg/day (1.28 kcal/mL and 6.3 g protein/100 mL) and delivered through a nasogastric tube. Throughout the ICU admission the nutrition prescription remained unchanged. During his ICU admission he had significant interruptions to the delivery of EN on 6 of the 10 days where EN was delivered. Interruption duration ranged from 3 to 14 hours and was mainly related to fasting for radiological and surgical procedures. Despite interruptions, nutrition adequacy ranged from 61% to 116%; delivery of prescribed energy exceeded 100% for each day of days 6–12. On days 1–5, underdelivery was associated with procedural interruptions; overdelivery during ICU admission was associated with increased propofol administration.

Robert was extubated on day 10 of his ICU stay and his nasogastric tube was removed. He remained in ICU for an additional 2 days and was prescribed a standard diet with ONS prescribed three times per day. Mobilising out of bed (sit-to-stand) first occurred on the day of ICU discharge and progressively increased during recovery on the ward. By hospital discharge he was eating 100% of meals (except dessert), was no longer consuming ONS and was able to ambulate independently including using stairs.

DISCUSSION

Critically ill patients often have increased nutritional requirements either as a result of pre-existing malnutrition or because of decreased nutritional intake that is insufficient to meet the increased energy expenditure typical in critical illness or injury. There are a number of key issues relating to nutritional status and the provision of nutrition that are central to this case study. These include trauma-related hypermetabolism, procedural interruptions, hypotension and shock requiring vasopressors.

Hypermetabolism and trauma: Metabolism during critical illness and injury can involve an ebb phase followed by a flow phase[42] However, in a recent prospective observational study of 55 patients admitted to the trauma ICU, heterogeneity in the degree of hypermetabolism was demonstrated.[212] For some time the 'one-size-fits-all' approach to nutrition support in critical illness and injury has been challenged and there has been increasing recognition that not all patients are the same. Several ICU nutrition guidelines recommend the use of indirect calorimetry to determine resting energy expenditure[41,50] and to use this data to guide nutrition prescription. This did not occur for this patient and instead a static equation (25 kcal/kg/day) was used to guide prescription of a standard polymeric formula (aiming for 2200 kcal/day).

Although the use of indirect calorimetry may have been beneficial for this patient, its use was precluded (at least early in the ICU stay) because of persistent bilateral pneumothoraxes, which interfere with measurement accuracy.[213] As these resolved, measuring energy expenditure using indirect calorimetry may have been beneficial because of the inaccuracy of predictive and static equations.[35,36] Without measurement it is difficult to know the patient's true resting energy expenditure and it is possible that the 25 kcal/kg/day may have underestimated requirements. Nevertheless, based on the available data Robert received in excess of his energy target given, it is recommended in the early acute phase to target 70% of estimated or measured energy expenditure and from days 3–7 (the late acute phase) the targets should be at 70% of estimated or 80–100% of measured energy expenditure.[52] Days where energy targets were not met were the days when significant interruptions in enteral feeding occurred. While most studies emphasise the detrimental impact of failing to achieve energy and protein targets, in this case study examples of overfeeding on a daily basis were evident, probably because of ongoing administration of propofol. Overfeeding is associated with increased insulin administration and this may, in part, explain the need for intravenous insulin for blood glucose control.

Surgical intervention: Repeated radiological and surgical interventions were required for ongoing assessment and injury management. As Robert remained intubated and mechanically ventilated, there was no need to discontinue enteral feeding prior to surgery. The repeated discontinuation of EN would have resulted in a significantly lower energy and protein adequacy and this would have a negative impact on long-term recovery. Maintaining lean body mass is critical to improved functional recovery following critical illness and patients for whom nutrition is optimised are more likely to be discharged home following hospitalisation.

Vasopressors: Hypotension and the use of vasopressors can reduce splanchnic perfusion and is sometimes perceived as a contraindication to EN. Enteral nutrients have been shown to increase gut blood flow, which allows the bowel to absorb nutrients during vasopressor therapy. There is insufficient evidence to suggest whether EN should continue or be withheld when vasopressors are being administered, with the results from a limited number of studies being inconsistent.[38] Individual patient assessment is required to guide clinical practice in this area. In this case study, EN was commenced despite vasopressor therapy and the patient did not exhibit any signs of gastric intolerance.

CASE STUDY QUESTIONS

1　What strategies can be used to ensure delivery of prescribed nutrition?
2　What considerations should be given to undertaking indirect calorimetry in a patient with chest injuries? Identify what assessments should be undertaken to ensure that performing this assessment is appropriate and likely to result in accurate measurement.
3　In the transition from EN to oral nutrition, what strategies could be used to ensure optimal nutrition intake during recovery?

RESEARCH VIGNETTE

McNelly AS, Bear DE, Connolly BA, et al. Effect of intermittent or continuous feed on muscle wasting in critical illness: a phase 2 clinical trial. Chest 2020;158(1):183–94.

Abstract

Background: Acute skeletal muscle wasting in critical illness is associated with excess morbidity and mortality. Continuous feeding may suppress muscle protein synthesis as a result of the muscle-full effect, unlike intermittent feeding, which may ameliorate it.

Research question: Does intermittent enteral feed decrease muscle wasting compared with continuous feed in critically ill patients?

Study design and methods: In a phase 2 interventional single-blinded RCT, 121 mechanically ventilated adult patients with multiorgan failure were recruited following prospective informed consultee assent. They were randomised to the intervention group (intermittent enteral feeding from six 4-hourly feeds per 24 h, $n = 62$) or control group (standard continuous enteral feeding, $n = 59$). The primary outcome was 10-day loss of rectus femoris muscle cross-sectional area determined by ultrasound. Secondary outcomes included nutritional target achievements, plasma amino acid concentrations, glycaemic control and physical function milestones.

Results: Muscle loss was similar between arms (-1.1% (95% CI, -6.1% to -4.0%); $P = 0.676$). More intermittently fed patients received 80% or more of target protein (odds ratio (OR) 1.52 (1.16–1.99); $P = 0.001$) and energy (OR 1.59 (1.21–2.08); $P = 0.001$). Plasma branched-chain amino acid concentrations before and after feeds were similar between arms on trial day 1 (71 micrometres (44–98 micrometres); $P = 0.547$) and trial day 10 (239 micrometres (33–444 micrometres); $P = 0.178$). During the 10-day intervention period, the coefficient of variation for glucose concentrations was higher with intermittent feed (17.84 (18.6–20.4)) versus continuous feed (12.98 (14.0–15.7); $P < 0.001$). However, days with reported hypoglycaemia and insulin usage were similar in both groups. Safety profiles, gastric intolerance, physical function milestones and discharge destinations did not differ between groups.

Interpretation: Intermittent feeding in early critical illness is not shown to preserve muscle mass in this trial despite resulting in a greater achievement of nutritional targets than continuous feeding. However, it is feasible and safe.

Trial registry: ClinicalTrials.gov; No.: NCT02358512; URL: https://www.clinicaltrials.gov.

Critique

Providing adequate nutrition during critical illness has been associated with improved patient outcomes,[214] although the impact on mortality has been difficult to demonstrate in high-quality RCTs. Ongoing research in nutrition in critical illness continues to address key issues for which additional evidence is needed, with priority areas identified for both paediatric[215] and adult[13] critically ill patients. For critical care nursing, attention is directed to the best strategies to support the delivery of prescribed EN. More than two decades ago the debate over continuous versus intermittent delivery of nutrition focused on issues of gastrointestinal tolerance,[216] aspiration,[217] changes to gastric pH[218] and increased glucose variability.[219] In this article by McNelly and colleagues,[220] the authors posit that continuous EN may suppress and intermittent EN may support muscle protein synthesis, with the primary outcome measure being the rectus femoris muscle cross area (RF_{CSA}), an outcome measure that is more likely to be influenced by a nutrition intervention than mortality, which has commonly been used in previous studies.[221]

The focus on muscle wasting is important because of the potential for this to impact functional recovery following critical illness. To address this question, the authors undertook an unblinded, phase 2 clinical trial in eight mixed ICUs in the United Kingdom, the multicentre design being a strength of this study. The inclusion criteria were set so that the patients most likely to benefit from nutrition support were identified, an important consideration when evaluation nutrition interventions.[51] Included were adult patients who: would be ventilated for more than 2 days, require EN via a nasogastric tube, demonstrated multiorgan failure, were expected to stay in ICU for more than 1 week and who were anticipated to survive for 10 or more days. Nutrition prescription was determined by the ICU dietitian, using predictive equations, the inaccuracy of which has been recognised in the literature.[36] After screening 3487 patients, 127 patients were randomised and allocated to either six 4-hourly feeds delivered over 3–5 minutes ($n = 62$) or continuous EN ($n = 59$). The sample size was based on an assumed reduction RF_{CSA} of 21.5% ($n = 58$) and the sample size doubled to account for dropout due to early death, recovery or protocol violation. This is an important consideration given that it is difficult to identify patients who are likely to remain in the study until day 10 and this could have a substantial impact on the study size if this sample size adjustment was not made. Of the 116 patients enrolled in the study, 63 (49%) had data available on day 10 of the study, underscoring the importance of the sample size adjustment. No difference in RF_{CSA} was observed between the intermittent and continuous groups (-1.1% (95% CI -6.1 to -4.0); $P = 0.676$). Adjusting for confounding factors including age, chronic disease, admission bicarbonate and PaO_2/FiO_2 ratio) did not change these results. Concentrations of plasma amino acids were not higher in the group fed intermittently, which may explain why an impact on physical function and health-related quality of life outcomes was not observed. Furthermore, the role of nutrition alone in maintaining muscle mass and function has been discussed in the literature, noting that nutrition in combination with exercise may be more beneficial.[222,223]

In RCTs, blinding to treatment allocation is designed to minimise bias. However, interventions such as this cannot be blinded to those delivering the intervention. However, the person performing the assessment of RF_{CSA} was blinded to treatment allocation, so minimising any risk of bias. One of the challenges in undertaking nutrition research in these groups is the difficulty in predicting length of stay. In this study the median duration of EN delivery was only 4 days (range 0–10 days) and this was observed in both groups. Consequently, the short duration of EN delivery may have been insufficient to impact the RF_{CSA}. Nutritional delivery was higher in the intermittently fed group than the continuously fed group for both protein (80.3% (95% CI, 77.3–83.4%) vs 69.9% (95% CI, 66.6–73.1%); $P < 0.001$) and energy (82.4% (95% CI, 79.2–85.6%) vs 72.5% (95% CI, 69.3–75.7%); $P < 0.001$). Interruptions to EN are a major contributing factor to inadequate nutrition delivery.[224] However, the number of interruptions were similar in both groups. What is not clear is whether compensation was made for interrupted continuous feeds to try to deliver the 24-hour goal volume. Similarly, interrupted intermittent feeding could have been delivered at a later time within the 24-hour period, contributing to improved nutritional intakes. Differences in nutritional delivery may perhaps not be observed if avoidable interruptions during continuous enteral feeding are minimised.

The implication of this research for nursing practice is significant. Perceptions regarding the safety of intermittent feeding were not substantiated in this study. Concerns with intermittent feeding include feeding intolerance and the potential for pulmonary aspiration.[217] However, in this study there were no observed differences in vomiting, use of prokinetics, gastric residual volumes >300 mL or diarrhoea. More glycaemic variability was observed in the patient group fed intermittently, which may require greater vigilance with monitoring of blood glucose and adjustment of insulin, if required. This would have an important impact on nursing workload, as was demonstrated in the NICE-SUGAR study.[225] For patients in the intermittent feeding group, nutrition was delivered by syringe bolus over 3–5 minutes; whether this was done manually is unclear and could have implications for nursing workload. In addition, more-frequent disconnection can potentially increase bacterial contamination,[226] and the associated undesired consequences of this.

More research in nutrition in critical illness is needed to fill important gaps. This study has extended what we know about the role that intermittent nutrition might play in the preservation of muscle mass in critically ill patients. Interdisciplinary collaboration in studies such as this can create opportunity to address aspects of enteral feeding practice of high relevance to nursing practice.

Learning activities

1   Review your patients' notes and calculate what their total daily caloric intake was for the previous day. Once you have obtained this figure, compare this with the prescribed intake. If patients have not received their total daily caloric intake, consider what factors may have contributed to this and how these might be overcome in future.

2   Review the notes of two medical and two elective surgical patients admitted to your ICU. Which patients demonstrated some evidence of pre-existing nutrition risk?

3   Should critically ill patients who have had gastrointestinal surgery not receive EN postoperatively?

4   Your patient has been in ICU for the past 14 days and is now ready to be discharged to the ward. During the patient's ICU stay there has been progressive loss of lean body mass. In handover to the nurses on the ward, what key points would you make to ensure that nutrition optimisation is a priority on the ward?

5   On admission to the ICU, a nasogastric tube is placed and its position confirmed on X-ray. Enteral feeding is subsequently commenced. What strategies do you take to ensure safe feeding throughout the patient's ICU stay?

6   During the initial admission period to ICU, your patient was not tolerating EN well. GRVs were high and the patient's gut was distended. PN has been the nutrition support strategy used for this patient and today the decision was made to re-introduce EN. How will you manage this transition from PN to EN?

Online resources

American Society for Parenteral and Enteral Nutrition (ASPEN), https://www.nutritioncare.org

Australasian Society for Parenteral and Enteral Nutrition (AuSPEN), https://www.auspen.org.au

British Dietetic Association (BDA), https://www.bda.uk.com

Critical Care Nutrition, https://www.criticalcarenutrition.com

European Society for Clinical Nutrition and Metabolism (ESPEN), https://www.espen.org

Further reading

Ayers P, Bobo ES, Hunt RT, et al, editors. ASPEN parenteral nutrition handbook. Silver Spring, MD: American Society for Parenteral and Enteral Nutrition; 2020.

Berger MM. Critical care nutrition therapy for non-nutritionists. New York: Springer; 2017.

Corkins MR, editor. The ASPEN pediatric nutrition support core curriculum. 2nd ed. Silver Spring, MD: American Society for Parenteral and Enteral Nutrition; 2015.

Farber P, Siervo M. Nutrition in critical care. Cambridge: Cambridge University Press; 2014.

Malone A, Nieman Carney L, Long Carrera A, et al. ASPEN enteral nutrition handbook. 2nd ed. Silver Spring, MD: American Society for Parenteral and Enteral Nutrition; 2019.

Rajendram R, Preedy VR, Patel VB, editors. Diet and nutrition in critical care. New York: Springer; 2020.

Seres DS, Van Way CW III, editors. Nutrition support for the critically ill. Champaign, IL: Humana Press; 2016.

References

1.   Batt J, Herridge M, Dos Santos C. Mechanism of ICU-acquired weakness: skeletal muscle loss in critical illness. Intensive Care Med 2017;43(12):1844–6.

2.   Schlenker ED. Proteins. In: Schlenker ED, Gilbert J, editors. Williams' essentials of nutrition and diet therapy. 12th ed. St Louis, MO: Mosby Elsevier; 2019, p. 68–83.

3.   McCance KL. Cellular biology. In: McCance KL, Huether S, editors. Pathophysiology. 8th ed. St Louis, MO: Mosby Elsevier; 2019, p. 1–46.

4.   Moonen H, Beckers KJH, van Zanten ARH. Energy expenditure and indirect calorimetry in critical illness and convalescence: current evidence and practical considerations. J Intensive Care 2021;9(1):8.

5. Sharma K, Mogensen KM, Robinson MK. Pathophysiology of critical illness and role of nutrition. Nutr Clin Pract 2019;34(1):12–22.

6. Preiser J-C, Ichai C, Orban J-C, et al. Metabolic response to the stress of critical illness. Br J Anaesth 2014;113(6):945–54.

7. Hudson L, Chittams J, Griffith C, et al. Malnutrition identified by Academy of Nutrition and Dietetics/American Society for parenteral and enteral nutrition is associated with more 30-day readmissions, greater hospital mortality, and longer hospital stays: a retrospective analysis of nutrition assessment data in a major medical center. JPEN J Parenter Enteral Nutr 2018;42(5):892–7.

8. Lew CCH, Yandell R, Fraser RJL, et al. Association between malnutrition and clinical outcomes in the intensive care unit: a systematic review [Formula: see text]. JPEN J Parenter Enteral Nutr 2017;41(5):744–58.

9. Mogensen KM, Horkan CM, Purtle SW, et al. Malnutrition, critical illness survivors, and postdischarge outcomes: a cohort study. JPEN J Parenter Enteral Nutr 2018;42(3):557–65.

10. Schuetz P, Seres D, Lobo DN, et al. Management of disease-related malnutrition for patients being treated in hospital. Lancet 2021;398(10314):1927–38.

11. McCartt J, Loszko A, Backes K, et al. Improving enteral nutrition delivery in the critically ill trauma and surgical population. JPEN J Parenter Enteral Nutr 2022;46(5):1191–7.

12. McClave SA, Taylor BE, Martindale RG, et al. Guidelines for the provision and assessment of nutrition support therapy in the adult critically ill patient: Society of Critical Care Medicine (SCCM) and American Society for Parenteral and Enteral Nutrition (A.S.P.E.N.). JPEN J Parenter Enteral Nutr 2016;40(2):159–211.

13. Arabi YM, Casaer MP, Chapman M, et al. The intensive care medicine research agenda in nutrition and metabolism. Intensive Care Med 2017;43(9):1239–56.

14. Correia M. Nutrition screening vs nutrition assessment: what's the difference? Nutr Clin Pract 2018;33(1):62–72.

15. Compher C, Chittams J, Sammarco T, et al. Greater protein and energy intake may be associated with improved mortality in higher risk critically ill patients: a multicenter, multinational observational study. Crit Care Med 2017;45(2):156–63.

16. Reber E, Gomes F, Vasiloglou MF, et al. Nutritional risk screening and assessment. J Clin Med 2019;8(7):1065.

17. Kondrup J, Rasmussen HH, Hamberg O, et al. Nutritional risk screening (NRS 2002): a new method based on an analysis of controlled clinical trials. Clin Nutr 2003;22(3):321–36.

18. de Vries MC, Koekkoek WK, Opdam MH, et al. Nutritional assessment of critically ill patients: validation of the modified NUTRIC score. Eur J Clin Nutr 2018;72(3):428–35.

19. Lee ZY, Heyland DK. Determination of nutrition risk and status in critically ill patients: what are our considerations? Nutr Clin Pract 2019;34(1):96–111.

20. Heyland DK, Dhaliwal R, Jiang X, et al. Identifying critically ill patients who benefit the most from nutrition therapy: the development and initial validation of a novel risk assessment tool. Crit Care 2011;15(6):R268.

21. Kalaiselvan MS, Renuka MK, Arunkumar AS. Use of nutrition risk in critically ill (NUTRIC) score to assess nutritional risk in mechanically ventilated patients: a prospective observational study. Indian J Crit Care Med 2017;21(5):253–6.

22. Moisey LL, Mourtzakis M, Kozar RA, et al. Existing equations to estimate lean body mass are not accurate in the critically ill: results of a multicenter observational study. Clin Nutr 2017;36(6):1701–6.

23. Price KL, Earthman CP. Update on body composition tools in clinical settings: computed tomography, ultrasound, and bioimpedance applications for assessment and monitoring. Eur J Clin Nutr 2019;73(2):187–93.

24. Moonen H, Van Zanten ARH. Bioelectric impedance analysis for body composition measurement and other potential clinical applications in critical illness. Curr Opin Crit Care 2021;27(4):344–53.

25. Lambell KJ, Tierney AC, Wang JC, et al. Comparison of ultrasound-derived muscle thickness with computed tomography muscle cross-sectional area on admission to the intensive care unit: a pilot cross-sectional study. JPEN J Parenter Enteral Nutr 2021;45(1):136–45.

26. Tatucu-Babet OA, Fetterplace K, Lambell K, et al. Is energy delivery guided by indirect calorimetry associated with improved clinical outcomes in critically ill patients? A systematic review and meta-analysis. Nutr Metab Insights 2020;13:1178638820903295.

27. Singer P, De Waele E, Sanchez C, et al. TICACOS international: a multi-center, randomized, prospective controlled study comparing tight calorie control versus liberal calorie administration study. Clin Nutr 2021;40(2):380–7.

28. Allingstrup MJ, Kondrup J, Perner A, et al. Indirect calorimetry in mechanically ventilated patients: a prospective, randomized, clinical validation of 2 devices against a gold standard. JPEN J Parenter Enteral Nutr 2017;41(8):1272–7.

29. De Waele E, Jonckheer J, Wischmeyer PE. Indirect calorimetry in critical illness: a new standard of care? Curr Opin Crit Care 2021;27(4):334–43.

30. Wischmeyer PE, Molinger J, Haines K. Point-counterpoint: indirect calorimetry is essential for optimal nutrition therapy in the intensive care unit. Nutr Clin Pract 2021;36(2):275–81.

31. McClave SA, Omer E. Point-counterpoint: indirect calorimetry is not necessary for optimal nutrition therapy in critical illness. Nutr Clin Pract 2021;36(2):268–74.

32. Schlein KM, Coulter SP. Best practices for determining resting energy expenditure in critically ill adults. Nutr Clin Pract 2014;29(1):44–55.

33. Walker RN, Heuberger RA. Predictive equations for energy needs for the critically ill. Respir Care 2009;54(4):509–21.

34. Bendavid I, Lobo DN, Barazzoni R, et al. The centenary of the Harris–Benedict equations: how to assess energy requirements best? Recommendations from the ESPEN expert group. Clin Nutr 2021;40(3):690–701.

35. Zusman O, Kagan I, Bendavid I, et al. Predictive equations versus measured energy expenditure by indirect calorimetry: a retrospective validation. Clin Nutr 2019;38(3):1206–10.

36. Tatucu-Babet OA, Ridley EJ, Tierney AC. Prevalence of underprescription or overprescription of energy needs in critically ill mechanically ventilated adults as determined by indirect calorimetry: a systematic literature review. JPEN J Parenter Enteral Nutr 2016;40(2):212–25.

37. Schorghuber M, Fruhwald S. Effects of enteral nutrition on gastrointestinal function in patients who are critically ill. Lancet Gastroenterol Hepatol 2018;3(4):281–7.

38. Wischmeyer PE. Enteral nutrition can be given to patients on vasopressors. Crit Care Med 2020;48(1):122–5.

39. Elke G, Hartl WH, Kreymann KG, et al. Clinical nutrition in critical care medicine - guideline of the German Society for Nutritional Medicine (DGEM). Clin Nutr ESPEN 2019;33:220–75.

40. Reintam Blaser A, Starkopf J, Alhazzani W, et al. Early enteral nutrition in critically ill patients: ESICM clinical practice guidelines. Intensive Care Med 2017;43(3):380–98.

41. Singer P, Blaser AR, Berger MM, et al. ESPEN guideline on clinical nutrition in the intensive care unit. Clin Nutr 2019;38(1):48–79.

42. van Zanten ARH, De Waele E, Wischmeyer PE. Nutrition therapy and critical illness: practical guidance for the ICU, post-ICU, and long-term convalescence phases. Crit Care 2019;23(1):1–10.

43. Krezalek MA, Yeh A, Alverdy JC, et al. Influence of nutrition therapy on the intestinal microbiome. Curr Opin Clin Nutr Metab Care 2017;20(2):131–7.

44. Pu H, Doig GS, Heighes PT, et al. Early enteral nutrition reduces mortality and improves other key outcomes in patients with major burn injury: a meta-analysis of randomized controlled trials. Crit Care Med 2018;46(12):2036–42.

45. Target Investigators for the ANZICS Clinical Trials Group; Chapman M, Peake SL, Bellomo R et al. Energy-dense versus routine enteral nutrition in the critically ill. N Engl J Med 2018;379(19):1823–34.

46. Reignier J, Boisrame-Helms J, Brisard L, et al. Enteral versus parenteral early nutrition in ventilated adults with shock: a randomised, controlled, multicentre, open-label, parallel-group study (NUTRIREA-2). Lancet 2018;391(10116):133–43.

47. Reintam Blaser A, Hiesmayr M. Enteral feeding, even when the gut does not feel very good? Curr Opin Clin Nutr Metab Care 2022;25:122–8.

48. Otani S, Coopersmith CM. Gut integrity in critical illness. J Intensive Care 2019;7:17.

49. Shukla A, Chapman M, Patel JJ. Enteral nutrition in circulatory shock: friend or foe? Curr Opin Clin Nutr Metab Care 2021;24(2):159–64.

50. Taylor BE, McClave SA, Martindale RG, et al. Guidelines for the provision and assessment of nutrition support therapy in the adult critically ill patient: Society of Critical Care Medicine (SCCM) and American Society for Parenteral and Enteral Nutrition (A.S.P.E.N.). Crit Care Med 2016;44(2):390–438.

51. Patel JJ, Martindale RG, McClave SA. Controversies surrounding critical care nutrition: an appraisal of permissive underfeeding, protein, and outcomes. JPEN J Parenter Enteral Nutr 2018;42(3):508–15.

52. Lambell KJ, Tatucu-Babet OA, Chapple LA, et al. Nutrition therapy in critical illness: a review of the literature for clinicians. Crit Care 2020;24(1):35.

53. Bendavid I, Zusman O, Kagan I, et al. Early administration of protein in critically ill patients: a retrospective cohort study. Nutrients 2019;11(1):106.

54. National Heart Lung, and Blood Institute Acute Respiratory Distress Syndrome (ARDS) Clinical Trials Network; Rice TW, Wheeler AP, Thompson BT, et al. Initial trophic vs full enteral feeding in patients with acute lung injury: the EDEN randomized trial. JAMA 2012;307(8):795–803.

55. Casaer MP, Mesotten D, Hermans G, et al. Early versus late parenteral nutrition in critically ill adults. N Engl J Med 2011;365(6):506–17.

56. Arabi YM, Aldawood AS, Haddad SH, et al. Permissive underfeeding or standard enteral feeding in critically ill adults. N Engl J Med 2015;372(25):2398–408.

57. Puthucheary ZA, Rawal J, McPhail M, et al. Acute skeletal muscle wasting in critical illness. JAMA 2013;310(15):1591–600.

58. Weijs PJM, Mogensen KM, Rawn JD, et al. Protein intake, nutritional status and outcomes in ICU survivors: a single center cohort study. J Clin Med 2019;8(1):43.

59. Mitchell A, Clemente R, Downer C, et al. Protein provision in critically ill adults requiring enteral nutrition: are guidelines being met? Nutr Clin Pract 2019;34(1):123–30.

60. Nicolo M, Heyland DK, Chittams J, et al. Clinical outcomes related to protein delivery in a critically ill population: a multicenter, multinational observation study. JPEN J Parenter Enteral Nutr 2016;40(1):45–51.

61. Preiser JC, Arabi YM, Berger MM, et al. A guide to enteral nutrition in intensive care units: 10 expert tips for the daily practice. Crit Care 2021;25(1):424.

62. Salciute-Simene E, Stasiunaitis R, Ambrasas E, et al. Impact of enteral nutrition interruptions on underfeeding in intensive care unit. Clin Nutr 2021;40(3):1310–17.

63. Heyland DK, Dhaliwal R, Wang M, et al. The prevalence of iatrogenic underfeeding in the nutritionally 'at-risk' critically ill patient: results of an international, multicenter, prospective study. Clin Nutr 2015;34(4):659–66.

64. Hoffmann M, Schwarz CM, Furst S, et al. Risks in management of enteral nutrition in intensive care units: a literature review and narrative synthesis. Nutrients 2020;13(1):82.

65. Segaran E, Lovejoy TD, Proctor C, et al. Exploring fasting practices for critical care patients – a web-based survey of UK intensive care units. J Intensive Care Soc 2018;19(3):188–95.

66. Kim H, Chang SJ. Implementing an educational program to improve critical care nurses' enteral nutritional support. Aust Crit Care 2019;32(3):218–22.

67. Huang J, Yang L, Zhuang Y, et al. Current status and influencing factors of barriers to enteral feeding of critically ill patients: a multicenter study. J Clin Nurs 2019;28(3–4):677–85.

68. Lapchmanan LM, Kee CM, Majid HBA, et al. Medical nutrition therapy; guidelines for critically ill adults. 2nd ed. Bulit Jalil, Kuala Lumpur: Persatuan Dietitian Malaysia; 2017.

69. Mesejo A, Vaquerizo Alonso C, Acosta Escribano J, et al. Guidelines for specialized nutritional and metabolic support in the critically-ill patient: update. Consensus SEMICYUC-SENPE: introduction and methodology. Nutr Hosp 2011;26(Suppl. 2):1–6.

70. Heyland DK, Dhaliwal R, Drover JW, et al,; Canadian Critical Care Clinical Practice Guidelines Committee. Canadian clinical practice guidelines for nutrition support in mechanically ventilated, critically ill adult patients. JPEN J Parenter Enteral Nutr 2003;27(5):355–73.

71. Heyland DK, Dhaliwal R, Patel J, et al. Systematic reviews 2021. Kingston, Ontario: Critical Care Nutrition; 2021. Available from: https://criticalcarenutrition.com/ccn-systematic-review. [Accessed 20 February 2023].

72. Compher C, Bingham AL, McCall M, et al. Guidelines for the provision of nutrition support therapy in the adult critically ill patient: the American Society for Parenteral and Enteral Nutrition. JPEN J Parenter Enteral Nutr 2022;46(1):12–41.

73. Rousseau AF, Losser MR, Ichai C, et al. ESPEN endorsed recommendations: nutritional therapy in major burns. Clin Nutr 2013;32(4):497–502.

74. Mehta Y, Mithal A, Kulkarni A, et al. Practice guidelines for enteral nutrition management in dysglycemic critically ill patients: a relook for Indian scenario. Indian J Crit Care Med 2019;23(12):594–603.

75. Prest PJ, Justice J, Bell N, et al. A volume-based feeding protocol improves nutrient delivery and glycemic control in a surgical trauma intensive care unit. JPEN J Parenter Enteral Nutr 2020;44(5):880–8.

76. Sachdev G, Backes K, Thomas BW, Si et al. Volume-based protocol improves delivery of enteral nutrition in critically ill trauma patients. JPEN J Parenter Enteral Nutr 2020;44(5):874–9.

77. Jiang L, Huang X, Wu C, et al. The effects of an enteral nutrition feeding protocol on critically ill patients: a prospective multi-center, before-after study. J Crit Care 2020;56:249–56.

78. Orinovsky I, Raizman E. Improvement of nutritional intake in intensive care unit patients via a nurse-led enteral nutrition feeding protocol. Crit Care Nurse 2018;38(3):38–44.

79. Marshall AP, Cahill NE, Gramlich L, et al. Optimizing nutrition in intensive care units: empowering critical care nurses to be effective agents of change. Am J Crit Care 2012;21(3):186–94.

80. Kozeniecki M, Pitts H, Patel JJ. Barriers and solutions to delivery of intensive care unit nutrition therapy. Nutr Clin Pract 2018;33(1):8–15.

81. Alkhawaja S, Martin C, Butler RJ, et al. Post-pyloric versus gastric tube feeding for preventing pneumonia and improving nutritional outcomes in critically ill adults. Cochrane Database Syst Rev 2015;2015(8):CD008875.

82. Liu Y, Wang Y, Zhang B, et al. Gastric-tube versus post-pyloric feeding in critical patients: a systematic review and meta-analysis of pulmonary aspiration-and nutrition-related outcomes. Eur J Clin Nutr 2021;75(9):1337–48.

83. Bond A, Czapran A, Lal S. Small bowel feeding: do you pay the price for bypassing the stomach? Curr Opin Clin Nutr Metab Care 2022;25(2):116–21.

84. Metheny NA, Krieger MM, Healey F, et al. A review of guidelines to distinguish between gastric and pulmonary placement of nasogastric tubes. Heart Lung 2019;48(3):226–35.

85. Miller KR, McClave SA, Kiraly LN, et al. A tutorial on enteral access in adult patients in the hospitalized setting. JPEN J Parenter Enteral Nutr 2014;38(3):282–95.

86. Blumenstein I, Shastri YM, Stein J. Gastroenteric tube feeding: techniques, problems and solutions. World J Gastroenterol 2014;20(26):8505–24.

87. Metheny NA, Stewart BJ, Mills AC. Blind insertion of feeding tubes in intensive care units: a national survey. Am J Crit Care 2012;21(5):352–60.

88. Berger MM, Reintam-Blaser A, Calder PC, et al. Monitoring nutrition in the ICU. Clin Nutr 2019;38(2):584–93.

89. Perlas A, Arzola C, Van de Putte P. Point-of-care gastric ultrasound and aspiration risk assessment: a narrative review. Can J Anaesth 2018;65(4):437–48.

90. Rowat AM, Graham C, Dennis M. Study to determine the likely accuracy of pH testing to confirm nasogastric tube placement. BMJ Open Gastroenterol 2018;5(1):e000211.

91. Heidarzadi E, Jalali R, Hemmatpoor B, et al. The comparison of capnography and epigastric auscultation to assess the accuracy of nasogastric tube placement in intensive care unit patients. BMC Gastroenterol 2020;20(1):196.

92. Kindopp AS, Drover JW, Heyland DK. Capnography confirms correct feeding tube placement in intensive care unit patients. Can J Anaesth 2001;48(7):705–10.

93. Brotfain E, Erblat A, Luft P, et al. Nurse-performed ultrasound assessment of gastric residual volume and enteral nasogastric tube placement in the general intensive care unit. Intensive Crit Care Nurs 2022;69:103183.

94. Powers J, Brown B, Lyman B, et al. Development of a competency model for placement and verification of nasogastric and nasoenteric feeding tubes for adult hospitalized patients. Nutr Clin Pract 2021;36(3):517–33.

95. Bourgault AM, Powers J, Aguirre L, et al. National survey of feeding tube verification practices: an urgent call for auscultation deimplementation. Dimens Crit Care Nurs 2020;39(6):329–38.

96. Bourgault AM, Upvall MJ, Nicastro S, et al. Challenges of de-implementing feeding tube auscultation: a qualitative study. Int J Nurs Pract 2022;28(2):e13026.

97. O'Connell F, Ong J, Donelan C, et al. Emergency department approach to gastric tube complications and review of the literature. Am J Emerg Med 2021;39:259.e5–7.

98. Powers J, Luebbehusen M, Aguirre L, et al. Improved safety and efficacy of small-bore feeding tube confirmation using an electromagnetic placement device. Nutr Clin Pract 2018;33(2):268–73.

99. Woon C. On track to the stomach!! Cortrak for the insertion of nasogastric tubes amongst neuroscience patients – how effective is it? Australas J Neurosci 2020;30(2):13–18.

100. Thong D, Halim Z, Chia J, et al. A systematic review and meta-analysis of the effectiveness of continuous versus intermittent enteral nutrition in critically ill adults. JPEN J Parenter Enteral Nutr 2022;46(6):1243–57.

101. Ma Y, Cheng J, Liu L, et al. Intermittent versus continuous enteral nutrition on feeding intolerance in critically ill adults: a meta-analysis of randomized controlled trials. Int J Nurs Stud 2021;113:103783.

102. De Lazzaro F, Alessandri F, Tarsitano MG, et al. Safety and efficacy of continuous or intermittent enteral nutrition in ICU patients: systematic review of clinical evidence. JPEN J Parenter Enteral Nutr 2022;46(3):486–98.

103. Stechmiller JK, Treloar D, Allen N. Gut dysfunction in critically ill patients: a review of the literature. Am J Crit Care 1997;6(3):204–9.

104. Nguyen T, Frenette AJ, Johanson C, et al. Impaired gastrointestinal transit and its associated morbidity in the intensive care unit. J Crit Care 2013;28(4):537.e11–17.

105. Deane AM, Ali Abdelhamid Y, Plummer MP, et al. Are classic bedside exam findings required to initiate enteral nutrition in critically ill patients: emphasis on bowel sounds and abdominal distension. Nutr Clin Pract 2021;36(1):67–75.

106. Sharma K, Mogensen KM, Robinson MK. Pathophysiology of critical illness and role of nutrition. Nutr Clin Pract 2019;34(1):12–22.

107. Wischmeyer PE. Overcoming challenges to enteral nutrition delivery in critical care. Curr Opin Crit Care 2021;27(2):169–76.

108. Reintam Blaser A, Preiser J-C, Fruhwald S, et al. Gastrointestinal dysfunction in the critically ill: a systematic scoping review and research agenda proposed by the Section of Metabolism, Endocrinology and Nutrition of the European Society of Intensive Care Medicine. Crit Care 2020;24(1):1–17.

109. Reintam Blaser A, van Zanten ARH. Electrolye disorders during the initiation of nutrition therapy in the ICU. Curr Opin Clin Nutr Metab Care 2021;24:151–8.

110. Yebenes JC, Campins L, Martinez de Lagran I, et al. Nutritrauma: a key concept for minimising the harmful effects of the administration of medical nutrition therapy. Nutrients 2019;11(8):1775.

111. Wang K, McIlroy K, Plank LD, et al. Prevalence, outcomes, and management of enteral tube feeding intolerance: a retrospective cohort study in a tertiary center. JPEN J Parenter Enteral Nutr 2017;41(6):959–67.

112. Blaser AR, Starkopf J, Kirsimagi U, et al. Definition, prevalence, and outcome of feeding intolerance in intensive care: a systematic review and meta-analysis. Acta Anaesthesiol Scand 2014;58(8):914–22.

113. Gimenes FRE, Baracioli F, Medeiros AP, et al. Factors associated with mechanical device-related complications in tube fed patients: a multicenter prospective cohort study. PLoS One 2020;15(11):e0241849.

114. Yasuda H, Kondo N, Yamamoto R, et al. Monitoring of gastric residual volume during enteral nutrition. Cochrane Database Syst Rev 2021;9:CD013335.

115. Elke G, Felbinger TW, Heyland DK. Gastric residual volume in critically ill patients: a dead marker or still alive? Nutr Clin Pract 2015;30(1):59–71.

116. Gungabissoon U, Hacquoil K, Bains C, et al. Prevalence, risk factors, clinical consequences, and treatment of enteral feed intolerance during critical illness. JPEN J Parenter Enteral Nutr 2015;39(4):441–8.

117. Reintam Blaser A, Deane AM, Preiser JC, et al. Enteral feeding intolerance: updates in definitions and pathophysiology. Nutr Clin Pract 2021;36(1):40–9.

118. Wang Z, Ding W, Fang Q, et al. Effects of not monitoring gastric residual volume in intensive care patients: a meta-analysis. Int J Nurs Stud 2019;91:86–93.

119. Reignier J, Mercier E, Le Gouge A, et al. Effect of not monitoring residual gastric volume on risk of ventilator-associated pneumonia in adults receiving mechanical ventilation and early enteral feeding: a randomized controlled trial. JAMA 2013;309(3):249–56.

120. Lew CCH, Lee Z-Y, Day AG, et al. Correlation between gastric residual volumes and markers of gastric emptying: a post hoc analysis of a randomized clinical trial. J Parent Enter Nutr 2022;46(4):850–7.

121. Marik PE. Enteral nutrition in the critically ill: myths and misconceptions. Crit Care Med 2014;42(4):962–9.

122. Juve-Udina ME, Valls-Miro C, Carreno-Granero A, et al. To return or to discard? Randomised trial on gastric residual volume management. Intensive Crit Care Nurs 2009;25(5):258–67.

123. Brotfain E, Erblat A, Luft P, et al. Nurse-performed ultrasound assessment of gastric residual volume and enteral nasogastric tube placement in the general intensive care unit. Intensive Crit Care Nurs 2022;69:103183.

124. Wen Z, Xie A, Peng M, et al. Is discard better than return gastric residual aspirates: a systematic review and meta-analysis. BMC Gastroenterol 2019;19(1):113.

125. Tatsumi H. Enteral tolerance in critically ill patients. J Intensive Care 2019;7:30.

126. Ladopoulos T, Giannaki M, Alexopoulou C, et al. Gastrointestinal dysmotility in critically ill patients. Ann Gastroenterol 2018;31(3):273–81.

127. Lewis K, Alqahtani Z, McIntyre L, et al. The efficacy and safety of prokinetic agents in critically ill patients receiving enteral nutrition: a systematic review and meta-analysis of randomized trials. Crit Care 2016;20(1):259.

120. Arabi YM, Reintam Blaser A, Preiser J-C, When and how to manage enteral feeding intolerance? Intensive Care Med 2019;45:1029–31.

129. Hill NE, Murphy KG, Singer M. Ghrelin, appetite and critical illness. Curr Opin Crit Care 2012;18(2):199–205.

130. Deane AM, Chapman MJ, Reintam Blaser A, et al. Pathophysiology and treatment of gastrointestinal motility disorders in the acutely ill. Nutr Clin Pract 2019;34(1):23–36.

131. Heyland DK, van Zanten ARH, Grau-Carmona T, et al. A multicenter, randomized, double-blind study of ulimorelin and metoclopramide in the treatment of critically ill patients with enteral feeding intolerance: PROMOTE trial. Intensive Care Med 2019;45(5):647–56.

132. Hay T, Bellomo R, Rechnitzer T, et al. Constipation, diarrhea, and prophylactic laxative bowel regimens in the critically ill: a systematic review and meta-analysis. J Crit Care 2019;52:242–50.

133. Dionne JC, Sullivan K, Mbuagbaw L, et al. Diarrhoea: interventions, consequences and epidemiology in the intensive care unit (DICE-ICU): a protocol for a prospective multicentre cohort study. BMJ Open 2019;9(6):e028237.

134. Reintam Blaser A, Deane AM, Fruhwald S. Diarrhoea in the critically ill. Curr Opin Crit Care 2015;21(2):142–53.

135. Sinha S, Lath G, Rao S. Safety of enteral nutrition practices: overcoming the contamination challenges. Indian J Crit Care Med 2020;24(8):709–12.

136. Boullata JI, Carrera AL, Harvey L, et al. ASPEN safe practices for enteral nutrition therapy [Formula: see text]. JPEN J Parenter Enteral Nutr 2017;41(1):15–103.

137. McClave SA, Lukan JK, Stefater JA, et al. Poor validity of residual volumes as a marker for risk of aspiration in critically ill patients. Crit Care Med 2005;33(2):324–30.

138. Nseir S, Le Gouge A, Lascarrou JB, et al. Impact of nutrition route on microaspiration in critically ill patients with shock: a planned ancillary study of the NUTRIREA-2 trial. Crit Care 2019;23(1):111.

139. McClave SA, DeMeo MT, DeLegge MH, et al. North American summit on aspiration in the critically ill patient: consensus statement. JPEN J Parenter Enteral Nutr 2002;26(6 Suppl.):S80–5.

140. Alvarez-Lerma F, Sanchez Garcia M; Task Force of Experts for Project "Zero VAP" in Spain. "The multimodal approach for ventilator-associated pneumonia prevention" – requirements for nationwide implementation. Ann Transl Med 2018;6(21):420.

141. Darawad MW, Sa'aleek MA, Shawashi T. Evidence-based guidelines for prevention of ventilator-associated pneumonia: evaluation of intensive care unit nurses' adherence. Am J Infect Control 2018;46(6):711–13.

142. Fetterplace K, Holt D, Udy A, et al. Parenteral nutrition in adults during acute illness: a clinical perspective for clinicians. Intern Med J 2020;50(4):403–11.

143. Harvey SE, Parrott F, Harrison DA, et al. Trial of the route of early nutritional support in critically ill adults. N Engl J Med 2014;371(18):1673–84.

144. Doig GS, Simpson F, Sweetman EA, et al. Early parenteral nutrition in critically ill patients with short-term relative contraindications to early enteral nutrition: a randomized controlled trial. JAMA 2013;309(20):2130–8.

145. Ridley EJ. Parenteral nutrition in critical illness: total, supplemental or never? Curr Opin Clin Nutr Metab Care 2021;24(2):176–82.

146. Heidegger CP, Berger MM, Graf S, et al. Optimisation of energy provision with supplemental parenteral nutrition in critically ill patients: a randomised controlled clinical trial. Lancet 2013;381(9864):385–93.

147. Casaer MP, Ziegler TR. Nutritional support in critical illness and recovery. Lancet Diabetes Endocrinol 2015;3(9):734–45.

148. Hellerman Itzhaki M, Singer P. Advances in medical nutrition therapy: parenteral nutrition. Nutrients 2020;12(3):717.

149. Bohl CJ, Parks A. A mnemonic for pharmacists to ensure optimal monitoring and safety of total parenteral nutrition: I AM FULL. Ann Pharmacother 2017;51(7):603–13.

150. Strachan S. Trace elements. Curr Anaesth Crit Care 2010;21(1):44–8.

151. Blanchette LM, Huiras P, Papadopoulos S. Standardized versus custom parenteral nutrition: impact on clinical and cost-related outcomes. Am J Health Syst Pharm 2014;71(2):114–21.

152. Gavin NC, Button E, Keogh S, et al. Does parenteral nutrition increase the risk of catheter-related bloodstream infection? A systematic literature review. JPEN J Parenter Enteral Nutr 2017;41(6):918–28.

153. Gavin NC, Button E, Castillo MI, et al. Does a dedicated lumen for parenteral nutrition administration reduce the risk of catheter-related blood stream infections? A systematic literature review. J Infus Nurs 2018;41(2):122–30.

154. Sugrue D, Jarrell AS, Kruer R, et al. Appropriateness of peripheral parenteral nutrition use in adult patients at an academic medical center. Clin Nutr ESPEN 2018;23:117–21.

155. Brodsky MB, Nollet JL, Spronk PE, et al. Prevalence, pathophysiology, diagnostic modalities, and treatment options for dysphagia in critically ill patients. Am J Phys Med Rehabil 2020;99(12):1164–70.

156. McIntyre M, Doeltgen S, Dalton N, et al. Post-extubation dysphagia incidence in critically ill patients: a systematic review and meta-analysis. Aust Crit Care 2021;34(1):67–75.

157. Brodsky MB, Levy MJ, Jedlanek E, et al. Laryngeal injury and upper airway symptoms after oral endotracheal intubation with mechanical ventilation during critical care: a systematic review. Crit Care Med 2018;46(12):2010–17.

158. Zuercher P, Moret CS, Dziewas R, et al. Dysphagia in the intensive care unit: epidemiology, mechanisms, and clinical management. Crit Care 2019;23(1):103.

159. Perren A, Zurcher P, Schefold JC. Clinical approaches to assess post-extubation dysphagia (PED) in the critically ill. Dysphagia 2019;34(4):475–86.

160. McIntyre M, Chimunda T, Koppa M, et al. Risk factors for postextubation dysphagia: a systematic review and meta-analysis. Laryngoscope 2022;132(2):364–74.

161. Brodsky MB, Huang M, Shanholtz C, et al. Recovery from dysphagia symptoms after oral endotracheal intubation in acute respiratory distress syndrome survivors. a 5-year longitudinal study. Ann Am Thorac Soc 2017;14(3):376–83.

162. Daly E, Miles A, Scott S, et al. Finding the red flags: swallowing difficulties after cardiac surgery in patients with prolonged intubation. J Crit Care 2016;31(1):119–24.

163. Petersen SJ, Tsai AA, Scala CM, et al. Adequacy of oral intake in critically ill patients 1 week after extubation. J Am Diet Assoc 2010;110(3):427–33.

164. Ridley EJ, Parke RL, Davies AR, et al. What happens to nutrition intake in the post–intensive care unit hospitalization period? An observational cohort study in critically ill adults. JPEN J Parenter Enteral Nutr 2019;43(1):88–95.

165. Chapple LS, Deane AM, Heyland DK, et al. Energy and protein deficits throughout hospitalization in patients admitted with a traumatic brain injury. Clin Nutr 2016;35(6):1315–22.

166. Moisey LL, Pikul J, Keller H, et al. Adequacy of protein and energy intake in critically ill adults following liberation from mechanical ventilation is dependent on route of nutrition delivery. Nutr Clin Pract 2021;36(1):201–12.

167. Rougier L, Preiser JC, Fadeur M, et al. Nutrition during critical care: an audit on actual energy and protein intakes. JPEN J Parenter Enteral Nutr 2021;45(5):951–60.

168. Ridley EJ, Chapple LS, Chapman MJ. Nutrition intake in the post-ICU hospitalization period. Curr Opin Clin Nutr Metab Care 2020;23(2):111–15.

169. Baldwin C, de van der Schueren MA, Kruizenga HM, et al. Dietary advice with or without oral nutritional supplements for disease-related malnutrition in adults. Cochrane Database Syst Rev 2021;12:CD002008.

170. Marshall AP, Lemieux M, Dhaliwal R, et al. Novel, family-centered intervention to improve nutrition in patients recovering from critical illness: a feasibility study. Nutr Clin Pract 2017;32(3):392–9.

171. Marshall AP, Wake E, Weisbrodt L, et al. A multi-faceted, family-centred nutrition intervention to optimise nutrition intake of critically ill patients: the OPTICS feasibility study. Aust Crit Care 2016;29(2):68–76.

172. Dickerson RN, Patel JJ, McClain CJ. Protein and calorie requirements associated with the presence of obesity. Nutr Clin Pract 2017;32(1 Suppl.):86S-93S.

173. Gallagher D, DeLegge M. Body composition (sarcopenia) in obese patients: implications for care in the intensive care unit. JPEN J Parenter Enteral Nutr 2011;35(5 Suppl.):21S-8S.

174. Dickerson RN. Metabolic support challenges with obesity during critical illness. Nutrition 2019;57:24–31.

175. Frankenfield DC, Ashcraft CM, Galvan DA. Prediction of resting metabolic rate in critically ill patients at the extremes of body mass index. JPEN J Parenter Enteral Nutr 2013;37(3):361–7.

176. Frankenfield DC. Obesity. In: Singer P, editor. Nutrition in intensive care medicine: beyond physiology. Basel, Switzerland: Karger; 2013, p. 144–53.

177. Al-Dorzi HM, Stapleton RD, Arabi YM. Nutrition priorities in obese critically ill patients. Curr Opin Clin Nutr Metab Care 2022;25(2):99–109.

178. Schetz M, De Jong A, Deane AM, et al. Obesity in the critically ill: a narrative review. Intensive Care Med 2019;45(6):757–69.

179. Luhr R, Cao Y, Soderquist B, et al. Trends in sepsis mortality over time in randomised sepsis trials: a systematic literature review and meta-analysis of mortality in the control arm, 2002–2016. Crit Care 2019;23(1):241.

180. Gyawali B, Ramakrishna K, Dhamoon AS. Sepsis: the evolution in definition, pathophysiology, and management. SAGE Open Med 2019;7:2050312119835043.

181. Evans L, Rhodes A, Alhazzani W, et al. Surviving sepsis campaign: international guidelines for management of sepsis and septic shock 2021. Intensive Care Med 2021;47(11):1181–247.

182. Khalid I, Doshi P, DiGiovine B. Early enteral nutrition and outcomes of critically ill patients treated with vasopressors and mechanical ventilation. Am J Crit Care 2010;19(3):261–8.

183. Fiaccadori E, Sabatino A, Barazzoni R, et al. ESPEN guideline on clinical nutrition in hospitalized patients with acute or chronic kidney disease. Clin Nutr 2021;40(4):1644–68.

184. Nystrom EM, Nei AM. Metabolic support of the patient on continuous renal replacement therapy. Nutr Clin Pract 2018;33(6):754–66.

185. Ronco C, Bellomo R, Kellum JA. Acute kidney injury. Lancet 2019;394(10212):1949–64.

186. Scheinkestel CD, Kar L, Marshall K, et al. Prospective randomized trial to assess caloric and protein needs of critically ill, anuric, ventilated patients requiring continuous renal replacement therapy. Nutrition 2003;19(11–12):909–16.

187. Yasuda H, Horibe M, Sanui M, et al. Etiology and mortality in severe acute pancreatitis: a multicenter study in Japan. Pancreatology 2020;20(3):307–17.

188. Lee PJ, Papachristou GI. New insights into acute pancreatitis. Nature Rev Gastroenterol Hepatol 2019;16:479–96.

189. Lee PJ, Papachristou GI. Management of severe acute pancreatitis. Curr Treat Options Gastroenterol 2020;18(4):670–81.

190. Li W, Liu J, Zhao S, Li J. Safety and efficacy of total parenteral nutrition versus total enteral nutrition for patients with severe acute pancreatitis: a meta-analysis. J Int Med Res 2018;46(9):3948–58.

191. Weinmann A. The surgical/trauma patient. In: Singer P, editor. Nutrition in intensive care medicine. Basel: Karger; 2013. p. 106–15.

192. Osland E, Yunus RM, Khan S, et al. Early versus traditional postoperative feeding in patients undergoing resectional gastrointestinal surgery: a meta-analysis. JPEN J Parenter Enteral Nutr 2011;35(4):473–87.

193. Guo F, Zhou H, Wu J, et al. Prospective study on energy expenditure in patients with severe burns. JPEN J Parenter Enteral Nutr 2021;45(1):146–51.

194. Klein GL. Disruption of bone and skeletal muscle in severe burns. Bone Res 2015;3:15002.

195. Lang TC, Zhao R, Kim A, et al. A critical update of the assessment and acute management of patients with severe burns. Adv Wound Care (New Rochelle) 2019;8(12):607–33.

196. Grammatikopoulou MG, Theodoridis X, Gkiouras K, et al. AGREEing on guidelines for nutrition management of adult severe burn patients. JPEN J Parenter Enteral Nutr 2019;43(4):490–6.

197. Carson JS, Khosrozadeh H, Norbury WB, et al. Nutritional needs and support for the burned patient. In: Herndon DN, Jones JH, editors. Total burn care. 5th ed. Philadelphia: Elsevier; 2018, p. 287–300.

198. Wise AK, Hromatka KA, Miller KR. Energy expenditure and protein requirements following burn injury. Nutr Clin Pract 2019;34(5):673–80.

199. Jeon J, Kym D, Cho YS, et al. Reliability of resting energy expenditure in major burns: comparison between measured and predictive equations. Clin Nutr 2019;38(6):2763–9.

200. Leung J, Ridley EJ, Cleland H, et al. Predictive energy equations are inaccurate for determining energy expenditure in adult burn injury: a retrospective observational study. ANZ J Surg 2019;89(5):578–83.

201. Rodriguez NA, Jeschke MG, Williams FN, et al. Nutrition in burns: Galveston contributions. JPEN J Parenter Enteral Nutr 2011;35(6):704–14.

202. Chen Z, Wang S, Yu B, et al. A comparison study between early enteral nutrition and parenteral nutrition in severe burn patients. Burns 2007;33(6):708–12.

203. Guo F, Zhou H, Wu J, et al. A prospective observation on nutrition support in adult patients with severe burns. Br J Nutr 2019;121(9):974–81.

204. Patel JJ, Martindale RG, McClave SA. Relevant nutrition therapy in COVID-19 and the constraints on its delivery by a unique disease process. Nutr Clin Pract 2020;35(5):792–9.

205. Correia M. Nutrition in times of Covid-19, how to trust the deluge of scientific information. Curr Opin Clin Nutr Metab Care 2020;23(4):288–93.

206. Chapple LS, Tatucu-Babet OA, Lambell KJ, et al. Nutrition guidelines for critically ill adults admitted with COVID-19: is there consensus? Clin Nutr ESPEN 2021;44:69–77.

207. Baker EH, Janaway CH, Philips BJ, et al. Hyperglycaemia is associated with poor outcomes in patients admitted to hospital with acute exacerbations of chronic obstructive pulmonary disease. Thorax 2006;61(4):284–9.

208. Lee TF, Drake SM, Roberts GW, et al. Relative hyperglycemia is an independent determinant of in-hospital mortality in patients with critical illness. Crit Care Med 2020;48(2):e115–22.

209. Stoudt K, Chawla S. Don't sugar coat it: glycemic control in the intensive care unit. J Intensive Care Med 2019;34(11–12):889–96.

210. Chase JG, Shaw G, Le Compte A, et al. Implementation and evaluation of the SPRINT protocol for tight glycaemic control in critically ill patients: a clinical practice change. Crit Care 2008;12(2):R49.

211. Holzinger U, Warszawska J, Kitzberger R, et al. Real-time continuous glucose monitoring in critically ill patients: a prospective randomized trial. Diabetes Care 2010;33(3):467–72.

212. Byerly S, Vasileiou G, Qian S, et al. Early hypermetabolism is uncommon in trauma intensive care unit patients. JPEN J Parenter Enteral Nutr 2022;46(4):771–81.

213. De Waele E, van Zanten ARH. Routine use of indirect calorimetry in critically ill patients: pros and cons. Crit Care 2022;26(1):123.

214. Zusman O, Theilla M, Cohen J, et al. Resting energy expenditure, calorie and protein consumption in critically ill patients: a retrospective cohort study. Crit Care 2016;20(1):367.

215. Tume LN, Valla FV, Floh AA, et al. Priorities for nutrition research in pediatric critical care. JPEN J Parenter Enteral Nutr 2019;43(7):853–62.

216. Ma Y, Cheng J, Liu L, et al. Intermittent versus continuous enteral nutrition on feeding intolerance in critically ill adults: a meta-analysis of randomized controlled trials. Int J Nurs Stud 2021;113:103783.

217. MacLeod JB, Lefton J, Houghton D, et al. Prospective randomized control trial of intermittent versus continuous gastric feeds for critically ill trauma patients. J Trauma 2007;63(1):57–61.

218. Gowardman J, Sleigh J, Barnes N, et al. Intermittent enteral nutrition – a comparative study examining the effect on gastric pH and microbial colonization rates. Anaesth Intensive Care 2003;31(1):28–33.

219. Bear DE, Hart N, Puthucheary Z. Continuous or intermittent feeding: pros and cons. Curr Opin Crit Care 2018;24(4):256–61.

220. McNelly AS, Bear DE, Connolly BA, et al. Effect of intermittent or continuous feed on muscle wasting in critical illness: a phase 2 clinical trial. Chest 2020;158(1):183–94.

221. Chapple LS, Ridley EJ, Chapman MJ. Trial design in critical care nutrition: the past, present and future. Nutrients 2020;12(12):3694.

222. Heyland DK, Day A, Clarke GJ, et al. Nutrition and Exercise in Critical Illness Trial (NEXIS Trial): a protocol of a multicentred, randomised controlled trial of combined cycle ergometry and amino acid supplementation commenced early during critical illness. BMJ Open 2019;9(7):e027893.

223. Heyland DK, Stapleton RD, Mourtzakis M, et al. Combining nutrition and exercise to optimize survival and recovery from critical illness: conceptual and methodological issues. Clin Nutr 2016;35(5):1196–206.

224. Peev MP, Yeh DD, Quraishi SA, et al. Causes and consequences of interrupted enteral nutrition: a prospective observational study in critically ill surgical patients. JPEN J Parenter Enteral Nutr 2015;39(1):21–7.

225. Bellomo R, Egi M. Glycemic control in the intensive care unit: why we should wait for NICE-SUGAR. Mayo Clin Proc 2005;80(12):1546–8.

226. Best C. Enteral tube feeding and infection control: how safe is our practice? Br J Nurs 2008;17(16):1036, 1038–41.

Gastrointestinal, metabolic and liver alterations

Andrea Marshall

Learning objectives

After reading this chapter, you should be able to:

- describe the changes in gastrointestinal physiology and metabolism associated with critical illness
- identify patients at risk for the development of stress ulcers and rationalise therapeutic interventions for their prevention
- identify patients at risk for the development of intra-abdominal hypertension and abdominal compartment syndrome and suggest management strategies to decrease intra-abdominal pressure
- describe the physiological changes that occur during diabetic ketoacidosis and rationalise assessment and treatment strategies
- discuss the effects of critical illness on hepatic function and evaluate the consequences of liver dysfunction
- describe the treatment of liver failure, including liver support therapies and transplantation.

Introduction

During episodes of critical illness, patients often experience disturbance in their metabolic and/or endocrine function. In the previous chapter, the changes to metabolism that occur during critical illness and the role of the gastrointestinal system in nutrition were outlined. The gastrointestinal system is also involved in many other important functions including immunity and protection.

Effective gastrointestinal function requires an adequate blood supply to ensure that oxygen and nutrients are available at the cellular level. However, in critical illness the splanchnic circulation may be compromised without overt signs being evident. This alteration in regional blood flow and tissue oxygen delivery can compromise normal metabolic and endocrine function.

In this chapter the effect of gastrointestinal physiology on critical illness is covered. Gastrointestinal dysfunction, including the development of stress-related mucosal diseases and of increased intra-abdominal pressure, is discussed. A major component of this chapter is dedicated to organ-specific gastrointestinal compromise including liver dysfunction, liver transplantation, alcoholic liver disease and pancreatitis. An overview of the assessment and management of diabetic ketoacidosis is also provided.

Gastrointestinal physiology

As described in Chapter 19, digestion and absorption of nutrients such as carbohydrates, amino acids, minerals and water are key functions of the gastrointestinal system. Other important roles of the gastrointestinal tract are immunity[1] and maintenance of the gut microbiome.[2]

Gastrointestinal dysfunction can occur in up to 60% of patients in the ICU.[3] The spectrum of gastrointestinal dysfunction is wide, with mild signs and symptoms represented as nausea, abdominal distention, reduced motility and/or ileus, which may contribute to malnutrition due to reduced nutritional delivery. More serious alterations in gastrointestinal function include breaches in mucosal integrity, increased intra–abdominal pressure, changes to the gut microbiome and impaired mesenteric perfusion. The relationship between the underlying mechanisms, the clinical effects, life-threatening conditions and clinical outcomes is detailed in Fig. 20.1.[4]

There are a number of different mechanisms by which the gastrointestinal system protects against the movement of substances (other than nutrients, water and electrolytes) into the systemic circulation and these are outlined in Table 20.1.[5–11]

Alterations to normal gastrointestinal physiology in critical illness

During critical illness, there are a number of alterations that can occur to gastrointestinal physiology. The intestinal epithelium consists of one layer of cells separating the gut lumen from the rest of the body. These cells are responsible for nutrient absorption, and important immune functions including a barrier to pathogens, secreting hormones, cytokines and antimicrobial peptides.[9] During critical illness, changes to gut epithelium, the immune system and gut microbiome may occur. Although nutrient absorption may be altered,[12,13] most critically ill patients appear to be able to tolerate enteral nutrition, making the clinical significance of impaired absorption unclear. Alterations in the defence mechanisms of the gastrointestinal tract may also occur and contribute to the development of multiple organ dysfunction in critical illness.[4] The changes to gut

---

FIGURE 20.1 Gastrointestinal dysfunction in critical illness.

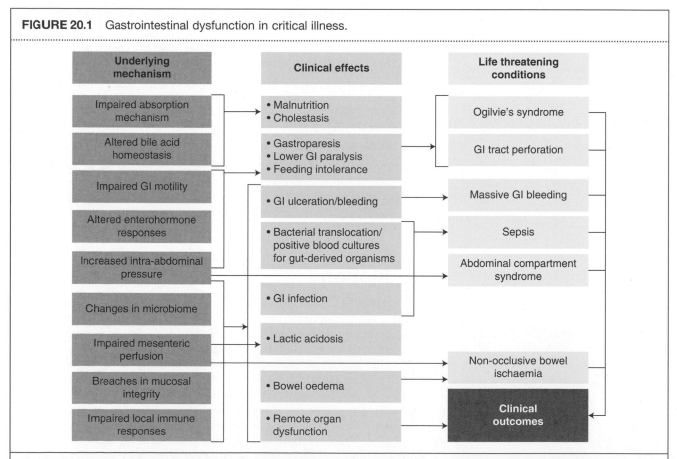

Source: Reintam Blaser A, Preiser J-C, Fruhwald S, et al. Gastrointestinal dysfunction in the critically ill: a systematic scoping review and research agenda proposed by the Section of Metabolism, Endocrinology and Nutrition of the European Society of Intensive Care Medicine. Crit Care 2020;24(1):1–17. (Licensed under Creative Commons Attribution 4.0.)

TABLE 20.1

Protective mechanisms of the gastrointestinal system and impacts of critical illness

MECHANISM	ACTION
Motility	Propels bacteria through the GI tract. In critical illness, motility may be altered because of enteric nerve impairment and altered smooth muscle function, inflammation (mediated by cytokines and nitric oxide), gut injury, hypoperfusion, medications (opioids, dopamine), electrolyte disturbances, hyperglycaemia, sepsis and increased intracranial pressure.[5]
Hydrochloric acid secretion	Contributes to gastric acidity and destroys bacteria. Parietal cells in the stomach produce hydrochloric acid and keep the intragastric environment relatively acidic (pH approx. 4.0). An acidic pH has bactericidal and bacteriostatic properties,[6] limiting overgrowth in the stomach.
Bicarbonate	Bicarbonate ions bind with hydrogen ions to form water and carbon dioxide, preventing the hydrogen ions (acid) from damaging the duodenal wall.[7]
Bile salts	Bile salts provide protection against bacteria by breaking down the liposaccharide portion of endotoxins, thereby detoxifying gram-negative bacteria in the gastrointestinal tract. The deconjugation of bile salts into secondary bile acids inhibits the proliferation of pathogens and may destroy their cell walls.[11]
Mucin production	Prevents the adhesion of bacteria to the wall of the GI tract. Mucous cells secrete large quantities of very thick, alkaline mucus (approximately 1 mm thick in the stomach). Glycoproteins present in the mucus prevent bacteria from adhering to and colonising the mucosal wall.[8]
Epithelial cell shedding	Limits bacterial adhesion. The mucosal lining of the entire gastrointestinal tract is composed of epithelial cells that create a physical barrier to bacterial invasion. These cells are replaced approximately every 3–5 days,[8] limiting bacterial colonisation.
Zona occludens (tight junctions surrounding each cell in the epithelial sheet)	The junctions between epithelial cells provide a barrier to microorganisms. Intermediate junctions (zonula adherens) function primarily in cell–cell adhesion, while the tight junctions (zonula occludens) limit the movement of bacteria and toxins across the gut wall.[9]
Gut-associated lymphoid tissue	Protection against bacterial invasion is provided by gut-associated lymphoid tissue, capable of cell-mediated and humoral-mediated immune responses.[9]
Kupffer cells	Kupffer cells in the liver and spleen provide a back-up defence against pathogens that cross the barrier of the gastrointestinal wall and enter the systemic circulation.[10]

function in critical illness are complex and there are probably many factors contributing to the development of gut dysfunction.

Gut permeability can change as a result of critical illness. Aetiological factors which may increase gut permeability include splanchnic hypoperfusion, decreased gastrointestinal motility and hypoxia.[14] Intestinal epithelial cells undergo accelerated programmed cell death, the tight junctions between epithelial cells are compromised and as a result microbes can permeate the barrier that is the intestinal wall.[9] Thinning of the mucus layer of the intestinal tract can also occur as a result of critical illness.[1] A thinner mucus layer can lead to autodigestion and destruction of the intestinal epithelium, which may allow pancreatic enzymes to enter intestinal lymphatic channels and this may result in tissue injury and multiple organ failure.[15]

More recently, significant attention has been focused on the gut microbiome and how changes in intestinal homeostasis can contribute to worsening clinical outcomes. While our understanding of the role of the gut microbiome is evolving, it is recognised that the microbial ecosystems of the gut changes substantially in critical illness. A healthy gut microbiome contributes to immune homeostasis, nutrient absorption and gut integrity. However, in critical illness the microbiota is disrupted and these changes can be caused by non-modifiable factors such as the patient's microenvironment, age and genetics. Smoking and alcohol consumption are also contributing factors that can contribute to changes after critical illness or injury.[2] Management of critical illness can also influence the gut microbiome. Pharmacological agents, such as antibiotics, opioids and proton pump inhibitors,[1] and nutritional support through enteral or parenteral nutrition, can also disrupt the 1000 different microbial species in the gut microbiome.[2] Physiological changes in critical illness together with treatment strategies may contribute to imbalance in the introduction, elimination and

TABLE 20.2

Ecological effects of critical illness on the gastrointestinal microbiome

PATHOPHYSIOLOGICAL PROCESSES	MICROBIAL IMMIGRATION	MICROBIAL ELIMINATION	ENVIRONMENTAL GROWTH CONDITIONS
Decreased oral intake	Decreased immigration of food-associated microbiota.[16]	No direct effect.	Shift to stress conditions of nutrient scarcity and altered nutritional substrate.[16]
Altered oropharyngeal microbiota	Increased immigration of Proteobacteria and potential pathogens.[17]	No direct effect.	No direct effect.
Intestinal dysmotility	No direct effect.	Decreased elimination, increased upper gastrointestinal community burden.	No direct effect.
Systemic hyperglycaemia and electrolyte disturbances	No direct effect.	Decreased elimination (intestinal dysmotility).[13]	No direct effect.
Gut hypoperfusion, reperfusion injury, impaired mucosal integrity	No direct effect.	Increased elimination via translocation to mesenteric lymphatics.[18]	Increased mucosal inflammation, increased free radical concentrations and nitrate availability,[20] shift from commensal anaerobes to Proteobacteria and select Firmicutes.[21]
Decreased bile salt concentration	No direct effect.	Decreased elimination of bile-sensitive species.[11]	Selective overgrowth of bile-sensitive species.[11]
Endogenous opioid production	No direct effect.	Decreased elimination (intestinal dysmotility).	Selective increase in virulence of opioid-responsive species,[22] disruption of stabilising commensal relationships.[23]
Endogenous catecholamine and inflammatory cytokine production	No direct effect.	Decreased elimination (intestinal dysmotility).[19]	Selective promotion of growth and virulence of potential pathogens,[18] increased mucosal inflammation via splanchnic hypoperfusion, decreased oxygen tension and pH.
Disruption of intestinal mucus layer	No direct effect.	Increased elimination via translocation to mesenteric lymphatics.[9]	Altered nutrient supply, altered oxygen gradients,[24] loss of mucus reservoir of antibacterial peptides.[25]
Impaired mucosal immunity: decreased IgA and defensing production	No direct effect.	Decreased elimination of potential pathogens, increased elimination via translocation to mesenteric lymphatics.[14]	Loss of growth inhibition for potential pathogens, decreased abundance of commensal Bacteroidetes.[26]

Source: Adapted from Dickson RP. The microbiome and critical illness. Lancet 2016;4:59–72.

reproduction of microbes and this may contribute to changes in the gut microbiome (Table 20.2).[9,11,13,14,16–26]

Stress-related mucosal damage

The reported incidence of stress-related mucosal damage is variable and complicated by variable definitions and difficulty in measurement of endpoints, and the heterogeneity of patient populations.[27] It is estimated that the majority of critically ill patients will develop evidence of stress-related mucosal erosion and subepithelial haemorrhage on endoscopy.[28] Occult abnormalities have been observed in approximately one-third of critically ill patients on mechanical ventilation; the most common of these are gastritis and mucosal erosion from the nasogastric tube.[29] Gastrointestinal bleeding occurs in 2–5% of patients[30] and is associated with worse patient outcomes.[31] The incidence of clinically significant bleeding – that is, bleeding associated with hypotension, tachycardia and a drop in haemoglobin level necessitating transfusion – is estimated to be 1% and 6%.[32] Over time the incidence of stress-related mucosal damage has continued to decrease and this is largely attributed to overall advances and improvements in the management of critically ill patients.[33] Aggressive fluid resuscitation, improved ventilatory management, which minimises increased lung pressures, and preferential use of enteral nutrition have probably all contributed to a reduced incidence of stress-related mucosal disease in the critically ill.[34]

Factors influencing the development of stress-related mucosal damage include splanchnic hypoperfusion, which may influence mucosal ischaemia and reperfusion injury.[35] The mucus–bicarbonate gel layer[24] and decreased prostaglandin levels, which impair mucus replenishment, and increased nitric oxide synthase contribute to reperfusion injury and cell death.[9] The protective mechanisms and factors that promote injury are detailed in Table 20.3.[6,9,11,36–40]

A number of risk factors are associated with the development of stress-related mucosal damage. These

---

TABLE 20.3

Factors contributing to stress-related mucosal disease

FACTORS	MECHANISM	ACTION
Protective mechanisms	Mucosal prostaglandins	Protect the mucosa by stimulating blood flow, mucus and bicarbonate production.[9] Stimulate epithelial cell growth and repair.
	Mucosal bicarbonate barrier	Forms a physical barrier to acid and pepsin, preventing injury to the epithelium.[6]
	Epithelial restitution and regeneration	Epithelial cells rapidly regenerate but the process is highly metabolic and may be impaired by physiological stress.[9]
	Mucosal blood flow	Mucosal blood flow helps remove acid from the mucosa, and supplies bicarbonate and oxygen to the mucosal epithelial cells.[36]
	Cell membrane and tight junctions	Tight junctions between mucosal epithelial cells prevent the back diffusion of hydrogen ions.[9]
Factors promoting injury	Acid	Gastric acid secretion may be a contributing factor to the development of stress-related mucosal injury, although gut ischaemia as a consequence of hypotension, use of vasoconstrictors or inflammatory mediators are also contributing factors.[37]
	Pepsin	May cause direct injury to the mucosa.[38]
	Mucosal hypoperfusion	Reduced mucosal blood flow results in reduced oxygen and nutrient delivery, making epithelial cells susceptible to injury.[39] Contributes to mucosal acid–base imbalances.
	Reperfusion injury	Nitric oxide, which causes vasodilation and hyperaemia, is released during hypoperfusion and results in an increase in cell-damaging cytokines.[40]
	Intramucosal acid–base balance	The mucus layer protects the epithelium and traps bicarbonate ions that neutralise acid, hence a decrease in bicarbonate secretion results in intramucosal acidosis and local injury.[6]
	Systemic acidosis	Results in increased intramucosal acidity.
	Free oxygen radicals	Generated as a result of tissue hypoxia, free oxygen radicals cause oxidative injury to the mucosa.[39]
	Bile salts	Bile salts reflux from the duodenum into the stomach and may have a role in stress-related damage, although the exact mechanism is uncertain.[11]
	Helicobacter pylori	Conflicting results exist about the role of *H. pylori* as a cause of stress-induced mucosal disease in the critically ill.[37]

Source: Reproduced from Marshall AP. The gut in critical illness. In: Carlson K, editor. AACN Advanced critical care nursing. Philadelphia: Elsevier; 2009, Table 29-3, with permission.

include, but are not limited to: shock where vasopressors or inotropes are required to maintain blood pressure, a need for intermittent or continuous renal replacement therapy, mechanical ventilation for more than 24 hours, acute coagulopathy, a history of coagulopathy within the previous 6 months, treatment with an anticoagulant and a history of chronic liver disease.[27,41]

Preventing stress-related mucosal damage

Prophylaxis for stress-related mucosal damage is often part of the care of the critically ill, although evidence demonstrating an added benefit when this therapy is applied to those patients who are not identified as at risk for developing stress-related mucosal damage is limited in both quantity and quality. The most frequently prescribed medications to prevent stress-related mucosal damage include proton pump inhibitors and histamine-2 receptor antagonists (H$_2$RA), the actions of which are depicted in (Fig. 20.2). The provision of enteral nutrition is another potential strategy to reduce stress-related mucosal damage.[42] The mechanism of action for these agents is detailed in Table 20.4.[6,41,43–45]

It is common for the majority of critically ill patients to receive some form of stress ulcer prophylaxis during their episode of critical illness, probably because of recommendations from influential groups such as the Surviving Sepsis Campaign continue to be made despite the recommendation being weak and based on moderate evidence.[46] With the risk for clinical substantial bleeding being low, it is important to consider whether stress ulcer prophylaxis is always warranted, especially considering that pharmacological therapy is not risk free and is associated with economic consequences.[47]

Two recent clinical trials have generated evidence which raises questions regarding the effectiveness of stress ulcer prophylaxis in reducing gastrointestinal bleeding and mortality in critically ill patients. In the European-based Stress Ulcer Prophylaxis in the Intensive Care Unit (SUP-ICU) trial, 3298 critically ill patients considered at risk of gastrointestinal bleeding were randomised to receive intravenous pantoprazole (40 mg) or placebo.[48] Clinically important bleeding was less frequently observed in those patients who received pantoprazole (relative risk (RR) 0.58; 95% confidence interval (CI) 0.40–0.86). However, this study did not demonstrate any difference in 90-day (RR 1.02; 95% CI 0.91–1.13); $P = 0.76$)[48] or 1-year mortality (RR 1.01; 95% CI 0.92–1.01).[49] There was also no difference observed for the composite outcome (clinically important bleeding, pneumonia, *C. difficile* infection, or myocardial ischaemia (RR 0.96; 95%

FIGURE 20.2 Mechanism of action of stress ulcer prophylaxis agents. ATPase = adenosine triphosphatase.

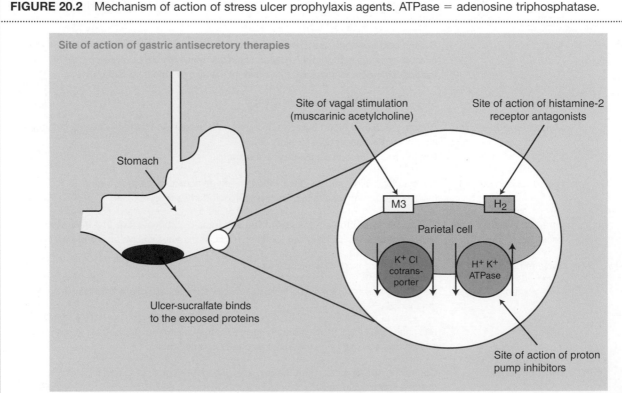

Source: Reproduced from Whitman Z, O'Neil DHR. Gastric disorders: modifications of gastric content, antacids and drugs influencing gastric secretions and motility. Anaesth Intensive Care Med 2017;19(1):25–9, with permission.

TABLE 20.4

Mechanism of action of stress ulcer prophylaxis

AGENT	MECHANISM OF ACTION	ADVERSE DRUG EFFECTS	CONSIDERATIONS
Proton pump inhibitors (PPIs): omeprazole esomeprazole pantoprazole lansoprazole dexlansoprazole rabeprazole	Irreversibly bind to the proton pump, effectively blocking all three receptors responsible for gastric acid secretion by the parietal cell. PPIs also limit vagally mediated gastric acid secretion.[43]	Nosocomial pneumonia, *Clostridium difficile* enteritis, myocardial ischaemia.	Changes in the gastric pH could lead to bacterial overgrowth.
Histamine-2 receptor antagonists: ranitidine cimetidine famotidine nizatidine	Inhibit the production of gastric acid by binding to the histamine-2 receptor on the basement membrane of the parietal cell.[44] Gastric acid secretion may still occur via stimulation of the acetylcholine or gastrin receptors in the parietal cells.[6]	Tachyphylaxis,[44] pneumonia.	Tolerance may develop within 48 hours.[6] Changes in the gastric pH could lead to bacterial overgrowth.
Enteral nutrition	Administration can buffer gastric acid and increase intragastric pH,[44] maintaining gastrointestinal barrier function and stimulating blood flow.[41]	Formula-specific intolerances.	For patients receiving enteral nutrition there may be no benefits to receiving stress ulcer prophylaxis.[45]

CI 0.83–1.11). The incidence of clinically important bleeding in patients receiving renal replacement therapy at any time during their ICU stay was similar to those who received the placebo.[50] However, in patients with increased disease severity (SAPS II >53) who received pantoprazole, the 90-day mortality was increased (RR 1.13; 95% CI 1.00–1.29), although some methodological weaknesses with this post hoc analysis are noted.[51]

The PEPTIC trial was a cluster crossover trial conducted at 50 ICUs in five countries where 26,982 intubated patients were randomised to receive either a proton pump inhibitor or a H_2 receptor antagonist.[52] There was no difference the number of patients who died at hospital by day 90 (risk ratio 1.05; 95% CI 1.00–1.10, $P = 0.054$). Clinically important upper gastrointestinal bleeding was lower in the PPI group (1.3%) than the H_2RA group (1.8%) (risk ratio, 0.73; 95% CI 0.57–0.92). Limitations of the trial include the significant crossover in the use of the assigned medication, where 4.1% of patients randomised to receive PPIs actually received H_2RAs and 20.1% of patients randomised to receive histamine-2 receptor blockers (H_2RBs) actually received PPIs.[52]

Recent systematic reviews on stress ulcer prophylaxis have also been conducted. The Cochrane review included randomised controlled trials (RCTs) and quasi-randomised controlled trials of critically ill patients admitted to ICU for >48 hours.[53] Any stress ulcer prophylaxis (PPIs, H_2RAs, sucralfate, antacids, prostaglandin analogues or anticholinergics) were compared with placebo or no intervention. Data suggest that the risk of clinically

important gastrointestinal bleeding was reduced (risk ratio 0.47; 95% CI 0.39–0.57), which represents a 10% reduction in gastrointestinal bleeding with any intervention. PPIs compared with H_2RAs were shown to be more effective in preventing clinically important upper gastrointestinal bleeding.[53] Barbateskovic and colleagues' systematic review of 42 trials and 6899 patients reported no difference in all-cause mortality with stress ulcer prophylaxis compared with placebo/no prophylaxis but was associated with a lower risk of any gastrointestinal bleeding.[54] More recently, Wang and colleagues undertook a systematic review of 72 RCTs (12,660 patients) that compared stress ulcer prophylaxis (PPIs, H_2RBs, or sucralfate) compared with placebo in adult critically ill patients.[55] In patients considered at high risk of gastrointestinal bleeding, both PPIs and H_2RAs reduced clinically important gastrointestinal bleeding (PPI – odds ratio (OR) 0.61; 95% CI 0.42–0.89; H_2RAs – OR 0.46; 95% CI 0.27–0.79). This review also suggested that the use of stress ulcer prophylaxis may increase the risk of pneumonia.[55] A subsequent and updated review by these authors,[56] which included data from the PEPTIC trial, supported the previous conclusions about a reduction in clinically important gastrointestinal bleeding in patients at increased risk with no impact on mortality.

The data available on stress ulcer prophylaxis in critically ill patients remain uncertain. Current international guidelines include weak recommendations for stress ulcer prophylaxis in critically ill patients at increased risk for clinically important gastrointestinal bleeding. Although also a weak recommendation, PPIs were favoured more than H_2RAs and it was recommended that sucralfate not be used.[57] When prescribing stress ulcer prophylaxis, it is important to identify those patients who are most likely to benefit as the potential economic benefit of avoiding non-beneficial treatments can be considerable.[58]

Practice tip

Proton pump inhibitors can potentially increase the risk of bacterial enteric infection. The mechanism of action is presumed to be a decrease in the gastric acid barrier or changes to the gut microbiome. Changes to the gut flora may result in the development of a *Clostridium difficile* infection. Consider *C. difficile* in patients who develop diarrhoea and for whom proton pump inhibitors are being used.[43]

Intra-abdominal hypertension and abdominal compartment syndrome

Intra-abdominal hypertension (IAH) and abdominal compartment syndrome have received increased attention in recent years and clinical research in this area is increasing. IAH occurs in nearly half of all intensive care patients and is an independent predictor of 28- and 90-day mortality.[59] The development of IAH is not confined to surgical patients or those with abdominal injury and is an important consideration for medical patients without abdominal conditions.

Aetiology

IAH and abdominal compartment syndrome can and do occur in a variety of patient populations.[60] Factors associated with IAH are numerous and can be grouped into three key categories: increased intra-abdominal volume, decreased abdominal compliance, or a combination of both.[61] The most significant risk factors include obesity, age, sepsis, abdominal infection, abdominal surgery, laparotomy, pancreatitis, hepatic failure, cirrhosis, gastrointestinal bleeding, ileus and liver dysfunction.[62] Risk factors that are more specific to critically ill patients include obesity, sepsis, abdominal surgery and ileus. Abdominal compartment syndrome is potentially fatal.[63] Consequently, it is imperative that all clinicians be aware of the underlying physiological changes, assessment and management in at-risk patients. Rates of IAH have decreased in recent years as increased recognition and early intervention have become more established in clinical practice.[64]

Practice tip

Patients who experience extra-abdominal septic shock are at increased risk of developing intra-abdominal hypertension, as are patients with sequential organ failure assessment (SOFA) scores higher than 7.[65]

Pathophysiology

Increased intra-abdominal pressure (IAP) results from an increase in pressure within the confined anatomical space of the abdominal cavity and can have a direct impact on many different body systems (Fig. 20.3). When IAP rises in this closed anatomical space, blood flow may be reduced and tissue viability threatened.[66]

This increase in pressure may result from causes such as intraperitoneal bleeding, peritonitis, ascites or distention of the gas-filled bowel. Clinical data show that increases in IAP result in physiological changes in vital organ function.[60] Early detection of increases in IAP can be challenging, and it is a sustained increase in abdominal pressure or the development of IAH that affects regional blood flow and impairs tissue perfusion, contributing to the development of multiple organ failure.[67] The pathophysiological consequences occur as a direct result of increased pressure within the abdominal cavity, resulting in vascular compression, direct compression of the organs and elevation of the diaphragm, which can falsely elevate intracardiac pressures.[68] A summary of the physiological changes associated with abdominal compartment syndrome is provided in Table 20.5.[60,68–71]

Normal intra-abdominal pressure

Clinical examination does not allow for accurate detection of increased IAP. The current gold standard for assessing IAP is measurement of intraurinary bladder pressure. In the spontaneously breathing patient, IAP is normally either atmospheric or subatmospheric. Mechanical ventilation, however, causes the IAP to increase near end-inspiration. After abdominal surgery, IAP may be increased slightly. The patient's clinical context must be considered when evaluating IAP. The most recent grading system for IAP is provided in Table 20.6.[72]

Measurement of intra-abdominal pressure

Measurement of pressure within the bladder has been validated as closely approximating IAP[73] and is the recommended standard approach for the measurement of intra-abdominal pressure.[61] This technique can, however, be influenced by the measurement technique. For example, air bubbles in the system and changes in transducer positions may influence pressure measurement, with wide variations in IAP being noted.[74]

There are a variety of techniques for measuring IAP described in the literature[75] and the direct peritoneal catheter measurement is the most ideal but not the most practical. IAP measurements should be performed when patients exhibit one or more of the risk factors, and the transbladder technique is the measurement technique recommended by the World Society of the Abdominal Compartment Syndrome.[72] The reliability of other methods, such as intragastric measurement, is not well demonstrated in clinical practice.

FIGURE 20.3   Systemic effects of intra-abdominal hypertension/abdominal compartment syndrome. AAP = abdominal perfusion pressure; CCP = cerebral perfusion pressure; CNS = central nervous system; CO = cardiac output, CVP = central venous pressure; GFR = glomerular filtration rate; ICP = intracranial pressure; ITP = intrathoracic pressure, $PaCO_2$ = partial pressure of CO_2 in the arterial blood; PaO_2 = partial pressure of oxygen in the arterial blood; PAW = peak airway pressure; PIP = peak inspiratory pressure; PAOP = pulmonary artery occlusion pressure; PRV = pulmonary vascular resistance; QS/QT = pulmonary shunt; SMA = superior mesenteric artery; SVR = systemic vascular resistance; VD/VT = dead space-to-tidal volume space.

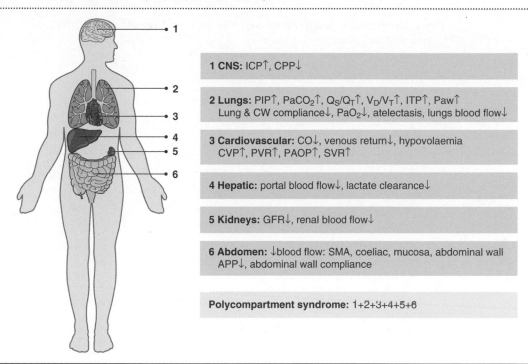

1 CNS: ICP↑, CPP↓

2 Lungs: PIP↑, $PaCO_2$↑, Q_S/Q_T↑, V_D/V_T↑, ITP↑, Paw↑
Lung & CW compliance↓, PaO_2↓, atelectasis, lungs blood flow↓

3 Cardiovascular: CO↓, venous return↓, hypovolaemia
CVP↑, PVR↑, PAOP↑, SVR↑

4 Hepatic: portal blood flow↓, lactate clearance↓

5 Kidneys: GFR↓, renal blood flow↓

6 Abdomen: ↓blood flow: SMA, coeliac, mucosa, abdominal wall
APP↓, abdominal wall compliance

Polycompartment syndrome: 1+2+3+4+5+6

Source: Reproduced from Pereira BM. Abdominal compartment syndrome and intra-abdominal hypertension. Curr Opin Crit Care 2019;25:688–96, Figure 2.

TABLE 20.5

Physiological changes associated with abdominal compartment syndrome

SYSTEM	PHYSIOLOGICAL EFFECTS
Respiratory[68,69]	Cephalad deviation of diaphragm leads to decreased lung and chest wall compliance. Peak inspiratory pressures increase. Functional residual volume and lung capacity are reduced, resulting in ventilation/perfusion mismatching. Hypoxia and hypercarbia may result, necessitating mechanical ventilation. Pulmonary vascular resistance increases.
Cardiovascular[68]	Inferior vena cava and portal vein compression results in decreased venous return. Decreased left ventricular compliance. Artificially increased right atrial pressure, pulmonary artery occlusion pressure. Decreased cardiac index. Elevated systemic vascular resistance from arteriolar vasoconstriction and increased intra-abdominal pressure (IAP).
Renal[70,71]	Oliguria (IAP 15–20 mmHg). Anuria (IAP >30 mmHg). May be a consequence of decreased cardiac output, compression of renal vessels, increased renal vascular resistance or redistribution of blood flow to renal medulla.

Continued

TABLE 20.5

Physiological changes associated with abdominal compartment syndrome—cont'd

SYSTEM	PHYSIOLOGICAL EFFECTS
Gastrointestinal[71]	Decreased splanchnic perfusion and tissue hypoxia.
	Increased GI mucosal acidosis.
	Reduced hepatic blood flow.
	Abnormalities in normal gut mucosal barrier function that may permit bacterial translocation.
	Decreased abdominal wall blood flow.
	Increased pressure on oesophageal varices may result in bleeding.
Neurological[60]	Increased intracranial pressure because of impaired venous return.

IAP = intra-abdominal pressure.

Source: Reproduced from Marshall AP. The gut in critical illness. In: Carlson K, editor. AACN Advanced critical care nursing. Philadelphia: Elsevier; 2009, Table 29-4, with permission.

TABLE 20.6

Intra-abdominal hypertension grading system[72]

GRADE	BLADDER PRESSURE (mmHg)	TREATMENT
I	12–15	Decompression is not indicated; continue monitoring.
II	16–20	Continue close monitoring, with treatment informed by the patient's clinical condition.
III	21–25	Assess for a trend in increased IAP measurements and identify any factors influencing measurement accuracy. Abdominal decompression (medical or surgical) is usually indicated.
IV	>25	Where a reliable and valid measurement above 25 mmHg is obtained, this constitutes a surgical emergency.

IAP = intra-abdominal pressure; mmHg = millimetres of mercury.

Source: Adapted from Kirkpatrick AW, Roberts DJ, De Waele J, et al. Intra-abdominal hypertension and the abdominal compartment syndrome: updated consensus definitions and clinical practice guidelines from the World Society of the Abdominal Compartment Syndrome. Intensive Care Med 2013;39(7):1190–206.

Practice tip

The transbladder technique is the most common method used for measuring IAP. Abdominal wall contraction can increase IAP and may not necessarily reflect an increase in intra-abdominal volume. While IAP measurement may be most reliable in sedated, mechanically ventilated patients, many patients in ICU may be awake and the degree of abdominal muscle contraction should be taken into consideration when undertaking IAP measurement.

IAP measurement should be accurate and reproducible. There are a number of commercial devices now available to aid the measurement of IAP; however, these are not required and a measurement system can easily be created from existing equipment normally available in most ICUs. The procedures for IAP measurement techniques may differ; however, the key principles for performing measurements are outlined in Table 20.7.[61,72,75–77]

Management of intra-abdominal hypertension and abdominal compartment syndrome

Surveillance for IAH and abdominal compartment syndrome requires close observation of the patient to identify potential risk factors and relevant changes to physiological parameters. For those patients who are at risk, close monitoring of IAP is required and pre-emptive measures are instituted. For example, a decision may be made to delay closure of the abdomen or to use an alternative means of abdominal content coverage. For the non-surgical patient, optimal resuscitation may be important in preventing IAH; overresuscitation needs to be avoided. The approach to managing the patient with IAH or abdominal compartment syndrome is dependent on their clinical presentation. The World Society of the Abdominal Compartment Syndrome has developed evidence-based management algorithms that are useful in guiding clinical management (Figs 20.4 and 20.5).[72]

TABLE 20.7

Key principles for measuring intra-abdominal pressure (IAP)[61,72,75]

	RECOMMENDATION
Measurement techniques	• IAP should be measured in mmHg. • Measurement should be recorded at end-expiration. • The transducer should be zeroed at the mid-axillary line at the level of the iliac crest. • Determine measurement 30–60 s after instillation of saline to allow bladder detrusor muscle to relax. • Monitor IAP every 4 h. Increase frequency of monitoring if IAP is greater than 20 mmHg. • Monitoring can be ceased when IAP is <12 mmHg for several hours and the patient is clinically improving.
Instillation volume	• A maximum of 25 mL sterile saline should be used as the instillation volume in adults. • In children the volume instilled should be 1 mL/kg with a minimum of 3 mL. • In infants under 4.5 kg the volume instilled should be 1 mL/kg.[76] • The temperature of saline should be as close to body temperature as possible to avoid bladder spasm.[77]
Patient position	• IAP should be measured in supine position, where possible. • IAP is significantly increased when the head of bed is elevated more than 20 degrees. • If head-of-bed elevation is required, consider the reverse Trendelenburg position during IAP measurement to minimise compression of the abdomen by the chest.

Source: Adapted from Kirkpatrick AW, Roberts DJ, De Waele J, et al. Intra-abdominal hypertension and the abdominal compartment syndrome: updated consensus definitions and clinical practice guidelines from the World Society of the Abdominal Compartment Syndrome. Intensive Care Med 2013;39(7):1190–206.

The critically ill patient with diabetes

Diabetes is a major cause of morbidity and mortality worldwide. The prevalence of diabetes internationally is rising. The prevalence is similar in males and females but highest in those aged 75–79 years. The prevalence is also higher in urban and high-income countries.[78] In 2019, diabetes was the ninth leading cause of death, with an estimated 1.5 million deaths directly caused by diabetes worldwide.[79] In 2021, an estimated 536.6 million people worldwide aged 20–79 had diabetes and this number is projected to increase to 783 million by the year 2045.[78] Reasons for this include an increase in the rates of obesity, physical inactivity, the ageing population, better detection of diabetes and longer survival of affected individuals.[80] Worryingly, reports of undiagnosed diabetes are on the increase, with almost one-in-two adults with diabetes being unaware of their status, meaning that an estimated 240 million people worldwide are living with undiagnosed diabetes.[81]

Aetiology of diabetes

Diabetes mellitus is a disorder of metabolism that is characterised by glucose intolerance. Diabetes is not a single disease per se, but a group of heterogeneous disorders where the aetiology of glucose disturbance is multifactorial.[82] The ongoing effect of poor glycaemic control can ultimately contribute to the development of end-organ damage. In the long term, diabetes is associated with increased morbidity and mortality, but acute complications of diabetes, such as diabetic ketoacidosis (DKA) and hyperosmolar hyperglycaemic state (HHS), may necessitate patient management in the ICU.

Acute complications of diabetes

DKA and HHS are two extremes of what can occur when a deficiency in insulin is present.[83] DKA is a metabolic derangement resulting from a relative or absolute insulin deficiency characterised by a previous diagnosis with diabetes or hyperglycaemia with a blood glucose level >200 mg/dL (>11.0 mmol/L), ketosis evidenced by raised blood ketone bodies (plasma beta-hydroxybutyrate ≥3.0 mmol/L) or ketonuria of more than 2+ on a standard urine ketone stick, and metabolic acidosis (pH <7.3) or serum bicarbonate of <15.0 mmol/L.[84] It is usually precipitated, in insulin- and non-insulin-dependent diabetics, by infection, other acute changes in the patient health or the omission (or inadequate dosing) of insulin.[85] It may also be the cause of the first presentation in new-onset diabetes. Additionally, DKA is increasingly being identified in patients with type 2 diabetes.[86]

HHS is seen more often in older patients with type 2 diabetes and is characterised by hyperglycaemia and the pathological consequences of extreme dehydration. Unlike DKA, where there is insufficient insulin, in HHS the insulin excretion is maintained, so lipolysis and ketoacidosis do not feature.[87] Although DKA and HHS are considered separate entities, DKA and HHS may coexist in about a third of cases, especially among older patients.[88]

DKA usually occurs much more quickly, with the onset of HHS being more insidious. Both complications are characterised by polyuria, polydipsia and weight loss.

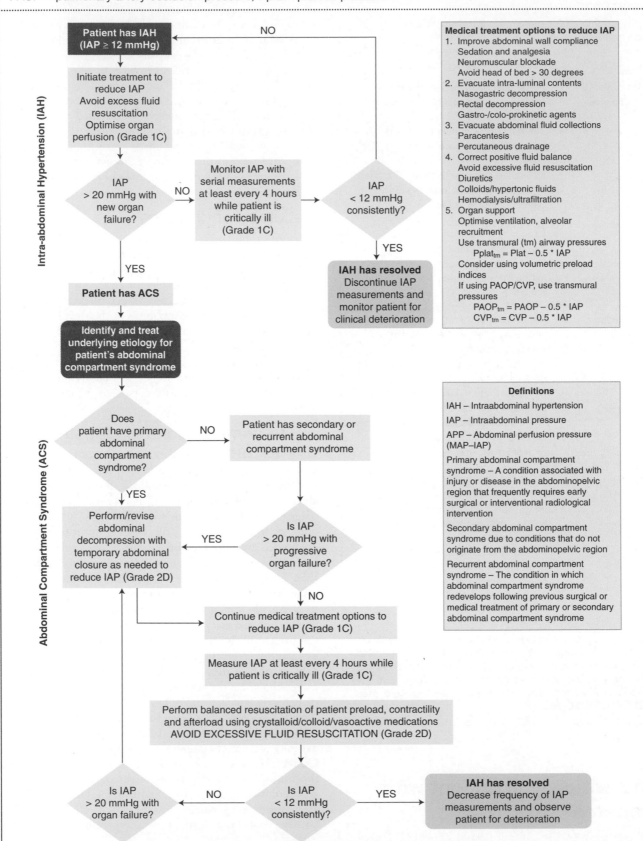

FIGURE 20.4 Intra-abdominal hypertension and abdominal compartment syndrome management algorithm. ACS = abdominal compartment syndrome; APP = abdominal perfusion pressure; CVP = central venous pressure; IAH = intra-abdominal hypertension; IAP = intra-abdominal pressure; mmHg = millimetres of mercury; PAOP = pulmonary artery occlusion pressure; Pplat= plateau pressure.

Intra-abdominal Hypertension (IAH)

Patient has IAH
(IAP ≥ 12 mmHg)

Initiate treatment to reduce IAP
Avoid excess fluid resuscitation
Optimise organ perfusion (Grade 1C)

IAP > 20 mmHg with new organ failure? — NO → Monitor IAP with serial measurements at least every 4 hours while patient is critically ill (Grade 1C) → IAP < 12 mmHg consistently?

YES ↓

Patient has ACS

Identify and treat underlying etiology for patient's abdominal compartment syndrome

IAP < 12 mmHg consistently? — YES → **IAH has resolved** Discontinue IAP measurements and monitor patient for clinical deterioration

Medical treatment options to reduce IAP
1. Improve abdominal wall compliance
   Sedation and analgesia
   Neuromuscular blockade
   Avoid head of bed > 30 degrees
2. Evacuate intra-luminal contents
   Nasogastric decompression
   Rectal decompression
   Gastro-/colo-prokinetic agents
3. Evacuate abdominal fluid collections
   Paracentesis
   Percutaneous drainage
4. Correct positive fluid balance
   Avoid excessive fluid resuscitation
   Diuretics
   Colloids/hypertonic fluids
   Hemodialysis/ultrafiltration
5. Organ support
   Optimise ventilation, alveolar recruitment
   Use transmural (tm) airway pressures
   $Pplat_{tm} = Plat - 0.5 * IAP$
   Consider using volumetric preload indices
   If using PAOP/CVP, use transmural pressures
   $PAOP_{tm} = PAOP - 0.5 * IAP$
   $CVP_{tm} = CVP - 0.5 * IAP$

Abdominal Compartment Syndrome (ACS)

Does patient have primary abdominal compartment syndrome? — NO → Patient has secondary or recurrent abdominal compartment syndrome

YES ↓

Perform/revise abdominal decompression with temporary abdominal closure as needed to reduce IAP (Grade 2D)

Is IAP > 20 mmHg with progressive organ failure? — YES → (Perform/revise abdominal decompression...)

NO ↓

Continue medical treatment options to reduce IAP (Grade 1C)

Measure IAP at least every 4 hours while patient is critically ill (Grade 1C)

Perform balanced resuscitation of patient preload, contractility and afterload using crystalloid/colloid/vasoactive medications
AVOID EXCESSIVE FLUID RESUSCITATION (Grade 2D)

Is IAP > 20 mmHg with organ failure? ← NO — Is IAP < 12 mmHg consistently? — YES → **IAH has resolved** Decrease frequency of IAP measurements and observe patient for deterioration

Definitions

IAH – Intraabdominal hypertension

IAP – Intraabdominal pressure

APP – Abdominal perfusion pressure (MAP–IAP)

Primary abdominal compartment syndrome – A condition associated with injury or disease in the abdominopelvic region that frequently requires early surgical or interventional radiological intervention

Secondary abdominal compartment syndrome due to conditions that do not originate from the abdominopelvic region

Recurrent abdominal compartment syndrome – The condition in which abdominal compartment syndrome redevelops following previous surgical or medical treatment of primary or secondary abdominal compartment syndrome

Source: Reprinted with permission of Springer Nature. Kirkpatrick AW, Roberts DJ, De Waele J, et al. Intra-abdominal hypertension and the abdominal compartment syndrome: updated consensus definitions and clinical practice guidelines from the World Society of the Abdominal Compartment Syndrome. Intensive Care Med 2013;39(7):1190–206.

FIGURE 20.5 Intra-abdominal hypertension (IAH) and abdominal compartment syndrome medical management algorithm. IAP = intra-abdominal pressure.

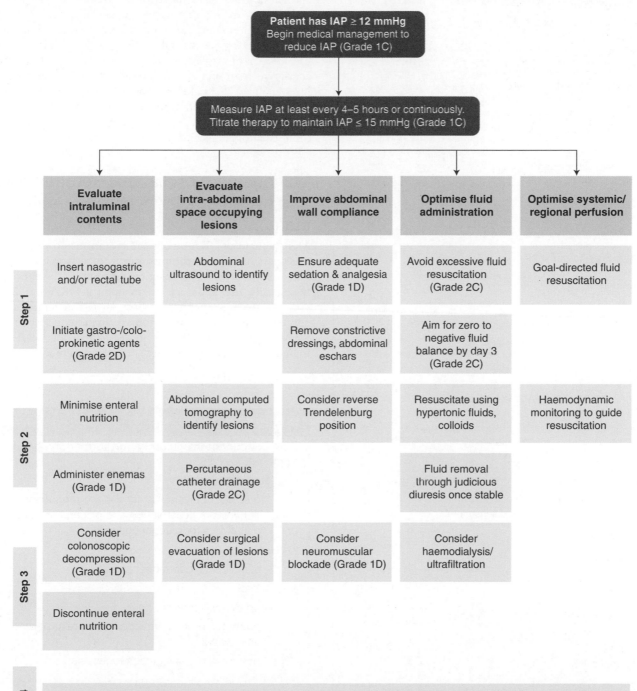

Source: Reprinted with permission of Springer Nature. Kirkpatrick AW, Roberts DJ, De Waele J, et al. Intra-abdominal hypertension and the abdominal compartment syndrome: updated consensus definitions and clinical practice guidelines from the World Society of the Abdominal Compartment Syndrome. Intensive Care Med 2013;39(7):1190–206.

Patients with DKA can also present with nausea and vomiting.[85,89] A comparison of DKA with HHS is provided in Table 20.8.[83,87,90,91]

TABLE 20.8
Comparison of presentation and electrolyte deficits in DKA and HHS[83,87,90,91]

PRESENTATION	DKA	HHS
Prodromal illness	Days	Weeks
Diabetes type	More common in T1D	More common in T2D
Coma	+ +	+ + +
Blood glucose	+ +	+ + +
Ketone	+ + +	0 or +
Acidaemia	+ + +	0 or +
Anion gap	+ +	0 or +
Osmolality	+ +	+ + +
Signs	Polydipsia Polyuria Weakness Weight loss Nausea Vomiting Abdominal pain	Polydipsia Polyuria Weakness Weight loss
Symptoms	Hypothermia Tachycardia Tachypnoea Kussmaul breathing Ileus Acetone breath Altered sensorium	Hypothermia Hypotension Tachycardia Altered sensorium

TYPICAL DEFICITS		
Total water (litres)	6	9
Water (mL/kg)	100	100–200
Na^+ (mmol/kg)	7–10	5–13
Cl^- (mmol/kg)	3–5	5–15
K^+ (mmol/kg)	3–5	4–6
PO_4 (mmol/kg)	5–7	3–7
Mg^{2+} (mmol/kg)	0.5–1.0	0.5–1.0
Ca^{2+} (mmol/kg)	0.5–1.0	0.5–1.0

T1D = type 1 diabetes; T2D = type 2 diabetes.

Pathophysiology

Inadequate production (or administration) of insulin to meet metabolic need (or a rise in metabolic demand resulting from the stress of infection, trauma or surgery, for instance) is associated with a rise in the secretion of the counterregulatory hormones glucagon, the catecholamines and cortisol[85,87] (Box 20.1). When insulin is deficient, hyperglycaemia results from gluconeogenesis, accelerated glycogenolysis and impaired glucose use by peripheral tissues. Lipase results in the breakdown of triglycerides into glycerol and free fatty acids, which are subsequently oxidised into ketone bodies in the liver.[91] As ketone bodies accumulate, serum bicarbonate concentration decreases and metabolic acidosis results. In HHS, insulin levels are higher and this inhibits ketogenesis and metabolic acidosis (Fig. 20.6).[91]

Management of diabetic ketoacidosis and hyperosmolar hyperglycaemic state

Management of DKA involves rehydration and electrolyte replacement, insulin administration, correction of acidosis and treatment of the precipitating factor.[85,89] Although historically the approach to managing DKA has been variable, there is evidence to suggest that a standardised approach can have a positive impact on patient outcome.[90]

Management of HHS is similar to that for DKA and includes: respiratory support; fluid replacement; insulin

BOX 20.1

Effects of counterregulatory hormones in diabetic ketoacidosis[85,87]

- Catecholamines:
  - promote lipolysis, resulting in the production of FFA and glycerol; FFA and glycerol used as precursors for gluconeogenesis.
- Glucagon:
  - stimulates gluconeogenesis.
- Cortisol:
  - promotes lipolysis
  - promotes protein breakdown and release of amino acids
  - promotes hepatic gluconeogenesis.

FFA = free fatty acids.
Source: Nyenwe EA, Kitabchi AE. The evolution of diabetic ketoacidosis: an update of its etiology, pathogenesis and management. Metabolism 2016;65(4):507–21.

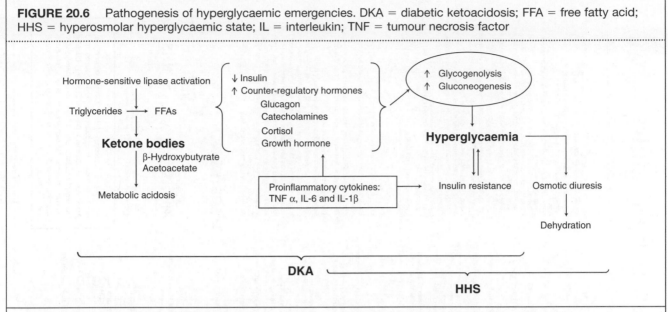

FIGURE 20.6 Pathogenesis of hyperglycaemic emergencies. DKA = diabetic ketoacidosis; FFA = free fatty acid; HHS = hyperosmolar hyperglycaemic state; IL = interleukin; TNF = tumour necrosis factor

Source: Reproduced with permission from Fayfman M, Pasquel FJ, Umpierrez GE. Management of hyperglycemic crises: diabetic ketoacidosis and hyperglycemic hyperosmolar state. Med Clin North Am 2017;101(3):587–606, Figure 1, p. 592.

treatment to turn off ketogenesis and the accompanying metabolic derangement; electrolyte replacement; monitoring for and prevention of complications of hypoglycaemia, hypokalaemia, hyperglycaemia and fluid volume overload; and patient teaching and support. Ongoing assessment of blood glucose levels is essential.[87]

Effectiveness of treatment is usually assessed by resolution of the acidosis (in DKA) and the control of hyperglycaemia. Regular testing of arterial blood gases, blood sugar and electrolytes (especially potassium) is vital until the blood sugar has stabilised and the ketosis and acidosis resolves.[91] Considering that fewer patients are now admitted to ICU with DKA and HHS, understanding the management of these patients is vital and protocols have been developed to guide practice.[90]

Blood ketones (beta-hydroxybutyrate) can now easily be measured using blood from a finger prick with a bedside handheld monitor. It has been suggested that blood ketone monitoring allows for insulin titration with reference to ketones in addition to usual blood sugar monitoring; however, point-of-care blood ketone monitoring remains subject to some measurement errors, whether the measurement is done in the laboratory or at the bedside.[92]

Comprehensive management of DKA is described in a recent clinical guideline by the Joint British Diabetes Societies Inpatient Care Group[90] and is summarised in Fig. 20.7. The treatment of HHS is detailed in the 2022 guideline by the same organisation.[93] Fig 20.8 provides a summary of the treatment approaches for HHS.

> **Practice tip**
>
> Sodium–glucose cotransporter-2 (SGLT2) inhibitors are relatively new drugs approved for diabetes. These drugs can increase the risk for DKA, which means that blood glucose levels may be normal or only mildly elevated, but patients may have increased ketone levels (euglycaemic ketoacidosis). Checking ketone levels in patients taking SGLT2 inhibitors should be undertaken to facilitate timely diagnosis.

Pancreatitis

The pancreas has many key endocrine and exocrine functions, regulating blood glucose through the production of the hormones insulin, glucagon and somatostatin, as well as producing enzymes to aid digestion in the gut. If pancreatic function is inhibited through injury or disease, this can have significant effects on systemic function.

In normal function, digestive enzymes are in an inactive form in the pancreas, becoming active only when in the presence of other substances found in the duodenum. Pancreatitis occurs when a known or unknown cause stimulates these digestive enzymes to become active while still inside the pancreas, leading to autodigestion of pancreatic tissue and inflammation. Common causes of acute pancreatitis are alcohol, gallstones, or this can often be idiopathic.[94,95] Pancreatitis is diagnosed by the presence

FIGURE 20.7 Single treatment pathway for diabetic ketoacidosis (DKA).

The Management of Diabetic Ketoacidosis in Adults

Where individuals aged 16–18 are managed by paediatric teams, the paediatric guidelines should be followed: https://www.bsped.org.uk/media/1798/bsped-dka-guideline-2020.pdf

Diagnostic criteria: all three of the following must be present
- capillary blood glucose above 11 mmol/L
- capillary ketones above 3 mmol/L or urine ketones ++ or more
- venous pH less than 7.3 and/or bicarbonate less than 15 mmol/L

BOX 1: Immediate management: time 0 to 60 minutes
(T=0 at time intravenous fluids are commenced)

If intravenous access cannot be obtained request critical care support immediately

Action 1: Commence 0.9% sodium chloride solution (use a large bore cannula) via an infusion pump
See Box 2 for rate of fluid replacement

Action 2: Commence a fixed rate intravenous insulin infusion (FRIII). (0.1units/kg/hr based on estimate of weight) 50 units human soluble insulin (Actrapid® or Humulin S®) made up to 50ml with0.9% sodium chloride solution. If patient normally takes long acting insulin analogue (glargine, detemir, degludec) continue at usual dose and time

Action 3: Assess patient
- Respiratory rate; temperature; blood pressure; pulse; oxygensaturation
- Glasgow Coma Scale
- Full clinical examination

Action 4: Further investigations
- Capillary and laboratory glucose
- Venous BG
- U&E and FBC
- Blood cultures
- ECG
- CXR
- MSU

Action 5: Establish monitoring regimen
- Hourly capillary blood glucose
- Hourly capillary ketone measurement if available
- Venous bicarbonate and potassium at 60 minutes, 2hours and 2 hourly thereafter
- 4 hourly plasma electrolytes
- Continuous cardiac monitoring if required
- Continuous pulse oximetry if required

Action 6: Consider and precipitating causes and treat appropria

---

HDU/level 2 facility and/or insertion of central line may be required in following circumstances (request urgent senior review)
- Young people aged 18–25 years
- Elderly
- Pregnant
- Heart or kidney failure
- Other serious co-morbidities
- Severe DKA by following criteria
  - Blood ketones above 6 mmol/L
  - Venous bicarbonate below 5 mmol/L
  - Venous pH below 7.1
  - Hypokalaemia on admission (below 3.5 mmol/L)
  - GCS less than 12
  - Oxygen saturation below 92% on air (Arterial blood gases required)
  - Systolic BP below 90 mmHg
  - Pulse over 100 or below 60 bpm
  - Anion gap above16 {Anion Gap = (Na⁺ + K⁺) – (Cl⁻ + HCO₃⁻)}

BOX 2: Initial fluid replacement

Restoration of circulating volume is priority
Systolic BP (SBP) below 90mmHg
Likely to be due to low circulating volume, but consider other causes such as heart failure, sepsis, etc.
- Give 500mls 0.9% sodium chloride solution over 10–15 minutes. If SBP remains <90mmHg repeat whilst awaiting senior input. Most people require between 500–1000mls given rapidly
- Consider involving the ITU / critical care team
- Once SBP is >90mmHg, give 1L 0.9% sodium chloride over the next 60 minutes. The addition of potassium is likely to be required in this second litre of fluid

Systolic BP on admission 90 mmHg and over
- Give 1L 0.9% sodium chloride over the first 60 minutes

Potassium level (mmol/L)	Potassium replacement mmol/L of infusion solution
> 5.5	Nil
3.5–5.5	40 mmol/L
< 3.5	senior review – additional potassium required

BOX 3: 60 minutes to 6 hours

Aims of treatment:
- Rate of fall of ketones of at least 0.5 mmol/L/hr OR bicarbonate rise 3 mmol/L/hrand blood glucose fall 3 mmol/L/hr
- Maintain serum potassium in normal range
- Avoid hypoglycaemia

Action 1: Re-assess patient, monitor vital signs
- Hourly blood glucose (lab blood glucose if meter reading 'HI')
- Hourly blood ketones if meter available
- Venous blood gas for pH, bicarbonate and potassium at 60 minutes, 2 hours and 2 hourly thereafter
- If potassium is outside normal range, re-assess potassium replacement and checkhourly. If abnormal after further hour seek immediate senior medical advice

Action 2: Continue fluid replacement via infusion pump as follows:
- 0.9% sodium chloride 1L with potassium chloride over next 2 hours
- 0.9% sodium chloride 1L with potassium chloride over next 2 hours
- 0.9% sodium chloride 1L with potassium chloride over next 4 hours
- Add 10% glucose 125ml/hr if blood glucose falls below 14 mmol/L
- **Consider** reducing the rate of intravenous insulin infusion to 0.05 units/ kg/hour when glucose falls below 14 mmol/L
More cautious fluid replacement in young people aged 18–25 years, elderly, pregnant, heart or renal failure. (Consider HDU and/or central line)

Action 3: Assess response to treatment
Insulin infusion rate may need review if
- Capillary ketones not falling by at least 0.5 mmol/L/hr
- Venous bicarbonate not rising by at least 3 mmol/L/hr
- Plasma glucose not falling by at least 3 mmol/L/hr
- Continue FRIII until ketones less than 0.6 mmol/L, venous pH >7.3 and/or venous bicarbonate over 18 mmol/L.
If ketones and glucose are not falling as expected always check the insulin infusion pump is working and connected and that the correct insulin residualvolume is present (to check for pump malfunction).
If equipment working but response to treatment is inadequate, increase insulin infusionrate by 1 unit/hr increments hourly until targets achieved.

Additional measures
- Regular observations and Early Warning Score (NEWS2)
- Accurate fluid balance chart, minimum urine output 0.5ml/kg/hr
- Consider urinary catheterisation if incontinent or anuric (not passed urine) by 60 minutes
- Nasogastric tube with airway protection if patient obtunded or persistently vomiting
- Measure arterial blood gases and repeat chest radiograph if oxygen saturation lessthan 92%
- Thromboprophylaxis with low molecular weight heparin
- Consider ECG monitoring if potassium abnormal or concerns about cardiac status

---

BOX 4: 6 to 12 hours

Aims:
- Ensure clinical and biochemical parameters are improving
- Continue IV fluid replacement
- Avoid hypoglycaemia
- Assess for complications of treatment e.g. fluid overload, cerebral oedema
- Treat precipitating factors as necessary

Action 1: Re-assess patient, monitor vital signs
- If patient not improving by criteria in Box 3, seek senior advice
- Continue IV fluid via infusion pump at reduced rate
  - 0.9% sodium chloride 1L with KCl over 4 hours
  - 0.9% sodium chloride with KCl over 6 hours
- Add 10% dextrose 125mls/hr if the glucose falls below 14 mmol/L
- **Consider** reducing the rate of intravenous insulin infusion to 0.05 units/ kg/hour when glucose falls below 14 mmol/L

Reassess cardiovascular status at 12 hours; further fluidmay be required
Check for fluid overload

Action 2 – Review biochemical and metabolic parameters
- At 6 hours check venous pH, bicarbonate, potassium, capillary ketones and glucose
- Resolution of DKA is defined at ketones <0.6 mmol/L AND venous pH >7.3 (do not use bicarbonate as a marker at this stage)
- Ensure a referral has been made to the diabetes team
- If DKA not resolved review insulin infusion (see BOX 3Action 3)
- If DKA resolved go to BOX 6

BOX 5: 12 to 24 HOURS

Expectation: By 24 hours the ketonaemia and acidosis should have resolved. Request senior review is not improving

Aim:
- Ensure that clinical and biochemical parameters are continuing to improve or are normal
- Continue IV fluid replacement if not eating and drinking
- If ketonaemia has cleared and the person is not eating or drinking, move to a variable rate intravenous insulin infusion (VRIII) as per local guidelines
- Reasses for complications of treatment, e.g. fluid overload, cerebral oedema
- Continue to treat precipitating factors
- Transfer to subcutaneous insulin if the person is eating and drinking normally and biochemistry is normal

Action 1 – Re-assess patient, monitor vital signs

Action 2 – Review biochemical and metabolic parameters
- At 12 hours check venous pH, bicarbonate, potassium, capillary ketones and glucose
- Resolution is defined as ketones <0.6 mmol/L, venous pH>7.3
- If not resolved review fluid Box 4 Action 1 and insulin infusion Box 3 Action 3

If DKA resolved go to Box 6

BOX 6: Resolution of DKA

Expectation: Patient should be eating and drinking and back on normal insulin
If DKA not resolved identify and treat the reasons for failure to respond. **This situation is unusual and requires senior and specialist input**

Transfer to subcutaneous insulin
Convert to subcutaneous regime when biochemically stable (capillary ketones less than 0.6 mmol/L AND pH over 7.3) and the patient is ready and able to eat. Do not discontinue intravenous insulin infusion until 30 minutes after subcutaneous short acting Insulin has been given Conversion to subcutaneous insulin should be managed by the Specialist Diabetes Team. If the team is not available use local guidelines. If the patient is newly diagnosed it is essential they are seen by a member of the specialist team prior to discharge
Arrange follow up with specialist team

FIGURE 20.8 Hyperosmolar hyperglycaemic state care pathway in adults.

JBDS-IP Joint British Diabetes Societies for Inpatient care

Hyperosmolar Hyperglycaemic State (HHS) care pathway in adults

Clinical features (all the below)

	A mixed picture of HHS and DKA occurs relatively frequently
1) Marked hypovolaemia	
2) Osmolality ≥320 mOsm/kg	
3) Marked hyperglycaemia (≥30 mmol/L)	
4) Wi:hout significant ketonaemia (≤3.0 mmol/L)	
5) Wi:hout significant acidosis (pH ≥7.3) and bicarbonate ≥15 mmol/L	

Aims of therapy

1) Improvement in clinical status and replacement of all estimated fluid losses by 24 hours
2) Gradual decline in osmolality: drop of 3–8 mOsm/kg/hr
3) Blood glucose: aim to keep to 10–15 mmol/L in the first 24 hours
4) Avoid hypoglycaemia and hypokalaemia
5) Prevent harm: VTE, osmotic demyelination, fluid overload, foot ulceration

Criteria for resolution of HHS: Holistic assessment of the following:

1) Clinical and cognitive status is back to the pre-morbid state
2) Osmolality <300 mOsm/kg
3) Hypovolaemia has been corrected (urine output ≥0.5 ml/kg/hr)
4) Blood glucose <15 mmol/L

Theme		0–60 minutes	60 minutes – 6 hours	6–12 hours	12–24 hours	24–72 hours
Clinical assessment and monitoring						
Clinical status / NEWS		History/Examination, NEWS, cardiac monitoring, urine output. Establish adequate intravenous lines (preferably 2 large bore IV cannules). Discuss with outreach/ICU team early if there are markers of high severity (see Table 1 overleaf)			Check for continuing improvement	
Precipitating cause(s)		Assess for precipitating cause(s): sepsis, diabetic foot infection, treatment omissions, vulnerable adult, vascular event (myocardial infarction, stroke)			Ongoing management of the precipitating cause(s)	Expect steady recovery, patient eating and drinking, and biochemistry as it was prior to HHS
Osmolality (VBG/blood) Measure/calculate (2xNa⁺) + Glucose + Urea		Check every hour for 6 hours. Until the urea is available, calculate using (2 x Na⁺ + glucose). Recalculate osmolality once urea is available, and then use (2 x Na⁺ + glucose + urea)		Check every 2 hours	Check every 4 hours (if no clinical improvement then check every 2 hours)	Ongoing management of the precipitating cause(s)
Aim for gradual decline of 3–8 mOsm/kg/hr						Replacement of all estimated fluid losses by 24 hours
How to interpret osmolality results		Check Figure 1 overleaf	Check Figure 1 overleaf	Check Figure 1 overleaf	Check Figure 1 overleaf	Individual BG target 6–10 mmol/L
Blood glucose (BG) (Aim for 10–15 mmol/L in the first 24 hours)		Fall in BG should be up to 5.0 mmol/L per hour (check Figure 2 overleaf for details)	Check every hour	Check every hour (check Figure 2 overleaf for details)	Check every hour (check Figure 2 overleaf for details)	
Interventions						
Intravenous fluids (0.9% saline) (In IV line 1) (caution in HF/CKD/BW <50 kg)		1 litre over 1 hour (caution in HF/CKD/BW <50 kg)	Aim for 2–3 litres positive balance by 6 hours	Aims for up to 6 litres positive balance by 12 hours	Reassess fluid balance to plan fluids replacement for the next 12 hours	Can be stopped if patient is eating and drinking
Insulin Infusion (FRIII 0.05 units/kg/hr using Actrapid®) (In IV line 2)		Use DKA guidelines if ketonaemia (>3.0 mmol/L) or ketonuria (≥2+). Start FRIII if ketonaemia (>1.0 – ≤3.0 mmol/L) or ketonuria (<2+)	Only commence if positive fluid balance and BG plateaued on repeated measurements (>3 occasions)		Rate may need adjustment to 1 unit/hr to achieve BG target 10–15 mmol/L	VRIII if not eating and drinking. Otherwise convert to subcutaneous insulin
Glucose infusion: 5% or 10% @ 125ml/hr (In IV line 2)		Not required at this stage	Only initiate if BG <14 mmol/L		Continue infusion at 125 ml/hr	Can be stopped if patient is eating and drinking
Potassium		Senior review / ICU outreach if potassium <3.5 or >6.0 mmol/L	Check Table 2 overleaf for potassium replacement guidelines	Check Table 2 overleaf for potassium replacement guidelines	Check Table 2 overleaf for potassium replacement guidelines	Check U&Es daily
Assessments and prevention						
Prevent harm		VTE prophylaxis (low molecular weight heparin). Assess for complications e.g. fluid overload, cerebral oedema, osmotic demyelination (deteriorating conscious level)				VTE prophylaxis until discharge. Daily feet checks
Prevent hypoglycaemia		Glucose 5% or 10% at 125 ml/hr if BG <14 mmol/L				Target BG 6–10 mmol/L
Prevent foot ulceration		Daily foot checks				Daily foot checks
Refer to the inpatient diabetes team early. Escalate management if there is clinical deterioration.						Review by inpatient diabetes team before discharge

Abbreviations: BG=blood glucose; BW=body weight; CKD=chronic kidney disease; FRIII=fixed rate intravenous insulin infusion; HF=heart failure; hr=hour; ICU=intensive care unit; IV=intravenous; kg=kilograms; NEWS=national early warning score; U&Es=urea and electrolytes; VBG=venous blood gas analysis; VRIII=variable rate intravenous insulin infusion; VTE=venous thromboembolism

@JBDSIP 2022

v1.41

Continued

JBDS-IP Joint British Diabetes Societies for inpatient care

Hyperosmolar Hyperglycaemic State (HHS) care pathway in adults

Figure 1: Managing osmolality changes during treatment of HHS

Calculated*/ Measured Osmolality	Sodium	Fluid status	Action
Decreasing by <3 mOsm/kg/hour	Increasing	Negative fluid balance and no signs of fluid overload	Increase rate of infusion of 0.9% saline
Decreasing at appropriate level (3-8 mOsm/kg/hour)	Increasing		Continue same rate of fluids
Decreasing >8 mOsm/kg/hour			Consider reducing infusion rate of IV fluids and/or insulin (if already commenced)
Increasing	Increasing	Negative fluid balance and no signs of fluid overload	Increase rate of infusion of 0.9% saline
		Adequate fluids balance	Consider switching to 0.45% saline at same rate

*Calculated osmolality (mOsm/kg) = (2xNa⁺) + Glucose + Urea

$$\text{*Calculated osmolality (mOsm/kg)} = (2 \times Na^+) + Glucose + Urea$$

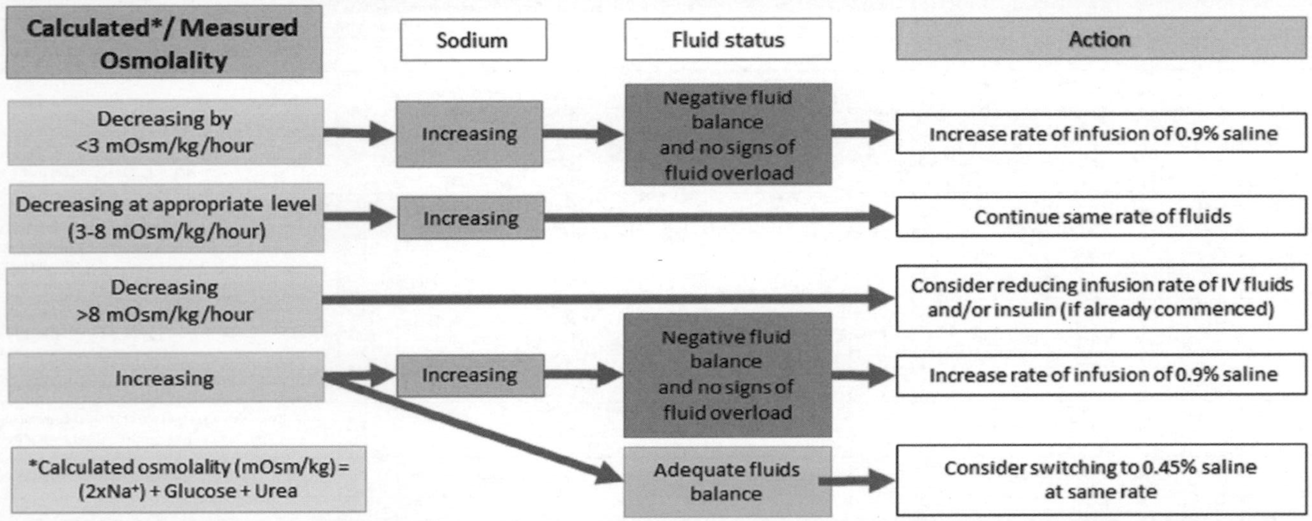

Figure 2: Managing glucose changes during treatment of HHS

Blood glucose	Fluid status	Action
Fall of blood glucose at a rate of up to 5 mmol/L per hour is ideal		
Blood glucose falling <5 mmol/L per hour	Negative fluid balance and no signs of fluid overload	Increase rate of infusion of 0.9% saline
	Adequate fluids balance	Commence Fixed Rate Insulin Infusion (FRIII) 0.05 units/kg/hour OR increase rate to 0.1 units/kg/hour (if already commenced) [convert to variable rate intravenous insulin infusion (VRIII) or sc insulin once HHS has resolved]
Blood glucose falling >5 mmol/L per hour		Check the rate of change in osmolality and consider reducing the rate of fluid replacement and/or IV insulin infusion rate

Table 1: Escalate to ICU/outreach if any of the following is present:

- Osmolality >350 mOsm/kg
- Sodium >160 mmol/L
- Venous/arterial pH <7.1
- Hypokalaemia (<3.5 mmol/L) or hyperkalaemia (>6 mmol/L) on admission
- Glasgow Coma Scale (GCS) <12 or abnormal AVPU (Alert, Voice, Pain, Unresponsive) scale
- Oxygen saturation <92% on air (assuming normal baseline respiratory function)
- Systolic blood pressure <90 mmHg
- Pulse >100 or <60 beats per minute
- Urine output <0.5 ml/kg/hour
- Serum creatinine >200 µmol/L and/or Acute kidney injury
- Hypothermia
- Macrovascular event such as myocardial infarction or stroke
- Other serious co-morbidity

Table 2: Potassium replacement guidelines

Potassium level in first 24 hours (mmol/L)	Potassium replacement in infusion solution
≥6.0	Senior review ICU/outreach
5.5-5.9	Nil
3.5-5.5	40 mmol/L
<3.5	Senior review ICU/Outreach. Additional potassium is required

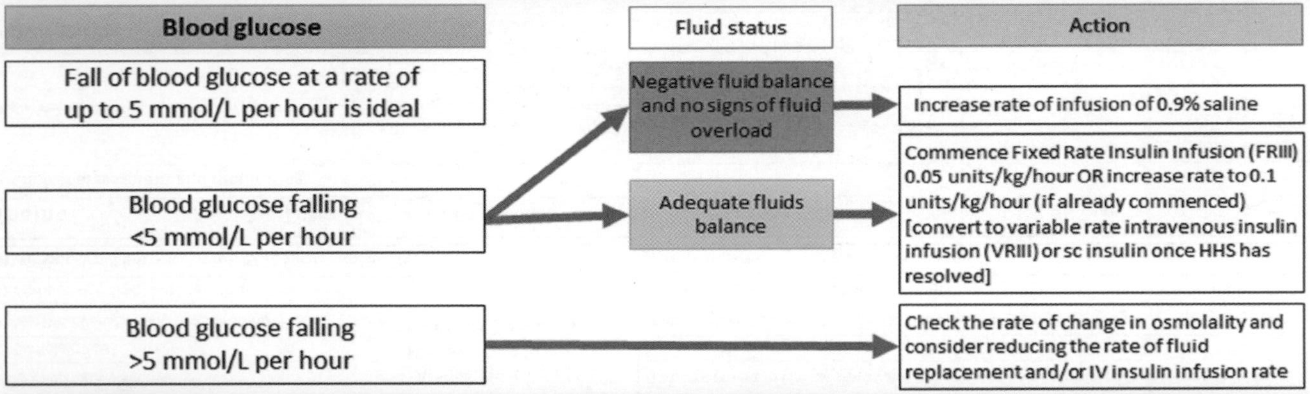

If the parameters in Figures 1 and 2 above are not met, seek specialist input early to help tailor the management according to the individual's need

v1.41

@JBDSIP 2022

of two of three of the following findings: abdominal pain consistent with the condition (acute, persistent, severe epigastric pain often radiating to the back), raised serum lipase or amylase (at least three times the upper limit of normal) and characteristic findings on contrast-enhanced computerised tomography scanning.[95]

Acute pancreatitis is subdivided into two types: interstitial oedematous pancreatitis and necrotising pancreatitis.[96] These are broadly differentiated by the condition of the pancreatic and surrounding tissues as inflamed or necrotic. There are two phases of the disease, early and late, with peaks of mortality at either point. The early phase is characterised by systemic inflammation, and the late phase when this persists longer than 1–2 weeks. Three classifications of severity are suggested, characterised by the presence of local or systemic complications and with increasing mortality (Table 20.9).[96,97]

All patients with organ failure or severe acute pancreatitis should be managed in a critical care setting.[95] Management focuses on monitoring vital organ function; supportive therapy with fluid resuscitation, analgesia and nutrition; and ongoing assessment to identify potential complications. Monitoring of vital organ function should incorporate abdominal pressure monitoring and strategies to decrease intra-abdominal pressure. Severe acute pancreatitis is one of the main causes of increased intra-abdominal pressure and abdominal compartment syndrome because of the capillary leak, massive fluid resuscitation and increased abdominal volume that occurs.[94] Acute pancreatitis should be managed with aggressive intravenous (IV) hydration to mitigate organ failure; currently there is no high-quality evidence for specific pharmacological interventions[94] and there is a dearth of evidence to inform optimal fluid resuscitation strategies in acute pancreatitis.[95] Similarly, there are no clear guidelines on the best strategies for managing pain, which is a predominant symptom in pancreatitis.[95] Early enteral nutrition is recommended in the recent ICU nutrition guidelines by the European Society of Enteral and Parenteral Nutrition.[98] The American Society of Enteral and Parenteral Nutrition also advocated for the use of enteral nutrition in the setting of severe acute pancreatitis, with delivery via a naso/orogastric tube in the first instance and with consideration of small bowel feeding if evidence of feed intolerance develops that cannot be managed through usual strategies.[99] Additional information on nutrition in critical illness is provided in Chapter 19.

Antibiotics may also be required for pancreatic or extrapancreatic infections. In the context of acute necrotising pancreatitis, early antibiotic therapy (within 72 hours of symptom onset or 48 hours of admission) may reduce mortality and the incidence of infected pancreatic necrosis.[100] Surgical intervention is reserved for the most severe cases and is not a recommended routine treatment strategy.

Liver dysfunction

The liver is responsible for a vast array of metabolic functions. It performs the vital functions of controlling metabolic pathways, participating in digestion, immunological protection, detoxifying chemicals and clearing toxins and drugs. This means that alterations to normal liver function can have broad-ranging consequences, from changes in metabolic processes (such as glucose homeostasis), failure to produce clotting factors (with resultant severe haemorrhage) to other organ effects such as brain, lung and kidney impairment and injury. Accordingly, liver dysfunction can impact substantially on the nursing care needs of the critically ill patient.

Related anatomy and physiology

The liver is the largest internal organ, weighing approximately 1200–1600 g in the adult. It receives approximately 25% of total cardiac output through a dual vascular supply consisting of the hepatic artery and portal vein. Approximately 75% of all hepatic blood flow arises from the portal vein, with the remaining 25% from the hepatic artery. Anatomically, the liver consists of four lobes: the major left and right lobes and the minor caudate and quadrate lobes. The right lobe is considerably larger than the left. Functionally, the liver is divided into eight segments, each with their own inflow and outflow blood supply and biliary drainage. Hepatic lobules, or liver *acini*, are small units consisting of a single or double layer of hepatocytes arranged in plates interspersed with capillaries (sinusoids) that receive inflowing blood from the portal and hepatic pathways. To protect the systemic circulation from the toxins absorbed from the intestines, the sinusoids are lined with macrophages known as Kupffer cells. The hepatic vein then drains effluent blood from the liver into the general circulation.

TABLE 20.9
Classifications of acute pancreatitis[96,97]

SEVERITY	CHARACTERISTICS
Mild acute pancreatitis	Absence of organ failure and absence of local or systemic complications Typically short and self-resolving.
Moderately severe acute pancreatitis	Transient organ failure or local or systemic complications in the absence of persistent organ failure (<48 h).
Severe acute pancreatitis	Persistent organ failure (>48 h) often with local and systemic complications.

Source: Reproduced from Banks PA, Bollen TL, Dervenis C, et al. Classification of acute pancreatitis – 2012: revision of the Atlanta classification and definitions by international consensus. Gut 2013;62(1):102-11, with permission of BMJ Publishing Group.

The liver is responsible for the synthesis and drainage system of bile (used in the breakdown and absorption of lipids from the intestine). Biliary salts are formed from multiple enzymatic reactions in the hepatocytes. Bile drains from the hepatocytes into bile ducts and then into the common hepatic duct, before passing into the gall bladder via the common bile duct.

The arrangement of the circulation to the liver with its rich vascular architecture enables it to perform the vital functions of carbohydrate, fat and protein metabolism; production of bile to aid in digestion; production, conjugation and elimination of bilirubin; immunological and inflammatory responses; glycogen storage; and detoxification of toxins and drugs. As the kidneys are responsible for the clearance of water-soluble toxins from the body, the liver clears protein-bound (largely albumin) toxins and excretes them into the gastrointestinal tract for elimination or reabsorption in water-soluble form for subsequent renal excretion.

Mechanisms of liver cell injury

Liver cell injury and death can occur either as a direct result of injury to the cell, resulting in cell necrosis, or as a result of cellular stress and the triggering of apoptotic pathways, leading to programmed cell death.[101] Major factors for the triggering of the apoptotic pathway are hypoxia causing ischaemia and reperfusion, reactive oxygen metabolites resulting from alcohol or drug ingestion, accumulation of bile acids resulting from cholestasis, and inflammatory cytokines such as tumour necrosis factor-alpha.[102] The apoptotic pathway results in the deconstruction of the cellular structure from the inside out, while necrosis results in cell rupture and release of cellular contents. Although these processes may overlap, it is thought that the apoptotic pathway is a way of preventing the inflammatory response that is triggered with cell necrosis. The activation of the inflammatory response results in secondary liver cell injury and contributes to the multiple organ dysfunction seen in liver failure.[102]

The degree and time course of liver cell damage from viral hepatitis depends on the immune response. Immune recognition and destruction of infected cells may result in either clearance of the virus or ongoing inflammation, cell death and fibrosis if the virus is not cleared. This process may progress over 20–40 years to cirrhosis and hepatocellular carcinoma.[103] Chronic excessive alcohol intake may also result in a slower chronic course of liver injury that eventually results in cirrhosis, liver failure or hepatocellular carcinoma.[104]

Liver cells may also be injured by the toxic effects of drugs or their metabolites, as in paracetamol overdose,[105] or by therapeutic doses of drugs such as non-steroidal anti-inflammatory drugs, phenytoin or antimalarial agents. Other poisoning from the ingestion of mushrooms (e.g. *Amanita phalloides*)[106] and from the use of recreational drugs such as ecstasy and amphetamines may result in liver cell death and liver failure.[107] Diseases of the biliary system, such as primary biliary cholangitis and primary sclerosing cholangitis, also result in liver dysfunction and failure.[108]

The liver has a remarkable regenerative capacity. After injury and necrosis, liver cells rapidly regenerate around areas of surviving cells to restore the lost tissue while maintaining homeostasis during hepatic regeneration.[109] However, with chronic injury, fibrosis or scarring occurs, resulting in the loss of the functional architecture and cell mass and ultimately in cirrhosis. Cirrhosis results in destruction of the normal liver vasculature, increased resistance to blood flow and back pressure into the portal circulation. Dilation of the venous system leading into the liver results in the formation of varices.[110]

Liver cell injury may occur to such a degree that a critical amount of hepatic necrosis results in the failure of the liver to maintain metabolic, synthetic and clearance functions, leading to death. Liver cell injury may also occur more slowly, giving rise to chronic liver injury.[111]

Epidemiology of viral hepatitis

Viral hepatitis affects hundreds of millions of people worldwide and is caused by five unrelated viruses which cause most of the global burden of viral hepatitis. Hepatitis B virus (HBV) and hepatitis C virus (HCV) are associated with significant morbidity, and most deaths from viral hepatitis are attributed to HBV and HCV.[112] Worldwide, the incidence of hepatitis B and C is estimated to be 330 million,[112] with the largest proportion (approximately 257 million) being people infected with hepatitis B. From 2010 to 2019 the overall global incidence of HBV has decreased from 1242 per 100,000 to 1002 per 100,000. A high mortality rate from hepatitis accounts for approximately 1.3 million deaths worldwide annually.[113] The highest incidence of acute HBV was reported for Western sub-Saharan Africa (2926.9/100,000) and Oceania (2328.6/100,000). Over time the prevalence of hepatitis B has decreased in some areas, probably because of public health measures and vaccination.[114] Regionally, the seroprevalence of hepatitis C varies, with the highest rates observed in Central, South and East Asia, North Africa and the Middle East.

In the same time period (2010–19), HCV initially declined then began to increase again in 2019. In 2019 the global incidence of HCV was 7.39 per 100,000.[113] The greatest decline in HCV incidence was observed in Western Europe, while the greatest increase was in East Asia. It should be noted, however, that approximately 25% of people with hepatitis C virus exposure have cleared the virus and are not chronically infected. Also, many patients can be cured of hepatitis C virus with newer therapies such as direct-acting antivirals; however, lack of access to antiviral therapy may limit the number of people who can be successfully treated and reducing newer infections is a major focus of health organisations.[115]

Alcohol-related liver disease

Alcohol-induced liver damage is an increasingly common cause of liver disease, particularly in the developed world.[116] The burden of alcohol-attributable diseases is significant. Globally it is estimated that there are 3 million alcohol-attributable deaths and 131.4 million disability-adjusted life-years, corresponding to 5.3% of all deaths and 5.0% of disability-adjusted life years. Alcohol use is a major risk factor for communicable, maternal, perinatal and nutritional diseases, non-communicable diseases and injury.[117] The mechanisms by which alcohol causes liver damage are complex and multifactorial.[118] The main factors involved in developing alcoholic fatty liver are increased production of toxic substances from alcohol metabolism, as well as ethanol having a direct effect on metabolic pathways.[119] In some individuals with alcoholic fatty livers, this will progress to a marked inflammatory stage, called alcoholic steatohepatitis (or alcoholic hepatitis). This is thought to be due to several other factors including acetaldehyde-induced toxic effects leading to oxidative stress (a byproduct of ethanol metabolism), the creation of reactive oxygen species (ROS) and the release of proinflammatory cytokines. Up to 44% of patients with severe alcoholic hepatitis die within 6 months after the onset of symptoms, so appropriate management is key.[120] Non-severe alcoholic hepatitis is also not without consequences and is associated with 13% mortality at 1 year.[121]

The onset of the clinical syndrome in alcoholic hepatitis is characterised by rapid-onset jaundice, fever, ascites and sarcopenia. Biochemically you would expect to find raised hepatic enzymes, raised white cell count, increased serum total bilirubin and a prolonged clotting time. The presence of a raised serum creatinine is a poor prognostic marker as it usually precedes renal failure and death.[119] Regular alcohol consumption of >20 g/d in females and >30 g/d in males where there are also clinical or biological abnormalities suggestive of liver injury is suggestive of alcoholic liver disease. There are several scoring systems including Maddrey's discriminant function, the Glasgow Alcoholic Hepatitis (GAH) score, the model for end-stage liver disease (MELD), the ABIC (**a**ge, serum **b**ilirubin, **i**nternational normalised ratio (INR) and serum **c**reatinine) score and the Lille model used for the assessment of severity of alcoholic hepatitis and to guide treatment, all using varied selections of biochemical markers (Table 20.10).[119]

The treatment of alcoholic hepatitis consists of the management of associated symptoms, as in any form of decompensated liver disease, and the mitigation of organ failure (Fig. 20.9). Any approach should include treatment of acute alcohol withdrawal syndrome (short-acting benzodiazepines) and the provision of adequate nutrition. Pharmacological treatment for alcoholic hepatitis is now led by corticosteroids, even though the benefit is short lived.[122] There are several potential therapies that are currently being explored which target malnutrition, intestinal dysbiosis, bile acid production, hepatocyte death, hepatocyte regeneration and life-threatening complications of the disease.[122] The effectiveness of these potential therapies will require ongoing high-quality research. There has been limited evidence for the use of liver transplantation for acute alcoholic hepatitis, but this is only in carefully selected patient groups who are not responding to medical therapy and has yet to be replicated on a wider scale.[123]

Acute and chronic liver failure

Liver dysfunction can be acute or chronic. Chronic liver disease is usually associated with cirrhosis and can develop from viral (hepatitis B and C), drug (alcohol), metabolic (Wilson's disease) or autoimmune (primary biliary cholangitis) conditions. Acute liver failure (ALF) is an

---

TABLE 20.10

Prognostic scores used in alcoholic hepatitis[119]

SCORE	BILIRUBIN	PT/INR	CREATININE/ UREA	LEUKOCYTES	AGE	ALBUMIN	CHANGE IN BILIRUBIN FROM DAY 0 TO DAY 7
Maddrey	+	+	−	−	−	−	−
MELD	+	+	+	−	−	−	−
GAHS	+	+	+	+	+	−	−
ABIC	+	+	+	−	+	+	−
Lille	+	+	+	−	+	+	+

ABIC = age, serum bilirubin and serum creatinine score; GAHS = Glasgow Alcoholic Hepatitis Score; INR = international normalised ratio; Maddrey = Maddrey discriminant function; MELD = model for end-stage liver disease.

Source: European Association for the Study of the Liver. Electronic address, easloffice@easloffice.eu; & European Association for the Study of the LIVER (2018, Jul). EASL clinical practice guidelines: management of alcohol-related liver disease. J Hepatol 2018;69(1):154–81.

FIGURE 20.9 Treatment algorithm in patients with suspected alcoholic hepatitis (AH). BW = body weight; DILI = drug-induced liver injury; GAHS = Glasgow Alcoholic Hepatitis Score; mDF = multi-drug fusion; NAC = N-acetylcysteine.

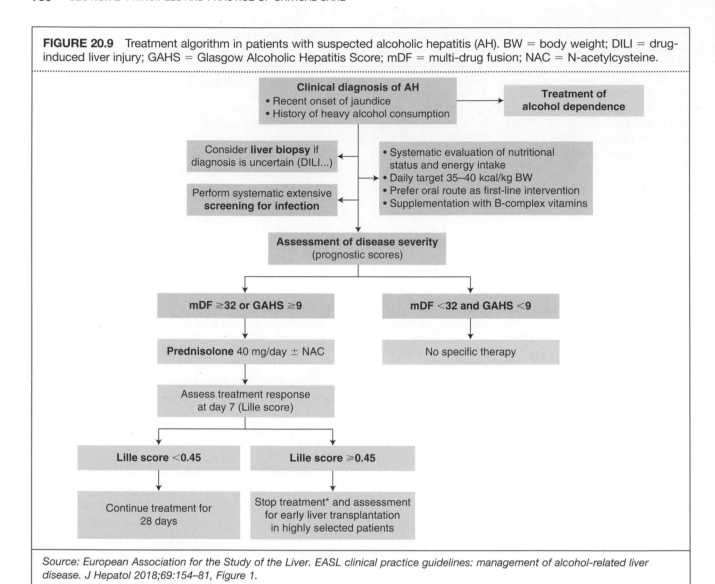

Source: European Association for the Study of the Liver. EASL clinical practice guidelines: management of alcohol-related liver disease. J Hepatol 2018;69:154–81, Figure 1.

uncommon condition associated with rapid liver dysfunction leading to jaundice, hepatic encephalopathy (HE) and coagulopathy.[124] Terminology for acute liver failure is not standardised and several terms have been proposed, including acute hepatic failure and fulminant hepatic failure. Historically, fulminant hepatic failure was used to refer to the rapid onset of liver failure accompanied by HE within 8 weeks of diagnosis in the absence of pre-existing liver disease.[101] Unfortunately, this was problematic because determining the onset of jaundice and encephalopathy is often difficult and coagulation results, such as the INR, are more reliable indicators of liver failure. It has also been proposed that 'hyperacute', 'acute' and 'subacute' liver failure should be used instead, with hyperacute liver failure referring to the development of encephalopathy within 7 days of the onset of jaundice, acute related to 8–28 days from jaundice to encephalopathy and subacute when encephalopathy occurs within 5–12 weeks of the onset of jaundice.[125] It has further been proposed

that acute and subacute hepatic failure should be used; however, universal acceptance of these terms has not occurred, with clinical use of all of the above terms.

ALF without pre-existing liver disease can result from drug reactions, toxins or viral infection, or from the effect on inflammatory mediators released in response to tissue injury. Liver failure can also occur as an acute decompensation of chronic liver disease, described as acute-on-chronic liver failure (ACLF) or as an end-stage decompensation in chronic liver failure. ACLF is a syndrome with heterogeneous definitions but is broadly characterised by severe acute hepatic dysfunction with associated extrahepatic organ failure and high short-term mortality, which can be precipitated by bacterial or viral infection, bleeding or intoxication and results in a severe clinical syndrome similar to that seen in ALF; however, osmotic compensatory mechanisms that fail in ALF tend to remain effective in ACLF, therefore making the development of intracranial hypertension less common.[126]

In ACLF, the function of the residual liver cell mass may be adequate to maintain hepatic homeostasis if the precipitating event can be treated, returning the patient to a compensated phase of their underlying disease. Definitions of ACLF differ internationally, although each definition recognised ACLF as being a distinct clinical entity.

End-stage decompensation of chronic liver failure represents irreversible deterioration with inadequate residual function to maintain homeostasis, and liver transplantation is the only long-term viable treatment. However, several studies have reported improvements in prognosis for patients with cirrhosis admitted to the ICU, and each patient's clinical situation should be considered rather than the presence of underlying chronic liver disease excluding these patients from ICU admission.[127]

Liver dysfunction is also a common consequence of critical illness and may be caused by inadequate perfusion leading to ischaemic injury or be a result of the inflammatory response in sepsis. Given the number of drugs that critically ill patients receive, the possibility of liver injury as a result of drug reactions and toxicity should always be considered.[128] Causes, definitions and key points can be seen in Fig. 20.10.[129]

Consequences of liver failure

The consequences of liver failure manifest as a syndrome of HE, renal dysfunction or hepatorenal syndrome (HRS), oesophageal and gastric varices, ascites, respiratory compromise, haemodynamic instability, susceptibility to infection, coagulopathy and metabolic derangement, with notable differences in presentation and treatment between acute (without pre-existing liver disease) and chronic presentations (Fig. 20.11).[128]

Hepatic encephalopathy

HE is a reversible neuropsychiatric complication due to metabolic dysfunction associated with liver disease.[130] The cerebral effects of liver failure may manifest as an altered sleep–wake cycle, mild confusion/disorientation, asterixis and coma. Patients with ACLF may develop a mild degree of cerebral oedema, while a differential feature of ALF is the risk of death from cerebral oedema and raised intracranial pressure.[131]

The mechanisms responsible for the development of HE are unclear, with both systemic and cerebral factors contributing to brain dysfunction (Fig. 20.12).[130] Raised ammonia levels resulting from the failure of the liver urea cycle are thought to be central to the pathogenesis. The raised ammonia levels disrupt the blood–brain barrier, which can lead to the development of cerebral oedema, a life-threatening complication in ALF. There are multiple ways in which increased ammonia levels contribute to HE including cellular swelling, inflammation, oxidative stress, mitochondrial dysfunction, disruption of cellular bioenergetics, altered pH and alterations in the membrane

FIGURE 20.10 Causes of liver insults, definitions and key points of intensive care acquired acute liver injury, hepatic dysfunction and acute liver failure. ALP = alkaline phosphatase; ALT = alanine aminotransferase; AST = aspartate aminotransferase; γ-GT = γ-glutamyl transpeptidase; ICG-PDR = indocyanine green plasma disappearance rate; INR = international normalised ratio.

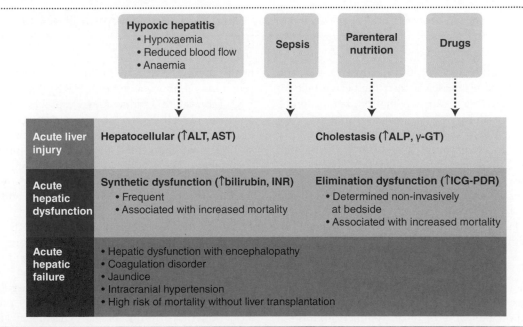

Source: Reproduced from Lescot T, Karvellas C, Beaussier M, Magder S. Acquired liver injury in the intensive care unit. Anesthesiology: The Journal of the American Society of Anesthesiologists 2012 Oct 1;117(4):898–904.

FIGURE 20.11 Liver as a trigger of organ injury and failure.

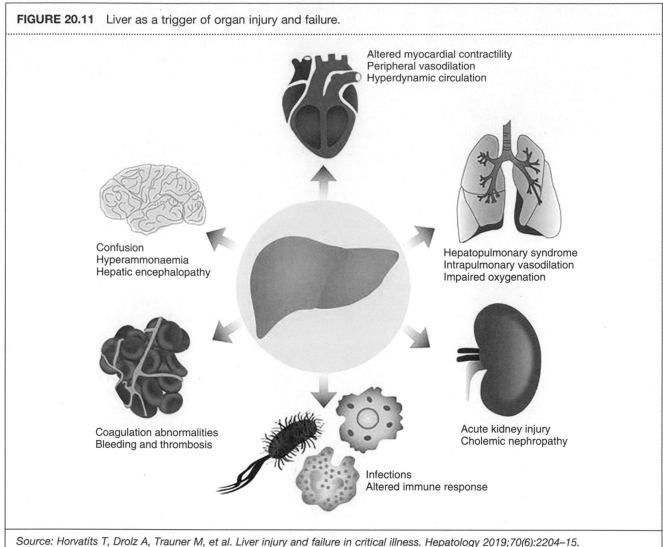

Altered myocardial contractility
Peripheral vasodilation
Hyperdynamic circulation

Confusion
Hyperammonaemia
Hepatic encephalopathy

Hepatopulmonary syndrome
Intrapulmonary vasodilation
Impaired oxygenation

Coagulation abnormalities
Bleeding and thrombosis

Acute kidney injury
Cholemic nephropathy

Infections
Altered immune response

Source: Horvatits T, Drolz A, Trauner M, et al. Liver injury and failure in critical illness. Hepatology 2019;70(6):2204–15.

potential.[132] In addition, ROS causing oxidative stress and inflammatory cytokine release can alter the permeability of the blood–brain barrier and can drive neuroinflammation.[130]

Traditionally HE has been classified using the West Haven criteria, a four-stage scale, according to the severity of clinical signs and symptoms (Table 20.11).[133] Although used in clinical practice, the West Haven criteria have poor sensitivity and no inherent metric component, with poor interobserver reliability. Classification of HE should incorporate the underlying context, severity, time course, precipitating factors and response and dependence on hypoammonemic treatments.[134]

Hepatorenal syndrome

HRS is the development of renal failure in patients with severe liver disease (acute or chronic), in the absence of any other identifiable cause of renal dysfunction; this is a diagnosis of exclusion and therefore acute kidney injury (AKI) should always be considered as the first potential cause of any renal dysfunction. AKI that develops rapidly

in the setting of ALF or ACLF is classified as HRS-AKI (previously known as type 1 HRS). Slowly progressing AKI (non-acute kidney injury), previously referred to as type 2 HRS, is now known as HRS-NAKI (Table 20.12).[135] The definition of AKI in cirrhosis has also been based on the Kidney Disease Improving Global Outcomes (KDIGO) serum creatinine criteria.[136] However, oliguria is also a sensitive and early marker for AKI in critically ill patients with cirrhosis and should also be considered.[137]

The pathophysiological features of HRS appear to be caused by an inflammatory response from the injured liver, resulting in upregulation of nitric oxide production that results in splanchnic vasodilation.[138] Splanchnic vasodilation results in redistribution of circulating blood volume and a lowered mean arterial pressure. The reduction in perfusion pressure results in an enhanced sympathetic nervous system response and local renal autoregulatory responses. The net result of these effects is a reduction in renal blood[137] (see Chapter 18).

FIGURE 20.12   Pathogenesis and pathophysiology of hepatic encephalopathy (HE). BBB = blood–brain barrier; ROS/RNS = reactive oxygen species/reactive nitrogen species; TIPS = transjugular intrahepatic portosystemic stent/shunt.

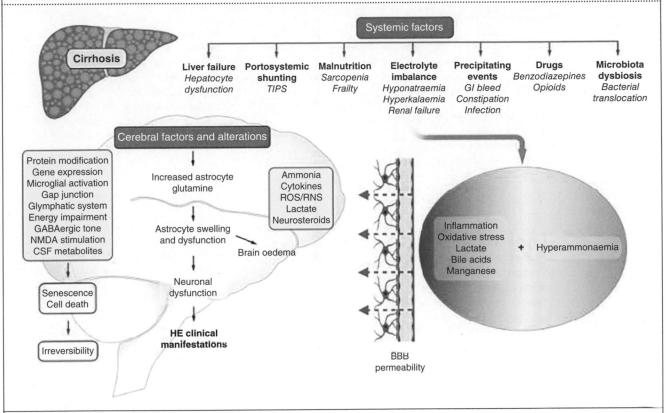

Source: Rose CF, Amodio P, Bajaj JS, et al. Hepatic encephalopathy: novel insights into classification, pathophysiology and therapy, J Hepatol 2020;73(6):1526–47, Figure 2.

Practice tip

Using lactate- or citrate-buffered substitution/dialysis fluid for renal replacement therapy in patients with very severe liver dysfunction should be undertaken with caution, as they may be unable to metabolise the lactate or citrate and could develop an increasing metabolic acidosis.

Varices and variceal bleeding

The development of varices and variceal bleeding arises from portal hypertension. This manifests when blood flowing from an area of high pressure (i.e. the cirrhotic liver) to areas of lower pressure (i.e. the collateral circulation, involving veins of the oesophagus, spleen, intestines and stomach) causes the tiny, thin-walled vessels to become engorged and dilated, forming varices that are vulnerable to gastric secretions, and resulting in rupture and haemorrhage.[139] Variceal haemorrhage is a major cause of acute decompensation and a reason for admission to the ICU. It is an acute clinical event characterised by severe gastrointestinal haemorrhage presenting as haematemesis, with or without melaena, and haemodynamic instability (tachycardia and hypotension).[140]

Practice tip

Coagulation state and the risk of trauma to varices should be carefully considered before insertion of nasogastric or orogastric tubes or suctioning of the upper airway. Trauma may result in epistaxis with significant bleeding or variceal bleeding.

Ascites

Ascites is one of the most common complications of cirrhosis, arising from the same pathophysiological mechanisms underlying the formation of varices (portal hypertension). In the ICU setting it becomes an issue when abdominal pressures rise, resulting in reduced cardiac output due to decreased venous return and renal impairment. Pressure on the diaphragm causes loss of lung volume, resulting in increased work of breathing and

TABLE 20.11

West Haven grading of hepatic encephalopathy[133]

	GRADE	CHARACTERISTICS
Covert	MHE	Psychometric or neuropsychological alterations of tests exploring psychomotor speed/executive functions or neurophysiological alterations without clinical evidence of mental change
	I	Trivial lack of awareness Euphoria or anxiety Shortened attention span Impaired performance of simple tests, e.g. addition
Overt	II	Lethargy or apathy Subtle personality changes Inappropriate behaviour
	III	Somnolence to semistupor, but unresponsive to verbal stimuli Confusion Gross disorientation
	IV	Coma: unresponsive to verbal or painful stimuli

TABLE 20.12

Definitions of hepatorenal syndrome[135]

	DEFINITION
HRS-AKI	• Increase in serum creatinine of ≥0.3 mg/dL within 48 h, *or*
	• Increase in serum creatinine ≥1.5 times from baseline (creatine value within previous 3 months, when available, may be used as baseline, and value closest to presentation should be used).
	• No response to diuretic withdrawal and 2-day fluid challenge with 1 g/kg/day of albumin 20–25%.
	• Cirrhosis with ascites.
	• Absence of shock.
	• No current or recent use of nephrotoxic drugs.

	• No signs of structural kidney injury:
	  ○ absence of proteinuria (>500 mg/day
	  ○ absence of haematuria (>50 RBCs per high-power field)
	  ○ normal findings on renal ultrasound.

HRS-NAKI (HRS-AKD)	• Estimated glomerular filtration rate of <60 mL/min/1.73 m² for <3 months in absence of other potential causes of kidney disease.
	• Percentage increase in serum creatinine <50% using last-available value of outpatient serum creatinine within 3 months as baseline value.
HRS-NAKI (HRS-CKD)	• Estimated glomerular filtration rate <60 mL/min/1.73 m³ for ≥3 months in absence of other potential causes of kidney disease.

AKD = acute kidney disease; AKI = acute kidney injury; CKD = chronic kidney disease; HRS = hepatorenal syndrome; NAKI = non-acute kidney injury; RBC = red blood cell.

Source: Adapted from Simonetto DA, Gines P, Kamath PS. Hepatorenal syndrome: pathophysiology, diagnosis, and management BMJ 2020;370:m2687.

compromised oxygenation. The presence of ascites can also lead to bacterial translocation from the gut, potentially causing spontaneous bacterial peritonitis and sepsis.[141]

Respiratory compromise

Patients with liver failure may have poor oxygen exchange, fluctuating Glasgow Coma Scale score that requires intubation for airway protection, and hepatopulmonary syndrome. Hepatopulmonary syndrome is found in up to 30% of patients with cirrhosis.[142] It is defined as heterogeneous pulmonary microvascular dilation resulting in impaired oxygenation, and it is generally assumed that vascular production of vasodilators, specifically nitric oxide, underlies the vasodilation in hepatopulmonary syndrome. It has also been hypothesised that the mechanisms that trigger hepatopulmonary syndrome are the same as those that result in the hyperdynamic circulation (low systemic vascular resistance and high cardiac output) seen in liver failure.[102,142] Other factors, such as pleural effusions or severe ascites, may impinge on ventilation.

Haemodynamic instability, susceptibility to infection, coagulopathy and metabolic derangement

A hyperdynamic, low-vascular-resistance picture, similar to that associated with sepsis, is seen in liver dysfunction. This probably results from the production, and reduction in clearance, of vasodilator substances (nitric oxide) from the inflammatory response of the injured liver cells. Sepsis may also be a complication of liver dysfunction because of the failure of the liver to produce acute-phase proteins and the impaired function of Kupffer cells, leading to a functional immunosuppression.[102]

Hepatocyte damage leads to a decreased production of the majority of clotting factors and, therefore, alters haemostatic function. However, conventional laboratory tests correlate poorly with actual occurrence of haemostatic complications; importantly, not only is the risk of bleeding elevated in liver dysfunction, but thrombosis can also occur.[102] The presence and severity of marked coagulopathy is a strong prognostic indicator.

Disordered metabolic function and failure of synthetic function can manifest as unstable blood glucose levels.

> **Practice tip**
>
> Patients in ALF or ACLF are at risk of hypoglycaemia, and blood glucose levels should be measured routinely.

Patient assessment

Early signs of the patient presenting with ALF are malaise, loss of appetite, fatigue, nausea, jaundice, bruising, bleeding, inflamed/enlarged liver, possibly epigastric and right-upper-quadrant pain, deranged liver function tests, fluctuating Glasgow Coma Scale score due to HE and high or low blood glucose levels.[143] Fluctuating blood glucose levels may require close monitoring, at least every 4 hours; patients may require insulin infusion or 10–50% dextrose infusion to maintain normoglycaemia. If ALF is suspected, admission to an ICU is recommended to monitor for further deterioration and provide supportive management and airway protection.

The patient presenting with ACLF will have similar symptoms but will present with other unique characteristics. Cirrhosis and portal hypertension will often lead to oesophageal and gastric varices, ascites, renal and pulmonary dysfunction, malnutrition, bone disease, sepsis, palmar erythema, spider naevi and feminisation in males.[144] If liver failure is suspected, investigating ingestion of hepatotoxic substances, such as paracetamol, steroids and ethanol, oral or intravenous recreational drug use and any recent travel that might have exposed the patient to viral infections is required. Early referral to specialist services, especially in ALF, is key to offering all treatment options.

Neurological considerations

Cerebral oedema is present in 80% of patients with grade IV encephalopathy and is the leading cause of death due to brain herniation.[145] Patients with cerebral oedema and raised intracranial pressure due to ALF are managed primarily as patients with acute head injury (see Chapter 17); however, there are important differences in pathophysiology that must be considered, as some treatment strategies used in acute brain injury may not be effective.

Assessment of liver function

Patients presenting with ALF require a careful history to establish the cause of liver injury. The well-known signs of chronic liver disease (e.g. palmar erythema, spider naevi and ascites) may not be present. Biochemical and haematological tests determine whether liver cell injury is occurring, with liver synthesis and clearance functions assessed by albumin level and prothrombin time and bilirubin level respectively.[146] These measures have been incorporated into a scoring system to determine liver dysfunction and prognostic information for liver transplantation suitability (MELD) (see later in this chapter under Liver transplantation). Liver function test values and indications are listed in Table 20.13.[147]

Treatment

ALF or ACLF therapy often involves the support and treatment of the consequences of liver failure, such as sepsis, encephalopathy, renal failure and coagulopathy (Table 20.14).[148–152] Treatments are usually directed to supportive therapy, depending on the severity of manifestation; liver transplantation may be required for patients who do not recover from ALF spontaneously, with approximately half of patients admitted with ALF receiving a liver transplant.[153]

Oesophageal balloon tamponade and transjugular intrahepatic portosystemic stent/shunt

When treatment of acute variceal bleeding is not successful with vasoactive drugs, fluid resuscitation and/or vessel ligation, alternative strategies such as balloon tamponade and transjugular intrahepatic portosystemic stent shunt (TIPSS) may be required. There are several types of balloon tamponade devices available on the market – the Sengstaken–Blakemore tube, the Linton tube and the Minnesota tube (Fig. 20.13)[154] – which can be inserted once the patient is intubated and resuscitated. The Sengstaken–Blakemore tube is a three-lumen tube with oesophageal and gastric balloons, and gastric aspiration port. The Minnesota tube adds a fourth lumen to allow oesophageal aspiration. The benefit of these tubes is that direct pressure can be applied to gastric and oesophageal varices by balloon inflation and traction. The Linton tube has one lumen for inflation of the pear-shaped gastric balloon and two additional lumens for oesophageal and gastric aspiration.

Prior to insertion (oral or nasal), balloons are lubricated, checked for leakage and the distance to the cardio-oesophageal junction is estimated (nose to ear, then to the xiphisternum). Once inserted, the gastric balloon is inflated with 50 mL air and pulled back until resistance is felt. The position (lying compressed against the cardio-oesophageal junction) is confirmed by X-ray. Then the gastric balloon is inflated according to the manufacturer's instructions and traction is applied with skin traction; the

TABLE 20.13
Liver function tests[147]

BLOOD TEST	NORMAL VALUE	DESCRIPTION
Alanine aminotransferase (ALT) and aspartate aminotransferase (AST)	ALT: <35 U/L AST: <40 U/L	• ALT and AST are enzymes that indicate liver cell damage; they are produced within the liver cells (hepatocytes) and leak out into the general circulation when the liver cells are damaged. • ALT is a more specific (but less sensitive) indication of liver inflammation. • In acute liver injury, ALT and AST may be elevated to the high 100s, even 1000s, of U/L. • In chronic liver damage, such as hepatitis or cirrhosis, there may be mild-to-moderate elevation (100–300 U/L). • ALT and AST are commonly used to measure the course of chronic hepatitis and the response to treatments.
Alkaline phosphatase (ALP) and gamma-glutamyl-transpeptidase (GGT)	ALP: 25–100 U/L GGT: males <50 U/L; females <30 U/L	• These are enzymes that indicate obstruction to the biliary system. • They are produced in the liver, or within the larger bile channels outside the liver. • GGT is used as the supplementary test to be sure that a rise in ALP is indeed coming from the liver or biliary tree. • A rise in GGT but normal ALP may indicate liver enzyme changes induced by alcohol or medications, causing no injury to the liver. • ALP and GGT are commonly used to measure bile flow obstructions due to disorders such as gallstones, a tumour blocking the common bile duct, biliary tree damage, alcoholic liver disease or drug-induced hepatitis.
Bilirubin	<20 micromol/L	• Results from the breakdown of red blood cells. Therefore, bilirubin is protein bound and circulates in the blood in an unconjugated form. The liver processes bilirubin to a water-soluble conjugated form that is excreted in the urine and faeces. • Liver injury or cholestasis results in an elevated bilirubin level. • Raised unconjugated bilirubin without an accompanying rise in conjugated bilirubin is consistent with red blood cell destruction (haemolysis). • Raised bilirubin levels result in jaundice. • In cases of chronic liver disease, bilirubin levels usually remain normal until significant damage occurs and cirrhosis develops. • In cases of acute liver failure (ALF), bilirubin levels will rise rapidly and result in marked jaundice; the degree of rise is indicative of the severity of illness.
Albumin	32–45 g/L	• Albumin is a major protein formed by the liver; it provides a gauge of liver synthetic function (i.e. albumin levels are lowered in liver disease).

Source: Pagana KD, Pagana TJ. Mosby's manual of diagnostic and laboratory tests. 3rd ed. St Louis, MO: Mosby Elsevier; 2006.

use of a weight (500 or 1000 mL IV fluid bag) attached to a rope occurs in some settings but the risk of tube migration is enhanced.[154] Nursing care of patients involves:

• sedation for comfort
• the head of the bed raised at least 30 degrees to facilitate gastric emptying and prevent aspiration
• ensuring that gastric/oesophageal ports are on free drainage, with regular monitoring of type and amount of drainage
• ensuring that correct traction is maintained, with regular checking of tube migration and checking the position at the nares/lips at regular intervals (4/24 hours).

Tamponade is generally maintained for 24 hours, then traction is removed and the balloon deflated to assess for further bleeding. If the patient is stabilised, endoscopy can be performed. If bleeding persists, the balloon(s) is/are re-inflated and traction reapplied.[155]

Once the patient has been stabilised, a TIPSS may be considered to control variceal haemorrhage. TIPSS is a metal expandable stent inserted to decompress the portal venous system, providing an artificial communication vessel between the portal and hepatic veins in the liver and alleviating portal pressure.[139]

Extracorporeal liver support

The aim of extracorporeal liver support therapy is to allow time for liver recovery or to provide support until a liver transplant is possible. There are two main types of extracorporeal liver support therapy, namely artificial (detoxification) and bioartificial devices (which provide

TABLE 20.14

Treatment of liver failure complications[124,135,149–153]

CONDITION	TREATMENT
Hepatic encephalopathy	• Treatment revolves around general supportive therapy until liver function recovers or liver transplant is undertaken. • Cerebral oedema and raised intracranial pressure are treated as for an acute head injury (see Chapter 17). • Reduce production and absorption of ammonia by preventing/controlling upper gastrointestinal bleeding. • Gastrointestinal administration of non-absorbable disaccharides such as lactulose or lactitol to remove ammonia from the blood and may be administered in conjunction with non-absorbable antibiotics such as rifaximin. • Continuous renal replacement therapy can also be useful in the removal of circulating ammonia. • As HE progresses, intubation may be required for airway protection. Mechanical ventilation strategies should target prevention of hypercapnia. Caution should be exercised when considering sedative and muscle relaxant agents for intubation in order to minimise increases in ICP.
Hepatorenal syndrome	• Liver transplant is the primary treatment for HRS-AKI in patients with cirrhosis. • If transplant is contraindicated or delayed, vasoconstrictors (e.g. terlipressin) may be effective in constricting the dilated splanchnic arterial bed, improving renal perfusion pressure and renal function. Vasoconstrictors may be given in association with intravenous albumin in order to increase intravascular volume. • Bacterial infections should be ruled out, although the benefit of antibiotics in established AKI-HRS is not evident.
Variceal bleeding	• A successful outcome, as in all cases of gastrointestinal haemorrhage, hinges on prompt resuscitation, haemodynamic support and correction of haemostatic dysfunction, preferably in the intensive care setting. • The patient is intubated for airway protection. • Adequate intravenous access in inserted, preferably large, wide-bore cannulas for rapid fluid resuscitation. • Haemodynamic instability is corrected with volume expanders initially and then blood products. • The source of bleeding is identified by endoscope, and varices are banded/ligated (latex bands placed around the varices to 'strangle' the vessel), or sclerotherapy or diathermy (heat used to cauterise a bleeding vessel) is used. • Terlipressin, vasopressin, somatostatin or octreotide infusions may be used to reduce portal circulation pressure. • Endoscopic band ligation after haemodynamic stabilisation within 6–12 hours of bleeding from eosphageal varices is detected. • Transjugular intrahepatic portosystemic shunt (TIPSS) may be used to lower portal pressure. • If bleeding is uncontrollable, a balloon tamponade device can be inserted.
Ascites	• Salt and water restrictions along with diuretic therapy are methods that have been used to control ascites in the preliminary phases of end-stage liver failure; however, in the intensive care setting these measures are impractical and usually unsuccessful. • Paracentesis is very effective at reducing ascites and is a simple procedure to remove fluid and an aid in diagnosis. • Correction of coagulopathy or thrombocytopenia should be considered when the international normalised ratio is greater than 2.5 or the platelet count is markedly reduced. • Paracentesis may aid in determining the cause of ascites (ascites-serum albumin gradient, ascitic cytology, microscopy and culture for acid-fast bacilli, chylous ascites) and in establishing or excluding primary or secondary peritonitis in patients with ascites (ascitic white cell and neutrophil count, culture). • Litres of ascites are normally removed, and the volume is replaced with IV concentrated albumin to prevent fluid shifts and hypotension. • Mean arterial pressures, central venous pressures, heart rate and urine output are carefully monitored during the procedure.

AKI = acute kidney injury; HE = hepatic encephalopathy; HRS = hepatorenal syndrome; ICP = intracranial pressure; IV = intravenous.

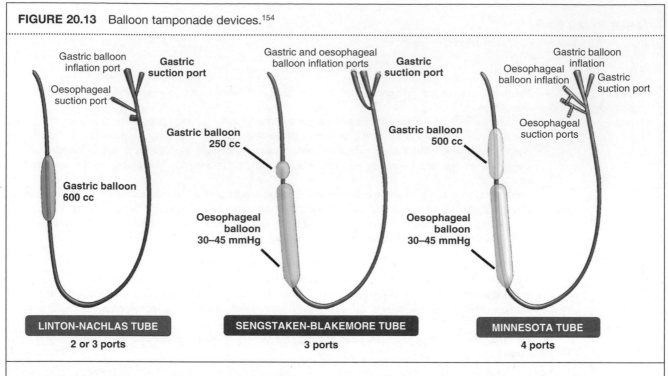

FIGURE 20.13 Balloon tamponade devices.[154]

Source: Bridwell RE, Long B, Ramzy M, et al. Balloon tamponade for the management of gastrointestinal bleeding. J Emerg Med 2022;62(4),545–58.

functional biological activity). The artificial devices are cell-free systems that use a combination of dialysis, mainly using albumin, and plasma exchange. These systems aim to reduce toxins and have been shown to reduce bilirubin and improve HE.[156] In contrast, bioartificial extracorporeal liver support devices are biological systems utilising either porcine hepatocytes or a human hepatoblastoma cell line to sustain temporary hepatic function; however, the construction and use of these devices is complex and has been limited to specialist centres. There are continuing challenges with extracting viable hepatic cells and incorporation into the bioreactors with which the extracorporeal circuits interface, thereby limiting their use.[157]

Despite much research, the clinical use of extracorporeal liver support therapies has been difficult owing to a lack of clinical guidelines about when to institute them and which types of patients should be selected, and technical considerations such as flow rate and duration of therapy have yet to be fully elucidated. The DIALIVE clinical trial evaluated safety as a primary endpoint and also examined clinical and pathophysiological effects and device performance in a recently completed RCT.[158] Although conducted in only 32 patients with ACLF with alcoholic cirrhosis, it was able to demonstrate that DIALIVE was safe and its use could significantly increase the proportion of patients resolving ACLF while reducing the time to resolution, forming a basis for a larger late-phase clinical trial. In many cases, the definitive treatment for severe

ALF is liver transplantation when irreversible liver injury has occurred.[153] However, extracorporeal liver support systems may provide sufficient liver support until transplantation is available.[156] To date, evidence suggests that artificial and bioartificial devices may be used for detoxification and biochemical improvements, but this is not accompanied by survival benefits. High-volume plasmapheresis is the only treatment to demonstrate a statistically significant improvement in transplant-free survival.[159]

Liver transplantation

Liver transplantation is the definitive treatment for patients suffering acute and chronic end-stage liver failure when other supportive critical care therapies have been exhausted. Over the past 20 years, survival after liver transplantation has improved, which has been related to better pretransplant and postoperative therapies and increases in intraoperative surgical refinement and management. This has also reduced time in critical care and reduced the overall hospital length of stay. For patients with acute liver failure, the 1-year survival rate following liver transplantation is 79% in Europe[160] and 84% in the United States.[161] Based on a systematic review and meta-analysis of research published up to 2020, the survival rate for children is highest at 1 year (86.62%) dropping to 68.60 at 10 years, although it is noted that survival rates increase when the study year is more recent.[162]

FIGURE 20.14   The model for end-stage liver disease (MELD/PELD) calculation. INR = international normalised ratio.

MELD

$(3.78 \times \log_e [\text{serum bilirubin*}]) + 11.20[\log_e \text{INR}] + 9.57[\log_e \text{serum creatinine*}] + 6.43$ (constant for liver disease aetiology)

PELD

$(0.436 \times \text{age†}) - (0.687 \times \log [\text{albumin\#}]) + (0.480 \times \log [\text{bilirubin*}]) + (1.857 \times \log [\text{INR}]) + (0.667 \times \text{growth failure‡})$

*   measured in mg/dL
\#   measured in g/dL
†   Age < 1 year = 1; all others = 0
‡   Values > 2 standard deviations from the norm = 1; all others = 0

Source: Reproduced from Protty MB, Haboubi HN, Yeoman AD. Changes in the Model of End-Stage Liver Disease (MELD) scores on day 7 predict mortality in acute on chronic liver disease: the delta-MELD project. J Hepatol 2017;55(1):S387.

Indications for transplantation

Indications for liver transplantation are patients with severe liver disease in whom alternative treatments have been exhausted. Categories consist of ALF, end-stage liver disease, metabolic liver disease and primary liver cancer.[163] Timing and patient selection are of critical importance, as this has contributed to the success of transplantation. Factors considered when assessing candidacy for transplantation include aetiology, age, liver failure scores, clinical picture and social support.[153] Retransplantation for any disorder is considered only in patients with acceptable predicted survival.

Contraindications for transplantation

Patients with extrahepatic malignancy and uncontrolled systemic infection where high-dose immunosuppressive therapy is contraindicated are not suitable for transplantation. Cardiovascular instability with increased vasopressor support is also a contraindication. In addition, patients with alcoholic liver disease with social instability and patients with inadequate or absent social support are relative contraindications owing to increased risk of non-adherence to immunosuppressive therapy.[153]

Recipient selection

Recipient selection for liver transplantation is of critical importance as it affects mortality, especially when determining patients with ALF. There are a variety of prognostic indicators and selection scoring systems, including the Kings College, Clichy, Child–Turcotte–Pugh, MELD and paediatric end-stage liver disease (PELD) scoring systems.[163–165] While there are different systems, most incorporate the severity of HE and coagulation status. The MELD score is a mathematical model that includes bilirubin, creatinine and the INR, which was originally devised to predict survival after TIPSS.[166] More-recent modifications of the MELD score to incorporate sodium as a key predictor of mortality

resulted in the MELD-Sodium (MELD-NA) score and this is now used to more accurately predict mortality, particularly in patients with low MELD scores.[167] The MELD/PELD score is an excellent predictor of mortality, especially in ALF (Fig. 20.14).[168] However, new strategies and methodologies are being explored that may improve future prognostication for transplant hepatology.[169]

Once the need for transplantation is established, the decision to allocate a donor liver to a patient is based on donor and recipient blood group, donor size and size of recipient, suitability of donor liver for splitting, severity of disease, matching of functional status of donor with severity of liver disease, and hepatitis B and C status of donor and recipient. Extensive testing and consultation are part of the liver transplant process. Clinical consultation occurs with hepatologists, clinical nurse consultants, social workers, dietitians, psychiatrists, psychologists and drug and alcohol professionals, if required.

Surgical techniques

Orthotopic liver transplantation

Orthotopic liver transplantation is the replacement of the diseased liver. It was pioneered in the 1960s and has been improved considerably owing to technical aspects of the surgery itself and enhanced haemodynamic stability during the procedure.[170]

Technical aspects of orthotopic liver transplantation are debated and largely based on personal experience and local protocols.[171] Two main techniques are used for orthotopic liver transplantation: portal bypass or the piggyback technique. Portal bypass occurs where an internal temporary portocaval shunt or external venovenous bypass is used.[172] In the piggyback technique, the recipient's inferior vena cava is left and the donor inferior vena cava is piggybacked onto the recipient's inferior vena cava. The advantages of this technique include haemodynamic stability during the anhepatic phase, reduced operating times and reduced use of blood products, enabling a shorter length of hospital stay.[172]

Split-liver transplantation

The disparity between the increasing number of people on transplant waiting lists and the shortage of donor livers available has led to several innovative strategies. Split-liver transplantation occurs when the donated organ is divided for two recipients, with the larger right segment to an adult and the smaller left lobe to a child.[173] The complication rate is higher in split-liver than in whole-liver transplants because of biliary leaks and anastomosis strictures. This technique has significantly reduced the number of children waiting for liver transplantation, although little impact has been made on adult waiting lists.[174]

Auxiliary liver transplantation

Auxiliary liver transplantation consists of implanting a segment of donor liver temporarily, to allow the recipient's native liver to recover. Once recovery has occurred, the donor liver may be removed, or immunosuppression ceased leading the implanted graft to atrophy. This approach is most useful in conditions known to cause reversible ALF (acute viral hepatitis, mushroom toxicity or drug-induced toxicity). This, therefore, potentially removes the long-term requirement for immunosuppression, and hence the associated complications.[175]

Adult living donor liver transplantation

Living donor liver transplantation is an established option for paediatric patients with end-stage liver disease; although it is also undertaken in adults, this remains relatively uncommon.[176] This technique involves removal of the left lobe from the live donor, usually the recipient's parent, which is then transplanted into the child. It is a relatively straightforward procedure, with little risk to the donor.[177] Survival may be superior in living donor liver transplantation compared with deceased donor liver transplantation and there may also be benefits for resource utilisation; however, these findings need to be confirmed in different contexts.[178]

Postoperative management

Initial management and nursing care

The initial postoperative care of liver transplant patients on return to critical care involves stabilisation, management of respiratory function, continuous haemodynamic monitoring and physical assessment, as with all critically ill surgical patients. Prolonged mechanical ventilation is usually not required unless otherwise indicated. Early extubation is associated with improved outcomes in this patient cohort[179] and extubation within a few hours after surgery is completed can be anticipated for most patients.[180] Oliguria is commonly related to intraoperative fluid losses and fluid shifts.

Once initial stabilisation is achieved, treatment is governed by clinical progress. Typically, the critical care stay for a routine postoperative liver transplantation does not exceed 24–48 hours; as long as physiological systems are maintained, discharge to the ward can be anticipated.

The initial postoperative care is similar for all liver transplant patients. However, progress, stability and discharge from critical care can be affected by the patient's preoperative condition and severity of liver failure. The unique pathophysiology inherent in the liver failure patient will predispose to varying effects on coagulopathy, cardiopulmonary, neurological, haemodynamic and metabolic functions.[180]

Blood loss and coagulopathy

The major risk during and postsurgery is massive blood loss, due to a combination of factors. The surgical process itself involves anastomosis of major arteries and veins, predisposing the patient to bleeding and hypovolaemia during surgery and anastomotic leaks postsurgery.[171] Patients are likely to be coagulopathic from hepatic synthetic dysfunction, leading to failure of synthetic clotting factors.[180] Assessment of coagulopathy in patients with end-stage liver disease is difficult when only standard laboratory tests are used. Viscoelastic tests can complement coagulation assessment and reflect the interaction between pro- and anticoagulants and platelets.[181] Correction of coagulopathy with blood products such as fresh frozen plasma, platelets, cryoprecipitate and factor VIIa may control minor postoperative bleeding,[182] but if bleeding continues an exploratory laparotomy may be required. Conversely, it is not desirable to overcorrect coagulopathy, owing to the potential for vascular complications such as hepatic artery thrombosis.[180] Careful monitoring is required to identify and manage hypotension, tachycardia, excessive blood loss from drains, falling haemoglobin, abdominal swelling and oozing from insertion sites. Thrombocytopenia is a common postoperative problem, with platelet counts often falling in the first week post-transplant. If platelet counts are low, a platelet transfusion may be necessary, especially prior to removal of drains, lines, cannulae and sheaths.

Cardiovascular

Cardiovascular complications are not uncommon for patients with end-stage liver disease and are a leading cause of death after liver transplantation; therefore, thorough preoperative cardiovascular evaluation is necessary.[183] In the postoperative period, haemodynamic instability in the early postoperative period may be due to hypovolaemia or haemorrhage. Treatment includes fluid boluses to increase preload and the initiation of inotropes may be necessary, with a low threshold for the introduction of advanced cardiac output monitoring. The patient may present with a hyperdynamic profile including a high cardiac output, low systemic vascular resistance and low mean arterial pressure,[184] although this usually reverses 1 week after transplantation.

Neurological

The most frequent neurological complications relate to patients with pre-existing HE. In ALF patients, cerebral oedema with raised intracranial pressure is common and, after liver transplantation, cerebral oedema may take up to 48 hours to subside. Therefore, continuation of preoperative measures to reduce intracranial pressure is necessary. These include elevating the head of the bed to 30 degrees; ensuring head, neck and body alignment; maintaining endotracheal tapes so they are not constrictive to allow venous return and prevent cerebral congestion; reducing neurological stimuli; and timing activities to prevent spikes in intracranial pressure (see Chapter 17).[184]

Respiratory

Pre-existing pulmonary complications associated with liver disease can affect postoperative recovery and need to be considered when weaning ventilation and maintaining adequate oxygenation. Most patients can be extubated shortly after ICU admission but this will depend on a number of other patient-related factors. Patients post-transplant often experience bi-basal collapse and consolidation, and are prone to infection, similar to other critical care patients who undergo complex surgical procedures that are extended.[185] Incentive spirometry, chest physiotherapy, early mobilisation and adequate pain relief are recommended, with early extubation the most effective intervention in reducing pulmonary complications.[185]

Gastrointestinal

Patients with end-stage liver disease often have malnutrition and bone disease, which may influence postoperative management. Fluid overload and ascites can quite often mask signs of malnutrition. Early nutrition is imperative in the postoperative period, and enteral feeding can supplement caloric needs (see Chapter 19). If caloric intake is inadequate, consultation with a dietitian will assist with enteral supplementation. Total parenteral nutrition is rarely required.

Renal

Renal dysfunction is a significant post-transplantation problem. Risk factors include pre-existing renal disease or HRS, intraoperative hypotension, extensive transfusion of blood products, nephrotoxic drugs such as cyclosporin and tacrolimus, sepsis and graft dysfunction.[184] HRS is reversible post-transplantation. Patients who are receiving renal support such as continuous renal replacement therapy usually require continuation of renal support postoperatively for a period of time until recovery of kidney function is evident (see Chapter 18).

Graft dysfunction and rejection

Retransplantation is required in 7–10% of liver transplants; the most common causes of early graft dysfunction are primary graft non-function and vascular complications.[186] The liver is the most tolerated of transplanted organs.

Immunosuppressive therapy has improved with the use of newer drugs and patients are most commonly placed on a combination of tacrolimus or cyclosporin and steroids.[187] In some stable, long-term patients, immunosuppressive therapy may be removed without graft rejection. For others, chronic allograft injury, late graft failure and adverse effects of antirejection therapy are ongoing problems.[186]

Although the liver is considered the organ that is best tolerated after transplantation, acute cellular rejection occurs in up to one-third of recipients, and chronic rejection occurs in approximately 3–17% of recipients.[188] Hyperacute rejection is rare,[188] and occurs because of formation of antibodies against the donor's major histocompatibility complex and can result in graft destruction.[189] Acute cellular rejection can occur in up to two-thirds of recipients, usually in the 6 weeks following transplantation.[190] Acute cellular rejection results from a T-cell-mediated inflammatory response and patients may be asymptomatic although some may become febrile, and have liver tenderness and non-specific malaise. Chronic rejection, usually preceded by a number of episodes of acute cellular rejection, results in progressive bile duct damage and may result in loss of the graft.[188]

Early allograft dysfunction occurs within 48 hours of transplantation, and is characterised by varying degrees of coma, renal failure, worsening coagulopathy, poor bile production, marked elevation in the liver enzymes and worsening acidosis. The cause of allograft dysfunction is not always known; possible causes are injury to the liver, either before or during the donor operation procedure, ischaemic-reperfusion injury or graft stenosis. Acute rejection is generally evident in the second week post-transplant and is generally suspected with an elevation in liver enzymes, a decline in bile quality (only if a T tube is present), occasional fever and tachycardia.

Primary graft non-function is defined as failure of the graft to function in the first postoperative week, but this can occur much more quickly. It is manifested by failure to regain consciousness, sustained elevated transaminases, increasing coagulopathy, acidosis and poor bile production. Causes include massive haemorrhagic necrosis, ischaemic-reperfusion injury and hepatic artery thrombosis.

Management of late complications

Re-admission to critical care after liver transplantation is not uncommon. Factors include cardiopulmonary dysfunction from infection or fluid overload, respiratory failure from collapse and consolidation, tachypnoea, recipient age, preoperative liver function, bilirubin, the amount of blood products administered intraoperatively, graft dysfunction, severe sepsis and postoperative surgical complications such as bleeding and biliary anastomotic leaks. Outcomes are affected by intraoperative and postoperative complications, renal failure, advanced liver disease and malnutrition.

Summary

The gastrointestinal system can become significantly compromised during critical illness. Alterations in the gastrointestinal system can also cause critical illness. The gastrointestinal system involves not just the gastrointestinal tract but also organs that support digestion including the pancreas and liver. Disruptions to the gastrointestinal system and normal gastrointestinal physiology can be altered during critical illness because of redistribution of blood flow away from the gut and other abdominal organs. Specifically, the gastrointestinal system can become hypoperfused and normal physiological processes responsible for digestion, absorption, immunity and protection become compromised.

Critically ill patients can be at risk of developing stress-related mucosal disease, although the incidence of clinically important bleeding remains relatively low. Nevertheless, it remains common practice to provide stress ulcer prophylaxis to critically ill patients, particularly for those patients considered at high risk. During critical illness, patients may also be at risk for the development of IAH, with approximately half of all ICU patients having increased IAP. Recognising potential risk factors for the development of IAH is essential so that monitoring can be commenced, and treatment initiated where necessary.

Critical illness can also result from the inability of the body to effectively use glucose in energy production. An increasing number of people worldwide have diabetes and when illness occurs this can precipitate significant alterations in blood glucose and result in the development of DKA or HHS. Because of the ensuing physiological derangements, these patients often need to be admitted to a critical care area for close monitoring and treatment until they are stabilised.

Liver dysfunction causing hepatocellular injury and death can occur from direct injury or cellular stress. This can be mediated via several avenues, such as metabolic disturbances, ischaemia, inflammatory processes or reactive oxygen metabolites from drug and alcohol ingestion. Acute failure can be acute or preceded by a chronic dysfunction. High rates of hepatitis B and C predispose individuals to chronic liver dysfunction that can lead to acute hepatic decompensation. While ALF is uncommon, patients who present are often critically ill. In addition, liver failure causes major disturbances in other body systems, often resulting in coagulopathy, cerebral oedema, HE, sepsis, renal failure and metabolic derangement. Therapy is usually directed at multiorgan support as extracorporeal liver support therapies are not sufficiently developed to sustain liver function during the acute phase.

Liver transplantation remains the definitive treatment option for acute-on-chronic liver failure patients when supportive multiorgan therapy is not sustainable. Pre-existing hepatic dysfunction and liver transplantation surgery can lead to a high risk of haemorrhage and coagulopathy postoperatively. Careful haematological management is required to control postoperative bleeding. Clinicians must ensure that patients receive appropriate haemodynamic management for hyperdynamic states and that measures to avoid rises in intracranial pressure are implemented.

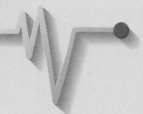

Case study

A 48-year-old female was admitted to the ICU after transfer from a local private hospital, with a history of nausea, vomiting and abdominal pain. Her admission weight was 72 kg and height was 156 cm (BMI 29.6). Her past medical history was unremarkable; alcohol intake was minimal. On examination she had abdominal tenderness in the right upper quadrant and epigastrium.

On admission the initial blood tests showed:

White blood cells	15.9 (4–11 × 10⁹/L)
Creatinine	55 (60–110 micromol/L)
Blood glucose	13.2 mmol/L
Lipase	1987 (0–160 U/L)
Amylase	796 (30–220 U/L)
Alkaline phosphatase	92 (30–110 U/L)
Lactate dehydrogenase	560 IU/L (120–250 U/L)
Alanine aminotransferase	809 (0–45 U/L)
Aspartate aminotransferase	253 (0–35 U/L)
Calcium	2.12 (2.10–2.60 mmol/L)
Bilirubin	70 (0–20 micromol/L)

She was diagnosed with gallstone pancreatitis and during her 7-week ICU stay she developed necrotising gallstone pancreatitis and intra-abdominal collections. Sepsis and systemic inflammatory response syndrome were evident throughout admission and she was administered multiple antibiotics to treat necrosis-associated infection. Respiratory failure was a feature during this admission, with invasive mechanical ventilation required several times during admission. Although extubation was possible on several occasions, she required endoscopy and cyst necrosectomy for removal of necrotic tissue. She developed acute kidney injury requiring dialysis and developed an intestinal ileus. Nutrition support was provided through a nasojejunal tube and she required administration of parenteral and enteral nutrition because of ongoing intolerance, despite use of prokinetic agents.

DISCUSSION

Severe acute pancreatitis is the most serious form of pancreatitis and is associated with a high morbidity and mortality. Initially the patient will exhibit a proinflammatory response, which results in systemic inflammatory response syndrome.[95] After the first few weeks an anti-inflammatory response occurs, which can lead to the development of multiple organ failure, as was the case for this patient, who exhibited respiratory, renal and gut failure. As the necrosis was associated with infection, this necessitated surgical removal of the tissue.

The nursing challenges associated with this patient included managing nutrition support. Although pancreatitis does not typically preclude the administration of enteral nutrition,[94] gastrointestinal inflammation and ileus made administration of enteral nutrition challenging; consequently, supplemental parenteral nutrition was added. Administration of enteral nutrition was also problematic because feeds were repeatedly stopped for endoscopy and removal of necrotic tissue.

Ongoing respiratory failure meant that mechanical ventilation was required. Pancreatitis can result in increased IAP and potentially higher than normal mean airway pressures, making it difficult to deliver adequate tidal volumes. Weaning from ventilation can be more difficult if the patient has decreased respiratory drive and increased work of breathing.

Prolonged ICU admission with nutrition inadequacy and long periods of immobility will impact functional recovery.

CASE STUDY QUESTIONS

1 When a patient is receiving enteral and parenteral nutrition simultaneously, how would you manage the transition enteral nutrition alone?
2 What consequences might prolonged critical illness have for longer-term functional recovery?
3 What complications of pancreatitis could occur and what assessments should be undertaken?

RESEARCH VIGNETTE

Ali Abdelhamid Y, Phillips LK, White MG, et al. Survivors of intensive care with type 2 diabetes and the effect of shared-care follow-up clinics. Chest 2021;159(1):174–85.

Abstract

Background: Follow-up clinics after ICU admission have demonstrated limited benefit. However, existing trials have evaluated heterogeneous cohorts and used physicians who had limited training in outpatient care.

Research question: What are the effects of a 'shared-care' intensivist–endocrinologist clinic for ICU survivors with type 2 diabetes on process measures and clinical outcomes 6 months after hospital discharge, and is it feasible to conduct a larger trial?

Study design and methods: This was a prospective, randomised, single-centre pilot study with blinded outcome assessment. Patients with type 2 diabetes who required ≥5 days of ICU care (mixed medical–surgical ICU) and survived to ICU discharge were eligible. Participants were randomised to attendance at the shared-care clinic 1 month after hospital discharge or usual care. Six months after hospital discharge, participants were assessed for outcomes including glycated haemoglobin, neuropathy, nephropathy, quality of life, return to employment, frailty and healthcare use. The primary outcome was participant recruitment and retention.

Results: During an 18-month period, 42 of 82 eligible patients (51%) were recruited. Four participants (10%) withdrew before assessment at 6 months and 11 (26%) died. At 6 months, only 18 of 38 participants who did not withdraw (47%) were living independently without support, and 24 (63%) required at least one subsequent hospital admission. In the intervention group ($n = 21$), 16 (76%) attended the clinic. Point estimates did not indicate that the intervention improved glycated haemoglobin (+5.6 mmol/mol; 95% CI −6.3 to 17; $P = 0.36$) or quality of life (36-Item Short Form Survey physical summary score, 32 (9) versus 32 (7); $P = 1.0$).

Interpretation: Outcomes for ICU survivors with type 2 diabetes are poor. Because of low participation and high mortality, a larger trial of a shared-care follow-up clinic in this cohort, using the present design, does not appear feasible.

Trial registry: Australian New Zealand Clinical Trials Registry (ANZCTR); No.: ACTRN12616000206426; URL: https://www.anzctr.org.au;

Critique

Glycaemic control in critical illness has long been a focus for critical care clinicians. Similarly, increased attention has been given to recovery following critical illness. In this article by Ali Abdelhamid and colleagues, they turn their attention to survivors of critical illness who had pre-existing type 2 diabetes. Type 2 diabetes affects up to one-third of adult patients admitted to the ICU.[191] Critical illness can exacerbate complications of diabetes including nephropathy and neuropathy.[192] Shared-care models in ambulatory patients with diabetes have been shown to limit complications, leading these authors to hypothesise that a similar model of shared-care involving intensivists and endocrinologists might improve long-term outcomes for survivors of critical illness who had pre-existing type 2 diabetes.

In this single-centre, pilot RCT, patients with type 2 diabetes who remained in the ICU for more than 5 days and were alive at ICU discharge were included in this study. Patients in the intervention group attended a shared-care clinic 1 month after hospital discharge. In preparation for the visit, patients were asked to record their blood glucose at least daily. Prior to the clinic visit a glycated haemoglobin (HbA$_{1c}$) blood test was conducted. During the clinic visit the endocrinologist reviewed the patient's blood glucose diary, adjusted oral hypoglycaemic agents and/or insulin, reviewed all medications and undertook a cardiovascular risk assessment with assessment of blood pressure, lipid profile and aspirin requirements determined in line with established guidelines. A personalised glycaemic target was established, and patients were assessed for complications of diabetes. The intensivist undertook a comprehensive assessment to identify any problems that may have developed as a result of critical illness including pain, airway complications, sensory changes, dysphagia, cognition or communication. Physical function was assessed with referral to the hospital's physiotherapy department, if needed. Psychological assessment was undertaken and, if evidence of anxiety or depression was identified, a referral to the hospital's psychology clinic was provided. Collaborative discussion between the endocrinologist and intensivist determined the need for further health professional referral or an additional clinic visit prior to the 6-month outcome visit. Clinic assessments were communicated to the patient's primary care physician.

As a pilot study, the primary outcome was feasibility, with a focus on recruitment (≥50% of eligible patients) and retention (≥80% of recruited patients) rates. Secondary outcomes included HbA$_{1c}$, hypoglycaemic awareness, neuropathy, nephropathy, health-related quality of life, frailty, employment and healthcare use. Participant satisfaction with ICU care and the follow-up clinic were included. Undertaking a pilot RCT is an important first step to assess the likelihood of a larger trial being successful but also to refine recruitment and retention strategies, evaluate intervention fidelity and assess the data collection strategies.[193]

A total of 82 patients met eligibility criteria and 42 agreed to participate. More patients in the intervention group were receiving insulin before the period of critical illness, the baseline HbA$_{1c}$ was higher and the median duration of mechanical ventilation was twofold greater. Approximately one-third of patients were mildly or moderately frail. Differences between the control and intervention groups may be attributed to the small sample size, which makes achieving equivalence at baseline more challenging.

Over the 18-month study period the recruitment rate was 51%. Declined participation was attributed to competing medical appointments (35%), failure to see benefit (33%) or fatigue/difficulty with travel (30%). There was a 90% retention rate in the study at 6 months. However, 11 (26%) of patients died before completing the outcome assessment;

consequently, data were available for only 62% of those patients who were enrolled. Retention in follow-up studies is challenging, particularly when the intervention is focused on the post discharge period[194] and it is possible that cognitive impairment may have impacted attendance and participation in the intervention. Incorporating cognitive assessment may have helped to determine whether this was an influencing factor, and purposefully including family members as part of the intervention may have assisted with attendance rates and completion of blood glucose recording. Family involvement in ongoing recovery following critical illness can be an important strategy, although this may be difficult to consistently enact for a number of reasons.[195]

The majority of patients attended the clinic alone and during the clinic visit medication changes, investigations and referrals to additional services frequently occurred. A number of complications of ICU admission were identified including voice changes, frozen joints, altered cosmesis, incontinence, fatigue and weakness. Half of patients required a mobility aid. Depression was identified for 3 (19%) participants and anxiety with depression identified for one patient (6%). One patient not already receiving treatment was referred to the general practitioner for follow-up.

Weight loss was observed in many participants and associated with increasing age. Nutrition intake data were not available in this study and nutritional compromise following hospital discharge may require longer-term attention to strategies to optimise nutrition, such as the use of oral nutrition supplements.[196] There was no difference in HbA_{1c} from baseline to 6 months or between the control and intervention groups. Acute kidney injury was observed in more than one-third of patients who required renal replacement therapy in the ICU. Five patients were dialysis dependent; three of these were patients who demonstrated a new progression to dialysis-dependent chronic renal failure. Less than half of participants were alive and living independently without formal supports at 6 months. Health-related quality of life was below that for an age-matched control population, but was similar for both the control and intervention groups. Healthcare use in the 6 months following ICU discharge was substantial. In the study design there was no adjustment made for comorbidities that may have existed prior to the episode of critical illness, and this may have influenced study findings.

A strength of this study is the collaborative nature of follow-up care between the endocrinologist and intensivist, with follow-up to other health professionals included as needed. The study methodology was equally strong, minimising potential biases and incorporating outcome measures that have been identified as important for survivors of critical illness.[197]

When developing future studies exploring the impact of a shared-care model, consideration should be given to interprofessional collaboration, frequency of follow-up, intervention co-design, inclusion of a patient–family dyad where possible and alternative strategies for intervention delivery so as to increase availability to those unable to attend in person. Attention should also be given to identifying patients most likely to benefit, such as those who are most likely to survive the 6 months following hospital discharge.

Learning activities

1   On your next clinical shift, identify what stress ulcer prophylaxis your patient is receiving (if any) and whether they have risk factors for the development of stress-related mucosal disease.

2   When you are next in the clinical area, consider the clinical presentations of the patients in the ICU and identify which patients might most benefit from IAP monitoring.

3   Compare and contrast the physiological changes that occur in DKA and HHS. How do these differences influence the management strategy for restoring normoglycaemia?

4   A patient with acute pancreatitis is admitted to ICU. On dietitian review, the recommendation is to commence enteral feeding via a nasogastric tube. Your experience has been that these patients require small bowel feeding or parenteral nutrition. What is the current evidence base for nutrition support for patients with pancreatitis?

5   What treatment strategies should you anticipate for a patient with alcoholic hepatitis?

6   What would make liver transplantation in patients with alcoholic hepatitis most successful?

Online resources

American Diabetes Association, https://www.diabetes.org/

Australian Diabetes Council, www.nfpfoundation.org.au/organisation/australian-diabetes-council

European Association for the Study of the Liver, https://easl.eu

European Society for Organ Transplantation (ESOT), https://esot.org/

International Diabetes Federation, https://www.idf.org/our-network/regions-members/europe/welcome.html

National Diabetes Education Program, https://www.ndep.nih.gov

Online MELD Calculator, https://optn.transplant.hrsa.gov/resources/allocation-calculators/meld-calculator/

The Australia and New Zealand Liver and Intestinal Transplant Registry, https://www.anzlitr.org/

The Transplantation Society of Australia and New Zealand (TSANZ), https://tsanz.com.au

World Society of the Abdominal Compartment Syndrome (WSACS), https://www.wsacs.org

Further reading

Friedman LS, Martin P. Handbook of liver disease. 4th ed. Philadelphia: Elsevier; 2017.

Holt RIG, Cockram C, Flyvbjerg A, et al. Textbook of diabetes. 5th ed. Hoboken: Wiley Blackwell; 2017.

McDonald D, Ackerman G, Khailova L, et al. Extreme dysbiosis of the microbiome in critical illness. Sphere 2016;1(4):e00199–16.

References

1. Otani S, Coopersmith CM. Gut integrity in critical illness. J Intensive Care 2019;7:17.

2. Miniet AA, Grunwell JR, Coopersmith CM. The microbiome and the immune system in critical illness. Curr Opin Crit Care 2021;27(2):157–63.

3. Asrani VM, Brown A, Huang W, et al. Gastrointestinal dysfunction in critical illness: a review of scoring tools. JPEN J Parenter Enteral Nutr 2020;44(2):182–96.

4. Reintam Blaser A, Preiser J-C, Fruhwald S, et al. Gastrointestinal dysfunction in the critically ill: a systematic scoping review and research agenda proposed by the Section of Metabolism, Endocrinology and Nutrition of the European Society of Intensive Care Medicine. Crit Care 2020;24(1):1–17.

5. Taylor RW. Gut motility issues in critical illness. Crit Care Clin 2016;32(2):191–201.

6. Whitman Z, O'Neil DHR. Gastric disorders: modifications of gastric content, antacids and drugs influencing gastric secretions and motility. Anaesth Intensive Care Med 2017;19(1):25–9.

7. Deane AM, Rayner CK, Keeshan A, et al. The effects of critical illness on intestinal glucose sensing, transporters, and absorption. Crit Care Med 2014;42(1):57–65.

8. Puleo F, Arvanitakis M, Van Gossum A, et al. Gut failure in the ICU. Semin Respir Crit Care Med 2011;32(5):626–38.

9. McClave SA, Lowen CC, Martindale RG. The 2016 ESPEN Arvid Wretlind lecture: the gut in stress. Clin Nutr 2018;37(1):19–36.

10. Zigmond E, Varol C. With respect to macrophages, judge the liver by its cover. Immunity 2017;47(2):219–21.

11. Begley M, Gahan CG, Hill C. The interaction between bacteria and bile. FEMS Microbiol Rev 2005;29(4):625–51.

12. Meng M, Klingensmith NJ, Coopersmith CM. New insights into the gut as the driver of critical illness and organ failure. Curr Opin Crit Care 2017;23(2):143–8.

13. Deane AM, Chapman MJ, Reintam Blaser A, et al. Pathophysiology and treatment of gastrointestinal motility disorders in the acutely ill. Nutr Clin Pract 2019;34(1):23–36.

14. de Jong PR, Gonzalez-Navajas JM, Jansen NJ. The digestive tract as the origin of systemic inflammation. Crit Care 2016;20(1):279.

15. Schmid-Schonbein GW, Chang M. The autodigestion hypothesis for shock and multi-organ failure. Ann Biomed Eng 2014;42(2):405–14.

16. David LA, Maurice CF, Carmody RN, et al. Diet rapidly and reproducibly alters the human gut microbiome. Nature 2014;505(7484):559–63.

17. Fox JG, Boutin SR, Handt LK, et al. Isolation and characterization of a novel Helicobacter species, "Helicobacter macacae," from rhesus monkeys with and without chronic idiopathic colitis. J Clin Microbiol 2007;45(12):4061–3.

18. Assimakopoulos SF, Triantos C, Thomopoulos K, et al. Gut-origin sepsis in the critically ill patient: pathophysiology and treatment. Infection 2018;46(6):751–60.

19. Dive A, Foret F, Jamart J, et al. Effect of dopamine on gastrointestinal motility during critical illness. Intensive Care Med 2000;26(7):901–7.

20. Winter SE, Winter MG, Xavier MN, et al. Host-derived nitrate boosts growth of E. coli in the inflamed gut. Science 2013;339(6120):708–11.

21. Honda K, Littman DR. The microbiome in infectious disease and inflammation. Annu Rev Immunol 2012;30:759–95.

22. Zaborina O, Lepine F, Xiao G, et al. Dynorphin activates quorum sensing quinolone signaling in *Pseudomonas aeruginosa*. PLoS Pathog 2007;3(3):e35.

23. Zaborin A, Smith D, Garfield K, et al. Membership and behavior of ultra-low-diversity pathogen communities present in the gut of humans during prolonged critical illness. mBio 2014;5(5):e01361–14.

24. Albenberg L, Esipova TV, Judge CP, et al. Correlation between intraluminal oxygen gradient and radial partitioning of intestinal microbiota. Gastroenterology 2014;147(5):1055–63.e8.

25. Meyer-Hoffert U, Hornef MW, Henriques-Normark B, et al. Secreted enteric antimicrobial activity localises to the mucus surface layer. Gut 2008;57(6):764–71.

26. Salzman NH, Hung K, Haribhai D, et al. Enteric defensins are essential regulators of intestinal microbial ecology. Nat Immunol 2010; 11(1):76–83.

27. Eaton P, Faulds M. Gastrointestinal dysfunction in the intensive care unit. Surgery 2021;39(10):684–9.

28. Barletta JF, Bruno JJ, Buckley MS, et al. Stress ulcer prophylaxis. Crit Care Med 2016;44(7):1395–405.

29. Ovenden C, Plummer MP, Selvanderan S, et al. Occult upper gastrointestinal mucosal abnormalities in critically ill patients. Acta Anaesthesiol Scand 2017;61(2):216–23.

30. Krag M, Perner A, Wetterslev J, et al. Prevalence and outcome of gastrointestinal bleeding and use of acid suppressants in acutely ill adult intensive care patients. Intensive Care Med 2015;41(5):833–45.

31. Reintam Blaser A, Poeze M, Malbrain ML, et al. Gastrointestinal symptoms during the first week of intensive care are associated with poor outcome: a prospective multicentre study. Intensive Care Med 2013;39(5):899–909.

32. Bardou M, Quenot JP, Barkun A. Stress-related mucosal disease in the critically ill patient. Nat Rev Gastroenterol Hepatol 2015;12(2): 98–107.

33. Barkun A, Bardou M. Proton-pump inhibitor prophylaxis in the ICU – benefits worth the risks? N Engl J Med 2018;379(23):2263–4.

34. Buendgens L, Tacke F. Do we still need pharmacological stress ulcer prophylaxis at the ICU? J Thorac Dis 2017;9(11):4201–4.

35. Gyires K, Feher A. Stress, neuropeptides and gastric mucosa. Curr Pharm Des 2017;23(27):3928–40.

36. Qin X, Sheth SU, Sharpe SM, et al. The mucus layer is critical in protecting against ischemia-reperfusion-mediated gut injury and in the restitution of gut barrier function. Shock 2011;35(3):275–81.

37. Kubicki M, Warrillo SJ. Gastrointestinal problems in intensive care. Anaesth Intensive Care Med 2018;19(3):93–7.

38. Allen A, Flemstrom G. Gastroduodenal mucus bicarbonate barrier: protection against acid and pepsin. Am J Physiol Cell Physiol 2005;288(1):C1–19.

39. Sertaridou E, Papaioannou V, Kolios G, et al. Gut failure in critical care: old school versus new school. Ann Gastroenterol 2015;28(3):309–22.

40. Santos RG, Quirino IE, Viana ML, et al. Effects of nitric oxide synthase inhibition on glutamine action in a bacterial translocation model. Br J Nutr 2014;111(1):93–100.

41. Al-Dorzi HM, Arabi YM. Prevention of gastrointestinal bleeding in critically ill patients. Curr Opin Crit Care 2021;27(2):177–82.

42. Ohbe H, Morita K, Matsui H, et al. Stress ulcer prophylaxis plus enteral nutrition versus enteral nutrition alone in critically ill patients at risk for gastrointestinal bleeding: a propensity-matched analysis. Intensive Care Med 2020;46(10):1948–9.

43. Schnoll-Sussman F, Niec R, Katz PO. Proton pump inhibitors: the good, gad, and ugly. Gastrointest Endosc Clin N Am 2020;30(2):239–51.

44. Plummer MP, Blaser AR, Deane AM. Stress ulceration: prevalence, pathology and association with adverse outcomes. Crit Care 2014;18(2):213.

45. Huang HB, Jiang W, Wang CY, et al. Stress ulcer prophylaxis in intensive care unit patients receiving enteral nutrition: a systematic review and meta-analysis. Crit Care 2018;22(1):20.

46. Evans L, Rhodes A, Alhazzani W, et al. Surviving Sepsis Campaign: international guidelines for management of sepsis and septic shock 2021. Crit Care Med 2021;49(11):e1063–143.

47. Marker S, Krag M, Moller MH. What's new with stress ulcer prophylaxis in the ICU? Intensive Care Med 2017;43(8):1132–4.

48. Krag M, Marker S, Perner A, et al. Pantoprazole in patients at risk for gastrointestinal bleeding in the ICU. N Engl J Med 2018;379(23): 2199–208.

49. Marker S, Krag M, Perner A, et al. Pantoprazole in ICU patients at risk for gastrointestinal bleeding-1-year mortality in the SUP-ICU trial. Acta Anaesthesiol Scand 2019;63(9):1184–90.

50. Schefold JC, Krag M, Marker S, et al. Outcomes of prophylactic pantoprazole in adult intensive care unit patients receiving dialysis: results of a randomized trial. Am J Nephrol 2019;50(4):312–19.

51. Marker S, Perner A, Wetterslev J, et al. Pantoprazole prophylaxis in ICU patients with high severity of disease: a post hoc analysis of the placebo-controlled SUP-ICU trial. Intensive Care Med 2019;45(5):609–18.

52. PEPTIC Investigators for the Australian and New Zealand Intensive Care Society Clinical Trials Group, Alberta Health Services Critical Care Strategic Clinical Network, the Irish Critical Care Trials Group; Young PJ, Bagshaw SM, Forbes AB, et al. Effect of stress ulcer prophylaxis with proton pump inhibitors vs histamine-2 receptor blockers on in-hospital mortality among ICU patients receiving invasive mechanical ventilation: The PEPTIC Randomized Clinical Trial. JAMA 2020;323(7):616–26.

53. Toews I, George AT, Peter JV, et al. Interventions for preventing upper gastrointestinal bleeding in people admitted to intensive care units. Cochrane Database Syst Rev 2018;6:CD008687.

54. Barbateskovic M, Marker S, Granholm A, et al. Stress ulcer prophylaxis with proton pump inhibitors or histamin-2 receptor antagonists in adult intensive care patients: a systematic review with meta-analysis and trial sequential analysis. Intensive Care Med 2019;45(2):143–58.

55. Wang Y, Ye Z, Ge L, et al. Efficacy and safety of gastrointestinal bleeding prophylaxis in critically ill patients: systematic review and network meta-analysis. BMJ 2020;368:l6744.

56. Wang Y, Ge L, Ye Z, et al. Efficacy and safety of gastrointestinal bleeding prophylaxis in critically ill patients: an updated systematic review and network meta-analysis of randomized trials. Intensive Care Med 2020;46(11):1987–2000.

57. Ye Z, Reintam Blaser A, Lytvyn L, et al. Gastrointestinal bleeding prophylaxis for critically ill patients: a clinical practice guideline. BMJ 2020;368:l6722.

58. Anstey MH, Litton E, Palmer RN, et al. Clinical and economic benefits of de-escalating stress ulcer prophylaxis therapy in the intensive care unit: a quality improvement study. Anaesth Intensive Care 2019;47(6):503–9.

59. Reintam Blaser A, Regli A, De Keulenaer B, et al. Incidence, risk factors, and outcomes of intra-abdominal hypertension in critically ill patients – a prospective multicenter study (IROI Study). Crit Care Med 2019;47(4):535–42.

60. Rogers WK, Garcia L. Intraabdominal hypertension, abdominal compartment syndrome, and the open abdomen. Chest 2018;153(1):238–50.

61. De Laet IE, Malbrain M, De Waele JJ. A clinician's guide to management of intra-abdominal hypertension and abdominal compartment syndrome in critically ill patients. Crit Care 2020;24(1):97.

62. Roberts DJ, Ball CG, Kirkpatrick AW. Increased pressure within the abdominal compartment: intra-abdominal hypertension and the abdominal compartment syndrome. Curr Opin Crit Care 2016;22(2):174–85.

63. Allen R, Sarani B. Evaluation and management of intraabdominal hypertension. Curr Opin Crit Care 2020;26(2):192–6.

64. Kimball EJ. Intra-abdominal hypertension and abdominal compartment syndrome: a current review. Curr Opin Crit Care 2021;27(2):164–8.

65. Pereira B, Dorigatti A, Melek M, et al. Septic shock patients admitted to the intensive care unit with higher SOFA score tend to have higher incidence of abdominal compartment syndrome – a preliminary analysis. Anaesthesiol Intensive Ther 2019;51(5):370–2.

66. Maluso P, Olson J, Sarani B. Abdominal compartment hypertension and abdominal compartment syndrome. Crit Care Clin 2016;32(2):213–22.

67. Fagoni N, Piva S, Marino R, et al. The IN-PANCIA study: clinical evaluation of gastrointestinal dysfunction and failure, multiple organ failure, and levels of citrulline in critically ill patients. J Intensive Care Med 2020;35(3):279–83.

68. Christensen M, Craft J. The cardio-respiratory effects of intra-abdominal hypertension: Considerations for critical care nursing practice. Intensive Crit Care Nurs 2018;44:53–8.

69. Tonetti T, Cavalli I, Ranieri VM, et al. Respiratory consequences of intra-abdominal hypertension. Minerva Anesthesiol 2020;86(8):877–83.

70. Pereira BM. Abdominal compartment syndrome and intra-abdominal hypertension. Curr Opin Crit Care 2019;25(6):688–96.

71. Gray S, Christensen M, Craft J. The gastro-renal effects of intra-abdominal hypertension: Implications for critical care nurses. Intensive Crit Care Nurs 2018;48:69–74.

72. Kirkpatrick AW, Roberts DJ, De Waele J, et al. Intra-abdominal hypertension and the abdominal compartment syndrome: updated consensus definitions and clinical practice guidelines from the World Society of the Abdominal Compartment Syndrome. Intensive Care Med 2013;39(7):1190–206.

73. Fusco MA, Martin RS, Chang MC. Estimation of intra-abdominal pressure by bladder pressure measurement: validity and methodology. J Trauma 2001;50(2):297–302.

74. Cheatham ML, Malbrain ML, Kirkpatrick A, et al. Results from the international conference of experts on intra-abdominal hypertension and abdominal compartment syndrome. II. Recommendations. Intensive Care Med 2007;33(6):951–62.

75. Lee RK, Gallagher JJ, Ejike JC, Hunt L. Intra-abdominal hypertension and the open abdomen: nursing guidelines from the abdominal compartment society. Crit Care Nurse 2020;40(1):13–26.

76. Defontaine A, Tirel O, Costet N, et al. Transvesical intra-abdominal pressure measurement in newborn: what is the optimal saline volume instillation? Pediatr Crit Care Med 2016;17(2):144–9.

77. Zou J, Zheng L, Shuai W, et al. Comparison of intra-abdominal pressure measurements in critically ill patients using intravesical normal saline at 15°C, 25°C, and 35°C. Med Sci Monit 2021;27:e932804.

78. Sun H, Saeedi P, Karuranga S, et al. IDF Diabetes atlas: global, regional and country-level diabetes prevalence estimates for 2021 and projections for 2045. Diabetes Res Clin Pract 2022;183:109119.

79. World Health Organization (WHO). Diabetes. Geneva: WHO; 2021. Available from: https://www.who.int. [Accessed 20 February 2023].

80. World Health Organization (WH0). Global report on diabetes. Geneva: WHO; 2016. Available from: https://www.who.int/publications/i/item/9789241565257. [Accessed 20 February 2023].

81. International Diabetes Federation (IDF). IDF Diabetes atlas. Brussels: IDF; 2021. Available from: https://diabetesatlas.org. [Accessed 20 February 2023].

82. Forouhi NG, Wareham NJ. Epidemiology of diabetes. Medicine 2019;47(1):22–7.

83. Dhatariya K. Diabetic ketoacidosis and hyperosmolar crisis in adults. Medicine 2018;47(1):46–51.

84. Dhatariya KK. Defining and characterising diabetic ketoacidosis in adults. Diabetes Res Clin Pract 2019;155:107797.

85. Long B, Willis GC, Lentz S, et al. Evaluation and management of the critically ill adult with diabetic ketoacidosis. J Emerg Med 2020;59(3):371–83.

86. Kamata Y, Takano K, Kishihara E, et al. Distinct clinical characteristics and therapeutic modalities for diabetic ketoacidosis in type 1 and type 2 diabetes mellitus. J Diabetes Complications 2017;31(2):468–72.

87. Long B, Willis GC, Lentz S, et al. Diagnosis and management of the critically ill adult patient with hyperglycemic hyperosmolar state. J Emerg Med 2021;61(4):365–75.

88. Anzola I, Gomez PC, Umpierrez GE. Management of diabetic ketoacidosis and hyperglycemic hyperosmolar state in adults. Expert Rev Endocrinol Metab 2016;11(2):177–85.

89. Dhatariya KK, Glaser NS, Codner E, et al. Diabetic ketoacidosis. Nat Rev Dis Primers 2020;6(1):40.

90. Dhatariya KK, Joint British Diabetes Societies for Inpatient Care. The management of diabetic ketoacidosis in adults – an updated guideline from the Joint British Diabetes Society for Inpatient Care. Diabet Med 2022;39(6):e14788.

91. Fayfman M, Pasquel FJ, Umpierrez GE. Management of hyperglycemic crises: diabetic ketoacidosis and hyperglycemic hyperosmolar state. Med Clin North Am 2017;101(3):587–606.

92. Kilpatrick ES, Butler AE, Ostlundh L, et al. Controversies around the measurement of blood ketones to diagnose and manage diabetic ketoacidosis. Diabetes Care 2022;45(2):267–72.

93. Dhatariya K, Haq M, Dashora U, et al. The management of hyperosmolar hyperglycaemic state (HHS) in adults. London: Joint British Diabetes Societies for Inpatient Care; 2022.

94. De Waele E, Malbrain M, Spapen HD. How to deal with severe acute pancreatitis in the critically ill. Curr Opin Crit Care 2019;25(2):150–6.

95. Sinonquel P, Laleman W, Wilmer A. Advances in acute pancreatitis. Curr Opin Crit Care 2021;27(2):193–200.

96. Colvin SD, Smith EN, Morgan DE, et al. Acute pancreatitis: an update on the revised Atlanta classification. Abdom Radiol (NY) 2020;45(5):1222–31.

97. Banks PA, Bollen TL, Dervenis C, et al. Classification of acute pancreatitis – 2012: revision of the Atlanta classification and definitions by international consensus. Gut 2013;62(1):102–11.

98. Singer P, Blaser AR, Berger MM, et al. ESPEN guideline on clinical nutrition in the intensive care unit. Clin Nutr 2019;38(1):48–79.

99. McClave SA, Taylor BE, Martindale RG, et al. Guidelines for the provision and assessment of nutrition support therapy in the adult critically ill patient: Society of Critical Care Medicine (SCCM) and American Society for Parenteral and Enteral Nutrition (A.S.P.E.N.). JPEN J Parenter Enteral Nutr 2016;40(2):159–211.

100. Ukai T, Shikata S, Inoue M, et al. Early prophylactic antibiotics administration for acute necrotizing pancreatitis: a meta-analysis of randomized controlled trials. J Hepatobiliary Pancreat Sci 2015;22(4):316–21.

101. Dong V, Nanchal R, Karvellas CJ. Pathophysiology of acute liver failure. Nutr Clin Pract 2020;35(1):24–9.

102. Krawitz S, Lingiah V, Pyrsopoulos NT. Acute liver failure: mechanisms of disease and multisystemic involvement. Clin Liver Dis 2018;22(2):243–56.

103. Piconese S, Cammarata I, Barnaba V. Viral hepatitis, inflammation, and cancer: A lesson for autoimmunity. J Autoimmun 2018;95:58–68.

104. Sharma P, Arora A. Clinical presentation of alcoholic liver disease and non-alcoholic fatty liver disease: spectrum and diagnosis. Transl Gastroenterol Hepatol 2020;5:19.

105. Rotundo L, Pyrsopoulos N. Liver injury induced by paracetamol and challenges associated with intentional and unintentional use. World J Hepatol 2020;12(4):125–36.

106. Ye Y, Liu Z. Management of Amanita phalloides poisoning: a literature review and update. J Crit Care 2018;46:17–22.

107. Garcia-Cortes M, Robles-Diaz M, Stephens C, et al. Drug induced liver injury: an update. Arch Toxicol 2020;94(10):3381–407.

108. Yokoda RT, Carey EJ. Primary biliary cholangitis and primary sclerosing cholangitis. Am J Gastroenterol 2019;114(10):1593–605.

109. Kitto LJ, Henderson NC. Hepatic stellate cell regulation of liver regeneration and repair. Hepatol Commun 2021;5(3):358–70.

110. Roehlen N, Crouchet E, Baumert TF. Liver fibrosis: mechanistic concepts and therapeutic perspectives. Cells 2020;9(4):875.

111. Grinspan LT, Verna EC. Chronic liver failure and hepatic cirrhosis. In: Wagener G, editor. Liver anesthesiology and critical care medicine. 2nd ed. Champaign, IL: Springer; 2018, p. 21–40.

112. Lanini S, Ustianowski A, Pisapia R, et al. Viral hepatitis: etiology, epidemiology, transmission, diagnostics, rreatment, and prevention. Infect Dis Clin North Am 2019;33(4):1045–62.

113. Veracruz N, Gish RG, Cheung R, et al. Global incidence and mortality of hepatitis B and hepatitis C acute infections, cirrhosis and hepatocellular carcinoma from 2010 to 2019. J Viral Hepat 2022;29(5):352–65.

114. Smith S, Harmanci H, Hutin Y, et al. Global progress on the elimination of viral hepatitis as a major public health threat: an analysis of WHO Member State responses 2017. JHEP Rep 2019;1(2):81–9.

115. Bailey JR, Barnes E, Cox AL. Approaches, progress, and challenges to hepatitis C vaccine development. Gastroenterology 2019;156(2):418–30.

116. Julien J, Ayer T, Bethea ED, et al. Projected prevalence and mortality associated with alcohol-related liver disease in the USA, 2019–40: a modelling study. Lancet Public Health 2020;5(6):e316–23.

117. Shield K, Manthey J, Rylett M, et al. National, regional, and global burdens of disease from 2000 to 2016 attributable to alcohol use: a comparative risk assessment study. Lancet Public Health 2020;5(1):e51–61.

118. Liu SY, Tsai IT, Hsu YC. Alcohol-related liver disease: basic mechanisms and clinical perspectives. Int J Mol Sci 2021;22(10):5170.

119. European Association for the Study of the Liver. EASL clinical practice guidelines: management of alcohol-related liver disease. J Hepatol 2018;69(1):154–81.

120. Hughes E, Hopkins LJ, Parker R. Survival from alcoholic hepatitis has not improved over time. PLoS One 2018;13(2):e0192393.

121. Bennett K, Enki DG, Thursz M, et al. Systematic review with meta-analysis: high mortality in patients with non-severe alcoholic hepatitis. Aliment Pharmacol Ther 2019;50(3):249–57.

122. Vergis N, Atkinson SR, Thursz MR. The future of therapy for alcoholic hepatitis – beyond corticosteroids. J Hepatol 2019;70(4):785–7.

123. Im GY, Cameron AM, Lucey MR. Liver transplantation for alcoholic hepatitis. J Hepatol 2019;70(2):328–34.

124. Stravitz RT, Lee WM. Acute liver failure. Lancet 2019;394(10201):869–81.

125. Cardoso FS, Marcelino P, Bagulho L, et al. Acute liver failure: an up-to-date approach. J Crit Care 2017;39:25–30.

126. Moreau R, Gao B, Papp M, et al. Acute-on-chronic liver failure: a distinct clinical syndrome. J Hepatol 2021;75(Suppl. 1):S27–35.

127. Zaccherini G, Weiss E, Moreau R. Acute-on-chronic liver failure: definitions, pathophysiology and principles of treatment. JHEP Rep 2021;3(1):100176.

128. Horvatits T, Drolz A, Trauner M, et al. Liver injury and failure in critical illness. Hepatology 2019;70(6):2204–15.

129. Lescot T, Karvellas C, Beaussier M, et al. Acquired liver injury in the intensive care unit. Anesthesiology 2012;117(4):898–904.

130. Rose CF, Amodio P, Bajaj JS, et al. Hepatic encephalopathy: novel insights into classification, pathophysiology and therapy. J Hepatol 2020;73(6):1526–47.

131. Liotta EM, Romanova AL, Lizza BD, et al. Osmotic shifts, cerebral edema, and neurologic deterioration in severe hepatic encephalopathy. Crit Care Med 2018;46(2):280–9.

132. Bosoi CR, Rose CF. Identifying the direct effects of ammonia on the brain. Metab Brain Dis 2009;24(1):95–102.

133. Conn HO, Leevy CM, Vlahcevic ZR, et al. Comparison of lactulose and neomycin in the treatment of chronic portal-systemic encephalopathy. A double blind controlled trial. Gastroenterology 1977;72(4 Pt 1):573–83.

134. Amodio P. Current diagnosis and classification of hepatic encephalopathy. J Clin Exp Hepatol 2018;8(4):432–7.

135. Simonetto DA, Gines P, Kamath PS. Hepatorenal syndrome: pathophysiology, diagnosis, and management. BMJ 2020;370:m2687.

136. Angeli P, Gines P, Wong F, et al. Diagnosis and management of acute kidney injury in patients with cirrhosis: revised consensus recommendations of the International Club of Ascites. Gut 2015;64(4):531–7.

137. Francoz C, Durand F, Kahn JA, et al. Hepatorenal syndrome. Clin J Am Soc Nephrol 2019;14(5):774–81.

138. Bernardi M, Moreau R, Angeli P, et al. Mechanisms of decompensation and organ failure in cirrhosis: from peripheral arterial vasodilation to systemic inflammation hypothesis. J Hepatol 2015;63(5):1272–84.

139. Alqahtani SA, Jang S. Pathophysiology and management of variceal bleeding. Drugs 2021;81(6):647–67.

140. Garcia-Tsao G, Abraldes JG, Berzigotti A, et al. Portal hypertensive bleeding in cirrhosis: Risk stratification, diagnosis, and management: 2016 practice guidance by the American Association for the Study of Liver Diseases. Hepatology 2017;65(1):310–35.

141. Ponziani FR, Zocco MA, Cerrito L, et al. Bacterial translocation in patients with liver cirrhosis: physiology, clinical consequences, and practical implications. Expert Rev Gastroenterol Hepatol 2018;12(7):641–56.

142. Fuhrmann V, Krowka M. Hepatopulmonary syndrome. J Hepatol 2018;69(3):744–5.

143. Montrief T, Koyfman A, Long B. Acute liver failure: a review for emergency physicians. Am J Emerg Med 2019;37(2):329–37.

144. Arroyo V, Moreau R, Jalan R. Acute-on-chronic liver failure. N Engl J Med 2020;382(22):2137–45.

145. Rose CF. What's new in our understanding of the pathogenesis of hepatic encephalopathy? Clin Liver Dis 2017;10(2):29–31.

146. Rajaram P, Subramanian R. Management of acute liver failure in the intensive care unit setting. Clin Liver Dis 2018;22(2):403–8.

147. Pagana KD, Pagana TJ, Pagana TN. Mosby's® diagnostic and laboratory tests reference. 16th ed. St Louis, MO: Elsevier; 2022.

148. Paugam-Burtz C, Levesque E, Louvet A, et al. Management of liver failure in general intensive care unit. Anaesth Crit Care Pain Med 2020;39(1):143–61.

149. European Association for the Study of the Liver. EASL clinical practice guidelines on the management of hepatic encephalopathy. J Hepatol 2022;77(3):807–24.

150. Gupta S, Fenves AZ, Hootkins R. The role of RRT in hyperammonemic patients. Clin J Am Soc Nephrol 2016;11(10):1872–8.

151. Pfisterer N, Unger LW, Reiberger T. Clinical algorithms for the prevention of variceal bleeding and rebleeding in patients with liver cirrhosis. World J Hepatol 2021;13(7):731–46.

152. Biggins SW, Angeli P, Garcia-Tsao G, et al. Diagnosis, evaluation, and management of ascites, spontaneous bacterial peritonitis and hepatorenal syndrome: 2021 practice guidance by the American Association for the Study of Liver Diseases. Hepatology 2021;74(2):1014–48.

153. Olivo R, Guarrera JV, Pyrsopoulos NT. Liver transplantation for acute liver failure. Clin Liver Dis 2018;22(2):409–17.

154. Bridwell RE, Long B, Ramzy M, Get al. Balloon tamponade for the management of gastrointestinal bleeding. J Emerg Med 2022;62(4):545–58.

155. Parbhu SK, Aldler DG. Endoscopic management of acute esophageal variceal bleeding. Tech Gastroint Endosc 2017;19(2):74–8.

156. Katarey D, Jalan R. Update on extracorporeal liver support. Curr Opin Crit Care 2020;26(2):180–5.

157. He YT, Qi YN, Zhang BQ, et al. Bioartificial liver support systems for acute liver failure: a systematic review and meta-analysis of the clinical and preclinical literature. World J Gastroenterol 2019;25(27):3634–48.

158. Agarwal B, Saliba F, Tomescue DR, et al. A multi-centre, randomized controlled study, to evaluate the safety and performance of the DIALIVE liver dialysis device in patients with acute on chronic liver failure (ACLF) versus standard of care (SOC) Gut 2021;70:A54.

159. Karvellas CJ, Subramanian RM. Current evidence for extracorporeal liver support systems in acute liver failure and acute-on-chronic liver failure. Crit Care Clin 2016;32(3):439–51.

160. Germani G, Theocharidou E, Adam R, et al. Liver transplantation for acute liver failure in Europe: outcomes over 20 years from the ELTR database. J Hepatol 2012;57(2):288–96.

161. Freeman RB Jr, Steffick DE, Guidinger MK, et al. Liver and intestine transplantation in the United States, 1997-2006. Am J Transplant 2008;8(4 Pt 2):958–76.

162. Ghelichi-Ghojogh M, Javanian M, Amiri S, et al. The survival rate of liver transplantation in children: a systematic review and meta-analysis. Pediatr Surg Int 2022;38(9):1177–86.

163. Mahmud N. Selection for liver transplantation: Indications and evaluation. Curr Hepatol Rep 2020;19(3):203–12.

164. Karvellas CJ, Francoz C, Weiss E. Liver transplantation in acute-on-chronic liver failure. Transplantation 2021;105(7):1471–81.

165. Wahid NA, Rosenblatt R, Brown RS Jr. A review of the current state of liver transplantation disparities. Liver Transpl 2021;27(3):434–43.

166. Malinchoc M, Kamath PS, Gordon FD, et al. A model to predict poor survival in patients undergoing transjugular intrahepatic portosystemic shunts. Hepatology 2000;31(4):864–71.

167. Mazumder NR, Atiemo K, Kappus M, et al. A comprehensive review of outcome predictors in low MELD patients. Transplantation 2020;104(2):242–50.

168. Protty MB, Haboubi HN, Yeoman AD. Changes in the model of end-stage liver disease (MELD) scores on day 7 predict mortality in acute on chronic liver disease: the delta-MELD project. J Hepatol 2017;55(1):S387.

169. Ge J, Kim WR, Lai JC, et al. "Beyond MELD" – emerging strategies and technologies for improving mortality prediction, organ allocation and outcomes in liver transplantation. J Hepatol 2022;76(6):1318–29.

170. Agopian VG, Petrowsky H, Kaldas FM, et al. The evolution of liver transplantation during 3 decades: analysis of 5347 consecutive liver transplants at a single center. Ann Surg 2013;258(3):409–21.

171. Czigany Z, Scherer MN, Pratschke J, et al. Technical aspects of orthotopic liver transplantation – a survey-based study within the Eurotransplant, Swisstransplant, Scandiatransplant, and British Transplantation Society Networks. J Gastrointest Surg 2019;23(3):529–37.

172. Doria C, Goldstein S, Marion IR. Orthotopic liver transplantation: surgical techniques. In: Doria C, editor. Contemporary liver transplantation organ and tissue transplantation. Champaign, IL: Springer; 2017, p. 29–56.

173. Hackl C, Schmidt KM, Susal C, et al. Split liver transplantation: current developments. World J Gastroenterol 2018;24(47):5312–21.

174. Perito ER, Roll G, Dodge JL, et al. Split liver transplantation and pediatric waitlist mortality in the United States: potential for improvement. Transplantation 2019;103(3):552–7.

175. Quadros J, Piedade C, Lopes MF. Auxiliary liver transplantation for management of acute liver failure in children – systematic review. Transplant Rev 2021;35(4):100631.

176. Iesari S, Inostroza Nunez ME, Rico Juri JM, et al. Adult-to-adult living-donor liver transplantation: the experience of the Universite Catholique de Louvain. Hepatobiliary Pancreat Dis Int 2019;18(2):132–42.

177. Soubrane O, Eguchi S, Uemoto S, et al. Minimally invasive donor hepatectomy for adult living donor liver transplantation: an international, multi-institutional evaluation of safety, efficacy and early outcomes. Ann Surg 2022;275(1):166–74.

178. Humar A, Ganesh S, Jorgensen D, et al. Adult living donor versus deceased donor liver transplant (LDLT Versus DDLT) at a single center: time to change our paradigm for liver transplant. Ann Surg 2019;270(3):444–51.

179. Tinguely P, Morare N, Ramirez-Del Val A, et al. Enhanced recovery after surgery programs improve short-term outcomes after liver transplantation – a systematic review and meta-analysis. Clin Transplant 2021;35(11):e14453.

180. Saner FH, Hoyer DP, Hartmann M, et al. The edge of unknown: postoperative critical care in liver transplantation. J Clin Med 2022;11(14):4036.

181. Carll T, Wool GD. Basic principles of viscoelastic testing. Transfusion 2020;60(Suppl. 6):S1–9.

182. Bezinover D, Dirkmann D, Findlay J, et al. Perioperative coagulation management in liver transplant recipients. Transplantation 2018;102(4):578–92.

183. Kwon HM, Hwang GS. Cardiovascular dysfunction and liver transplantation. Korean J Anesthesiol 2018;71(2):85–91.

184. Amaral B, Vicente M, Pereira CSM, et al. Approach to the liver transplant early postoperative period: an institutional standpoint. Rev Bras Ter Intensiva 2019;31(4):561–70.

185. Griffiths SV, Conway DH, Investigators P-C, et al. What are the optimum components in a care bundle aimed at reducing post-operative pulmonary complications in high-risk patients? Perioper Med 2018;7:7.

186. Jeffrey AW, Delriviere L, McCaughan G, et al. Excellent contemporary graft survival for adult liver retransplantation: an Australian and New Zealand registry analysis from 1986 to 2017. Transplant Direct 2019;5(8):e472.

187. Di Maira T, Little EC, Berenguer M. Immunosuppression in liver transplant. Best Pract Res Clin Gastroenterol 2020;46–47:101681.

188. Kok B, Dong V, Karvellas CJ. Graft dysfunction and management in liver transplantation. Crit Care Clin 2019;35(1):117–33.

189. Hale DA. Basic transplantation immunology. Surg Clin North Am 2006;86(5):1103–25, v.

190. Rodriguez-Peralvarez M, Rico-Juri JM, Tsochatzis E, et al. Biopsy-proven acute cellular rejection as an efficacy endpoint of randomized trials in liver transplantation: a systematic review and critical appraisal. Transpl Int 2016;29(9):961–73.

191. Plummer MP, Bellomo R, Cousins CE, et al. Dysglycaemia in the critically ill and the interaction of chronic and acute glycaemia with mortality. Intensive Care Med 2014;40(7):973–80.

192. Krinsley JS. Is it time to rethink blood glucose targets in critically ill patients? Chest 2018;154(5):1004–5.

193. Eldridge SM, Lancaster GA, Campbell MJ, et al. Defining feasibility and pilot studies in preparation for randomised controlled trials: development of a conceptual framework. PLoS One 2016;11(3):e0150205.

194. Bloom SL, Stollings JL, Kirkpatrick O, et al. Randomized clinical trial of an ICU recovery pilot program for survivors of critical illness. Crit Care Med 2019;47(10):1337–45.

195. Davidson JE, Aslakson RA, Long AC, et al. Guidelines for family-centered care in the neonatal, pediatric, and adult ICU. Crit Care Med 2017;45(1):103–28.

196. van Zanten ARH, De Waele E, Wischmeyer PE. Nutrition therapy and critical illness: practical guidance for the ICU, post-ICU, and long-term convalescence phases. Crit Care 2019;23(1):368.

197. Needham DM, Sepulveda KA, Dinglas VD, et al. Core outcome measures for clinical research in acute respiratory failure survivors. An international modified Delphi Consensus study. Am J Respir Crit Care Med 2017;196(9):1122–30.

Chapter 21

Pathophysiology and management of shock

Margherita Murgo, Elizabeth Papathanassoglou

Learning objectives

After reading this chapter, you should be able to:

- describe the clinical manifestations of shock
- differentiate the various shock states
- describe principles of shock management
- discuss endpoints of resuscitation
- identify appropriate monitoring for a patient with shock
- review and evaluate care for a patient with a specific shock type.

Introduction

Shock is an altered physiological state that affects the functioning of every cell and organ system in the body. It is a complex syndrome reflecting changing blood flow to body tissues with accompanying cellular dysfunction and eventual organ failure. Shock presents as a result of imbalance of oxygen supply and demand[1] and impaired nutrient delivery to the tissue:[2,3]

- when compensatory mechanisms can no longer respond to decreases in tissue perfusion
- when nutrient uptake is impaired at the cellular level.

While the cause of shock may be multifactorial, treatment focuses on optimising tissue perfusion and oxygen delivery. Shock is often classified according to the primary underlying mechanism: a disruption of intravascular blood volume, impaired vasomotor tone or altered cardiac contractility.[2] The shock syndrome is one of the most pervasive manifestations of critical illness present in intensive care patients.

Early detection and management of shock to reverse pathological processes improves patient outcomes.[4] Shock is a medical emergency and although the traditional hallmark is hypotension – where the systolic blood pressure is <90 mmHg – this can be a late or misleading sign which should be monitored in context to the patient.[5] Use of clinical assessment tools is useful for the early identification of specific types of shock, such as hypovolaemic or septic.

However, no single tool can apply to all types of shock.[6] It is therefore critical that other signs and symptoms are identified early by frequent observations to detect a patient's deteriorating state and respond before irreversible shock ensues.[7] No single vital sign is adequate in determining the level or extent of shock, nor is there a specific laboratory test that diagnoses the cause of shock. The Australian Commission on Safety and Quality in Health Care has issued a national consensus statement on recognising and responding to acute physiological deterioration which includes shock states.[8] The statement includes essential elements of clinical assessment, diagnosis, escalation of care, rapid response systems and interprofessional communication, as well as organisational prerequisites including leadership, education, audit and quality of care.

The statement identifies that patient assessment should include as a minimum: respiratory rate, oxygen saturation, heart rate, blood pressure, temperature, level of consciousness and new-onset confusion or behaviour change. In this chapter an overview of the pathophysiology of shock, the commonly described categories and associated pathologies, along with appropriate monitoring and interventions for managing a patient in shock, are described.

Pathophysiology

Shock is a state of reduced end-organ oxygenation due to a mismatch between tissue oxygen delivery and demand.[9] Shock is classified by aetiology:[1,10] hypovolaemic, cardiogenic, distributive and obstructive (Fig. 21.1). Each

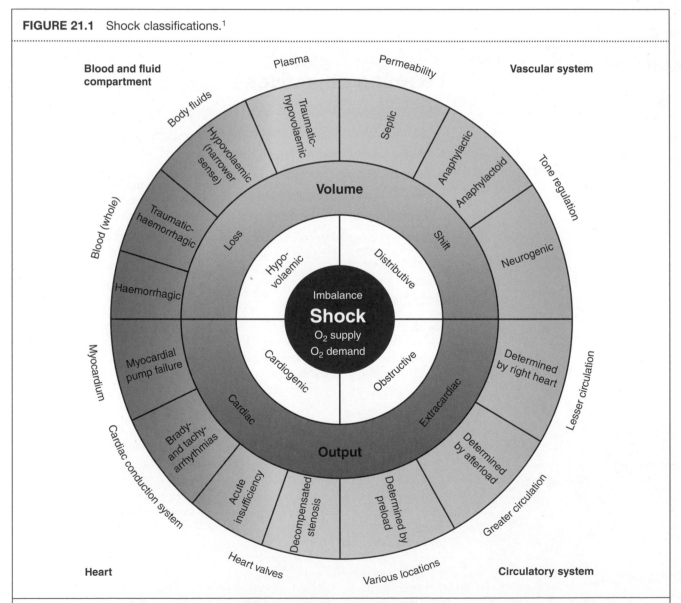

FIGURE 21.1 Shock classifications.[1]

Source: Standl T, Annecke T, Cascorbi I, et al. The nomenclature, definition and distinction of types of shock. Dtsch Arztebl Int 2018;115(45):757–68.

TABLE 21.1
Shock types

SHOCK TYPE	MAIN CHARACTERISTIC
Hypovolaemic	A reduction in circulating blood volume through haemorrhage or dehydration or plasma fluid loss.
Cardiogenic	Pump failure (impaired cardiac contractility) usually as a result of myocardial infarction.
Obstructive	Characterised by blockage of circulation to the tissues by impedance of outflow or filling in the heart (e.g. due to cardiac tamponade or pulmonary emboli).
Distributive	A maldistribution of circulation from sepsis, anaphylaxis or neurogenic injury.

Source: Adapted from Manji RA, Wood KE, Kumar A. The history and evolution of circulatory shock. Crit Care Clin 2009;25:1–29, with permission.

type has a specific mechanism of action that leads to altered tissue perfusion and oxygen and nutrient uptake at the cellular level[11] (Table 21.1).[12] In practice, it is common for different shock types to be existent in the same presentation; for example, a patient with septic shock might also be hypovolaemic and/or have myocardial dysfunction. The signs of tissue perfusion, types of shock and cardiac changes are depicted in Fig. 21.2.[13]

Shock occurs when there is an inability of the body to meet metabolic demands of the tissues.[11] Hypoperfusion (decreased blood flow to the tissues) results in cellular dysfunction as the cell enters anaerobic metabolism, resulting in drastically decreased adenosine triphosphate (ATP) production. The shortage in ATP supply disturbs ionic homeostasis resulting in calcium influx intracellularly and, eventually, cellular death. Additionally, leakage of intracellular contents extracellularly activates an inflammatory cascade, which results in organ damage.[14] At this point, adaptive responses can no longer accommodate circulatory changes.[11]

Adaptive responses in shock are moderated via numerous 'sensors' throughout the thorax and large vessels in particular, which detect subtle changes in pressure (baroreceptors) or biochemical changes (chemoreceptors). These receptors feedback to the hypothalamus, which regulates, through the pituitary gland and adrenal cortex, the release of a number of hormones including antidiuretic hormone and adrenocorticotrophic hormone to target organs such as the kidney and adrenal glands. In response to hypotension and hypovolaemia, the heart rate and myocardial contractility are increased, and peripheral blood arterioles and venules constrict owing to sympathetic stimulation by the cardiac and vasomotor centres in the lower pons and medulla oblongata. Parasympathetic vagal

nerves modulate the heart rate, whereas sympathetic spinal cord peripheral nerves control the basal tone of the entire circulation. Catecholamines released by the sympathetic system (noradrenaline (norepinephrine) and adrenaline (epinephrine)) activate α_1-receptors, while activation of β_1- and α_1-receptors in heart and blood vessels decreases acetylcholine release.[15]

The adrenal cortex mediates the mineral and glucocorticoid response to counter the developing effects of shock. This concurrent direct feedback stimulates the sympathetic nervous system to act on blood vessel tone, particularly the arterioles, and organs such as the adrenal gland and kidney to respond via the release of endogenous catecholamines, mineral and glucocorticoids (aldosterone, cortisol) and the renin–angiotensin–aldosterone system. Concomitant activation of the renin–angiotensin–aldosterone system results in synthesis of angiotensin II, a powerful vasoconstrictor that further potentiates the reduction in peripheral blood vessel capacity.

Collectively, these responses form a sympatho–endocrine–adrenal axis that moderates the systemic response to shock. The axis maintains blood perfusion of vital organ systems and combines with the inflammatory response to limit local and systemic tissue damage, ultimately conferring a survival advantage. Combined responses include profound vasoconstriction, oligoanuria (fluid retention), redirection of blood flow to vital organs, hyperglycaemia, immunomodulation and procoagulation. This universal response to impending shock is particularly effective in compensating for loss of circulating blood volume, but may be counterproductive when heart failure occurs or when the peripheral tissues' ability to extract oxygen is compromised, as in distributive shock states.

As adaptive responses fail, the cardiac output becomes insufficient to provide adequate organ perfusion despite increasing tissue oxygen consumption (see Chapters 9 and 10). Normally the ratio of oxygen delivery to oxygen consumption is 5:1. When oxygen delivery decreases, tissues increase their rate of oxygen extraction. However, when the ratio of oxygen delivery to consumption falls to 2:1, oxygen consumption becomes 'delivery dependent', meaning that the tissues cannot increase oxygen extraction any further, resulting in oxygen debt.[16]

Tissue and organ hypoperfusion may also exist despite a relatively normal cardiac output and may not be immediately clinically evident. This results from microcirculatory shunting and in maldistribution of blood flow to some tissues while other areas receive more blood flow than needed and this is often referred to as distributive shock.[17] This response is typical of the shock types that affect vasomotor tone – for example, septic, neurogenic and anaphylactic shock. Maldistribution may leave some organ systems ischaemic for long periods, leading to persistent organ dysfunction and failure.[17] There is also evidence of persistent mitochondrial dysfunction despite normalisation of perfusion and oxygenation – a condition previously termed 'cytopathic hypoxia'.[18] Excessive signalling by proinflammatory and gaseous mediators,

FIGURE 21.2 Types of shock: (**A**) signs of tissue perfusion; (**B**) types of shock; (**C**) cardiac changes. CVP = central venous pressure; SvO_2 = mixed venous oxygen saturation.

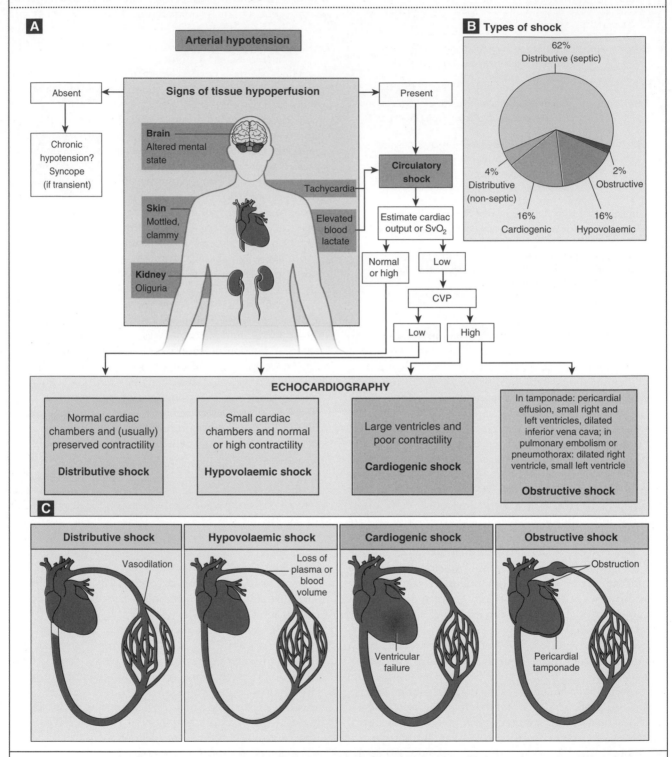

FIGURE 21.3 Blood lactate and shock.

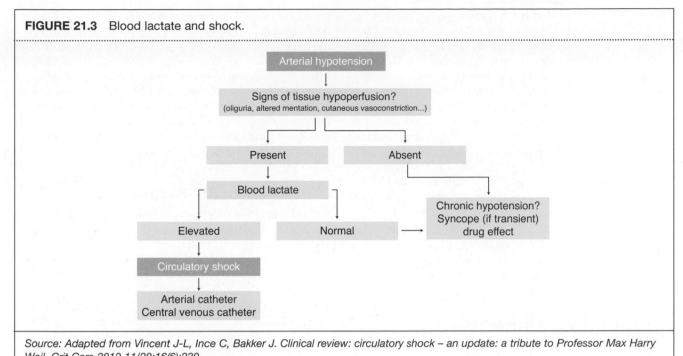

Source: Adapted from Vincent J-L, Ince C, Bakker J. Clinical review: circulatory shock – an update: a tribute to Professor Max Harry Weil. Crit Care 2012 11/20;16(6):239.

such as nitric oxide (NO), carbon monoxide (CO) and tumour necrosis factor-alpha (TNF-α), impede the ability of the mitochondria to use oxygen for ATP production, leading to decreased oxygen extraction.[19]

ATP stores become depleted as a result of this impaired mitochondrial oxygen utilisation[20] interfering with electron transport and metabolism. NO is associated with vascular relaxation and is a major contributor to alterations in microvasculature and capillary leak in sepsis.[21]

Organ systems have varying responses in shock and are not measured directly. While macrocirculation can be assessed through measurements of blood pressure and cardiac output, the effectiveness of microcirculation, which is crucial for organ function, is not readily assessable.[22]

Often surrogate markers of global hypoperfusion are used to indicate the severity of shock. Mixed venous oxygen saturation lactate and acid–base disturbances, such as an increase in strong ion gap, have been suggested as early markers of mitochondrial dysfunction and cellular hypoperfusion[23] (Fig. 21.3).[12] Surrogate biochemical markers of hypoperfusion (pH, serum lactate and standard base excess) assess acidaemia and provide some insight into the degree of shock.[24] Lactate, a strong anion with basal production of approximately 20 mmol/kg,[25] is a product of metabolism.[26] Increased levels are present in tissue hypoxia, hypermetabolism, decreased lactate clearance, inhibition of pyruvate dehydrogenase and activation of inflammatory cells, all characteristics of developing shock (Table 21.2[25]). Increased lactate production is a warning sign of impending organ failure, as it is indicative of anaerobic metabolism. Blood lactate levels have been directly linked to deteriorating patient

TABLE 21.2

Hyperlactataemia in critical illness

MECHANISMS	SERUM LEVELS	CAUSES
Increased glycolysis	Lactate >5 mmol/L and pH <7.35 (normal lactate <2 mmol/L)	Hypoxaemia Anaemia Hypoperfusion
Decreased clearance	Severe hyperlactataemia (>10 mmol/L) is associated with high ICU mortality (78.2%)	Shock Sepsis CPR

Source: Adapted from Kushimoto S, Akaishi S, Sato T, et al. Lactate, a useful marker for disease mortality and severity but an unreliable marker of tissue hypoxia/hypoperfusion in critically ill patients. Acute Med Surg 2016;3(4):293–97. doi: 10.1002/ams2.207.

outcomes in shock.[27] Serum concentrations greater than 5 mmol/L in the setting of metabolic acidosis are indicative of high mortality.[26] In patients with septic shock, monitoring of serum lactate levels is recommended to guide resuscitation efforts.[28]

As the shock state worsens and the body fails to compensate, organ systems begin to fail. This is complicated by 'capillary leak' or increased microvascular permeability that leads to interstitial oedema due to alterations to the vascular endothelium. Many immune mediators including circulating cytokines, oxygen-free radicals and activated neutrophils alter the structure of the endothelial cells, and damage the endothelial glycocalyx.[29]

The endothelial glycocalyx prevents the endothelium from inflammatory activation, but when it is degraded the endothelium is exposed to cytokine binding, which initiates an inflammatory and coagulation cascade.[29] Moreover, endothelial cytoskeleton alterations create space to allow larger intravascular molecules to cross into the extravascular space, with proteins and water moving from the intravascular space into the interstitium.[23] This response mechanism improves the supply of nutrient-rich fluid to the site of injury; however, systemically, fluid shifts lead to hypovolaemia, impaired organ function and development of acute organ injury such as acute kidney injury.[30] This developing organ injury is the precedent to organ failure (see Chapter 22).

The next sections of this chapter describe the general assessment and management of shock, different classifications of shock and specific management principles to avoid or limit tissue injury and the eventual progression to organ failure.

Patient assessment

Critically ill patients often exhibit signs of tissue hypoxia as a result of cardiovascular disturbances that may be observed through clinical examination.[31] Table 21.3 provides an overview of the physiological changes in shock. Therapy is targeted to maintain oxygen delivery to vital organs in order to prevent ischaemia and cell death.[32] Ideally, organ systems and tissues should be monitored individually; however, global measures, such as perfusion pressure, cardiac output and oxygen delivery, are commonly used as surrogates to assist in treatment decision making.[3,33] Patient assessment and haemodynamic monitoring,

including calculation of cardiac output, are used to differentiate shock states and assess progress in relation to treatment.[33] Cardiac output, and its derivatives, is seen by many clinicians as an important assessment of shocked patients as it is a major determinant of oxygen delivery.[3] Critically ill patients are frequently assessed, with continuous monitoring usually required. Clinical estimations of cardiac output from physical examination alone can be unreliable and patient status may change quickly.[34] Therefore, invasive techniques are most commonly used in critical care (see also Chapter 9).

Non-invasive assessment

Perfusion status is determined clinically using gross organ function such as mental status, urine output and peripheral warmth and colour (Fig. 21.4).[34] Basic physical assessment of the cardiovascular and central nervous systems and renal function is essential when assessing a patient at risk of shock. Subtle changes in mentation, urine output, heart rate and capillary refill are all signs of physiological compensation in response to altered tissue perfusion associated with shock.[34] Regular tracking of these vital signs and trend monitoring through careful documentation can alert clinicians to impending deterioration in the shock state.[8] The shock index is also an easy bedside calculation (HR/SBP (heart rate/systolic blood pressure)) and has been used as a predictive screening tool for shock states.[4] Normal values range between 0.5 and 0.7, with shock indicated as the value increases.[35]

Level of consciousness may deteriorate; an early sign may be anxiety, and progress to restlessness, delirium, agitation or coma; in children this is more difficult to assess but is signified by behaviour changes. Other

---

TABLE 21.3

Physiological changes in shock

SHOCK CLASSIFICATION	CARDIAC OUTPUT	SYSTEMIC VASCULAR RESISTANCE	CAPILLARY CIRCULATION	PULMONARY CAPILLARY PRESSURE	PULMONARY VASCULAR RESISTANCE
Hypovolaemic	↓	↑	↓	↓	↑
Cardiogenic	↓	↑	↓	↑	↑
Distributive:					
• septic	↑	↓	↓	↓	↑
• anaphylactic	↓	↓	↓	↓	↓
• neurogenic	↓/NC	↓	↓	↓	↑
Obstructive	↓	↓	↓	↑	↑

↑ = increase; ↓ = decrease; NC = no change.

FIGURE 21.4 Windows for assessment.

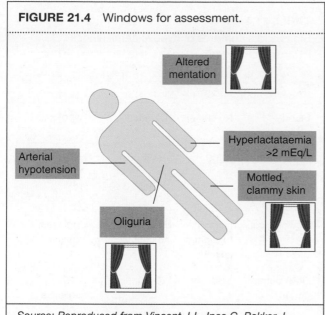

Source: Reproduced from Vincent J-L, Ince C, Bakker J. Clinical review: circulatory shock – an update: a tribute to Professor Max Harry Weil. Crit Care 2012;16(6):239.

assessment findings include cool, clammy skin, postural hypotension, tachycardia and decreased urine output.[36] The reliability of these measures may vary, particularly where multiple assessments by different clinicians are performed. In the ICU, continuous electrocardiograph monitoring and invasive monitoring techniques are employed to assist in the objective assessment of changes in cardiovascular state.[37] Reliable and accurate non-invasive clinical assessment techniques of estimating cardiac output are useful,[34] allowing assessment of patients without invasive monitoring, or used to verify accuracy of invasive devices.

Haemodynamic status and assessing fluid responsiveness using non-invasive methods is possible and important. Passive leg raises to 45°C for several minutes induces a fluid bolus without the associated risk of administering fluid to assess volume status.[38] Clinical ultrasound is used for assessment of inferior vena cava (IVC) collapsibility during respiration to assess volume status.[39] However, a recent meta-analysis of studies assessing the use of IVC diameter as a measure of fluid responsiveness highlighted study heterogeneity and found the method unreliable.[40]

Invasive assessment

Invasive assessment allows for real-time measurement of clinical variables so that patient responses to interventions can be monitored and quickly changed if required.[41] Continuous assessment of heart rate and blood pressure by an intra-arterial catheter enables circulatory access for frequent blood sampling. This provides the ability to assess serum lactate levels, electrolytes and blood gas estimation, including pH. It is also possible to measure pulse pressure and stroke volume variation, determined via algorithms

with proprietary technologies.[38,41] These measures may be useful in assessing fluid responsiveness.[42]

The indicator dilution method using a thermal (thermodilution) signal (cold or hot) was traditionally the customary clinical standard for measuring cardiac output in the ICU.[3,38,41] This was achieved by placement of a pulmonary artery catheter, or a central line, in conjunction with a thermistor-tipped arterial cannula (transpulmonary aortic thermodilution).[41] Other invasive techniques measure cardiac output continuously using pulse contour or arterial pressure analysis and ultrasound Doppler methods using an oesophageal probe.[41] All methods have degrees of invasiveness, can be time consuming to yield measurements of acceptable accuracy,[41] may be expensive and are not without risk of complications.[43] The pulmonary artery catheter is a controversial assessment tool, and the risk associated with the invasive device versus benefits for the measurement of cardiac output should be considered during use.[44]

Another invasive assessment approach is the continuous estimation of mixed venous oxygen saturation using a light-emitting sensor in a pulmonary artery catheter. As tissue oxygen delivery fails to meet demand and oxygen extraction rises, the residual oxygen content of blood returning to the lungs will fall; in effect, this is a surrogate indicator of failure to meet body tissue oxygen demand. This technology was used in the landmark study by Rivers and colleagues,[45] which protocolised resuscitation after deterioration of septic shock in the emergency department (ED) and was part of a goal-directed approach to managing patients. This single-centre study was the subject of much interest for its outcomes, with goal-directed resuscitation being assessed in several major multicentre studies to verify findings within an international context and varying approaches to critical care delivery.[46]

Management principles

Patients require monitoring, assessment and interventions that optimise oxygen delivery to improve outcomes.[38,41] Managing a patient in shock focuses on treating the underlying cause, and restoration and optimisation of organ perfusion. General management strategies should not be overlooked. This includes supportive care and risk minimisation to prevent hospital-acquired complications.[47] Using mnemonics to remember routine elements of care can support clinician decision making and ensure complex care is remembered when patients are critically ill. It allows all members of the workforce to participate in standard approaches.[48] A daily 'FASTHUG',[49] or one of its many iterations, helps ensure daily assessment and interventions in priority areas, which improves the quality of care for patients in the ICU (see Practice tip below). However, interventions should be assessed for their applicability to individual patients to ensure they are required and align with the patient's goals of care.[50] Clinical management of patients with different types of shock is discussed separately below.

Practice tip

'FASTHUG' mnemonic

- **F**eeding (prevent malnutrition, promote adequate caloric intake)
- **A**nalgesia (reduce pain; improve physical and psychological wellbeing)
- **S**edation (titrate to the 3Cs – calm, cooperative, comfortable)
- **T**hromboembolic prophylaxis (prevent deep vein thrombosis)
- **H**ead of bed elevated (up to 45 degrees to reduce reflux and VAP)
- **U**lcer prophylaxis (to prevent stress ulceration)
- **G**lycaemic control (to maintain normal blood glucose levels)

Source: Vincent J-L. Give your patient a fast hug (at least) once a day. Crit Care Med 2005;33:1225–9.

TABLE 21.4

Signs and symptoms of hypovolaemic shock

PARAMETER	MILD (15–30% LOSS)	MODERATE (30–40% LOSS)	SEVERE (>40% LOSS)
Blood pressure	No change	Lowered	Hypotensive
Pulse (bpm)	≥100	≥120	≥140
Respirations (breaths/min)	>20	>30	>40
Neurological	Normal to slightly anxious	Mildly anxious to confused	Confused, lethargic
Urine output (mL/h)	>30	20–30	5–15, negligible
Capillary refill	Normal	Reduced, >4 s	Reduced, >4 s

Source: Hooper N, Armstrong TJ. Shock, hemorrhagic. Treasure Island, FL: StatPearls Publishing; 2018. Available from: https://www.ncbi.nlm.nih.gov/books/NBK470382/. CC BY 4.0.

Hypovolaemic shock

Hypovolaemia is a common primary cause of shock and a factor in other shock states. Insufficient circulating blood volume is the underlying mechanism, leading to decreased cardiac output and altered tissue perfusion.[1] Death related to haemorrhage is more likely in the first few hours after injury but improvements in trauma systems has reduced mortality.[51] The most obvious cause is direct injury to vessels leading to haemorrhage, but there are more insidious causes such as dehydration from prolonged vomiting or diarrhoea, sepsis and burns.[52] Haemorrhagic shock accounts for a considerable proportion of hypovolaemic shock,[53,54] with trauma and gastrointestinal haemorrhage significant contributors.[55] Mortality is high for patients when significant haemorrhage begins outside of acute care.[54,55] Trauma-induced coagulopathy leading to multiple organ dysfunction increases mortality. It is also important to consider other types of shock, as differential diagnoses to ensure the correct treatment of the patient.[36]

Hypovolaemic shock is often classified as mild, moderate or severe, depending on the amount of volume loss (Table 21.4[56]). As the shock state worsens, associated compensatory mechanisms will be more pronounced, and hypovolaemic shock may deteriorate to multiple organ dysfunction syndrome if poor oxygen delivery is prolonged[54] (see Chapter 22).

Clinical manifestations

Symptoms of haemorrhage may not be present until more than 15% of blood volume is lost, and will deteriorate as the shock state worsens.[57] Blood volume is approximately 7% of body weight, although estimating blood or plasma loss may be difficult as dilutional effects of resuscitation fluids may be evident when assessing haemoglobin and haematocrit.[56] As the body compensates for the reduced circulating volume, widespread vasoconstriction occurs in most body systems apart from the heart and central nervous system. Systemic vascular resistance rises markedly in an attempt to retain a viable circulatory system; this accounts for many of the signs and symptoms associated with circulatory compensation. Observations may include an increase in diastolic blood pressure and narrowing pulse pressure before systolic blood pressure drops.[56] As tissues are starved of oxygen and nutrients over a prolonged ischaemic time, local mediators are released as part of the inflammatory responses, leading to organ microvasculature vasodilation, and capillaries reopen to maintain oxygen delivery and reduce hypoxia.[56] This is a hallmark of developing multiple organ dysfunction syndrome. It is important to assess for trauma-induced coagulopathy, which may occur through consumption of coagulation factors and haemodilution from resuscitation fluids. In the presence of acidosis and hypothermia, coagulopathy has high mortality,[54] often termed the lethal triad (see Fig. 21.4).[58]

Patient management

There are recommendations that relate to the management of specific causes of hypovolaemia. Clinical management is nuanced but focuses on minimising fluid loss and careful restoration of circulating blood volume once the airway and breathing are secure. In general, for trauma and major bleeding, damage control resuscitation is recommended.[54,58]

General care priorities

More than one large-bore intravenous cannulae are usually inserted and lost circulating volume is replaced by a fluid appropriate to the clinical circumstances to achieve haemodynamic endpoints, such as a mean arterial pressure (MAP) >65 mmHg. Body heat can be lost rapidly owing to blood loss, the rapid infusion of room temperature fluids and exposure in the prehospital setting or during repeated physical examination. It is therefore important to institute measures to maintain patient temperature >35°C to avoid coagulopathies and loss of thermoregulation. The aim is to ameliorate the lethal triad. Oxygen may be administered to prevent hypoxaemia[59] and a urinary catheter aseptically inserted to monitor urine output.[60,61]

Critical care nurses must be efficient and practised at initial patient assessment to establish the degree of compensation occurring in a hypovolaemic patient. Fig. 21.5 highlights clinical manifestations of haemorrhage. Careful consideration of a patient's clinical picture will establish a hierarchy and priority of needs. Hospitals in Australia, and in other areas internationally, must have rapid response systems that trigger escalation of care to appropriate levels when a patient deteriorates.[50] However, nurses are in a position to institute first-line management, such as establishing intravenous access, if this is a skill within their scope of practice. There are also many protocols and guidelines available to guide initial fluid resuscitation where a patient has indications of inadequate circulating blood volume. Although such guidelines might vary slightly, they often aim to restore circulating blood volume through the administration of fluid boluses.[62] Balanced crystalloids are recommended[52,63] although normal saline 0.9% is reported as one of the most popular resuscitation fluids.[62] The volume is dependent on the clinical circumstances of the patient.[52,64] Critical bleeding

and massive transfusion protocols (Fig. 21.6) should also be available to guide patient management. BloodSafe Australia (https://www.bloodsafelearning.org.au) has lessons available on this issue. Vasopressors and inotropes may be required to support perfusion in some circumstances.[54]

Fluid resuscitation

Fluid resuscitation is a first-line treatment for hypovolaemic shock;[63] providing fluid volume increases preload and therefore cardiac output and organ perfusion. Fluid bolus is often triggered when patients are hypotensive and have low urine output, tachycardia, skin mottling and high lactate.[62] Both crystalloids and colloids are used as resuscitation fluids and, given that they have had different effects in different critically ill patients with different shock aetiology,[62,63] fluid therapy should be managed in the same way as prescribing medication after consideration of the risks and benefits of a selected fluid.

Giving a fluid challenge is not always appropriate; the determining factors, given current evidence, usually include assessment of volume responsiveness[63] and whether the infusion will not be deleterious, causing overload, fluid shifts and organ injury and perpetuating inflammatory responses.[62,64] The fluid type, volume, rate and targeted endpoints should be documented; and often this is structured as a bolus dose in volume to achieve a measured haemodynamic variable. Table 21.5 lists some of the frequently used resuscitation fluids and their compositions.[65] When massive transfusion is required, attention should be given to product selection, and this should be guided by an evidence-based protocol. Fluid infused usually reflects fluid loss. For example, in burns, plasma replacement might be warranted; in massive haemorrhage, fresh blood may be indicated. There has been a recent systematic review of a bundle of care for haemorrhagic shock to assess the impact of concordance with guidelines and patient outcomes[59] (Box 21.1[66]).

Minimum volume resuscitation

Much of the knowledge around major trauma and haemorrhage has come from military research and management of 'field trauma'.[58] The early use of blood products, haemostatic agents and low fluid volume during damage control resuscitation confers a survival benefit.[58] Maintaining a systolic blood pressure of approximately 90 mmHg, in the absence of traumatic brain injury, is beneficial as clotting factors are not diluted and the remaining blood volume retains its viscosity.[67] Selection of the appropriate fluid for surgical management and 'permissive hypotension' (deliberate limiting or minimising resuscitation until after adequate surgical control of haemorrhage)[54,58] will be assessed by the multidisciplinary team. This restrictive fluid regimen is a process linked to damage control surgery. The goal of this management strategy is to maintain the systolic blood pressure endpoint using blood products in an effort to limit coagulopathy,[58] and stopping the haemorrhage through direct pressure, tamponade devices and other techniques.[54,68] Definitive surgical repair is undertaken after

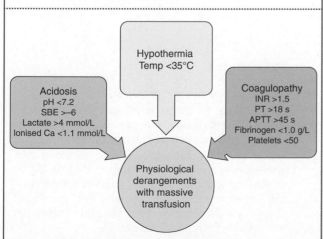

FIGURE 21.5 Physiological derangements during haemorrhage/massive transfusion. APTT = activated partial thromboplastin time; Ca = calcium; INR = international normalised ratio; PT = prothrombin time; SBE = standard base excess.

FIGURE 21.6   Massive transfusion protocol. APTT = activated partial thromboplastin time; Ca = calcium; FFP = fresh frozen plasma; INR = international normalised ratio; PT = prothrombin time; RBC = red blood cells.

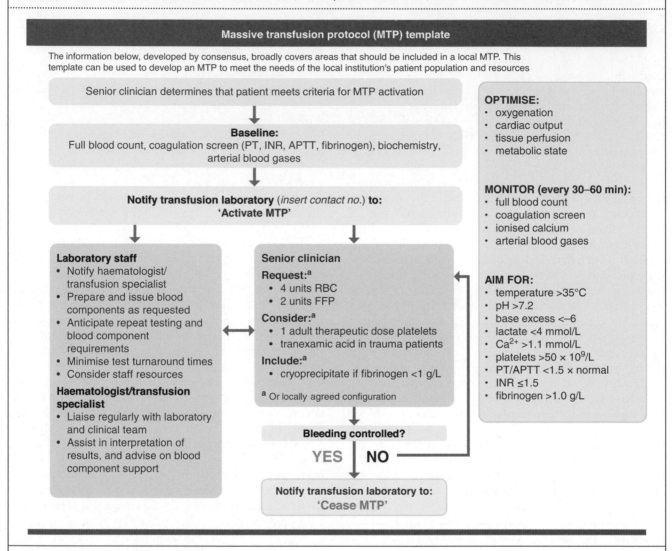

Massive transfusion protocol (MTP) template

The information below, developed by consensus, broadly covers areas that should be included in a local MTP. This template can be used to develop an MTP to meet the needs of the local institution's patient population and resources

Senior clinician determines that patient meets criteria for MTP activation

Baseline:
Full blood count, coagulation screen (PT, INR, APTT, fibrinogen), biochemistry, arterial blood gases

Notify transfusion laboratory (*insert contact no.*) **to:** 'Activate MTP'

Laboratory staff
- Notify haematologist/ transfusion specialist
- Prepare and issue blood components as requested
- Anticipate repeat testing and blood component requirements
- Minimise test turnaround times
- Consider staff resources

Haematologist/transfusion specialist
- Liaise regularly with laboratory and clinical team
- Assist in interpretation of results, and advise on blood component support

Senior clinician
Request:[a]
- 4 units RBC
- 2 units FFP

Consider:[a]
- 1 adult therapeutic dose platelets
- tranexamic acid in trauma patients

Include:[a]
- cryoprecipitate if fibrinogen <1 g/L

[a] Or locally agreed configuration

Bleeding controlled?
YES | NO

Notify transfusion laboratory to: 'Cease MTP'

OPTIMISE:
- oxygenation
- cardiac output
- tissue perfusion
- metabolic state

MONITOR (every 30–60 min):
- full blood count
- coagulation screen
- ionised calcium
- arterial blood gases

AIM FOR:
- temperature >35°C
- pH >7.2
- base excess <–6
- lactate <4 mmol/L
- Ca^{2+} >1.1 mmol/L
- platelets >50 × 10^9/L
- PT/APTT <1.5 × normal
- INR ≤1.5
- fibrinogen >1.0 g/L

Source: National Blood Authority. http://www.blood.gov.au.

bleeding is controlled and coagulopathies, temperature and acid–base disturbances are corrected in the ICU.[54]

Blood transfusions should be considered in concert with the clinical circumstances. The consensus practice point set out by the National Blood Authority guidelines considers that it is likely to be appropriate to administer red cells in patients with haemoglobin levels less than 70 g/L.[69] Use of medications such as recombinant factor VII in trauma patients requiring massive transfusion is not recommended by the Australian National Blood Authority guidelines for critical bleeding massive transfusion.[70] However, 1 gram of tranexamic acid should be administered as a bolus within 3 hours of injury, followed by 1 gram over 8 hours in acutely bleeding, critically ill patients.[69]

Practice tip

Fluid bolus in high-risk groups
- Care should be taken when administering fluid bolus to all patients with particular attention to high-risk groups such as older patients.
- Assess regularly for signs of fluid overload and pulmonary oedema including: shortness of breath, orthopnoea, bibasal auscultation of fine end-inspiratory crackles, oedema and increased central venous pressure. Escalate signs of distress immediately for medical review.

TABLE 21.5
Resuscitation fluids

VARIABLE	HUMAN PLASMA	4% ALBUMIN	COLLOIDS — HYDROXYETHYL STARCH 10% (200/0.5)	HES 6% (450/0.7)	HES 6% (130/0.4)	HES 6%	HES 6% (130/0.42)	HES	4% SUCCINYLATED MODIFIED FLUID GELATIN	3.5% UREA-LINKED GELATIN	CRYSTALLOIDS 0.9% SALINE	COMPOUNDED SODIUM LACTATE	BALANCED SALT SOLUTION
Trade name		Albumex	Hemohes	Hextend	Voluven	Volulyte	Venofundin	Tetraspan	Gelofusine	Haemaccel	Normal saline	Hartmann's or Ringer's lactate	Plasmalyte
Colloid source		Human donor	Potato starch	Maize starch	Maize starch	Maize starch	Potato starch	Potato starch	Bovine gelatin	Bovine gelatin			
Osmolarity (mOsm/L)	291	250	308	304	308	286	308	296	274	301	308	280.6	294
Sodium (mmol/L)	135–145	148	154	143	154	137	154	140	154	145	154	131	140
Potassium (mmol/L)	4.5–5.0			3.0		4.0		4.0		5.1		5.4	5.0
Calcium (mmol/L)	2.2–2.6			5.0				2.5		6.25		2.0	
Magnesium (mmol/L)	0.8–1.0			0.9		1.5		1.0					3.0
Chloride (mmol/L)	94–111	128	154	124	154	110	154	118	120	145	154	111	98
Acetate (mmol/L)	1–2					34		24					27
Lactate (mmol/L)				28								29	
Malate (mmol/L)								5					
Gluconate (mmol/L)													23
Bicarbonate (mmol/L)	23–27												
Octanoate (mmol/L)		6.4											

Note: to convert the values for potassium to milligrams per decilitre, divide by 0.2558. To convert the values for calcium to milligrams per decilitre, divide by 0.250. To convert the values for magnesium to milligrams per decilitre, divide by 0.4114.

Source: Lira A, Pinsky M. Choices in fluid type and volume during resuscitation: impact on patient outcomes. Ann Intensive Care 2014;4:38. Springer. CC BY 4.0.

BOX 21.1

Resuscitation from haemorrhagic shock

- Commence massive transfusion protocol.

- Upon arrival, measure lactate and/or base deficit.

- In a 1:1:1 ratio, transfuse packed red blood cells, platelets and plasma.

- Upon arrival, measure coagulopathy using viscoelastic techniques.

- Avoid large-volume crystalloid resuscitation (no more than 3 L over 6 hours).

Source: Adapted from Shafi S, Collinsworth AW, Richter KM, et al. Bundles of care for resuscitation from hemorrhagic shock and severe brain injury in trauma patients – translating knowledge into practice. J Trauma Acute Care Surg 2016;81(4):780–94.

Fluid type

The scientific rationale for using colloids over crystalloids as a resuscitation fluid is to preserve plasma oncotic pressure, retaining fluid in the intravascular space using far less volume.[62] This rationale has not been supported by the research, however, and debate continues particularly for subgroups.[62,64,71] If moderate-to-severe hypovolaemia is suspected, blood is often used to improve oxygen-carrying capacity. Further dilution of blood by volume expanders increases hypoxia, otherwise known as isovolaemic anaemia, and red cells are usually required. Use of isotonic saline as a volume expander is common, although resuscitation with large volumes of saline solutions can be associated with hyperchloraemic acidosis[62] and haemodilution.[63] Blood and blood components are usually considered necessary where patients exhibit signs of moderate-to-severe haemorrhage. There is no perfect resuscitation fluid, and selection is guided by patient condition and the type of fluid lost; a goal-directed, rather than aggressive, approach is usually suggested.[63]

Blood and blood products

There are a number of factors to consider when administering large amounts of blood products. Massive transfusion is defined as replacement of a patient's total blood volume in less than 24 hours or 50% of blood volume in 4 hours.[70] This equates to approximately 10 units of packed red blood cells, although there are inconsistent descriptions in the literature and newer estimations are more sensitive.[72] A number of complications following massive transfusion can be evident, such as transfusion reactions, coagulopathies, hypothermia and sepsis.[70] Massive transfusion is also associated with high mortality,[72] with human errors such as misidentification and incorrect blood component to patient also a significant risk during high-stress situations.

Patients receiving massive blood transfusions require careful monitoring for signs of volume overload, metabolic derangements, hypothermia, citrate toxicity, hyperkalaemia and coagulopathies because clotting factors are often depleted. Dilution and clotting factor consumption cause microvascular bleeding, often manifesting as oozing from multiple sites even after surgical correction (disseminated intravascular coagulation).[73] A recent meta-analysis assessed whether administration of fresher blood decreased mortality in critically ill patients. This was based on the hypothesis that shorter storage would reduce 'storage lesion' and harm to patients. It found the age of red cells does not affect outcome of critically ill patients.[74]

The National Blood Authority in Australia Critical Care module suggests a restrictive blood transfusion strategy.[69] This is supported by a National Safety and Quality Health Service Standard related to blood management.[50] The standard requires health services to optimise conserving the patient's own blood, document decisions about transfusion, prescribe in alignment with national criteria and report adverse events.[50] The current version of the Critical Care Module in the national guidelines outlines the deleterious effects of blood transfusion and makes clear recommendations about when red cells and other blood products are appropriate for use.[69]

Leukocyte depletion occurs during donation in many countries including Australia. This decreases up-regulation of the inflammatory immune response associated with transfusion. Internationally, there are a number of organisations that produce guidelines for blood transfusion. The Council of Europe has published a high-level guide on the preparation of and quality assurance on the use of blood components. The Australian National Blood Authority has published six comprehensive and easy-to-use clinical practice guidelines (see Practice tip).

Practice tip

Blood product usage

Keeping up to date can be assisted by using abbreviated recommendations and tools for use at the bedside. For example, the National Blood Authority (Australia) website has guidelines on critical bleeding/massive transfusion (see Online resources) which are currently being updated. Similar resources are available from other jurisdictions such as Canada, the United Kingdom and the United States of America. Always refer back to your local policies and guidelines before patient intervention.

The Australian National Blood Authority critical bleeding/massive transfusion guideline makes clear recommendations about blood product use during haemorrhage.[70] See Fig. 21.6 for the massive transfusion protocol template.

Fluid resuscitation in burns

Major burns are a special circumstance for fluid resuscitation. Thermal injury leads to systemic inflammation that increases capillary permeability and third spacing.[75] Patients with significant burns are usually aggressively fluid resuscitated during the first 24 hours after injury. A formula (e.g. Parkland) is often used to determine the volume of fluid to be administered to achieve haemodynamic endpoints.[71]

Cardiogenic shock

Cardiogenic shock manifests as circulatory failure from cardiac dysfunction, and is reflected in a low cardiac output (cardiac index <1.8 L/min/m^2 without support and <2.2 L/min/m^2 with support),[76] hypotension (systolic blood pressure <90 mmHg), severe pulmonary congestion and high central vascular filling pressures (pulmonary artery occlusion pressure >18 mmHg).[77]

Cardiogenic shock is commonly associated with acute myocardial infarction[78] and manifests when 40% or more of the left ventricle is ischaemic.[78] It is also related to mechanical disorders (e.g. acute cardiac valvular dysfunction or septal defects), deteriorating cardiomyopathies or congestive cardiac failure[78] and trauma. Cardiogenic shock can also occur as a result of obstruction or inhibition of left ventricular ejection, also referred to as obstructive shock, such as pulmonary embolus, dissecting aneurysm or cardiac tamponade[1] (see Chapter 10). Myocardial depression from non-cardiac causes such as sepsis, acidosis, myocardial depressant factor, hypocalcaemia or drug impact may be so severe as to present as cardiogenic shock.

Incidence has been estimated at 3% of patients presenting with acute myocardial infarction. Mortality is high (25–50%),[79] given that death from acute myocardial infarction overall is 7%. Wider distribution of interventional cardiac revascularisation services has probably improved outcomes for patients who present early in the course of their acute disease.[78] Current timing recommendations for treating myocardial infarction with ST elevation with primary percutaneous coronary intervention include a door-to-balloon time of 90 minutes or less to improve outcomes.[80]

Clinical signs include poor peripheral perfusion, tachycardia, hypotension, arrhythmia, weak pulse and other signs of organ dysfunction such as confusion, agitation, oliguria, cool extremities, peripheral oedema, jugular venous distention and dyspnoea, many of which are present in hypovolaemic shock.[78]

Compensatory mechanisms are conflicting, as cardiac workload is increased on an already-failing heart, yet cardiac muscle oxygen delivery may be compromised. A careful but rapid assessment of the clinical history is helpful in differentiating the precipitant cause of this shock.

Managing patients with heart failure as a result of cardiogenic shock can be challenging and is often undertaken simultaneously with preparation for definitive treatment. Maintaining perfusion is difficult, as compensatory mechanisms usually cause further harm to the heart. While judicious administration of fluid is considered in terms of optimising remaining cardiac function, administration of pharmacological agents that reduce cardiac workload and improve function is paramount: dobutamine for inotropic and afterload-reducing effects via vasodilation[76] and morphine to reduce pain, improve coronary perfusion and reduce oxygen demand. Treatment of the underlying cause is critical and may include surgery to repair obstruction to flow or percutaneous resolution of a coronary artery blockage. See Chapter 10 for a more detailed discussion of the management of acute myocardial infarction and heart failure.

Obstructive shock is a result of an obstruction to blood flow in the heart or large vessels and is not as common as other types of shock.[1] It has a similar clinical presentation to cardiogenic shock and is associated with a low cardiac output due to extracardiac processes inhibiting circulatory flow. The two main types are associated with impedance to cardiac filling from causes such as tension pneumothorax and cardiac tamponade and factors that increase afterload such as aortic dissection or massive pulmonary embolus.[1] Examples of conditions that can lead to obstructive shock are provided in Table 21.6. Obstructive shock may be temporarily treated by maintaining preload with fluid resuscitation until definitive intervention can be performed to remove the obstruction to forward blood flow.

Clinical manifestations

The clinical features of cardiogenic shock are reflective of congestive cardiac failure, although with greater severity[76] (Box 21.2). Other symptoms consistent with the cause of the cardiogenic shock may also be present, including chest pain and ST-segment changes, murmurs, features of pericardial tamponade and arrhythmias.

In the absence of invasive monitoring, the profile of hypotension, peripheral hypoperfusion and severe pulmonary and venous congestion is evident, although this 'classic' profile is not universal. On initial examination, approximately 30% of patients with shock of left ventricular aetiology will have no pulmonary congestion and an estimated 9% will have no hypoperfusion.[81]

In acute left ventricular myocardial infarction, the structural or contractile abnormality impairs systolic performance, resulting in incomplete left ventricular emptying. This results in subsequent progressive congestion of first the left atrium, then the pulmonary circulation, right ventricle, right atrium and finally the venous circulation.[79] When invasive haemodynamic monitoring is available, changes that may be observed include decreased cardiac output and increased systemic resistance and myocardial oxygen demand (Fig. 21.7).

A patient with cardiogenic shock is also assessed and monitored for their oxygen delivery and tissue oxygen requirements. Systemic oxygen delivery falls in proportion to a declining cardiac output and is further exacerbated as hypoxaemia develops with pulmonary oedema. Initially,

TABLE 21.6
Obstructive shock types

TYPE	DESCRIPTION	SIGNS	AETIOLOGY	TYPICAL MANAGEMENT
Cardiac tamponade	Acute circulatory failure secondary to compression of the heart chambers by a pericardial effusion.	Anxiety, hypotension, chest pain, tachypnoea, pulsus paradoxus, tachycardia, high CVP.	Pericardial injury, aortic dissection, trauma, post-cardiac surgery and rarely infective causes. Symptoms include right-sided diastolic collapse.	Pericardial drainage
Tension pneumothorax	Progressive build-up of air within the pleural space by allowing air in but not out; pressure in the pleural space pushes the mediastinum to the opposite side, obstructing venous return to the heart.	Deviated trachea away from the affected side, hyperexpansion on the side of the pneumothorax with little air movement and distended neck veins.	Penetrating chest injury, blunt trauma, hospital procedures such as insertion or removal of central lines, lung biopsy.	Needle thoracostomy as soon as possible (large cannula inserted to the 2nd intercostal space at the mid-clavicular line); however this procedure is not without complications and it has been suggested that the diagnosis should be confirmed on X-ray prior to the procedure, and a pleural drain will be required after.
Pulmonary embolism	Thrombotic occlusion of a pulmonary artery.	Increases right-sided afterload, enlarges RV and deviates septum to left, decreasing left ventricular volume and compliance.	Shortness of breath, chest pain, haemoptysis.	Thrombolysis or surgical embolectomy.

CVP = central venous pressure; RV = right ventricle.
Source: Adapted from Bodson L, Bouferrache K, Vieillard-Baron A. Cardiac tamponade. Curr Opin Crit Care 2011;17:416–24.

BOX 21.2

Clinical features of cardiogenic shock

- Low cardiac output and hypotension
- Poor peripheral perfusion – pale, cool, clammy peripheries
- Oliguria
- Altered mentation, restlessness and anxiety
- Tachycardia and arrhythmias
- Pulmonary congestion with widespread inspiratory crackles and hypoxaemia (perhaps with frank pulmonary oedema)
- Dyspnoea and tachypnoea
- Respiratory alkalosis (hyperventilation) or acidosis (respiratory fatigue)
- Lactic acidosis
- Distended neck veins, elevated jugular venous pressure

oxygen consumption may be sustained by an increase in tissue oxygen extraction ratio.[16] A quarter of delivered oxygen is extracted by tissues but, as delivery falls, tissues extract proportionally more oxygen to meet metabolic needs. Oxygen consumption can therefore be sustained until the severity of oxygen delivery deficit exceeds the ability to increase extraction. Maximal extraction is approximately 50%, and consumption falters when oxygen delivery falls to around 500–600 mL/min (cardiac index <2.2 L/min/m^2).[78] While use of a pulmonary artery catheter is a well-described measure of severity in cardiogenic shock, there is no evidence of improved patient outcomes.[78,82]

Once oxygen consumption falls, subsequent anaerobic metabolism leads to lactic acidosis.[83] Progressive tissue ischaemia and injury ensue, along with worsening metabolic acidosis unless oxygen delivery can be restored. Myocardial contractile performance continues to deteriorate when myocardial ischaemia develops, or when existing ischaemia or infarction extends, leading to a vicious cycle of ischaemia and dysfunction.

FIGURE 21.7 Sequence of haemodynamic changes in cardiogenic shock.

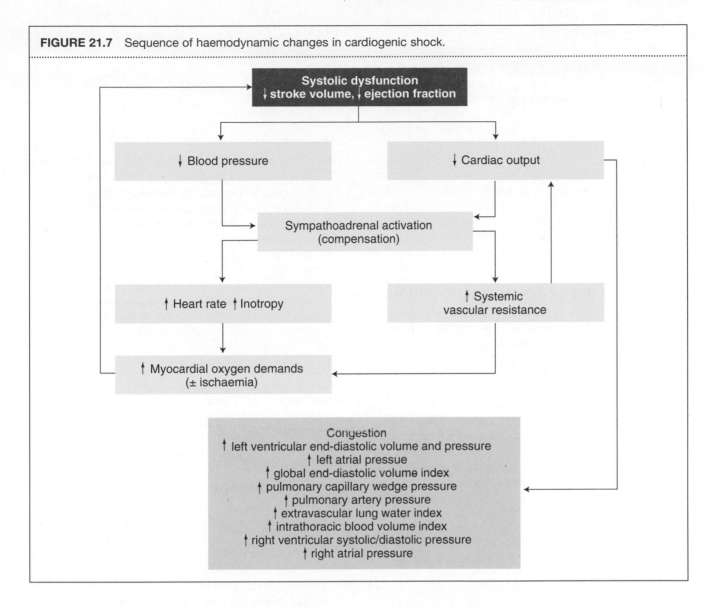

Compensatory responses effective in hypovolaemic shock are initially advantageous, but may ultimately be counterproductive when cardiogenic shock is due to myocardial infarction:[78]

- Tachycardia offsets low stroke volume but increases myocardial oxygen consumption and decreases diastolic duration, reducing coronary perfusion time.

- Vasoconstriction limits the severity of hypotension but increases resistance to left ventricular emptying and may contribute to worsening of the cardiac output, in particular when cardiogenic shock is due to contractile dysfunction.

- An increase in cardiac workload to overcome the rise in systemic afterload increases myocardial oxygen demand, which cannot be met owing to coronary artery occlusion.

- Developing pulmonary congestion is no longer contained within the pulmonary capillary and moves into the alveolar capillary space, creating pulmonary

oedema, further impeding oxygen delivery to the circulation.

Patient management

Treatment of cardiogenic shock includes haemodynamic management, respiratory and cardiovascular support, biochemical stabilisation and reversal or correction of the underlying cause. This complex presentation requires a coordinated approach to the multiple aspects of care of a patient with cardiogenic shock.

A rapid response to impending deterioration associated with cardiogenic shock includes repeated assessment and measures to optimise oxygen supply and demand. Frequent, thorough assessment of the patient's status is essential, and should focus on:

1 identification of patients at risk of physiological deterioration

2 assessment of the severity of shock and identification of the organ or system dysfunction

3 assessment of the impact of treatment

4 identification of the complications of treatment.

Assessment follows a systematic approach and is conducted as often as indicated by the patient's condition, centring on the cardiovascular system as well as related systems that cardiac function influences, including the respiratory, renal, neurological and integumentary systems.

Typical treatment regimens require preload reduction, augmentation of contractility with intravenous inotropes and afterload manipulation.[76] These aspects are undertaken concurrently owing to the potential severity of cardiogenic shock. Endotracheal intubation with mechanical ventilation is implemented, if necessary, but the need for mechanical ventilation is associated with an increase in mortality.[78]

Optimising oxygen supply and demand

As cardiogenic shock is associated with an imbalance of oxygen supply and demand throughout the body, measures to optimise this balance by increasing oxygen supply and decreasing demand are essential (Box 21.3).

Preload management

Preload reduction relieves pulmonary congestion, reduces myocardial workload and improves contractility, which is in part impaired by overstretched ventricles. Careful assessment of patient fluid status is necessary[82] prior to either the administration of small aliquots of fluid to enhance deteriorating myocardial function or enhanced diuresis to reduce circulating blood volume. Any fluid offloading is balanced against the risk of excessive blood volume depletion and depression of cardiac output and blood pressure. Desired endpoints of therapy may include a reduction in right atrial, pulmonary artery and pulmonary artery occlusion pressures, or improvements in

---

BOX 21.3

Managing oxygen supply and demand

Strategies to increase oxygen supply include:

- positioning the patient upright to promote optimum ventilation by reducing venous return and lessening pulmonary oedema; this strategy may contribute to hypotension
- administering oxygen, continuous positive airway pressure and bilevel positive airway pressure support as required.

Strategies to reduce oxygen demand include:

- limiting physical activity
- implementing measures to reduce patient anxiety, including communication, explanation and analgesic and sedative medications. Avoid those medications that are cardiodepressive.

---

intrathoracic blood volume, global end–diastolic volume and extravascular lung water, depending on available monitoring equipment.

Practice tip

Measures to reduce preload include:

- sitting a patient up with their legs either hanging over the side of the bed or in a dependent position
- intravenous diuretics administered as an intermittent bolus or, if necessary, as a continuous infusion
- venodilation (glyceryl trinitrate infusions at 10–200 micrograms/min titrated to blood pressure)[76]
- ultrafiltration (may be considered to rapidly reduce circulating volume)
- respiratory support with continuous positive airway pressure (indicated for pulmonary relief, with the additional benefit of reducing venous return).

Additional measures to reduce pulmonary hypertension may be employed. Appropriate analgesia is useful to lessen anxiety and oxygen demands during cardiogenic shock and may offer additional benefits by reducing pulmonary artery pressure and pulmonary oedema. Other treatment options include correction of hypercapnoea, if present, and nitric oxide by inhalation.

Inotropic therapy

Intravenous positive inotropes promote myocardial contractility to improve cardiac output and blood pressure.[76] Currently available inotropes are not uniform in their beneficial effect on cardiac output and blood pressure because of additional vasoactive actions (either vasodilation or constriction) (Table 21.7[76,84]). Selection of an inotropic agent is therefore partly based on inotropic potency as well as the desired effect on vascular resistance:

- vasodilation in addition to inotropy (inodilator effect) favours cardiac output, but may compromise blood pressure[85]
- vasoconstriction in addition to inotropy (inoconstrictor effect) improves blood pressure but may at times compromise left ventricular emptying and cardiac output.

All inotropes present a paradox in the treatment of cardiogenic shock, as they have the potential to increase heart rate and myocardial oxygen demands, and increase the frequency of arrhythmias.[16] Monitoring is used to identify heart rate, rhythm and the development of ST-segment or T-wave changes. The best regimen for cardiogenic shock has not been established. There is controversy about using drug combinations with opposing effects; however, there is evidence that using dilators and pressors together is superior to the use of inopressors alone.[76,82] The vasodilation seen with inodilator agents

TABLE 21.7

Vasoactive agents

DRUG	ACTIONS	DOSE RANGE	PHYSIOLOGICAL EFFECTS	NURSING CONSIDERATIONS
Dobutamine[76]	α_1-agonist β_1-agonist β_2-agonist	0.5–1 micrograms/kg/min	Inotropy Vasodilation ↑↑ Cardiac output ↑ Blood pressure ↑ Heart rate	CVC administration. Arrhythmia risk. Excess dilation may cause hypotension. Frequently used in cardiogenic and septic shock.
Dopamine	Dopaminergic β_1-agonist α-agonist (at higher doses)	'Inotropic' dose: 5–10 micrograms/kg/min 'High' dose: 10–20 micrograms/kg/min	Mainly inotropic ↑ Blood pressure ↑ Cardiac output Vasoconstriction dominates ↑↑ Blood pressure	CVC administration. Tachycardia. Arrhythmia risk. Risk peripheral vascular compromise.
Levosimendan[84]	Calcium sensitiser	Loading: 6–12 micrograms/kg over 10 min Infusion: 0.05–0.2 micrograms/kg/min (max 24–48 h use)	Inotropy Vasodilation ↑↑ Cardiac output	Tachycardia. Arrhythmia risk. Risk hypokalaemia. Risk Q-T prolongation. Excess dilation may cause hypotension. Half-life: 5 days.
Adrenaline	Sympathomimetic α-agonist β_1-agonist β_2-agonist	1–20 micrograms/min or higher	Potent inotrope and constrictor ↑ Cardiac output ↑↑ Blood pressure ↑↑ Heart rate	Tachycardia common. Arrhythmia risk. Risk peripheral vascular compromise. Myocardial work.
Milrinone	Phosphodiesterase inhibitor	Loading: 50–75 micrograms/kg Infusion: 0.375–0.75 micrograms/kg/min	Inotropy Potent vasodilator ↑↑ Cardiac output ↓ Blood pressure	Vasodilation may be marked. Observe for hypotension. Used in cardiogenic shock refractory to other agents.
Noradrenaline	Sympathomimetic α-agonist β_1-agonist Little effect on β_2-receptors	1–20 micrograms/min or higher	Potent inotrope and constrictor ↑↑ Blood pressure ↑ Coronary artery blood flow	Reflex bradycardias. Arrhythmia risk. Risk peripheral vascular compromise.
Vasopressin	Vascular (V-1) receptors Renal (V-2) receptors	0.1–0.4 micrograms/min	Inotropy ↑ SVR ↑Vasoconstriction	Check liver function. Requires renal adjustment. May decrease SV and CO.

CVC = central venous catheter; SVR = systemic vascular resistance; ↑ = increase; ↓ = decrease.

Sources: Adapted from Manolopoulos PP, Boutsikos I, Boutsikos P, et al. Current use and advances in vasopressors and inotropes support in shock. J Emerg Crit Care Med 2020;4;20. Heringlake M, Alvarez J, Bettex D, et al. An update on levosimendan in acute cardiac care: applications and recommendations for optimal efficacy and safety. Exp Rev Cardiovasc Ther 2021;19(4):325–35.

may reduce both preload and afterload, leading to more effective myocardial pumping and an increased cardiac output. The effect on blood pressure is variable, as the opposing actions of increased contractility and vasodilation are not uniform in potency and occur with differing effects between patients. By reducing afterload, left ventricular emptying is favoured, with a reduction in cardiac contractility reducing myocardial oxygen demand. In a large study of more than 900 patients with cardiogenic shock requiring a vasopressor agent to maintain perfusion, short-term mortality was improved when a dilator was part of the medication regimen.[86]

Inoconstrictors constrict the vasculature, resulting in increased preload and afterload while also increasing myocardial contractility.[87] These increases, particularly in afterload, generally result in a raised blood pressure, but the impact on cardiac output is less predictable. An increase in cardiac output is often seen with these agents, but the increase in afterload may become limiting to left ventricular emptying when there is significant contractile impairment. Inoconstrictors are therefore generally selected when the afterload and resultant blood pressure are more severely compromised than the cardiac output. Vasoconstriction also further increases myocardial work and myocardial oxygen demand, and may worsen ischaemia.[86]

Dobutamine has traditionally been the inodilator of choice,[76] although evidence for levosimendan, a calcium-sensitising agent, suggests improved outcomes.[84] The slow onset of action time of levosimendan (hours) makes it a less suitable drug for acute resuscitation; other inotropes are therefore currently used initially and, if required, levosimendan is introduced later. The long half-life (>5 days) of levosimendan confers a lasting impact on contractility after cessation of the infusion. Milrinone is also an effective inodilator,[76] but excessive vasodilation may contribute to significant hypotension; in practice, a concurrent vasoconstrictor (e.g. noradrenaline) may be administered. Close management of intravascular fluid volume is critical when using these agents.

Dopamine and adrenaline are the major agents in the inoconstrictor class and are more effective at raising blood pressure than inodilators. Both agents also increase cardiac output, but when there is significant impairment of contractility the increase in afterload may cause cardiac output to suffer. Importantly, inoconstrictors increase myocardial work and oxygen demands, raise heart rate and increase the risk of tachyarrhythmias; these impacts are stronger with adrenaline than for dopamine.[78]

Afterload control

Specific management of afterload, independent of contractility, is sometimes necessary, although caution is needed as the maintenance of blood pressure often provides little scope for further afterload reduction. Arteriodilators such as sodium nitroprusside reduce afterload and increase cardiac output, although with limitations due to hypotension.[88] The introduction of oral angiotensin-converting enzyme inhibitors is recommended as soon as possible after stabilisation of the patient with infarct-related cardiogenic shock.[89]

Adjunctive therapies

A range of adjunctive therapies is available for refractory shock, when first-line treatments are ineffective, and can include the use percutaneous mechanical circulatory support devices, which are now used more frequently[90] – these include the intra-aortic balloon pump (IABP) and extracorporeal membrane oxygenation (ECMO). Initiation of mechanical ventilation and correction of metabolic disturbances are also key interventions. These strategies are discussed below in relation to cardiogenic shock.

There is evidence that the early use of assistive devices may be preferable to inotropes and vasopressors in reducing cardiac workload in cardiogenic shock.[78] Mechanical assist devices also support coronary perfusion and circulation during procedures that treat causes of cardiogenic shock and are an option for patients who cannot be stabilised solely on medical treatment.[91] There is evidence that their use leads to improved survival.[78]

Intra-aortic balloon pumping

Low cardiac output, pulmonary congestion, reduced MAP and myocardial ischaemia from cardiogenic shock may all be improved by the introduction of IABP therapy (see Chapter 12). Balloon inflation during diastole raises MAP and promotes coronary and systemic blood flow, while balloon deflation in advance of systole reduces afterload. This afterload reduction improves cardiac output and reduces left ventricular systolic pressure, lessening the oxygen demands of the ischaemic ventricle by reducing the necessary contractile force of the left ventricle. However, IABP has not been shown to improve outcomes from patients with early revascularisation and optimal medical management.[82,92] The IABP-SHOCK trial had some limitations, with a high crossover rate, relatively small sample size and variable insertion timing.[90]

Extracorporeal membrane oxygenation

ECMO is an accepted treatment of cardiac failure when persistent shock is evident despite adequate fluid resuscitation and administration of vasopressors and inotropes.[82] There is a survival benefit in patients with cardiogenic shock.[93] ECMO is defined as the temporary use of a modified cardiopulmonary bypass circuit for support of patients with potentially reversible cardiac and/or respiratory failure.[93] ECMO provides a mechanism for gas exchange as well as cardiac support, thereby allowing for recovery from existing disease. This therapy is complex and should be provided in centres where adequate facilities and human resources are available to ensure optimal implementation.[93] There are recommendations set for use of ECMO on the Extracorporeal Life Support Organisation website (see Online resources). Management of the patient receiving ECMO is complex. Often, more than one nurse is required to provide support in the first 24 hours. Large-bore catheters are used to ensure adequate extracorporeal circulation. Apart from the infective risk, disconnection poses a risk of rapid exsanguination. While ECMO provides cardiac support and gas exchange, it is vital to continue to promote recovery by maintaining cardiac function and reducing the risk of complications.

Ventricular assist devices

These devices are rapidly implantable to support one or both ventricles.[91] Research has shown that left ventricular assist devices increase cardiac output and improve coronary blood flow. The mechanism draws blood from the left ventricle across the aortic valve and into the ascending aorta.[94] There are significant risks with their use, however.[95] Long-term outcomes indicate that use of these devices is similar to that of IABP.[96]

Respiratory support

Varying degrees of pulmonary oedema accompany cardiogenic shock, causing hypoxaemia due to intrapulmonary shunt, decreased compliance and increased work of breathing. Hyperventilation with respiratory alkalosis may initially compensate for hypoxaemia and lactic acidosis, but fatigue during this increased work of breathing may cause patient progression to hypoventilation and respiratory acidosis. Oxygen is administered for hypoxaemia, but the response may be limited as the primary gas exchange defect is an intrapulmonary shunt. Oxygen should be used with care as it increases coronary vascular resistance. Non-invasive ventilatory approaches such as high-flow nasal cannula may be sufficient, but intubation and mechanical ventilation may be required in the acute phase of treatment.[78] Continuous positive airway pressure at conventional levels of 5–15 cmH$_2$O is well established as a support for the spontaneously breathing patient with pulmonary oedema.[97] This respiratory support strategy improves hypoxaemia, decreases the work of breathing, reduces left ventricular afterload and provides additional benefit by impeding venous return, an effect that may lessen pulmonary congestion. These benefits are weighed against the potential for hypotension.

If hypoventilation and dyspnoea continue despite the use of continuous positive airway pressure, non-invasive bilevel positive airway pressure may be considered. Additional pressure support is applied during inspiration, above existing baseline pressure, which improves inspiratory efficiency, with increased tidal volume and reduced work of breathing.[97] Endotracheal intubation and ventilation should be undertaken when neither strategy above results in improvement, or when the patient continues to deteriorate or tire. Many clinicians prefer to intubate and ventilate early, even in the absence of a specific respiratory need, in order to decrease the cardiovascular demands of the greater ventilatory effort. However, this approach is controversial as mechanical ventilation is associated with poorer patient outcomes and disturbs cardiovascular balance, as it exerts changes to intrathoracic pressures, particularly at inspiratory initiation.

Ventilation strategies largely reflect those for other compliance disorders such as adult respiratory distress syndrome and are described in more detail in Chapter 15. Initially, full mechanical ventilation with little or no contribution from the patient is appropriate to correct arterial blood gases and lessen the cardiovascular demands of the ventilatory burden. Subsequent reduction of ventilatory support, as the patient's respiratory ability improves, follows conventional processes.

Biochemical normalisation

Frequent biochemistry measurement is necessary to detect and monitor the following aspects of care:

- arterial blood gases to identify the adequacy of ventilation and oxygenation and the presence of metabolic acidosis
- lactic acid measurement to assess the level of shock and changes in patient response to treatment
- hypokalaemia or hypomagnesaemia with aggressive diuretic use
- hyperkalaemia due to severe acidosis, especially in the presence of renal failure
- hyperglycaemia due to the stress response to acute illness, and in response to sympathomimetic administration
- a decline in bicarbonate levels owing to pH buffering, although replacement therapy is not routinely undertaken unless the arterial pH is life threatening
- urea and creatinine to detect the onset of acute renal failure due to renal hypoperfusion.

Renal replacement therapies may be used for fluid and electrolyte control when renal function suffers or as a strategy for unloading fluid from the circulation (see Chapter 18).

Sepsis and septic shock

Sepsis is a leading cause of admission to ICU and has an associated high mortality. In Australia, between 2013 and 2018, 1.8% of hospitalised patients had a diagnosis of sepsis, of whom 12% died in hospital, exhibiting a 11 times higher risk of dying than non-sepsis patients. The incidence of sepsis was highest among the youngest patients.[98] Notably, the incidence of sepsis is higher in Indigenous peoples and in the tropical Northern Territory, where sepsis rates are substantially higher than for temperate Australia, the United States and Europe.[99] Sepsis occurs in response to infection and can lead to organ system dysfunction and circulatory shock, resulting in high morbidity and mortality rates for hospitalised patients. Sepsis is a very complex syndrome with a heterogeneous clinical presentation that poses several challenges for its early detection and treatment.[100]

New definitions published in 2016 highlight the complex pathophysiology of sepsis and septic shock.[101] Sepsis is a life-threatening organ dysfunction resulting from a dysregulated host response to infection.[101] Septic shock is defined as a subset of sepsis in which circulatory, cellular and metabolic alterations are associated with a higher mortality rate than sepsis alone.[101] The use of the systemic inflammatory response syndrome (SIRS) criteria to identify sepsis was identified as not clinically useful, as SIRS criteria can be present in many hospitalised patients, including those who never develop infection. A study of 1,171,797 patients from 172 ICUs in Australia and New

Zealand over a 14-year timeline found that, among 109,663 who had infection and organ failure, 13,278 (12.1%) did not have SIRS criteria indicative of sepsis, highlighting that 1 in 8 patients admitted with infection and new organ failure had high rates of organ failure with significant morbidity and mortality despite not meeting the SIRS criteria for the definition of sepsis.[102]

The third consensus definition task force recommended that the terms sepsis syndrome, septicaemia and severe sepsis be eliminated. New criteria for identifying organ dysfunction in the ICU was outlined including use of the Sequential (sepsis-related) Organ Failure Assessment (SOFA) score. Variables required to calculate the SOFA include the PaO_2/FiO_2 ratio, the Glasgow Coma Scale score, MAP, serum creatinine or urine output, bilirubin level, platelet count, and type, dose and rate of vasopressor therapy. Organ dysfunction is identified as being represented by an increase in the SOFA score of 2 points or more.[101] Sepsis screening tools are recommended for the early identification of sepsis, within or outside the ICU. These may be based on manual scoring or automated electronic data capture. There are several tools, including SOFA, the National Early Warning Score (NEWS) and the Modified Early Warning Score (MEWS). Although their diagnostic and predictive value varies, machine learning applications may enhance their performance.[103,104] The Australian Clinical Care Standard recommends time critical management using a clinical pathway that supports early recognition.[105]

A 2020 World Health Organization report identified that, although the age-standardised incidence and mortality of sepsis shows a decline since 1990, sepsis remains a major cause of morbidity and fatality worldwide, with a high health-related burden in sub-Saharan Africa, Oceania, south Asia, east Asia and southeast Asia.[106] In Australian ICUs, there are approximately 48,000 admissions to hospital annually with sepsis as the main reason, of which at least 1400 die. Of survivors, many are left with a permanent disability or impaired function, such as cognitive, physical or psychological.[107]

The Surviving Sepsis Campaign

The Surviving Sepsis Campaign is an international collaborative formed after the Barcelona Declaration in 2002 to reduce the mortality of sepsis by 25% over a 5-year period. The aims included increasing awareness and developing treatment guidelines for severe sepsis and shock, including a comprehensive list of graded recommendations (now in its sixth edition).[28] Worldwide Sepsis Day occurs on 13 September each year to continue the push for improving outcomes.

The most recent update of the 'Surviving Sepsis Campaign guidelines' was published in 2021 and outlines evidence-based recommendations for the management of sepsis and septic shock.[28] However, some bundles based on previous versions of the guidelines were developed then refuted, so it is important for critical care nurses to continuously update knowledge as further evidence

becomes available. An example of a refuted bundle relates to tight glycaemic control. The recommendation in the Surviving Sepsis guidelines supported tight glycaemic control in earlier versions.[108] However, the NICE-SUGAR study subsequently concluded that measures to maintain a blood glucose level of <10 mmol/L increased mortality particularly in relation to severe hypoglycaemia.[109] A meta-analysis of 26 ICU-related 'tight glycaemic control' studies suggested that the practice could increase the risk to ICU patients.[110] The 2021 version of the Surviving Sepsis Campaign recommends initiating insulin therapy at a glucose level of ≥10 mmol/L, and identifies the need for optimal glycaemic control protocols to be developed for diabetic and non-diabetic patients, and medical and surgical patients.[28]

Clinical manifestations

Septic shock results when infectious agents or infection-induced mediators in the bloodstream produce haemodynamic compromise. Primarily a form of distributive shock, it is characterised by ineffective tissue oxygen delivery and extraction associated with endothelial damage, inappropriate peripheral vasodilation and mitochondrial dysfunction despite preserved or increased cardiac output.[111] Hypovolaemia is also associated with septic shock because of the characteristic increased vasodilation. This presents a clinical picture of a warm, pink and apparently well-perfused patient in the early stages of septic shock with an elevated cardiac output, in contrast to that seen in hypovolaemic or cardiogenic shock patients. The central pathophysiological characteristic of sepsis is a systemic inflammatory response. Therefore, early signs will typically include: fever, or hypothermia, temperature lower than 36°C; elevated heart rate >90 beats per minute in adults; respiratory rate >20 breaths per minute in adults. If severe sepsis with organ dysfunction ensues, signs and symptoms may progress to altered mentation, hypoxia/cyanosis, oliguria and/or anuria, and/or ileus. If septic shock develops, hypotension will follow. At early 'compensated' stages of shock, blood pressure may still be normal, but signs of distributive shock may be apparent – such as warm extremities and fast capillary refill (less than 1 second), a presentation described as 'warm shock'.[112] However, cellular dysfunction in the presence of a failing compensatory process will ultimately lead to cellular membrane damage, loss of ion gradients, leakage of lysosomal enzymes, proteolysis due to activation of cellular proteases and reductions in cellular energy stores that may result in cell death. Once enough cells from vital organs have reached this stage, shock becomes irreversible, and death can occur despite eradication of the underlying septic focus. A recent Australian Commission on Safety and Quality in Health Care report identified that more than one-third of hospitalised patients with sepsis experience multiple organ dysfunction, of which the most common was renal dysfunction.[98]

Endothelial activation and damage are crucial factors in multiorgan dysfunction. Aberrant endothelial responses in sepsis include defects in vasoregulation, most notably vasodilation due to nitric oxide release, and increased vascular permeability, inflammation and coagulation.[111] The effect of sepsis and septic shock on the cardiovascular system is profound; the haemodynamic hallmark is generalised arterial vasodilation with an associated decrease in systemic vascular resistance. Arterial vasodilation is mediated in part by cytokines that up-regulate the expression of inducible nitric oxide synthase in the vasculature. Vascular response to the vasodilatory effect of nitric oxide and the activation of ATP-sensitive potassium channels combine to cause closure of the voltage-gated calcium channels in the cell membrane. As the vasoconstrictor effect of noradrenaline and angiotensin II depends on open calcium channels, lack of response to these pressor hormones that are central to compensatory mechanisms in shock can occur, with the inevitable failure of delivery of oxygen to the functional mitochondria, resulting in lactic acidosis in patients with sepsis.[113] With high circulating levels of endogenous vasoactive hormones during sepsis, down-regulation of their receptors occurs.

Early identification and diagnosis

Sepsis is a very complex syndrome with heterogeneous clinical presentation that poses several challenges for its early detection and treatment.[100] Where a patient can respond cogently during history and physical assessment, timelines of the infective process should be documented. Sites considered as infective sources include decubitus ulcers, invasive lines, drains, wounds, sinuses, ears, teeth, throat, chest, blood, lungs, back, abdomen, perianal, genital/urinary tract, bones and joints. More-invasive sampling may include bronchioalveolar lavage, cerebral spinal fluid, pleural fluid, abdominal collections or biopsy of other sites as clinically appropriate. X-rays, computerised tomography scans and surgical consultation will also be a priority.

Patient management

Despite the importance of early detection of sepsis, there is no consensus on a gold standard screening tool.[114] The 2021 Surviving Sepsis guidelines recommend against the use of the quick Sequential Organ Failure Assessment (qSOFA) as the sole screening tool, because of low sensitivity.[103] In Australia, rapid response systems are embedded[8] and when aggregated scoring systems are used they possess the sensitivity to identify deteriorating patients with sepsis.[114] Many services use pathways like the SEPSIS KILLS pathway,[115] which aligns with the principles set out in the Australian Sepsis Clinical Care Standard.[105]

As with other forms of shock, initial management includes not only acting to correct physiological deterioration, by initiating fluid management and frequent observation and assessment, but also addressing the underlying cause of sepsis through source (of infection) control. Goal-directed therapy includes prevention of

tissue hypoxia, typically through rigorous fluid resuscitation with crystalloids to achieve specific haemodynamic endpoints, such as a central venous pressure of 8–12 mmHg, MAP of >65 mmHg and urine output >0.5 mL/kg/h. Vasopressor and inotropic therapy may then be added to maintain adequate perfusion pressure; noradrenaline is the vasopressor of choice because of its vasoconstrictor effects.[28]

Initial resuscitation

Sepsis and septic shock are medical emergencies and require immediate resuscitation.[28] In the 2021 Surviving Sepsis guidelines, initial resuscitation with 30 mL/kg of intravenous crystalloids is commenced immediately upon recognition of sepsis. As most patients require continued fluid administration, there is a risk of fluid overload, which may result in prolonged ventilation, acute kidney injury and increased mortality. An initial assessment and ongoing re-evaluation of the response to treatment are paramount. Heart rate, central venous pressure and systolic blood pressure are often poor indicators of fluid status, and dynamic measures are recommended to assess the need for additional fluid resuscitation and predicting those patients who are likely to respond to a fluid challenge by increasing stroke volume. Dynamic measures include passive leg raising combined with cardiac output measurement, and the effect of fluid challenges and increases in intrathoracic pressure induced by mechanical ventilation on stroke volume, systolic pressure or pulse pressure.[28]

An initial target MAP of 65 mmHg is recommended over higher MAP targets in patients with septic shock requiring vasopressors. Resuscitation is recommended to normalise lactate in patients with elevated lactate levels as a marker of tissue hypoperfusion.[113]

The 2021 Surviving Sepsis guidelines recommend use of capillary refill time, along with other measures, to guide resuscitation.[28] Capillary refill time is a readily available measure, even in low-resource settings. Normal capillary refill time is less than 2 seconds. One study demonstrated that normalising capillary refill time was superior to normalising lactate levels with regard to the effectiveness.[116]

Minimum continuous monitoring also includes electrocardiogram, blood pressure, pulse oximetry and other measures to assess preload and volume responsiveness, along with regular assessment of lactate, oxygenation and markers of inflammation and coagulation.

Source control and antimicrobial therapy

Identifying and removing the source of infection and treating the infection with appropriate antimicrobial therapy are the mainstays of therapy for a patient with sepsis. In a recent US study, genitourinary, lower respiratory and systemic fungal infections were the most common sites of infection in sepsis, with intra-abdominal, lower respiratory and biliary tract infections exhibiting the highest mortality rates.[117] In Australia, an earlier study identified that the most prevalent site of primary infection is pulmonary, followed by abdominal, together accounting for approximately 70% of cases.[118]

To provide patients with appropriate antimicrobial treatment, obtaining appropriate samples prior to instigating empirical antimicrobial therapy is the clinical standard, although any prescribed treatment should not be delayed as time to antibiotic administration is important in severe sepsis.[119] Blood cultures should be obtained immediately but should not delay antimicrobial therapy.[105] Blood cultures should be drawn percutaneously and through vascular access devices when appropriate. In a large retrospective study, every additional hour to effective antimicrobial initiation in the first 6 hours after onset of hypotension was associated with >7% decrease in survival.[119] The new recommendations stratify the course of action according the certainty of sepsis.[28] When sepsis is not certain, more time for assessment is allowed. When there is high certainty for sepsis, antimicrobial therapy should be initiated immediately, ideally within 1 hour. Diagnostic investigation should be limited to 3 hours, after which administration of antimicrobials should be initiated. If, however, sepsis is unlikely, antimicrobials should not be started. The new sepsis guidelines recommend continuous re-evaluation and assessment for alternative diagnoses.[28] In case a non-infectious aetiology is either confirmed or strongly suspected, empirical antimicrobials should be discontinued without the need to complete a short course of antimicrobials.[120] To prevent the risks of unwarranted antimicrobials or inappropriate antibiotic coverage, the 2021 guidelines stratify recommendations according to the perceived likelihood of multidrug-resistant organisms, methicillin-resistant *Staphylococcus aureus* and fungal infections.

Optimising dosage to achieve a therapeutic concentration is also important. Current practice depends on the mechanism of action of the antibiotic. For example, glycopeptides are often continuously infused to maintain a serum concentration above the minimum inhibitory concentration and therefore kill microbes more effectively. More recently there has been evidence that beta-lactams should also be infused.[121] Beta-lactams are time dependent and the concentration needs to be four times higher than the minimum inhibitory concentration in order to have efficacy.[122] The new Surviving Sepsis guidelines include a weak recommendation for prolonged infusion of beta-lactams after an initial bolus.[28]

Aminoglycosides have an effect through rapid administration to reach target concentrations and have a 'post-antibiotic effect'.

Haemodynamic support and adjunctive therapy

A range of drug therapies aimed at supporting and ameliorating the signs and symptoms of septic shock is available and, while inotropes in particular provide an important adjunct in managing the acute shock phase, other drug therapies remain controversial.

Fluid therapy in sepsis

Nurses' role in assessing responses to fluid resuscitation, and in patients' haemodynamic status, is paramount. Fluid resuscitation with crystalloid or colloid fluids has long been controversial in the critical care literature. In the 2021 sepsis guidelines, crystalloids are recommended over colloids as the first-line fluid, with albumin recommended for those patients receiving large volumes of crystalloids. It is recommended not to use gelatins, based on the higher risk for kidney damage and anaphylaxis, costs and unclear advantage for survival.[120,123,124]

Moreover, for resuscitation, balanced crystalloids, known as chloride-restrictive or buffered solutions, are recommended over normal saline, 0.9% sodium chloride, to prevent adverse effects.[125] Although the administration of normal saline solution has been standard practice for decades, potential adverse effects include hyperchloraemic metabolic acidosis, acute kidney injury and increased inflammation. Additionally, a meta-analysis has shown that balanced crystalloids were associated with improvements in survival compared with saline.[126] However, the BaSICS trial did not find a difference in 90-day mortality with intravenous fluid bolus treatment using a balanced solution versus saline solution.[127] Another area of controversy for the resuscitation of septic shock is the use of restrictive versus liberal fluid strategy for the first 24 hours of resuscitation. The 2021 sepsis guidelines did not make a recommendation on this point, but two large ongoing trials are expected to shed light on the relative merits of these approaches.[128,129]

Irrespective of fluid selection, the disruption of the vascular bed in early septic shock through widespread vasodilation results in increased capillary permeability and rapidly developing interstitial oedema. Large amounts of fluid can be administered without seemingly improving oxygen delivery while adding to developing generalised oedema that further impairs cellular delivery of oxygen and nutrients. Fluid resuscitation alone is therefore of limited value in septic shock and other measures must be considered.

Inotropes and vasopressors

Inotropes and vasopressors must be initiated when fluid resuscitation is not effective in restoring tissue perfusion. Critical care nurses manage and titrate fluid and vasopressor/inotrope therapy. For adults with septic shock who require vasopressors, an initial target MAP of 65 mmHg is recommended over higher MAP targets.[28] Invasive monitoring of arterial blood pressure is recommended as a basis for titration of vasopressors; therefore, assuring placement of an arterial catheter is necessary. To avoid delay in restoring MAP, the 2021 guidelines recommend starting vasopressor infusion from a peripheral vein until central venous access is secured.[28] Although there is a potential risk of extravasation and ischaemia at the site of infusion when peripheral catheters are used,[130] a delay of initiation of vasopressors until a central catheter is secured can increase the risk for injury and infection. Therefore, based on evidence on the low complication rate with peripheral vasopressors,[130,131] and the detrimental effects of delayed vasopressor therapy, vasopressors can be initiated from a peripheral vein proximal to the antecubital fossa. If, however, their infusion needs to be prolonged, it can be switched to a central vein. Adverse effects are less likely within the first 6 hours of peripheral infusion.[131]

Noradrenaline is the first-line agent for septic shock. To avoid escalation of the noradrenaline dose, vasopressin can be added. Adrenaline is recommended as a third vasopressor agent, or dobutamine, if there is persistent low cardiac output. Levosimendan is not recommended for persistent low cardiac output because of the lack of benefit, related risks and increased costs.[28,120]

Administration of vasopressin in vasodilatory shock may help maintain blood pressure despite the relative ineffectiveness of other vasopressor hormones.[76] Specifically, arginine vasopressin may inactivate the KATP channels and thereby lessen vascular resistance to noradrenaline and angiotensin II. The early use of vasopressin in combination with noradrenaline may help reduce adrenergic side-effects.[132] The sites of major arterial vasodilation in sepsis – the splanchnic circulation, the muscles and the skin – are vascular beds that contain abundant arginine vasopressin receptors. In sepsis, vasopressin stores are quickly depleted. Administration of exogenous arginine vasopressin (0.04–0.06 units/min) can raise blood pressure by 25–50 mmHg by returning plasma concentrations of antidiuretic hormones to their earlier high levels.[133]

Corticosteroids

The use of corticosteroid therapy in severe sepsis remains controversial. A meta-analysis has shown administration of systemic corticosteroids can accelerate the resolution of shock[134] (see Chapter 22). Moreover, administration of corticosteroids is associated with more vasopressor-free days. However, the effect of corticosteroids on mortality is not clear, and they may be associated with increased neuromuscular weakness.[28] The Surviving Sepsis guidelines recommend not using intravenous hydrocortisone to treat adult septic shock patients if adequate fluid resuscitation and vasopressor therapy are able to restore haemodynamic stability. However, for adults with septic shock with an ongoing requirement for a dose of noradrenaline or adrenaline ≥0.25 micrograms/kg/min for at least 4 hours after initiation to maintain the target MAP, there is a weak recommendation to use intravenous hydrocortisone at a dose of 200 mg/d given as 50 mg intravenously every 6 hours or as a continuous infusion.[28]

Supportive therapy

The 2021 Surviving Sepsis guidelines outline several areas of supportive therapy including red blood cell transfusion, renal replacement therapy, stress ulcer prophylaxis, deep vein thrombosis prophylaxis and nutritional support. A restrictive red blood cell transfusion approach is recommended only when the haemoglobin concentration decreases to <7.0 g/dL However, consideration of additional factors, such as acute myocardial ischaemia, severe hypoxaemia or acute haemorrhage is required for decisions around red blood cell transfusion. The 2021 Surviving Sepsis guidelines do not include specific recommendations for blood product administration.[28]

Critically ill patients have an increased risk of gastrointestinal mucosal injury owing to a sustained stress response; hence, stress ulcer prophylaxis with either proton pump inhibitors or histamine-2 receptor antagonists is recommended for patients with sepsis or septic shock.[28] However, a recent meta-analysis indicated a higher risk of recurrent *Clostridioides (Clostridium) difficile* infections with proton pump inhibitors.[135] See Chapter 20 for further discussion about stress ulcer prophylaxis.

In adults with sepsis or septic shock, pharmacological venous thromboembolism prophylaxis is recommended unless there are contraindications. Low molecular weight heparin appears to be superior to unfractionated heparin for the prevention of deep vein thrombosis.[136] The 2021 guidelines advise against using mechanical intermittent pneumatic compression and/or graduated stockings, based on a recent randomised clinical trial which found no difference in the rates of deep vein thrombosis, pulmonary embolism and mortality.[137] Moreover, an international consensus statement identified a number of adverse events associated with mechanical venous thromboembolism prophylaxis, including skin irritation, discomfort and pain, and rare but severe adverse events such as soft tissue and nerve injury.[138] However, in patients where pharmacological prophylaxis is contraindicated, mechanical venous thromboembolism prophylaxis may be beneficial. The Surviving Sepsis guidelines recommend either continuous or intermittent renal replacement therapy for patients with sepsis and acute kidney injury. Recent meta-analyses have shown no differences in patient outcomes when the two modalities are compared.[139] For adult patients with sepsis or septic shock who can be fed enterally, the guidelines suggest early initiation of enteral nutrition, within 72 hours. The early administration of enteral nutrition may contribute to gut integrity and prevention of translocation of bacteria, possibly attenuating the inflammatory response and insulin resistance.[140] See Chapter 20 for further detail about nutrition support in critical illness. The evidence about temperature management in shock states and sepsis is conflicting and it should be managed depending on the clinical circumstances.[141] Fever is an adaptive response to infection and is beneficial in activating various immune responses. The HEAT trial[142] explored whether permissive hyperthermia through avoidance of paracetamol in known or suspected infection in ICU improves survival to 28 days. The intervention and control groups had similar outcomes.[143]

Patients who survive septic shock typically face a protracted recovery, facing the physical, psychological, social and cognitive effects of a prolonged ICU stay. Patients face many rehabilitation challenges as well as the long-term complications of sepsis. The 2021 Sepsis guidelines recommend that the goals of care should be addressed early on, within the first 72 hours, with patients and/or families. Also, treatment plans should incorporate palliative care principles and, as appropriate, end-of-life care planning. As critical care nursing promotes patient- and family-centred care, addressing the needs of families and providing ongoing information and support are essential.

Septic shock in patients with COVID-19 infection

During the coronavirus disease 2019 (COVID-19) pandemic, a high percentage of COVID-19 patients in ICU developed shock. In these patients, shock is associated with organ failure, through underlying mechanisms that remain unclear. It has been proposed that the pathophysiology of COVID-19-related shock may have distinct characteristics compared with typical septic shock.[144] The Surviving Sepsis Campaign published guidelines for critically ill adult patients with COVID-19 in March 2020; however, since then our understanding and management of COVID-19 continues to evolve.[145] As COVID-19 patients may develop any type of shock, including septic (distributive), cardiogenic, hypovolaemic and obstructive, early recognition and differentiation are paramount. Noradrenaline may be used to optimise perfusion until identification of the underlying pathophysiology.[146] Acute cardiac injury, indicated by an elevated troponin level, has been common in COVID-19 patients, with causes including stress cardiomyopathy and myocarditis.[147] Obstructive shock has been associated with coagulopathies, often despite prophylactic anticoagulation. In patients with sudden haemodynamic and respiratory deterioration, acute pulmonary embolism should be suspected.[146]

Anaphylaxis

Anaphylaxis is the most severe, potentially life-threatening form of an allergic or hypersensitivity reaction,[148,149] which is often underrecognised and improperly treated before ICU admission.[148–150] It is a systemic syndrome often involving two or more organs including skin/mucous membranes, airways, and cardiovascular and/or gastrointestinal systems.[151] The Australian Commission on Safety and Quality in Health Care has issued a clinical care standard determining clinical pathways that should be in place at healthcare services. These include an assessment protocol, protocol for intramuscular administration of adrenaline, appropriate monitoring and processes for protocol adherence and clinicians' competence.[152] Anaphylaxis is mostly immunoglobulin E mediated.[153] Food-induced anaphylaxis has been defined by the National Institute of Allergy and Infectious Diseases as a serious allergic reaction that is rapid in onset, typically

mediated by immunoglobulin E, involving systemic mediator release from sensitive mast cells and basophils.[154] Food-induced anaphylaxis is being increasingly studied owing to increasing prevalence because of both genetic and unspecified environmental factors.[155] Food anaphylaxis has the same mechanism and clinical manifestations as other allergens, with sensitised mast cells and basophils. Exercise-induced anaphylaxis and food-dependent, exercise-induced anaphylaxis are rare but potentially life-threatening syndromes depending on the temporal association of allergen ingestion and exercise. Food-dependent, exercise-induced anaphylaxis develops when the ingestion of sensitising food is combined with exercise. Although the underlying mechanisms are not fully understood, increased gastrointestinal permeability and redistribution of blood flow, as well as dehydration, may play a role.[156]

Allergies are common; however, anaphylaxis appears rare.[157] In Australia the incidence of severe anaphylaxis is among the highest in developed countries.[158] Although data are sporadic in the literature, 0.01–0.02% of the general population is affected.[153] Anaphylaxis appears more common in Western countries, with a rising incidence,[154,159] but this may be related to better reporting mechanisms. The prevalence of allergy with anaphylaxis has been documented to be as high as 7% in Australian children, with insect stings, oral medications or food the most often cited causes. However, in one study, less than 1% of the population actually suffered an anaphylactic reaction manifesting with generalised multisystem allergic reaction, including evidence of airway involvement, rashes and gastrointestinal and cardiovascular dysfunction.[160] A recent Australian study reported a 9-fold rise in annual food anaphylaxis admission rates between 1998 and 2019, with an average rate of 18.2 per 100,000 population and the highest rates in those younger than 1 year.[161] There have been more than 100 food allergens identified, but there are a few responsible for most reactions and this differs based on geographical location and cannot always be explained by genetic factors.[155] The International Collaboration in Asthma, Allergy and Immunology is developing consensus guidelines to support management.[162]

The diagnosis of anaphylaxis is based on clinical criteria. The World Allergy Organization published diagnostic criteria based on clinical parameters (Box 21.4).[163] The gold standard laboratory test is serum total tryptase during the acute phase followed by a baseline measurement (≥24 h). Although increased total mast cell tryptase is diagnostic, it might not always be present; therefore, the diagnosis must be clinical.[151]

Clinical manifestations

The allergic response is via a host mast-cell reaction mediated by immunoglobulin E,[163] and antibody produced in response to the allergen that is attached to basophils (mast cells). Once sensitised to an allergen, subsequent

---

BOX 21.4

Diagnostic criteria for anaphylaxis

1 Acute onset of an illness (over minutes to several hours) involving skin, mucosal tissue or both (for example, generalised hives, pruritus or flushing, swollen lips/tongue/uvula), plus *either*:

  a respiratory compromise (for example, dyspnoea, wheeze/bronchospasm, stridor, reduced peak expiratory flow rate, hypoxaemia)

  b reduced blood pressure (BP) or associated symptoms of end-organ dysfunction (for example, hypotonia [circulatory collapse], syncope, incontinence), *or*

2 **Two** or more of the following that occur rapidly after exposure to a likely allergen for that patient (minutes to several hours):

  a involvement of the skin/mucosal tissue (e.g. generalised hives, itch/flush, swollen lips/tongue/uvula)

  b respiratory compromise (e.g. dyspnoea, wheeze/bronchospasm, stridor, reduced peak expiratory flow rate, hypoxaemia)

  c reduced BP or associated symptoms of end-organ dysfunction (e.g. hypotonia, syncope, incontinence)

  d persistent GI symptoms (e.g. crampy abdominal pain, vomiting), *or*

3 Age-related decrease in systolic BP or a greater than 30% decrease from baseline after exposure to a known allergen for that patient (minutes to several hours):

  a 1 month to 1 year: systolic BP of less than 70 mmHg

  b 1–10 years: systolic BP of less than (70 mmHg plus twice the age)

  c 11 years to adult: systolic BP of less than 90 mmHg or greater than 30% decrease from baseline.

---

exposure may lead to an anaphylactic reaction in affected individuals. One suggested mechanism is that subsequent exposure leads to mast-cell–allergen complexes and the release of histamine.[164] Reactions to an allergen cannot be predicted, however, and subsequent exposure may lead to either an amplified or a lesser response. The specific pathophysiology and immune cells and mediators can vary greatly depending on individual circumstances.[165] There may be an initial reaction, which subsides with treatment over about 24 hours, but a second or rebound reaction has also been described occurring up to 8–10 hours after initial exposure to an allergen.[163]

Exposure to an allergen causes release of histamine and other mediators, with subsequent vasodilation and increased microvascular permeability – a distributive form of shock. Histamine peaks at 5–10 minutes and is metabolised rapidly, returning to baseline within 60 minutes. Other mediators have a sustained effect.[153] This makes histamine a poor clinical biomarker for anaphylaxis. The antigen–antibody reaction may directly damage vascular walls, while release of vasoactive mediators, such as histamine, serotonin, bradykinins and prostaglandins, triggers a systemic response, resulting in vasodilation and increased capillary permeability, with widespread loss of fluid into the interstitial space and hypovolaemia. Blood pressure and cardiac output/index may fall with a compensatory rise in heart rate. Severe bronchospasm may also occur from mediator-induced bronchial oedema and pulmonary smooth muscle contraction. Abdominal pain is thought to be due to the inflammation of Peyer's patches, which are clusters of lymphatic tissue containing B lymphocytes located in the mucosa and submucosa of the small intestine.[164]

A list of signs and symptoms for anaphylaxis appears in Table 21.8. It is thought that anaphylaxis is sometimes misdiagnosed because up to 20% of presentations do not have obvious cutaneous signs.[154] Anaphylaxis should be considered when there are two or more organ systems involved. There is a high mortality in patients with asthma and those on beta-blocker or angiotensin-converting enzyme inhibitor medications.[166] These medications may limit the effectiveness of adrenaline therapy. Age and pre-existing lung disease are the most important factors in relation to severity; older people and those with asthma or airways disease have a higher risk of a life-threatening reaction.[164]

Patient management

Initial management

Diagnosis of an anaphylactic reaction requires an appropriate assessment and history, including acute onset, history of allergic reaction and initial measures instituted to support airway, breathing and circulation. Removal of the causative agent, if possible, and treatment within 30 minutes of exposure to an allergen result in improved outcomes.

The Australasian Society of Clinical Immunology and Allergy have produced guidelines for the acute management of anaphylaxis[167] and online training is also available (see Online resources). These guidelines are broadly applicable in critical care units. See the Practice tip for a list of suggested anaphylaxis emergency equipment.

Measures to assess and support airway, breathing and circulation are important, considering the rapid impact of circulating mediators and potential decline in respiratory and cardiovascular function. Securing the airway and providing high oxygen concentration is vital, as most anaphylactic-related deaths are due to asphyxiation.[153] Adrenaline is recommended as first-line drug treatment[153,164] and in a recent systematic review the

TABLE 21.8
Symptoms of allergic reactions

ORGAN SYSTEM	IMMEDIATE SYMPTOMS	DELAYED SYMPTOMS
Cutaneous	Erythema Pruritus Urticaria Morbilliform eruption Angioedema	Erythema Flushing Pruritus Morbilliform eruption Angio-oedema Eczematous rash
Ocular	Pruritus Conjunctival erythema Tearing Periorbital oedema	Pruritus Conjunctival erythema Tearing Periorbital oedema
Upper respiratory	Nasal congestion Pruritus Rhinorrhoea Sneezing Laryngeal oedema Hoarseness Dry staccato cough	
Lower respiratory	Cough Chest tightness Dyspnoea Wheezing Intercostal retractions Accessory muscle use	Cough, dyspnoea, wheezing
GI (oral)	Angio-oedema of the lips, tongue or palate Oral pruritus Tongue swelling	
GI (lower)	Nausea Colicky abdominal pain Reflux Vomiting Diarrhoea	Nausea Abdominal pain Reflux Vomiting Diarrhoea Haematochezia Irritability and food refusal with weight loss (young children)
Cardiovascular	Tachycardia (occasionally bradycardia in anaphylaxis) Hypotension Dizziness Fainting Loss of consciousness	
Miscellaneous	Uterine contractions Sense of 'impending doom'	

Source: Adapted from Simons FER, Ardusso LRF, Bilò MB, et al. International consensus on (ICON) anaphylaxis. World Allergy Organization Journal 2014;7(1):1-19. doi: 10.1186/1939-4551-7-9.

Practice tip

Anaphylaxis emergency box[167]

- Adrenaline 1:1000 (consider adrenaline autoinjector availability in rural locations for initial administration by nursing staff)
- 1-mL syringes; 22–25 G needles (25-mm length) are recommended for intramuscular injections for all ages (consistent with Australian immunisation handbook)
- Oxygen, airway equipment, including rebreather oxygen masks, nebuliser masks and suction defibrillator
- Manual blood pressure cuff
- Intravenous access equipment (including large-bore cannulae)
- At least 3 litres of normal saline
- A hands-free phone to allow healthcare providers in remote locations to receive instructions while keeping hands free for resuscitation

evidence suggested prompt use of adrenaline to reduce the risk of death.[149]

Administration is usually via intramuscular injection (to the vastus lateralis muscle or mid–outer thigh) as it leads to a more rapid increase in plasma concentration than subcutaneous administration.[149] The first dose is often given using the patient's own injecting device (e.g. Epipen or Anapen) for common food and venom allergies as they are more likely to occur out of hospital. Subsequent doses are usually required once a patient is in hospital. The Australasian Society of Clinical Immunology and Allergy suggests intramuscular adrenaline in the doses suggested in Table 21.9.[168] A 2021 update of the evidence for the emergency management of anaphylaxis, by the Resuscitation Council of the UK, emphasises repeating intramuscular adrenaline doses after 5 minutes if symptoms do not resolve.[169] After 2–3 doses of adrenaline, if there is an inadequate response or patient deterioration then intravenous adrenaline infusion must start. Infusions should be administered through a dedicated line, infusion pump and antireflux valves as possible.[167] Intravenous doses of adrenaline depend on the severity and condition of the patient. If the patient is unresponsive and life support algorithms are in play, the dose of adrenaline is 1 milligram, as per the International Liaison Committee on Resuscitation Guidelines, and the algorithms for cardiopulmonary resuscitation are followed for subsequent dosing. The dose of adrenaline administered in anaphylaxis for patients who have not been managed with advanced life support algorithms is more controversial. When a continuous infusion is required for ongoing symptom management, it is suggested that an adrenaline infusion be prepared and administered at a dose of 0.1 micrograms/kg/min with titration to maintain the desired blood

TABLE 21.9

Adrenaline dosages chart

....

Adrenaline is the first-line treatment of anaphylaxis and acts to reduce airway mucosal oedema, induce bronchodilation, induce vasoconstriction and increase strength of cardiac contraction.

Give INTRAMUSCULAR INJECTION (IMI) OF ADRENALINE (1:1000) into outer mid thigh (0.01 mg per kg up to 0.5 mg per dose) without delay using an adrenaline autoinjector if available OR adrenaline ampoule and syringe, as follows.

AGE (YEARS)	WEIGHT (KG)	VOL. ADRENALINE 1:1000	ADRENALINE AUTOINJECTOR
~<1	<7.5 kg	0.1 mL	Not available
~1–2	10	0.1 mL	7.5a–20 kg (~<5 yrs) 0.15 mg device (e.g. EpiPen Jr)
~2–3	15	0.15 mL	
~4–6	20	0.2 mL	
~7–10	30	0.3 mL	>20 kg (~>5 yrs) 0.3 mg device (e.g. EpiPen)
~10–12	40	0.4 mL	
~>12 and adults	>50	0.5 mL	

a Whilst 10–20 kg was the previous weight guide for a 0.15-mg adrenaline autoinjector device, a 0.15-mg device may now also be prescribed for an infant weighing 7.5–10 kg by health professionals who have made a considered assessment. Use of a 0.15-mg device for treatment of infants weighing 7.5 kg or more poses less risk, particularly when used without medical training, than use of an adrenaline ampoule and syringe.

Source: Reproduced with permission from the Australasian Society of Clinical Immunology and Allergy (ASCIA). The latest version of the source document can be found here: https://www.allergy.org.au/hp/papers/acute-management-of-anaphylaxis-guidelines.

pressure. The same monitoring as for any patient on an adrenaline infusion should be used, including continuous blood pressure.[168]

Aggressive fluid resuscitation (20 mL/kg) is also usually required,[168] as the intravascular blood volume may quickly be depleted by up to 70%. The type of fluid used in resuscitation can vary and, if a colloid is being administered to the patient and there is no known other trigger for the reaction, the colloid should cease as it may be responsible.[168] A maximum of 50 mL/kg in the first 30 minutes is suggested for persistent hypotension.[168]

Airway management

Early elective intubation is recommended for patients with airway oedema, stridor or any oropharyngeal swelling. Patients with airway swelling and/or angio-oedema are at high risk for rapid deterioration and respiratory compromise.[168] Late presentation to hospital or delayed intubation when airway swelling is present may mean that intubation and other emergency airway procedures may be extremely difficult. Multiple attempts at intubation increase laryngeal oedema or cause trauma to the airway. Early recognition of the potentially difficult airway allows planning for alternative airway management by experts in difficult airways.

Adjunctive support

The updated guidelines on the acute management of anaphylaxis by the Resuscitation Council of the UK include recommendations against the routine use of corticosteroids and antihistamines.[169] This recommendation is based on evidence that routine use of corticosteroids may be harmful, and associated with increased morbidity in acute anaphylaxis.[170] However, corticosteroids may be used as a third-line agent for underlying asthma or shock. Corticosteroids may also be beneficial for refractory anaphylaxis despite two doses of intramuscular adrenaline, and anaphylaxis with poorly controlled asthma. In such cases, corticosteroids are used as an adjunct to adrenaline and inotropes/vasopressor agents. Beta-2 agonists (such as salbutamol) may be used as adjuncts for lower respiratory symptoms after initial treatment with intramuscular adrenaline.[169]

Glucagon and noradrenaline may be required for patients on beta-blockers who may have resistant severe hypotension and bradycardia.[171] Glucagon exerts positive inotropic and chronotropic effects, independently of catecholamines, while atropine may reverse bradycardia.[172] Vasopressin and other vasopressors such as metaraminol are suggested where shock is refractory to adrenaline.[153] Given that a second reaction (biphasic) may occur after the initial allergic response, monitoring should continue for up to 48 hours.[153] It is suggested that antihistamines are not used in the initial emergency treatment for anaphylaxis, as they are not effective in treating respiratory or cardiovascular symptoms and they do not improve survival.[173] Moreover, H_1-antihistamine-related sedation may obscure the symptoms of anaphylaxis, and an intravenous bolus may cause hypotension.[174]

Preventative care

There is no current cure for anaphylaxis. Individuals with known allergies are taught avoidance of allergens as a first line, and then to have a management plan for inadvertent exposure including the use of emergency kits with adrenaline for intramuscular injection (Epipen).[162,168] Antihistamines are also used in food allergy to manage non-severe reactions. Recent advances in immune-modulating pharmacological agents, including allergen-specific immunotherapy and biological therapies (mostly monoclonal antibodies), appear to improve patient outcomes.[175] Desensitisation therapy may also reduce severity of symptoms and therefore improve quality of life.[176]

Neurogenic/spinal shock

Neurogenic shock is a form of distributive shock caused by loss of vasomotor (sympathetic) tone from disruption to or inhibition of neural output. It may develop in patients with cervical and high thoracic spinal cord injury. Characteristics include a systolic blood pressure <90–100 mmHg and a heart rate <80 bpm without other obvious causes.[177] Note that the heart rate is within otherwise-accepted normal limits. Neurogenic shock must be differentiated from hypovolaemic shock, which is often associated with tachycardia. Neurogenic shock is most often described as a triad of hypotension, bradycardia and hypothermia. However, the precise mechanisms are unknown.[178] The primary cause is a spinal cord injury above T6, secondary to disruption of sympathetic outflow from T1–L2 and to unopposed vagal tone, leading to decreased vascular resistance and associated vascular dilation and increased activity below the injury level.[179] It may also develop after anaesthesia, particularly spinal, cerebral medullary ischaemia or when there is spinal cord complete or partial injury above the mid-thoracic region (thoracic outflow tract).

Spinal shock is a subclass of neurogenic shock, with a transient physiological (rather than anatomical) reflex depression of cord function below the level of injury and associated loss of sensorimotor functions. Incidence has been reported in 14% of patients presenting to the ED within 2 hours of injury, predominantly[180] affects up to 20% of patients with cervical damage and lasts up to 5 weeks after an injury.[179] Spinal shock can also occur with a spinal cord laceration or contusion, and is associated with varying degrees of motor and sensory deficit (see also Chapters 17 and 23). Trauma is frequently the reason for primary injury,[180] with traffic accidents, assault, falls at work and sport the most common causes and a 4:1 ratio of males to females.[181] Simultaneous injuries may also be responsible for haemodynamic compromise,[180] and neurogenic shock with hypotension may have multiple aetiologies.[178] Haemorrhagic shock in combination with neurogenic shock has a poor outcome.

Clinical manifestations

Inhibited sympathetic outflow results in dominance of the parasympathetic nervous system, with a reduction in systemic vascular resistance and lowered blood pressure. Preload to the right heart is reduced, which lowers stroke volume and subsequent cardiac output/index. The usual response to reduction in cardiac output (a raised heart rate) does not occur owing to the parasympathetic nervous system and blockage of sympathetic compensatory responses, and the patient may be bradycardic and hypotensive,[179] with their skin warm and dry.

In spinal shock there may be an initial rise in blood pressure due to release of catecholamines, followed by hypotension,[179] which usually resolves within 24 hours.[181] Flaccid areflexic paralysis,[181] including that of the bladder and bowel, is observed and sustained priapism may also develop. Symptoms may last hours to days, until the reflex arcs below the level of injury begin to regain function. This is a result of damage to the spinal cord, and obvious manifestations include pale, cold skin above the site of injury and warm, pink skin below it. Anhidrosis (absence of sweating) may be present. Heart rate may be slow, requiring intervention.

Secondary injury may occur from impaired vasomotor tone, ischaemia, thrombosis, increased permeability, inflammation and cellular dysfunction. Spinal cord oedema occurs 3–6 days after injury and may lead to a shocked state.[181]

Patient management

The extent of injury, whether complete (no sensory or motor function) or incomplete (some sensory or motor function), determines clinical medical management. Priority focuses on airway, breathing and circulation. The riskiest time is the first 7–10 days after injury.[182]

Treatment involves early surgical decompression and fixation, vasopressors to enhance spinal cord perfusion and reduce secondary injury, and corticosteroids.[183] Haemodynamic support is required and is usually provided in an escalating manner with fluid first followed by pharmacological agents to maintain targets. Haemodynamic support with vasopressors to maintain a systolic blood pressure <90 mmHg and MAP >85–90 mmHg are recommended.[182] In patients with spinal cord injury, optimisation of MAP correlates with better recovery.[184] Noradrenaline is the vasopressor of choice as it appears to maximise the benefit to the spinal cord compared with phenylephrine and dopamine.[183,185] Spinal surgery has better outcomes when performed within 24 hours of the trauma.[179]

Initial stabilisation and neck immobilisation

After neck and torso stabilisation, the patient with confirmed or suspected spinal cord injury is placed in a position that supports spinal precautions (neutral neck positioning with immobilisation), with spinal boards removed within 20 minutes if possible. Immobilisation may be achieved with sandbags on either side of the head, the use of collars and log rolling.[181] Caution for spinal instability remains despite medical imaging clearance, because of the potential for spinal ligament damage. The patient is positioned supine, with their legs in alignment with the torso.

Elevation of the head may cause pooling of blood in the lower limbs, exacerbating hypotension,[179] and makes the patient sensitive to sudden position changes. It is important to note that, while this is a standard practice, it also may cause additional unintended issues for the patient such as discomfort, occipital pressure areas and impaired respiratory function. These precautions also inhibit airway interventions and increase the risk of aspiration and raised intracranial pressure.[181]

Spinal cord pressure monitoring and corticosteroids

Invasive epidural and intrathecal pressure monitoring have emerged as approaches to directly assess spinal perfusion. Elevated intraspinal pressure accounts for lower spinal perfusion pressures and is associated with secondary spinal cord injury.[186] In clinical studies, spinal perfusion pressures <50 mmHg have been associated with poor neurological recovery.[187] However, more work is needed to understand the clinical significance of intraspinal pressure and its role as a therapeutic target. Corticosteroid therapy remains controversial as a neuroprotective treatment for acute spinal cord injury. Methylprednisolone does not appear to improve patient outcomes at the acute phase, and is associated with a number of complications, including infections and gastrointestinal bleeding. Current guidelines do not recommend the use of steroids for acute spinal cord injury.[188]

Fluid therapy

Loss of sympathetic outflow requires close cardiac and haemodynamic monitoring for bradycardia and hypotension. Cardiovascular complications such as hypotension, bradycardia and arrhythmias are common after spinal cord injury.[179] Symptomatic bradycardia is treated and may require cardiac pacing if the patient is unresponsive to atropine. Therapies include fluid resuscitation with the addition of inotropes, if necessary, to improve vasomotor function. This increases preload and maintains a MAP >80–85 mmHg[182] to restore spinal cord perfusion and to prevent secondary neuronal hypoperfusion.[189] This higher (supranormal) MAP may be targeted to improve recovery and prevent secondary injuries.[189] Volume expansion with colloids and crystalloids or blood products will vary depending on the patient's situation; however, subgroup analysis in the

SAFE trial indicated that colloids and hypotonic solutions may not be the best options.[190]

TABLE 21.10
Respiratory muscle innervation by cord level

CORD LEVEL INNERVATION	ACCESSORY MUSCLE
C3–C5 (mostly C4)	Diaphragm
C6	Serratus anterior Latissimus dorsi Pectoralis
T1–11	Intercostals
T6–L1	Abdominals

Respiratory support

Respiratory insufficiency is common[191] and, as such, respiratory function is closely monitored to prevent or minimise atelectasis, pneumonia and secretion retention. The level of injury is indicative of the potential for respiratory muscle weakness (Table 21.10). The diaphragm is innervated by the phrenic nerve (originating at C3–C5); any injury above C3 leads to complete respiratory muscle paralysis and patients will require ventilatory support.[192] Incomplete injuries between C3 and C5 may also require ventilation initially but subsequently recover some respiratory function. Intubation is complicated by any spinal cord injury as airway interventions cause some level of spinal movement, and respiratory failure is an independent predictor of mortality in spinal cord injury.[181] Coughing, and therefore secretion clearance, is reliant on 'expiratory muscles' and, for patients with injuries that interfere with abdominal and intercostal muscle function, careful monitoring of the work of breathing and secretion clearance should be initiated. There will be varying levels of decreased respiratory function with substantially reduced lung volumes.

Adjunctive support

Hypothermia may be present, resulting from dilated peripheral blood vessels allowing radiant loss of heat. A patient is monitored for core temperature changes, and external warming devices may be required.

Paralytic ileus is a concern in the acute phase of injuries above T5, where disruption of integrative innervation pathways leads to unmodulated colonic functioning[193] and peristaltic hypomotility. Ileus may lead to respiratory compromise and should be managed. The patient should remain 'nil by mouth' and treatment includes gastric decompression, adequate intravenous hydration and electrolyte balance. Drug therapy with prokinetics, probiotics, aperients and intravenous neostigmine or lignocaine has been reported to be useful.

Pressure care is attended every second hour and, where Jordan frames are used, slats should be removed between uses. The patient is susceptible to deep venous thrombosis,[179] which is a particularly high risk when spinal cord injury is involved, so sequential calf compression devices and other prophylaxis such as anticoagulants are initiated early with D–dimers monitored regularly.

Resuscitation endpoints

Endpoints of resuscitation in shock states are similar but will differ depending on the cause. Table 21.11 outlines some of the discussed targets.

TABLE 21.11

Resuscitation endpoints

PARAMETER	TARGETS/RECOMMENDATIONS	PRECAUTIONS
Blood pressure	Target diastolic blood pressure ≥65 mmHg. Target systolic blood pressure >90 mmHg as soon as possible.	This target may be higher depending on pre-morbid state and specific organ requirements such as closed head injury or haemorrhagic shock.
Urine output	Target ≥0.5 mL/h.	
Serum lactate levels	There is evidence that serum lactate is a clear marker for outcome in patients.[25] There have been suggestions that any patient with a lactate >4 should be managed in a critical care environment. Improving lactate levels to 'normal' is associated with improved survival.	For patients presenting to emergency with a suspicion of sepsis it should be measured and assessed in the first hour.
Arterial base deficit	In combination with lactate base deficit in shock, is related to oxygen transport imbalance at the cellular level and it is a good marker with lactate level for adequacy of resuscitation.	A high base deficit (≥4) is indicative of abnormal oxygen utilisation and patients have a higher mortality.
Oxygen monitoring	Monitoring of oxygen saturation is readily available and required when any shock state is suspected. It is important to assess oxygen requirements even in the setting of acceptable oxygen saturation, as increasing requirement is indicative of deterioration. *P/F* ratio may be used as a guide to assess the level of dysfunction, given that the normal result is approximately 500 (100/0.21). Oxygenation should also be assessed through arterial blood gas sampling, and utilisation assumptions may be made by comparing with a venous sample.	A *P/F* ratio <250 in the presence of high supplemental oxygen should be regarded as indicative of serious respiratory dysfunction. Any patient requiring maximum oxygen support should be investigated.
Mixed venous oxygen saturation	Normal mixed venous oxygen saturation levels are between 60% and 80%. It may be used to guide resuscitation but is an invasive method of monitoring. Haemoglobin should be measured in conjunction with this variable.	A reduced mixed venous saturation indicates increasing extraction and worsening shock state. High levels may be seen that may be indicative of cellular dysfunction in relation to oxygen extraction.
End-tidal carbon dioxide	End-tidal carbon dioxide monitors usually provide both numeric and graphic waveform displays of the concentration using non-invasive measurement of exhaled carbon dioxide. End-tidal carbon dioxide is an estimate of the patient's alveolar ventilation status. 'Stat cap' devices are standard on resuscitation trolleys for supporting confirmation of endotracheal tube placement by quickly establishing whether carbon dioxide is exhaled.	End-tidal carbon dioxide monitoring is unreliable in the setting of increased ventilation perfusion mismatch with worsening arterial carbon dioxide retention and increased peripheral carbon dioxide production.

TABLE 21.11

Resuscitation endpoints—cont'd

PARAMETER	TARGETS/RECOMMENDATIONS	PRECAUTIONS
Preload	Preload should be maximised without overstretching. Usually this is achieved using fluid bolus in shock states (refer to the relevant sections).	Where preload is leading to congestion and cardiac failure, pharmacotherapy and ventilator support may be required.
Right ventricular end-diastolic volume index	Provides a clinical estimate of right ventricular preload and has a normal adult parameter of 60–100 mL/m^2. Observing for changes with fluid challenge may support resuscitation by providing information about volume responsiveness.	
Afterload	Afterload reduction strategies are employed in many shocked states to improve cardiac output as increased afterload increases the work of the myocardium. Afterload is affected by vascular resistance. Calculations for SVR are used to measure afterload.	During shock states, resistance is increased through constriction and oxygen and energy are required for function.
Contractility	Contractility is not easily measured clinically, but the improvement would be observed usually by increased cardiac output or other surrogate measures with the addition of inotropes.	
Temperature	Thermoregulation is an essential homeostatic mechanism. Many critically ill patients will have an elevated temperature. The literature is variable about management of temperature in different shock states.	Treatment of temperature may differ between shock states particularly in relation to patients with traumatic brain injury, sepsis and post-cardiac arrest.

P/F ratio = partial pressure of oxygen-to-fraction of inspired oxygen ratio (PaO$_2$/FiO$_2$); SVR = systemic vascular resistance.

Summary

Shock is a generic term describing a syndrome and pervasive set of life-threatening symptoms that requires time-critical interventions to improve survival. The pathophysiological changes associated with shock feature a complex interaction of compensatory mechanisms that attempt to sustain perfusion and oxygen delivery to the vital organ systems of the body. These protective responses are particularly strong in supporting cerebral perfusion and combine responses from the sympathetic nervous, endocrine and adrenal/renal systems. As shock develops, cellular dysfunction occurs in response to the release of a large collection of systemic and local inflammatory mediators, which inevitably overwhelm cell function and lead to diffuse organ injury if shock continues unabated. The classification system described here differentiates shock into categories including hypovolaemic, cardiogenic, obstructive and distributive; classification is dependent on aetiology. Distributive shock states result in impaired oxygen and nutrient delivery to the tissues as a result of failure of the vascular system (the blood distribution system). While there may be additional factors (e.g. infection) beyond simple failure to provide sufficient perfusion to the capillary bed due to widespread vascular dilation, the common factor for all underlying causes of distributive shock is widespread failure of the vasculature. Categories of distributive shock include sepsis, anaphylaxis and neurogenic shock.

Assessment is required to distinguish the type of shock to support appropriate treatment decisions, targeting the cause and managing associated symptoms. Critical care nurses are in a position to provide clinical assessment and first-line emergency management of the various shock states. Collaborative integrated care is important to provide the patient with the best possible outcome using a coordinated comprehensive care plan.

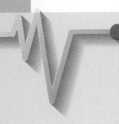

Case study

Janine is an independent 49-year-old First Nations woman who presented to the local medical service with respiratory symptoms that had persisted for several days. She was diagnosed with a viral upper respiratory infection and went home with her family with instructions to stay hydrated. Over the next few days, she felt worse but was reluctant to attend the hospital because of her bad experiences in the past. She became agitated so her family brought her to the local hospital. On assessment she met the criteria for the sepsis pathway.

Janine is 94 kg and has a history of type 2 diabetes, hypertension and depression. Initial observations in the emergency department included a blood pressure of 128/75 mmHg, heart rate of 112 bpm, temperature of 38.2°C and respiratory rate of 22 breaths/min, with an oxygen saturation of 92% on room air. Routine blood tests were ordered, and a bolus of intravenous fluid was administered in line with the hospital guidance. Intravenous antibiotics were administered, and blood cultures and lactate (1.8 mmol/L) were taken in the department within the first 6 hours of presentation. The next set of observations included a temperature of 38.9°C. The emergency department was busy, and Janine was transferred to the medical assessment unit pending admission.

The next morning Janine was reviewed on the ward round and continued to have a high respiratory rate and required 8 L of oxygen/min to sustain saturations >94%. Her observations included an increased temperature of 38.5°C and blood pressure of 110/68 mmHg. An initial chest X-ray showed left lower lobe consolidation. A note was made by the medical team in the medical record to revise antibiotics following blood culture results.

A medical review was urgently requested by the nurse as, although observations were not triggering a rapid response as part of family escalation, they had expressed concern about Janine's condition.

On assessment by the admitting team, a referral was made to the ICU. Janine was transferred to ICU for ongoing management of respiratory sepsis. She received non-invasive ventilation to maintain oxygen saturations >94%. Eventually invasive ventilation was required along with noradrenaline to support blood pressure. Blood glucose levels were difficult to manage, and she required an insulin infusion. Janine was in ICU for 5 days and improved enough to return to the ward. She was in hospital for 14 days. Janine required another hospital admission for sepsis within 6 months of the first episode and had ongoing fatigue, and impaired cognitive and physical functions which reduced her quality of life.

DISCUSSION

This case study demonstrates a common sepsis presentation. Respiratory sepsis accounts for about 50% of ICU sepsis admissions. In Australia the Closing the Gap initiatives include 17 national socioeconomic targets including long and healthy lives for Aboriginal and Torres Strait Islander peoples.

People who survive sepsis may experience cognitive impairment. The impacts of sepsis on physical function include reduced fitness and deconditioning, all of which contribute to loss of independence and reduced quality of life in survivors. Aboriginal and Torres Strait Islander peoples have poorer health outcomes than other Australians and their sepsis incidence is higher than that of other Australians. It is important when considering sepsis programs that they are inclusive, codesigned and include triggers to recognise sepsis in diverse populations. It has been suggested that reducing sepsis in Aboriginal and Torres Strait Islander populations requires reducing risk factors and addressing inequities that have health implications.

CASE STUDY QUESTIONS

1 Identify risk factors for Janine.
2 List the signs and symptoms of sepsis.
3 How could Janine's initial care have been optimised?
4 What is the current guidance for empirical antimicrobials in respiratory sepsis?
5 What opportunities exist to improve Janine's outcomes in the post-acute phase?

RESEARCH VIGNETTE

Florens N, Chabert B, Stevic N, et al. Adjusting mean arterial pressure alarms improves the time spent within blood pressure targets in patients with septic shock: a quasi-experimental study. Aust Crit Care. 2021;34(4):358–62.

Abstract

Background: Noradrenaline is the first-line vasoactive drug in septic shock. As underdosages or overdosages can be harmful for patients, it seems useful to maintain the MAP within preset bounds.

Objectives: We sought to assess whether adjusted MAP alarms could improve MAP control in patients with septic shock.

Methods: We conducted a quasi-experimental before-and-after study. During two consecutive periods, data on MAP control were obtained from patients with septic shock ($n = 50$/period) treated with noradrenaline over more than 24 hours. The noradrenaline administration protocol, including prescription of the MAP target range (e.g. 65–75 mmHg), was identical during the two periods. During the first period (control group), the preset alarms of the monitor were used (i.e. low and high systolic blood pressure alarms set at 90 and 160 mmHg respectively). During the second period, adjusted MAP alarms were implemented, with upper and lower bounds corresponding to the prescribed MAP target range (MAP-Alarm group). The primary endpoint was the percentage of time outside the desired MAP target range during the first 24 hours of noradrenaline infusion.

Results: Baseline characteristics were not significantly different. The primary endpoint was significantly lower in the MAP-Alarm group than in the control group ($25 \pm 13\%$ versus $51 \pm 18\%$, respectively; $P < 0.01$). MAP was higher than the target $14 \pm 11\%$ of the time in the MAP-Alarm group, versus $37 \pm 17\%$ in the control group ($P < 0.01$) and lower than the target $11 \pm 9\%$ of the time in the MAP-Alarm group, versus $21 \pm 22\%$ in the control group ($P < 0.05$). There was no significant difference between the two groups with regard to the dose of noradrenaline, duration of noradrenaline administration and survival.

Conclusions: These results suggest that adjusting MAP alarms to the desired MAP target range could dramatically improve the percentage of time spent within MAP targets in patients with septic shock, but does not reduce exposure to noradrenaline.

Critique

MAP below a threshold of approximately 60 mmHg is associated with decreased organ perfusion.[194] In a large retrospective study involving 110 US hospitals, it was reported that the longer the time MAP was 65 mmHg, the higher the risk of mortality, acute kidney and myocardial injury.[195] However, as this study was retrospective it did not differentiate between refractory hypotension that could not be corrected with vasoactive medications and permissive hypotension, where MAP values below 65 mmHg were acceptable for some patients. Increasing MAP improves blood flow and tissue perfusion. Although previous SSC guidelines recommended targeting a MAP of greater than 65 mmHg, the 2021 Surviving Sepsis guidelines strongly recommend an initial target MAP of 65 mmHg over higher MAP targets for adults with septic shock on vasopressors.[28] This recommendation was based on a large randomised controlled trial in ICU patients with septic shock aged 65 years or older.[196] A 'permissive hypotension' group, where MAP was kept between 60 and 65 mmHg, was compared with a 'usual care' group that received vasopressors to achieve MAP $\geq$65 mmHg. The 90-day mortality in both groups was similar, but the 'permissive hypotension' group received significantly less vasopressors.

There is no recommendation for the upper MAP limit; however, the benefits of raising MAP must be balanced against the potential side effects of vasoactive medications. MAP should be kept within narrow limits by tightly titrating doses of noradrenaline and other vasoactive medications as needed, which is a very important and time- and decision making-intensive nursing task. Practically, maintaining MAP within predefined targets can be challenging.

In this study, Florens and colleagues reported that using MAP-specific alarms with upper and lower limits corresponding to the prescribed MAP range helped achieve optimal MAP levels for a significantly greater percentage of time, which according to the evidence presented above is expected to result in better tissue perfusion and less organ dysfunction. These findings highlight a practical evidence-based way to implement the 2021 Surviving Sepsis guidelines recommendation regarding tight control of MAP values and improve the quality of care. However, these findings need to be regarded in light of some limitations of this study. The study was a 1-year quasi-experimental before-and-after observational cohort study conducted, in a 15-bed ICU, as a quality improvement program. As such, it lacks the rigour of randomised controlled trials and has high risk of bias, by virtue of being a before–after comparison at a single centre. Moreover, although the authors report results regarding MAP, they do not present any clinical data, complications or adverse effects in the study cohorts.

In conclusion, given the effect of MAP on organ perfusion, and its potential association with organ dysfunction and mortality, it is important to continue exploring ways to optimise MAP monitoring and titration of vasoactive medications according to MAP targets. It is also essential to clarify the relationship between MAP levels and patient outcomes through well-controlled studies. MAP monitoring and MAP-specific alarms can be part of quality improvement initiatives for ICU patients with sepsis and septic shock.

Learning activities

1   What are the implications for antibiotic-dosing patients receiving renal replacement therapies?
2   What assessments are important to obtain for a patient presenting with signs of hypoperfusion?
3   What are the common management strategies for all shock types?
4   What are the important considerations for managing care at the end of life?

Online resources

American College of Surgeons Trauma Quality Improvement Program, https://www.facs.org/media/zcjdtrd1/transfusion_guildelines.pdf

American Heart Association, https://www.heart.org

American Heart Association, Quality improvement, https://www.heart.org/en/professional/quality-improvement

Anaphylaxis NHS, https://www.nhs.uk/conditions/anaphylaxis/

Association for the Advancement of Blood & Biotherapies, https://www.aabb.org/

Australasian Society of Clinical Immunology and Allergy, Anaphylaxis resources, https://www.allergy.org.au/health-professionals/anaphylaxis-resources

Australasian Society of Clinical Immunology and Allergy, Anaphylaxis training for health professionals: https://www.allergy.org.au/hp/hp-e-training/ascia-anaphylaxis-e-training-for-health-professionals

Australian and New Zealand Anaesthetic Allergy Group, https://anzaag.com

Australian Commission on Safety and Quality in Health Care, Acute anaphylaxis clinical care standard, 2021, https://www.safetyandquality.gov.au/standards/clinical-care-standards/acute-anaphylaxis-clinical-care-standard

Australian Sepsis Network, https://www.australiansepsisnetwork.net.au/

Canadian Blood Services, https://professionaleducation.blood.ca/en/transfusion/clinical-guide/massive-hemorrhage-and-emergency-transfusion

Extracorporeal life support organization: https://www.elso.org/Home.aspx

JAMA Network, Trauma and injury, https://jamanetwork.com/collections/42136/trauma-and-injury

Joint United Kingdom (UK) Blood Transfusion and Tissue Transplantation Services Professional Advisory Committee, https://www.transfusionguidelines.org/transfusion-handbook/7-effective-transfusion-in-surgery-and-critical-care/7-3-transfusion-management-of-major-haemorrhage

National Blood Authority Australia, https://www.nba.gov.au

National Sepsis Program, https://www.safetyandquality.gov.au/our-work/national-sepsis-program

NSW Institute for Trauma and Injury Management, https://www.aci.health.nsw.gov.au/get-involved/institute-of-trauma-and-injury-management/clinical/trauma-guidelines/Guidelines

Patient Blood Management Guidelines, https://www.blood.gov.au/pbm-guidelines

Spinal Cord Injuries Australia: https://scia.org.au/

Surviving Sepsis Campaign, https://www.sccm.org/SurvivingSepsisCampaign/Home

Traumatic Brain Injury, https://www.traumaticbraininjury.com/

World Allergy Organization, https://www.worldallergy.org

World Health Organization, Spinal cord injury, https://www.who.int/news-room/fact-sheets/detail/spinal-cord-injury

Further reading

Australian Commission on Safety and Quality in Health Care (ACSQHC). The national consensus statement recognising and responding to acute physiological deterioration. Sydney, NSW: ACSQHC, 2021. Available from: https://www.safetyandquality.gov.au/our-work/recognising-and-responding-deterioration/recognising-and-responding-acute-physiological-deterioration/national-consensus-statement-essential-elements-recognising-and-responding-acute-physiological-deterioration

Stettler GR, Moore EE, Nunns GR, et al. Rotational thromboelastometry thresholds for patients at risk of massive transfusion. J Surg Res 2018;228:154–9.

References

1. Standl T, Annecke T, Cascorbi I, et al. The nomenclature, definition and distinction of types of shock. Dtsch Arztebl Int 2018;115(45):757–68. doi: 10.3238/arztebl.2018.0757.

2. Kislitsina ON, Rich JD, Wilcox JE, et al. Shock – classification and pathophysiological principles of therapeutics. Curr Cardiol Rev 2019;15(2):102–13. doi: 10.2174/1573403x15666181212125024.

3. Cecconi M, De Backer D, Antonelli M, et al. Consensus on circulatory shock and hemodynamic monitoring. Task force of the European Society of Intensive Care Medicine. Intensive Care Med 2014;40(12):1795–815. doi: 10.1007/s00134-014-3525-z.

4. Al Aseri Z, Al Ageel M, Binkharfi M. The use of the shock index to predict hemodynamic collapse in hypotensive sepsis patients: a cross-sectional analysis. Saudi J Anaesth 2020;14(2):192–99. doi: 10.4103/sja.SJA_780_19.

5. Kearney F, Moore A. Evaluation of hypotension. BMJ Best Practice. London: BMJ Publishing Group; 2022. Available from: https://bestpractice.bmj.com/topics/en-us/1196. [Accessed 22 February 2023].

6. Kamikawa Y, Hayashi H. Equivalency between the shock index and subtracting the systolic blood pressure from the heart rate: an observational cohort study. BMC Emerg Med 2020;20(1):87. doi: 10.1186/s12873-020-00383-2.

7. Strehlow MC. Early identification of shock in critically ill patients. Emerg Med Clin North Am 2010;28(1):57–66, vii. doi: 10.1016/j.emc.2009.09.006.

8. Australian Commission on Safety and Quality in Health Care (ACSQHC). National consensus statement: essential elements for recognising and responding to acute physiological deterioration. 3rd ed. Sydney, NSW: ACSQHC; 2021.

9. Stratton S. Evaluation of shock. BMJ Best Practice. London: BMJ Publishing Group; 2022. Available from: https://bestpractice.bmj.com/topics/en-us/779. [Accessed 22 February 2023].

10. Bloom JE, Andrew E, Dawson LP, et al. Incidence and outcomes of nontraumatic shock in adults using emergency medical services in Victoria, Australia. JAMA Netw Open 2022;5(1):e2145179. doi: 10.1001/jamanetworkopen.2021.45179.

11. Kowalski A, Brandis D. Shock resuscitation. Treasure Island, FL: StatPearls Publishing; 2022. Available from: https://www.ncbi.nlm.nih.gov/books/NBK534830/. [Accessed 22 February 2023].

12. Vincent J-L, Ince C, Bakker J. Clinical review: circulatory shock – an update: a tribute to Professor Max Harry Weil. Crit Care 2012;16(6):239. doi: 10.1186/cc11510.

13. Vincent JL, De Backer D. Circulatory shock. N Engl J Med 2013;369(18):1726–34. doi: 10.1056/NEJMra1208943.

14. Patel S, Holden K, Calvin B, et al. Shock. Crit Care Nurs Q 2022;45(3):225–32. doi: 10.1097/cnq.0000000000000407.

15. Bonanno FG. Physiopathology of shock. J Emerg Trauma Shock 2011;4(2):222–32. doi: 10.4103/0974-2700.82210.

16. Lim HS. Cardiogenic shock: failure of oxygen delivery and oxygen utilization. Clin Cardiol 2016;39(8):477–83. doi: 10.1002/clc.22564.

17. Smith N, Lopez RA, Silberman M. Distributive shock. Treasure Island, FL: StatPearls Publishing; 2022. Available from: https://www.ncbi.nlm.nih.gov/books/NBK470316/. [Accessed 22 February 2023].

18. Ince C, Mik EG. Microcirculatory and mitochondrial hypoxia in sepsis, shock, and resuscitation. J Appl Physiol (1985) 2016;120(2):226–35. doi: 10.1152/japplphysiol.00298.2015.

19. Zhu Z, Chambers S, Zeng Y, et al. Gases in sepsis: novel mediators and therapeutic targets. Int J Mol Sci 2022;23(7):3669. doi: 10.3390/ijms23073669.

20. Nagar H, Piao S, Kim CS. Role of mitochondrial oxidative stress in sepsis. Acute Crit Care 2018;33(2):65–72. doi: 10.4266/acc.2018.00157.

21. Fortin CF, McDonald PP, Fülöp T, et al. Sepsis, leukocytes, and nitric oxide (NO): an intricate affair. Shock 2010;33(4):344–52. doi: 10.1097/SHK.0b013e3181c0f068.

22. Janotka M, Ostadal P. Biochemical markers for clinical monitoring of tissue perfusion. Mol Cell Biochem 2021;476(3):1313–26. doi: 10.1007/s11010-020-04019-8.

23. Hubens WHG, Vallbona-Garcia A, de Coo IFM, et al. Blood biomarkers for assessment of mitochondrial dysfunction: an expert review. Mitochondrion 2022;62:187–204. doi: 10.1016/j.mito.2021.10.008.

24. Bou Chebl R, El Khuri C, Shami A, et al. Serum lactate is an independent predictor of hospital mortality in critically ill patients in the emergency department: a retrospective study. Scand J Trauma Resusc Emerg Med 2017;25(1):69. doi: 10.1186/s13049-017-0415-8.

25. Kushimoto S, Akaishi S, Sato T, et al. Lactate, a useful marker for disease mortality and severity but an unreliable marker of tissue hypoxia/hypoperfusion in critically ill patients. Acute Med Surg 2016;3(4):293–97. doi: 10.1002/ams2.207.

26. Foucher CD, Tubben RE. Lactic shock. Treasure Island, FL: StatPearls Publishing; 2022. Available from: https://www.ncbi.nlm.nih.gov/books/NBK470202. [Accessed 22 February 2023].

27. Zhang Z, Xu X. Lactate clearance is a useful biomarker for the prediction of all-cause mortality in critically ill patients: a systematic review and meta-analysis*. Crit Care Med 2014;42(9):2118–25. doi: 10.1097/ccm.0000000000000405.

28. Evans L, Rhodes A, Alhazzani W, et al. Surviving sepsis campaign: international guidelines for management of sepsis and septic shock 2021. Intensive Care Med 2021;47(11):1181–247. doi: 10.1007/s00134-021-06506-y.

29. Uchimido R, Schmidt EP, Shapiro NI. The glycocalyx: a novel diagnostic and therapeutic target in sepsis. Crit Care 2019;23(1):16. doi: 10.1186/s13054-018-2292-6.

30. Kellum JA, Romagnani P, Ashuntantang G, et al. Acute kidney injury. Nature Rev Dis Primers 2021;7(1):52. doi: 10.1038/s41572-021-00284-z.

31. Abe H, Semba H, Takeda N. The roles of hypoxia signaling in the pathogenesis of cardiovascular diseases. J Atheroscler Thromb 2017;24(9):884–94. doi: 10.5551/jat.RV17009 .

32. Messina A, Calabrò L, Pugliese L, et al. Fluid challenge in critically ill patients receiving haemodynamic monitoring: a systematic review and comparison of two decades. Crit Care 2022;26(1):186. doi: 10.1186/s13054-022-04056-3.

33. Kaufmann T, van der Horst ICC, Scheeren TWL. This is your toolkit in hemodynamic monitoring. Curr Opin Crit Care 2020;26(3):303–12. doi: 10.1097/mcc.0000000000000727.

34. Hiemstra B, Koster G, Wiersema R, et al. The diagnostic accuracy of clinical examination for estimating cardiac index in critically ill patients: the Simple Intensive Care Studies – I. Intensive Care Med 2019;45(2):190–200. doi: 10.1007/s00134-019-05527-y.

35. Koch E, Lovett S, Nghiem T, et al. Shock index in the emergency department: utility and limitations. Open Access Emerg Med 2019;11:179–99. doi: 10.2147/oaem.S178358.

36. Haseer Koya H, Paul M. Shock. Treasure Island, FL: StatPearls Publishing; 2022. Available from: https://www.ncbi.nlm.nih.gov/books/NBK531492. [Accessed 22 February 2023].

37. Mtaweh H, Trakas EV, Su E, et al. Advances in monitoring and management of shock. Pediatr Clin North Am 2013;60(3):641–54. doi: 10.1016/j.pcl.2013.02.013.

38. Russell A, Rivers EP, Giri PC, et al. A physiologic approach to hemodynamic monitoring and optimizing oxygen delivery in shock resuscitation. J Clin Med 2020;9(7):2052. doi: 10.3390/jcm9072052.

39. Weekes AJ, Tassone HM, Babcock A, et al. Comparison of serial qualitative and quantitative assessments of caval index and left ventricular systolic function during early fluid resuscitation of hypotensive emergency department patients. Acad Emerg Med 2011;18(9):912–21. doi: 10.1111/j.1553-2712.2011.01157.x.

40. Orso D, Paoli I, Piani T, et al. Accuracy of ultrasonographic measurements of inferior vena cava to determine fluid responsiveness: a systematic review and meta-analysis. J Intensive Care Med 2020;35(4):354–63. doi: 10.1177/0885066617752308.

41. Saugel B, Vincent JL. Cardiac output monitoring: how to choose the optimal method for the individual patient. Curr Opin Crit Care 2018;24(3):165–72. doi: 10.1097/mcc.0000000000000492.

42. Rathore A, Singh S, Lamsal R, et al. Validity of pulse pressure variation (PPV) Compared with stroke volume variation (SVV) in predicting fluid responsiveness. Turk J Anaesthesiol Reanim 2017;45(4):210–17. doi: 10.5152/tjar.2017.04568.

43. Evans DC, Doraiswamy VA, Prosciak MP, et al. Complications associated with pulmonary artery catheters: a comprehensive clinical review. Scand J Surg 2009;98(4):199–208. doi: 10.1177/145749690909800402.

44. Suess EM, Pinsky MR. Hemodynamic monitoring for the evaluation and treatment of shock: what is the current state of the art? Semin Respir Crit Care Med 2015;36(6):890–8. doi: 10.1055/s-0035-1564874.

45. Rivers E, Nguyen B, Havstad S, et al. Early goal-directed therapy in the treatment of severe sepsis and septic shock. N Engl J Med 2001;345(19):1368–77. doi: 10.1056/NEJMoa010307.

46. Nguyen HB, Jaehne AK, Jayaprakash N, et al. Early goal-directed therapy in severe sepsis and septic shock: insights and comparisons to ProCESS, ProMISe, and ARISE. Crit Care 2016;20(1):160. doi: 10.1186/s13054-016-1288-3.

47. Australian Commission on Safety and Quality in Health Care (ACSQHC). Hospital-acquired complications information kit. Sydney, NSW: ACSQHC; 2018.

48. Yartsev A. Elements of routine care in the ICU: FASTHUG. Sydney, NSW: Alex Yartsev; 2018. Available from: https://derangedphysiology. com/main/required-reading/miscellaneous-topics/Chapter%201.0.0/elements-routine-care-icu-fasthug. [Accessed 22 February 2023].

49. Vincent JL. Give your patient a fast hug (at least) once a day. Crit Care Med 2005;33(6):1225–9. doi: 10.1097/01.ccm.0000165962.16682.46.

50. Australian Commission on Safety and Quality in Health Care (ACSQHC). National safety and quality health service standards. 2nd ed. Sydney, NSW: ACSQHC; 2021.

51. Brohi K, Gruen RL, Holcomb JB. Why are bleeding trauma patients still dying? Intensive Care Med 2019;45(5):709–11. doi: 10.1007/s00134-019-05560-x.

52. Taghavi S, Nassar A, Askari R. Hypovolemic shock. Treasure Island, FL: StatPearls Publishing; 2022. Available from: https://www.ncbi.nlm. nih.gov/books/NBK513297/. [Accessed 22 February 2023].

53. Cannon JW. Hemorrhagic shock. N Engl J Med 2018;378(4):370–9. doi: 10.1056/NEJMra1705649.

54. Spahn DR, Bouillon B, Cerny V, et al. The European guideline on management of major bleeding and coagulopathy following trauma: fifth edition. Crit Care 2019;23(1):98. doi: 10.1186/s13054-019-2347-3.

55. Gipson JS, Wood EM, Cole-Sinclair MF, et al. Major haemorrhage fatalities in the Australian national coronial database. Emerg Med Australas 2018;30(3):382–8. doi: 10.1111/1742-6723.12915.

56. Hooper N, Tyler JA. Hemorrhagic shock. Treasure Island, FL: StatPearls Publishing; 2021. Available from: https://www.ncbi.nlm.nih.gov/ books/NBK470382/. [Accessed 22 February 2023].

57. Johnson AB, Burns B. Hemorrhage. Treasure Island, FL: StatPearls Publishing; 2022. Available from: https://www.ncbi.nlm.nih.gov/books/ NBK542273/. [Accessed 22 February 2023].

58. Leibner E, Andreae M, Galvagno SM, et al. Damage control resuscitation. Clin Exp Emerg Med 2020;7(1):5–13. doi: 10.15441/ceem.19.089.

59. Lang E, Neuschwander A, Favé G, et al. Clinical decision support for severe trauma patients: machine learning based definition of a bundle of care for hemorrhagic shock and traumatic brain injury. J Trauma Acute Care Surg 2022;92(1):135–43. doi: 10.1097/ta.0000000000003401.

60. Blumlein D, Griffiths I. Shock: aetiology, pathophysiology and management. Br J Nurs 2022;31(8):422–8.

61. Gardner E. Deprescribing in end-of-life care. Br J Community Nurs 2019;24(10):474–77. doi: 10.12968/bjcn.2019.24.10.474.

62. Finfer S, Myburgh J, Bellomo R. Intravenous fluid therapy in critically ill adults. Nature Rev Nephrol 2018;14(9):541–57. doi: 10.1038/s41581-018-0044-0.

63. Casey JD, Brown RM, Semler MW. Resuscitation fluids. Curr Opin Crit Care 2018;24(6):512–18. doi: 10.1097/mcc.0000000000000551.

64. Marik PE, Byrne L, van Haren F. Fluid resuscitation in sepsis: the great 30 mL per kg hoax. J Thorac Dis 2020;12(Suppl. 1):S37–47. doi: 10.21037/jtd.2019.12.84.

65. Lira A, Pinsky MR. Choices in fluid type and volume during resuscitation: impact on patient outcomes. Ann Intensive Care 2014;4:38. doi: 10.1186/s13613-014-0038-4.

66. Shafi S, Collinsworth AW, Richter KM, et al. Bundles of care for resuscitation from hemorrhagic shock and severe brain injury in trauma patients – translating knowledge into practice. J Trauma Acute Care Surg 2016;81(4):780–94. doi: 10.1097/ta.0000000000001161.

67. Jiang S, Wu M, Lu X, et al. Is restrictive fluid resuscitation beneficial not only for hemorrhagic shock but also for septic shock? a meta-analysis. Medicine 2021;100(12):e25143. doi: 10.1097/md.0000000000025143.

68. Ball CG. Damage control resuscitation: history, theory and technique. Can J Surg 2014;57(1):55–60. doi: 10.1503/cjs.020312.

69. National Blood Authority (NBA). Patient blood management guidelines: module 4 – critical care. Canberra, ACT: NBA; 2013.

70. National Blood Authority (NBA). Patient blood management guidelines: module 1 critical bleeding/massive transfusion. Canberra, ACT: NBA; 2011.

71. Ramesh GH, Uma JC, Farhath S. Fluid resuscitation in trauma: what are the best strategies and fluids? Int J Emerg Med 2019;12(1):38. doi: 10.1186/s12245-019-0253-8.

72. Moore SA, Raval JS. Massive transfusion: a review. Ann Blood 2022;7:18. doi: 10.21037/aob-22-3.

73. Papageorgiou C, Jourdi G, Adjambri E, et al. Disseminated intravascular coagulation: an update on pathogenesis, diagnosis, and therapeutic strategies. Clin Appl Thromb Hemost 2018;24(9_suppl):8s–28s. doi: 10.1177/1076029618806424.

74. Zhang W, Yu K, Chen N, et al. Age of red cells for transfusion and outcomes in critically ill patients: a meta-analysis. Transfus Med Hemother 2019;46(4):248–55. doi: 10.1159/000498863.

75. Nielson CB, Duethman NC, Howard JM, et al. Burns: pathophysiology of systemic complications and current management. J Burn Care Res 2017;38(1):e469–e81. doi: 10.1097/bcr.0000000000000355.

76. Manolopoulos PP, Boutsikos I, Boutsikos P, et al. Current use and advances in vasopressors and inotropes support in shock. J Emerg Crit Care Med 2020;4:20.

77. Hernandez-Montfort JA, Miranda D, Randhawa VK, et al. Hemodynamic-based assessment and management of cardiogenic shock. US Cardiol Rev 2022;16:e05. doi: 10.15420/usc.2021.12.

78. Vahdatpour C, Collins D, Goldberg S. Cardiogenic shock. J Am Heart Assoc 2019;8(8):e011991. doi: 10.1161/jaha.119.011991.

79. Jones TL, Nakamura K, McCabe JM. Cardiogenic shock: evolving definitions and future directions in management. Open Heart 2019;6(1):e000960. doi: 10.1136/openhrt-2018-000960.

80. Park J, Choi KH, Lee JM, et al. Prognostic implications of door-to-balloon time and onset-to-door time on mortality in patients with ST-segment-elevation myocardial infarction treated with primary percutaneous coronary intervention. J Am Heart Assoc 2019;8(9):e012188. doi: 10.1161/jaha.119.012188.

81. Menon V, White H, LeJemtel T, et al. The clinical profile of patients with suspected cardiogenic shock due to predominant left ventricular failure: a report from the SHOCK Trial Registry. SHould we emergently revascularize Occluded Coronaries in cardiogenic shocK? J Am Coll Cardiol 2000;36(3 Suppl A):1071–6. doi: 10.1016/s0735-1097(00)00874-3.

82. Shah AH, Puri R, Kalra A. Management of cardiogenic shock complicating acute myocardial infarction: a review. Clin Cardiol 2019;42(4):484–93. doi: 10.1002/clc.23168.

83. Matyukhin I, Patschan S, Ritter O, et al. Etiology and management of acute metabolic acidosis: an update. Kidney Blood Press Res 2020;45(4):523–31. doi: 10.1159/000507813

84. Heringlake M, Alvarez J, Bettex D, et al. An update on levosimendan in acute cardiac care: applications and recommendations for optimal efficacy and safety. Expert Rev CardiovascTher 2021;19(4):325–35. doi: 10.1080/14779072.2021.1905520.

85. Allen JM. Understanding vasoactive medications: focus on pharmacology and effective titration. J Infus Nurs 2014;37(2):82–6. doi: 10.1097/nan.0000000000000022.

86. Pirracchio R, Parenica J, Resche Rigon M, et al. The effectiveness of inodilators in reducing short term mortality among patient with severe cardiogenic shock: a propensity-based analysis. PLoS One 2013;8(8):e71659. doi: 10.1371/journal.pone.0071659.

87. Nativi-Nicolau J, Selzman CH, Fang JC, et al. Pharmacologic therapies for acute cardiogenic shock. Curr Opin Cardiol 2014;29(3):250–7. doi: 10.1097/hco.0000000000000057.

88. Hottinger DG, Beebe DS, Kozhimannil T, et al. Sodium nitroprusside in 2014: a clinical concepts review. J Anaesthesiol Clin Pharmacol 2014;30(4):462–71. doi: 10.4103/0970-9185.142799.

89. Herman LL, Padala SA, Ahmed I. Angiotensin converting enzyme inhibitors (ACEI). Treasure Island, FL: StatPearls Publishing; 2022. Available from: https://www.ncbi.nlm.nih.gov/books/NBK431051/. [Accessed 22 February 2023].

90. Miller PE, Solomon MA, McAreavey D. Advanced percutaneous mechanical circulatory support devices for cardiogenic shock. Crit Care Med 2017;45(11):1922–9. doi: 10.1097/ccm.0000000000002676.

91. Ni hlci T, Boardman HMP, Baig K, et al. Mechanical assist devices for acute cardiogenic shock. Cochrane Database Syst Rev 2020;6(6):CD013002.

92. Wan YD, Sun TW, Kan QC, et al. The effects of intra-aortic balloon pumps on mortality in patients undergoing high-risk coronary revascularization: a meta-analysis of randomized controlled trials of coronary artery bypass grafting and stenting era. PLoS One 2016;11(1):e0147291. doi: 10.1371/journal.pone.0147291.

93. Makdisi G, Wang IW. Extra corporeal membrane oxygenation (ECMO) review of a lifesaving technology. J Thorac Dis 2015;7(7):E166–76. doi: 10.3978/j.issn.2072-1439.2015.07.17.

94. Weil BR, Konecny F, Suzuki G, et al. Comparative hemodynamic effects of contemporary percutaneous mechanical circulatory support devices in a porcine model of acute myocardial infarction. JACC Cardiovasc Interv 2016;9(22):2292–303. Available from: https://doi.org/10.1016/j.jcin.2016.08.037.

95. Schrage B, Ibrahim K, Loehn T, et al. Impella support for acute myocardial infarction complicated by cardiogenic shock. Circulation 2019;139(10):1249–58. doi: 10.1161/circulationaha.118.036614.

96. Karami M, Eriksen E, Ouweneel DM, et al. Long-term 5-year outcome of the randomized IMPRESS in severe shock trial: percutaneous mechanical circulatory support vs. intra-aortic balloon pump in cardiogenic shock after acute myocardial infarction. Eur Heart J Acute Cardiovasc Care 2021;10(9):1009–15. doi: 10.1093/ehjacc/zuab060.

97. Masip J, Peacock WF, Price S, et al. Indications and practical approach to non-invasive ventilation in acute heart failure. Eur Heart J 2018;39(1):17–25. doi: 10.1093/eurheartj/ehx580.

98. Li L, Sunderland N, Rathnayake K, et al. Sepsis epidemiology in Australian public hospitals, a nationwide longitudinal study (2013–2018). Infection Dis Health 2021;26:S9. doi: 10.1016/j.idh.2021.09.032.

99. Davis JS, Cheng AC, McMillan M, et al. Sepsis in the tropical Top End of Australia's Northern Territory: disease burden and impact on Indigenous Australians. Med J Aust 2011;194(10):519–24. doi: 10.5694/j.1326-5377.2011.tb03088.x.

100. Caraballo C, Jaimes F. Organ dysfunction in sepsis: an ominous trajectory from infection to death. Yale J Biol Med 2019;92(4):629–40.

101. Singer M, Deutschman CS, Seymour CW, et al. The third international consensus definitions for sepsis and septic shock (Sepsis-3). JAMA 2016;315(8):801–10. doi: 10.1001/jama.2016.0287.

102. Kaukonen KM, Bailey M, Pilcher D, et al. Systemic inflammatory response syndrome criteria in defining severe sepsis. N Engl J Med 2015;372(17):1629–38. doi: 10.1056/NEJMoa1415236.

103. Schorr C, Odden A, Evans L, et al. Implementation of a multicenter performance improvement program for early detection and treatment of severe sepsis in general medical-surgical wards. J Hosp Med 2016;11(Suppl. 1):S32–9. doi: 10.1002/jhm.2656.

104. Islam MM, Nasrin T, Walther BA, et al. Prediction of sepsis patients using machine learning approach: a meta-analysis. Comput Methods Programs Biomed 2019;170:1–9. doi: 10.1016/j.cmpb.2018.12.027.

105. Australian Commission on Safety and Quality in Health Care (ACSQHC). Sepsis clinical care standard. Sydney, NSW: ACSQHC; 2022.

106. Rudd KE, Johnson SC, Agesa KM, et al. Global, regional, and national sepsis incidence and mortality, 1990–2017: analysis for the Global Burden of Disease Study. Lancet 2020;395(10219):200–11. doi: 10.1016/s0140-6736(19)32989-7.

107. Australian Commission on Safety and Quality in Health Care (ACSQHC). Sepsis survivorship: a review of the impacts of surviving sepsis for Australian patients. Sydney, NSW: ACSQHC; 2020.

108. Van den Berghe G, Schetz M, Vlasselaers D, et al. Clinical review: intensive insulin therapy in critically ill patients: NICE-SUGAR or Leuven blood glucose target? J Clin Endocrinol Metab 2009;94(9):3163–70. doi: 10.1210/jc.2009-0663.

109. Finfer S, Chittock D, Li Y, et al. Intensive versus conventional glucose control in critically ill patients with traumatic brain injury: long-term follow-up of a subgroup of patients from the NICE-SUGAR study. Intensive Care Med 2015;41(6):1037–47. doi: 10.1007/s00134-015-3757-6.

110. Griesdale DE, de Souza RJ, van Dam RM, et al. Intensive insulin therapy and mortality among critically ill patients: a meta-analysis including NICE-SUGAR study data. CMAJ 2009;180(8):821–7. doi: 10.1503/cmaj.090206.

111. Fernández-Sarmiento J, Schlapbach LJ, Acevedo L, et al. Endothelial damage in sepsis: the importance of systems biology. Front Pediatr 2022;10:828968. doi: 10.3389/fped.2022.828968.

112. Mahapatra S, Heffner AC. Septic shock. Treasure Island, FL: StatPearls Publishing; 2022. Available from: https://www.ncbi.nlm.nih.gov/books/NBK430939/. [Accessed 22 February 2023].

113. Lee SM, An WS. New clinical criteria for septic shock: serum lactate level as new emerging vital sign. J Thorac Dis 2016;8(7):1388–90. doi: 10.21037/jtd.2016.05.55.

114. Australian Commission on Safety and Quality in Health Care (ACSQHC). Review of trigger tools to support the early identification of sepsis in healthcare settings. Sydney, NSW: ACSQHC; 2021.

115. Li L, Rathnayake K, Green M, et al. Comparison of the quick Sepsis-related Organ Failure Assessment and adult sepsis pathway in predicting adverse outcomes among adult patients in general wards: a retrospective observational cohort study. Intern Med J 2021;51(2):254–63. doi: 10.1111/imj.14746.

116. Fernando SM, Tran A, Taljaard M, et al. Prognostic accuracy of the quick sequential organ failure assessment for mortality in patients with suspected infection: a systematic review and meta-analysis. Ann Intern Med 2018;168(4):266–75. doi: 10.7326/m17-2820.

117. Chou EH, Mann S, Hsu TC, et al. Incidence, trends, and outcomes of infection sites among hospitalizations of sepsis: a nationwide study. PLoS One 2020;15(1):e0227752. doi: 10.1371/journal.pone.0227752.

118. Finfer S, Bellomo R, Lipman J, et al. Adult-population incidence of severe sepsis in Australian and New Zealand intensive care units. Intensive Care Med 2004;30(4):589–96. doi: 10.1007/s00134-004-2157-0.

119. Strich JR, Heil EL, Masur H. Considerations for empiric antimicrobial therapy in sepsis and septic shock in an era of antimicrobial resistance. J Infect Dis 2020;222(Suppl. 2):S119–31. doi: 10.1093/infdis/jiaa221.

120. Schorr C, Seckel M, Papathanassoglou E, et al. Nursing implications of the updated 2021 Surviving Sepsis Campaign guidelines. Am J Crit Care 2022;31(4):329–36.

121. Taccone FS, Laterre PF, Dugernier T, et al. Insufficient β-lactam concentrations in the early phase of severe sepsis and septic shock. Crit Care 2010;14(4):R126. doi: 10.1186/cc9091.

122. Dulhunty JM, Roberts JA, Davis JS, et al. A protocol for a multicentre randomised controlled trial of continuous beta-lactam infusion compared with intermittent beta-lactam dosing in critically ill patients with severe sepsis: the BLING II study. Crit Care Resusc 2013;15(3):179–85.

123. Annane D, Siami S, Jaber S, et al. Effects of fluid resuscitation with colloids vs crystalloids on mortality in critically ill patients presenting with hypovolemic shock: the CRISTAL randomized trial. JAMA 2013;310(17):1809–17. doi: 10.1001/jama.2013.280502.

124. Rochwerg B, Alhazzani W, Gibson A, et al. Fluid type and the use of renal replacement therapy in sepsis: a systematic review and network meta-analysis. Intensive Care Med 2015;41(9):1561–71. doi: 10.1007/s00134-015-3794-1.

125. Semler MW, Kellum JA. Balanced crystalloid solutions. Am J Respir Crit Care Med 2019;199(8):952–60. doi: 10.1164/rccm.201809-1677CI.

126. Rochwerg B, Alhazzani W, Sindi A, et al. Fluid resuscitation in sepsis: a systematic review and network meta-analysis. Ann Intern Med 2014;161(5):347–55. doi: 10.7326/m14-0178 .

127. Zampieri FG, Machado FR, Biondi RS, et al. Effect of intravenous fluid treatment with a balanced solution vs 0.9% saline solution on mortality in critically ill patients: the BaSICS randomized clinical trial. JAMA 2021;326(9):1–12. doi: 10.1001/jama.2021.11684.

128. Meyhoff TS, Hjortrup PB, Møller MH, et al. Conservative vs liberal fluid therapy in septic shock (CLASSIC) trial-Protocol and statistical analysis plan. Acta Anaesthesiol Scand 2019;63(9):1262–71. doi: 10.1111/aas.13434.

129. Self WH, Semler MW, Bellomo R, et al. Liberal versus restrictive intravenous fluid therapy for early septic shock: rationale for a randomized trial. Ann Emerg Med 2018;72(4):457–66. doi: 10.1016/j.annemergmed.2018.03.039.

130. Medlej K, Kazzi AA, El Hajj Chehade A, et al. Complications from administration of vasopressors through peripheral venous catheters: an observational study. J Emerg Med 2018;54(1):47–53. doi: 10.1016/j.jemermed.2017.09.007.

131. Loubani OM, Green RS. A systematic review of extravasation and local tissue injury from administration of vasopressors through peripheral intravenous catheters and central venous catheters. J Crit Care 2015;30(3):653.e9–17. doi: 10.1016/j.jcrc.2015.01.014.

132. Ukor IF, Walley KR. Vasopressin in vasodilatory shock. Crit Care Clin 2019;35(2):247–61. doi: 10.1016/j.ccc.2018.11.004.

133. Shi R, Hamzaoui O, De Vita N, et al. Vasopressors in septic shock: which, when, and how much? Ann Transl Med 2020;8(12):794. doi: 10.21037/atm.2020.04.24.

134. Rygård SL, Butler E, Granholm A, et al. Low-dose corticosteroids for adult patients with septic shock: a systematic review with meta-analysis and trial sequential analysis. Intensive Care Med 2018;44(7):1003–16. doi: 10.1007/s00134-018-5197-6.

135. D'Silva KM, Mehta R, Mitchell M, et al. Proton pump inhibitor use and risk for recurrent *Clostridioides difficile* infection: a systematic review and meta-analysis. Clin Microbiol Infect 2021;16:S1198-743X(21)00035-5. doi: 10.1016/j.cmi.2021.01.008. Online ahead of print.

136. Alhazzani W, Lim W, Jaeschke RZ, et al. Heparin thromboprophylaxis in medical-surgical critically ill patients: a systematic review and meta-analysis of randomized trials. Crit Care Med 2013;41(9):2088–98. doi: 10.1097/CCM.0b013e31828cf104.

137. Arabi YM, Al-Hameed F, Burns KEA, et al. Adjunctive intermittent pneumatic compression for venous thromboprophylaxis. N Engl J Med 2019;380(14):1305–15. doi: 10.1056/NEJMoa1816150.

138. Rabe E, Partsch H, Morrison N, et al. Risks and contraindications of medical compression treatment –a critical reappraisal. An international consensus statement. Phlebology 2020;35(7):447–60. doi: 10.1177/0268355520909066.

139. Zhao Y, Chen Y. Effect of renal replacement therapy modalities on renal recovery and mortality for acute kidney injury: a PRISMA-compliant systematic review and meta-analysis. Semin Dial 2020;33(2):127–32. doi: 10.1111/sdi.12861.

140. McClave SA, Heyland DK. The physiologic response and associated clinical benefits from provision of early enteral nutrition. Nutr Clin Pract 2009;24(3):305–15. doi: 10.1177/0884533609335176.

141. Doyle JF, Schortgen F. Should we treat pyrexia? And how do we do it? Crit Care 2016;20(1):303. doi: 10.1186/s13054-016-1467-2.

142. Young PJ, Weatherall M, Saxena MK, et al. Statistical analysis plan for the HEAT trial: a multicentre randomised placebo-controlled trial of intravenous paracetamol in intensive care unit patients with fever and infection. Crit Care Resusc 2013;15(4):279–86.

143. Young P, Saxena M, Bellomo R, et al. Acetaminophen for fever in critically ill patients with suspected infection. N Engl J Med 2015;373(23):2215–24. doi: 10.1056/NEJMoa1508375.

144. Hutchings SD, Watchorn J, Trovato F, et al. Microcirculatory, endothelial, and inflammatory responses in critically ill patients with COVID-19 are distinct from those seen in septic shock: a case control study. Shock 2021;55(6):752–58. doi: 10.1097/shk.0000000000001672.

145. Alhazzani W, Møller MH, Arabi YM, et al. Surviving Sepsis Campaign: guidelines on the management of critically ill adults with coronavirus disease 2019 (COVID-19). Intensive Care Med 2020;46(5):854–87. doi: 10.1007/s00134-020-06022-5.

146. Fox S, Vashisht R, Siuba M, et al. Evaluation and management of shock in patients with COVID-19. Cleve Clin J Med 2020. doi: 10.3949/ccjm.87a.ccc052.

147. Madjid M, Safavi-Naeini P, Solomon SD, et al. Potential effects of coronaviruses on the cardiovascular system: a review. JAMA Cardiol 2020;5(7):831–40. doi: 10.1001/jamacardio.2020.1286.

148. Nurmatov UB, Rhatigan E, Simons FE, et al. H_2-antihistamines for the treatment of anaphylaxis with and without shock: a systematic review. Ann Allergy Asthma Immunol 2014;112(2):126–31. doi: 10.1016/j.anai.2013.11.010.

149. Dhami S, Panesar SS, Roberts G, et al. Management of anaphylaxis: a systematic review. Allergy 2014;69(2):168–75. doi: 10.1111/all.12318.

150. Sundquist BK, Jose J, Pauze D, et al. Anaphylaxis risk factors for hospitalization and intensive care: a comparison between adults and children in an upstate New York emergency department. Allergy Asthma Proc 2019;40(1):41–7. doi: 10.2500/aap.2019.40.4189.

151. Beck SC, Wilding T, Buka RJ, et al. Biomarkers in human anaphylaxis: a critical appraisal of current evidence and perspectives. Front Immunol 2019;10:494. doi: 10.3389/fimmu.2019.00494.

152. Australian Commission on Safety and Quality in Health Care (ACSQHC). Acute anaphylaxis clinical care standard. Sydney, NSW: ACSQHC; 2021.

153. Kanji S, Chant C. Allergic and hypersensitivity reactions in the intensive care unit. Crit Care Med 2010;38(Suppl. 6):S162–8. doi: 10.1097/CCM.0b013e3181de0c99.

154. Sampson HA, Muñoz-Furlong A, Campbell RL, et al. Second symposium on the definition and management of anaphylaxis: summary report – Second National Institute of Allergy and Infectious Disease/Food Allergy and Anaphylaxis Network symposium. J Allergy Clin Immunol 2006;117(2):391–7. doi: 10.1016/j.jaci.2005.12.1303.

155. Berin MC, Sampson HA. Mucosal immunology of food allergy. Curr Biol 2013;23(9):R389–400. doi: 10.1016/j.cub.2013.02.043.

156. Barg W, Medrala W, Wolanczyk-Medrala A. Exercise-induced anaphylaxis: an update on diagnosis and treatment. Curr Allergy Asthma Rep 2011;11(1):45–51. doi: 10.1007/s11882-010-0150-y.

157. Anagnostou K, Turner PJ. Myths, facts and controversies in the diagnosis and management of anaphylaxis. Arch Dis Child 2019;104(1):83–90. doi: 10.1136/archdischild-2018-314867.

158. Liu FC, Chiou HJ, Kuo CF, et al. Epidemiology of anaphylactic shock and its related mortality in hospital patients in Taiwan: a nationwide population-based study. Shock 2017;48(5):525–31. doi: 10.1097/shk.0000000000000899.

159. Turnbull JL, Adams HN, Gorard DA. Review article: the diagnosis and management of food allergy and food intolerances. Aliment Pharmacol Ther 2015;41(1):3–25. Available from: https://doi.org/10.1111/apt.12984.

160. Boros CA, Kay D, Gold MS. Parent reported allergy and anaphylaxis in 4173 South Australian children. J Paediatr Child Health 2000;36(1):36–40. doi: 10.1046/j.1440-1754.2000.00444.x.

161. Mullins RJ, Dear KBG, Tang MLK. Changes in Australian food anaphylaxis admission rates following introduction of updated allergy prevention guidelines. J Allergy Clin Immunol 2022;150(1):140–5.e1. doi: 10.1016/j.jaci.2021.12.795.

162. Simons FER, Ardusso LRF, Bilò MB, et al. International consensus on (ICON) anaphylaxis. World Allergy Organ J 2014;7(1):1–19. doi: 10.1186/1939-4551-7-9.

163. Simons FE, Ardusso LR, Bilò MB, et al. World allergy organization guidelines for the assessment and management of anaphylaxis. World Allergy Organ J 2011;4(2):13–37. doi: 10.1097/WOX.0b013e318211496c.

164. Brown SG. Clinical features and severity grading of anaphylaxis. J Allergy Clin Immunol 2004;114(2):371–6. doi: 10.1016/j.jaci.2004.04.029.

165. Reber LL, Hernandez JD, Galli SJ. The pathophysiology of anaphylaxis. J Allergy Clin Immunol 2017;140(2):335–48. doi: 10.1016/j.jaci.2017.06.003.

166. Turner PJ, Jerschow E, Umasunthar T, et al. Fatal anaphylaxis: mortality rate and risk factors. J Allergy Clin Immunol Pract 2017;5(5):1169–78. doi: 10.1016/j.jaip.2017.06.031.

167. Australasian Society of Clinical Immunology and Allergy (ASCIA). Acute management of anaphylaxis. Sydney, NSW: ASCIA; 2021. Available from: https://allergy.org.au/hp/papers/acute-management-of-anaphylaxis-guidelines/. [Accessed 22 February 2023].

168. Australasian Society of Clinical Immunology and Allergy (ASCIA). ASCIA HP guidelines – acute management of anaphylaxis. Sydney, NSW: ASCIA; 2023.

169. Dodd A, Hughes A, Sargant N, et al. Evidence update for the treatment of anaphylaxis. Resuscitation 2021;163:86–96. doi: 10.1016/j.resuscitation.2021.04.010.

170. Campbell DE. Anaphylaxis management: time to re-evaluate the role of corticosteroids. J Allergy Clin Immunol Pract 2019;7(7):2239–40. doi: 10.1016/j.jaip.2019.07.005.

171. Tang AW. A practical guide to anaphylaxis. Am Fam Physician 2003;68(7):1325–32.

172. Murakami Y, Kaneko S, Yokoyama H, et al. Successful treatment of severe adrenaline-resistant anaphylactic shock with glucagon in a patient taking a beta-blocker: a case report. JA Clin Rep 2021;7(1):86. doi: 10.1186/s40981-021-00490-4.

173. Shaker MS, Wallace DV, Golden DBK, et al. Anaphylaxis – a 2020 practice parameter update, systematic review, and Grading of Recommendations, Assessment, Development and Evaluation (GRADE) analysis. J Allergy Clin Immunol 2020;145(4):1082–123. doi: 10.1016/j.jaci.2020.01.017.

174. Randall KL, Hawkins CA. Antihistamines and allergy. Aust Prescr 2018;41(2):41–5. doi: 10.18773/austprescr.2018.013.

175. van de Veen W, Akdis M. The use of biologics for immune modulation in allergic disease. J Clin Invest 2019;129(4):1452–62. doi: 10.1172/jci124607.

176. de Silva D, Rodríguez Del Río P, de Jong NW, et al. Allergen immunotherapy and/or biologicals for IgE-mediated food allergy: a systematic review and meta-analysis. Allergy 2022;77(6):1852–62. doi: 10.1111/all.15211.

177. Dave S, Cho JJ. Neurogenic shock. Treasure Island, FL: StatPearls Publishing; 2022. Available from: https://www.ncbi.nlm.nih.gov/books/NBK459361/. [Accessed 22 February 2023].

178. Summers RL, Baker SD, Sterling SA, et al. Characterization of the spectrum of hemodynamic profiles in trauma patients with acute neurogenic shock. J Crit Care 2013;28(4):531.e1–5. doi: 10.1016/j.jcrc.2013.02.002.

179. Hagen EM. Acute complications of spinal cord injuries. World J Orthop 2015;6(1):17–23. doi: 10.5312/wjo.v6.i1.17.

180. Guly HR, Bouamra O, Lecky FE. The incidence of neurogenic shock in patients with isolated spinal cord injury in the emergency department. Resuscitation 2008;76(1):57–62. doi: 10.1016/j.resuscitation.2007.06.008 .

181. Stevens RD, Bhardwaj A, Kirsch JR, et al. Critical care and perioperative management in traumatic spinal cord injury. J Neurosurg Anesthesiol 2003;15(3):215–29. doi: 10.1097/00008506-200307000-00009.

182. Ryken TC, Hurlbert RJ, Hadley MN, et al. The acute cardiopulmonary management of patients with cervical spinal cord injuries. Neurosurgery 2013;72(Suppl. 2):84–92. doi: 10.1227/NEU.0b013e318276ee16.

183. Karsy M, Hawryluk G. Modern medical management of spinal cord injury. Curr Neurol Neurosci Rep 2019;19(9):65. doi: 10.1007/s11910-019-0984-1.

184. Hawryluk G, Whetstone W, Saigal R, et al. Mean arterial blood pressure correlates with neurological recovery after human spinal cord injury: analysis of high frequency physiologic data. J Neurotrauma 2015;32(24):1958–67. doi: 10.1089/neu.2014.3778.

185. Streijger F, So K, Manouchehri N, et al. A direct comparison between norepinephrine and phenylephrine for augmenting spinal cord perfusion in a porcine model of spinal cord injury. J Neurotrauma 2018;35(12):1345–57. doi: 10.1089/neu.2017.5285.

186. Yang CH, Quan ZX, Wang GJ, et al. Elevated intraspinal pressure in traumatic spinal cord injury is a promising therapeutic target. Neural Regen Res 2022;17(8):1703–10. doi: 10.4103/1673-5374.332203.

187. Squair JW, Bélanger LM, Tsang A, et al. Spinal cord perfusion pressure predicts neurologic recovery in acute spinal cord injury. Neurology 2017;89(16):1660–7. doi: 10.1212/wnl.0000000000004519.

188. Hurlbert RJ, Hadley MN, Walters BC, et al. Pharmacological therapy for acute spinal cord injury. Neurosurgery 2013;72(Suppl. 2):93–105. doi: 10.1227/NEU.0b013e31827765c6.

189. Miko I, Gould R, Wolf S, et al. Acute spinal cord injury. Int Anesthesiol Clin 2009;47(1):37–54. doi: 10.1097/AIA.0b013e3181950068.

190. Finfer S, Bellomo R, Boyce N, et al. A comparison of albumin and saline for fluid resuscitation in the intensive care unit. N Engl J Med 2004;350(22):2247–56. doi: 10.1056/NEJMoa040232.

191. Johnson KG, Hill LJ. Pulmonary management of the acute cervical spinal cord injured patients. Nurs Clin N Am 2014;49(3):357–69. doi: 10.1016/j.cnur.2014.05.009.

192. Alizadeh A, Dyck SM, Karimi-Abdolrezaee S. Traumatic spinal cord injury: an overview of pathophysiology, models and acute injury mechanisms. Front Neurol 2019;10:282. doi: 10.3389/fneur.2019.00282.

193. Baumann A, Audibert G, Klein O, et al. Continuous intravenous lidocaine in the treatment of paralytic ileus due to severe spinal cord injury. Acta Anaesthesiol Scand 2009;53(1):128–30. doi: 10.1111/j.1399-6576.2008.01787.x.

194. Asfar P, Radermacher P, Ostermann M. MAP of 65: target of the past? Intensive Care Med 2018;44(9):1551–52. doi: 10.1007/s00134-018-5292-8.

195. Maheshwari K, Nathanson BH, Munson SH, et al. The relationship between ICU hypotension and in-hospital mortality and morbidity in septic patients. Intensive Care Med 2018;44(6):857–67. doi: 10.1007/s00134-018-5218-5.

196. Lamontagne F, Richards-Belle A, Thomas K, et al. Effect of reduced exposure to vasopressors on 90-day mortality in older critically ill patients with vasodilatory hypotension: a randomized clinical trial. JAMA 2020;323(10):938–49. doi: 10.1001/jama.2020.0930.

Chapter 22

Multiple organ dysfunction syndrome

Melanie Greenwood, Alison Juers

Learning objectives

After reading this chapter, you should be able to:

- define the common terminology related to multiple organ dysfunction syndrome
- describe the related pathophysiology of multiple organ dysfunction syndrome
- identify the clinical manifestations of multiple organ dysfunction syndrome
- identify patients at risk of developing multiple organ dysfunction, including predictors of mortality
- initiate appropriate monitoring, care planning and evaluation strategies for the patient with multiple organ dysfunction in relation to the current evidence base
- discuss treatment strategies that promote homeostasis in the patient with multiple organ dysfunction syndrome.

Introduction

Multiple organ dysfunction syndrome (MODS) remains common, resource intensive and the most frequent cause of death in the intensive care.[1–5] MODS is essentially an iatrogenic critical care disease whereby the provision of support for failing organs permits survival of patients that may have otherwise succumbed to their illness and further unintended organ insult is permitted to progress.[1] The term MODS describes a continuum of physiological derangements and subsequent dynamic alterations in organ function that may occur during a critical illness.[1] Multiple organ failure was a term commonly used, but is somewhat misleading as normal physiological function can, in most cases, be restored in survivors of a critical illness who have temporary organ dysfunction.[2,3] Although the syndrome affects many organs, it also affects physiological systems such as the haematological, immune and endocrine systems. MODS therefore more accurately describes altered organ function in a critically ill patient who requires medical and nursing interventions to achieve homeostasis.[1,2]

MODS is associated with widespread endothelial and parenchymal cell injury because of hypoxic hypoxia, direct cytotoxicity, apoptosis, immunosuppression and coagulopathy.[1] The inflammatory response, tissue hypoxia, immune and cellular metabolic dysregulations, and endothelial and microvascular dysfunction are a result of cytokine storms that affect various organs in the body causing structural and tissue changes, which generally manifest as lung, kidney or liver dysfunction.[6,7] The clinical changes in the patient with developing MODS may result in:[8,9]

1 increasing volume requirements and mild respiratory alkalosis, accompanied by oliguria and hyperglycaemia

2 tachypnoea, hypocapnia and hypoxaemia, with moderate liver dysfunction and possible haematological abnormalities

3 developing shock with azotaemia, acid–base disturbances and significant coagulation abnormalities

4 vasopressor dependence with oliguria or anuria, ischaemic colitis and lactic acidosis.

Cellular damage in various organs in patients who develop MODS begins with the onset of local injury that is then compounded by activation of the innate immune system. This includes a combination of pattern recognition, receptor activation and release of mediators at the microcellular level, leading to episodes of hypotension or hypoxaemia and secondary infections.[6–8] The primary therapeutic goal for nursing and medical staff is prompt, definitive control of the source of infection or proinflammation[9] and early recognition of pre-existing factors that may lead to subsequent organ damage away from the initial site of injury. This pre-emptive therapy is instituted to maintain adequate tissue perfusion and prevent the onset of MODS. Recognition and response to early signs of clinical deterioration are therefore important to minimise further organ dysfunction.[10]

In this chapter the pathophysiology of inflammatory and infective conditions that may lead to multiple organ dysfunction is described. System responses and specific organ dysfunction are discussed, expanding on the dialogue in previous chapters, particularly Chapter 20. Assessment of the severity of MODS and nursing considerations in the treatment of the MODS patient are presented.

Pathophysiology

The syndrome of multiple organ dysfunction is most closely related to an outcome of sepsis, which is described in Chapter 21; however, it may have many other causes, such as trauma[11] or failure of the gut.[12] MODS is a state characterised by aberrant cellular responses involving multiple organ systems and sequential processes. The pathogenesis of MODS is complex, simultaneously involving every cell type, neurohormonal axis and organ system.[10]

In brief, alterations in tissue perfusion and oxygenation at the level of the microcirculation can result in dysfunction of organs.[1] Hypoxic hypoxia results from altered metabolic regulation of tissue oxygen delivery, which contributes to further organ dysfunction. Microcirculatory injury, as a result of lytic enzymes and vasoactive substances (nitric oxide, endothelial growth factor), is compounded by the inability of erythrocytes to navigate the septic microcirculation. Mitochondrial electron transport is affected by endotoxins in sepsis, nitric oxide and tumour necrosis factor-alpha (TNF-α), leading to disordered energy metabolism (Fig. 22.1).[13,14] This causes cytopathic or histotoxic anoxia.[10] This context of impaired oxygen utilisation where oxygen delivery is normal[1,2,10] results from diminished mitochondrial production of cellular energy – adenosine triphosphate (ATP) – despite normal or even supranormal intracellular oxygen levels.[14] Cellular hypoxia increases free radicals, further compounding oxidative stress, which results in calcium entering the endoplasmic reticulum and mitochondria, leading to cell death.[15] Cytopathic hypoxia appears resistant to resuscitation measures, and may ultimately worsen already-existing organ dysfunction. During sepsis or ischaemia, mitochondria respond by facilitating cell death rather than the restoration of homeostasis.[15]

Apoptosis is normal physiological programmed cell death and is the main mechanism to eliminate dysfunctional cells.[16] It involves chromatin condensation, membrane blebbing, cell shrinkage and subsequent breakdown of cellular components into apoptotic bodies. This normally orderly process is deranged in critical illness, leading to tissue or organ bed injury and MODS. Proinflammatory cytokines released in sepsis may delay apoptosis in activated macrophages and neutrophils, whereas in other tissues, such as gut endothelium, accelerated apoptosis occurs.[13,17]

In contrast, necrosis is a form of cell death characterised by cellular swelling and loss of membrane integrity as a result of hypoxia or trauma. Necrosis has been termed 'cellular energy crisis'[18] and is unregulated, resulting in loss of membrane sodium/potassium/ATPase pumps. This loss leads to cell swelling, rupture and spillage of intracellular contents into surrounding regions, creating collateral damage.[18] Necrosis can therefore involve significant amounts of tissue and organ bed damage. Apoptosis differs from necrosis in that it does not seem to involve the recruitment of inflammatory cells or mediators to complete its task. Activation of an enzyme cascade systematically cleaves proteins and degrades the cell's nuclear deoxyribonucleic acid (DNA), the end result being death of the cell. This requires energy from mitochondria; if not available, necrosis of the cell occurs. Apoptosis and necrosis are processes important to understand in relation to future MODS research.[18]

Epigenetic control is involved in the modulation of inflammation, and its dysregulation can contribute to cell damage and organ dysfunction.[19] Increased concentrations of cell-free plasma DNA are present in various clinical conditions such as stroke, myocardial infarction and trauma – a likely result of accelerated cell death. Maximum plasma DNA concentrations correlate significantly with acute physiology and chronic health evaluation (APACHE) II scores and maximum sequential organ failure assessment (SOFA) scores (described later in this chapter), with

FIGURE 22.1 Pathophysiology of cellular dysfunction.

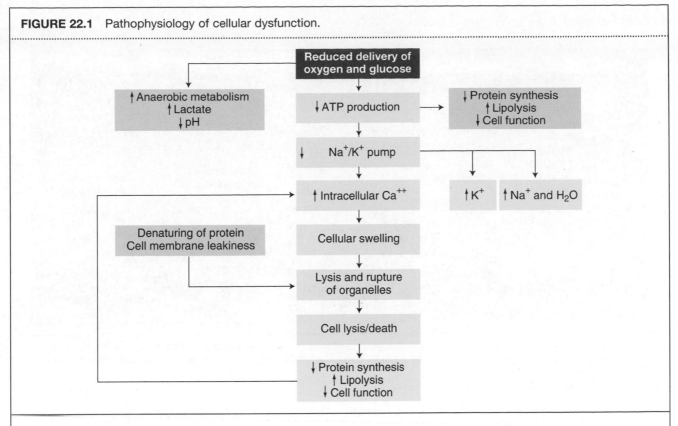

Source: McCance KL, Grey TC. Altered cellular and tissue biology. In: Pathophysiology: the biologic basis for disease in adults and children. 9th ed. St Louis: Mosby; 2022.

cell-free plasma DNA concentrations higher in hospital non-survivors than in survivors. Targeting epigenetics, particularly DNA as an independent predictor of mortality, can represent novel therapeutic approaches to prevent MODS in critical disease.[19]

Other cellular organelles may also exhibit pathological reactions in MODS. In ischaemia/reperfusion, endoplasmic reticulum loses its ability to process proteins, which induces the expression of heat-shock proteins,[20] affecting transcription of proteins necessary for organ-specific functions. For example, liver cell metabolism, renal cell function or cardiac cell contractility may be affected.[20] This has led to the concept of a mode of hibernation[7,15,21] of cells at the expense of survival of the whole organism.[21]

Cellular communication is also altered in MODS. Cells normally communicate through highly interactive bidirectional neural networks.[22] The endothelium acts as a communication interface between cells, organs and systems and is involved in orchestration of systemic responses, including haemodynamic regulation, inflammation and coagulation; oxygen and nutrient delivery; oxidative stress; and sensing of psychological stress and neuroendocrine alterations.[7,8,10] In critical illness, endothelia release molecules that trigger the immune and neuroendocrine systems to produce a generalised inflammatory response.[8] The combination of the pathophysiological processes

involved with the development of MODS, compensatory mechanisms and the effect on target organs and systems is now discussed.

Systemic response

After an overwhelming incident such as trauma, breaches in intestinal integrity, sepsis or non-infectious inflammation, a complex range of interrelated reactions occurs that results in a cascade of responses. The complex host response generated involves the inflammatory immune systems, hormonal activation and metabolic derangements, resulting in multiple organ system involvement.[6,7,10,11] These host responses are initially adaptive to maintain nutrient perfusion to the tissues; however, eventually organ systems become dysfunctional and fail, and the body is no longer able to maintain homeostasis[10] (Fig. 22.2).

Initially, proinflammatory mediators are released locally to fight foreign antigens and promote wound healing. Anti-inflammatory mediators are also released to down-regulate the initial response to the insult.[23] If the local defence system is overwhelmed, inflammatory mediators appear in the systemic circulation and recruit additional leukocytes to the area of damage. Cytokine release syndrome (CRS) is an uncontrolled systemic inflammatory response which attacks multiple systems

FIGURE 22.2 Progression of SIRS-sepsis-shock-MODS.[13]

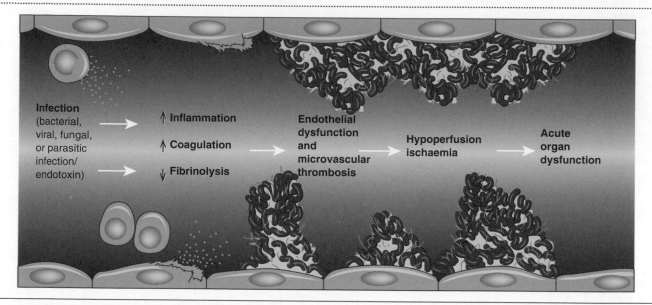

Source: Cheek DJ, Martin LL, Morris SE. Shock, multiple organ dysfunction syndrome, and burns in adults. In: Rogers J, editor. McCance & Huether's pathophysiology: the biologic basis for disease in adults and children. 9th ed. St Louis, MO: Mosby Elsevier; 2022, with permission.

and organs.[6] A whole-body stress response ensues, further compounding the situation. If the proinflammatory mediators and the anti-inflammatory response are imbalanced, the patient may develop systemic inflammatory response syndrome (SIRS) and subsequent immunological dissonance of organ dysfunction.[2,19,23]

Regardless of the trigger event, lymphocytes (T cells, B cells, natural killer cells) and macrophages are activated by cytokines (cellular signalling agents) to commence the inflammatory or anti-inflammatory response. A number of interleukins (IL) have been identified as key cytokines in proinflammatory (e.g. IL-1, IL-6) or anti-inflammatory (e.g. IL-10, IL-6, IL-4) responses. IL-6 is unique in that it has both pro- and anti-inflammatory properties.[23] The inflammatory response results in clinical signs of hypoperfusion, culminating in shock.

Intracellular transcription factors, in particular nuclear factor kappa B, are important in innate and adaptive immunity,[23,24] as they regulate the transcription of genes involved in the inflammatory and acute stress response, leading to expression of TNF-α, interleukins and tissue factor.[2,22] Nuclear factor kappa B therefore plays an important role in response pathways in critical states including hypoxia, ischaemia, haemorrhage, sepsis, shock and MODS.[23,25]

The inflammatory cascade activates a number of prostaglandins and leukotrienes that also have pro- and anti-inflammatory effects. Thromboxane A₂ plays a role in the acute phase, in part due to stimulation of platelet aggregation, leading to microvascular thrombosis and tissue injury;[23] it may also play a role in pulmonary bronchoconstriction and myocardial depression.

The specific pathophysiological concepts of inflammation, oedema and infection are discussed below.

Inflammation

Inflammation is part of innate immunity, a generic response to injury, and is normally an excellent mechanism to localise injury and promote healing.[25–28] The basis of this immune response is recognition of, and an immediate response to, an invading pathogen without necessarily having previous exposure to that pathogen.[27] Neutrophils, macrophages, natural killer cells, dendrites, coagulation and complement are the principal active components of the innate host response.[27] Compensatory anti-inflammatory response syndrome and SIRS produce cardiovascular shock, altered homeostasis, apoptosis, organ dysfunction and immune suppression.[23]

The classic signs of inflammation are:

- pain
- oedema
- erythema and heat (from vasodilation)
- leukocyte accumulation and capillary leak.[27]

Nitric oxide and prostaglandins (e.g. prostacyclin) are the primary mediators of vasodilation and inflammation at the injury site.[6,27] Injured endothelium produces molecules that attract leukocytes and facilitate movement to the tissues. White blood cells accumulate by margination (adhesion to endothelium during the early stages of inflammation) and neutrophils accumulate at the injury site, where rolling and adherence to binding molecules on the endothelium occurs with eventual movement across the endothelium into the tissues.[27] Different blood components therefore escape the intravascular space and occupy the interstitial space, where they play the main role in successive phases of the inflammatory response. The endothelium therefore plays a bidirectional mediating role between blood flow and the interstitial space where inflammation mainly takes place.[23] Macrophages, neutrophils and monocytes are responsible for phagocytosis and the production of toxic free radicals to kill invading pathogens.[15] The complement system, a collection of 30 proteins circulating in the blood, is also activated, with plasma and membrane proteins acting as adjuncts to inflammatory and immune processes.[27] When activated by inflammation and microbial invasion, these processes facilitate lysis (cellular destruction) and phagocytosis (ingestion) of foreign material.[7,27]

Dysfunction of organ systems often persists after the initial inflammatory response diminishes; this is largely unexplained, although dysoxia (abnormal tissue oxygen metabolism and utilisation) has been implicated.[7,14] Hypoxia induces release of IL-6, the main cytokine that initiates the acute-phase response. After reperfusion of ischaemic tissues, tissue and neutrophil activation forms reactive oxygen species (e.g. hydrogen peroxide) as a byproduct. These strong oxidants damage other molecules and cell structures that they come into contact with,[16,27] resulting in water and sodium infiltrate and cellular oedema.

Oedema

Oedema occurs as a consequence of alterations to tissue endothelium, with increased microvascular permeability or 'capillary leak'. As noted earlier, many mediators, including circulating cytokines, oxygen free radicals and activated neutrophils, alter the structure of endothelial cells, enabling larger molecules such as proteins and water to cross into the extravascular space.[6,27] This response mechanism improves supply of nutrient-rich fluid to the site of injury but, if this becomes systemic, fluid shifts can lead to hypovolaemia or third-spacing (interstitial oedema), or affect other organs (e.g. acute lung injury, acute kidney injury).[27]

Infection and immune responses

Infection exists when there is one of the following: positive culture, serology,[28,29] the presence of polymorphonuclear leukocytes in a normally sterile body fluid except blood, or clinical focus of infection such as perforated viscus or pneumonia.[29] The immune response to infection has both non-specific and specific actions, with inflammation and coagulation responses intricately linked in sepsis pathophysiology.[27–31] Tissue injury and the production of inflammatory mediators lead to:

- coagulation via the expression of tissue factor and factor VIIa complex (tissue factor pathway)[28]
- coagulation amplification via factors Xa and Va, leading to massive thrombin formation and fibrin clots (common coagulation pathway).[10,32]

Note that blood cell injury or platelet contact with endothelial collagen initiates the contact activation pathway.[28]

Procoagulation

Tissue factor is a procoagulant glycoprotein-signalling receptor,[10,28] expressed when tissue is damaged or cytokines are released from macrophages or the endothelium[32] (Fig. 22.3). Prothrombin is formed, leading

---

FIGURE 22.3 Tissue factor pathway. IL = interleukin; PAI = plasminogen activator inhibitor; TAFI = thrombin activatable fibrinolysis inhibitor; TNF = tumour necrosis factor.

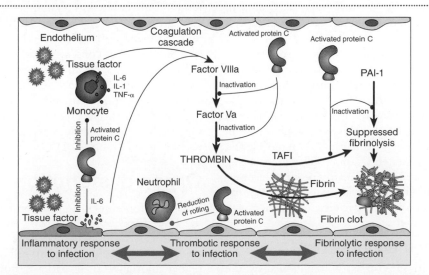

Source: Adapted from Rogers J, editor. McCance & Huether's pathophysiology: the biologic basis for disease in adults and children. 9th ed. St Louis, MO: Mosby Elsevier; 2022, with permission.

to thrombin and fibrin generation from activated platelets. Resulting clots are stabilised by factor XIII and thrombin-activatable fibrinolysis inhibitor (TAFI).[32] Fibrinolysis is a homeostatic process that dissolves clots via the plasminogen–tissue plasminogen activator–plasmin pathway (involving antithrombin, activated protein C and tissue factor pathway inhibitor). Activated protein C:[33]

- reduces inflammation by decreasing TNF-α and nuclear factor kappa B production
- reduces thrombin production when activated via thrombin–thrombomodulin complexes (anticoagulant action)
- inhibits thrombin-activatable fibrinolysis inhibitor and plasminogen activator inhibitor-1 (profibrinolytic action).[33]

Activated protein C is consumed in severe sepsis, and thrombomodulin is unable to activate protein C, promoting a proinflammatory, prothrombotic state.[33]

Endocrine response

Physiological changes are triggered as a normal response to a stressor. In a critically ill patient, however, chronic activation of the stress response, including the hypothalamic–pituitary–adrenal axis and the sympathetic–adrenal–medullary axis, results in ongoing production of glucocorticoid hormones and catecholamines.[34,35] This response interferes with the regulation of cytokine-producing immune cells, leading to immune dysfunction. Other compensatory mechanisms are instigated in an attempt to maintain supply and perfusion to organs.[1,2]

These homeostatic mechanisms are activated through positive- or negative-feedback systems to counteract stress. When stress is extreme or prolonged, these normal homeostatic mechanisms may be insufficient and a patient may respond through a sequence of physiological changes called the stress response. The stress response occurs in three stages: the alarm reaction, the resistance reaction and exhaustion (Fig. 22.4).[13]

The alarm reaction (flight-or-fight response)[33] is initiated when stress is detected, increasing the amount of glucose and oxygen available to the brain, skeletal muscle and heart. Two-thirds of total blood volume is also redistributed to support central circulation.[34] A rise in glucose production and the breakdown of glycogen in skeletal muscle increases circulating glucose levels, providing an immediate energy source. The long-lasting second stage is a resistance reaction, involving hypothalamic, pituitary and adrenal hormone release.[35,36] Response exhaustion occurs when these physiological changes can no longer maintain homeostasis.

Compensatory mechanisms

Internal equilibrium (homeostasis) is maintained by the nervous and endocrine systems, and these work symbiotically with other compensatory mechanisms, such as endothelial cells, to maintain cellular perfusion. The nervous system responds rapidly to maintain homeostasis by sending impulses to organs to activate neurohormonal responses (see Chapters 16 and 21). Autonomic dysfunction reflects 'uncoupling' of neutrally mediated organ interactions in MODS[15] characterised by heart rate, baroreflex and chemoreflex variability. Endothelins (ET-1, ET-2, ET-3) are potent vasoconstrictors produced by endothelial cells that regulate arterial pressure.[15] The endocrine system works in a slow and sustained manner by secreting hormones, which travel via the blood to end-organs.

An initial acute-adaptive response is activated when an insult or stress occurs. For example, the body senses a disruption of blood flow through baroreceptor and chemoreceptor reflex actions: baroreceptors located in the carotid sinus detect changes in arterial pressure,[32] while chemoreceptors colocated with the baroreceptors detect oxygen, carbon dioxide and hydrogen ion concentration. When alterations are sensed, the cardiovascular centre in the brain adjusts autonomic outflow accordingly.[32] In a patient with decreased tissue perfusion, there is increased peripheral vasoconstriction, contractility and heart rate. Blood flow is shunted to the vital organs (brain, heart, lungs), and away from less vital areas such as the gastrointestinal system, skin and reproductive organs.[32] Important hormonal regulators of blood flow are also activated from decreased blood flow to the kidneys, including adrenocorticotrophic hormone and the renin–angiotensin–aldosterone system (see Chapter 18). Adrenal medullary hormones, adrenaline (epinephrine) and noradrenaline (norepinephrine), vasopressin (antidiuretic hormone) and atrial natriuretic peptide also regulate blood flow to maintain adequate circulation and tissue oxygenation.[36]

Arterial pressure is a major determinant of tissue perfusion as it forces blood through the regional vasculature.[36] Hypotension (systolic blood pressure <90 mmHg or mean arterial pressure (MAP) <70 mmHg) results from either low systemic vascular resistance or a low cardiac output.[36] Glomerular filtration falls, leading to reduced urine output; low cerebral blood flow results in an altered level of consciousness, and other manifestations reflect low-flow states in other organ systems. To maintain oxygen supply, respirations and heart rate increase to meet organ oxygenation demands.[32] Heart rate variability is suggested as a strong predictor of mortality in MODS.[37] Organ dysfunction ensues if balance is not sufficiently re-established (Table 22.1).

Organ dysfunction

Organ dysfunction is a common clinical presentation in the ICU (Fig. 22.5).[1,2] Patients with dysfunction in the respiratory, cardiovascular, hepatic or metabolic systems are 50% more likely to require ICU treatment and have a higher mortality than patients not requiring intensive care.[38] As each additional organ becomes dysfunctional, prognosis deteriorates.[1,2] Timely identification of organ dysfunction is therefore critical, as early diagnosis and

FIGURE 22.4 Actions of the stress response.[13] ACTH = adrenocorticotrophic hormone; ADH = antidiuretic hormone; CRH = corticotrophin-releasing hormone; IGF-I = insulin-like growth factor I; PMN = polymorphonuclear leukocyte.

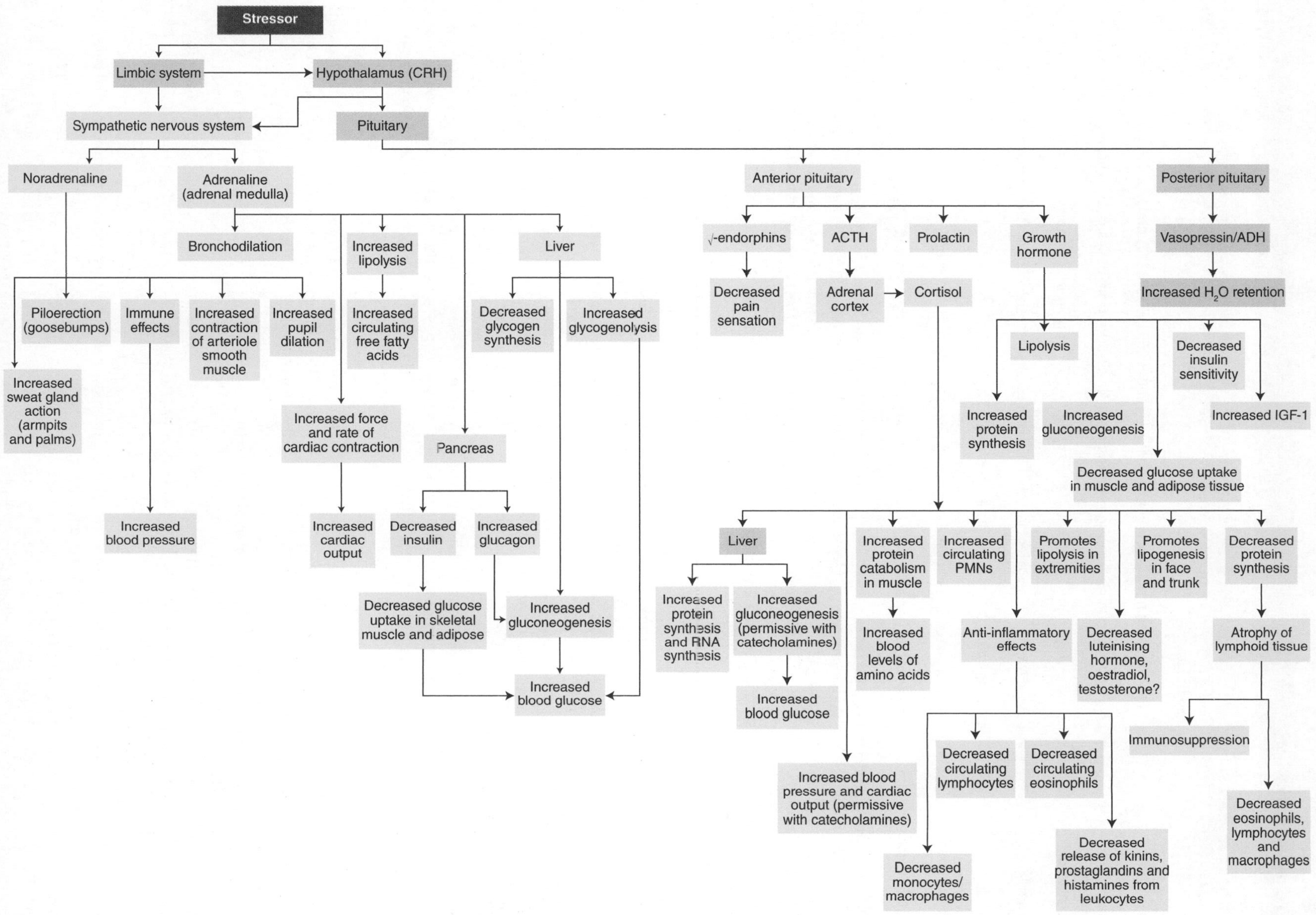

Source: Adapted from Rogers J, editor. McCance & Huether's pathophysiology: the biological basis for disease in adults and children. 9th ed. St Louis: Mosby Elsevier; 2022, with permission.

TABLE 22.1

Acute organ dysfunction[31,65,123,124]

ORGAN SYSTEM	CLINICAL PARAMETERS
Cardiovascular	Patient requires vasopressor support for systolic BP <90 mmHg or MAP <70 mmHg for 1 h despite fluid bolus.
Respiratory	Patient requires mechanical ventilation: *P/F* ratio <250, PEEP >7.5 cmH$_2$O.
Renal	Low urine output <0.5 mL/kg/h; raised creatinine >50% from baseline or requiring acute dialysis.
Haematological	Low platelet count (<1,000,000/mm^3) or APTT/PTT >upper limit of normal.
Metabolic	Low pH with increased lactate (pH <7.3 and plasma lactate >upper limit of normal).
Hepatic	Liver enzymes >2 × upper limit of normal.
Central nervous	Altered level of consciousness/reduced Glasgow Coma Scale score.
Gastrointestinal	Translocation of bacteria, possible elevated pancreatic enzymes and cholecystitis.

APTT = Activated partial thromboplastin time; BP = blood pressure; MAP = mean arterial pressure; PEEP = peak end-expiratory pressure; *P/F* = PaO$_2$/FiO$_2$ = partial pressure of arterial oxygen/fraction of inspired oxygen; PTT = partial thromboplastin time.

Sources: Asim M, Amin F, El-Menyar A. Multiple organ dysfunction syndrome: contemporary insights on the clinicopathological spectrum. Qatar Med J 2020;2020(1):22; Caraballo C, Jaimes F. Organ dysfunction in sepsis: an ominous trajectory from infection to death. Yale J Biol Med 2019;92(4):629–40; Leone M, Asfar P, Radermacher P, et al. Optimizing mean arterial pressure in septic shock: a critical reappraisal of the literature. Crit Care 2015;19(1):101; Singer M, Deutschman CS, Seymour CW, et al. The Third International Consensus definitions for sepsis and septic shock (Sepsis-3). JAMA 2016;315(8):801–10.

intervention reduce damage and improve recovery in organ systems.[2,4] The organ systems that most commonly fail are the pulmonary and cardiovascular system.[3,4] Organ and system dysfunctions are a result of hypoperfusion, inflammation, cellular dysfunction and oedema. Dysfunctions of the cardiovascular (Chapters 10 and 11), respiratory (Chapter 14), renal (Chapter 18) and hepatic and gastrointestinal systems (Chapter 20) have been addressed previously. The next sections address the haematological, endocrine and metabolic systems. Neurological dysfunction is also common in the patient with MODS, and complements previous discussions in Chapter 17.

Haematological dysfunction

Inflammatory responses and disseminated intravascular coagulation (DIC) have pivotal and synergistic roles in the development of MODS.[1,16] Elevated cytokines, particularly IL-6, IL-8 and IL-10, correlate with coagulation parameters and the development of intravascular coagulation.[39] The coagulopathy present in MODS results from deficiencies of coagulation system proteins such as protein C, antithrombin III and tissue factor inhibitors.[16,39] Inflammatory mediators initiate direct injury to the vascular endothelium, releasing tissue factor, triggering the tissue factor pathway (extrinsic coagulation cascade) and accelerating thrombin production.[39] Coagulation factors are activated as a result of endothelial damage, with binding of factor XII to the subendothelial surface and

activation of factors VIII, X, XI and XII, calcium and phospholipid.[39] The final pathway is the production of thrombin, which converts soluble fibrinogen to fibrin. Fibrin and aggregated platelets form intravascular clots.

Inflammatory cytokines also initiate coagulation through the activation of tissue factor, a principal activator of coagulation. Endotoxins increase the activity of inhibitors of clot breakdown (fibrinolysis). Levels of protein C and endogenous activated protein C are decreased in sepsis; this inhibits coagulation cofactors Va and VIIa and acts as an antithrombotic in the microvasculature.[39]

Microvascular thrombosis that leads to MODS results from two major syndromes: thrombotic microangiopathy and DIC. Thrombotic microangiopathy is characterised by formation of microvascular platelet aggregates and occasionally fibrin formation. Typically, there is history of injury to the microvascular endothelium (e.g. thrombotic thrombocytopenic purpura, haemolytic uraemic syndrome, haemolytic anaemia, elevated liver enzymes and low platelet syndromes of pregnancy or antiphospholipid antibody syndrome).[40] Thrombotic microangiopathy usually presents with normal coagulation profiles such as prothrombin times and partial thromboplastin time.[40]

DIC results from widespread activation of tissue factor-dependent coagulation, insufficient control of coagulation and plasminogen-mediated attenuation of fibrinolysis.[40,41] This leads to the formation of fibrin clots,

FIGURE 22.5   Pathogenesis of multiple organ dysfunction syndrome.[32]

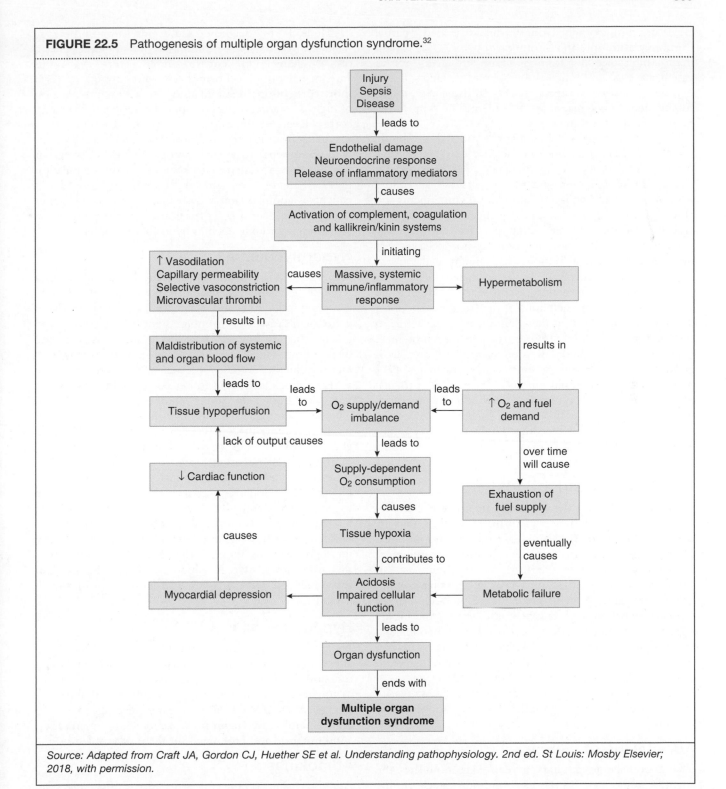

Source: Adapted from Craft JA, Gordon CJ, Huether SE et al. Understanding pathophysiology. 2nd ed. St Louis: Mosby Elsevier; 2018, with permission.

consumption of platelets and coagulation proteins, occlusion of the microvasculature and resultant reductions in cellular tissue oxygen delivery.[41] DIC is most commonly a result of trauma or sepsis and is an exaggerated response to normal coagulation, aimed at limiting infection and exsanguination and promoting wound healing.[40]

Thrombocytopenia (a platelet count of <80,000/ mm³ or a decrease of ≥50% over the preceding 3 days) signifies haematological failure,[41] with leukocytopenia/ cytosis, markers of coagulation and DIC also present.[1,41] Treatment is supportive and aimed at removing the triggering insults. Clinical biomarkers include a simultaneous rise in prothrombin time, the activated partial thromboplastin time and thrombocytopenia.[41,42] A patient may exhibit bleeding from puncture sites (e.g. invasive vascular access) and mucous membranes including bowel or upper gastrointestinal tract. Bruising or other subcutaneous petechiae may be evident. The skin should be protected from trauma.

Primary therapy is directed at the cause of the insult, with SIRS, ischaemia, uraemia, hepatotoxins and sources of infection, injury or necrosis managed concurrently. Aggressive resuscitation includes crystalloid or colloid administration and replacement of blood components and clotting factors using packed cells, platelets, cryoprecipitate and fresh frozen plasma. Endpoints for haemoglobin, platelets and coagulation levels have not been agreed upon and replacement is therefore individualised.[42]

The role of heparin or fractionated heparin is controversial in the presence of sepsis, particularly in those with overt thromboembolism or extensive fibrin deposition, such as in purpura fulminans or ischaemia in the extremities.[43] Administration of activated protein C in its role as inhibitor of the coagulation cascade is controversial. A review of four studies involving 4911 participants (4434 adults and 477 paediatric patients) identified no reduction in risk of death (28-day mortality) in adult participants with severe sepsis, but was associated with a higher risk of bleeding.[44] Effectiveness was not associated with the degree of severity of sepsis[44] and, therefore, activated protein C is no longer recommended.

Endocrine dysfunctions

Numerous endocrine derangements are noted in critically ill patients, including abnormalities in thyroid, adrenocortical, pancreas, growth and sex hormones.[45] Critical illness-related corticosteroid insufficiency (CIRCI) is associated with more-frequent use of vasopressors and increased mortality.[35] A high thyrotrophin level is an independent predictor of non-survival in critically ill patients, while subclinical hypothyroidism has significant negative effects on cardiac function and haemodynamic instability.[35,46] Hyperglycaemia is a marker of severity of illness and predictor of poor outcome in non-diabetic patients.[46] Leptin, an adipokine, increases early in sepsis and trauma, correlating with illness severity and contributing to the proinflammatory pathogenesis of MODS.[26]

Adrenal insufficiency

The hypothalamic–pituitary–adrenal axis modulates the adaptive response to stressors[46] through catecholamine secretion, cytokine activation and vasopressin release. CIRCI may affect the balance of anti-inflammatory and pro-inflammatory processes.[46,47] Adrenal insufficiency is present in a high proportion of patients with sepsis, septic shock, bleeding or multiple trauma.[35,45–47] Adrenal insufficiency as a cause of shock should be considered in any patient with hypotension with no signs of infection, cardiovascular disease or hypovolaemia.

Methods to diagnose acute adrenal insufficiency include: (1) a single random cortisol level check, or a change in cortisol level after exogenous adrenocorticotrophic hormone is administered, or (2) a short corticotrophin stimulation test with administration of high-dose adrenocorticotrophic hormone. A change in cortisol level ($\leq$9 micrograms/dL) is considered indicative of adrenal insufficiency. It is, however, argued that patients with severe sepsis may have appropriate cortisol levels but not the reserve function to respond to the stimulation test.[47] Evaluation of adrenal function in critically ill patients is complex and assays of free cortisol levels offer an advantage over total cortisol levels in the presence of low binding proteins such as hypoalbuminaemia.[47,48]

Hyperglycaemia

Hyperglycaemia is common in critically ill patients as a result of stress-induced insulin resistance and accelerated glucose production, and excessive circulating levels of glucagon, growth hormone, sympathomimetics and glucocorticoids (see Chapter 19). An increased caloric intake from parenteral or enteral nutrition may also increase glucose levels. Hyperglycaemia as a stress response in septic shock is thought to be an adaptive and beneficial response, though in some studies maintaining blood glucose at less than 10 mmol/L resulted in 10% reduction in 90-day mortality.[49] Hyperglycaemia has undesirable effects such as fluid imbalance, immune dysfunction, promoting inflammation, abnormalities in granulocyte adherence, chemotaxis, phagocytosis and intracellular killing.[35,46] Resulting associations between severe hyperglycaemia and adverse clinical outcomes have been reported in observational studies.[49–51] Meta-analysis of randomised controlled trials of intensive insulin therapy for septic patients showed no reduction in mortality;[51] therefore, lower target blood sugar levels are not recommended for managing glycaemia in critically ill patients.

Hypocalcaemia

Hypocalcaemia is common in patients with MODS[52] and affects myocardial contractility and neuromuscular functions. The link between neuromuscular changes such as polyneuropathy or polymyopathy and critical illness has not been established beyond early investigations into corticosteroid use, neuromuscular-blocking medication administration and prolonged mechanical ventilation.[52]

Adipokines

Adipose tissue is an endocrine organ that plays an important role in immunity and metabolism affecting the function of multiple organs through the secretion of adipokines (hormones and cytokines). Adipokines, which are bioactive proteins produced by adipocytes and cells of the immune system, exert their effect on metabolism, immunity and inflammation through endocrine, paracrine and autocrine secretion.[26] There is a link between increased circulating adipokines, in particular blood resistin and visfatin, and severe inflammation and critical illness, which are associated with poor outcomes.[26]

Neurological dysfunction

Evidence has highlighted that multiple organ dysfunction can result from severe traumatic brain injury or subarachnoid haemorrhage (see Chapter 17). Cardiovascular and respiratory dysfunction contribute to mortality in approximately two-thirds of all deaths following severe traumatic brain injury.[53] In non-traumatic subarachnoid haemorrhage the incidence and importance of life-threatening conditions from non-neurological physiology has been identified, including lethal arrhythmias, myocardial ischaemia and dysfunction and neurogenic pulmonary oedema.[54] The cause of cardiovascular and respiratory organ dysfunction following these acute, severe neurological events is associated with dysfunction of the sympathetic nervous system. Beta-blockers may modulate the sympathetic storm resulting from severe neurological injury; however, they have no impact upon survival.[55]

Critically ill patients may develop a syndrome of neuromuscular dysfunction characterised by generalised muscle weakness and an inability to wean successfully from mechanical ventilation. ICU-acquired weakness, including critical illness neuromyopathy syndromes, has been associated with risk factors including hyperglycaemia, SIRS, sepsis, MODS, renal replacement therapy, glucocorticoids, neuromuscular-blocking agents and catecholamine administration.[56,57] The risk of ICU-acquired weakness is nearly 50% in patients with sepsis, MODS or protracted ventilation,[57] with short-term survival uncertain. Addressing high blood glucose levels may be a potential strategy for decreasing ICU-acquired weakness.[6,58]

Survivors of sepsis-induced multiple organ dysfunction may also suffer long-term cognitive impairment, including alterations in memory, attention, concentration and/or global loss of cognitive function.[58] The participation of the brain during sepsis is poorly understood; septic encephalopathy affects approximately one-third of septic patients.[57,58] In Chapter 6 the physical, psychological and cognitive sequelae for survivors of a critical illness during their recovery are described.

Multiple organ dysfunction

MODS contributes to significant morbidity, mortality and use of intensive care resources worldwide.[2–4] This has certainly been highlighted by the COVID-19 pandemic, with patients suffering from severe COVID presenting more commonly with MODS.[59] Indeed, greater than 90% of intensive care deaths are due to MODS either directly or indirectly.[1] Patients with MODS have an increased ICU length of stay when compared with high-risk patients without multiple organ involvement[60–63] and very high 5-year mortality.[63,64] Mortality and length of stay are proportional to the number of dysfunctional organs and the severity of dysfunction.[2,65,66] Post-traumatic

MODS increases with age, severity of injury, gender (increased incidence in males), presence of traumatic brain injury, massive transfusion (>6 units packed red blood cells), coagulopathy, thrombocytopenia, hypotension on admission and hyperlactataemia.[5,67] The epidemiology of MODS, however, is difficult to accurately establish, given the broad spectrum of organ dysfunction that presents in the heterogeneous ICU population.[1] North American and Australian studies in post-injury organ failure indicate a reduction in incidence.[68] Decreasing incidence of early-onset MODS in non-cardiac emergency surgical admissions in Finland has also been observed.[69] Internationally, a reduction in MODS-related mortality is reported;[60,69] however, data from the developing world remain scant. A study of the relationship between multiorgan dysfunction and COVID-19 severity identified that patients with a history of organ dysfunction have a greater risk of developing severe COVID-19, and in turn COVID-19 can promote acute multiorgan dysfunction.[59] Post-injury MODS mortality rates are between 11% and 27%.[6,70–72] This overall decrease in mortality is occurring despite increasing patient acuity and may reflect improvements in the delivery of critical care.[64,73]

Scoring systems

Organ dysfunction can be a consequence of a primary insult or a secondary insult due to circulating mediators (e.g. the patient with acute lung injury from pneumonia who also has renal dysfunction or failure as a consequence). This is sometimes quantified by scoring systems used for assessment of MODS severity and predicting mortality, but also explored as clinical management tools.[2,11,74–77] These systems have been tested and modified to assess organ dysfunction severity and prognosis in an effort to identify patients who will benefit most from timely clinical intervention.[11] Scoring systems such as APACHE, simplified acute physiology score and mortality probability models account for information relating to a 24-hour cycle of patient data (commonly in the first 24 hours of admission), but do not account for the dynamic nature of many of the factors that affect clinical outcomes, potentially limiting their use for early MODS diagnosis and intervention.

Specific instruments designed to assess organ dysfunction or failure include the SOFA score, the more trauma-specific Denver multiple organ failure score, the Marshall multiple organ dysfunction score, the predisposition, infection, response and organ dysfunction (PIRO) score and the logistic organ dysfunction score (Table 22.2).[30,65,74,77,78] The Denver score appears to be more specific for detecting trauma-related MODS; however, the SOFA score demonstrates greater sensitivity.[77–79] SOFA scores uses the worst values for six commonly measured clinical parameters within a 24-hour period: PaO_2/FiO_2 (P/F ratio), an index that may be used to characterise acute respiratory distress syndrome; platelet count; bilirubin level; mean arterial blood pressure ± inotropic support; Glasgow Coma Scale score; and

TABLE 22.2

Sequential organ failure assessment (SOFA) score[30,73,125,126]

SOFA SCORE	0	1	2	3	4
Respiration PaO_2/FiO_2	>400	≤400	≤300	≤200[a]	≤100[a]
Coagulation platelets × $10^3/mm^3$	>150	≤150	≤100	≤50	≤20
Liver bilirubin	<1.2 mg/dL >20 micromol/L	1.2–1.9 20–32	2.0–5.9 33–101	6.0–11.9 102–204	>12.0 >204
Cardiovascular hypotension	MAP >70 mmHg	MAP <70 mmHg	Dopamine ≤5 or dobutamine (any dose)[b]	Dopamine >5 or adrenaline ≤0.1 or noradrenaline ≤0.1[b]	Dopamine >15 or adrenaline >0.1 or noradrenaline >0.1[b]
CNS Glasgow Coma Scale	15	13–14	10–12	6–9	<6
Renal creatinine or urine output	<1.2 mg/dL <110 micromol/L	1.2–1.9 110–170	2–3.4 171–299	3.5–4.9 300–440 or <500 mL/day	>5.0 >440 or <200 mL/day

[a]With respiratory support.

[b]Adrenergic agents administered for at least 1 h (doses in micrograms/kg per min).

FiO_2 = fraction of inspired oxygen; MAP = mean arterial pressure; micromol/L = micromols per litre; PaO_2 = partial pressure of arterial oxygen.

Sources: Seymour CW, Liu VX, Iwashyna TJ, et al. Assessment of clinical criteria for sepsis: for the Third International Consensus definitions for sepsis and septic shock (Sepsis-3). JAMA 2016;315(8):762–74; Evans L, Rhodes A, Alhazzani W, et al. Surviving sepsis campaign: international guidelines for management of sepsis and septic shock 2021. Crit Care Med 2021;49(11):e1063–143; Hutchings L, Watkinson P, Young J, et al. Defining multiple organ failure after major trauma: a comparison of the Denver, Sequential Organ Failure Assessment and Marshall scoring systems. J Trauma Acute Care Surg 2017;82(3):534–41; Sun GD, Zhang Y, Mo SS, et al. Multiple organ dysfunction syndrome caused by sepsis: risk factor analysis. Int J Gen Med. 2021;14:7159–64.

creatinine concentration or urine output. A score greater than 3 or higher indicates single-organ dysfunction, with a total score of >5 or 2 or more single-organ dysfunctions indicative of MODS.[75] A rise in the baseline SOFA score (assumed to be zero in the absence of known organ dysfunction) of greater than or equal to 2 points signifies acute organ dysfunction in the setting of infection.[31] Many variations of SOFA-based models have emerged in the literature, including modification of the neurological component utilising the Richmond Agitation–Sedation scale to assess the neurological component more accurately, which is often problematic in the intubated, sedated patient.[79] SOFA scoring has the advantage of ease of use, as the clinical and laboratory data required are routinely available. Overall, there is no one universally accepted gold standard scoring system, with different systems used in MODS research. Although scoring systems have been useful for assessment of MODS severity, no system has been able to consistently predict MODS outcomes.[2,3] Given that the majority of scoring systems were developed over 25 years ago, it can be argued that updated systems that reflect current understanding of MODS need to be developed.[66]

Other factors

Biomarkers such as lactate, base deficit and platelet count are being studied as indicators of occult hypoperfusion and severity of organ dysfunction.[31,80,81] Blood lactate levels are routinely collected in the early stage of ICU admission, supporting early resuscitation as a management strategy to prevent organ dysfunction. Serial lactate scores may, therefore, be appropriate to guide optimal oxygen delivery in early resuscitation, with hyperlactataemia a sign of impending organ dysfunction.[31,82] With the production of point-of-care lactate analysers, pre-hospital lactate levels may also identify patients predisposed to MODS and influence care delivery.

Other biomarkers that are being explored include matrix metalloproteinases (MMPs), key mediators in inflammation, N-terminal peptide of proatrial/brain natriuretic peptide, which correlated with MODS score in trauma patients, early plasma high-mobility group box 1 (HMGB1) levels, which have demonstrated correlation with SOFA scores in post-cardiac arrest patients, and anti-inflammatory proteins IL-IRA and CC-16 in severely injured trauma patients.[2,72] Higher initial serum procalcitonin levels have shown promise in predicting the development of MODS, although procalcitonin levels are cleared by continuous renal replacement therapy and need to be interpreted with caution in patients receiving this therapy.[83,84] Prospective, well-controlled studies are, however, needed to confirm the role of biomarkers in MODS management.[2,83]

Variations in the human DNA sequences can affect the way a person responds to disease. Epigenetic research focuses upon modulation of inflammation and immunity. Researchers have studied the gene code for plasminogen activator inhibitor 1, which is a key element in the inhibition of fibrinolysis and is active during acute inflammation[18,85] (the gene most studied is found at the 4G/5G insertion/ deletion loci), and have found that different aspects bind as either a repressor (5G) or an activator (4G) protein. For example, the 4G allele (position on the gene) of the 4G/5G gene sequence variation has been associated with increased susceptibility to community-acquired pneumonia and increased mortality in cases of severe pneumonia. It has also been reported to affect the risk of developing severe outcomes and higher mortality in meningococcal sepsis and trauma.[19,85] In trauma, damage-associated molecular patterns are released into the extracellular and vascular compartments. Mitochondrial DNA is a damage-associated molecular pattern and a potential activator of the immune response to trauma, identification of which raises its potential for therapeutic modulation.[19] Among critically ill patients with severe sepsis due to pneumonia, carriers of the plasminogen activator inhibitor 1 4G/5G genotypes have higher risk for MODS and septic shock.[86] In future, identification of genetic factors may assist selection of appropriate therapy for the patient at risk. Experimental *BRCA1* gene therapy research is showing early promising results on key cellular processes involved in stimulating DNA repair and cellular defence.[87,88]

Patient management

To date there is no aetiological treatment for MODS. This is not surprising given the complexity of the pathophysiological changes that occur with MODS and our evolving understanding of the syndrome.[2] Improvement in patient survival with MODS is thought to be due to improved identification of patients predisposed to MODS, improved shock and critical care management, awareness of secondary insults and a better understanding of the risk factors associated with MODS. Current prevention and management strategies therefore focus on identifying at-risk patients via informed clinical assessment, scoring systems and biomarkers, efficient shock resuscitation, timely treatment of infection or injury, exclusion of secondary inflammatory insults and organ support to allow time for the immune response to dampen or resolve.[2,11,31,79]

Effective shock resuscitation

For the critically injured patient, shock resuscitation includes permissive hypotension (with a higher arterial

---

BOX 22.1

Surviving Sepsis Campaign

The Surviving Sepsis Campaign is an international collaborative formed in 2003 to reduce the mortality of sepsis. Guidelines for the management of severe sepsis and shock were updated in 2021 and offer a comprehensive list of graded recommendations to care for these patients.[81] Many of the recommendations for practice have implications for critical care nurses and the multidisciplinary team (see Online resources).

Source: Adapted from Evans L, Rhodes A, Alhazzani W et al. Surviving Sepsis Campaign: international guidelines for management of sepsis and septic shock: 2021. Crit Care Med 2021;49(110):e1063–143.

---

pressure for traumatic brain-injured patients) and reversal of hypothermia, coagulopathy and acidosis. Additionally, damage control surgery, judicious volume replacement and transfusion of blood products reduces the likelihood of MODS development.[88]

A number of interventions have been recommended to reduce mortality for patients with MODS due to sepsis. The Surviving Sepsis Campaign international guidelines are based on clinical evidence graded according to the quality of evidence available (Box 22.1). The fifth version of the guidelines, released in 2021, emphasises sepsis and septic shock as medical emergencies, recommending a minimum of 30 mL/kg intravenous crystalloid resuscitation within the first 3 hours of sepsis-induced hypoperfusion, aiming for a MAP of 65 mmHg in shocked patients needing vasopressors. Further fluid resuscitation is guided by ongoing thorough clinical assessment and normalisation of elevated lactate levels.[81] See Chapter 21 for further discussion of resuscitation in shock.

Early treatment of injury/infection

In the severely injured patient, damage control surgery controls haemorrhage, minimising protracted resuscitation-associated acidosis and coagulopathy. Moreover, inflammatory mediator release is attenuated. Subsequent debridement of non-viable or infected tissue reduces the likelihood of the development of MODS from sepsis, which is often a delayed presentation in the trauma patient.[88]

Timely treatment of infection in the patient with sepsis or septic shock is critical in the prevention and management of MODS. In the septic patient, the incidence of early acute kidney injury increases with delays in antimicrobial therapy from the onset of hypotension,[89] as does acute lung injury.[90] Mortality increases for every hour's delay in administration of the first appropriate antimicrobials.[91] The Surviving Sepsis Campaign guidelines recommend empirical, broad-spectrum IV antimicrobials be commenced as soon as possible and within 1 hour of identification of sepsis or septic shock.[81] While there has been conjecture regarding optimal timing, subsequent, high-quality studies reinforce the mortality benefit of early antimicrobial therapy particularly in septic shock.[92–98]

As early antimicrobial administration may be difficult to achieve, given competing patient management priorities (e.g. airway management, volume resuscitation, vasopressor administration), systems must be developed to promote early administration.[99–103] Nurses are in a pivotal position to ensure that these guidelines or processes are developed, implemented and evaluated.

Practice tip

Tips for promoting early antimicrobial administration in severe sepsis/septic shock:[81,100–104]

- Sepsis protocol in use recognising sepsis as a time-dependent emergency.[105]
- Ensure antimicrobial therapy is given high priority in sepsis protocol.
- Do not delay antimicrobial administration if there is difficulty in sampling blood cultures (cultures need to be collected within 45 minutes of diagnosis of severe sepsis or septic shock).
- Ensure adequate supply of antimicrobials in the emergency department and ICU that fit local colonisation patterns.
- Utilise STAT orders for initial antimicrobial administration.
- Administer appropriate antibiotics that can be given via intravenous push versus longer infusion.
- Plan efficient sequencing of antimicrobial administration. Consider simultaneous delivery via multiple vascular access.
- Consider intraosseous access for first-dose antimicrobial administration.
- Emphasise education of staff on the significance of early administration of an initial antimicrobial.
- Consider other potential barriers to early antimicrobial administration in your facility, e.g. critically analyse communication strategies within healthcare teams.

Combination antibiotic therapy may offer a survival benefit in septic shock, but may be deleterious to patients with a low mortality risk.[103] Certainly, antibiotic overuse and misuse is of concern, given the emergence of antibiotic resistance.[92,93] Other factors that can lead to antibiotic failure in the critically ill include increased volume of distribution secondary to expanded extracellular volume, transient increased drug clearance due to elevated cardiac output (early sepsis) and increased free-drug levels secondary to reduced serum albumin. Maximum antibiotic dosage levels on day 1 of therapy, guided by predicted volume of distribution, are therefore recommended in life-threatening infections, as inadequate antibiotic

penetration can occur owing to impaired vascularity of infected tissue (inhibits delivery of antibiotic), antibiotic antagonism (uncommon but possible with combination therapy) and coexisting unrecognised bacterial infection.[81,106] Subsequent antibiotic dosing must be guided by drug clearance. This will be influenced by the associated organ dysfunction.[106] Nursing assessment of patient response to antibiotic therapy (resolution or exacerbation of signs of sepsis) and surveillance for sites of unrecognised infection are also important.

Source control (e.g. abscess drainage, removal of infected necrotic tissue or potentially infected device) is also an essential aspect of infection control and should be implemented as soon as practicable after diagnosis of sepsis. The method of source control chosen should always involve a risk/benefit analysis, as source control interventions can exacerbate complications.[93] Nurses play a pivotal role in identification of an infection source via astute ongoing patient assessment.[101,105]

Steroid therapy

As septic shock is a major complication of infectious processes, the relationship among the immune, coagulation and neuroendocrine systems has been explored.[7,35,106] The role of corticosteroids in the treatment of septic shock has led to a number of trials that suggested some survival benefit for low-dose corticosteroid therapy. More research is required, however, because of conflicting findings from individual studies.

A meta-analysis which included 50 randomised controlled trials demonstrated that corticosteroid therapy for sepsis increased the incidence of the vasopressor-free days, ventilation-free time, shock reversal at days 7 and 28, and adverse events such as hyperglycaemia and hypernatraemia.[107] The Surviving Sepsis guidelines recommend the use of intravenous corticosteroids in patients with septic shock after adequate fluid resuscitation and ongoing use of vasopressors (noradrenaline ≥ 0.25 micrograms/kg/min for at least 4 hours after initiation to maintain the target MAP) without haemodynamic stability.[81,108]

Therapy with corticosteroids at a physiological dose, rather than a high dose, followed observations that patients with septic shock who had a reduced response to corticotrophin were more likely to have increased mortality, and that pressor response to noradrenaline may be improved by the administration of hydrocortisone.[108] A trial exploring steroid use in sepsis demonstrated reduced vasopressor requirements and early lower mortality, but found no difference in 1-year survival. A multicentre trial to address whether hydrocortisone therapy reduces mortality (ADRENAL) demonstrated that hydrocortisone administration did not improve survival in patients with septic shock.[109] Among patients with septic shock receiving positive pressure ventilation, a continuous infusion of hydrocortisone did not result in lower 90-day mortality than placebo.[109] Shock reversal was shorter in patients who received a hydrocortisone infusion (200 mg/d) compared with placebo, with more ventilator-free days, decreased length of stay in intensive care and it was noted that there were fewer blood transfusions in the hydrocortisone group.[109]

Long-term treatment with corticosteroids may result in an inadequate response of the adrenal axis to subsequent stress such as infection, surgery or trauma, with resulting onset or worsening of shock.[110] Critical illness alters cortisol metabolism and function; for example, renal dysfunction may prolong the half-life of circulating cortisol, and inflammatory cytokines may increase glucocorticoid receptor affinity. Corticosteroid administration is associated with increased neuromuscular weakness, plus hyperglycaemia, and may affect patient outcomes, necessitating insulin to normalise blood glucose levels. A multicentre trial (Corticosteroids and Intensive Insulin Therapy for Septic Shock (COIITS))[111] demonstrated that intensive insulin therapy (aiming for a glucose level 4.5–6.0 mmol/L) did not improve in-hospital mortality for patients treated with hydrocortisone and oral fludrocortisones for septic shock.

Exclusion of secondary insults and organ support

Prevention of secondary inflammatory insults and organ support include a broad range of interventions including use of massive transfusion protocols,[112] recognition of abdominal compartment syndrome via urine catheter manometry,[113] lung-protective ventilation, early nutritional support, glycaemic monitoring, haemodynamic support using vasopressors and extracorporeal organ support such as renal replacement therapy, plasma exchange and extracorporeal membrane oxygenation (ECMO).[2,81] Managing multiple extracorporeal organ supports is complex and compounds the issues of vascular access, maintenance of blood flows to the circuits and prevention of circuit failure due to clotting.[114] This has led to the development of a singular extracorporeal device that can offer multiple organ support therapies (e.g. ADVanced Organ Support (ADVOS)).[115] While results from small, uncontrolled clinical trials and observational studies have been encouraging, larger prospective trials are required.[116] Routine evidence-based measures are also

essential, including hygiene; bowel management; pressure area, mouth and eye care; and other processes of care (e.g. FASTHUG; see Chapter 21).

Awareness of the latest evidence that underpins management of these complex patients is important. Nurses play a key role in prevention of secondary insults by delivery of thorough, coordinated and timely nursing care.[99] Despite this, there is a surprising dearth of literature specifically addressing the complex nursing care required by a MODS patient. These patients require highly skilled nurses who are able to balance competing priorities via ongoing patient assessment, care planning, monitoring and evaluation. MODS patients are also associated with increased nursing workload, with implications for staffing.[69,117] Contemporary research is focusing on homogeneous subgroups of critically ill patients in an effort to refine MODS treatment, as opposed to heterogeneous groups where treatment impacts may be hidden by patient diversity.[117–126] However, when survival has been achieved in the MODS patient, treatment pivots towards effective rehabilitation to reduce long-term sequelae of the disease and improve quality of life. Unfortunately, there is a distinct lack of quality evidence in relation to rehabilitation interventions in MODS patients.[118] The complex care required to nurse the MODS patient is highlighted in the clinical case study.

> ### Practice tip
>
> Tips for detecting haematological dysfunction in the patient with MODS[65,122]
>
> - Monitor the skin for significant bruising or petechiae.
> - Check the sites of invasive devices such as arterial, central venous access or urinary catheters for bleeding.
> - Test urine or faeces for occult blood.
> - Note oral bleeding during mouth care or from the nose when nasal cleansing.
> - Detect progressive changes in coagulation or platelet profiles.

Summary

Multiple organ dysfunction is a common presentation to critical care units across the world. Critical care nurses require high-level knowledge of pathophysiology and early recognition of failure of individual organs and the antecedents to the development of organ failure. The pathophysiological consequence of the inflammatory response as a consequence of conditions such as trauma, gut failure, disease and sepsis requires understanding of individual organ function and responses to stressors. This is so that pre-emptive strategies can be initiated to prevent further organ failure and support individual organs. Patients with MODS are complex patients to manage, requiring highly skilled nursing care that involves vigilant assessment, planning of intervention priorities, monitoring and ongoing treatment evaluation. Well-developed time management skills are required to include all routine cares and required treatment. Balancing care priorities begins on patient presentation as highlighted by the importance of initial resuscitation, early antimicrobial therapy and advanced haemodynamic support.

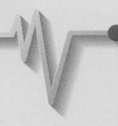

Case study

Mrs Kelly, aged 70, presented to hospital via ambulance transfer at 09:00 h with increased swelling and pain 1 month post right total knee replacement. She lived at home with her husband and had been unwell for 2 days with fever and pain at the surgical site. Her wound had one small section of non-union when the dressing was removed 2 weeks postoperatively, which she treated with application of betadine. She did not wish to present to her local hospital and her transfer via ambulance was delayed owing to COVID-19 demands. It was noted that she was allergic to penicillin (rash).

On admission to the orthopaedic ward, Mrs Kelly was alert and orientated, although in significant pain. Her vital signs at 10:05 h were within normal limits, with the exception of BP 92/62 mmHg (weight 52 kg). She was reviewed by her surgeon, who planned a return to the operating theatre for washout in the evening and requested infectious diseases (ID) review. IV access was secured, and urgent bloods taken: white cell count (WCC) 9.6 ($3.5-10 \times 10^9$/L), neutrophils 8.27 ($1.5-8.0 \times 10^9$/L), C-reactive protein (CRP) 326 (<5 mg/L), erythrocyte sedimentation rate (ESR) 52 (1–30 mm/h), creatinine 81 (45–90 micromol/L), alanine amino transferase (ALT) 101 (5–30 U/L). The ID physician examined the patient at 13:15 h and ordered blood cultures, commencement of IV fluids, IV vancomycin once theatre samples from the infected joint had been collected and to be notified if her systolic blood pressure (SBP) was <90 mmHg.

The patient's vital signs were next taken at 14:25 h where it was noted BP had fallen to 84/44 mmHg. The ID physician was notified, who requested commencement of IV vancomycin 1.5 g; it was commenced at 14:45 h. The patient's BP at 14:45 h remained low at 87/45 mmHg and a clinical review by the ICU RMO was requested. Clinical review was delayed owing to a concurrent medical emergency team call; Mrs Kelly was reviewed at 15:40 h and transferred to ICU at 16:20 h (day 0).

On arrival in ICU, Mrs Kelly remained alert and orientated but in severe pain. She was hypotensive (BP 70/50 mmHg); other vital signs were within normal limits, SpO$_2$ was 96% on room air. Fluid resuscitation was commenced with a total of 1 L colloid and 1 L crystalloid administered, with no improvement in BP. A PICC and arterial line were inserted and noradrenaline by intravenous injection (IVI) was commenced to maintain MAP at >60 mmHg. Initial arterial blood gas (ABG) results showed a lactate of 1.9 (0–2.2 mmol/L). Patient-controlled analgesia fentanyl was added plus a ketamine infusion for pain control. At 18:30 h, IV vancomycin 1 g was administered as it was determined that only 500 mg of the dose commenced in the ward had been administered. IV lincomycin 600 mg was administered at 20:00 h. Vasopressin IVI was added to reduce increasing noradrenaline requirements. The patient was transferred to operating theatre at 20:15 h and returned to ICU intubated and ventilated at 00:00 h (day 1) post-knee washout, synovectomy and insert exchange. Copious pus was noted in the joint space and surrounding soft tissues, with the poor quality of the surrounding tissues suggestive of infection beyond 2 days.

Oxygenation requirements remained minimal post-op at an FiO$_2$ of 0.3. A creatinine rise to 121 micromol/L in the setting of acidaemia (bicarbonate 18 (22–28 mmol/L)) indicated non-oliguric acute kidney injury. A stress dose of hydrocortisone 50 mg was given and echocardiography requested to exclude septic cardiomyopathy. Adrenaline IV hydrocortisone was added to keep MAP >65 mmHg. Onset of atrial fibrillation 110 bpm was noted at 05:00 h. A central venous line was inserted and IV amiodarone commenced. Atrial flutter with a variable block developed (ventricular rate 38 bpm – Fig. 22.6) after administration of only 20 mL of amiodarone, so the infusion was ceased. Echocardiography revealed an ejection fraction of <20% with a dilated left ventricle and severe global hypokinesis. Low-normal systolic function was noted in the right ventricle, in addition to moderate mitral and tricuspid valve regurgitation. *Staphylococcus aureus* was detected in the blood cultures and gram-positive cocci in the theatre samples sensitive to cefalotin; IV vancomycin was ceased and IV cephazolin added (tolerated prior admission). The patient was now coagulopathic: INR 1.8 (0.8–1.2), prothrombin time 19 s (8–14), activated partial prothrombin time 47 s (23–28), fibrinogen 5.62 g/L (1.8–4.2); IV vitamin K 10 mg was administered. The patient's husband was informed of the patient's critical condition and the likelihood that she may not survive her illness. Nasogastric feeds and mechanical thromboprophylaxis were commenced.

At 16:30 h the patient had a 7-second episode of ventricular standstill followed by a period of ventricular escape beats (Fig 22.7). This responded to inotrope titration. A further two episodes occurred requiring brief cardiac compression and instigation of external pacing. IV atropine 600 micrograms was administered followed by commencement of an isoprenaline IVI and cessation of pacing.

FIGURE 22.6   Atrial flutter with a variable block.

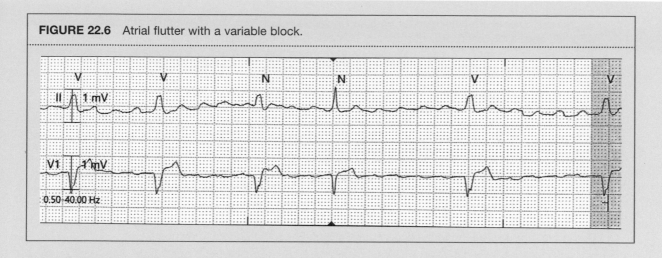

FIGURE 22.7   Ventricular standstill followed by a period of ventricular escape beats.

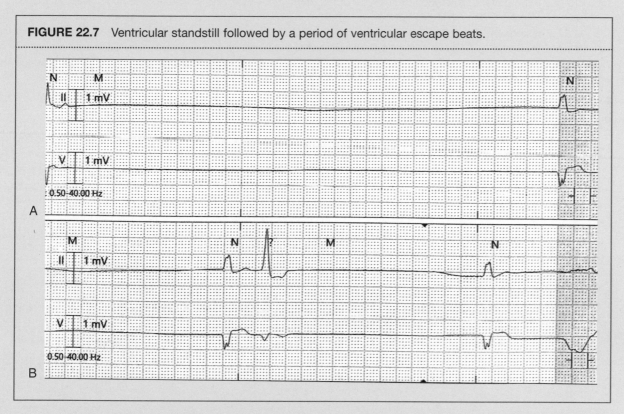

By day 2 in ICU, IVI vasopressin and adrenaline has been weaned off, with noradrenaline requirements reducing. Creatinine levels had normalised and spontaneous diuresis was noted. Sedation was reduced and Mrs Kelly started responding to verbal commands.

A rise in the WCC to 34 was noted on day 3 in ICU. The knee remained painful to touch; however, there was no evidence of cellulitis or exudate and the surgeon considered source control to be adequate. Mrs Kelly's coagulation profile had normalised and subcutaneous heparin was commenced. Her ECG remained in atrial flutter, however, with a 2:1 block. Stat IV digoxin was administered for rate control with effect. Extubation was delayed owing to concerns that the left ventricle would decompensate on removal of positive-pressure ventilation and to await results of repeat echocardiography.

Day 4 echocardiography was marginally improved; however, severe systolic left ventricular dysfunction remained (ejection fraction 25–30%). WCC had decreased to 26, CRP to 128 and Hb was 79 (120–160 g/L); 1 unit of packed cells was administered. The patient was extubated at 10:00 h and was agitated and aggressive. She received haloperidol 1 mg and midazolam 1 mg with effect, although she remained anxious at times and mildly confused. Her primary complaint was back pain (pre-existing), which was managed with continued fentanyl infusion and addition of regular gabapentin and prn tapentadol IR. Noradrenaline infusion was successfully weaned off. She was commenced on an oral diet.

On day 5 the patient was notably less confused; however, she experienced two episodes of rapid atrial fibrillation treated with further stat IV digoxin and magnesium plus regular oral digoxin and metoprolol. Her heart rate remained elevated at 110–120 bpm on day 6 and oral amiodarone was added with a reduction in digoxin dose. On day 6 in ICU, Mrs Kelly became febrile to 38°C, her knee was noted to be painful and tissue surrounding the wound was warm to touch.

Her temperature persisted on day 7 and CRP had risen to 185. Given the optimisation of her cardiac status, a decision was made to prioritise source control and return to operating theatre for a washout, debridement and insert exchange of the wound. The joint was inflamed but not obviously infected. Necrotic tissue surrounding the joint was debrided. Further blood cultures were taken intraoperatively and lines changed. A vac dressing was added to the large wound deficit. She returned to ICU extubated.

On day 8 the patient remained febrile (38.9°C). Vancomycin was added to extend antibiotic cover. A further unit of packed cells was administered for Hb 78. She returned to theatre for a washout and change of VAC dressing. On day 9 *Serratia marcescens* was cultured from wound and blood cultures, in addition to methicillin-sensitive *S. aureus*: therefore, IV cephazolin was ceased and meropenem added on review of sensitivities. Mrs Kelly continued to improve and was transferred to the ward on day 12 for further plastics management of her wound deficit.

DISCUSSION

Sepsis is a time-critical emergency that can result in MODS. This case study highlights how delays to treatment, specifically time to first dose of antibiotics, can easily occur. In Mrs Kelly's case there was a delay in presentation due to a lack of awareness by Mrs Kelly and her husband about sepsis, delay in presentation due to pandemic pressures on the ambulance system, delay in treatment due to knowledge deficit of nursing staff who did not initiate more-frequent patient assessment from admission or commence the Sepsis emergency flow chart, delay in treatment due to internal pressure on the medical emergency team, delay in first-dose antibiotic administration – antibiotics that could be given via IV bolus were not ordered, and delay in identifying that the dose of antibiotic had not been completed because of competing priorities in the ICU. Despite this the patient did make a full recovery; however, she had a significantly extended stay in hospital.

CASE STUDY QUESTIONS

1   Identify the organs and body systems that failed in the case of Mrs Kelly.
2   Review the recommendations for preparation and administration of IV vancomycin, IV lincomycin and IV cephazolin, noting which drugs can be administered via IV bolus.
3   Develop a care plan for Mrs Kelly on admission to ICU. Ensure that you include routine care as well as care specifically targeted at organ support. Discuss your plan with an experienced colleague.

RESEARCH VIGNETTE

Soussi S, Sharma D, Jüni P, et al. Identifying clinical subtypes in sepsis-survivors with different one-year outcomes: a secondary latent class analysis of the FROG-ICU cohort. Crit Care 2022;26:114.

Abstract

Background: Late mortality risk in sepsis survivors persists for years, with high re-admission rates and low quality of life. The present study seeks to link the clinical sepsis survivors' heterogeneity with distinct biological profiles at ICU discharge and late adverse events using an unsupervised analysis.

Methods and findings: In the original FROG-ICU prospective, observational, multicentre study, ICU patients with sepsis on admission (Sepsis-3) were identified ($n = 655$). Among them, 467 were discharged alive from the ICU and included in the current study. Latent class analysis was applied to identify distinct sepsis survivors, clinical classes using readily available data at ICU discharge. The primary endpoint was 1-year mortality after ICU discharge. At ICU discharge, two distinct subtypes were identified (A and B) using 15 readily available clinical and biological variables. Patients assigned to subtype B (48% of the studied population) had more-impaired cardiovascular and kidney functions, haematological disorders and inflammation at ICU discharge than subtype A. Sepsis survivors in subtype B had significantly higher 1-year mortality compared with subtype A (respectively, 34% vs 16%, $P < 0.001$). When adjusted for standard long-term risk factors (e.g. age, comorbidities, severity of illness, renal function and duration of ICU stay), subtype B was independently associated with increased one-year mortality (adjusted hazard ratio (HR) = 1.74 (95% CI 1.16–2.60); $P = 0.006$).

Conclusions: A subtype with sustained organ failure and inflammation at ICU discharge can be identified from routine clinical and laboratory data and is independently associated with poor long-term outcome in sepsis survivors.

Critique

The researchers set the background for the study by drawing attention to how improvements in critical care have decreased hospital mortality in septic patients. With the decrease in mortality, survival from sepsis has increased, resulting in more patients discharged from hospital with the sequelae of critical illness. Preventative measures for sepsis-related lowered quality of life are limited by an incomplete understanding of the causal mechanisms of post-sepsis syndrome. The current understanding of post-sepsis survivors and their long-term adverse events is therefore poorly understood, and the researchers were seeking to identify hidden subtypes of sepsis survivors at intensive care discharge using clinical and laboratory parameters. The researchers used a primary endpoint of all-cause mortality 1 year after discharge, with secondary outcomes measured at 3 and 6 months after intensive care discharge, re-admission with the first year after intensive care discharge and health-related quality of life (Short Form-36). Clinical and biological data were recorded at inclusion and discharge, along with severity scores and Charlson age–comorbidity index. The Charlson age–comorbidity index combines 19 medical conditions with age. Routine biological data was also collected including circulating markers for inflammation, cardiovascular and renal data at two set points – inclusion to the study and at ICU discharge.

The researchers found two sepsis survivor classes (subtype A and subtype B), which were derived from 15 clinical and biological data. When adjusted for standard risk factors such as age, comorbidities, length of stay in intensive care, severity of illness and renal function, subtype B was independently associated with worse kidney function, anaemia, coagulopathy and increased inflammation. Furthermore, subtype B patients showed elevated markers of cardiovascular injury and had increased 1-year mortality after intensive care unit discharge and higher mortality at 3 months.

The study provides a novel approach suggesting that persistent inflammation and worsening organ dysfunction, mainly in the heart and kidney, in stabilised sepsis survivors may be associated with increased mortality and worsening underlying pathology. Persistent inflammation accelerates atherosclerosis, plaque rupture and cardiovascular death, while the prolonged immunosuppression is likely to be related to post-sepsis syndrome-associated infections.

The strength of the study is the availability of detailed data collected at discharge from the ICU and 1-year outcomes. Limitations are that data were collected from the years 2011–13, and since then there have been changes in the management of sepsis survivors. The researchers identified that internal validity of data could have been improved, though large data sets were obtained. Also, the population studied had sepsis diagnosed within 24 hours of admission, which did not capture patients who developed sepsis during their hospital admission. The causal relationships between subtypes and long-term outcomes in sepsis survivors requires further research.

Learning activities

1 Identify five key elements essential in managing the patient with emergent MODS.

2 Outline four strategies that may facilitate the prevention of MODS.

3 Identify eight strategies that aim to minimise secondary insult and provide organ support for the MODS patient.

4 Organ dysfunction is associated with reduced cellular oxygenation. What are some of the ways in which cellular oxygen delivery can be disrupted?

5 What are the four key systemic pathophysiological responses that contribute to the development of MODS?

6 There are different scoring systems available to identify MODS and the SOFA score is one of the most common. What variables are used when determining a SOFA score?

Online resources

The Institute for Healthcare Improvement (IHI) is a non-profit organisation for advancing the quality and value of health care. Search the site for sepsis-related information about improving care and severe sepsis bundles, https://www.ihi.org

The Surviving Sepsis Campaign guidelines webpage provides access to full text documents, references, presentations, updated position statements and tools related to the guidelines, https://www.sccm.org/SurvivingSepsisCampaign/Home

The US National Institutes of Health Clinical Trials Registry. Search the site for current trials in MODS, https://www.clinicaltrials.gov

Further reading

Alsina M, Martin-Ancel A, Alarcon-Allen A, et al. The severity of hypoxic-ischaemic encephalopathy correlates with multiple organ dysfunction in the hypothermia era. Pediatr Crit Care Med 2017;18(3):234–40.

Estenssoro E. The central nervous system as an indicator of multiple organ dysfunction: a mini-review. J Organ Dysfunct 2007;3:3–6.

Hu Q, Hao C, Tang S. From sepsis to acute respiratory distress syndrome (ARDS): emerging preventive strategies based on molecular and genetic researches. Biosci Rep 2020;40(5):BSR20200830.

Poulose V, Koh J, Tay TR, et al. A randomised pilot study of parenteral glutamine supplementation in severe sepsis. Crit Care Shock 2017;20(3):61–7.

Van Wessen KJP, Leenen LPH. Reduction in mortality rates of postinjury multiple organ dysfunction syndrome: a shifting paradigm? A prospective population-based cohort study. Shock 2018;49(1):33–8.

Yadav H, Harrison AM, Hanson AC, et al. Improving the accuracy of cardiovascular component of the Sequential Organ Failure Assessment Score. Crit Care Med 2015;43(7):1449–57.

Zhao P-y, Xia Y, Tao Z-B, et al. Global research status of multiple organ dysfunction syndrome during 2001–2021: a 20-year bibliometric analysis. Front Med 2022;9:814381.

References

1. Marshall J, Deutschman C. The multiple organ dysfunction syndrome: syndrome, metaphor and unsolved clinical challenge. J Int Care Med 2020;35(12):1564–75.

2. Gourd N, Nikitas N. Multiple organ dysfunction syndrome. J Int Care Med 2020;35(12):1564–75.

3. Cole E, Gillespie S, Vulliamy P, et al. Multiple organ dysfunction after trauma. Br J Surg 2020;107(4):402–12.

4. Jansson, M, Ohtonen PP, Syrjäiä HP, et al. Changes in the incidence and outcome of multiple organ failure in emergency non-cardiac surgical admissions: a 10-year retrospective observational study. Minerva Anaestesiol 2021;87(2):174–83.

5. Krishnamoorthy V, Temkin N, Barber J, et al; Transforming Clinical Research and Knowledge in TBI (TRACK-TBI) Investigators. Association of early multiple organ dysfunction with clinical and functional outcomes over the year following traumatic brain injury: a transforming research and clinical knowledge in traumatic brain injury study. Crit Care Med 2021;49(10):1769–78.

6. Chen P, Tang Y, He W, et al., Potential pathophysiological mechanisms underlying multiple organ dysfunction in cytokine release syndrome. Mediators Inflamm 2022;2022:7137900.

7. Kozlov AV, Grillari J. Pathogenesis of multiple organ failure: the impact of systemic damage to plasma membranes. Front Med 2022;9:1–12.

8. Zhao W, Li H, Li J, et al. The mechanism of multiple organ dysfunction syndrome in patients with COVID-19. J Med Virol 2022;94(5):1886–92.

9. Ricci Z, Robmagnoli S, Ronco C, et al. From continuous renal replacement therapies to multiple organ support therapy. Contrib Nephrol 2018;194:155–69.

10. Jarczak D, Kluge S, Nierhaus A. Sepsis – pathophysiology and therapeutic concepts. Front Med (Lausanne) 2021;8(628302):1–22.

11. Rendy L, Sapan H, Kalesarran L. Multiple organ dysfunction syndrome (MODS) prediction score in multi-trauma patients. Int J Surg Open 2017;8:1–6.

12. Chen P, Billiar T. Gut microbiota and multiple organ dysfunction syndrome (MODS). Ad Exp Med Biol 2020;1238:195–202.

13. McCance K, Huether S, Brashers V, et al. Pathophysiology: the biologic basis for disease in adults and children. 9th ed. St Louis, MO: Mosby Elsevier; 2022.

14. Panditrao M, Panditrao M. Optimising oxygen delivery in sepsis: a review. AUJMSR 2019;1(1):8–15.

15. Toro-Perez J, Rodrigo R. Contribution of oxidative stress in the mechanisms of postoperative complications and multiple organ dysfunction syndrome. Redox Rep 2021;26(1):35–44.

16. Cheng Z, Abrams ST, Toh J, et al. The critical roles and mechanisms of immune cell death in sepsis. Front Immunol 2020;11(1918):1–10.

17. Spapen HD, Jacobs R, Honoré PM. Sepsis-induced multi-organ dysfunction syndrome – a mechanistic approach. J Emerg Crit Care Med 2017;1(10):1–17.

18. D'Arcy M. Cell death: a review of the major forms of apoptosis, necrosis and autophagy. Cell Biol Int 2019;43:582–92.

19. Crimi E, Cirri S, Benincasa G, et al. Epigenetics mechanisms in multiorgan dysfunction syndrome. Anaesth Analg 2019;129(5):1422–132.

20. Bautista-Carbajal P, Duarte-Molina P, Contla-Martinez II, et al. Extracellular heat shock protein 70 is a mortality predictor in patients with septic shock and is associated with the APACHE II and SOFA scores, and the pro-inflammatory immune response. World Acad Sci J 2021;3(30):1–8.

21. Graetz T, Hotchkiss R. Preventing organ failure in sepsis – the search continues. Nat Rev Nephrol 2017;13(1):5–6.

22. Picollet-D'hahan N, Zuchowska A, Lemeunier I, et al. Multiorgan-on-a-chip: a systemic approach to model and decipher inter-organ communication. Trends Biotechnol 2021;39(8):788–810.

23. Doganyigit Z, ErogluE, Akyuz E. Inflammatory mediators of cytokines and chemokines in sepsis: from bench to bedside. Hum Exp Toxicol 2022;41:1–11.

24. Eichhorn T, Linsberger I, Laukova L, et al. Analysis of inflammatory mediator profiles in sepsis patients reveals that extracellular histones are strongly elevated in nonsurvivors. Mediators Inflamm 2021;2021:8395048.

25. Liu, T, Zhang L, Joo D, et al. NF-κB signaling in inflammation. Signal Transduct Target Ther 2017;2:17023.

26. Haupt J, Krysiak N, Unger M, et al. The potential of adipokines in identifying multiple trauma patients at risk of developing multiple organ dysfunction syndrome. Eur J Med Res 2021;26(1):1–10.

27. Siddall E, Khatri M, Radhakrishnan J. Capillary leak syndrome: etiologies, pathophysiology, and management. Kidney Int 2017;92(1):37–46.

28. Landen N, Li D, Stahle M. Transition from inflammation to proliferation: a critical step during wound healing. Cell Mol Life Sci 2016;73(20):3861–85.

29. Klein Klouwenberg, PM, Cremer OL, van Vught LA, et al. Likelihood of infection in patients with presumed sepsis at the time of intensive care unit admission: a cohort study. Crit Care 2015;19(1):319.

30. Seymour CW, Liu VX, Iwashyna TJ, et al. Assessment of clinical criteria for sepsis: for the Third International Consensus definitions for sepsis and septic shock (Sepsis-3). JAMA 2016; 315(8):762–74.

31. Singer M, Deutschman CS, Seymour CW, et al. The Third International Consensus definitions for sepsis and septic shock (Sepsis-3). JAMA 2016;315(8):801–10.

32. Craft J, Gordon C, Huether S, et al. Alterations of cardiovascular function across the lifespan. In: Huether SE, McCance KL, editors. Understanding pathophysiology. Sydney, NSW: Mosby; 2018, p. 648.

33. Simmons J, Pittet JF. The coagulopathy of acute sepsis. Curr Opin Anaesthesiol 2015;28(2):227–36.

34. Sharma K, Morgensen K, Robinson M. Pathophysiology of critical illness and role of nutrition. Nutr Clin Pract 2018;34(1):12–22.

35. Widmer A, Schuetz P. Endocrine dysfunction during sepsis – are changes in hormone levels a physiological adaptation or a therapeutic target? J Lab Precis Med 2018;3(61):1–6.

36. Belfiore A, LeRoith D. Principles of endocrinology and hormone action. New York: Springer; 2018, p. 1–794.

37. de Castilho FM, Ribeiro ALP, Nobre V, et al. Heart rate variability as predictor of mortality in sepsis: a systematic review. PLoS One 2018;13(9):e0203487.

38. Lambden S, Laterre PF, Levy MM, et al. The SOFA score – development, utility and challenges of accurate assessment in clinical trials. Crit Care 2019;23(1):374.

39. Wang J, Yang X, Li Y, et al. Specific cytokines in the inflammatory cytokine storm of patients with COVID-19-associated acute respiratory distress syndrome and extrapulmonary multiple-organ dysfunction. Virol J 2021;18(117):1–12.

40. Wada T, Shiraishi A, Gando S, et al. Disseminated intravascular coagulation immediately after trauma predicts a poor prognosis in severely injured patients. Sci Rep 2021;11(1):11031.

41. Gando S, Fujishima S,Saitoh D, et al. The significance of disseminated intravascular coagulation on multiple organ dysfunction during the early stage of acute respiratory distress syndrome. Thromb Res 2020;191:15–21.

42. Sang Y, Roest M, de Laat B, et al. Interplay between platelets and coagulation. Blood Rev 2021;46:100733.

43. Fu S, Yu S, Wang L, et al. Unfractionated heparin improves the clinical efficacy in adult sepsis patients: a systematic review and meta-analysis. BMC Anesthesiol 2022;22(1):28.

44. Tuttle KM, McDonald MD, Anderson EJ. Re-evaluating biologic pharmacotherapies that target the host response during sepsis. Int J Mol Sci 2019;20(23):6049.

45. Wasyluk W, Wasyluk M, Zwolak A. Sepsis as a pan-endocrine illness – endocrine disorders in septic patients. J Clin Med 2021;10(10):2075.

46. Annane D, Pastores S, Rochwerg B, et al. Guidelines for the diagnosis and management of critical illness-related corticosteroid insufficiency (CIRCI) in critically ill patients (part I): Society of Critical Care Medicine (SCCM) and European Society of Intensive Care Medicine (ESICM) 2017. Intensive Care Med 2017;43(12):2078–88.

47. Hamrahian A, Fleseriu M. Evaluation and management of adrenal insufficiency in critically ill patients: disease state review. Endocr Pract 2017;23(6):716–25.

48. Annane D, Renault A, Brun-Buisson C, et al. Hydrocortisone plus fludrocortisone for adults with septic shock. N Engl J Med 2018;378(9):809–18.

49. Wernly B, Lichtenauer M, Hoppe U, et al. Hyperglycemia in septic patients: an essential stress survival response in all, a robust marker for risk stratification in some, to be messed with in none. J Thorac Dis 2016;8(7):e621–4.

50. van Vught LA, Wiewel MA, Klein Klouwenberg PM, et al. Admission hyperglycemia in critically ill sepsis patients: association with outcome and host response. Crit Care Med 2016;44(7):1338–46.

51. Bohé J, Abidi H, Brunot V,et al. Individualised versus conventional glucose control in critically-ill patients: the CONTROLING study – a randomized clinical trial. Intensive Care Med 2021;47(11):1271–83.

52. Pal R, Ram S, Zohmangaihi D, et al. High prevalence of hypocalcemia in non-severe COVID-19 patients: a retrospective case–control study. Front Med (Lausanne) 2021;7:590805.

53. Krishnamoorthy V, Komisarow JM, Laskowitz DT, et al. Multiorgan dysfunction after severe traumatic brain injury: epidemiology, mechanisms, and clinical management. Chest 2021;160(3):956–64.

54. Kurtz P, Taccone FS, Bozza FA, et al. Systemic severity and organ dysfunction in subarachnoid hemorrhage: a large retrospective multicenter cohort study. Neurocrit Care 2021;35(1):56–61.

55. Sadi L, Sjölin G, Ahl Hulme R. Beta-blockade is not associated with improved outcomes in isolated severe extracranial injury: an observational cohort study. Scand J Trauma Resusc Emerg Med 2021;29(1):132.

56. Czempik PF, Pluta MP, Krzych ŁJ. Sepsis-associated brain dysfunction: a review of current literature. Int J Environ Res Public Health 2020;17(16):5852.

57. Sekino N, M. Selim M, Shehadah A. Sepsis-associated brain injury: underlying mechanisms and potential therapeutic strategies for acute and long-term cognitive impairments. J Neuroinflammation 2022;19(1):101.

58. Manabe T, Heneka MT. Cerebral dysfunctions caused by sepsis during ageing. Nature Rev Immunol 2022;22(7):444–58.

59. Wu T, Zuo Z, Kang S, et al. Multi-organ dysfunction in patients with COVID-19: a systematic review and meta-analysis. Aging Dis 2020;11(4);874–94.

60. Van Wessen KJP, Leenen LPH. Reduction in mortality rates of postinjury multiple organ dysfunction syndrome: a shifting paradigm? A prospective population-based cohort study. Shock 2018;49(1):33–8.

61. Soo A, Zuege DJ, Fick GH, et al. Describing organ dysfunction in the intensive care unit: a cohort study of 20,000 patients. Crit Care 2019;23(1):186.

62. Brogan J, Fazzari M, Philips K, et al. Epidemiology of organ failure before and during COVID-19 pandemic surge conditions. Am J Crit Care 2022;31(4):283–92.

63. Gritte RB, Souza-Siqueira T, Curi R, et al. Why septic patients remain sick after hospital discharge? Front Immunol 2021;11:605666.

64. Rudd KE, Johnson SC, Agesa KM, et al. Global, regional, and national sepsis incidence and mortality 1990–2017: analysis for the Global Burden of Disease Study. Lancet 2020;395(10219):200–11.

65. Asim M, Amin F, El-Menyar A. Multiple organ dysfunction syndrome: contemporary insights on the clinicopathological spectrum. Qatar Med J 2020;2020(1):22.

66. Marshall J. Measuring organ dysfunction. Med Klin Intensivmed Notfmed 2020;115(S1):S15–20.

67. Baez A. Development of multiple organ dysfunction syndrome in older and younger adult trauma patients. Int J Crit Illn Inj Sci 2019;9(1):21–4.

68. Sauaia A, Moore FA, Moore EE. Postinjury inflammation and organ dysfunction. Crit Care Clin 2017;33(1):167–91.

69. Jansson M, Ohtonen P, Syrjala H, et al. The proportion of understaffing and increased nursing workload are associated with multiple organ failure: a cross sectional study. J Adv Nurs 2020;76:2113–24.

70. Pedersen PB, Henriksen DP, Brabrand M, et al. Organ failure, aetiology and 7-day all-cause mortality among acute adult patients on arrival to an emergency department: a hospital-based cohort study. Eur J Emerg Med 2021;28(6):448–55.

71. Kleinfled D, Tuip-de Boer A, Hollman M, et al. Early increases in anti-inflammatory biomarker is associated with the development of multiple organ dysfunction syndrome in severly injured trauma patients. Trauma Surg Acute Care Open 2019;4:e000343. doi: 10.1136/tsaco-2019-000343.

72. Rhee C, Klompas M. Sepsis trends: increasing incidence and decreasing mortality, or changing denominator? J Thorac Dis 2020;S89–100.

73. Hutchings L, Watkinson P, Young J, et al. Defining multiple organ failure after major trauma: a comparison of the Denver, Sequential Organ Failure Assessment and Marshall scoring systems. J Trauma Acute Care Surg 2017;82(3):534–41.

74. Vogel J, Liao M, Hopkins E, et al. Prediction of postinjury multiple-organ failure in the emergency department: development of the Denver Emergency Department Trauma Organ Failure Score. J Trauma Acute Care Surg 2014;76(1):140–5.

75. Anami E, Grion C, Cardoso L, et al. Serial evaluation of SOFA score in a Brazilian teaching hospital. Intensive Crit Care Nurs 2010;26(2):75–82.

76. Frolich M, Wafaisade A, Mansuri A, et al. Which score should be used for posttraumatic multiple organ failure? Comparison of the MODS, Denver- and SOFA-Scores. Scand J Trauma Resusc Emerg Med 2016;24(1):130.

77. Dewar D, White A, Attia J, et al. Comparison of post injury multiple-organ failure scoring systems: Denver versus Sequential Organ Failure Assessment. J Trauma Acute Care Surg 2014;77(4):624–9.

78. Vasilevskis E, Pandharipande P, Graves A, et al. Validity of a modified sequential organ failure assessment score using the Richmond Agitation–Sedation scale. Crit Care Med 2016;44(1):138–46.

79. Oh DH, Kim MH, Jeong WY, et al. Risk factors for mortality in patients with low lactate level and septic shock. J Microbiol Immunol Infect 2019;52(3):418–25.

80. Villar J, Short JH, Lighthall G. Lactate predicts both short- and long-term mortality in patients with and without sepsis. Infect Dis (Auckl) 2019;12:1178633719862776.

81. Evans L, Rhodes A, Alhazzani W, et al. Surviving sepsis campaign: international guidelines for management of sepsis and septic shock 2021. Crit Care Med 2021;49(11):e1063–43.

82. AlRawahi AN, AlHanai FA, Doig CJ, et al. The prognostic value of serum procalcitonin measurements in critically injured patients: a systematic review. Crit Care 2019;23(1):390.

83. Honore P, David C, Attou R, et al. Procalcitonin to allow early detection of sepsis and multiple organ failure in severe multiple trauma: beware of some confounders. Crit Care 2020;24:9.

84. Falcão-Holanda RB, Brunialti MKC, Jasiulionis MG, et al. Epigenetic regulation in sepsis, role in pathophysiology and therapeutic perspective. Front Med (Lausanne) 2021;8:685333.

85. Engoren M, Jewll ES, Douville N, et al. Genetic variants associated with sepsis. PLoS One 2022;17(3):e0265052.

86. Benz D, Balogh ZJ. Damage control surgery: current state and future directions. Curr Opin Crit Care 2017;23(6):491–7.

87. Teoh H, Quan A, Creighton AK, et al, BRCA1 gene therapy reduces systemic inflammatory response and multiple organ failure and improves survival in experimental sepsis. Gene Ther 2013;20:51–61.

88. Mas-Celis F, Olea-López J, Parroquin-Maldonado JA. Sepsis in trauma: a deadly complication. Arch Med Res 2021;52(8):808–16.

89. Peerapornratana S, Manrique-Caballero CL, Gómez H, et al. Acute kidney injury from sepsis: current concepts, epidemiology, pathophysiology, prevention and treatment. Kidney Int 2019;96(5):1083–99.

90. Sauer A, Peukert K, Putensen C, et al. Antibiotics as immunomodulators: a potential pharmacologic approach for ARDS treatment. Eur Respir Rev 2021;30(162):210093.

91. Martínez ML, Plata-Menchaca EP, Ruiz-Rodríguez JC, et al. An approach to antibiotic treatment in patients with sepsis. J Thorac Dis 2020;12(3):1007–21.

92. Ko BS, Choi SH, Kang GH, et al. Time to antibiotics and the outcome of patients with septic shock: a propensity score analysis. Am J Med 2020;133(4):485–91.e4.

93. Whiles B, Deis A, Simpson S. Increased time to initial antimicrobial administration is associated with progression to septic shock in severe sepsis patients. Crit Care Med 2017;45(4):623–9.

94. Liu V, Fielding-Singh V, Greene J, et al. The timing of early antibiotics and hospital mortality in sepsis. Am J Respir Crit Care Med 2017;196(7):856–63.

95. Kethireddy S, Bilgili B, Sees A, et al. Culture-negative septic shock compared with culture-positive septic shock: a retrospective cohort study. Crit Care Med 2018;46(4):506–12.

96. Pruinelli L, Westra B, Yadav P, et al. Delay within the 3-hour Surviving Sepsis Campaign guideline on mortality for patients with severe sepsis and septic shock. Crit Care Med 2018;46(4):500–5.

97. Kalil A, Johnson D, Lisco S, et al. Early goal-directed therapy for sepsis: a novel solution for discordant survival outcomes in clinical trials. Crit Care Med 2017;45(4):607–14.

98. Asner SA, Desgranges F, Schrijver IT, et al. Impact of the timeliness of antibiotic therapy on the outcome of patients with sepsis and septic shock. J Infect 2021;82(5):125–34.

99. Kleinpell R, Blot S, Boulanger C, et al. International critical care nursing considerations and quality indicators for the 2017 Surviving Sepsis Campaign guidelines. Intensive Care Med 2019;45(11):1663–6.

100. Amaral A, Fowler R, Pinto R, et al. Patient and organizational factors associated with delays in antimicrobial therapy for septic shock. Crit Care Med 2016;44(12):2145–53.

101. deBoisblanc B. It is about time: antibiotic delays in the treatment of septic shock. Crit Care Med 2016;44(12):2279–80.

102. Leisman D, Wie B, Doerfler M, et al. Association of fluid resuscitation initiation within 30 minutes of severe sepsis and septic shock recognition with reduced mortality and length of stay. Ann Emerg Med 2016;68(3):298–311.

103. Sjövall F, Perner A, Hylander Møller M. Empirical mono- versus combination antibiotic therapy in adult intensive care patients with severe sepsis – a systematic review with meta-analysis and trial sequential analysis. J Infect 2017;74(4):331–44.

104. Hagel S, Bach F, Brenner T, et al. Effect of therapeutic drug monitoring-based dose optimization of piperacillin/tazobactam on sepsis-related organ dysfunction in patients with sepsis: a randomized controlled trial. Intensive Care Med 2022;48(3):311–21.

105. Bleakley G, Cole M. Recognition and management of sepsis: the nurse's role. Br J Nurs 2020;29(21):1248–51.

106. Markwart R, Saito H, Harder T, et al. Epidemiology and burden of sepsis acquired in hospitals and intensive care units: a systematic review and meta-analysis. Intensive Care Med 2020;46(8):1536–51.

107. Liang H, Song H, Zhai R, et al. Corticosteriods for treating sepsis in adult patients: a systematic review and meta-analysis. Front Immunol 2021;12(709155):1–17.

108. Mirza M, Zafar M, Siddiqui M, et al. Role of steroids in critically-ill sepsis patients: a review article and literature to review. J Community Hosp Intern Med Perspect 2021;11(6):825–9.

109. Venkatesh B, Finfer S, Cohen J, et al. Adjunctive glucocorticoid therapy in patients with septic shock. N Engl J Med 2018;378(9):797–808.

110. Gibbison B, López-López JA, Higgins JPT, et al. Corticosteroids in septic shock: a systematic review and network meta-analysis. Crit Care 2017;21(1):78.

111. Annane D, Bellissant E, Bollaert P, et al. Corticosteroids for treating sepsis. Cochrane Database Syst Rev 2015;(12):CD002243.

112. Anand T, Ramnanan R, Skinner R, et al. Impact of massive transfusion and aging blood in acute trauma. Am Surg 2016;82(10):957–9.

113. Kakisis JD. Abdominal compartment syndrome. Caution: contents under pressure. Eur J Vasc Endovasc Surg 2019;58(5):680.

114. Huber W, Garibay A. Options in extracorporeal support of multiple organ failure. Med Klin Intensivmed Notfmed 2020;115(Suppl. 1):S28–36.

115. Fuhrmann V, Weber T, Roedl K et al. Advanced organ support (ADVOS) in the critically ill: first clinical experience in patients with multiple organ failure. Ann Intensive Care 2020;10:96. doi: 10.1186/s13613-020-00714-3.

116. Acharya M, Berger R, Popov A-F. the role of the ADVanced Organ Support (ADVOS) system in critically ill patients with multiple organ failure. Artif Organs 2022;46:735–46.

117. Dierkes AM, Aiken LH, Sloane DM, et al. Hospital nurse staffing and sepsis protocol compliance and outcomes among patients with sepsis in the USA: a multistate cross-sectional analysis. BMJ Open 2022;12(3):e056802.

118. Arienti C, Lazzarini S, Pollini E, et al. Effectiveness of rehabilitation interventions in adults with multi-organ dysfunction syndrome: a rapid review. J Rehabil Med 2021;53:jrm00221.

119. Pedersen PB, Hrobjartsson A, Nielsen DL, et al. Prevalence and prognosis of acutely ill patients with organ failure at arrival to hospital: a systematic review. PLoS One 2018;13(11):e0206610.

120. Bouza C, López-Cuadrado T. Epidemiology and trends of sepsis in young adults aged 20–44 years: a nationwide population-based study. J Clin Med 2020;9(1):77.

121. Rohde J, Odden A, Bonham C, et al. The epidemiology of acute organ system dysfunction from severe sepsis outside of the intensive care unit. J Hosp Med 2013;8(5):243–7.

122. Spahn DR, Bouillon B, Cerny V, et al. The European guideline on management of major bleeding and coagulopathy following trauma: fifth edition. Crit Care 2019;23(1):98.

123. Caraballo C, Jaimes F. Organ dysfunction in sepsis: an ominous trajectory from infection to death. Yale J Biol Med 2019;92(4):629–40.

124. Leone M, Asfar P, Radermacher P, et al. Optimizing mean arterial pressure in septic shock: a critical reappraisal of the literature. Crit Care 2015;19(1):101.

125. Sun GD, Zhang Y, Mo SS, et al. Multiple organ dysfunction syndrome caused by sepsis: risk factor analysis. Int J Gen Med 2021;14:7159–64.

126. Xiao K, Liu B, Guan W, et al. Prognostic analysis of elderly patients with multiple organ dysfunction syndrome undergoing invasive mechanical ventilation. J Healthc Eng 2020;6432048.

Specialty practice

Chapter 23

Emergency presentations

Wayne Varndell, Pauline Calleja

Learning objectives

After reading this chapter, you should be able to:

- describe the uniqueness of the emergency care environment
- describe the different international triage models and outline the development of Australasian triage models
- discuss the process of initial patient assessment and triage nursing practice
- integrate emergency nursing principles and practice for emergency care
- describe the various roles of extended nursing practice in the emergency setting
- describe the principles and practice of patient preparation for retrievals or transfers
- discuss the principles for the management of disaster victims in the emergency department (ED)
- discuss the initial nursing management of common presentations to the ED, including respiratory or neurological dysfunction, chest pain, abdominal pain, poisoning, envenomation, submersion and heat illness.

Introduction

Emergency nursing practice encompasses many varied clinical presentations. This chapter provides an overview of emergency care provided to patients treated within an emergency department (ED) and is not specific to patients who are critically ill. In many hospitals, critical care nurses are required at times to move between the ED, ICU, and cardiac and recovery units. This chapter therefore aims to aid critical care nurses who may deliver patient care within the emergency care setting. Please read in conjunction with Chapters 24 and 25, which describe the management of additional common presentations to the ED: trauma and resuscitation emergencies, respectively. Chapter 1 contains information on extended nursing roles relevant to emergency nursing.

In this chapter the organisational systems and processes of care in an ED environment, including triage, specifics of ED extended practice nursing roles, multiple casualties/disaster management and transport/retrieval of critically ill patients, are described. Details of a select group of the most common emergency presentations and conditions related to critical care practice are then discussed. The initial clinical assessment and incidences of these common presentations are outlined, and the likely diagnoses associated with these presentations and their initial management in the ED are identified. Ongoing management of these selected conditions is covered in this chapter.

Emergency nursing practice encompasses the holistic care of individuals of all ages who present with perceived or actual physical and/or mental health alterations and of all levels of acuity. These presentations are often undiagnosed and require a range of prompt symptomatic and definitive interventions. Emergency clinical practice is usually unscheduled, episodic and acute in its nature, and therefore is unique in the demands it places on clinicians.[1] In many instances the emergency nurse is the first clinical contact with an acutely ill or injured patient.[1,2]

Background

Emergency nursing is unique, in that it involves the care of patients with health problems that are often undiagnosed on presentation but perceived as sufficiently acute by the individual to warrant seeking emergency care in the hospital setting or to be unable to be managed by chronic care services. As patients present with signs and symptoms rather than medical diagnoses, refined assessment skills are paramount in determining level of acuity and urgency of the patient to facilitate assessment in a safe and timely manner. Many skills required by emergency nurses are based on a broad foundation of knowledge that serves as a guide in collecting information, making observations, evaluating data, and sorting and analysing relevant information to inform decision making.[1,2] This foundation enables an emergency nurse to communicate appropriately with other healthcare team members, and to implement appropriate independent and collaborative nursing interventions.[3,4]

Emergency nurses are specialists in acute episodic nursing care, and their knowledge, skills and expertise encompass almost all other nursing specialty areas. Emergency nurses, therefore, possess a unique body of knowledge and skill sets to manage a wide variety of presentations across all age groups; this includes familiarity with general physical and emotional requirements of each age group as these relate to their presenting health needs.[2] ED nurses work collaboratively with pre-hospital emergency personnel, doctors and other healthcare providers and community agencies to provide patient care.[4,5] Roles in the ED include triage, direct patient care, patient flow, collaborative care delivery, providing emotional support during crises, documenting and arranging ongoing care, admission to the hospital, transfer to another healthcare facility or discharge into the community, often within time-pressured deadlines.[5,6] Triage ensures that patients are managed in order of clinical urgency, and that ED resources such as staff, equipment and treatment area are applied appropriately.[7]

History of triage

Triage was first described in 1797 during the Napoleonic wars by Surgeon Marshall Larrey, Napoleon's chief medical officer, who introduced a system of sorting casualties that presented to the field dressing stations. His aims were military rather than medical, however, so the highest priority was given to soldiers who had minor wounds and could be returned quickly to the battle lines with minimal treatment.[8]

The documented use of triage was limited until World War I, when the term was used to describe a physical area where sorting of casualties was conducted, rather than a description of the sorting or triage process itself.[8] Triage continued to develop into a formalised assessment process, with subsequent adoption of initial categorising of patient urgency and acuity within most civilian EDs.[8]

International approaches to triage

The triage process has evolved internationally, particularly over the past two decades. Four main triage scales are available and, although used in the country in which they were developed, they have also been implemented or adapted in other health services. The Canadian Emergency Department Triage and Acuity Scales (CTAS),[9] the Manchester Triage Scale (MTS)[10] and the Australasian Triage Scale (ATS)[11,12] are the most common five-level triage scales used, with the ATS being reported as the most reliable,[13,14] although debate exists about how reliability is measured[15] and some contexts rely on other factors to determine suitability, preferring the MTS.[16,17] In the United States of America (USA), three-level triage scales have historically been used but, due to poorer performance compared with five-level triage scales,[16] the five-level triage scales are now recommended for use across the USA (e.g. the Emergency Severity Index (ESI) or the CTAS). Newer triage systems have been developed, such as the Taiwan Triage and Acuity Scale,[18] the Danish Emergency Process Triage,[19] the Soterion Rapid Triage System[20] and the 4-tier South African Triage Scale designed specifically for low- to middle-income countries and rural settings.[21]

Characteristics of the ATS, CTAS, MTS and ESI five-level triage scales are presented in Table 23.1.[22] Although somewhat similar, there are variations in some respects such as timeframes for which a person should wait to see a doctor. For example, the ESI does not define expected time intervals to doctor evaluation, and not all scales are adapted to specific populations, such as paediatrics, or settings, such as rural environments. The MTS differs from the ATS, CTAS and ESI in that it uses an algorithm approach that now includes 53 presenting complaints to derive a triage score. The other systems use a slightly different approach where a combination of observation, history taking and physical examination facilitates the nurse's judgement to apply a triage score. Updates to and

TABLE 23.1

Comparison of characteristics of the CTAS, ATS, ESI and MTS 5-level triage scales

CRITERION	CTAS	ATS	ESI	MTS
Time to triage assessment	10 min	NS	NS	NS
Time to nurse assessment	Based on initial triage	NS	NS	NS
Time to doctor assessment	Immediate/15/30/60/120 min	Immediate/10/30/60/120 min	NS	Immediate/10/60/120/240 min
Fractile response time (CTAS)/performance threshold (MTS)	I-98, II-95, III-90, IV-85, V-80	I-100, II-80, III-75, IV-70, V-70	NS	NS
Pain scale	10-point scale	NS	>7/10 *consider* up-triage to ESI level 2.	A major factor considered for each chief complaint.
Paediatrics	Used in CTAS	NS but generally recognised.	Paediatric VS criteria included to help determine ESI level 2 vs 3; fever criteria for <24 months included.	Not addressed in the algorithm.
Sentinel diagnoses	Yes	Yes	Not used.	52 chief complaints vs sentinel diagnosis.
Expected admission rates	Specified	Defined using actual data from multiple sites.	Benchmarking data available.	NS
Education implementation material	Web-based training available for a fee.	Emergency Education Triage Kit (ETEK) Workbook, resource book and quick reference guide website: https://www.health.gov.au/internet/main/publishing.nsf/Content/casemix-ED-triage+Review+Fact+Sheet+Documents	2012 edition of the Implementation handbook Emergency Severity Index (ESI): a triage tool for emergency departments website: https://www.ahrq.gov/professionals/systems/hospital/esi/index.html	Published manual: Mackway-Jones K, Marsden J, Windle J, editors. Emergency triage. Manchester Triage Group. 3rd ed. Plymouth: Wiley Blackwell; 2013
Rural setting	Yes	NS	NS	NS
Additional comments			Uses acuity to identify level 1 and 2 patients, and resources to identify levels 3–5.	Algorithmic approach that uses 52 chief complaint-based flow charts; the triage nurse then continues an algorithmic approach and assesses life threat, pain, haemorrhage, consciousness level, temperature and acuteness for each chief complaint.

Note: National ATS performance thresholds have since been revised to: 100%, 80%, 75%, 70%, 70%.[24] In NSW, ATS 2 and ATS 3 have been further revised to 95% and 85% respectively.[25]

ATS = Australasian Triage Scale; CTAS = Canadian Emergency Department Triage and Acuity Scales; ESI = Emergency Severity Index; MTS = Manchester Triage Scale; NS = not specified; VS = vital sign.

Source: Adapted from Fernandes CM, Tanabe P, Gilboy N, et al. Five-level triage: a report from the ACEP/ENA Five-level Triage Task Force. J Emerg Nurs 2005;31(1):39–50; quiz 118, with permission.

computerisation of previous guidelines have been undertaken over the years. Educational materials to support each of the scales are available. An international triage scale has been proposed but requires development and testing.[23]

Development of triage processes: focus on Australia and New Zealand

Australia is a world leader in the development of emergency triage and patient classification systems. Because other triage systems (CTAS, MTS, ESI) have primarily been adapted from the Australian system,[24–26] the focus here is on the development of the Australian and New Zealand ATS. Since the late 1960s, a number of locally developed triage systems were developed and implemented; in the early 1990s a unified scale was proposed. The National Triage Scale (NTS) was subsequently tested and demonstrated to have the essential characteristics of utility, reliability and validity, with subsequent studies showing higher levels of accuracy in predicting patient admission[27–29] and mortality[27–29] compared with CTAS, MTS and ESI. In 1993, the NTS was adopted by the Australasian College for Emergency Medicine and subsequently renamed the ATS, as it was implemented in most EDs in Australia and New Zealand (Table 23.2).[30]

The process of triage

All patients presenting to an ED should be triaged on arrival by a suitably experienced and trained registered nurse.[31] This assessment represents the first clinical contact and the commencement of care in the department. The ideal features of a triage area are: a well-signposted location close to the patient entrance, the ability to conduct examination and primary treatment of patients in privacy, close proximity to the acute treatment and resuscitation areas, and appropriate resources including an examination table, thermometer, a sphygmomanometer, stethoscope, glucometer and pulse oximetry.[31] Access to emergency equipment, communication devices (such as a telephone and emergency buzzer), standard precaution equipment (such as gloves and handwash) and paper/electronic recording facilities are also important.

As the first clinician in the ED to interview the patient, the triage nurse gathers and documents information from the patient, family and friends or pre-hospital emergency personnel. Professional maturity is required to manage the stress inherent in dealing with an acutely ill patient and family members (under significant stress themselves) while rapidly making an informed judgement on priorities of care for a wide range of clinical problems.[32]

The triage nurse receives and records information about the patient's reason for presentation to the ED, beginning with a clear statement of the complaint, followed by historical information and related relevant details such as time of onset, duration of symptom/s and what aggravates or relieves the symptom/s. A brief, focused physical assessment including vital signs may be undertaken to identify the urgency and severity of the condition, and may be collected as part of the triage process to inform decision making.[33] Triage assessment generally should be no longer than 2–5 minutes, balancing speed and thoroughness.[31] From the information collected from the patient, the triage nurse determines their level of clinical urgency and assigns a 1–5 ATS category.[31] The patient must be then allocated to an appropriate area within the ED for care to be delivered.[34]

Patients with acute conditions that threaten life or limb receive the highest priority while those with minor illness or injury are assigned a lower priority. It may not be possible to categorise the patient correctly in all instances, and it is better to conservatively allocate priority to ensure the patient is seen sooner if the triage category is unclear.[12] Importantly, a triage allocation can be altered at any time.[31] If a patient's condition changes while awaiting medical assessment/treatment, or if additional relevant information becomes available that impacts on the patient's urgency, the patient should be retriaged to a category that reflects the determined urgency. Frequent, ongoing observation and assessment of patients is, therefore, routine practice following the initial triage assessment.[34]

> **Practice tip**
>
> Triage decisions must be accurate, ensure the patient's safety and be reproducible across clinicians and departments. The decision regarding triage urgency should not be clouded by factors other than the patient's clinical condition.[35]

The premise for a triage decision is that utilisation of valuable healthcare resources should provide the greatest benefit for those most in need, and that persons in need of urgent attention always receive that care.[33] Triage encompasses the entire body of emergency nursing practice, and nurses complete a comprehensive triage education program prior to commencing this role, and should be actively engaged in continual professional development activities to maintain consistency of triage practice.[12,36]

Triage categories

After triage assessment is undertaken on arrival, patients are allocated one of five triage categories depending on the triage scale used (see Tables 23.1 and 23.2). Prompt assessment of airway, breathing, circulation and disability remains the cornerstone of patient assessment in any clinical context, including triage.[37]

Triage assessment

Patient assessment at triage has three major components: quick, systematic and dynamic. Speed of assessment is required in life-threatening situations, with the focus on airway, breathing, circulation and disability, and a quick

TABLE 23.2

Australasian Triage Scale (ATS) category characteristics[30]

ATS CODE	TYPICAL DESCRIPTION
1	Immediately life threatening (or imminent risk of deterioration).
	Patients are critically ill and require immediate transfer to a resuscitation area for initial resuscitation, with no delay at triage. The majority will arrive by ambulance, and will be suffering from:
	multi-trauma
	shock
	unconsciousness
	ongoing seizure
	extreme dyspnoea
	cardiorespiratory arrest
	severe behavioural disorder/immediate threat.
2	Imminently life threatening.
	Patients 'at high risk' of critical deterioration or have very severe pain from any cause. Assessment and treatment need to commence within 10 min for:
	chest pain or other symptoms suggestive of myocardial ischaemia, pulmonary embolism or aortic dissection
	important time-critical treatment (e.g. thrombolysis, antidote)
	severe abdominal pain or other symptoms suggestive of ruptured aortic aneurysm
	severe dyspnoea from any cause
	altered levels of consciousness
	acute stroke
	sepsis with physiological compromise
	fever, rash, headache, suggestive of sepsis or meningitis
	severe skeletal trauma such as femoral fractures or limb dislocations
	very severe pain from any cause (practice mandates the relief of pain or distress within 10 min)
	severe agitation, threat to self or others
3	Potentially life-threatening or situational urgency.
	Patients have significant illness or injury and should have assessment and treatment commenced within 30 min of presentation. Typical patients include those with:
	moderately severe pain from any cause (e.g. abdominal pain, acute headache, renal colic), but not suggestive of critical illness; practice mandates relief of severe discomfort or distress within 30 min
	symptoms of significant infections (e.g. lung, renal)
	moderate injury (e.g. Colles' fracture, severe laceration without active haemorrhage)
	head injury, with transient loss of consciousness
	persistent vomiting/dehydration
	moderately severe pain requiring analgesia.
4	Potentially serious.
	The patient's condition may deteriorate, or adverse outcome may result, if assessment and treatment is not commenced within 1 h of arrival. Patients have moderate symptoms, symptoms of prolonged duration or acute symptoms of low-risk pre-existing conditions, including:
	minor acute trauma (e.g. sprained ankle)
	minor head injury, no loss of consciousness
	mild haemorrhage
	earache or other mildly painful conditions.
	Practice mandates relief of discomfort or distress within 1 hour.
	There is a potential for adverse outcome if time-critical treatment is not commenced within 1 h.
	Likely to require complex work-up and consultation and/or inpatient management.
5	Less urgent.
	The patient's condition is minor or chronic; acute symptoms of minor illness, symptoms of chronic disease or with a duration of greater than 1 week. Symptoms or clinical outcome will not be significantly affected if assessment and treatment are delayed up to 2 h from arrival. Examples include:
	chronic lower back pain with mild symptoms
	minor wounds: small abrasion/minor lacerations
	most skin conditions
	clinical administrative presentations (e.g. results review, medical certificates, repeat prescriptions).

Source: Adapted from Australasian College for Emergency Medicine. Guidelines on the implementation of the Australasian Triage Scale in Emergency Departments Australia: Australasian College for Emergency Medicine; 2016.

decision on what level of intervention is required. A systematic approach to assessment is used for all patients in all circumstances, to ensure reproducibility. Finally, the triage assessment must be dynamic, in that several aspects can be undertaken at once, and acknowledges that a patient's condition can change rapidly after initial assessment. Various assessment models are available, but fundamentally they all include components of observation, history taking, primary survey and secondary survey.[38]

Patient history/interview

The triage interview provides the basis for data gathering and clinical decision making regarding patient acuity. After an introduction, the triage nurse asks person-specific, open-ended questions. Use of close-ended questions or summative statements enables clarification and confirmation of information received, and a means of checking understanding by the patient.[39] Privacy is important to ensure that the patient is comfortable in answering questions of a personal nature. Most EDs need to balance providing an area that is private and accessible with one safe for staff to work in relative isolation.

A large component of the triage assessment may be based on subjective data, which are then compared and combined with objective data obtained through the senses of smell, sight, hearing and touch to determine a triage category. Although not required during every triage episode to reach an accurate decision, vital signs such as pulse, blood pressure, respiratory rate, oxygen saturation, temperature and blood glucose level can be measured to assist in estimating urgency.[40] Additional investigations that are surplus to requirement to make a triage decision should be avoided in order to ensure that triage does not in itself become a barrier to the patient accessing care.

Primary survey

While taking a patient history, the triage nurse also simultaneously conducts a primary survey. As noted earlier, airway, breathing, circulation and neurological function are observed. If any major problem is observed (or a patient is identified as ATS category 1 or 2), the interview is ceased and the patient is transferred immediately to the acute treatment or resuscitation area.[40]

Focused clinical assessment

A secondary survey, involving a focused, systematic physical examination, is conducted after the patient history and primary survey have been completed. This examination is not comprehensive but rather focuses on the presenting complaint while avoiding tunnel vision and wrong conclusions. Remember that the patient may not be able to lie down or be exposed for an examination in the triage area and may be distressed. The triage process should reflect a system of rapid assessment that is reproducible and adaptable to a variety of presentations. The secondary survey may be performed by the triage nurse if time permits, or by another registered nurse who may be able to initiate appropriate investigations (such as

X-rays) or initial management (such as analgesia), according to hospital protocols. Further information regarding advanced practice roles, such as the clinical initiatives nurse, is presented in Chapter 1.

> **Practice tip**
>
> The triage physical assessment should be quick, accurate and concise, focusing on the presenting complaint.

Approaches to triage assessment

A range of approaches to nursing assessment is applicable to triage assessments (Table 23.3).[41] A body systems approach enables systematic examination of each body system to discover abnormalities (i.e. in the central nervous system, cardiovascular system, respiratory system, gastrointestinal system, etc).[42] Detailed descriptions of systems assessment are available elsewhere in the text.[43]

Triage assessment of specific patient groups

While triage assessment is a complex process for a range of patient presentations, some specific groups are more demanding, such as mental health, paediatric, older and mass casualty patients.

Mental health presentations

Patients with psychiatric problems presenting to an ED should be triaged, assessed and treated as for other

---

TABLE 23.3

Aids to triage assessment[41]

MNEMONIC	COMPONENTS
SOAPIE	Subjective data
	Objective data
	Assessment (to enable formulation of a ...)
	Plan (that is ...)
	Implemented (and ...)
	Evaluated (as to its success)
AMPLE	Allergies
	Medications
	Past medical history
	Last food and fluids ingested
	Environmental factors and events leading to presentation
PQRST	Provoking or Precipitating factors
	Quality and quantity (severity) of the symptom
	Region/radiation
	Symptoms associated
	Time of onset and duration of episode, and treatment

TABLE 23.4

Examples of a mental health triage tool[39]

ATS		OBSERVATION	ACTION
1	Immediate	Severe behavioural disorder with immediate threat of dangerous violence to self or others.	Provide continuous visual observation in safe environment. Ensure adequate personnel to provide restraint/detention.
2	Emergency	Severe behavioural disturbance with probable risk of danger to self and others.	Provide continuous visual observation in safe environment. Use defusing techniques. Ensure adequate personnel to provide restraint/detention.
3	Urgent	Moderate behavioural disturbance or severe distress with possible danger to self and others.	Provide safe environment, frequent visual observations every 10 min.
4	Semi-urgent	Semi-urgent mental health problem with no immediate risk to self or others.	Regular visual observations at a maximum of every 30 min.
5	Non-urgent	No behavioural disturbance or acute distress with no danger to self or others.	Regular visual sighting at a maximum of 1-h intervals.

ATS = Australasian Triage Scale.

Source: Adapted from Department of Health and Aged Care. Emergency triage education kit. Department of Health and Aged Care 2013. Available from: http://www.health.gov.au/internet/main/publishing.nsf/Content/casemix-ED-triage+Review+Fact+Sheet+Documents.

presenting patients, with particular attention to appropriate initial medical assessment and management.[44]

Resources outlining specific mental health triage category descriptors are readily available and relate specific aspects of mental health presentation with clinical urgency and triage categories (Table 23.4)[39] including an outline of suggested responses, such as patient placement requirements based on the level of risk and urgency.[44] Although the triage process has the same underlying principles, factors associated with mental health presentations may vary between geographical settings and countries where there are differences in health system structure, financing and sociocultural contexts.[45,46]

Paediatric presentations

Children presenting to the ED are assessed and assigned a triage category as for adults, although vital differences in paediatric anatomy, physiology and clinical presentations should be considered (see Chapter 27). The reliance on information from parents or primary carers and their capacity to identify deviations from normal are important, particularly in supporting recognition of often-subtle indicators of serious illness in infants and young children. Paediatric triage resources are available to assist in identifying physiological alterations and applying a triage category based upon identified physiological discriminators.[47,48]

Practice tip

A short time is a long time in the life of a child; children may develop serious illness in a much shorter time than for an adult.

Older persons

With the ageing population globally, there is a trend towards an increase in the use of emergency services by older persons.[49] Age has been shown to be independently associated with short-term mortality following an ED visit.[50] While older persons should be triaged according to their presenting complaint, this can be complicated by various factors that may increase the risk of being undertriaged.[51,52] It is therefore important to consider additional comorbidities, place of residence, medications and cognitive function when triaging older adults.[52] Evidence-based recommendations and policy guidelines for the management of older persons in the ED are available, with additional recommendations provided by key organisations.[53–55] Important points to remember when triaging the older person include the following:[56,57]

- Older persons have an increased medical complexity and nursing dependency.
- Be attuned to the potential signs of elder abuse, and the presence of pressure sores.
- Note the use of aids such as hearing aids, glasses and walking sticks that assist with activities of daily living.
- The older person (particularly if from an aged care facility) may have an advanced medical directive that should be used to ensure their wishes are respected in the event of a life-threatening illness.

Practice tip

When triaging older people, important considerations include other illnesses they may have, where they live, medications they are on and changes in their cognitive function.

Extended clinical skills

Within the ED, there has been an evolution of clinical roles and skill set for nurses. This has come about largely in response to an increasing number of emergency presentations, and to improve performance in patient flow, waiting times, length of stay and patient satisfaction.[58,59] Within the ED, new clinical roles, as discussed in more detail in Chapter 1, mean that registered nurses with extended clinical skills and knowledge can progress patient assessment and management through nurse-initiated radiology and nurse-initiated analgesia.

Nurse-initiated radiology

Nurse-initiated radiology ordering enables radiological investigations of extremities,[60] joints such as hips and shoulders, and the chest according to clinical protocols that list inclusion and exclusion criteria[60] based on findings from the patient's history and clinical examination. The inclusion criteria reflect well-established clinical indicators. Although nurse-initiated radiology ordering is often undertaken as an extended triage nurse function, it can be performed by any accredited nurse. The use of nurse-initiated radiology, especially in association with extremity injuries, is safe and accurate, reducing both waiting time and department transit time and improving both patient and staff satisfaction.[60,61]

Nurse-initiated analgesia

Although pain is a common complaint in many patients presenting to the ED, timeliness, adequacy and appropriateness of analgesia administration have been suboptimal and contribute to poor patient satisfaction.[58] Consequently, many EDs have developed nurse-initiated analgesia protocols, standing orders or pathways to enable designated emergency nurses to implement analgesia regimens before medical assessment. These protocols are locally derived and note patient inclusion and exclusion criteria for managing mild, moderate or severe pain in both adult and paediatric patients, and often include administration of an antiemetic. A numerical pain rating scale or a visual analogue scale is used to direct the type and route of analgesia administration. Severe pain protocols outline intravenous (IV) narcotic administration, including incremental and total maximum administration dosages. After administration of the initial dose, the administering nurse gives subsequent doses in response to patient assessment of pain score and vital signs (pulse, blood pressure and respiratory rate). Protocols directed towards moderate and minor pain may include either single or incremental IV or oral analgesia. Nurse-initiated analgesia protocols are safe and effective, shortening the time that ED patients wait for analgesia, which should assist in improving patient outcomes and satisfaction.[58,61]

Retrievals and transport of critically ill patients

The care of an acutely ill patient often includes transport, either within a hospital to undergo tests and procedures or between hospitals to receive a higher level of care or access a hospital bed. The movement of critically ill patients places the patient at a higher risk of complications during the transport period[62,63] because of condition changes, inadequate availability of equipment or support from other clinicians, or the physical environment in the transport vehicle. For this reason, the standard of care during any transport must be equivalent to, or better than, that at the referring clinical area.[63,64] Safe transport of patients requires planning and stabilisation by staff with appropriate skills and experience.[62,64] This section focuses on the movement of critically ill patients between hospitals.

Retrievals

Although there are a variety of retrieval or transport models, most retrieval teams comprise doctors, nurses and paramedics with specialised training in critical care. The skills of the escort personnel need to match the acuity of the patient so that personnel can respond to whatever clinical problems are presented.[65] Therefore, retrieval team staff members need to deliver high-level critical care equal to the standard of the receiving centre but also need to be familiar with the challenges associated with working outside the hospital environment. Standards and guidelines for the transport of critically ill patients have been established by multiple professional associations.[65,66] There is now significant evidence that trauma systems impact positively on patient outcomes and in particular reduce the odds of mortality for critically ill patients who have their inter-hospital transfer coordinated by a central retrieval organisation.[67]

When transporting an unstable patient, it is essential that a minimum of two people focusing solely on the clinical care aspects of the patient are present, in addition to other staff transporting the patient and equipment. The transport team leader is usually a medical officer with advanced training in critical care medicine or, for the transport of critical but stable patients, a registered nurse with critical care experience. The precise composition of the transport team can depend on the clinical circumstances in each case. The skill set includes advanced cardiac life support, arrhythmia interpretation and treatment, and emergency airway management; where possible a specialised team focused only on transporting critically ill patients ensures better patient outcomes and fewer adverse events.[68]

Preparing a patient for inter-hospital transport

Adequate and considered preparation for the transport of a critically ill patient from one hospital area to another should be appropriately planned and not compromised by undue haste. Appropriate evaluation and stabilisation are required to ensure patient safety during transport, including assessment of airway, breathing, circulation and suitable IV access as well as safety of staff and assets.[69]

If potential airway compromise is suspected, careful consideration should be given to an elective intubation prior to transport rather than an emergency airway intervention in a moving vehicle, airborne aircraft or a radiology department. A laryngeal mask airway is not an acceptable method of airway management for critically ill patients undergoing transport because of the problems associated with movement.[69] A nasogastric or orogastric tube is inserted in all patients requiring mechanical ventilation, and especially prior to aeromedical transport.

Fluid resuscitation and inotropic support are initiated prior to transporting the patient. Planning for the trip needs to include adequate reserves of blood or other IV fluid for use during transport. If the patient is combative or uncooperative, the use of sedative and/or neuromuscular blocking agents and analgesia may be indicated, and in some cases will preclude certain types of transport at specific times of the day (e.g. patients at high risk for behavioural challenges may not be transported aeromedically at night unless sedated and paralysed, owing to the risk to staff and patient). A syringe pump with battery power is the most appropriate method for delivering medications for sedation and pain relief. A urinary catheter is inserted for transports of extended duration and all unconscious patients.[69]

Equipment essential for transport includes:

- equipment for airway management, sized appropriately and transported with each patient (check for operation before transport)
- portable oxygen source of adequate volume to provide for the projected time frame, with enough of a reserve as a contingency in case of unexpected delays (this reserve requirement will depend on the type of retrieval, patient needs and retrieval distance)
- non-rebreather mask and bag–valve–mask with oxygen reservoir of the appropriate size
- handheld spirometer for tidal volume measurement
- available high-pressure suction
- basic resuscitation drugs and supplemental medications, such as sedatives and narcotic analgesics (considered in each specific case) and other drugs as required for the patient presentation when transporting from rural/remote locations owing to limited assets in these locations
- a transport monitor, displaying electrocardiogram (ECG) and heart rate, oxygen saturation, end-tidal carbon dioxide (CO_2) and as many invasive channels as required for pressure measurements, with defibrillation capability

- any infection prevention control equipment required, with specific communication to receiving area of actual or probable infectious status.[70]

All equipment batteries should be charged and, if extended transport is likely, spare batteries or alternative power sources need to be checked; additionally, retrieval conditions may impact operation of equipment, so ensuring equipment guidelines for operation are known and accounted for is an important safety consideration.

The patient's identification bracelet should be checked and verified, medical records and relevant information such as laboratory and radiology findings are copied for the receiving facility, and other documentation includes initial medical evaluation and medical officer to medical officer communication, with the names of the accepting doctors and the receiving hospital.[69]

Patient monitoring during transport

Critically ill patients undergoing transport receive the same level of monitoring as they would have in a critical care unit. Monitoring equipment should be selected for its reliable operation under transport conditions, as monitoring can be difficult during transport; the effects of motion, noise and vibration can make even simple clinical observations (e.g. chest auscultation or palpation) difficult, if not impossible. Due to the risk of transporting ventilated patients, the monitor should have a capacity for storing and reproducing patient bedside data and printouts during transport.[69] An appropriate transport ventilator provides full ventilatory support, monitors airway pressure with a disconnect alarm and should have adequate battery and gas supply for the duration of transport.[69] Adverse events during transport of critically ill patients fall into three categories: (1) equipment dysfunction or dislodgement, including but not limited to ECG lead disconnection, loss of battery power, loss of IV access, accidental extubation, occlusion of the endotracheal tube or exhaustion of oxygen supply (at least one team member should be proficient in operating and troubleshooting all equipment); (2) physiological deteriorations related to the critical illness; and (3) transport team-related incidents including incorrect placement of patient on trolley, fall of patient from trolley during transport, incorrect transport destination and unplanned transport time delay or extension.[68,71] Mechanisms for audit, quality improvement and teaching purposes should be in situ to allow for feedback, performance review and service improvements.[64]

Respiratory presentations

Patients with respiratory dysfunction are common presentations to the ED and are seen across all age groups. Respiratory symptoms can be associated with a broad range of underlying pathologies. This section will discuss the initial assessment and treatment of several common respiratory diseases seen in the ED. Chapter 14

> **BOX 23.1**
>
> **Signs and symptoms commonly associated with respiratory presentations**[72]
>
> - Shortness of breath
> - Dyspnoea (painful or difficulty breathing)
> - Decreased SaO_2
> - Cyanosis
> - Alteration in respiratory rate – tachypnoea/bradypnoea
> - Alterations in respiratory depth or pattern
> - Use of accessory muscles
> - Intercostal and/or subcostal recession
> - Inability to speak in full sentences
> - Wheeze
> - Stridor (upper airway respiratory disorders)
> - Alterations in level of consciousness
> - Anxiety/feeling of impending doom

provides more-detailed information regarding respiratory diseases.

Presenting symptoms and incidence

Patients presenting with respiratory complaints may display a range of symptoms. These symptoms will vary based upon the age of the patient, the underlying cause of the symptoms and the severity of the underlying condition. A list of frequently encountered respiratory signs and symptoms can be found in Box 23.1.[72]

Shortness of breath or dyspnoea is a frequent symptom or complaint on presentation to the ED. Respiratory presentations are not isolated to any one specific patient population or age group and are frequently encountered in patients across the lifespan. Dyspnoea, while commonly associated with respiratory conditions such as asthma, pneumonia, chronic obstructive pulmonary disease and cardiac conditions, has multiple aetiologies and can be caused by disease in almost any organ system.[72] Shortness of breath is a significant symptom and is commonly associated with the need for hospital admission.

Assessment, monitoring and diagnostics

On arrival, patients with respiratory complaints should be quickly assessed utilising a systematic approach to determine whether there is any potentially life-threatening disturbance to the airway, breathing or circulation that requires immediate medical assessment and/or resuscitative intervention.

Initial assessment should include a thorough history focused on the presenting complaint/s. A detailed history may often identify the underlying process; however, the emergency clinician should maintain a high index of suspicion of other potential causes during the initial assessment.[72,73] The history should focus on the nature of symptoms, the timing of the onset of symptoms, associated features, the possibility of trauma or aspiration and the past medical history, especially the presence of chronic respiratory conditions. After obtaining a history, a physical assessment of the respiratory system should be undertaken (see Chapter 13 for a detailed description of respiratory physical assessment).

Patients with significant respiratory symptoms are best managed in an acute monitored bed or resuscitation area of the ED. A set of observations including heart rate, respiratory rate, blood pressure, temperature and oxygen saturation should be completed, and the patient's heart rate and oxygen saturation can be continuously monitored. Pulse oximetry plays an important role in the monitoring of the patient with a respiratory complaint. The recognition of hypoxaemia is significantly improved with the use of pulse oximetry.[74]

IV access should be obtained, and venous blood samples may be collected for full blood count, urea, electrolytes and creatinine where clinically indicated. A chest X-ray (CXR) should be ordered in most instances. The CXR is one of the most useful investigations in the patient with a respiratory presentation. Interpretation of the CXR will not distinguish between all possible underlying pathologies and may appear normal in some instances. Therefore, interpretation of the CXR should always be performed in light of the clinical history and other examination findings.[75] An arterial blood gas (ABG) test may be indicated in patients with a significant respiratory presentation. The ABG will provide useful information that assists in identifying alterations to oxygenation, ventilation and acid–base status.[75] In many cases, a venous blood gas can be gained in lieu of ABG to avoid arterial trauma and a painful procedure for the patient. Venous blood gas values of PCO_2, pH and HCO_3^- can be interpreted to estimate the corresponding arterial values to inform decision making as if an ABG has been gained.[76] Further, in critically ill patients a venous blood gas may be used to detect and diagnose acid–base disturbances with reasonable diagnostic accuracy, even in shock states, compared with the ABG.[76] Spirometry or peak flow measurements may also be utilised in the assessment of the patient. Peak expiratory flow rate, forced vital capacity and forced expiratory volume in 1 second are useful in determining the nature of the underlying respiratory condition and, when the values are compared with predicted normal values, are useful in determining severity.[75] These tests are, however, effort and technique dependent and the patient who is acutely short of breath may not be able to perform them. The use of spirometry may be further restricted in patients with infectious respiratory diseases (e.g. coronavirus disease 2019 (COVID-19)).[77]

Oxygen therapy should be commenced early in patients presenting with signs of acute respiratory compromise, including patients known to have chronic obstructive pulmonary disease. Patients with acute hypoxia require oxygen. The often-mentioned complications associated with oxygen, especially in the patient with known chronic obstructive pulmonary disease, are uncommon. Such complications are concentration and time dependent, having a slow onset, which allows time for monitoring with pulse oximetry, blood gas analysis and clinical review.[55]

Patient diagnoses and management

Common diagnoses related to patients who present with shortness of breath include asthma, respiratory failure and pneumonia.[78]

Asthma

Asthma is a very common reason for patients presenting to Australasian EDs. Just over 1 in 10 people in Australia have asthma (2.7 million, 10.7% of the total population), with people born in Australia being twice as likely to have asthma compared to overseas (12.6% versus 6.0%).[79] Asthma is a chronic inflammatory disease of the airways in which many cells and cellular elements play a role, including mast cells, eosinophils, T lymphocytes, macrophages, neutrophils and epithelial cells. The inflammatory changes cause recurrent episodes of wheezing, breathlessness, chest tightness and coughing associated with widespread reversible air-flow obstruction of the airways. This air-flow obstruction or excessive narrowing is a result of airway smooth muscle contraction and swelling of the airway wall due to smooth muscle hypertrophy, inflammatory changes, oedema, goblet cell and mucous gland hyperplasia and mucus hypersecretion.[80,81]

Normally, airways widen during inspiration and narrow in expiration. In asthma, the above responses combine to

severely narrow or close the lumen of the bronchial passages during expiration, with altered ventilation and air trapping.[80,81] The causes of asthma are related to many factors, including allergy,[82] infection (increased reaction to bronchoconstrictors such as histamine), irritants (e.g. noxious gases, fumes, dusts, dust mites, powders) and heredity, although the exact role or importance of any hereditary tendency is difficult to assess.[80]

A patient usually has a history of previous asthma attacks. Near-fatal asthma is defined as a person who is exhausted, with severe dyspnoea, and unable to speak, with a silent chest.[83] Common risk factors that a patient may experience a future fatal or near-fatal asthma exacerbation include a recent history of poor asthma symptom control, and a prior history of a previous near-fatal asthma exacerbation requiring endotracheal intubation, mechanical ventilation and intensive care admission.[84] Often, an acute episode follows a period of exercise or exposure to a noxious substance, or a known allergen. The onset of the asthma may be characterised by vague sensations in the neck or pharynx, tightness in the chest with breathlessness, a loose but non-productive cough with difficulty in raising sputum, and difficulty breathing, particularly on expiration, with increasing severity as the episode continues; apprehension and tachypnoea may follow as the patient becomes hypoxic, with audible wheezing.[80,81,83,84]

The characteristics and initial assessment of acute mild, moderate and severe/life-threatening asthma in adults are outlined in Table 23.5.[81] The associated clinical management guidelines for acute asthma are outlined in Table 23.6. Be alert to the high-risk patient whose ability to ventilate is impaired: this is a life-threatening condition. Such patients will exhibit an inability to talk, central

TABLE 23.5

Initial assessment and characteristics of acute asthma[81]

	SEVERITY OF ATTACK		
SYMPTOMS	MILD/ MODERATE	SEVERE	SEVERE OR LIFE THREATENING
Able to talk in	Sentences	Unable to finish sentence in one breath.	
Physical exhaustion	No	Use of accessory muscles neck and intercostal. Tracheal tug or subcostal recession.	Exhaustion or collapse. May have paradoxical chest wall movement.
Pulse oximetry (room air)	>94%	90–94%	<90%
Level of consciousness	Normal	May be agitated, obvious respiratory distress.	Reduced conscious level.
Wheeze intensity	Variable	Moderate–soft.	Often soft or absent.
Central cyanosis	Absent	May be present.	Cyanosis present.

Source: Adapted from National Asthma Council Australia. Asthma Management Handbook 2022. Available from: https://www.asthmahandbook.org.au/.

TABLE 23.6

Initial clinical management in acute asthma

	MILD	MODERATE	SEVERE OR LIFE THREATENING
Hospital admission necessary	Probably not.	Likely to be required.	Yes, arrange immediate transfer to high-level care.
Oxygen	High flow of at least 8 L/min, titrated to maintain SaO$_2$ >90%, preferably >94%. Monitor effect by oximetry. Frequent measurement of arterial blood gases in severe asthma if not responding.		
Beta-2-agonist via a metered-dose inhaler and spacer *or* nebulised solution with 8 L/min O$_2$	Salbutamol 4–12 puffs via spacer. Repeat dose every 20–30 min for first hour if needed or sooner if needed.	Salbutamol 8–12 puffs *or* salbutamol 5 mg nebule if patient cannot breathe through spacer. Repeat dose every 20 min for first hour or sooner if needed.	Salbutamol 10 mg via continuous nebulisation.
Ipratropium bromide metered-dose inhaler via spacer *or* nebulised solution	If poor response, add 8 puffs via spacer.	If poor response, add 8 puffs via spacer or 500 micrograms nebule via nebuliser added to nebulised salbutamol. Give dose every 20 min for first hour, then repeat every 4–6 h as required.	If poor response, add 8 puffs via spacer or 500 micrograms nebule via nebuliser added to nebulised salbutamol. Give dose every 20 min for first hour, then repeat every 4–6 h as required.
Steroids	Yes, oral prednisolone 37.5–50 mg.	Yes, oral prednisolone 37.5–50 mg. If oral route not possible, hydrocortisone 100 mg IV every 6 h.	IV hydrocortisone 100 mg 6-hourly.
Other agents	Not indicated.	Not indicated.	For life-threatening and no response, magnesium sulfate 10 mmol IV infusion over 20 min may help.
CXR (and other investigations	Not usually necessary.	Not necessary unless focal signs present, or no improvement with therapy.	Necessary if no response to initial therapy or suspect pneumothorax/infection. Check for hypokalaemia.
Observations	Regular.	Continuous.	Continuous.

Source: Adapted from National Asthma Council Australia. Asthma Management Handbook 2022. Available from: https://www. asthmahandbook.org.au/.

cyanosis, tachycardia, use of respiratory accessory muscles, a silent chest on auscultation and possibly a history of previous intubation for asthma.[80,81,83,84]

Acute respiratory failure

Acute respiratory failure exists when the lungs do not provide sufficient gas exchange to meet the body's need for oxygen consumption, carbon dioxide elimination or both. Acute respiratory failure results from a number of causes.[85] When alveolar ventilation decreases, arterial oxygen tension falls and carbon dioxide rises. The rise in arterial carbon dioxide produces increased serum carbonic acid and pH falls, resulting in respiratory acidosis.[85] If uncorrected, low arterial oxygen combines with low cardiac output to produce diminished tissue perfusion and tissue hypoxia. Anaerobic metabolism results in increased lactic acid, aggravating the acidosis caused by carbon dioxide retention. In the process, a wide range of symptoms

develop, involving the central nervous and cardiovascular systems.[81] Arterial blood gases confirm the diagnosis, with hypercarbia and a partial pressure of carbon dioxide in the arterial blood >45 mmHg and hypoxaemia evidenced by a partial pressure of oxygen in the arterial blood <60 mmHg, and a pH <7.35 evident. A CXR identifies the specific lung disease.[85]

Clinical management focuses on correction of hypercapnia, treatment of hypoxaemia, correction of acidosis and identification and correction of the specific cause[85] (see Chapter 14). For a spontaneously breathing patient, administer oxygen by a Venturi mask (24%) or nasal cannula. Adjust oxygen therapy, according to ABG findings at 15–20-minute intervals, to achieve a partial pressure of oxygen in the arterial blood (PaO$_2$) of 85–90 mmHg. For a patient with inadequate respiratory effort, non-invasive ventilation may be instituted (see Chapter 15). In an apnoeic situation, initiate ventilatory assistance with bag–mask ventilation (see Chapter 15) prior to endotracheal intubation, and then commence mechanical ventilation.

Pneumonia

Pneumonia is an acute inflammatory condition of lung tissue caused by a variety of viral and bacterial organisms, fungi and parasites.[86] These organisms cause an inflammatory response from the cells involved in the affected segment of lung tissue. Pneumonia may occur in previously healthy patients, but more often it is associated with conditions that impair the body's defence mechanisms[87] (see Chapter 14). The predominant symptoms associated with pneumonia are a combination of cough, chest pain (usually pleuritic), dyspnoea, fever (with or without chills) and mucoid, purulent or bloody sputum, with an abrupt or gradual onset.[86] Common findings on physical exam include tachypnoea, fever, tachycardia, possible cyanosis, diminished respiratory excursion due to pleuritic pain, end-respiratory crackles or rales on auscultation with bronchial breathing over areas of consolidation[86,87] (see Chapter 14).

Investigations include a CXR, which may reveal varying infiltrates – interstitial, segmental or lobar. The CXR, however, may initially be clear until later in the illness and following adequate rehydration.[72] Venous blood samples will be analysed to identify a raised white cell count (i.e. leukocytosis). Blood cultures and sputum cultures will also be acquired to assist in identifying the causative organism. Blood gases will assist in determining the degree of impaired gas exchange. Hypoxaemia and often hypocarbia may be present.[86]

Initial treatment involves administration of oxygen therapy via face mask. Oxygen therapy should be evaluated frequently in response to pulse oximetry values. Treatment will routinely require IV fluid therapy to ensure adequate hydration, and administration of antibiotics orally or parenterally in accordance with existing antibiotic guidelines or suspected infective agent (see Chapter 14). Ventilatory support may be required in some cases; in spontaneously breathing patients, non-invasive ventilation via a face mask should be utilised before invasive ventilation. Mechanical ventilation is not normally required unless there is some underlying cardiopulmonary disease.[86]

Chest pain presentations

Chest pain or chest discomfort is a common presenting complaint to the ED and can be associated with a number of different clinical conditions, several of which are associated with life-threatening pathology.[88] The identification of cardiac-related chest pain is important. During an initial assessment it may be difficult to differentiate between non-cardiac and cardiac causes of chest discomfort based on pain characteristics such as intensity, location, radiation and other associated symptoms.[89] Therefore, it is important to consider any presentation in which chest pain is a feature as cardiac in origin until a cardiac cause has been ruled out or another cause has been confirmed.

Description of presenting symptoms and incidence

The incidence of acute chest pain presentations appears to be increasing as patients are more aware of the importance of early treatment for myocardial infarction owing to public awareness campaigns.[89] In American EDs in 2022, over 7.6 million people presented with chest pain as their primary complaint.[90] The pain or discomfort associated with chest pain presentations is often described in a variety of ways in terms of onset, intensity, duration and radiation (Table 23.7).[91]

Up to 30% of patients who will go on to be diagnosed with an acute coronary syndrome (ACS) may present with a number of these associated symptoms but without chest pain.[92,93] These patients tend to be elderly, female, diabetic and non-white minorities. Therefore, it is important to consider the possibility of a cardiac presentation in patients presenting with these associated symptoms even in the absence of chest pain.[90]

Assessment, monitoring and diagnostics

Any patient presenting with a complaint of chest pain requires urgent assessment, generally within 10 minutes of arrival to the ED. Any patient with evidence of a

TABLE 23.7
Features of chest pain[91,107]

CHEST PAIN FEATURE	DESCRIPTION
Description	Typical: pressure, a weight on the chest, tightness, constriction about the throat, an aching feeling Less typical: epigastric, indigestion, stabbing, pleuritic, sharp
Onset	Unprovoked or gradual With physical exertion or emotional stress
Intensity	Mild to severe
Radiation	To one or both arms, neck, jaw or back
Associated symptoms	Shortness of breath, nausea, vomiting, weakness, dizziness, anxiety, feeling of impending doom, palpitations, diaphoresis

Source: Adapted from Dagiely S. An algorithm for triaging commonly missed causes of acute abdominal pain. J Emerg Nurs 2006;32(1):9; with permission

disturbance to airway, breathing or circulation requires close monitoring, immediate medical assessment and resuscitative interventions. The initial assessment should include a 12-lead ECG and a history of the presenting complaint, including an evaluation of the pain utilising a systematic approach. The ECG should be rapidly evaluated for the presence of ST-segment elevation or a new left bundle branch block suggestive of an acute myocardial infarction (AMI) so that time-critical treatment can be initiated. If the initial ECG is non-diagnostic and symptoms continue, repeat ECGs should be performed at 15-minute intervals.[90,94]

The patient should have cardiac monitoring commenced in order to identify any life-threatening arrhythmias. Supplemental oxygen should also be commenced in patients with SaO_2 <90%, patients in respiratory distress and those presenting high-risk features for hypoxia. Supplemental oxygen use for patients without hypoxia has not been proven to cause benefit or harm but has the disadvantages of cost and discomfort for the patient.[95] An IV cannula should be inserted and routine venous blood samples collected for troponin T or troponin I, which are cardiac enzymes that, when elevated, suggest myocardial injury. Cardiac enzymes are usually repeated within 6 hours of ED presentation.[96] A physical examination should also be performed. The physical examination may be of limited value in identifying cardiac causes of the pain but will be beneficial in identifying non-cardiac causes of the pain or complications associated with cardiac-related conditions.[89,90] The examination should also include assessment of the abdomen, as a number of significant abdominal complaints may also present with chest pain as a feature.[94] A CXR should also be performed in order to identify any potential causes for the patient's pain.

Patient diagnoses and management
Acute coronary syndromes

Chest pain of cardiac origin results from reduced or obstructed coronary blood flow, commonly due to atherosclerosis, although coronary artery spasm or an embolism may also be involved.[97] Angina, whether stable or unstable, is a temporary condition in which there is no damage to the myocardial cells. A time-critical obstruction results in death or necrosis of a segment of myocardial cells, resulting in an AMI.[94]

ACS collectively describes unstable angina and AMI. In 2020, coronary heart disease was the single leading cause of death in Australia, accounting for 10% of all deaths. Compared with non-Indigenous Australians, Indigenous Australians have a higher prevalence of coronary heart disease[98] and had 1.4 times the out-of-hospital death rate.[99] It is the leading cause of premature death and disability in both Australia and New Zealand, although death rates have fallen since the 1960s. ACS is a common life-threatening condition seen in the ED and therefore represents an important area of clinical practice

in the ED. Chapters 10 and 11 provide additional information about presentations of cardiac dysfunction, including pathophysiology, clinical manifestations and treatment of cardiac conditions. This section summarises clinical management processes in the ED.[97]

The initial management of patients with suspected ACS involves risk stratification and rapid identification of patients with AMI, initiation of antithrombotic therapy and identification of suitability for reperfusion therapy.[90,97] Reperfusion therapy consists of the administration of thrombolytic drugs with or without percutaneous coronary intervention (angioplasty ± stent). Percutaneous coronary intervention is generally available only to patients in larger centres where there is access to such resources. If percutaneous coronary intervention is not available, suitable patients should be managed with thrombolysis.[90]

The ongoing management in the ED for patients with ACS includes oxygen therapy in patients with SaO_2 <93%,[96] administration of aspirin 300 mg – if not already administered by pre-hospital personnel – and pain relief. Pain relief management generally includes the administration of IV morphine in small incremental doses. Pain relief may also include the administration of nitrates initially via the sublingual route; however, if pain persists despite IV morphine, the administration of IV nitrates may be indicated.[97] The patient and family should also be provided reassurance, information and emotional support.

Patients without initial evidence of AMI are subsequently stratified into high-, intermediate- and low-risk groups based upon the presence of a number of clinical features associated with the presentation, including the significance and duration of pain, ECG findings, past history, cardiovascular disease risk factors and cardiac enzyme results.[97] Specific ongoing treatment and management is then guided by the associated risk pathway.[88]

Thoracic aortic dissection

Thoracic aortic dissection (TAD) occurs when there is a tear in the intimal layer of the vessel wall. Blood passes through the tear, separates the intima from the vessel media or adventitia and results in a false channel. Shear forces lead to dissection propagation as blood flows through the false channel.[94] The incidence of TAD is quite low; ACS is 80 times more common. Identification of this life-threatening condition in the patient presenting with chest pain is important, as patients often require immediate surgery. TAD is most commonly seen in men aged 50 to 70 years who have a history of hypertension. Other risk factors include Marfan's disease and other connective tissue disorders, cocaine or ecstasy use, pregnancy and aortic valve replacement.[100] TAD is associated with an acute and sudden onset of severe pain that is maximal at symptom onset. Pain is usually located in the midline and may be present in the back and rarely radiates. The pain is often described as sharp, tearing or ripping in nature.[100] Patients may also have pulse deficits or blood pressure differences (>20 mmHg) between the upper arms. CXR will be abnormal in 80–90% of cases, with a widened mediastinum seen in nearly 70% of cases.[101] However, in under 20% of patients with aortic dissection it may be unremarkable.[102] While patients commonly have the diagnosis confirmed using contrast computed tomography (CT), emergency physicians increasingly use bedside ultrasound to rapidly evaluate the abdominal aorta for aneurysm (sensitivity 67–80% and specificity 99–100%).[103] The management of TAD is aimed at aggressive control of blood pressure and pulse with sodium nitroprusside and beta-blockers, relief of pain with narcotic analgesia, and referral and/or transport to cardiothoracic services for definitive surgical intervention.[101]

Abdominal symptom presentations

Acute abdominal pain is one of the most common presenting complaints, accounting for 5–10% of all presentations to the ED.[104] Despite sophisticated diagnostic modalities, identifying the specific cause for the presenting abdominal pain will not be found in 25% of patients discharged from ED, and between 30 and 40% of admitted patients.[105] About one-third of adult patients aged over 65 who present with acute abdominal pain will require surgical intervention and/or hospital admission.[105]

Common causes in the elderly include cholecystitis, diverticular disease, bowel obstruction and gastroenteritis.[106] Elderly patients are more likely to have catastrophic illnesses rarely seen in younger patients, including mesenteric ischaemia, leaking or ruptured abdominal aortic aneurysm and myocardial infarction, with up to one-third requiring surgical intervention.[105] Presentations by elderly patients are often complicated by delays in seeking medical attention, atypical presentations, associated medical conditions and comorbidities, medications and cognitive function.

Assessment, monitoring and diagnostics

Patients presenting with abdominal pain are assessed quickly for any disturbance to airway, breathing or circulation requiring close monitoring, immediate medical assessment and/or resuscitative interventions. Abnormal vital signs are suggestive of clinically significant abdominal pain.[106] A thorough history includes location and timing of onset; quantity, quality and radiation of pain; and associated symptoms, previous history and general state of health. A complaint-specific history and physical examination is performed for a differential diagnosis.[105] Physical assessment includes visual inspection of the abdomen with the patient in a supine position, followed by auscultation, then gentle palpation and percussion of all four quadrants of the abdomen, working towards the area

of reported pain.[105] While location of the pain is important, it can be misleading, as various pathological processes can localise to different areas of the abdomen (Fig. 23.1).[107] An ECG is considered to rule out myocardial ischaemia or infarction, as some cardiac patients may present with upper abdominal pain as the predominant symptom. Myocardial ischaemia may also be caused by the physiological stress of the intra-abdominal pathology.[106]

Administration of narcotic analgesia in acute abdominal pain does not hinder assessment or obscure abdominal findings, or cause increased morbidity or mortality, and may allow for a better abdominal examination.[106] Incremental doses of a narcotic can minimise pain but not palpation tenderness. Analgesics enable relaxation of the patient's abdominal muscles and decrease anxiety, potentially improving information obtained from the physical examination.[108]

Venous blood samples are collected for full blood count, urea, electrolytes, creatinine, liver function tests and lipase.[105] A dipstick urinalysis can suggest specific disease. For example, leukocytes, nitrites and/or blood in the urine can suggest a urinary tract infection and haematuria can suggest renal colic, but should be considered in the context of other clinical findings and formal microscopy.[105] Women of child-bearing age with abdominal pain provide the challenge of a broader range of potential causative pathologies. History and physical examination are unreliable in determining pregnancy. If pregnancy or a pregnancy-related disorder is possible, a urine beta-human chorionic gonadotrophin (β-HCG) test is performed. Test sensitivity is extremely high; a positive finding occurs within a few days of conception, and accuracy is comparable to blood sampling. An ectopic pregnancy may be missed if pregnancy is not considered; an ectopic pregnancy is extremely unlikely if the β-HCG result is negative.[109]

Patient diagnoses and management

Common abdominal diagnoses for acute abdominal pain are abdominal aortic aneurysm, appendicitis and bowel obstruction.

Abdominal aortic aneurysm

Abdominal aortic aneurysm is more likely to develop in men than women, is a common cause of death in all patients over the age of 65 years and is responsible for 0.8% of all deaths.[110] The traditional presentation is acute pain in the back, flank or abdomen, with hypotension and a palpable pulsatile abdominal mass in the older patient. Missed diagnoses primarily occur because physical examination is frequently unreliable.[101] The distal aorta is subject to the greatest changes in arterial pressure and biomechanical stress, hence the majority of abdominal aortic aneurysms are found below the renal arteries.[110] Many patients with dissecting abdominal aortic aneurysm are misdiagnosed with renal colic because of haematuria present, no palpable pulsatile mass and flank pain.[101] Other common misdiagnoses include diverticulitis,

FIGURE 23.1 An algorithm for triaging commonly missed causes of acute abdominal pain.[107] AAA = abdominal aortic aneurysm; β-HCG = beta-human chorionic gonadotrophin; RLQ = right lower quadrant.

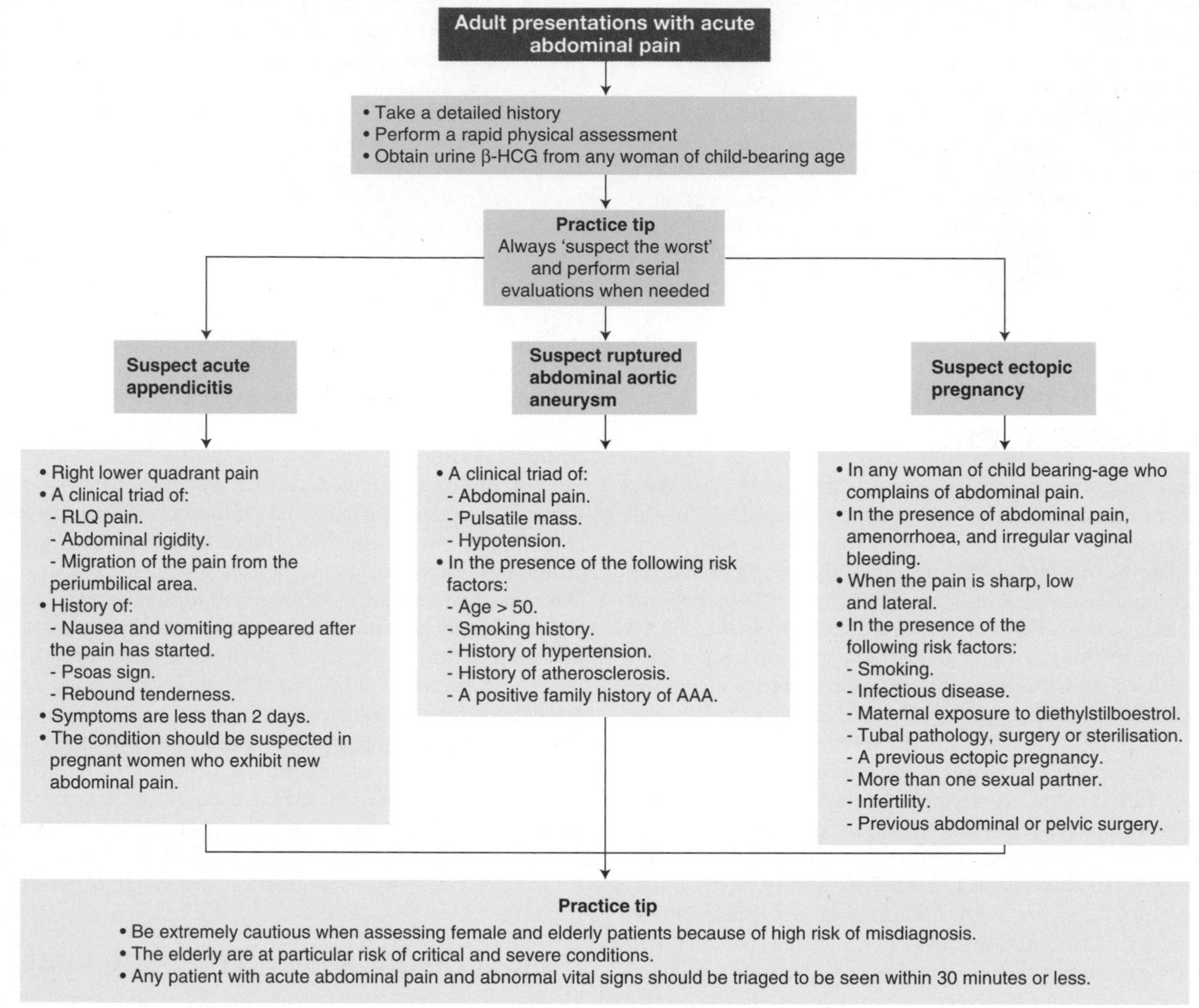

Adult presentations with acute abdominal pain

- Take a detailed history
- Perform a rapid physical assessment
- Obtain urine β-HCG from any woman of child-bearing age

Practice tip
Always 'suspect the worst' and perform serial evaluations when needed

Suspect acute appendicitis

- Right lower quadrant pain
- A clinical triad of:
  - RLQ pain.
  - Abdominal rigidity.
  - Migration of the pain from the periumbilical area.
- History of:
  - Nausea and vomiting appeared after the pain has started.
  - Psoas sign.
  - Rebound tenderness.
- Symptoms are less than 2 days.
- The condition should be suspected in pregnant women who exhibit new abdominal pain.

Suspect ruptured abdominal aortic aneurysm

- A clinical triad of:
  - Abdominal pain.
  - Pulsatile mass.
  - Hypotension.
- In the presence of the following risk factors:
  - Age > 50.
  - Smoking history.
  - History of hypertension.
  - History of atherosclerosis.
  - A positive family history of AAA.

Suspect ectopic pregnancy

- In any woman of child bearing-age who complains of abdominal pain.
- In the presence of abdominal pain, amenorrhoea, and irregular vaginal bleeding.
- When the pain is sharp, low and lateral.
- In the presence of the following risk factors:
  - Smoking.
  - Infectious disease.
  - Maternal exposure to diethylstilboestrol.
  - Tubal pathology, surgery or sterilisation.
  - A previous ectopic pregnancy.
  - More than one sexual partner.
  - Infertility.
  - Previous abdominal or pelvic surgery.

Practice tip
- Be extremely cautious when assessing female and elderly patients because of high risk of misdiagnosis.
- The elderly are at particular risk of critical and severe conditions.
- Any patient with acute abdominal pain and abnormal vital signs should be triaged to be seen within 30 minutes or less.

Source: Dagiely S. An algorithm for triaging commonly missed causes of acute abdominal pain. J Emer Nurs 2006;32(1):9.

gastrointestinal haemorrhage, AMI and musculoskeletal back pain.[110] Abdominal aortic aneurysms are surgically repaired more than any other type of aneurysm. Unless a patient receives immediate resuscitation and surgical intervention, 90% of patients with a ruptured abdominal aortic aneurysm will die; however, even with surgery the mortality rate is still 50%.[110]

Appendicitis

Appendicitis is the most common acute abdominal pain presentation worldwide that requires a surgical intervention. The peak incidence is in the second and third decades of life, with an overall incidence of around 1.9 per 1000 persons per year.[111] About 7% of people in Western countries will have appendicitis during their lifetime.[111] Along with pain (usually in the right lower quadrant), other presenting symptoms may include nausea and vomiting.[112] Imaging increases diagnostic accuracy and aims to decrease the negative appendectomy rate. CT is the preferred modality of imaging; however, in children and pregnant women, abdominal ultrasound is preferred.[105] Appendicitis can mimic almost all acute abdominal pain presentations, and during the initial ED visit it is frequently misdiagnosed as gastroenteritis, pelvic inflammatory disease or urinary tract infection.[112] Although it is a well-studied disease, appendicitis continues to be difficult to diagnose in ED because of its varied presentations. Elderly patients require careful consideration because of associated comorbidities[111,113] and women of child-bearing age are commonly misdiagnosed owing to anatomical changes associated with pregnancy. Treatment includes management of pain-related symptoms and provision of IV hydration. In low-risk patient groups, earlier use of antibiotics may successfully resolve the issue in up to 90% of cases, without the need for surgical removal of the appendix.[113] In the context of free perforation of the appendix, the definitive treatment is emergency appendectomy.[111]

Practice tip

Elderly patients require careful consideration because of associated comorbidities and age-related changes to their response to illness.

Bowel obstruction

A bowel obstruction commonly results from impaired peristaltic movement, hernias, adhesions and neoplasms.[114] Presentation includes poorly localised colicky pain that increases in intensity and location, with subsequent abdominal swelling and vomiting of faecal fluid.[115] Management may be conservative (management of symptoms, placement of a nasogastric tube for gastrointestinal decompression and IV fluid therapy and electrolyte replacement); however, all patient suspected of a complicated bowel obstruction (e.g. complete obstruction, perforation, necrosis) should have abdominal exploration in the operating theatre.[116]

Ectopic pregnancy

An ectopic pregnancy is implantation outside the uterus, most commonly in the fallopian tubes, Ectopic pregnancy occurs at a rate of about 11 per 1000 pregnancies, with the incidence thought to be higher in developing countries.[117] Presenting symptoms can include lower abdominal pain that can become severe, feeling faint, bleeding and shoulder tip pain. There are three approaches to management of ectopic therapy including surgery, methotrexate, and expectant management for a small proportion of women. Emergency surgery is indicated in the event of haemodynamic instability, or signs of impending or active rupture of the ectopic mass.[117]

Acute stroke

Cerebrovascular disease is highly prevalent in developed countries. In some countries that have seen continuing industrialisation (such as Asia and Africa) the increasingly unhealthy lifestyle is being reflected in diseases including cerebrovascular disease.[35] In China, which has the greatest burden of stroke in the world, the incidence (115 per 100,000 person-years) is relatively low, but the incidence and mortality rates are amongst the highest in the world.[60] In Australia, cerebrovascular disease is the third-largest cause of death.[99]

The two general stroke classifications are as follows:

- Ischaemic strokes are precipitated by disrupted blood flow to an area of the brain as a result of arterial occlusion, and occur in up to 62% of all stroke incidences,[118] with similar pathophysiology and treatment modalities to that of AMI.[119] From an ED perspective, serious long-term disability can be minimised if ischaemic stroke is recognised and treated promptly (<4.5 hours).[120]

- Haemorrhagic strokes are caused by rupture of a blood vessel, which produces bleeding into the brain parenchyma, and account for 28% of all incident strokes.[118] (Chapter 17 details the pathophysiological processes.)

For patients diagnosed with an ischaemic stroke, approximately 13% will die within the first 30 days,[121] with 12% having permanent disability requiring care in a nursing home or other long-term facility.[122]

Assessment, monitoring and diagnostics

Symptoms of stroke are common amongst patients presenting to the ED; presenting signs vary from profound alterations in level of consciousness and limb hemiplegia to mild symptoms affecting speech, cognition or coordination. Symptoms may include confusion, dizziness, ataxia, visual disturbances, dysphasia or receptive and expressive aphasia, dysphagia, weakness and numbness or tingling of the face, arm or leg, which is usually unilateral.[119] Many disorders resemble a stroke presentation so emergency clinicians must quickly determine whether another condition is responsible for the patient's neurological deficits. Other conditions include postictal phase following seizures, migraine with neurological deficits, hypoglycaemia or hyperglycaemia, systemic infections, brain tumours, hyponatraemia and hepatic encephalopathy.[123]

The aims of the initial contact phase with the patient is to ensure medical stability, to reverse any contributing conditions to the patient's problem, to identify the pathophysiological basis for the presenting neurological symptoms, and to identify whether patients experiencing an ischaemic stroke will be suitable for thrombolytic therapy.[123] The focus of initial assessment is airway, breathing, circulation and disability. Of note, for airway assessment, stroke symptoms include altered muscle function affecting swallowing and speech functions. A patient with a Glasgow Coma Scale (GCS) score of 9 or less may require intubation to protect and secure the airway.[124] The patient's breathing pattern should be assessed and continually monitored. Supplemental oxygen should be provided to hypoxic patients to maintain oxygen saturation >94%; however, it should be avoided in non-hypoxic stroke victims.[119] Hypertension is common, with the increase improving any cerebral ischaemia so this should not be lowered unless dangerously high or contraindicated.[123] Hypotension or dehydration decreases cerebral blood flow and perfusion and should be corrected, though fluid replacement is instituted with caution. Vital signs are documented every 15 minutes during drug therapy in order to identify changes suggestive of internal bleeding. Maintaining blood pressure at <185/110 mmHg during fibrinolytic infusion decreases the risk of intracerebral haemorrhage.[125]

A thorough assessment of neurological disability should be undertaken, including a GCS (see Chapter 16). An ECG is recorded to detect any abnormal rhythm such as atrial fibrillation, which may be associated with stroke presentation.[126] IV access is obtained to administer medication and collect blood for electrolytes, haematology and coagulation studies. Assessment of blood glucose will rule out hypoglycaemia or hyperglycaemia as a cause of the presenting symptoms. Abnormal glucose levels adversely affect cerebral metabolism.[127] After obvious alternative diagnoses are excluded, a brain CT scan determines whether a stroke is haemorrhagic or ischaemic in origin. While a new-onset ischaemic stroke may not be evident for up to 24 hours, blood in the cranial cavity will be apparent immediately. Patients with any sign of haemorrhage are excluded for fibrinolytic therapy.[120]

Management

Acute ischaemic stroke management includes timely administration of a fibrinolytic agent in appropriately selected patients (Box 23.2),[120] which facilitates reperfusion, minimises tissue damage and reduces long-term stroke sequelae. Longer times between symptom onset and fibrinolytic infusion are associated with higher rates of morbidity and mortality.[120] Early presentation is therefore essential to instigate appropriate assessments and investigations, including CT scanning, and then thrombolytic administration and still fall within the narrow treatment window. Acute stroke unit care, with specialised teams dedicated to the rapid assessment and management of presentations, can significantly reduce death and disability[123] (see Chapter 17).

Overdose and poisoning

Poisoning is a common clinical presentation throughout the world. Worldwide up to 9% of deaths are related to drug and alcohol misuse in the age group between 15 and 29.[128] Suicide is a global issue and over 700,000 people die from suicide annually.[129] It is the fourth leading cause of deaths in young people aged 15–19 years. The most common forms of suicide include ingestion of pesticide, hanging and from firearms.[129] In Australia, 2019–22 data reveal that 24% of injury causing deaths were from suicide.[99] In Australia, males are 3–4 times more likely to die from suicide, while females are more likely to attempt suicide or present to hospital as a result of intentional self-harm.[130] Another difference for Australia is that, while suicide is the leading cause of death for 15–19 year olds, suicide rates are highest for men aged 40–44 years, 50–54 years and ≥85 years.[130]

The usual types of poisoning encountered as ED presentations include self-poisoning with prescribed drugs

---

BOX 23.2

Criteria for administering fibrinolytic therapy in ischaemic stroke[120]

Inclusion criteria (all must be positive):

- Age ≥18 years
- Clinical diagnosis of ischaemic stroke with measurable neurological deficit
- Time of symptom onset <4.5 h minimum and well established

Exclusion criteria (all must be negative):

- Evidence of intracranial haemorrhage on non-contrast head CT
- Only minor or rapidly improving stroke symptoms
- High suspicion of subarachnoid haemorrhage, even with normal CT
- Active internal bleeding
- Known bleeding condition, including but not limited to platelets <100,000/mm³
- Patient received heparin within 48 h and had an elevated activated PTT
- Current use of oral anticoagulants (e.g. warfarin)
- Recent use of anticoagulant and elevated INR (>1.5) or prothrombin time (>15 s)
- Intracranial surgery or serious head trauma, or previous stroke within 3 months
- Major surgery or serious trauma within 14 days
- History of intracranial haemorrhage, arteriovenous malformation, or aneurysm
- Witnessed seizure at stroke onset
- Recent AMI
- Systolic blood pressure >185 mmHg or diastolic blood pressure >110 mmHg at time of treatment

AMI = acute myocardial infarction; CT = computed tomography; INR = international normalised ratio; PTT = partial thromboplastin time

---

and ingestion of illicit drugs and common dangerous substances (e.g. detergents, cleansers, psychotropic agents, analgesics, insecticides, paracetamol, aspirin).[131] A range of artificial and naturally occurring substances can produce acute poisoning. The toxicity of a substance depends on numerous factors, such as dose, route of exposure and the victim's pre-existing conditions. Poisoning, whether intentional or unintentional, can occur at any time, and may involve single or multiple substances.[131]

The vast amount of knowledge required concerning all poisons prompted the development of poison control information centres to provide specific information and guidance for healthcare providers and the general public on the management of a poisoned patient, to collect statistics on toxic substances and to educate the public on the prevention or recognition of toxic exposures. Other initiatives to limit the incidence and severity of acute poisoning include the control of drugs, specific information on labels, the introduction of blister packs and enforced safety standards such as childproof caps.[131]

Assessment, monitoring and diagnostics

The poisoned patient may present with a wide range of clinical features from no symptoms through to a life-threatening condition or the potential to deteriorate rapidly, and should always be assessed immediately. Triage decisions should be based on the potential for rapid deterioration and the need for urgent intervention. Resuscitation may be necessary before any further definitive care can be commenced. The priorities of care for all patients include the assessment and maintenance of an airway, adequate ventilation and circulation.[132] Successful resuscitation may require removal of the toxin, counteraction of the poisoning by an antidote if available, and the treatment or support of symptoms.[132] It is extremely important to note that many drugs, such as paracetamol, may have limited initial effects but serious, potentially fatal consequences if not treated in a timely manner.[133]

An accurate history is often the most significant aid in directing care. If a history is unobtainable or uncertain, there are several general guidelines that may prove helpful for dealing with the patient who has an altered mental state or consciousness level[132,134] (Table 23.8).

Poisoning should always be considered when dealing with a patient who has a sudden-onset, acute illness. If there is a strong suspicion of poisoning, a clinician should attempt to compare the patient's presentation with symptoms caused by the suspected toxin and the likelihood of exposure.

Accidental poisonings are the commonest cause of medical emergencies in the paediatric patient population. Childhood ingestions tend to be accidental and to involve a single substance. Intentional poisonings occur more often with adults, and are more likely to involve multiple substances.[130,132] Poisonings in the aged population are often complicated by coexisting medical conditions which may exaggerate the effects or impair the excretion of the substances involved. Adult women attempt suicide with poisons more often than men, but men's suicide intentions are associated with a higher mortality rate.[130,132,135]

Practice tip

Poisonings in the aged population are often complicated by coexisting medical conditions which may exaggerate the effects or impair excretion of the substances involved.[135]

TABLE 23.8

Acronyms outlining potential causes of altered levels of consciousness[132,134]

ACRONYM	CAUSE	ACRONYM	CAUSE
T	Trauma	A	Alcohol/Acidosis
I	Infection	E	Endocrine
	Insulin (hypo-/hyperglycaemia)		Encephalopathy
P	Psychosis		Electrolyte abnormality
	Porphyria		Epilepsy
	Poisoning	I	Insulin/diabetes
S	Seizure		Infection
	Syncope	O	Oxygen: hypoxia of any cause
	Space-occupying lesion		Opiates/Overdose
	Stroke	U	Uraemia/Untherapeutic underdose of medication

Previous history

Patients with existing medical conditions often have multiple medications that could be either intentionally or unintentionally ingested. The use of multiple drugs may cause untoward reactions. A patient with a history of depression may attempt suicide with psychotropic drugs. A quick onset and acute illness or condition should raise the level of suspicion of poisoning, especially if there is no history of previous signs or symptoms that suggests another cause.

Suspected toxin

Rescue personnel, family or friends should bring any container, plant product or suspected toxin with the patient to the hospital, as long as the substance presents no risk of contamination to the person retrieving it. A child's play area should be inspected for possible sources of toxins.[132]

Time of poisoning

History should include time of exposure, onset of symptoms and time since treatment began. Often many patients cannot provide an accurate history and so questioning of support friends and family is essential.[136]

However, this is still not always accurate.[137] Alcohol is the most common drug ingested with other intentional self-poisonings, and can potentiate a range of medication effects and increase the incidence of vomiting and potential aspiration.[112,132,137] Poisonings in children tend to be accidental, until they reach teenage years.[137,138] In adults, recent research shows a specific pattern of poisoning, occurring most often around 18:00 hours; when poisoning agents are taken alongside alcohol, this usually occurs later in the evening, at around 20:00 hours.[139] There is further research to be undertaken to understand the timing pattern of deliberate self-harm poisonings and time of day related to diurnal patterns and the impact that alcohol has on deliberate poison ingestion.[139]

A thorough assessment may provide clues about an unconscious, uncooperative or suspicious presentation. Assess for respiratory effort, skin colour, pupil size and reactivity, reflexes and general status. Auscultation of the lung fields, the apical pulse and presence of active bowel sounds provide a baseline for further assessment and clues about current problems. Check blood pressure as often as necessary to determine cardiovascular stability. Percuss the thorax and abdomen to detect accumulations of fluid or air.[132,136] Needle marks, pill fragments, uneaten leaves or berries or drug paraphernalia assist in diagnosis.[132,136] The presence of pressure areas on the skin may indicate how long the patient has been unresponsive. Any odours are important to note. An oily–garlicky or kerosene-like smell may be due to pesticides.[140] Other odours may indicate chronic medical disorders (e.g. fruity odour with diabetic ketoacidosis) or neglect of personal hygiene.

Practice tip

Odours are important to note, as they may reflect not only poisoning but other medical disorders; for example, a fruity odour may reflect diabetic ketoacidosis.

Toxicology screens include an analysis of serum and urine to determine the presence and amount of a substance. Laboratory levels are helpful but must be considered according to the nature of the substance and its rate of metabolism. Serum electrolytes, non–electrolytes, osmolality, ABGs and urine electrolytes are used to determine the patient's overall status or response to therapy. Continuous cardiac monitoring supplemented with a 12-lead ECG or invasive monitoring devices may be required to help provide symptomatic care.[132]

Initial and ongoing care of the victim follows three principles:[132,137]

1 preventing further absorption of the toxin
2 enhancing elimination of absorbed toxin from the body
3 preventing complications by providing symptomatic or specific treatments, including psychiatric management.

Management: preventing toxin absorption

Ingested poisons are best removed while still in the upper gastrointestinal tract when possible. Emesis and gastric lavage were used in the past to empty the stomach, although a significant body of evidence now suggests that these are relatively ineffective and effectiveness decreases rapidly after 1 hour.[132,137] Both the patient and the substance should be evaluated for appropriateness of gastric emptying.[132]

The patient's consciousness level, gag reflex and ability to vomit while protecting the airway from aspiration should be considered. Any central nervous system depressants can obtund the protective gag or cough reflex. If the ingested substance has a rapid onset of action, such as with benzodiazepines, it is safer to avoid emetics because of the risk of a sudden fall in the level of consciousness.[132,137]

Ingested poisons

Evaluate the substance ingested to determine whether gastric emptying is appropriate. The physical properties of a drug may make it more responsive to a particular type of gastric emptying. For example, the antimuscarinic effect of tricyclic antidepressants on gut motility can prolong gastrointestinal absorption, increasing plasma levels.[141] Also, consider the effects of substances on tissue. Corrosives, such as acids, alkalis and iron supplements, produce irritation and tissue breakdown when in contact with the skin or mucous membranes. Recognition is important, as therapy may cause further injury. Emesis could be contraindicated, and a lavage tube may further traumatise injured tissue.[137] Ipecac syrup and vomiting are generally ineffective against a substance with an antiemetic property, such as phenothiazines.[137] Waiting for emesis also causes further delay in definitive treatment. Other substances have natural emetic qualities if taken in sufficient doses and can also have other immediate effects that complicate the severity of the patient condition (e.g. hand soaps and liquid soap detergents can cause emesis but also oropharyngeal irritation, such as oedema of the tongue and respiratory symptoms).[142]

Evaluate other substances on an individual basis. There are situations, however, when the amount, character or additional chemicals present make it necessary to remove the ingested substance from the stomach. Occasionally, therapy is based on the reported amount taken or time since ingestion. Time since ingestion is important to rule out the benefit of therapy. The stomach tends to empty its contents after 1 hour, unless a substance that slows gastric motility has been ingested. For example, narcotics can slow peristalsis and may be found in the stomach several hours after ingestion.[132] A patient may also underreport the dosage to avoid an obviously unpleasant experience. Although conservative management with observation is appropriate in certain situations, the risk of not treating might be greater in others.[132] If a large number of tablets or pills are consumed at one time, they may clump together in the stomach and form a mass that is too large to pass out of the pylorus (e.g. aspirin).[143]

Once a substance enters the lower gastrointestinal tract, it can be absorbed into the mesenteric circulation. As absorption can vary according to substance, slow-release characteristics, rate of peristalsis and the presence of other substances, it is possible for a poison to be present in the bowel for an extended period of time. If intestinal motility can be stimulated or the toxin permanently bound until excretion, then further absorption is reduced.[132] Activated charcoal is a refined product with an enormous surface area that binds to a large range of substances to enhance elimination, and is the most effective decontaminating agent currently available if ingested within 1 hour of poisoning.[132,137] Unfortunately, not all poisons ingested can be bound by charcoal, such as alcohol, corrosives, hydrocarbons and heavy metals.[132,137]

Inhaled poisons

A patient poisoned by inhalation of toxic gases or powders should be removed from the source as soon as it is safe to do so.[132] The history of a patient suspected of an inhaled poison should include time of exposure, the duration of exposure, the onset of symptoms, suspected inhalant and time since treatment began.

Staff involved in direct care of the patient should take precautions to avoid unprotected contact to reduce the risk of self-contamination with unknown substances. For many inhaled poisons, clothing may contain significant amounts of the poison and serve as a continuous source of the toxin. Contaminated linen and clothes should be removed carefully, sealed in a bag and destroyed.[132]

Contact poisons

Contact poisons are dangerous because of their ability to enter the body via the skin or mucous membranes. All clothing and all of the toxic substance should be carefully removed, preferably with an irrigating and neutralising solution. Precautions to avoid direct skin contact and reduce the risk of self-contamination should be used.[137] Clothing may contain significant residual amounts of the poison and serve as a continuous source of the toxin. Contaminated linen and clothes should be sealed in a bag and destroyed.[132]

Management: enhancing elimination of the toxin from blood

After a substance has entered the bloodstream, it is normally excreted from the body either in an unchanged form or after liver metabolism and detoxification. Various metabolic byproducts are eliminated in the bile and faeces or urine. The administration of large volumes of IV solutions and/or diuretics can enhance urinary excretion of substances by increasing the filtration process by forcing diuresis. Enhanced secretion can also occur by inhibiting absorption in the renal tubules or by stimulating the secretion of substances into the urine.[132,137]

Alkalinisation of urine

Manipulation of the absorption or secretion process of a drug can be assisted by chemically altering the structure of some substances. All substances break down into ions at a specific pH for that substance. Altering the pH of urine with acidifying or alkalising drugs allows the poison to be forced into an ionic state and then excreted in the urine. This ion-trapping process is effective only for substances that are primarily eliminated by the kidneys[132,137] – for example, salicylates and tricyclic antidepressants.[137,141]

Haemodialysis or haemoperfusion

If a dangerous amount of a poison is present or if renal failure is evident, haemodialysis may be used to enhance excretion, particularly with poisoning from salicylates, ethylene glycol, methanol, lithium, phenobarbital and chlorates; haemoperfusion may be used on specialist advice for severe poisoning with barbiturates, chloral hydrate and theophylline.[137] Dialysis is effective only in removing substances that are reversibly bound to serum proteins, or not stored in body fat. This is a highly invasive approach and is normally reserved for life-threatening cases (see Chapter 18 for further discussion).[137]

Management: preventing complications and specific symptomatic care

Supportive care is the key element in managing an acutely poisoned patient. Once a patient has either ingested or been exposed to many poisons, there are limited options other than to treat the symptoms as they appear or become clinically significant (Table 23.9).[132,133,136–138,140,141,143]

Antidotes act to antagonise, compete with or override the effects of the poison, although few specific antidotes exist for toxins (Table 23.10).[132,137] In some cases, an absorbed toxin can be rendered benign by the use of an antidote (e.g. the interaction between naloxone and opiates). For chelating agents, such as desferrioxamine for iron poisoning, a non-toxic compound is formed that is then safely eliminated from the body.[144] The effect of an antidote may be only temporary if the antidote has a shorter half-life than the poison. Most antidotes are given either in a specific dose or at a response-to-dose rate. For many poisonings, symptomatic care involves support and protection of vital organ systems. Routine and frequent physical assessment of respiratory, cardiovascular and renal function enables identification of potential problems. If large volumes of fluids or drugs that alter serum pH are administered, the patient's electrolyte and acid–base balance are also monitored.[132]

A poisoning may be the physical manifestation of an emergency or crisis that requires emotional support. A patient may have underlying emotional conflict/s or mental health problems, regardless of whether the poisoning was intentional or accidental. Psychological care is, therefore, an important component for all patients presenting with poisoning.[132,137] Many facilities offer the services of a mental health worker while the patient is still in the ED. If the

TABLE 23.9

Summary of the management of poisoning victims[132,133,136–138,140,141,143]

AIM	ACTION
Prevent absorption of toxin.	• Ingested toxins: activated charcoal is the most effective method of reducing adsorption. • Inhaled toxins: remove victim from source of contamination and administer oxygen or provide fresh air. • Contact toxins: remove any substances from the body surface, preferably with copious amounts of irrigating fluid. Remove clothing and place in a sealed bag to reduce vapour hazards. Use special caution with corrosive materials and pesticides.
Enhance elimination of the toxin from the blood.	Ingested or injected toxins: administer an antidote or antagonist if available (e.g. naloxone for opiates; flumazenil for benzodiazepines). Employ forced diuresis, for acidification or alkalinisation of the urine; and haemodialysis.
Prevent complications by providing symptomatic or specific treatment.	Carefully monitor all vital systems. Continually reassess patient for changes or response to therapy. Administer antidotes as prescribed. Provide symptomatic care as needed for: cardiac arrhythmias, CNS depression or stimulation, fluid and electrolyte imbalances, acid–base disturbances, renal function, effects of immobility.

TABLE 23.10

Common emergency antidotes[132,137]

POISONING	ANTIDOTE
Benzodiazepines	Flumazenil
Beta-blockers	Glucagon, atropine
Calcium channel blockers	Calcium, glucagon, high-dose insulin euglycaemic therapy
Opioids	Naloxone
Paracetamol	Acetylcysteine
Organophosphates	Atropine and pralidoxime
Tricyclic antidepressants	Sodium bicarbonate
Carbon monoxide	Oxygen
Insulin	Dextrose
Digoxin	Digoxin antibodies (DigiFab™)
Cyanide	Sodium nitrate, sodium thiosulfate, dicobalt edetate, hydroxocobalamin
MDMA	Dantrolene
Methanol, ethylene glycol	Ethanol, fomepizole
Warfarin	Vitamin K, prothrombin complex concentrate, FFP

FFP = fresh frozen plasma; MDMA = 3,4-methylenedioxy methamphetamine.

patient's condition is stable and the poisoning has not altered their mental state, early intervention is appropriate.

For adult patients, the desire for treatment is not as important as the way treatment is received. Even though patients may initially refuse care, if approached in a non-threatening way and given some form of control they will usually consent to care. If threatened with force or restraints, they are placed in the position of either submitting to coercion or resisting therapy to 'protect' themselves. A paediatric patient may be too young either to fully understand or to effectively cooperate with staff.

Central nervous system depressants

Many common medications are capable of depressing levels of consciousness, thought processes or important regulatory centres located within the central nervous system (CNS). The clinical findings associated with CNS alteration can vary a great deal from drug class to class or within the same drug family, as physical effects are dependent on the chemical structure of the drug, the dose, the route of exposure, any other co-ingested drugs and the rate of drug metabolism. In addition, the chemical structure and/or purity of illicit drugs may be affected by variations or deliberate aberrations in the manufacturing process.[145] Drugs in this section include sedatives, hypnotics, tranquillisers and narcotics.

Assessment

The predominant observed effect is an altered level of CNS function.[145] A spectrum of physical findings is possible with the selective action of the specific drug on inhibitory or excitatory centres of the brain; effects can vary from mild euphoria to convulsions, or mild sedation to coma, dependence, addiction and tolerance. Narcotics constrict the pupil, and some patients experience nausea and vomiting due to a stimulation of the chemoreceptor trigger zone in the medulla.[145]

A narcotic overdose is distinctive, with a set of readily identifiable features. These features include a decreased respiratory rate and tidal volume, constriction of the pupil, hypotension and an altered level of consciousness.[137,145,146] Other factors may, however, affect these findings, as outlined in Box 23.3.[132,146]

Patients with an altered level of consciousness are subject to injury from decreased sensory ability or prolonged immobilisation and should receive pressure area care regularly.

Effects of multiple drug use

A patient who ingests a combination of drugs may experience toxicity because of additive or synergistic effects.[145] Illicitly produced drugs will most likely have had substances added (e.g. glucose powders, icing sugar, talcum powder) to dilute or 'cut' them, to increase the volume of their supply and hence the profit to the supplier.[147,148] Users may also intentionally inject other drugs (e.g. antihistamines, amphetamines, benzodiazepines) to modify or potentiate the effects of narcotics.[145,148]

Potential for acute or active infections

The use of non-sterile solutions and equipment and the sharing of injection equipment significantly increase the likelihood of acute or active infections. Frequent exposure and a depressed immune response also predispose a patient to severe infections, such as hepatitis, osteomyelitis, infective bacterial endocarditis and encephalitis/meningitis.[145]

Management

General principles apply for the management of a patient with ingestion of a toxic substance with a reduced level of consciousness. Prevent continued absorption by administering activated charcoal for oral ingestions and provide symptomatic care (Table 23.11).[132,137,141,149]

Central nervous system stimulants

CNS stimulants increase the activity of the reticular activating system, promoting a state of alertness and affecting the medullary control centres for respiratory and cardiovascular function. Many illegal stimulants are poorly manufactured, with no guarantee of purity or consistency in dosage. The possibility of overdose is therefore always present, producing profound CNS excitation.[137,145] Commonly used stimulants include amphetamines, dexamphetamine, methylphenidate, lysergic acid diethylamide (LSD), phencyclidine (PCP), caffeine, cocaine and methamphetamines.[145,146,147]

Assessment

Both psychological and physical symptoms are produced. A patient may demonstrate repetitive, non-purposeful movements, grind their teeth and appear suspicious of or paranoid about others. Physiological stimulation causes an increase in metabolism, with flushing, diaphoresis, hyperpyrexia, pupillary dilation and vomiting evident. Dizziness, loss of coordination, chest pains, palpitations or abdominal cramps may also occur. During the acute phase of poisoning, severe intoxication and loss of rational mental functioning may lead individuals to behave irrationally and even attempt suicide. Anxiousness and a general state of tension may also lead the affected person to attempt to harm others.[150] Death is possible from cardiovascular collapse or as a sequel to convulsions and acute drug toxicity.[146,151,152]

Management

If a patient has ingested the drug, emesis or lavage is of little value, and an individual risk–benefit assessment is required. Gastric emptying may precipitate more-severe agitation with a concomitant rise in blood pressure, pulse rate and metabolism.[150] Activated charcoal and cathartics may be administered to promote elimination. Ongoing emergency management includes:[150]

- support of vital functions
- reduction of external stimulation by placing the patient in a quiet, non-threatening environment where a supportive person can attempt to calm and 'talk the person down' while observing for untoward reactions
- sedation when necessary, although it is not desirable to give more medications in a precarious situation; sedation may be needed to control seizures or keep the patient from self-harm.

Practice tip

Note that there are no specific antidotes for CNS stimulants.

TABLE 23.11

Assessment and management of specific drug overdoses[132,137,141,149]

TYPE OF POISONING	GENERAL MANAGEMENT	ANTIDOTE	CLINICAL CONSIDERATIONS
CNS depressants (morphine, heroin, methadone, oxycodone)	Supportive care of airway, breathing, circulation.	Naloxone hydrochloride (Narcan™); specific reversal agent.	Action of naloxone may be much shorter than the duration of effect of the drug; the patient may need to be observed for return of unconsciousness.
CNS stimulants	Supportive care of airway, breathing, circulation.	Benzodiazepines may be used to reduce symptoms.	Reduce stimulation in the surrounding environment; monitor cardiovascular status and temperature.[132,137,146,149]
Salicylate	Observe for hyperventilation and acid–base disturbances.	Nil; charcoal may be used.	Monitor electrolyte changes and increases in fever.
Paracetamol	Careful history required to determine time and amount taken; initially vague symptoms.	Acetylcysteine	Antidote must be given within the specified time range; consider the effects of other drugs (i.e. paracetamol and codeine combinations); monitor for signs of hepatotoxicity.
Carbon monoxide	Supportive care of airway, breathing, circulation.	High concentrations of oxygen therapy	Hyperbaric oxygen may be required; monitor carboxyhaemoglobin; oxygen saturation monitors will give erroneously high readings.
Organophosphates	Decontamination; supportive care of airway, breathing, circulation.	Pralidoxime chloride; benzodiazepines	Maintain careful decontamination and personal safety considerations.

Amphetamines and designer drugs

Amphetamines and designer drugs have been drugs of abuse for several years. Originally, many of them were designed and introduced as anaesthetic agents, decongestants or for other legitimate purposes. Amphetamines are chemically related to adrenaline (epinephrine) and are like catecholamines, with a similar CNS response.[150] Amphetamines are synthetic sympathomimetic drugs; they are available in oral, intranasal or IV forms; crystalline rock forms such as 'ice' are smoked.[151] Death may occur from overdose, self-mutilation or dangerous activities such as diving or walking on roads.

Assessment

Depending on the dose, route and time since exposure, a person exhibits characteristic behavioural and physical changes. With high-dose intoxication, the patient has pronounced CNS involvement – altered levels of consciousness, seizure activity or a loss of protective gag, corneal and swallow reflexes. Nystagmus is a classic sign, along with hypertension and an elevated body temperature. A significant rise in arterial pressure presents a risk for intracerebral haemorrhage.[150] One of the distinguishing features of amphetamines is their ability to produce coma without affecting respirations.[151] The patient may risk dehydration and renal failure if muscle breakdown has

occurred. Hyperthermia and seizures must be aggressively managed.[150] Hyperthermia is a significant contributing factor to morbidity and mortality.[150]

Lower-dose intoxications do not produce unconsciousness but typically cause behavioural patterns that reflect depersonalisation and distorted perceptions of events or other people. The patient's physical and mental responses may be dulled and slow, or abusive and delusional. Intoxication is marked by paranoid thoughts, with the patient responding to therapeutic or friendly gestures with behaviours ranging from apprehension to aggressive hostility. To avoid stimulating the patient and thereby intensifying the behaviour, a quiet environment should be provided for initial assessment and treatment, although this is often difficult in the ED.[150]

> **Practice tip**
>
> Noxious environmental stimulation such as bright lighting, loud noises and activity can provoke these patients to become anxious and uncooperative.

Management

Gastric emptying is normally ineffective owing to delays in seeking treatment. If a patient presents early, activated charcoal and cathartics are useful in preventing further absorption. Noises, sights and sounds provoke paranoid ideation and may present a risk to staff and other patients. 'Talking down' is usually not successful and probably serves only to exacerbate the situation. If the patient is demonstrating hostile or self-abusive forms of behaviour, chemical restraints may be needed to protect him/her and any others present. The use of physical restraints is not without danger, and they should never be used as a substitute for a more desirable environment. If the threat of danger or psychosis is significant, sedatives such as diazepam or haloperidol may be necessary to control the patient's behaviour. IV diazepam is also used to control frequent seizure activity, and along with hyperthermia should be aggressively managed.[150] If behaviour or hyperthermia remains significantly dangerous to patient or staff, intubation and paralysis may be required.[150]

Salicylate poisoning

Aspirin is the commonest form of salicylate in the home and is found in many over-the-counter medications, such as combination analgesic and topical ointments.[153] Aspirin may be ingested orally, absorbed through the rectal mucosa, or applied to the skin in topical preparations. Under normal circumstances, the kidneys serve as the principal organ of excretion. In Australia, salicylate poisoning is relatively uncommon, because of public preference for paracetamol as the preferred analgesic and antipyretic.[153] The three common types of aspirin overdose are: accidental ingestion (more common in young children), intentional ingestion (more common in adults) and chronic toxicity (occurs in any age group).[143]

Assessment, monitoring and diagnostics

Intentional or accidental ingestion is straightforward, with a clear history of poisoning. Chronic toxicity is, however, often unrecognised.[153] Many individuals are not aware of correct dosages, may combine multiple drugs, each of which contains aspirin, or may have impaired excretion due to dehydration. The symptoms of chronic aspirin overdose include dehydration, lethargy and fever and resemble the original problem being treated, and some people will continue treating themselves with aspirin for these symptoms. Chronic toxicity has a higher mortality than acute ingestion.[153]

Toxicity may result if aspirin is ingested in amounts greater than 150 mg/kg, with severe toxicity at >300 mg/kg and potentially fatal levels from >500 mg/kg.[153] Aspirin toxicity can result in tachypnoea, fever, tinnitus, disorientation, coma and convulsions. Acid–base disturbances arise from a direct stimulatory effect on the respiratory centre in the CNS. An increased rate and depth of respirations causes hypocarbia and respiratory alkalosis, with renal compensation by bicarbonate elimination. However, salicylates also alter metabolic processes, resulting in metabolic acidosis. Blood gases can therefore reflect acidosis, alkalosis or a combination of the two.

Aspirin interferes with cellular glucose uptake, causing initial hyperglycaemia. Cellular levels of glucose become depleted, and the patient then demonstrates hypoglycaemic effects, particularly those related to the CNS. Later, serum levels may be either normal or hypoglycaemic.[153] Patients may be nauseated and vomit after ingestion, causing fluid and electrolyte imbalance.[143] Aspirin use is also associated with local tissue irritation and gastrointestinal bleeding. Normal platelet function is altered by aspirin, with an increased tendency for bleeding. Concomitant use of anticoagulants increases the risk of haemorrhage.[143]

Management

Absorption can be reduced with activated charcoal. Repeat doses should be given for patients with signs of ongoing absorption.[137] Urine alkalisation and forced diuresis can significantly increase elimination, as salicylates are weak acids excreted by the kidneys. Haemodialysis is reserved for extreme cases with profound acidosis, high blood levels, persistent CNS symptoms or renal failure.[137]

As salicylates have no known specific antidote,[153] supportive therapy includes prevention of dehydration by carefully monitoring fluid output and providing adequate fluid replacement and monitoring serum electrolytes for imbalance and replacing as needed. Evaluate arterial blood gases to determine whether the patient continues to have an effect from aspirin toxicity or is not responding to therapy. Temperature elevations should be controlled with external cooling methods if fever develops.

Paracetamol poisoning

The incidence of paracetamol (also known as acetaminophen) toxicity is associated with approximately half of all Australasian toxic ingestions, owing in part to its common availability as an analgesic/antipyretic agent.[154] The drug is absorbed in the stomach and small bowel, with 98% metabolised by the liver using one of two mechanisms: most is via a pathway that breaks down into non-toxic byproducts; the second hepatic pathway usually metabolises about 4% of the drug but the process has a toxic byproduct. The liver is capable of detoxifying the toxic byproduct by combining it with a naturally occurring substance, glutathione. In an overdose or when the minor pathway has already been stimulated (e.g. concomitant barbiturate use), more paracetamol is metabolised by the secondary pathway and the toxic byproduct accumulates, quickly consuming the available glutathione and resulting in liver tissue destruction.[154,155]

Assessment, monitoring and diagnostics

The amount of paracetamol ingested is best determined from the patient history, as serum levels, although helpful, can be easily distorted. A nomogram is used to plot measured levels against time after ingestion as a relative indicator of toxicity. A relatively small dose of 200 mg/kg or 10 g (whichever is less) of paracetamol is considered to be toxic.[154,155]

TABLE 23.12

Phases of toxic damage resulting from an excess of paracetamol[132,137,154,155]

PHASE	TIME FRAME	SYMPTOMS	TREATMENT
Phase 1	First 24 h	Vague symptoms of nausea, vomiting and malaise.	Activated charcoal in first 2 hours, serum investigations; if indicated. Commence acetylcysteine infusion.
Phase 2	24–48 h	Vague symptoms subside; onset of right upper quadrant pain due to hepatic injury; urine output may decrease as paracetamol potentiates the effect of antidiuretic hormone; liver enzymes, bilirubin, proteins and clotting studies may be abnormal.	Follow guidelines for continued evaluation of serum levels and corresponding treatment with acetylcysteine infusion.
Phase 3	60–72 h	Liver impairment becomes more obvious, with jaundice, coagulation defects, hypoglycaemia and hepatic encephalopathy; renal failure or cardiomyopathy may also occur; death from hepatic failure occurs in approximately 10% of severe overdose.	Liver transplant may be considered.

Liver function studies are helpful to recognise the development of hepatic dysfunction or damage. These include liver enzymes, serum bilirubin, protein, prothrombin time, partial thromboplastin time and platelets.[156] Three phases of toxic damage resulting from excess paracetamol are presented in Table 23.12.[132,137,154,155]

Management

Absorption can be reduced with activated charcoal when the patient presents to hospital early; however, following periods of 2 hours or greater ingestion-activated charcoal is unlikely to be very effective. Haemodialysis with a charcoal dialysate has been used in an attempt to remove unchanged paracetamol from the liver, but this does not remove the toxic byproduct. Forced diuresis is also not effective, because little paracetamol (only about 2%) is removed by the kidneys.[154]

The specific therapy for paracetamol poisoning is administration of the antidote, acetylcysteine, which is structurally similar to glutathione and binds to the toxic byproduct. When given within 24 hours of an acute ingestion, acetylcysteine is effective in preventing hepatic damage.[154,155]

Carbon monoxide poisoning

Carbon monoxide is a gaseous byproduct of incomplete fuel combustion and is present where there is a flame in a confined space with improper ventilation or air exchange. Levels of carbon monoxide can accumulate rapidly, and the gas is dangerous as it is colourless, odourless, tasteless and non-irritating.[157] Common sources of carbon monoxide are faulty radiant heaters, kerosene lamps, cooking stoves, engine exhausts and fireplaces. Acute carbon monoxide poisoning is the commonest form of successful poisoning in three of the world's most developed countries.[157,158]

Assessment, monitoring and diagnostics

Haemoglobin has a 210–240-fold greater affinity for carbon monoxide than for oxygen and shifts the oxygen–haemoglobin curve to the left (see Chapter 13). As carbon monoxide displaces oxygen from red blood cells, the patient experiences hypoxaemia and hypoxia.[137,157,158] Headache, nausea and vague pains are often experienced at onset of poisoning, and the patient may feel increasingly tired and sleepy, have difficulty concentrating and fail to recognise the onset of poisoning. With higher levels of inhalation, the patient may be tachypnoeic, tachycardic and experience loss of consciousness. A characteristic red colour presents in the lips with skin flushing.[157,158] The most important factors in determining carbon monoxide poisoning are a history of exposure with an elevated blood carboxyhaemoglobin level.[157,158]

Management

As CO is an inhaled toxin, the patient should be removed from the contaminated environment to prevent further absorption and allowed to breathe fresh air until 100% oxygen can be administered, although this may be ineffective because of the bond between carbon monoxide and haemoglobin. High-flow, high-concentration oxygen administration will, however, substantially reduce the half-life of carbon monoxide.[157] Hyperbaric oxygenation is used to treat severe cases of carbon monoxide poisoning, as pressurised oxygen reduces the half-life of the carboxyhaemoglobin molecule and shortens the duration of its effects.[157] Mild-to-moderate poisoning can be managed without the use of hyperbaric oxygen, as hyperbaric oxygenation is not available at every facility. Treatment depends on carboxyhaemoglobin serum levels, time since exposure, transport time to the hyperbaric chamber and the clinical symptoms of the patient.[157,158]

Patients should be monitored for adverse effects of hypoxia, as they may have convulsions, cardiac arrhythmias and acid–base disturbances.

Corrosive acids

Several substances are discussed here owing to their similar ability to cause local tissue injury. Some common acids involved in toxic emergencies are acetic acid (vinegar), carbolic acid (phenol disinfectants), chlorine (swimming pools, sanitising agents), hydrochloric acid (pools, cleaning agents), hydrofluoric and oxalic acid (laundry agents), sodium bisulfate (toilet cleaning agents that become acidic when added to water) and sulfuric acid (car battery acid).

Ingested corrosives can produce immediate or late life-threatening complications. In general, acids cause burn-like injuries.[159,160] Patients who ingest corrosive agents can show signs of tachycardia, hypotension and tachypnoea.[159] Life-threatening complications can present, with ulceration and perforation of oral and oesophageal mucosa, presenting a danger for haemorrhage and mediastinitis, and patients may also show signs of dyspnoea, chest pain, fever, subcutaneous emphysema and on auscultation a pleural rub.[159] Certain corrosive agents, like hydrofluoric acids, can have a direct effect on cardiovascular deterioration as they cause hypocalcaemia, which may present as changes to the QT interval, torsades des pointes or other arrhythmias.[160]

Assessment

Physical findings are site specific and relate to the type of exposure: ingestion, inhalation or contact (Table 23.13).[159,160] Ingested acids present as burns to the mouth and pharynx. Patients able to vocalise complain of pain, gastric irritation with vomiting and haematemesis. Fumes from an ingested substance may cause pneumonitis. Contact burns of skin or eyes are similar to other types of burns, with a sharply defined blister or wound, inflammation, pain and ulceration. Hypotension and cardiovascular collapse are also possible when damage occurs to underlying vital structures.[159,160]

Inhalation irritates respiratory tissues, producing direct damage, oedema and alterations in ventilation. Patients may initially experience coughing, choking, gasping for air and increased respiratory secretions. Clinicians should assess and monitor any obvious tissue injury, impaired respiratory function and subsequent effects of hypoxia and pulmonary oedema, which may occur up to 6–8 hours later.[159,160] ABGs, ventilation studies, serial CXRs and frequent physical assessments are used to monitor for changes.

Management

Contaminated clothing should be removed to prevent recontamination; care should be taken to ensure staff are not contaminated and exposed in this process. Patients with external contamination should be washed thoroughly to remove any remaining surface material that may come into contact with treating staff. For acid contact with skin

TABLE 23.13

Summary of assessment and management of acid and alkali exposure[159,160]

	CORROSIVE ACIDS OR CORROSIVE ALKALIS
Assessment	• Burns to skin, mouth, pharynx or oesophagus. • Gastric irritation with nausea and vomiting. • Continuous cardiac monitoring.
Management	• Airway. • Breathing. • Circulation. • Decontamination.
Prevent absorption	• Do not induce vomiting. • Remove contaminated clothing. • Flush the skin with copious amounts of water. • If early enough, may be able to aspirate and evacuate stomach contents to limit absorption (<1 hour after ingestion).
Enhance elimination	• Administer chelating agents if they exist, such as calcium gluconate or magnesium containing antacids for hydrofluoric acid.
Symptomatic management	• Protect burnt skin with sterile dressings. • Monitor respiratory status.

or eyes, begin immediate flushing with a non-reactive liquid and continue to do so for at least 15 minutes to guarantee complete removal. In most cases, water will be the safest and best available liquid. Provide skin or eye protection with a sterile dressing.[159]

For ingested acids, emesis should not be attempted, as the substance will cause additional damage when ejected from the stomach. A gastric tube may also cause structural damage by penetrating or irritating friable tissues; however, if it is less than 1 hour since ingestion, a small-bore nasogastric tube may be used to aspirate fluid from the stomach.[159] Do not attempt to neutralise the acid, as this may result in a chemical reaction and generate heat as a byproduct, with potential further burning and damage to the patient.[159] Suctioning of oral secretions should be done carefully and with as much visualisation of tissues as possible.

Corrosive alkalis

Alkalis produce tissue destruction on contact by interacting with tissue component fats and proteins and producing necrotic tissue. Erosion of the oesophagus and stomach occurs if ingested orally, and peritonitis or mediastinitis may develop as sequelae. Late effects are similar to those produced by acids. Oesophageal strictures due to scarring are common after ingestion. About 25% of patients who ingest a strong alkali will die from the initial insult.[160]

Skin contact and ingestion are the commonest types of injury from an alkali; however, ingestion is the most immediately life-threatening form of contact. Alkalis involved in toxic emergencies include many substances found around the house, such as detergents and cleaning agents that contain ammonia, cement and builder's lime, low-phosphate detergents, dishwasher detergents that contain sodium carbonate and laundry bleaches that contain sodium hypochlorite.[160]

Assessment

The immediate response to ingestion is increased secretions, pain, vomiting or haemoptysis. Signs of perforation include fever, respiratory difficulty or peritonitis. Approximately 98% of patients develop strictures.[160] Alkalis and skin contact produce a soap-like substance because of the interaction with tissue fats, giving a slimy, soapy feeling.[160]

Management

Induced vomiting or gastric lavage should not be attempted for ingested alkalis, as these will be neutralised by stomach acid. Lavage tubes may cause further tissue damage.[160] External contact with alkalis necessitates copious irrigation of the point of contact. Continue irrigation for at least 15 minutes; in the case of the eye, irrigation may be necessary for up to 30 minutes. Cover all wounds after irrigation with sterile dressings to reduce the risk of infection.

A patient should be nil by mouth until an inspection of the mouth and throat is conducted to determine the amount and extent of burns. Consultation with a toxicologist will help drive management of ingested chemicals and so should be given priority.

Petroleum distillates

Petroleum distillates are common substances. Typical petroleum products are benzene, fuel oils, petrol, kerosene, lacquer diluents, lubricating oil, mineral oil, naphthalene, paint thinners and petroleum spirits. Toxicity depends on route of exposure (ingestion or aspiration), volatility (ease with which the substance evaporates), viscosity (density or thickness), amount ingested and presence of other toxins.[161]

Products with a low viscosity are more likely to be aspirated and can quickly spread over the lung surface. Substances with low viscosity and high volatility – for example, benzene, kerosene and turpentine – are toxic even in low doses and death can be sudden, particularly for intentional inhalants.[161] Mortality is increased if an additional toxic substance is present, or if accidental aspiration occurs.[161]

Assessment

Aspiration causes pneumonitis with low-grade fever, tachypnoea, coughing, choking, gagging and pulmonary oedema as a late effect.[161] As petroleum distillates are fat solvents and rapidly cross the lipid-rich cell membrane, nerve tissue is especially sensitive to injury. A patient may exhibit local effects, such as depressed nerve conduction, or varied central effects, such as feelings of well-being, headache, tinnitus, dizziness, visual disturbances, through to respiratory depression, altered levels of consciousness, convulsions and coma.[137,161]

Management

In the awake and alert patient, the decision to treat is based on the physical properties of the substance, the likelihood of aspiration or other complications and the amount consumed.[137,161] When preventing absorption, careful consideration needs to be given to gastric emptying, as induced vomiting or gastric lavage should be avoided.

The patient's respiratory status should be immediately assessed for possible aspiration. A patient who is coughing, has cyanosis or appears hypoxic may have aspirated or developed chemical pneumonitis.[161] If the patient is lethargic or unconscious, an endotracheal tube must be placed for adequate airway protection, although this heightens the risk of aspiration as hydrocarbons adhere to the tube and increase the risk of chemical pneumonitis.[137]

Organophosphates

Organophosphates are a large and diverse group of chemicals used in domestic, industrial and agricultural settings (e.g. insecticides, herbicides).[162] The primary effect of organophosphates is binding and inactivation of acetylcholinesterase, a neurotransmitter that metabolises acetylcholine.[162]

Organophosphates can be absorbed through the skin, ingested or inhaled. Although most patients become symptomatic soon after ingestion, the onset and duration of action depend on the nature and type of compound, the degree and route of exposure, the mode of action of the compound, its lipid solubility and rate of metabolic degradation.[162]

Mortality from intentional ingestion of organophosphates causing poisoning accounts for 30% of deaths from successful suicides globally.[163] While intentional deaths using pesticides (in particular organophosphates) are rare now because of governmental control and restriction of these formulations, herbicide exposure is still fairly common and more particularly in agricultural areas.[163] Common complications include respiratory distress, seizures and aspiration pneumonia, with respiratory failure the commonest cause of death.[162]

Assessment, monitoring and diagnostics

The clinical findings of organophosphate poisoning can be divided into three broad categories: muscarinic effects, nicotinic effects and effects on the CNS.[162] Common

TABLE 23.14

Types of paralysis that may result from organophosphate poisoning[163–165]

TYPE	ONSET	PRESENTATION	DURATION OF SYMPTOMS
Type 1	Occurs shortly after exposure.	Acute paralysis secondary to persistent depolarisation at the neuromuscular junction.	
Type 2	24–96 h after resolution of acute cholinergic poisoning.	Paralysis and respiratory distress. Proximal muscle groups are involved, with relative sparing of distal muscle groups.	Up to 3 weeks
Type 3	2–3 weeks after exposure to large doses of certain organophosphates.	Distal muscle weakness with relative sparing of the neck muscles, cranial nerves and proximal muscle groups.	Up to 12 months

muscarinic manifestations are summarised by the mnemonic SLUDGE: **S**alivation, **L**acrimation, **U**rination, **D**efecation, **G**I upset, **E**mesis.[164,165] Other symptoms include bradycardia, hypotension, bronchospasm, cough, abdominal pain, blurred vision, miosis and sweating. Nicotinic effects include muscle fasciculations, cramping, weakness and diaphragmatic failure. Autonomic effects include hypertension, tachycardia, pupillary dilation and pallor.

CNS effects include anxiety, restlessness, confusion, ataxia, seizures, insomnia, dysarthria, tremors, coma and paralysis. The three types of paralysis that may result from organophosphate poisoning are described in Table 23.14.[163–165]

Laboratory diagnosis is based on the measurement of cholinesterase activity using either erythrocyte or plasma levels; erythrocyte cholinesterase is more accurate, but plasma cholinesterase is easier to test and is more widely available. Erythrocyte acetylcholinesterase is found in the grey matter of the CNS, red blood cells, peripheral nerve and muscle. Plasma cholinesterase circulates in plasma and is found in the white matter of the CNS, pancreas and heart.[164,165]

Management

Initial priorities in managing organophosphate poisoning are airway, breathing and circulation, incorporating D for danger, as organophosphates also present considerable risk to staff caring for the patient, especially during the initial phases of management. All of the patient's clothing should be removed and considered as hazardous waste. The patient's decontamination with soap and water is a priority, as soap with a high pH breaks down organophosphates.[162,165] Staff must use personal protective equipment, such as neoprene or nitrile gloves, and gowns are worn when decontaminating patients. Charcoal cartridge masks for respiratory protection may be useful, although evidence suggests that the nosocomial risk to staff may not be as significant as was once thought and basic universal precautions may be sufficient.[162] Intubation is commonly required after significant exposure, owing to

respiratory distress from laryngospasm, bronchospasm or severe bronchorrhoea. Continuous cardiac monitoring and an ECG are used to check for bradycardias. Activated charcoal is used for gastric decontamination for those patients who have ingested organophosphate. The mainstay of treatment is atropine and pralidoxime, with a benzodiazepine used for seizure control.[162] Atropine blocks acetylcholine receptors and halts the cholinergic stimulation. Very large doses of atropine are usually required, 1–2 g IV, which are repeated if muscle weakness is not relieved or the signs of poisoning recur. Clearing of bronchial secretions is the endpoint of atropine administration, not pupil size nor the absolute dose.[165] Pralidoxime hydrochloride reactivates acetylcholinesterase and is effective at restoring skeletal muscle function but is less effective at reversing muscarinic signs. Over time, the bond between organophosphate and cholinesterase becomes permanent and the effectiveness of pralidoxime diminishes.[165] Benzodiazepines are clinically indicated through their binding to specific receptor sites, potentiating the effects of gamma-aminobutyrate and facilitating inhibitory transmitters for management of seizures.[145]

Envenomation

Venomous animals can be land based or marine based, and their distribution ranges from broad to very specific locations. Exposure of humans to venom produces a large and varied range of symptomatology, which often results in an emergency presentation.[156] It is, therefore, important for critical care nurses to be familiar with the types of potentially venomous animals inhabiting the catchment area of their health setting. From a first aid perspective, it is vital that nurses are familiar with the presentation and management of specific life-threatening or injury-causing envenomation, including the use of antivenom when one exists. Most countries have local poison information centres for advice from expert toxicologists (see Online resources). Common envenomations across Australia and New Zealand are described below.

Redback/katipo spider bite

Description and incidence

The redback spider (*Latrodectus hasseltii*) is found throughout Australia but more commonly in temperate regions. Tasmania has the lowest frequency of reported bites, whereas areas around southern New South Wales to southern Queensland produce significant numbers of bites and envenomations.[166] The redback spider is easily identifiable by the presence of a red, orange or brownish stripe on its characteristic black, globular abdomen. The female is much larger than the male; generally, only the female is considered dangerous. Juveniles are smaller, more variably coloured and may lack any spots or stripes. Bites from both male and juvenile spiders may result in symptoms, although these tend to be less significant than bites from females.[166]

The redback spider has also become established outside Australia, including in New Zealand.[166] Although bites are rare, small populations of redback spiders have been reported in New Zealand in Central Otago (South Island) and New Plymouth (North Island) since the early 1980s.[167] The only other venomous spider in New Zealand is the katipo (*Latrodectus katipo*) from the same genus as the redback. The katipo has a black, rounded body, slender legs and a red stripe on the abdomen. Symptoms of katipo spider bite are similar to those of the redback spider and, where indicated, redback antivenom is used to treat bites.[166]

A redback spider bite is a frequent cause for ED presentations and the most clinically significant spider bite in Australia.[168] Most bites are minor, with either minimal or no symptoms and requiring no antivenom. In approximately 20% of cases, significant envenomation occurs and antivenom administration is generally indicated, although death is extremely unlikely in untreated cases. Redback antivenom is no longer recommended for use in Australia; however, some controversy exists about this recommendation in paediatric patients.[169,170]

Clinical manifestations

Envenomation by a redback spider is known as latrodectism; the venom contains excitatory neurotoxins that stimulate release of catecholamines from sympathetic nerves and acetylcholine from motor nerve endings.[166] Signs and symptoms associated with a significant envenomation are distinctive, and diagnosis is by clinical findings. Initially, there is a minor sting at the bite site, where the spider may or may not have been seen. Over the first hour, the bite becomes progressively painful to severe, spreading proximally with and involving swollen and tender local lymph nodes. Localised sweating at the bite site or limb or generalised sweating may appear, associated with hypertension and malaise. Pain eventually becomes generalised and may be expressed as chest, abdominal, head or neck pain suggestive of other acute conditions such as myocardial infarction.[166]

Progression of symptoms generally occurs in less than 6 hours but may take up to 24 hours. People with minor untreated bites may experience symptoms for several weeks.[166] Other less common signs and symptoms include local piloerection, nausea, vomiting, headache, fever, restlessness/insomnia, tachycardia and neurological symptoms such as muscle weakness or twitching.[166]

Assessment

Patients presenting with pain from a bite who have the offending spider with them are straightforward in terms of initial assessment. Identification of the spider is confirmed, and a history of the event obtained, including the time of the bite and any first aid initiated. A brief assessment of the bite site and the involved limb is undertaken, including the extent of pain, presence of sweating and painful tender lymph nodes, and a baseline set of vital signs. Patients are then placed in a suitable area for medical assessment and ongoing observation.[166]

Adult patients presenting with vague limb pain, or preverbal children who are 'distressed' and 'cannot be settled', may be unaware that they have been bitten by a redback. The pain may not have been felt at the time of the bite and no spider may have been seen. Thorough history taking, physical assessment and knowledge of the effects of latrodectism enable detection of a suspected spider bite.[166]

Management

There is no recommended definitive first aid for a redback spider bite. Application of cold packs to the bite site and administration of simple analgesia, such as paracetamol, may assist with local pain relief. The use of a pressure immobilisation bandage is not necessary, as symptom progression is slow and not life threatening, and will cause further pain only in the affected limb. Remove any pressure bandage that was applied during first aid after identification of the spider is confirmed.[166]

Administration of redback antivenom is no longer recommended (even though it is still available, controversy about this continues); however, pain should be treated with simple analgesics first and proceeding to opioid analgesia if required.[166] Opioid analgesia may not always control pain; however, further research is being undertaken to investigate pain control options for these patients.[166]

Practice tip

Observations for the development or progression of symptoms of a redback envenomation focus on development of local pain that spreads proximally and increases in intensity, development of sweating (either local or generalised) and hypertension.

Funnel-web spider bite

Description and incidence

Funnel-web spiders are the most venomous spiders to humans worldwide, and Australian funnel-web spiders

(*Atrax* or *Hadronyche* genera) are found primarily along the east coast. The Sydney funnel-web spider (*Atrax robustus*) is found mainly around Sydney, while other species are found in eastern New South Wales and central and southern Queensland. The spider is large, black or dark brown and approximately 3 cm long in the body. Male spiders have smaller bodies and are significantly more toxic than females.[166]

Clinical manifestations

Funnel-web spider bites are potentially rapidly lethal; however, only 10–20% of bites result in systemic envenomation, with the majority being minor and not requiring antivenom.[171] The bite is extremely painful, and fang marks are likely to be seen. Signs and symptoms of systemic envenomation may appear within 10–30 minutes, and include perioral tingling and tongue fasciculation, increased salivation, lacrimation; piloerection, sweating; nausea, vomiting, headache; hypertension, tachycardia; dyspnoea, pulmonary oedema; irritability; and decreased consciousness and coma.[171] Regardless of the presence of symptoms, all possible funnel-web spider bites are managed as a medical emergency.[156]

Assessment

Patients with suspected funnel-web spider bites are rapidly assessed for the presence of any signs and symptoms of envenomation and allocated an ATS triage category of 1–3, based on presenting symptoms. A pressure immobilisation bandage is applied if this was not done during initial first aid.[166] Patients with signs of envenomation are moved to a resuscitation area for immediate treatment, including urgent antivenom administration and management of the clinical effects of envenomation. Monitoring and assessment for potentially serious manifestations focus on:

- airway compromise due to decreased level of consciousness, requiring airway protection with an airway adjunct or endotracheal intubation
- breathing for respiratory compromise due to pulmonary oedema, requiring continuous positive airway pressure or intubation/ventilation with positive end-expiratory pressure (see Chapter 15)
- circulatory compromise due to profound hypotension, although a late sign with hypertension more commonly seen, requires IV access and volume replacement. Circulatory compromise/failure may lead to cardiac arrest requiring cardiopulmonary resuscitation (see Chapter 25).

All patients require full monitoring with constant one-to-one observation. A patient with no signs of envenomation on arrival has a detailed history taken regarding the circumstances of the bite, the time of bite, a description of the spider and any first aid undertaken. The patient is then regularly assessed for any symptoms suggesting systemic envenomation. After thorough medical assessment, if there are no signs of systemic envenomation, any first aid such as a pressure immobilisation bandage is removed, and the patient observed for 6 hours. With no diagnostic test for funnel-web spider envenomation and no venom detection procedure available, clinical diagnosis is based on the history and symptoms.[166]

Management

For signs of systemic envenomation, two vials of funnel-web spider antivenom are administered slowly IV over 15–20 mintes.[156,166] Premedication is not required, although the patient is observed closely for anaphylaxis.[156] More antivenom after 15–30 minutes may be required until all major symptoms have resolved.[166] The antivenom dose for children is the same as the adult dose.[156] First aid measures such as a pressure immobilisation bandage can be removed after antivenom administration and the symptoms have stabilised; this may take several hours.[166] Serum sickness from antivenom should be monitored for up to 14 days after administration.[156,166]

Snake bites

Worldwide there are a variety of snakes that have the capacity to envenomate humans and cause life-threatening clinical features; broadly, these snakes fall into three groups: elapids, pit vipers and cobras. Australia has elapids (front-fanged), and have significance for medical care, New Zealand has no snakes requiring medical intervention when in contact with humans.[172] This section will focus on the life-threatening Australasian elapid species.

Description and incidence

Australasia is inhabited by many snakes (over 140 recognised snakes from 30 different species, 25% of all known venomous snakes, and 40% of all dangerous front-fanged snakes or elapids).[173] New Zealand has no known venomous terrestrial snakes.[172] Australian venomous snakes are found in both rural areas and residential and metropolitan areas, especially when in close proximity to bushland and in periods of drought. Snake bite envenoming constituted 15% of admissions in Australian hospitals between 2000 and 2013.[174] Mortality rates associated with those hospitalised with snake venom were twice as high as those associated with other envenomations (e.g. arthropod envenomation).[174] Despite this, Australia has very few poor outcomes associated with snakebite compared with other countries, and this is related to our advanced treatment (antivenom development, research and detection abilities), accessibility to treatment and education about snakes and envenomation.[175]

Clinical manifestations

The majority of snake bites do not result in significant envenomation.[173] Bites are generally recognised by the patient at the time because of associated pain, although some bites are unrecognised. The bite site may show minimal to obvious signs of punctures or scratches, with accompanying swelling and bruising. Multiple bites are

TABLE 23.15

Characteristics and clinical manifestations of snake venom[173,177,178]

TOXIN	EFFECTS	SIGNS AND SYMPTOMS
Neurotoxin	Blocks transmission at the neuromuscular junctions, causing skeletal and respiratory muscle flaccid paralysis, presynaptic and/or postsynaptic.	Ptosis (drooping of upper eyelids) Diplopia (double vision) Ophthalmoplegia (partial or complete paralysis of eye movements) Fixed, dilated pupils Muscle weakness Respiratory weakness, paralysis
Haemotoxin	Causes coagulopathies, resulting in either: defibrination with low-fibrinogen, unclottable blood, but usually with a normal platelet count *or* direct anticoagulation with normal fibrinogen and platelet count. Both cause an elevated prothrombin ratio and international normalised ratio.	Bleeding from bite wounds Bleeding at venipuncture sites Haematuria
Myotoxin	Causes myolysis, resulting in generalised destruction of skeletal muscles with high serum creatine kinase and leading to myoglobinuria and occasionally severe hyperkalaemia.	Muscle weakness Muscle pain on movement Red or brown urine, which tests positively to blood

possible and are generally associated with major envenomation. Australian snake venoms contain various toxins that are responsible for the systemic effects (Table 23.15).[173,176,177,178] Renal damage may occur as a consequence of myoglobinuria from severe rhabdomyolysis or haemoglobinuria associated with coagulopathies, leading to acute renal failure (see Chapter 18).[176]

Assessment

Patients presenting with snake bite(s) are allocated a high priority for assessment and treatment even if they appear well on arrival. Patients who present without effective first aid measures (the application of a pressure immobilisation bandage and splint) have these applied immediately.[156,172] The pressure immobilisation bandage is applied with a broad (15-cm) bandage, commencing over the bite site with the same pressure that would be used for a sprained ankle. The bandage is then extended to cover the whole limb, including fingers/toes, and the limb is splinted and immobilised.[156] Correct application of the pressure bandage is important, as any benefit is lost with bandages that are too loose, not applied to the whole limb or with no splinting or immobilisation.[156] Elasticised bandages are superior to crepe bandages in obtaining and maintaining adequate pressure. Do not wash the wound prior to applying the pressure immobilisation bandage, as swabbing of the bite site is used when performing venom detection.[156] The patient should not mobilise in order to minimise distribution of any injected venom. Once applied, the pressure immobilisation bandage is not

removed until the patient is in a healthcare location that is stocked with antivenom.[156,172]

> **Practice tip**
>
> Pressure immobilisation may be contraindicated or ineffective in bites from exotic snake species (e.g. vipers and some cobras). Many of these non-Australasian species of snake have venoms that cause local tissue destruction. Pit vipers and cobras can both cause extensive localised tissue damage and therefore pressure immobilisation can make this worse. Immobilisation is the mainstay of first aid.[179]

A brief and focused history explores the time and circumstances of the bite, a description of the snake (colour, length), geographical location and the application of any first aid. The patient is assessed for general symptoms including headache, nausea, vomiting, abdominal pain, collapse, convulsions and anxiety, although these alone do not indicate envenomation.[172] Additional signs and symptoms include blurred or double vision, slurred speech, muscle weakness, respiratory distress, bleeding from the bite site or elsewhere, and pain and swelling at the bite site and associated lymph nodes.[172]

Patients with suspected snake bite are located in an acute area with full monitoring available, with symptomatic patients placed in a resuscitation area. The patient requires insertion of IV access devices and collection of blood for pathology tests including full blood count, urea, electrolytes, creatine, creatinine kinase and full coagulation studies. Unnecessary venipunctures should be avoided, including sites where it may be difficult to control bleeding should it occur. Healthcare settings without ready access to pathology services may need to perform whole blood clotting time testing at the bedside to assess for any coagulopathy; however, point-of-care testing is not accurate in these cases and therefore, where possible, the patient should be retrieved to the nearest centre for testing as soon as possible.[156,172]

All probable snake bites require observation for at least 12 hours, as some serious symptoms may be delayed.[172] Patients should be assessed for tachycardia, hypotension or hypertension, and falling oxygen saturation, altered respiratory rate, forced vital capacity or peak expiratory flow rate, indicating respiratory muscle paralysis. Frequent neurological observations focus on identification of muscle weakness and paralysis; clinicians should note any ptosis, diplopia, dysphagia, slurred speech, limb weakness or altered levels of consciousness. An indwelling catheter should be inserted for close monitoring of urine output and presence of any myoglobin in urine.[172]

In the past a bedside snake venom detection kit has been used at the bite site or with a urine sample to determine the type of snake; however, this is no longer routinely recommended, and all patients who are showing signs of envenomation should be treated for such with either polyvalent or geography-indicated antivenom, without waiting for test results.[156,172] If the patient is not showing signs of envenomation, a swab is taken of the bite site. A swab of the washings from the bite area is collected by leaving the pressure immobilisation bandage on and creating a window over the bite site to expose the bitten area. Additional to swabs, blood tests checking for changes to clotting times should also be taken.[156,172] Point-of-care testing should not be used to determine changes to clotting times as they are not reliable in relation to snake envenomation (e.g. ISTAT testing).[156]

Practice tip

Whole blood clotting time is performed by drawing 1 mL venous blood and placing it in a glass test tube. If the blood has not clotted within 20 minutes, a coagulopathy is likely to exist, suggesting envenomation; however, this test still can fail to identify 20% of cases likely to require antivenom.[180]

In patients with known snake bite and systemic envenomation, antivenom administration is required if there is any degree of paralysis, significant coagulopathy, any myolysis (myoglobinuria or creatinine kinase >500 micrograms per litre), unconsciousness and/or convulsions.[172] In an asymptomatic patient with normal pathology and a negative laboratory test, it is likely that envenomation has not occurred. In this case, the pressure immobilisation

bandage can be removed under close observation in a resuscitation area (but only in a hospital with laboratory testing ability).[156] The patient is fully re-evaluated including repeat blood tests, assessing coagulation parameters, within 1–2 hours after removal of the pressure bandage. If the patient's condition remains unchanged, further observation and repeat blood tests at 6 and 12 hours are required. Patients with no evidence of envenomation after 12 hours may be discharged.[172]

Management

A patient with evidence of systemic envenomation requires antivenom administration; monovalent antivenom is used in preference to polyvalent antivenom when the identity of the snake species is known. Polyvalent antivenom is a mixture of all monovalent antivenoms, and is therefore used for severe envenomation where the identity of the snake is unknown and the patient's condition does not allow time for a snake venom detection kit result, or where there is insufficient monovalent antivenom available.[172] Expert advice from a poison information centre may assist in identifying the snake, based on known habitats and distribution as well as presenting symptoms. Antivenom is always administered IV in a diluted strength of 1:10 (or less if volume is a concern) via an infusion. Administration is commenced slowly while observing for signs of any adverse reaction. The infusion rate can be increased if no reaction occurs, with the whole initial dose administered over 15–20 minutes. The dose will vary depending on the type of antivenom, type of snake and number of bites; while current recommendations is to use only one vial of antivenom ever,[172] controversy about this is present because of two deaths in 2015 and 2016 where higher doses of antivenom might have impacted on patient outcomes.[181] Therefore, some guidelines start with use of one vial and then advise that more may be given depending on the clinical situation.[156] Use of premedication before antivenom administration is controversial; at present the antivenom manufacturer does not recommend any premedication to reduce the chance of anaphylaxis. However, what is agreed on is that clinicians should be prepared to treat anaphylaxis, with adrenaline at the ready.[156,172]

When the patient's condition has stabilised after the initial dose of antivenom, the pressure immobilisation bandage is removed, with continuous close observation for any clinical deterioration caused by the release of venom contained by the pressure bandage. If deterioration is evident, treatment by a clinical toxicologist and in critical care settings is required.[172] Patients without signs of deterioration still require ongoing observation in a high-dependency unit/intensive care unit and repeat testing of coagulation at 6, 12 and 24 hours after antivenom administration. Ongoing observation and pathology studies should occur for at least 24 hours.[172]

In children, management for snake bite is similar, with antivenom dosages the same as for an adult. Dilution volume can be reduced (from 500 mL to 250 mL) for children or those at risk of fluid overload.[156]

Box jellyfish envenomation

Chironex fleckeri (box jellyfish) is one of the world's most dangerous venomous animals.[182] The jellyfish is a cubic (box-shaped) bell measuring 20–30 cm across and weighing up to 6 kg and, as it is transparent in water, it can be difficult to identify. The tentacles are covered with millions of stinging nematocysts, each a spring-loaded capsule that contains a penetrating thread that discharges venom. Threads are 1 mm in length and capable of penetrating the dermis of adult skin. The tentacles also produce a sticky substance that promotes adherence to a victim's skin, causing some tentacles to be torn off and remain attached to the person, where the nematocysts remain active.[183]

Description and incidence

Most stings occur during the summer months (December, January) in the tropical waters of northern Australia, from Gladstone in Queensland around to Broome in Western Australia, on hot, calm and overcast days when the jellyfish moves from the open sea to chase prey in shallow water. The exact incidence of stings is difficult to determine, but they are common in children, with recent deaths occurring in children from rural or remote areas of Australia.[184,185] There have been more than 80 confirmed deaths from envenomation by *Chironex fleckeri* in Australia,[186] of which the last 12 were children.[178]

Clinical manifestations

Most stings are minor, with clinically significant stings occurring from larger jellyfish. Stings generally occur on the lower half of the body and are characterised by immediate and severe pain. Pain increases in severity and may cause victims, especially children, to become incoherent. While mechanisms of toxicity remain poorly understood, death is thought to occur from central respiratory failure, or cardiotoxicity leading to atrioventricular conduction disturbances or paralysis of cardiac muscle.[178]

Multiple linear lesions, which characteristically appear in a cross-hatched pattern, are seen on the area where tentacle contact occurs. A pattern of transverse bars is usually seen along the lesions, along with an intense acute inflammatory response, initially as a prompt and massive appearance of wheals, followed by oedema, erythema and vesicle formation, which can lead to partial- or full-thickness skin death.[178,183]

Assessment

Patients presenting to ED after potential box jellyfish sting are easily diagnosed based on the history, the presence of pain and their skin lesions as outlined above. Generally, some form of pre-hospital management or first aid will have been instituted. On arrival, patients with signs of clinically significant stings, alteration in consciousness, cardiovascular or respiratory function, or those with severe pain are seen immediately.

Management

Treatment focuses on appropriate first aid, administration of adequate pain relief, symptomatic management of cardiovascular and respiratory effects and the administration of box jellyfish antivenom when indicated. While the Australian Resuscitation Council recommends that first aid measures include liberal application of vinegar to the sting area for 30–60 seconds, this is being questioned by researchers as not being well evidenced,[183] and although some treatment focuses include heat or ice application,[156] researchers question this as there is no evidence to support the application of ice. Vinegar has been thought to inactivate the undischarged nematocysts, and is still recommended so removal of any remaining tentacles should occur prior to vinegar to prevent further envenomation.[156] However, some emerging research contradicts this belief, although this is not conclusive yet.[183] Clinical practice for mild stings includes application of ice packs and simple oral analgesia, after the application of vinegar. Patients with moderate-to-severe pain require IV narcotic analgesia. For patients with continuing severe pain, antivenom is administered along with continued parenteral analgesia.[156,183]

Patients are observed for the development of cardiorespiratory symptoms, including arrhythmias. Management focuses on specific clinical effects, ranging from oxygen administration and IV fluid resuscitation through to intubation/mechanical ventilation or cardiopulmonary resuscitation.[156] Antivenom is indicated in patients with cardiorespiratory instability, cardiac arrest or severe pain unrelieved by narcotic analgesia. Antivenom is carried by pre-hospital personnel, and administration may occur prior to ED presentation. A 20,000-unit ampoule of box jellyfish antivenom is diluted in 100 mL normal saline or Hartmann's solution[183] and administered IV, starting slowly but then, if there are no concerns, increasing the rate to administer over 5–10 minutes.[156] The number of ampoules used varies with clinical status: at least one for cardiorespiratory instability and up to six for a cardiac arrest.[183]

Pressure immobilisation bandage application is not recommended.[183] Some research has suggested an adjunct role for magnesium sulfate (0.2 mmol/kg up to 10 mmol, over 15 minutes IV) in management for patients not responding to antivenom.[183]

Irukandji envenomation

The Irukandji is a small marine jellyfish, with stinging tentacles capable of causing intense pain and catecholamine release.[187]

Description and incidence

Irukandji syndrome has an incidence of continuing research and is caused by marine envenomation by the *Carukia Barnesi* jellyfish (Irukandji) encountered in far northern and northwestern areas of Australia. Death is uncommon and attributed to cerebral haemorrhage, and is associated with other comorbid conditions; however, Irukandji syndrome is a potentially life-threatening emergency and should be treated in a resuscitation environment.[156]

Assessment

People stung by an Irukandji may have no symptoms initially, and experience a latent time period, but may develop symptoms up to 1 hour after being stung.[183] Irukandji syndrome produces clinical features of severe lower back pain, chest pain, muscle cramps, blood pressure lability, tachycardia, shortness of breath, difficulty breathing, diaphoresis, restlessness, vomiting and anxiety.[156,183] A patient with suspected Irukandji envenomation is placed in an acute area with full monitoring available. In rural and remote environments, all should be transferred to a hospital with critical care capability.[156]

Management

The mainstays of patient management are pain control and symptom management. Application of vinegar has been part of first aid treatment but, due to delay in the presentation of symptoms following a sting, this may be of limited value. Evidence is emerging indicating that washing the area with either fresh or salt water may also be effective. Pain is severe, and large repeat doses of opioid analgesia may be required; if requirements for opioids are very high, fentanyl is considered.[183] There is anecdotal evidence that magnesium sulfate may have a role in the management of Irukandji syndrome not responsive to the above treatments, but this remains unproven, and clonidine is also being trialled with promising results.[183] For patients who are in a hypertensive crisis, glyceryl trinitrate is used, initially sublingually; however, an infusion may be required.[156]

Ciguatera

Ciguatera is a type of seafood poisoning caused by the consumption of fish, especially certain tropical reef fish, which contain one or more naturally occurring neurotoxins from the family of ciguatoxins. Ciguatera is reported as the most common form of seafood poisoning in the world, and is considered a mild non-fatal disease, affecting at least 50,000 people every year.[188] In Australia, there have been numerous outbreaks of ciguatera poisoning in many areas of the country including New South Wales.[189]

Ciguatera toxins (ciguatoxins) are among the deadliest poisons known.[190] These heat-stable toxins originate from a microorganism that attaches to certain species of algae in tropical areas around the world; these toxins become altered after ingestion by progressively larger fish up the food chain.[190]

Clinical manifestations and diagnosis

Ciguatera poisoning typically presents as an acute gastrointestinal illness, followed by a neurological illness with classical symptoms of heat and cold reversal of sensation that may last for a few days after consumption of contaminated fish,[188] but symptoms usually commence between 1 and 6 hours after ingestion[183] (Table 23.16).[190]

A patient may become sensitive to repeated exposure to ciguatoxins; additional exposure to poisoning from ciguatera may be more severe than the first episode. Importantly, patients exposed to ciguatera suffer recurrences following the consumption of seemingly innocuous foods (e.g. nuts, nut oils, caffeine, alcohol or animal protein foods), with relapses months or years after the initial poisoning.[190]

Diagnosis is made on a patient's history and clinical features: consumption of fish followed by an acute gastrointestinal and neurological illness. There is no conclusive diagnostic test for the presence of ciguatoxins.[190]

TABLE 23.16
Symptoms of ciguatera[190]

GASTROINTESTINAL	NEUROLOGICAL	CARDIOVASCULAR	OTHER SYMPTOMS
Abdominal pain	Paraesthesia in extremities and around the mouth, tingling, burning and pain	Bradycardia	Dermatitis
Nausea		Tachycardia	Rash
Vomiting		Hypotension	Arthralgia and myalgia
Diarrhoea	Painful extremities	Hypertension	General weakness
	Paradoxical temperature reversal where hot feels cold and cold feels hot	Arrhythmia	Salivation
	Temperature sensitivity		Dyspnoea
	Vertigo		Neck stiffness
	Dental pain where teeth feel loose		Headache
	Blurred vision		Ataxia
	Tremor		Sweating
			Metallic taste in the mouth

Management

Treatment of ciguatera poisoning is supportive care and symptom management. Mannitol is no longer recommended; therefore, IV fluids and analgesics are the mainstay of treatment, and avoidance of alcohol, which is known to exacerbate symptoms, is recommended.[156,183]

Scombroid fish poisoning

Scombroid poisoning is a form of food poisoning caused by the combination of inadequately cooled fish and the bacterial decomposition of the fish flesh resulting in a release of histamine.[183] The active component of scombrotoxin is histamine. The main groups of fish associated with this type of poisoning are the Scombridae – that is, tuna and mackerel; however, other fish such as mahi-mahi have also been known to have illness-causing potential. Scombrotoxin is not affected by the cooking process, and therefore cooked fish with scombrotoxin can still cause posioning.[191]

Clinical manifestations and diagnosis

People normally start feeling unwell about 30 minutes after eating fish affected with scombrotoxin, with flushing, development of a rash and urticaria.[183] This may be followed by more profound symptoms such as tachycardia, pounding headaches, difficulty breathing and collapse due to hypotension.[192]

Management

Patients must be managed as per anaphylactoid reactions,[183] which if not managed can lead to death. The mainstays of treatment are controlling the histamine reaction with antihistamines and supportive nursing care for symptoms. Histamine-2 receptor blockers have been shown to be useful for up to 24 hours following the development of symptoms.[183,193] This prolonged treatment allows the scombrotoxin to be eliminated from the patient's system. In rare cases, if symptoms are severe and resistant to antihistamines, drugs such as intramuscular adrenaline and low-dose pressors may play a role in management.[193]

Drowning

Description and incidence

Drowning is the process of experiencing respiratory impairment due to submersion or immersion in a liquid. Non-fatal drowning is generally defined as survival, at least temporarily, after suffocation by submersion in a liquid medium. Near-drowning is now an obsolete term.[194,195] Submersion incidents are often preventable events associated with significant mortality and morbidity in both adults and children, usually necessitating an ED presentation and subsequent hospital admission. Drowning is the third leading cause of accidental death worldwide, and accounts for up to 7% of all injury-related deaths.[196] Worldwide, there are an estimated 236,000 drowning deaths annually, with children, males and those with increased access to water most at risk.[196] Over half of the world's drowning occurs in the Western Pacific region, and is 27 to 32 times higher than rates seen in European countries.[196] The location of drowning varies from country to country. In the USA, artificial pools and natural bodies of freshwater were common drowning locations, particularly for children.[197] In Australia, drowning often occurs in rivers and creeks (26%), at the beach (22%) or in the ocean (15%).[198] A bimodal distribution of deaths is seen in children, with a peak in the toddler age group (0–4 years) and a second peak in young adult males (20–24 years).[199]

It is estimated that, for every drowning death, there are 4–5 non-fatal drowning hospital admissions and 14 ED presentations.[200,201] Non-fatal drowning is also associated with high-impact injuries, especially boating or personal watercraft incidents and shallow-diving-related injuries. While cervical spinal cord injury is uncommon in non-fatal drowning (0.5%), assessment for signs of injury and consideration of mechanism should be included.[202]

Clinical manifestations

The sequence of events in drowning has been identified primarily by animal studies, highlighting an initial phase of panic struggling, some swimming movements and sometimes a surprise inhalation. There may be aspiration of small amounts of water at this time that produces laryngospasm for a short period. Apnoea and breath holding occur during submersion and are often followed by variable amount of aspiration of fluid, followed by apnoea. This leads to severe hypoxia, loss of consciousness and disappearance of airway reflexes, resulting in further water moving into the lungs prior to death.[195]

Approximately 80–90% of submersion victims aspirate water into the lungs because of loss of airway reflexes and laryngospasm. Approximately 10–15% of victims have sustained laryngospasm, and no detectable amount of water will be aspirated, with the resulting injury secondary to anoxia. The terms 'dry' and 'wet' drowning were discarded at the World Congress on Drowning.[203] Pre-existing medical conditions predisposing a person to drowning which should be considered during management include seizures, arrhythmia (especially torsades de pointes associated with long Q–T interval), coronary artery disease, depression, cardiomyopathy (dilated or hypertrophic obstructive), hypoglycaemia, hypothermia, intoxication and trauma.[195]

Pulmonary manifestations after aspiration of fresh or salt water differ, as fresh water is hypotonic and when aspirated moves quickly into the microcirculation across the alveolar–capillary membrane. With freshwater aspiration, surfactant is destroyed, producing alveolar instability, atelectasis and decreased lung compliance and resulting in marked ventilation/perfusion mismatching.[195] In contrast, salt water has 3–4 times the osmolality of blood and, when aspirated, draws damaging protein-rich fluid from the plasma into the alveoli, resulting in both interstitial and alveoli oedema, with associated

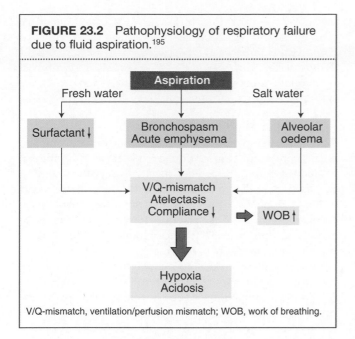

FIGURE 23.2 Pathophysiology of respiratory failure due to fluid aspiration.[195]

V/Q-mismatch, ventilation/perfusion mismatch; WOB, work of breathing.

bronchospasm and subsequent shunting and ventilation/perfusion mismatch.[202]

Despite these different physiological effects from aspirated fresh and salt water, the resulting clinical manifestation is the same: profound hypoxaemia secondary to ventilation/perfusion mismatch with intrapulmonary shunting (Fig. 23.2).[195] Patients with evidence of fluid aspiration often progress to develop severe acute respiratory distress syndrome within a very short time.[203] No significant effects on electrolytes are noted in humans, as rarely more than 10 mL/kg and commonly no more than 4 mL/kg of water are aspirated, while clinically significant electrolyte disturbances occur when over 22 mL/kg have been aspirated.[204]

Cardiovascular effects are influenced by the extent and duration of hypoxia, derangement of acid–base status, the magnitude of the stress response and hypothermia.[195] Ventricular arrhythmias and asystole may result from hypoxaemia and metabolic acidosis. Acute hypoxia results in release of pulmonary inflammatory mediators, which increase right ventricular afterload and decrease contractility.[204] Hypotension is commonly seen resulting from volume depletion secondary to pulmonary oedema, intracompartmental fluid shifts and myocardial dysfunction.[203]

Severe hypoxic and ischaemic injury is the most important factor related to outcome and subsequent quality of life. Other factors influencing the extent of injury include water temperature and submersion time, stress during submersion and coexisting cardiovascular and neurological disease.[205] Prediction of death · or persistent vegetative state in the immediate period after non-fatal drowning varies widely. Patients awake or with only blunted consciousness on presentation usually survive without neurological sequelae. A third of patients admitted in coma or after cardiopulmonary resuscitation will survive neurologically intact or with only minor deficits, while the remaining two-thirds of patients will either die or remain in a vegetative state.[195]

Hypothermia is a well-documented feature in submersion victims.[205] Incidents of submersion times of greater than 15 minutes where victims recovered with a good neurological outcome all occurred in very cold water (<10°C). While the exact mechanisms in these outcomes are unclear, acute cold submersion hypothermia may be protective against cerebral insult by: very rapid cooling in victims with low levels of subcutaneous fat who have aspirated a large amount of very cold water, induced muscle paralysis leading to minimal struggling and very little oxygen depletion, and the heart gradually slowing to asystole in the presence of profound hypothermia.[202,205] In these cases, prolonged resuscitative efforts may be warranted, including active and aggressive rewarming interventions, which should not be abandoned until the patient has been rewarmed to at least 32°C.[195]

Assessment

Continuously monitor heart rate, blood pressure and oxygen saturation, and assess neurological status, including any seizure activity. Deterioration is evident with a falling level of consciousness, a high alveolar–arterial gradient, respiratory failure evidenced by a partial pressure of carbon dioxide in the arterial blood >45 mmHg or worsening blood gas results.[203] Caution should be taken to avoid activities that may cause a rise in intracranial pressure. A 12-lead ECG identifies any arrhythmias that result from acidosis and hypoxia rather than electrolyte abnormalities. The patient should be managed conventionally (see Chapter 11).[202] All patients require serial CXR, as lung fields often worsen in the first few hours. In clinically significant submersions, the CXR will typically show bilateral infiltrates undifferentiated from other causes of pulmonary oedema.

Management

The condition of the patient, the environment and the skill of the attending rescue personnel will influence pre-hospital management of the post-submersion patient, and the adequacy of initial basic life support at the scene is the most important determinant of outcome.[202] A Heimlich manoeuvre should not be performed in an attempt to remove aspirated water, as it is ineffective and likely to promote aspiration of gastric contents. Supplemental oxygen 100% is administered as soon as possible.[205]

For patients presenting to the ED in cardiac arrest, active resuscitation measures continue (see Chapter 25). Duration of submersion is potentially a better predictor of outcome, with less than 6 minutes showing the highest rate (88.2%) of survival, compared with water temperature.[206] The focus of management for patients with spontaneous circulation includes respiratory support and the correction of hypoxia, neurological assessment and maintenance of optimal cerebral perfusion, cardiovascular support and maintenance of haemodynamic stability, correction of hypothermia and management of other associated injuries.

All patients require 100% supplemental oxygen via a non-rebreathing mask initially, unless mechanical ventilation is required. Indications for endotracheal intubation include inability to maintain own airway, PaO_2 <60 mmHg or SpO_2 <90% despite high flow oxygen, PCO_2 >50 mmHg.[205] Patients without any respiratory symptoms should be observed for 6–12 hours, until there is a normal CXR, no signs of respiratory distress and normal oxygen saturation on room air.[195] Alert patients unable to maintain adequate oxygenation should be considered for continuous positive airway pressure or bilevel positive airway pressure prior to intubation provided they are able to maintain their own airway, with its effect on circulation monitored closely (see Chapter 15).

While cerebral oedema and intracranial hypertension is often seen in hypoxic neuronal injury, only general supportive measures are recommended as there is insufficient evidence to indicate that invasive intracranial pressure monitoring and related management improve outcomes.[195] Any seizures should be promptly treated with appropriate measures (see Chapter 17). Acute respiratory distress syndrome should be managed with non-invasive ventilation if possible.[205] Barbiturate-induced coma or corticosteroids is not recommended as there is no evidence of improvement in outcome.[205]

Cardiovascular support may require a multifaceted approach, initially by improving hypoxia and correcting circulating volume. Hypotensive patients require rapid volume expansion (crystalloid or colloid) and an indwelling catheter for hourly urine measurement. Patients with persistent cardiovascular compromise may require inotropic support in conjunction with invasive haemodynamic monitoring.[203]

Patients presenting with associated high-impact or shallow-diving mechanisms should have cervical spine immobilisation instituted with the application of a rigid cervical collar, especially for complaints of neck pain or an altered level of consciousness (see Chapter 17). The management of hypothermia and rewarming methods outlined below are appropriate for the management of non-fatal drowning.

Hypothermia

Description and incidence

Hypothermia is a core body temperature that is lower than 35°C and occurs with exposure to low ambient temperatures that are influenced by low environmental temperatures, humidity, wind velocity, extended exposure time or cold water immersion.[207] Cold injury is a common occurrence in those climates with cooler ambient conditions; however, when body heat is lower than the surrounding environmental conditions, it can easily develop so it is not an uncommon problem in Australia and New Zealand, despite the relatively warm

weather zones in the former. The very young and very old are most susceptible to injury.[207] A normal core temperature of 37°C has a variation of 1–2°C. Temperature maintenance is essential for normal homeostatic functioning, and normal adaptive mechanisms can respond to reductions in ambient temperature.

Clinical manifestations

When skin temperature is reduced after exposure to the cold, sympathetic stimulation occurs causing peripheral vasoconstriction, decreased skin circulation and shunting of blood centrally to vital organs. Blood pressure, heart rate and respiratory rate rise, and shivering (involuntary clonic movements of skeletal muscle) stimulates metabolic activity to produce heat and blood flow to striated muscles to maintain a normal core temperature. If continued exposure to cold occurs, these compensatory functions fail, and hypothermia results.[208]

Ambient temperatures need not be particularly low, as other contributing factors such as wind or a person having wet clothing may be significant. A patient with a decreased level of consciousness may present with hypothermia after lying on a cool surface. As a person's core temperature drops, progressive cardiac abnormalities occur; normal sinus rhythm may progress to sinus bradycardia, T-wave inversion, prolonged P–R and Q–T intervals, atrial fibrillation and ventricular fibrillation. A QRS abnormality, the Osborn wave, represented by a positive deflection at the junction of the QRS and ST segments, is frequently described as being characteristic of cold injury.[209]

Metabolic acidosis and blood-clotting abnormalities are common, as well as hypoglycaemia, which occurs because of depletion of glycogen stores caused by excessive shivering. Hyperglycaemia can be present because of inhibition of insulin action due to the lowered temperature.[207] The physiological alterations that accompany lowering of core temperature to below 30°C are summarised in Table 23.17.[207-209]

Management

A patient with severe hypothermia may appear dead: cold, pale, stiff, with no response to external stimulation. However, successful resuscitation of patients has occurred at temperatures as low as 17°C, owing to the low body temperature protecting vital organs from hypoxic injury.[209] This is reflected in the anecdotal phrase, 'patients are not dead until they are warm and dead'; however, a core temperature of <15°C or K^+ >12 mmol/L is considered unsalvageable.[207] In most cases, resuscitation should continue until the patient's core temperature reaches 32°C.[210]

> **Practice tip**
>
> Removing wet clothing and drying the patient is an extremely important first aid measure for a cold, wet patient to prevent further cooling.

TABLE 23.17

Physiological effects of hypothermia[207–209]

PHYSIOLOGICAL EFFECTS	DEGREE OF HYPOTHERMIA		
	MILD (32–35°C)	MODERATE (28–32°C)	SEVERE (<28°C)
General metabolic	Shivering Raised oxygen consumption Hyperkalaemia	Raised oxygen consumption Acidosis	Normal metabolic functions fail
Cardiac	Vasoconstriction Tachycardia Increased cardiac output	Atrial arrhythmias Bradycardia	Ventricular arrhythmias Decreased cardiac output
Respiratory	Tachypnoea Bronchospasm	Decreased respiratory drive	Apnoea
Neurological	Confusion Hyperreflexia	Lowered level of consciousness Hyporeflexia	Coma Absent reflexes
Coagulation	Platelet dysfunction Impaired clotting enzyme function Increased blood viscosity	Increased haematocrit	Lower bleeding times due to failure of clotting systems

Passive external rewarming (PER) is the preferred treatment in patients with mild hypothermia (32–35°C). In PER, wet clothing is removed, then the patient is covered with blankets or other forms of insulation, producing a reduction in heat loss, and allowing the patient's intrinsic heat production to rewarm them.

Active external warming is indicated for moderate-to-severe hypothermia (32–28°C). Shunting of cold peripheral blood to the core may lead to further chilling of the myocardium and ventricular fibrillation.[207] Therefore, rewarming of the trunk should be commenced before that of the extremities in order to minimise core temperature afterdrop with associated acidaemia and hypotension related to arterial vasodilation.[208] External warming using warm blankets, forced warm air blankets and heat packs in contact with the patient's body should raise body temperature by approximately 2.5°C per hour.[209] Inhalation rewarming with oxygen warmed to 42–46°C is also effective, as around 10% of metabolic heat is lost through the respiratory tract.[210]

If a patient's core temperature is <28°C, 'core rewarming' is indicated. This approach is favoured, as experimental evidence indicates that return to normal cardiovascular function is more rapid with temperature rises of up to 7.5°C per hour.[207] A number of invasive internal warming options are available, including peritoneal lavage, although the most effective of all internal methods is cardiopulmonary bypass, as it transfers heat at a rate several times faster than any other methods available, that being approximately 7.5°C per hour. While the technique is efficient, it is obviously more invasive and carries associated risks, and so is reserved for profoundly hypothermic patients.[209]

> **Practice tip**
>
> Always measure the blood glucose of hypothermic patients to exclude hypoglycaemia as a reason for an altered conscious state.

Hyperthermia and heat illness

Description and incidence

Potentially one of the more significant environmental fears expressed by many scientists is the issue of climate change and the consequence of heat-related illness worldwide. Global temperatures have increased because of climate change, leading to events such as recurrent prolonged hot weather days which have recently caused numerous deaths through Europe, the USA and Australia, and scientists are predicting that the events will become more common.[211] Heat-related illness is common in Australia and represents a significant public health risk, although there are only limited deaths compared with what has happened in the USA and Europe.[207]

Heat-related illness can affect any age group; however, it is the very young, because of their larger surface area, reduced sweating capacity and inability to access their own fluids, and the older person, who may have fluid restrictions because of other health reasons or is taking medications that affect the capacity to sweat, and a tendency to layer clothing, who are at the highest risk. The other vulnerable group is those in the younger age bracket undertaking physical activity during hot weather periods, whether because of work or during sports.[212]

Alterations in thermoregulatory function cause varying degrees of heat illness, categorised as three types: heat cramps, heat exhaustion and heat stroke.[212] Excessive exposure to heat substantially increases fluid and electrolyte losses from the body.[213] The loss of both fluids and electrolytes in addition to impaired organ function leads to the complications of heat illnesses. Factors contributing to heat illness include elevated ambient temperature, increased heat production due to exercise, infection and drugs such as amphetamines, phenothiazines or other stimulants.[213]

Clinical manifestations

Environmental heat illness is more likely to develop when the ambient temperature exceeds 32–35°C and the humidity is greater than 70%.[214] Assessment of the patient's physical state and vital signs including GCS provides some evidence of hypovolaemia and potential or impending shock.

Heat exhaustion is a more severe form of heat illness and is associated with severe water or salt depletion due to excessive sweating; the patient's temperature may range between normal and below 40°C.[214] Combined water and salt losses cause muscle cramps, nausea and vomiting, headache, dizziness, weakness, fainting, thirst, tachycardia, hypotension and profuse sweating, but with normal neurological function.

Heat stroke is the most severe and serious form of heat-related illness, with temperatures above 41°C and impaired neurological function. Heat stroke is a profound disturbance of the body's heat-regulating ability, and is often referred to as 'sunstroke', although it relates to the body's inability to dissipate heat, loss of sweat function and severe dehydration rather than actual sun exposure.[212]

Management

Initial management of the hyperthermic patient focuses on airway, breathing and circulation, correction of urgent physiological states such as hypoxia, severe potassium imbalances and acidosis. A heat-stressed patient can have large fluid losses and require prompt fluid resuscitation, preferably isotonic sodium chloride solution. Total water deficit should be corrected slowly; half of the deficit is administered in the first 3–6 hours, with the remainder over the next 6–9 hours.[214]

Rapid cooling is the second priority: lowering core temperature to less than 38.9°C within 30 minutes improves survival and minimises end-organ damage.[213] Non-invasive external methods of cooling include removal of clothing and covering the patient with a wet, tepid sheet. Ice packs can be placed next to the patient's axillae, neck and groin. Invasive cooling measures such as iced gastric lavage and cardiopulmonary bypass are reserved for the patient who fails to respond to conventional cooling methods.[213] Core body temperature should be monitored using a continuous rectal or tympanic probe.

Multiple patient triage/disaster

Disaster triage is a process designed to provide the greatest benefit to multiple patients when treatment resources and facilities are limited. Disaster triage systems differ from the routine triage system used within the ED (e.g. the ATS, MTS): system care is focused on those victims who may survive with proper therapy, rather than on those who have no chance of survival or who will live without treatment. The system was first devised during war as a method of managing large numbers of battlefield casualties. Today it is applicable for treating multiple victims of illness or injury outside and within the hospital setting. Variations exist between states and countries regarding disaster victim triage classifications. It is, therefore, important to be familiar with local plans and policy.

Triage of mass victims may be necessary in common situations – for example, vehicle collisions with multiple occupants – as well as other large-scale disasters, such as earthquakes, floods, bushfires, damaging storms, public transport incidents or explosions. The principles of triage vary little, though the methods used to communicate triage information and to match victims with available resources may differ. Triage at the scene of a major incident or disaster is commenced by the first qualified person to arrive, most commonly an ambulance officer of the first responding team. This person is initially responsible for performing immediate primary surveys on all victims and for determining and communicating the numbers and types of resources needed to provide initial care and transport.[215]

In Australia, New Zealand, the UK and the USA, disaster systems have up to five triage categories (depending on jurisdictional and local protocols), usually with corresponding colours. Despite slight variation, the aim is similar: to provide the best level of care and ensure the highest number of survivors. Those who are mortally injured but alive may be given a low treatment priority, though this will almost certainly ensure their death. These decisions are, therefore, best made by an experienced doctor. In a situation with a large number of casualties, one or more doctors should be present at the site to lead the triage effort. Further, it is not within the scope of practice of non-physician emergency personnel to pronounce a patient dead, but properly trained ambulance or rescue personnel can recognise the signs of death for the purposes of triage until doctors can formally declare death.[216]

Emergency department response to an external disaster: receiving patients

Disasters may produce mass victims on a scale that means routine processes and practices in the ED and hospital will be overwhelmed. The ED response to an external disaster forms part of the overall hospital response, outlined in a hospital disaster plan. The ED response plans also sit within the larger context of other health disciplines where there is a consideration of the prevention of, preparedness for, response to and recovery from the health problems arising from a disaster.[217,218] These plans are reviewed regularly for currency and practised for preparedness. The following aspects form part of ED planning and response to receiving patients from an external disaster.

Department preparation

If the disaster site is close to the hospital, a significant number of disaster victims will self-evacuate from the site and arrive at the hospital without any pre-hospital triage, treatment or decontamination before any formal notification has been received. In this instance the ED will need to declare the incident and commence the notification process required.[215,217] The ED may be quickly overwhelmed with arriving patients. On notification of a disaster response, a number of key positions should be allocated (medical coordinator, nursing coordinator, triage nurse, medical triage officer). These personnel are senior staff with specific disaster training and knowledge of the hospital's disaster plan.[215,217] Nursing and medical coordinators are responsible for allocating staff to specific duties; all designated roles are outlined on action cards available for staff to read prior to commencing their roles.

The capacity of the ED to accommodate a large influx of patients needs to be maximised.[219] Patients currently in the department are reviewed for a decision to admit. Patients requiring admission are transferred out of the department to a suitable location in the hospital. Patients suitable for discharge or referral to their local medical officer, including patients with minor complaints currently waiting, should be discharged or referred to community resources. A small number of patients may need to remain in the ED, and their care will need to be prioritised in conjunction with arriving disaster victims.[220]

Areas of the department are designated to accommodate the expected severity of the victims (e.g. resuscitation room for priority 1 patients, observation areas for priority 2). Walking wounded casualties with relatively minor injuries and who are unlikely to require admission to hospital are best accommodated in a treatment area outside the ED, as this reduces congestion and increases the capacity for more significantly injured victims to be managed.[220]

Additional staff members are notified from the current staff lists to participate in the disaster management. Staff members are allocated to teams to manage bed spaces within designated treatment areas. Additional staff from outside the ED may be deployed to assist; these staff should be teamed with routine ED staff because of their familiarity with the layout and location of equipment and other resources.[219] It is important to recognise the need to replace staff to avoid fatigue, especially in incidents of a protracted nature. Therefore, not all staff should be called in initially. Where possible, staff members who usually work together on a daily basis should work in teams during the disaster period.[215,220]

Triage and reception

Routine, day-to-day triage and reception processes will be ineffective when receiving large numbers of disaster victims. A registration process for disaster victims generally involves collecting minimal personal information from the patients, where possible, and the allocation of a prepared disaster hospital number used for identification and ordering investigations.[221] Triage assessments will often be undertaken by both a medical officer and a nurse, and the process will be brief and focused.[222] Most victims will have been allocated a triage tag in the field, but are re-evaluated for any changes, as their condition may have deteriorated. Triage assessment is based on observations of the nature and extent of the victims' injuries.[222] Patients present in the ED prior to disaster notification are considered part of the disaster event and triaged in the same manner.

Treatment

Treatment provided during a disaster will not reflect routine practices; priorities focus on resuscitation, identification of serious injuries, identification of patients requiring urgent surgery and stabilisation of patients for transfer out of the ED. The best overall outcomes during a disaster are achieved when the routine principles of resuscitation and management are adapted to reflect the resources available.[217,220]

Transfer from the ED

Patients are triaged, stabilised and transferred out to the operating theatre or other clinical areas as soon as possible using designated transfer staff and a coordinated process outlined in the hospital plan. This will maintain the effectiveness and efficiency of the department as victims continue to arrive. During and after the incident, opportunity for staff to debrief is an important aspect to manage staff psychosocial well-being.[215]

Chemical, biological and radiological events

The prospect of chemical, biological or radiological terrorism, especially an event that causes mass casualties, poses a significant challenge to healthcare systems. The use of infectious organisms or toxic compounds by terrorists can have both immediate and long-term effects.[223] Since the Japanese doomsday cult Aum Shinrikyo released sarin nerve gas on the Tokyo subway in March 1995, killing 12 people, terrorist incidents and hoaxes involving toxic or infectious agents have been on the rise. The ease of obtaining non-nuclear radioactive material may mean that 'dirty bombs'[215] are more likely to be used as an explosive device. The availability and the impact of chemical and biological threat materials are both relatively high, with potentially devastating impact.[223] Because biological and chemical agents are so dissimilar, each category will be dealt with separately, but there are common elements or characteristics.

Chemical agents

Chemical agents are super-toxic chemicals used for the purpose of poisoning victims. They are similar to hazardous industrial chemicals, but hundreds of times more toxic.[215,224] For example, the 1995 sarin attack in Tokyo caused 1039 injuries and at least 4000 people had psychogenic symptoms.[224] Sarin is approximately 60 times more toxic than methylisocyanate. To put this in perspective, a leak of methylisocyanate from a factory in Bhopal, India, in 1984 caused 200,000 people to be affected, with 10,000 severely affected and 3300 deaths.[225] Relatively small quantities of a military grade chemical agent could have the same capability to produce large numbers of casualties (symptomatic and psychological).[223]

Table 23.18[215,224] provides a summary of the more common chemical agents, their effects, clinical presentations and treatments. It needs to be stressed that specialised personal protective equipment (PPE) and specialist training are required to manage these situations.[215,224]

Biological agents

The use of biological weapons is not a recent concept. Biological agents have the longest history of use, dating back to the 14th century.[226] Biological agents are living organisms or toxins that have the capacity to cause disease in people, animals or crops. Toxins are a special type of poisonous chemical categorised as biological agents because they were created by living organisms. They generally behave like chemical agents and serve the same function: to poison people.

Biological agents are relatively inexpensive to produce and have the potential to be devastating in their effects. Organisms such as anthrax, plague and smallpox have been the agents of greatest concern from the perspective of potential terrorist use.[226] Table 23.19 presents an outline of biological agents, clinical presentations and treatments.[215,226]

Radiological agents

Radiological materials can pose both an acute and a long-term hazard to humans. In many ways, they behave like some of the chemical agents in that they cause cellular damage. A major difference is that radiological agents do not necessarily have to be inhaled or come into contact with the skin to do damage. While radiological incidents have resulted in death from radiation sickness, with very few exceptions, the vast majority of cases simply require decontamination and monitoring.[227]

The deployment of a nuclear weapon would be catastrophic, as evidenced by events such as that in Hiroshima, or industrial accidents, as occurred at Chernobyl. Although very different, both events produced immediate injury and produced long-term effects of ionising radiation on large populations. The event of highest risk is likely to be a 'dirty bomb' that combines conventional explosives with any available radioactive source.[227]

Psychological effects

A chemical, biological or radiological terrorism incident may or may not result in mass casualties and fatalities as intended. However, large numbers of psychological casualties are very likely and, therefore, regardless of the effectiveness of the attack and number of people actually exposed to the agent, there will most likely be a mass casualty situation.[215,228] The psychological implications of chemical and biological weapons may be worse than the physical ones. Chemical and biological weapons are weapons of terror; part of their purpose is to wreak destruction via psychological means by inducing fear, confusion and uncertainty in everyday life. The long-term

---

TABLE 23.18

Summary of common chemical agents, effects, clinical presentations and treatments[215,224]

TYPE OF CHEMICAL	EFFECT	EXAMPLE	CLINICAL PRESENTATION	ANTIDOTES/TREATMENT
Nerve agent	Inhibits the activation of acetylcholinesterase.	Sarin VX Soman Tabun	Muscarinic and nicotinic signs	Atropine 2-Pyridine aldoxime methyl chloride Benzodiazepines
Blood agents	Binds with cytochrome oxidase, causing hypoxia.	Cyanide	Hypoxia	Cyanide kit Sodium nitrite Sodium thiosulfate
Vesicants	Chemical burns.	Mustard gas Lewisite	Burns and blisters	Decontamination with soap and water
Pulmonary agents	Irritation to the respiratory tract.	Chlorine phosgene	Respiratory distress Pulmonary oedema	Oxygen

TABLE 23.19

Summary of biological agents, clinical presentations and treatments[215,223,224]

BIOLOGICAL GROUP	EXAMPLE	CLINICAL PRESENTATION	TREATMENT
Virus	Smallpox (variola)		Supportive care
Bacteria	Anthrax (*Bacillus anthracis*)	Inhalational • Respiratory failure • Widened mediastinum • Severe sepsis	Antibiotics
	Plague (*Yersinia pestis*)	Pneumonic plague • Respiratory failure • Haemoptysis • Painful lymph nodes	Antibiotics
Toxin	Botulism (*Clostridium botulinum*)		Supportive care Botulism immune globulin

social and psychological effects of an episode of chemical or biological attack, real or suspected, would be as damaging as the acute ones, if not more so.[228]

Major challenges for chemical, biological or radiological responders

A well-delivered chemical or biological event would be catastrophic and exposure for emergency workers likely, as occurred previously when 110 staff developed signs and symptoms of exposure following the 1995 sarin attack in Tokyo.[229]

To protect staff, there must be clear procedures for dealing with potentially exposed or contaminated patients. This begins with proper assessment of a patient in need of isolation or decontamination and includes understanding of what PPE is appropriate and the capability of staff to use the PPE effectively. Emergency personnel must also have immediate access to the PPE that they need to limit their risk of exposure. However, the issue is complex: advanced levels of PPE require training and special skills to be used safely. Decontamination of patients with chemical exposure is a high-risk activity for untrained staff.[224]

Summary

An overview of important emergency systems and processes, outlining the practice of initial assessment and prioritisation of patients presenting to the ED through triage, has been provided in this chapter. The role of the emergency nurse in the initial assessment, intervention and management of the patient has been described. The initial ED management of common emergency presentations was outlined, reflecting current practice and based on the latest available evidence.

The emergency environment is dynamic, and it was beyond the scope of this chapter to describe the full extent of emergency nursing practice and the clinical entities that are frequently managed. It is therefore important for a critical care nurse to be familiar with the content provided in the other chapters in this text, as well as other resources. As noted at the beginning of this chapter, other common presentations to the ED, such as trauma and cardiorespiratory arrest, are described in Chapters 24 and 25.

Emergency nursing is a demanding specialty area of practice, as are all areas of specialty practice. The challenges with emergency nursing come with the volumes of predicable patient groups, changing demographics in the community and the unpredictable or unusual presentations and volume of presentations. Emergency nurses need to prepare themselves with a broad knowledge base, adaptability to change and resilience to meet these demands.

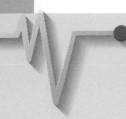

Case study

15 OCTOBER 2022

16:00 h: Patient Tarryn Rogers, a 29-year-old female, presented to the ED with urinary tract infection symptoms of dysuria, oliguria and back pain, for the past 8 days. At triage, she did not appear to be distressed, and reported an onset of mild-to-moderate suprapubic abdominal pain and dysuria 2 days previously. There was no compromise to airway, breathing or circulation; her temperature was 37.3°C and the remaining vital signs were within normal parameters. Capillary blood glucose was 6.3 mmol/L. She was allocated an ATS category 4 (to be seen within 1 h) and placed in the reception area while awaiting assessment.

16:30 h: While awaiting initial assessment by the treating doctor, a registered nurse (RN) initiated relevant investigations and analgesia. Early acquisition of relevant investigations means that information necessary to make a treatment or diagnostic decision will be at hand at the earliest possible time. The RN obtained blood samples for full blood count, electrolytes, urea and creatinine, and a mid-stream urine sample to complete urinalysis including β-HCG. Paracetamol 1 g and ural (urinary alkaliniser) for analgesia were administered.

17:15 h: Tarryn was reviewed by a doctor. On clinical exam, she had moderate tenderness over her suprapubic region on palpation, mild left flank pain on percussion of the costovertebral angle, bowel sounds were present and the abdomen was soft. There was no evidence of rebound guarding. McBurney's and Rovsing signs were negative. Visual examination did not reveal evidence of hernia or any scars from previous abdominal surgeries. She did not have nausea or vomiting, bowel actions were normal, there was no vaginal discharge, and she had not been sexually active for the past 3 months. Her last menstrual period was 3 weeks ago, and of normal duration and volume. Past medical history included type 2 diabetes, and two previous urinary tract infections in the past 12 months. She had no previous pregnancies. She reported urinary discomfort with increased frequency of passing small amounts of urine over the past 8 days and had attended her general practitioner (GP) 2 days ago, who prescribed trimethoprim. Her white cell count was 12×10^9/L; other bloods were normal. Mid-stream urine was sent for microscopy, culture and sensitivity (MC&S) testing. Urinalysis was positive for leukocytes, protein, blood and nitrates. Her urinary β-HCG was negative.

After discussion with an emergency consultant, a decision was made to not conduct a CT scan because of the uncomplicated nature of the patient's presentation, her young age and low risk features. The attending doctor explained to the patient that the pain and symptoms were most likely due to a urinary tract infection but may also progress upwards to involve the kidney (pyelonephritis). The most prudent course recommended was to treat empirically with an alternative oral antibiotic ciprofloxacin, follow up MC&S results with the GP, and monitor for any worsening symptoms. It was confirmed that Tarryn had support at home, and someone who could transport her easily back to the ED if necessary. A repeat set of vital signs were taken that confirmed that blood pressure, pulse, respiratory rate and temperature were within normal parameters. The patient was discharged home with an information leaflet explaining the signs and symptoms of concern that would require her to return to the ED.

17 OCTOBER 2022

10:45 h: Tarryn re-presented to triage 2 days later with worsening flank pain, fever, nausea and vomiting. In triage she was alert and interacting, her blood pressure was 100/72 mmHg, heart rate was 111 bpm, she had dry mucous membranes, her respiration rate was 17 breaths/min, SaO$_2$ was 98% on room air, tympanic temperature was 38.3°C, and her pain was rated 7/10. She was allocated an ATS category 3, to be seen within 30 minutes, and a non-monitored bed requested from the nurse unit manager for ongoing management of the patient.

11:10 h: On reaching a bed, the RN responsible for Tarryn's ongoing care obtained a full set of vital signs. Tarryn's blood pressure was 99/66 mmHg, her heart rate 112 bpm, respiratory rate 20 breaths/min, SaO$_2$ 98% on room air, and temperature was 38.8°C.

A peripheral IV catheter was inserted, and bloods taken for electrolytes, renal function and full blood count. A mid-stream urine was requested. The patient stated that her pain rated 9/10. The RN initiated analgesia of oxycodone 5 mg and paracetamol 1 g for pain management, and metoclopramide 10 mg IV for nausea and vomiting. The RN advised the patient to remain nil by mouth while waiting to be seen by either the treating doctor or the nurse practitioner.

12:00 h: A history and physical assessment were completed by the treating doctor. Tarryn described that initially the pain was suprapubic, then progressed to the left flank. She had not felt like eating overnight and had developed nausea and vomiting overnight. On assessment, the doctor found an acute tender left flank on percussion of the costovertebral angle. The treating doctor made a working diagnosis of pyelonephritis. She was prescribed IV fluids (1 L over 8 hours) and gentamicin while awaiting the results of outstanding blood and urine tests.

12:50 h: Diagnostic tests were still outstanding. Tarryn notified the nurse that she felt worse. On review by the RN, a deterioration in vital signs was also noted; her blood pressure was 72/51 mmHg, heart rate 136 bpm, respiratory rate 26 breaths/min, SaO_2 98% on room air, and temperature 39.2°C. Her deteriorating condition was escalated to the nurse unit manager and senior doctor for urgent review, and the patient was moved to a resuscitation bay for closer management and observation of possible septic shock secondary to pyelonephritis.

On review by the senior doctor, the following interventions were commenced:

- A second intravascular catheter was inserted.
- A fluid challenge was commenced at 20 mL/kg.
- Additional investigations including a venous blood gas and two independent sets of blood cultures were obtained.

Her previous blood work was reviewed and showed a greatly elevated white blood cell count of $22 \times 10^9/L$; stage 1 acute renal failure, blood sugar level of 11.8 mmol/L and level lactate of 3.1 mmol/L. A request was made for urgent renal and review for urosepsis. The treating doctor performed a bedside ultrasound and noticed several cavities within the left kidney. Following renal consultation, IV antibiotics were changed to piperacillin-tazobactam in the absence of susceptibility data from MC&S.

13:45 h: Tarryn improved following fluid bolus with repeat vital signs and her blood pressure was now 100/75 mmHg, heart rate 110 bpm, respiratory rate 18 breaths/min and SaO_2 98% on room air. She was considered stable enough to undergo an urgent CT of the abdomen, which identified three abscesses within the left kidney. Two of the abscesses were under 5 mm; however, the third was 11 mm and would require draining.

Tarryn was admitted to the high-dependency unit for ongoing IV antibiotics, drainage of the 11-mm renal abscess and observation. On day 5 of Tarryn's admission the MC&S urine results obtained on Tarryn's first presentation were positive for *Escherichia* (i.e. *E. coli*), which was resistant to trimethoprim, ciprofloxacin and ampicillin.

CASE STUDY QUESTIONS

1. Tarryn presents twice to the ED with a presenting complaint of abdominal pain. What features influenced the triage nurse to allocate a different triage category for the second presentation?
2. On Tarryn's initial presentation, she is sent home without having definitive imaging via a CT abdomen that could possibly have identified a diagnosis of renal abscesses. Why did the treating consultant decide against a CT abdomen on her first visit to the ED?
3. During management of the same disease process, Tarryn is at different times managed in three different areas of the ED. Why is this?
4. During Tarryn's second presentation, she clinically deteriorates. What are the clinical manifestations of severe sepsis and septic shock that she exhibited?
5. An IV fluid bolus and targeted antibiotics are administered. What does each of these interventions seek to achieve?
6. Why was an urgent abdominal CT not undertaken until Tarryn's vital signs had improved?

RESEARCH VIGNETTE

Cornish S, Klim S, Kelly A. Is COVID-19 the straw that broke the back of the emergency nursing workforce?
Emerg Med Australas 2021;33(6):1095–99[230]

Abstract

Background: The emergency nursing workforce is at risk of shortages that will impact patient care both internationally and in Australia. This risk is a focus for workforce retention studies, workforce modelling and intervention studies. It is known that the environment that emergency nurses work within can impact on burnout and intention to leave the profession or the discipline of emergency nursing. Other factors impacting on retention of emergency nurses is leadership, a lack of support systems appropriate to emergency nurses' needs and feeling undervalued and disempowered. The COVID-19 pandemic has impacted all of these factors and it is unknown what this means for future retention of the emergency nursing workforce.

Objectives: The aim of the study was to explore Australian emergency nurses' intentions to leave after the first year of the SARS-CoV-2 (COVID-19) pandemic.

Design: Online descriptive survey.

Setting: Australia.

Participants: Emergency nurses in Australia.

Methods: A voluntary online survey, recruited to via social media platforms, professional organisation memberships and invitations to nurse unit managers and ED leaders, and no incentives offered to participants. Sub-survey analysis: there were 69 items in six sections including participant characteristics, life at home, the work environment, nursing practice, career intentions, perceptions of nursing with some free text options. There is no known number of emergency nurses in Australia (data is not recorded or collected).

Results: There were 392 completed surveys from 537 log-ins, and 528 participants completed some or all of the survey questions. Of these, 398 participants completed questions related to future intentions for their career. Most respondents were from Victoria (52.3%), with New South Wales second (22.4%) and the nurses from other states and territories making up the rest of the 25% of respondents. Almost half (48.2%) of participants reported they were intending to leave emergency nursing within 5 years. Nurses who worked in EDs that provided care for COVID-19 patients were more likely to leave, although having provided care for a COVID-19 patient was not associated with intention to leave emergency nursing. No other demographic or cohort factors were associated with intention to leave (e.g. age (excluding nurses >60 years), higher specialist qualifications, or years of ED experience). Other factors associated with intention to leave were related to the nurses' experience, including feeling disconnected from emergency colleagues, support systems and the organisation since the onset of the pandemic.

Conclusions: At this single time point, approximately 1 year post pandemic commencement, a significant number of emergency nurses reported an intention to leave the discipline of emergency nursing.

Critique

This paper described the intentions of emergency nurses to leave their discipline area at a single time point, a year after the COVID-19 pandemic commenced. Previous research both domestically and internationally shows concerning results for ED nurse turnover and intention to leave. In Australia a main concern about being able to interpret research like this is that we do not collect data about numbers of emergency nurses, and that definitions for what is classed as an emergency nurse is not as clear cut as for other areas of specialisation. For example, in rural and remote areas, EDs are staffed by all nurses in the hospital or clinic, not by specific staff employed solely for that discipline area. While data can be collected to identify higher degree qualifications specific to emergency nursing, there is not a requirement to possess these qualifications to work in the ED, and not all nurses who obtain higher qualifications are working in that discipline area. Additionally, while there are two emergency nursing-specific professional organisations in Australia, not all nurses who work in emergency care are members.

This study methodology used snowball sampling, advertising on social media sites, convenience sampling of one of the two emergency nursing professional organisations through invitations to the membership, and direct contact with nurse unit managers and ED leaders. What is not known is whether all departments across Australia were contacted to share invitations with their staff, and reporting of ethics approvals did not create any clarity in this regard. Perhaps only Victorian EDs were contacted, and this may explain the higher participant numbers from Victoria. Alternatively, perhaps the author's home state and contacts in this field have influenced this overrepresentation from Victorian nurses (or underrepresentation from other states and territories). We also have not been told whether the other professional emergency nursing organisation in Australia was considered as part of the recruitment strategy.

Results are concerning in that nearly half of the sampled nurses intend to leave their discipline field in the next 5 years; however, the authors do note limitations in relation to the timing of the study (a single time point), and that with no denominator for the sample it is hard to show potential turnover data, a low response rate to the survey, and that attitudes of intention to leave may fluctuate over time and in response to how the pandemic and management of this and the workforce proceeds.

Unfortunately, the pandemic has impacted on issues that were already known internationally and in Australia to impact on nurses' decisions to leave emergency nursing. Feeling disconnected from colleagues, support systems and their organisation have been significantly impacted on by management approaches for COVID-19. This includes the impact of PPE on feeling connected to colleagues and patients, the move to online rather than in-person non-clinical meetings, local managers being required to work offsite rather than in-department, and social interactions being severely constrained or stopped for long periods of time. This is also a concern for the future, where models of working may not necessarily return to pre-COVID face-to-face approaches.

In addition, the risk of personal illness, and bringing the virus home to families, including those who are at high risk, mandated vaccination, public concern about contamination and who is responsible for this were influential in nurses feeling stressed about their profession. Additionally, the rapid, constant change to management of clinical approaches and guidelines without time for collaboration and input from frontline staff changed the work environment constantly and significantly. Previous protective factors such as years of experience in emergency nursing and possession of higher qualifications were not found to impact in this study.

Overall, this is an example of a study that has significant limitations in methodology as it is reported, but whose results can be seen as a potential barometer of a single viewpoint in time. This study cannot be considered as transferable or a representative view of emergency nurses across Australia for intention to leave; however, it shows the need for further studies in this field, with considerations for design (e.g. longitudinal approaches) and recruitment methodology (which may have been more robust but cannot be identified from what was reported). Additionally, this study shows a gap and need for improvement for what data we collect about numbers of nurses in specialist discipline areas such as emergency, and how we shape future working models for staff, managers and organisations, and of course retention strategies for emergency nurses.

Learning activities

1   Review your local guidelines for treatment and management of sepsis.

2   Relevant imaging can help guide a future treatment plan or surgical intervention; however, it may also represent an unacceptable risk as it is a difficult environment for resuscitation if there is a sudden clinical deterioration. What would be considered minimum physiological parameters for safe transport to imaging?

3   In abdominal pain presentations, patients may experience 'visceral' and/or 'somatic' pain depending upon which structures are involved in the disease process. Which structures experience these different types of pain, and how do they differ in symptoms?

Online resources

American Emergency Nurses Association, https://www.ena.org

Australasian College for Emergency Medicine, https://www.acem.org.au

Australian College of Emergency Nursing, https://acen.com.au

Australian Institute of Health and Welfare, https://www.aihw.gov.au

Australian Venom Research Unit, https://biomedicalsciences.unimelb.edu.au/sbs-research-groups/biochemistry-and-pharmacology-research/AVRU-Australian-venom-research-unit

Best Bets, https://bestbets.org

Clinical Toxicology Resources, Women's and Children's Hospital, Adelaide, http://toxinology.com

College of Emergency Nursing Australasia, https://www.cena.org.au

College of Emergency Nursing New Zealand, https://www.nzno.org.nz/groups/colleges/college_of_emergency_nurses

Commonwealth Serum Laboratories Antivenom Handbook eMedicine, https://www.emedicine.com

National Asthma Council of Australia, https://www.nationalasthma.org.au

New Zealand Health Information Service, https://www.healthnavigator.org.nz

New Zealand Ministry of Health, https://www.moh.govt.nz

Poisons Information Australia, telephone: 131126, https://www.health.gov.au/contacts/poisons-information-centre

Poisons Information New Zealand, telephone: 0800 POISON or 0800 764766, https://poisons.co.nz

The Cochrane Centre, https://www.cochrane.org

Further reading

White J. A clinician's guide to Australian venomous bites and stings: incorporating the updated CSL Antivenom Handbook; 2013. CSL Ltd. Available from: https://www.toxinology.com/fusebox.cfm?staticaction=generic_static_files/cgavbs_avh.html. [Accessed 25 February 2023].

References

1. Ju QY, Huang LH, Zhao XH, et al. Development of evidence-based nursing-sensitive quality indicators for emergency nursing: a Delphi study. J Clin Nurs 2018;27(15-16):3008–19.

2. Fry M, Shaban RZ, Considine J. Chapter 1. Emergency nursing in Australia and New Zealand. In: Curtis K, Ramsden C, Shaban RZ, et al, editors. Emergency and trauma care for nurses and paramedics. 3rd ed. Chatswood, NSW: Elsevier; 2019, p. 3–16.

3. O'Shay S. 'The chronicle of nightmares': emergency nurses' frontstage and backstage communication in the emergency department. Health Commun 2022; Apr 19:1–12. doi: 10.1080/10410236.2022.2062835. Online ahead of print.

4. Hettinger AZ, Benda N, Roth E, et al. Ten best practices for improving emergency medicine provider–nurse communication. J Emerg Med 2020;58(4):581–93.

5. Pun JKH, Matthiessen CMIM, Murray KA, et al. Factors affecting communication in emergency departments: doctors and nurses' perceptions of communication in a trilingual ED in Hong Kong. Int J Emerg Med 2015;8(1):48.

6. Cameron M, Shaw V, Parsons M. Expanding the emergency nurse role to meet demand: nurse and physician perspectives. Emerg Nurse 2020;28(6):26–33.

7. Moon S-H, Cho I-Y. The effect of competency-based triage education application on emergency nurses' triage competency and performance. Healthcare (Basel) 2022;10(4):596.

8. Nakao H, Ukai I, Kotani J. A review of the history of the origin of triage from a disaster medicine perspective. Acute Med Surg 2017; 4(4):379–84.

9. Canadian Association of Emergency Physicians (CAEP). The Canadian Triage and Acuity Scale: combined adult/paediatric education program: participant manual (v2.5b). Ottawa, ON: CAEP; 2013. Available from: https://ctas-phctas.ca/wp-content/uploads/2018/05/participant_manual_v2.5b_november_2013_0.pdf. [Accessed 25 February 2023].

10. Mackway-Jones K, Marsden J, Windle J. Emergency triage: Manchester Triage Group. 3rd ed. Chichester, West Sussex, UK: John Wiley and Sons Limited; 2014.

11. Australasian College for Emergency Medicine (ACEM). Guidelines on the implementation of the Australasian Triage Scale in emergency departments. Melbourne, VIC: ACEM; 2016. Available from: https://acem.org.au/getmedia/51dc74f7-9ff0-42ce-872a-0437f3db640a/G24_04_Guidelines_on_Implementation_of_ATS_Jul-16.aspx. [Accessed 25 February 2023].

12. College of Emergency Nursing Australasia (CENA). Position statement: triage and the Australasian Triage Scale. Beaumaris, VIC: CENA; 2015. Available from: https://www.cena.org.au/public/118/files/Governance/CENA-Position-Statement-Triage-and-the-Australasian-Triage-Scale.pdf. [Accessed 25 February 2023].

13. van der Wulp I, van Stel HF. Calculating kappas from adjusted data improved the comparability of the reliability of triage systems: a comparative study. J Clin Epidemiol 2010;63(11):1256–63.

14. Hinson JS, Martinez DA, Cabral S, et al. Triage performance in emergency medicine: a systematic review. Ann Emerg Med 2019;74(1):140–52.

15. Farrohknia N, Castrén M, Ehrenberg A, et al. Emergency department triage scales and their components: a systematic review of the scientific evidence. Scand J Trauma Resusc Emerg Med 2011;19:42.

16. Krey J. Triage in emergency departments. Comparative evaluation of 4 international triage systems. Med Klin Intensivmed Notfallmed 2016;111(2):124–33.

17. Parenti N, Reggiani MLB, Iannone P, et al. A systematic review on the validity and reliability of an emergency department triage scale, the Manchester Triage System. Int J Nurs Stud 2014;51(7):1062–9.

18. Ng CJ, Yen ZS, Tsai JC, et al. Validation of the Taiwan triage and acuity scale: a new computerised five-level triage system. Emerg Med J 2011;28(12):1026–31.

19. Kongensgaard FT, Fløjstrup M, Lassen A, et al. Are 5-level triage systems improved by using a symptom based approach? – a Danish cohort study. Scand J Trauma Resusc Emerg Med 2022;30(1):31.

20. Maningas PA, Hime DA, Parker DE, et al. The Soterion Rapid Triage System: evaluation of inter-rater reliability and validity. J Emerg Med 2006;30(4):461–9.

21. Dalwai M, Valles P, Twomey M, et al. Is the South African Triage Scale valid for use in Afghanistan, Haiti and Sierra Leone? BMJ Global Health 2017;2(2):e000160.

22. Fernandes CM, Tanabe P, Gilboy N, et al. Five-level triage: a report from the ACEP/ENA Five-level Triage Task Force. J Emerg Nurs 2005;31(1):39–50; quiz 118.

23. Jelink GA. Towards an international triage scale. Eur J Emerg Med 2001;8(1):1–2.

24. Australasian College for Emergency Medicine (ACEM). Triage. Melbourne, VIC: ACEM; 2022. Available from: https://acem.org.au/Content-Sources/Advancing-Emergency-Medicine/Better-Outcomes-for-Patients/Triage. [Accessed 25 February 2023].

25. NSW Government. Premier's priorities – data information sheet. Sydney, NSW: NSW Government; 2022. Available from: https://www.nsw.gov.au/sites/default/files/2020-11/Improving-service-levels-in-hospitals-data-information-sheet.pdf. [Accessed 25 February 2023].

26. FitzGerald G, Jelinek GA, Scott D, et al. Emergency department triage revisited. Emerg Med J 2010;27(2):86–92.

27. Van Gerven R, Delooz H, Sermeus W. Systematic triage in the emergency department using the Australian National Triage Scale: a pilot project. Eur J Emerg Med 2001;8(1):3–7.

28. Dent A, Rofe G, Sansom G. Which triage category patients die in hospital after being admitted through emergency departments? A study in one teaching hospital. Emerg Med 1999;11(2):68–71.

29. Doherty SR, Hore CT, Curran SW. Inpatient mortality as related to triage category in three New South Wales regional base hospitals. Emerg Med (Fremantle) 2003;15(4):334–40.

30. Australasian College for Emergency Medicine (ACEM). Guidelines on the implementation of the Australasian Triage Scale in emergency departments. Melbourne, VIC: ACEM; 2016. [Accessed 25 February 2023].

31. Australasian College for Emergency Medicine (ACEM). Guidelines on the implementation of the Australasian Triage Scale in emergency departments. Melbourne, VIC: ACEM; 2016. Available from: https://acem.org.au/getmedia/51dc74f7-9ff0-42ce-872a-0437f3db640a/G24_04_Guidelines_on_Implementation_of_ATS_Jul-16.aspx. [Accessed 25 February 2023].

32. Hodge A, Hugman A, Varndell W, et al. A review of the quality assurance processes for the Australasian Triage Scale (ATS) and implications for future practice. Australas Emerg Nurs J 2013;16:21–9.

33. Burgess L, Kynoch K, Hines S. Implementing best practice into the emergency department triage process. Int J Evid Based Healthc 2019;17(1):27–35.

34. College of Emergency Nursing Australasia (CENA). Patients awaiting care in the ED. Beaumaris, VIC: CENA; 2022. Available from: https://www.cena.org.au/public/118/files/Position%20Statements/CENA-Position-Statement-Patients-awaiting-care-in-the-ED.pdf. [Accessed 25 February 2023].

35. Gorick H. Factors that affect nurses' triage decisions in the emergency department: a literature review. Emerg Nurse 2022;30(3):14–19.

36. Thawley A, Aggar CW, N. The educational needs of triage nurses. Health Educ Pract 2020;3(1):26–38. doi: 10.33966/hepj.3.1.14121.

37. Varndell W, Hodge A, Fry M. Triage in Australian emergency departments: results of a New South Wales survey. Australas Emerg Care 2019;22(2):81–6.

38. College for Emergency Nursing Australasia (CENA). Triage and the Australasian Triage Scale. Beaumaris, VIC: CENA; 2012. Available from: https://www.cena.org.au/public/118/files/Governance/CENA-Position-Statement-Triage-and-the-Australasian-Triage-Scale.pdf. [Accessed 25 February 2023].

39. Australian Government Department of Health and Aging. Emergency triage education kit. Canberra, ACT: Department of Health; 2013. Available from: https://www.health.gov.au/resources/collections/emergency-triage-education-kit?utm_source=health.gov.au&utm_medium=callout-auto-custom&utm_campaign=digital_transformation. [Accessed 25 February 2023].

40. Australian Government Department of Health and Aging. Recommended triage method: Australian Government; 2013. Available from: https://www1.health.gov.au/internet/publications/publishing.nsf/Content/triageqrg~triageqrg-method. [Accessed 25 February 2023].

41. Hodge A, Varndell W, editors. Professional transitions in nursing. Sydney, NSW: Routledge; 2018.

42. Moura BRS, Oliveira GN, Medeiros G, et al. Rapid triage performed by nurses: Signs and symptoms associated with identifying critically ill patients in the emergency department. Int J Nurs Pract 2022;28(1):e13001.

43. Curtis K, Ramsden C, Shaban R, et al, editors. Emergency and trauma care for nurses and paramedics. 3rd ed. Sydney, NSW: Elsevier; 2019.

44. Mental Health and Drug and Alcohol Office. Mental health triage policy. Sydney, NSW: NSW Government; 2012. Available from: https://www1.health.nsw.gov.au/pds/ActivePDSDocuments/PD2012_053.pdf. [Accessed 25 February 2023].

45. Dragovic M, Pascu V, Hall T, et al. Emergency department mental health presentations before and during the COVID-19 outbreak in Western Australia. Australas Psychiatry 2020;28(6):627–31.

46. Australian Institute of Health and Welfare (AIHW). Mental health services in Australia. Canberra, ACT: AIHW; 2022. Available from: https://www.aihw.gov.au/reports/mental-health-services/mental-health-services-in-australia/report-contents/hospital-emergency-services. [Accessed 25 February 2023].

47. Malyon L, Williams A, Ware RS. The emergency triage education kit: improving paediatric triage. Australas Emerg Nurs J 2014;17(2):51–8.

48. Magalhães-Barbosa MC, Robaina JR, Prata-Barbosa A, et al. Reliability of triage systems for paediatric emergency care: a systematic review. Emerg Med J 2019;36(4):231.

49. Vilpert S, Monod S, Jaccard Ruedin H, et al. Differences in triage category, priority level and hospitalization rate between young-old and old-old patients visiting the emergency department. BMC Health Serv Res 2018;18(1):456.

50. Ruge T, Malmer G, Wachtler C, et al. Age is associated with increased mortality in the RETTS-A triage scale. BMC Geriatr 2019;19(1):139.

51. Wachelder JJH, Stassen PM, Hubens LPAM, et al. Elderly emergency patients presenting with non-specific complaints: characteristics and outcomes. PLoS One 2017;12(11):e0188954.

52. Puig-Campmany M, Blázquez-Andión M, Ris-Romeu J. Triage tools: a cautious (and critical) view towards their use in old patients. Eur Geriatr Med 2022;13(2):319–22.

53. Colwell C. Geriatric trauma: initial evaluation and management. UpToDate; 2022. Available from: https://www.uptodate.com/. [Accessed 25 February 2023].

54. Australasian College for Emergency Medicine (ACEM). Care of older persons in the emergency department. Melbourne, VIC: ACEM; 2020. Available from: https://acem.org.au/getmedia/bfd84f83-fcb2-492a-9e66-47b7896e5c70/Policy_on_the_Care_of_Older_Persons_in_the_ED. [Accessed 25 February 2023].

55. Lucke JA, Mooijaart SP, Heeren P, et al. Providing care for older adults in the Emergency Department: expert clinical recommendations from the European Task Force on Geriatric Emergency Medicine. Eur Geriatr Med 2022;13(2):309–17.

56. McCabe JJ, Kennelly SP. Acute care of older patients in the emergency department: strategies to improve patient outcomes. Open Access Emerg Med 2015;7:45–54.

57. Arendts G, Lowthian J. Demography is destiny: an agenda for geriatric medicine in Australasia. EMA 2013;25(3):271–8.

58. Varndell W, Fry M, Elliott D. Quality and impact of nurse-initiated analgesia in the emergency department: a systematic review. Int Emerg Nurs 2018;40:46–53.

59. Varndell W, Topacio M, Hagness C, et al. Nurse-performed focused ultrasound in the emergency department: a systematic review. Australas Emerg Care 2018;21(4):121–30.

60. Considine J, Shaban RZ, Curtis K, et al. Effectiveness of nurse-initiated X-ray for emergency department patients with distal limb injuries: a systematic review. Eur J Emerg Med 2019;26(5):314–22.

61. Burgess L, Kynoch K. Effectiveness of nurse-initiated interventions on patient outcomes in the emergency department: a systematic review protocol. JBI Database Syst Rev Implement Rep 2017;15(4):873–81.

62. Hunt D. Transfer of the critically ill adult patient. Surgery (Oxford) 2018;36(4):166–70.

63. Bourn S, Wijesingha S, Nordmann G. Transfer of the critically ill adult patient. BJA Educ 2017;18(3):63–8.

64. Eiding H, Kongsgaard UE, Olasveengen TM, et al. Interhospital transport of critically ill patients: a prospective observational study of patient and transport characteristics. Acta Anaesthesiol Scand 2022;66(2):248–55.

65. Australasian College for Emergency Medicine (ACEM), Australian and New Zealand College of Anaesthetists, College of Intensive Care Medicine of Australia and New Zealand. Guidelines for transport of critically ill patients. Melbourne, VIC: ACEM; 2018. Available from: https://acem.org.au/getmedia/0daba691-5e60-4a88-b6a8-24f2af3e5ebf/Guidelines_for_the_Transport_of_Critically_Ill_Patients. [Accessed 25 February 2023].

66. Goldhill D, Gemmell L, Lutman D, et al. Association of Anaesthetists of Great Britain and Ireland guideline. Interhospital transfer. London: AAGBI; 2009. Available from: http://www.aagbi.org/sites/default/files/interhospital09.pdf. [Accessed 25 February 2023].

67. Kennedy MP, Gabbe BJ, McKenzie BA. Impact of the introduction of an integrated adult retrieval service on major trauma outcomes. Emerg Med J 2015;32(11):833–9.

68. Hu Y, Shi D, You L, et al. Intrahospital transport of critically ill patients: a survey of emergency nurses. Nurs Crit Care 2021;26(5):326–32.

69. Australasian College for Emergency Medicine (ACEM), Australian and New Zealand College of Anaesthetists, College of Intensive Care Medicine of Australia and NewZealand. Guidelines for transport of critically ill patients. Melbourne, VIC: ACEM; 2015. Available from: https://acem.org.au/getmedia/0daba691-5e60-4a88-b6a8-24f2af3e5ebf/Guidelines_for_the_Transport_of_Critically_Ill_Patients. [Accessed 25 February 2023].

70. Yousuf B, Sujatha KS, alfoudri H, et al. Transport of critically ill COVID-19 patients. Intensive Care Med 2020;46(8):1663–4.

71. Salt O, Akpınar M, Sayhan MB, et al. Intrahospital critical patient transport from the emergency department. Arch Med Sci 2020;16(2):337–44.

72. Marshall K. Breathlessness: causes, assessment and non-pharmacological management. Nurs Times 2020;116(9):24–6.

73. Kuzniar T. Assessment of dyspnea. BMJ Best Practice. London: British Medical Journal; 2022. Available from: https://bestpractice.bmj.com/topics/en-gb/862. [Accessed 25 February 2023].

74. Chan ED, Chan MM, Chan MM. Pulse oximetry: understanding its basic principles facilitates appreciation of its limitations. Respir Med 2013;107(6):789–99.

75. Orr B, Roberts J. Respiratory emergencies: the acutely breathless patient. In: Fulde S, Fulde G, editors. Emergency medicine the principles of practice. 7th ed. Sydney, NSW: Elsevier; 2020, p. 216–38.

76. Schrauben SJ, Negoianu D, Costa C, et al. Accuracy of acid–base diagnoses using the central venous blood gas in the medical intensive care unit. Nephron 2018;139(4):293–8.

77. McGowan A, Laveneziana P, Bayat S, et al. International consensus on lung function testing during the COVID-19 pandemic and beyond. ERJ Open Res 2022;8(1):00602–2021.

78. Stapczynski J. Respiratory distress. In: Tintinalli J, Stapczynski J, Ma J, et al, editors. Emergency medicine: a comprehensive study guide. 9th ed. American College of Emergency Physicians. New York: McGraw-Hill; 2019, p. 425–31.

79. Australian Bureau of Statistics (ABS). Asthma. Belconnen, ACT: ABS; 2022. Available from: https://www.abs.gov.au/statistics/health/health-conditions-and-risks/asthma/latest-release#:~:text=Just%20under%202.7%20million%20people,(9.5%25%20and%207.9%25). [Accessed 25 February 2023].

80. Goto TH, K. Acute asthma and status asthmaticus. In: Tintinalli J, Stapczynski J, Ma J, et al, editors. Emergency medicine: a comprehensive study guide. 9th ed. American College of Emergency Physicians. New York: McGraw-Hill; 2019, p. 461–6.

81. National Asthma Council Australia. Asthma management handbook. Melbourne, VIC: National Asthma Council; 2022. Available from: https://www.asthmahandbook.org.au/. [Accessed 25 February 2023].

82. Fanta C, Cahill K. Acute exacerbations of asthma in adults: emergency department and inpatient management. UpToDate; 2022. Available from: https://www.uptodate.com/contents/acute-exacerbations-of-asthma-in-adults-emergency-department-and-inpatient-management. [Accessed 25 February 2023].

83. McMurray A, Cunningham S, Fleming L. Defining near fatal asthma – an international eDelphi study. Eur Respir J 2019;54(Suppl. 63):PA949.

84. Madison J, Irwin R. Identifying patients at risk of fatal asthma: UpToDate; 2022. Available from: https://www.uptodate.com/contents/identifying-patients-at-risk-for-fatal-asthma. [Accessed 25 February 2023].

85. Bates C. Chronic obstructive pulmonary disease. In: Tintinalli J, Stapczynski J, Ma J, et al, editors. Emergency medicine: a comprehensive study guide. 9th ed. American College of Emergency Physicians. New York: McGraw-Hill; 2019, p. 467–72.

86. Anderson E, French S, Maloney G. Community-acquired pneumonia, aspiration pneumonia, and noninfectious pulmonary infiltrates. In: Tintinalli J, Stapczynski J, Ma J, et al, editors. Emergency medicine: a comprehensive study guide. 9th ed. American College of Emergency Physicians. New York: McGraw-Hill; 2019, p. 439–48.

87. Pessoa E, Bárbara C, Viegas L, et al. Factors associated with in-hospital mortality from community-acquired pneumonia in Portugal: 2000–2014. BMC Pulm Med 2020;20(1):18.

88. Cullen L, Greenslade JH, Hawkins T, et al. Improved Assessment of Chest pain Trial (IMPACT): assessing patients with possible acute coronary syndromes. Med J Aust 2017;207(5):195–200.

89. Smith L, Mahler S. Chest pain. In: Tintinalli J, Stapczynski J, Ma J, et al, editors. Emergency medicine: a comprehensive study guide. 9th ed. American College of Emergency Physicians. New York: McGraw-Hill; 2019, p. 329–33.

90. Hollander J, Chase M. Evaluation of the adult with chest pain in the emergency department: UpToDate; 2022. Available from: https://www.uptodate.com/contents/evaluation-of-the-adult-with-chest-pain-in-the-emergency-department. [Accessed 25 February 2023].

91. Parsonage WA, Cullen L, Younger JF. The approach to patients with possible cardiac chest pain. Med J Aust 2013;199(1):30–4.

92. DeVon HA, Burke LA, Vuckovic KM, et al. Symptoms suggestive of acute coronary syndrome: when is sex important? J Cardiovasc Nurs 2017;32(4):383–92.

93. Isaksson RM, Brulin C, Eliasson M, et al. Older women's prehospital experiences of their first myocardial infarction. J Cardiovasc Nurs 2013;28(4):360–9.

94. Saccasan P, Whelan A. The approach to the patient with chest pain or dyspnoea. In: Fulde S, Fulde G, editors. Emergency medicine the principles of practice. 7th ed. Sydney, NSW: Elsevier; 2020, p. 157–75.

95. Hofmann R, James SK, Jernberg T, et al; DETO2X–SWEDEHEART Investigators. Oxygen therapy in suspected acute myocardial infarction. N Engl J Med 2017;377(23):1240.

96. Chew D, Scott IA, Cullen L, et al. National Heart Foundation of Australia and New Zealand: Australian clinical guidelines for the management of acute coronary syndromes 2016. Med J Aust 2016;205(3):128–33.

97. Maruno K. Acute coronary syndromes. In: Fulde S, Fulde G, editors. Emergency medicine the principles of practice. 7th ed. Sydney, NSW: Elsevier; 2020, p. 176–88.

98. Gardiner FW, Rallah-Baker K, Dos Santos A, et al. Indigenous Australians have a greater prevalence of heart, stroke, and vascular disease, are younger at death, with higher hospitalisation and more aeromedical retrievals from remote regions. eClinicalMedicine 2021;42.

99. Australian Institute of Health and Welfare (AIHW). Deaths in Australia. Canberra, ACT: AIHW; 2022. Available from: https://www.aihw.gov.au/reports/life-expectancy-death/deaths-in-australia/contents/leading-causes-of-death. [Accessed 25 February 2023].

100. Bautz B, Schneider JI. High-risk chief complaints i: chest pain-the big three (an update). Emerg Med Clin North Am 2020;38(2):453–98.

101. Johnson G, Prince L. Aortic dissection and related aortic syndromes. In: Tintinalli J, Stapczynski J, Ma J, et al, editors. Emergency medicine; a comprehensive study guide. American College of Emergency Physicians. 9th ed. New York: McGraw-Hill; 2019, p. 412–14.

102. Khan IA, Nair CK. Clinical, diagnostic, and management perspectives of aortic dissection. Chest 2002;122(1):311–28.

103. Fojtik JP, Costantino TG, Dean AJ. The diagnosis of aortic dissection by emergency medicine ultrasound. J Emerg Med 2007;32(2):191–6.

104. Australian Institute of Health and Welfare (AIHW). Emergency department care activity. Canberra, ACT: AIHW; 2022. Available from: https://www.aihw.gov.au/reports-data/myhospitals/intersection/activity/ed. [Accessed 25 February 2023].

105. Kendall J. Evaluation of the adult with abdominal pain in the emergency department. UpToDate; 2022. Available from: https://www.uptodate.com/contents/evaluation-of-the-adult-with-abdominal-pain-in-the-emergency-department. [Accessed 25 February 2023].

106. Masneri D, O'Brien M. Acute abdominal pain. In: Tintinalli J, Stapczynski J, Ma J, et al, editors. Emergency medicine: a comprehensive study guide. 9th ed. American College of Emergency Physicians. New York: McGraw-Hill; 2019, p. 473–80.

107. Dagiely S. An algorithm for triaging commonly missed causes of acute abdominal pain. J Emer Nurs 2006;32(1):9.

108. Muntlin A, Carlsson M, Safwenberg U, et al. Outcomes of a nurse-initiated intravenous analgesic protocol for abdominal pain in an emergency department: a quasi-experimental study. Int J Nurs Stud 2011;48(1):13–23.

109. Day R, Fordyce J. Approaches to abdominal pain. In: Cameron P, Little M, Mitra B, et al, editors. Textbook of adult emergency medicine. 5th ed. Edinburgh: Elsevier; 2020, p. 302–8.

110. Murphy A. Aneurysms. In: Cameron P, Little M, Mitra B, et al, editors. Textbook of adult emergency medicine. 5th ed. Edinburgh: Elsevier; 2020, p. 259–61.

111. Banerjee A. Acute appendicitis. In: Cameron P, Little M, Mitra B, et al, editors. Textbook of adult emergency medicine. 5th ed. Edinburgh: Elsevier; 2020, p. 333–5.

112. DeKoning E. Acute appendicitis. In: Tintinalli J, Stapczynski J, Ma J, et al, editors. Emergency medicine: a comprehensive study guide. 9th ed. American College of Emergency Physicians. New York: McGraw-Hill; 2019, p. 523–6.

113. Smink D, Soybel D. Management of acute appendicitis in adults. UpToDate; 2022. Available from: https://www.uptodate.com/contents/management-of-acute-appendicitis-in-adults. [Accessed 25 February 2023].

114. Price T. Bowel obstruction. In: Tintinalli J, Stapczynski J, Ma J, et al, editors. Emergency medicine: a comprehensive study guide. 9th ed. American College of Emergency Physicians. New York: McGraw-Hill; 2019, p. 530–1.

115. Yates K. Bowel obstruction. In: Cameron P, Little M, Mitra B, et al, editors. Textbook of adult emergency medicine. 5th ed. Edinburgh: Elsevier; 2020, p. 309–11.

116. Bordeianou L, Yeh DD. Etiologies, clinical manifestations, and diagnosis of mechanical small bowel obstruction in adults. UpToDate; 2022. Available from: https://www.uptodate.com/contents/etiologies-clinical-manifestations-and-diagnosis-of-mechanical-small-bowel-obstruction-in-adults?search=bowel%20obstruction&source=search_result&selectedTitle=1~150&usage_type=default&display_rank=1#H1. [Accessed 25 February 2023].

117. Tan G. Ectopic pregnancy and bleeding in early pregnancy. In: Cameron P, Little M, Mitra B, et al, editors. Textbook of adult emergency medicine. 5th ed. Edinburgh: Elsevier; 2020, p. 576–8.

118. Caplan L. Stroke: etiology, classification, and epidemiology. UpToDate; 2022. Available from: https://www.uptodate.com/contents/stroke-etiology-classification-and-epidemiology?search=Stroke:%20Etiology,%20classification,%20and%20epidemiology&source=search_result&selectedTitle=1~150&usage_type=default&display_rank=1. [Accessed 25 February 2023].

119. Go S. Stroke ansyndromes. In: Tintinalli J, Stapczynski J, Ma J, et al, editors. Emergency medicine: a comprehensive study guide. 9th ed. American College of Emergency Physicians. New York: McGraw-Hill; 2019, p. 1119–36.

120. Oliveira-Filho J, Samuels O. Approach to reperfusion therapy for acute ischemic stroke: UpToDate; 2022. Available from: https://www.uptodate.com/contents/approach-to-reperfusion-therapy-for-acute-ischemic-stroke. [Accessed 25 February 2023].

121. Zhang R, Wang Y, Fang J, et al. Worldwide 1-month case fatality of ischaemic stroke and the temporal trend. Stroke Vasc Neurol 2020;5(4):353.

122. Clery A, Bhalla A, Bisquera A, et al. Long-term trends in stroke survivors discharged to care homes: the South London Stroke Register. Stroke 2020;51(1):179–85.

123. Aguirreberrena G. Neurological emergencies. In: Fulde S, Fulde G, editors. Emergency medicine the principles of practice. 7th ed. Sydney, NSW: Elsevier; 2020, p. 262–84.

124. Munroe B, Hutchinson C. Patient assessment and essentials of care. In: Curtis K, Ramsden C, Shaban RZ, et al, editors. Emergency and trauma care for nurses and paramedics. 3rd ed. Chatswood, NSW: Elsevier; 2019, p. 243–80

125. Kim SM, Woo HG, Kim YJ, et al. Blood pressure management in stroke patients. J Neurocrit Care 2020;13(2):69–79.

126. Uphaus T, Grings A, Groschel S, et al. Automatic detection of paroxysmal atrial fibrillation in patients with ischaemic stroke: better than routine diagnostic workup? Eur J Neurol 2017;24:990–4.

127. Oliveira-Filho J, Mullen M. Initial assessment and management of acute stroke. UpToDate; 2022. Available from: https://www.uptodate.com/contents/initial-assessment-and-management-of-acute-stroke?search=Initial%20assessment%20and%20management%20of%20acute%20stroke&source=search_result&selectedTitle=1~150&usage_type=default&display_rank=1. [Accessed 25 February 2023].

128. Finnell JT. Alcohol-related disease. In: Walls RM, Hockberger RS, Gausche-Hill M, editors. Rosen's emergency medicine: concepts and clinical practice. 10th ed. Philadelphia, PA: Elsevier; 2023, p. 1846–60.

129. World Health Organization (WHO). Suicide. Geneva: WHO; 2021 Available from: https://www.who.int/news-room/fact-sheets/detail/suicide. [Accessed 25 February 2023].

130. Australian Institute of Health and Welfare (AIHW). Australia's health 2022: in brief. Canberra, ACT: AIHW; 2022. Available from: https://www.aihw.gov.au/reports/australias-health/australias-health-2022-in-brief/summary. [Accessed 25 February 2023].

131. Sellors K. Poisoning and overdose. In: Fulde S, Fulde G, editors. Emergency medicine the principles of practice. 7th ed. Sydney, NSW: Elsevier; 2020, p. 285–319.

132. Meehan TJ. Care of the poisoned patient. In: Walls R, Hockberger RS, Gausche-Hill M, editors. Rosen's emergency medicine: concepts and clinical practice. 10th ed. Philadelphia: Elsevier; 2023, p. 1827–36.

133. Locci C, Cuzzolin L, Capobianco G, et al. Paracetamol overdose in the newborn and infant: a life-threatening event. Eur J Clin Pharmacol 2021;77(6):809–15.

134. Wikibooks. Emergency medicine/altered mental status. 2019. Available from: https://en.wikibooks.org/wiki/Emergency_Medicine/Altered_mental_status. [Accessed 25 February 2023].

135. Beauchamp GA, Carey JL, Adams T, et al. Sex differences in poisonings among older adults: an analysis of the Toxicology Investigators Consortium (ToxIC) Registry, 2010 to 2016. Clin Ther 2018;40(8):1366–74.e8.

136. Abhilash KPP. Emergency medicine. Delhi: Jaypee Brothers Medical Publishers; 2018.

137. Wyatt JP, Taylor RG, de Wit K, et al. Oxford handbook of emergency medicine. Oxford, UK: Oxford University Press; 2020.

138. Gunja N. Poisoning. In: Cameron P, editor. Textbook of paediatric emergency medicine. 3rd ed. Chatswood, NSW: Elsevier; 2019, p. 465–78.

139. Chitty KM, Kirby K, Osborne NJ, et al. Co-ingested alcohol and the timing of deliberate self-poisonings. Aust N Z J psychiatry 2018;52(3):271–8.

140. Menezes RG, Rizwan T, Khan A, et al. Homicidal pesticide poisoning – an overview. Forensic Sci Rev 2021;33(1):67–78.

141. Ferri FF. Tricyclic antidepressant overdose. In: Ferri's clinical advisor. Philadelphia: Elsevier; 2022, p. 1501.e11–13.

142. De Pralormo S, Brunet M, Marquis A, et al. Ingestion of bar soap may produce serious injury: clinical effects and risk factors. Clin Toxicol (Phila) 2019;57(5):356–61.

143. Hatten BW. Aspirin and nonsteriodal agents. In: Walls R, Hockberger RS, Gausche-Hill M, editors. Rosen's emergency medicine: concepts and clinical practice. 10th ed. Philadelphia: Elsevier; 2023, p. 1867–83.

144. Therapeutic Guidelines. Iron poisoning. Melbourne, VIC: Therapeutic Guidelines; 2021. Available from: https://tgldcdp.tg.org.au/quideLine?guidelinePage=Toxicology+and+Toxinology&frompage=etgcomplete. [Accessed 25 February 2023].

145. Minns AB, Clark RF. Substance abuse. In: Walls R, Hockberger RS, Gausche-Hill M, editors. Rosen's emergency medicine: concepts and clinical practice. 9th ed. Philadelphia: Elsevier; 2018, p. 1823–8.e1.

146. Shukla L, Ghadigaonkar DS, Murthy P. Poisoning with drugs of abuse: identification and management. Indian J Crit Care Med 2019; 23(Suppl. 4):S296–304.

147. Chary MA, Ericksen TB. Cocaine and other sympathomimetics. In: Walls R, Hockberger RS, Gausche-Hill M, et al, editors. Rosen's emergency medicine: concepts and clinical practice. 10th ed. Philadehia: Elsevier; 2023, p. 1906–16.

148. Australian Government. What are drugs? Canberra, ACT: Australian Government; 2019. Available from: https://www.health.gov.au/health-topics/drugs/about-drugs/what-are-drugs. [Accessed 25 February 2023].

149. Parrott AC. Why all stimulant drugs are damaging to recreational users: an empirical overview and psychobiological explanation. Hum Psychopharmacol 2015;30(4):213–24.

150. Hoggett KA. Drugs of abuse. In: Cameron P, Little M, Mitra B, et al, editors. Textbook of adult emergency medicine. 5th ed. Edinburgh: Elsevier; 2020, p. 773–7.

151. Vivolo-Kantor AM, Hoots BE, Seth P, et al. Recent trends and associated factors of amphetamine-type stimulant overdoses in emergency departments. Drug Alcohol Depend 2020;216:108323.

152. Gladden RM, O'Donnell J, Mattson CL, et al. Changes in opioid-involved overdose deaths by opioid type and presence of benzodiazepines, cocaine, and methamphetamine - 25 states, July–December 2017 to January–June 2018. MMWR Morbid Mortal Wkly Rep 2019;68(34):737–44.

153. Graudins A, Green D. Salicylate. In: Cameron P, Little M, Mitra B, et al, editors. Textbook of adult emergency medicine. 5th ed. Edinburgh: Elsevier; 2020, p. 760–2.

154. Graudins A, Wong A. Paracetamol. In: Cameron P, Little M, Mitra B, et al, editors. Textbook of adult emergency medicine. 5th ed. Edinburgh: Elsevier; 2020, p. 756–60.

155. Chiew AL, Reith D, Pomerleau A, et al. Updated guidelines for the management of paracetamol poisoning in Australia and New Zealand. Med J Aust 2020;212(4):175–83.

156. Queensland Health, Royal Flying Doctor Service (Queensland section). Primary clinical care manual. 11th ed. Cairns: Office of Rural and Remote Health, Queensland Government; 2022.

157. Buckley NA. Carbon monoxide. In: Cameron P, Little M, Mitra B, et al, editors. Textbook of adult emergency medicine. 5th ed. Edinburgh: Elsevier; 2020, p. 798–801.

158. Meadan CW, Nelson LS. Inhaled toxins. In: Walls R, Hockberger RS, Gausche-Hill M, editors. Rosen's emergency medicine: concepts and clinical practice. 10th ed. Philadelphia: Elsevier; 2023, 1940–7.

159. Graudins A, Alfred S. Hydrofluoric acid. 2020. In: Cameron P, Little M, Mitra B, et al, editors. Textbook of adult emergency medicine. 5th ed. Edinburgh: Elsevier; 2020, p. 781–3.

160. Hoyte C. Caustics. In: Walls R, Hockberger RS, Gausche-Hill M, editors. Rosen's emergency medicine: concepts and clinical practice. 10th ed. Philadelphia: Elsevier; 2023, p. 1900–5.

161. Wang GS, Buchanan JA. Hydrocarbons. In: Walls R, Hockberger RS, Gausche-Hill M, editors. Rosen's emergency medicine: concepts and clinical practice. Philadelphia, PA: Elsevier. 10th ed. 2023, p. 1935–9.

162. Roberts DM, Bode M. Pesticides. 2020. In: Cameron P, Little M, Mitra B, et al, editors. Textbook of adult emergency medicine. 5th ed. Edinburgh: Elsevier; 2020, p. 784–8.

163. Osborne NJ, Cairns R, Dawson AH, et al. Epidemiology of coronial deaths from pesticide ingestion in Australia. Int J Hyg Environ Health 2017;220(2):478–84.

164. Roberts DM. Pesticides. In: Cameron P, Jelinek G, Kelly A, et al, editors. Textbook of adult emergency medicine. 4th ed. Edinburgh: Elsevier; 2014, p. 1017–23.

165. Welker K, Thompson TM. Pesticides. In: Walls R, M., Hockberger RS, Gausche-Hill M, editors. Rosen's emergncy medicine: concepts and clinical practice. 10th ed. Philadelphia, PA: Elsevier; 2023, p. 1962–71.

166. Isbister GK. Spider bite. 2020. In: Cameron P, Little M, Mitra B, et al, editors. Textbook of adult emergency medicine. 5th ed. Edinburgh: Elsevier; 2020, p. 827–30.

167. Bryan SA, van Heezik Y, Vink CJ, et al. Invasive redback spiders (Latrodectus hasseltii) threaten an endangered, endemic New Zealand beetle (Prodontria lewisii). J Insect Conserv 2015;19(5):1021–7.

168. Isbister GKFMD, Page CBMF, Buckley NAFMD, et al. Randomized controlled trial of intravenous antivenom versus placebo for latrodectism: the second Redback Antivenom Evaluation (RAVE-II) Study. Ann Emerg Med 2014;64(6):620–8.e2.

169. Cocks J. Response to Re: Redback spider bites in children in South Australia: a 10-year review of antivenom effectiveness. Emerg Med Australas 2022;34(2):298–9.

170. Downes MA, Lovett CJ, Berling I, et al. Re: Redback spider bites in children in South Australia: A 10-year review of antivenom effectiveness. Emerg Med Australas 2022;34(2):297–8.

171. Kilham HA, Isbister GK. Australian funnel-web spider envenoming. J Paediatr Child Health 2020;56(12):1843–5.

172. Isbister GK. Snakebite. 2020. In: Cameron P, Little M, Mitra B, et al, editors. Textbook of adult emergency medicine. 5th ed. Edinburgh: Elsevier; 2020, p. 819–23.e1.

173. Australian Venom Research Unit. Snakebite in Australia. Parkville, VIC: University of Melbourne; 2018.

174. Welton RE, Williams DJ, Liew D. Injury trends from envenoming in Australia, 2000–2013. Intern Med J 2017;47(2):170–6.

175. Zdenek CN. 7 reasons Australia is the lucky country when it comes to snakes. London: The Conversation Media Group; 2022. Available from: https://theconversation.com/7-reasons-australia-is-the-lucky-country-when-it-comes-to-snakes-175188. [Accessed 25 February 2023].

176. Welton RE, Liew D, Braitberg G. Incidence of fatal snake bite in Australia: a coronial based retrospective study (2000–2016). Toxicon (Oxford) 2017;131:11–15.

177. Mackessy SP. Handbook of venoms and toxins of reptiles. Milton, MA: CRC Press; 2021.

178. Murray L, Little M, Pascu O, et al. Toxicology handbook. Chatswood, NSW: Elsevier Australia; 2015. Available from: https://www.clinicalkey.com.au/dura/browse/bookChapter/3-s2.0-C20140004121. [Accessed 25 February 2023].

179. White J. Exotic snakebite. 2020. In: Cameron P, Little M, Mitra B, et al, editors. Textbook of adult emergency medicine. 5th ed. Edinburgh: Elsevier; 2020, p. 824–7.

180. Ratnayake I, Shihana F, Dissanayake DM, et al. Performance of the 20-minute whole blood clotting test in detecting venom induced consumption coagulopathy from Russell's viper (Daboia russelii) bites. Thromb Haemost 2017;117(3):500–7.

181. Tibballs J. Australian snake antivenom dosing: what is scientific and safe? Anaesth Intensive Care 2020;48(2):129–33.

182. Seymour JE. Are we using the correct first aid for jellyfish? Med J Aust 2017;206(6):249–50.

183. Seymour JE, Pereira P. Marine injury, envenomation and poisoning 2020. In: Cameron P, Little M, Mitra B, et al, editors. Textbook of adult emergency medicine. 5th ed. Edinburgh: Elsevier; 2020, p. 831–4.

184. Tiemensma M, Currie BJ, Byard RW. Fatal jellyfish envenoming – pediatric and geographic vulnerabilities. J Forensic Sci 2021;66(5):2006–9.

185. Guardian staff. Teenager dies after box jellyfish sting at Queensland beach. Guardian. 2022 28th February 2022. Available from: https://www.theguardian.com/australia-news/2022/feb/28/teenager-dies-after-box-jellyfish-sting-at-queensland-beach. [Accessed 25 February 2023].

186. Baile S. Box jellyfish in Australia – 9 facts about the world's deadliest jellyfish. Diamond Creek, VIC: Expedition Australia; 2019. Available from: https://www.expeditionaustralia.com.au/2019/07/box-jellyfish-in-australia-9-facts-about-the-worlds-deadliest-jellyfish/. [Accessed 25 February 2023].

187. Isoardi KZ, Isbister GK. Poisoning by venomous animals. Medicine 2020;48(3):220–3.

188. Perkins A. Marine poisonings, envenomations, and trauma. In: Kellerman RD, Bope ET, editors. Conn's current therapy [e-book]. Philadelphia: Elsevier; 2018, p. 1243–7.

189. Farrell H, Murray SA, Zammit A, et al. Management of ciguatoxin risk in Eastern Australia. Toxins 2017;9(11):367.

190. Friedman MA, Fernandez M, Backer LC, et al. An updated review of ciguatera fish poisoning: clinical, epidemiological, environmental, and public health management. Marine Drugs 2017;15(3):72.

191. Hungerford JM. Histamine and scombrotoxins. Toxicon (Oxford) 2021;201:115–26.

192. Gonzalez JM, McGhee S, Ortega J. Facial flushing, nausea, sweating, and palpitations after eating fish. J Nurse Practitioners 2021;17(8):1042–4.

193. Feng C, Teuber S, Gershwin ME. Histamine (Scombroid) Fish poisoning: a comprehensive review. Clin Rev Allergy Immunol 2015;50(1):64–9.

194. Meisenheimer E, Bevis Z, Tagawa C, et al. Drowning injuries: an update on terminology, environmental factors, and management. Curr Sports Med Rep 2016;15(2):91–3.

195. Chandy D, Weinhouse G. Drowning (submersion injuries): UpToDate; 2021 [updated August 19th 2021. Available from: https://www.uptodate.com/contents/drowning-submersion-injuries. [Accessed 25 February 2023].

196. World Health Organization (WHO). Drowning. Fact sheet. Geneva: WHO; 2021. Available from: https://www.who.int/news-room/fact-sheets/detail/drowning. [Accessed 25 February 2023].

197. Centers for Disease Control and Prevention (CDC). Drowning prevention. Atlanta, GA: CDC; 2022. Available from: https://www.cdc.gov/drowning/facts/index.html.

198. Royal Life Saving Australia. National drowning report 2021. Broadway, NSW: Royal Life Saving Australia; 2022. Available from: https://www.royallifesaving.com.au/__data/assets/pdf_file/0007/50110/RLS_NationalDrowningReport2021_LR.pdf. [Accessed 25 February 2023].

199. Australian Institute of Health and Welfare (AIHW). Drowning and submersion. Canberra, ACT: AIHW; 2022. Available from: https://www.aihw.gov.au/reports/injury/drowning-and-submersion. [Accessed 25 February 2023].

200. Gaida F, Gaida J. Infand and toddler drowning in Australia: patterns, risk factors and prevention recommendations. J Paediatrics Child Health 2016;52:923–7.

201. Martinez FE, Hooper AJ. Drowning and immersion injury. Anaesth Intens Care Med 2014;15(9):420–3.

202. Mountain D. Drowning. In: Cameron P, Little M, Mitra B, et al, editors. Textbook of adult emergency medicine. 5th ed. Edinburgh: Elsevier; 2020, p. 719–23.

203. Robinson K. Drowning. In: Fulde S, Fulde G, editors. Emergency medicine the principles of practice. 7th ed. Sydney, NSW: Elsevier; 2020, p. 861–9.

204. Shepherd S. Submersion injury, near drowning. Patient; 2010. http://www.patient.co.uk/. [Accessed Dec 2014; no longer available online].

205. Cantwell G, Verive M. Drowning treatment and management 2021 [updated 21 October 2021. Available from: https://emedicine.medscape.com/article/772753-treatment. [Accessed 25 February 2023].

206. Quan L, Mack CD, Schiff MA. Association of water temperature and submersion duration and drowning outcome. Resuscitation 2014;85(6):790–4.

207. Fulde G. Hypothermia and hyperthermia. In: Fulde S, Fulde G, editors. Emergency medicine the principles of practice. 7th ed. Sydney, NSW: Elsevier; 2020, p. 897–910.

208. Rogers I. Hypothermia. In: Cameron P, Little M, Mitra B, et al, editors. Textbook of adult emergency medicine. 5th ed. Edinburgh: Elsevier; 2020, p. 702–5.

209. Zafren K, Mechem C. Accidental hypothermia in adults. UpToDate; 2022. Available from: https://www.uptodate.com/contents/accidental-hypothermia-in-adults?search=Accidental%20hypothermia%20in%20adults&source=search_result&selectedTitle=1,150&usage_type=default&display_rank=1. [Accessed 25 February 2023].

210. Tsuei B, Kearney P. Hypothermia in the trauma patient. Injury 2005;35(1):7–15.

211. Gamage PJ, Finch CF, Fortington LV. Document analysis of exertional heat illness policies and guidelines published by sports organisations in Victoria, Australia. BMJ Open Sport Exerc Med 2020;6(1):e000591.

212. Rogers I. Heat-related illness. In: Cameron P, Little M, Mitra B, et al, editors. Textbook of adult emergency medicine. 5th ed. Edinburgh: Elsevier; 2020, p. 700–1.

213. Mechem C. Severe non-exertional hyperthermia (classic heat stroke) in adults: UpToDate; 2022. Available from: https://www.uptodate.com/contents/severe-nonexertional-hyperthermia-classic-heat-stroke-in-adults?search=Severe%20non-exertional%20hyperthermia%20(classic%20heat%20stroke)%20in%20adults:%20&source=search_result&selectedTitle=1~150&usage_type=default&display_rank=1. [Accessed 25 February 2023].

214. LoVecchio F. Heat emergencies. In: Tintinalli J, Ma J, Yealy D, et al, editors. Emergency medicine: a comprehensive study guide. 9th ed. American College of Emergency Physicians. New York: McGraw-Hill; 2019, p. 1345–9.

215. Samarasinghe I, Wassertheil J. Mass casualty incidents, chemical, biological and radiological hazard contingencies. In: Fulde S, Fulde G, editors. Emergency medicine the principles of practice. 7th ed. Sydney, NSW: Elsevier; 2020, p. 911–54.

216. Wieteska S, editor. Major incident medical management and support: the practical approach at the scene. 3rd ed. Sydney, NSW: Wiley-Blackwell; 2012.

217. Affairs DfH. Australian disaster resilience handbook collection: Australian emergency management arrangements (Third Edition). Canberra: DHA; 2019.

218. Markenson D, Losinsik S. Hospital and emergency department preparedness. In: Veenema T, editor. Disaster nursing and emergency preparedness: for chemical, biological, and radiological terrorism, and other hazards. 4th ed. New York: Springer; 2018, 51–66.

219. Veenema T. Essentials of disaster planning. In: Veenema T, editor. Disaster nursing and emergency preparedness: for chemical, biological, and radiological terrorism, and other hazards. 4th ed. New York: Springer; 2018, p. 1–22.

220. Hendrickson R, Horowitz B. Disaster preparedness. In: Tintinalli J, Stapczynski J, Ma J, et al, editors. Emergency medicine: a comprehensive study guide. 9th ed. American College of Emergency Physicians. New York: McGraw-Hill; 201, p. 19–24.

221. Romig L, Brooke L. Disaster triage. In: Veenema T, editor. Disaster nursing and emergency preparedness: for chemical, biological, and radiological terrorism, and other hazards. 4th ed. New York: Springer; 2018, p. 379–98.

222. Howard PK, Foley AL. Disaster triage – are you ready? J Emerg Nurs 2014;40(5):515–17.

223. Croddy E, Ackerman G. Biological and chemical terrorism: a unique threat. In: Veenema t, editor. Disaster nursing and emergency preparedness: for chemical, biological, and radiological terrorism, and other hazards. 4th ed. New York: Springer; 2018, p. 465–82.

224. Loden J, Kice S, Benitez J. Chemical agents of concern. In: Veenema T, editor. Disaster nursing and emergency preparedness: for chemical, biological, and radiological terrorism, and other hazards. 4th ed. New York: Springer; 2018, p. 483–506.

225. Varma. D, Guest. I. The Bhopal accident and methyl isocyanate toxicity. J Toxicol Environ Health 1993;40(4):513–29.

226. Pigot D, Kazzi Z, Nafziger S. Biological agents of concern. In: Veenema T, editor. Disaster nursing and emergency preparedness: for chemical, biological, and radiological terrorism, and other hazards. 4th ed. New York: Springer; 2018, p. 507–24.

227. Karam A. Radiological incidents and emergencies. In: Veenema T, editor. Disaster nursing and emergency preparedness: for chemical, biological, and radiological terrorism, and other hazards. 4th ed. New York: Springer; 2018, p. 569–90.

228. Carlson S, Meeker E, Plum K, Veenema T. Management of the psychosocial effects of disasters. In: eenema T, editor. Disaster nursing and emergency preparedness: for chemical, biological, and radiological terrorism, and other hazards. 4th ed. New York: Springer; 2018, p. 167–78.

229. Okumura T, Hisaoka T, Yamada A, et al. The Tokyo subway sarin attack – lessons learned. Toxicol Appl Pharmacol 2005;207(2 Suppl.):471–6.

230. Cornish S, Klim S, Kelly AM. Is COVID19 the straw that broke the back of the emergency nursing workforce? Emerg Med Australas 2021;33(6):1095–9.

Chapter 24

Trauma management

Catherine Bell, Kerstin Prignitz Sluys

Learning objectives

After reading this chapter, you should be able to:

- identify the benefits and limitations of an organised trauma system
- describe the rationale for a systematic approach to the patient who has sustained injuries
- discuss the benefits of appropriate management of the patient with serious injury and/or multitrauma
- describe the acute management of the patient with multiple serious fractures
- describe the acute management of patients with burn injuries, abdominal injuries and chest trauma
- describe the nurse's role in managing the trauma patient undergoing damage-control resuscitation.

Introduction

Injuries continue to be a major public health concern worldwide, whether measured by years of productive life lost, prolonged or permanent disability, or financial cost. The Global Burden of Diseases, Injuries, and Risk Factor Study (GBD 2019) estimated that injuries accounted for 8% of total deaths annually.[1] In adolescents aged 10–24 years, road injuries (ranked first), self-harm (third) and interpersonal violence (fifth) were among the top causes of premature deaths and disability-adjusted life-years; similarly, deaths as a result of road injuries were ranked first in the 25–45-year group.

The epidemiology of injury differs with severity. The majority of injured patients requiring admission to an ICU are those with serious injuries associated with motor vehicles, motorbikes and pedestrian collisions. Falls, self-inflicted injuries and assaults are less common, but still lead to critical care admission. A significant proportion of injured patients admitted to critical care have experienced neurotrauma (see Chapter 17), while other common injuries include multiple fractures and injury to internal organs in the thorax and abdomen.

The systematic organisation of trauma systems, major changes in practice and delivery of time-critical interventions have made the traditional boundaries between pre-hospital emergency medical service and hospital-based emergency, surgery, radiology and intensive care services more seamless, improving the survival of trauma patients in recent years. Consequently, a greater number of patients with severe multiple injuries are now admitted to critical care units. These patients generally require complex nursing care, often for lengthy periods, both within the ICU and beyond. The common traumatic injuries that result in admission to adult critical care and the principles of management are outlined in this chapter. Paediatric trauma is covered in Chapter 27. The terms 'injury' and 'trauma' are used interchangeably in this text.

Trauma systems and processes

The establishment of trauma systems in middle- to high-income countries has been found to reduce mortality, improve patient outcomes and reduce costs[2] because of the consistent operational components that are included. Each system is organised to meet the local requirements, including economic development and social structures available. Trauma systems are an organised and integrated approach to care delivery for the injured person from the site of injury, appropriate hospital or trauma facility that has the capacity to care for the person through rehabilitation and return to ideal functioning. The operational components in a trauma system should include injury prevention, pre-hospital care, acute care facilities and post-hospital care, appropriate human resources and evaluation.

There have been two systems developed, initially an exclusive system and subsequently in 1991 an inclusive system. In exclusive systems all injured patients are referred to a centralised healthcare facility, bypassing the resources of other healthcare facilities in the region. The disadvantages of this are that non-designated centres become deskilled, while the designated centres may also become overwhelmed by increased volume of admissions. In inclusive systems, all healthcare facilities within a region are involved in the care of the injured patient within the capabilities of their resources and proximity. Referral to high-level trauma centres for the most severely injured patients is the objective and relies on intra-hospital transport service support.[2] Both systems consist of a public health model that is designed to reduce morbidity and mortality.

Dedicated care provided in a major trauma centre has been reported to improve outcomes in the USA, Canada, Australia and UK, with an established relationship between trauma centre volume and outcomes, although inclusive trauma systems that have a lower volume of trauma admissions have also demonstrated improved outcomes.

Pre-hospital care

There is a wide variation in the level of pre-hospital care that is provided, ranging from basic life support (BLS) to advanced life support (ALS),[3] with the principle of delivering quality patient care for the briefest period of time post injury while facilitating rapid transport to hospital. Globally, there is a wide range of pre-hospital trauma care, including non-existent, BLS provided by emergency medical service (EMS), non-physician advanced life support,[3] physician and/or pre-hospital nurse ALS. Within each system, the skill level of the EMS providers can vary, with BLS providers able to initiate minimally invasive care and focus primarily on prompt transportation of the patient, and those with ALS skills able to provide advanced level interventions such as intubation, administration of intravenous (IV) fluids and medications.

Three principles of pre-hospital trauma care include examination and recognition of injuries with potential to cause rapid decompensation, triage if there are multiple victims and stabilisation and transport to a hospital capable of coping with identified injuries.[4]

Pre-hospital care is a fundamental element of an organised trauma system with an agreed triage process at each step of the patient's journey. The elements of the pre-hospital system include:

1 EMS transport system, including paramedic-, physician- or nurse-led care

2 triage protocols and coordinated dispatch including communication between EMS and hospitals

3 appropriate transport platforms, and agreed protocols for hospital designation, trauma bypass and inter-hospital transfer.[5]

Incorporated with appropriate pre-hospital triage and transport is the need to implement BLS including airway, breathing and haemorrhage control. There are generally two models of pre-hospital care of the trauma patient, commonly referred to as either 'scoop and run' or 'stay and play'. The first relies on minimal interventions, BLS and quick transport, while the second includes ALS interventions which may delay transport to higher levels of care. Both concepts remain controversial and the relationship between survival and scene time remains unclear.[6] These concepts follow on from the 'Golden Hour', first articulated in the 1970s when it was considered that mortality decreased if patients receive definitive care within 60 minutes of injury, although evidence remains inconsistent.[7,8] The first hour post injury represents the first peak in trimodal distribution of mortality in the trauma population.[9] Advances in pre-hospital management such as resuscitative endovascular balloon occlusion of the aorta (REBOA), massive transfusion and helicopter emergency medical services (HEMS) may be influencing survival and challenging the previously held dogma.[7]

Transport of the critically ill trauma patient

As suggested by the Golden Hour principle, trauma is a time-sensitive condition. Transport of the trauma patient includes primary transport directly to the trauma centre, as well as secondary transport or retrieval from one healthcare facility to another for specialty services.

In most developed countries, primary transportation of the injured patient is by road ambulance or helicopter, although other modes of transport are widely used worldwide, such as private vehicles or police cars. Randomised trials comparing road and helicopter transport are few; however, reviews in England and the USA have demonstrated a 15% risk-adjusted mortality reduction when transported via HEMS, with similar results reported in a study in the Netherlands.[10]

Secondary transfer of trauma patients between healthcare facilities can occur via ground or air EMS. Air EMS is either helicopter or fixed wing depending on available services, distance and weather conditions. Secondary transfer of an injured person may occur for clinical reasons, such as specialist availability or the requirement for higher levels of care, or for non-clinical reasons such as bed availability. Factors that can influence the choice of transport vehicle for the trauma patient include:

- nature of trauma
- possible clinical impact of the transport environment
- urgency of intervention
- distances involved
- number of retrieval personnel and volume of accompanying equipment
- road transport times and road conditions
- weather conditions and aviation restrictions
- aircraft landing facilities
- range and speed of vehicle.[11,12]

General principles related to the transport of critically ill and injured patients are covered in Chapter 23.

Trauma reception

Reception of the trauma patient at the emergency department (ED) is generally performed by the triage nurse, with patients managed in designated resuscitation areas and received by a trauma team. In the severely injured patient, a multidisciplinary team receives the patient and commences assessment and treatment concurrently.

Healthcare systems generally use triage to establish the appropriate destination for an injured patient based on severity of injury and facility resources to prevent over- or under-triage of patients. The three phases of triage for the injured patient include the pre-hospital dispatch of an ambulance or pre-hospital care resources, assessment by the first clinician at the scene and then in the ED on patient arrival at the healthcare facility.[13,14] One of the

confounders in triage is the lack of consensus on what is defined as a 'major trauma', which in turn may lead to suboptimal care provision related to the over-triage or under-triage of patients to trauma centres or other healthcare facilities. The other identified confounder is EMS provider initial clinical assessment and familiarity with local service providers impacting destination decisions rather than adherence to guidelines.[14]

In a mass-casualty incident, triage may be performed in the field. Despite documented benefits, such as shorter ED time, ED to computed tomographic imaging time, ED to operating room time and improved survival, having a trauma team is not universal, even within advanced trauma systems.[12]

In the ED, the trauma team receives the patient after a comprehensive, clear handover that is heard by the entire team. The importance of a handover from the pre-hospital teams or paramedics cannot be overestimated.

The formal process of triage provides a means of categorising patients based on threat to life, including rapid, standardised initial assessment and prioritisation. Although there are many different triage systems in use, those with widespread adoption and published evidence include the Australasian Triage Scale (ATS), the Canadian Triage and Acuity Scale (CTAS), the Emergency Severity Index (ESI), the Manchester Triage Scale (MTS) and the South African Triage Scale (SATS), with shared core concepts of identifying and prioritising patients with time-sensitive care needs, a five-level classification scheme endorsed by the American College of Emergency Physicians (ACEP) and Emergency Nursing Association, set targets for physician review and provider group consensus while universally relying on subjective judgement by trained triage providers.[15] See Chapter 23 for further description of the ATS.

The triage nurse may be the first healthcare professional with contact with the family/next of kin. Consideration should be given to appropriate communication and meeting their needs.

Trauma teams

The purpose of the trauma team is to provide a coordinated and collaborative approach by relevant specialists to the injured patient in a designated resuscitation area. Despite the perceived benefits of having a trauma team, they are not available in all hospitals. Some hospitals have developed two- or three-tiered activation criteria that incorporate information such as haemodynamic parameters, mechanism of injury, injuries sustained and age.[14] The pre-notification of arrival by the EMS and activation of the trauma team is an essential component of a well-organised trauma system (Table 24.1).[16] Activation mechanisms within the triage tools used can lead to over-triage, which results in the trauma team being overutilised and consequently impacting on other patients within the emergency department or healthcare facility. Conversely, under-triage potentially results in the appropriate team members who are needed not being available, which may delay life-saving treatment,

TABLE 24.1

Criteria for activation of trauma team

PHYSIOLOGICAL CRITERIA	INJURY CRITERIA	MECHANISM	OTHER
Respiratory rate <10 or >30 per min. Systolic BP <100 mmHg (<75 mmHg for child). Oxygen saturation <90%. GCS <13.	Penetrating injuries. Amputation. Suspected spinal injury. Burns >20%. Pelvic fracture. Significant injuries involving more than one body region.	Ejected from vehicle. Fall >3 m. Explosion. Pedestrian impact >30 kph. Prolonged extrication time.	Pregnancy. Age <16 or >55. Significant comorbidity. All inter-hospital transfers.

Sources: Adapted from Cameron P. Trauma. In: Cameron P, Jelinek G, Kelly A-M et al, editors. Textbook of adult emergency medicine. 4th ed. Elsevier; 2015, p. 71–162, Table 3.1.1;[17] Victoria T. Trauma Victoria: major trauma guidelines and education – Victorian state trauma system. Victoria: Victorian Department of Health; 2018. Available from: https://trauma.reach.vic.gov.au.[12]

making the accuracy of triage vital for both the injured person and the healthcare facility.[17]

The trauma team consists of different members of specialty units such as emergency medicine, surgery, nursing, anaesthesia, intensive care and support staff, who all contribute to the assessment and management of the patient. It is well established that effective leadership in trauma teams has an important role in patient outcomes and optimal team functioning, with several attributes found to be of importance to those performing the role of trauma team leader who is responsible for overseeing the resuscitation of the injured person, including formulating a definitive plan and ensuring that additional investigations are undertaken. These attributes include communication, experience or expertise, situational awareness, management of the team and task delegation, and having clear and confident decision making.[18] There are several elements that can affect the team's efficiency or clinical outcomes and, as such, the team leader role should include:

- preparing the team
- receiving handover
- directing the team and responding to information
- debriefing the team
- talk with the patient's family/friend.[11]

Primary survey

Priorities of care are similar to those in all health settings and often based on Advanced Trauma Life Support (ATLS) principles outlined by the American College of Surgeons (see Chapter 23). The components of care will often occur simultaneously rather than sequentially and are designed to identify immediately life-threatening injuries, and treat them in a prioritised sequence, based on the patient's physiology at the time.[11]

The evaluation of patients after trauma must be rapid, systematic and organised, and include:

- airway with cervical spine precautions
- breathing

- circulation with control of external haemorrhage
- disability, including brief neurological assessment
- exposure/environment, including prevention of hypothermia when removing clothing
- prevention of complications or further compromise.

Adjuncts used in the primary survey include continuous ECG monitoring, pulse oximetry, carbon dioxide (CO_2) monitoring (if indicated) and arterial blood gases (ABGs).

Compromise to airway and breathing may result from direct injury, for example to the trachea, or indirectly through decreased level of consciousness. Compromise to circulation is usually a result of significant blood loss although it may occur from injuries, such as cardiac contusions in chest trauma, or the patient's pre-existing disease. The primary survey should be repeated if there is any clinical deterioration, including reassessment of any interventions undertaken to ensure they remain effective.[19]

Secondary survey

Following primary survey and stabilisation of the life-threatening problems, patients should undergo a secondary survey (see Chapter 23). This is a systematic examination of the body regions to identify injuries that have not yet been recognised. It is essential that both the front and the back of the patient, as well as areas covered by clothing, are examined during this process. Consideration of the patient's past medical history, allergies, medications, last meal time and mechanism of injury, if known, is important during the secondary survey, although this can be challenging in the patient with altered conscious state.[19] Adjuncts to the secondary survey include diagnostic tests, such as additional X-rays, computed tomography scans[12] or angiography.

Tertiary survey

A tertiary survey should be conducted upon the arrival of trauma patients in the ICU, or soon after. The purpose of this third survey is to identify injuries that have not yet been detected, assess initial response to treatment, and plan assessment and management strategies for future care.

The tertiary survey consists of another head-to-toe physical examination, assessment of the patient's condition in the context of their earlier condition and the treatment that has been administered, a full review of all diagnostic information gained so far, and acquisition of the patient's past health history if available. A systematic approach minimises the number of injuries that are not identified during the first 24 hours of care. It is also important to repeat the tertiary survey after the patient regains consciousness and begins to mobilise. Joint injuries may become apparent only during weight-bearing movements.

Radiological and other investigations

The radiographer is a vital member of the trauma team and is essential in expediting investigations such as chest, cervical spine or pelvis that are often required in the resuscitation area. Other X-rays are rarely beneficial or change the course of treatment; however, depending on injuries identified they may be requested.

If the patient is sufficiently stable after the secondary survey, more extensive investigation in the radiology department should be undertaken, including whole-body/pan-scan computed tomography (CT), which has become standard practice in many trauma centres and has been shown to have a high sensitivity and low rate of missed injuries.[20] The patient should be accompanied and monitored by appropriately skilled multidisciplinary clinicians during all transfers for investigation.

It is essential that clinicians consider investigations carefully, to ensure that all necessary imaging is undertaken, but not delay urgent interventions such as surgery. Required investigations will depend on the examinations undertaken as part of the secondary survey, the treatment that has already been administered and the current condition of the patient.

Focused assessment with sonography for trauma

The focused assessment with sonography for trauma (FAST) is generally used during the secondary survey, particularly where abdominal trauma is suspected. The FAST exam is not designed to detect solid organ injuries, or injuries to the intestine, mesentery, diaphragm or any retroperitoneal haemorrhage that may be associated with pelvic fractures; however, it has been shown to have 85–96% sensitivity, approaching 100% sensitivity in the hypotensive patient when examining for free fluid. It is used in nearly all level 1 trauma centres and is part of the Advanced Trauma Life Support (ATLS) algorithms.

The scope of the FAST has expanded to the extended FAST (e-FAST) and has been shown to be as accurate in detecting a haemothorax or pneumothorax as a chest X-ray (CXR), with current guidelines published by the American College of Emergency Physicians.[21]

The abdomen is scanned in four zones:

* pericardial
* Morison's pouch (right upper quadrant, between the liver and kidney)
* splenorenal (left upper quadrant/perisplenic space; blood will usually collect around the spleen), and
* pelvis (the pouch of Douglas/rectovesicular space; blood usually pools behind the bladder).[22]

A FAST scan generally takes 1–2 minutes when performed by an experienced, credentialled clinician. Findings are regarded as positive (fluid (blood) observed), negative or equivocal. Technical difficulties can be experienced owing to body habitus, the presence of bowel gas, pneumoperitoneum or pneumomediastinum.[22] While a positive FAST is useful in identifying whether a patient should receive urgent surgical intervention, a negative FAST does not rule out significant abdominal trauma. The FAST exam can produce a false-positive result, particularly if there is misinterpretation of fluid-filled bowel as free fluid, or a false-negative result if the scan is performed soon after the injury and the volume of free fluid is small.[23] Where a patient is undergoing a prolonged trauma resuscitation phase, there may be an indication to repeat the FAST after 20 minutes. The National Institute for Health and Care Excellence[24] released guidelines in 2016 recommending that FAST be omitted entirely if the patient is going to have CT imaging, which is a more sensitive and specific test for intra-abdominal injury; however, taking an unstable patient to the CT scan can result in catastrophe and delays in definitive management, in which case diagnosis should include physical examination, FAST and any radiographical imaging if time allows.[25] Diagnostic peritoneal lavage (DPL) is indicated when other methods of investigation (FAST, CT) are not available, and has been removed as a first-line diagnostic tool in ATLS protocols. Unlike FAST and CT scans, DPL can only be performed once.[26]

Common clinical presentations

Trauma generally occurs to a specific area of the body (e.g. the chest or the head) or consists of an injury caused by a specific external cause (e.g. burns). This section has been arranged according to these specific types of injury, including skeletal, chest, abdominal and burns. Specific considerations relating to penetrating injuries have been covered separately, although the majority of care for patients with penetrating injuries will follow the principles of the area of injury. For example, a patient with a penetrating injury of the abdomen will generally be cared for in the same way as all patients with abdominal trauma.

Patients with multi/poly-trauma will also be cared for according to the principles of care for each specific injury, although consideration of priorities is essential. Care should follow the common principles of airway, breathing and circulation as developed by the American College of Surgeons over 30 years ago,[11] hence concentrating on respiratory and circulatory compromise first, before the treatment of other injuries. The relative importance of other injuries, for example neurological trauma or skeletal trauma, will vary for each individual patient and will be dependent on the physiological impact of the injuries. Neurological and spinal cord injury are reviewed in Chapter 17.

Mechanism of injury

Mechanism of injury describes how energy from an external force is transferred to a person, resulting in physical injury. Kinetic energy is energy in motion and can be classified as blunt or penetrating. The principles of kinetic energy associated with blunt trauma are generally those of acceleration and deceleration forces that can lead to shearing or compression injuries, while penetrating injury is proportional to the velocity of the object striking tissue and the associated energy dissipation leading to either permanent or temporary cavitation.[11] In addition to kinetic energy, there is thermal energy in the form of chemical agents, cold, heat and radiation. Injuries are also commonly classified based on intentionality. Unintentional injuries result typically from road traffic injuries, falls, fire and burn injuries, poisoning and drowning. Intentional injuries result from interpersonal violence (assault), suicide and collective violence (war).[27]

The most common mechanisms of injury are either blunt or penetrating injury. The third, less common mechanism of injury is blast injury, usually due to explosions related to industrial or recreational accidents or terrorist acts. The mechanisms of blast injuries include:

- primary blast injury – blast overpressure reaches the person and transmitted forces exert their effects on the body, causing direct tissue damage
- secondary blast injury – created by debris that is physically displaced by the blast overpressure
- tertiary blast injury – caused when the person is physically displaced by the force of the peak overpressure and blast winds leading to blunt traumatic injuries being sustained
- quaternary blast injury – miscellaneous blast injuries caused directly by the explosion including injuries such as burns, or toxic substance exposure
- quinary blast injury – a hyperinflammatory state manifested by hyperpyrexia, diaphoresis, low central venous pressure (CVP) and positive fluid balance.[28]

The mechanism of injury is recognised as affecting both survival and requirements for admission to ICU.

Generic principles of management of the injured patient

Nursing care of trauma patients is characterised by the need to integrate practices directed towards limiting the impact of the injury, and healing injuries to multiple body areas is a complex process. The delivery of critical care services is a coordinated, multidisciplinary approach. This section outlines the principles of care relevant to all trauma patients, including positioning, mobilisation and damage control resuscitation.

Positioning and mobilisation

Positioning and mobilisation can be a significant challenge, especially in those patients with multiple injuries that create competing needs. Positioning refers to the alignment and distribution of the patient in the bed, for example supine, Fowler, semi-recumbent or prone. In addition to these fundamental nursing postures, there is positioning of the limbs (i.e. elevated arms and legs). Mobilisation refers to the movement of joints by the patient to shift from one place to another. This movement may be restricted to rolling within the bed, or moving out of the bed.

The principles of positioning and mobilisation are generally not different from those in other critically ill patients, and should incorporate the need to:

- promote the patient's comfort
- maintain the patient's and staff members' safety
- prevent complications
- facilitate delivery of care.

Difficulty in positioning and mobilisation is often experienced when there is concern for the stability of the patient's spine, in particular the cervical spine in the unconscious patient. Specific protocols such as the NEXUS criteria and the Canadian C-Spine Rule are used for confirming the absence of injury to the cervical spine, and potentially eliminating the need for imaging in appropriate patients.[29] These tools evaluate the neck only and, depending on injury mechanism and patient assessment, motion restriction of the rest of the spine may be required. Patients are considered at extremely low risk of cervical spine injury if the following criteria are met:

- no midline cervical spine tenderness
- no focal neurological deficit
- no evidence of intoxication
- no painful distracting injuries
- no altered mental status.[29]

For patients who exhibit any of the above criteria, a clinical examination is unreliable and radiographic assessment is advised. The debate continues as to whether these protocols should be used in any patient who is unconscious, intoxicated or complaining of cervical soreness or abnormal neurology. The following principles should be incorporated into confirming the presence or absence of injury:

- Obtain a detailed history of the injury wherever possible, including specific investigation of mechanisms of injury that might exert force on the cervical spine. A high index of suspicion should remain, particularly in the setting of injuries often associated with cervical spine injury, including craniofacial trauma, rib fractures, pneumothoraces and damage to the great vessels and/or trachea.

- Undertake plain X-rays of the full length of the spine, interpreted by a radiologist. A helical or multidetector CT scan can reliably rule out injury; however, use is subject to availability.[30]

- Where any abnormality exists in clinical or radiological assessment, or the patient remains unconscious, a CT or MRI may be undertaken, and this must be reported by a radiologist.

- A correctly fitted rigid collar should remain in place only until the patient is appropriately reviewed and the chance of a cervical spine injury is eliminated. If a rigid collar is required for more than 4 hours, a semi-rigid collar (e.g. Philadelphia) should be used.

- Maintain appropriate pressure area care to areas under the rigid collar as well as the usual pressure points until cervical clearance is gained.

The practice of maintaining a patient in a rigid collar for days without active attempts to gain cervical clearance should be avoided at all costs. Adverse events of rigid cervical collars include:

- increased intracranial pressure related to pressure on neck veins

- unnecessary movement of unstable fractures that can occur with the fitting and application of a collar, discomfort and pain

- pressure injuries and tissue necrosis

- restricting mouth opening

- difficulty swallowing, airway compromise and aspiration.[31]

The two methods available for moving the trauma patient are staff manual handling and lifting hoists. Generally, trauma patients can be log-rolled as frequently as required for nursing care (Table 24.2). Any restrictions to patient positioning and weight bearing because of injuries or physiological status must be considered through this process; it is essential that care be taken to prevent any worsening of injuries due to handling of the patient. Although the benefits of immobilisation of the cervical spine have not been demonstrated through research, it is a practice that is supported by years of cumulative trauma and triage clinical experience and should be used to prevent worsening of injuries. Knowledge of the position restrictions for each limb, including all weight-bearing joints and the vertebrae, is imperative to avoid secondary iatrogenic injury. Certain injuries will impose position and mobility restrictions (Table 24.3).

Damage-control resuscitation

Uncontrolled post-traumatic bleeding is the leading cause of potentially preventable death, accounting for up to 40% of deaths related to trauma in the civilian setting. In the last decade, resuscitation of the haemorrhaging patient has undergone significant changes, resulting in the concept of

---

TABLE 24.2
Spinal precautions

ACTION	RATIONALE	RATIONALE	METHOD
Head hold	To maintain the cervical spine in a neutral position during any position change.	To prevent flexion, extension and lateral head tilting during any movement.	1 Nurse holds head from head of bed – the head is held firmly by placing one hand around the patient's jaw with fingers spread to cup the jaw and hold the endotracheal tube as necessary. The forearm is used to support the side of the head. 2 Nurse holds head from side of bed – nurse stands on side of bed that the patient will be rolled towards. One hand is placed firmly under the patient's occiput. Ensure nurse is in a position to support the weight of the head. 3 The other hand holds the jaw and endotracheal tube as necessary. The patient is rolled onto the forearm of the nurse holding the head, which completes the biomechanical support for the head, immobilising the cervical spine during the rolling.
Log roll	To maintain the entire spine in anatomical alignment position during any position change.	To prevent rotational torsion on the spinal column by minimising twisting of the craniocervical, cervicothoracic and thoracolumbar junctions of the spinal column.	The patient is rolled in one smooth motion with assistants supporting the shoulder and pelvic girdles. Another assistant supports the legs so the patient moves in one plane. The patient is rolled in one smooth motion, with the nurse holding the head issuing the command to start and stop the manoeuvre.

TABLE 24.3

Position and mobility restrictions in trauma patients

TYPE OF INJURY	RESTRICTIONS
Traumatic brain injury	• Nurse head up 15–30 degrees. • Side-lying as tolerated. • Full tilt on bed if cervical spine not yet cleared of injury. • Occasionally nursed flat if ICP is problematic.
Facial trauma	• Generally nurse in head-elevated position to reduce swelling, using either full bed tilt or back rest elevation.
Chest trauma	• Nurse in varying positions from semi-Fowler to side-lying. • Postural drainage (head down) usually beneficial if not contraindicated by other injuries (e.g. head or facial).
Abdominal trauma	• Nurse in varying positions from semi-Fowler to side-lying. • Preferable to have some degree of hip flexion when lying supine to reduce abdominal suture line tension.
Pelvic trauma	• Position restrictions are dependent on severity of fracture(s), use of external fixateurs and degree of stabilisation. • Some patients may sit out of bed and ambulate with external pelvis fixateur in situ. • Position restrictions require regular review, as changed or loss of fixation may affect recovery.
Extremity trauma	• Significant position restrictions may include limb elevation, avoidance of side-lying or limited movement.

ICP = intracranial pressure.

damage–control resuscitation (DCR). DCR refers to management bundles for resuscitation designed to rapidly identify the sources of bleeding, followed by immediate interventions to minimise blood loss, restore tissue perfusion and achieve haemodynamic stability.[32] DCR starts pre-hospital and continues intra-hospital through the emergency room, operating room and the ICU.

Pre-hospital time should be minimised and trauma patients in haemorrhagic shock should be transported directly to a hospital in a trauma system for surgical interventions. The use of local direct pressure in combination with topical haemostatic agents is recommended to enhance bleeding control in the pre-surgical setting. Tourniquet is recommended on uncontrolled arterial bleeding from crushed extremity injuries, traumatic amputations, penetrating injuries and blast injuries and should be left in place until surgical control of the bleeding has been achieved. Pelvic binders, correctly placed, should be used in the pre-surgical setting if a pelvic fracture is suspected.[33] Adequate ventilation, oxygenation and patent airway is of essence and normoventilation is recommended with a $PaCO_2$ of 5.0–5.5 kPa (35–40 mmHg) to avoid vasoconstriction, decreased cerebral blood flow and impaired tissue perfusion. In bleeding patients, the early use of protective ventilation with low tidal volume (around 6 mL/kg) and moderate positive end–expiratory pressure (PEEP) is recommended to avoid acute respiratory distress syndrome.[28] Only in imminent cerebral herniation should hyperventilation-induced hypocapnia be used.[32] Intravenous morphine is recommended to be the first-line analgesic; the dose should be adjusted as needed to achieve adequate pain relief.[24,32]

Aggressive fluid replacement to maintain tissue oxygenation in haemorrhaging patients has been found to increase the hydrostatic pressure on wounds, dislodge blood clots and cause dilution of coagulation factors and hypothermia in the traumatised patient. To avoid the adverse effects of early aggressive volume replacement, DCR aims to achieve a lower-than-normal blood pressure called 'permissive hypotension'.[32] A target systolic blood pressure (SBP) of 80–90 mmHg is recommended, not as an endpoint but until surgical control of the haemorrhage is obtained. In patients with severe traumatic brain injury (TBI) (Glasgow Coma Scale (GCS) ≤8) and spinal injuries, permissive hypotension is contraindicated as an adequate perfusion pressure is essential for tissue oxygenation of the injured central nervous system (CNS). In these patients, a mean arterial blood pressure (MAP) above 80 mmHg should be maintained. In acute life-threatening situations when blood pressure cannot be maintained by adequate volume resuscitation, vasopressors may also be required to maintain targeted arterial pressure. If the patient continues to have a poor response to fluid resuscitation, cardiac dysfunction should be suspected and assessed promptly.[32]

The principles of DCR include:[34]

- minimisation of isotonic crystalloid solutions
- permissive hypotension
- transfusion of a balanced ratio of blood products
- goal-directed correction of coagulopathy.

Upon admission to the hospital, the initial assessment should focus on the bleeding using a combination of patient's physiological status, mechanism of injury, anatomical injury severity and the patient's response to initial DCR. The following bundle is used intra-hospital through the emergency room, operating room and the ICU.

Intra-hospital bundle

- Full blood count, prothrombin time,[35] platelet count, fibrinogen, calcium, viscoelastic testing (VEM), lactate and/or base deficit and pH assessed within the first 15 minutes and repeatedly monitored as indicated
- Immediate intervention applied in patients with haemorrhagic shock and an identified source of bleeding unless initial resuscitation measures are successful.
- Immediate further investigation undertaken using FAST, multi-slice CT (MSCT), whole-body CT (WBCT) or immediate surgery if massive intra-abdominal bleeding is present in patients presenting with haemorrhagic shock and an unidentified source of bleeding.
- Damage-control surgery applied if shock or coagulopathy are present.
- DCR concept continued until bleeding source is identified and controlled.
- Restrictive erythrocyte transfusion strategy (haemoglobin 70–90 g/dL).

Coagulopathy

About one-third of all bleeding trauma patients show signs of early acute coagulopathy upon arrival to hospital. These patients have a significant increase in multiple organ failure and death in comparison with patients with similar injuries in the absence of coagulopathy.[32] Early acute coagulopathy resulting from a combination of tissue injury, bleeding-induced shock, inflammatory changes and the activation of anticoagulant and fibrinolytic pathways is displayed in Fig. 24.1. The severity of the coagulopathy is affected by environmental and clinical interventions that result in or contribute to hypothermia, dilution from transfusion of crystalloids and blood products, acidaemia, hypoperfusion and coagulation factor consumption. Brain injury and pre-hospital fluid administration are known to modify coagulopathy in addition to individual patient-related factors including age, genetic background, underlying disease and premedication such as oral anticoagulants and antiplatelet agents.[32]

Standard coagulation monitoring includes prothrombin time,[35] activated partial thromboplastin time (APTT), platelet counts and fibrinogen. The international normalised ratio (INR) should be included in the measurement and repeated as required. Fibrinogen is the first coagulation factor to reach a critical low concentration during activation of coagulation in bleeding and studies have shown that early detection and prompt correction improve morbidity and mortality. Blood coagulation and fibrinolysis can be measured using traditional laboratories or a viscoelastic method (thrombelastography (TEG) or rotational thromboelastometry (ROTEM)) preferably at bedside (point-of-care testing).[32]

Supplement of fibrinogen can be administered as fresh frozen plasma (FFP), or pathogen-inactivated FFP, cryoprecipitate or fibrin concentrate.[34] Tranexamic acid prevents fibrinolysis and is recommended to be administered within 3 hours of injury. Management of haemorrhage should be carefully monitored to ensure that blood transfusion is appropriate, as it is associated with significant risks, including overload, allergic reactions and trauma-related transfusion-related acute lung injury (TRALI),[36] acute respiratory distress syndrome (ARDS)[28] and multiple organ dysfunction syndrome (MODS). The risk for TRALI, inflammatory-mediated pulmonary oedema resulting in hypoxia within hours of transfusion, is highest with transfusion of plasma.[34]

Targeted care to reduce bleeding may be referred to as a *coagulation bundle*:[32]

- tranexamic acid administered as early as possible
- acidosis, hypothermia and hypocalcaemia treated
- fibrinogen maintained at 1.5–2 g/L
- platelets maintained at >100 × 10⁹/L
- prothrombin complex concentrate administered in patients pretreated with warfarin or direct-acting oral coagulants (until antidotes are available).

Hypothermia

Hypothermia is defined as a core temperature <35°C[37] and is associated with acidosis and coagulopathy, also known as the 'lethal triad', leading to higher morbidity and mortality. Even in subtropical environments, hypothermia is identified in approximately two-thirds of major trauma cases during the pre-hospital[37] or in-hospital phase of care.

Uncontrolled causes of hypothermia can be endogenous or accidental. Endogenous causes include metabolic dysfunction with decreased heat production or central nervous system dysfunction with insufficient thermo-regulation, such as in neurological trauma. Dermal dysfunction (e.g. a burn) is another endogenous cause of hypothermia.

Accidental hypothermia can occur without thermoregulatory dysfunction, and generally occurs as a result of environmental exposure either at the injury site, during transport to, or between, healthcare facilities, as a result of aggressive fluid resuscitation[37] or during prolonged surgical procedures. The pathophysiological

FIGURE 24.1 Factors, both pre-existing and trauma related, that contribute to traumatic coagulopathy.

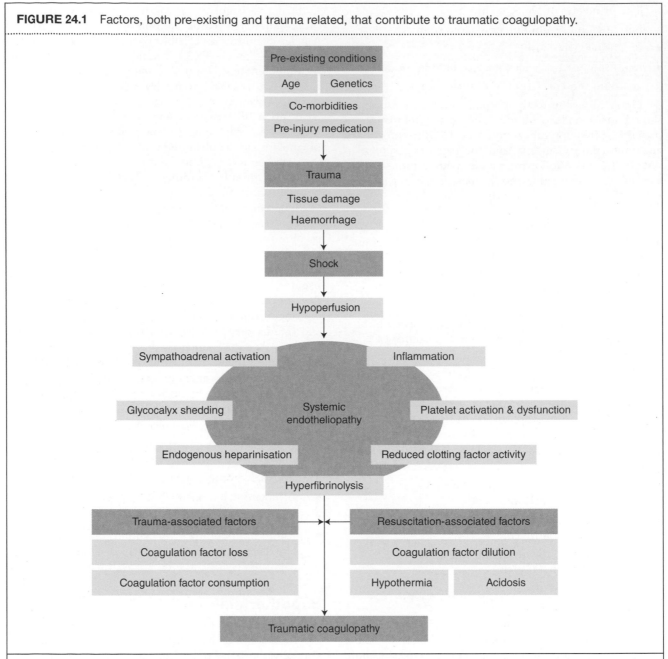

Sources: Adapted from Brohi K. Trauma induced coagulopathy. J R Army Med Corps 2009;155(4):320–2; Hess JR, Brohi K, Dutton RP, Hauser CJ, Holcomb JB, Kluger Y, Mackway-Jones K, Parr MJ, Rizoli SB, Yukioka T, et al. The coagulopathy of trauma: a review of mechanisms. J Trauma 2008;65(4):748–54; Chang R, Cardenas JC, Wade CE, Holcomb JB. Advances in the understanding of trauma-induced coagulopathy. Blood 2016;128(8):1043–9; Stensballe J, Henriksen HH, Johansson PI. Early haemorrhage control and management of trauma-induced coagulopathy: the importance of goal-directed therapy. Curr Opin Crit Care 2017;23(6):503–10; Caspers M, Maegele M, Frohlich M. Current strategies for hemostatic control in acute trauma hemorrhage and trauma-induced coagulopathy. Expert Rev Hematol 2018;11(12):987–95; Spahn DR, Bouillon B, Cerny V, Coats TJ, Duranteau J, Fernandez-Mondejar E, Filipescu D, Hunt BJ, Komadina R, Nardi G, et al. Management of bleeding and coagulopathy following major trauma: an updated European guideline. Crit Care 2013;17(2):R76.'

changes associated with hypothermia vary depending on the severity and are outlined in Chapter 23. Of relevance, shivering leads to increased oxygen consumption and acidosis, platelet dysfunction leads to impaired clotting and fibrinolysis, while haemorrhage reduces the circulating volume, which in turn may lead to a reduction in core body temperature and hypoperfusion of tissues. Hypoperfusion may cause hypoxia and subsequent production of lactic acid, which in turn slows the clotting cascade allowing haemorrhage to continue.[38] Studies have shown that these patients require more blood products and have an 80% increased risk of mortality.[32]

Measures to prevent and reduce hypothermia and the risk of hypothermia-induced coagulopathy include:

- removing wet clothing
- ensuring the patient is adequately covered to avoid additional heat loss
- warming IV fluids
- using forced air warming or electrical warming blankets
- limiting crystalloid infusion
- monitoring and maximising oxygenation
- treating and preventing respiratory acidosis
- permissive hypotension, except in traumatic brain injury
- finding and stopping the bleeding, remembering that other bleeding sites may be present
- increasing the surrounding temperature.[38]

In extreme cases of hypothermia, methods of rewarming such as cardiopulmonary bypass and peritoneal dialysis or lavage might be used.

Practice tip

Check whether trauma patients are on anticoagulant or antiplatelet agents, particularly those patients who have chronic disease or are elderly. If patients are taking these medications, be on the alert for complications associated with coagulopathy.

Damage-control surgery

The goals of controlling haemorrhage and prevention of contamination while limiting the stress of surgery to the patient are the underlying principles of DCS. Initially, DCS was used for injuries sustained in the abdomen but this has now expanded to include thoracic, skeletal and vascular injuries. The first surgical intervention in thoracic trauma with bleeding is the insertion of chest tubes followed by damage-control thoracotomy. Patients with pelvic injuries and retroperitoneal bleeding may need external compression by pelvic binder, retroperitoneal packing and urgent radiological angioembolisation for control of the bleeding; although the use of REBOA has also been suggested, one meta-analysis demonstrated worse survival trends.[39,40] In massive haemorrhage with continued bleeding, aortic cross-clamping or REBOA can be life saving. In REBOA, a flexible catheter is placed by a vascular surgeon into the femoral artery and manoeuvred into the aorta, inflating a balloon at its tip to stop blood flow beyond the balloon. The times the balloon can be inflated differ depending on the placement.[39,41]

The term 'damage-control orthopaedics' includes long-bone fractures stabilised with external fixateurs

rather than primary definitive surgeries (osteosynthesis), preventing patients from secondary procedure-related trauma. Definitive orthopaedic surgeries can be performed after 4–14 days when the patients have stabilised.

Patients presenting with the following conditions are recommended for damage-control surgery:[32]

- severely injured patients presenting with deep haemorrhagic shock, signs of ongoing bleeding and coagulopathy
- severely injured patients with coagulopathy, hypothermia (≤34°C), acidosis (pH ≤7.2), an inaccessible major venous injury with a need for time-consuming procedures or concomitant injury outside the abdomen.

DCS is performed in the following stages and with a multidisciplinary approach:[32,42]

- Stage 1 – surgery: operative time should be as short as possible with the primary goal to stop bleeding, reduce contamination and provide adequate end-organ perfusion. Angioembolisation may be required during this phase.
- Stage 2 – resuscitation: completed generally in ICU and includes rewarming, correction of metabolic acidosis and coagulation disorders, optimising ventilation and haemodynamics.
- Stage 3 – definitive surgery: relaparotomy and definitive surgical repair, which generally occurs after 48 hours to lower the risk of rebleeding.
- Stage 4 – reconstructive: particularly in patients with open abdomens or extremities that have open wounds requiring grafting, or skin closure after tissue healing has occurred.

Nursing a patient who undergoes DCS requires recognition of the principles and aims of the surgery, as well as flexibility in the care of the patient after the initial surgery but before definitive surgery. When the patient is admitted to the ICU postoperatively, the standard mechanisms for the treatment of hypothermia, acidosis and coagulopathy, as discussed above, should be implemented. After DCS, patients may also have an open abdomen with temporary dressings or skeletal fractures with external fixateurs in situ and may require multiple return trips to the operating room to achieve final closure.

Deep venous thrombosis (DVT) and pulmonary embolism (PE), collectively known as hospital-acquired venous thromboembolism (VTE) is a life-threatening complication with an incidence of up to 50% following trauma related to immobility and the acute-phase response. PE is the third leading cause of death in those who survive beyond the third day. It is recommended that within 24 hours, after bleeding has been controlled, pharmacological thromboprophylaxis should be administered. This may be applied in combination with the use of early mechanical thromboprophylaxis with intermittent pneumatic compression (IPC) or early mechanical thromboprophylaxis with antiembolic stockings.[43]

Skeletal trauma

Skeletal trauma involves injury to the bony structure of the body. Although skeletal injuries alone rarely result in the patient being admitted to critical care, damage to surrounding blood vessels and nerves, as well as potential complications such as fat embolism syndrome[44] and rhabdomyolysis, may cause the patient to become seriously ill. Patients with skeletal trauma who require admission to ICU include those with multiple injuries, severe pelvic fractures (often associated with significant blood loss), long-bone fractures (often associated with fat embolism syndrome (FES)) and thoracic injuries such as flail segment. A small number of people with crush injuries that cause significant damage to muscles, often resulting in rhabdomyolysis, also require admission to the ICU because of the risk of kidney injury.[45]

In Australia and the European Union, approximately 50% of all trauma patients requiring admission to a hospital have fractures caused by falls and road traffic incidences.[46,47]

Pathophysiology

Bone is composed of an organic matrix with three main components: organic matrix, inorganic mineral content, mineral salts and water. This composition forms the framework for bones, which are hardened through the deposit of the calcium and other minerals around fibres. Mineral salts are deposited between gaps in the collagen laces and once the gaps are filled they crystallise and cause the tissues to harden in a process called ossification.[48]

A fracture is simply defined as a break in the continuity of a bone and generally occurs when there is force applied that exceeds the tensile or compressive strength of the bone. Fracture classification includes:

- complete or incomplete
- linear, oblique, spiral or transverse
- open or closed.

Initial fracture management includes the following:

- Identification of fractures during primary and secondary survey along with limb assessment for vascular injuries, including the presence or absence of distal pulses.
- Adequate analgesia is vital, along with reduction of deformity and splintage to reduce bleeding and pain. Traction may be used if the injury is above the knee.
- Irrigation of open wounds is not recommended; however, saline-soaked gauze under an occlusive dressing is recommended until surgical review can occur.[49] Surgical principles include debridement and lavage, stabilisation which often includes external fixation and tissue closure.[50]

Definitive fracture management includes:

- immediate stabilisation to reduce swelling, support the fracture and prevent bone ends penetrating the skin or entrapping nerves or vessels
- surgical planning
- stabilisation including casts, external fixation, interlocking nails, plates or screws (internal fixation).[51]

Fat embolism

Fat embolism occurs when fat enters the circulation and it may or may not have clinical manifestations. Fat embolism syndrome (FES) presents with respiratory, neurological or dermatological features and is a little-understood complication of trauma. It may occur in patients who have experienced a fracture of a long bone, particularly if multiple fractures or fractures to the middle or proximal parts of the femur are experienced. Fractures to the pelvis can also lead to a fat embolism. The incidence of FES is low (<1–2.2%).[44] FES consists of fat in the blood circulation associated with an identifiable pattern of clinical signs and symptoms that include hypoxaemia, neurological symptoms and a petechial rash. Patients generally present 12–72 hours after they have experienced a relevant fracture and often require admission to a critical care unit for assessment and treatment, including mechanical ventilation.[44]

Internationally, there continues to be disagreement regarding the pathophysiological changes associated with FES, although there is general consensus on the following principles. It has been accepted that there is a mechanical component to the changes that take place in FES, where fat is physically forced into the venous system and causes physical obstruction of the vasculature.[52] Although marrow pressure is normally 30–50 mmHg, it can be increased up to 800 mmHg during intramedullary reaming (the process where the medullary cavity of the bone is surgically enlarged to fit a surgical implant such as a tibial nail), consequently reaching a pressure significantly above pressures throughout the vasculature.

A second theory, associated with the biochemical changes that occur during trauma, proposes that trauma is associated with a higher level of circulating free fatty acids, which triggers a cascade of inflammatory and thrombotic events causing aggregation of molecules which damages the pulmonary endothelial cells, causing alveolar oedema and possibly haemorrhage which may progress to acute lung injury, ARDS and respiratory failure.[52]

Rhabdomyolysis

Rhabdomyolysis is a potentially life-threatening condition and is caused by either acquired or inherited factors. It is characterised by primary (mechanical) or secondary (metabolic) skeletal muscle injury, resulting in cell death and the release of byproducts into the circulation that are potentially toxic or can lead to complications such as acute kidney injury (AKI). Traumatic injuries account for less than 20% of causes for rhabdomyolysis development.

Patients with multitrauma, crush injuries involving the torso or extremities and those with compartment syndrome are at highest risk.[53] Mortality in patients with rhabdomyolysis is reported to be between 7.2% and 14%.[54]

Rhabdomyolysis occurs from the breakdown of muscle fibres resulting in the distribution of the cellular contents of the affected muscle throughout the circulation and occurs during the reperfusion of injured muscle. There are two phases of injury that are essential for the development of rhabdomyolysis: the first is when muscle ischaemia occurs and the second is with reperfusion of the injured muscle. The length of time that muscle is ischaemic affects the development of rhabdomyolysis, with periods of less than 2 hours generally not producing permanent damage, whereas periods longer than 2 hours can result in irreversible anatomical and functional changes.[55] Presentation varies widely across patient groups and ranges from asymptomatic elevated creatinine kinase (CK) to life-threatening conditions with electrolyte disturbances, cardiac arrhythmias, acute renal failure and disseminated intravascular coagulation.[56]

Treatment principles include the identification and release of any compartment syndrome; however, aspects such as IV fluid resuscitation, despite the low evidence surrounding its use, is recommended in the Eastern Association for the Surgery of Trauma (EAST) guidelines. The administration of bicarbonate or mannitol remains controversial, with the EAST guidelines recommending against their use.[57]

Clinical manifestations

Common forms of skeletal trauma include the following:

- *Long-bone fractures* – the long bones are the humerus, radius, ulna, femur, tibia and fibula. Fractures of these bones can carry a high level of morbidity, especially if they involve a joint such as a trimalleolar fracture of the ankle (distal tibia and fibula). In many cases, definitive surgical management is required, with internal fixation.

- *Dislocations* – all joints are at risk of traumatic dislocation, depending on the mechanism of injury. Dislocations can be limb threatening if they cause neurovascular compromise. Reduction of traumatic dislocation is a medical emergency.

- *Open fractures (compound)* – any break in the skin that communicates directly with the fracture is classified as an open fracture. Open fractures carry a high infection risk; irrigation and debridement should be performed within 24 hours.[49]

- *Traumatic amputation* – amputation refers to an avulsion in which the affected limb or body appendage is completely separated from the body. This can occur when a digit or extremity is sheared off by either mechanical or severing forces – for example, amputation of a thumb by a bandsaw. Traumatic amputations vary in severity and ongoing

compromise, with a clean-cut amputation more likely to be successfully reattached than a crushed extremity. Criteria that inform the surgical decision-making process include: the amount of tissue loss; location on the body at the connection site; damage to underlying and surrounding tissues, bones, nerves, tendons/muscles and vessels; and condition of the amputated part.

- *Fractures of the pelvis* – the pelvis is the largest combined bony structure in the body and serves to provide an essential supporting framework for ambulation and protection of pelvic organs. Major blood vessels and nerves traverse the pelvic bones, supplying the lower limbs and pelvic organs. Therefore, injury to any part of the pelvis is serious. The three bones that comprise the pelvic ring are the two innominate bones (ilium and pubic rami) and the sacrum. Due to its reinforced structure, the amount of force required to fracture the pelvis is substantial. Fractures of the pelvis can affect one or both sides of the pelvis and be stable or unstable. A variety of classification systems exist to describe the severity of pelvic fractures, the most common being the Tile classification (Fig. 24.2).[58,59]

- *Fractures of the spinal column* (see also Chapter 17) – the spinal column includes all the bony components in the cervical, thoracic and lumbar vertebral regions. Fractures of the vertebra are common in trauma patients, but the actual incidence of fracture without spinal cord injury in multitrauma patients is not well described. Not all fractures cause vertebral column instability with the subsequent risk of spinal cord damage. A spinal column fracture will be diagnosed as mechanically stable or unstable and this will affect the positioning and possible activity of the patient.

- *Discoligamentous injuries of the spinal column* (see also Chapter 17) – the soft tissue components of the spinal column include the spinal cord, the intervertebral discs and the spinal ligaments. An injury to the spinal column can disrupt one or more of these structures with or without fracture. These injuries can be highly unstable, and the nurse must be vigilant with spinal precautions and the fitting and management of the patient requiring a rigid cervical collar or semirigid cervical collar.

Patient management

There are several major considerations for the nurse managing the critically ill patient with skeletal trauma. These include appropriate assessment as well as application of traction, management of any amputated parts, and stabilisation of pelvic fractures and spine precautions. These latter aspects of care will be conducted in collaboration with medical and allied health colleagues.

Bones are very vascular structures and can be the cause of substantial blood loss in the trauma patient. The critical care nurse should therefore be cognisant of the potential

FIGURE 24.2 Classification of pelvic fractures.

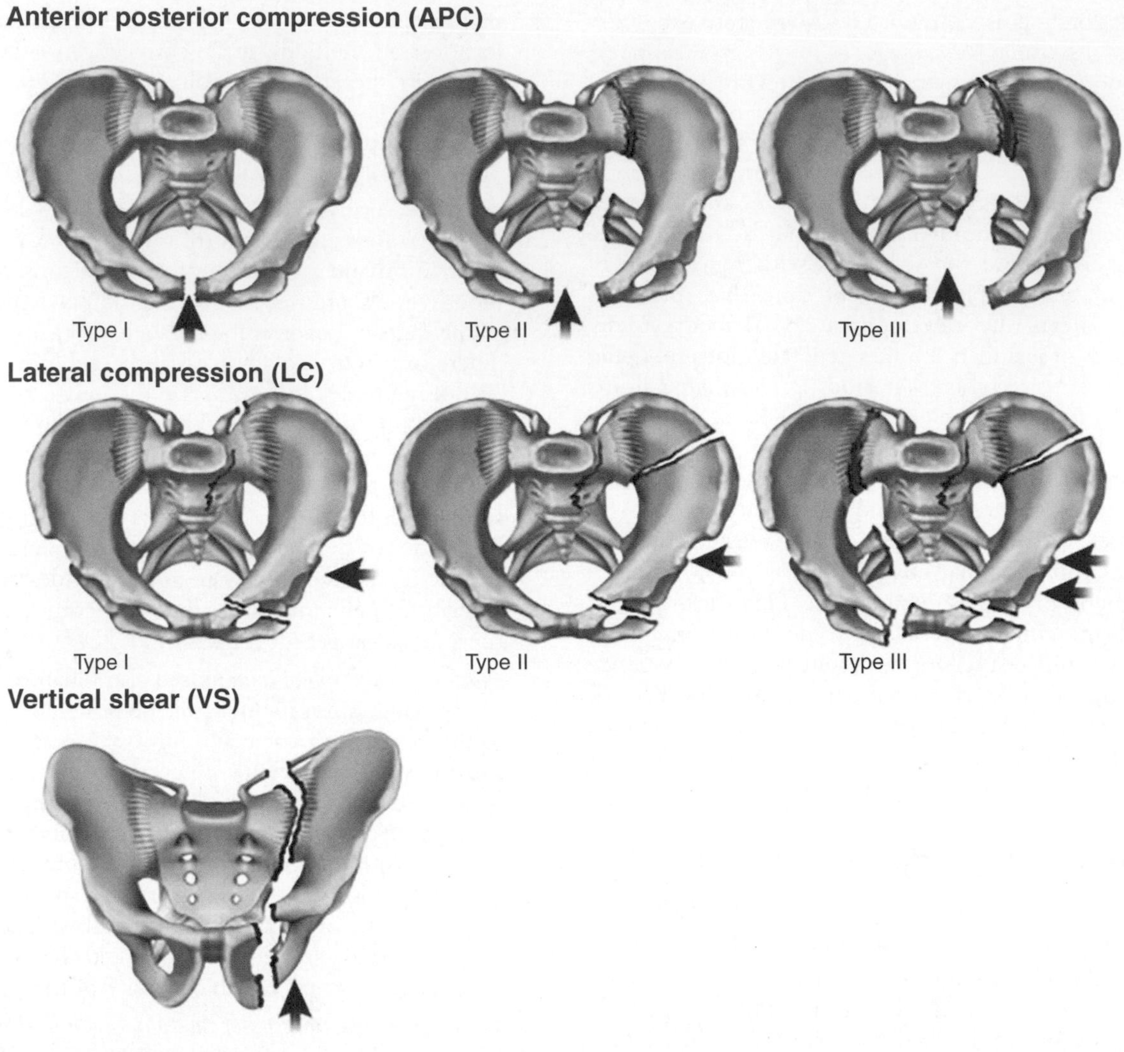

Anterior posterior compression (APC)

Type I   Type II   Type III

Lateral compression (LC)

Type I   Type II   Type III

Vertical shear (VS)

Sources: Gray A, Chandler H, Sabri O. Pelvic ring injuries: classification and treatment. Orthop Trauma 2018;32(2):80–90, Figure 2;[58] Ziran NM, Smith WR Pelvic fractures. In: Smith W, Stahel P, editors. Management of musculoskeletal injuries in the trauma patient. New York: Springer; 2014, p. 143–64.[59]

for extensive blood loss in common fractures (Table 24.4).[60] Given the potential for extensive blood loss, as well as the frequent close proximity of nerves and blood vessels to bones, neurovascular assessment of the patient with skeletal trauma is essential (Table 24.5).

Splinting

The purpose of splinting is to align and immobilise the bone, which alone has remarkable haemorrhage control properties, is a potentially life-saving intervention and is generally undertaken by nursing staff. Every fractured bone that has not undergone definitive orthopaedic management requires splinting. Examples of intermediate stabilisation of fractures include the following:

- *Positioning of injured limbs* – all patients who have a splint in situ may need to have it elevated to promote venous return and minimise tissue oedema. In the ICU the trauma patient will often be nursed flat, with the bed on tilt for a head-elevation position. In these circumstances, the injured dependent limb must be elevated on pillows. Care must be taken to ensure that elevation does not place pressure on any part of the limb; for example, a hand sack made from a pillowcase tied to an IV pole should not be used, as it places direct pressure on the path of the median nerve and can cause an iatrogenic neurapraxia.

- *Wooden/air splints* – are padded appliances that are strapped to the injured limb. Ideally, no patient should remain in wooden splints for longer than 4 hours, as pressure may build up on pressure points.

- *Plaster backslab* – limbs with fractures will often swell as a physiological response to injury; a plaster backslab composed of layered plaster of paris is the preferred treatment, as it accommodates swelling and can easily be loosened by nursing staff at any time of day. It is imperative that this be adequately padded within the limitations of providing structural support

to the limb. Poorly made or ill-fitting backslabs can cause major complications, such as pressure sores or displacement of fractures.

- *Traction* – may be required as part of fracture management, and involves the application of a pulling force to fractured or dislocated bones. There are three types of traction:
  - skeletal, where traction pins are anchored into the bone (i.e. Steinmann pin)
  - skin, where the body is gripped, as in the use of slings and bandages
  - manual, applied by a clinician pulling on a body part, such as in the reduction of dislocation. It may also be applied to maintain the traction during nursing care manoeuvres such as log-rolling or repositioning of the traction.

The principles of traction are to achieve alignment of bones while preventing complications. Remember that incorrectly applied traction is painful and can exacerbate the injury. The following should guide management of the patient with traction:

1 The grip or hold on the body must be adequate and secure.

2 Provision for counter-traction must be made.

3 Minimise friction.

4 Maintain the line and magnitude of the pull, once correctly established.

5 Frequently check the apparatus and the patient to ensure that: (1) the traction set-up is functioning as

---

TABLE 24.4

Potential blood loss caused by fractures

	ESTIMATED BLOOD LOSS WITH VARIOUS TYPES OF FRACTURES (IN LITRES)
Ankle	0.5 to 1.5
Elbow	0.5 to 1.5
Femur	1 to 2
Hip	1.5 to 2.5
Humerus	1 to 2
Knee	1 to 1.5
Pelvis	1.5 to 4.5
Tibia	0.5 to 1.5

Source: Orthopedic trauma www.rn.org® reviewed December 2020, expires December, 2022. Provider information and specifics available on our website. Unauthorised distribution prohibited. ©2020 rn.org®, S.A., rn.org®, LLC by Wanda Lockwood, RN, BA, MA.

TABLE 24.5

Neurovascular observations of the skeletal trauma patient[a]

OBSERVATION	PROCESS	COMMENTS
Skin colour	State the skin colour of the area inspected as it compares with the unaffected part. NB: distal limb pulses may be difficult to palpate in the injured limb; a warm pink limb is a perfused limb.	Pink: normal perfusion. Pale: reduced perfusion. Dusky, purple or cyanotic discoloration: usually indicating significantly reduced perfusion. Demarcated: a distinct line where the skin colour changes to dusky (usually follows the vessel path).
Skin temperature to touch	State the ambient temperature of the skin to touch as it compares with normally perfused skin at room temperature.	Normal: not discernibly cold to touch. Reduced skin temperature indicates reduced perfusion.
Voluntary movement	The patient should be able to move the non-immobilised distal part of any injured limb (i.e. fingers and toes of a plastered limb).	It is important to assess range of motion where that is possible, provided this will not aggravate the injury. Reduced movement may indicate compromise to either the nerve or blood supply to the limb.
Sensation	The patient should be able to report normal sensation to touch.	Sensation should be assessed in nerve distributions (i.e. all fingers and toes). Reduced sensation may indicate compromise to either the nerve or blood supply to the limb.

[a] Note: should be undertaken on all injured limbs both pre- and postoperatively as required

planned, and (2) the patient is not suffering any pain or further injury as a result of the traction treatment.

Traumatic amputations

Traumatic amputation is the separation of a limb or appendage from the body. During the pre-hospital phase, any amputated body part should be wrapped in a clean or sterile (if available) cloth and placed in a plastic, waterproof bag inside an insulated cooler with ice. It is important that the ice does not come into direct contact with the amputated part. When managed using these principles, the amputated part may be viable for up to 6–12 hours before reattachment. Depending on any additional injuries, and the cardiovascular status of the patient, surgery for limb salvage will be scheduled as soon as possible.

Postoperative management will be guided by the type of surgery that was performed – specifically, whether or not amputation occurred. Principles of postoperative care include:

- appropriate positioning of the affected limb, usually based on surgical orders
- frequent neurovascular observations, particularly observing for reperfusion injury, which manifests as an acute compartment syndrome or vascular trashing of distal vessels from a clot
- implementing changes in treatment initiated in response to altered perfusion in a timely manner
- psychological support to assist the patient in dealing with the injury.

Pelvic stabilisation

Pelvic fractures occur in approximately 10% of patients with blunt trauma and can be uncomplicated, requiring no surgical intervention, or they can be serious enough to be the primary cause of death from exsanguination. The mortality rate from pelvic fracture ranges from 5% to 20% and is mainly attributed to exsanguinating haemorrhage in young patients and multiorgan failure in elderly patients.[61] Variability in mortality rates have been reported as low as 7.3% in the UK and up to 46% in Japan in patients with bleeding pelvic fractures and associated injuries. Pelvic fractures are associated with a long-term decrease in physical functioning, problems undertaking activites of daily life (ADLs) and associated with adverse psychological health.[62]

Appropriate assessment and management of pelvic fractures should encompass diagnostic evaluation, non-invasive pelvis stabilisation, abdominal evaluation, perineum and genitalia assessment and the requirement for surgical intervention and angiography.[62]

The initial management of the patient with a fractured pelvis involves assessment and splinting. Assessment should encompass the following two aspects:

1 haemodynamic status – to identify signs of ongoing blood loss and determine fluid resuscitation requirements
2 stability of the pelvic ring – assessed via clinical examination and diagnostic imaging. Palpation and inspection of the anterior and posterior pelvis for signs of trauma, including tenderness in the conscious patient, is generally adequate.

The orthopaedic surgeon may undertake further clinical assessments including signs of acetabular fracture, pain on movement and instability on adduction along with a vascular and neurological exam including motor function, reflexes and sensation, as there is a high incidence of lumbosacral plexus injuries. 'Springing' of the pelvis is not recommended as it does not reliably predict pelvic fractures and may cause further bleeding.[62]

Nursing staff may conduct these assessments under appropriate specialist guidance in a setting such as remote area trauma nursing or via tele-health consultation.

Non-invasive pelvic binding, in the form of either a bedsheet or a proprietary pelvic binder, may make a significant impact on patient morbidity and mortality. Such a manoeuvre will stabilise the pelvis and assist in approximating bleeding vessels, thereby assisting in haemostasis[62] (Fig. 24.3).[63]

Pelvic binders are temporary devices, and ideally not left in situ for longer than 4 hours. If a patient is to remain in the binder longer than 4 hours (maximum 24 hours), nursing staff must take care to minimise pressure and a management plan agreed upon.[62]

Conscious patients should be advised to report signs of increasing pressure, such as positional paraesthesia. Increasing abdominal swelling may indicate a need to reposition the binder. Position restrictions should be

FIGURE 24.3 Application of a pelvic binder.

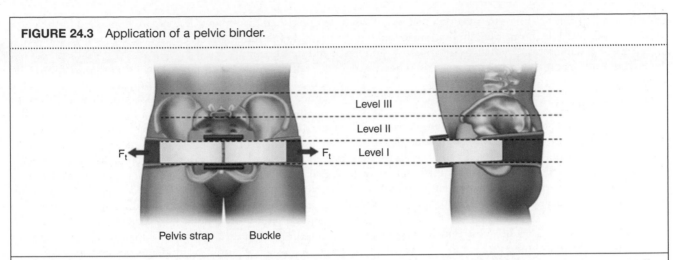

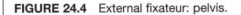

Level III

Level II

F_t Level I

Pelvis strap   Buckle

Source: Hong S-K, Kim DK, Jeon SR. Primary management of polytrauma. Singapore: Springer Singapore; 2019, p. 93–114, Figure 7.2.[63]

FIGURE 24.4 External fixateur: pelvis.

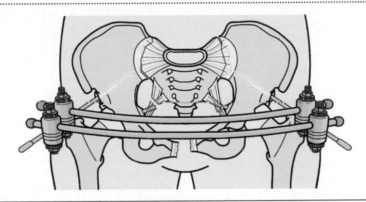

Source: Mostafa AMHAM, Kyriacou H, Chimutengwende-Gordon M, Khan WS. An overview of the key principles and guidelines in the management of pelvic fractures. Journal of Perioperative Practice 2021;31(9):341–8. doi: 10.1177/1750458920947358.[62]

clarified by all members of the healthcare team, especially if the patient will be in the binder for a lengthy period. The patient may be able to be log-rolled and side-lie with a pelvic binder in situ. Release of a pelvic binder should be undertaken only with caution and as part of definitive care (e.g. within the operating theatre), with all relevant members (particularly the orthopaedic or trauma surgeon) of the healthcare team present.

Invasive pelvic fixation uses an external fixateur (Fig. 24.4) to achieve pelvic stabilisation if definitive surgery cannot be performed. The application of an external bridging frame (either anterior or posterior) to stabilise the pelvis may be an interim or definitive treatment measure that may be in situ for days or weeks.[62] Current recommendations for pelvic ring definitive surgery is within 72 hours of the patient being physiologically stable if associated injuries allow.[62] Patients in external fixation may be permitted to mobilise, although the extent of mobilisation will depend on the stability of the fracture.

While the external fixateur is in place, the following nursing care is required:

- *Pin site care* – the pin sites are usually cleaned with isotonic saline and left open unless there is a large amount of exudate, in which case they may be covered with dry absorbent dressing; care should be taken to identify gaping or stretched skin around the site, as this may require surgical intervention.

- *Analgesia* – this is based on patient reports of pain and taking into account planned activities such as mobilisation and physiotherapy.

- *Mobilisation* – this is based on stability of the pelvis, and in consultation with the surgeon.

- *Patient education* – particularly regarding the safety of the procedure and mobilisation and rehabilitation plans.

Pelvic embolisation involves interventional radiology to control haemorrhage in patients with pelvic fractures. Because of the large arteries that traverse the pelvis, arterial bleeding can be the cause of substantial blood loss in 10–20% of cases. The timing of embolisation, particularly in relation to stabilisation, remains controversial, and is dependent on the availability of appropriately trained staff and resources.

Chest trauma

Chest trauma is recognised as a severe, potentially life-threatening form of injury that may require admission to critical care. Chest trauma covers a broad array of injuries and severity, and ranges from relatively minor injuries (e.g. abrasions and fracture of a single rib) to major, immediately life-threatening injuries (e.g. cardiac rupture or tension pneumothorax).

Approximately 10–15% of chest injuries will require admission to hospital for more than 24 hours, with approximately 15% of those requiring admission to ICU, more than 50% requiring mechanical ventilation and nearly 50% of patients requiring chest tube insertion.[64]

Blunt force mechanism secondary to road traffic accidents, falls, crush or blast injuries has been reported as accounting for over 90% of thoracic injuries.[64,65] Mortality related to blunt chest trauma ranges from 9% to 60%; however, it is the second leading cause of death after head injury in road traffic accidents.[66] Consideration of age when evaluating chest trauma is important as often older patients have more injuries and serious complications in comparison with a younger or paediatric population because of differences in bone density and elasticity as we age.[67] One review of blunt thoracic injury mortality reported a fourfold increase in mortality in patients over 65 years compared with younger patients, with risk factors identified as the development of pneumonia, respiratory complications and ICU admission for hypoxaemia.[68]

Chest trauma injuries are the third most common injury in multitrauma patients, following head and extremities trauma, and are at significant risk of developing respiratory failure or other life-threatening complications such as airway obstruction, tension pneumothorax and massive haemothorax. Even patients who present with no immediate life-threatening respiratory complications are at high risk of developing respiratory failure if injuries are not identified and appropriately managed.[68]

Penetrating injuries are often related to gunshot or stabbing injuries and present with direct lung or organ injury that often requires operative intervention,[65] but can be associated with road traffic accidents, impalement related to falls or blast injuries with shrapnel present.

Pre-hospital death is usually associated with injuries to the heart or major vessels causing disruption of the respiratory or circulatory systems, or both.[65] Those who survive to hospital may still have life-threatening injuries that require immediate intervention and, as such, they require rapid assessment, diagnosis and treatment.

Pathophysiology

The chest or thoracic cavity is made up of two structures: a bony cavity consisting of the ribs, sternum, scapulae and clavicles, and the muscular structure of the respiratory muscles and diaphragm. The organs contained in the chest include the lungs, airways, heart, blood and lymph vessels and oesophagus.

Chest trauma can be separated into injury to the thoracic structure including the ribs and diaphragm; injury to the lung, airways and associated tissue; injury to the heart and associated tissue; and injury to the vascular or digestive system located in the chest. Physiological consequences of thoracic trauma are hypoxia, hypercarbia and acidosis. Contusions, haematomas and alveolar collapse, or changes in intrathoracic pressure related to injury, can lead to hypoxia and metabolic acidosis. Hypercarbia is associated with insufficient ventilation and causes respiratory acidosis related to changes in intrathoracic pressure relationships, depressed levels of consciousness[11] or insufficient respiratory function secondary to pain. The other consequence is the combined effect on both the cardiovascular and respiratory functions due to hypovolaemia causing hypoperfusion and shock, generally related to blood loss.

Chest trauma includes the following:

- *Rib fractures* – these occur in up to 20% of trauma admissions and are an independent predictor of injury. Associated with other injuries such as haemothorax, pneumothorax and pulmonary contusions, often they are a source of severe pain and increased pulmonary complications. With each fracture, in older patients the risk of pneumonia increases by 27% and mortality by 19%.[65]

- *Flail chest* – comprising <1% of patients with rib fractures,[69] the diagnosis should be both radiological and through physical examination. A radiographic flail is when three or more ribs are fractured in two or more places. A clinical flail is when there is paradoxical chest wall movement, which can lead to hypoventilation and respiratory failure. Flail chest can also occur with separation of the costochondral junction[67] or when there are three or more consecutive fractures with a concomitant sternal fracture.[69] Up to 80% of patients with flail chest will require ICU admission, with 60% requiring mechanical ventilation.[70]

  Usually such fractures occur in the anterior or lateral sections of the rib cage, where there is less muscle protection. The significant impact of this injury is paradoxical movement of the flail segment during spontaneous ventilation, so that when a patient inspires, the flail segment moves inwards with the negative intrapleural pressure instead of expanding with the rib cage. In the mechanically ventilated patient this paradoxical movement may not be as evident. Compromised respiratory function is caused by the increased work of breathing that this ineffective flail segment creates, as well as the contused lung that normally occurs underneath the flail segment along with the severe pain and tenderness.

- *Diaphragmatic injuries* – these generally occur when there has been a significant rise in intra-abdominal pressure associated with transmission of force through abdominal viscera or laterally resulting in shearing tears. Diaphragmatic injuries are present in 0.8–8% of patients, with blunt trauma and 10–15% related to penetrating wounds, with 12–63% undiagnosed on initial presentation and with 70–75% occurring on the left side and 23% on the right side.

The right hemidiaphragm is thought to be congenitally stronger and protected by the liver. When the rupture is sufficiently large, protrusion of the abdominal contents into the thoracic space is likely, resulting in cardiac and respiratory compromise. Operations for other abdominal injuries may reveal a diaphragmatic tear, with the treatment being a direct repair.[71]

- *Pulmonary contusion* – this is bruising to the lung tissue, usually as a result of mechanical force. This bruising is followed by diffuse haemorrhage and interstitial and alveolar oedema, resulting in impaired gas exchange due to shunting, and leading to hypoxia and increased oxygen requirements. This injury is often associated with rib fractures; respiratory failure may develop over time rather than instantaneously. Pulmonary contusions represent up to 75% of injured patients; significant blunt chest trauma has up to 25% mortality.[67] These contusions can be caused by motor vehicle accidents, high-velocity missile wounds or high-energy shock waves from explosions in the air and water.

- *Pneumothorax* – this is accumulation of air between the visceral and parietal pleura, which occurs with both blunt and penetrating mechanisms and is seen in 40–50% of thoracic trauma. A pneumothorax can be divided into three types: simple (or closed), communicating (or open) or tension:
  - A simple or closed pneumothorax indicates that there is no communication with the atmosphere, and results from a fractured rib puncturing the lung parenchyma; however, it may also occur when impact occurs at full inspiration and the glottis is closed, leading to increased intra-alveolar pressure and subsequent rupture.
  - Open pneumothoraces, also known as 'sucking chest wound', generally occur in the setting of penetrating trauma, where air is able to move from the external atmosphere to the pleural space during inspiration and if untreated leads to tension pneumothorax and potentially death. Treatment consists of an occlusive dressing sealed on three sides to allow air to escape but preventing air from entering the wound.
  - A tension pneumothorax occurs when air is not able to escape from the pleural space, leading to mediastinal displacement resulting in decreased venous return and compression on the opposite lung.[65] Clinical presentation includes severe dyspnoea and air hunger in the awake patient through to cardiovascular collapse.[72] With the use of imaging modalities such as CT scan, the

phenomenon of occult pneumothorax (pneumothorax detected on CT scan that was not diagnosed on X-ray) has appeared. A review by the Western Trauma Association found that approximately 10% of occult pneumothoraces could be observed safely and up to 80% in the ventilated patient group.[73]

- *Haemothorax* – this is accumulation of blood in the pleural space after blunt or penetrating chest trauma. In blunt injuries the source of blood is most commonly from fractured ribs and adjacent lung laceration, although injury to the blood vessels or cardiac injuries may also be the cause.[67] With penetrating injuries, haemothorax is related to direct injury to the lung, arteries, heart or major blood vessels in the thoracic cavity. Breath sounds are usually reduced on the side of the haemothorax; percussion is noted to be dull rather than hyper-resonant[65] unless it is a haemopneumothorax, and there may be evidence of tracheal deviation away from the affected side. Small haemothoraces (<200 mL blood) may not be apparent on clinical or radiological investigation, although respiratory compromise is likely to be present. Massive haemothorax is defined as more than 1500 mL[65] and causes circulatory compromise from hypovolaemia, vena cava compression and hypoxaemia; it requires operative control of the bleeding. Initial management of a haemothorax is the insertion of a chest tube to allow for drainage of the accumulated blood.[67] Optimal evacuation of residual clots and breakdown of adhesions and loculated effusions are important to prevent complications such as empyema or fibrothorax and can be achieved using a surgical approach in the later phase of care.[67]

- *Cardiac trauma* – myocardial contusion is the most common outcome of blunt cardiac injury; however, this can lead to arrhythmias and impaired myocardial function. Other injuries include rupture of the heart wall, septum or valves or damage to the coronary arteries.[72] The right side of the heart is most commonly injured, probably as a result of the anterior placement of this side of the heart in the thorax, although more than half the patients with a blunt cardiac trauma experience injury to multiple cardiac chambers. Motor vehicle crashes account for 50% of blunt cardiac injuries, followed by pedestrians struck by vehicles, motorcyclists and falls greater than 6 m. The incidence of myocardial injury in blunt chest trauma ranges from 15% to 75%, so a high level of suspicion is necessary when assessing these patients.

- *Aortic injuries* – injuries to the brachiocephalic, left subclavian or right subclavian branches of the aorta are associated with high mortality at the scene. Minor aortic injuries usually involve a small intimal tear with small periaortic haematoma, while significant injuries include the intima and full thickness of media with associated high risk of rupture. Aortic transection and rupture are associated with >80% mortality within the first 30 minutes of injury; those who do survive to hospital frequently have a significant injury and if left untreated have a 50% mortality in the first 7 days.[74] A widened mediastinum on CXR is a sign of aortic dissection; however, thoracic CT scan with IV contrast is the gold standard for diagnosis for those patients who survive to hospital. Pharmacotherapy to stabilise and prevent progression should be considered, although thoracic endovascular aortic repair (TEVAR) is recommended if anatomically feasible, or open surgical repair.[74]

- *Tracheobronchial injuries* – these tend to occur as a result of direct blunt trauma and in close proximity to the carina. They are relatively rare, with a reported incidence rate between 2% and 3% of trauma patients, with 30–80% mortality pre-hospital due to asphyxia, tension pneumothorax or other injuries to heart and major vessels; however, mortality drops to approximately 9–20% in those who survive to hospital.[75,76] Common symptoms include tachypnoea, respiratory distress and haemoptysis, along with extending subcutaneous emphysema. Lower airway injuries cause pneumothorax, with massive air leak through intercostal catheters (ICCs), so lung re-expansion cannot occur, and pneumomediastinum, while complete transection can lead to airway occlusion.[77] If suspicious for tracheobronchial injury, a CT and/ or bronchoscopy should be undertaken.[76]

Clinical manifestations

Injuries to the thoracic cavity can manifest according to the structures and systems involved (Table 24.6). When multiple organs and systems are involved, the combined injuries pose an increased threat to life.

TABLE 24.6

Clinical manifestations of chest trauma

SYSTEM	MANIFESTATION	MANIFESTATION
Respiratory • Airways • Lungs • Diaphragm	Any sign of respiratory compromise, noting that serial observations are an important indicator of imminent decompensation.	Abnormal respiratory rate (≤12 or >20 breaths/min). Abnormal chest wall movement, including asymmetrical chest wall expansion. Reduced breath sounds. Obstructed airway. Hypoxia (<94%). Hypercarbia. Apnoea. Dyspnoea. Haemoptysis. Crepitus/surgical emphysema.
Cardiovascular • Heart • Great vessels	Circulatory insufficiency resulting in decreased tissue perfusion.	Abnormal heart rate (<60 or >100 bpm). Arrhythmia. In severe cases, pulseless electrical activity (see Chapter 11). Pulsus alternans. Decreased cardiac output. Lowered blood pressure (systolic <100 mmHg). Reduced peripheral perfusion. Confusion and reduced consciousness level. Interscapular or retrosternal pain.
Gastrointestinal • Oesophageal rupture	Perforation and contamination of mediastinum.	Crepitus. Haemopneumothorax. Pain – chest and abdominal. Cough. Stridor. Bleeding. Sepsis (late).
Systemic • Air embolism	May occur in response to injury of a vessel that traverses an air space; manifestations will vary depending on location and associated injuries.	Varied depending on location, but may include: • focal neurological sign • cardiac deterioration.

Patient management

Given the underlying structures of heart, lungs and great vessels, chest trauma can cause rapid deterioration in the patient. Ongoing and thorough assessment, particularly in relation to the signs and symptoms outlined in Table 24.6, is essential. Other essential aspects of care include patient positioning and management of pain relief and consideration for forced vital capacity (FVC) evaluation to assess lung capacity and response to interventions.

Assessment

Initial assessment in the ED should be conducted on an ongoing basis, with formal documentation of these findings occurring every few minutes until stabilisation. The frequency of ongoing assessment will then be based on the patient's condition, but is likely to be needed every 15 minutes initially, reducing to hourly with transfer to the critical care unit. Signs of chest trauma that represent life-threatening emergencies include the following:

- *Cardiac tamponade* – as blood collects in the pericardium, the venous return to the heart is impeded, resulting in reduced cardiac output. Signs of cardiac tamponade include:
  - anxiety and agitation
  - elevated heart rate
  - muffled heart sounds
  - reducing pulse pressure, with falling systolic blood pressure (BP) and rising diastolic BP
  - increased preload (CVP and/or pulmonary capillary wedge pressure (PCWP))
  - distended neck veins
  - signs of reduced cardiac output, including lower level of consciousness, poor peripheral perfusion and reduced urine output.
- *Tension pneumothorax* – in this the lung/s collapse as the pleural space fills with air that cannot escape (Fig. 24.5). As the volume of air grows with each breath, the thoracic cavity contents are compressed or pushed against the opposite side of the chest. Signs of tension pneumothorax include:
  - elevated heart rate
  - increased respiratory rate
  - hypotension
  - decreased air entry, particularly over the affected lung, with possible asymmetrical lung expansion
  - hyper-resonant percussion sounds
  - tracheal deviation
  - distended neck veins
  - surgical emphysema.[78]

Practice tip

Unexplained hypotension in a patient with chest trauma may indicate a tension pneumothorax; an urgent CXR is required for diagnosis.

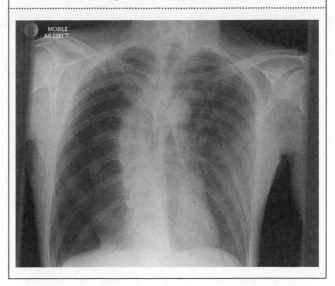

FIGURE 24.5 Right tension pneumothorax.

Positioning

Early mobilisation can prevent the complications of prolonged bed rest and immobility and assist with chest physiotherapy. Patients should be nursed side to side and in a variety of positions, including sitting upright. They should be mobilised as soon as their injuries permit, but this may be limited by pain. Mobilisation can improve tidal volumes, optimise functional residual capacity, enhance ventilation/perfusion matching and facilitate secretion clearance.[79]

Care must be taken to accommodate the increased work of breathing that is associated with injuries to the lungs. Supplemental oxygen will assist the patient's exercise tolerance. Further, if the patient is mechanically ventilated, additional mechanical support (i.e. transient increase in pressure support) may be applied to assist the patient's exercise tolerance. Being unable to catch their breath is a terrifying experience that may result in increased anxiety for patients and should be avoided wherever possible.

Pain relief

The principles of managing pain in chest trauma patients are similar to those for other patients, with effective pain management being a major determinant of maintaining adequate spontaneous breathing. Early escalation of interventions and frequent review of management strategies are essential and may assist in avoiding mechanical ventilation in the less-severe group of chest trauma patients, so effective deep breathing and coughing must be promoted. A variety of approaches exist, including systemic analgesia and regional techniques that may be used concurrently (see Chapter 6).

Systemic analgesia includes oral, intravenous (intermittent, continuous or patient-controlled analgesia (PCA)), intramuscular and transdermal analgesia. It may cause sedation, respiratory and cough suppression and delirium, which can impact on patient cooperation and physiotherapy participation.

Regional analgesia includes epidurals, thoracic paravertebral block, intercostal nerve block, myofascial plane blocks such as serratus anterior block and erector spinae blocks.[72]

Non-pharmacological means such as the use of supplemental oxygen, breathing exercises, massage, relaxation and diversion techniques should also be considered.

Surgical management of injury

Surgical intervention in patients with chest trauma includes repair of any tears, ruptures and lacerations that result from blunt or penetrating injury. The emergency thoracotomy has proved beneficial in a select group of patients with penetrating trauma and less than 15 minutes of cardiopulmonary resuscitation, with several guidelines outlining indications and criteria including those published by the Joint Trauma System (JTS), the Western Trauma Association (WTA), the Eastern Association for the Surgery of Trauma (EAST) and the American College of Surgeons.[77] A meta-analysis of mortality by mechanism of injury found a 92.8% rate in blunt injuries versus 78.7% for penetrating injuries in ED, with differences also found between trauma centres in the US versus other international trauma centres (92.9% versus 72.3%).[80]

While different techniques are used in different settings, the main access to the thoracic cavity is via a left thoracotomy, a midline sternotomy or a 'clamshell' incision. The 'clamshell' incision allows access to both thoracic cavities, the lower mediastinum and heart.[81] Initial assessment of the patient will determine the need for a thoracotomy in either the ED or the operating room. All staff members working in trauma reception that have the capacity for emergency thoracotomy should be familiar with the equipment and process for this procedure. Postoperative nursing care of these patients should follow the same principles as for patients who have undergone routine cardiothoracic surgery.

Although not indicated in the unstable patient, the utilisation of video-assisted thoracoscopic surgery (VATS) in the relatively stable patient post-initial resuscitation allows for evacuation of clotted haemothorax or decortication of empyema. Surgical repair of rib fractures is being used more globally and was conditionally recommended by EAST in 2017 as it can reduce mortality, length of stay, incidence of pneumonia and need for tracheostomy.[72]

Chest drainage

Insertion of an ICC drains the air and/or blood from between the pleura, resulting in re-instatement of the negative intrapleural pressure and re-inflation of the underlying lung.

The principles of chest drainage include the following:

1 The lungs are encased in a potential space. The visceral pleura attaches to the parietal pleura via surface tension, creating a negative intrapleural pressure and attaching the lung to the chest wall. During inspiration, the rib cage moves out and the diaphragm contracts and moves down, increasing the size of the intrathoracic space. Air moves from an area of higher pressure in the environment to an area of lower pressure within the lungs along a pressure gradient.

2 An ICC is inserted into the pleural space, passing between the ribs.

3 The drainage system and seal provide an ongoing means of removing air and/or fluid from the pleural space, while preventing air from the atmosphere entering via the ICC. If the traditional glass bottle system is being used, the seal is provided by placing the distal end of the ICC under water (usually 2 cm). The catheter should not be placed under excessive levels of water, as this creates resistance and will limit air and fluid escaping from the pleural space.

4 Suction is often added to the drainage system to promote drainage of fluid.

Care of the chest trauma patient with intercostal drainage is directed towards ensuring sterility and patency of the system and assessing the amount and type of drainage, as well as the impact on the patient (Table 24.7). Additional considerations include the following:

• ICC may be positional, or alternatively haemo/ pneumothoraces may be loculated. Repositioning of the patient may be necessary or consideration of

---

TABLE 24.7

Assessment of chest drainage

CHARACTERISTIC	DESCRIPTION
Water seal	Ensure there is sufficient water in the water seal chamber.
Bubbling	Continued bubbling indicates an air leak.
Drainage	Observe the nature and volume of fluid exudate (NB: >1500 mL stat or 200/mL/h for 2–4 h; surgical exploration may be required).
Patency	Ensure the intercostal catheter is not blocked; remove any blood clots.
Swinging	Oscillation of fluid in the ICC confirms patency, as this reflects the changes in intrapleural pressure with respiration; such oscillation should continue even when the lung has re-expanded.
Suction	If suction is ordered, check the appropriate level is being delivered.

replacing the existing catheter. The catheter should not be advanced into the pleural space once initial insertion is complete.

- Side-lying or lifting the patient, especially with a frame, may kink or disconnect the ICC.
- Surgical emphysema around the site of the ICC may dislodge the tip of the catheter out of the pleural cavity as the emphysema swells. Ongoing assessment, including a CXR, is required to confirm the position of the ICC.
- Movement of the patient, including sitting upright, will assist with fluid drainage; the volume of drainage should be assessed after moving the patient.
- Monitoring of respiratory function should continue after removal of the ICC, along with consideration for repeat CXR, to detect recollection of air or fluid.

> **Practice tip**
>
> Fresh, brightly coloured blood drained from the ICC indicates continued active bleeding, whereas dark blood usually indicates older blood that has been resting in the pleural space for some time.

Ventilatory support

Ventilatory support is often required for patients with chest trauma (see Chapter 15 for general principles). The following specific considerations apply:

- *Non-invasive ventilation* – care should be taken based on associated injuries, with contraindications including fractured base of skull or facial fractures.
- *Intubation* – haemoptysis is relatively common in patients with lung injury, and care must be taken to ensure removal of blood clots from the ETT. Heated, humidified air and regular suctioning will assist with maintaining ETT patency.
- *Airway injury* – initiation of positive-pressure ventilation in the chest trauma patient may identify damage to a small airway that previously went unnoticed (damage to a large airway will usually have been detected early in the assessment phase). Treatment will depend on the severity and location of the rupture, but usually requires decompression of the pleura with an ICC, possibly surgical intervention and advanced respiratory support such as independent lung ventilation.
- *Use of tracheostomy* – this may be required for patients with injury to the trachea and is managed using the same principles as with any patient with a tracheostomy.

Allied health interventions

Physiotherapy is generally required for chest trauma patients. The primary aspects of care include chest physiotherapy, given that mechanical ventilation may be for extended periods of time, as well as mobility exercises. Occupational therapy may offer diversionary activities or communication alternatives in ventilated patients. Social work may assist with counselling financial and social concerns. Early referral of selected patients to allied health professionals has the potential to significantly influence patient outcome and reduce family stressors.

Abdominal trauma

Abdominal trauma presents unique challenges to clinicians due to the abdominal cavity's high diversity of organs and structures. The abdomen is the third most commonly injured region of the body, with an associated abdominal injury present in approximately 10–20% of all trauma admissions and mortality reported to be around 20%. In the USA, stab and gunshot wounds predominate, while in Australia and most European countries blunt trauma is more common.[82,83] Management of abdominal injuries includes ruling out life-threatening haemorrhage, physical examination and imaging, with patients who are haemodynamically unstable requiring aggressive fluid resuscitation and evaluation for surgical exploration, as delayed operative management by more than 10 minutes has an associated threefold increase in mortality.[25] Therefore, the need for early, accurate diagnosis and treatment is paramount. Although gunshot wounds are not as common as stabbing injuries, they do account for 90% of penetrating trauma mortality, especially in the USA.[84]

Penetrating injury commonly involves the small intestine, colon and liver, whereas blunt trauma includes tears, laceration or rupture to liver, spleen, mesenteric artery or great vessels, renal, bladder, diaphragm, gastric or pancreas.[85] Indications for immediate exploration include hypotension, peritonitis and evisceration, otherwise serial examination may be sufficient. In blunt abdominal trauma the spleen is the organ that is most commonly injured, with the liver being the second most common,[85] while injury to the hollow viscous organs is relatively uncommon in comparison.

Recent advances in diagnostic and treatment techniques for abdominal trauma have seen an increased emphasis on non-operative management for solid organ injury, with increased use of angioembolisation. Non-operative management should be considered in haemodynamically stable patients, with an emphasis on close patient monitoring and regular laboratory examinations, potentially including ICU or high-dependency care.[82]

Pathophysiology

The abdominal cavity consists of a range of tissues and organ structures, including musculoskeletal, solid and hollow organs, vessels and nerves. Musculoskeletal structures include the major abdominal muscle groups forming the abdominal wall, as well as the lumbar vertebrae and pelvis. Solid organs include the liver, spleen, pancreas, kidneys and adrenal glands (and ovaries in women). Hollow organs include the stomach, small and large intestines, gall bladder and bladder (and uterus in women). Finally, the vessels and nerves include a complex array of all abdominal blood vessels (arterial and venous), lymphatics and nerves including neural plexuses and the spinal cord. Traumatic abdominal injuries are classified as being extraperitoneal, intraperitoneal and/or retroperitoneal. Importantly, a patient can have any mix or multiples of these. The classification of injury guides clinical decision making.

The pathophysiology of abdominal trauma is largely related to the structure(s) injured. Careful serial assessments are essential to identify changing clinical manifestations. The most common clinical manifestation of abdominal trauma is haemorrhage[25] and/or signs of an acute abdomen, such as pain, tenderness, rigidity and bruising. Importantly, these are life-threatening signs and require immediate surgical intervention.

The most significant sign of abdominal trauma in the conscious patient is thought to be pain, either immediate or delayed; the injured person who presents with altered mental state from either a TBI, drugs, alcohol or metabolic disturbances cannot be assessed for pain. Other signs of abdominal injury include dizziness, nausea and vomiting, and dyspnoea related to irritation of the peritoneum or obstruction.[84] Inspection may elicit evidence of abrasions, bruising, obvious penetrating injury, distended abdomen or specific bruising that may raise the suspicion of a retroperitoneal injury. Palpation may elicit pain, guarding or distention of the abdomen which could be indicative of haemorrhage. Auscultation can be used to note the presence or absence of bowel sounds, although this is a more significant sign if serial assessments are made.[12]

Where hollow viscus perforation has occurred, repeated clinical examination plus or minus serial imaging is required for decision making. Abdominal bruising reflective of a seatbelt pattern is reported to be associated with an 8–23% incidence of hollow viscus injury.[86] Other signs of abdominal trauma can be related to the structure that has been injured. For example, haematuria demonstrates trauma to some part of the urinary tract, including the kidneys.

A key aspect with any abdominal injury is that the superficial injury does not always reflect what lies below. For example, it is not possible to be certain of the trajectory that a bullet took after it passed through the skin.

Contusion/laceration

Sudden deceleration of moving body tissues can result in laceration or haemorrhage into the tissues (contusion). This is related to the tearing of the tissues that occurs from inertia, or the tendency of tissues to resist changes in speed or direction (e.g. to keep moving forwards when the body has stopped moving, resulting in a tearing action to the tissues). Any structure in the abdomen is susceptible to this type of injury. Commonly, the liver and spleen are the worst-affected organs, largely related to a seatbelt injury in motor vehicle collisions. Laceration of a solid

organ can be a minor injury that is appropriately monitored and managed conservatively or non-operatively; alternatively, a similar injury can lead to exsanguination (e.g. a liver laceration into the hilum that involves the inferior vena cava). Hollow viscous organs can be contused, as can the mesentery and peritoneum.

Perforation

Full-thickness injury, or perforation, to a hollow viscus organ is life threatening. Perforation of the intestine can result in peritoneal soiling and ischaemic bowel. Small intestinal injuries constitute more than half of all blunt intestinal injuries, the second most common region being the colon; the left colon is more commonly injured than the right or transverse colon. Full-thickness perforations are less common than serous or seromuscular tears. Importantly, patients with this type of abdominal trauma can present late (by days). If presenting late, the usual clinical manifestations are pain, peritonitis and sepsis, along with an associated increase in mortality and morbidity

Secondary injury: abdominal compartment syndrome

The abdominal viscera are highly vascular and subject to vascular engorgement during massive fluid resuscitation. Where this occurs, there is an acute rise in intra-abdominal pressure (IAP). The World Congress of Abdominal Compartment Syndrome (WSAC), now known as WSAC – the Abdominal Compartment Society, defined intra-abdominal hypertension (IAH) as an IAP less than 12 mmHg without physiological derangement, and abdominal compartment syndrome[77] was defined as IAP greater than 20 mmHg with new organ dysfunction or failure. Compromise of respiratory function and compression of the abdominal organs causes organ dysfunction and may lead to the development of systemic inflammatory response syndrome (SIRS) and multiorgan failure.[87] This is a surgical emergency and the abdominal cavity requires decompression immediately; however, the resultant open abdomen is seen as a potential risk to life. The incidence of ACS has declined over time, probably as a result of an increased index of suspicion, early recognition and DCR techniques including judicious use of crystalloids in resuscitation and the use of 'open abdomen' and negative pressure dressings. Case reports indicate an ACS incidence of 4–8% in critically ill patients.[87]

Prediction of ACS is related to the pattern of injury (catastrophic blunt or penetrating injury with shock), pathophysiology (hypothermia, acidosis or coagulopathy), surgical approach of haemorrhage control, haemostatic resuscitation and restriction of crystalloid administration. See Chapter 20 for a detailed review of ACS including IAP monitoring and subsequent management.

Patient management

Recent trends have seen an increasing use of non-operative care of patients with abdominal injury. In these patients, monitoring for deterioration is essential, as is the

TABLE 24.8

Common signs of abdominal injury

SIGN	DESCRIPTION	SUSPECTED INJURY
Grey Turner's sign	Blueish discoloration of the lower abdomen and flanks 6–24 h after onset of bleeding.	Retroperitoneal haemorrhage.
Kehr's sign	Left shoulder-tip pain caused by diaphragmatic irritation.	Splenic injury, although can be associated with any intra-abdominal bleeding.
Cullen's sign	Bluish discoloration around the umbilicus.	Pancreatic injury, although can be associated with any peritoneal bleeding.
Coopernail's sign	Ecchymosis of scrotum or labia.	Pelvic fracture or pelvic organ injury.

Source: Wright JA. Seven abdominal assessment signs every emergency nurse should know. J Emerg Nurs October 1997:446–50.

ability to activate surgery and care for patients accordingly. Care of patients after abdominal trauma also includes effective diagnosis, surgical or radiological interventions and associated care. DCS is now a mainstay in management.

With the high use of non-operative management techniques for solid organ injury, the role of monitoring of patients with abdominal trauma is pivotal. Nurses must be cognisant of the clinical signs of abdominal injury, especially haemorrhage, and act on these immediately (Table 24.8). Specific aspects of nursing care for patients after abdominal trauma include pain management, monitoring and postoperative care. Patients often experience severe pain as a result of both the primary trauma and any surgical intervention for repair (see Chapter 6).

Vital sign monitoring is a mainstay of nursing management in patients with abdominal trauma, and all patients should have appropriate monitoring (as outlined in trauma reception). It is also essential that patients receive a urinalysis after incurring abdominal trauma in order to identify trauma to the urinary system.

Postoperative management of trauma laparotomy is the same as in any abdominal surgical procedure. The specific nursing care elements will depend on which organ has been injured and the surgical procedure undertaken. Careful attention must be paid to general nursing care elements for all patients (see Chapter 5).

Postoperative feeding and bowel care should be discussed with the healthcare team and plans made early to avoid delays and adverse events such as constipation (see Chapter 19 for principles of feeding). A paralytic ileus is a common manifestation of the critically ill abdominal trauma patient. Ensuring that the gut is decompressed, with a functional enterogastric tube that is correctly positioned, is essential. Because constipation is a common problem, early intervention and implementation of a bowel care protocol for trauma should be considered (see Chapter 5).

Diagnosis in the trauma setting consists of a thorough clinical assessment, the potential use of FAST, DPL,

abdominal CT and laparotomy or laparoscopy. Clinical assessment may reveal clinical signs such as skin bruising, lacerations, signs of abdominal rigidity and guarding. The various locations of clinical signs are clues to potential abdominal injury. The results of this phase of the investigation will determine what additional diagnostic tests are undertaken.

Diagnostic peritoneal lavage

DPL is a procedure that can be undertaken rapidly to assess for intra-abdominal bleeding, although it is frequently used only where FAST or CT is not available. Unlike FAST and CT scans, DPL can be performed only once.[26]

Disadvantages of DPL include:

- not organ specific
- high false-negative rate
- high level of invasiveness and associated complications
- inability to detect retroperitoneal, diaphragm or iatrogenic injuries
- potential interference with the interpretation of subsequent CT scans.

Abdominal computed tomography

Abdominal CT is recognised as having high sensitivity and specificity in the setting of intra-abdominal injury and is therefore accepted as a diagnostic mainstay,[83] particularly for patients with blunt trauma who are haemodynamically stable, and may be useful in determining the disposition of the patient. The main exception to this is where the results of a FAST examination are positive and the patient is taken to surgery urgently. The specific protocols vary depending on the suspected injuries; however, in most scans IV contrast is administered, with delay phase imaging used for suspected renal, ureteric or bladder injuries.

Debate exists as to the role of oral contrast as it does not increase the yield of axial imaging, can result in unnecessary delays and is not without risk in the trauma patient who must remain supine and immobilised in a cervical collar.[25] It is essential that nursing assessment for the risk of aspiration be conducted and strategies to manage the vomiting patient planned. If patients have a wide-bore enterogastric tube in situ, consider aspirating this to reduce the risk of aspiration. Any supine patient given radiographic contrast should not be left unattended, and there should be sufficient staff members available at short notice to roll the patient onto their side if they vomit. The healthcare team should discuss the risk of vomiting prior to ordering the test so that an informed decision can be made regarding the risk:benefit ratio on an individual case basis.

Laparotomy/laparoscopy

The role and indications for diagnostic operations such as laparotomy/laparoscopy is well described in the literature, and is essential to aid diagnosis (laparoscopy) and provide appropriate treatment to control haemorrhage and repair organ injury (laparotomy). When this procedure is considered appropriate, rapid but safe transit to the operating room should be undertaken. As the consequences of missed or delayed diagnosis of abdominal injury can be catastrophic for the patient, opening the peritoneal cavity to exclude injury in selected cases is a necessity. One meta-analysis demonstrated a decrease in therapeutic laparotomy from 69% to 47.5%, while therapeutic laparoscopy increased from 7.2% to 22.7%.[88]

Indications for emergency laparotomy in blunt trauma include:

- peritonism
- free air under the diaphragm
- significant gastrointestinal haemorrhage
- hypotension with a positive FAST scan
- increasing abdominal pain
- high-grade solid organ injuries if embolisation is not available
- physiological deterioration.[11,25]

Indications for emergency laparotomy in penetrating trauma include:

- penetrating abdominal trauma plus hypotension
- peritonism
- free air
- evisceration
- gunshot wounds traversing the peritoneum.[11]

Embolisation

Interventional radiology and angioembolisation can help to evaluate and potentially treat bleeding and control pseudoaneurysms and traumatic arteriovenous fistula, and is generally considered as an adjunct to non-operative management of abdominal injuries,[89] especially where bleeding occurs in areas considered difficult to access. Failure to control bleeding or unsuccessful cannulation owing to pathological or anatomical variations can occur and the patient may progress to laparotomy for definitive management. Via an arterial approach, commonly the left femoral artery, the interventional radiologist can insert cannulae to identify arterial blushes (bleeders). Once identified, the vessel can be ligated via mechanical coiling or blocked chemically.[89]

The patient undergoing embolisation for the control of haemorrhage requires meticulous monitoring including haemoglobin, and an ability to respond immediately to signs of hypovolaemic shock should the patient rebleed.

Management of the patient with an open abdomen

In cases of severe abdominal trauma, the patient may be returned to the ICU with an open abdomen, covered with a temporary wound-closure system. There are various types of open abdominal dressings including standard wound packing secured with clear adhesive dressing, negative-pressure wound therapy (NPWT) and dynamic closure techniques that are used in conjunction with NPWT. A review and meta-analysis of NPWT and dynamic closure techniques found it to be superior in closing the open abdomen and in reducing the fistula rate.[90] NPWT prevents uncontrolled evaporative loss and secondary bacterial contamination, reduces heat loss and allows early detection of bleeding. The principal aim of the dressing is to provide coverage for the contents of the peritoneum, or where there is a need for repeated opening of the abdomen. Ultimately, the aim is to close the skin as soon as possible when the patient's physiological status normalises. The benefit of the open abdomen approach is that it can avoid the development of intra-abdominal hypertension or ACS by avoiding increased intra-abdominal pressure.[91] Another challenge for the patient with the open abdomen is the potential for the development of enteroatmospheric fistulas when fascial closure is not achieved, and there is a requirement for late reconstructive therapy.

The primary aims of managing a patient with an open abdomen includes minimising complications of prolonged immobility, observing for signs of ongoing ACS, restoring the patient's physiology to normal and supporting the patient and family through a psychologically distressing time. Understandably, both the patient and their family can be distressed by the appearance of an open abdomen. There are no specific position restrictions for a patient with an open abdomen, but haemodynamic status is often labile so care must be taken with side-lying and hygiene care. Nutritional support is another aspect of recovery. Patients with open abdomen post DCS are hypermetabolic and current evidence supports early feeding to meet nutritional needs.[90] Consideration of parenteral nutrition should be discussed if there is an associated bowel injury; however, the initiation of enteral nutrition has been found to lead to higher abdominal closure rates, lower fistula rates and a reduction of mortality in patients with an open abdomen.[92]

Splenic injuries

The spleen is the solid organ most commonly injured in blunt trauma, with the degree of injury ranging from a small subcapsular haematoma to hilar devascularisation. Its location (under the ribs) makes it vulnerable to secondary injury from fractured ribs. Splenic injury should always be suspected in patients who have sustained a direct blow to the abdomen, as it is a large organ. The most common sign of splenic injury is pain over the left upper quadrant; however, haemodynamic instability, severe abdominal pain and symptoms of peritonitis may be present, but the lack of signs and symptoms does not rule out splenic injury. The Organ Injury Scale (OIS) was revised in 2018 to include imaging criteria and pathological criteria. The Spleen OIS has five grades designed to aid classification and management[93] (Table 24.9). Complications associated with blunt spleen injury include significant bleeding after initial management. General complications from angiography relate to vascular access and include retroperitoneal haematoma, pseudoaneurysm, arteriovenous fistula formation, peripheral nerve injury, thrombosis, dissection and distal embolisation.[94]

The spleen comprises more than 25% of the total lymphoid mass, making it the largest lymphoid organ in

---

TABLE 24.9

Spleen Injury Scale

AAST GRADE	AIS SEVERITY	IMAGING CRITERIA (CT FINDINGS)	OPERATIVE CRITERIA	PATHOLOGICAL CRITERIA
I	2	Subcapsular haematoma <10% surface area.	Subcapsular haematoma <10% surface area.	Subcapsular haematoma <10% surface area.
		Parenchymal laceration <1 cm depth.	Parenchymal laceration <1 cm depth.	Parenchymal laceration <1 cm depth.
		Capsular tear.	Capsular tear.	Capsular tear.
II	2	Subcapsular haematoma 10–50% surface area; intraparenchymal haematoma <5 cm.	Subcapsular haematoma 10–50% surface area; intraparenchymal haematoma <5 cm.	Subcapsular haematoma 10–50% surface area; intraparenchymal haematoma <5 cm.
		Parenchymal laceration 1–3 cm.	Parenchymal laceration 1–3 cm.	Parenchymal laceration 1–3 cm.
III	3	Subcapsular haematoma >50% surface area; ruptured subcapsular or intraparenchymal haematoma ≥5 cm.	Subcapsular haematoma >50% surface area or expanding; ruptured subcapsular or intraparenchymal haematoma ≥5 cm.	Subcapsular haematoma >50% surface area; ruptured subcapsular or intraparenchymal haematoma ≥5 cm.
		Parenchymal laceration >3 cm depth.	Parenchymal laceration >3 cm depth.	Parenchymal laceration >3 cm depth.
IV	4	Any injury in the presence of a splenic vascular injury or active bleeding confined within splenic capsule.	Parenchymal laceration involving segmental or hilar vessels producing >25% devascularisation.	Parenchymal laceration involving segmental or hilar vessels producing >25% devascularisation.
		Parenchymal laceration involving segmental or hilar vessels producing >25%, devascularisation.		
V	5	Any injury in the presence of splenic vascular injury with active bleeding extending beyond the spleen into the peritoneum.	Hilar vascular injury which devascularises the spleen.	Hilar vascular injury which devascularises the spleen.
		Shattered spleen.	Shattered spleen.	Shattered spleen.

Source: Spleen Organ Injury Scale – 2018 Revision; Feliciano DV. A review of "Changes in the management of injuries to the liver and spleen" (2005). Am Surg 2021;87(2):212–18.[93]

the body with the primary function of assisting with immunity, especially against encapsulated organisms. Therefore, patients who have had a splenectomy are at risk of infections, particularly encapsulated organisms.[95] As these patients have a lifetime increased risk of infection, they require careful education surrounding the risks and the importance of follow-up immunisations, which should be in accordance with either the US Center for Disease Control and Prevention (CDC) or professional organisations that assist with the prevention of disease. These patients should be encouraged to seek medical attention promptly to decrease the risk of severe infection. The current recommendation for pre-discharge immunisations includes:

- pneumococcal vaccine
- meningococcal vaccines
- influenza vaccine.

The patient may also be commenced on antibiotic prophylaxis and should be advised to wear a medi-alert disk or card and consult specialist travel advice when travelling.[95]

Liver injuries

Liver injuries should be suspected in anyone with injury to the lower chest or abdomen owing to its size and location, which make it susceptible to injury.[96] Liver injuries range from minor to life threatening, with the most common cause of morbidity and mortality in the acute phase related to haemorrhage.[97] Mortality rates vary from 9% to 42% for patients admitted with liver injuries.[98]

Injuries to the liver are classified according to mechanism and grade by the American Association for the Surgery of Trauma (AAST), with a five-level injury scale[93] (Table 24.10). Most grade I–III injuries can be managed non-operatively, whereas grade IV–VI injuries often require operative management. According to the WEST guidelines, 72.8% of grade IV injuries and 62.6% of grade V injuries have been successfully managed non-operatively. Non-operative management should be undertaken only when there are appropriate monitoring capabilities, such as high-dependency unit or ICU, available for serial clinical evaluations and operating room and surgical capabilities available for urgent laparotomy if the patient deteriorates. In the non-operatively managed patient, repeat CT or surgery should be considered if there is increased abdominal pain, jaundice or clinical signs of bleeding. Patients who are haemodynamically unstable require surgical review and urgent laparotomy; however, if stable then the gold standard for diagnosis of liver injuries is CT scan with contrast.[97]

ICU admission is in the context of optimising resuscitation, correction of haemostasis, treating any progressive organ failure and facilitating serial clinical examinations.

Early complications of liver injury relate to hypoperfusion or massive transfusions, with severe injuries leading to biliary fistula, peritonitis/biliary ascites, pseudoaneurysms, biochemical abnormalities, altered coagulation and, rarely, liver failure.[97] In high-grade injury, complication rates are reported between 12% and 14%.[92] Complications associated with angioembolisation include hepatic necrosis, gall-bladder necrosis, bile leak and abscess formation.

Penetrating injuries

Penetrating trauma refers to the piercing of the skin by a foreign object, which is largely localised to a single body region. Exceptions to this may occur – for example, with firearm wounds if there are multiple bullet-entry wounds or multiple knife-stab sites. The most common examples include knife and gunshot wounds, although solid objects such as fences, signposts and tools can cause penetrating trauma.

Caution must be taken when caring for patients with penetrating injury to prevent injury to staff. This is particularly important when the patient presents with a knife in situ or a large, protruding foreign object in their body. It should also be noted that some penetrating trauma occurs as a result of a criminal act, and it is essential to observe rules governing forensic evidence. Police should be notified by the senior clinician involved in providing care.

Clinical manifestations

The clinical manifestations of penetrating injuries are dependent on where in the body the penetrating injury has occurred, the underlying organs and the amount of force and dispersion caused by the injury. For example, a high-velocity bullet will cause substantial tissue damage in a wider area than just the bullet's track. The clinical manifestations of penetrating trauma can be divided into two broad types:

1 *conspicuous* – where the penetrating article is grossly visible (e.g. a shard of glass, a branch or a knife); care must be taken not to focus solely on the visible cause of injury but to continue to undertake a systematic trauma assessment

2 *inconspicuous* – where the penetrating article is not immediately visible and may become apparent only during the systematic trauma assessment of the patient (e.g. with gunshot wounds and projectiles); in these injuries the visual signs on the external skin may not reflect the catastrophic injury underlying it (e.g. ventricle lacerations or serious vascular injury).

Patient management

Patients with penetrating injury will be cared for based on the severity and area of injury they have sustained. Surgical intervention is usually more urgent than that seen with blunt injury, as bleeding may be occurring from a ruptured organ or vessel either into a body cavity or externally. For this reason, the incidence of procedures such as laparotomy and thoracotomy is high in patients with a penetrating injury.

TABLE 24.10

Liver Injury Scale

AAST GRADE	AIS SEVERITY	IMAGING CRITERIA (CT FINDINGS)	OPERATIVE CRITERIA	PATHOLOGICAL CRITERIA
I	2	Subcapsular haematoma <10% surface area.	Subcapsular haematoma <10% surface area.	Subcapsular haematoma <10% surface area.
		Parenchymal laceration <1 cm.	Parenchymal laceration <1 cm depth capsular tear.	Parenchymal laceration <1 cm depth capsular tear.
II	2	Subcapsular haematoma 10–50% surface area; intraparenchymal hematoma <10 cm in diameter.	Subcapsular haematoma 10–50% surface area; intraparenchymal hematoma <10 cm in diameter.	Subcapsular haematoma 10–50% surface area; intraparenchymal hematoma <10 cm in diameter.
		Laceration 1–3 cm in depth and ≤10 cm.	Laceration 1–3 cm in depth and ≤10 cm length.	Laceration 1–3 cm in depth and ≤10 cm length.
III	3	Subcapsular haematoma >50% surface area; ruptured subcapsular or parenchymal haematoma.	Subcapsular haematoma >50% surface area or expanding; ruptured subcapsular or parenchymal haematoma.	Subcapsular haematoma >50% surface area; ruptured subcapsular or intraparenchymal haematoma.
		Intraparenchymal haematoma >10 cm.	Intraparenchymal haematoma >10 cm.	Intraparenchymal haematoma >10 cm.
		Laceration >3 cm depth.		
		Any injury in the presence of a liver vascular injury or active bleeding contained within liver parenchyma.	Laceration >3 cm in depth.	Laceration >3 cm in depth.
IV	4	Parenchymal disruption involving 25–75% of a hepatic lobe.	Parenchymal disruption involving 25–75% of a hepatic lobe.	Parenchymal disruption involving 25–75% of a hepatic lobe.
		Active bleeding extending beyond the liver parenchyma into the peritoneum.		
V	5	Parenchymal disruption >75% of hepatic lobe.	Parenchymal disruption >75% of hepatic lobe.	Parenchymal disruption >75% of hepatic lobe.
		Juxtahepatic venous injury to include retrohepatic vena cava and central major hepatic veins.	Juxtahepatic venous injury to include retrohepatic vena cava and central major hepatic veins.	Juxtahepatic venous injury to include retrohepatic vena cava and central major hepatic veins.

Source: Liver Injury Scale – 2018 revision; Feliciano DV. A review of "Changes in the management of injuries to the liver and spleen" (2005). Am Surg 2021;87(2):212–18.[93]

In Australia, Germany and many other European countries the incidence of penetrating trauma represents a minority, unlike the USA where larger volumes of this type of trauma are experienced; as such, management of this particular group can be challenging.[99]

In the emergency setting the following considerations are generally unique to the patient with a penetrating injury:

- Stabilise the foreign object. This may require padding and/or taping an object, for example a knife, to ensure minimal movement and prevent further damage until definitive care can remove the object.

- Care for the patient in a non-standard position. This will be dependent on how and where any foreign object is protruding from the body. For example, it may be necessary to care for a patient in the side-lying or prone position until the object is removed.

- Minimise volume resuscitation: this describes the practice of resuscitating a patient only sufficiently to maintain adequate perfusion to essential organs until definitive repair of the wound can be undertaken. Reduced volume of IV fluids may be associated with more-favourable outcomes.[99]

- Provide psychosocial care of the patient and family. It is possible that patients with penetrating injury will need specific psychosocial care, particularly when the injury occurred as a result of assault.

Burns

Burns are the fourth most common type of trauma worldwide, with the majority of burns being minor and not requiring treatment; however, major burns have significant morbidity unless treated appropriately because of the rapid development of organ failure and death.[100] Burn injuries can be caused by friction, radiation, cold, chemicals or electricity, with most being caused by heat from fire or hot liquids. The degree of injury depends on the source and the duration of contact. An understanding of these changes will assist with planning appropriate care for this group of patients.

Worldwide, approximately 90% of burns occur in low- and middle-income areas in comparison with high-income countries, which are seeing a downward trend in burn injuries. The World Health Organization (WHO) estimates there are 11 million burn injuries annually, 180,000 of which are fatal.[101] Patients who are admitted to specialised critical care services have been found to have an associated reduction in hospital mortality.

Patients with burn injuries have unique challenges in regard to fluid resuscitation, metabolic stress, infections complicating burn recovery, along with abnormal drug pharmacology, severe pain, psychological stress, prolonged critical care and hospital stays, multiple surgical procedures, use of skin substitutes, and extensive rehabilitation.

In general terms, assessment is based on the size, depth and anatomical site of the injury, mechanism of injury and the presence of coexisting conditions. Outcomes for burns patients have improved with improvement of surgical treatment, intensive care management strategies and multidisciplinary team input.

All patients with a serious burn injury should be referred to a specialised burns unit that is staffed and equipped appropriately to manage burns owing to the physical and psychological impact it has. Burns associations that have implemented referral criteria include the American Burns Association, the National Health Service in the UK, the Australian and New Zealand Burn Association (ANZBA), the European Burns Association and others such as in the Netherlands the Dutch Burn Foundation, which uses criteria adopted from the Emergency Management of Severe Burns (EMSB)[102] (Box 24.1).[103]

Pathophysiology

The skin is the largest organ in the human body and accounts for 15% of its weight. It has multiple purposes, including protection from infection, regulation of body heat and function as a vapour barrier.

The skin consists of three layers: the epidermis, the dermis and subcutaneous tissue:

- *Epidermis* – this layer is characterised by having regenerative ability.

BOX 24.1

Criteria for treatment in a specialised burn centre

- Burns greater than 10% total body surface area (TBSA)
- Burns greater than 5% TBSA in children
- Full-thickness burns greater than 5% TBSA
- Burns of special areas – face, hands feet, genitalia, perineum, major joints and circumferential limb or chest burns
- Burns with inhalation injury
- Electrical burns
- Chemical burns
- Burns with pre-existing illness
- Burns associated with major trauma
- Burns at the extremes of age – young children and the elderly
- Burn injury in pregnant women
- Non-accidental burns

Source: https://anzba.org.au/care/referral-criteria/ and adapted from ABA – Shetty P, Cox C, Javia V. Inappropriate transfer of burn patients. Ann Plast Surg 2021;86(1):29–34.[103]

- *Dermis* – the dermis has no regenerative ability, but because the glands, vessels and follicles are lined with epidermis, burns that involve this layer may still regenerate.
- *Subcutaneous* tissue – this layer has no regenerative ability (Fig. 24.6).

Local changes

Once the cause of the burn has been removed, response in the local tissues may lead to injury in deeper zones. Those local changes include the zones of coagulation, stasis and hyperaemia (Fig. 24.7)[104] and the specific changes are outlined below.

- *Zone of coagulation:* this occurs at the point of maximum damage. Irreversible tissue loss occurs in this zone as a result of coagulation of the constituent proteins, which requires debridement.
- *Zone of stasis:* this is the immediate area surrounding the necrosis, and has a moderate degree of insult with decreased tissue perfusion. Tissue in this zone is potentially salvageable if sufficient resuscitation is achieved to increase tissue perfusion.
- *Zone of hyperaemia:* this is the outermost zone. Tissue in this zone will usually recover and is generally not at risk of further necrosis unless there are prolonged or severe periods of hypotension, infection or oedema.

FIGURE 24.6 Depth of burn.

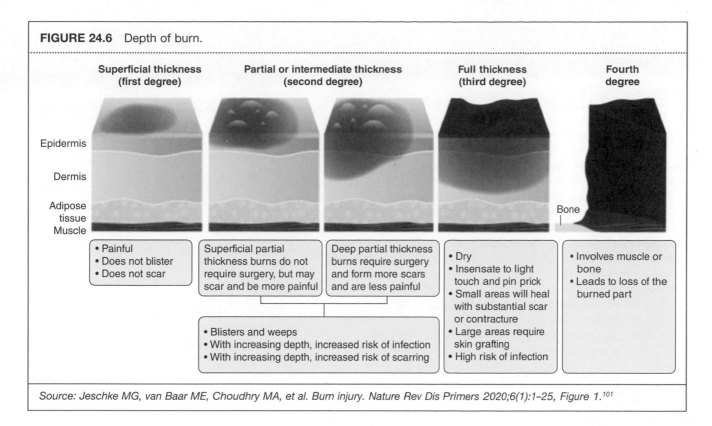

Superficial thickness (first degree)	Partial or intermediate thickness (second degree)	Full thickness (third degree)	Fourth degree

• Painful
• Does not blister
• Does not scar

Superficial partial thickness burns do not require surgery, but may scar and be more painful

Deep partial thickness burns require surgery and form more scars and are less painful

• Blisters and weeps
• With increasing depth, increased risk of infection
• With increasing depth, increased risk of scarring

• Dry
• Insensate to light touch and pin prick
• Small areas will heal with substantial scar or contracture
• Large areas require skin grafting
• High risk of infection

• Involves muscle or bone
• Leads to loss of the burned part

Source: Jeschke MG, van Baar ME, Choudhry MA, et al. Burn injury. Nature Rev Dis Primers 2020;6(1):1–25, Figure 1.[101]

FIGURE 24.7 Zone of burn damage.

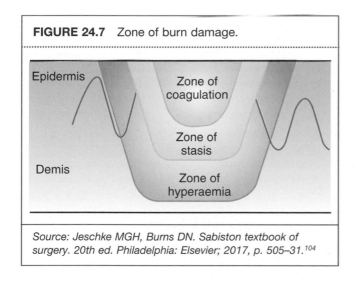

Source: Jeschke MGH, Burns DN. Sabiston textbook of surgery. 20th ed. Philadelphia: Elsevier; 2017, p. 505–31.[104]

FIGURE 24.8 Systemic changes that occur with burn injury.

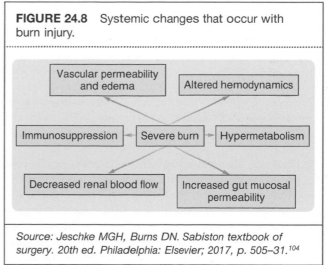

Source: Jeschke MGH, Burns DN. Sabiston textbook of surgery. 20th ed. Philadelphia: Elsevier; 2017, p. 505–31.[104]

Systemic changes

Similar to other traumatic injuries, burn injury triggers an inflammatory process due to cell destruction; however, in burns this process can be triggered multiple times after initial resuscitation, which can lead to organ dysfunction and death. Distributive shock also occurs, leading to compromised tissue perfusion and oxygen delivery as a result of capillary leakage, which contributes to profound tissue oedema and fluid accumulation. A hypermetabolic state after injury is typically observed owing to the release of stress hormones[101] (Fig. 24.8).

Inhalation injury

Inhalation injury relates to the transfer of hot gas or toxic products into the airway. leading to airway oedema, bronchospasm secondary to aerosolised irritants, small airway obstruction and alveolar flooding due to disruption to the epithelium, with the consequences generally evident in the first 24 hours post injury. Suspicion for inhalation injury should occur when patients present with facial burns, singed nasal hairs or eyebrows, wheezing or stridor, carbonaceous sputum, hoarseness or anxiety; however, bronchoscopy to identify subglottal damage is essential.[105] Bronchoscopic criteria for confirmation of an inhalation injury is not well defined, despite an existing grading system. Damage to the airway causes increased mucous production, oedema, mucosal ulceration and haemorrhage. Airway obstruction is related to oedema causing narrowed passageways impeding air flow. Damage to lung parenchyma further results in pulmonary oedema and potentially acute respiratory distress syndrome.[28,106]

The specific changes are dependent on the types of substances inhaled at the time of injury. If coarse smoke particles are inhaled, these will primarily be deposited in the upper tracheobronchial tree, while fine smoke particles will usually be lodged in the alveoli. In carbon monoxide poisoning there are commonly mental status changes, varying from headache to coma, or the classic 'cherry red cyanosis', which may be obscured by soot or burns. Upper airway injury is characterised by progressive airway occlusion, pharyngeal or supraglottic oedema and facial swelling, and is generally identified in patients with early respiratory distress, stridor or hypoxaemia.

A carboxyhaemoglobin of >10% within the first hour post-injury is strongly indicative of inhalation injury and cyanide poisoning, especially when there is lactic acidosis, abnormal haemodynamics and reduced GCS.[107] Assume that carbon monoxide poisoning has occurred in patients trapped in enclosed areas, with caution required in interpreting oxygen saturation levels.

Other than traditional ventilation strategies, extracorporeal life support could be considered as a respiratory support option, although the evidence clarifying benefits and limitations is limited, largely because of the small sample sizes (extracorporeal life support is discussed further in Chapter 15).[108,109]

Electrocution injuries

Reported rates of electrical burns are 4–5%, with the hands being the most common source point, followed by the head.

There are three types of electrical burn injury: true electrical injury by current flow, arc injury from the electrical arc as it passes from the source to an object, and flame injury from ignition of clothing or surroundings.

Evaluation should include ECG, cardiac enzymes, urinalysis and CT scan if there is loss of consciousness. Consideration for continuous cardiac monitoring should occur if it is a high-voltage source; however, if the patient is stable and blood tests are within normal limits then discharge can occur.

Management of external burns sustained from an electrical current is the same as for other burn injuries.[110]

Clinical manifestations

The most prominent clinical manifestations of burn injury are the dermal signs of injury. Burn depth is classified by the degree of injury in the epidermis, dermis, subcutaneous fat and underlying structures.

1 *First-degree burn:* epidermal burns are painful, erythematous and blanch to touch. Skin is pink to red in colour and intact, an example being sunburn. Healing occurs within 7 days. Treatment is aimed at comfort using agents such as aloe, or simple pain relief such as oral non-steroidal anti-inflammatory agents.

2 *Second-degree burn:* superficial partial-thickness burn injury involves the epidermal and superficial dermal layers caused by scald injuries and flash flame burns. Skin is erythematous, painful, blanches to touch and often blisters. This degree of burn injury will re-epithelialise in 7–14 days. After healing, these burns may have a slight skin discoloration.

3 *Mid-dermal partial-thickness injuries:* these extend a part way into the dermis. They have a large zone of damaged non-viable tissue extending into the dermis, with damaged but viable tissue at the base. Preservation of the damaged but viable tissue (particularly in the initial period following injury) is pivotal to preventing burn wound progression. As some of the nerve endings remain viable, pain is present but is less severe when compared with superficial burns. Similarly, as some of the capillaries remain viable, capillary return is present, albeit delayed. Skin appears pale and mottled, does not blanch but is painful to pin-prick. Healing takes 2–5 weeks, often with severe scarring.

4 *Deep partial-thickness burns:* these extend into the deep dermal layer. The tissue is a characteristic pink to pale ivory in appearance. It can also have a blotchy red base due to extravasation of red blood cells (RBC). The underlying tissue does not blanch, and the hair is easily removed; sensation is reduced. These burns usually take in excess of 3 weeks to heal and are managed with surgical excision and closure.

5 *Third-degree burn:* full-thickness burns destroy both layers of skin (epidermis and dermis) and may penetrate more deeply into underlying structures. Appearance is characterised by a hard, leathery eschar that is painless and black, white or cherry red. These injuries require excision and skin grafting, otherwise they heal by re-epithelialisation from the wound edges.[100]

Assessment of the total body surface area (TBSA) of burns

The extent of injury is best described using the percentage of the TBSA that sustained burns. The measurement of burn surface area is important during the initial management of people with burns for estimating fluid requirements and determining the need for transfer to a burns service. Erythema should not be included when calculating burn area.

There are two frequently used methods that provide a reproducible estimation of the area of surface area burns. These are as follows:

- *Rule of nines* – for the adult population, the most widely known and easily applied method of

FIGURE 24.9 Diagram of the 'rule of nines'. (A) Adult. (B) Child.

Adult body Part	% of total BSA
Arm	9%
Head	9%
Neck	1%
Leg	18%
Anterior trunk	18%
Posterior trunk	18%

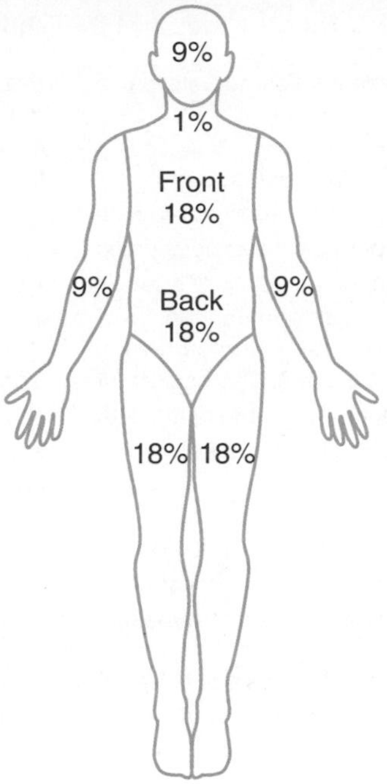

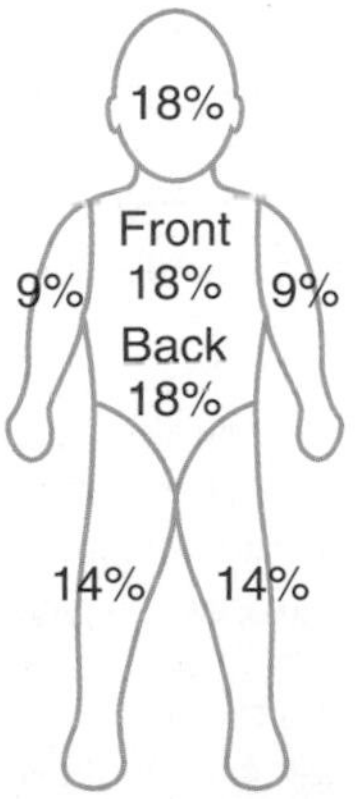

Child body Part	% of total BSA
Arm	9%
Head and neck	18%
Leg	14%
Anterior trunk	18%
Posterior trunk	18%

Source: Jeschke MGH, Burns DN. Sabiston textbook of surgery. 20th ed. Philadelphia: Elsevier; 2017, p. 505–31.[104]

Patient management

Initial assessment is the same for all traumatic injuries, including the minimisation of hypothermia and hyperkalaemia along with the immediate priorities of care (outlined below); however, fluid resuscitation is vital in the first 24 hours in this patient population (Table 24.11). Beyond 24 hours the general principles of care for the critically ill patient are the same, including wound management (discussed below) (Fig. 24.10).

Emergency principles of care

The principles of care, once the danger has been removed, are to stop the burning process and to cool the wound to minimise the burden of injury, using either running water, wet towels or saline-soaked gauze. Burns cooled for 20 minutes show greater re-epithelisation than other cooling times.[12] The wound and the patient should then be covered to reduce risk of hypothermia. Adequate analgesia must be provided early in patient care.

Airway

Burns localised to the face and mouth, or with presence of carbonaceous sputum (sputum with signs of smoke or charcoal), may indicate an airway burn and contribute to localised oedema, which poses a greater risk for airway compromise.

All patients with burn injury require supplemental oxygen. Upper airway obstruction may develop rapidly, and respiratory status is continually monitored. Classic signs of obstruction including stridor, dyspnoea and hoarse voice warrant immediate intubation and should be considered early, as worsening oedema can make intubation difficult. Airway stability is mandatory for safe transfer.

Breathing

Carbonaceous pulmonary secretions are a hallmark of airway injury. Dyspnoea and tachypnoea are signs of respiratory distress, while pulmonary oedema will often ensue with airway burns.

Circulation

Evaluation of circulating blood volume can be difficult in severely burned patients, especially those who may have accompanying injuries. The massive interstitial and intracellular fluid shifts associated with acute burn injury will deplete circulating volume and result in shock if uncorrected. Fluid resuscitation aims to prevent shock and to support organ function, while avoiding the complications of over- or underadministration of fluid such as compartment syndrome. Fluid resuscitation should commence as indicated when there is >20% TBSA in adults.[12] Early IV cannulation (with two wide-bore cannulae) and the administration of high-volume fluids must begin immediately.[11] There are multiple formulas available to calculate fluid replacement; however, the Parkland formula is most widely used. The most common is crystalloid fluid, in conjunction with colloids such as albumin or plasma, administered at 2 mL/kg/% TBSA as per the modified Parkland formula. Half

estimating TBSA is the 'rule of nines' (Fig. 24.9). The principle of this assessment method is that most areas of the body constitute 9% (or multiples of 9%) of the TBSA.

- *Palmar surface* – the surface area of a patient's palm (including fingers) is about 1% TBSA. This method of estimating TBSA is yet to be validated. The palmar surface method can be used to estimate relatively small burns (<15% of total surface area) or very large burns (>85%, when unburnt skin is counted), but is inaccurate for medium-sized burns. This method is seen as crucial in evaluating burns of mixed distribution.[111]

TABLE 24.11

Acute nursing care after burn injury (first 24 hours)

ELEMENT OF CARE	MINOR BURN INJURY (<10%)	MAJOR BURN INJURY	CRITICALLY ILL
Fluid replacement	Generally not fluid loaded.	Fluid replacement as per relevant formula.	Major fluid replacement.
Need for intubation and mechanical ventilation	Supplemental oxygen therapy. Only if airway burns are suspected or comorbidities require it.	Supplemental oxygen therapy. Intubation and mechanical ventilation may be required with analgesia and in burns shock. Any airway burn in this group requires intubation.	Mandatory.
Respiratory and cardiovascular observations	Hourly TPR, BP, SpO$_2$ adapted according to patient status.	Continuous ECG, SpO$_2$, temperature, urine output (hourly observations if not continuously monitored).	Continuous invasive haemodynamic, respiratory and urine output monitoring, including core temperature
Neurovascular observations	Assess neurovascular status of circumferential burns to chest and limbs (including fingers and toes).	Assess neurovascular status of circumferential burns to chest and limbs (including fingers and toes).	Assess neurovascular status of circumferential burns to chest and limbs (including fingers and toes).
Analgesia	Continuous, intermittent or patient-controlled (if patient capable) analgesia ± conscious sedation for dressings.	Continuous IV analgesia ± conscious sedation for dressings.	Continuous IV analgesia + sedation.
Arterial blood gas, serum potassium; chloride and haemoglobin	Baseline and as indicated by patient's condition.	Baseline and as indicated by patient's condition.	Baseline and minimum 4-hourly depending on patient's condition, including temperature and ventilatory requirements.
Haematology	Baseline and as indicated by patient's condition.	Baseline and as indicated by patient's condition, noting that more frequent assessment will be needed if coagulopathy is present.	Baseline and as indicated by patient's condition, noting that more frequent assessment will be needed if coagulopathy is present.
Feeding	Oral intake should be monitored and encouraged.	Enteral or oral intake should commence within 24 h of injury (NB: burns of >20% TBSA require enteral feeding).	Enteral feeding should commence within 24 h of injury.
General burn dressings	Primary debridement undertaken by nursing staff with theatre debridement if indicated due to burn depth. Burn escharotomy as indicated (unlikely unless circumferential injury).	Primary debridement undertaken by nursing staff with theatre debridement if indicated due to burn depth. Burns escharotomy as indicated (likely with circumferential injury).	Primary debridement undertaken by nursing staff with theatre debridement if indicated due to burn depth. Burns escharotomy as indicated (highly likely).

BP = blood pressure; ECG = electrocardiogram; IV = intravenous; SpO$_2$ = peripheral oxygen saturation; TBSA = total body surface area; TPR = temperature, pulse, respiration.

of the calculated fluid should be administered in the first 8 hours post injury and the remainder over the next 16 hours. A meta-analysis of burn resuscitation outcomes indicated that use of colloids enables the infusion of a lower total cystalloid in the first 24 hours, which assists in preserving the endothelial microvasculature and reducing fluid leak and oedema, also reducing the risk of abdominal compartment syndrome.[101] Volume replacement should be adjusted to maintain adequate urine output, monitoring of organ perfusion or invasive monitoring including central venous pressure, transoesophageal echocardiogram and pulmonary artery catheterisation, if available. The use of

FIGURE 24.10 Phases of burns care.

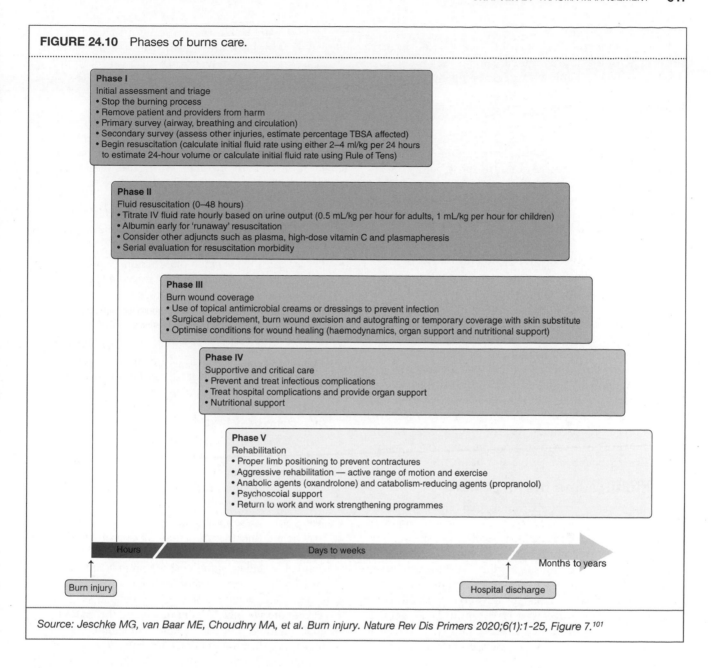

Phase I
Initial assessment and triage
- Stop the burning process
- Remove patient and providers from harm
- Primary survey (airway, breathing and circulation)
- Secondary survey (assess other injuries, estimate percentage TBSA affected)
- Begin resuscitation (calculate initial fluid rate using either 2–4 ml/kg per 24 hours to estimate 24-hour volume or calculate initial fluid rate using Rule of Tens)

Phase II
Fluid resuscitation (0–48 hours)
- Titrate IV fluid rate hourly based on urine output (0.5 mL/kg per hour for adults, 1 mL/kg per hour for children)
- Albumin early for 'runaway' resuscitation
- Consider other adjuncts such as plasma, high-dose vitamin C and plasmapheresis
- Serial evaluation for resuscitation morbidity

Phase III
Burn wound coverage
- Use of topical antimicrobial creams or dressings to prevent infection
- Surgical debridement, burn wound excision and autografting or temporary coverage with skin substitute
- Optimise conditions for wound healing (haemodynamics, organ support and nutritional support)

Phase IV
Supportive and critical care
- Prevent and treat infectious complications
- Treat hospital complications and provide organ support
- Nutritional support

Phase V
Rehabilitation
- Proper limb positioning to prevent contractures
- Aggressive rehabilitation — active range of motion and exercise
- Anabolic agents (oxandrolone) and catabolism-reducing agents (propranolol)
- Psychoscoial support
- Return to work and work strengthening programmes

Hours   Days to weeks   Months to years

Burn injury   Hospital discharge

Source: Jeschke MG, van Baar ME, Choudhry MA, et al. Burn injury. Nature Rev Dis Primers 2020;6(1):1-25, Figure 7.[101]

invasive monitoring capability will be based on cardiovascular status, the need for inotropic support, the extent of the burn and the potential for infection. One meta-analysis showed slightly lower, but not significant, mortality in those with invasive monitoring in selected high-risk patients.[35]

Recommended urine output goals are 0.3–0.5 mL/kg/h in adults,[35] 0.5–1 mL/kg/h in patients <30 kg and 1–2 mL/kg/h in children.[112] Ideally, urine output should be measured via indwelling catheters; however, this is not always practical in some geographical locations.

The evolution of 'fluid creep' has been reported, caused by over-resuscitation, which increases the risk of respiratory insufficiency, cardiac failure and abdominal and extremity compartment syndrome.[100]

Patients with circumferential full-thickness burn injury may require escharotomies because of the extensive oedema and the inelasticity of burn eschar. Delayed capillary return, a cool limb and increased pain manifest earlier than loss of palpable pulse.

Minimising hypothermia

Treatment strategies, such as cooling the burn and administering high–volume fluid replacement, exposure of wounds following injury and during dressing changes, place the patient at high risk of hypothermia. Continuous temperature monitoring is essential, and strategies to maintain normothermia should be implemented immediately. Strategies include minimising exposure, warming fluids and warming the patient's environment. Warm blankets and heated humidified supplemental oxygen are valuable adjuncts along with consideration for invasive IV catheters with capability for warming or cooling, if available.

Hyperkalaemia

Cell destruction from the burn injury can result in high serum potassium levels, which should be monitored closely. Metabolic acidosis will exacerbate the hyperkalaemia, as intracellular exchange of hydrogen ions with potassium ions takes place.

Nutrition

Burns induce a hypermetabolic response after 96 hours, which can last up to 36 months post injury. Stress hormones such as catecholamines, glucocorticoids and glucagon are released and can cause increased BP, peripheral insulin resistance and breakdown of glycogen, proteins and lipids resulting in increased body temperature, increased total body protein loss and muscle-wasting which can result in organ dysfunction and death.[101] Supplemental feeding is mandatory and should commence as soon as possible following severe burn injuries. A meta-analysis of seven randomised controlled trials showed that mortality, gastrointestinal haemorrahage, sepsis, pneumonia, renal failure and hospital length of stay were all reduced in patients commenced on enteral nutrition within 24 hours.[113] Due to gastrointestinal complications such as delayed gastric emptying or ileus, enteral nutrition may not be feasible and parenteral nutrition should be started; however, there is a greater risk for complications in burns patients receiving parenteral nutrition, which can include gastrointestinal haemorrhage, pneumonia, renal failure sepsis, *Pseudomonas* bacteraemia and death.[114]

The multitrauma burns patient

The combination of traumatic injury and burn injury often occurs in high-energy motor vehicle accidents, industrial accidents or trauma associated with explosives. These patients present with a wide variety of severity and patterns, depending on the mechanism of injury. Treatment of many traumatic injuries takes priority over definitive burn care, and early operation and repair are advised as fresh burns are initially thought to be free of bacteria. Optimal management is achieved through balancing the conflicting treatment requirements for each injury as discussed below:

- *Spinal injury* – if the patient has potential spinal injuries in addition to the burn, spinal precautions must be maintained; however, cervical collars should not be used over a burnt neck or upper chest because of the potential for swelling and subsequent restriction. If a collar is used, changing it to an appropriate size as the swelling worsens or goes down is essential.

- *Skeletal injury* – skin traction cannot be used in a patient with burn injury; this will necessitate the use of an external fixateur or early internal fixation, which has an associated higher risk of infection.

Burn dressings

Mitigating infection is the primary aim of good burns nursing. The greatest challenge is minimising the risk for cross-contamination, and patients should be nursed in a single room where possible. Burn dressings present a physical challenge, particularly when large areas of the body are affected.

The traditional burn dressing in the ICU is undertaken as a surgically clean technique. The following is a guide to specific aspects of burn management:

- *Debridement* – the excision of dead skin. Gentle scrubbing is generally used to remove loose tissue and burst blisters. Forceps and scissors may be required to lift and remove smaller areas of tissue. Extensive areas of debridement will usually be undertaken in the operating room.

- *Blisters* – small blisters should be left intact whereas large blisters may be aspirated or deroofed during debridement, although it should be noted that evidence regarding blister management is poor. Blisters over joints that are restricting movement should also be debrided.

- *Escharotomy* – this is an incision through the eschar and does not involve opening muscle fascia. The escharotomy immediately relieves the compression and is a limb-/life-saving surgical manoeuvre. The escharotomy is dressed as a burn to prevent infection.

- *Skin grafts* – these are required to cover skin defects. They may be full-thickness or partial-thickness grafts and may be harvested from the patient or obtained from a cadaver donor. Regardless of the type of skin graft, nursing care remains the same, with the aim being to maximise adherence. Specific nursing care of the graft site includes leaving the site intact and immobilising the graft site, applying the appropriate wound care regimen, preventing shearing injury to the graft site and minimising the risk for infection. With autografts, wound care will also be required for the donor site.

- *Skin substitutes* – these can be catagorised as biological substitutes, synthetic substitutes, or a combination of both. Synthetic skin substitutes are free from any risk of disease transmission; however, there are only a few available.

Summary

Caring for the trauma patient is increasingly challenging, as the age distribution of those being injured has expanded from the young and healthy population to include older patients who are living longer. Patients across the age and health continuum can experience significant ongoing compromise to their health and quality of life. Care of the trauma patient presents the critical care nurse with multiple challenges. With the introduction of trauma systems, the outcome and survival of injured patients has improved dramatically. The severity of injury and patient outcome are dependent on effective pre-hospital care, resuscitation, definitive surgical management on arrival at the hospital and intensive care. Principles of resuscitation of the trauma patient are the same as for all patients, with a primary, secondary and tertiary survey being undertaken, and maintenance or correction of airway, breathing and circulation taking precedence. Prevention of the 'lethal triad' of acidosis, hypothermia and coagulopathy has the potential to significantly influence patient outcome. Consideration of the specific injury, with its resultant pathophysiological changes, is necessary to care effectively for patients with abdominal, chest, multiple or burn injuries.

Case study

Michael, a 62-year-old male, was involved in an accident when the car he was travelling in at high speed collided with a tree. At the scene he was hypotensive and GCS 3, his bilateral lower limbs and right wrist were deformed, and there was also evidence of flail chest and unequal chest wall movement. He was extricated from the car after 35 minutes with a cervical collar in situ, IV access was established, bilateral finger thoracostomy was performed and he was transferred by HEMS to the closest trauma centre.

EMERGENCY DEPARTMENT

Trauma team activation and massive transfusion activation were initiated before Michael's arrival. On presentation his vital signs were: heart rate 140, respiratory rate absent (bag-valve mask ventilation was in place), BP 86/40, SpO_2 73% on 15 L, GCS 3 with pupils 4 mm and non-reactive, temperature 35.0°C; ABG: pH 7.07, PO_2 46, PaO_2 121, bicarbonate 13, SaO_2 97%, Hb 85, glucose 10.3 and lactate 11.5.

Primary survey concluded:

- airway: patent, not protected
- cervical collar in situ – unknown injuries
- breathing: no spontaneous breaths; no tracheal deviation; proceeded to rapid sequence intubation
- circulation: absent; pulseless electrical activity (PEA) arrest on transfer to trolley, 6 mg adrenaline; left resuscitative thoracotomy; left rapid infusion line inserted; return of spontaneous circulation after 5 minutes eFAST: negative
- ECG: sinus rhythm
- disability: open left femur fracture.

Secondary survey results were:

- GCS 3 – pupils 4 mm and non-reactive
- cervical collar in situ
- bilateral finger thoracostomy – converted to intercostal catheter insertion
- left resuscitation thoracotomy
- ETT with equal chest expansion
- abdomen soft, not distended
- limbs: open left distal femur fracture, obvious deformity right distal femur and right distal radius/wrist.

Investigations and injuries diagnosed:

- bilateral rib fracture 2–9, sternal fracture, moderate bilateral pneumothoraces, pulmonary contusions, left axilla bleeding, retrosternal haematoma
- contrast extravasation to bilateral flanks, lateral abdominal wall, epigastric region, epigastric and pelvic free fluid
- left neck of femur fracture, left superior and inferior pubic rami fracture, bilateral L2–L4 transverse process fractures, bilateral distal femur comminuted fractures, right tibial plateau fracture
- angiography: demonstrated bleeding into both thighs, multifocal active.

Past medical history included: hypertension, depression and spinal stenosis.

Medications were Targin and perindopril.

Total blood products administered included: 16 RBC, 6 FFP, 5 cryoprecipitate, 2 pooled platelets.

OPERATING THEATRE

The patient was transferred to operating theatre after multidisciplinary discussion on priorities of management; temperature on transfer was 34.1°C.

Initial orthopaedic surgery comprised external fixation applied to bilateral legs, and negative-pressure dressing applied to bilateral open wounds. The cardiothoracic team followed and controlled bleeding from the left intercostal artery, closed the thoracostomy wound and inserted three ICCs. The general surgery team proceeded to trauma laparotomy for omental bleeding with intraoperative hypoxia and haemodynamic instability, which stabilised after new ICC insertion. A negative-pressure wound device was applied because of concerns for ACS related to fluid resuscitation.

Total transfusion of blood products from arrival in theatre was 24 RBC, 7 pooled platelets, 24 FFP and 23 cryoprecipitate.

ICU MANAGEMENT

On arrival in ICU, Michael's condition was critical and required ongoing fluid resuscitation and replacement of blood products including 5 RBC, 2 FFP and 1 pooled platelets. Total fluid infused in first 12 hours was 16 L; the total measured output was 2.2 L leading to a fluid balance 14 L positive (1 L crystalloid).

Michael was intubated and remained sedated and mechanically ventilated. Results were: GCS 3 – pupils 4 mm and non-reactive; initial ABG pH 7.35, PCO_2 34, PaO_2 81, bicarbonate 18, SaO_2 97%, Hb 113, glucose 8.8, lactate 7.2; K^+ 3.0, temperature 35.8°C.

Haemodialysis was commenced as urine output <10 mL/h, and evidence of rhabdomyolysis with CK 45,000, with normal renal indices initially.

A family discussion was held to share current condition and concerns about potential recovery.

Days 2–26: There were ongoing concerns regarding a poor GCS. MRI of the brain on day 2 demonstrated watershed infarction. To assess neurology, sedation was ceased and analgesia reduced to fentanyl 20 micrograms/h.

Parenteral nutrition was commenced as per the general surgeon's request for the patient to remain nil orally; however, enteral nutrition was commenced on day 5.

After 3 days of nil sedation, Michael was eye opening to painful stimuli, with no peripheral responses to pain.

On day 3, Michael was returned to theatre for definitive closure of his abdominal wound. Repeat CT brain demonstrated nil new changes. The family were updated regarding concerns for recovery from neurological injury; however, they indicated that despite his history of depression they felt he would wish to be given the opportunity for best recovery he could make. Quality of life issues were discussed.

On day 8, the patient was returned to the operating theatre for fixation of the left neck of femur fracture and right distal radius fracture as he was demonstrating increasing hypertension and tachycardia in response to pain.

On day 15, Michael was eye opening, withdrawing bilateral upper limbs to painful stimuli, and a decision was made to proceed to tracheostomy to facilitate respiratory weaning from mechanical ventilation. This was successfully achieved by day 24 of Michael's admission. Ongoing operative fixation of severely comminuted distal femur fractures continued.

On day 26 he was transferred to ward level care and planning for rehabilitation was commenced.

CASE STUDY QUESTIONS

1 Discuss the components of the 'DCR and surgery' and three stages in relation to this patient's initial presentation and disposition post-ED.

2 Discuss serial abdominal assessment in the intensive care environment and contributing factors for the development of ACS in this patient.

3 Discuss potential complications and considerations for patients requiring massive blood transfusion. What investigations can assist in targeting blood product replacement?

4 Discuss rhabdomyolysis and the contributing factors in relation to Michael and the clinical management that can be initiated to prevent renal damage.

RESEARCH VIGNETTE

Cole E, Gillespie S, Vulliamy P, et al. Multiple organ dysfunction after trauma. J Br Surg 2020;107(4):402–12.

Abstract

Background: The nature of multiple organ dysfunction syndrome (MODS) after traumatic injury is evolving as resuscitation practices advance and more patients survive their injuries to reach critical care. The aim of this study was to characterise contemporary MODS subtypes in trauma critical care at a population level.

Methods: Adult patients admitted to major trauma centre critical care units were enrolled in this 4-week point-prevalence study. MODS was defined by a daily total Sequential Organ Failure Assessment (SOFA) score of more than 5. Hierarchical clustering of SOFA scores over time was used to identify MODS subtypes.

Results: Some 440 patients were enrolled, of whom 245 (55·7%) developed MODS. MODS carried a high mortality rate (22·0% versus 0·5% in those without MODS; $P < 0.001$) and 24·0% of deaths occurred within the first 48 hours after injury. Three patterns of MODS were identified, all present on admission. Cluster 1 MODS resolved early with a median time to recovery of 4 days and a mortality rate of 14·4%. Cluster 2 had a delayed recovery (median 13 days) and a mortality rate of 35%. Cluster 3 had a prolonged recovery (median 25 days) and high associated mortality rate of 46%. Multivariable analysis revealed distinct clinical associations for each form of MODS; 24-hour crystalloid administration was associated strongly with cluster 1 ($P = 0.009$), traumatic brain injury with cluster 2 ($P = 0.002$) and admission shock severity with cluster 3 ($P = 0.003$).

Conclusion: Contemporary MODS has at least three distinct types based on patterns of severity and recovery. Further characterisation of MODS subtypes and their underlying pathophysiology may lead to future opportunities for early stratification and targeted interventions.[115]

Critique

MODS is associated with poor outcome for trauma patients, and continues to place high demands on critical care and other healthcare resources. The nature of MODS seems to be changing; more recent research has found differences in patterns of onset, severity and outcome, challenging earlier theories. The main outcome in this study was to define the occurrence and pattern of MODS by using the SOFA total score. A SOFA score of 6 or more affecting two or more organs was used to define the onset of MODS. TBI was diagnosed when the Abbreviated Injury Score (region head) was ≥3. The results show that over half of the patients developed MODS, with a high mortality rate compared with those without MODS. Three subtypes of MODS were identified. The first subtype ($n = 167$) with early resolving MODS was associated with crystalloid use in the first 24 hours after injury. The second subtype ($n = 54$) with longer-resolving MODS was associated with TBI and appeared to have a separate clinical trajectory not limited to the CNS component of the SOFA score alone. The third subtype ($n = 24$) with the prolonged form of MODS was associated with shock severity on admission; a weak association was found with crystalloid administration, and no association was found with the volume of blood products. Overall, patients who received less than 1.5 L of crystalloids in the first 24 hours resolved MODS in a shorter time and had shorter critical care days.

This point-prevalence study has several strengths. Patients were included from all adult regional level 1 trauma centres in Great Britain in the era of contemporary damage-control resuscitation. Robust statistical analysis was used including post-hoc tests and was well described and discussed. The authors also acknowledged and discussed the shortcomings thoroughly. The unsupervised hierarchical clustering analysis was used to identify MODS subtypes. The clustering analysis is a form of explorative data analysis in which observations are divided into different groups that share common characteristics. 'Unsupervised' means that the number of clusters was not specified in advance. In this study, the number of clusters was selected in advance based on adequate cluster size for analyses. The authors suggest future studies with larger cohorts of patients.

Early and accurate identification of trauma patients at risk for MODS post-injury is of outmost importance. Contemporary damage control resuscitation recommends avoiding crystalloids to prevent proinflammatory effects on coagulation and the endothelium. Modern damage-control resuscitation with personalised resuscitations (individual blood product ratios based on point of care testing) and hybrid angiography operating suites can further improve the survival of severely injured patient.[32] Future research needs to develop prediction models that can identify patients at risk early in their clinical course. Critical care nurses, using their clinical expertise, should be aware of the administration of crystalloids prior to and after the admission to critical care within the first 24 hours to possibly improve trauma patients' safety and outcome.

Learning activities

1 Review your local guidelines for DCR and massive transfusion protocol. Reflect on the balance between timely and adequate resuscitation for patients, which saves lives, and the need to avoid blood product waste and morbidities associated with massive transfusion.

2 Discuss the benefits for the trauma patient with or without TBI of combining pharmacological thromboprophylaxis with mechanical thromboprophylaxis.

3 Outline the strengths and weaknesses of inclusive and exclusive trauma systems and the impact on staff training and management of the trauma patients in each.

4 Outline the components of a trauma system including discussion on the elements of pre-hospital system and key attributes of the team leader in the ED during resuscitation.

Further reading

Biswadev M, Wood EM, Reade MC. Whole blood for trauma resuscitation? Injury 2022;53(5):1573–5.

Cannon JW, Kahn MA, Raja AS, et al. Damage control resuscitation in patients with severe hemorrhage: a practice management guideline from the Eastern Association for the surgery of trauma. J Trauma Acute Care Surg 2017;82(2):605–17.

Mathews ZR, Koyfman A. Blast injuries. J Emerg Med 2015;49(2):573–87.

Spahn DR, Boullion B, Cerny V, et al. The European guideline on management of major bleeding and coagulopathy following trauma, 5th edn. Crit Care 2019;23:98. doi: 10.1186/s13054-019-2347-3.

References

1. GBD 2019 Diseases and Injuries Collaborators. Global burden of 369 diseases and injuries in 204 countries and territories, 1990–2019: a systematic analysis for the Global Burden of Disease Study 2019. Lancet 2020;396(10258):1204–22.

2. David JS, Bouzat P, Raux M. Evolution and organisation of trauma systems. Anaesth Crit Care Pain Med 2019;38(2):161–7.

3. Wisborg T, Castren M, Lippert A, et al. Training trauma teams in the Nordic countries: an overview and present status. Acta Anaesthesiol Scand 2005;49(7):1004–9.

4. Diakomi M. Prehospital fluid resuscitation, pain relief and stabilization. In: Pikoulis E, editor. Emergency medicine, trauma and disaster management. Cham, Zug: Springer Link; 2021. p. 19–24.

5. Nasr A, Saavedra Tomasich F, Collaço I, et al. The trauma golden hour a practical guide. 1st ed. 2020. Cham, Zug: Springer International Publishing; 2020.

6. Berkeveld E, Popal Z, Schober P, et al. Prehospital time and mortality in polytrauma patients: a retrospective analysis. BMC Emerg Med 2021;21(1):1–78.

7. Okada K, Hisashi M, Saito N, et al. Revision of 'golden hour' for hemodynamically unstable trauma patients: an analysis of nationwide hospital-based registry in Japan. Trauma Surg Acute Care Open 2020;5(1):e000405.

8. Hsieh S-L, Hsiao C-H, Chiang W-C, et al. Association between the time to definitive care and trauma patient outcomes: every minute in the golden hour matters. Eur J Trauma Emerg Surg 2021;48(4):2709–16. doi: 10.1007/s00068-021-01816-8.

9. Michaels D, Pham H, Puckett Y, et al. Helicopter versus ground ambulance: review of national database for outcomes in survival in transferred trauma patients in the USA. Trauma Surg Acute Care Open 2019;4(1):e000211.

10. Beaumont O, Lecky F, Bouamra O, et al. Helicopter and ground emergency medical services transportation to hospital after major trauma in England: a comparative cohort study. Trauma Surg Acute Care Open 2020;5(1):e000508.

11.   Surgeons ACo. ATLS: advanced trauma life support – student course manual. 10th ed. Chicago, IL: American College of Surgeons; 2018.

12.   Victoria T. Trauma Victoria: major trauma guidelines & education – Victorian state trauma system. Victoria. Melbourne, VIC: Victorian Department of Health; 2018. Available from: https://trauma.reach.vic.gov.au. [Accessed 25 February 2023].

13.   Varghese M. Prehospital trauma care evolution, practice and controversies: need for review. Int J Inj Contr Saf Promot 2020;27(1):69–82.

14.   Morris RS, Karam BS, Murphy PB, et al. Field-triage, hospital-triage and triage-assessment: a literature review of the current phases of adult trauma triage. J Trauma Acute Care Surg 2021;90:e138–45.

15.   Hinson JS, Martinez DA, Cabral S, et al. Triage performance in emergency medicine: a systematic review. Ann Emerg Med 2019;74(1):140–52.

16.   Schwing L, Faulkner T, Bucaro P, et al. Trauma team activation: accuracy of triage when minutes count. J Trauma Nurs 2019;26(4):208–14. doi: 10.1097/JTN.0000000000000450.

17.   Cameron P. Trauma. In: Cameron P, Jelineck G, Kelly A-M, et al, editors. Textbook of adult emergency medicine. 4th ed. Philadelphia: Elsevier; 2014. p. 71–162.

18.   Kassam FC, Alexander R, Evans, D, et al. What attributes define excellence in a trauma team? A qualitative study. Can J Surg 2019;62:450–3.

19.   James D, Pennardt AM. Trauma care principles. StatPearls. Treasure Island, FL: StatPearls Publishing; 2023. Available from: https://pubmed.ncbi.nlm.nih.gov/31613537/. [Accessed 25 February 2023].

20.   Yoong S, Kothari R, Brooks A. Assessment of sensitivity of whole body CT for major trauma. Eur J Trauma Emerg Surg 2019;45(3):489–92.

21.   Shwe S, Witchey L, Lahham S, et al. Retrospective analysis of eFAST ultrasounds performed on trauma activations at an academic level-1 trauma center. World J Emerg Med 2020;11(1):12.

22.   Bloom BA, Gibbons RC. Focused assessment with sonography for trauma. StatPearls. Treasure Island, FL: StatPearls Publishing; 2021. Available from: https://pubmed.ncbi.nlm.nih.gov/29261902/. [Accessed 25 February 2023].

23.   Desai N, Harris T. Extended focused assessment with sonography in trauma. BJA Educ 2018;18(2):57–62.

24.   National Institute for Health and Care Excellence (NICE). Major trauma: assessment and initial management. NG39 NG. London: NICE; 2016. Available from: https://www.nice.org.uk/guidance/ng39. [Accessed 25 February 2023].

25.   Brenner M, Hicks C. Major Abdominal trauma: critical decisions and new frontiers in management. Emerg Med Clin 2018;36(1):149–60.

26.   Taylor DA, Sherry SP, Sing RF. Interventional critical care: a manual for advanced care practitioners. 2nd ed. Cham, Zug: Springer; 2021, p. 351–4.

27.   World Health Organization (WHO). Children's environmental health. Injuries. Geneva: WHO; 2018. Available from: https://www.who.int/health-topics/children-environmental-health#tab=tab_1. [Accessed 25 February 2023].

28.   Boling B, Karakashian AL. Blast injuries. Glendale, CA: Cinahl Information Systems; 2019. Available from: https://www.ebscohost.com/assets-sample-content/NRCP-Blast-Injuries-Quick-Lesson.pdf. [Accessed 25 April 2023].

29.   Naik A, Kotecha H, Singh SK, et al. Canadian C-spine rule (CCR) versus National Emergency X-Radiography Utilization Study (NEXUS) for screening cervical spine injury. Int J Orthop Sci 2021;7:787–9.

30.   Garg B, Ahuja K. C-spine clearance in poly-trauma patients: a narrative review. J Clin Orthop Trauma 2021;12(1):66–71.

31.   Stanton D, Hardcastle T, Muhlbauer D, et al. Cervical collars and immobilisation: a South African best practice recommendation. African J Emerg Med 2017;7(1):4–8.

32.   Spahn DR, Bouillon B, Cerny V, et al. The European guideline on management of major bleeding and coagulopathy following trauma. Crit Care 2019;23(1):1–74.

33.   Rudloff MI, Triantafillou KM. Management of pelvic ring injuries in unstable patients. Orthop Clin North Am 2016;47(3):551–63.

34.   Chang R, Holcomb JB. Optimal fluid therapy for traumatic hemorrhagic shock. Crit Care Clin 2017;33(1):15–36.

35.   Gupta A, Asirvatham E, Reddy K, et al. Fluid resuscitation in adult burns. Curr Med Issues 2021;19(2):103–9.

36.   Australian & New Zealand Burns Association (ANZBA). ANZBA Referral criteria. Albany Creek, QLD: ANZBA; 2013. Available from: https://anzba.org.au/care/referral-criteria/. [Accessed 25 February 2023].

37.   van Veelen MJ, Brodmann Maeder M. Hypothermia in trauma. Int J Environ Res Public Health 2021;18(16):8719.

38.   Kadapamannil D, Rajan S. Hypothermia in prehospital polytrauma victims: an overlooked companion. Res Opin Anesth Intensive Care 2020;7(4):223.

39.   Granieri S, Frassini S, Cimbanassi S, et al. Impact of resuscitative endovascular balloon occlusion of the aorta (REBOA) in traumatic abdominal and pelvic exsanguination: a systematic review and meta-analysis. Eur J Trauma Emerg Surg 2022;48(5):3561–74.

40.   Vaidya R, Waldron J, Scott A, et al. Angiography and embolization in the management of bleeding pelvic fractures. J Am Acad Orthop Surg 2018;26(4):e68.

41.   Morrison JJ, Galgon RE, Jansen JO, et al. A systematic review of the use of resuscitative endovascular balloon occlusion of the aorta in the management of hemorrhagic shock. J Trauma Acute Care Surg 2016;80(2):324–34.

42.   Leibner E, Andreae M, Galvagno Jr SM, et al. Damage control resuscitation. Clin Exp Emerg Med 2020;7(1):5–13. Available from: https://doi.org/10.15441/ceem.19.089.

43.   Paydar S, Sabetian G, Khalili H, et al. Management of deep vein thrombosis (DVT) prophylaxis in trauma patients. Bull Emerg Trauma 2016;4(1):1.

44.   Timon C, Keady C, Murphy C. Fat embolism syndrome – a qualitative review of its incidence, presentation, pathogenesis and management. Malays Orthop J 2021;15(1):1.

45.   Cabral BMI, Edding SN, Portocarrero JP, et al. Rhabdomyolysis. Disease-a-Month 2020;66(8):101015.

46. Eurosafe. Injuries in the European Union 2012–2014. 6th ed. Amsterdam: Luxembourg Institute of Health; 2016. [Available from: http://www.eurosafe.eu.com/key-actions/injury-data/reports. [Accessed 25 February 2023].

47. Australian Institute of Health and Welfare (AIHW). Injury. Canberra, ACT: AIHW; 2018. Available from: https://www.aihw.gov.au/reports-statistics/health-conditions-disability-deaths/injury/overview. [Accessed 25 February 2023].

48. Nursing Times. Skeletal system 1: the anatomy and physiology of bones: Nursing Times; 2020. [Available from: https://www.nursingtimes.net/clinical-archive/orthopaedics/skeletal-system-1-the-anatomy-and-physiology-of-bones-27-01-2020/. [Accessed 25 February 2023].

49. Eccles S. Standards for the management of open fractures. Oxford, England: Oxford University Press; 2020.

50. Diwan A, Eberlin KR, Smith RM. The principles and practice of open fracture care, 2018. Chin J Traumatol 2018;21(04):187–92.

51. Nixon AJ, Auer JA, Watkins JP. Principles of fracture fixation. In: Nixon AJ, editor. Equine fracture repair. New York: John Wiley; 2019, p. 127–55.

52. Fukumoto LE, Fukumoto KD. Fat embolism syndrome. Nurs Clin North Am 2018;53(3):335–47.

53. Kodadek L, Carmichael II SP, Seshadri A, et al. Rhabdomyolysis: an American Association for the Surgery of Trauma Critical Care Committee clinical consensus document. Trauma Surg Acute Care Open 2022;7(1):e000836.

54. Khu YL, Lewis B, Blackshaw L, et al. Aetiologies and factors associated with poor clinical outcomes in rhabdomyolysis: a retrospective cohort study in an Australian trauma centre. Intern Med J 2021;51(2):264–7.

55. Bosch X, Poch E, Grau JM. Rhabdomyolysis and acute kidney injury. New Engl J Med 2009;361(1):62–72.

56. Wafaisade A, Paffrath T, Lefering R, et al. Patterns of early resuscitation associated with mortality after penetrating injuries. Br J Surg 2015;102(10):1220–8.

57. Sawhney JS, Kasotakis G, Goldenberg A, et al. Management of rhabdomyolysis: a practice management guideline from the Eastern Association for the Surgery of Trauma. Am J Surg 2022;224(1 Pt A):196–204.

58. Gray A, Chandler H, Sabri O. Pelvic ring injuries: classification and treatment. Orthop Trauma 2018;32(2):80–90.

59. Ziran NM, Smith WR. Pelvic fractures. In: Smith WR, Stahel PF. Management of musculoskeletal injuries in the trauma patient: New York: Springer; 2013, p. 143–64.

60. Lockwood W. Orthopaedic trauma. RN.org; 2020. Available from: https://www.rn.org/courses/coursematerial-267.pdf. [Accessed 25 February 2023].

61. Abdelrahman H, El-Menyar A, Keil H, et al. Patterns, management, and outcomes of traumatic pelvic fracture: insights from a multicenter study. J Orthop Surg Res 2020;15(1):1–11.

62. Mostafa AM, Kyriacou H, Chimutengwende-Gordon M, et al. An overview of the key principles and guidelines in the management of pelvic fractures. J Perioper Pract 2021;31(9):341–8.

63. Hong S-K, Kim DK, Jeon SR. Primary management of polytrauma. 1st ed. Singapore: Springer Singapore; 2019.

64. Hajjar WM, Al-Nassar SA, Almutair OS, et al. Chest trauma experience: incidence, associated factors, and outcomes among patients in Saudi Arabia. Pak J Med Sci 2021;37(2):373–8.

65. Flood L, Roodenburg B. Chest trauma. Anaesth Intensive Care Med 2020;21(8):397–401.

66. Eghbalzadeh K, Sabashnikov A, Zeriouh M, et al. Blunt chest trauma: a clinical chameleon. Heart 2018;104(9):719.

67. Dogrul BN, Kiliccalan I, Asci ES, et al. Blunt trauma related chest wall and pulmonary injuries: an overview. Chin J Traumatol 2020;23(3):125–38.

68. Yadollahi M, Arabi AH, Mahmoudi A, et al. Blunt thoracic injury mortality and clinical presentation. Trauma Monthly 2018;23(4).

69. Daskal Y, Paran M, Korin A, et al. Multiple rib fractures: does flail chest matter? Emerg Med J 2021;38(7):496–500.

70. de Moya M, Mayberry J. Rib Fracture management a practical manual. 1st ed. Cham, Zug: Springer International Publishing; 2018.

71. Abdellatif W, Chow B, Hamid S, et al. Unravelling the mysteries of traumatic diaphragmatic injury: an up-to-date review. Can Assoc Radiol J 2020;71(3):313–21.

72. Kim M, Moore JE. Chest trauma: current recommendations for rib fractures, pneumothorax, and other injuries. Curr Anesthesiol Rep 2020;10(1):61–8.

73. de Moya M, Brasel KJ, Brown CVR, et al. Evaluation and management of traumatic pneumothorax: a Western Trauma Association critical decisions algorithm. J Trauma Acute Care Surgery 2022;92(1):103–7.

74. Ryaan E-A, O'Brien D, Bozso SJ, et al. Blunt cardiac trauma: a narrative review. Mediastinum 2021;5:28.

75. Welter S, Essaleh W. Management of tracheobronchial injuries. J Thorac Dis 2020;12(10):6143.

76. Schibilsky D, Driessen A, White WJ, et al. Traumatic tracheobronchial injuries: incidence and outcome of 136.389 patients derived from the DGU traumaregister. Sci Rep 2020;10(1):1–7.

77. Rieth A, Varga E, Kovács T, et al. Contemporary management strategies of blunt tracheobronchial injuries. Injury 2021;52:S7–14.

78. Jalota R, Sayad E. Tension pneumothorax. Treasure Island, FL: Statpearls Publishing; 2020. Available from: https://pubmed.ncbi.nlm.nih.gov/32644516/. [Accessed 25 February 2023].

79. Aswegen Hv, Reeve J, Beach L, et al. Physiotherapy management of patients with major chest trauma: results from a global survey. Trauma 2020;22(2):133–41.

80. Liu A, Nguyen J, Ehrlich H, et al. Emergency resuscitative thoracotomy for civilian thoracic trauma in the field and emergency department settings: a systematic review and meta-analysis. J Surg Res 2022;273:44–55.

81. Farooqui AM, Cunningham C, Morse N, et al. Life-saving emergency clamshell thoracotomy with damage-control laparotomy. BMJ Case Rep 2019;12(3):e227879.

82. Goedecke M, Kühn F, Stratos I, et al. No need for surgery? patterns and outcomes of blunt abdominal trauma. Innov Surg Sci 2019;4(3):100–7.

83. Bouzat P, Valdenaire G, Gauss T, et al. Early management of severe abdominal trauma. Anaesth Crit Care Pain Med 2020;39(2):269–77.

84. Rishall ML, Puskarich MA. Abdominal trauma. In: Walls RH, Hockberger R, Gausche-Hill M, et al, editors. Rosen's emergency medicine: concepts and clinical practice. 10th ed. Philadelphia: Elsevier; 2023, p. 398–412.

85. Lockwood W. Abdominal trauma. RN.org; 2020. Available from: https://www.rn.org/courses/coursematerial-10000.pdf. [Accessed 25 February 2023].

86. Barmparas G, Patel DC, Linaval NT, et al. A negative computed tomography may be sufficient to safely discharge patients with abdominal seatbelt sign from the emergency department: a case series analysis. J Trauma Acute Care Surg 2018;84(6):900–7.

87. Lewis M, Benjamin ER, Demetriades D. Intra-abdominal hypertension and abdominal compartment syndrome. Curr Probl Surg 2021;58(11):100971.

88. Ki Y-J, Jo Y-G, Park Y-C, et al. The efficacy and safety of laparoscopy for blunt abdominal trauma: a systematic review and meta-analysis. J Clin Med 2021;10(9):1853.

89. Al-Thani H, Abdelrahman H, Barah A, et al. Utility of angioembolization in patients with abdominal and pelvic traumatic bleeding: descriptive observational analysis from a level 1 trauma center. Ther Clin Risk Manag 2021;17:333–43.

90. Sava J, Alam HB, Vercruysse G, et al. Western Trauma Association critical decisions in trauma: management of the open abdomen after damage control surgery. J Trauma Acute Care Surg 2019;87(5):1232–8.

91. Crumley C. Abdominal negative pressure wound therapy devices for management of the open abdomen: a technologic analysis. J Wound Ostomy Continence Nurs 2022;49(2):124–7.

92. Coccolini F, Ivatury R, Sugrue M, et al. Open abdomen a comprehensive practical manual. 1st ed. Cham, Zug: Springer International Publishing; 2018.

93. Feliciano DV. A review of "Changes in the management of injuries to the liver and spleen" (2005). Am Surg 2021;87(2):212–18.

94. Tran S, Wilks M, Dawson J. Endovascular management of splenic trauma. Surg Pract Sci 2022:100061. doi: 10.1016/j.sipas.2022.100061.

95. Garden OJ, Parks RW. Principles and practice of surgery. 7th ed. Edinburgh: Elsevier; 2018.

96. Thurman P. Abdominal injuries. In: McQuillan KA, Makic MBF, editors. Trauma nursing: from resuscitation through rehabilitation. 5th ed. Philadelphia: Elsevier; 2020, p. 553–74.

97. Hetherington A, Cardoso FS, Lester EL, et al. Liver trauma in the intensive care unit. Curr Opin Crit Care 2022;28(2):184–9.

98. Afifi I, Abayazeed S, El-Menyar A, et al. Blunt liver trauma: a descriptive analysis from a level I trauma center. BMC Surg 2018;18(1):1–9.

99. Committee on Emergency Medicine IC, C TMotGTSWAwk-kdPTLRLCFMMMBMBBP. Patterns of early resuscitation associated with mortality after penetrating injuries. J Br Surg 2015;102(10):1220–8.

100. Greenhalgh DG. Management of burns. New Engl J Med 2019;380(24):2349–59.

101. Jeschke MG, van Baar ME, Choudhry MA, et al. Burn injury. Nature Rev Dis Primers 2020;6(1):1–25.

102. Van Yperen DT, Van Lieshout EM, Nugteren LH, et al. Adherence to the emergency management of severe burns referral criteria in burn patients admitted to a hospital with or without a specialized burn center. Burns 2021;47(8):1810–17.

103. Shetty P, Cox C, Javia V. Inappropriate transfer of burn patients. Ann Plast Surg 2021;86(1):29–34. doi: 10.1097/SAP.0000000000002464.

104. Jeschke MGH, Burns DN. Sabiston textbook of surgery. 20th ed. Philadelphia: Elsevier; 2017, p. 505–31.

105. Galeiras R, Seoane-Quiroga L, Pertega-Diaz S. Prevalence and prognostic impact of inhalation injury among burn patients: a systematic review and meta-analysis. J Trauma Acute Care Surg 2020;88(2):330–44.

106. Shubert J, Sharma S. Inhalation injury. Statpearls. Treasue Island, FL: Statpearls Publishing; 2018. Available from: https://pubmed.ncbi.nlm.nih.gov/30020633/. [Accessed 25 February 2023].

107. Foncerrada G, Culnan DM, Capek KD, et al. Inhalation injury in the burned patient. Ann Plast Surg 2018;80(3 Suppl 2):S98–105.

108. Chiu Y-J, Ma H, Liao W-C, et al. Extracorporeal membrane oxygenation support may be a lifesaving modality in patients with burn and severe acute respiratory distress syndrome: Experience of Formosa Water Park dust explosion disaster in Taiwan. Burns 2018;44(1):118–23.

109. Szentgyorgyi L, Shepherd C, Dunn KW, et al. Extracorporeal membrane oxygenation in severe respiratory failure resulting from burns and smoke inhalation injury. Burns 2018;44(5):1091–9.

110. Bounds EJ, Khan M, Kok SJ. Electrical burns. Statpearls. Treasue Island, FL: Statpearls Publishing; 2022. Available from: https://pubmed.ncbi.nlm.nih.gov/30137799/. [Accessed 25 February 2023].

111. Kim E, Drew PJ. Management of burn injury. Surgery (Oxford) 2022;40(1):62–9.

112. Chad LM, Howard AW. Management of burn injuries. Trauma Rep 2019;20(1). Available from: https://www.reliasmedia.com/articles/143698-management-of-burn-injuries. [Accessed 25 February 2023].

113. Pu H, Doig GS, Heighes PT, et al. Early enteral nutrition reduces mortality and improves other key outcomes in patients with major burn injury: a meta-analysis of randomized controlled trials. Crit Care Med 2018;46(12):2036–42.

114. Masch JL, Bhutiani N, Bozeman MC. Feeding during resuscitation after burn injury. Nutr Clin Pract 2019;34(5):666–71.

115. Cole E, Gillespie S, Vulliamy P, et al. Multiple organ dysfunction after trauma. Br J Surg 2020;107(4):402–12.

Chapter **25**

Resuscitation

Trudy Dwyer, Jennifer Dennett, Margaret Nicholson

Learning objectives

After reading this chapter, you should be able to:

- identify the benefits of a universal approach to resuscitation systems
- discuss the importance of basic life support in the context of advanced life support
- describe the safety precautions of defibrillation
- discuss the principles of therapeutic hypothermia
- discuss indications, actions and routes of administration of medications used in advanced life support
- outline the treatment algorithm for both shockable and non-shockable rhythms
- outline the nurse's role in facilitating family presence during an arrest.

Introduction

The continuum of critical illness for an individual can span the period before and beyond hospital admission. Resuscitation is often required outside the critical care environment. The 'cardiac arrest' team has evolved to use a more proactive, early-intervention approach, utilising a range of rapid response systems and instruments to detect deterioration in patients' clinical status (see Chapter 3). It is well recognised that improved outcomes from cardiac arrest are dependent on early recognition and initiation of the 'chain of survival'.[1] This chapter introduces the resuscitation systems and processes in both the pre-hospital and the in-hospital settings. The chain of survival provides a framework for the management of the person experiencing cardiac arrest and resuscitation in specific circumstances. The chapter expands on the final link in the chain, advanced life support (ALS), to outline advanced airway management, rhythm recognition, administration of medications and post-resuscitation care. Resuscitation involves many moral and ethical issues, such as family presence during resuscitation, deciding when to cease or initiate resuscitation and near-death experiences.

Cardiac arrest

Coronary heart disease (CHD) is the leading cause of death in most industrialised countries, with over half of these being due to sudden cardiac

KEY WORDS
....

advanced life
   support
capnography
cardiac arrest
cardiopulmonary
   resuscitation
out-of-hospital
   cardiac arrest
resuscitation
return of
   spontaneous
   circulation
   (ROSC)
sudden cardiac
   arrest

arrest (SCA).[2,3] Despite advances in CHD management, the survival rate from cardiac arrest is reported to be around 10%.[2–5] Survival after SCA is dependent on the presenting rhythm, early defibrillation, effective cardiopulmonary resuscitation, early ALS and post-resuscitation care.[5,6] Cardiac arrest has typically been categorised by the location of the event: out-of-hospital cardiac arrest (OHCA) or in-hospital cardiac arrest (IHCA).[2] Traditionally, the presenting rhythm with the majority of witnessed OHCA SCAs was ventricular fibrillation (VF) hence bystander cardiopulmonary resuscitation and early defibrillation were the focus of resuscitation efforts.[2,6,7] But, over time, the incidence of patients who have an OHCA presenting with VF is decreasing and that of those with shockable rhythm is increasing, possibly secondary to the modification of risk factors or interventions that shorten VF/pulseless ventricular tachycardia (pVT) duration, such as the use of cardiovascular drugs or implantable cardioverter-defibrillators.[8] Early interventions are now directed to uninterrupted CPR.

Incidence/aetiology of cardiac arrests

The prevalence of CHD varies worldwide; therefore, estimates of the incidence of SCA are difficult to obtain.[9] There are many factors that contribute to cardiac arrest. In adults, the most common cause of cardiac arrest is a primary cardiac event,[10,11] with coronary artery disease accounting for up to 90% of all victims.[12,13] CHD is the most likely cause of death in those over 35 years of age, in comparison with non-cardiac causes such as drowning, acute airway obstruction or trauma for people less than 35 years of age.[13] While causes of cardiac arrest are numerous, most often it is associated with VF triggered by an acutely ischaemic or infarcted myocardium or primary electrical disturbance.[3]

Acute myocardial infarction is the most common precursor to cardiac arrest. In victims of trauma, drug overdose and drowning, the predominant cause of cardiac arrest is asphyxia. Cardiac arrest in children is less common and even more rarely sudden,[14,15] with the common causes being trauma, congenital heart disease, long QT syndrome, drug overdose, hypoxia and hypothermia. The most common arrhythmia in infants is bradycardia; prognosis is especially poor if asystole is present.[14,16] Chest compression should be started if the pulse is less than 60/minute with poor perfusion.[16] While the aetiology of OHCA is predominantly due to CHD, the aetiology of IHCA differs. Table 25.1 lists some of the common aetiologies of IHCA.

Pathophysiology

In SCA with cardiac origin, it is believed that myocardial ischaemia leads to ventricular irritability and the progression from pVT to VF and ultimately asystole.[17] After the onset of VF (in animal studies), carotid arterial blood flow continues for approximately 4 minutes even in the absence of cardiac compressions, as coronary perfusion

---

TABLE 25.1

Aetiology of in-hospital cardiac arrest[2]

COMMON	LESS COMMON
Hypoxia	Cardiac tamponade
Acute coronary syndrome	Hypothermia
Arrhythmias	Pneumothorax
Hypovolaemia	Pulmonary emboli
Sepsis/infection	Toxins
Heart failure	Electrolyte disturbances

---

pressure (the pressure gradient between the aorta and the right atrium) falls over this period.[17] This initial phase is characterised by minimal ischaemic injury, and it is during this time that defibrillation is most likely to result in the restoration of a perfusing rhythm, while initiation of effective cardiac compressions will increase the coronary perfusion pressure.[17]

Progression of the cardiac arrest beyond 4 minutes results in accumulation of toxic metabolites, depletion of high-energy phosphate stores and the initiation of ischaemic cascades.[17] Increasing probability of irreversible cellular injury exists where a cardiac arrest extends for longer than 10 minutes, and the return of a spontaneous circulation during this period may initiate a reperfusion injury[17] (see Chapter 11 for further discussion).

Resuscitation systems and processes

Since the rediscovery of the effectiveness of closed-chest CPR in 1960 and its subsequent widespread adoption, CPR has saved the lives of many, potentially ensuring years of productive life.[18,19] The International Liaison Committee on Resuscitation (ILCOR), formed in 1992, promotes global discussion and consistency of guidelines between these international resuscitation councils, providing a consensus mechanism for near-continuous review of resuscitation science.[19]

Survival of arrests

Despite advances in resuscitation and technology, the survival to hospital discharge rates remain variable, at around 10% for OHCAs and 26% for IHCAs.[4,20] Factors associated with higher rates of mortality for adults are: age over 80 years, unwitnessed arrest, delays before commencing CPR, delayed defibrillation (pre-shock pauses) and delays prior to resumption of CPR (post-shock pauses) and non-ventricular tachycardia/fibrillation rhythm.[21] While the outcome statistics for children following IHCA are better than for OHCA, only one-third of children with IHCA will survive to discharge with optimal neurological function.[15] Marked differences in the inclusion criteria and outcome definitions may, however, also explain the wide variations in survival rates from cardiac arrests. In recognition of these variations, international guidelines such as the Utstein guidelines[21] have been implemented to consistently document, monitor and compare OHCAs and in-hospital resuscitation.

IHCA survival to hospital discharge rates are reportedly around 20–30%.[22] The majority of IHCA cardiac arrests are men (58–62%), have an initial rhythm that is predominantly (70%) non-shockable (i.e. asystole/pulseless electrical activity) and 22% have a shockable initial rhythm (ventricular tachycardia or ventricular fibrillation).[2,23,24] Many factors such as age, time of day, presence or absence of morbidity before or during the hospital admission, absence of 'not-for-resuscitation' orders, quality of the CPR, asystole and non-ICU location contribute to the in-hospital survival rates.[24–26]

Chain of survival

To optimise a person's chance of survival, the 'chain of survival' strategy has been developed,[27] which represents a sequence of events that must occur as quickly as possible: early recognition, early CPR, early defibrillation and post-resuscitation care (Fig. 25.1). These time-sensitive, sequential actions optimise a cardiac arrest victim's chances of survival. Communities with integrated links along this chain have demonstrated higher survival rates after OHCA than those with deficiencies in these links.[26]

Early recognition of cardiac arrest

The chain of survival begins with early recognition of a medical emergency and the activation of a rapid response system.[2,28] However, the chain of survival has not always been adequate when a cardiac arrest occurs in the hospital, including lack of early recognition, timeliness or availability of equipment or staff.[25,29] Two-thirds of IHCAs are potentially avoidable, with up to 50–84% of all IHCAs demonstrating evidence of deterioration in the 6–8 hours preceding the arrest.[30,31] Early-warning scoring systems (EWS) use (score) the patient's routinely measured physiological measurements (vital signs) to facilitate early recognition of the deteriorating patient. When the patient's score reaches a predetermined threshold, the EWS triggers the clinician to escalate care.[32–35] Patient scores and trigger thresholds vary across health sectors (Table 25.2). There is variable evidence that the implementation of an EWS reduces hospital mortality, or respiratory or cardiac arrests[3,36,37] (see Chapter 3 for further discussion). To further facilitate earlier activation of the rapid response teams, many hospitals have implemented systems for family and patients to directly escalate and activate a care process on a patient's behalf.[38]

Basic life support

When a patient is considered to be in potential or actual arrest, a primary and secondary survey should be conducted in the DRSABCD sequence:[39]

- **D**anger – check for danger (hazards or risks to safety).
- **R**esponsive – check for response (responsive/unconscious).
- **S**end – send for help.
- **A**irway – open the airway. Airway assessment is undertaken to establish a patent airway while maintaining cervical spine support (if injury is suspected).
- **B**reathing – check breathing. Breathing includes the assessment and establishment of breathing, noting rate, pattern and chest movement.
- **C**PR – start CPR. Give 30 chest compressions (almost 2 compressions/second) followed by 2 breaths.
- **D**efibrillation – attach an automated external defibrillator as soon as available and follow its prompts.

Continue CPR until responsiveness and normal breathing return. Ideally, these interventions are performed simultaneously or in rapid sequence and will take no longer than 60–90 seconds to complete. This systematic approach correlates closely with the actions of health professionals when a patient collapses in the in-hospital environment (Fig. 25.2).

FIGURE 25.1 Chain of survival.[26]

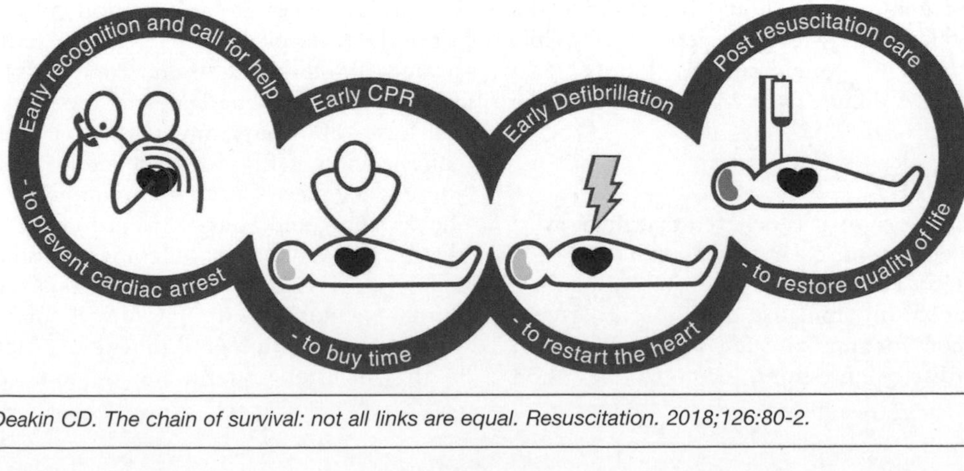

Source: From Deakin CD. The chain of survival: not all links are equal. Resuscitation. 2018;126:80-2.

TABLE 25.2

Early calling criteria[33–35]

AREA	ADULTS	CHILDREN 0–12 MONTHS	1–8 YEARS
Airway	Threatened	Threatened	Threatened
Breathing	All respiratory arrests RR <8 RR >27 SpO$_2$ <90%	All respiratory arrests RR <20 RR >50 Grunting respirations SpO$_2$ <90%	All respiratory arrests RR <15 RR >35 SpO$_2$ <90%
Circulation	All cardiac arrests PR <50 PR >130 Systolic BP <90	All cardiac arrests PR <100 PR >180 Systolic BP <50 Capillary return >4 seconds Marked pallor	All cardiac arrests PR <90 PR >160 Systolic BP <80
Neurology	Sudden fall in the level of consciousness (fall in the Glasgow Coma Scale score of ≥2 points) Repeated or prolonged seizures	Floppy Unresponsive Depressed conscious level Prolonged seizures	Floppy Unresponsive Depressed conscious level Prolonged seizures
Other	Any patient you are seriously worried about who does not fit the above criteria		

Note: These values are a guide and vary with different organisations. Always adhere to facility policy.

BP = blood pressure; PR = pulse rate; RR = respiratory rate.

FIGURE 25.2   Life support flow chart for the in-hospital patient.[36] ABCDE = airway, breathing, circulation, disability, exposure; ALS = advanced life support; BLS = basic life support; CPR = cardiopulmonary resuscitation; IV = intravenous; RRT = rapid response team.

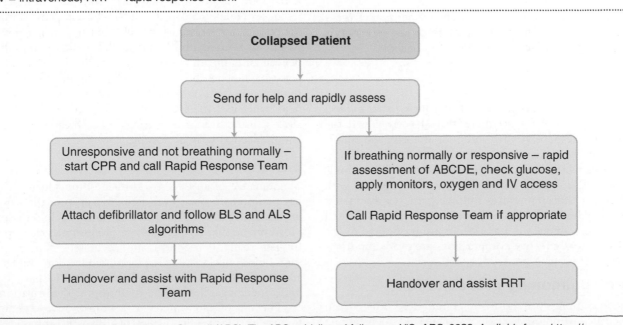

Source: From Australian Resuscitation Council (ARC). The ARC guidelines. Melbourne, VIC: ARC; 2022. Available from: https://resus.org.au/the-arc-guidelines/.

Airway

Recognition of airway obstruction includes listening for inspiratory (stridor), expiratory or grunting noises. The work of breathing can be assessed by the respiratory rate, intercostals, subcostal or sternal recession, use of accessory muscles, tracheal tug or flaring of the alae nasi. Nasal flaring is especially evident in infants with respiratory distress. Noisy breathing is obstructed breathing, but the volume of the noise is not an indicator of the severity of respiratory failure. Should obstruction to air flow be detected, then the airway should be opened using either of these manoeuvres: the head-tilt and chin-lift or jaw thrust. Assess a person's airway without turning them onto the side unless the airway is obstructed with fluid (vomit or blood) or submersion injuries.[39]

The airway of the infant differs from that of the older child or adult in that the infant has a large head and tongue and small mouth, and the larynx is narrower, shorter, more anterior and acutely angled[17] (see Chapter 27). The airway of an infant is also more cartilaginous and can be easily occluded when the neck is hyperextended; in addition, the large tongue can easily fall back to obstruct the pharynx.[40] Hence, the head of an infant should be maintained in the neutral position, whereas a child aged 1–8 years will require the 'sniffing position', with varying degrees according to age. The chin-lift and head-tilt manoeuvres may be used in children to obtain the appropriate positioning for age. Jaw thrust may be used if the head-tilt/chin-lift is contraindicated.[40] Do not use the finger sweep to clear the airway of an infant, as this may result in damage to the delicate palatal tissues and cause bleeding, which can worsen the situation. Use of finger sweep can force foreign bodies further down into the airway.[40] Suction is more useful for removing vomitus and secretions.

Practice tip

In paediatric patients, both cuffed and non-cuffed endotracheal tubes are acceptable for use in infants and children undergoing emergency intubation.[1]

Breathing

To assess for the presence of breathing, look, listen and feel for breath sounds for no more than 10 seconds. If the person is unresponsive with absent or abnormal breathing, call for help and commence compressions immediately. Agonal gasps are not to be considered normal breathing. Typically, the arterial blood may remain saturated with oxygen for several minutes following the cardiac arrest and, as cerebral and myocardial cell oxygenation is limited more by the absence of cardiac output as opposed to the reduced PaO_2, effective compressions are more important initially than rescue breaths.[27]

Cardiopulmonary resuscitation

Cardiac compressions should be commenced if the victim is unconscious, unresponsive, not moving and not breathing normally. Where possible, change the person delivering the compressions every 2 minutes. Pulse check by lay rescuers and health professionals in basic life support (BLS) is not recommended. Assessment of effective chest compression by healthcare professionals may be made by continuous end-tidal CO_2 ($ETCO_2$) monitoring. For CPR to be effective, the patient should be flat, supine and on a firm surface. The chest should be compressed in the midline over the lower half of the sternum, which equates to the 'centre of the chest', at a depth of >5 cm (adults), 5 cm (children) and 4 cm (infants). Equal time should be spent in compression as spent on the release,[36] with a rate of 100–120 compressions per minute for adults, infants and children, the rate rising to 120/min for the newborn.[27,36] CPR should be initiated when the heart rate is <60 beats per minute (bpm) for the newborn[14] and the small child and <40 bpm for the large child with poor perfusion (not responding). Performed correctly, external cardiac compressions (ECC) can produce a systolic blood pressure peak of 60–80 mmHg (in adults) and a cardiac output of 20–30% of normal.[27,41] With external chest compressions it takes time to reach optimal levels of coronary perfusion pressure and, ultimately, blood flow. Any interruption to chest compressions therefore decreases the coronary perfusion pressure and resultant blood flow, ultimately reducing survival.[42] After 30 compressions the airway should be opened and two breaths given.[43]

Survival potentially improves when an individual receives a higher number of chest compressions during CPR, even if the person receives fewer ventilations. Because of this, it is recommended that a 30:2 compression-to-ventilation ratio is used in adults, children and infants regardless of the number of rescuers, and 3:1 for neonates. Having noted this, in paediatric settings where staff have specialty basic life support/advanced life support (BLS/ALS) training, the compression ratio changes to 15:2 and a ratio of 3:1 for the newborn with any number of rescuers (Table 25.3). In the out-of-hospital environment the rescuer not only may be reluctant to initiate mouth-to-mouth resuscitation,[44] but will also take 8 seconds to deliver one breath.[45] When a rescuer is reluctant to perform rescue breaths, ECC without expired air resuscitation (EAR) should be encouraged, as the generally held belief is that ECC alone is better than no CPR at all.[46,47] In the healthcare setting, rescue breaths should be commenced as soon as possible.

Evaluation during resuscitation

Maintenance of an effective cardiac output during CPR has traditionally been evaluated by palpating the carotid or femoral pulse in adults (the brachial in children). However, neither lay persons nor professionals can rapidly (in less than 10 seconds) and accurately perform this step. Pulse checks are not recommended for evaluation after defibrillation until 2 minutes of CPR have been performed, regardless of the rhythm post-defibrillation.

The use of capnometry as a non-invasive technique for monitoring the effectiveness of CPR is recommended.[12]

TABLE 25.3

CPR for adults, children and infants[1]

AGE	AIRWAY	COMPRESSION (CPR)	1 OR 2 PERSONS
Infants <1 year	Jaw support or chin-lift (no head-tilt)	Two fingers or two overlying thumbs on the lower end of the sternum with hands encircling the chest (preferred), 100–120 beats/min	30:2 PALS 15:2 (2 rescuers)
Younger child: 1–8 years	Head-tilt more than infants but less than adults	Heel of one hand, 100–120 beats/min	30:2 PALS 15:2 (2 rescuers)
Older child: 9–14 years	Head-tilt	Two hands, 100–120 beats/min	30:2 PALS 15:2 (2 rescuers)
Adult	Head-tilt	Two hands, 100–120 beats/min	30:2

PALS = paediatric advanced life support.

TABLE 25.4

Augment compression devices[53–55]

DEVICE	DESCRIPTION
Active compression–decompression (ACD-CPR)	• Utilises a small portable device to compress and decompress the chest ('plunger method'). • Enhances ventilation and venous return by raising the negative intrathoracic pressure, which facilitates venous return, priming the heart for subsequent compressions.
Interposed abdominal compression (IAC) combined with CPR (IAC-CPR)	• Force applied to the abdomen during the recoil please of chest compression. • Results in increased resistance in the descending aorta, raising the coronary perfusion pressure.
Non-invasive automated chest compression device (e.g. AutoPulse®)	• Utilises a load-distributing band (LDB) to compress the anterior chest. • The device is built around a backboard that contains a motor. • The motor tightens or loosens LDB around the patient's chest.

As the partial pressure of the $ETCO_2$ concentration correlates with pulmonary blood flow during CPR, the adequacy of resuscitation efforts is evaluated by measuring this parameter. $ETCO_2$ also correlates with cardiac output, return of spontaneous circulation (ROSC) and outcomes in cardiac arrest.[48,49] A mean $ETCO_2$ of 20 mmHg or above has been associated with survival from cardiac arrest, while a mean $ETCO_2$ <10 mmHg is associated with poor outcomes.[49] A rise in $ETCO_2$ during CPR may indicate increased probability of defibrillation success, the ROSC and survival to hospital discharge.[50–51] Having noted this, hyperventilation during CPR is not recommended and may be harmful. Clinical studies show that rescuers consistently hyperventilate patients during a cardiac arrest.[51]

Devices to augment compression

As ECC supplies only 15–30% of normal cardiac output[52] and 15% of normal cerebral blood flow, various mechanical CPR devices have been trialled to improve cardiac compression.[53–55] While no mechanical adjunct is currently recommended,[56] a few of the devices are outlined in Table 25.4. There is, however, a growing incidence of the use of some of these devices in the pre-hospital environment and in situations where it is difficult to provide high-quality compressions such as during transport, prolonged cardiac arrests or where manual compression may compromise user safety.[54–56] These devices should be used in a properly supervised program and the users should be well trained.[55,56]

Practice tip

When ventilating a patient without an advanced airway, ventilation should be continued at a ratio of 30 compressions to 2 ventilations.[56]

Defibrillation

While CPR has been associated with improved survival to discharge from hospital, it cannot be substituted for the definitive treatment of early defibrillation of a shockable rhythm.[57] It is thought that CPR will supply sufficient oxygen to the brain and heart until defibrillation is available.

Precordial thump

A precordial thump is a single, sharp blow delivered with a clenched fist to the mid-sternum of a victim's chest from a height of 25–30 cm above the sternum.[7,58,59] The mechanical energy generated by the precordial thump may generate a few joules, and therefore is applied within the first few seconds of onset of a monitored pVT rhythm, and is no longer recommended for VF as it has a very low success rate at conversion to a perfusing rhythm.[58,59] Because of the very low success rate and the brief period for application, delivery of the thump must not delay accessing help or a defibrillator. A precordial thump may be used in monitored and witnessed pVT arrest while awaiting the arrival of the defibrillator.[36]

It should not be used in patients with unwitnessed cardiac arrest or those with recent sternotomy or chest trauma.[59]

Electrical defibrillation

Defibrillation is the passage of a current of electricity through a fibrillating heart to simultaneously depolarise the mass of myocardial cells and allow them to repolarise uniformly to an organised electrical activity.[12]

> **Practice tip**
>
> An automatic external defibrillator (AED) should be applied as soon as possible so that a shock can be given if appropriate.[60]

There are two types of external defibrillators: the manual external defibrillator and the automatic external defibrillator. Most manual defibrillators have AED capacity. The manual defibrillator, in manual mode, requires the user to be able to immediately and accurately recognise arrhythmias and make the decision whether to initiate defibrillation or not. In comparison, the AED automatically detects and interprets the rhythm without relying on the user's recognition of arrhythmias. AEDs can be operated in both manual and semiautomatic mode. When using an AED, the user determines whether the person is unresponsive, not breathing and without signs of life.[57,60] The AED requires only three to four steps to operate: (1) turn power on, (2) place self-adhesive electrodes on a victim's chest, (3) rhythm analysis follows (hands-off period), and (4) then (if advised by the machine) press the shock button; in some devices this step

is also automated. The AED will automatically interpret the cardiac rhythm and, if VF/pVT is present, will advise the operator to provide a shock.

Health professionals with expertise in rhythm recognition may reduce the 'hands-off' period using a manual defibrillator.[61,62] The combined pre-shock and the post-shock pause ideally should be less than 5 seconds.[12] This can be achieved by continuing compressions while the defibrillator is charging and resuming chest compressions immediately after the delivery of the shock. Use of the AED should not be restricted to trained personnel.[62] Members of the public should be encouraged to use AEDs in the event of a cardiopulmonary arrest.[60,62] This public access to early defibrillation has seen the placement of defibrillators in aircraft, casinos and cricket grounds, with non-medical personnel such as police, flight attendants, security guards, family members and even children successfully initiating early defibrillation.[62] The effectiveness of training non-traditional out-of-hospital first responders to use the AED has improved survival to discharge rates.[20,62] Similarly, IHCA also occur in any area, and all healthcare workers should be capable of initiating early defibrillation.[12] While BLS does not have to include the use of adjunctive equipment, the use of AEDs by persons with education in their use is supported and should be taught. Fig. 25.2 outlines the integration of defibrillation with BLS.

> **Practice tip**
>
> Pads are placed on the exposed chest in an anterior–lateral position, some devices require pads to be placed in an anterior–posterior position.[60]

For 90% of people in VF, return of a perfusing rhythm will occur after a single shock. However, it is rare that a pulse will be palpable with the perfusing rhythm; hence the immediate resumption of chest compressions in the post-shock period is supported.[12] Failure to successfully convert VF after the single-shock strategy may indicate the need for a period of effective CPR (30:2) for 2 minutes and rhythm reanalysis, followed by shock if indicated.[12] A single-shock strategy is now recommended for all patients in cardiac arrest requiring defibrillation for VF or pVT.[60] Not all of the electrical energy delivered during defibrillation will traverse the myocardium. The optimum defibrillation energy level is that which sufficiently abolishes the arrhythmia to enable the return of an organised rhythm, with minimal myocardial damage.[12,63] Other biphasic energy levels may be used providing there are relevant clinical data for a specific defibrillator to suggest that an alternative energy level provides adequate shock success.[1,64] If the initial shock is unsuccessful, subsequent shocks should be delivered at the initial dose, or higher energy levels may be selected.[12] In children, 4 J/kg is recommended for the initial and subsequent shocks.[12,40,65] Where paediatric defibrillation

TABLE 25.5

Factors contributing to the success or failure of defibrillation[68–70]

SUCCESS	FAILURE	PRECAUTIONS
• VF duration • Early defibrillation (if VF <3 min) • Initial CPR (if VF >3 min) • Presenting rhythm (pVT/VF) • Paddle/pad size and placement • Use of self-adhesive pads	• Inadequate contact with the chest (excessive chest hair). • Faulty positioning of the paddles. • Synchronise button in the 'on' position, flat battery or fractured lead. • Positioning over bone/fat or breast tissue, chest size. • Drying out of gel conduction pads. • Patient factors: acidosis, hypoxia, electrolyte imbalance, drug toxicity, hypothermia. • Time of respiration (best delivered at end-expiration) • PEEP and auto-PEEP (air-trapping) should be minimised. • Paddles/electrodes too small (8–12 cm electrodes for adults).	• Place defibrillation electrodes at least 8 cm away from ECG electrodes, or implantable medical devices, pacemakers, vascular access devices. • Remove medication patches, wipe the area before applying defibrillation electrodes. • Do not defibrillate unless all are clear of the bed/patient. • Do not charge/discharge paddles in the air. • Do not have the patient in contact with metal. • Do not allow oxygen to flow onto the patient during delivery of the shock (at least 1 m from the patient). • Ensure the chest is dry. • Do not use electrode gels and pastes as these can spread between the paddles and potentially spark.

ECG = electrocardiogram; PEEP = peak end-expiratory pressure; VF = ventricular fibrillation; VT = ventricular tachycardia.

pads are not readily available, standard adult AEDs and pads are suitable for use in children older than 8 years. Ideally, for children between 1 and 8 years, paediatric pads and an AED with paediatric capability should be used.[1,40] These pads are placed as per the adult methodology ensuring the pads do not touch, which may necessitate anterior–posterior pad placement.

The importance of early, uninterrupted chest compressions and early defibrillation are well promulgated in the ILCOR guidelines.[12] As the length of time from collapse is difficult to estimate accurately, it is imperative that rescuers perform quality chest compressions until the defibrillator is both available and charged.[46,66,67] Table 25.5 outlines some of the common factors contributing to the success or failure of defibrillation.[57,68–70]

Advanced life support

Basic life support provides about 20–30% of normal cardiac output and a fraction of inspired oxygen (FiO_2) of 0.1–0.16. Consequently, a significant number of patients rely on the provision of ALS for survival. ALS extends BLS to provide the knowledge and skills essential for the initiation of early treatment and stabilisation of people post-cardiac arrest. Advanced skills traditionally include defibrillation, advanced airway management and the administration of resuscitation drugs. Algorithms for management of cardiopulmonary arrest (Figs 25.3 and 25.4) outline the two decision paths, also referred to as the shockable and non-shockable treatment algorithms in ALS: (1) defibrillation and CPR for pVT/VF (shockable) and (2) identifying and treating the underlying cause for non-VT/VF (non-shockable).

Advanced airway management

A person with signs of acute hypoxia should be administered oxygen at the highest possible concentration, including initially during CPR.[43] Oxygen should never be withheld for fear of adverse effects, as rescue breaths provide an inspired oxygen concentration of only 15–18%.[56] The administration of oxygen alone does not result in adequate ventilation and, as such, the establishment of an effective airway is paramount. Airway management is essential in the performance of CPR, and may be administered using a variety of techniques. These may include: compression-only CPR with high-flow oxygen by face mask, rescue breathing (bag–mask ventilation) and insertion of a supraglottic airway device that does not require laryngoscopy or tracheal intubation.[71] The choice of advanced airway adjunct is determined by the availability of equipment, the skills of the personnel and the success rate of endotracheal (ET) intubation[71–74] (see Table 25.6 and Chapter 15).

The endotracheal tube (ETT) is considered the 'gold standard' for airway management in a cardiac arrest, as it protects the airway, assists effective ventilation, ensures delivery of high concentrations of oxygen and eases suctioning. However, currently there is no evidence that ETT is superior to supraglottic airway in terms of either neurological outcomes or survival.[71] It is vital that CPR is not interrupted for more than 5 seconds during attempts at ET intubation. Waveform capnography or an oesophageal detector device should be applied to confirm the correct placement of supraglottic airway or ETT.[12,71]

$ETCO_2$ should be used to monitor the quality of the CPR. Given the limitations noted in Table 25.6, a variety

FIGURE 25.3 Advanced life support flow chart.[1] ABCDE = airway, breathing, circulation, disability, exposure; CPR = cardiopulmonary resuscitation; ETT = endotracheal tube; IV/IO = intravenous/intraosseous; LMA = laryngeal mask airway; SpO$_2$ = peripheral capillary oxygen saturation

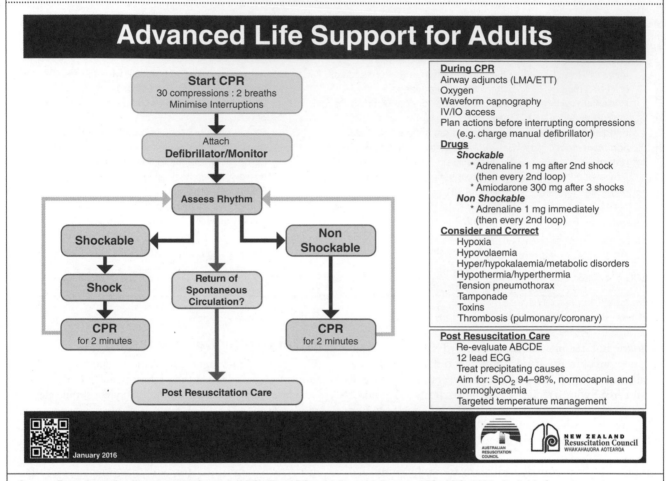

Source: From Australian Resuscitation Council (ARC). The ARC guidelines. Melbourne, VIC: ARC; 2022. Available from: https://resus.org.au/the-arc-guidelines/.

of adjunct airway/ventilation management devices are available, such as: bag–mask ventilation (BMV), supraglottic airways devices such as the laryngeal mask airway (LMA) and the classic laryngeal mask airway, the oesophageal–tracheal airway (Combitube) and the i-gel®. The benefit of the supraglottic airway devices is that they are easily inserted without interruption to chest compressions. Currently, there is no evidence to support the routine use of any particular advanced adjunct airway devices.[71] Healthcare professionals trained to use supraglottic airway devices (e.g. LMA) may consider their use for airway management during cardiac arrest and as a backup or rescue airway in a difficult or failed tracheal intubation.

Once an airway has been established, continue chest compressions, without interruption, and ventilate the lungs at a rate of approximately 6–10 ventilations a minute. All delivered breaths should be timed with release of compression for effective delivery of the breath. Minimise the likelihood of excessive ventilation by delivering one breath during the relaxation phase of every 15th compression.[36]

Rhythms

There is an association between the initial cardiac arrhythmias and survival to discharge after SCA. Cardiac arrest rhythms can be divided into two subsets:

1 VF and pVT
2 non-VF/pVT incorporating asystole and pulseless electrical activity (PEA).

The most common arrhythmias observed in SCA are pVT and VF, with 60–85% of all patients initially presenting with these lethal arrhythmias.[6] In-hospital PEA occurs as the initial rhythm in approximately 44–60% of cases[75,76] and the overall survival to discharge rate is 9%.[76] Bradycardia (41%) followed by asystole are the most common arrest arrhythmias in children.[75] In the paediatric population, their hearts respond to prolonged severe hypoxia and acidosis by progressive bradycardia leading to asystole.[12] Despite reported ROSC rates of around 76%, survival to hospital discharge in children remains low, at 38%.[76]

FIGURE 25.4 Advanced life support for infants and children flow chart.[1] ABCDE = airway, breathing, circulation, disability, exposure; CPR = cardiopulmonary resuscitation; ETT = endotracheal tube; IV/IO = intravenous/intraosseous; LMA = laryngeal mask airway; SpO$_2$ = peripheral capillary oxygen saturation

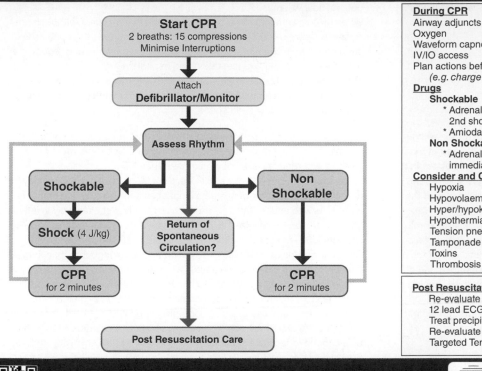

Advanced Life Support for Infants and Children

Start CPR
2 breaths: 15 compressions
Minimise Interruptions

Attach **Defibrillator/Monitor**

Assess Rhythm

Shockable

Non Shockable

Shock (4 J/kg)

Return of Spontaneous Circulation?

CPR for 2 minutes

CPR for 2 minutes

Post Resuscitation Care

During CPR
Airway adjuncts (*LMA/ETT*)
Oxygen
Waveform capnography
IV/IO access
Plan actions before interrupting compressions
  (*e.g. charge manual defibrillator to 4 J/kg*)
Drugs
  Shockable
    * Adrenaline 10 micrograms/kg after
      2nd shock (*then every 2nd loop*)
    * Amiodarone 5 mg/kg after 3 shocks
  Non Shockable
    * Adrenaline 10 micrograms/kg
      immediately (*then every 2nd loop*)
Consider and Correct
  Hypoxia
  Hypovolaemia
  Hyper/hypokalaemia/metabolic disorders
  Hypothermia/hyperthermia
  Tension pneumothorax
  Tamponade
  Toxins
  Thrombosis (*pulmonary/coronary*)

Post Resuscitation Care
  Re-evaluate ABCDE
  12 lead ECG
  Treat precipitating causes
  Re-evaluate oxygenation and ventilation
  Targeted Temperature Management

 January 2016

 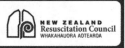 **NEW ZEALAND** Resuscitation Council WHAKAHAUORA AOTEAROA

Source: From Australian Resuscitation Council (ARC). The ARC guidelines. Melbourne, VIC: ARC; 2022. Available from: https://resus.org.au/the-arc-guidelines/.

TABLE 25.6

Adjuncts used during resuscitation[1,12,72–74]

AIRWAY TYPE	DESCRIPTION	PRACTICE CONSIDERATIONS
Oropharyngeal (Guedel's) airway	Conforms to the curve of the palate, moving the tongue forward away from the posterior pharyngeal wall. Sizes from 000 to 5.	Incorrect size or placement may contribute to airway obstruction by pushing the tongue back into the pharynx. Unlike adult insertion, the insertion of the oropharyngeal airway in infants and young children is inserted right-way-up; a tongue depressor or laryngoscope should be used to aid insertion.
Nasopharyngeal airway	Soft tube inserted into the nasopharynx.	Use with caution in patients with head injuries. With the exception of infant's head-tilt, jaw support or jaw thrust is still necessary when using either the oropharyngeal or the nasopharyngeal airway.

Continued

TABLE 25.6
Adjuncts used during resuscitation—cont'd

AIRWAY TYPE	DESCRIPTION	PRACTICE CONSIDERATIONS
Bag–valve–mask (BVM) systems	A self-inflating bag that may be connected to a face mask, laryngeal mask airway or endotracheal tube (ETT).	BVMs are often inappropriately used and offer no protection to the airway. Two-person technique is preferable. Single-person BVM ventilation may result in a poor seal around the patient's mouth and the delivery of less than optimal tidal volumes.[12] When using a BVM, it is best performed using two rescuers, although not always possible. As the airway is not protected, smaller tidal volumes with supplementary oxygen can provide adequate oxygenation and reduce the risk of gastric inflation, regurgitation and aspiration. The mask should be used right-way-up with children and upside-down with infants. The soft circular mask is preferred for infants, as it provides an excellent seal with low dead space.
Laryngeal mask airway (LMA)	Consists of a tube with an elliptical cuff fitted at the distal end that inflates in the hypopharynx around the posterior perimeter of the larynx. The LMA is inserted orally using a blind technique so that the distal end of the mask abuts against the base of the hypopharynx, behind the cricoid cartilage, and the cuff is inflated to form an airtight seal around the larynx.	The LMA is used as a first-line adjunct when endotracheal intubation is not available. The LMA is easier to insert than a Combitube, more rapidly inserted and requires less equipment than the ETT. When used as a first-line airway device, the LMA provides a clear airway with a significantly lower risk of gastric overinflation and regurgitation than the BVM.[12] As with adults, the LMA can be used safely and effectively in infants.[72] LMA: size 1 for <5 kg; size 1.5, 5–10 kg; size 2, 10–20 kg; size 2.5, 20–30 kg; size 4, 50–70 kg; size 5, 70–100 kg; size 6, >100 kg. Use in newborns over 34 weeks gestation and weighing more than 2 kg.[72] Complications of LMA include gastric aspiration, partial airway obstruction, coughing or gastric insufflation. Some types of LMA have a gastric port which enables insertion of an orogastric tube to deflate and empty the stomach of contents so avoiding aspiration of gastric contents. An intubating LMA (Fastrach™) is also available and this type of LMA is used as a conduit to facilitate intubation. Contraindications include patients unable to open their mouths adequately, pharyngeal pathology, airway obstruction at or below level of the larynx, low pulmonary compliance or high airway resistance, or increased risk of aspiration.
Oesophageal–tracheal Combitube (ETC)	The ETC is a double-lumen airway with proximal and distal cuffs that is passed into the oesophagus.	It is effective in maintaining an airway when performed by unskilled personnel and is a suitable alternative to tracheal intubation. The ETC enables ventilation, whether it is positioned in the oesophagus or the trachea. Only one size needed for most adults.
Laryngeal tube (LT)	Airway tube with a small oesophageal cuff and a larger pharyngeal cuff. The distal tip is positioned in the upper oesophagus.	Use is comparable to classic LMA and LMA ProSeal™.[73]
i-gel®	The cuff of the i-gel is made of gel and does not require inflation.	Very easy to insert with minimal training.[12] Enables continuous chest compression without interruption for ventilation.[74]
Endotracheal tube (ETT)	During intubation, direct application of firm pressure to the cricoid cartilage is required to compress the oesophagus between the trachea and vertebral column and minimise/prevent regurgitation of gastric contents.	Endotracheal intubation is a difficult skill to acquire and maintain. In addition to routine clinical methods, ETT placement can be confirmed by either measurement of $ETCO_2$ or use of an oesophageal detector; the latter is more reliable in a non-perfusing rhythm (Class IIb). Immediate complications associated with intubation include oesophageal intubation, right main bronchi intubation, or ETT occlusion (kinking, sputum, cuff, blood).

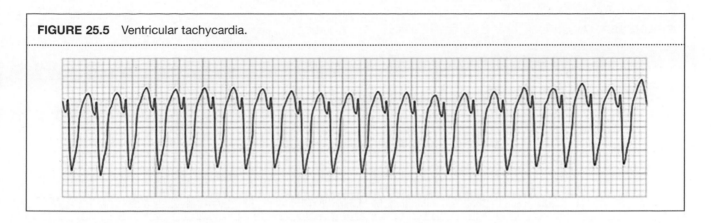

FIGURE 25.5   Ventricular tachycardia.

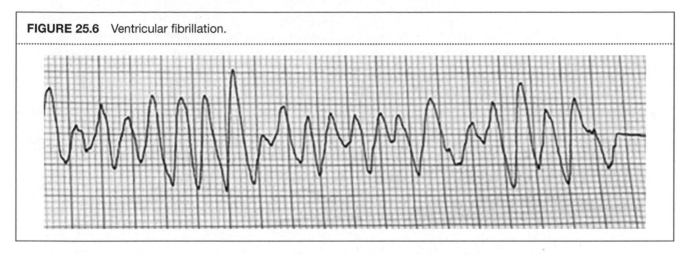

FIGURE 25.6   Ventricular fibrillation.

Ventricular fibrillation and pulseless ventricular tachycardia

As previously noted, the only intervention shown to unequivocally improve long-term survival after a VF or pVT arrest is prompt and effective BLS, uninterrupted chest compressions and early defibrillation.[12] pVT and VF rhythms are displayed in Figs 25.5 and 25.6. Energy levels and subsequent shocks are equivalent for both VF and pVT.

Non-VF/pVT

Non–VF/pVT arrhythmias include PEA and asystole. PEA reflects dissociation between the heart's electrical and mechanical activities. It is important to note that PEA may present as any rhythm normally compatible with a pulse (e.g. sinus rhythm, sinus tachycardia/bradycardia). PEA is characterised by a stroke volume insufficient to produce a palpable pulse, despite electrical activity. The survival rate for PEA/asystole averages 5%.[77] Management of PEA includes identifying and correcting reversible causes, summarised as the four Hs and four Ts in Table 25.7.

Careful confirmation of asystole (Fig. 25.7) on two leads and the absence of a palpable pulse are essential when making the decision to manage asystole. When an in-hospital arrest has an initial rhythm of asystole, survival to discharge has been reported as 11%.[75]

TABLE 25.7

Causes of pulseless electrical activity[1,2]

THE FOUR HS	THE FOUR TS
• Hypoxia	• Tamponade
• Hypovolaemia	• Tension pneumothorax
• Hypo/hyperthermia	• Toxins/poisons/drugs
• Hypo/hyperkalaemia and metabolic disorders	• Thrombosis: pulmonary/ coronary

Medications administered during cardiac arrest

Resuscitation drugs can be administered during a cardiac arrest using a variety of routes including peripheral and central veins or intraosseously. Administration by the central venous route remains the optimal method, but the decision to access peripheral versus central cannulation will depend on the skill of the operator. Peripheral venous cannulation is the quickest and easiest method; however, the patient in cardiac arrest may have inaccessible peripheral veins.[78] Should a decision be made to insert a central line during a cardiac arrest, this must not take

FIGURE 25.7 Asystole.

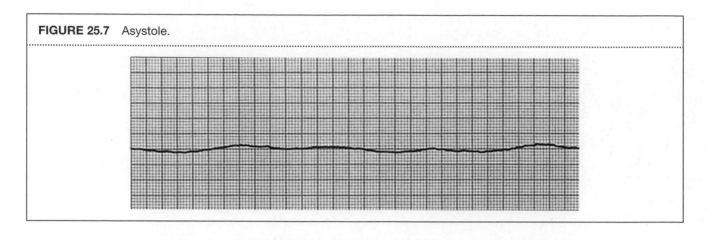

precedence over defibrillation attempts, CPR or airway maintenance. Intravenous medications should be flushed with 20–30 mL (adults) of an isotonic solution followed by at least 1 minute of continuous ECCs. Where there is difficulty accessing a peripheral vein, selected medications may be administered via an intraosseous (IO) route.[78]

IO is preferred if intravenous access is not possible. Insertion sites include (1) proximal tibia (2–3 cm below the tibial tuberosity), (2) distal tibia (proximal to the medial malleolus), (3) distal femur (midline, 2–3 cm above external condyle), (4) proximal humerus and (5) sternum. IO infusion involves the insertion of a metal needle using a drill into the bone marrow and provides a rapid, safe and reliable access to the circulation. The marrow sinusoids of the long bones are a non-collapsible venous system in direct connection with the systemic circulation, allowing drugs to reach the central circulation as quickly as medications injected into central veins. Intraosseal access is safe and effective for use in patients of all age groups.[78] General blood specimens such as biochemistry values, blood cultures, haemoglobin and cross-match studies can also be taken from the marrow at cannulation, but must be sent to the pathology department for analysis and not put through arterial blood gas machines.

Practice tip

Tibial and humerus IO routes are as effective as central venous routes in administering medications during CPR, reaching maximum blood concentrations in less than 2 minutes.

Vasopressors such as adrenaline (epinephrine) and vasopressin have been used as adjuncts in cardiac arrests to improve the success of CPR.[79–81] While there is no evidence to show that the routine use of any vasopressor during a cardiac arrest will increase survival to discharge from hospital, adrenaline is still recommended.[82] Findings from randomised controlled trials have challenged the use of adrenaline in OHCA.[80,83] OHCA patients who receive a standard dose of adrenaline do demonstrate improved

likelihood of ROSC[83] and it improves survival to discharge in patients with non-shockable rhythm.[81]

The optimal dose of adrenaline in the pre-hospital and in-hospital settings remains unclear. Current recommendations propose that 1 mg should be administered for pVT/VF following the second shock and then every second loop thereafter. For asystole and PEA, administer 1 mg of adrenaline in the initial loop, then every second loop (Table 25.8).[1]

The optimal role and exact benefit of antiarrhythmic medications in cardiac resuscitation is yet to be fully elucidated, but they have very little, if any, role to play in the treatment of cardiac arrests.[12] The common antiarrhythmic drugs include amiodarone, magnesium, atropine and calcium (see Table 25.8). Amiodarone is the leading antiarrhythmic medication because its safety and efficacy have been demonstrated. There is no evidence of improved survival with the use of atropine in a cardiac arrest with asystole or PEA.[23] Calcium chloride has little use in the management of arrhythmias unless caused by hyperkalaemia, hypocalcaemia or hypermagnesaemia, or an overdose of calcium channel-blocking drugs. Sodium bicarbonate is no longer administered routinely,[84] as it may cause hypernatraemia, hyperosmolality and intracellular acidosis from the rapid ingress of CO_2 generated from its dissociation. However, it is recommended if the cardiac arrest is associated with hyperkalaemia or tricyclic antidepressant overdose.[12]

There are insufficient data to support the routine use of magnesium in cardiac arrests,[82] except if torsades de pointes is suspected.[12,84] Thrombolytics should not be routinely administered in a cardiac arrest, but they may be considered in adults with proven or suspected pulmonary embolism or acute thrombotic aetiology.[12] Following the administration of the fibrinolytic medication, CPR should be continued for at least 30 minutes before the termination of CPR, and consideration given to continuing it for 60–90 min.[78]

During peri-arrest, strategies should be initiated to prevent the development of serious peri-arrest arrhythmias. Whenever possible, arterial blood gases, serum electrolytes and a 12-lead ECG should be obtained to assist with

TABLE 25.8

Medications used during resuscitation[1]

| ACTION | INDICATIONS | DOSE | | ADVERSE EVENTS |
		ADULTS	PAEDIATRIC	
Adrenaline is a catecholamine that increases aortic diastolic pressure and coronary artery perfusion by producing arteriolar vasoconstriction. It may facilitate defibrillation by improving myocardial blood flow during CPR. Traditionally the first-line medication for the treatment of VF and refractory pVT, adrenaline has not demonstrated improved outcomes after cardiac arrest and has been associated with post-resuscitation myocardial dysfunction.	VF and pVT resistant to the three initial counter-shocks after the second shock and then every second loop PEA and asystole.	VF and pVT: 1 mg after the second shock then after every second loop. PEA and asystole: 1 mg in the initial loop, then every second loop.	VF and pVT: 10 micrograms/kg after the second shock then after every second loop. PEA and asystole: 10 micrograms/kg immediately, then every second loop.	Tachyarrhythmia: hypertension, coronary vasoconstriction, increased myocardial oxygen consumption.
Amiodarone is a class III antiarrhythmic agent, characterised by an ability to delay action potential, thereby initiating a more regular heart rate. Amiodarone also directly affects smooth muscle and blocks calcium channels and alpha-adrenergic receptors, resulting in coronary and peripheral arterial vasodilation and a reduction in afterload and systemic blood pressure.	pVT/VF after the third shock refractory to three shocks. Polymorphic pVT and wide complex tachycardia of uncertain origin. Control of haemodynamically stable VT when cardioversion is unsuccessful (in the presence of LV dysfunction). Adjunct to electrical cardioversion of SVT. Prophylaxis of recurrent VF/pVT.	Initial bolus dose: 300 mg in 20 mL dextrose. A further 150 mg could be considered for refractory cases. *Peri-arrest:* an infusion of 15 mg/kg over 24 h may be commenced.	Initial dose: 5 mg/kg bolus over 2 min, which may be repeated to a maximum of 300 mg. *Peri-arrest:* IV infusion 5–15 µg/kg/min as continuous infusion (max of 1.2 g in 24 h).	Vasodilation and hypotension, bradycardia, heart block. May have negative inotropic effects. Use with caution in renal failure. Avoid use in torsades de pointes and other causes of prolonged Q–T.
Magnesium is a major intracellular cation resulting in smooth muscle relaxation and membrane stabilisation.	Torsades de pointes with or without a pulse; cardiac arrest associated with digoxin toxicity. Failure of defibrillation and adrenaline to reverse VF and pVT. Documented hypokalaemia or hypomagnesaemia.	Bolus dose: 5 mmol. *Peri-arrest:* may be followed by infusion of 20 mmol infused over 4 h.	IV or IO bolus: 0.1–0.2 mmol/kg. May be followed by an infusion of 0.3 mmol/kg over 4 h.	Hypotension with rapid administration. Use with caution if renal failure present. Muscle weakness, paralysis and respiratory failure. Tachycardia and excitement.
Calcium is essential to nerve and muscle impulse formation and excitation.	Not recommended for routine administration in cardiac arrest. Consider administration for: hypocalcaemia, hyperkalaemia, overdose of calcium blockers.	Bolus dose: 5–10 mL 10% calcium chloride (6.8 mmol).	0.2 mL/kg 10% calcium chloride, or 0.7 mL/kg 10% calcium gluconate via IV.	Calcium is incompatible with a range of medications and may precipitate in IV lines. Tissue necrosis with extravasation may occur.

Continued

TABLE 25.8

Medications used during resuscitation—cont'd

ACTION	INDICATIONS	DOSE		ADVERSE EVENTS
		ADULTS	PAEDIATRIC	
Sodium bicarbonate (NaHCO$_3$) is an alkaline agent that may be used to correct an acidosis. Routine administration of sodium bicarbonate for treatment of in-hospital and out-of-hospital cardiac arrest is not recommended.	Correcting a metabolic acidosis (pH <7.1), or base deficit of ≤10 or after 15 min; preexisting hyperkalaemia; tricyclic antidepressant overdose and urinary alkalinisation in overdose; or hypoxic lactic acidosis.	Bolus dose: 1 mmol/kg administered over 2–3 min, then as guided by arterial blood gases. As NaHCO$_3$ is incompatible with many medications, it should be administered by a separate line or flushed before and after administration.	0.5–1 mmol/kg via IV or IO administered over 2–3 min.	Should not be routinely administered. Alkalosis, hypernatraemia, hyperosmolality, paradoxical cerebral acidosis, depressed cardiac contractility and metabolic acidosis.
Potassium is an electrolyte essential for cell membrane stabilisation that is occasionally used in ALS.	Persistent documented VF, suspected hypokalaemia or hypomagnesaemia, and cardiac arrest associated with digoxin toxicity.	Slow bolus: 5 mmol.	0.03–0.07 mmol/kg via slow administration IV or IO. *Peri-arrest:* 0.2 mmol/kg/h as a continuous infusion; dilute with at least 50 times its volume and mix well, as can be fatal; 0.2–0.5 mmol/kg/h to a max of 1 mmol/kg if hypokalaemia severe but not immediately life-threatening.	Hyperkalaemia with bradycardia, hypotension with possible asystole and extravasation may lead to tissue necrosis.

ALS = advanced life support; ECC = external cardiac compression; IO = intraosseous; LV = left ventricular; PEA = pulseless electrical activity; SI = sinoatrial; SVT = supraventricular tachycardia; VF = ventricular fibrillation; VT = ventricular tachycardia.

Source: Adapted from Australian Resuscitation Council (ARC). ANZCOR guidelines. Victoria, Australia: Australian Resuscitation Council. Melbourne, VIC: ARC; 2018. Available from: https://resus.org.au/the-arc-guidelines/.

determining the precise rhythm and appropriate medical interventions.[16] The presence or absence of adverse signs and symptoms will dictate interventions.

Interventions can broadly be divided into three options for immediate treatment:

1 antiarrhythmics (refer to *peri-arrest* in Table 25.8)

2 electrical cardioversion

3 cardiac pacing.

Common peri-arrest arrhythmias and interventions are covered in Chapter 11. Antiarrhythmic interventions such as medications, physical manoeuvres and electrical therapies may be proarrhythmic.[16] These proarrhythmic interventions alter the cardiac depolarisation and/or repolarisation, lengthening or shortening the QT and predisposing to fatal arrhythmias.[85]

Fluid resuscitation

Fluid resuscitation may be considered if hypovolaemia is suspected as a possible cause of the cardiac arrest.[86] Sodium chloride (0.9%) is the most widely used fluid. It is used as a rapid infusion in the initial stages of resuscitation (at least 20 mL/kg). However, there is insufficient evidence to support or refute the routine administration of fluids during a cardiac arrest in the absence of hypovolaemia.[86]

Temporary cardiac pacing

During a cardiac arrest, temporary cardiac pacing may be required for sustained symptomatic bradycardia that is unresponsive to medical intervention. Two types of temporary cardiac pacing are utilised during a cardiac arrest: transvenous (invasive) and transcutaneous (external, non-invasive). As most current defibrillators have the capacity to pace, transcutaneous pacemakers are generally used in an arrest situation.

Ultrasound imaging

Ultrasound imaging has been shown to have some benefit in the detection and diagnosis of reversible causes of arrest including cardiac tamponade, pulmonary embolism, pneumothorax, aortic dissection and hypovolaemia. Placement of the probe at the subxiphoid position prior to stopping for planned rhythm assessment will facilitate views within 10 seconds and minimise chest compression interruptions.[20] While the use of imaging has not been shown to improve outcome, absence of heart motion on sonography during resuscitation is highly predictive of death.[20]

Special conditions

Although not common, there are some clinical presentations that require special considerations in a cardiac arrest scenario; these include pregnancy, electrical injuries and drowning. The principles of airway, breathing and circulation remain the same, but modifications must be made because of the physiological changes that occur.

Pregnancy

Healthy pregnant women can develop subtle clinical signs of clinical deterioration which may be mistaken for discomfort of pregnancy. Where these changes go undetected, the woman's clinical state can rapidly move to a worse clinical state, increasing risk of morbidity for the woman and/or her baby.[87] While rare, cardiac arrest in the pregnant woman is the leading cause of maternal death.[88] Precipitants include pulmonary embolism, sepsis, trauma, peripartum haemorrhage, amniotic fluid embolism, eclamptic seizure, congenital and acquired cardiac disease, myocardial infarction, subarachnoid haemorrhage, poisoning/self-harm and cerebral aneurysm.[88–92] The best outcome for both mother and the fetus in the setting of maternal cardiac arrest is likely to be achieved by timely resuscitation or delivery by caesarean section.[88]

The principles of airway, breathing and circulation remain the same, but modifications must be made because of the physiological changes that occur with normal pregnancy.[88] A number of factors may need to be considered when resuscitating a pregnant woman. If the fundus height is at or above the level of the umbilicus (approximately 20 weeks of gestational age), aortocaval compression may result in a fall in cardiac output of up to 25%.[90,92] During CPR, the mother may be placed in the left lateral tilt (15–30 degrees)[91] or supine with a pillow under the right buttock, to displace the uterus from the inferior vena cava, facilitating venous return and cardiac output.[90–92] Often, the angle of the tilt is overestimated, potentially reducing the quality of the chest compressions.[92] The uterus may also be manually and gently displaced to the left to remove caval compression.[92] While ventilation-to-compression ratios remain the same for a pregnant woman, chest compression may be complicated by flaring of the ribs, raised diaphragm, obesity and breast hypertrophy.[89]

The superior displacement of stomach contents by the gravid uterus and a relaxed cardiac sphincter contribute to an increased risk of gastric aspiration in the pregnant woman.[89] Because of this increased risk, cricoid pressure should be applied until after the airway is protected by a cuffed tracheal tube.[92] Tracheal intubation should be attended to early on, using a short-handled laryngoscope[93] or with a blade mounted at more than 90 degrees,[92] as airway anatomy is altered with the larynx more anterior and superior, while the pharyngeal mucosa is slightly oedematous and friable.[92] A tracheal tube a size smaller than one normally chosen for a similar-sized non-pregnant woman may be used because of potentially narrower airways secondary to oedema or swelling.[89] Defibrillation energy, drug doses and administration are in accordance with ALS guidelines.[91,92]

If maternal cardiac arrest occurs in the labour ward, operating room or emergency department and BLS and ALS measures are unsuccessful, the uterus should be emptied by surgical (scalpel) intervention within 4–5 minutes.[92] Maternal resuscitation may not be possible until the fetus is removed. Successful resuscitations have occurred after prompt surgical intervention.[92] Refer to Chapter 28 for additional information about critical illness and pregnancy.

Practice tip

Personal protective equipment (PPE) should be used according to the perceived risk in the local setting. Follow local infection prevention and control guidelines and if there is a risk of exposure to blood and body fluids then a mask and protective eyewear should be included.

Electrical injuries

Electrical burn injuries and lightning injuries are similar in that they occur infrequently, commonly cause widespread acute and delayed tissue damage and can arrest the heart and respiratory centre. Burn injuries are discussed in Chapter 24. This section focuses on the cardiac arrest situation. High-voltage electrocution is associated with a high incidence of cardiac arrest and these incidents carry a relatively high incidence of morbidity and mortality.[93] Immediate CPR and ALS in this cohort is often successful given the high incidence of shockable rhythms.[93] The most common cause of death with lightning injury is cardiac arrest due to VF, asystole or respiratory arrest.[94]

Because of the potential for cardiac injuries, all patients should be admitted for cardiac monitoring after they experience a lightning strike.

A lightning strike may result in asystole followed by spontaneous return of circulation. If ventilation is initiated early and severe hypoxia does not ensue, a patient's chance of recovery should be better.[94] Initial response of BLS should always begin with D (danger) – that is, avoidance of injury to the rescuer. Ensure that the environment is safe for rescuers by disconnecting the electrical supply, where possible, without touching the patient. Where high-voltage lines (power lines) are in contact with the person or the vehicle, no attempt should be made to extricate the person from the vehicle until the situation is deemed safe by an authorised electricity supply person. Once the environment is safe, commence BLS resuscitation. The neck and spine should be protected, as there may be trauma.

In lightning victims, emphasis is on the immediate resuscitation of those who appear unresponsive. Respiratory arrest may be prolonged owing to paralysis of the medullary respiratory centre; if not corrected, cardiac arrest secondary to hypoxia ensues. Fixed, dilated pupils should not be used as a poor prognosis of outcome, as victims can benefit from prolonged resuscitation without major sequelae.[94]

Drowning

General issues in managing drowning presentations are discussed in Chapter 23. This section focuses on resuscitation of a cardiorespiratory arrest. Hypoxia and acute lung injury from drowning result in respiratory arrest that, if not corrected, may proceed to a cardiac arrest.[95] A patient's emotional state, associated diseases, previous hypoxia and water temperature all influence this progression.

The primary goal of initial intervention is the relief of hypoxaemia and restoration of cardiovascular stability.[95,96] Resuscitation of drowning victims follows BLS guidelines, with commencement as soon as practical. While rescue breathing may commence while the victim is still in the water, provided it is safe for the rescuer, in-water resuscitation does increase rescue time.[96] As drowning victims may have swallowed considerable amounts of water, vomiting and aspiration of gastric contents can be a major problem during resuscitation. To minimise the risks of inhalation, abdominal compression, the Heimlich manoeuvre and attempts to drain water from the lungs are not recommended. Instead, the victim should be placed on the side for the initial assessment of airway and breathing.[95] Cardiac arrest in these victims is secondary to hypoxia, so compression-only CPR is likely to be less effective compared with CPR with rescue breaths.[96] Once experienced personnel arrive, ALS and administration of oxygen should be initiated. The principles of respiratory support and ventilation are discussed in Chapter 15, and treatment of the sequelae of a drowning victim is discussed in Chapter 23.

Extracorporeal CPR (eCPR)

Extracorporeal CPR (eCPR) is the provision of an artificial circulation via extracorporeal membrane oxygenation (ECMO) (see Chapter 15) in patients who have refractory cardiac arrest where the cause is potentially reversible. This rescue therapy is complex and is not universally available; however, eCPR is increasingly being used in both OHCA and IHCA and is a feasible option; it should be considered in an early-stage CPR and in certain situations where implementation teams are available.[97]

Resuscitation teams

Resuscitation teams should be organised to ensure that the individual skills of each member are used effectively and efficiently.[98] The exact composition of the resuscitation team will vary between organisations, but generally the team should possess the following skills:[96]

- advanced airway management and intubation skills
- intravenous access skills including central venous access
- defibrillation and external pacing abilities
- medication administration skills
- post-resuscitation skills.

As members of a resuscitation team in the hospital generally do not work together but come from all areas of the hospital, the team should have a designated leader. The team leader gives direction and guidance, assigns tasks and makes clinical decisions without directly performing specific procedures.[16,98] The leader should engender the team's trust. Where leaders initiate structure within the arrest team, members not only work together better, they also perform the tasks of resuscitation more quickly and more effectively.[98] The leader nominates the roles of arrest team members. Roles of team members include airway management, chest compression, medication administration (including IV access), documentation of events and care of family members. The team leader should be responsible for post-resuscitation transfer, documentation, communicating with family members and healthcare professionals and debriefing of the team.[98]

The resuscitation scenario is both complex and stressful for all participants. Often, participants express feelings that too many people are involved, with no one person in control. Unfortunately, the concept of the multidisciplinary team, where all members' contributions are equally respected, is generally not evident in the literature.[98] In addition, while nurses already present at a cardiac arrest in the hospital setting may be willing and competent to perform CPR, they may be prevented from doing so because of the arrival of the cardiac arrest team.[98,99]

Post-resuscitation phase

The aim of post-resuscitation care is the maintenance of cerebral and myocardial perfusion and the return of a patient to a state of best possible health. Resuscitation does not cease with the return of spontaneous circulation. ROSC after cardiac arrest does not always equate to a positive outcome for the patient. High mortality rates have been attributed to ischaemic–reperfusion injury to multiple organs that are involved with whole-of-body ischaemia during cardiac arrest.[100] The reperfusion responses that occur following successful resuscitation are termed post-cardiac arrest syndrome. The syndrome comprises hypoxic–ischaemic brain injury, post-cardiac arrest myocardial dysfunction, the systemic ischaemia/reperfusion response and the persistent precipitating pathology.[101] Coordinated care and specific interventions initiated in the post-arrest phase can influence outcomes.[101] Immediate post-resuscitation care, coronary angiography, treatment of seizures, blood pressure control, adequate urine output (1 mL/kg/h), normal or decreasing plasma lactate and temperature control are a few of the targeted objectives of care.[101]

Temperature control in adults after cardiac arrest

During cardiac arrest, prolonged global ischaemia coupled with inadequate reperfusion during the immediate post-resuscitation period can lead to severe cerebral hypoxic injury.[102] Temperature control as part of the post-cardiac arrest management provides significant survival benefit as well as improved cardiac and neurological function.[102] Several cooling techniques are described in Box 25.1.[102–104]

Temperature control cooling consists of the induction, maintenance and rewarming phases.[105] ILCOR recommends that unconscious adult patients with spontaneous circulation after a cardiac arrest should be cooled to maintain a targeted temperature between 32°C and 36°C for 12–24 hours with any initial rhythm.[102] However, recent reviews of the literature challenge the benefits of targeted hypothermia,[103,105] therefore it is recommended to refer to local policy and guidelines for temperature targets. It is important to note that shivering should be avoided, as should fever, for at least 72 hours.[104]

Blood glucose levels should be monitored frequently in the post-cardiac arrest phase and providers should treat

hyperglycaemia (>10 mmol/L) with insulin while avoiding hypoglycaemia.[105]

Near-death experiences

While there is no single definition of this phenomenon, a near-death experience has been described as *'a profound psychological event including transcendental and mystical elements, typically occurring to individuals close to death or in situations of intense physical or emotional danger'*.[106] Contemporary literature is relabelling this phenomenon as *'recalled experience of death'*.[107] Experiences have typically depicted as predominantly pleasurable, and included altered time perception, memories of light (described as brilliant, unusual or mystical), meeting deceased relatives, out-of-body sensations, feelings of the presence of a deity, joy and peace.[106–108] While reported experiences are consistent, many of these studies are heterogeneous with targeted populations, and experiences may vary between cultures.[109] People report the experiences as life transforming, contributing to changes in behaviours, attitudes and beliefs for the individual.[110] After-effects of a near-death experience include absence of fear of death, an appreciation for life, a more spiritual view of life, less regard for material wealth and/or a heightened chemical sensitivity.[110] These changes in attitudes do not diminish with time.[110] The incidence of near-death experiences after cardiac arrest is reported at 10–18%, with a mean age at resuscitation being around 60 years.[110–111] Hence, an awareness of the incidence of near-death experiences and of the cultural differences and needs of the person with a reported near-death experience is essential post-cardiac arrest. Chapter 7 provides more information about family and cultural care.

Special considerations

The chapter to this point primarily has focused on the physiological considerations of resuscitation to achieve the goal of preservation of cellular function. However, this outcome is achieved in only a minority of cases.[22–24] Decision making around the initiation of CPR and resuscitation interventions and the progression and termination of resuscitation involves a multitude of factors.

Family presence during an arrest

The practice of family members witnessing resuscitation has become more evident over time. This shift in practice has been attributed to increasing patient autonomy and the presence of family at a cardiac arrest in popular television shows. This has contributed to public support, and family members requesting – and expecting – to be present.[112] Indeed, professional resuscitation bodies recommend that family should be afforded the opportunity to be present.[112,113] However, translating these recommendations into practice varies among healthcare personnel and across cultures.[114] Cited concerns are that the family may stress or distract the work of the resuscitation team, medicolegal implications and concern about an adverse psychological impact on the parents/family.[115] Contrary to these beliefs,

---

BOX 25.1

Cooling techniques post-cardiac arrest[102–104]

External:

- Cooling blankets/pads, ice packs, wet towels, cooling devices, mattress or cooling helmets

Internal:

- Transnasal evaporating cooling
- IV administration of cold fluids
- IV heat-exchange device
- Peritoneal and pleural lavage (not generally used)

there is limited evidence that family members interfere with the performance of the resuscitation team.[115]

Where families are provided with the option of being present, a staff member should be identified to have sole responsibility of (1) focusing on and supporting the family, (2) collaborating with the resuscitation team and family, considering family context, (3) the needs of the family post-resuscitation and (4) the needs of surrounding patients.[116] In-patients who witness a resuscitation of another patient do find it a stressful experience and may require follow-up care.[117] Chapter 7 is dedicated to family and cultural care, providing additional information about family support.

Ceasing CPR

The decision to cease CPR is often difficult; continuing CPR beyond 30 minutes without ROSC is usually futile unless the arrest was compounded by hypothermia, submersion in cold water, lightning strike, drug overdose or other identified and treatable conditions such as intermittent VF/pVT.[16] Prolonging resuscitation for more than 60 minutes may be beneficial for a severely hypothermic child victim of near-drowning. Pupillary signs should not be used as a predictor of outcome in infants and children, as 11–33% of children with non-reactive pupils have survived long term after CPR.[17] It is important to have eliminated all causes as far as possible.

Termination of resuscitation is a multifactorial process, influenced by provider comfort and experience, patient prognosis and the patient's desires, wishes and values. Organisational issues such as the local culture, protocols, resources and guidelines will all impact on termination decisions. With scientific advances such as ECMO as a bridge for refractory VF and evidence-based protocols becoming more widely implemented, current impressions of termination decisions will change over time.[118,119] It is appropriate to invite suggestions from team members, to ensure that all members are comfortable with a decision to stop the resuscitation attempt.[16] Ultimately, terminating CPR is equivalent to a determination of death, and must be made by a doctor. In some out-of-hospital circumstances it may be the paramedical staff who make this decision to stop CPR, essentially terminating resuscitation.[120] Because of this need, termination of resuscitation guidelines have been developed for use in the out-of-hospital setting. One prospectively validated termination of resuscitation guideline is the 'basic life support termination of resuscitation rule', which may be adopted to guide the termination of pre-hospital CPR in adults.[25] This validated rule is described below.

In the pre-hospital setting, stop CPR if there is:

- no ROSC

and

- no shocks are administered

and

- the arrest is not witnessed by emergency medical-services personnel.

Otherwise, the rule recommends transportation to the hospital, in accordance with routine practice.[121]

Legal and ethical considerations

Burgeoning technology in the 1960s enabled the support of oxygenation and circulation for people whose illnesses would have been lethal just a few years before. Traditionally, enthusiasm for restoration of life led healthcare workers to routinely initiate CPR for all patients who died in hospital.[122] Unfortunately, this led to inappropriate resuscitation attempts and the realisation of the economic, medical and ethical burden to society when survivors had a resultant poor quality of life.[123,124] In the 1970s, growing concern about inappropriate application of CPR and patients' rights led authors to suggest means of forgoing resuscitation and involving patients in decision making. Traditionally, the decision to initiate or withhold CPR was often made by the treating medical team in the absence of the patient or family.[125,126]

Hospital personnel responded by developing procedures for withholding CPR through the documentation of 'do not attempt to resuscitate' orders, doctor's orders for life-sustaining treatment, advance directives or living wills[126,127] (see Chapter 4). For patients or their surrogates to meaningfully participate in decision making about CPR and limitation-of-treatment orders, they must have some understanding of survival rates and adverse effects associated with such interventions.[126] Consequently, much debate has ensued over the right of a person to forgo treatment.

Based on research findings, some propose that, while patients want to be involved in CPR decision making and want some form of advance directive, their knowledge is limited and often derived from television dramas.[126,128] Understanding of quality of life, morbidity and other outcomes after CPR strongly influences their preferences.[129,130] Most patients, and indeed healthcare workers, commonly hold unrealistic expectations of CPR success,[128] and will often reverse their preference for commencing CPR once they are informed of the true probability of survival, functional status and quality of life after resuscitation. When compared with the general public, survivors following cardiac arrest generally assess their quality of life as good 12 months post-arrest.[130] Regardless of this, healthcare workers continue to demonstrate a reluctance to discuss CPR options with patients.[131,132] Despite open discussion, variations in the timing of the orders, poor documentation and communication can result in CPR being inappropriately commenced.[127] Conversely, and contrary to medical and nursing opinions, some people choose CPR even when they have a terminal illness, coma or serious disability.[129]

Standardised orders for limitations on life-sustaining treatments (e.g. do not attempt to resuscitate) should be considered to decrease the incidence of futile resuscitation attempts and to ensure that adult patients' wishes are honoured. These orders should be specific, detailed, transferable across healthcare settings and easily understood.

Processes, protocols and systems should be developed that fit within local cultural norms and legal limitations to allow providers to honour patients' wishes about resuscitation efforts.[25] With the exception of a zero-survival rate, there remains no formal consensus on 'do not attempt to resuscitate' decision-making practices or the termination of resuscitation. While researchers have attempted to develop prognostic indicators for cardiac arrest outcome, moralists would argue that the use of such prognostic tools alone reflects utilitarianism, and that they should never be used in isolation of the input of the patient and healthcare team.[133]

Summary

Outcomes for patients after in-hospital SCA remain poor. Successful management of a patient following SCA depends largely on the timely implementation of the chain of survival. Nurses should understand the role of the chain of survival in the resuscitation of the person following cardiac arrest. The chain emphasises the importance of early recognition and intervention, continuous uninterrupted compressions and the early use of the defibrillator as a BLS skill. Understanding when to start, when to continue and when to stop are equally important and are influenced by multiple factors. Including the patient's wishes in decision making is of utmost importance to ensure that futile resuscitation attempts are avoided. Despite the plethora of research on the topic of resuscitation, there is much we still need to investigate and learn from.

Case study

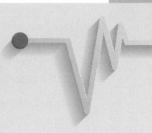

On a Tuesday evening you arrived for your night shift and are caring for Alice, a 74-year-old lady with squamous cell carcinoma to the base of the tongue requiring a partial glossectomy and floor-of-mouth reconstruction with a free flap and formation of tracheostomy, the flap taken from her R forearm with dressing to remain intact for 5 days. A size 7.5 Portex tracheostomy tube was in situ, the cuff to remain inflated overnight with pressure support ventilation, PS 10, PEEP 7, FiO_2 40%. Alice had been weaned from ventilator support during the day and is now tolerating high-flow therapy with the cuff on the tracheostomy tube deflated by the head and neck team. Alice had been sitting out in the chair during the day. Her respiratory rate (RR) was 18, SpO_2 96% on 38% FiO_2, heart rate (HR) was 90. Her pain score was 4–5/10. Alice was transferred back to bed with two nurses assisting. Alice did not complain of any pain and her vital signs have remained stable.

An hour into the shift Alice started to pluck at the linen on her bed and her HR started to increase. Alice tugged on her tracheostomy tube and coughed; on suctioning there was no evidence of sputum plugging, nor any sputum to be suctioned and the end-tidal CO_2 trace reading was 36 and RR was 24, with SpO_2 93% with an increase in FiO_2 to 45%. It was thought that Alice may have postoperative atelectasis and delirium. Alice had another large cough and pointed to her neck. A senior nurse was immediately called to the bed area to assist with suctioning and the senior doctor was contacted to attend urgently.

Alice was removed from the ventilator tubing and a bag resuscitator was applied directly to her tracheostomy tube with 100% FiO_2 delivered. Alice was difficult to ventilate via the tracheostomy tube and became hypoxic rapidly, gasping for breath. There was a decision made to put Alice back onto the ventilator. Alice went into cardiac arrest with signs of subcutaneous emphysema (swelling) over her trachea and face. With chest compressions continuing, Alice's tracheostomy tube was removed and an endotracheal tube was inserted orally. Alice required three cycles of CPR with no shocks required, PEA and adrenaline 1 mg administered. Pleural decompression was performed bilaterally into the second intercostal space, mid-clavicle and ROSC was achieved. Bilateral intercostal catheters were inserted and Alice stabilised. The ENT team arrived and re-inserted the tracheostomy tube, and noted that a false lumen was present. The tracheostomy tube had migrated into a false passage causing subcutaneous emphysema to develop.

CASE STUDY QUESTIONS

1 What was the probable cause of the cardiac arrest when considering the 4Hs and Ts (hypoxia; hypovolaemia; hyper/hypokalaemia/metabolic disorders; hypothermia/hyperthermia tension pneumothorax; tamponade; toxins; thrombosis (pulmonary/coronary))?
2 Was there evidence of 1 H and 1 T?
3 Why didn't 100% oxygen delivery increase oxygen saturations?
4 Why did pleural decompression immediately cause ROSC?
5 What are the first steps in identifying a tracheostomy emergency?
6 Was there another way to deliver oxygen to this patient?
7 Why is it important to have the airway algorithm appropriate to the patient at the bedside?

RESEARCH VIGNETTE

Hsu CH, Considine J, Pawar RD, et al. Cardiopulmonary resuscitation and defibrillation for cardiac arrest when patients are in the prone position: a systematic review. Resusc Plus 2021;8:100186.[136]

Abstract

Aim: To perform a systematic review of CPR and/or defibrillation in the prone position compared with turning the patient supine prior to starting CPR and/or defibrillation.

Methods: The search included PubMed, Embase, Web of Science, Cochrane, CINAHL Plus, and medRxiv on 9 December 2020. The population included adults and children in any setting with cardiac arrest while in the prone position. The outcomes included arterial blood pressure and end-tidal capnography during CPR, time to start CPR and defibrillation, return of spontaneous circulation, survival and survival with favourable neurological outcome to discharge, 30 days or longer. ROBINS-I was performed to assess risk of bias for observational studies.

Results: The systematic review identified 29 case reports (32 individual cases), two prospective observational studies and two simulation studies. The observational studies enrolled 17 patients who were declared dead in the supine position and reported higher mean systolic blood pressure from CPR in prone position (72 mmHg vs 48 mmHg, $P < 0.005$; 79 ± 20 mmHg vs 55 ± 20 mmHg, $P = 0.028$). One simulation study reported a faster time to defibrillation in the prone position. Return of spontaneous circulation and survival to discharge or 30 days were reported in adult and paediatric case reports. Critical risk of bias limited our ability to perform pooled analyses.

Conclusions: We identified a limited number of observational studies and case reports comparing prone versus supine CPR and/or defibrillation. Prone CPR may be a reasonable option if immediate supination is difficult or poses unacceptable risks to the patient.

Critique

Background: The benefits of prone positioning ventilation to improve oxygenation in patients with severe respiratory failure and its subsequent increased use in COVID-19 pandemic are well documented.[134–137] In the event of cardiac arrest, the standard recommendation is to deliver CPR and/or defibrillation in the supine position.[138] However, supinating a ventilated, critically ill patient in a hurry comes with the potential risk of tube displacement and/or delays commencing CPR.[135] These concerns, coupled with low-level evidence suggesting that prone CPR may be feasible if an advanced airway is already in place, saw some organisations seeking a review of treatment recommendations.

The International Liaison Committee on Resuscitation, when making treatment recommendations, undertakes rigorous systemic reviews (SRs) of existing evidence to inform all new Consensus on Science and Treatment Recommendations (CoSTR).[139] This SR was aimed at reviewing evidence to compare starting CPR and/or defibrillation in the prone position versus turning the patient supine.

SRs and meta-analyses are considered essential tools when summarising evidence both reliably and accurately. The SR presented provided sufficient transparency and key information to allow the readers to critically judge the available evidence.[140] The review protocol was registered with the Prospective Register of Systematic Reviews (PROSPERO #CRD42021230691) and was available in the supplemental material. The study reported was framed using the PICOST format and the review process followed the Preferred Reporting Items for Systemic Reviews and Meta-Analyses (PRISMA) guidelines.[140]

A variety of relevant databases were used to conduct the review, including PubMed, CINAHL plus, Web of Science, Embase and Cochrane. Due to the nature of the treatment intervention being investigated and the paucity of evidence case series, case reports and small non-RCTs were included. Using a predefined data extraction tool, two reviewers independently screened and extracted data. Where weak or moderate agreement[141] occurred between reviewers ($\kappa < 0.60$) a third reviewer was engaged. Next, four investigators assessed the extracted studies for methodological quality and risk of bias. Case reports and observational studies were assessed using respectively the modified Murad and colleagues' tool or the ROBINS-I tool.[142]

Of 945 studies included in the first level of screening, following removal of 862 duplicates ($\kappa = 0.66$) 83 full studies were screened. Of the 32 papers included in the final review (κ for full text papers = 0.94), 29 were case reports (describing 32 individual cases), 2 were prospective non-randomised studies and 1 was a simulation study. Because of the critical risk of bias in these studies, the investigators opted to not undertake a meta-analysis.

The majority of patients from the case reports ($n = 31$: 19 adult and 12 paediatric) were in the prone position in the operating room and one was in the prone position in the ICU. In 22 of the cases (12 adults and 11 children), CPR was commenced in the prone position. Two observational studies involving 17 patients, who were reported as deceased following conventional CPR, found a significantly higher mean systolic blood pressure with CPR in the prone position compared with CPR in the supine position (72 mmHg vs 48 mmHg, $P < 0.005$).[143,144] The authors do caution that this finding has very low certainty of evidence.

Return of spontaneous circulation was reported in 22/23 adult cases and 4/9 paediatric cases. There were no explicitly reported favourable neurological outcomes (in adult or paediatric cases) for either survival to hospital discharge or outcome at 30 days or longer. Implicit favourable neurological outcomes were reported in 15 cases (eight adult and seven paediatric cases). There was explicit reporting of survival to discharge in 13 adult and 11 paediatric cases.

While commencing CPR/defibrillation in the supine position remains gold standard and is known to be effective, the increasing number of critically ill patients requiring prone positioning has warranted the investigation of best evidence to inform treatment recommendations around initiating CPR/defibrillation when the patient is in the prone position. This SR found there is limited high-level evidence to determine whether the delivery of chest compressions/ defibrillation in the prone position or immediate supination is more beneficial. It did however find low-level evidence suggesting prone compressions potentially produce higher arterial blood pressure and adequate cardiac output. However, this evidence is at extremely high risk of bias.

The final treatment recommendation

Commencing CPR in the prone position may be a reasonable approach if the patient has an advanced airway in place and immediate supination is not feasible (e.g. because of patient size, intravenous lines) or poses a significant patient risk (good practice statement).

Defibrillating a patient in a prone position who is in a shockable rhythm is reasonable (good practice statement).

Immediate supination is recommended for patients who don't have an advanced airway in situ (strong recommendation, very low certainty of evidence) or where there is a primary airway problem (i.e. dislodged ETT). Invasive monitoring and $ETCO_2$ will assist the clinician to determine the efficacy of compressions in the prone position and assist decision making about when to perform supination (good practice statement).

Learning activities

1 What is the percentage range of cardiac output when providing effective external cardiac compression?
2 What are the initial three priorities in sudden cardiac arrest?
3 Identify the stage in the ALS flow chart when adrenaline is administered.
4 How does the medical emergency team system reduce the incidence of cardiopulmonary arrests?
5 What is the dose of adrenaline for adults if given via the intraosseous route?
6 What is the rationale for targeted temperature management in adults after cardiac arrest?

Online resources

American Heart Association (AHA), https://www.heart.org

Australian Resuscitation Council (ARC), https://resus.org.au

Division of Pediatric Emergency Medicine (CPEM), https://med.nyu.edu/departments-institutes/emergency-medicine/divisions/pediatric-emergency-medicine

European Resuscitation Council (ERC), https://www.erc.edu

International Liaison Committee on Resuscitation (ILCOR), https://ilcor.org

New Zealand Resuscitation Council (NZRC), https://www.resus.org.nz

Further reading

Mentzelopoulos SD, Couper K, Van de Voorde P, et al. European Resuscitation Council Guidelines 2021: ethics of resuscitation and end of life decisions. Resuscitation 2021;161:408–32.

Mølgaard RR, Jørgensen L, Christensen EF, et al. Ambivalence in nurses' use of the early warning score: a focussed ethnography in a hospital setting. J Adv Nurs 2022;78(5):1461–72.

Nolan JP, Ornato JP, Parr MJ, et al. Resuscitation highlights in 2020. Resuscitation 2021;162:1–10.

Schwalbach KT, Yong SS, Wade RC, et al. Impact of intraosseous versus intravenous resuscitation during in-hospital cardiac arrest: a retrospective study. Resuscitation 2021;166:7–13.

References

1. Australian Resuscitation Council (ARC). The ARC guidelines. Melbourne, VIC: ARC; 2022. Available from: https://resus.org.au/the-arc-guidelines/. [Accessed 15 February 2023].

2. Allencherril J, Lee PYK, Khan K, et al. Etiologies of in-hospital cardiac arrest: a systematic review and meta-analysis. Resuscitation 2022; 175:88–95.

3. Al-Khatib SM, Stevenson WG, Ackerman MJ, et al. 2017 AHA/ACC/HRS guideline for management of patients with ventricular arrhythmias and the prevention of sudden cardiac death: a report of the American College of Cardiology/American Heart Association Task Force on Clinical Practice Guidelines and the Heart Rhythm Society. J Am Coll Cardiol 2018;72(14):e91–220.

4. Virani SS, Alonso A, Benjamin EJ, et al. on behalf of the American Heart Association Council on Epidemiology and Prevention Statistics Committee and Stroke Statistics Subcommittee. Heart disease and stroke statistics – 2020 update: a report from the American Heart Association. Circulation 2020;141:e139–596.

5. Andrew E, Nehme Z, Wolfe R, et al. Long-term survival following out-of-hospital cardiac arrest. Heart 2017;103(14):1104–10.

6. Holmgren C, Bergfeldt L, Edvardsson N, et al. Analysis of initial rhythm, witnessed status and delay to treatment among survivors of out-of-hospital cardiac arrest in Sweden. Heart 2010;96:1826–30.

7. Wah W, Wai KL, Pek PP, et al. Conversion to shockable rhythms during resuscitation and survival for out-of hospital cardiac arrest. Am J Emerg Med 2017;35(2):206–13.

8. Berdowski J, Berg RA, Tijssen JGP, et al. Global incidences of out-of-hospital cardiac arrest and survival rates: systematic review of 67 prospective studies. Resuscitation 2010;81(11):1479–87.

9. Herlitz J, Engdahl J, Svensson L, et al. Can we define patients with no chance of survival after out-of-hospital cardiac arrest? Heart 2004;90(10):1114–18.

10. Australian Institute of Health and Welfare (AIHW). Australia's health 2022. Australia's health series no. 12. Canberra, ACT: AIHW; 2022. Available from: https://www.aihw.gov.au/reports/australias-health/australias-health-2022-data-insights/about [Accessed 15 February 2023].

11. Müller D, Agrawal R, Arntz H-R. How sudden is sudden cardiac death? Circulation 2006;114(11):1146–50.

12. Soar J, Bottiger BW, Carli P, et al. European resuscitation council guidelines 2021: Adult advanced life support. Resuscitation 2021;161:115–51.

13. Herlitz J, Svensson L, Engdahl J, et al. Characteristics of cardiac arrest and resuscitation by age group: an analysis from the Swedish Cardiac Arrest Registry. Am J Emerg Med 2007;25(9):1025–31.

14. Manley BJ, Owen LS, Hooper SB, et al. Towards evidence-based resuscitation of the newborn infant. Lancet 2017;389(10079):1639–48.

15. Meert K, Telford R, Holubkov R, et al. Paediatric in-hospital cardiac arrest: factors associated with survival and neurobehavioural outcome one year later. Resuscitation 2018;124:96–105.

16. Van de Voorde P, Turner NM, Djakow J, et al. European resuscitation council guidelines. 2021: paediatric life support. Resuscitation 2021;161:327–87.

17. Lurie K, Nemergut E, Yannopoulos D, et al. The physiology of cardiopulmonary resuscitation. Anesth Analg 2016;122(3):767–83.

18. Olasveengen TM, de Caen AR, Mancini ME, et al. International consensus on cardiopulmonary resuscitation and emergency cardiovascular care science with treatment recommendations summary. Resuscitation 2017;121:201–14.

19. Perkins GD, Neumar R, Monsieurs KG, et al. The International Liaison Committee on Resuscitation – review of the last 25 years and vision for the future. Resuscitation 2017;121:104–16.

20. Shuvy M, Morrison LJ, Koh M, et al. Long-term clinical outcomes and predictors for survivors of out-of-hospital cardiac arrest. Resuscitation 2017;112:59–64.

21. Perkins GD, Jacobs IG, Nadkarni VM, et al. Cardiac arrest and cardiopulmonary resuscitation outcome reports: update of the Utstein Resuscitation Registry Templates for Out-of-hospital Cardiac Arrest: a statement for healthcare professionals from a task force of the International Liaison Committee on Resuscitation (American Heart Association, European Resuscitation Council, Australian and New Zealand Council on Resuscitation, Heart and Stroke Foundation of Canada, InterAmerican Heart Foundation, Resuscitation Council of Southern Africa, Resuscitation Council of Asia); and the American Heart Association Emergency Cardiovascular Care Committee and the Council on Cardiopulmonary, Critical Care, Perioperative and Resuscitation. Resuscitation 2015;96:328–40.

22. Lauridsen KG, Djärv T, Breckwoldt J, et al. Pre-arrest prediction of survival following in-hospital cardiac arrest: a systematic review of diagnostic test accuracy studies. Resuscitation 2022;179:141–51.

23. Andersen LW, Holmberg MJ, Berg KM, et al. In-hospital cardiac arrest: a review. JAMA 2019; 321(12):1200–10.

24. Veerappa S, Orosz J, Bailey M, et al. Epidemiology of in-hospital cardiac arrest patients admitted to the intensive care unit in Australia: a retrospective observational study. Intern Med 2023:1–8. doi: 10.1111/imj.16007. Online ahead of print.

25. Soar J, Mancini M, Bhanji F, et al. On behalf of the education, implementation, and teams chapter collaborators. Part 12: education, implementation, and teams: 2010 International Consensus on Cardiopulmonary Resuscitation and Emergency Cardiovascular Care Science with Treatment Recommendations. Resuscitation 2010;81:e288–330.

26. Deakin CD. The chain of survival: not all links are equal. Resuscitation 2018;126:80–2.

27. Merchant RM, Topjian AA, Panchal AR, et al. Adult basic and advanced life support, pediatric basic and advanced life support, neonatal life support, resuscitation education science, and systems of care writing groups. Part 1: executive summary: 2020 American Heart Association guidelines for cardiopulmonary resuscitation and emergency cardiovascular care. Circulation 2020;142(16 Suppl. 2):S337–57.

28. McGaughey J, O'Halloran P, Porter S, et al. Early warning systems and rapid response to the deteriorating patient in hospital: a systematic realist review. J Adv Nurs 2017;73(12):2877–91.

29. Smith GB. In-hospital cardiac arrest: is it time for an in-hospital 'chain of prevention'? Resuscitation 2010;81(9):1209–11.

30. Lafonte M, Cai J, Lissauer ME. Failure to rescue in the surgical patient: a review. Curr Opin Crit Care 2019;25(6):706–11.

31. Kause J, Smith G, Prytherch D, et al. A comparison of antecedents to cardiac arrests, deaths and emergency intensive care admissions in Australia and New Zealand, and the United Kingdom – the ACADEMIA study. Resuscitation 2004;62(3):275–82.

32. Sprogis S, Currey J, Considine J, et al. Physiological antecedents and ward clinician responses before medical emergency team activation. Crit Care Resusc 2017;19(1):50–6.

33. Le Lagadec D, Dwyer T. Scoping review: the use of early warning systems for the identification of in-hospital patient at risk of deterioration. Aust Crit Care 2017;30(4):211–18.

34. Campbell V, Conway R, Carey K, et al. Predicting clinical deterioration with Q-ADDS compared to NEWS, Between the Flags, and eCART track and trigger tools. Resuscitation 2020;153:28–34.

35. Le Lagadec MD, Dwyer T, Browne M. Patient deterioration in Australian regional and rural hospitals: is the Queensland adult deterioration detection system the criterion standard? J Patient Saf 2021;17(8):e1879–83.

36. Australian Resuscitation Council (ARC). ARC guideline 11.1 – introduction to and principles of in-hospital resuscitation. Melbourne, VIC: ARC; 2019. Available from: https://resus.org.au/the-arc-guidelines/. [Accessed 15 February 2023].

37. Smith GB, Prytherch DR, Meredith P, et al. The ability of the National Early Warning Score (NEWS) to discriminate patients at risk of early cardiac arrest, unanticipated intensive care unit admission, and death. Resuscitation 2013;84(4):465–70.

38. Guinane J, Hutchinson AM, Bucknall T. Patient perceptions of deterioration and patient and family activated escalation systems – a qualitative study. J Clin Nurs 2018;27(7–8):1621–31.

39. Australian Resuscitation Council (ARC). ANZCOR guideline 4 – airway. Melbourne, VIC: ARC; 2021. Available from: https://resus.org.au/the-arc-guidelines/. [Accessed 15 February 2023].

40. Australian Resuscitation Council (ARC). ANZCOR guideline 12.2 – paediatric advanced life support (PALS). Melbourne, VIC: ARC; 2021. Available from: https://resus.org.au/the-arc-guidelines/. [Accessed 15 February 2023].

41. Wyckoff MH, Aziz K, Escobedo MB, et al. Part 13: neonatal resuscitation. Circulation 2015;132(18 Suppl. 2):S543–60.

42. Berg R, Saunders A, Kern K, et al. Adverse hemodynamic effects of interrupting chest compressions for rescue breathing during cardiopulmonary resuscitation for ventricular defibrillation cardiac arrest. Circulation 2001;104:2465–70.

43. Nolan J, Ornato J, Parr M, et al. Resuscitation highlights in 2016. Resuscitation 2017;114:A1–7.

44. Dwyer T. Psychological factors inhibit family members' confidence to initiate CPR. Prehosp Emerg Care 2008;12(2):157–61.

45. Assar D, Chamberlain D, Colquhoun M, et al. Randomised controlled trial of staged teaching for basic life support: skill acquisition at bronze stage. Resuscitation 2000;45:7–15.

46. Olasveengen TM, Semeraro F, Ristagno G, et al. European resuscitation council guidelines 2021: basic life support. Resuscitation 2021;161:98–114.

47. Bobrow B, Spaite D, Berg R, et al. Chest compression-only CPR by lay rescuers and survival from out-of-hospital cardiac arrest. JAMA 2010;304(3):1447–54.

48. Crickmer M, Drennan IR, Turner L, et al. The association between end-tidal CO_2 and return of spontaneous circulation after out-of-hospital cardiac arrest with pulseless electrical activity. Resuscitation 2021;167:76–81.

49. Abella BS. High-quality cardiopulmonary resuscitation: current and future directions. Curr Opin Crit Care 2016;22(3):218–24.

50. Paiva EF, Paxton JH, O'Neil BJ. The use of end-tidal carbon dioxide ($ETCO_2$) measurement to guide management of cardiac arrest: a systematic review. Resuscitation 2018;123:1–7.

51. Paxton JH, O'Neil BJ. CPR capnography: it's not where you've been, but where you're going. Resuscitation 2022;181:121–2.

52. Delguercio L, Feins N, Cohn J, et al. Comparison of blood flow during external and internal cardiac massage in man. Circulation 1965; 31(Suppl. 1):171–80.

53. Chiang CY, Lim KC, Lai PC, et al. Comparison between prehospital mechanical cardiopulmonary resuscitation (CPR) devices and manual CPR for out-of-hospital cardiac arrest: a systematic review, meta-analysis, and trial sequential analysis. J Clin Med 2022;11(5):1448.

54. Kahn PA, Dhruva SS, Rhee TG, et al. Use of mechanical cardiopulmonary resuscitation devices for out-of-hospital cardiac arrest, 2010–2016. JAMA Network Open 2019;2(10):e1913298.

55. Karasek J, Blankova A, Doubková A, et al. The comparison of cardiopulmonary resuscitation-related trauma: mechanical versus manual chest compressions. Forensic Sci Int 2021;323:110812.

56. Australian Resuscitation Council (ARC). ANZCOR guideline 11.6 – equipment and techniques in adult advanced life support. Melbourne, VIC: ARC; 2016. Available from: https://resus.org.au/the-arc-guidelines/. [Accessed 15 February 2023].

57. Australian Resuscitation Council (ARC). ANZCOR guideline 7 – automated external defibrillation in basic life support. Melbourne, VIC: ARC; 2021. Available from: https://resus.org.au/the-arc-guidelines/. [Accessed 15 February 2023].

58. Nehme Z, Andrew E, Bernard SA, et al. Treatment of monitored out-of-hospital ventricular fibrillation and pulseless ventricular tachycardia utilising the precordial thump. Resuscitation 2013;84(12):1691–6.

59. Australian Resuscitation Council (ARC). ANZCOR guideline 11.3 – precordial thump and fist pacing. Melbourne, VIC: ARC; 2011. Available from: https://resus.org.au/the-arc-guidelines/. [Accessed 15 February 2023].

60. Australian Resuscitation Council (ARC). ANZCOR guideline 11.4 – electrical therapy for adult advanced life support. Melbourne, VIC: ARC; 2016. Available from: https://resus.org.au/the-arc-guidelines/. [Accessed 15 February 2023].

61. Tomkins WGO, Swain AH, Bailey M, et al. Beyond the pre-shock pause: the effect of prehospital defibrillation mode on CPR interruptions and return of spontaneous circulation. Resuscitation 2013;84(5):575–9.

62. Brooks SC, Clegg GR, Bray J, et al. Optimizing outcomes after out-of-hospital cardiac arrest with innovative approaches to public-access defibrillation: a scientific statement from the International Liaison Committee on Resuscitation. Circulation 2022;145(13):e776–801.

63. Morrison LJ, Henry RM, Ku V, et al. Single-shock defibrillation success in adult cardiac arrest: a systematic review. Resuscitation 2013;84(11):1480–6.

64. Wang C-H, Huang C-H, Chang W-T, et al. Biphasic versus monophasic defibrillation in out-of-hospital cardiac arrest: a systematic review and meta-analysis. Am J Emerg Med 2013;31(10):1472–8.

65. Ali U, Bingham R. Current recommendations for paediatric resuscitation. BJA Educ 2018;18(4):116–21.

66. Chan PS, Krumholz HM, Spertus JA, et al. Automated external defibrillators and survival after in-hospital cardiac arrest. JAMA 2010; 304(19):2129–36.

67. Christenson J, Andrusiek D, Everson-Stewart S, et al. Chest compression fraction determines survival in patients with out-of-hospital ventricular fibrillation. Circulation 2009;120(13):1241–7.

68. Ristagno G, Li Y, Gullo A, et al. Amplitude spectrum area as a predictor of successful defibrillation. In: Gullo A, editor. Anaesthesia and pharmacology of intensive care emergency medicine A.P.I.C.E., Proceedings of the 23rd Annual Meeting – International Symposium on Critical Care Medicine. Milan: Springer; 2011, p. 141–60.

69. Monteleone PP, Borek HA, Althoff SO. Electrical therapies in cardiac arrest. Emerg Med Clin North Am 2012;30(1):51–63.

70. Morley P. Cardiopulmonary resuscitation. In: Harley I, Hore P, editors. Anaesthesia: an introduction. 5th ed. East Hawthorn, VIC: IP Communications; 2012; p. 174–89.

71. Mohamed BA. Airway management during cardiopulmonary resuscitation. Curr Anesthesiol Rep 2022;12:363–72.

72. Trevisanuto D, Cavallin F, Nguyen LN, et al. Supreme laryngeal mask airway versus face mask during neonatal resuscitation: a randomized controlled trial. J Pediatr 2015;167(2):286–91.e1.

73. Yamaga S, Une K, Kyo M, et al. Gas insufflation in the stomach during cardiopulmonary resuscitation using laryngeal tube ventilation in comparison with bag-valve-mask ventilation. Circulation 2012;126(Suppl. 21):A295.

74. Soar J. Which airway for cardiac arrest? Do supraglottic airways devices have a role? Resuscitation 2013;84(9):1163–4.

75. Norvik A, Unneland E, Bergum D, et al. Pulseless electrical activity in in-hospital cardiac arrest – a crossroad for decisions. Resuscitation 2022;176:117–24.

76. Frazier ME, Brown SR, O'Halloran A, et al. Risk factors and outcomes for recurrent paediatric in-hospital cardiac arrest: retrospective multicenter cohort study. Resuscitation 2021;169:60–6.

77. Ambinder DI, Patil KD, Kadioglu H, et al. Pulseless electrical activity as the initial cardiac arrest rhythm: importance of preexisting left ventricular function. J Am Heart Assoc 2021;10(13):e018671.

78. Australian Resuscitation Council (ARC). ANZCOR Guideline 11.5 – medications in adult cardiac arrest. Melbourne, VIC: ARC; 2016. Available from: https://resus.org.au/the-arc-guidelines/. [Accessed 15 February 2023].

79. Mentzelopoulos SD, Zakynthinos SG, Siempos I, et al. Vasopressin for cardiac arrest: meta-analysis of randomized controlled trials. Resuscitation 2012;83(1):32–9.

80. Perkins GD, Ji C, Deakin CD, et al. A randomized trial of epinephrine in out-of-hospital cardiac arrest. N Engl J Med 2018;1–11.

81. Fernando SM, Mathew R, Sadeghirad B, et al. Epinephrine in out-of-hospital cardiac arrest – a network meta-analysis and subgroup analyses of shockable and non-shockable rhythms. Chest 2023;S0012-3692(23)00165-4. doi: 10.1016/j.chest.2023.01.033. Online ahead of print.

82. Berg KM, Soar J, Andersen LW, et al. Adult advanced life support: 2020 International consensus on cardiopulmonary resuscitation and emergency cardiovascular care science with treatment recommendations. Circulation 2020;142(16 Suppl. 1):S92–139.

83. Jacobs IG, Finn JC, Jelinek GA, et al. Effect of adrenaline on survival in out-of-hospital cardiac arrest: a randomised double-blind placebo-controlled trial. Resuscitation 2011;82(9):1138–43.

84. Panchal AR, Bartos JA, Cabañas JG, et al. Part 3: adult basic and advanced life support: 2020 American Heart Association guidelines for cardiopulmonary resuscitation and emergency cardiovascular care. Circulation 2020;142(16 Suppl. 2):S366–468.

85. Pitcher D, Nolan J. Peri-arrest arrhythmias. London: Resuscitation Council UK; 2015. Available from: https://www.resus.org.uk/resuscitation-guidelines/peri-arrest-arrhythmias/. [Accessed 15 February 2023].

86. Australian Resuscitation Council (ARC). ANZCOR guideline 11.2 – protocols for adult advanced life support. Melbourne, VIC: ARC; 2018. Available from: https://resus.org.au/the-arc-guidelines/. [Accessed 15 February 2023].

87. Ebert L, Massey D, Flenady T, et al. Midwives' recognition and response to maternal deterioration: a national cross-sectional study. Birth 2022;1:1–11. doi: 10.1111/birt.12665. Online ahead of print.

88. Enomoto N, Yamashita T, Furuta M, et al. Effect of maternal positioning during cardiopulmonary resuscitation: a systematic review and meta-analyses. BMC Pregnancy Childbirth 2022;22(1)159.

89. Stokes N, Kikucki J. Management of cardiac arrest in the pregnant patient. Curr Treat Options Cardiovasc Med 2018;20(7):57.

90. Lipman S, Cohen S, Einav S, et al. The Society for Obstetric Anesthesia and Perinatology consensus statement on the management of cardiac arrest in pregnancy. Anesth Analg 2014;118(5):1003–16.

91. Australian Resuscitation Council (ARC). ANZCOR guideline 11.10 – resuscitation in special circumstances. Melbourne, VIC: ARC; 2011. Available from: https://resus.org.au/the-arc-guidelines/. [Accessed 15 February 2023].

92. Lavonas EJ, Drennan IR, Gabrielli A, et al. Part 10: special circumstances of resuscitation. Circulation 2015;132(18 Suppl. 2):S501–18.

93. Keyloun JW, Travis TE, Johnson LS, et al. An unusual presentation of inhalation injury in a patient with high voltage electrical injury: a case report. Int J Surg Case Rep 2020;77:357–61.

94. Rotariu EL, Manole MD. Cardiac arrest secondary to lightning strike: case report and review of the literature. Pediatr Emerg Care 2020;36(1):e18–20.

95. Szpilman D, Morgan PJ. Management for the drowning patient. Chest 2021;159(4):1473–83.

96. Bierens J, Abelairas-Gomez C, Furelos RB, et al. Resuscitation and emergency care in drowning: a scoping review. Resuscitation 2021; 162:205–17.

97. Koen TJ, Nathana®l T, Philippe D. A systematic review of current ECPR protocols. A step towards standardisation. Resusc Plus 2020;3:100018.

98. Hunziker S, Johansson AC, Tschan F, et al. Teamwork and leadership in cardiopulmonary resuscitation. J Am Coll Cardiol 2011;57(24):2381–8.

99. Mølgaard RR, Jørgensen L, Christensen EF, et al. Ambivalence in nurses' use of the early warning score: a focussed ethnography in a hospital setting. J Adv Nurs 2021;78(5):14611472.

100. Dalessio L. Post-cardiac arrest syndrome. AACN Adv Crit Care 2020;31(4):383–93.

101. Nolan JP, Sandroni C, Böttiger BW, et al. European resuscitation council and European society of intensive care medicine guidelines 2021: post-resuscitation care. Resuscitation 2021;161:220–69.

102. Australian Resuscitation Council (ARC). ANZCOR Guideline 11.8 – targeted temperature management (TTM) after cardiac arrest. Melbourne, VIC: ARC; 2016. Available from: https://resus.org.au/the-arc-guidelines/. [Accessed 15 February 2023].

103. Shrestha DB, Sedhai YR, Budhathoki P, et al. Hypothermia versus normothermia after out-of-hospital cardiac arrest: a systematic review and meta-analysis of randomized controlled trials. Ann Med Surg 2022;74:103327.

104. Bray JE, Cartledge S, Finn J, et al. The current temperature: a survey of post-resuscitation care across Australian and New Zealand intensive care units. Resusc Plus 2020;1–2:100002.

105. Australian Resuscitation Council (ARC). ANZCOR Guideline 11.7 – post-resuscitation therapy in adult advanced life support. Melbourne, VIC: ARC; 2022. Available from: https://resus.org.au/the-arc-guidelines/. [Accessed 15 February 2023].

106. Quinn RJ. Sentiment analysis of web scraped near-death experience narratives. J Near-Death Stud 2020;38(3):157–79.

107. Parnia S, Post SG, Lee MT, et al. Guidelines and standards for the study of death and recalled experiences of death – a multidisciplinary consensus statement and proposed future directions. Ann N Y Acad Sci 2022;1511(1):5–21.

108. Cassol H, Pétré B, Degrange S, et al. Qualitative thematic analysis of the phenomenology of near-death experiences. PLoS One 2018; 13(2):e0193001.

109. Pistoia F, Mattiacci G, Sarà M, et al. Development of the Italian version of the Near-Death Experience Scale. Front Hum Neurosci 2018;12:45.

110. Greyson B. Persistence of attitude changes after near-death experiences: do they fade over time? J Nerv Ment Dis 2022;210(9):692–6.

111. Van Lommel P, Van Wees R, Meyers V, et al. Near-death experience in survivors of cardiac arrest: a prospective study in the Netherlands. Lancet 2001;358(9298):2039–45. doi: 10.1016/S0140-6736(01)07100-8.

112. Dwyer TA. Predictors of public support for family presence during cardiopulmonary resuscitation: a population-based study. Int J Nurs Stud 2015;52:1064–70.

113. McLean J, Gill FJ, Shields L. Family presence during resuscitation in a paediatric hospital: health professionals' confidence and perceptions. J Clin Nurs 2016;25(7–8):1045–52.

114. Lederman Z, Baird G, Dong C, et al. Attitudes of Singapore emergency department staff towards family presence during cardiopulmonary resuscitation. Clin Ethics 2017;12(3):124–34.

115. Dainty KN, Atkins DL, Breckwoldt J, et al. Family presence during resuscitation in paediatric and neonatal cardiac arrest: a systematic review. Resuscitation 2021;162:20–34.

116. Douma MJ, Graham TA, Ali S, et al. What are the care needs of families experiencing cardiac arrest?: a survivor and family led scoping review. Resuscitation 2021;168:119–41.

117. Fiori M, Latour JM, Los F. 'Am I also going to die, doctor?' A systematic review of the impact of in-hospital patients witnessing a resuscitation of another patient. Eur J Cardiovasc Nurs 2017;16(7):585–94.

118. Stub D, Bernard S, Pellegrino V, et al. Issues in establishing the refractory out-of-hospital cardiac arrest treated with mechanical CPR, hypothermia, ECMO and early reperfusion (CHEER) study. Heart Lung Circ 2012;21(1):S163.

119. Richardson AS, Tonna JE, Nanjayya V, et al. Extracorporeal cardiopulmonary resuscitation in adults. Interim guideline consensus statement from the extracorporeal life support organization. ASAIO J 2021;67(3):221–8.

120. Adams BD, Benger J. Should we take patients to hospital in cardiac arrest? BMJ 2014;349:g5659.

121. Morrison LJ, Eby D, Veigas PV, et al. Implementation trial of the basic life support termination of resuscitation rule: reducing the transport of futile out-of-hospital cardiac arrests. Resuscitation 2014;85(4):486–91.

122. Lynn J, Gregory CO. Regulating hearts and minds: the mismatch of law, custom and resuscitation decisions. J Am Geriatr Soc 2003;51(10):1502–3.

123. Bossaert LL, Perkins GD, Askitopoulou H, et al. European Resuscitation Council Guidelines for Resuscitation 2015: section 11. The ethics of resuscitation and end-of-life decisions. Resuscitation 2015;95:302–11.

124. Salins NS, Pai SG, Vidyasagar M, et al. Ethics and medico legal aspects of 'not for resuscitation'. Indian J Palliat Care 2010;16(2):66–9.

125. Mills A, Walker A, Levinson M, et al. Resuscitation orders in acute hospitals: a point prevalence study. Australas J Ageing 2017;36(1):32–7.

126. Sritharan G, Mills AC, Levinson MR, et al. Doctors' attitudes regarding not for resuscitation orders. Aust Health Rev 2018;41(6):680–7.

127. Mockford C, Clarke B, Field R, et al. A systematic review of do-not-attempt-cardiopulmonary-resuscitation (DNACPR) orders: summarising the evidence around decision making and implementation. Resuscitation 2014;85:S85.

128. Scquizzato T, Gazzato A, Semeraro F, et al. Cardiac arrest reported in newspapers: a new, yet missed, opportunity to increase cardiopulmonary resuscitation awareness. Resuscitation 2021;160:68–9.

129. Yuen JK, Reid MC, Fetters MD. Hospital do-not-resuscitate orders: why they have failed and how to fix them. J Gen Intern Med 2011;26(7):791–7.

130. Smith K, Andrew E, Lijovic M, et al. Quality of life and functional outcomes 12 months after out-of-hospital cardiac arrest. Circulation 2015;131(2):174–81.

131. Sharma RK, Jain N, Peswani N, et al. Unpacking resident-led code status discussions: results from a mixed methods study. J Gen Intern Med 2014;29(5):750–7.

132. Hart J, Kerlin M. Interpreting 'Do not resuscitate': a cautionary tale of physician influence. Ann Am Thorac Soc 2017;14(4):491–2.

133. Gobert F, Le Cam P, Guérin C. Buying time to save a life: a 3-month 'call in the dark for awareness'. Intensive Care Med 2016;42(10):1634–6.

134. Hsu CH, Considine J, Pawar RD, et al. Cardiopulmonary resuscitation and defibrillation for cardiac arrest when patients are in the prone position: a systematic review. Resusc Plus 2021;8:100186. doi: 10.1016/j.resplu.2021.100186.

135. Richards H, Robins-Browne K, O'Brien T, et al. Clinical benefits of prone positioning in the treatment of non-intubated patients with acute hypoxic respiratory failure: a rapid systematic review. Emerg Med J 2021;38(8):594–9.

136. Nolan JP, Ornato JP, Parr MJ, et al. Resuscitation highlights in 2020. Resuscitation 2021;162:1–10.

137. Weiss TT, Cerda F, Scott JB, et al. Prone positioning for patients intubated for severe acute respiratory distress syndrome (ARDS) secondary to COVID-19: a retrospective observational cohort study. Br J Anaesth 2021;126(1):48–55.

138. Berg K, Hsu CH, Considine J, et al, on behalf of the Advanced Life Support, Basic Life Support and Paediatric Life Support Task Forces at the International Liaison Committee on Resuscitation (ILCOR). Cardiopulmonary resuscitation and defibrillation for cardiac arrest when patients are in the prone position consensus on science with treatment recommendations. Brussels, Belgium: International Liaison Committee on Resuscitation (ILCOR) Advanced Life Support and Basic Life Task Forces, 2021 February 08. Available from: https://ilcor.org. [Accessed 15 February 2023].

139. Perkins GD, Morley PT, Nolan JP, et al. International Liaison Committee on Resuscitation: COVID-19 consensus on science, treatment recommendations and task force insights. Resuscitation 2020;151:145–7.

140. Page MJ, McKenzie JE, Bossuyt PM, et al. The PRISMA 2020 statement: an updated guideline for reporting systematic reviews. BMJ 2021;372:n71.

141. McHugh ML. Interrater reliability: the kappa statistic. Biochem Med 2012;22(3):276–82.

142. Murad MH, Sultan S, Haffar S, et al. Methodological quality and synthesis of case series and case reports. BMJ Evid Based Med 2018;23(2):60–3.

143. Mazer SP, Weisfeldt M, Bai D, et al. Reverse CPR: a pilot study of CPR in the prone position. Resuscitation 2003;57(3):279–85.

144. Wei J, Tung D, Sue SH, et al. Cardiopulmonary resuscitation in prone position: a simplified method for outpatients. J Chin Med Assoc 2006;69(5):202–6.

Chapter 26

Postanaesthesia recovery

Julie Cussen, Ulrica Nilsson

Learning objectives

After reading this chapter, you should be able to:

- describe the principles of immediate postoperative respiratory and cardiovascular management
- discuss the assessment and management of respiratory-related complications following surgery and general anaesthesia
- discuss the assessment and management of non-respiratory complications following surgery and general anaesthesia
- discuss the principles and possible complications of central neural blockade
- describe principles of managing postoperative pain
- discuss the signs, symptoms and treatment for anaesthetic complications such as malignant hyperthermia, and inadvertent hypothermia, delayed awakening and postoperative delirium.

Introduction

In 1751, realising that postoperative patients were vulnerable, the first postanaesthetic care unit (PACU) was created.[1] By the 1940s the importance of recovering from anaesthesia was recognised. Areas close to the operating theatre were created, allowing patients leaving the operating theatre to be closely monitored for signs of respiratory failure so that appropriate management could be instituted.[1] Today, perianaesthesia nursing is recognised as a specialty in its own right and postgraduate education opportunities exist to support nurses to develop expertise in this area.

While surgical techniques and anaesthetic medications have changed exponentially, the primary purpose of immediate postanaesthesia/postoperative care, whether provided in the PACU or the ICU, has altered little in the last 70 years. The focus remains on critical evaluation and stabilisation of patients after surgery, with an emphasis on anticipation and prevention of complications arising from either the anaesthetic or the surgical procedure.[2] While this chapter is titled 'Postanaesthesia recovery' it is worth noting that patients are also recovering from their own specific surgical procedure, which may require specific assessment and management.

The Australian National Consensus Statement on essential elements for recognising and responding to clinical deterioration[3] reports that measurable physiological abnormalities occur prior to adverse events such as cardiac arrest and death and suggests that early recognition of changes in a patient's condition, followed by prompt and effective treatment, can minimise poor outcomes. While the mortality in surgical patients has fallen in the last decade, mainly as a result of effective recognition and treatment of patient deterioration, failures in this process are still occurring.[4] The understanding of such failures may be the driving force behind some patients being admitted to the ICU or high-dependence unit following surgery, especially if they require ongoing high-level assessment and management. Postoperative patients who are not critically ill may also be recovered in the ICU after hours, and it is this group of patients to which this chapter is directed. In this chapter a brief overview of nursing the patient in the period following surgery and anaesthesia is provided, with the focus being on the recovery of non-critically ill patients.

In this chapter we will review anaesthesia and commonly used anaesthetic agents, postanaesthesia nursing care and assessment and management of specific postoperative complications. We acknowledge that postanaesthesia care nursing is a specialty in its own right and that this chapter will provide an overview. We encourage readers to refer to the end of this chapter for further reading about this specialty.

Introduction to anaesthesia

There are five components to anaesthesia. These include hypnosis, analgesia, muscle relaxation, sympatholysis and amnesia.[5] As a result of improvements in pharmacological agents used in anaesthesia, we now see patients emerging from anaesthesia in minutes rather than hours and, consequently, patients can be discharged from perianaesthesia care more quickly. Critical care nurses, whether they specialise in postanaesthesia recovery or not, need a thorough understanding of the pharmacology related to anaesthesia as this underpins patient assessment and management.

Phases of anaesthesia

There are four stages to anaesthesia that a critical care nurse should recognise and consider when undertaking patient assessment. Stage I (analgesia) may be described as the 'induction stage' from the beginning of induction of general anaesthesia to loss of consciousness. This is the lightest level of anaesthesia and, although there is sensory and mental depression, patients can often obey commands, breathe normally and maintain protective reflexes.[5] Stage II (excitement or delirium) begins with loss of consciousness and ends when a regular breathing pattern starts and the eyelid reflex is lost. Responses such as vomiting and laryngospasm can also occur in this stage, although with newer anaesthetic agents most patients move through this stage quickly.

Stage III (surgical anaesthesia) has four 'planes': plane 1, regular spontaneous breathing, constricted pupils and central gaze; however, eyelid and swallow reflexes usually disappear; plane 2, intermittent cessations of respiration, loss of corneal and laryngeal reflexes; plane 3, referred to as 'true surgical anaesthesia' because it is ideal for most surgeries; this plane is marked by complete relaxation of intercostal and abdominal muscles; and plane 4, irregular respirations, paradoxical rib-cage movement and diaphragmatic paralysis resulting in apnoea. Patients in stage III anaesthesia will not respond when a surgical incision is made. In stage III, patients will have sensory depression, loss of recall, depressed reflexes and some evidence of skeletal muscle relaxation. Swallowing, retching and vomiting reflexes disappear sequentially during induction and reappear in the same order during emergence from anaesthesia.[5]

During recovery from anaesthesia, if the patient is breathing using diaphragmatic muscles but does not have intercostal muscle involvement, they are probably still in stage III of anaesthesia. Lack of muscle tone, particularly in the jaw and abdomen, also suggests that the patient is in stage III anaesthesia. As the anaesthesia lightens, respiration will have a normal rate and rhythm.[5]

Stage IV anaesthesia (overdose) lasts from when respiration stops to failure of the circulatory system and is lethal without cardiovascular and respiratory support. Determining the stage of anaesthesia cannot be done by assessing any single parameter.[5] Rather, all clinical signs should be considered in relation to the patient's clinical condition and the particular anaesthetic agent used.[5]

Anaesthetic agents

Once referred to as the 'art of anaesthesia', modern anaesthesia now rests firmly on scientific foundations; however, the practice still remains a mixture of science and art.[6] The aim of good anaesthesia is to provide the safest anaesthetic, in the lightest plane possible, which allows a given procedure to be performed while the patient is pain free. This is why other medications, such as muscle relaxants, will be given in conjunction with anaesthetic agents so that muscle relaxation can occur at a lighter stage of anaesthesia.

Non-opioid agents

Non-opioid intravenous agents include non-barbiturates, barbiturates and sedatives. Non-opioid drugs interact with gamma-aminobutyric acid (GABA), an inhibitory neurotransmitter in the brain, with the specific actions being drug dependent.

Non-barbiturates

Propofol is the most frequently used intravenous induction agent in the Western world.[7] It produces rapid loss of consciousness with no accumulation in tissues, leading to quick recovery. Propofol also decreases laryngeal reflexes, making it particularly suitable for smooth insertion of supraglottic airways (SGAs) including laryngeal masks compared with other induction agents.[7] Adverse effects include pain on injection, which is mitigated by the addition of lignocaine (lidocaine), apnoea on induction, hypotension due to a reduction in systemic vascular resistance and myocardial depression, and extraneous muscle movements not thought to be epileptiform. The depressant effect of propofol on the respiratory system may result in airway and ventilatory support being required for those patients who are not already intubated and ventilated.

> ### Practice tip
>
> Propofol administered to older adult patients can result in a significant drop in blood pressure. Therefore, this group of patients should be carefully monitored.

Etomidate is a short-acting hypnotic agent without any analgesic effects. Although not available in all countries, and not licensed for use in Australia, etomidate is used in many countries, especially for intubation of critically ill patients, mainly because of the minimal cardiovascular effects of the drug.[8] Etomidate causes only a slight increase in heart rate and slight decrease in blood pressure. Cardiac index and peripheral vascular resistance are not significantly influenced, and the drug does not seem to be arrhythmogenic. Controversy does exist around the use of single bolus dose etomidate for anaesthetic induction because of the higher incidence of adrenal suppression.[9] However, there is no broad consensus of the effect of such suppression on patient outcome.[10]

Barbiturate

The barbiturate thiopental dominated intravenous anaesthesia until the mid 1980s, when propofol was introduced.[11] Thiopentone provides rapid, smooth induction but delayed recovery, has poor analgesic properties and is associated with side effects such as laryngospasm and arrhythmias.[12]

> ### Practice tip
>
> Obese patients administered thiopental sodium may have delayed wakening because the drug is highly fat soluble.

Inhalation anaesthesia

Assessing emergence from inhalation anaesthesia requires an understanding of the pharmacological effects of these agents, and an overview of their characteristics. A brief summary of these agents is provided in Table 26.1. These agents are essentially depressant drugs, and some are more likely to affect myocardial and respiratory function than others.

> ### Practice tip
>
> Encouraging deep breathing during the recovery period is essential to promote removal of inhalation gases.

Opioids

Analgesia is fundamental to recovery from surgery and opioids continue to be the cornerstone of perioperative analgesia. Advances in pharmacology and molecular biology have led to the development of many different types of opioids and recognition and classification of opioid receptors.[13] Historically, general anaesthesia has relied almost exclusively on opioids administered as intermittent boluses or as a continuous infusion to manage nociception intraoperatively and pain postoperatively.[14] While opioids are the most effective antinociceptive agents, they can have undesirable side effects and an overreliance on opioids has contributed to an opioid abuse epidemic.[15] For almost 30 years the concept of opioid sparing, or multimodal analgesia, to reduce overreliance on opioids has been widely practised.[13] However, it is important to recognise that opioids are effective analgesics and have an important role in multimodal pain management in carefully selected and closely monitored patients.[16] Effective opioid stewardship includes the administration of sufficient opioid analgesia to facilitate recovery while minimising the risk of opioid-related harm.[17] Opioids are an important agent in the anaesthetic process and the postoperative period, with their main purpose being to provide analgesia. Opioids also enhance the effectiveness of inhaled anaesthetics, allowing lower doses to be provided. In the postoperative period, opioids are commonly administered to alleviate pain associated with the surgical process. Opioids, whether they are natural or synthetic substances, bind to receptors producing a morphine-like or opioid agonist effect.[18]

Opioid receptors include the mu (μ), delta (δ) and kappa (κ) receptors located in the central nervous system, mostly in the brainstem and spinal cord. The mu receptors, specifically the mu-1 receptors, are responsible for supraspinal analgesia effects when stimulated. When mu-2 receptors are stimulated hypoventilation, bradycardia, physical dependence, euphoria and ileus can occur.

Common opioid drugs used intra- and postoperatively for pain relief include morphine and fentanyl. Pethidine is no longer commonly used for long-term pain relief due to the accumulation of normeperidine over time, which can result in central nervous system toxicity.[19]

> ### Practice tip
>
> Morphine is metabolised by the liver and the metabolites are excreted by the kidneys so the analgesic and sedating effects can be prolonged and potentially dangerous for patients with renal failure.

Opioid-sparing and opioid-free anaesthesia

The opioid crisis in the United States (US) and Canada has resulted in increasing overdose death rates and contributed to a decline in average US life expectancy.[20] It is the result of a problem that has emerged over a long

TABLE 26.1

Common inhalation anaesthetic agents

	CHARACTERISTICS
Isoflurane	Reduces systemic arterial blood pressure and systemic vascular resistance. Heart rate increased during recovery. Produces respiratory depression. Produces skeletal muscle relaxation in a dose-related fashion. Does not sensitise the myocardium to catecholamines compared with halothane so fewer arrhythmias are observed. Patient awakens 15–30 min following termination of anaesthetic gas but may be longer if surgery exceeds 45–60 min.
Sevoflurane	Emergence from anaesthesia occurs in minutes. Decreases blood pressure and systemic vascular resistance. A respiratory depressant. Does not increase risk of arrhythmias. Can increase intracranial pressure in a dose-related manner.
Desflurane	Extremely rapid emergence. Dose-related decrease in blood pressure. Low rate of cardiac arrhythmias. Irritates respiratory tract and induces coughing. May induce laryngospasm. Almost totally eliminated by the respiratory system.
Nitrous oxide	No side effects unless hypoxia is present. Non-toxic and non-irritating. Can be administered alone or in combination with other agents. Diffusion hypoxia can occur when not enough nitrous oxide is removed from the lungs at the end of the surgical procedure.

Source: Drain CB. Inhalation anesthesia. In: Odom-Forren J, editor. Drain's perianesthesia nursing: a critical care approach. 7th ed. St. Louis, MO: Elsevier; 2018, p. 260–71.

period,[21] with the US Department of Health 2016–17 data estimating that 2.1 million people have opioid use disorder (OUD).[22] Strategies to minimise the use of perioperative opioids include regional anaesthesia techniques and multimodal pharmacological techniques.[22]

Regional anaesthetic techniques include:

- neuraxial blocks (epidural and spinal analgesia)
- upper extremity blocks (interscalene, supraclavicular/infraclavicular, bier, axillary brachial plexus)
- truncal blocks (transverse abdominis plane (TAP), paravertebral, intercostal nerve block)
- lower extremity blocks (saphenous nerve, femoral nerve, ankle block).
  Multimodal pharmacological therapy includes:
- non-steroidal anti-inflammatory drugs (acetaminophen, ketorolac),
- gabapentenoids (gabapentin, pregabalin)
- N-methyl-D-aspartate receptor antagonists (ketamine)
- alpha-2 adrenergic agonists (clonidine, dexmedetomidine)

- glucocorticoids (dexamethasone)
- local anaesthetics (lignocaine).

Spinal and epidural opioid administration

Opioids can be administered as part of either spinal or epidural anaesthesia. In spinal anaesthesia, drugs are administered into the cerebral spinal fluid that surrounds the spinal cord, and puncture of the dura is required for this administration. In contrast with epidural administration, the drugs are delivered outside the dura.[23] Administration of morphine (0.1–0.2 mg) directly into the spinal fluid results in a maximal concentration within 5–10 minutes; the duration of action is 80–200 minutes. In contrast, a higher dose of morphine is required when administered into the epidural space (5 mg), with pain relief in effect within 30–60 minutes that can last up to 24 hours. Additional morphine can be administered via the epidural route if required to a maximum of 10 mg in 24 hours. Fentanyl and sufentanil can also be administered epidurally and are more suited for continuous infusion. When intrathecal or epidural opioids are administered, close observation of the patient, particularly respiratory and conscious state, is essential as there may be delayed respiratory depression. Caution should also be taken with additional opioid administration during the first 24 hours as the half-life of opioids administered via these routes is increased.

Opioid antagonists

Should opioid-induced respiratory depression occur in the postanaesthesia period, an opioid antagonist might be needed. Naloxone is a pure opioid antagonist that reverses the depressant effects of the drug and is usually administered in a titrated fashion, assessing patient response. A dose of 0.1–0.2 mg is usually sufficient. The onset of action is quick and occurs within 1–2 minutes of administration; the half-life is 30–80 minutes.[24] After 3–5 minutes, if reversal is still not achieved, additional doses of naloxone can be administered.[18]

Benzodiazepines and benzodiazepine antagonists

Benzodiazepines are sedatives that depress the limbic system and may cause some cortical depression.[25] They interact with GABA, the inhibitory neurotransmitter, causing decreased orientation through a hypnotic effect, retrograde amnesia, anxiolysis and skeletal muscle relaxation.[25] The hypnotic action of benzodiazepines is enhanced by the effects of opiates and barbiturates.

Midazolam is the most popular benzodiazepine used in anaesthesia and critical care and has a wide variety of uses including procedural sedation and induction of anaesthesia. Low-dose midazolam can be administered preoperatively to provide anxiolysis, sedation and amnesia and, although generally considered safe, it may cause delayed recovery due to residual drowsiness and amnesia and is associated with emergence delirium and cognitive dysfunction.[26] Midazolam has onset of action of 3–5 minutes, but an elimination half-life of 2–6 hours so can cause prolonged post-procedure sedation.[27] Enhanced recovery protocols recommend avoidance of routine benzodiazepine premedication in favour of more-targeted use for specific clinical outcomes.[26]

Practice tip

Midazolam does not affect intracranial pressure and, therefore, can safely be used in patients with intracranial pathology or who are undergoing neurosurgery.

If required, the pharmacological effects of benzodiazepines can be reversed. Flumazenil is a benzodiazepine agonist that should be administered intravenously in 0.1-mg increments to avoid rapid reawakening. The usual dose is 0.4 mg and the maximum amount administered should be no more than 1.0 mg.[25] The drug takes effect within 5 minutes of administration and has a duration of action between 1 and 2 hours.

Practice tip

Flumazenil has a shorter duration of action than most benzodiazepines so patients should be carefully assessed for resedation after the initial dose is administered. If signs of resedation are evident, additional flumazenil can be administered every 20 minutes to a maximum dose of 3.0 mg in a 1-hour period.

Butyrophenones

As sedative agents, butyrophenones such as haloperidol and droperidol produce a state of profound calm and immobility where the patient appears to be pain free and dissociated from their surroundings. Butyrophenone use in anaesthesia is, however, uncommon. Haloperidol is rarely used because of its long duration of action and high incidence of extrapyramidal side effects. Droperidol in the perioperative period is largely used for its antiemetic and sedative effects.

Practice tip

Some patients who have received droperidol report feeling terrified and unable to express how they feel while also having an outward appearance of being very calm. In the postanaesthesia period, it is important that support is provided to patients even if they appear calm.

Droperidol is known to potentiate the action of barbiturates and opioids with some effects lasting as long as 10–12 hours.[25] Nurses should constantly assess the patient for signs of respiratory depression. In the postanaesthesia period, regular stimulation of the patient and encouragement of deep breathing is necessary as patients can drift back to sleep and have slow and/or shallow respirations. In some instances, patients who have received droperidol have become apnoeic.[25]

Neuromuscular blocking agents

Since the 1940s, neuromuscular blocking agents have been used as pharmacological agents in anaesthesia. Although not all patients will require neuromuscular blockade during anaesthesia, these agents may be given to facilitate endotracheal intubation. Muscle relaxation is also indicated to facilitate some surgical procedures, such as abdominal surgery, in ophthalmic surgery to relax extraocular muscles, and to facilitate mechanical ventilation. Nurses who are responsible for the assessment and management of the postoperative patient should understand the physiology of neuromuscular transmission and mechanism of action of the various neuromuscular blocking agents that may be used in anaesthesia.

The neuromuscular junction has three components: the motor nerve fibre, the synaptic cleft and the motor endplate of striated muscle (Fig. 26.1). Neuromuscular

FIGURE 26.1 Neuromuscular junction.[5]

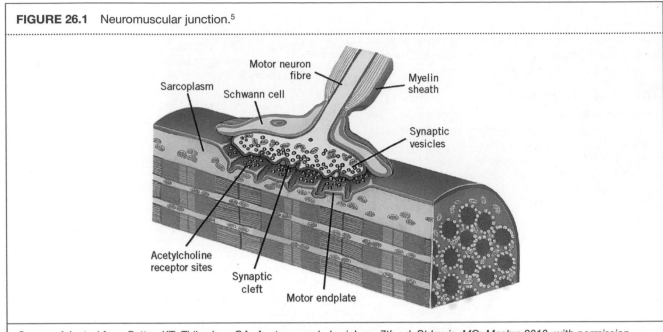

Source: Adapted from Patton KT, Thibodeau GA. Anatomy and physiology. 7th ed. St Louis, MO: Mosby; 2010, with permission.

transmission is predominantly dependent on acetylcholine (ACh), as the natural transmitter.[28] ACh receptors are located on the motor end-plate and, when bound to ACh, membrane channels open and this results in an influx of sodium ions, causing depolarisation of the motor end-plate membrane. Potassium ions exit, causing repolarisation, allowing the membrane potential to again become negative. These sequences allow muscle contraction to occur. ACh is broken down by acetylcholinesterase, which is present in the synaptic cleft, and is metabolised before the excited muscle returns to its resting state. The broken-down ACh elements are then used for the manufacture of new ACh molecules in the nerve terminal ending.

Non-depolarising neuromuscular blocking agents

Non-depolarising neuromuscular blocking agents block the action of ACh at the postsynaptic receptor sites in the neuromuscular junction (Fig. 26.2) by competing with ACh at these binding sites and blocking neuromuscular transmission.[28] There are many different types of non-depolarising neuromuscular blocking agents.[29] Although the end effect of these agents is similar, their pharmacological effects differ in relation to onset of action, duration of effect and excretion (Table 26.2).

Residual neuromuscular block is a complication that can occur following use of neuromuscular blockade[29] and can result in adverse respiratory complications.[30] Pharmacological reversal of neuromuscular block can be used when the effects of the neuromuscular blocking agent remain present at the end of the surgery. Conventional reversal of neuromuscular blockade involves administration of an anticholinesterase. Anticholinesterase inhibits the action of cholinesterases that inactivate ACh, hence

potentiating the effects of the neurotransmitter ACh, and helps restore skeletal muscle activity.[29] Anticholinesterases stimulate the muscarinic receptors and elicit side effects including bradycardia, arrhythmias and bronchospasm as well as nausea and vomiting. For this reason, antimuscarinic agents such as atropine or glycopyrrolate must be administered at the same time as the reversal agent.[29] The expanded array of neuromuscular blockade reversal agents now allows for fast and complete reversal and the reduction of postoperative complications from residual block.[31]

Sugammadex is also used to reverse the effect of neuromuscular blockade, specifically when the agents rocuronium and vecuronium are used. Sugammadex is the first selective neuromuscular drug-binding agent and reverses the effect of the neuromuscular blocking drugs through encapsulation. Hypersensitivity to sugammadex can occur within the first 5 minutes following administration and, as such, patients receiving this drug should be closely monitored for signs of drug-induced hypersensitivity.[32]

> ### Practice tip
>
> When patients return from surgery, review their anaesthetic record to see whether a neuromuscular blocking agent has been used and, if it was, whether a reversal agent was given.
>
> If sugammadex is given to a female patient of child-bearing years, and this patient was using a hormonal contractive agent, such as the contraceptive pill, vaginal ring, implant or intrauterine system or device, the patient should be advised to take additional contraceptive precautions for 7 days following sugammadex administration.[33]

FIGURE 26.2 **(A)** Normal muscle contraction.
(B) Neuromuscular blockade.

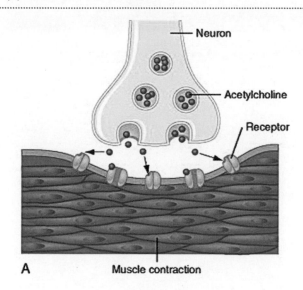

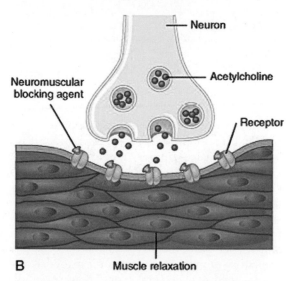

Source: Adapted from Siedlecki SL. Pain and sedation. In: Carlson K, editor. Advanced Critical Care Nursing. St Louis, MO: Saunders; 2009, Figure 4-13, p. 79, with permission.

Depolarising neuromuscular blocking agents

Suxamethonium, also known as succinylcholine, is the only depolarising neuromuscular blocking agent used in anaesthesia and has a rapid onset of effect and an ultrashort duration of action.[34] It is most often used in rapid sequence induction for the purpose of endotracheal intubation. Suxamethonium works at the site of the ACh receptor and causes persistent depolarisation at the motor endplate.[35] Patients administered suxamethonium demonstrate muscle fasciculations because of the sudden increase in ACh at the motor endplate.

Suxamethonium administration of 1 mg/kg results in complete neuromuscular suppression in around 60 seconds. The very rapid onset of paralysis remains its true advantage as a patient can be intubated almost immediately. Suxamethonium administration can induce hyperkalaemia so its use in patients with electrolyte disorders, such as those with severe burns or diabetic ketoacidosis, is not recommended.[34] The duration of action of suxamethonium is relatively short as the drug is hydrolysed rapidly by plasma pseudocholinesterase. Paralysis associated with administration of suxamethonium usually lasts only 5–10 minutes. Some patients may have reduced pseudocholinesterase activity. This can be an acquired deficiency that might be associated with liver disease, severe anaemia, malnutrition, prolonged pyrexia, pregnancy and renal dialysis. Congenital deficiencies in pseudocholinesterase are relatively uncommon.

Practice tip

Patients with either acquired or congenital pseudocholinesterase deficiency may remain paralysed for prolonged periods of time and may require mechanical ventilation for up to 48 hours.

Factors influencing neuromuscular blocking agents

There are a number of factors that can influence neuromuscular blocking agents. Many of these include drug interactions and alterations in electrolyte balance (see Table 26.3).[36] Dehydration can also increase the sensitivity to skeletal muscle relaxants because of increased neuromuscular excitability, slowed renal function and drug excretion and increased plasma concentration of the relaxant. Acid–base balance can also influence neuromuscular blockade where acidosis and increased carbon dioxide levels result in a stronger effect of the neuromuscular blocking agent pancuronium.[35] Hypothermia can antagonise the effect of neuromuscular blocking agents, as with pancuronium, or can potentiate the effect as seen with suxamethonium. Prior to extubation of a patient following a relaxant anaesthesia, the anaesthetist may use 'train-of-four' where the level of neuromuscular block is assessed using a peripheral nerve stimulator.

TABLE 26.2

Pharmacological overview of commonly used non-depolarising neuromuscular blocking agents

	VECURONIUM BROMIDE	ATRACURIUM BESYLATE	CISATRACURIUM BESYLATE	ROCURONIUM BROMIDE
Dose for intubation (mg/kg)	0.08–0.1	0.4–0.5	0.1–0.2	0.1
Intubation to relaxation time (min)	2.5–3.0	2.0–2.5	2.8–3.4	1.0–2.0
Dose for muscle relaxation (mg/kg)	0.05–0.06	0.2–0.5	2.5	0.6–1.0
Recovery time (min)	30–60	30–45	55–75	30–90
Reversible	Yes	Yes	Yes	Yes
Time to reversal (after initial dose, in min)	25–80 (dose-dependent)	20–35	10–15	5–10
Cumulative effects	Slight	No	No	No
Fasciculations and muscle soreness	None	No	No	No
Risk of histamine release	None	Minimal	No	No
Cardiovascular effects	None	Few	None	None

Source: Adapted from Drain CB. Neuromuscular blocking agents. In: Odom-Forren J, editor. Drain's perianesthesia nursing: a critical care approach. 7th ed. St Louis, MO: Elsevier; 2018, p. 297–315, with permission.

Non-steroidal anti-inflammatory drugs

Non-steroidal anti-inflammatory drugs (NSAIDs) are routinely used in enhanced recovery after surgery (ERAS) programs as they are considered a potent opioid-sparing analgesic without undesired side effects such as nausea or sedation.[37] Postoperative pain caused by inflammation depends on prostaglandin E2 synthesised by cyclo-oxygenase (COX) in neural cells.[38] Traditional NSAIDs act through peripheral inhibition of COX-1 and COX-2 enzymes, inhibiting the synthesis of prostaglandins, mediators of inflammation and vasodilation.[39] NSAIDs include ibuprofen, parecoxib, indomethacin, ketorolac and diclofenac.

Practice tip

A recent meta-analysis comparing codeine and NSAIDs for postoperative pain in outpatient surgery found that patients report better pain scores, better global assessments and fewer adverse effects when their postoperative pain is treated with NSAIDs than with codeine.[40]

Dissociative anaesthetics

Ketamine produces a dissociative state of hypnosis and analgesia. It can be used for induction and maintenance of anaesthesia, and has a rapid onset and relatively rapid offset. It has sympathomimetic effects that preserve cardiac function and has minimal effect on respiration. It is used primarily for its analgesic properties. Ketamine is associated with significant adverse psychological effects from larger doses.[41] Ketamine selectively blocks pain conduction and perception yet does not depress those parts of the central nervous system not involved in pain transmission and perception. When patients are administered ketamine, they experience profound analgesia and unconsciousness, but respiratory function is usually not impaired. Ketamine also causes increased cerebral blood flow so should be avoided in those patients at risk of developing increased intracranial pressure.[42]

Of particular importance to the nurse managing a postoperative patient who has received ketamine is an understanding that psychic aberrations can occur on emergence from anaesthesia. Patients can experience vivid dreaming with or without psychomotor activity. They can appear confused or irrational and hallucinate. If the patient does have augmented psychomotor responses and irrational behaviour, medications such as dexmedetomidine or a benzodiazepine can be administered.

Practice tip

Ketamine can be used as a sole anaesthetic agent for paediatric patients who appear to be less prone to psychic disturbances.

TABLE 26.3

Drug–drug interactions[36]

DRUG	INTERACTION	RESULT	MECHANISM
Antihypertensive drugs			
Propranolol	Inhalation anaesthetics	Bradycardia, hypotension	Additive effect.
	Lignocaine	Enhanced negative inotropic effect	Propranolol reduces liver blood flow and lignocaine clearance.
	Heparin	Myocardial depression	Heparin increases free fatty acids, which displace propranolol from plasma protein binding sites, leading to increased free propranolol.
Lignocaine	Non-depolarising muscle relaxants	Increased duration of neuromuscular blockade	Synergistic effect.
Digitalis	Suxamethonium/succinylcholine	Arrhythmias	Direct effect or caused by hyperkalaemia that can be induced by succinylcholine.
	Thiazide diuretics	Increased potassium excreted by kidneys	Combined effect of two drugs on kidneys promotes potassium excretion.
Quinidine	Digitalis	Can produce digitalis intoxication	Decreased digitalis clearance and increased concentration of digitalis.
	Myasthenia gravis plus skeletal muscle relaxants	Postoperative respiratory depression	Blockade of ACh receptors at neuromuscular postsynaptic membrane.
Antibiotics			
Neomycin Streptomycin Dihydrostreptomycin Polymyxin A Polymyxin B Colistin Viomycin Paromomycin Kanamycin Lincomycin Gentamicin Tetracycline	Non-depolarising skeletal muscle relaxants	Potentiate non-depolarising muscle relaxants, respiratory depression	Neuromuscular blockade caused by reduction in amplitude of endplate potential.
Opioids			
Morphine Fentanyl Sufentanil Remifentanil	Inhalation anaesthetics	Potentiation, respiratory and cardiovascular depression	Depressant effects of inhalation anaesthetics and opioids are additive.
Pethidine/meperidine	Inhalation anaesthetics	Potentiation, respiratory and cardiovascular depression	Depressant effects of inhalation anaesthetics and opioids are additive.
	Enovid Norinyl	Birth control pill potentiates pethidine/meperidine	Excess female sex hormones with oral contraceptive therapy, which may slow metabolism of pethidine/meperidine.
	MAOI	MAOI interacts with pethidine/meperidine metabolite	Type I: seizures Type II: hypotension

Continued

TABLE 26.3

Drug–drug interactions—cont'd

DRUG	INTERACTION	RESULT	MECHANISM
Sympathomimetic amines			
Adrenaline	Inhalation anaesthetics	Cardiac arrhythmias	Anaesthetic agents may sensitise myocardium to endogenous and exogenous catecholamines.
Electrolytes			
Increased extracellular potassium	Skeletal muscle relaxants	Increased resistance to depolarisation and greater sensitivity to non-depolarising muscle relaxants	Acute increase in extracellular potassium increases endplate transmembrane potential, thus causing hyperpolarisation.
Decreased extracellular potassium	Skeletal muscle relaxants	Increased effects of depolarising muscle relaxants and increased resistance to non-depolarising muscle relaxants	Acute decrease in extracellular potassium lowers resting endplate transmembrane potential.
Increased calcium levels	Non-depolarising skeletal muscle relaxants	Decreased response	Calcium increases release of ACh and enhances excitation–contraction coupling mechanism.
Magnesium ions	Muscle relaxants	Potentiation	Magnesium ions cause partial muscle relaxation by blocking release of ACh.
Calcium chloride	Digitalis	Additive effect on heart	High concentrations of calcium inhibit positive inotropic actions of digitalis and potentiate digitalis toxicity.
Miscellaneous			
Frusemide Thiazide Ethacrynic acid	Non-depolarising skeletal muscle relaxants	Intensified neuromuscular block	Electrolyte imbalance (hypokalaemia).
Procaine Lignocaine	Non-depolarising and depolarising skeletal muscle relaxants	Enhanced neuromuscular blockade	Decreased end-plate potential.
Lithium	Non-depolarising and depolarising skeletal muscle relaxants	Potentiated neuromuscular blockade	Lithium ions are substituted for sodium ions at presynaptic level.
Chlorpromazine	Non-depolarising skeletal muscle relaxants	Enhanced neuromuscular blockade	Potentiation of neuromuscular blockade.
All inhalation anaesthetics	Non-depolarising skeletal muscle relaxants	Augment block in dose-dependent manner	Central nervous system depression or presynaptic inhibition of ACh.
Insulin	Corticosteroids, oral contraceptives, loop and thiazide diuretics	Reduction in effects	Insulin antagonises effects.
Hydrocortisone Dexamethasone Prednisone	Phenobarbital	Decreased effect of the steroids	Increased metabolism.

ACh = acetylcholine.

Source: Adapted from Nagelhout JJ. Basic principles of pharmacology. In: Odom-Forren J, editor. Drain's perianesthesia nursing: a critical care approach. 7th ed. St Louis, MO: Elsevier; 2018, p. 243–59, with permission.

Drug interactions

Many patients undergoing anaesthesia will be taking medications in addition to those required for surgery and anaesthesia. Whenever two or more drugs are given to a patient, there is a potential for drug interactions to occur (Box 26.1).[43] Such interactions can have a potentially negative effect on the patient, and knowledge of these interactions will help guide nursing assessment (Table 26.3).[36]

BOX 26.1

Monoamine oxidase inhibitors[43]

The interaction of this class of drug with common anaesthetic agents is important to recognise. Although monoamine oxidase inhibitors (MAOI) are not as commonly used as in the past, many patients may still be prescribed these for management of depression. MAOIs inhibit *N*-demethylase and therefore decrease the breakdown of pethidine/meperidine. A type I response to this drug interaction includes seizures, agitation, rigidity and hyperpyrexia. A Type II response includes hypotension, respiratory depression and coma.

Source: Adapted from Rasool F, Ghafoor R, Lambert DG. Antidepressants and antipsychotics: anaesthetic implications. Anaesth Intensive Care Med 2014;15(7):314–17.

Practice tip

Some antibiotics such as gentamicin can potentiate non-depolarising muscle relaxants and make reversal of these agents more difficult.

Local and regional anaesthesia

Local anaesthesia works by blocking nerve conduction so that the patient does not feel painful stimuli. Local anaesthetics work by binding to sodium channels, preventing a conformational change and the influx of Na^+ and depolarisation slows, preventing depolarisation and transmission of the neuronal action potential.[44] A second mechanism may also cause disruption of the ion channel when local anaesthetic molecules are incorporated into the cell membrane (Fig. 26.3). The sensitivity to local anaesthetics depends on the nerve fibres, with sensitivity increased for the smaller nerve fibres. Myelinated fibres are also blocked before non–myelinated fibres if they are of the same diameter. Assessment and management of the patient receiving local or regional anaesthesia is provided later in this chapter.

FIGURE 26.3 Mechanism of action for local anaesthesia. **(A)** Transmission of the pain message to the central nervous system through depolarisation of the axon of a sensory nerve cell. **(B)** Blocking of the action potential in a sensory nerve cell through blocking of the sodium channel by local anaesthetic drugs.

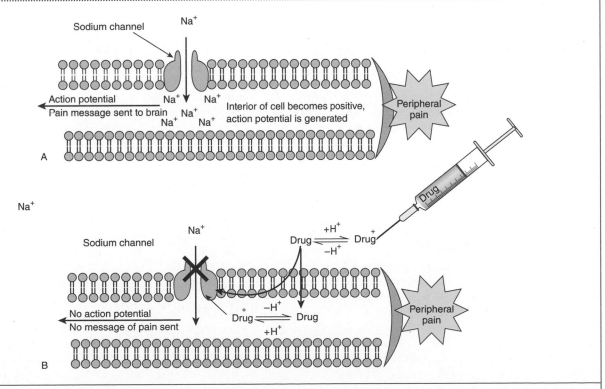

Source: Adapted from Friel CJ, Eliadi C, Pesaturo KA. Local anesthetic use in perioperative areas. Perioper Nurs Clin 2010;5:203–14, with permission.

Assessment and management in the postoperative period

The postoperative recovery is divided into three stages: early recovery, or phase I; intermediate recovery, or phase II; and late recovery, which may be referred to as phase III.[45] During phase I the patient is closely monitored in the PACU, high-dependency unit (HDU) or ICU until fully awake from anaesthesia and motor functions and protective reflexes are regained.[45]

When caring for a patient immediately after surgery, it is essential that the nurse has a full understanding of the possible complications of each individual procedure that has been performed. If a nurse is allocated a patient and does not understand the surgical procedure they must ask, possibly at the time of anaesthetic handover, to gain an understanding of what complications might occur in their patient. It is beyond the scope of this text to discuss all possible procedural complications. However, some examples of specific complications include: water intoxication and/or sodium depletion in surgery that flushes large amounts of saline solution or water under pressure (e.g. transurethral resection of the prostate (TURP), endometrial ablation); upper airway obstruction following surgery under the muscle layer of the neck (thyroidectomy, parotid cyst); postpartum haemorrhage (post-lower uterine segment caesarean section) requiring assessment with fundal height measurements; specific vascular observations for patients following free-flap surgery (deep inferior epigastric perforators (DIEP) or transverse rectus abdominis myocutaneous (TRAM)), not just observing for arterial vascularity but also venous engorgement; and cervical shock in gynaecological patients that causes a fall in both blood pressure and heart rate.

Anaesthetic handover

Handover is an important component that will help guide postoperative assessment and management and a critical stage in surgical patient care. There is no standardised and agreed approach to handover; however, it is recognised that some form of standard process is required.[46] A formal handover will be provided by the treating anaesthetist to the nurse who will be caring for the patient at the time of transfer of care. The quality of the handover must be such that it allows the nurse to safely assume responsibility for the patient. It is important for nurses to understand

this process, knowing what information needs to be gleaned from the handover as they accept responsibility for the patient's care. In some hospitals there is also a nursing handover from the perioperative nurse that may provide information about the surgical procedure, dressing, drain tubes and any notable intraoperative events. The handover therefore plays a crucial role in determining the patient's future care plan. There are a variety of different handover tools available internationally, many of which incorporate similar elements. For example, the SBAR mnemonic is used to guide handover through discussion of the:

Situation

Background

Assessment

Recommendation.

The Australian and New Zealand College of Anaesthetists recommended the ISOBAR acronym, which represents:

Identification to ensure that the patient is correctly identified

Situation, including current clinical status and patient-centred care requirements

Observations – latest observations

Background and history

Assessment and **a**ctions to establish an agreed management plan

Responsibility and **r**isk management.[46]

Consistency in the handover method will help enhance its quality so it is important to know which approach is used in your hospital.

In the PACU it is common to use discharge criteria to assess the patient's readiness for transfer to a lower acuity nursing area. These are based on assessments using the patient baseline as a comparison; some are numeric based whereas others are not. The Aldrete scoring system is a commonly used numeric tool that assesses activity, respiration, circulation, consciousness and oxygen saturation using scoring points 0, 1 or 2, maximum total score 10, with 10 indicating the best possible condition.[47] Transition from the PACU to the phase II step-down unit requires a scoring of 9 or higher in the Aldrete scoring system (Table 26.4). Patients undergoing surgery with local anaesthesia usually proceed immediately to phase II recovery. In phase II recovery, patients are still cared for at the day surgery unit or surgical ward but are not monitored as closely as in phase I.[48]

Respiratory assessment and management

Immediately after surgery, patients are susceptible to events that can compromise adequacy of ventilation and oxygenation, so airway and respiratory management skills are fundamental for nursing staff caring for this group.[49] Postoperative patients are predisposed to hypoxaemia due to incomplete lung re-expansion, reduced chest wall and

TABLE 26.4
The modified Aldrete scoring system

CRITERIA	POINT VALUE
Consciousness	
Fully awake	2
Arousable	1
Not responding	0
Oxygenation	
SpO$_2$ >94% on room air	2
SpO$_2$ >90% on oxygen	1
SpO$_2$ <90% on oxygen	0
Mobility	
Able to move four extremities on command	2
Able to move two extremities on command	1
Able to move zero extremities on command	0
Breathing	
Able to breathe deeply	2
Dyspnoea	1
Apnoea	0
Circulation	
Systemic BP ± 20% of the preanesthetic level	2
Systemic BP between 20% and 49% of the preanesthetic level	1
Systemic BP ± 50% of the preanesthetic level	0

Maximum score: 10; discharge score ≥9.
Source: Aldrete J, Kroulik D. A postanesthetic recovery score. Anesthesia & Analgesia 1970;49:924–34.

diaphragmatic activity caused by surgical injury and pain, consequences of haemodynamic impairment and residual effects of anaesthetic medications. This includes residual neuromuscular blockade and other effects related to narcotics, sedatives, hypnotics and inhalational gases.[49] This can cause decreased rate and depth of breathing, which contributes to alveolar hypoventilation and consequently results in increased levels of carbon dioxide and decreased levels of oxygen in the blood and atelectasis. Postoperative shivering may also increase oxygen consumption, thereby increasing the risk of hypoxaemia. Prolonged hypoxaemia may promote serious consequences, including arrhythmias, myocardial ischaemia and cognitive dysfunction.[50]

Respiratory depression is more common among patients who have had general rather than spinal anaesthesia. Obstructive sleep apnoea (OSA) is associated with increased risk following general anaesthesia and this prevalence may be increasing as the rates of obesity (a known risk factor for OSA) among the surgical population have increased dramatically over the last several decades. Assessment of the patient's respiration includes respiratory rate and oxygen saturation. A respiratory depression event is occurring if hypoventilation (three episodes of <8 respirations per minute), apnoea (episode of apnoea ≥10 seconds) or hypoxaemia (three episodes of oxyhaemoglobin desaturations as measured by pulse oximetry (<90% with or without nasal cannula)) is present.[51] More accurate and detailed assessment of gas exchange requires arterial blood gas analysis. Depending on the nature of the surgical intervention, some patients may require a more detailed respiratory assessment that incorporates inspection, palpation, percussion and auscultation as well as capnography to assess end-tidal carbon dioxide. It is important to have a detailed knowledge and understanding of the respiratory system and how to assess the respiratory function of postanaesthesia patients. For a detailed discussion of respiratory assessment and monitoring, see Chapter 13.

Assessment and management of the airway

A complication seen in the immediate postanaesthesia period is airway obstruction.[30] The depressant effects of anaesthesia can mean that the postoperative patient is not able to protect or maintain a patent airway. Signs that the patient might have an airway obstruction include increased respiratory effort, respiratory muscle retraction, abnormal breath sounds and signs of altered gas exchange. In many cases, opening the airway by tilting the head backwards and extending the neck (if not contraindicated) can help to restore airway patency. Artificial airways may be used to prevent obstruction that occurs when the patient's tongue and epiglottis fall back on the posterior pharyngeal wall.

All airway complications are serious as they all, in some way or another, obstruct the airway to varying degrees and put the patient at risk of decreased oxygenation and possible hypoxia. These complications can be from an upper airway obstruction such as laryngeal spasm, subglottic oedema or lower airway obstruction such as bronchospasm and non-cardiogenic pulmonary oedema. They may result from a simple problem, such as poor mandibular positioning where the tongue falls back obstructing the airway, to a complete laryngeal spasm with no air entry.[30] Any of these problems can cause life-threatening hypoxia if not rectified immediately.

Some patients may leave the operating theatre with a supraglottic airway, for example a laryngeal mask, and this can be removed once they are awake and able to open their mouth and maintain their own airway. Others may have an endotracheal tube in situ, which may be the reason for their transfer to the ICU or HDU. In an intubated patient a systematic approach to determining whether the patient is ready to be extubated should be implemented and should include assessing whether the patient is fully reversed, awake, cooperative and able to follow commands. The patient should be normothermic and, if airway oedema is suspected, an endotracheal tube leak test should be performed where the cuff is deflated and breathing assessed prior to tube removal. A medical officer needs to be available at extubation should immediate re-intubation be required (see Chapter 15).

Assessment and management of ventilatory capacity and oxygenation

The altered respiratory rate and depth that may occur as a result of anaesthesia require focused assessment and understanding of the ways in which anaesthetic agents can influence both ventilator capacity and oxygenation in the postoperative period. In a large cohort study designed to compare the accuracy of different methods of modelling vital signs and trends for detecting clinical deterioration, data were collected for 269,999 medical and surgical admissions across five hospitals.[52] Respiratory rate was identified as the best predictor of clinical deterioration. Similar findings were observed in a large Canadian observational study by Kellett and colleagues, who reported that the respiratory rate increased most in non-survivors.[53] While any change in vital signs is important to assess in the early postoperative period, the pharmacological agents used intra- and postoperatively can have a significant impact on respiratory function.

The use of oxygen therapy has been under some debate, and in recent years the free use of oxygen is being questioned and routine supplemental oxygen administration to prevent hypoxaemia may not be necessary in most postoperative patients.[50] Patients with normal respiratory function and an oxygen saturation >94% on room air administration of supplemental oxygen may mask the symptoms of poor respiration function. In contrast, the World Health Organization (WHO)[54] has recommended that adult patients who have undergone general anaesthesia with endotracheal intubation for surgical procedures should receive supplemental oxygen at a fraction of inspired oxygen of 80% and, if feasible, that this continue for 2–6 hours postoperatively to reduce the risk of surgical site infections. In short, the free use of oxygen therapy should be replaced with a specific assessment of oxygen requirements for each individual patient. Nevertheless, this has generated considerable controversy, especially regarding selection of studies, statistical analysis and insufficient analysis of potentially negative effects of hyperoxaemia due to high oxygen administration.[50]

Because respiratory effort can be compromised, almost all postoperative patients will receive supplemental oxygen, and with all patients the amount of oxygen received should be guided by the patient's clinical condition and assessment of arterial oxygen saturation. Some patients may require respiratory support in the postoperative period and will remain intubated and ventilated for a period of time after surgery. If patients require ongoing mechanical ventilation, they may require admission to ICU. For a detailed understanding of patients requiring mechanical ventilation and ongoing respiratory support, see Chapter 15.

Cardiovascular assessment and management

In the postanaesthesia period, assessment of cardiovascular function will be frequently undertaken, with monitoring of blood pressure and heart rate. Detailed description of cardiovascular assessment is provided in Chapter 9. Postoperative patients are at risk of developing cardiovascular complications as they will have generally had some degree of blood loss, will have been administered anaesthetic medications, or have temperature changes that may have altered vascularity. For example, central neural blockage will cause vascular vasodilation and interference to the body's sympathetic responses, which can lead to hypotension. Conversely, hypertension can be present when patients experience pain.

Hypotension can be transient or more sustained. Transient hypotension can occur in relation to drug administration. Conversely, more-sustained hypotension and the development of shock can occur in relation to blood loss or from an altered distribution of flow that occurs secondary to sympathetic blockade and vasodilation that can occur in regional anaesthesia. Decreased cardiac output might be seen in some patients and could be related to decreased preload that occurs in hypovolaemia or decreased cardiac output secondary to myocardial injury contractility as a result of either myocardial injury or cardiac output and vasodilatory states.[30] Shock is characterised by a decrease in blood pressure (20–30% decrease from the patient's baseline) and an increase in heart rate, and is not an uncommon occurrence in postoperative patients.[30] Cardiovascular compromise that results from blood and fluid loss can lead to hypovolaemic shock. Specific assessment and management strategies for the patient with shock are provided in Chapter 21.

> **Practice tip**
>
> Inadvertent hypothermia will cause vasoconstriction that may mask a low circulating blood volume.

Fluid and electrolyte balance

Overhydration in postoperative patients has been associated with a delayed return of bowel function, postoperative ileus, postoperative nausea and vomiting, and increased length of stay.[55] Conversely, underhydration (i.e. hypovolaemia), if undetected, may lead to postoperative complications including acute kidney injury, surgical site infections, sepsis and delirium, as well as prolonged hospital stay.[55] The primary goals of fluid management in the immediate postoperative phase are to maintain adequate intravascular volumes, left ventricular filling pressures, cardiac output, blood pressure and the delivery of oxygen to the tissues.[56] Normal concentrations of electrolytes and body fluids are vital to maintain the physiological function of all bodily systems.[56] The goals and strategies for volume replacement are patient dependent and should take into consideration the preoperative condition of the patient, cardiovascular and renal status, and intraoperative fluid losses.[56] It is recommended to assess postoperative hydration status routinely and manage accordingly during the recovery.

Venous thromboembolism prophylaxis

Venous thromboembolism (VTE) prophylaxis is essential as postoperative deaths from deep vein thrombosis (DVT) and subsequent pulmonary embolism are not uncommon. Risk factors for VTE are: age $\geq$60 years, obesity (body mass index $\geq$40 kg/m^2), preoperative immobilisation, chronic venous insufficiency, active or in-treatment cancer, one or more significant medical comorbidities (such as heart disease, metabolic, endocrine or respiratory pathologies, acute infectious diseases or inflammatory conditions), use of hormone replacement therapy, thrombophilia or a personal or family history of DVT/pulmonary embolism, current pregnancy or puerperium, and surgery lasting at least 120 minutes.[57]

Recommendations for thromboprophylaxis in patients with no to low risks are general and include early mobilisation and optimal hydration. In patients at high risk of developing VTE, anticoagulant prophylaxis with subcutaneous heparin is recommended as well as early mobilisation and optimal hydration. A pneumatic pressure device is either commenced intraoperatively (as in the case of some orthopaedic surgeries where a tourniquet was used) or continued from the intraoperative phase, and is recommended in patients with an increased bleeding risk. Thromboembolism deterrent antiembolism stockings should be checked to ensure they are fitted correctly, and anticoagulant prophylaxis must be ordered and administered. A preoperative screening tool for VTE can be used to guide practice, and individual surgeons' preferences for VTE prophylaxis may be consulted.[57,58]

Pain assessment and management

Experiencing postoperative pain has been found to be the most common fear of surgical patients.[59] Inadequate pain relief has been shown to alter the body's metabolic responses, which can delay recovery, extend hospital length of stay, increase morbidity rates and potentially lead to the development of a chronic pain state.[60] Conversely, effective pain control reduces postoperative complications, facilitates rehabilitation and provides a more rapid recovery from surgery.[61] Effective pain management is underpinned by assessment and quick response. Self-reporting subjective pain scales represent the standard of postoperative pain

assessment, allowing patients to report pain using a unidimensional scale of numbers or words. Commonly used to evaluate pain intensity, the visual analogue scale, verbal rating scale and numerical rating scale are valid, reliable and suitable for use in monitoring postoperative pain in patients who are able to self-report.[62] For a detailed discussion on pain assessment and pain management, see Chapter 7. More information on pain medications is also provided in Chapter 7 and earlier in this chapter in the discussion on anaesthetic drugs.

No perfect analgesic drug exists, and it is firmly believed that adequate pain relief requires more than one analgesic, and this approach is referred to as 'multimodal analgesia' and is considered an essential component of care. Multimodal analgesia involves choosing drugs that act on different parts of the anatomical pain pathways and includes a mix of narcotic and non-narcotic analgesics, patient-controlled analgesia, central neural blockade and peripheral nerve blocks. Paracetamol (acetaminophen) has become a main feature of multimodal pain relief in moderate to severe pain and also helps reduce nausea in postoperative patients.[62]

Tramadol is also an effective agent for pain relief. Tramadol binds to mu-opioid receptors and also inhibits the reuptake of serotonin and noradrenaline (norepinephrine).[63] Tramadol can be administered intravenously and is also available in oral and rectal preparations. The primary advantage of tramadol is the relative lack of respiratory depression, an important consideration in the immediate postoperative period.[63] An oral controlled-release tablet containing both oxycodone-hydrochloride and the opioid antagonist naloxone is also available.[63] Existing evidence suggests that better knowledge of different routes of administration of analgesics, their indications and limitations can provide the most appropriate management of acute pain and prevent the development of chronic pain.[61,64]

Two categories of non-steroidal anti-inflammatory drugs are available: non-selective, which inhibit both COX-1 and COX-2 pathways (e.g. ibuprofen, naproxen, ketorolac, diclofenac); and selective, which inhibit only COX-2 (e.g. celecoxib).[65] However, concerns remain regarding the risk of complications, including acute kidney injury and anastomotic leak.[62] Opioids have long been the cornerstone treatment for moderate and severe postoperative pain. There is, however, tension between their benefit and threat to optimal postoperative recovery. The α-2 receptor agonists clonidine and dexmedetomidine can be used to treat postoperative pain. Clonidine and dexmedetomidine reduce opiate use but with a risk for sedation and hypotension.[62]

Patient-controlled analgesia

Patient-controlled analgesia (PCA) has been shown to decrease total opioid consumption and increase patient and nurse satisfaction in postoperative patients. In the postoperative and critical care setting, patients have not experienced an increased incidence of adverse events.[66] The patient is also able to anticipate activities such as rolling or coughing that are associated with increases in pain and is able to self-administer a narcotic bolus prior to the activity in order to manage any pain that might occur.[67] Following a loading dose of analgesia, the PCA pump is programmed based on the patient's needs and the pharmacokinetics of the drug being administered. The parameters programmed into the PCA pump include the bolus dose and a lockout interval. This allows the patient to attain immediate analgesia, with the lockout interval preventing acute increases in the amount of drug delivered.[68]

Regional anaesthesia

Regional anaesthesia is a broad term to describe nerve blocks that block a region, for example arm blocks or femoral blocks. It involves injecting a local anaesthetic near major nerve bundles. To improve the accuracy of drug delivery, selected nerves can be located using ultrasound guidance or a nerve stimulator.[69]

Central neural blockade: epidural/spinal

Central neural blockade or neuraxial anaesthesia is a generic term for epidural, spinal, epidural–spinal or caudal anaesthesia,[44] which blocks pain during a surgical procedure. Many of the medications used in epidural or spinal anaesthesia can continue to provide pain relief in the postoperative period, with local anaesthetic agents having differing durations of action. Local anaesthetic agents with adrenaline may be given if a longer duration of action is required.[44] When intrathecal or epidural opioids are administered, close observation of the patient, particularly the patient's respiratory rate and conscious state, are essential as there may be delayed respiratory depression.[68]

Practice tip

The two most popular positions for epidural and spinal blockade are the 'sitting position', where the patient rolls forward and pushes their back outwards like an 'angry cat', and the 'lateral decubitus' position, where the patient is in a lateral position assuming the 'fetal position'.[44] Both positions allow easier needle access between the vertebrae and are chosen by the anaesthetist. The most important factors that affect the level of neural blockade following spinal anaesthesia are the baricity of the anaesthetic solution, the drug dose, the specific site of injection and the position of the patient at the time of insertion and immediately after injection.[70] Postoperatively, the patient may be seated.

Practice tip

Patients who have received a spinal blockade will have a greater motor block than those with an epidural. This is because the local anaesthetic is injected into the subarachnoid space with the cerebrospinal fluid (CSF) where the spinal nerves are not myelinated, providing a denser motor block.

Care of the patient following epidural or spinal anaesthesia requires an understanding of the possible complications associated with this type of anaesthesia. A wide range of complications can occur including high spinal block, hypotension, bradycardia, spinal and epidural haematoma, post-dural puncture headache, nausea and vomiting, urinary retention and transient neurological symptoms.[44] In addition to normal postoperative observations, continual assessment for possible complications should be maintained, including: observation of the epidural catheter site for bleeding, catheter migration, swelling or redness; discussion with the patient regarding the onset of pain or tenderness at the catheter site; and protective care and observation of anaesthetised limbs.[44] Attention to pressure area care is essential; ensure that the patient is not lying on drain tubing or exposed to heat or cold packs while the block is still in effect as these will not be felt by the patient, so increasing the risk of injury.

High spinal block

Assessing dermatomes after spinal and epidural anaesthesia is important in order to identify any exaggerated dermatome spread that can occur (Fig. 26.4).[63] Signs and symptoms may include dyspnoea, numbness or weakness in the upper extremities, nausea that often precedes hypotension and bradycardia.[63] Reduced doses of medications are necessary for select patients in whom a

---

FIGURE 26.4 Dermatomes.

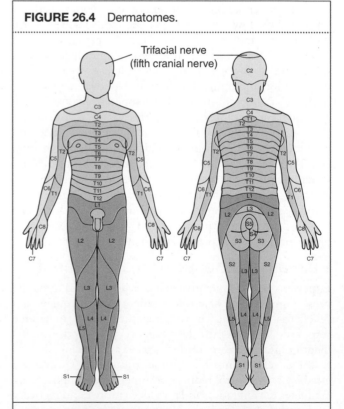

Source: Adapted from Nagelhout J, Plaus K. Nurse anesthesia. 4th ed. St Louis, MO: Saunders; 2010, with permission.

normal dose might be excessive. Blocking of the cardiac sympathetic fibres from T1 to T4 may cause loss of chronotropic and inotropic drive and a fall in cardiac output, which results in hypotension and bradycardia requiring urgent medical attention.[63]

Careful assessment of dermatome levels must be performed. Ice is often used to assess sensory block as hot and cold sensations pass along the same pathway as pain. Central neural blockade blocks not only sensory fibres but also motor function and sympathetic outflow. Continuous assessment of the level of motor blockade using the Bromage score should be performed (Table 26.5).[71,72]

The level of differential blockade is judged by finding the level of sensory block with temperature sensitivity and recognising that the sympathetic block may be two or more segments higher. Motor blockade will be approximately two segments lower.[70] Sympathetic cardiac accelerator fibres arise from T1 to T4 (at and above mid-nipple level). Close monitoring of heart rate and blood pressure should be initiated when the sensory block is sitting around T6 because of the potential for sympathetic

TABLE 26.5
Modified Bromage score[71]

SCORE	CRITERIA
1	Complete block (unable to move feet or knees).
2	Almost complete block (able to move feet only).
3	Partial block (just able to move knees).
4	Detectable weakness of hip flexion while supine (full flexion of knees).
5	No detectable weakness of hip flexion while supine.
6	Able to perform partial knee bend.

Note: This modified Bromage score differs from the original score by including two additional criteria. The other substantial difference is that the original Bromage score[73] began with grade I, which was free movement of legs and feet, whereas in this modified Bromage scale score, 1 is complete block.

Source: Adapted from Breen TW, Shapiro T, Glass B et al. Epidural anesthesia for labor in an ambulatory patient. Anesth Analg 1993;77(5):919–24, with permission

outflow to be blocked.[70] A block at T1–T4 may produce profound bradycardia and hypotension from arterial dilation and venous pooling.[70] Consequently, a significant fall in cardiac output may occur without the body being able to compensate through the usual sympathetic responses. This change in patient condition should be treated as a medical emergency and treatment for shock implemented. Bradycardia can be treated with atropine and hypotension with fluid resuscitation therapy and/or vasopressors.[70] High spinal blocks can affect respiratory muscles, so ongoing assessment of respiratory function should be initiated and airway support provided as required.

Spinal or epidural haematoma

Both epidural and spinal haematomas are more likely to occur in patients who have abnormal coagulation levels, either disease related or as a result of pharmacological therapies.[70] Consequently, coagulation studies must be performed prior to neuraxial anaesthesia being considered, as changes in clotting profiles are an absolute contraindication to insertion of these blocks. Clotting status must also be performed prior to removal of the catheter, and strict guidelines exist for removal in patients who are receiving prophylactic anticoagulants,[70] with recommendations specific to the anticoagulation medication used.

Epidural haematoma can lead to compression of the spinal nerves, causing various degrees of irreversible damage. The symptoms of haematoma include sharp back and leg pain with a motor weakness and/or sphincter dysfunction.[70] Recognition of these symptoms can be delayed until after the effect of the anaesthesia has dissipated. In the event of such symptoms, it is vital to call for immediate medical assistance. Rapid neurological imaging such as a computed tomography or magnetic resonance imaging scan should be performed to assess the location, size and extent of the haematoma, as neurological outcomes are vastly improved if decompression occurs within 8–12 hours.[70]

Post-dural puncture headache

Post-dural puncture headache is not an uncommon complication of interventional neuraxial blockade[73,74] and is a common complication of spinal anaesthesia in the obstetric population.[75] If either a spinal or epidural needle accidentally tears the dura enough to cause CSF to leak out, this may cause a post-dural puncture headache.[73,74]

Conservative management of this condition includes assisting the patient with full bed rest, maintaining adequate hydration and assisting the administering of prescribed medications such as analgesics and caffeine. An autologous blood patch/epidural blood patch can be used to manage post-dural puncture headaches.[76] This is done by taking autologous blood and injecting it into the epidural space where the tear has occurred. The blood covers the area of dural puncture and prevents further leakage of CSF.[76]

Management of nausea and vomiting

Postoperative nausea and vomiting are a concern for patients and clinicians alike and affect as many as one-third of patients receiving anaesthesia. As the most undesirable postoperative complication, postoperative nausea and vomiting also can contribute to complications such as wound dehiscence, aspiration, increased intracranial pressure and increased cardiovascular demand. For some patients, deep breathing, a cool cloth on the forehead and reassurance can help assist with nausea; however, for most postoperative patients, pharmacological interventions will be necessary. Common pharmacological agents for the management of nausea and vomiting are listed in Table 26.6.

Thermoregulation

Anaesthesia and the operating suite environment provide the perfect storm for the development of inadvertent hypothermia, with the cold environment, exposure, opened body cavities, suppression of the thermoregulation

---

TABLE 26.6

Pharmacological interventions for postoperative nausea and vomiting

DRUG (RECEPTOR SITE AFFINITY)	DOSE[a]	DURATION OF ACTION	ADVERSE EFFECTS	COMMENTS AND RECOMMENDATIONS FOR USE
Droperidol (dopamine)	Adult: 0.625–1.25 mg IV Paediatric: 20–50 micrograms/kg IV (children ≥2 years)	12–24 h	Sedation, hypotension, EPS	Higher doses and doses that are repeated too soon can cause sedation, EPS and QT prolongation.
Prochlorperazine (dopamine)	Adult: 5–10 mg IM or IV; 25 mg PR Paediatric:[b] 0.13 mg/kg IM; 0.2 mg/kg PO 2–3 times daily; 0.1 mg/kg 3–4 times daily PR	2–6 h IV, IM, PO; 12 h PR	Sedation, hypotension, EPS	Effective first-line agent.
Promethazine (dopamine, histamine, ACh)	Adult: 6.25–25 mg IM, IV or PR Paediatric (≥2 years of age): 0.25–0.5 mg/kg IV, IM, PR[c]	4 h	Sedation, hypotension, EPS	Good for patients with motion sickness or undergoing surgery affecting vestibular apparatus.
Diphenhydramine (histamine, ACh)	Adult: 12.5–50 mg IM, IV Paediatric (≥2 years of age): 1 mg/kg IV or PO (maximum, 25 mg for <6 years of age)	4–6 hours	Sedation, dry mouth, blurred vision, urinary retention	Good for patients with motion sickness or undergoing surgery affecting vestibular apparatus.
Metoclopramide (dopamine)	Adult: 10–20 mg IV Paediatric: 0.15–0.25 mg/kg	6–8 h	Sedation, hypotension, EPS	Increases gastric motility; good if nausea or vomiting is from gastric stasis; reduce dose to 5 mg in renal impairment; consider diphenhydramine to prevent EPS in children.
Ondansetron (serotonin)	Adult: 4 mg IV; 4–8 mg ODT or wafer Paediatric: 0.05–0.1 mg/kg	Up to 24 h	Headache, lightheadedness, constipation	Much more effective for vomiting than nausea; 2 mg may be sufficient to treat PONV in PACU.
Granisetron (serotonin)	Adult: 1 mg IV over 30 s Paediatric: N/A	Up to 24 h	Headache, lightheadedness	Much more effective for vomiting than nausea.
Palonosetron (serotonin)	Adult: 0.075 mg IV	24 h	Headache, constipation	Prolonged duration of action; given immediately before induction of anaesthesia.

TABLE 26.6

Pharmacological interventions for postoperative nausea and vomiting—cont'd

DRUG (RECEPTOR SITE AFFINITY)	DOSE[a]	DURATION OF ACTION	ADVERSE EFFECTS	COMMENTS AND RECOMMENDATIONS FOR USE
Hyoscine/ scopolamine (ACh)	Adult: 1.5 mg transdermal patch Paediatric: N/A	72 h[d]	Sedation, dry mouth, visual disturbances, dysphoria, confusion, disorientation, hallucinations	Good for patients with motion sickness or undergoing surgery affecting vestibular apparatus; apply 4 h before exposure.
Dexamethasone	Adult: 4–10 mg IV Paediatric: 0.5–1 mg/kg	Up to 24 h	Watch blood sugar in patients with diabetes; watch for fluid retention, especially in cardiac patients	Generally well tolerated in healthy patients; may take time (hours) to work – administer before induction of anaesthesia.
Aprepitant	Adult: 40 mg PO 1–3 h before anaesthesia	Up to 24 h	Generally well tolerated	Oral prophylaxis only; caution with patients taking warfarin; can reduce effectiveness of oral contraceptives.

[a] Unless otherwise indicated, paediatric doses should not exceed the adult dose for each antiemetic agent.

[b] Children weighing more than 10 kg or older than 2 years of age only. Change from IM to PO as soon as possible. With administration PR, dosing interval varies from 8 to 24 h depending on child's weight.

[c] Maximum of 12.5 mg in children younger than 12 years.

[d] Remove after 24 h when used to prevent or treat PONV. Instruct patient to wash the patch site and hands thoroughly.

ACh = acetylcholine; ECG = electrocardiogram; EPS = extrapyramidal symptoms, such as motor restlessness or acute dystonia; IM = intramuscular; IV = intravenous; ODT = orally disintegrating tablets; PACU = postanaesthesia care unit; PO = orally; PONV = postoperative nausea and vomiting; PR = per rectum.

Source: Adapted from O'Brien D. Postanesthesia care complications. In: Odom-Forren J. 7th ed. Drain's perianesthesia nursing: a critical care approach. St Louis, MO: Elsevier; 2018, p. 398–416, with permission.

centre and medications that cause vasodilation. Inadvertent or unplanned hypothermia is defined as a core temperature below 36°C[77] and is divided into three categories: mild (34–36°C), moderate (30–34°C) and severe (≤30°C). Unlike the exposure hypothermia discussed in Chapter 23, inadvertent or unplanned hypothermia generally falls within the mild range. Sequelae of this condition may include infection, sepsis, impaired wound healing, adverse cardiac events, shock, altered drug metabolism, shivering, impaired coagulation, delayed postoperative recovery and increased postoperative discomfort. In elective operations there is a fourfold increase in mortality and a doubled complication rate, with sepsis and stroke being the most increased.[78] The pathophysiological effects of hypothermia include a left oxyhaemoglobin shift, increased oxygen requirements and the ability of vasoconstriction to mask a low circulating blood volume. Recognising these effects, nursing care should include rewarming the patient, providing supplemental oxygen and close monitoring of blood pressure during rewarming because of the potential for the patient to decrease their systolic blood pressure as vasoconstriction is reversed. It is mandatory to assess and monitor the patient's temperature. Postoperative

hypothermia should be treated by the administration of convective or conductive heat until normothermia is achieved and continued until the patient's body temperature is greater than 36°C[78] (see Chapter 23).

> **Practice tip**
>
> During rewarming, patients with inadvertent hypothermia may initially decrease their body temperature before it starts to rise. This does not mean that the first temperature reading was inaccurate; rather, it is an indication of a phenomenon called 'after fall' that occurs when rewarming hypothermic patients.

Voiding and urinary retention

Postoperative urinary retention (POUR), an inability to void, is a frequent postoperative complication which can result in bladder overdistention. Decreasing the risk for overdistention of the bladder is an important patient safety issue. The bladder damage is, to a large extent, an avoidable healthcare-related injury caused by inadequate bladder-monitoring routines. Consequences of POUR

TABLE 26.7
Urinary retention assessment

AMOUNT RETAINED	ACTION
100–150 mL	Assess again after 3 h.
150–300 mL	Assess again after 2 h.
300–400 mL	Assess again after 1 h.
>400 mL	Intermittent, or indwelling catheter.

include increased patient discomfort and pain, an increased risk of urinary tract infections, increased length of stay in hospital, increased medical costs and, for severely acute POUR, permanent detrusor muscle damage.[79] Factors associated with POUR include procedure duration, intraoperative fluid administration, regional anaesthesia and opioid administration.[80] Anaesthesia affects micturition in several ways. During spinal anaesthesia the nerves necessary for spontaneous micturition are blocked and the spinal block has to regress below dermatome S3 before voluntary control over the urethral sphincter returns.[81] General anaesthetics cause bladder atony by interfering with the autonomic regulation of detrusor tone. Sedative-hypnotics and volatile anaesthetics suppress detrusor contraction and the micturition reflex. Reported bladder volume limits vary from 400 to 600 mL.[81] To detect urinary retention, a portable ultrasound scanner to monitor bladder volume is a non-invasive, safe and time-saving method. Action taken is dependent on the amount of urine which is retained in the bladder (Table 26.7). POUR is managed with urethral catheterisation.

The postoperative bariatric patient

The prevalence of obesity is increasing[82] and therefore management of the bariatric or obese patient in the postoperative period warrants detailed discussion. Bariatric patients undergoing anaesthesia will have particular needs in the postanaesthesia period, irrespective of the surgical procedure. For example, the higher incidence of cardiovascular disease means that careful electrocardiographic monitoring should be implemented during recovery from anaesthesia. Assessment of haemodynamic status is important, as it is with any postoperative patient, and accurate measurement of blood pressure is contingent on the use of appropriately sized blood pressure cuffs.

Bariatric patients are also at increased risk for resedation because many anaesthetic drugs are lipophilic and metabolised more slowly by obese patients. Because of increased respiratory compromise, opioids should be used with caution and multimodal treatments are encouraged including the use of non-steroidal anti-inflammatory agents, PCA, local anaesthesia or oral analgesia and the epidural route for analgesia.[83]

Specific assessment and management relative to the bariatric patient include consideration for the prevention of venothromboembolism and pressure injuries. Proper fitting of compression stockings should be monitored so that a tourniquet effect of the stockings is avoided. Knowledge of the surgical procedure and intraoperative positioning will help guide assessment of the patient for signs of intraoperative pressure injury. Intravenous access should be monitored closely, as initiating intravenous access can be challenging in this patient group.

Bariatric patients have an increased risk of extubation failure[84] and the most important consideration in the postoperative period is the assessment of respiratory function. There is a direct correlation between the degree of obesity a patient suffers and the risk and rate of pulmonary complications.[83,85] Airway management may be difficult and hazardous because of anatomical features such as a large tongue and excessive pharyngeal and palatal soft tissue impairing vision and making mask ventilation awkward.

Bariatric patients have impaired oxygen reserve and often have comorbidities resulting in impaired respiratory mechanics during ventilation and increasing the risk of postoperative pulmonary complications.[84] With a reduced functional residual capacity further decreased by supine positioning and general anaesthesia, atelectasis is commonly observed during intraoperative ventilation.[84] Strategies that may improve postoperative outcomes of bariatric patients include the use of higher levels of positive end-expiratory pressure (PEEP), preoxygenation with continuous positive airway pressure (CPAP) followed by PEEP and intraoperative recruitment manoeuvres.[84] Postoperatively, the bariatric patient should be placed in a head-elevated/semi-seated position. The safety and efficacy of CPAP or non-invasive positive pressure ventilation (NIPPV) are well established in the perioperative period and may be considered after extubation. These modalities impede upper airway obstruction, reduce hypoventilation and atelectasis, improve gas exchange and respiratory function and decrease breathing effort.[84] Appropriate airway management, anaesthetic management and adequate ventilation strategy that extends beyond the immediate postextubation period may improve postoperative outcomes for bariatric patients.[84]

Assessment and management of specific postoperative complications

Laryngospasm

Laryngospasm is an airway emergency occurring most commonly during intubation or extubation and is defined as the sustained closure of the vocal cords, as a primitive protective airway reflex to prevent aspiration after a stimulus.[86] It is more common in young paediatric patients than in adults and is most common in infants 1–3 months old.[87] Laryngeal spasm can result in an incomplete or complete airway obstruction,[30,88] with the latter being more uncommon. Prevention of this condition includes extubating patients either deeply paralysed or fully reversed (but not in between), and causes include fluid or secretions on the vocal cords.[86]

Treatment includes gentle positive-pressure ventilation. If hypoxia develops, propofol in a subhypnotic dose usually breaks the spasm; otherwise paralysis with intravenous suxamethonium (0.5–1 mg/kg) or rocuronium (0.4 mg/kg) and controlled ventilation may be required.[86]

Signs and symptoms of laryngeal spasm include inspiratory stridor, dyspnoea, a distressed/sweating patient and an upper airway noise on auscultation. As postoperative patients generally have supplemental oxygen, these symptoms may or may not include a decrease in oxygen saturations in mild laryngeal spasm. Treatment of this condition will include sitting the patient up to facilitate ventilation, supplemental oxygen, gentle suctioning of the upper airway and providing airway support as required.[30,88] It is important to reassure the patient, as anxiety can exacerbate the condition.

Non-cardiogenic pulmonary oedema

Pulmonary oedema may be defined simply as increased total lung water. Non-cardiogenic pulmonary oedema is where increased lung water occurs in the absence of a cardiac aetiology. In the postanaesthesia period, non-cardiogenic pulmonary oedema can occur because of upper airway obstruction such as laryngospasm, bolus dosing with naloxone, reversal of neuromuscular blockade or significant hypoxia.[30] In young athletic males, non-cardiogenic pulmonary oedema may occur in relation to the generation of negative intrathoracic pressure during an upper airway obstruction as the diaphragm contracts against a closed or semi-closed glottis.[89] The severity of pulmonary oedema corresponds to the degree to which high negative inspiratory pressures are generated.[89] Symptoms usually occur within 1 hour of the upper airway obstruction, but may present as much as 6 hours later.[30] The patient may then develop sudden respiratory distress, tachypnoea, cough, shortness of breath, sudden decrease in oxygen saturation and the classic sign of pink, frothy sputum.[30] Vital signs may or may not change.

Rapid diagnosis and treatment are essential to alleviate this respiratory complication. Treatment of this condition includes providing supplemental oxygenation. Continuous positive airway pressure can be used and, if the patient requires airway management, they may be intubated and mechanically ventilated with positive end-expiratory pressure.[30] For further information on oxygenation and caring for an intubated patient, see Chapter 15.

Subglottic oedema/ post-intubation croup

Subglottic oedema or post-intubation croup is a complication that occurs later than laryngospasm but will almost always appear within 3 hours following extubation.[87] Although this condition can occur in adults, it is most commonly seen in the 1–4-year-old age group.[30] The risk of developing subglottic oedema can be lessened in children by allowing a slight gas leak around the endotracheal tube.[87]

Signs and symptoms of subglottic oedema include inspiratory stridor, retractions, hoarseness, crowing respiration and a croup-like cough, and a patient who is apprehensive and restless. Humidified oxygen may help reduce airway swelling and nebulised racemic adrenaline can also help reduce subglottic oedema. If additional treatment is required, a helium–oxygen mixture can be used or dexamethasone administered.[30]

Bronchospasm

Bronchospasm is a lower airway obstruction, characterised by spasmodic smooth muscle contraction that causes narrowing of the bronchi and bronchioles.[30] Generally, bronchospasm will occur in patients with a pre-existing pulmonary illness such as asthma or chronic obstructive pulmonary disease, but it may also develop in healthy patients in the presence of allergy, anaphylaxis or pulmonary aspiration. For this reason, if a patient without pulmonary pathology develops bronchospasm, a high degree of suspicion should be employed by the nurse to ensure that the underlying cause is not allergic or due to pulmonary aspiration.

Signs and symptoms of bronchospasm include coughing, a distinct wheeze upon auscultation, noisy shallow respiration, chest retractions, use of accessory muscles, prolonged expiratory phase of respiration, hypertension and tachycardia. The nurse should sit the patient up, provide assisted oxygen, call for medical assistance and reassure the patient.

Initial management of this patient will include removal of the identified cause if possible,[30] and treatment will depend on the cause, specific symptoms and severity of the bronchospasm. This may include humidified oxygen, administration of a beta$_2$-adrenergic agonist, intubation and intermittent positive-pressure ventilation and perhaps antibiotics. Antihistamines and steroids may also be required.[30]

Aspiration pneumonitis

Mendelson syndrome – aspiration of gastric content that results in a severe pulmonary complication – was first reported in the 1940s.[90] Preoperative patient preparation, including fasting, is aimed at minimising the risk of aspiration. Pregnant women, obese patients, patients with gastro-oesophageal reflux disease and non-fasting patients are all at increased risk of aspiration pneumonitis.[63]

Clinical progression after aspiration varies widely, from no and very mild symptoms to bronchopneumonia and possible development of acute respiratory distress syndrome.[63] The severity of progression is increased by several factors including the aspirate pH, quantity of aspirate and the presence of solid particles.[63] Symptoms include tachypnoea, tachycardia, cough and possible bronchospasm.[63] While this condition may be dramatic in onset, it can also be insidious in nature. Bronchospasm that occurs in a healthy patient should be investigated further.[63]

Postoperative delirium

Elderly people are at an increased risk of developing postoperative delirium (POD). The incidence of POD varies widely but is reported to be 10%–60%, with the highest rates occurring in elderly. POD is characterised by a fluctuating disturbance in attention and awareness that develops over a short period of time (hours to days) with disorganised thinking, features of inattention and fluctuating level of consciousness, representing acute brain dysfunction. In clinical practice, delirium can be classified into three subtypes based on psychomotor behaviour: hyperactive, hypoactive or mixed. Hyperactive delirium presents with agitation, restlessness and hypervigilance. Patients with hypoactive delirium are lethargic with slowed mentation and decreased movement. Importantly, care providers are much more likely to miss a diagnosis of delirium in patients with hypoactive features. Emergence delirium refers to psychomotor agitation that occurs as the patient emerges from a general anaesthesia. Early diagnosis is important to treat the condition.[91] Recommended tools to assess POD include the 4AT,[92] the Nursing Delirium Symptom Checklist (Nu-DESC) and the Confusion Assessment Method for Intensive Care Unit (CAM-ICU). Regular use of a validated screening tool is critical in ensuring that delirium is not left undiagnosed.[92]

Care to decrease the risk of POD includes strategies to orient the patient in time and place, regular communication and explanation about what is happening; give the patient time to understand and respond, keep things simple and rephrase if necessary. A supportive environment including letting the patient sit upright if possible and minimising unnecessary noise, letting the patient use their own spectacles and hearing aids and starting with early mobilisation are also recommended strategies. It is also important to avoid, identify and treat hypoxia, hypotension, pain, hypothermia, signs of infection, urinary retention and inability to void.[93] If POD arises, assessment, identification and management of underlying causes such as pain, infection, constipation, hypothermia, urinary retention, dehydration and metabolic derangement must be undertaken. To date, there are limited pharmacological options for the treatment of POD, but antipsychotics are a first-line treatment for agitation.[91]

Delayed awakening

Time to emerge from anaesthesia is variable between patients and may depend on a multitude of factors including the type of anaesthesia and the length of surgery. Occasionally, the time for a patient to awake may be longer than expected and this could be due to a plethora of factors.[30]

Delayed emergence may occur in a patient who was recovering in the ICU or may be the reason for an admission to ICU. The most common cause of delayed awakening is prolonged effect from anaesthesia and associated medications, but it could also be due to metabolic complications including hypoglycaemia, hyponatraemia, hypocalcaemia, hypomagnesaemia, hypercarbia, hypoxia, hypothermia, hypovolaemia or neurological injury.[30] A full neurological assessment will be required[30] using the Glasgow Coma Scale (GCS). The primary management is always in support of airway, breathing and circulation while the cause is sought.

Malignant hyperthermia

Malignant hyperthermia is a rare, catastrophic, often fatal syndrome that is triggered by volatile anaesthetic agents and suxamethonium.[94] It is an uncommon disorder with autosomal dominant inheritance, involving abnormal skeletal muscle calcium metabolism.[94] Although its pathogenesis is relatively well understood, there is wide variability in the time of onset and the presentation of clinical signs and symptoms.[95] Most cases of malignant hyperthermia occur within 30 minutes of anaesthesia and therefore will be seen and treated in the operating suite. In some circumstances the delayed onset or wrongly identified early clinical manifestation has hindered timely recognition and treatment.[96] Patients presenting with febrile illness after surgery should be assessed for malignant hyperthermia. This is a particularly important consideration for those patients who are discharged home after surgery but re-present to the hospital emergency department.

Early symptoms of malignant hyperthermia include tachycardia, tachypnoea, sweating, rise in end-tidal carbon dioxide levels, hyperthermia, and involuntary contraction of skeletal muscle which may manifest as masseteric muscle spasm in the early stage.[96]

The treating medication, dantrolene sodium, is a skeletal muscle relaxant that decreases the amount of calcium released by the sarcoplasmic reticulum, reversing the pathophysiology of malignant hyperthermia (Box 26.2).[95–98]

Transferring care of the postoperative patient: discharge to an inpatient ward

Without question, the immediate postoperative period will require high-quality, safe nursing care to detect and/or prevent serious complications. Many factors affect the patient's response to anaesthesia and surgery; therefore the length of stay for each patient will vary.

For this reason, most PACUs have discharge criteria that involve a thorough assessment of the patient's vital signs, pain, conscious state, nausea and vomiting, and escalation of a care plan prior to patient discharge from the PACU.[99] These criteria are used to determine when a patient is ready to be discharged to the ward and can be used in the ICU when non-critically ill patients are in ICU recovering from anaesthesia (Table 26.8). Critically ill postoperative patients will have their discharge managed by the ICU clinician team.

BOX 26.2

Management of malignant hyperthermia[97,98]

- Stop trigger agents immediately.
- Administer 100% oxygen and hyperventilate.
- Call for help – press emergency bell.
- Contact the operating theatre to get specialised help from an anaesthetist.
- Obtain sodium dantrolene, the treating agent, and administer 2.5 mg/kg with no upper dose limit.
- Notify pharmacy department to replenish stores of sodium dantrolene.
- Use aggressive cooling to prevent the patient reaching the thermal critical level of >40.6°C.
- Assist in associated management of arrhythmias and electrolyte imbalance.
- Assess cardiac function, urine output and colour (urinary catheterisation may be required).

Sources: Hooper VD. Care of the patient with thermal imbalance. In: Odom-Forren J, editor. Drain's perianesthesia nursing: a critical care approach. 7th ed. St Louis, MO: Elsevier; 2018, p. 763–73; Hirshey Dirksen S, Van Wicklin S, Ledrut Mashman D et al. Developing effective drills in preparation for a malignant hyperthermia crisis. AORN 2013;97(3):330–52.

TABLE 26.8

Discharge criteria for the postoperative patient

Conscious state	Conscious and able to respond appropriately to verbal stimuli.
Respiratory function	Able to protect his or her own airway. Has a cough reflex. Respiratory rate must be greater than 12 breaths/min. Oxygen saturation should be >94% on room air and assessed at least 10 min after oxygen discontinued. Need for supplemental oxygen should be determined by medical team for those patients who do not have an oxygen saturation >94% on room air.
Cardiovascular function	Vital signs need to be within normal limits and considered in relation to the patient's preoperative vital signs. Heart rate and blood pressure should be within 20% of preoperative.
Temperature	Patient's core temperature should be between 36°C and 37°C.
Pain	The patient should be pain free or have pain at a manageable level.
Nausea and vomiting	The patient should be free from nausea and vomiting. Patients with persistent nausea may return to the ward after liaison with medical staff and appropriate ongoing management in place.
Wound care	Dressings should be dry and intact. Drains should be labelled with amount, date and time. Drainage should be assessed to ensure excessive drainage is not present. Women who have had a lower caesarean section will have their fundal height assessed. The fundal height should be equal to or less than the level of the umbilicus. Per vaginal (PV) loss must be assessed in both gynaecological and obstetric patients, ensuring that the blood loss is within normal limits.
Neurological and neurovascular observations	Should be within normal limits.
Documentation	Nursing documentation completed legibly in ink. Ensure medical staff members have written up appropriate notes and orders.

Summary

In conclusion, patients who have received anaesthesia and undergone surgical procedures are vulnerable to a multitude of different complications. Although they may not be critically ill, patients who are transferred to the ICU immediately following surgery require close monitoring and observation. Respect for, and knowledge and understanding of, such complications will allow the nurse to provide a safer postoperative journey.

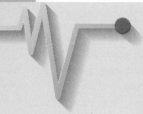

Case study

Mrs Stella Cohen was a 75-year-old patient who presented to the ICU following coronary artery grafting surgery. Her past history included severe coronary artery disease and angina, non-insulin-dependent diabetes and periods of depression. She has no history of dementia, and she does not smoke and does not abuse alcohol or other substances.

Mrs Cohen received a full relaxant general anaesthetic and had an uneventful operative period and was safely transferred to the ICU at 19:30 hours. She remained intubated and ventilated overnight and was extubated in the morning the day after surgery. She did well immediately after the extubation, with some pain but no sign of confusion noted by the ICU nurses. Her blood pressure was 120/80 mmHg, her heart rate was 90 bpm and oxygen saturation was 98%. During the night, Mrs Cohen developed acute confusion including disorientation. The GCS score was 15. The temperature was 37.2°C but had a transient peak to 38.4°C the day before. She never required intubation, sedation or pressors. Her confusion persisted throughout her 4-day ICU stay, and psychiatric evaluation led to a diagnosis of delirium, which cleared slowly as her medical condition stabilised. Mrs Cohen went to a skilled nursing facility and then home, where no further delirium was noted.

DISCUSSION

Delirium, defined as an acute decline in attention and cognition, represents a serious complication in patients after anaesthesia and surgery and is predictive of mortality at 6 months in ICU patients. Postoperative delirium is characterised by a fluctuating disturbance in attention and awareness that develops over a short period of time (hours to days), with disorganised thinking, features of inattention and a fluctuating level of consciousness, representing acute brain dysfunction. In clinical practice, delirium can be classified into three subtypes based on psychomotor behaviour: hyperactive, hypoactive or mixed. Hyperactive delirium presents with agitation, restlessness and hypervigilance. Patients with hypoactive delirium are lethargic with slowed mentation and decreased movement. Importantly, care providers are much more likely to miss a diagnosis of delirium in patients with hypoactive features. Diagnosis in the postsurgical setting is based on validated clinical scales. The CAM-ICU patients scale has been validated in medical and coronary ICU patients as a reliable tool to detect delirium. The Nursing Delirium Screening Scale (Nu-DESC) includes five items scored 0–2: disorientation, inappropriate behaviour, inappropriate communication, illusions/hallucinations and psychomotor retardation. Delirium is indicated by a score ≥2. The Nu-DESC can be useful as an additional tool to pain scores for ensuring patient comfort and restoration of postoperative brain function in the PACU/ICU.[100,101]

The pathophysiology of delirium remains poorly understood; hypotheses suggest that neuroinflammation, ACh deficiencies and neurotransmitter impairments are related to patients' acute brain dysfunction. Genetic factors have also been identified as risk factors for developing postoperative delirium in the elderly. The ageing brain exhibits both quantitative and qualitative changes in neuronal circuitry that could account for the greater sensitivity of older patients to delirium.[100,101]

CASE STUDY QUESTIONS

1   Describe the hypothetical mechanisms for postoperative delirium.
2   Discuss the risk factors for postoperative delirium in relation to the patient described in this case study.
3   Describe the symptoms of postoperative delirium.
4   How can delirium be assessed? Give examples of the type of scales.

RESEARCH VIGNETTE

Malik KM, Imani F, Beckerly R, et al. Risk of opioid use disorder from exposure to opioids in the perioperative period: a systematic review. Anesthesiol Pain Med 2020;10(1):e101339.

Abstract

Opioid use disorder (OUD), a major source of morbidity and mortality globally, is regularly linked to opioids given around the time of surgery. The perioperative period, however, is markedly heterogeneous, with the diverse providers using opioids distinctively, and the various drivers of opioid misuse at play dissimilarly, throughout the perioperative period. The risk of OUD may, therefore, be different from opioids given at the various phases of perioperative care, and the ensuing recommendations for their use may also be dissimilar. Systematic search and analysis of the pertinent literature, following the accepted standards, showed an overall increased risk of misuse from the perioperative opioids. However, the analysed studies had significant methodological limitations, and were constrained mainly to the outpatient phase of the perioperative period. Lacking any data, this risk, therefore, is unknown for the intraoperative and postoperative recovery periods. Consequently, no firm recommendations can be extended to anaesthesia providers generally managing these perioperative stages. Furthermore, with significant methodological limitations, the current recommendations for opioid use after surgery are also arbitrary. Therefore, though proposals for perioperative opioid use are formulated in this article, substantive recommendations would require clear delineation of these risks, while avoiding the limitations noted in this review.

Critique

Almost 60% of individuals presenting for surgery are opioid naïve (i.e. have not received opioids in the 30 days prior to surgery). Yet almost 10% of the opioid naïve end up in *new persistent opioid use*, meaning that continuation of opioid use takes place beyond the immediate postoperative period over a longer period than intended, so-called opioid use disorder.

There is also concern that poorly controlled acute postoperative pain can hasten the transition to chronic pain conditions and persistent postoperative opioid use. Consequently, it is necessary to balance the desire to limit opioid supply with the need to provide adequate analgesia.[102] The availability of opioids for analgesic purposes varies substantially across the globe and it is not surprising that countries that have much higher prescribing rates for opioids, such as in North America, Western Europe and Australia, have greater rates of non-medical use and opioid overdose deaths.[103]

In this review the overall risk of new OUD varied significantly from as low as 0.09% to as high as 13%. The highest rates of opioid misuse were reported in subsets of patients undergoing spinal (23.6%) and orthopaedic surgeries (13.7%). The possible risk of OUD seems to be greater when opioids were given at the postoperative stage, especially in the late stage. When administrating opioids intraoperatively, the risk for OUD was low.

Not all patients who develop OUD are the same. New persistent opioid use after surgery probably represents a constellation of many different phenomena, which is difficult to discern without additional context from the patient.[104] Individual risk factors for OUD include male sex, externalising disorders in childhood, poor school performance, low commitment to education and non-completion of secondary education. In addition, there is increasing recognition of the potential importance of co-occurring mental disorders, such as depression and post-traumatic stress disorder (PTSD), and physical health problems, such as chronic non-cancer pain, in the development of OUD, both in and outside the context of medical treatment. These risk factors often co-occur, which increases the risk for OUD.[103] To measure these risk factors such as depression, physical and mental health and PTSD preoperatively, in order to capture persons that are in risk for OUD, would be preferable. Further, opportunities to provide psychiatric support may also affect postoperative opioid use. One suggested model is a multidisciplinary program that incorporates psychological support as part of a broader platform of interventions to prevent chronic postsurgical pain. Implementing evidence-based standards to encourage responsible opioid prescribing while also promoting effective pain management for patients after surgery is also one way to decrease the risk of OUD.[105]

The perioperative period is heterogeneous, with the diverse providers using opioids individually. The risk of OUD may, therefore, be different from opioids given at the various phases of perioperative care, and the ensuing recommendations for their use may also be contradictory.

The authors undertook a systematic review of the literature reporting the risk of OUD from opioids given perioperatively. They searched three major databases, PubMed, Medline and Embase, using search terms; however, the precise search strategy was not detailed, so preventing accurate replication of this search. If the search terms were limited to 'perioperative', 'postoperative' and 'preoperative' combined with 'opioids' AND 'addiction', it is possible that some relevant studies may have been overlooked. Backward citation searching was used to identify any articles which may have been missed when searching the databases. Only studies published in English were included, introducing a language bias, which is common in published systematic reviews. The focus was on published clinical studies, which would have increased the applicability to clinical practice. It is unclear whether a single author or multiple authors undertook the screening of articles and data extraction. The approach to data analysis was also not specified.

This systematic review includes 17 articles, all of which used retrospective and observational study designs. There were significant limitations noted for the included studies, including variability in how OUD was defined, and accepted standards for ascertaining OUD were not met for most studies. Underreporting of conditions which may have predisposed the patients to substance use disorders was attempted for some studies; nevertheless, underreporting was likely.

There was diversity in the types of surgical patients such as caesarean delivery, hand surgery, gynaecology surgeries, hip and knee surgeries, urological surgeries, bariatric surgeries, same-day surgeries and 'major elective' surgery.

Because the overall strength of evidence is low, recommendation made by the author need to be cautiously interpreted. One recommendation was to wean patients off opioids and to employ alternative non-opioid therapies prior to the hospital discharge after surgery. Others were to endorse opioids of appropriate type and quantity commensurate with the type of surgery and the expected duration of post-surgical pain, to closely monitor the patient's opioid consumption, and to preferentially use non-opioid analgesics. Overall, in view of the substantial risks posed by OUD, and the utility of perioperative opioids, any substantive recommendations can be offered only if the risk of OUD is clearly delineated for the various perioperative stages.

Learning activities

1　Subglottic oedema occurs mainly in young children but can also be observed in adults. Subglottic oedema may be observed as long as 3 hours postextubation. What signs and symptoms might you observe in the patient with subglottic oedema?

2　What type of strategies could be used to minimise the use of perioperative opioid?

3　Bariatric patients undergoing surgery warrant special consideration. What specific assessment might you undertake for this specific patient group?

4　What action should be taken if the amount of urine is 300–400 mL retained in the bladder?

5　What strategies could you use to manage emergence delirium?

Online resources

American Association of Nurse Anaesthesiology, https://www.aana.com/

American Society of Anesthesiologists, https://www.asahq.org

American Society of PeriAnesthesia Nurses, https://www.aspan.org

Association of Anaesthetists of Great Britain and Ireland, https://anaesthetists.org

Association of Perioperative Registered Nurses, https://www.aorn.org

Australian College of Operating Room Nurses, https://www.acorn.org.au

International Federation of Perioperative Nurses, https://www.ifpn.world

Operating Room Nurses Association of Canada, https://www.ornac.ca

Perioperative Nurses College of New Zealand Nurses Organisation, https://www.nzno.org.nz/groups/colleges_sections/colleges/perioperative_nurses_college

Further reading

British Journal of Anaesthetic and Recovery Nursing.

Journal of PeriAnesthesia Nursing.

Odom-Forren J, editor. Drain's perianesthesia nursing: a critical care approach. 7th ed. St Louis, MO: Elsevier; 2018.

Hamlin L, Davies M, Richardson-Tench M, et al. Perioperative nursing: an introduction. 2nd ed. Sydney: Elsevier; 2016.

References

1. American Society of PeriAnesthesia Nurses (ASPAN). ASPAN's history. Cherry Hill, NJ: ASPAN; 2012. Available from: https://www.aspan.org/About/About-ASPAN/ASPAN-History. [Accessed 25 February 2023].

2. Schick L. Assessment and monitoring of the perianesthesia patient. In: Odom-Forren J, editor. Drain's perianesthesia nursing: a critical care approach. 7th ed. St Louis, MO: Elsevier; 2018, p. 357–84.

3. Australian Commission on Safety and Quality in Health Care (ACSQHC). National safety and quality health service standards. Sydney, NSW: ACSQHC; 2021, p. 67–72.

4. Massa S, Wu J, Wang C, et al. Interprofessional training and communication practices among clinicians in the postoperative ICU handoff. Jt Comm J Qual Patient Saf 2021;47(4):242–9.

5. Drain. Inhalation anesthesia. In: Odom-Forren J, editor. Drain's perianesthesia nursing: a critical care approach. St Louis, MO: Elsevier; 2018, p. 260–71.

6. Butterworth J, Mackey D, Wasnick J. The practice of anesthesiology. In: Butterworth J, Mackey D, Wasnick J, editors. Morgan and Mikhail's clinical anesthesiology. 7th ed. New York: McGraw-Hill; 2022, p. 1–6.

7. Ode K. Intravenous anaesthetic agents. Anaesth Intensive Care Med 2019;20(2):118–25.

8. Raeder J. Procedural sedation in ambulatory anaesthesia: what's new? Curr Opin Anesthesiol 2019;32(6):743–8.

9. Yao Y-t, He L-x, Fang N-x, et al. Anesthetic induction with etomidate in cardiac surgical patients: a PRISMA-compliant systematic review and meta-analysis. J Cardiothorac Vasc Anesth 2021;35(4):1073–85.

10. Dalia AA, Raines DE. Etomidate and adrenocortical suppression: should we take the concerns to heart? J Cardiothorac Vasc Anesth 2021;35(4):1086–8.

11. Cascella M. Rise and decline of the barbiturate methitural for intravenous anesthesia: a systematic search and narrative synthesis. J Anesth Hist 2021;7(1):11–16.

12. Gaddam NR, Kelkar VP, Kulkarni SJ, et al. A comparative study of propofol, thiopentone sodium, and ketofol as induction agents for electro convulsive therapy. J Anaesthesiol Clin Pharmacol 2021;37(4):554.

13. Fawcett WJ, Ljungqvist O, Lobo DN. Perioperative opioids – reclaiming lost ground. JAMA Surg 2021;156(11):997–8.

14. Brown EN, Pavone KJ, Naranjo M. Multimodal general anesthesia: theory and practice. Anesth Analg 2018;127(5):1246.

15. Egan TD. Are opioids indispensable for general anaesthesia? Br J Anaesth 2019;122(6):e127–35.

16. Cooney M. Opioid analgesics. In: Cooney M, Quinlan-Colwell A, editors. Assessment and multimodal management of pain: an integrative approach. St Louis, MO: Elsevier; 2021, p. 222–302.

17. Levy N, Quinlan J, El-Boghdadly K, et al. An international multidisciplinary consensus statement on the prevention of opioid-related harm in adult surgical patients. Anaesthesia 2021;76(4):520–36.

18. Drain C. Opioid intravenous anesthetics. In: Odom-Forren J, editor. Drain's perianesthesia nursing: a critical care approach. 7th ed. St Louis, MO: Elsevier; 2018, p. 284–96.

19. Baldo BA, Rose MA. The anaesthetist, opioid analgesic drugs, and serotonin toxicity: a mechanistic and clinical review. Br J Anaesth 2020;124(1):44–62.

20. Redfield RR. CDC Director's media statement on US life expectancy. Washington, DC: CDC Newsroom Releases; 2018.

21. Brown R, Morgan A. The opioid epidemic in North America: implications for Australia. Trends & Issues in Crime and Criminal Justice no. 578. Canberra, ACT: Australian Institute of Criminology; 2019, p. 1–15.

22. Everson M, McLain N, Collins MJ, et al. Perioperative pain management strategies in the age of an opioid epidemic. J PeriAnesth Nurs 2020;35(4):347–52.

23. Arslantas R. Spinal anesthesia: applications to cesarean section and pain. In: Rajendram R, Patel VB, Preedy VR, et al, editors. Features and assessments of pain, anaesthesia, and analgesia. London: Elsevier; 2022. p. 381–9.

24. Howlett C, Gonzalez R, Yerram P, et al. Use of naloxone for reversal of life-threatening opioid toxicity in cancer-related pain. J Oncol Pharmacy Pract 2016;22(1):114–20.

25. Drain C. Nonopioid intravenous anesthetics. In: Odom-Forren J, editor. Drain's perianesthesia nursing: a critical care approach. 7th ed. St Louis, MO: Elsevier; 2018. p. 272–83.

26. Joshi GP. General anesthetic techniques for enhanced recovery after surgery: Current controversies. Best Pract Res Clin Anaesthesiol 2021;35(4):531–41.

27. Pastis NJ, Yarmus LB, Schippers F, et al. Safety and efficacy of remimazolam compared with placebo and midazolam for moderate sedation during bronchoscopy. Chest 2019;155(1):137–46.

28. Fagerlund MJ, Jeevendra Martyn, J A. Neuromuscular physiology and pharmacology. In: Gropper MAMDP, editor. Miller's anesthesia. 9th ed. Philadelphia: Elsevier; 2020, p. 333–53.e2.

29. Murphy G, De Boer HD, Eriksson LI, et al. Reversal (antagonism) of neuromuscular blockade. In: Gropper MAMDP, editor. Miller's anesthesia. 9th ed. Philadelphia: Elsevier; 2020, p. 832–64.e5.

30. O'Brien D. Postanesthesia care complications. In: Odom-Forren J, editor. Drain's perianesthesia nursing: a critical care approach. 7th ed. St Louis, MO: Elsevier; 2018, p. 398–416.

31. Groudine SB, Minkowitz HS, Valentine DL. Real-world experience with neuromuscular blockade reversal. J Clin Anesth 2017;42:102.

32. de Kam P-J, Nolte H, Good S, et al. Sugammadex hypersensitivity and underlying mechanisms: a randomised study of healthy non-anaesthetised volunteers. Br J Anaesth 2018;121(4):758–67.

33. Williams R, Bryant H. Sugammadex advice for women of childbearing age. Anaesthesia 2018;73(1):133–4.

34. Brull SJ, Meistelman, C. Pharmacology of neuromuscular blocking drugs. In: Gropper MAMDP, editor. Miller's anesthesia. 9th ed. Philadelphia: Elsevier; 2020, p. 792–831.e8.

35. Drain C. Neuromuscular blocking agents. In: Odom-Forren J, editor. Drain's perianesthesia nursing: a critical care approach. 7th ed. St Louis, MO: Elsevier; 2018, p. 297–315.

36. Nagelhout J. Basic principles of pharmacology. In: Odom-Forren J, editor. Drain's perianesthesia nursing: a critical care approach. 7th ed. St Louis, MO: Elsevier; 2018, p. 243–59.

37. Chen Q, Chen E, Qian X. A narrative review on perioperative pain management strategies in enhanced recovery pathways – the past, present and future. J Clin Med 2021;10(12):2568.

38. Zhang Z, Xu H, Zhang Y, et al. Nonsteroidal anti-inflammatory drugs for postoperative pain control after lumbar spine surgery: a meta-analysis of randomized controlled trials. J Clin Anesth 2017;43:84–9.

39. Schoenbrunner AR, Joshi GP, Janis JE. Multimodal analgesia in the aesthetic plastic surgery: concepts and strategies. Plast Reconstr Surg Glob Open 2022;10(5):e4310.

40. Choi M, Wang L, Coroneos CJ, et al. Managing postoperative pain in adult outpatients: a systematic review and meta-analysis comparing codeine with NSAIDs. CMAJ 2021;193(24):E895–905.

41. Vuyk J, Sitsen E, Reekers M. Intravenous anesthetics. In: Gropper MAMDP, editor. Miller's anesthesia. 9th ed. Philadelphia: Elsevier; 2020, p. 638–79.e10.

42. Bell RF, Kalso EA. Ketamine for pain management. Pain Rep 2018;3(5):e674.

43. Rasool F, Ghafoor R, Lambert DG. Antidepressants and antipsychotics: anaesthetic implications. Anaesth Intensive Care Med 2014; 15(7):314–17.

44. Nagelhout J. Local anaesthetics. In: Odom-Forren J, editor. Drain's perianesthesia nursing: a critical care approach. 7th ed. St Louis, MO: Elsevier; 2018, p. 329–43.

45. Liu Y, Qiu Y, Fu Y, et al. Evaluation of postoperative recovery: past, present and future. Postgrad Med J 2022: postgradmedj-2022-141652. doi: 10.1136/postgradmedj-2022-141652. Online ahead of print.

46. Wang XL, He M, Feng Y. Handover patterns in the PACU: a review of the literature. J Perianesth Nurs 2021;36(2):136–41.

47. Aldrete JA, Kroulik D. A postanesthetic recovery score. Anesth Analg 1970;49(6):924–34.

48. Nilsson U, Gruen R, Myles P. Postoperative recovery: the importance of the team. Anaesthesia 2020;75:e158–e64.

49. Wright S. Assessment and management of the airway. In: Odom-Forren J, editor. Drain's perianesthesia nursing: a critical care approach. 7th ed. St Louis, MO: Elsevier; 2018, p. 417–30.

50. Suzuki S. Oxygen administration for postoperative surgical patients: a narrative review. J Intensive Care 2020;8(1):1–6.

51. Laporta ML, Sprung J, Weingarten TN. Respiratory depression in the post-anesthesia care unit: Mayo Clinic experience. Bosnian J Basic Med Sci 2021;21(2):221.

52. Churpek MM, Adhikari R, Edelson DP. The value of vital sign trends for detecting clinical deterioration on the wards. Resuscitation 2016;102:1–5.

53. Kellett J, Murray A, Woodworth S, et al. Trends in weighted vital signs and the clinical course of 44,531 acutely ill medical patients while in hospital. Acute Med 2015;14(1):3–9.

54. Allegranzi B, Bischoff P, de Jonge S, et al. New WHO recommendations on preoperative measures for surgical site infection prevention: an evidence-based global perspective. Lancet Infect Dis 2016;16(12):e276–87.

55. Nelson G, Bakkum-Gamez J, Kalogera E, et al. Guidelines for perioperative care in gynecologic/oncology: Enhanced Recovery After Surgery (ERAS) Society recommendations – 2019 update. Int J Gynecol Cancer 2019;29(4):651–68.

56. Malina D. Fluid and electrolytes. In: Odom-Forren J, editor. Drain's perianesthesia nursing: a critical care approach. 7th ed. St Louis, MO: Elsevier; 2018, p. 199–214.

57. Golemi I, Adum JPS, Tafur A, et al. Venous thromboembolism prophylaxis using the Caprini score. Disease-a-Month 2019;65(8):249–98.

58. Afshari A, Ageno W, Ahmed A, et al. European guidelines on perioperative venous thromboembolism prophylaxis: executive summary. Eur J Anaesthesiol 2018;35(2):77–83.

59. Ertürk EB, Ünlü H. Effects of pre-operative individualized education on anxiety and pain severity in patients following open-heart surgery. Int J Health Sci 2018;12(4):26.

60. Yang MMH, Hartley RL, Leung AA, et al. Preoperative predictors of poor acute postoperative pain control: a systematic review and meta-analysis. BMJ Open 2019;9(4):e025091.

61. Puntillo F, Giglio M, Varrassi G. The routes of administration for acute postoperative pain medication. Pain Ther 2021;10(2):909–25.

62. Small C, Laycock H. Acute postoperative pain management. Br J Surg 2020;107(2):e70–80.

63. Foran P. Postanaesthesia nursing care. In: Sutherland-Fraser S, Davies M, Richardson-Gillespie BM, et al, editors. Perioperative nursing – an introduction. 3rd ed. Sydney, NSW: Elsevier; 2022, p. 415–46.

64. Ruetzler K, Blome CJ, Nabecker S, et al. A randomised trial of oral versus intravenous opioids for treatment of pain after cardiac surgery. J Anesth 2014;28(4):580–6.

65. Pasero C. Pain mamgement. In: Odom-Forren J, editor. Drain's perianesthesia nursing: a critical care approach. 7th ed. St Louis, MO: Elsevier; 2018, p. 431–55.

66. Papa L, Maguire L, Bender M, et al. Patient controlled analgesia for the management of acute pain in the emergency department: a systematic review. Am J Emerg Med 2022;51:228–38.

67. McKeen MJ, Quraishi SA. Clinical review of intravenous opioids in acute care. J Anesthesiol Clin Sci 2013;2(1):1.

68. Mitra S, Carlyle D, Kodumudi G, et al. New advances in acute postoperative pain management. Curr Pain Headache Rep 2018;22(5):1–11.

69. Australian and New Zealand College of Anaesthetists (ANZCA). Types of anaesthesia. Melbourne, VIC: ANZCA; 2020. Available from: https://www.anzca.edu.au/getattachment/d23b786d-e485-4e5b-a4b4-e6a8f9686172/Types-of-anaesthesia. [Accessed 25 February 2023].

70. Butterworth J, Mackey D, Wasnick J. Spinal, epidural amd caudal blocks. In: Butterworth J, Mackey D, Wasnick J, editors. Morgan and Mikhail's clinical anesthesiology. 7th ed. New York: McGraw-Hill Medical; 2022, p. 965–1006.

71. Breen TW, Shapiro T, Glass B, et al. Epidural anesthesia for labor in an ambulatory patient. Anesth Analg 1993;77(5):919–24.

72. Bromage PR. Epidural analgesia. Philadelphia: WB Saunders Company; 1978.

73. Kim JE, Kim SH, Han RJW, et al. Postdural puncture headache related to procedure: incidence and risk factors after neuraxial anesthesia and spinal procedures. Pain Med 2021;22(6):1420–5.

74. Shaparin N, Gritsenko K, Shapiro D, et al. Timing of neuraxial pain interventions following blood patch for post dural puncture headache. Pain Physician 2014;17(2):119–25.

75. FitzGerald S, Salman M. Postdural puncture headache in obstetric patients. Br J General Pract 2019;69(681):207–8.

76. Ioscovich A, Giladi Y, Fuica RL, et al. Anesthetic approach to postdural puncture headache in the peripartum period: an Israeli national survey. Acta Anaesthesiol Scand 2018;62(10):1460–5.

77. Link T. Guidelnes in practice: hypothermia prevention. AORN J 2020;111(6):653–66.

78. Simegn GD, Bayable SD, Fetene MB. Prevention and management of perioperative hypothermia in adult elective surgical patients: a systematic review. Ann Med Surg 2021;72:103059.

79. Cremins M, Vellanky S, McCann G, et al. Considering healthcare value and associated risk factors with postoperative urinary retention after elective laminectomy. Spine J 2020;20(5):701–7.

80. Scott AJ, Mason SE, Langdon AJ, et al. Prospective risk factor analysis for the development of post-operative urinary retention following ambulatory general surgery. World J Surg 2018;42(12):3874–9.

81. Brouwer TA, van Roon EN, Rosier PFWM, et al. Postoperative urinary retention: risk factors, bladder filling rate and time to catheterization: an observational study as part of a randomized controlled trial. Perioper Med 2021;10(1):2.

82. Gurka MJ, Filipp SL, DeBoer MD. Geographical variation in the prevalence of obesity, metabolic syndrome, and diabetes among US adults. Nutr Diabetes 2018;8(1):1–8.

83. Clifford T. Care of the patient undergoing bariatric surgery. In: Odom-Forren J, editor. Drain's perianesthesia nursing: a critical care approach. 7th ed. St Louis, MO: Elsevier; 2018, p. 656–63.

84. Carron M, Safaee Fakhr B, Ieppariello G, et al. Perioperative care of the obese patient. Br J Surg 2020;107(2):e39–55.

85. Mendonça J, Pereira H, Xará D, et al. Obese patients: respiratory complications in the post-anesthesia care unit. Revista Portuguesa de Pneumologia (English ed.) 2014;20(1):12–19.

86. Silva CR, Pereira T, Henriques D, et al. Comprehensive review of laryngospasm. Update in Anaesthesia: J Anesth Crit Care 2020;35:15–8.

87. Butterworth J, Mackey D, Wasnick J. Airway management. In: Butterworth J, Mackey D, Wasnick J, editors. Morgan and Mikhail's clinical anesthesiology. 7th ed. New York: McGraw-Hill Medical; 2022, p. 307–44.

88. Drain C. The respiratory system. In: Odom-Forren J, editor. Drain's perianestheia nursing: a critical care approach. 7th ed. St Louis, MO: Elsevier; 2018, p. 155–88.

89. Toukan Y, Gur M, Bentur L. Negative pressure pulmonary edema following choking on a cookie. Pediatr Pulmonol 2016;51(7):E25–7.

90. Ciardulli A, Saccone G, Anastasio H, et al. Less-restrictive food intake during labor in low-risk singleton pregnancies: a systematic review and meta-analysis. Obstet Gynecol 2017;129(3):473–80.

91. Jin Z, Hu J, Ma D. Postoperative delirium: perioperative assessment, risk reduction, and management. Br J Anaesthesia 2020;125(4):492–504.

92. Rengel KF, Pandharipande PP, Hughes CG. Postoperative delirium. La Presse Médicale 2018;47(4):e53–64.

93. Nilsson U, Bergman L. "Never the same" after surgery: postoperative delirium and early postoperative cognitive decline. J PeriAnesth Nurs 2021;36(3):321–2.

94. Chan TY, Bulger TF, Stowell KM, et al. Evidence of malignant hyperthermia in patients administered triggering agents before malignant hyperthermia susceptibility identified: missed opportunities prior to diagnosis. Anaesth Intensive Care 2017;45(6):707–13.

95. Zhou J, Nozari A, Bateman B, et al. Neuromuscular disorders including malignant hyperthermia and other genetic disorders. In: Gropper MA, editor. Miller's anesthesia. 9th ed. Philadelphia, Elsevier; 2020. p. 1113–44.

96. Bin X, Wang B, Tang Z. Malignant hyperthermia: a killer if ignored. J PeriAnesth Nurs 2022;37(4):435–44.

97. Hooper VD. Care of the patient with thermal imbalance. In: Odom-Forren J, editor. Drain's perianesthesia nursing: a critical care approach. 7th ed. St Louis, MO: Elsevier; 2018, p. 763–73.

98. Hirshey Dirksen SJ, Van Wicklin SA, et al. Developing effective drills in preparation for a malignant hyperthermia crisis. AORN J 2013;97(3):329–53.

99. Australian and New Zealand College of Anaesthetists (ANZCA). Position statement on the post-anesthesia care unit. Melbourne, VIC: ANZCA; 2020. Available from: https://www.anzca.edu.au/getattachment/7045495a-0f12-4464-852c-b93c0453e1ed/PS04(A)-Position-statement-on-the-post-anaesthesia-care-unit. [Accessed 25 February 2023].

100. Oh S-T, Park JY. Postoperative delirium. Korean J Anesthesiol 2019;72(1):4–12.

101. Safavynia SA, Arora S, Pryor KO, et al. An update on postoperative delirium: clinical features, neuropathogenesis, and perioperative management. Curr Anesthesiol Rep 2018;8(3):252–62.

102. Alexander JC, Patel B, Joshi GP. Perioperative use of opioids: current controversies and concerns. Best Pract Res Clin Anaesthesiol 2019;33(3):341–51.

103. Strang J, Volkow ND, Degenhardt L, et al. Opioid use disorder. Nature Rev Dis Primers 2020;6(1):1–28.

104. Bicket MC, Lin LA, Waljee J. New persistent opioid use after surgery: a risk factor for opioid use disorder? Ann Surg 2022;275(2):e288–9.

105. Neuman MD, Bateman BT, Wunsch H. Inappropriate opioid prescription after surgery. Lancet 2019;393(10180):1547–57.

Chapter 27

Paediatric considerations in critical care

Tina Kendrick, Anne-Sylvie Ramelet

Learning objectives

After reading this chapter, you should be able to:

- consider and anticipate the specific needs of critically ill infants, children and their families
- describe common conditions that lead to critical illness in infants and children
- apply and analyse age-appropriate assessment, monitoring and management of critically ill infants and children
- interpret age-appropriate parameters and care required by critically ill infants and children who require ventilation
- apply psychological and emotional care required by critically ill infants and children, and their families
- consider the family members as partners in their child's care and decisions.

Introduction

This chapter focuses on specific considerations for the care of critically ill infants and children experiencing, or at risk of experiencing, common life-threatening conditions. These include respiratory diseases common in the paediatric population, major trauma, shock and sepsis. It is aimed at the critical care nurse who encounters paediatric patients occasionally and, while not designed to meet all the needs of specialist paediatric critical care nurses, it provides a summary of the assessment, monitoring and care required by critically ill children. A systems approach has been used in this chapter for convenience, although paediatrics is a specialty defined by age rather than body systems.

Not only will children experience different patterns of illness and injury in comparison with adults, but their behavioural and physiological responses to illness will also differ. It is important that the child's primary caregiver, who will usually be a parent (the term used throughout this chapter), is included in planning many aspects of care. While members of the critical care team are expert in management of critical illness, parents are generally the experts on their child. They can provide their child's health history and know how best to settle their child in addition to knowing what their 'normal' behaviours are. For these reasons, parents are valuable partners of the team and their concern should never be ignored or downplayed.

Children account for over 6% of all ICU admissions in Australia and New Zealand, representing a figure of 2.12 admissions per 1000 children, a slightly higher figure than in the UK and Republic of Ireland (1.43/1000).[1] In 2018, fewer children required invasive or non-invasive ventilation than previous years, with around 36% of admissions requiring intubation, and just over 45% receiving non-invasive ventilation.[1]

The age distribution of children in paediatric ICUs (PICUs) has remained the same for many years, with 2018 Australasian data showing that children under the age of 5 years represent almost 64% of admissions, with 54.8% under 12 months of age and 35% of all ICU admissions.[1] Boys represent almost 57% of children admitted to ICUs. Increasing numbers of chronically critically ill children, defined as those staying in ICU for 14 days and longer or two or more stays in the last year, account for around one-third of a unit's bed census, and have prolonged length of stay (LOS) up to five times higher than patients without chronic critical care illness. Reduced mortality rates and improved management have resulted in the changing population within PICUs.[2]

The impact of the severe acute respiratory syndrome coronavirus-2 (SARS-CoV-2) pandemic on the paediatric population has been different to that in the adult population, with fewer children experiencing severe disease and hence reduced mortality rates. The impact on the clinical environment and clinical practice, and in particular the effects of limited access to family and visitors, has been a major cultural difference within the PICU. Use of technology has been possible in some settings to facilitate family contact, particularly when restricted visiting has occurred; however, the impact of sick parents and family, interrupted education and isolation from friends and family caused by lockdowns is yet to be explored. In this chapter, we highlight where relevant the influence of the SARS-CoV-2 virus and pandemic on both clinical conditions and clinical care of children.

Anatomical and physiological considerations in children

Children require age-appropriate and developmentally appropriate care. An appropriate range of paediatric equipment is required to assess, monitor and treat all ages and sizes of infants and children. General considerations, based on differences between children and adults, are described with specific differences detailed using a systems approach. The terms 'infants' and 'children' are used throughout the remainder of this chapter. 'Infants' are aged up to 12 months, and 'children' are aged between 1 and 16 years. A number of general considerations, based on anatomical and physiological differences from adults, need to be considered for the critically ill child.

- Children and infants have increased surface area-to-volume ratio compared with adults, which leads to increased heat loss and insensible fluid losses, placing them at increased risk of developing hypothermia and dehydration. Providing an environment that maintains the infant and small child's body temperature is essential. Avoid exposing infants and children more than necessary; use warming blankets, open-care systems for all newborns and infants under 4 kg, and overhead heaters when exposure is unavoidable. Temperature monitoring is essential when using any heating devices to avoid iatrogenic thermal injury.

- Lower glycogen stores and increased metabolic rate predispose infants to hypoglycaemia. Medication doses and fluid requirements are calculated on age and kilograms of body weight. Weight of infants and children should therefore be estimated as accurately as possible. There are several length-based tapes that can be used to estimate weight, with those that incorporate body habitus outperforming other methods of weight estimation.[3]

- Fluid requirements are based on body weight and aim to ensure adequate hydration while preventing fluid overload. Maintenance intravenous (IV) fluids for infants and young children typically require the addition of glucose.[4] Without compelling evidence in favour of balanced versus unbalanced IV fluids in children, 0.9% sodium chloride is still recommended for fluid boluses in paediatric resuscitation.[5] Table 27.1 provides a guide for maintenance fluid requirements of children based on body weight.[6]

- Excluding the newborn period, normal values for all blood gas and serum electrolyte levels are the same as adult levels. Creatinine and urea levels will vary with age.

Practice tip

To estimate weight, use the Broselow™ tape measure in the following way: (1) place the tape so the red arrow is positioned at the top of the child's head; (2) align the tape parallel to the side of the child, who must be lying in a supine position; (3) extend the legs straight; (4) bend the ankle so the toes are pointing straight up. Look at the weight in the coloured areas directly under the bottom of the foot. The tape can also be used to indicate ideal body weight for drug dosing in bariatric children.

Practice tip

If paediatric oxygen masks are not available, an adult-sized mask, including a partial non-rebreather mask, can be used in an emergency. Place the nose section under the child or infant's chin in the 'upside-down' position.

TABLE 27.1

Guide to maintenance fluids in healthy children

For each of the first 10 kg body weight: 100 mL/kg/day (approx. 4 mL/kg/h)
+ for each of the second 10 kg of body weight: 50 mL/kg/day (approx. 2 mL/kg/h)
+ for every subsequent kg of body weight: 20 mL/kg/day (approx. 1 mL/kg/h)
Most unwell children and those receiving humidification of gases should receive 2/3 maintenance fluids

WEIGHT (KG)	mL/H	TOTAL (mL/DAY)
4	16	400
6	25	600
8	33	800
10	41	1000
12	46	1100
14	50	1200
16	54	1300
18	58	1400
20	62	1500
25	66	1600
30	75	1700
35	70	1800
40	79	1900
50	87	2100

Source: Adapted from The Royal Children's Hospital, Melbourne Fluid Calculator.[6]

TABLE 27.2

Target cerebral perfusion pressure (CPP) and intracranial pressure (ICP) by age[9,10]

AGE	DESIRABLE MINIMUM CPP (mmHG)	DESIRABLE MINIMUM ICP (mmHG)
Neonates <1 month	>40	<2
Infants 1–12 months	>45	5
Children 1–6 years	>50	6–13
Children 7–10 years	>55	Up to 15
Children over 10 years	>60 mmHg	Up to 15

Source: Adapted from Woods KS, Horvat CM, Kantawala S, et al. Intracranial and cerebral perfusion pressure thresholds associated with inhospital mortality across pediatric neurocritical care. Pediatr Crit Care Med 2021;22(2):135–46; The Sydney Children's Hospitals Network. Severe traumatic brain injury – PICU – practice guideline. Sydney, NSW: The Sydney Children's Hospitals Network; 2021, p. 1–15.

Central nervous system

Many central nervous system functions, such as locomotion and hand–eye coordination, take months to years to fully develop. Cerebral cortex functions are particularly underdeveloped, with myelination of all major nerve tracts continuing throughout infancy.[7] Consequently, assessment and management priorities will be dictated by the level of neurological maturity of the infant or child. The plasticity inherent in the brain of the infant may compensate for injury more readily than in older children and adults in some circumstances, with other areas of the infant's brain taking over function. Because the eight cranial bones are not yet fused, infants' skulls cope with both birth and ongoing growth, which is greatest in the first 2 years of life. In the first year, the cartilaginous sutures fuse at two points to form the posterolateral fontanelle. The larger anterior fontanelle closes during the second year as bone is laid down. By around 5 years of age, the sutures of the child's skull are completely fused.[8] However, the thinner skull will provide less protection to underlying tissues than the adult skull.

While slow rises in intracranial volume may be accommodated over time in children under 3 years of age, they will usually be accompanied by growing head circumference, making routine measurement of head circumference in children under 3 years of age an important assessment. However, the less rigid skull of the older child will not compensate for acute rises in intracranial volume, and the child will display symptoms of neurological compromise.[9] Normal ranges of intracranial pressure (ICP) and cerebral perfusion pressure (CPP) are lower than in adults, reaching adult range by adolescence. Age-related values commonly used to guide treatment are displayed in Table 27.2.[9,10]

Cardiovascular system

Infants produce both fetal and adult haemoglobin up to 6 months of age, when levels of fetal haemoglobin (approximately 60–70% up to this point) fall rapidly and production of adult haemoglobin predominates.[8] Fetal haemoglobin allows greater amounts of oxygen to be carried for any given PaO_2 in utero and in infancy. Circulating blood volume per kilogram decreases with age; in the infant, circulating volume is approximately 85 mL/kg, with total body water accounting for 70% of body mass, adjusting to the adult values of 65 mL/kg and total body water of 60%.[8] The apex beat is heard at the fourth intercostal space, mid-clavicle and, by around

7 years of age, the left ventricle has grown and the apex beat can be heard at the fifth intercostal space, as in adults. An infant's cardiac output is approximately 500 mL/min, which, relative to body weight, is about twice that of an adult.[8] Heart rate is a major determinant of cardiac output in infants and young children, who have limited ability to increase stroke volume. Tachycardia is an early sign of distress, but bradycardia is an ominous sign in infants and young children, as they are more dependent on a high heart rate to maintain cardiac output. In infants, bradycardia of 60/min and below requires resuscitation.

Arterial blood pressure should be appropriate for age, weight and clinical condition. While mean arterial pressure is generally used, systolic blood pressure is the trigger for many acute warning systems.[11] Monitoring blood pressure using correct cuff sizes is important because incorrect cuff size is a common cause of inaccurate blood pressure readings in children. Diastolic blood pressure is recorded at Korotkoff sound 5 (K5); age-related parameters for mean blood pressure are displayed in Table 27.3.[12]

Paediatric considerations for cardiovascular assessment

Cardiovascular assessment in children includes clinical parameters that are similar to those observed in adults. The normal values are, however, age and weight dependent. Indirect evidence of poor systemic perfusion in infants may include:[13]

- feeding difficulties
- abdominal distention
- fluid imbalances
- temperature instability
- hypoglycaemia
- hypocalcaemia
- apnoea.

Neurological changes with poor systemic perfusion in children are irritability, then disorientation or lethargy. Clinical signs of reduced cardiac output, typically seen in shock, are similar to adults.[14] Age-related parameters for heart rate and respiratory rate are displayed in Table 27.4.

Respiratory system

The child's respiratory system, including airways, continues to mature until at least 8 years of age; therefore, the paediatric airway is described and managed differently from the adult's. Structural and mechanical differences predispose infants and young children to respiratory compromise. Respiratory compromise leading to apnoea and even respiratory arrest is a relatively common occurrence in the paediatric population, although specific incidences of occurrence have not been determined.

The newborn's larynx is just one-third of the diameter of the adult larynx.[8] In combination with narrow nasal passages and obligatory nose-breathing up to 5–6 months of age, infants may experience respiratory distress if nasal passages become oedematous or contain secretions such as mucus or blood. With the airway of an infant measuring around 6 mm in diameter at the level of the cricoid, obstruction is more likely than in adults. The paediatric airway is characterised and differentiated from an adult airway by the following features (Figs 27.1 and 27.2):[8,15]

- short maxilla and mandible
- large tongue
- floppy epiglottis
- shorter trachea
- more acute angle of airway, particularly notable when attempting to visualise with a laryngoscope
- a more cephalad larynx that moves distally as the neck grows
- a cricoid ring that is the narrowest portion of the airway[15]
- smaller lower airways, less developed with fewer alveoli
- true alveoli not present until 2 months, with full complement developed by around 8 years of age
- little smooth muscle present in airways
- little collateral ventilation in airways, as the pores of Kohn and canals of Lambert are not fully developed until about 3–4 years of age.

Paediatric respiratory assessment

The thoracic cavity of infants and children is characterised by a highly compliant thin chest wall, with poorly

---

TABLE 27.3
Age-related ranges for mean blood pressure[12]

AGE	MEAN BP (mmHG)
Term newborn	40–60
3 months	45–75
6 months	50–90
1 year	50–90
3 years	50–90
7 years	60–90
10 years	60–90
12 years	65–95
14 years	65–95

Source: Adapted from Hillgruber RJ, Lutskov P, West NC, et al. Blood pressure nomograms for children undergoing general anesthesia, stratified by age and anesthetic type, using data from a retrospective cohort at a tertiary pediatric center. J Clin Monit Comput 2022;36(6):1667–77.

TABLE 27.4

Age-related heart and respiratory rates

AGE	RESPIRATORY RATE 50TH CENTILE	RESPIRATORY RATE RANGE 10TH–90TH CENTILE	HEART RATE 50TH CENTILE	HEART RATE RANGE 10TH–90TH CENTILE
Birth–<3 months	35	27–47	142	123–165
3–<6 months	31	25–42	135	118–155
6–9 months	29	24–38	131	115–151
10–<12 months	28	23–36	127	111–150
12–<18 months	26	22–33	124	107–149
18–<24 months	25	21–31	120	103–145
2–<3 years	24	20–30	117	99–38
3–<4 years	24	20–28	111	94–131
4–<6 years	23	20–27	105	88–126
6–<8 years	22	20–26	100	81–122
8–<12 years	20	18–24	94	77–116
12–<15 years	20	16–24	86	69–106
15–<16 years	20	16–23	83	66–103

Source: Adapted from O'Leary F, Hayen A, Lockie, F, Peat J. Defining normal ranges and centiles for heart and respiratory rates in infants and children: a cross-sectional study of patients attending and Australian tertiary hospital paediatric emergency department. Arch Dis Child 2015;100:733–37.

FIGURE 27.1   Anatomy of the adult airway.

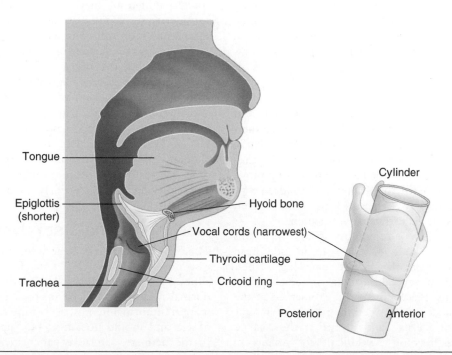

Source: Courtesy Susan Gilbert.

FIGURE 27.2 Anatomy of the paediatric airway.

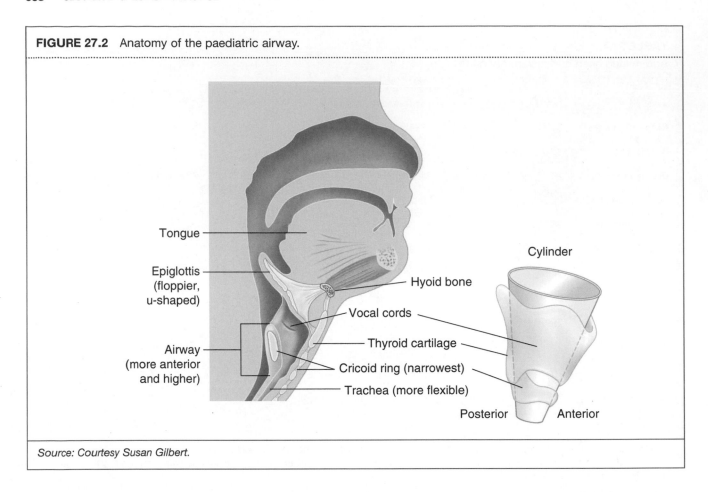

Tongue

Epiglottis
(floppier,
u-shaped)

Hyoid bone

Vocal cords

Thyroid cartilage

Airway
(more anterior
and higher)

Cricoid ring (narrowest)

Trachea (more flexible)

Cylinder

Posterior   Anterior

Source: Courtesy Susan Gilbert.

developed intercostal and accessory muscles. The diaphragm is the most important muscle for infants and children in respiration, with abdominal muscles also used. The compliant chest wall prevents generation of high intrathoracic pressures, meaning that infants and young children are unable to significantly increase tidal volume; rather, they increase minute volume by breathing faster. This means that tachypnoea is a normal response to illness in infants and children, and a slowing respiratory rate in children may indicate impending collapse rather than clinical improvement.[16]

Assessing airway patency is important. Talking and crying indicate that the infant or child is maintaining their own airway. Adventitious airway noises in children include wheezing, stridor and grunting. In infants, grunting may be heard and is an attempt by the baby to produce positive end-expiratory pressure (PEEP). Infants and children who are grunting, gasping or unconscious need urgent assessment for possible endotracheal intubation.

Other observed signs of respiratory distress in infants and children up to about 8 years old include head bobbing in infants, nasal flaring and paradoxical chest movement observed in several locations on the chest and known as recessions. Recessions can be observed at the costal margin, or subcostal; between the ribs, or intercostal; at the sternum, or sternal; and at the trachea, called tracheal tug. Oral feeding is difficult for infants in

moderate-to-severe respiratory distress owing to limitations associated with sucking and breathing at the same time. In addition, tachypnoea greater than 60–80 breaths/min may lead to vomiting and aspiration; therefore, enteral nutrition may not be possible initially, so consideration of intravenous therapy is essential until enteral nutrition can commence.[17]

Diagnosis of an upper or lower respiratory illness may be made, using the history of the symptoms from the parent or the child when age-appropriate, in conjunction with physical assessment of the child. Assessment of the rate, rhythm, effort and pattern of breathing according to age as well as colour and agitation should be undertaken. Just as heart rate is used to increase cardiac output, children compensate to maintain oxygenation for some time by breathing more rapidly until they become fatigued, when they are likely to become hypoxic and ultimately apnoeic.

Gastrointestinal tract dysfunction

There are few differences between the child's and adult's gastrointestinal tract (GIT) outside the neonatal period, although a palpable liver below the costal margin is a normal finding. It will be up to 3 cm below the costal margin in normal infants, decreasing to 1 cm by 4–5 years of age, and should no longer be palpable in adolescents. In the neonate, a relative pancreatic amylase deficiency means utilisation of starches is less effective. Fats are also absorbed less well, which is the reason why higher-fat milks such as cow's milk are not ideal for infants. Protein synthesis and storage is, however, enhanced in the neonate.[7]

As the infant liver is not completely mature at birth, gluconeogenesis is deficient, causing low and unstable blood sugar level in the first weeks of life. The infant is therefore reliant on fat stores until normal feeding is established.[8] Formation of plasma proteins and clotting factors are likely to be inadequate in the first weeks of life; therefore, all newborns in Australasia and many other areas of the world are given vitamin K shortly after birth to prevent bleeding. Blood glucose monitoring and provision of early nutrition are essential aspects of care, especially for infants. Children normally have increased metabolic demands to achieve growth but have fewer energy stores than adults.

Other systems and considerations

The following section presents the paediatric considerations of the genitourinary, musculoskeletal and integumentary systems.

Genitourinary system

The small developing pelvic bones of infants and young children cause adult pelvic organs, such as the bladder, to be located in the lower abdominal cavity. Urine output in children is calculated in mL/kg body weight/h. In infants with immature kidney function and limited ability to conserve water, urine output should be 1–2 mL/kg/h. In the first month of life, infants have limited capacity to concentrate urine to only 1.5 times their plasma osmolality, whereas adults concentrate their urine to 3–4 times plasma osmolality. The higher metabolic rate of infants produces twice the acid that an adult will, leading to a tendency to acidosis in critical illness.[7] By 6 months of age, normal urine output should be 1 mL/kg/h, and by adolescence 0.5–1 mL/kg/h is considered normal.

Catheterisation is generally required in critically ill infants and children for accurate hourly measurement of urine output. Where this is not possible, particularly where small sizes of indwelling catheters are not readily available, weighing nappies will provide an interim estimate of urine output. Inserting feeding tubes in place of a urinary catheter is not recommended.

Practice tip

Where catheterisation is not possible, nappies can be weighed to estimate urine output. Use an indelible marker to record the dry weight of a disposable nappy on the nappy itself. This weight is then subtracted from the nappy's wet weight to give an estimate of volume, with 1 g equivalent to 1 mL.

Musculoskeletal system

Children have less-developed musculature than adults, with less protection from external forces that collide with the child. Conversely, a child's skeleton is more cartilaginous than adults and therefore more pliable. As a result, rib fractures rarely accompany chest trauma in children whereas lung contusions are common.[18] The skeleton in children changes from less cartilaginous in nature at infancy to complete ossification and adult features during adolescence, so daily calcium requirements increase over childhood and adolescence.[7]

Integumentary system

Infants have a thinner epidermis, dermis and subcutaneous tissue than adults, which will continue to mature. This results in a greater susceptibility to absorption of chemicals, injury from adhesive tapes and any shearing force and loss of water and heat, particularly in the newborn period.[8] Critically ill children are more likely to develop pressure injuries on the occiput, ear, sacrum, heel or thigh, with pressure injuries in children often associated with equipment pressing or rubbing on the skin. The Braden QD Scale can assess both immobility-related and device-related pressure injury risk in children.[19] This scale is based on the Braden Q Scale used in PICUs, and includes nine subscales: mobility, activity, sensory perception, skin moisture, tissue perfusion and oxygenation, friction and shear, total number of diagnostic or therapeutic devices, whether devices could be repositioned and whether underlying skin was protected.[19]

Developmental considerations

Admission to ICU is very stressful both for paediatric patients and for their family.[20] The stressors, combined with the effects of critical illness, can lead to disturbances in normal child development and attachment. The psychological needs of children and families are not always met, and can differ between mothers and fathers.[21–23] This is especially true for prolonged-stay PICU patients.[24,25] Factors that affect the psychosocial well-being of a critically ill child include loss of usual routines and self-control, family presence and role, family and friends' visits, comfort and the ICU environment.[26] The consequences and psychological effects can last for 1 year after the PICU stay.[27]

Knowledge and understanding of developmental psychology can help nurses to assess and plan care for the critically ill child. Identification of internal strengths, external supports and environmental modification can facilitate coping and reduce stress in these children.[28] Parental support is an important coping mechanism of infants and children during periods of stress. Strategies to facilitate coping in children of all ages include:

- facilitating parental presence at all times, including during invasive procedures and resuscitation[29,30]
- maintaining normal routines and rituals as much as possible, including story reading, music,[31,32] bedtime

routines, presence of favourite toys[33] and a comforting object from home[34]

- promoting sleep by reducing environmental noise[35]
- providing appropriate analgesia and sedation[35]
- providing opportunities for play and activities unrelated to treatment.[33]

Erikson's psychosocial theory is helpful for understanding childhood development.[36] This theory asserts that people experience eight 'psychosocial crisis stages' that significantly affect their development and personality. The first five stages are presented below.

Infants (stage 1)

The first year of life is concerned with developing a sense of trust, laying a foundation for all future relationships.[37,38] The affective exchanges between infant and the primary caregiver provide a foundation for neurological development and lead to the creation of neural networks (particularly in the right hemisphere) that will influence the infant's personality and relationships with others throughout life.[39] Generally, up to the age of 6 months, infants are able to cope with limited separation from their mothers; however, changes to usual routines create anxiety and stress. From about 6 to 18 months of age, separation is the major fear, with changes to usual routine and environment resulting in anxiety. Experience of adversity such as PICU hospitalisation in early life can disrupt social learning and cause adjustment problems.[40] Therefore, critically ill infants require parental presence and the maintenance of normal routines, including breastfeeding, as much as is practicable.

Toddlers (stage 2)

The toddler period, between 1 and 3 years of age, is a time for establishing autonomy and independence. Control over bodily functions, increasing the ability to communicate, the ability to view the self as separate from others and the ability to tolerate brief separation from the mother are all developmental characteristics during this period. Toddlers tend to be egocentric in how they view the world, so illness, procedures and separation from parents may be perceived as punishment.[38] Their thinking processes include transduction, animism and ritual. Transductive thinking allows a child to link unrelated objects or events, such as separation and endotracheal suction if suction occurs after the parent leaves the room. Animism attributes lifelike traits to inanimate objects, so the ventilator may become a hissing monster, or monitoring leads may be trying to trap them. Many toddlers have varying levels of ritual or sameness, including always eating off the same plate or a security toy or blanket. Regression, or loss of recently acquired skills such as toileting, may also occur during critical illness, creating further distress. When caring for critically ill toddlers, encourage parental presence and maintain as many of the usual rituals and routines as possible to facilitate coping.

Pre-school children (stage 3)

Children from 3 to 5 years of age fall into the pre-school period of development. It is characterised by discovery, inventiveness, curiosity and the development of culturally and socially acceptable behaviour.[37] Pre-schoolers generally verbalise their needs reasonably well. While thought processes become less ritualistic and negative, pre-school children are still egocentric and experience emerging magical thinking; hence ideas about causality and linking events may be faulty. Fears, both real and imagined, are prevalent during this period.[37] For example, fears of monsters or being hurt may occur. They may also feel guilty as a result of illness. There is, however, greater understanding of the passage of time, so parents can leave the pre-schooler for defined short periods.[37] Hospitalisation remains difficult, but pre-schoolers can understand their diagnostic and therapeutic procedures, and when they receive age-appropriate and concrete information they feel more prepared as they know what to expect.[37,41]

School-age children (stage 4)

Children from 5 to 11 years are usually referred to as being of school age. This period represents a widening of the sphere of influence from parents/family to include the school environment and peers. A transition from egocentric thinking to concrete operations occurs,[42] with children becoming more independent and achievement-oriented for their sense of self-worth.[43] They understand that an object may change its appearance but retain its qualities. For example, if some water is poured into a differently shaped glass, the volume remains the same, even though its appearance has changed. In the ICU, school-aged children may have a distorted or fantasy-laden view, and will need concrete explanations. Sicker children are less able to cope with the ICU environment and are more likely to regress, which can have a significant impact on their sense of self-worth.[43] Modesty and privacy are imperative at this age.[44] Preadolescence occurs between 10 and 11 years, and represents a time of turmoil and emotional upheaval.[42]

Adolescents (stage 5)

Adolescence is considered a time of transition from childhood to adulthood. It is typically represented by children aged 12–18 years, or teenagers. Internal changes relate to emotional upheaval, search for autonomy and transition of thought process from concrete to abstract, so they can imagine possible outcomes without actually experiencing them. External changes relate to physical changes, such as the emergence of secondary sex characteristics, with a related preoccupation with bodily functions and image.[38]

A goal in adolescence is to develop an integrated sense of self, achieved through managing the conflicting demands of family and peers. Peer identity is essential to psychological growth and development, as is the gradual shift from family to peer orientation. Peer groups provide a way for adolescents to self-evaluate and to bolster self-esteem.[45]

Adolescents also target authority figures with retaliation and defiance. Conversely, adolescents will seek out non-parental adults, such as a teacher or relative, to obtain approval and acceptance. Existing psychopathology in the adolescent negatively affects parental and peers' relationships as well as autonomy. It is therefore important to adapt care to adolescents' needs in a way they can express and modulate their emotions.[46]

Family issues and consent

When children are admitted to an ICU, the whole family is affected by the hospitalisation. Parents' psychological reactions to their child's life-threatening situation include stress, anxiety and depression, but are not associated with illness type.[47] Around 30% of parents will experience acute and post-traumatic stress after PICU discharge, up to months later.[47,48] Therefore, health professionals need to pay particular attention to parents who present those symptoms. Early screening for psychological stress to identify risk and provide specialised psychological support is recommended.[48] Parents and siblings of children who die in hospital need special support from nursing and medical staff and to be allowed to stay at the bedside if they wish.[49] Follow-up consultations may be required.[50]

Family-centred care (FCC) provides a framework for the care of children and their family in hospital, and is discussed in Chapter 8. Care based on an equal relationship between family and healthcare professionals, parental presence and participation in care, and open and honest information is recommended.[51] Critically ill children are particularly vulnerable to short- and long-term emotional and psychological sequelae, but parental presence and participation in care can make a difference.

Parents need to feel involved in their child's care, and this includes the need for information, communication, understanding the child's illness and being part of the decision-making process.[51] Family-centred rounds can reduce PICU LOS, and improve workflow.[52] Particular attention to communication should be paid to parents who are non-native language speakers, with regular use of interpreters to avoid interpretation errors.[53] A partnership between staff and parents is the ideal situation, but parents often need to be reminded how to maintain the parental role and how they can effectively care for both their child's and their own psychological health.[54] Parents should be allowed to be present during potentially stressful situations such as endotracheal suction, cannulation and resuscitation if they choose to, provided that adequate support from a nurse or another designated healthcare worker is given, as it can increase parental satisfaction and coping.[29] Being present at the end of their child's life may help parents through their grieving process.[55] Not allowing parents to be present during procedures is a form of paternalism that goes against the principle of patient- and family-centred care (PFCC).[56] Parents should, however, be informed of their right to leave if they wish.[30]

Consent and assent

Except for emergency treatment, parents or legal guardians need to consent to all aspects of medical care, including preventive, diagnostic or therapeutic measures for children. The legal age of consent differs between jurisdictions, and is 18 years in major European countries and some states of Australia. However, children also gain legal rights to agree for their own medical treatment, as they get older. Children aged ≥16 years can consent to medical treatment like adults in many countries, such as the UK, Switzerland, Germany, Belgium, France, Quebec and Spain.[57,58] This is also the case in New South Wales and South Australia, where the legal age for consent is 14 and 16 years respectively.[59] Informed assent is described as providing permission for procedures when a child is not legally authorised or lacks sufficient understanding to provide informed consent but has the emotional maturity and intellectual capacity to agree to procedures; this usually appears at around 12 years old.[60] To be considered competent, young people must be able to understand the nature of the decision as well as the consequences of making or not making the decision.[60] Whenever possible, it is recommended to obtain the child's assent for treatment or procedures. Children, even when deemed not competent, have the right to be informed and, when appropriate, to be asked for their permission. However, refusal of treatment by a child has no legal bearing when a parent has consented. Importantly, parents may also refuse to consent and, in that case, laws and legal mechanisms for resolving disputes may be used.[60] It should be noted that consenting to medical treatment differs from consenting to research participation; the legislation regarding the latter varies greatly across countries.[61,62]

Pain, sedation, delirium and withdrawal

Critically ill infants and children are particularly exposed to painful procedures, invasive monitoring devices and treatments that require pain relief and sedation for their comfort. Nevertheless, deep sedation can result in the patient developing delirium and benzodiazepine withdrawal, especially when high-dose or prolonged administration is provided.[63] Unrelieved pain and delirium have been associated with short- and long-term physiological and psychological complications, including increased risk of mortality and morbidity.[64] Prevention of procedural pain is important not only to avoid pain-related complications and emotional trauma, but also to facilitate the procedure.[65] The optimal level of sedation varies for each patient and will be dependent on the underlying diagnosis and severity of illness. An evidence-based guideline for best practice of analgesia, sedation and delirium has recently been established for children.[34] An individualised daily sedation level targeted to the child's clinical status is recommended to help maintain children in a comfortable state without compromising haemodynamic and respiratory status, while minimising other undesirable effects of analgesics and sedatives.[34,66] Unlike in adult ICU patients, sedation interruption to sedation protocolisation is not recommended in children, as it failed to show any improvement in patient outcome.[34] A benzodiazepine-sparing analgesia/sedation protocol using opiate and dexmedetomidine infusions as first-line sedation showed some benefits when compared with continuous benzodiazepine infusions, including decrease in opiate withdrawal, duration of mechanical ventilation and PICU LOS.[67] Some children are difficult to sedate; preliminary work has shown those children require three or more sedation classes, have suspected delirium, and unplanned extubation and device removal.[68] They often need other sedation adjuvants.[69]

When the provision of analgesics and sedatives is necessary to keep children comfortable, there is a risk for withdrawal of these drugs when given over a prolonged period of time and when receiving several sedative agents.[70] Prevalence rates of withdrawal syndrome in PICU patients receiving benzodiazepines and/or opioids for 5 or more days varied greatly between 20% and 85%, but has tended to decrease in the last decade, with rates below 50%.[70] Screening for iatrogenic withdrawal syndrome should be initiated between days 3 and 5 when high opioid and benzodiazepine doses are used.[34] Some evidence suggests that prevention of withdrawal should be initiated as early as after 3 days of treatment with opioids and sedatives.[71]

Delirium is highly prevalent in critically ill children (up to 34%), with the hypoactive subtype of delirium being the most prevalent (46–81%).[72] Risk factors for developing delirium include administration of cumulative doses of benzodiazepines and opioids, and the number of psychotropic agents used, but are also associated with intellectual disability, increased mechanical ventilation duration and some organ failures.[72,73] Early screening for delirium upon admission and throughout PICU discharge is strongly recommended as a prerequisite for appropriate interventions and minimising associated complications.[34]

Assessment

The assessment of pain, sedation, delirium and withdrawal in children is particularly challenging, because all of these symptoms have overlapping behavioural cues.[74] Although several sources should be used to accurately assess pain in non-communicative children,[75] validated observation measurement tools remain the best methods and are recommended for use in daily practice to monitor and document pain intensity, level of sedation, presence of delirium and signs of withdrawal.[74] To assess acute and postoperative pain, the PICU Multidimensional Assessment Pain Scale (PICU-MAPS),[76] the COMFORT behaviour scale[77] and the modified Faces Legs Activity Cry Consolability (FLACC) scale[78] are recommended. In children able to self-report (from 6 years old), pain can be assessed using the Numeric Rating Scale, the Visual Analogue Scale, the Oucher Scale or the Wong–Baker Faces pain scale.[34] To assess non-pain-related distress and sedation, the COMFORT scale, the COMFORT behaviour scale, the State Behavioural Scale (SBS) and the Richmond Agitation–Sedation Scale are the tools that have the strongest psychometric properties and clinical utility to evaluate the level of sedation in infants and children in ICU.[34] The evaluation of withdrawal should be performed when opioids and/or benzodiazepines are administered for 3–5 days and longer, using valid tools, such as the Withdrawal Assessment Tool (WAT-1)[34,79,80] and the Sophia Observation Withdrawal Symptoms scale.[80] Finally, delirium can be assessed with the Paediatric Confusion Assessment Method – Intensive Care Unit (pCAM-ICU),[34] the Sophia Observation Withdrawal Symptoms – Paediatric Delirium scale (SOS-PD) and the Cornell Assessment for Pediatric Delirium (CAPD).[34,81,82]

Management

Pharmacological and non-pharmacological approaches to manage pain, sedation, delirium and withdrawal are recommended.[34,83] Painful procedures should be minimised when possible. Some non-pharmacological therapies have been shown to be beneficial alone in managing mild pain or in combination with drug therapy in infants and young children. These therapies include non-nutritive sucking (e.g. finger or pacifier) with or without sucrose for infants up to 4 months.[34,84] Recent evidence shows sweet solutions (24–30% sucrose and 25% glucose) have a positive analgesic effect in infants up to 12 months during immunisation and nasogastric tube insertion.[84] After 12 months there is no effect.[85] Art therapy such us music, painting or storytelling, verbal and non-verbal communication between nurses and children, other forms of distraction and unlimited parental presence in the ICU are non-pharmacological approaches to decrease postoperative pain.[86]

Pharmacological treatment in children is challenging as their drug responses differ from adults because of age-related differences. Therefore, pharmacological treatment of pain, sedation and delirium should be tailored to the child's need and condition. Continuous opioid infusions are used at the lowest effective dose and minimum duration, based on regular pain assessment. The addition of acetaminophen and a non-steroidal anti-inflammatory drug is recommended in early postoperative analgesia and to decrease opioid requirements.[34] Fentanyl is not recommended in children with low cardiac output, and fentanyl boluses (>5 micrograms/kg) may cause chest wall rigidity.[82] Remifentanyl (a synthetic opioid with a 3–4-minute half-life) is ideal for children with renal or hepatic dysfunction, and for supporting rapid titration with minimal patient haemodynamic changes.[82] Although there is no consensus on sedation management, midazolam remains the first-choice sedative for children.[65] However, dexmedetomidine, an α_2-receptor agonist, is recommended as primary agent for sedation in postoperative cardiac children expected to be extubated early.[34,82,87,88]

Dexmedetomidine demonstrated better analgesia and less shivering and agitation in PICU children than routine analgesia and sedation,[88] decreased the need for opioids and sedative drugs, and helped reduce withdrawal syndrome and delirium.[34,89] The most frequent adverse effects reported with dexmedetomidine have been bradycardia in around 8% of children[88] and hypotension, but these effects can be resolved with dose reduction, intravenous fluid bolus and careful monitoring.[90] In children older than 1 year, propofol may be effective and safe for short-term sedation only in acute respiratory failure and minor ICU procedures (at doses of 1–2 mg/kg).[91,92] Its use as a continuous infusion should be limited to trained personnel,[92] at doses less than 4 mg/kg/h (67 micrograms/kg/min) during the periextubation period and administered for less than 48 hours in order to minimise the risk of propofol-related infusion syndrome.[34,82,92] Children with neuromuscular blockade agent (NMBA) treatment should have the lowest dose required, adequate sedation and analgesia, and be monitored with train-of-four and clinical assessment to determine depth of neuromuscular blockade.[34] Cisatracurium is most commonly used because of its rapid spontaneous recovery of neuromuscular function.[82]

Upper airway obstruction

Upper airway obstruction is common in infants and young children for two major reasons: the anatomical size of the airway and the frequency of respiratory infections experienced in early childhood. Congenital structural abnormalities and infections as well as foreign body aspiration are the three categories of causes of upper airway obstruction in children. Upper airway obstruction and infections have been associated with SARS-CoV-2 infection, and testing for the virus should be considered.[93]

General description and clinical manifestations

General indicators of respiratory distress will be present in a child suffering from upper airway obstruction. Specific clinical signs of upper airway obstruction in children include:

- a longer inspiratory phase with an unchanged expiratory phase
- stridor on inspiration
- chest wall recessions
- lower respiratory rate
- in infants, head bobbing and nasal flaring
- hoarseness
- drooling of saliva.[94]

The aim is to assess the child without causing further distress, as a crying, agitated child can further increase the degree of obstruction and work of breathing, leading to respiratory collapse. Observing and listening to the child's symptoms without disturbing them will provide important clues about the level and degree of obstruction the child is experiencing. The paediatric assessment triangle (PAT) is a useful and widely used tool to facilitate rapid assessment of the child's appearance, work of breathing and skin circulation.[95] Stridor indicates obstruction in the upper airway, while wheeze is suggestive of lower airway disease. When stridor is also associated with a barking cough, it is likely to be croup. A softer stridor in a child who looks systemically unwell may indicate epiglottitis. When a previously well child presents with a sudden onset of stridor, it is likely to indicate foreign body aspiration, and eliciting the history of a sudden choking episode can clarify the diagnosis.[96]

Congenital airway abnormalities

Congenital structural abnormalities of the airway are present at birth; depending upon severity of obstruction, they may take hours to months to become apparent. These include laryngomalacia, laryngeal web, tracheomalacia and vascular rings. These infants and children require referral to a specialist paediatric centre for ongoing management and, if they develop respiratory infections, are likely to become compromised much more easily than children with normal airways.

Laryngomalacia is the most common cause of stridor in the newborn period. Stridor is produced by flaccid, soft laryngeal cartilage and aryepiglottic folds that collapse into the glottis on inspiration.[97] An inspiratory stridor, usually high-pitched, will be present. It may be intermittent, may decrease when the patient is placed prone with the neck extended, may increase with agitation and is usually present from birth or the first weeks of life. The infant's cry is usually normal. Feeding problems may be associated with increased respiratory distress. Laryngoscopy confirms the laryngomalacia diagnosis. Treatment is supportive, with only a small proportion of infants requiring airway reconstructive surgery. Where respiratory distress interferes with feeding and growth, a tracheostomy may be indicated.[97]

A laryngeal web is made of membrane that typically spreads between the vocal cords, with an inspiratory stridor present soon after birth. Diagnosis is confirmed by laryngoscopy. Treatment involves lysis in the case of thin membranous webs, whereas a tracheostomy may be required for a thicker fibrotic web.[98] Laryngeal webs can also develop after contracting illnesses such as diphtheria or after traumatic injuries in both children and adults.[98]

Tracheomalacia and tracheobronchomalacia involve malformed cartilage rings, with lack of rigidity and an oval shape to the lumen. Secondary tracheomalacia is associated with prolonged intubation and prematurity, and presents within the first year of life.[99] Malacias are characterised by wheezing and stridor on expiration, with collapse of the tracheal or bronchial lumen. Diagnosis is confirmed by fluoroscopy and bronchoscopy, which demonstrate tracheal collapse on expiration. As the infant grows, cartilaginous development improves the airway by about 2 years of age, but a number of children will require airway stenting or reconstructive surgery.[99]

Vascular rings result from congenital malformations of the intrathoracic great vessels, resulting in compression of the airways.[100] Infants present with stridor at birth or within the first few weeks of life. Other symptoms include wheezing, cough, cyanosis, recurrent bronchopulmonary infections and dysphagia. Diagnosis may be confirmed by computed tomography (CT) scan, magnetic resonance imaging (MRI) scan or endoscopy, which reveals indentations secondary to the extrinsic pressure of the vasculature. The anatomy of the vascular malformations is determined by angiography. Treatment is surgical correction of the vascular malformation.[100]

Monitoring and diagnostics

Initial monitoring and diagnostic studies for infants and children with upper airway obstruction are ideally of a non–invasive nature, to avoid distress. Pulse oximetry is a non–invasive method of monitoring oxygenation. Arterial blood gases are performed only when absolutely necessary, as this may increase the child's distress and so worsen the degree of obstruction. Continuous ECG monitoring is also indicated.

Lateral airway X-rays are unlikely to be helpful in the setting of croup and epiglottitis and, when they are likely to involve separating the child from a parent, are potentially harmful and not recommended.[101] When there is a less dramatic presentation of the infant or child, or when the diagnosis is not clear, as in the case of an inhaled foreign body, a chest X-ray may be diagnostic.

Practice tip

Close direct observation from a short distance away is an ideal nursing practice, accompanied by non-invasive monitoring. Ideally, the critical care nurse will be positioned to hear the child's stridor. Blood sampling, cannulation and other invasive procedures should be left until the airway has been secured, the child has been anaesthetised or the airway obstruction is resolving.

Managing the paediatric airway

A child's airway may be managed in various ways. Simple positioning may be all that is required. Children will often assume an upright sitting position and may become more distressed if placed into the supine position; therefore, when possible, the best position for an infant or child with upper airway obstruction may be sitting on their parent's lap. Because of the anatomy and physiology of the respiratory tract, avoid extending the head of infants. Chin-lift and jaw-thrust are useful airway adjuncts in children to maintain an airway and to facilitate use of a bag–valve–mask. It may be necessary to use an oropharyngeal airway or nasopharyngeal airway, laryngeal

masks and endotracheal intubation in an unconscious or sedated infant.[94]

Intubation

Intubation may be required to manage airway obstruction.[94] The introduction of paediatric-specific endotracheal tubes (ETTs) with a microcuff and markings to ensure correct placement below the glottis has seen the replacement in many settings of uncuffed ETTs with cuffed ETTs.[102] Cuffed ETTs facilitate ventilation when a leak is undesirable, including in the child with facial and airway burns, for volume ventilation strategies, when using inhaled nitric oxide and for high-frequency ventilatory strategies such as oscillation ventilation. Equipment necessary for paediatric airway management, including intubation, is shown in Fig. 27.3. Fig. 27.4 shows a range of sizes of uncuffed ETTs, 2.5–5.5 mm, that should be available in 0.5-mm increments, while cuffed ETTs are available in sizes from 3 mm through to 9 mm. Selecting the correct ETT size includes having the recommended tube size plus tubes that are 0.5 mm larger and smaller than calculated. For children over 1 year of age, several formulae exist to calculate appropriate tube sizes, but the age-based and the fifth fingernail width-based predictions of ETT size remain the most commonly used.[103] Table 27.5 provides a sizing guide for ETTs, suction catheters and nasogastric tubes for infants and children.[104,105]

Practice tip

To calculate ETT tube size and length, use the following guides from the 2021 Australian and New Zealand Resuscitation Guidelines:[104]

- *for term newborns ≥3 kg:* size 3.0 mm or 3.5 mm (uncuffed tubes) or 3.0 mm (cuffed tubes)
- *for infants up to 6 months:* size 3.5 mm or 4.0 mm (uncuffed tubes) or 3.5 mm (cuffed tubes)
- *for infants 7–12 months:* size 4.0 mm (uncuffed tubes) or 3.5 mm (cuffed tubes)
- *for children over 1 year:* uncuffed tubes, size (mm) = age (years)/4 + 4; cuffed tubes, size (mm) = age (years)/4 + 3.5.

The commonest method used to intubate children is a modified rapid-sequence method. Rapid-sequence intubation is performed when the child may have a full stomach and is at risk of aspiration during intubation.[106] For children, the modification of technique involves bag–mask ventilation prior to intubation to prevent the occurrence of hypoxia.[107] It involves the practically simultaneous administration of sedative medication and a muscle relaxant immediately before intubation.[106] The main advantages of this method include avoidance of hypoxia, good airway visualisation with a relaxed jaw, open immobile vocal cords and elimination of all movement including gagging and coughing.[106] Careful consideration of appropriate induction agents is required

FIGURE 27.3 Paediatric intubation equipment.

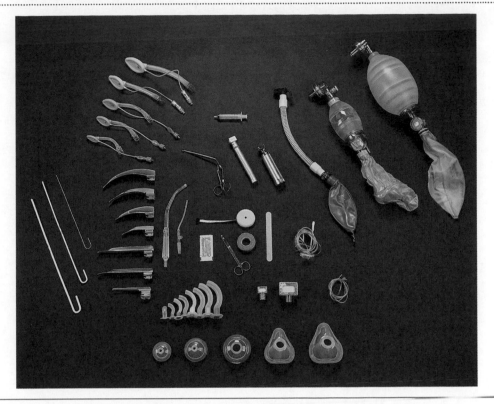

Source: Courtesy Paul de Sensi. With kind permission from Sydney Children's Hospital Network (SCHN).

FIGURE 27.4 Range of sizes in paediatric cuffed and uncuffed ETTs.

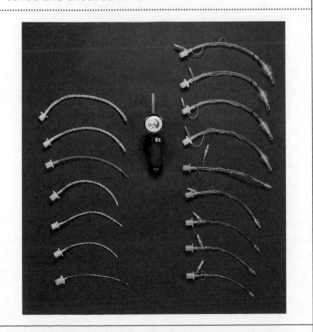

Source: Courtesy Paul de Sensi. With kind permission from Sydney Children's Hospital Network (SCHN).

for children with haemodynamic instability or a head injury/raised ICP as agents such as thiopentone, propofol and midazolam may not be appropriate or require dose modification.

Specific conditions affecting the upper airway

Bacterial and viral infections of the upper airway are common in children. Croup is the most common infection causing upper airway obstruction in children. Epiglottitis is now rarely seen in countries where immunisation against *Haemophilus influenzae* type b (Hib) was introduced into the immunisation schedule. However, it has not disappeared, and adults are now more likely than children to die from epiglottitis.[108] It is important to distinguish epiglottitis from croup in order to initiate appropriate management.[108] Other less common infectious causes of upper airway obstruction seen in young children include bacterial tracheitis and retropharyngeal abscess. Diseases thought to have disappeared, such as Lemierre's syndrome[109] and diphtheria, have not been completely eradicated, with resurgences seen in recent years, particularly in resource-poor countries.[110]

Infection of the lymphoid tissue around the nodes draining the nasopharynx, sinuses and eustachian tubes

TABLE 27.5

Endotracheal tube (ETT), suction catheter and nasogastric tube (NG) sizes for infants and children

AGE	WEIGHT (KG)	ETT SIZE (MM ID)	AT GUM (cm)	AT NOSE (cm)	ETT SUCTION CATHETER (FG)	GASTRIC TUBE (FG)
0 (term newborn)	2>3	3.0 (U)	6	7.5	5	6
0 (term newborn)	>3	3.0–3.5 (U) 3.0 (C)	8.5	10.5	6	8
0–6 months	3.5–5	3.5 (U)	9	11	6–7	8
3–12 months	6–9	3.5	10	12	6–7	8
1 year	10–12	4.0	11	14	8	8
2 years	13–14	4.5	12	15	8	10
3 years	14–15	4.5	13	16	8	10
4–5 years	16–19	5.0	14	17	8–10	12
6–7 years	20–23	5.5	15	19	10	12
8–9 years	24–29	6.0	16	20	10–12	12
10–11 years	30–37	6.5	17	21	12	14
12–13 years	38–49	7.0	18	22	12–14	16
14+ years	50–60	7.5	19	23	14	16
Adult	>60	8–9	20–21	24–25	14	16

FG = French gauge; ID = internal diameter; U = uncuffed; C = Cuffed.

Source: Adapted from Australian & New Zealand Councils on Resuscitation. ANZCOR Guideline 12.2 – paediatric advanced life support (PALS). Australian & New Zealand Council on Resuscitation; 2021; Shann F. Drug doses. 17th ed. Parkville, VIC: Royal Children's Hospital; 2017.[104,105]

may cause pus to accumulate in the retropharyngeal space, leading to a retropharyngeal abscess. Presenting symptoms include a history of upper respiratory tract infection (URTI), sore throat, fever, toxic appearance, meningismus, stridor, dysphagia and difficulty handling secretions.[111] Diagnosis is usually made on airway imaging or bronchoscopy. Treatment involves surgical drainage and antibiotic administration.[111] Short-term intubation may be required until swelling has resolved following surgery.

Croup

Croup (laryngotracheobronchitis) is the most common infective cause of upper airway obstruction in children aged 6 months to 6 years, with peak incidence at 2 years.[112] Croup is used to describe a set of symptoms caused by acute swelling causing obstruction in the upper airway (larynx, trachea and bronchi) from inflammation and oedema, caused mostly by the parainfluenza or influenza viruses, and is most commonly seen in winter months.[113] Croup has also been associated with the

SARS-CoV-2 pandemic in children.[114] Recent advances in croup management have been responsible for a fall in the number of children requiring hospitalisation and intubation. Possible complications of croup include respiratory failure, respiratory arrest, hypoxic damage, secondary bacterial infection, acute pulmonary oedema, persistence or recurrence.[113]

Clinical manifestations

Croup is characterised by a barking or seal-like cough, inspiratory stridor and hoarse voice.[94] The severity of croup is assessed based on increased respiratory rate, increased heart rate, altered mental state, work of breathing and stridor. Stridor at rest is noted in moderate-to-severe croup and is often quite loud. If a child's stridor becomes softer but the work of breathing remains increased, it should be treated as an emergency as the obstruction may become more severe. The symptoms of croup are listed and compared with those of epiglottitis in Table 27.6. Diagnosis is made on physical assessment and the history of the illness.

TABLE 27.6

Clinical features of croup and epiglottitis

	CROUP	EPIGLOTTITIS
Aetiology	Viral	Bacterial
Age	6 months–3 years	Infancy through adulthood
Onset	Subacute (over days)	Acute (over hours)
Fever	Mild (<38°C)	Severe (>38.5°C)
Cough	Present (often barking or seal-like)	May be present
Drooling	Absent	Present
Activity	Distressed	Lethargic
Colour	Pale/sick	Toxic
Obstruction	+++	+
Stridor	Inspiratory, high-pitched	Expiratory snore
Sore throat	Uncommon	Common
Position	Any	Tripod; sitting up
Course	Gradual worsening or improvement	Unpredictable; fatal if not treated
Season	Autumn–winter	Throughout the year

Source: Adapted from Lee DR, Lee CH, Won YK, et al. Clinical characteristics of children and adolescents with croup and epiglottitis who visited 146 emergency departments in Korea. Korean J Pediatr 2015;58(10):380–5.

Management

Management of croup depends on the severity of the upper airway obstruction. Children with moderate-to-severe croup should be given face-mask oxygen and allowed to adopt the position that they find most comfortable. Strategies such as positioning the child in a parent's lap and holding the face mask close to their face may limit their distress and can have beneficial effects on oxygenation.[112]

Practice tip

If placement of a face mask to deliver oxygen causes increased agitation and worsens respiratory distress in young children, have the parent hold the mask near their child's face and increase the flow rate. 'Blow-over' oxygen will increase oxygen saturation and, as the child settles, mask or nasal cannulae can be reintroduced.

The use of steroids in combination with nebulised adrenaline (epinephrine) is responsible for significant improvement of symptoms in children within 12 hours of administration, abating the need for intubation in the vast majority of cases.[115] Nebulised adrenaline is efficacious in reducing airway inflammation, with effects seen within 5 minutes and lasting up to 2 hours. Although nebulisers can be repeated, the benefits lessen with subsequent treatments. Adrenaline does not alter the course of croup. Steroids will be effective within 2 hours and effects last for up to 24 hours.[115]

Epiglottitis

Epiglottitis is inflammation of the epiglottis, frequently involving surrounding structures, with the classic description of a swollen, cherry-red, softened and floppy epiglottis, which tends to fall backwards, obstructing the airway.[116] Obstruction also occurs circumferentially, from the oedematous, inflamed aryepiglottic folds surrounding the larynx. It is typically caused by Hib and, since the introduction of childhood immunisation programs to protect against Hib infection in many countries, the incidence has dropped significantly. Interestingly, adults are more likely to die from epiglottitis than children.[108] Hib infection can cause meningitis, septicaemia, septic arthritis and cellulitis as well as epiglottitis. The disease process and development of major symptoms progress rapidly over a few hours and an untreated child may become acutely obstructed. A child will make a full recovery without sequelae if diagnosis and treatment are appropriate and timely.

Clinical manifestations

The child with epiglottitis presents looking unwell with a fever and is unable to swallow secretions, drooling saliva and refusing to talk or swallow. The child may maintain an upright position, usually leaning with the head extended, supporting a sitting position with the arms stretched out behind in what is known as the tripod position. Hypoxaemia is usually present. Sudden respiratory arrest followed by cardiac arrest can occur unpredictably. Cardiac arrest is likely to be asystolic in rhythm owing to either vagal stimulation or hypoxia secondary to airway obstruction.[117]

Management

The most important aspect in the management of epiglottitis is rapid diagnosis and minimal handling of the child until an airway is in place. Children with epiglottitis require urgent intubation because acute airway obstruction followed by cardiac arrest is a potential hazard. Thus, the aim of nursing management at this time is to keep the child as calm as possible until the airway is secured.[117] The child should be nursed propped up with pillows or on a parent's lap while arrangements are made for intubation. Procedures such as cannulation and examination of the throat should be avoided until the child's airway is secure.[117]

Prophylaxis with antibiotics is required for families and household contacts if there is an infant under 12 months of age and/or a child in the household under the age of 5 years who is not fully immunised.

Foreign body aspiration

Aspiration of a foreign body into the upper airway or upper oesophagus is another relatively common cause of obstruction in children. Infants tend to swallow food items such as nuts and seeds, while toddler-aged children tend to swallow coins, teeth, etc.[96] An inhaled foreign body is likely to have a rapid onset with no previous symptoms. Sometimes the diagnosis is missed for days, weeks or even months, and the child's symptoms may be non-specific, such as a cough with or without blood-stained sputum.[96] Ingestion or aspiration of magnets and button batteries has increased in recent years. Button batteries cannot be easily discerned from coins on X-ray; however, if lodged in the airway or oesophagus, they can cause ulceration rapidly, and it is recommended they be removed within 2 hours.[118] Batteries in the stomach will usually be passed through the GIT uneventfully. Magnets pose a problem when more than one is ingested or aspirated and should be removed via endoscopy regardless of whether the child is asymptomatic.[118]

Clinical manifestations

Sudden onset of coughing, gagging and an audible stridor in a previously well infant or child is suggestive of an inhaled foreign body.[96] However, an accurate history – such as a recent coughing or choking episode – is the most sensitive factor in making a diagnosis of inhaled foreign body.

Management

Management will depend on the location and level of the aspirated foreign body, as it may have lodged in the pharynx, oesophagus, larynx, trachea or bronchial tree. Coughing is encouraged for mild airway obstruction.[11] Up to five back blows may be successful in dislodging the foreign body, which may be followed by up to five chest thrusts and back blows.[11] Direct laryngoscopy and removal of a foreign body using Magill forceps may be required for an acute episode when back blows and chest thrusts have been unsuccessful. When the foreign body has lodged below the carina, diagnosis and definitive treatment usually consist of removal of the foreign body via a bronchoscopy under general anaesthesia.[96]

The child experiencing lower airway disease

Lower airway disease in children is a common reason for admission to ICU. Infants under 12 months usually present with bronchiolitis or pneumonia. Asthma is more common in older children, but infants nearing 12 months of age may develop asthma and there is often confusion between bronchiolitis and asthma at this age. Bronchiolitis and asthma are commonly seen in children, and the management of each condition is discussed below. National and worldwide clinical guidelines for these conditions have been developed and are continually updated.[119–121]

SARS-CoV-2 in children

More recently, the SARS-CoV-2 pandemic has affected a minority of children.[122,123] The SARS-CoV-2 infection is less severe in children than in adults,[122–125] with less than 0.1% of total deaths occurring in children, mostly those under 5 years of age.[125] A severe paediatric form of SARS-CoV-2 infection is caused by activation of the cytokine storm, involving hyperinflammatory markers, such as TNF-α, interleukin-1β and 6, and interferon-α, causing pulmonary cell damage and progression towards pneumonia, acute respiratory distress and multisystem inflammatory syndrome in children (MIS-C).[123,126,127] MIS-C is also known as paediatric inflammatory multisystem syndrome temporally associated with COVID-19 (PIMS-TS).[128,129] It occurs when inflammation is generalised owing to a non-neutralising IgG antibody and a cytokine storm.[123]

Specific risk factors for MIS-C in children are not yet fully established.[130] However, one study found that older ages in children and adolescents (median 10 years), comorbidities such as asthma, seizure disorder, obesity or body mass index >20, developmental delay and diabetes are risk factors in developing MIS-C.[126]

Clinical manifestations

In this context, MIS-C is the main focus in PICU. It affects a broader age range,[131] especially school-aged children (median age 8–10 years).[130] Studies have reported clinical manifestations such as:

- systemic inflammation symptoms (myalgias, lymphadenitis or lymphadenopathy, and persistent fever).[127,130,131]
- gastrointestinal symptoms (abdominal pain, diarrhoea, nausea, vomiting).[127,130,131]
- mucocutaneous changes (rash, conjunctivitis, acral peeling, lip swelling, strawberry tongue or erosions).[127,130,131]
- neurological symptoms (headache, altered mental status, focal deficits and meningismus).[130,131]
- cardiopulmonary symptoms (cardiac dysfunction, vasoactive support, chest pain, respiratory distress, dyspnoea and requirement for mechanical ventilation).[126,130,131]
- laboratory findings: low level of lymphocytes, platelets and albumin; high level of neutrophils, lactate dehydrogenase, alanine transaminase, aspartate transaminase, C-reactive protein, procalcitonin, ferritin, erythrocyte sedimentation rate, interleukin-6, D-dimer, fibrinogen, B-type natriuretic peptide and troponin.[127]

Some MIS-C manifestations are similar to Kawasaki disease. Differences in features include age over 5 years, myocardial depression, and neurological, gastrointestinal and shock symptoms, which are not common in Kawasaki disease.[127,128,130,131] Also, some laboratory findings in PIMS-TS differ in Kawasaki disease (troponin and brain natriuretic peptide increase, lymphopenia and thrombocytopenia).[127,130,131]

Assessment and patient management

The diagnosis of PIMS-TS should be made on case definition items: age <18 years, persistent fever, elevated inflammation biomarkers, cardiac enzymes, coagulation and fibrinolytic test, single or multiorgan dysfunction,[128] gastrointestinal symptoms and cardiac manifestations (i.e. electrocardiograph abnormalities such as atrial and ventricular tachycardia, QT prolongation, heart blocks and changes with ST-segment and T-wave),[127] and positive result in SARS-CoV-2 PCR, serology or antigen test, or COVID-19 exposure in the previous 4 weeks. Other probable causes need to be considered.[128]

Treatment includes symptom management, respiratory support, steroids.[130] Intravenous immunoglobulin is also recommended.[127,129,130,131] Adjuncts with a proinflammatory cytokine inhibitor (Anakinra or tocilizumab), and tumour necrosis factor blocking agents (infliximab) are recommended in refractory PIMS-TS.[127,131] Aspirin may also be considered in coronary artery aneurysms.[127,128,131]

When severe isolation measures are practised, alternative options must be put in place to allow communication with families and provide necessary family-centred care, as well as communication and rounding with the healthcare team, virtual visiting for extended family members, and psychological support to children and their parents.[132]

Bronchiolitis

Viral bronchiolitis in infancy is characterised by obstruction of the small airways, resulting in air trapping and respiratory distress in infants less than 12 of age. It is the commonest severe respiratory infection of infancy, although the course is usually mild to moderate, and is self-limiting, usually requiring no treatment.[120] Severe infection represents less than 5% of all cases, though representing 13% of total PICU admissions.[133] Measures such as social distancing and use of masks undertaken for SARS-CoV-2 have also reduced acute bronchiolitis cases.[134] Bronchiolitis is usually associated with prematurity, infants under 3 months of age and cardiac and pulmonary comorbidities.[133,135–137]

Respiratory syncytial virus (RSV) causes between 59 and 70% of bronchiolitis cases.[134] Other viruses include rhinovirus, bocavirus, parainfluenza virus types 1, 2 and 3, influenza B, human metapneumovirus, enterovirus, adenovirus types 1, 2 and 5 and *Mycoplasma*.[133,134,137] RSV invades the epithelial cells of the bronchioles, spreading via syncytia which are created when host cell membranes fuse with neighbouring cells. This results in shedding and destruction of the epithelium and mucus production, leading to small airway blockage and the clinical features of bronchiolitis.[138]

Bronchiolitis occurs in the colder months as it proliferates at low temperatures.[133] In Australia and New Zealand most cases of bronchiolitis occur between late autumn and early spring, with a peak in winter.[139] There is a paradoxical relationship between the incidence of RSV and other viral pathogens causing bronchiolitis. RSV epidemics occur when other respiratory pathogen epidemics are diminishing, and vice versa.[140] Nevertheless, there were changes in the incidence peak of bronchiolitis during the pandemic of COVID-19. In Europe the peak between 2020 and 2021 was in May, with a mean temperature of 23°C,[133] while in Australia the peak was in December, in the summer season.[139,140] This dynamic over the peak of bronchiolitis disease coincided with the reduction of isolation measures and the global spread of a new virus.[133,139–141]

Clinical manifestations

Bronchiolitis is a clinical diagnosis, and non-isolation of a causative viral agent does not exclude the diagnosis. The typical clinical features of bronchiolitis start with URTI symptoms such as rhinorrhoea and an irritating cough. In more-serious illness, infants develop a persistent cough, chest recessions, tachypnoea, wheeze, crackles, fever and poor feeding.[121] Severe cases of bronchiolitis, in addition to the above symptoms, can develop dyspnoea, hypoxia (oxygen saturation in room air <92%), fever over 39°C, persistent crackles, respiratory acidosis (pH <7.3), apnoea and cyanotic events.[121,142,143] Other signs such as pulmonary infiltrates, hyperinflation and atelectasis are apparent on chest X-ray.[143] In very young, premature or low-birth-weight infants, apnoea is often the presenting symptom, which then develops into severe respiratory distress. Exhaustion and failure to maintain adequate oxygen saturation are signs of impending respiratory failure.[121] The clinical course of bronchiolitis is usually 7–10 days; however, the effects of severe illness may last much longer.

Assessment and patient management

Initial assessment includes assessment of signs and symptoms to determine severity of illness, including indications for admission to ICU.[120]

- *mild:* normal behaviour and feeding, tachypnoea, nil to mild chest wall retraction, and O_2 saturations >92%
- *moderate:* intermittent irritability, increased respiratory rate, moderate chest wall retractions, tracheal tug, nasal flaring, O_2 saturations 90–92%, may have brief apnoea and reduced feeding
- *severe:* increasing irritability, lethargy, fatigue, increase or decrease in respiratory rate, marked chest wall retractions, tracheal tug, grunting, nasal flaring, O_2 saturations <90%, frequent or prolonged apnoea, and inability to feed.

Hospitalised infants should be tested for respiratory viruses, particularly SARS-CoV-2, RSV and influenza.[121] Management of infants presenting with bronchiolitis depends upon illness severity. Mild cases can be managed in the ED and may be suitable for discharge.[120] Those with moderate bronchiolitis must be observed in the emergency department. They require hourly observations, continuous cardiorespiratory and oxygen saturation monitoring, temperature, respiratory support starting with low-flow oxygen initially, and escalating to heated humidified high-flow oxygen via nasal cannulae (HHFNC) in presence of hypoxia and increased work of breathing (oxygen saturation <92%). Infants should be nursed with the head elevated, minimal handling and psychosocial support if required.[121] If not feeding adequately, provision of hydration and nutrition is required.

Non-invasive ventilation support such as continuous positive airway pressure (CPAP) may be required, including for those infants who do not respond within 90 minutes on HHFNC.[120,121] ICU admission is required for severe cases where there is no improvement and there are persistent desaturations, and significant or recurrent apnoeas associated with desaturations. In addition to moderate level care and increased ventilatory support, closer monitoring via blood gas analysis, other blood work for electrolyte and haematological monitoring are required, along with inflammatory markers such as C-reactive protein (CRP) and septic work-up and chest X-ray.[120,121] Prone positioning and minimising the impact of procedures on the infant are also important, especially in infants less than 3 months of age. Chest physiotherapy is not indicated and nasal suction only as clinically indicated. There is no role for medications such as glucocorticoids, antibiotics or nebulised agents such as hypertonic saline, adrenaline or beta-2 agonists.[120]

Asthma

Asthma is a chronic, diffuse and reversible obstruction of the lower respiratory tract. Its aetiology is generally due to inflammation and is characterised by mucosal and immune system dysfunction.[119,144] There is a complex interaction between bronchial wall cells, inflammatory mediators and the nervous system. The chronic inflammatory process causes narrowing of bronchial airways, obstructing air flow. This leads to episodes of wheezing, breathlessness and chest tightening that are usually reversible. Consequently, a modification of compliance of the lungs increases the work of breathing.[145]

Asthma is a multifactorial disease. Some studies have identified many variants of genes associated with asthma susceptibility, including *CD52*,[146,147] *CDHR3* and *GSDMB*.[148] In addition, environmental factors (air pollution, parental smoking, animal allergens, dust mites, mould),[145] eczema and low levels of vitamin D have all been strongly correlated with asthma.[148] Male gender is also a risk factor.[146] Once asthma has developed, there are triggers that may precipitate an attack, including viral illnesses, particularly respiratory viruses, and environmental factors.[149]

Asthma is one of the commonest paediatric presentations to emergency departments (EDs) and its worldwide prevalence is growing, with differences among various populations.[150] A study in 204 countries estimated the global prevalence of asthma at 24%.[151] The current disease rate in children is 7.9% in the USA,[152] 9.4% in the European Union,[153] and 8.3% in Australia.[151]

Clinical manifestations

ICU admission is required when children present in respiratory failure with an asthma exacerbation that is not responding to conventional treatment.[154] These exacerbations can be due to viral infection and allergy,[144] demographic characteristic (pre-school age, low income, black race, Hispanic ethnicity and minority), seasonal patterns, bacterial infections and environmental factors as well as psychological factors such as stress.[155] Other factors such as obesity and genetic predisposition may be important in reacting to beta-2 agonist therapy.[144,155] Arterial blood gas analysis usually reveals mild respiratory alkalosis and hypoxaemia initially; however, more-severe asthma may show combined respiratory and metabolic acidosis and hypercapnia as the child tires and is unable to eliminate carbon dioxide (CO_2).[156] The severity of the exacerbation is classified as: mild with absent or low increase in work of breathing, moderate with marked increase in work of breathing, and severe with tachypnoea (>30/min), pulse rate >120 bpm, hypoventilation (SpO_2<90%), severe chest retractions and marked increase in work of breathing that alters behaviour of the child.[119,144]

Patient assessment and management

Assessment of asthma is based on severity classifications.[144] There are many scores available to assist in determining the severity of asthma, including the Asthma Control Questionnaire, the Asthma Control Test and the Asthma Exacerbation Clinical Score, which can predict the risk of exacerbation.[156] Whatever method is used, assessments should be frequent and the response to treatment recorded.

Asthma management should be personalised, following a care cycle of assessing, adjusting and reviewing steps for individual patient needs.[119] The broad management aims in severe asthma include: maintaining oxygenation (to achieve SpO_2 >92%), rapid bronchodilation,[154] treating any cardiovascular compromise,[119] and continuous monitoring.[144] In children with severe asthma, consider symptom control, risk factors, lung function and comorbidities.[119] Hypoxaemia results from ventilation/perfusion (V/Q) mismatch due to lower airway obstruction,[156,157] hypoventilation, hypercarbia and pulmonary vasoconstriction related to acidosis.[156] Hypoxaemia can result in further bronchoconstriction, hypotension, systemically-reduced oxygen availability, increased myocardial oxygen consumption and neurological symptoms such as agitation, confusion or decreased level of consciousness.

Bronchodilators may worsen hypoxaemia through worsening V/Q mismatch or bronchoconstriction, due to the hyperosmolarity of the nebulised solution.[158] In addition, rapid changes to the compliance of the airways together with hyperexpanded lungs may result in airway collapse. Oxygen delivery is achieved by high-flow oxygen mask with a reservoir bag. All nebuliser therapy should be oxygen driven. However, if hypoxaemia persists despite maximal bronchodilator therapy and oxygen administration, mask CPAP may be considered.[154,159]

Beta-2 agonists, anticholinergics and steroids form the foundation of acute severe asthma management, but for children over 40 kg and those who have reached puberty it may be more appropriate to administer IV adrenaline. Beta-2 agonists act by relaxing bronchial smooth muscle, improving mucociliary transport and inhibiting mediator release. In severe to life-threatening asthma, inhaled short-acting beta-2 agonists combined with an anticholinergic are recommended as they improve lung function, decrease side effects such as nausea and tremor and decrease the risk for hospital admission if treated early. Adverse effects of beta-2 agonist administration include hypokalaemia, tachycardia, tremors, agitation and hyperglycaemia. Mild lactic acidosis may also occur. Intravenous salbutamol infusion should be considered when there is severe, life-threatening asthma refractory to inhaled treatment. Inhaled salbutamol may be discontinued once IV infusion has commenced, but should be re-established before ceasing the infusion. In acute severe episodes, salbutamol is usually given every 20 minutes; if there is little response, continuous nebuliser therapy may be required.[154,159] Ipratropium bromide is used in combination with salbutamol for severe exacerbations.[119,144] In this instance, a feeding tube is inserted into the nebuliser and the chamber replenished as it empties. Anticholinergics, in combination with beta-2 agonists, improve lung function by augmenting the action of beta-2 agonists, blocking irritant receptors and bronchodilation of larger airways.[155]

Corticosteroids may be used earlier in children with allergic asthma and risk factors.[144] They decrease airway inflammation, enhance the effects of beta-2 agonists and reduce mucus production. Oral and intravenous methods of administration are equally effective. The effects of systemic steroids are apparent within 3–4 hours of administration, with maximal benefit achieved within 6–12 hours. There is little evidence to support giving inhaled steroids during an acute episode, and their use is not recommended in combination with salbutamol.[159]

Magnesium sulfate promotes smooth muscle relaxation by inhibiting uptake of calcium. Intravenous magnesium sulfate has demonstrated efficacy in acute severe asthma, but there is a modest benefit of inhaled magnesium sulfate combined with a beta-2 agonist.[144,154,159]

Intravenous aminophylline is a bronchodilator, improving diaphragmatic contractility, and is a central respiratory stimulant. It has shown some benefit with regard to improved lung function in severe asthma that is unresponsive to inhaled bronchodilators and steroids, with the benefit being dependent on appropriate dosage.[154,159] However, the narrow therapeutic window and side effects of induced nausea and/or vomiting represent a risk of complication, so its use should be limited to managing severe asthma not responsive to other agents.[160]

Ventilation may be required when there is profound hypoxaemia, severe muscle fatigue or decreased level of consciousness, and no or limited response to standard therapy.[159] However, as asthmatic children are at higher risk of complications such as barotrauma and air trapping, there is a higher risk of death associated with ventilation in this group of patients.[161] Non-invasive ventilation (NIV) is the first choice, with some evidence that it rapidly corrects gas exchange abnormalities, assists with respiratory muscle fatigue and can avoid intubation.[154,159] The absolute contraindications for NIV include: cardiac/respiratory arrest, severe encephalopathy, haemodynamic instability, facial surgery/deformity, absence of protective airway reflexes, severe respiratory distress with paradoxical abdominal muscles or thoracic muscle use, severe upper gastrointestinal bleeding, nausea or vomiting, unstable arrhythmia and upper airway obstruction. Relative contraindications for NIV are facial surgery/deformity/trauma, and inability to maintain upper airway patency.[162]

Intubation may be necessary when signs of deterioration are present, such as elevated CO_2 levels, exhaustion, alteration of mental status, haemodynamic instability and refractory hypoxaemia.[154,159] Because of high airway pressures, a cuffed ETT should be used. When using invasive ventilation, it is recommended to maintain adequate oxygenation, accept permissive hypercapnia (maintaining pH at or above 7.2), and use prolonged expiratory times, a slow breath rate (reducing air trapping), and a PEEP below the level of auto-PEEP (to reduce work of breathing).[159]

Children with acute severe asthma will often have a raised metabolic rate and increased insensible losses, together with reduced oral intake. With increased intrathoracic pressure from air trapping, even mild dehydration may compromise cardiac output. Therefore, adequate fluid replacement is necessary. In addition, pulmonary secretions will thicken and plug the airways if fluid intake is inadequate. IV fluids should be provided until the child's condition and oral intake improve.[163]

Asthma does not increase the risk of SARS-CoV-19, and asthmatic children infected with SARS-CoV-2 tend to be asymptomatic and can continue taking their prescribed asthma medicines. Where possible, due to the risk of aerosol-related viral transmission, it is recommended to avoid the use of nebulisers.[119,144]

Nursing the ventilated child

Principals of mechanical ventilation were covered in Chapter 15. Issues such as gastric decompression, adequate analgesia and sedation and undertaking steps to prevent accidental extubation are similar to those for adults.

Specific considerations for ventilating infants and children include the following:

- Providing oxygenation before, during and after suctioning with 100% O_2. The child's clinical status is monitored throughout the procedure.[164]

- Heated humidification is recommended in children, although there is no evidence to suggest any type of humidification, but children have limited respiratory reserve and are prone to airway blockage.[165]

- Equipment should fit the child's size to avoid unnecessary dead space.

- Endotracheal suctioning should be performed only when clinically indicated and normal saline instillation is not recommended.[164,166]

- To prevent iatrogenic atelectasis, the suction catheter size should be less than or equal to two-thirds the internal diameter of the ETT. Suction pressure should be limited to 60 mmHg (8 kPa) for infants, and up to 200 mmHg (27 kPa) for adolescents. A suction regulator is useful to monitor the amount of applied negative pressure, as too much can result in atelectasis.[166]

- Cuffed and uncuffed endotracheal tubes are appropriate for infants. Cuffed tubes are used increasingly. As the patient's position affects ETT cuff pressure, it should be monitored and adjusted as required after mobilisation.

- Restraints may be required to limit the movement of the child, with the aim of preventing accidental extubation rather than maintaining the child in an immobile state. Restraints may be physical, such as arm boards or hand ties; or chemical, such as sedation.

A decision-making tool can assist nurses to make appropriate decisions in performing endotracheal suction in children.[164,167]

Modes of ventilation

There are many modes of ventilation (see Chapter 15). This section includes information specifically related to paediatric ventilation. As with adults, arterial blood gases should be taken about 15–20 minutes after initiating mechanical ventilation.

Volume ventilation in children

Typically, volume ventilation is not used in infants under 5 kg owing to the small tidal volumes that risk being lost in the distensible tubing and leaking around the ETT. In addition, most volume ventilators do not have a constant fresh gas flow, so the infant must work harder to trigger a breath. Some of the newer models of ventilator have attempted to overcome these problems. Steps in beginning volume ventilation for a child are as follows:[168]

1 Set a tidal volume of 5–8 mL/kg. This is a protective lung strategy approach and can be increased if needed to a maximum of 9–10 mL/kg.

2 Set the rate at 20 breaths/min for infants and younger children. This is lower than physiological for infants, but the slightly larger tidal volumes will compensate. For older children and adolescents, 10–14/min.

3 Set the FiO_2 at <0.5 and titrate according to oxygen saturation and blood gases.

4 Set the PEEP at 5–8 cmH_2O. This is slightly higher than physiological.

5 Set the trigger sensitive enough to allow the infant or child to trigger a breath without working too hard. If a continuous fresh gas flow is available, this is preferable. If autocycling occurs, decrease the trigger-setting sensitivity gradually until the autocycling stops.

Pressure ventilation in children

The pressure ventilation mode is most commonly used in infants weighing less than 5 kg or with children who have a large leak around an uncuffed ETT. Steps in beginning pressure ventilation for a child are as follows and should be based on arterial blood gases:[168]

1 Set the peak inspiratory pressure (PIP) at 18–20 cmH_2O.

2 Set the PEEP at 4–6 cmH_2O (rarely exceeds 7 cmH_2O).

3 Set the rate at 20 breaths/min.

4 Set the FiO_2 at <0.6 and titrate according to oxygen saturation and blood gases.

5 Set the trigger sensitivity to trigger a breath without autotriggering. Most pressure ventilators have a constant fresh gas flow, which allows the child to breathe spontaneously without increased effort.

Non-invasive ventilation

NIV refers to ventilatory support without an artificial airway in the trachea (see Chapter 15). As in adults, NIV may be used to reduce the need for intubation in children. Its use in children is safe and effective for the treatment of acute respiratory failure, acute viral bronchiolitis, neuromuscular disease and asthma.[168]

High-frequency oscillatory ventilation

High-frequency oscillatory ventilation (HFOV) uses supraphysiological ventilatory rates and tidal volumes less than anatomical dead space to accomplish gas exchange. Typical ventilator rates are 3–15 Hz or 180–600 breaths/min (1 Hz = 60 breaths). HFOV is primarily used in managing infants and children with diffuse alveolar or interstitial disease requiring high peak distending pressures. Goals include maximising alveolar recruitment, minimising barotrauma and providing adequate alveolar gas exchange.[169]

HFOV is delivered primarily by a specialised ventilator that uses a diaphragm piston unit to actively move gas into and out of the lung, and a non-compliant breathing circuit. A major difference between HFOV and other forms of ventilation is that there is active expiration with oscillation, versus passive expiration for conventional ventilation. Unlike conventional ventilation, which uses bulk flow to deliver gas to the lungs, using smaller than dead space tidal volumes utilises the mechanisms of pendelluft, Taylor dispersion, asymmetrical velocity profiles, cardiogenic mixing and, to a very limited extent, bulk flow.[169] These are all terms that describe the distribution of gas when rapid rates and tiny volumes are used.

Ventilation is dependent on amplitude (a determinant of tidal volume) much more than rate. With oscillation ventilation, lowering frequency (Hz) improves CO_2 removal. This is thought to occur because the oscillating diaphragm is able to move through a greater distance, therefore increasing tidal volume by providing more inspiratory time and a longer expiratory time.

The principal determinants of oxygenation are the same as those for conventional ventilation. Therefore, as with conventional ventilation, the alveoli must be open and prevented from collapsing if hypoxaemia is to be corrected. HFOV theoretically achieves this through delivering a high mean airway pressure without imposing a large tidal volume, but there is insufficient evidence to promote its use over conventional ventilation in children and infants.

The child experiencing shock

A detailed description of shock is given in Chapter 21, with specific paediatric considerations addressed here.

Hypovolaemic and septic shock (also termed distributive shock) are the most common types of shock in children. Cardiogenic shock is rare and is seen mainly after open-heart surgery, severe myocarditis or cardiomyopathy and in untreated shock. The infant with an undiagnosed congenital heart defect, in particular lesions that rely on the ductus arteriosus – known as duct-dependent lesions – can present collapsed and in shock in the first weeks of life as the duct closes.[170] As infants and children presenting in hypovolaemic shock are likely to respond to fluid resuscitation alone, they may not require transfer to a specialist paediatric centre. However, children presenting with septic shock or cardiogenic shock will require transfer to a specialist paediatric centre for ongoing management, and early contact should be made to initiate goal-directed therapy as soon as possible. Those children who do not respond to fluid volume alone will require invasive haemodynamic monitoring and possible pharmacological intervention.

Sepsis is a leading cause of death in infants and children worldwide.[171,172] The mortality rate for septic shock in children ranges from 4% to as high as 50% in resource-restricted countries.[171,172] Sepsis remains a significant source of critical illness and mortality globally in infants and children, with the incidence of sepsis accounting for over half of cases.[173] Early detection of sepsis in children has been the focus in many countries, as failure to recognise it is directly correlated with mortality. There is further work to enhance awareness of recognition of sepsis by parents and prior to hospitalisation, since there is still no reliable single test for sepsis.[173] Sepsis in children

TABLE 27.7	
Organisms causing sepsis in newborns, infants and children	
AGE GROUP	COMMON ORGANISMS CAUSING SEPSIS
Newborns	Group B beta-haemolytic streptococci
	Enterobacteriaceae (such as *E. coli*)
	Listeria monocytogenes
	Herpes simplex virus
	Staphylococcus aureus
	Neisseria meningitidis
Infants	*Haemophilus influenzae*
	Streptococcus pneumoniae
	Staphylococcus aureus
	Neisseria meningitidis
Children	*Staphylococcus aureus*
	Neisseria meningitidis
	Streptococcus pneumoniae
	Enterobacteriaceae

Source: Adapted from Maloney PM. Sepsis and septic shock. Emerg Med Clin North Am 2013;31:583–600.

follows a similar trajectory to that in adults, namely refractory shock leading to death in the first 3 days, with later deaths after 3 days attributable to multiple organ dysfunction, and neurological and respiratory failure following treatment withdrawal.[174]

Causes of septic shock in infants and children are often different from those in adolescents and adults. The commonest infecting organisms are often age related and are listed in Table 27.7. Meningococcal sepsis remains the leading cause of septic shock in developed countries such as Australia and New Zealand. In resource-limited countries, leading causes of fatal sepsis include diarrhoeal diseases, malaria, lower respiratory tract infections and HIV/AIDS.[172]

Clinical manifestations

There are many similarities between children and adults in the clinical manifestations of shock (see Chapter 21). Guidelines for children published in 2020 have removed the emphasis previously placed on inflammatory response and instead incorporate organ dysfunction markers specific to children, recognising that, in children, sepsis is associated with life-threatening organ dysfunction resulting from a dysregulated response to infection.[171]

Clinical features of evolving septic shock in children include:

- abnormal temperature (high or low)
- altered neurological status
- altered perfusion – peripheral vasodilation *or* vasoconstriction with delayed capillary refill time – before hypotension develops

- abnormal white cell count – may be low in the neonate and then high in all other paediatric age groups
- abnormal heart rate and respiratory rate for age (high or low)
- two of the following: unexplained metabolic acidosis, increased lactate, oliguria.[14]

Systemic hypotension is not necessary to make the diagnosis of septic shock in children. Tachycardia in the absence of fever is a more reliable sign than hypotension, as up to 25% of the child's circulating volume may be lost before hypotension occurs. Hypotension is hence a late sign in children and may indicate late decompensated shock, particularly following fluid delivery.[174]

One other specific factor for children that is not relevant in the adult population is a higher risk of sepsis in preterm infants and in infants with cardiac defects or chronic lung disease.[175]

Patient assessment and diagnostics

Assessment of the child with shock is based on clinical assessment, with less reliance on biochemical testing than in adult shock.[171] Ideally, shock should be diagnosed before hypotension occurs. Hypothermia or hyperthermia and altered neurological status, which provides information about cardiac output and perfusion pressure, and peripheral vasodilation (warm shock) or vasoconstriction with capillary refill >3 seconds (cold shock) are clinical signs of shock in children.[14]

Careful respiratory and cardiovascular assessment is required, as described in this chapter and Chapters 11 and 13. Monitoring of children experiencing shock is the same as for adults (see Chapter 21). It consists of continuous monitoring of heart rate, intra-arterial blood pressure, SvO_2 saturation, quality of peripheral pulses, capillary refill, level of consciousness, temperature and urine output as indirect measures of cardiac output as well as serial blood gas, lactate and electrolyte analysis, with potential to use a stroke index in children once they are admitted to ICU.[176] Diagnosis of septic shock can be difficult in children. When present, non-blanching rash is a specific sign of meningococcal septicaemia.[177]

Practice tip

As rash may be less visible in dark-skinned children, check the soles of the feet, the palms of the hands and conjunctivae in these children.

A certain proportion of children will present with non-specific symptoms or signs of infection, such as fever, vomiting, lethargy, irritability or headache, and the condition may be difficult to distinguish from other less serious infections.[13] Laboratory testing of samples of blood, urine, stool, sputum, cerebrospinal fluid and any obvious wounds or lesions is standard practice in adults and children.

Patient management

The use of screening tools in acutely unwell children is aimed at the early recognition of shock. Rapid institution of appropriate goal-directed therapy and targeting the causative agent remain the mainstays of managing septic shock in children, as in adults. Goal-directed therapies such as oxygen therapy, fluid resuscitation, maintenance of acceptable blood pressure and institution of pharmacological treatment and other supportive treatments to achieve therapeutic goals are practised in managing shock in children, and are linked to better outcomes.[171]

Large amounts of fluid may be required by children despite peripheral oedema or absence of overt fluid loss. The most recent recommendations for fluid boluses recommend differing approaches for health systems with access to ICU and those systems without ICU access.[171] Where access to ICU is readily available, aggressive fluid resuscitation and antibiotics in the first hour before development of hypotension is linked to improved mortality in children with hypovolaemic and septic shock.[171] In resource-limited environments where access to ICU is not available and a child is not hypotensive, it is recommended that only maintenance fluids be commenced and boluses avoided.[171,172]

Intravascular access in children can be difficult, and umbilical venous access in newborns and intraosseous access in children can be used before the placement of central lines.[14] Regardless of type, intraosseous needles all allow rapid access to the intramedullary capillary network, facilitating delivery of fluids, drugs and blood products. The preferred site in infants and children is the proximal tibia, 2–3 cm below the tibial tuberosity.[175] Once sited, a syringe must be attached to aspirate and correct placement ascertained. Fluid boluses can then be given via syringe into the intramedullary space with the aim of restoring circulating volume, which will in turn facilitate venous access with improvement of peripheral perfusion.[175]

Similarly to adults, after appropriate volume resuscitation has been given and symptoms of shock are not resolving or hypotension is developing, inotropes and vasopressors are recommended. Inotropic drugs that are recommended in children include adrenaline (epinephrine) and noradrenaline (norepinephrine).[178] Vasodilators, including sodium nitroprusside or nitroglycerine, are used to recruit microcirculation; type III phosphodiesterase inhibitors are used to improve cardiac contractility.[178] The use of hydrocortisone has not been shown to change outcome in septic shock in children and is not recommended.[171] For refractory shock that is not responding to maximal therapy, but thought to be reversible, extracorporeal life support may be considered. Extracorporeal membrane oxygenation (ECMO) is increasingly used for critically ill infants and children with other forms of shock such as cardiogenic shock, including in the postoperative cardiothoracic surgical patient, and, increasingly, for out-of-hospital cardiac arrest patients.[179]

Extracorporeal membrane oxygenation

Extracorporeal membrane oxygenation is an alternative method of providing ventilatory and/or cardiac support for newborns, infants and children, as well as adults.[180] When used to support ventilation, ECMO allows the lungs to rest and heal. Ventilation settings are reduced to minimal in order to minimise the iatrogenic effects of positive pressure. There are two main methods of ECMO: venovenous and venoarterial. Venoarterial (VA) ECMO is more common in infants and children than the alternative – venovenous (VV) ECMO – largely because of the increased risk of limb ischaemia associated with large-bore cannulas in veins, such as the internal jugular or femoral vein.[179] Use of paediatric femoral venoarterial ECMO reduces the risk of limb ischaemia in infants and children.[180] Alternative placements of cannulas for venoarterial ECMO after cardiothoracic surgery are the right atrium and aorta. Venoarterial ECMO allows support of both circulation and ventilation. Essentially, blood is drained from the 'venous' line, pumped through a membrane to oxygenate the blood and remove CO_2, then returned through a filter via the 'arterial' cannula.[181] Further details regarding ECMO and ECMO systems are discussed in Chapter 15.

Infants and children are considered for ECMO if they have potentially reversible lung or cardiac injury, or shock that has not responded to conventional therapies. Contraindications include irreversible brain or central nervous system (CNS) injury, immunodeficiency or severe coagulopathy, or where infant vessel size would prohibit the placement of a cannula. Long-term outcomes continue to improve; however, further longer-term outcome studies are required.[179] ECMO centres need to maintain their competence by performing the procedure often. The SARS-CoV-2 pandemic has further increased interest in ECMO for children.[180] A recent meta-analysis of ECMO use in paediatric sepsis has suggested that survival rates of almost 60% warrant early consideration of ECMO in the management of refractory septic shock.[181]

The child experiencing acute neurological dysfunction

There are many reasons why an infant or child can present with an acute episode of neurological dysfunction. Common presentations to an ICU include meningitis,[182] encephalitis, seizures and encephalopathy (see also Chapter 17). Assessment and recognition of the clinical features and management of the various causes of neurological dysfunction in children are the keys to achieving good outcomes.

Neurological assessment

To assess a child's level of consciousness, several different scales can be used. The Glasgow Coma Scale (GCS) is commonly used, but the Paediatric Glasgow Coma Scale is more appropriate for children under 2 years. Another reliable scale is the Paediatric Full Outline of Unresponsiveness (FOUR) score; it includes four parameters (eye response, motor response, pupil reflexes and breathing) rated on a 0–4 scale, giving a possible score of between 0 (completely unresponsive) and 16. The FOUR score and the GCS are both able to predict in-hospital morbidity and poor outcome at the end of hospitalisation.[183]

Other neurological assessment parameters include the following:

- Pupils – assess size, reaction and symmetry.
- Posture – abnormal flexion posturing, often referred to as decorticate posturing, is a flexion response of the arms with either flexion or extension of the legs, while abnormal extension posturing, often referred to as decerebrate posturing, is an extension response of all limbs, where arms rotate externally. Both abnormal flexion and extension posturing in a previously normal child may indicate raised intracranial pressure.
- Meningism – this is indicated by neck stiffness in a child ≥2 years of age, and full/bulging fontanelle in an infant.[184]

Seizures

Seizures are covered in Chapter 17. The various aetiologies of seizures in children include febrile convulsions, CNS infection such as meningitis or encephalitis, metabolic imbalances, drugs, trauma or epilepsy. Seizures in children are common, with up to 10% of children having an unprovoked seizure without recurrence.[186] Seizure incidence fluctuates from 33.3 to 82 per 100,000 children per year, with the highest cases in the first year of life, and decreases in teenage years.[185] Febrile convulsions are associated with temperature >100.9°F (>38.3°C) and occur in 3–5% of children, commonly between the ages of 6 months and 5 years, without a history of epilepsy or evidence of an intracranial infection.[185] They can be simple (generalised and occur once in a 24-hour period, lasting less than 5 minutes), complex (focal or localised to a specific part of the body, lasting 15–30 minutes or recurring within a 24-hour period), or develop into status epilepticus (lasting more than 30 minutes).[185]

Patient management

Management of the paediatric patient with seizures is similar to management of the adult and includes early administration of midazolam, second-line agents such as phenytoin and levetiracetam, and barbiturate if seizures are refractory (see Chapter 17); there are, however, some specific paediatric considerations.[185]

The paediatric patient suffering seizures is more susceptible than an adult to hypoglycaemia. Hypoglycaemia may lead to secondary brain injury during and after seizures. Blood glucose levels should always be checked in children suffering from seizures and intravenous fluids containing glucose should be administered.[187]

Care of the seizing or post-ictal child is generally supportive, and includes monitoring for signs of ongoing seizures, administration of appropriate anticonvulsants and regular assessment of neurological function. In young infants, seizures may be difficult to determine and may include stiffening, staring and lip smacking rather than obvious clonic activity.[185] Continuous electroencephalogram monitoring is therefore recommended for non-convulsive seizures performed during both wakefulness and sleep. The objective of EEG is to assess abnormalities that might suggest a focal lesion.[185,188]

Meningitis

Meningitis is an acute inflammation of the meninges that usually develops over 1–2 days. A fulminant form of meningitis caused by *Neisseria meningitidis*, responsible for invasive meningococcal disease (IMD), may develop over several hours. Organisms causing bacterial meningitis vary by age group. In infants under 3 months of age, group b *Streptococcus*, *E. coli*, *Streptococcus pneumoniae* and *Listeria* are the most likely agents.[189] In children over 3 months of age, meningococcus, *Haemophilus influenzae* type b and *S. pneumoniae* are more common.[190] The commonest causes of viral meningitis in infants and children include herpes simplex virus and the enteroviruses.[190,191] Tuberculous meningitis, while still rare, is becoming more common, particularly in immigrant families or those who recently travelled to affected areas.[192] Bacterial meningitis continues to have a poorer outcome than other forms of meningitis, despite advances in therapy.[189]

Incidence

Data on the incidence of meningitis are limited to the major bacterial types, particularly for infants and children over 2 months of age. Hib, meningococcal and pneumococcal infections are notifiable.[193] The mortality rate of meningococcal meningitis in children is lower than in adults and increases with associated sepsis.[194] However, IMD-related complications, such as hearing loss, chronic renal failure cognitive impairment and psychological problems, occur more frequently in children than in adults.[195]

Meningococcus is the main cause of meningitis in children. Specific strains tend to be prevalent in different regions of the world, with serogroups A, B, C, W-135, Y and X the current strains responsible for almost all invasive meningococcal disease.[194] In Europe, the Americas and Oceania, serogroups B, C and Y have caused most cases. Serogroup A has been associated with the highest incidence (up to 1000 per 100,000 cases), causing large outbreaks of meningococcal disease in sub-Saharan Africa and Asia, while serogroups W-135 and X have emerged more recently and are responsible for major disease outbreaks in sub-Saharan Africa.[196] Available vaccines differ around the world based on the prevalent strains, so recent overseas travel and place of vaccination should be obtained in the history.

The incidence of invasive pneumococcal disease has significantly dropped in developed regions such as Europe, North America and Australia since the introduction of routine vaccination and decreased hospitalisation rate.[197] Incidence in Australia has ranged from 6 to 8 per 100,000, with most cases in the under-5-years and over-70-years age groups.[198] Risk factors include extreme prematurity, chronic lung disease, trisomy 21 (Down syndrome), diabetes, indigenous status and immunocompromised children.[198,199] Clinical manifestations or symptoms vary with the age of the child, duration of the illness and history of antibiotic use for the current illness. Case fatality ratio fluctuates between regions of the world (600,000 deaths worldwide),[200] but is lower in high-income countries (12–80%), with higher rates in low- and middle-income countries.[200]

Patient management

Initial management of the infant or child with meningitis includes assessment and management of the airway, breathing, circulation and disability.[188] Rapid antibiotic therapy is recommended and is likely to decrease case fatality.[200,201] Once the initial resuscitation has been completed, consideration should be given to correcting any biochemical abnormalities. In particular, blood sugar level should be checked and corrected in the early management phase. Once meningitis is suspected, a lumbar puncture (LP) is generally performed to confirm diagnosis, but if the child is haemodynamically unstable or has ongoing seizures, problems with ventilation or signs of raised intracranial pressure, the LP should be delayed and blood cultures obtained.[202]

While steroid use in meningitis has some benefit in reducing morbidity in adults,[203] there is no evidence to recommend use in children. Infants and children with meningitis require intensive care management when there is a reduced level of consciousness and respiratory and/or circulatory compromise. The broad aims of management are to support ventilation and circulation while preventing secondary brain injury. Regular assessment and monitoring of associated risks such as seizures, syndrome of inappropriate antidiuretic hormone secretion (SIADH) or cerebral salt wasting and sepsis is essential.

Encephalitis

The most common type of encephalitis in children is acute viral encephalitis, and the most common causative agent is herpes simplex virus (HSV).[204] Left untreated, HSV is almost uniformly fatal, with over half of survivors experiencing significant long-term morbidity. Other causes of encephalitis in children include:[201,205]

- enteroviruses (e.g. enterovirus 71, coxsackievirus, polio and echovirus)
- varicella zoster virus
- Epstein–Barr virus
- cytomegalovirus
- adenovirus
- rubella
- measles

- Murray Valley encephalitis (MVE) virus
- Kunjin virus
- West Nile virus.

Worldwide, the incidence of acute encephalitis ranges between 3.5 and 7.4 cases per 100,000 children, with a mortality rate around 6%.[206] Children under 1 year of age are at higher risk of developing encephalitis. Other risk factors include immune dysfunction and exposure to risk animals, or specific geographic location.

Encephalitis symptoms are similar to meningitis, but often with a much slower onset. Progressively worsening headache, fever and decreased level of consciousness or behavioural changes characterise encephalitis. Focal neurological signs and seizures may indicate involvement of the meninges or spinal cord.[207]

Patient management

Prompt administration of aciclovir (acyclovir) is warranted to all patients with clinical symptoms suggesting encephalitis because of the high mortality and morbidity rates.[205] Other viruses are also treated with aciclovir. Intensive care management involves supporting ventilation and managing neurological complications such as seizures and cerebral oedema. If the child is unconscious on presentation, the disease course will be more severe.

Gastrointestinal and renal considerations in children

Many critically ill infants and children are at risk of developing complications involving the kidney and the GIT.

Acute kidney injury (AKI) is increasingly identified and is associated with increased length of stay, increased morbidity and increased mortality.[208] A prospective multicentre study[209] using the Kidney Disease Improving Global Outcomes (KDIGO) acute kidney injury definitions and staging found that the incidence of AKI in critically ill children and young adults is significant, occurring in around 25% of patients in ICU within the first week of admission. AKI in combination with significant accumulation of fluid further worsens outcome.[210] Identified risk factors for developing AKI include: exposure to nephrotoxic medications, organ and bone marrow transplantation, shock, organ dysfunction and following congenital cardiac surgery.[209,211] Critically ill children, similar to adults, require monitoring of kidney function by both serial serum creatinine and urine output, as creatinine monitoring alone may miss up to two-thirds of those with AKI.[209] Consequently, continuous renal replacement therapy (CRRT) should be considered earlier in management than has previously been the case and is discussed in Chapter 18. Persistent AKI is associated with fluid accumulation and a worse outcome; therefore children experiencing AKI will benefit from prompt transfer to a specialty PICU to commence CRRT as soon as AKI is suspected.[211]

The child's GIT will need protection from developing ulceration and bleeding in critical illness. The incidence of GI bleeding is notably decreasing.[212] Recent studies have shown that some patient groups in PICU may be at greater risk, such as those placed onto ECMO.[213] Clinically significant bleeding causing haemodynamic instability or requiring transfusion is reported to be rare in children in PICUs.[214] The same treatments can be used in both children and adults, with no one agent, dose or regimen standing out as better for minimising bleeding and ulceration or leading to fewer complications such as pneumonia.[215]

Nutritional considerations

The aims of nutrition in critically ill children are twofold. First, children are at particular risk of malnutrition because they are growing and have greater energy requirements for their weight and less storage capacity than adults. Second, children are at particular risk of developing protein–calorie malnutrition, which can lead to immunodysfunction, increased risk of infections, morbidity and death in those children with organ dysfunction.[216] Morbidity and mortality are also associated with malnutrition in children admitted to the PICU – both obese and underweight children are at risk.[217] Nutritional status should be monitored as soon as practical, ideally within the first 24 hours of admission and regularly while in PICU.[216]

Nutrition is also important in maintaining gut mucosa integrity, preventing the development of hypo- and hyperglycaemia, assisting with maintenance of immune function and modulating the immune response as well as providing energy.[217] Identified barriers to achieving adequate enteral nutrition for critically ill children worldwide include: withholding of feeds for procedures or surgery, lack of access to dietitians, particularly after hours and at weekends, fluid restrictions that are routine practice in the ICU, and delays in commencing transpyloric tube placement/confirmation, as well as a lack of education on optimising nutrition.[218] In order to minimise delays and/or restrictions, use of feeding protocols and liberalising fluids where possible to maximise enteral nutrition should be considered.[216]

When caring for critically ill infants and children, nutrition to support growth needs to be considered. Ideally, enteral feeding of critically ill children should commence within 12–24 hours of admission to ICU, but may not be achievable until the child is transferred to a specialist centre.[217] It may not be appropriate to commence feeds if the child requires transfer, surgery or intubation. A dietitian should be consulted to advise on appropriate enteral feeding formulas for children, in addition to organising caloric supplementation of feeds.[217] The dietitian can advise on handling of human milk while in hospital for breastfeeding mothers, who will need to express milk when the infant is not yet feeding orally or to provide milk for tube feeding. In addition, dietitians can assess the child's energy requirements and the amount of feed required to meet needs, as both under- and overfeeding have been identified as issues in the PICU.[216,217] The evidence for additives in enteral feeding is not clear-cut in children, and therefore routine supplementation for critically ill infants and children is not common practice.

Intravenous therapy for children

Until enteral feeding is established, critically ill infants and children will require maintenance IV fluids. Traditionally, hypotonic fluids – fluids containing a concentration of sodium lower than normal serum sodium – have been administered as maintenance fluids. However, hypotonic fluids have no role in the management of critically ill infants and children, as they are responsible for iatrogenic hyponatraemia in hospitalised children.[4,219] For critically ill children, the capacity to excrete additional free water is often impaired. In addition, some common conditions seen in the ICU, including pain, nausea and infections of the CNS, the GIT, the lung and post-surgery, increase secretion of antidiuretic hormone (ADH), so promoting the retention of water.[220] The risk of developing cerebral oedema is increased in children, who also have increased body tissue water content, and studies indicate that there is an increased risk of developing acute hyponatraemia leading to seizures.[220]

Newborn infants up to around 1 month of age will require a higher concentration of glucose, up to 10%. It has been common paediatric practice to use only 500-mL IV bags in children for safety reasons; however, 1 L bags are more common. In the modern era across Westernised countries, use of volumetric IV pumps and burettes has been standard paediatric practice.

Infants and children generally require added glucose in IV fluids. In infants under 3 months of age, glucose concentration is increased to at least 5% and up to 10%. The addition of potassium chloride into maintenance fluids is common, particularly in fasting children, and requires serial monitoring of serum potassium. The use of balanced IV fluids is thought to be associated with a reduced incidence of hyperchloraemia compared with 0.9% sodium chloride; however, a recent systematic review and meta-analysis has failed to demonstrate this.[5]

For fluid resuscitation in infants and children, the use of glucose-containing IV fluids is contraindicated, and 0.9% sodium chloride remains a safe resuscitation fluid of choice across the life span, including in the delivery suite for newborn fluid resuscitation.[220]

Glucose control in children

The predisposition to hypoglycaemia in children has meant that aggressive treatment of hyperglycaemia is not commonplace in critically ill children. The most recent systematic review and meta-analysis including 6 studies involving over 4000 children showed no difference in outcomes and an increase in hypoglycaemia incidence and severity in the tight glucose control arms.[221] Monitoring for hypoglycaemia continues to be an important assessment parameter, particularly in sicker children who require ventilatory support, inotropic support and where enteral feeding may be contraindicated. Hypoglycaemia may be an indicator of worsening organ function; therefore, further research needs to focus on the safety of insulin therapy in the non-diabetic critically ill child before aggressive routine management of hyperglycaemia can be recommended.[221]

Liver disease in children

Acute liver failure is relatively rare in children. It arises as a primary problem in children from countries where viral hepatitis is endemic and is associated with paracetamol overdose and chronic liver disorders, toxins, autoimmune disease, malignancies, vascular and biliary tree malformations as well as unidentified causes.[222] Chapter 20 contains more detail on liver function and dysfunction. There are varying severities and forms of liver failure. Infants and children experiencing fulminant hepatic failure and hepatic encephalopathy, regardless of underlying cause, are critically ill and require transfer to a specialist PICU for ongoing management and possible liver transplantation. The mortality rate is strongly linked to the development of cerebral oedema and intracranial hypertension, and is reported to be as high as 50% where cerebral oedema occurs.[223] Promising work with auxiliary liver transplant of partial livers and preservation of the native liver in predominantly older children with infections or toxic causes of their liver failure has demonstrated recovery of the native liver and subsequent withdrawal of immunosuppressive agents.[224] Many critically ill infants and children are at risk of developing some degree of liver dysfunction; therefore, liver function of all critically ill children requires careful monitoring and management. Clinical manifestations and management of infants and children with liver failure are similar to those of adults.

Paediatric trauma

Trauma is a leading cause of death in children and young adults in high-income countries; in middle and low-income countries it is second only to deaths from infections.[172,225] The approach to management of trauma in children is the same as in adults. See Chapter 24 for details on trauma systems and trauma management. While some evidence from North America indicates that specialist paediatric trauma centres produce better outcomes for injured children,[226] the largely spread-out and relatively small population distribution in Australia, New Zealand and many other countries means that children will often be treated initially in adult settings.

Incidence and patterns of injury in children

Injury is a leading cause of death in all children aged over 1 year across the world and represents half of all deaths in children 10 years and older.[227] As sociodemographic circumstances improve, injury burden decreases; however, road traffic injuries, burns and drowning kill many children,[228] while falls remain a leading cause of presentation to EDs worldwide.[227] Children living in regional and rural areas have increased rates of traumatic injuries and deaths from trauma, as do children from lower socioeconomic backgrounds with crowded living conditions.[227]

Injury patterns in children differ from adults, with traumatic brain injury, blunt trauma and more diffuse injuries more common in children. There is a bimodal injury pattern associated with age, with peak incidence occurring in children aged 1–4 years and a second peak during adolescence and young adulthood, reflecting the different activities associated with each group.[229] Infants and young children have a decreased sense of danger and reduced ability to protect themselves, while adolescents have increased exposure to higher risk activities in conjunction with exposure to alcohol, drugs and motor vehicles.[230] Time of day and seasonal factors play a role in childhood injury, with children more likely to be injured at the end of the school day and during summer months, when the incidence of drowning increases.[228]

Injury-related deaths in children are highest in the transport deaths category, followed by falls, drowning and assault.[230] Motor vehicle accidents involving children over 4 years old as passengers, pedestrians or cyclists are the commonest cause of injury in Australian children.[231] Trauma associated with the use of all-terrain vehicles, such as quad bikes, is common, particularly in rural areas.[232] For children 14 years and younger, falling from one level to another, such as falling from a window, was the most common form of falls-related injury.[231,232]

Drowning is another leading cause of death in children, with more than 175,000 children drowning worldwide each year. In low- and middle-income countries across Southeast Asia and the Western Pacific, higher rates of drowning occur and are associated with playing, washing or collecting water from open bodies of water.[230] In wealthier countries such as Australia, drownings in this age group peak in the summer months and are more likely to be linked to recreational activities.[231] Boys outnumber girls in this category, with two-thirds being boys. Children under 5 years are more likely to drown by falling into backyard swimming pools, while older children (5–14 years) drown during planned swimming or other recreational activities in pools and open waterways such as dams and rivers.[233]

In Europe, drowning is associated with lower socioeconomic status, with a greater number of deaths by drowning in the poorer parts of eastern and southern Europe compared with western Europe. In low-income countries, the incidence remains high, with deaths from drowning having the highest mortality rate.[227]

Risk factors

The kinetic forces involved in injury are associated with a more diffuse injury pattern and a greater incidence of multiple trauma in children, as more of the child's body is subjected to the traumatic forces.[226] Children generally have less subcutaneous fat and musculature, providing less protection to the liver, kidneys and spleen, leading to a higher incidence of lung contusions and abdominal trauma.[226] In addition, the relatively large head size of the infant, particularly, and the child leads to a high incidence of head injury.

Primary survey and resuscitation

Initial stabilisation of children who have experienced a traumatic injury is likely to have occurred in the field. Once at the hospital, the primary survey is conducted to assess for, detect and stabilise the child with life-threatening injuries. Undertaking a primary survey and resuscitation uses the same structured approach in children and adults. Chapters 23 and 24 cover emergency presentations and trauma management; however, specific paediatric considerations are highlighted below.

Children sustaining trauma to the head, just as adults, are managed with cervical spine precautions including a collar, until the spine has been radiologically and clinically cleared.[226] A selection of paediatric collars should be available and the measuring guide used to ensure a good fit. As the collar can cause neck flexion in infants and small children, the child's torso may need to be elevated with a folded blanket to maintain a neutral neck position. The head and neck are usually immobilised, with head blocks (e.g. rolled towels) placed on either side of the head to maintain in-line stabilisation and prevent movement. The combative, uncooperative child will not tolerate this, and the actions are likely to increase the child's agitation and movement. Critical care nurses can position themselves to maintain in-line stabilisation while talking and soothing the child or, ideally, where parents are present seek their assistance to console their child. Specific paediatric trauma boards are available that are designed to maintain the child's head in a neutral position, but are generally used only in pre-hospital settings.

Fluid resuscitation is a controversial area of practice in paediatric trauma, where therapies have been generally less well studied than in adults. However, in a haemodynamically unstable child, including the child with a traumatic brain injury at risk of secondary brain injury from hypotension, fluid resuscitation of 20 mL/kg of 0.9% saline followed by reassessment is recommended.[226] Close monitoring of heart rate is essential.[226] If more than 20 mL/kg are required, immediate surgical assessment for bleeding is indicated, as excessive administration of crystalloid fluids can be harmful and impact on outcome.[234]

Exposure of the child, with temperature control, is necessary to assess the child completely for injuries. As hypothermia can develop quickly in children, overhead heating sources and blankets are ideally used to keep the child warm. Hypothermia in trauma patients is associated with increased risk for coagulopathy and mortality, as in adults, so providing warmth is essential in paediatric trauma nursing care.[226] The child's right to privacy and dignity should also be considered and exposure minimised.

Secondary survey

Undertaking a secondary survey is similar in children and adults and is described in Chapters 23 and 24. Specific paediatric considerations are highlighted below.

In children, particularly those under 1 year of age, if injuries and the accompanying history do not seem to match, non-accidental injury should be considered and noted. History should be obtained from the child where possible, from any witnesses to the accident and from ambulance officers if they attended. Parents or caregivers will provide details of the child's past medical history, any medications and any known allergies.

Specific conditions

Specific injuries that are seen in children are discussed briefly under the headings of traumatic brain injury, chest trauma and abdominal trauma. Obtaining an accurate history of the accident or events leading up to an injury is useful in determining the type of injuries that children may have sustained. Regardless of aetiology, where a child has been involved in a motor vehicle accident (MVA) or sustained a fall, there are likely to be multiple injuries and the situation should be treated as such until other injuries have been considered and excluded.[226]

Traumatic brain injury

Traumatic brain injury (TBI) is a leading cause of deaths and injury worldwide in children. In developing regions such as Asia and Africa, TBI is increasing as the population has increased access to motor vehicles.[227] In Australia and other wealthy economies, children experience the greatest number of head injuries of any age group.[227,235] TBI is often associated with MVAs where the child is a vehicle occupant, a pedestrian or a cyclist, and with falls and with near-drowning. TBI is described in detail in Chapter 17.

Age and gender are the most significant risk factors for TBI, with peak incidence in the 0–4-years group and in males.[228,236] Other factors to consider in children are the increased tendency of the immature brain of children to experience disruption of the blood–brain barrier and, unlike adults, for an increased cerebral blood volume to lead to cerebral oedema owing to higher brain water content.[237]

While there are guidelines for the management of paediatric brain injury,[238] the limitations of the paediatric research evidence that underpinned these has led to reliance on less-rigorous studies and ongoing dependence on expert consensus and extrapolation from adult research evidence.[238] As the clinical manifestations of TBI in children are very similar to those in adults, management is also very similar. The practice of hyperventilation should be avoided unless there is immediate risk of herniation, as it is associated with regional cerebral ischaemia.[238]

The modified GCS for children has previously been described in this text and should be used when assessing children. Indications for ICP monitoring in children include all infants and children with a severe head injury, which equates to a GCS score of 8 or below that persists

following adequate cardiopulmonary resuscitation, and those children who present with abnormal motor posturing and hypotension.[239] Combined with invasive haemodynamic monitoring, targeted therapy to manage both ICP and CPP remains an important part of treatment. While thresholds for treating intracranial hypertension in children have not been studied, it has been known since the 1980s that prolonged intracranial hypertension or high ICP levels will worsen outcome. An ICP of 20 mmHg is considered high in children, with 15 mmHg considered high in infants. ICPs of these values are the usual cut-off points and are likely to be treated with the aim of lowering ICP while maintaining an adequate CPP.[239] Target CPP for various ages is listed in Table 27.2.

Diagnosis

Diagnostic techniques and clinical management of children with TBI mirror those in adults (see Chapter 17). The smaller size of children means that diagnostics such as mixed cerebral venous saturation and direct brain oxygen saturation are not common practice in paediatrics, with further work required in direct brain oxygen saturation to determine utility and parameters.[239] A high index of suspicion for spinal injuries in paediatric TBI should be maintained, as spinal cord injury without radiological abnormality on plain X-rays and CT is a feature of paediatric spinal injury.[226] While CT scans are available in more centres than MRI, they involve radiation exposure to the young spine and miss spinal cord injury without radiological abnormality. MRI is more effective in determining spinal cord injury than CT and, as it involves no radiation exposure, is the investigation of choice to determine spinal injury in children.[240]

Treatment

Several of the therapies used in the treatment of the child with severe head injury are controversial, as they have lacked sufficient scientific rigour when the small number of studies were evaluated to make clear, high-quality evidence recommendations.[238] Essentially, treatment of TBI in children is identical to adult management: minimising intracranial hypertension and maintaining optimal CPP while preventing secondary injury from hypoxia, hypercarbia and hypotension, while reducing the risk of iatrogenesis from treatment. Hyperglycaemia that persists beyond 48 hours of the injury is associated with a worse outcome; however, studies are yet to be undertaken to determine whether this is modifiable with the use of tight glycaemic control.[238]

Hypothermia has not been shown to make a difference in outcome in children with hypoxic–ischaemic brain injury as it has in newborns and adults. Moderate hypothermia (temperature maintained at 32–34°C) has been studied in children with disappointing results; therefore, the current recommendation is that a core temperature of 35–38°C should be targeted.[239] The use of decompressive craniectomy for early indications of herniation, ongoing neurological deterioration or development of intractable intracranial hypertension that is refractory to maximal treatment such as drainage of cerebrospinal fluid (CSF), sedation and barbiturates has demonstrated improved mortality and functional recovery for some children.[239]

Outcomes from TBI in children are associated with the severity of the initial injury and the presence and control of secondary brain injury, as in adults. Hypotension and hypoxia prior to hospital admission are strongly linked to mortality and poor functional outcome, with some emerging evidence that hypertension and hyperglycaemia in the first 24 hours may also predict poor outcomes at 1-year post-injury.[239]

Chest trauma

Thoracic injuries in children rarely occur in isolation with traumatic injuries and are often accompanied by head and neck injuries. There is some evidence that blunt thoracic injuries are indicative of a more severe injury and are associated with higher mortality.[241] Injury to the heart and great vessels, in particular, is associated with higher mortality. The combination of head injury and thoracic injury is also known to have higher mortality. Most chest injuries in children are sustained as a consequence of MVAs.[242] The pattern of injury in children is predominantly one of blunt trauma. Lung contusions are the commonest thoracic injury seen in children.[243] As the rib cage is much more compliant in children, ribs are rarely broken, but they can damage underlying structures such as the lungs, so pulmonary contusions, pneumothorax and haemothorax are often seen. The clinical manifestations, approach to assessment, monitoring and management of children sustaining thoracic trauma are similar to those in adults, and are discussed in Chapter 24. Children with thoracic injuries are generally managed in a specialist trauma centre equipped to manage children.[243]

Abdominal trauma

Abdominal trauma in children is a leading cause of death when combined with head injury.[244] Blunt trauma from MVAs is the most common mechanism of injury, but bicycle handlebars may also inflict a significant injury. The liver and spleen are the most commonly injured organs in abdominal trauma and can usually be managed non-surgically in the haemodynamically stable child.[244] The abdominal organs are relatively large in children, with less musculature and a more compliant ribcage, meaning that there can be injury to underlying organs with no apparent external injury.[244] Blunt trauma is common, while penetrating injury is less common, resulting from gunshot and stab wounds. These injuries are associated with older children and adolescents, though a thinner body wall may result in greater underlying organ damage, particularly if the flank is penetrated.[245]

During the primary survey, the child's abdomen should be exposed and may reveal signs such as bruising from bicycle handles, tyre marks, abrasions or contusions.

Abdominal distention is a less reliable sign in children, as distention may be from air that is swallowed from pain and crying. However, as in adults, the primary survey may not include the abdomen if other immediately life-threatening injuries are present, such as thoracic and/or head injuries. These injuries will take precedence, so it may not be until the secondary survey can be undertaken that abdominal injuries are considered. The monitoring and management of children sustaining abdominal trauma results in fewer splenectomies and surgical intervention than in adults.[244] Further details of managing abdominal trauma are discussed in Chapter 24.

More-judicious use of both CT scanning and surgery is practised in paediatric trauma centres, due to increased concerns regarding radiation exposure to children and experience with conservative management of abdominal trauma.[244,246] Clinical indicators determine the need for a CT scan of the abdomen, including children with multiple injuries, gross haematuria with a minor injury and children with haemodynamic instability with no obvious source of blood loss. Diagnostic peritoneal lavage has largely ceased with the increasing utility of, and expertise with, focused ultrasound in trauma (FAST) in EDs, and the recent development of contrast-enhanced ultrasound is becoming a preferred investigation to detect injuries in the abdomen.[244] Monitoring of blood in urine is a simple, useful technique to detect bladder and kidney injuries. Management of abdominal trauma generally requires only haemodynamic and laboratory monitoring in conjunction with supportive therapies such as fluid replacement, monitoring of urine output and pain management with the aim of detecting signs of haemorrhage.[244]

Post-intensive care syndrome in children

Post-intensive care syndrome has also been described in children (PICS-p), with many children surviving critical illness with multiple complications across the health domains of the PICS-p.[247] More conditions have been associated with this syndrome, including worsening multidimensional impairments and failure in social reconstruction, with persistence of multidimensional symptoms extending beyond hospital discharge and up to 1 year after critical illness.[248,249] Risk factors for children and parents have been identified, including possible triggering factors such as younger age, chronic comorbidities, mechanical ventilation, invasive procedures, PICU LOS, delirium, iatrogenic withdrawal, use of sedative and vasoactive medications, ECMO, renal replacement therapies, internalising behaviours, neurodevelopmental disorders, Indigenous status and minority groups. Parents and/or family member risk factors include socioeconomic status, education level, history of mental illness and distress.[250–252]

Clinical manifestations

The manifestations of PICS-p are heterogeneous and wide ranging because of the multiple components involved. The frequency of PICS-p can vary according to the domain affected. The physical domain has been affected in up to 63% of children, cognitive disability in up to 73%[21,253] and psychological disorders among older children in up to 88%,[21] with up to 32% reporting post-traumatic stress disorder, hyperactivity and depression (self-identified).[251] Social domain affectation has reported as between 36% and 67%.[253]

Common symptoms in the physical domain include fatigue, sleep disturbances, reduced quality of life, loss of muscle mass and weight, diminished sensation, muscle weakness associated with polyneuromyopathy, neurological function, pain, heart function and lung function. Feeding problems also occur (dysphagia or dependence on parenteral nutrition).[251,252,254] Cognitive manifestations include deficits in attention, memory, processing speed, language, weakened visuospatial functions and intellectual disability.[251,252,254] Psychological symptoms are linked with changes in self-esteem and include delusional memories or fears, hallucinations, depression and post-traumatic stress disorder (PTSD).[21,251,252,254] Social manifestations in children include isolation of children, school absenteeism, inadequate educational support and falling grades. In addition, parents have social affectation with parental stress, loss of employment of one parent, financial problems, anxiety and moderate–severe depression.[251,252,254]

Patient assessment

To date, there is little in-hospital or post-PICU discharge follow-up to assess potential complications of the PICS-p, and there are no consensus recommendations for clinical practice and follow-up consultations for PICU patients.[250,255] There are a list of recommended instruments to measure PICS-p in PICU survivors, but these have been mainly limited to research.[256] Implementation of an ICU-liberation bundle seems to be the best prevention against PICS-p to date; however, further research is needed to demonstrate its benefit.[257]

Summary

Critically ill infants and children have several anatomical and physiological differences that predispose them to different types of critical illness when compared with adults. Children's relative physiological and psychological immaturity means that their needs may be different from adults when critically ill. Family support is important and parental presence should be allowed at all times. Patterns of disease may differ from adults – for example, a high incidence of respiratory illness and a predisposition to sustaining multiple trauma – but children have a lower incidence of sepsis, heart failure, liver failure and SARS-CoV-2 than adults. The need for specialised nursing and medical care as well as adapted equipment means that many critically ill children will require transfer to a specialist paediatric centre.

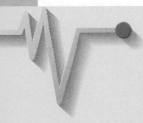

Case study

You are reviewing a 4-month-old male infant, weighing 7 kg, in your emergency department (ED) as the ED team are concerned about his work of breathing. Oliver's parents tell you that he has been well and feeding normally, has recently had his 4-month vaccinations and is normally breastfed. Two days ago he developed a runny nose, a fever to 38°C and occasional cough. His 3-year-old sister had a cold a week ago and has recovered. Yesterday Oliver's cough worsened and he was feeding more frequently but only for short periods. Today he appears very congested, is unsettled and irritable and having difficulty feeding, so his concerned parents brought him to the ED. He arrived and was triaged around 90 minutes ago. The ED doctor has seen him briefly and respiratory virus testing was undertaken for SARS-CoV-19, RSV and other respiratory viruses.

On examination, you notice that he is breathing rapidly at 70 breaths/minute, has intercostal and subcostal recessions and nasal flaring. His heart rate is 146/min and his capillary refill is 3–4 seconds. The ED nurse tells you that his oxygen saturation when he presented 90 minutes ago was sitting continuously at 89–91%, his respiratory rate was 80–90 breaths/minute and he was occasionally grunting. Oliver was commenced on low-flow oxygen therapy via nasal cannulae at 1 L/min. Since then his saturations have been 91–94%; however, he remains tachypnoeic, tachycardic and unsettled.

The ED doctor and nurse decide to insert a peripheral cannula, take bloods, including venous blood gas, commence intravenous maintenance fluids after providing a fluid bolus of 160 mL of 0.9% sodium chloride and commence humidified high-flow oxygen via nasal cannula at 2 L/kg/min) with FiO_2 of 35%.

After a further 10 minutes where Oliver's work of breathing continues to increase, it is decided that he should be intubated, placed on a ventilator and moved to the PICU for ongoing management.

Following 48 hours of intubation and positive pressure ventilation, Oliver is successfully extubated. While in PICU he has received sedation and analgesia, received intravenous fluids and then commenced on enteral feeding until 4 hours ago when feeds ceased prior to extubation. Following extubation, Oliver was placed onto low-flow oxygen therapy to maintain oxygen saturations of 92–94%. This was weaned off overnight. At 6 hours post-extubation, Oliver was given a comfort breast feed, which he took well, and then continued to feed regularly. The next morning Oliver was discharged to the ward. After 24 hours, Oliver was discharged home.

CASE STUDY QUESTIONS

1 Which respiratory virus is the most common cause of bronchiolitis in infants?
2 Describe a preferred approach to intubation of a collapsed child. Calculate the appropriate ETT size for Oliver.
3 Oliver will be kept fasted and feeds will commence after 6 hours. While on IV fluids only, calculate how much maintenance fluids per hour you should run Oliver's fluids at to deliver two-thirds maintenance (humidification is in progress).
4 After 6 hours, you commence enteral nutrition for Oliver. What are your considerations when providing enteral feeds? What would be the best form of enteral nutrition to provide?
5 How will you assess Oliver's level of sedation while he is intubated and ventilated?
6 Consider how you will ensure ongoing communication and connection with Oliver and his parents.

RESEARCH VIGNETTE

Yagiela LM, Edgar CM, Harper FWK, et al. Parent post-traumatic growth after a child's critical illness. Front Pediatr 2022;10:989053. doi: 10.3389/fped.2022.98905.

Abstract

Objective: Post-traumatic growth is the experience of a positive change after a traumatic event. Our objective is to characterise the factors associated with post-traumatic growth in parents after a child's PICU admission.

Study design: A cross-sectional survey study examining post-traumatic growth and select independent variables in parents 1 year after a child's ≥72 h PICU admission for an acute illness or injury. The study was completed in parents of children discharged alive from a tertiary care PICU from 1 January 2017 to 31 December 2017. A mixed-effects linear regression model was built to evaluate the association of post-traumatic stress, anxiety, depression, resiliency, family function and child function with post-traumatic growth.

Results: Eighty-two parents of 52 children discharged alive in 2017 completed the survey. Fifty-two percent were ≥35 years and 64.3% were mothers. The median age of their children was 2.8 years (interquartile range (IQR) 0.5–11.3) with a median hospital stay of 12 days (IQR 6–20). Moderate-to-high levels of post-traumatic growth occurred in 67.1% of parents. Increased hospital length of stay (beta coefficient (β coeff) 0.85; $P = 0.004$, 95% confidence interval (CI) 0.27, 1.43) and parent post-traumatic stress symptoms (β coeff 1.04; $P = 0.006$, 95% CI 0.29, 1.78) were associated with increased post-traumatic growth, and increased parent depression symptoms (β coeff −1.96; $P = 0.015$; 95% CI −3.54, −0.38) with decreased post-traumatic growth.

Conclusion: Longer child hospital stays and increased parent post-traumatic stress symptoms were associated with increased post-traumatic growth, while increased depression was associated with less post-traumatic growth. The impact of future PICU parent psychosocial interventions on parents may be best assessed using a dual outcome focused on reducing negative mental health symptoms while concurrently promoting skills to facilitate parent adaptation and post-traumatic growth.

Critique

This study addresses an important issue that is poorly investigated in families with a child in paediatric intensive care. The introduction states the problem of parental post-traumatic stress in PICU and offers a definition of post-traumatic growth. The rationale for the study is well formulated and it identified the gap in this concept in the US population. The authors argue that a broader understanding of parental post-traumatic growth and how modifiable factors can impact post-traumatic growth will inform the development of PICU-based psychosocial interventions to better target parental emotional needs. The aim and objectives of the study align with the problem statement and are clearly stated.

The methods present the design and participants of the study. The authors conducted a cross-sectional survey study, which is consistent with the research aim. The population was focused on parents of children discharged from the PICU who face complex changes in children's growth and development after a critical illness. The sampling technique and sample size calculation were not described. The authors invited all participants who met the selection criteria, although only 18% agreed to participate and completed the online survey (link sent by email). This response rate is relatively low and could have introduced sampling bias. The authors indicated a primary outcome (post-traumatic growth) and, according to the literature, they assessed independent variables related to parent and child conditions that could explain the primary outcome. These included demographics and health characteristics, and functional status in children. Anxiety, depression, post-traumatic stress, resiliency and family functioning were measured in parents. The authors used validated instruments to evaluate all study outcomes and employed rigorous statistical analysis methods. The research followed the ethical guidelines and complied with most quality requirements according to its study design.

The results show the reality experienced by parents, as the majority (67%) have moderate-to-high levels of post-traumatic growth. Moreover, it was associated with children's health condition (length of stay and rehospitalisation), and with demographic (male gender and age ≥35 in parents), economic (employment, income >$20,000/year) and psychological factors (post-traumatic stress symptoms and parent depression). Although parents' resiliency and family functioning did not affect post-traumatic growth, the authors reported few parents (21%) with high resiliency and 13–41% of parents with unhealthy family functioning.

The results found are relevant to clinical practice because they give important suggestions for developing preventive interventions for parents and their children in the ICU. Further, the ICU health team can make efforts to reduce the length of stay and increase psychological and emotional support. Therefore, paediatric ICU health care should be extended to parents for better long-term outcomes that positively impact society.

To evaluate the methodological quality of survey studies, you can refer to the CROSS guideline: a consensus-based checklist for reporting of survey studies – the equator network (https://www.equator-network.org).

Learning activities

The questions below relate to the following scenario.

You are reviewing a 5-year-old girl, Emma, in the paediatric ward who was admitted from ED following a febrile seizure. On investigation, she was found to have pneumonia, and it is day 2 of admission. Emma has increased work of breathing and the paediatric nurses are concerned. She is lying flat in the bed, looks distressed, and is crying and calling out for her mother. She has moderate-to-severe respiratory distress and is receiving low-flow oxygen therapy of 3 L/min via nasal prongs. Monitoring shows an oxygen saturation of 93%, respiratory rate of 34 breaths/min and heart rate of 110 bpm and you consider her work of breathing to be moderate to severe respiratory distress. Emma has a peripheral intravenous cannula in her left hand. Her mother arrives as you begin your assessment. You note that when you touched Emma's arm she felt hot.

1 Consider your approach to assessing Emma. What are some immediate nursing interventions you could perform that may console her and improve her work of breathing while you perform your assessment?

2 When you perform an axillary temperature recording, you notice her temperature is 38.6°C. Would you stop your assessment at this point to administer any medication? If so, which one?

3 Outline your next steps in your review of Emma's worsening condition. Are there important aspects of history you need to consider before escalating Emma's treatment?

4 If you are thinking of escalating respiratory therapy, what options are available in your hospital? Where is the best place now for Emma to be nursed?

5 Emma needs intravenous fluids commenced. She has a cannula that was used for antibiotics 90 minutes ago. Calculate Emma's maintenance IV fluid rate.

Online resources

Extracorporeal Life Support Organization (ELSO), a free non-profit consortium of healthcare centres, researchers and industry who provide guidelines and position statements regarding ECMO for children and adults, https://www.elso.org

Online weight-based maintenance fluid calculator from Royal Children's Hospital, Melbourne, https://www.rch.org.au/clinicalguide/forms/fluids-calculator/

OPENPediatrics, a free, open access online resource for the paediatric critical care community, https://www.openpediatrics.org

References

1. Australian and New Zealand Intensive Care Society (ANZICS). Report of the Australian and New Zealand Paediatric Intensive Care Registry 2018. Melbourne, VIC: ANZICS; 2019.

2. Shappley R, Noles D, Spentzas T. Pediatric chronic critical illness: validation, prevalence, and impact in a children's hospital. Pediatr Crit Care Med 2021;22(12):e636–9.

3. Young KD, Korotzer NC. Weight estimation methods in children: a systematic review. Ann Emerg Med 2016;68(4):441–51.e10.

4. Torres SF, Iolster T, Schnitzler EJ, et al. Hypotonic and isotonic intravenous maintenance fluids in hospitalised paediatric patients: a randomised controlled trial. BMJ Paediatr Open 2019;3(1):e000385.

5. Lehr AR, Rached-d'Astous S, Barrowman N, et al. Balanced versus unbalanced fluid in critically ill children: systematic review and meta-analysis. Pediatr Crit Care Med 2022;23(3):181–91.

6. The Royal Children's Hospital Melbourne. Clinical practice guidelines fluid calculator. Melbourne, VIC: RCHM; 2022.

7. Guyton A, Hall J. Fetal and neonatal physiology. In: Hall JE, Hall ME, editors. Guyton and Hall textbook of medical physiology. 14th ed. Philadelphia: Saunders; 2020, p. 1061–70.

8. Blackburn S. Maternal, fetal & neonatal physiology: a clinical perspective. St Louis, MO: Elsevier Saunders; 2018.

9. Woods KS, Horvat CM, Kantawala S, et al. Intracranial and cerebral perfusion pressure thresholds associated with inhospital mortality across pediatric neurocritical care. Pediatr Crit Care Med 2021;22(2):135–46.

10. The Sydney Children's Hospitals Network. Severe traumatic brain injury – PICU – practice guideline. Sydney, NSW: Sydney Children's Hospitals Network; 2021, p. 1–15.

11. Van de Voorde P, Turner NM, Djakow J, et al. European Resuscitation Council guidelines 2021: paediatric life support. Resuscitation 2021;161:327–87.

12. Hillgruber RJ, Lutskov P, West NC, et al. Blood pressure nomograms for children undergoing general anesthesia, stratified by age and anesthetic type, using data from a retrospective cohort at a tertiary pediatric center. J Clin Monit Comput 2022;36(6):1667–77.

13. Emr B, Alcamo A, Carcillo J, et al. Pediatric sepsis update: how are children different? Surg Infect 2018;19(2):176–83.

14. Walker SB, Conlon TW, Zhang B, et al. Clinical signs to categorize shock and target vasoactive medications in warm versus cold pediatric septic shock. Pediatr Crit Care Med 2020;21(12):1051–8.

15. Holzki J, Brown K, Carroll R, et al. The anatomy of the pediatric airway: has our knowledge changed in 120 years? A review of historic and recent investigations of the anatomy of the pediatric larynx. Pediatr Anaesth 2018;28(1):13–22.

16. Friedman M, Nitu M. Acute respiratory failure in children. Pediatr Ann 2018;47(7):e268–73.

17. Iyer R, Bansal A. What do we know about optimal nutritional strategies in children with pediatric acute respiratory distress syndrome? Ann Transl Med 2019;7(19):510.

18. Reynolds SL. Pediatric thoracic trauma: recognition and management. Emerg Med Clin N Am 2018;36(2):473–83.

19. Curley M, Hasbani N, Quigley S, et al. Predicting pressure injury risk in pediatric patients: the Braden QD Scale. J Pediatr 2018;192:189–95e2.

20. Alzawad Z, Lewis F, Kantrowitz-Gordon I, et al. A qualitative study of parents' experiences in the pediatric intensive care unit: riding a roller coaster. J Pediatr Nurs 2020;51:8–14.

21. Ko MSM, Poh PF, Heng KYC, et al. Assessment of long-term psychological outcomes after pediatric intensive care unit admission: a systematic review and meta-analysis. JAMA Pediatr 2022;176(3):e215767.

22. Alzawad Z, Lewis F, Walker A. Parents' challenges beyond the pediatric intensive care unit: fraying at the seams while balancing between two worlds, home and hospital. Children (Basel) 2022;9(2):267.

23. Nelson LP, Lachman SE, Goodman K, et al. Admission psychosocial characteristics of critically ill children and acute stress. Pediatr Crit Care Med 2021;22(2):194–203.

24. Ercin-Swearinger H, Lindhorst T, Curtis J, et al. Acute and posttraumatic stress in family members of children with a prolonged stay in a PICU: secondary analysis of a randomized trial. Pediatr Crit Care Med 2022;23(4):306–14.

25. Ramelet AS. Long-stay paediatric intensive care unit patients: a minority deserving special attention. Nurs Crit Care 2020;25(3):138–9.

26. Grandjean C, Ullmann P, Marston M, et al. Sources of stress, family functioning, and needs of families with a chronic critically ill child: a qualitative study. Front Pediatr 2021;9:740598.

27. Rennick JE, Knox AM, Treherne SC, et al. Family members' perceptions of their psychological responses one year following pediatric intensive care unit (PICU) hospitalization: qualitative findings from the caring intensively study. Front Pediatr 2021;9:724155.

28. Coats H, Bourget E, Starks H, et al. Nurses' reflections on benefits and challenges of implementing family-centered care in pediatric intensive care units. Am J Crit Care 2018;27(1):52–8.

29. Committee ENACPG, Vanhoy M, Horigan A, et al. Clinical practice guideline: family presence. J Emerg Nurs 2019;45(1):76 e1–29.

30. Bettencourt A, Gorman M, Mullen J. Pediatric resuscitation. Crit Care Nurs Clin N Am 2021;33(3):287–302.

31. Garcia Guerra G, Joffe A, Sheppard C, et al. Music use for sedation in critically ill children (MUSiCC trial): a pilot randomized controlled trial. J Intensive Care 2021;9(1):7.

32. Rennick JE, Stremler R, Horwood L, et al. A pilot randomized controlled trial of an intervention to promote psychological well-being in critically ill children: soothing through touch, reading, and music. Pediatr Crit Care Med 2018;19(7):e358–66.

33. Claus M, Maia E, Oliveira A, et al. A inserção do brincar e brinquedo nas práticas de enfermagem pediátrica: pesquisa convergente assistencial. Escola Anna Nery 2021;25(3):e20200383.

34. Smith HAB, Besunder JB, Betters KA, et al. 2022 Society of Critical Care Medicine clinical practice guidelines on prevention and management of pain, agitation, neuromuscular blockade, and delirium in critically ill pediatric patients with consideration of the ICU environment and early mobility. Pediatr Crit Care Med 2022;23(2):e74–110.

35. Calandriello A, Tylka J, Patwari P. Sleep and delirium in pediatric critical illness: what is the relationship? Med Sci (Basel) 2018;6(4):90.

36. Erikson E. Identity and the life cycle. New York: Norton & Company; 1994.

37. Erskine R. Child development in integrative psychotherapy: Erik Erikson's first three stages. Int J Integrative Psychother 2019;10:11–34.

38. Maree JG. The psychosocial development theory of Erik Erikson: critical overview. Early Child Dev Care 2021;191(7–8):1107–21.

39. Samdan G, Kiel N, Petermann F, et al. The relationship between parental behavior and infant regulation: a systematic review. Dev Rev 2020;57:100923.

40. Fonagy P, Campbell C. Future directions in personality pathology. Curr Opin Psychol 2021;37:145–51.

41. Hockenberry M, Wilson D, Rodgers C. Wong's essentials of pediatric nursing. 11th ed. St Louis, MO: Elsevier; 2021, p. 1168.

42. Piaget J. The child's conception of the world: a 20th-century classic of child psychology. Lanham, MD: Rowman & Littlefield Publishers; 2007.

43. Jepsen S, Haahr A, Eg M, et al. Coping with the unfamiliar: how do children cope with hospitalization in relation to acute and/or critical illness? A qualitative metasynthesis. J Child Health Care 2019;23(4):534–50.

44. Hao Y, Hong S, Su Y. Chinese children showed self-deprecating modest behavior at ages of 7–8. Social Dev 2021;30(4):994–1005.

45. National Academies of Sciences, Engineering, and Medicine. The promise of adolescence: realizing opportunity for all youth. Backes EP, Bonnie RJ, editors. Washington, DC: National Academies Press; 2019.

46. Sharp C. Adolescent personality pathology and the alternative model for personality disorders: self development as nexus. Psychopathology 2020;53(3-4):198–204.

47. Abela K, Wardell D, Rozmus C, et al. Impact of pediatric critical illness and injury on families: an updated systematic review. J Pediatr Nurs 2020;51:21–31.

48. Iwata M, Han S, Hays R, et al. Predictors of depression and anxiety in family members 3 months after child's admission to a pediatric ICU. Am J Hosp Palliat Care 2019;36(10):841–50.

49. Youngblut JM, Brooten D. What children wished they had/had not done and their coping in the first thirteen months after their sibling's neonatal/pediatric intensive care unit/emergency department death. J Palliat Med 2021;24(2):226–32.

50. Butler A, Copnell B, Hall H. When a child dies in the PICU: practice recommendations from a qualitative study of bereaved parents. Pediatr Crit Care Med 2019;20(9):e447–51.

51. Terp K, Weis J, Lundqvist P. Parents' views of family-centered care at a pediatric intensive care unit-a qualitative study. Front Pediatr 2021;9:725040.

52. Lopez M, Vaks Y, Wilson M, et al. Impacting satisfaction, learning, and efficiency through structured interdisciplinary rounding in a pediatric intensive care unit: a quality improvement project. Pediatr Qual Saf 2019;4(3):e176.

53. Khan A, Yin HS, Brach C, et al. Association between parent comfort with english and adverse events among hospitalized children. JAMA Pediatr 2020;174(12):e203215.

54. Nelson LP, Lachman SE, Li SW, et al. The effects of family functioning on the development of posttraumatic stress in children and their parents following admission to the PICU. Pediatr Crit Care Med 2019;20(4):e208–15.

55. Ramelet AS, Bergstraesser E, Grandjean C, et al. Comparison of end-of-life care practices between children with complex chronic conditions and neonates dying in an ICU versus non-ICUs: a substudy of the Pediatric End-of-LIfe CAre Needs in Switzerland (PELICAN) project. Pediatr Crit Care Med 2020;21(5):e236–46.

56. Hansson J, Hornfeldt A, Bjorling G, et al. The healthcare staffs' perception of parents' participation in critical incidents at the PICU: a qualitative study. Nurs Rep 2021;11(3):680–9.

57. National Health Service (NHHS) UK. Consent to treatment. London: NHS; 2019. Available from: https://www.nhs.uk/conditions/consent-to-treatment/. [Accessed 25 February 2023].

58. Swiss Centre of Expertise in Human Rights (SCHR). La position de l'enfant face au traitement médical [Child's position in medical treatment]. Zurich: SCHR; 2018. Available from: https://skmr.ch/fr/publications-documentations/artikel/die-stellung-des-kindes-bei-einer-medizinischen-behandlung. [Accessed 25 February 2023].

59. National Health and Medical Research Council (NHMRC). National statement on ethical conduct in human research 2007 (Updated 2018). Canberra, ACT: NHMRC; 2018. p. 110. Available from: https://www.nhmrc.gov.au/about-us/publications/national-statement-ethical-conduct-human-research-2007-updated-2018#block-views-block-file-attachments-content-block-1. [Accessed 25 February 2023].

60. Grootens-Wiegers P, Hein I, van den Broek J, et al. Medical decision-making in children and adolescents: developmental and neuroscientific aspects. BMC Pediatr 2017;17(1):120.

61. National Health and Medical Research Council (NHMRC). National statement on ethical conduct in human research 2007 (updated 2018). Canberra, ACT: NHMRC; 2018, p. 30–2. Available from: https://www.nhmrc.gov.au/about-us/publications/national-statement-ethical-conduct-human-research-2007-updated-2018#block-views-block-file-attachments-content-block-1. [Accessed 25 February 2023].

62. Lepola P, Needham A, Mendum J, et al. Informed consent for paediatric clinical trials in Europe. Arch Dis Child 2016;101(11):1017–25.

63. Zuppa AF, Curley MAQ. Sedation, analgesia and neuromuscular blockade in pediatric critical care: overview and current landscape. Pediatr Clin North Am 2017;64(5):1103–16.

64. Patel AK, Bell MJ, Traube C. Delirium in pediatric critical care. Pediatr Clin North Am 2017;64(5):1117 32.

65. Baarslag M, Allegaert K, Knibbe C, et al. Pharmacological sedation management in the paediatric intensive care unit. J Pharm Pharmacol 2017;69(5):498–513.

66. Aydin S, Ofori-Amanfo G, Ushay H. Sedation and analgesia following pediatric heart surgery – less may be more. Critical Care Med 2018; 46(1):170–2.

67. Shildt N, Traube C, Dealmeida M, et al. "Difficult to sedate": successful implementation of a benzodiazepine-sparing analgosedation-protocol in mechanically ventilated children. Children 2021;8(5):348.

68. Lebet RM, Asaro LA, Zuppa AF, et al. Face and content validity of variables associated with the difficult-to-sedate child in the paediatric intensive care unit: a survey of paediatric critical care clinicians. Aust Crit Care 2018;31(3):167–73.

69. Taffarel P, Bonetto G, Jorro Baron F, et al. Sedation and analgesia in patients on mechanical ventilation in pediatric intensive care units in Argentina. Arch Argent Pediatr 2018;116(2):e196–203.

70. Best KM, Wypij D, Asaro LA, et al. Patient, process, and system predictors of iatrogenic withdrawal syndrome in critically ill children. Crit Care Med 2017;45(1):e7–15.

71. da Silva P, Reis M, Fonseca T, et al. Opioid and benzodiazepine withdrawal syndrome in PICU patients: which risk factors matter? J Addict Med 2016;10(2):110–16.

72. Semple D, Howlett MM, Strawbridge JD, et al. A systematic review and pooled prevalence of delirium in critically ill children. Critical Care Med 2022;50(2):317–28.

73. Ricardo Ramirez C, Alvarez Gomez ML, Agudelo Velez CA, et al. Clinical characteristics, prevalence, and factors related to delirium in children of 5 to 14 years of age admitted to intensive care. Med Intensiva (Engl ed.) 2019;43(3):147–55.

74. Harris J, Ramelet A-S, van Dijk M, et al. Clinical recommendations for pain, sedation, withdrawal and delirium assessment in critically ill infants and children: an ESPNIC position statement for healthcare professionals. Intensive Care Med 2016;42(6):972–86.

75. Barney C, Andersen R, Defrin R, et al. Challenges in pain assessment and management among individuals with intellectual and developmental disabilities. Pain Rep 2020;5(4):e821.

76. Ramelet AS, Rees NW, McDonald S, et al. Clinical validation of the Multidimensional Assessment of Pain Scale. Pediatr Anaesth 2007;17(12):1156–65.

77. Ista E, van Dijk M, Tibboel D, et al. Assessment of sedation levels in pediatric intensive care patients can be improved by using the COMFORT "behavior" scale. Pediatr Crit Care Med 2005;6(1):58–63.

78. Lempinen H, Polkki T, Kyngas H, et al. Feasibility and clinical utility of the Finnish version of the FLACC pain scale in PICU. J Pediatr Nurs 2020;55:211–16.

79. Zaccagnini M, Ataman R, Nonoyama ML. The Withdrawal Assessment Tool to identify iatrogenic withdrawal symptoms in critically ill paediatric patients: a COSMIN systematic review of measurement properties. J Eval Clin Pract 2021;27(4):976–88.

80. Avila-Alzate J, Gomez-Salgado J, Romero-Martin M, et al. Assessment and treatment of the withdrawal syndrome in paediatric intensive care units: systematic review. Medicine (Baltimore) 2020;99(5):e18502.

81. Bosch-Alcaraz A, Luna-Castano P, Garcia-Soler P, et al. Level of discomfort in critically ill paediatric patients and its correlation with sociodemographic and clinical variables, analgosedation and withdrawal syndrome. COSAIP multicentre study (Phase 2). Ann Pediatr (Engl ed) 2021;95(6):397–405.

82. Egbuta C, Mason K. Current state of analgesia and sedation in the pediatric intensive care unit. J Clin Med 2021;10(9):1847.

83. Di Nardo M, Boldrini F, Broccati F, et al. The LiberAction Project: implementation of a pediatric liberation bundle to screen delirium, reduce benzodiazepine sedation, and provide early mobilization in a human resource-limited pediatric intensive care unit. Front Pediatr 2021;9:788997.

84. Peng HF, Yin T, Yang L, et al. Non-nutritive sucking, oral breast milk, and facilitated tucking relieve preterm infant pain during heel-stick procedures: a prospective, randomized controlled trial. Int J Nurs Stud 2018;77:162–70.

85. Trottier ED, Doré-Bergeron M-J, Chauvin-Kimoff L, et al. Managing pain and distress in children undergoing brief diagnostic and therapeutic procedures. Paediatr Child Health 2019;24(8):509–21.

86. Sabeti F, Mohammadpour M, Pouraboli B, et al. Health care providers' experiences of the non-pharmacological pain and anxiety management and its barriers in the pediatric intensive care units. J Pediatr Nurs 2021;60:e110–16.

87. Mondardini MC, Daverio M, Caramelli F, et al. Dexmedetomidine for prevention of opioid/benzodiazepine withdrawal syndrome in pediatric intensive care unit: interim analysis of a randomized controlled trial. Pharmacotherapy 2022;42(2):145–53.

88. Lin Y, Zhang R, Shen W, et al. Dexmedetomidine versus other sedatives for non-painful pediatric examinations: a systematic review and meta-analysis of randomized controlled trials. J Clin Anesth 2020;62:109736.

89. Sperotto F, Mondardini MC, Dell'Oste C, et al. Efficacy and safety of dexmedetomidine for prolonged sedation in the PICU: a prospective multicenter study (PROSDEX). Pediatr Crit Care Med 2020;21(7):625–36.

90. Chan J, Shariff Uddin I, Hui Chaw S, et al. Hemodynamic response of high- and low-dose dexmedetomidine of pediatric in general anesthesia: a systematic review and meta-analysis of randomized controlled trials. Asian J Anesthesiol 2021;59(1):7–21.

91. Xiao Z, He T, Jiang X, et al. Effect of dexmedetomidine and propofol sedation on the prognosis of children with severe respiratory failure: a systematic review and meta-analysis. Transl Pediatr 2022;11(2):260–9.

92. Filho E, Riechelmann M. Propofol use in newborns and children: is it safe? A systematic review. J Pediatr (Rio J) 2020;96(3):289–309.

93. Bharathan S, Swami V, Bidari L. Airway obstruction in children with COVID-19 presenting with stridor. Pediatr Infect Dis 2022;4(2):62–4.

94. Eskander A, de Almeida J, Irish J. Acute upper airway obstruction. N Engl J Med 2019;381(20):1940–9.

95. Ma X, Liu Y, Du M, et al. The accuracy of the pediatric assessment triangle in assessing triage of critically ill patients in emergency pediatric department. Int Emerg Nurs 2021;58:101041.

96. Antón-Pacheco J, Martín-Alelú R, López M, et al. Foreign body aspiration in children: treatment timing and related complications. Int J Pediatr Otorhinolaryngol 2021;144:110690.

97. Clark C, Kugler K, Carr M. Common causes of congenital stridor in infants. JAAPA 2018;31(11):36–40.

98. Kou YF, Rutter MJ. Laryngeal webs and laryngotracheoesophageal clefts: state of the art. Semin Pediatr Surg 2021;30(3):151056.

99. Kamran A, Zendejas B, Jennings R. Current concepts in tracheobronchomalacia: diagnosis and treatment. Semin Pediatr Surg 2021;30(3):151062.

100. Worhunsky DJ, Levy BE, Stephens EH, et al.. Vascular rings. Semin Pediatr Surg 2021;30(6):151128.

101. Patwari PP, Sharma GD. Common pediatric airway disorders. Pediatr Ann 2019;48(4):e162–8.

102. Dariya V, Moresco L, Bruschettini M, et al. Cuffed versus uncuffed endotracheal tubes for neonates. Cochrane Database Syst Rev 2022;1:CD013736.

103. Kanaris C, Murphy P. Fifteen-minute consultation: intubation of the critically ill child presenting to the emergency department. Arch Dis Child Educ Pract Ed 2022;107(5):330–7.

104. Australian & New Zealand Councils on Resuscitation (ANZCOR). ANZCOR guideline 12.2. Paediatric advanced life support (PALS). Australian & New Zealand Council on Resuscitation; 2021. Available from: https://resus.org.au/new-and-revised-guidelines-and-editorial-changes/. [Accessed 25 February 2023].

105. Shann F. Drug doses. 17th ed. Parkville, VIC: Royal Children's Hospital; 2017.

106. Sulton CD, Middlebrooks LS, Taylor T. The pediatric airway and rapid sequence intubation. Pediatr Emerg Med Rep 2020;25(1). Available from: https://www.reliasmedia.com/articles/145479-the-pediatric-airway-and-rapid-sequence-intubation. [Accessed 25 February 2023].

107. Overmann KM, Boyd SD, Zhang Y, et al. Apneic oxygenation to prevent oxyhemoglobin desaturation during rapid sequence intubation in a pediatric emergency department. Am J Emerg Med 2019;37(8):1416–21.

108. Allen M, Meraj T, Oska S, et al. Acute epiglottitis: analysis of U.S. mortality trends from 1979 to 2017. Am J Otolaryngol 2021;42(2):102882.

109. Repper DC, Arrieta AC, Cook JE, et al. A case of Lemierre syndrome in the era of COVID-19: all that glitters is not gold. Pediatr Infect Dis J 2020;39(12):e445–7.

110. Exavier M-M, Paul Hanna M, Muscadin E, et al. Diphtheria in children in northern Haiti. J Trop Pediatr 2018;65(2):183–7.

111. Akhavan M. Ear, nose, throat: beyond pharyngitis: retropharyngeal abscess, peritonsillar abscess, epiglottitis, bacterial tracheitis, and postoperative tonsillectomy. Emerg Med Clin 2021;39(3):661–75.

112. Quraishi H, Lee DJ. Recurrent croup. Pediatr Clin N Am 2022;69(2):319–28.

113. Pound CM, Knight BD, Webster R, et al. Predictors of hospitalization for children with croup: a population-based cohort study. Hosp Pediatr 2020;10(12):1068–77.

114. Venn AMR, Schmidt JM, Mullan PC. A case series of pediatric croup with COVID-19. Am J Emerg Med 2021;43:287.e1–3.

115. Venn AMR, Schmidt JM, Mullan PC. Pediatric croup with COVID-19. Am J Emerg Med 2021;43:287.e1–3.

116. Gates A, Gates M, Vandermeer B, et al. Glucocorticoids for croup in children. Cochrane Database Syst Rev 2018; 8(8):CD001955.

117. Davies I, Jenkins I. Paediatric airway infections. BJA Educ 2017;17(10):341–5.

118. Baiu I, Melendez E. Epiglottitis. JAMA 2019;321(19):1946.

119. Lee JH. Foreign body ingestion in children. Clin Endosc 2018;51(2):129–36.

120. Reddel HK, Bacharier LB, Bateman ED, et al. Global initiative for asthma strategy 2021: executive summary and rationale for key changes. Am J Respir Crit Care Med 2022;205(1):17–35.

121. O'Brien S, Borland ML, Cotterell E, et al. Australasian bronchiolitis guideline. J Paediatr Child Health 2019;55(1):42–53.

122. National Institute for Health and Care Excellence (NICE). Bronchiolitis in children: diagnosis and management. London: NICE; 2021, p. 26.

123. Cui X, Zhao Z, Zhang T, et al. A systematic review and meta-analysis of children with coronavirus disease 2019 (COVID-19). J Med Virol 2021;93(2):1057–69.

124. Parisi GF, Indolfi C, Decimo F, et al. COVID-19 pneumonia in children: from etiology to management. Front Pediatr 2020;8:616622.

125. Ludvigsson JF. Systematic review of COVID-19 in children shows milder cases and a better prognosis than adults. Acta Paediatr 2020;109(6):1088–95.

126. World Health Organization (WHO). Child mortality (under 5 years). Geneva: WHO: 2022. Available from: https://www.who.int/news-room/fact-sheets/detail/levels-and-trends-in-child-under-5-mortality-in-2020. [Accessed 25 February 2023].

127. Bhalala US, Gist KM, Tripathi S, et al. Characterization and outcomes of hospitalized children with coronavirus disease 2019: a report from a multicenter, viral infection and respiratory illness universal study (coronavirus disease 2019) registry. Crit Care Med 2022;50(1):e40–51.

128. Waseem M, Shariff MA, Tay ET, et al. Multisystem inflammatory syndrome in children. J Emerg Med 2022;62(1):28–37.

129. Schlapbach LJ, Andre MC, Grazioli S, et al. Best practice recommendations for the diagnosis and management of children with pediatric inflammatory multisystem syndrome temporally associated with SARS-CoV-2 (PIMS-TS; multisystem inflammatory syndrome in children, MIS-C) in Switzerland. Front Pediatr 2021;9:667507.

130. Soomann M, Wendel-Garcia PD, Kaufmann M, et al. The SARS-CoV-2 pandemic impacts the management of Swiss pediatric intensive care units. Front Pediatr 2022,10:761815.

131. Rubens JH, Akindele NP, Tschudy MM. Acute covid-19 and multisystem inflammatory syndrome in children. BMJ 2021;372:n385.

132. Jonat B, Gorelik M, Boneparth A, et al. Multisystem inflammatory syndrome in children associated with coronavirus disease 2019 in a children's hospital in New York City: patient characteristics and an institutional protocol for evaluation, management, and follow-up. Pediatr Crit Care Med 2021;22(3):e178–91.

133. Rose L, Yu L, Casey J, et al. Communication and virtual visiting for families of patients in intensive care during the COVID-19 pandemic: a UK national survey. Ann Am Thorac Soc 2021;18(10):1685–92.

134. Kenmoe S, Kengne-Nde C, Ebogo-Belobo JT, et al. Systematic review and meta-analysis of the prevalence of common respiratory viruses in children < 2 years with bronchiolitis in the pre-COVID-19 pandemic era. PloS One 2020;15(11):e0242302.

135. Linssen RS, Teirlinck AC, van Boven M, et al. Increasing burden of viral bronchiolitis in the pediatric intensive care unit; an observational study. J Crit Care 2022;68:165–8.

136. Guitart C, Bobillo-Perez S, Alejandre C, et al. Bronchiolitis, epidemiological changes during the SARS-CoV-2 pandemic. BMC Infect Dis 2022;22(1):84.

137. Mount MC, Ji X, Kattan MW, et al. Derivation and validation of the critical bronchiolitis score for the PICU. Pediatr Crit Care Med 2022;23(1):e45–54.

138. Guitart C, Alejandre C, Torrus I, et al. Impact of a modification of the clinical practice guide of the American Academy of Pediatrics in the management of severe acute bronchiolitis in a pediatric intensive care unit. Med Intensiva (Engl ed) 2021;45(5):289–97.

139. Simpson J, Loh Z, Ullah MA, et al. Respiratory syncytial virus infection promotes necroptosis and HMGB1 release by airway epithelial cells. Am J Respir Crit Care Med 2020;201(11):1358–71.

140. Yeoh DK, Foley DA, Minney-Smith CA, et al. Impact of coronavirus disease 2019 public health measures on detections of influenza and respiratory syncytial virus in children during the 2020 Australian winter. Clin Infect Dis 2021;72(12):2199–202.

141. Foley D, Phuong L, Peplinski J, et al. Examining the interseasonal resurgence of respiratory syncytial virus in Western Australia. Arch Dis Child 2022;107(3):e7.

142. Li Y, Johnson EK, Shi T, et al. National burden estimates of hospitalisations for acute lower respiratory infections due to respiratory syncytial virus in young children in 2019 among 58 countries: a modelling study. Lancet Respir Med 2021;9(2):175–85.

143. Na'amnih W, Kassem E, Tannous S, et al. Incidence and risk factors of hospitalisations for respiratory syncytial virus among children aged less than 2 years. Epidemiol Infect 2022;150:e45.

144. Kadmon G, Feinstein Y, Lazar I, et al. Variability of care of infants with severe respiratory syncytial virus bronchiolitis: a multicenter study. Pediatr Infect Dis J 2020;39(9):808–13.

145. Moral L, Asensi Monzo M, Julia Benito JC, et al. Pediatric asthma: the REGAP consensus. An Pediatr (Engl ed) 2021;95(2):125 e1–11.

146. Sinyor B, Perez LC. Pathophysiology of asthma. StatPearls.Treasure Island, FL: StatPearls Publishing; 2022. Available from: https://pubmed.ncbi.nlm.nih.gov/31869060/. [Accessed 25 February 2023].

147. Han Y, Jia Q, Jahani P, et al. Genome-wide analysis highlights contribution of immune system pathways to the genetic architecture of asthma. Nat Commun 2020;11(1):1776.

148. Chang D, Hunkapiller J, Bhangale T, et al. A whole genome sequencing study of moderate to severe asthma identifies a lung function locus associated with asthma risk. Sci Rep 2022;12(1):5574.

149. Eliasen A, Pedersen C, Rasmussen M, et al. Genome-wide study of early and severe childhood asthma identifies interaction between CDHR3 and GSDMB. J Allergy Clin Immunol 2022;150(3):622–30.

150. Holmdahl I, Filiou A, Stenberg Hammar K, et al. Early life wheeze and risk factors for asthma – a revisit at age 7 in the GEWAC-cohort. Children (Basel) 2021;8(6):488.

151. Dharmage S, Perret J, Custovic A. Epidemiology of asthma in children and adults. Front Pediatr 2019;7:246.

152. Safiri S, Carson-Chahhoud K, Karamzad N, et al. Prevalence, deaths, and disability-adjusted life-years due to asthma and its attributable risk factors in 204 countries and territories, 1990–2019. Chest 2022;161(2):318–29.

153. Stern J, Pier J, Litonjua AA. Asthma epidemiology and risk factors. Semin Immunopathol 2020;42(1):5–15.

154. Selroos O, Kupczyk M, Kuna P, et al. National and regional asthma programmes in Europe. Eur Respir Rev 2015;24(137):474–83.

155. Boeschoten S, de Hoog M, Kneyber M, et al. Current practices in children with severe acute asthma across European PICUs: an ESPNIC survey. Eur J Pediatr 2020;179(3):455–61.

156. Navanandan N, Hatoun J, Celedon JC, et al. Predicting severe asthma exacerbations in children: blueprint for today and tomorrow. J Allergy Clin Immunol Pract 2021;9(7):2619–26.

157. Vasileiadis I, Alevrakis E, Ampelioti S, et al. Acid–base disturbances in patients with asthma: a literature review and comments on their pathophysiology. J Clin Med 2019;8(4):563.

158. Taytard J, Lacin F, Nguyen TLT, et al. Children with uncontrolled asthma and significant reversibility might show hypoxaemia. Eur J Pediatr 2020;179(6):999–1005.

159. Williams DM, Rubin BK. Clinical pharmacology of bronchodilator medications. Respir Care 2018;63(6):641–54.

160. Mahesh S, Ramamurthy MB. Management of acute asthma in children. Indian J Pediatr 2022;89(4):366–72.

161. Zafar G, Zulfiqar H. Aminophylline. StatPearls.Treasure Island, FL: StatPearls Publishing; 2022. Available from: https://www.ncbi.nlm.nih.gov/books/NBK545175/#article-17463.s5. [Accessed 25 February 2023].

162. Battisti A, Haftel A, Murphy-Lavoie H. Barotrauma. StatPearls.Treasure Island, FL: StatPearls Publishing; 2022. Available from: https://www.ncbi.nlm.nih.gov/books/NBK482348/. [Accessed 25 February 2023].

163. Sequera-Ramos L, Garcia-Marcinkiewicz A, Riva T, et al. Noninvasive ventilation in children: a review for the pediatric anesthesiologist. Pediatr Anaesth 2022;32(2):262–72.

164. Kantor D, Hirshberg E, McDonald M, et al. et al. Fluid balance Is associated with clinical outcomes and extravascular lung water in children with acute asthma exacerbation. Am J Respir Crit Care Med 2018;197(9):1128–35.

165. Schults J, Charles K, Long D, et al. The paediatric airway suction (PAWS) appropriateness guide for endotracheal suction interventions. Aust Crit Care 2022;35(6):651–60.

166. Gillies D, Todd D, Foster J, et al. Heat and moisture exchangers versus heated humidifiers for mechanically ventilated adults and children. Cochrane Database Syst Rev 2017(9):CD004711.

167. Blakeman T, Scott J, Yoder M, et al. AARC clinical practice guidelines: artificial airway suctioning. Respir Care 2022;67(2):258–71.

168. Davies K, Bulsara M, Ramelet A-S, et al. Reliability and criterion-related validity testing (construct) of the endotracheal suction assessment tool (ESAT©). J Clin Nurs 2018;27(9–10):1891–900.

169. Egbuta C, Easley R. Update on ventilation management in the pediatric intensive care unit. Pediatr Anesth 2022;32(2):354–62.

170. Miller AG, Scott BL. 2021 Year in review – pediatric mechanical ventilation. Respir Care 2022;67(11):1476–88.

171. Lal N, Varshney T. The collapsed newborn in the emergency department. BJA Educ 2018;18(8):254–8.

172. Weiss SL, Peters MJ, Alhazzani W, et al. Surviving Sepsis campaign international guidelines for the management of septic shock and sepsis-associated organ dysfunction in children. Pediatr Crit Care Med 2020;21(2):e52–106.

173. Assies R, Snik I, Kumwenda M, et al. Etiology, pathophysiology and mortality of shock in children in low (middle) income countries: a systematic review. J Trop Pediatr 2022;68(4):fmac053.

174. Harley A, Schlapbach L, Johnston A, et al. Challenges in the recognition and management of paediatric sepsis – the journey. Australas Emerg Care 2022;25(1):23–9.

175. Schlapbach LJ, Straney L, Bellomo R, et al. Prognostic accuracy of age-adapted SOFA, SIRS, PELOD-2, and qSOFA for in-hospital mortality among children with suspected infection admitted to the intensive care unit. Intensive Care Med 2018;44(2):179–88.

176. Hilarius K, Skippen P, Kissoon N. Early recognition and emergency treatment of sepsis and septic shock in children. Pediatr Emerg Care 2020;36(2):101–6.

177. Singh Y, Villaescusa JU, da Cruz EM, et al. Recommendations for hemodynamic monitoring for critically ill children – expert consensus statement issued by the cardiovascular dynamics section of the European Society of Paediatric and Neonatal Intensive Care (ESPNIC). Crit Care 2020;24(1):620.

178. Brady R. Meningococcal infections in children and adolescents: update and prevention. Adv Pediatr 2020;67:29–46.

179. Lee E-P, Wu H-P, Chan O-W, et al. Hemodynamic monitoring and management of pediatric septic shock. Biomed J 2022;45(1):63–73.

180. Erdil T, Lemme F, Konetzka A, et al. Extracorporeal membrane oxygenation support in pediatrics. Ann Cardiothorac Surg 2019;8(1):109–15.

181. Cashen K, Regling K, Saini A. Extracorporeal membrane oxygenation in critically ill children. Pediatr Clin North Am 2022;69(3):425–40.

182. Ramanathan K, Yeo N, Alexander P, et al. Role of extracorporeal membrane oxygenation in children with sepsis: a systematic review and meta-analysis. Crit Care 2020;24(1):684.

183. Wainwright MS, Guilliams K, Kannan S, et al. Acute neurologic dysfunction in critically ill children: the PODIUM consensus conference. Pediatrics 2022;149(1 Suppl. 1):S32–8.

184. Almojuela A, Hasen M, Zeiler FA. The Full Outline of UnResponsiveness (FOUR) score and its use in outcome prediction: a scoping review of the pediatric literature. J Child Neurol 2019;34(4):189–98.

185. Mihai CM, Chisnoiu T, Cambrea CS, et al. Neurological manifestations found in children with multisystem inflammatory syndrome. Exp Ther Med 2022;23(4):261.

186. Fine A, Wirrell E. Seizures in children. Pediatr Rev 2020;41(7):321–47.

187. Schiller K, Avigdor T, Kortas A, et al. Monitoring glucose concentrations in children with epilepsy on a ketogenic diet. Healthcare (Basel) 2022;10(2):245.

188. Vassilopoulos A, Mohammad S, Dure L, et al. Treatment approaches for functional neurological disorders in children. Curr Treat Options Neurol 2022;24(2):77–97.

189. Erickson T, Munoz F, Troisi C, et al. The epidemiology of meningitis in infants under 90 days of age in a large pediatric hospital. Microorganisms 2021;9(3):526.

190. Mwenda JM, Soda E, Weldegebriel G, et al. Pediatric bacterial meningitis surveillance in the World Health Organization African Region using the invasive bacterial vaccine-preventable disease surveillance network, 2011–2016. Clin Infect Dis 2019;69(Suppl. 2):S49–57.

191. Mathew S, Al Khatib HA, Al Ansari K, et al. Epidemiology profile of viral meningitis infections among patients in Qatar (2015–2018). Front Med (Lausanne) 2021;8:663694.

192. du Preez K, Jenkins H, Donald P, et al. Tuberculous meningitis in children: a forgotten public health emergency. Front Neurol 2022;13:751133.

193. Walls T, Cho V, Martin N, et al. Vaccine impact on long-term trends in invasive bacterial disease in New Zealand children. Pediatr Infect Dis J 2018;37(10):1041–7.

194. Di Pietro G, Biffi G, Castellazzi M, et al. Meningococcal disease in pediatric age: a focus on epidemiology and prevention. Int J Environ Res Public Health 2022;19(7):4035.

195. Huang L, Heuer O, Janssen S, et al. Clinical and economic burden of invasive meningococcal disease: evidence from a large German claims database. PloS One 2020;15(1):e0228020.

196. Parikh SR, Campbell H, Bettinger JA, et al. The everchanging epidemiology of meningococcal disease worldwide and the potential for prevention through vaccination. J Infect 2020;81(4):483–98.

197. Lochen A, Croucher NJ, Anderson RM. Divergent serotype replacement trends and increasing diversity in pneumococcal disease in high income settings reduce the benefit of expanding vaccine valency. Sci Rep 2020;10(1):18977.

198. Department of Health. Invasive pneumococcal disease (IPD) laboratory case definition (LCD). Canberra, ACT: Australian Government; 2020.

199. Malo JA, Ware RS, Lambert SB. Estimating the risk of recurrent invasive pneumococcal disease in Australia, 1991–2016. Vaccine 2021;39(40):5748–56.

200. Scelfo C, Menzella F, Fontana M, et al. Pneumonia and invasive pneumococcal diseases: the role of pneumococcal conjugate vaccine in the era of multi-drug resistance. Vaccines (Basel) 2021;9(5):420.

201. Erickson T, Muscal E, Munoz F, et al. Infectious and autoimmune causes of encephalitis in children. Pediatrics 2020;145(6):e20192543.

202. Bedetti L, Lugli L, Marrozzini L, et al. Safety and success of lumbar puncture in young infants: a prospective observational study. Front Pediatr 2021;9:692652.

203. Hsieh D, Lai Y, Lien C, et al. Nationwide population-based epidemiological study for outcomes of adjunctive steroid therapy in pediatric patients with bacterial meningitis in Taiwan. Int J Environ Res Public Health 2021;18(12):6386.

204. Zhang S-Y. Herpes simplex virus encephalitis of childhood: inborn errors of central nervous system cell-intrinsic immunity. Hum Genet 2020;139(6):911–18.

205. Toczylowski K, Bojkiewicz E, Barszcz M, et al.. Etiology, clinical presentation and incidence of infectious meningitis and encephalitis in Polish children. J Clin Med 2020;9(8):2324.

206. Saxena R, Chakraborti A. Half a century with pediatric viral encephalitis. Indian Pediatr 2020;57(15):957–8.

207. Armangue T, Spatola M, Vlagea A, et al. Frequency, symptoms, risk factors, and outcomes of autoimmune encephalitis after herpes simplex encephalitis: a prospective observational study and retrospective analysis. Lancet Neurol 2018;17(9):760–72.

208. de Galasso L, Picca S, Guzzo I. Dialysis modalities for the management of pediatric acute kidney injury. Pediatr Nephrol 2020;35(5):753–65.

209. Kaddourah A, Basu R, Bagshaw S, et al; AWARE Investigators. Epidemiology of acute kidney injury in critically ill children and young adults. N Engl J Med 2017;376(1):11–20.

210. Gist K, Selewski D, Brinton J, et al. Assessment of the independent and synergistic effects of fluid overload and acute kidney injury on outcomes of critically ill children. Pediatr Crit Care Med 2020;21(2):170–7.

211. Alobaidi R, Anton N, Burkholder S, et al. Association between acute kidney injury duration and outcomes in critically ill children. Pediatr Crit Care Med 2021;22(7):642–50.

212. Al-Dorzi H, Arabi Y. Prevention of gastrointestinal bleeding in critically ill patients. Curr Opin Crit Care 2021;27(2):177–82.

213. O'Halloran CP, Andren KG, Mecklosky J, et al. Mortality and factors associated with hemorrhage during pediatric extracorporeal membrane oxygenation. Pediatr Crit Care Med 2020;21(1):75–81.

214. Goyer I, Lacotte E, Montreuil J, et al. Proton pump inhibitor use and associated infectious complications in the PICU: propensity score matching analysis. Pediatr Crit Care Med 2022;23(12):e590–4. doi: 10.1097/PCC.0000000000003063.

215. Duffett M, Chan A, Closs J, et al. Stress ulcer prophylaxis in critically ill children: a multicenter observational study. Pediatr Crit Care Med 2020;21(2):e107–13.

216. Tume LN, Valla FV, Joosten K, et al. Nutritional support for children during critical illness: European Society of Pediatric and Neonatal Intensive Care (ESPNIC) metabolism, endocrine and nutrition section position statement and clinical recommendations. Intensive Care Med 2020;46(3):411–25.

217. Kratochvíl M, Klučka J, Klabusayová E, et al. Nutrition in pediatric intensive care: a narrative review. Children 2022;9(7):1031.

218. Tume LN, Eveleens RD, Verbruggen SCAT, et al. Barriers to delivery of enteral nutrition in pediatric intensive care: a world survey. Pediatr Crit Care Med 2020;21(9):e661–71.

219. S A. Hypotonic versus isotonic maintenance fluid administration in the pediatric surgical patient. Semin Pediatr Surg 2019;28(1):43–6.

220. Feld L, Neuspiel D, Foster B, et al. Clinical practice guideline: maintenance intravenous fluids in children. Pediatrics 2018;142(6):e20183083.

221. Chen L, Li T, Fang F, et al. Tight glycemic control in critically ill pediatric patients: a systematic review and meta-analysis. Crit Care 2018;22(1):57.

222. Montrief T, Koyfman A, Long B. Acute liver failure: a review for emergency physicians. Am J Emerg Med 2019;37(2):329–37.

223. Squires JE, Alonso EM, Ibrahim SH, et al. North American Society for Pediatric Gastroenterology, Hepatology, and Nutrition position paper on the diagnosis and management of pediatric acute liver failure. J Pediatr Gastroenterol Nutr 2022;74(1):138–58.

224. Quadros J, Piedade C, Lopes MF. Auxiliary liver transplantation for management of acute liver failure in children – systematic review. Transplant Rev 2021;35(4):100631.

225. Troeger CE, Khalil IA, Blacker BF, et al. Quantifying risks and interventions that have affected the burden of diarrhoea among children younger than 5 years: an analysis of the Global Burden of Disease Study 2017. Lancet Infect Dis 2020;20(1):37–59.

226. Hannon M, Middelberg L, Lee L. The initial approach to the multisystem pediatric trauma patient. Pediatr Emerg Care 2022;38(6):290–8.

227. Haagsma JA, James SL, Castle CD, et al. Burden of injury along the development spectrum: associations between the socio-demographic index and disability-adjusted life year estimates from the Global Burden of Disease Study 2017. Inj Prev 2020;26(Suppl. 2):i12–26.

228. Adeloye D, Bowman K, Chan K, et al. Global and regional child deaths due to injuries: an assessment of the evidence. J Glob Health 2018;8(2):021104.

229. Henley G, Harrison J. Hospitalised farm injury, Australia: 2010–11 to 2014–15: Canberra, ACT: Australian Institute of Health and Welfare; 2018.

230. Bradshaw C, Bandi A, Muktar Z, et al. International study of the epidemiology of paediatric rrauma: PAPSA research study. World J Surg 2018;42(6):1885–94.

231. Australian Institute of Health and Welfare (AIHW). Injury in Australia. Canberra, ACT: AIHW; 2022. Available from: https://www.aihw.gov.au/reports/injury/injury-in-australia. [Accessed 25 February 2023].

232. Henley G, Harrison J. Hospitalised farm injury, Australia, 2010–2011 to 2014–2015. Canberra, ACT: Australian Institute of Health and Welfare, Flinders University; 2018. Report No.: INJCAT 189. Available from: https://www.aihw.gov.au/getmedia/279bb48f-d2fe-47b9-823c-63cdb2a1a3cf/aihw-injcat-189.pdf.aspx?inline=true. [Accessed 25 February 2023].

233. Royal Life Saving Society Australia. The national drowning report 2022. Sydney: Royal Life Saving Australia; 2022.

234. Zhu H, Chen B, Guo C. Aggressive crystalloid adversely affects outcomes in a pediatric trauma population. Eur J Trauma Emerg Surg 2021;47(1):85–92.

235. Dahl H, Andelic N, Lovstad M, et al. Epidemiology of traumatic brain injury in children 15 years and younger in South-Eastern Norway in 2015–16. Implications for prevention and follow-up needs. Eur J Paediatr Neurol 2021;31:70–7.

236. Chong S, Dang H, Ming M, et al. Traumatic brain injury outcomes in 10 Asian pediatric ICUs: a pediatric acute and critical care medicine Asian network retrospective study. Pediatr Crit Care Med 2021;22(4):401–11.

237. Amagasa S, Tsuji S, Matsui H, et al. Prognostic factors of acute neurological outcomes in infants with traumatic brain injury. Childs Nerv Syst 2018;34(4):673–80.

238. Kochanek PM, Tasker RC, Carney N, et al. Guidelines for the management of pediatric severe traumatic brain injury, third edition: update of the Brain Trauma Foundation guidelines, executive summary. Pediatr Crit Care Med 2019;20(3):280–9.

239. Kochanek PM, Tasker RC, Bell MJ, et al. Management of pediatric severe traumatic brain injury: 2019 consensus and guidelines-based algorithm for first and second tier therapies. Pediatr Crit Care Med 2019;20(3):269–79.

240. Brown P, Munigangaiah S, Davidson N, et al. A review of paediatric cervical spinal trauma. Surgery (Oxford) 2020;38(9):495–9.

241. Ugalde IT, Chan HK, Mendez D, et al. Computed tomography of the chest in younger pediatric patients with thoracic blunt trauma rarely changes surgical management. West J Emerg Med 2022;23(3):324–33.

242. Evans L, Aarabi S, Durand R, et al. Torso vascular trauma. Semin Pediatr Surg 2021;30(6):151126.

243. Bird R, Braunold D, Matava C. Chest trauma in children – what an anesthesiologist should know. Pediatr Anaesth 2022;32(2):340–5.

244. Chaudhari P, Rodean J, Spurrier R, et al. Epidemiology and management of abdominal injuries in children. Acad Emerg Med 2022;29(8):944–53.

245. Lynch T, Kilgar J, Al Shibli A. Pediatric abdominal trauma. Curr Pediatr Rev 2018;14(1):59–63.

246. Alzahem A, Soundappan S, Cass D. The predictors for positive yield abdominal computed tomography in pediatric abdominal trauma. Pediatr Emerg Care 2020;36(10):e543–8.

247. Manning JC, Pinto NP, Rennick JE, et al. Conceptualizing post intensive care syndrome in children-the PICS-p framework. Pediatr Crit Care Med 2018;19(4):298–300.

248. Yuan C, Timmins F, Thompson DR. Post-intensive care syndrome: a concept analysis. Int J Nurs Stud 2021;114:103814.

249. Gayat E, Cariou A, Deye N, et al. Determinants of long-term outcome in ICU survivors: results from the FROG-ICU study. Crit Care 2018;22(1):8.

250. Long DA, Fink EL. Transitions from short to long-term outcomes in pediatric critical care: considerations for clinical practice. Transl Pediatr 2021;10(10):2858–74.

251. Woodruff AG, Choong K. Long-term outcomes and the post-intensive care syndrome in critically ill children: a North American perspective. Children (Basel) 2021;8(4):254.

252. Choong K. Post-intensive care syndrome – the paediatric perspective. ICU Manag Pract 2020;4:288–91.

253. Chaiyakulsil C, Opasatian R, Tippayawong P. Pediatric postintensive care syndrome: high burden and a gap in evaluation tools for limited-resource settings. Clin Exp Pediatr 2021;64(9):436–42.

254. Tang M, Xu M, Su S, et al. Post-intensive care syndrome in children: a concept analysis. J Pediatr Nurs 2021;61:417–23.

255. Manning JC, Scholefield BR, Popejoy E, et al. Paediatric intensive care follow-up provision in the United Kingdom and Republic of Ireland. Nurs Crit Care 2021;26(2):128–34.

256. Fink E, Maddux A, Pinto N, et al. A core outcome set for pediatric critical care. Crit Care Med 2020;48(12):1819–28.

257. Walz A, Canter MO, Betters K. The ICU liberation bundle and strategies for implementation in pediatrics. Curr Pediatr Rep 2020;8(3):69–78.

Chapter 28

Pregnancy and postpartum considerations

Wendy Pollock, Alison James

Learning objectives

After reading this chapter, you should be able to:

- identify the core physiological adaptations of pregnancy pertinent to critical care nursing
- describe the antenatal assessment that would be required when caring for a woman 28 weeks pregnant in ICU
- describe the priorities of management for a postpartum woman admitted to ICU with preeclampsia
- outline the standard postnatal care required by a woman in ICU for the 48 hours following birth
- discuss the principles of cardiac arrest management during pregnancy
- consider the resources and equipment available in your workplace that are specifically required for the care of pregnant and postpartum women.

Introduction

The admission of a pregnant or postpartum woman to an ICU can extend ICU staff beyond their comfort zone. Pregnant and postpartum women undergo substantial physiological adaptations. Nursing staff members also need to consider the fetus and be aware of, and manage, obstetric conditions. This chapter provides an overview of the epidemiology of critical illness in pregnancy, describes the physiological adaptations of pregnancy and the puerperium, outlines some key medical conditions and their interaction with pregnancy and describes the major obstetric conditions that are associated with critical illness. Additionally, we include guidance on specific practices related to caring for pregnant and postpartum women in ICU. Research into critical care obstetrics is expanding; however, at times the evidence being drawn on remains dated.

Epidemiology of critical illness in pregnancy

Most women experience a healthy, normal pregnancy and the development of critical illness associated with pregnancy is usually sudden and unexpected. Approximately 1 in 220 births to 1 in 450 births in high-income countries

KEY WORDS

antenatal assessment

asthma during pregnancy

breastfeeding

cardiac disease

critical illness in pregnancy

fetal well-being

obstetric haemorrhage

postpartum care

severe acute maternal morbidity

severe preeclampsia

results in a maternal ICU admission, making up approximately 1–1.5% of the ICU population; more than three-quarters of admissions occur following the birth of the baby.[1-3] However, there are increasing numbers of women with comorbidities having children and this may lead to higher rates of ICU admission. Furthermore, some groups of women are more likely to have a maternal ICU admission; for example, in the UK, black women are more likely than white women to be admitted to an ICU, as are Indigenous and migrant women in Australia.[3-5] Admission of a pregnant woman to ICU is infrequent and more likely to relate to a non-obstetric diagnosis such as pneumonia. Conversely, in postpartum women, a condition directly associated with pregnancy is more common – usually preeclampsia or obstetric haemorrhage.[1]

Pregnant and postpartum admissions to ICU are usually short, with most lengths of stay less than 24 hours. There is variation in the threshold for admission to an ICU, as many women do not receive specific ICU interventions. In general, about one-third of women who experience severe acute maternal morbidity are admitted to the ICU.[6] It is feasible that admission to ICU could be avoided by up-skilling midwifery services to provide an intermediate level of care.[7] Furthermore, with early identification of clinical deterioration and timely, appropriate intervention, it is feasible that up to 40% of maternal ICU admissions are potentially preventable.[8] In developed countries, the mortality of pregnant and postpartum women admitted to ICU is relatively low, at around 3%, compared with the 15% mortality observed in the regular ICU population.[1]

Practice tip

Any maternal death or death of a woman during pregnancy or within 42 days of having been pregnant should be reported to the relevant authority, even if the pregnancy is not thought to have contributed to the cause of death.

Adapted physiology of pregnancy

The physiological changes that occur during pregnancy influence the majority of body systems, commence shortly after conception and enable changes that facilitate fetal and uterine growth, and prepare the woman for birth and lactation. The physiological changes described in this chapter relate to women with singleton pregnancies who are not in labour. Where multiple pregnancy occurs, physiological adaptations may be exaggerated and labour brings further changes to the adapted physiology, such as increased cardiac output.[9] The normal physiological changes of pregnancy differ from woman to woman, depending on factors such as maternal age, health and genetic influences. The uterus and breasts undergo major changes during pregnancy and are described in detail in

physiology and midwifery textbooks such as Maternal, fetal, and neonatal physiology: a clinical perspective and Myles textbook for midwives.[10,11]

The puerperium (also referred to as the postnatal or postpartum period) commences after the placenta and membranes are expelled, when there is a sharp drop in the placental hormones including progesterone and oestrogens.[10] The puerperium is usually defined as 6 weeks, during which time the body systems gradually return to the pre-pregnant or near-pre-pregnant state.[12] Lactation will become established, where the mother chooses to breastfeed.

Haematological system
Blood volume and red cells

Total blood volume, plasma volume and red cell mass increase during pregnancy.[10] Plasma volume increases by 40–50%, and, although there is an increase in red cell production, it is not enough to keep up with the increase in plasma volume, resulting in a reduction in measured haemoglobin, often referred to as haemodilutional anaemia.[13,14] Overall, total blood volume increases by 1500–1600 mL and this is required to accommodate the metabolic demands of the developing fetus, and prepares the woman for normal blood loss associated with birth (<500 mL). Pregnant women are renowned for being able to maintain stable vital signs, with blood losses as much as 1500 mL before acutely deteriorating.[15]

Blood clotting and haemostasis

Both elements of the haemostatic system (coagulation and fibrinolysis) activate during pregnancy. Pregnancy is termed a hypercoagulable state, due to an increase in clotting factors II, VIII and IX, an increase in fibrinogen and fibrin degradation products, and a decrease in some naturally occurring anticoagulants.[16] There is also venous stasis and microscopic vascular damage, and both pregnant and postnatal women are at increased risk of venous thromboembolism (VTE).[17] The changes occurring to the haemostatic system are summarised in Table 28.1.[16,18,19] Of note, gestational thrombocytopenia (defined as platelets of 80–150 × 10^9/L) occurs in 6–8% of healthy pregnant women and generally has no negative impact on the woman or fetus.[20]

Cardiovascular system
Anatomical and ECG changes

The heart undergoes anatomical change during pregnancy including left ventricular hypertrophy. Cross-sectional areas of the aortic, pulmonary and mitral valves increase by 12–14%.[21] Electrocardiography (ECG) changes may include atrial/ventricular ectopics, Q waves in lead II, III and AVF, ST-segment changes, T-wave inversion in lead III and left-axis deviation.[22] ECG interpretation should take into account the pregnant woman's cardiovascular risk factors and presenting symptoms.

TABLE 28.1

Haemostatic changes during pregnancy[16,18,19]

HAEMOSTATIC COMPONENT	CHANGES DURING PREGNANCY
Platelets	
Count	Unchanged
Lifespan	Unchanged
Clotting factors	
Factors VII, VIII and IX	Increased
von Willebrand factor	Increased
Fibrinogen (factor I)	Doubles by term
Other clotting factors	Mainly unchanged
Fibrinolysis	
D-dimer level	Progressively increases during pregnancy By term, level >0.5 mg/L common

Heart rate, stroke volume and cardiac output

Peripheral vasodilation occurs from 5 weeks' gestation, stimulated by progesterone and endothelium-dependent factors including nitric oxide, which also vasodilates the placental vessels.[23–25] There is a subsequent 25–40% decrease in systemic vascular resistance (SVR).[26] The maternal heart rate increases by about 10 beats per minute (bpm), peaking in the third trimester.[27] Stroke volume increases between 18% and 32%, beginning as early as 8 weeks' gestation.[28] Cardiac output increases during the first and second trimesters, peaking at 30–40% over non-pregnant values towards the end of the second trimester (~6 L/min), although this increase may not be linear.[26] Furthermore, cardiac output measurement depends on the device used and our understanding of cardiac output during pregnancy is still evolving.[9]

Blood pressure

Blood pressure (BP) begins dropping as early as 6–8 weeks' gestation, with the lowest levels recorded during the second trimester and returning to pre-pregnancy measurements near term. Normal BP ranges are 95–139 systolic and 55–89 diastolic, based on the 3rd and 97th centiles of BP measurements of over 1000 women.[27]

Aortocaval compression and supine hypotension

After 20 weeks' gestation, a woman lying flat on her back may experience supine hypotension, secondary to aortocaval compression, with reduction in venous return, cardiac output and placental blood flow.[29] Cardiac stroke volume can be reduced by as much as 70% and a pregnant woman of ≥20 weeks' gestation should not be nursed flat on her back.[25] A left lateral lying position of 15–30 degrees results in improved maternal cardiac output and may be achieved with the use of a wedge/pillows, or tilted if on a theatre table or spinal board.[30] Left manual uterine displacement is advocated during cardiopulmonary resuscitation (CPR) to facilitate optimal chest compressions.[29]

Postpartum cardiovascular changes

Heart rate returns to pre-pregnancy levels by 10 days postpartum while blood pressure has normally returned to pre-pregnancy levels by term and does not change during the puerperium.[25] The first few days of the puerperium are associated with a significant diuresis, resulting in the haemoconcentration of blood. Therefore, the risk of thromboembolism is higher during the postpartum period than during pregnancy. Appropriate risk assessment and prophylactic measures should be implemented to reduce the risk of VTE.[31]

Post birth, cardiac output increases as approximately 500 mL of blood is autotransfused from the now-contracted uterus back into the maternal circulation At this point in the postpartum phase, stroke volume is increased while the maternal heart rate is often slowed.[32] For most women, the immediate postpartum elevation in cardiac output lasts only 48 hours. By 2 weeks postpartum, many haemodynamic parameters have returned to pre-pregnancy levels for most women, although some have been recorded as remaining above pre-pregnancy levels at 12 months postpartum, including cardiac output.[25,33]

Respiratory system

The respiratory system undergoes widespread adaptation from early pregnancy, with effects on the airway through to gaseous exchange at the alveolar level evident, including variation to 'normal' parameters when interpreting arterial blood gas results. These changes support the increased metabolic demands of pregnancy.[34]

Changes to the upper airways and thorax

Normal physiological changes of pregnancy include generalised vasodilation of the upper airway vasculature, increased neck circumference due to fat deposition and an increase in mucosal oedema.[35] These physiological changes are thought to be responsible for the symptoms of rhinitis, nasal stuffiness and epistaxis that are more common in pregnancy.[35] Changes also occur to the chest wall, with relaxation of ligaments resulting in outward-flaring of the lower ribs and a 50% increase in the subcostal angle.[10] The diameter and the circumference of the thorax increase by 2 cm and 5–7 cm, respectively.[35] These physical changes are thought to cause the diaphragm to rise by 4 cm before there is additional pressure from the enlarging uterus.[34]

Respiratory muscle function does not change significantly during pregnancy and rib cage compliance is unaltered. The functional residual capacity (FRC) is reduced by 10–30%, making the pregnant woman more vulnerable to hypoxaemia during any apnoeic period.[34] Chest X-ray interpretation is unchanged during pregnancy.[36] Overall, oxygen requirements increase by up to 33% at term.[29]

Changes to the physiology of breathing

From 5 weeks' gestation, multiple factors increase respiratory drive. Elevated progesterone levels are thought to lower the $PaCO_2$ threshold in the respiratory centre, resulting in hyperventilation.[37] Minute ventilation (MV) begins to increase soon after conception, peaking at 40–50% above pre-conception level at term (7.5–10.5 L/min). The increase in minute ventilation is achieved by a 30–50% increase in tidal volume (e.g. an increase of 200 ± 50 mL at term), without any increase in respiratory rate.[35] Consequently, normal arterial blood gas values are different in pregnancy (Table 28.2). The reduced $PaCO_2$ level enables fetal CO_2 to passively cross the placenta for maternal excretion. PaO_2 normally increases by 10 mmHg, although the PaO_2 level is affected by posture, particularly as the pregnancy progresses.[38] Later in pregnancy the supine position can reduce PaO_2 by 10 mmHg compared with the same woman in the sitting position.[39] The kidneys compensate for the lowered $PaCO_2$ by increasing bicarbonate excretion to maintain a normal pH.[35] Normal oxygen saturation in pregnancy demonstrates a slight reduction in SpO_2 as the pregnancy progresses, with a normal value ranging from 94 to 100%.[27]

Hyperventilation of pregnancy is associated with a feeling of breathlessness in up to 70% of healthy pregnant women.[40] Consequently, distinguishing 'physiological dyspnoea' from 'pathological dyspnoea' (e.g. developing cardiomyopathy or pulmonary embolism) can present a challenge in pregnancy and requires careful investigation.

Postpartum respiratory changes

Complete resolution of the spirometry and arterial blood gas changes occurring in pregnancy is accomplished by 5 weeks postpartum,[38] although the daily transition of these parameters over the first week postpartum is not

---

TABLE 28.2

Key physiological changes in pregnancy

PARAMETER	CHANGE DURING PREGNANCY	PARAMETER	CHANGE DURING PREGNANCY
Cardiovascular system		**Respiratory system**	
Heart rate	↑ 10–20 bpm	Respiratory rate	Unchanged
Stroke volume	↑ 18–32%	Tidal volume	↑ 30–50%
Blood pressure:		Minute volume	↑ 40–50%
Systolic	↓ 5–10 mmHg	Oxygen consumption	↑ 15–20%
Diastolic	↓ 10–25 mmHg	Arterial blood gas analysis values:	
Cardiac output	↑ 30–50%	PaO_2	80–110 mmHg
Systemic vascular resistance	↓ up to 40%	$PaCO_2$	28–32 mmHg
Central arterial and venous pressures	Unchanged	pH	7.40–7.45
		HCO_3^-	18–21 mmol/L
Haematological system		SaO_2	≥95%
Blood volume	↑ 1200–1600 mL	Vital capacity	Unchanged
Plasma volume	↑ 30–50%	Functional reserve capacity	↓ 17–20% (from 1.7 L to 1.35 L)
Red blood cells	↑ 20–30%	Lung compliance	Unchanged
White blood cells	↑ 100–300%	**Renal system**	
Platelets	Up to 20% decrease but count remaining within normal limits	Glomerular filtration rate	↑ 40–50%
		Serum urea and creatinine	↓
Fibrinogen	↑ 100%	Urine output	Unknown
Serum albumin level	↓ 10–15%	Proteinuria	<300 mg/day

known. One very old study reported that CO_2 levels took between 2 and 5 days to return to normal non-pregnant values postpartum.[41] Rapid changes to the $PaCO_2$ level will contribute to the development of acidaemia, which may be clinically relevant around the time of delivery or in the early postpartum phase if the woman has an active disease state or experiences a complication such as severe postpartum haemorrhage.

Renal system

The smooth muscle of the renal pelvises, calyces, ureters and urethra dilates during early pregnancy largely because of the effects of progesterone. Each kidney lengthens by approximately 1–1.5 cm because of dilation, associated mild hydronephrosis and increased vascularity.[35] Widespread dilation causes urinary stasis and increased likelihood of urinary tract infection.[10] Acute pyelonephritis is a common renal complication and is associated with preterm labour.[42]

The glomerular filtration rate (GFR) increases by 40–50%, peaking by the end of the first trimester, with some reduction towards non-pregnant levels over the third trimester.[43] The increase in GFR may result in glycosuria and proteinuria.[43] Glycosuria does not accurately reflect blood sugar levels and is unhelpful in monitoring diabetes.[10] Proteinuria, up to 300 mg per 24 hours, is considered normal in pregnancy. Conversely, the high GFR results in lowered mean serum levels of both urea and creatinine; a plasma urea level exceeding 4.9 mmol/L and plasma creatinine level higher than 75 micromol/L should be viewed as abnormal and indicative of potential renal impairment requiring investigation.[44] There is a reduction in normal serum sodium level, from 140 to 136 mmol/L, and a reduction in plasma osmolality from 290 to 280 mOsmol/kg.

Postpartum renal changes

The most significant postpartum renal change is the diuresis that occurs during the first 3 days. This diuresis serves to offload the additional blood volume that the woman has had circulating for the duration of the pregnancy. There has been little examination of 'normal urine output', with the standard 0.5 mL/kg/h reported as a minimum acceptable level; however, a true 'normal' level is likely to be closer to 0.8 mL/kg/h.[45] Moreover, 30 mL/h is often accepted as the minimum amount regardless of the woman's weight.[46] Creatinine levels are within the normal non-pregnancy range within 24 hours postpartum, while the lower urea levels remain for at least 48 hours.[44] The bladder returns to the pelvis in the early postpartum period as the uterus and other organs resume their pre-pregnancy position.

Gastrointestinal system and liver

The enlarging uterus pushes abdominal organs aside, making assessment and diagnosis of an acute abdomen difficult and changes landmarks for surgical incisions.[47] For example, the appendix is progressively displaced upwards and laterally from McBurney's point at the third month, reaching the level of the iliac crest by late pregnancy.[48] Pregnant women with prior abdominal surgery and adhesions are also more predisposed to intestinal obstruction.[49]

Due to the effects of progesterone and the mechanical presence of the enlarging uterus, there is delayed gastric emptying, decreased cardiac sphincter tone and raised intra-abdominal pressure, which predisposes women to heartburn and increases their risk of aspiration.[35] Bowel peristalsis slows, from the effects of progesterone, commonly resulting in constipation; this slowing of peristalsis, along with pressure from the gravid uterus on the pelvic vasculature, also contributes to haemorrhoids.

Hepatobiliary changes in pregnancy

There is no significant increase in hepatic arterial blood flow during pregnancy. However, blood flow to the liver supplied by the portal vein doubles,[50] which may have an impact on oral medication metabolism. Changes in hepatic enzymes responsible for drug metabolism may alter the pharmacokinetics of some medications (e.g. more-rapid clearance of nifedipine).[51] Serum albumin levels reduce to 30–40 g/L for the majority of pregnancy, with levels as low as 25 g/L normal during the second postpartum day.[44] This low albumin level reduces colloid osmotic pressure, contributing to the presence of oedema, which is common in pregnancy.

The general smooth muscle vasodilation affects the hepatobiliary ducts, resulting in sluggish bile motility and delayed emptying of the gall bladder. These changes lead to an increased incidence of cholelithiasis and cholecystitis during pregnancy.[47]

Changes in white blood cells and the immune system

The immune system in pregnancy is dynamic, changing from proinflammatory, to anti-inflammatory and back to proinflammatory according to the stage of pregnancy.[52] Pregnant women have increased innate immune system activity (non-specific response) and a lowered adaptive immune system (specific antibody response), with pregnant women more vulnerable to some infections, such as malaria and varicella.[53,54] Pregnant women are often in contact with small children and potentially have an increased exposure to various infections. The white blood cell number increases throughout pregnancy, peaking at around 30 weeks' gestation, when a normal level may be as high as $15–25 \times 10^9$/L.[44]

The placenta and membranes
Placental development

The placenta develops from the trophoblastic layer of the fertilised ovum and is completely formed and functioning 10 weeks following fertilisation. The chorionic villi attach to the uterine wall via the decidua. The result is an interface

FIGURE 28.1 The maternal–placental interface.

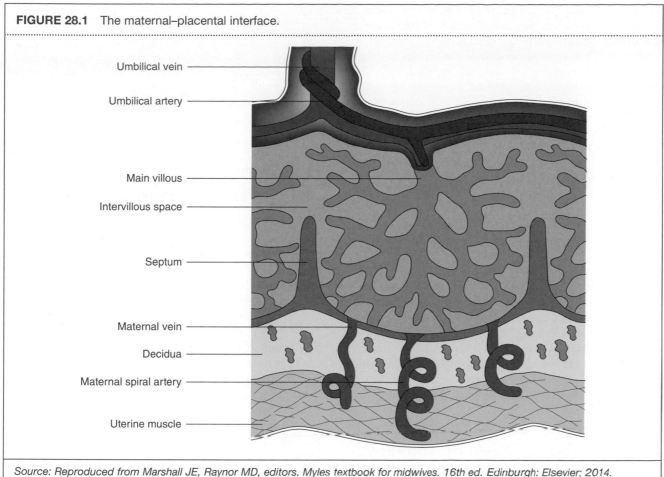

Umbilical vein

Umbilical artery

Main villous

Intervillous space

Septum

Maternal vein

Decidua

Maternal spiral artery

Uterine muscle

Source: Reproduced from Marshall JE, Raynor MD, editors. Myles textbook for midwives. 16th ed. Edinburgh: Elsevier; 2014.

whereby maternal blood fills a space in which the nutritive villi float and are bathed in the maternal blood (Fig. 28.1). The blood drains back into the maternal circulation via maternal sinuses and the endometrial veins. Approximately 150 mL of maternal blood, replenished three to four times per minute, bathe the villi in the intervillous space. The chorionic villi maximise the available surface area to optimise the exchange of products across the maternal–placental interface. By term, this surface area is said to be as large as 13 m². Initially, four layers of cells separate the maternal blood from the fetal blood, reducing to three after 20 weeks' gestation; these cell layers are collectively referred to as the 'placental membrane' or 'placental barrier'. Damage to villi, such as a threatened abortion or blunt trauma, can enable fetal haemoglobin and squames to enter the maternal circulation, leading to rhesus (RH) isoimmunisation or, rarely, amniotic fluid embolism.

Functions of the placenta

The placenta provides six major functions to sustain the pregnancy and fetus: respiration, nutrition, storage, excretion, protection and endocrine.[11] Fetal lungs are filled with amniotic fluid and all oxygenation and removal of carbon dioxide must be provided via the placenta. Fetal haemoglobin has a slightly different structure to adult haemoglobin and

has a higher affinity for oxygen. Both oxygen and carbon dioxide cross the placental membrane by simple diffusion. Nutrients are actively transported across the placental membrane, with the placenta able to select the substances needed by the fetus, even at the expense of the mother if necessary.[11] The placenta is able to store glucose by converting it to glycogen and reconverting it to glucose as required and also stores iron and some fat-soluble vitamins.

The placental membrane operates as a barrier between the maternal and fetal circulations and provides a limited protective function. Generally, few bacteria can cross the placenta, although viruses can cross readily. The placenta produces large volumes of hormones including progesterone, oestrogens, placental lactogen, chorionic gonadotrophin, growth factors, cytokine vasoactive substances, placental growth hormone, thyrotrophin and corticotrophin.[10] The placenta does not have a nerve supply, so all activities regulated by the placenta must be undertaken by other mechanisms (e.g. chemical changes, hormonal changes).

Impaired utero-placental gaseous exchange

Effective gas exchange across the placental membrane depends on sufficient maternal blood pressure and adequate O_2 and CO_2 gradients for passive diffusion to occur. In response to hypoxaemia, a fetal brain-sparing mechanism goes into effect that increases fetal arterial pressure and redirects blood delivery to the main organs, namely the brain, heart and adrenal glands.[55] This centralisation of fetal blood flow is more apparent in response to maternal hypoxaemia than to reduced utero-placental blood flow. Whether the fetus will die in utero or survive, and the degree of any neurological compromise, depends on the degree and duration of asphyxia, the recurrent nature of asphyxia and the degree to which the fetus is able to compensate for the asphyxia.

Clinical implications of the physiological adaptations of pregnancy

The normal physiological adaptations of pregnancy may explain the so-called 'minor discomforts' of pregnancy, including constipation, varicose veins, indigestion, breathlessness and fatigue. The adaptations influence the majority of body systems (see Table 28.2) and must be taken into consideration when monitoring physiological parameters, interpreting investigation results and planning treatment for the critically ill woman (Table 28.3).

Recognition of clinical deterioration in pregnant and postpartum women

The physiological adaptations of pregnancy may make early recognition of clinical deterioration more challenging. For example, with 30–40% more cardiac output and 40–50% more circulating volume, substantial blood loss occurs before there are changes in vital signs, such as heart rate and blood pressure. Additionally, pregnancy and childbirth are considered normal life events in young, healthy women; serious complications occur rarely, which can lead to complacency. The implementation of system-wide standards on the early recognition of clinical deterioration has resulted in a reduction of cardiac arrest-related admission to ICU.[56] Despite the UK Confidential Enquiry into Maternal Deaths recommending the use of maternity-modified early-warning systems since 2007, few countries have a nationally agreed system in place. Ireland is one country with a well-established national maternity early-warning system, demonstrating that it is possible.[57] Furthermore, recent work identifying normal vital signs, taking into account the physiology of pregnancy, may support progress in the development of national maternity early-warning systems more broadly.[27] Pregnant and postpartum women do experience clinical deterioration in hospital, with about 10% of medical emergency team (MET) calls resulting in the women requiring admission to ICU.[58] Critical care nurses who attend maternity MET calls should be appropriately educated on the unique elements of the maternity population.

> ### Practice tip
>
> Be aware that high systolic blood pressure may not be listed as a vital sign criterion to trigger a MET call in general hospitals that apply generic vital sign criteria to the maternity population[59] – yet high systolic blood pressure is highly relevant in the maternity population and the pregnancy condition preeclampsia.

Diseases and conditions unique to pregnancy

There are a number of conditions unique to pregnancy that might cause a woman to become critically ill and result in admission to ICU, including preeclampsia, obstetric haemorrhage, amniotic fluid embolism and peripartum cardiomyopathy. These conditions are discussed in detail below.

Preeclampsia

The umbrella term 'hypertension disorders of pregnancy' describes myriad conditions in pregnancy where hypertension is a major feature, with the definition for hypertension during pregnancy: systolic BP ≥ 140 mmHg and/or diastolic BP ≥ 90 mmHg.[60,61] These hypertensive conditions include gestational hypertension, chronic hypertension and preeclampsia, which incorporates eclampsia, and haemolysis, elevated liver enzymes and low platelets (HELLP) syndrome (Table 28.4).[60,62] Comprehensive descriptions of these conditions and their management have been published by the UK's National Institute for Health and Care Excellence (NICE) and the Society of Obstetric Medicine Australia and New Zealand (SOMANZ).[60,62] Another useful resource is the California Maternity Quality Care Collaborative Improving Health Care Response to Hypertensive Disorders of Pregnancy Toolkit (2021), available at https://www.cmqcc.org/resources-tool-kits/toolkits/HDP.[63]

Preeclampsia is a progressive, multisystem disorder consisting of variable clinical features related to endothelial cell dysfunction, occurring in response to toxins released from the placenta. The indication for ICU admission is usually related to organ dysfunction.[64] Preeclampsia remains a leading cause of maternal death in both developed and developing countries,[65] and a primary reason for ICU admission in developed countries during pregnancy, birth and the postnatal period.[66]

Aetiology

The placenta is strongly implicated in the cause of preeclampsia; its removal is the only definitive treatment for the condition. Theories explaining the pathophysiology of preeclampsia include immune maladaptation, abnormal trophoblast embedding, endothelial activation and excessive inflammatory response, and a genetic susceptibility. Additionally, it is postulated that there may be alternative pathophysiology for early-onset (<34 weeks) disease

TABLE 28.3

Clinical relevance of physiological adaptations in pregnancy

EFFECTS OF THE NORMAL PHYSIOLOGY OF PREGNANCY	CLINICAL IMPLICATIONS
Cardiovascular system	
Increased likelihood of: • venous stasis • varicose veins • deep vein thrombosis • haemorrhoids • swollen ankles.	Consider use of thromboprophylaxis.
Potential for aortocaval compression from about 20 weeks' gestation.	Avoid nursing the woman flat on her back, e.g. tilt bed if unable to nurse woman on her side or use pillows/wedges to obtain a lateral tilt of 15–30 degrees but full left lying is best. CPR and haemodynamic measurements should be done with a left lateral tilt. Manual displacement of the uterus is an alternative way to relieve aortocaval compression during CPR.
Haemodynamic stability despite large blood loss. Sudden deterioration.	Be alert to subtle signs of haemodynamic compromise.
Respiratory system	
Nasal passages more likely to bleed on instrumentation (e.g. nasal intubation, nasogastric insertion). More likely to bleed from the gums. More prone to hypoxaemia during apnoea, e.g. when being intubated. All pregnant women are considered to have a high-risk airway: • especially if the woman has preeclampsia • particularly if the woman is obese. More likely to develop pulmonary oedema. Diaphragm raised by about 5 cm.	Nasal-tracheal intubation is not usually an option. Have a doctor experienced with intubation on hand when a pregnant woman is being intubated. Ensure that the artificial airway is protected and guard against accidental extubation. Review the 'failed intubation' protocol in the ICU. Pre-oxygenate with 100% O_2 prior to intubation or suctioning unless contraindicated. Titrate fluid resuscitation carefully – especially in women with severe preeclampsia. Check diaphragm location prior to ICC insertion for haemothorax/pleural effusion.
Gastrointestinal system	
Pregnant women are more likely to: • aspirate • develop constipation • present with advanced signs and symptoms of acute abdomen, e.g. appendicitis, bowel obstruction. • Pregnant women have additional and specific nutritional needs.	Maintain cricoid pressure, if instructed, throughout CPR and intubation until the person obtaining an artificial airway instructs its release. Chart bowel actions and ensure a bowel management strategy is implemented. Early consideration of non-obstetric causes of an acute abdomen. Consult with a dietitian early to ensure that the woman receives adequate nutrition during ICU admission.
Renal system	
Progesterone and relaxin cause relaxation and dilation of smooth muscles. Renal calyces and renal pelvis become distended. Ureters and urethra are elongated, dilated and have reduced peristalsis. Stasis of urine and increased risk of ascending infection. Acute pyelonephritis is associated with preterm labour. Bladder is displaced into the abdominal cavity after the first trimester.	Minimise use of indwelling urinary catheter. Renal impairment may be signified by lower serum urea and creatinine levels than in non-pregnancy. Some glycosuria and proteinuria are normal in pregnancy. The bladder is at risk of traumatic injury in the second and third trimesters.

CPR = cardiopulmonary resuscitation; ICC = intercostal catheter.

TABLE 28.4

Definitions of conditions characterised by hypertension in pregnancy[60,62]

TERM	DEFINITION
Hypertension in pregnancy Severe hypertension	Systolic BP ≥140 mmHg and/or a diastolic BP ≥90 mmHg. Systolic BP >160 mmHg or a diastolic BP >110 mmHg.
Chronic hypertension	Hypertension presenting in the first 20 weeks or that existed prior to the pregnancy without an apparent underlying cause.
Gestational hypertension	Hypertension arising after 20 weeks' gestation and resolving by 3 months postpartum. No evidence of any other feature of the multisystem disorder preeclampsia.
Preeclampsia	Hypertension after 20 weeks' gestation in combination with one or more of the following: • proteinuria (urine protein:creatinine ratio of 30 mg/mmol or more or albumin:creatinine ratio of 8 mg/mmol or more, or at least 1 g/L [2+] on dipstick testing). Other organ dysfunction: • renal insufficiency: creatinine 90 micromol/L or more • haematology abnormalities – thrombocytopenia, disseminated intravascular coagulation or haemolysis • liver involvement (elevated transaminases (alanine aminotransferase or aspartate aminotransferase over 40 IU/litre) with or without right upper quadrant or epigastric abdominal pain) • neurological complications including eclampsia, clonus, altered metal condition, severe headaches, visual scotomata (repeating) • uteroplacental dysfunction including fetal growth restriction, stillbirth or umbilical artery doppler waveform analysis that is abnormal.
Eclampsia	Generalised tonic–clonic seizures, not caused by epilepsy or other disease, and occurring ≥20 weeks' gestation, during labour or in the postpartum.
HELLP syndrome	A form of severe preeclampsia, although hypertension may not be present. Diagnosis of HELLP syndrome is made by the presence of the following three criteria: 1 Haemolysis: characteristic peripheral blood smear and serum lactate dehydrogenase (LDH) >600 U/L or serum total bilirubin ≥1.2 mg/dL 2 Elevated liver enzymes: serum alanine aminotransferase (ALT) ≥70 micromol 3 Low platelet count: <100 × 10^9/L (and/or falling from previous results).

DIC = disseminated intravascular coagulopathy; HELLP = haemolysis-elevated liver enzymes and low platelets.

compared with later-onset disease (Box 28.1).[67,68] The contribution of each component and whether they are relevant in all cases of preeclampsia are not known.

Early-onset preeclampsia (<34 weeks) is associated with impaired remodelling of the uterine spiral arteries and abnormal placental implantation. It is thought that maternal–fetal immune maladaptation could be the main cause for this superficial placentation.[68] Placental flow defects are detected as early as 12 weeks in some women who go on to develop preeclampsia.[69] In late-onset preeclampsia (≥34 weeks), growth of the placental villi have reached their functional limit, resulting in intervillous hypoxia and leading to syncytiotrophoblast stress.[70] Placental ischaemia and reperfusion with subsequent oxidative stress have been regarded as major pathogenetic drivers in both pathways. Further, a number of antiangiogenic factors are considered centrally responsible for the endothelial dysfunction and maternal organ injury.[71] The excessive systemic inflammatory response and associated endothelial dysfunction and enhanced vascular reactivity result in widespread vasospasm that precedes the onset of clinical signs, such as hypertension. Other common clinical manifestations in preeclampsia include enhanced endothelial cell permeability and platelet aggregation, explaining the increased likelihood of oedema and thrombosis.[72]

In summary, preeclampsia presents after 20 weeks' gestation, but the foundation for the disease may relate to abnormal placentation early in the first trimester.

Risk factors

Several maternal characteristics are associated with an increased likelihood for the development of preeclampsia; these include:[68]

• nulliparity

• age ≥40 years

Theories on the pathophysiology of preeclampsia[67,68]

Placentation and the immune theory of preeclampsia:
- Maternal–fetal (paternal) immune maladaptation.
- Superficial abnormal placentation.
- Impaired spiral artery remodelling.

Placental debris hypothesis: syncytiotrophoblast shedding:
- Increased syncytiotrophoblast shedding.
- Placental ischaemia and reperfusion with subsequent oxidative stress.
- Increased circulating levels of inflammatory cytokines, corticotrophin-releasing hormone, free-radical species and activin A.

Endothelial activation and inflammation:
- Enhanced vascular sensitivity to angiotensin II and noradrenaline (norepinephrine) with vasoconstriction and hypertension.
- A fall in production/activity of vasodilator prostaglandins, especially prostacyclin and nitric oxide.

Genes, the genetic-conflict hypothesis and genetic imprinting:
- Susceptibility genes, many of which interact with the maternal cardiovascular or haemostatic system, or with the regulation of maternal inflammatory responses.
- Early-onset (<34 weeks) and late-onset (≥34 weeks) disease.
- Early-onset disease is underpinned by abnormal placentation – incomplete spiral artery remodeling.
- Late-onset disease demonstrates a placenta that is stressed and beginning to fail as placental growth has reached its functional limits.
- Abnormal placental perfusion and the release of antiangiogenic factors such as SFlt-1 with decreased placental growth factor are the common outcomes of all underlying causes.

- pre-existing medical conditions including diabetes, chronic hypertension, chronic renal disease and antiphospholipid antibodies
- preeclampsia in a prior pregnancy, particularly if it presented prior to 34 weeks
- family history of preeclampsia, particularly on the maternal side of the family
- multiple pregnancy, e.g. twins
- body mass index >30 kg/m² prior to pregnancy.

High priority is placed on early and accurate diagnosis of preeclampsia in order to reduce fetal and maternal morbidity and mortality. Identifying women at moderate-to-high-risk of preeclampsia is important, as low-dose aspirin administered from 14–16 weeks' gestation, usually up to 37 weeks or birth, has been shown to significantly reduce the development of the condition.[73] Prediction of women at risk of developing preeclampsia in the first trimester accompanying maternal and fetal risk factors include biochemical risk screening for pregnancy-associated plasma protein A (PAPP-A) and placental growth factor (PlGF), and uterine artery pulsatility index (UTPI) measurement.[74] Nevertheless, research investigating how preeclampsia may be prevented continues.

Incidence

The global incidence of preeclampsia is reported to be 1.0% to 5.6%, with the incidence of eclampsia ranging from 0.1% to 2.7% although these estimates may be conservative.[75] The incidence of eclampsia in developed countries has reduced since the routine use of magnesium sulfate has been adopted; in the UK the rate is about three cases of eclampsia for every 10,000 births[76] while in Australia and New Zealand it is closer to two cases for every 10,000 births.[77] In Latin America the incidence of eclampsia is 17/10,000 births, while in Egypt it is 115/10,000 births.[78,79] However, there is variation in eclampsia even in high-income areas, which is considered to reflect the quality of care.[80] The incidence of HELLP syndrome is reported to be between 0.25% and 0.67% of all pregnancies.[81,82] Preeclampsia is one of the most common indications for ICU admission, at approximately one ICU admission for every 1000 deliveries.[1]

Clinical presentation and diagnosis

The clinical presentation of preeclampsia is often subtle, resulting in delayed diagnosis and treatment. Common symptoms include feeling 'generally unwell', headache, heartburn, nausea and vomiting and oedema: all non-specific symptoms experienced by many pregnant women who do not have preeclampsia. Severe preeclampsia is associated with severe headache, hyperreflexia, visual disturbances, severe epigastric pain, right upper quadrant pain and, rarely, acute blindness. Diagnosis is made when the woman has hypertension (BP ≥140/90) in association with evidence of multisystem involvement (Box 28.2).[60,62,67] Severe preeclampsia is diagnosed when the BP is ≥160/110 in association with multisystem involvement.[60] Additionally, eclampsia and HELLP syndrome are considered severe variants of preeclampsia even if the woman is normotensive.[83]

This clinical diagnosis has replaced the traditional triad of signs of hypertension, proteinuria and oedema, in accordance with increased understanding of the multisystem nature of the disease. Common investigations include urea, creatinine and electrolytes, full blood examination, liver function tests and spot urine protein/creatinine ratio. Additional tests, such as coagulation

BOX 28.2

Diagnostic features of preeclampsia[60,62,67]

Hypertension $\geq$140/90[a] accompanied by one or more of the following:

- Renal involvement:
  - significant proteinuria: dipstick proteinuria subsequently confirmed by spot urine protein/creatinine ratio $\geq$30 mg/mmol, albumin:creatinine ratio $\geq$8 mg/mmol, or >300 mg protein in a 24-h urine collection
  - where albumin:creatinine ratio used instead of protein:creatinine ratio for preeclampsia diagnosis 8 mg/mmol
  - acute kidney injury (creatinine $\geq$90 micromol/L).
- Haematological involvement:
  - thrombocytopenia ($<$100 $\times$ 10^9/L)
  - haemolysis
  - DIC.
- Liver involvement:
  - raised serum transaminases (including ALT or AST >40 IU/litre).
- Right upper quadrant, epigastric/abdominal pain.
- Neurological involvement:
  - eclampsia
  - hyperreflexia/sustained clonus
  - severe headache
  - visual disturbances (e.g. blindness, unabating visual scotomata)
  - cerebral haemorrhage
  - altered mental status.
- Cardiac involvement:
  - pulmonary oedema.
- Uteroplacental involvement:
  - fetal growth restriction
  - angiogenic irregularities
  - abnormal umbilical artery Dopplers
  - abruption.

[a]Although hypertension is usually a component of diagnosis, it is not always present, especially in women with an atypical presentation, such as HELLP syndrome.

studies, may be required as indicated by the clinical condition. Intrauterine fetal growth restriction is a sign of placental involvement and timely investigation into fetal well-being will be indicated.

The presentation of preeclampsia is usually restricted to women $\geq$20 weeks' gestation when placental development is complete, unless they have a coexisting condition that is known to be associated with a $<$20 weeks' presentation of preeclampsia including hydatidiform mole, multiple pregnancy, fetal triploidy, severe maternal renal disease or antiphospholipid antibody syndrome.[62] Importantly, preeclampsia should resolve within 3 months postpartum.

Most first eclamptic seizures occur during pregnancy (42–45%), with 19–24% occurring during labour and 33–36% postpartum.[84] The majority of postpartum eclampsia occurs in the first 48 hours, although eclampsia may occur up to 2–3 weeks postpartum – even in women with no evidence of preeclampsia during pregnancy. Despite the nomenclature, eclampsia can occur without any preceding signs and symptoms of preeclampsia. In the UK Obstetric Surveillance System (UKOSS) eclampsia study, only 38% of women had established hypertension and proteinuria in the week preceding the eclamptic fit and 21% of women had no sign or symptom prior to the first eclamptic fit.[84] HELLP syndrome commonly presents during pregnancy, with about 30% postpartum.[85] Most women admitted to ICU with a diagnosis of preeclampsia have usually delivered prior to transfer, and require support for complications of preeclampsia – for example, acute kidney injury, disseminated intravascular coagulopathy (DIC), pulmonary oedema – and fluid management. Once the placenta is delivered, most women improve within 24–48 hours; however, in particular, women with HELLP syndrome may experience a worsening of the condition in the first 48 hours postpartum. Uncontrolled hypertension remains a major concern and is associated with cerebral haemorrhage, one of the dominant causes of death in women with preeclampsia.

Management priorities

The management of women with severe preeclampsia is focused on stabilising the woman's condition, optimal timing of delivery of the baby (and placenta) and preventing complications of the condition. Women with eclampsia and HELLP syndrome require the same treatments as other women with severe preeclampsia, even though they may or may not have the same degree of hypertension.[62] Additionally, steroids were thought to have been useful for the treatment of HELLP syndrome but this is probably not the case (Box 28.3).[86]

Control of hypertension

Obtaining control of high blood pressure remains a priority not only to improve organ perfusion but also to minimise the risk of cerebral haemorrhage.[87] Both systolic and diastolic pressures are important, and care should be taken to ensure a gradual lowering of blood pressure as a rapid drop can compromise fetal well-being. There is no evidence for the superiority of any specific antihypertensive, although there is some evidence that diazoxide may result in a potentially harmful rapid drop in the woman's blood pressure and that ketanserin may not be as effective as hydralazine.[88] Intravenous labetalol has replaced IV hydralazine as the most common drug used to treat very high blood pressure in many countries, though both are commonly used. Be mindful that labetalol is less effective for women of black African or Caribbean origins and will need replacement with an alternative.[89]

Prevention and treatment of eclampsia

Eclampsia is a generalised tonic–clonic seizure in the setting of preeclampsia – though it may also be the first presenting sign with hypertension and proteinuria developing following the first seizure. Magnesium sulfate has received the most attention as an anticonvulsant in preeclampsia, with its mechanism of action thought to be connected to the release of prostacyclin from the endothelium, reversing the vasoconstriction that is the basis of the disease.[90,91] Magnesium is the anticonvulsant of choice to prevent and treat eclampsia and is superior to anticonvulsant drugs.[92] Magnesium has been shown to halve the likelihood of eclampsia.[92] A common magnesium regimen is:[63]

- Give a 4-g IV loading dose over 15–20 minutes.
- Administer an ongoing infusion of 1 g/h.
- Give an additional 2-g IV loading dose over 5 minutes to treat a recurrent eclamptic seizure; if possible, take bloods for magnesium prior to administering the bolus dose.
- Continue infusion until 24 hours following delivery or 24 hours following the last eclamptic fit, whichever occurs later.

Elevated serum magnesium levels will depress deep tendon reflexes and the respiratory rate, ultimately leading to cardiac arrest.

The suggested antidote to magnesium sulfate toxicity is 1 g of calcium gluconate (or chloride) IV (10 mL of 10% solution).[63] Monitoring of the urine output is mandatory, given this medication is excreted mainly via the renal system. Ongoing clinical assessment must also include continual oxygen saturation monitoring, respiratory rate and hourly deep tendon reflexes, which combined should identify potentially toxic magnesium

levels in the patient who is breathing spontaneously. There is no consensus regarding the therapeutic serum magnesium concentrations to prevent eclampsia or cause magnesium toxicity. Winter and colleagues (2017), in their UK Practical obstetric multi professional training (PROMPT) manual, suggest a therapeutic range of 2–4 mmol/L.[30] Should a woman on a magnesium infusion experience an eclamptic seizure, the first drug of choice is more magnesium. Otherwise, management of an eclamptic seizure is the same as for any other generalised tonic–clonic seizure, remembering the importance of left lateral positioning post seizure during pregnancy to relieve aortocaval compression.

Optimal fluid management

Careful titration of intravenous fluid is required to optimise plasma volume and organ perfusion without causing pulmonary oedema.[93] Central venous pressure is universally accepted as unhelpful for guiding fluid management in preeclampsia. Transthoracic echocardiography (TTE) has demonstrated impaired diastolic function in women with preeclampsia and is advocated by some to guide fluid management.[94]

Thromboprophylaxis

Preeclampsia is an independent risk factor for thromboembolic disease and due consideration must be made of the need for thromboprophylaxis (in the absence of any contraindications) for women in the ICU.[95]

Betamethasone

When severe preeclampsia is diagnosed prior to 34 weeks' gestation, the woman is normally prescribed steroids to promote fetal lung maturity and surfactant production.[62]

Optimal timing of delivery

Women with severe preeclampsia can be cured only by delivery, regardless of gestation. Consequently, a woman with severe preeclampsia is usually stabilised (hypertension controlled and magnesium sulfate commenced) and arrangements made for delivery. Ideally, women <34 weeks' gestation should be transferred to a high-level referral obstetric centre prior to delivery.

Subsequent pregnancy and long-term cardiovascular health

Women who have experienced preeclampsia are eight times more likely to experience preeclampsia again in a subsequent pregnancy than women who did not experience preeclampsia in their first pregnancy.[96] It seems that earlier-onset preeclampsia and more-severe disease are related to risk of recurrence. Some treatments (e.g. low-dose aspirin) have shown benefit in reducing the likelihood of recurrence in select high-risk groups.[73] Importantly, women who have experienced preeclampsia are twice as likely to die from cardiovascular disease later in life, and so preeclampsia is an important risk factor for cardiovascular disease development.[97]

Obstetric haemorrhage

Obstetric haemorrhage is a generic term indicating that there is bleeding from the uterus or genital tract in a pregnant or postpartum woman. It may be used when a woman experiences early-pregnancy bleeding (e.g. prior to 20 weeks' gestation) and also if she has experienced either antepartum (>20 weeks' gestation and prior to birth) or postpartum (after birth of the baby) haemorrhage. The past decade has seen an increase in both the incidence and the severity of haemorrhage, with more women requiring a blood transfusion for postpartum haemorrhage than in the past.[98] Major obstetric haemorrhage is a common reason for postpartum women to be admitted to ICU, at 0.7/1000 deliveries.[1] Unfortunately, there is no agreed terminology for major obstetric haemorrhage; for example, maternal/obstetric and massive/major/severe are often used interchangeably. Furthermore, definition of a 'major obstetric haemorrhage' is variable and may include >1500 mL blood loss, >2500 mL blood loss, a drop of >4 g/L Hb, >4 units of red blood cells (RBCs) transfused within 4 hours, or a need for non-RBC blood products or >8 units of RBCs transfused within 24 hours. Regardless, major obstetric haemorrhage is often sudden and unexpected, and is frequently associated with an acute coagulopathy. Early recognition and treatment of major obstetric haemorrhage is vital to ensure the best outcome for mother and fetus. A repeated finding in maternal death reviews is a delay by obstetric providers in recognising the severity of haemorrhage and consequent deterioration in the maternal condition.[99]

The common causes of antepartum and postpartum haemorrhage are described below, with common management strategies presented at the end of the section.

Antepartum haemorrhage

The definition of antepartum haemorrhage (APH) varies around the world. In the UK, APH is defined as bleeding from the genital tract, occurring from 24 weeks of pregnancy and prior to the birth of the baby, while bleeding prior to 24 weeks' gestation is classified as a threatened miscarriage.[100] Contrastingly, the Australian definition of APH is bleeding from the genital tract after the 20th week of pregnancy and before the onset of labour.[101] APH occurs in 3–5% of all pregnancies and is a cause of maternal and fetal morbidity and mortality.[102] The two main known causes of APH are placental abruption and placenta praevia.[11] However, for many women, the cause of an APH may never be determined and this is designated 'antepartum haemorrhage of unknown origin'.[102]

Placental abruption (or abruptio placentae)

Placental abruption is premature separation (i.e. before the birth of the baby) of a normally sited placenta from the uterine wall, and has an incidence of 0.26–0.8%.[102] It results from bleeding into the decidua basalis of the placenta with haematoma formation and resultant placental separation.[103] Bleeding associated with placental abruption may be revealed (i.e. it is visible per vagina (PV)), such as when the placenta partially separates along an edge of the placenta. However, bleeding may also be concealed (i.e. no blood loss is visible PV) where the centre part of the placenta detaches, leaving the placental edges attached.[34] Risk factors for placental abruption include previous abruption, preeclampsia, blunt trauma (e.g. car crash, domestic violence), a sudden reduction in uterine volume (e.g. after delivery of the first baby in a twin pregnancy), cocaine use and smoking.[103]

As the amount of visible blood loss may be disproportionate to the actual amount of bleeding that has occurred in placental abruption, careful assessment of maternal physiological parameters, clinical history and assessment of fetal well-being is vital. Placental abruption is often accompanied by abdominal pain, back pain where there is a posteriorly-situated placenta and contractions.[104] Moderate abruptions (blood loss ≥1000 mL) may necessitate urgent delivery by caesarean section, owing to the presence of fetal distress and maternal physiological compromise.[34] Where a significant proportion of the placenta has separated and the abruption is severe, a woman may present with hypovolaemic shock, severe abdominal pain, a hard or woody uterus on palpation (couvelaire uterus), DIC and intrauterine fetal death.[34] Where fetal death has occurred, vaginal delivery may be advocated and, in the majority of cases, only women with severe placental abruptions are admitted to ICU.

Placenta praevia

Placenta praevia occurs when part or the whole placenta is situated over (major) or alongside (minor) the cervical os. Placenta praevia has an incidence of 3% at term.[102] The lower uterine segment does not fully form until 28–32 weeks' gestation, and the shearing stress as the lower uterine segment forms may precipitate detachment of the placenta from the uterine wall causing maternal bleeding. Bleeding can occur at any time, is usually painless (unlike moderate/severe placental abruptions) and may be torrential. Placenta praevia is a main cause of APH, accounting for 30% of all cases.[105] Management is dictated by the estimated blood loss, maternal condition, fetal well-being and whether the bleeding is ongoing.

Morbidly adherent placenta – placenta accreta spectrum

Morbidly adherent placenta is a serious complication where the placental villi abnormally invade the myometrium; there

---

BOX 28.4

Categories of morbidly adherent placenta[106]

- Placenta accreta: the placenta is abnormally adherent to the uterine lining.
- Placenta increta: the placenta invades the uterine muscle (myometrium).
- Placenta percreta: the placenta grows through the myometrium and into adjacent structures, such as the bladder and ureters.

BOX 28.5

Causes of postpartum haemorrhage characterised by the '4 Ts'[111]

Tone:
- Uterine atony
- Functional or anatomical distortion of the uterus (e.g. bicornuate uterus, fibroids)

Tissue:
- Retained placental products
- Abnormal placenta

Trauma:
- Cervical and genital tract damage during delivery
- Uterine inversion

Thrombin:
- Coagulation disorders

Source: Adapted from NSW Health. Maternity – prevention, detection, escalation and management of postpartum haemorrhage (PPH). Sydney, NSW: Department of Health; 2017.

---

are three types with increasing severity termed accreta, increta and percreta (Box 28.4).[106] The main risk factors for morbidly adherent placenta are a prior caesarean section and placenta praevia.[107] When relevant risk factors are present, screening for morbidly adherent placenta using ultrasound and/or magnetic resonance imaging (MRI) may be undertaken prior to elective caesarean section, although there is debate as to the most effective diagnostic method.[107] Placental tissue can be very invasive and may infiltrate local structures such as the bladder. Many women with morbidly adherent placenta undergo emergency hysterectomy at the time of caesarean section, as a means to remove the placenta and control bleeding.[107] Alternative management is to deliver the baby by caesarean section and leave the placenta in situ to be reabsorbed, where feasible to do so (conservative management).[108] Morbidly adherent placenta can cause catastrophic haemorrhage and maternal mortality; a coordinated multidisciplinary approach is required prior to delivery in order to minimise complications.[107] Due to the rising caesarean section rate, morbidly adherent placenta is more common than in the past and contributes to the increase seen in emergency hysterectomy and massive blood transfusion.[109]

Practice tip

Read a woman's operation report if she has a diagnosis of placenta accreta to identify the extent to which the placental tissue has invaded local structures, such as the bladder, ureters and bowel. For example, the bladder is often affected and a cystotomy may have been required to separate the placenta from the bladder.

Postpartum haemorrhage

Postpartum haemorrhage (PPH), a major cause of maternal death in developed and developing countries, is defined as ≥500 mL blood loss from the genital tract after the birth of the baby. The incidence and severity of PPH are increasing in developed countries.[98,110] PPH rates commonly sit at around 10% of all births, although they may be as high as 25% in some jurisdictions. As outlined earlier, severe PPH lacks an agreed definition. Consequently, the incidence of severe PPH varies depending on how it has been defined. Additionally, PPH is classified according to the timing of the haemorrhage in relation to the birth. Primary PPH occurs within the first 24 hours after birth, whereas secondary PPH occurs from 24 hours up to 6 weeks following birth. Primary PPH is often caused by uterine atony, while secondary PPH is more likely to be associated with retained products and associated infection.

The causes of PPH are varied and have been classified by the 'four Ts': tone, tissue, trauma and thrombin (Box 28.5).[111] The cause of PPH should be identified and targeted with specific management, in conjunction with the general principles of haemorrhage management.

Severe obstetric haemorrhage management priorities

The vast majority of women admitted to ICU with obstetric haemorrhage will be transferred following birth, and are therefore postpartum on admission to ICU. As with any major haemorrhage (see Chapter 21), the principles of treatment are:

- to restore an adequate circulating volume and maintain oxygen and perfusion to vital organs
- to obtain haemostasis and correct coagulopathy
- to prevent complications.

All maternity providers should have a 'massive transfusion protocol' that outlines action and escalation of care for massive bleeding.[112] Maternity adaptations from a standard massive transfusion protocol include consideration for early triggering of the protocol given the common underestimation of blood loss and ability for the maternity patient to initially maintain haemodynamic stability despite large blood loss, aim to maintain a higher level of fibrinogen (>2.0 g/L) and avoidance of permissive hypotension while the uterus remains in situ.[112]

Maintaining circulating volume, oxygenation and perfusion

Accurate estimation of blood loss is difficult, as bleeding can be concealed, and blood loss may be mixed with amniotic fluid making accurate estimation a challenge, potentially leading to an underestimation of fluid resuscitation needs. Furthermore, peripartum women are at an increased risk of acute pulmonary oedema, which further complicates fluid resuscitation, especially for women who have preeclampsia.[93] Standard resuscitation fluids, such as Hartmann's or normal saline, should be infused according to routine practice for the non-obstetric haemorrhage. Access to O-negative blood is important to maintain oxygen-carrying capacity while waiting for cross-matched blood. Adaption of a massive transfusion protocol may be necessary; permissive hypotension is not an acceptable strategy while the uterus is in situ, as an acidotic, poorly oxygenated uterus will not contract.[112]

Practice tip

Keep in mind the following:

- Serum albumin levels decrease in normal pregnancy, with the lowest levels recorded in the early postpartum period.[44]
- Central venous pressure (CVP) and pulmonary artery pressure (PAP) can be interpreted the same as for non-obstetric patients (as long as the woman does not have preeclampsia).

Achieving haemostasis and correct coagulopathy

Specific interventions to control bleeding include radiological arterial embolisation or balloon occlusion of the internal iliac arteries, uterine compression suture (e.g. B-Lynch suture), use of an intrauterine balloon tamponade (e.g. Bakri balloon) and emergency hysterectomy. Women may need to return to theatre for abdominal packing for ongoing 'ooze' that may continue after a hysterectomy. Many women with severe obstetric haemorrhage in ICU have developed DIC that requires treatment with the appropriate blood products.[113]

Patient blood management guidelines have been developed by the Australian National Blood Authority, with Module 1 (critical bleeding), Module 4 (critical care) and Module 5 (obstetrics and maternity) of most relevance.[112,114,115] Fibrinogen is usually doubled by the end of pregnancy, and low fibrinogen levels are associated with increasing severity of PPH.[113] Use of fibrinogen concentrate for the treatment of PPH is of increasing interest. Point-of-care devices that examine the quality of the clot, such as thromboelastography (TEG) and rotational thromboelastometry (ROTEM), are frequently used to guide management of obstetric haemorrhage.[116] These point-of-care devices enable a more targeted approach to haemostatic resuscitation and have demonstrated a reduction in blood component usage with the use of fibrinogen concentrate.[117]

Tranexamic acid has shown some benefit in the management of PPH and administration is recommended as soon as possible after the haemorrhage is recognised.[118] Recombinant factor VIIa has been used successfully in the management of severe obstetric haemorrhage and may be considered for use in the management of the bleeding woman in accordance with the massive transfusion protocol. Treatment is more likely to be effective if administered before the woman becomes hypothermic and acidotic.[119]

Preventing complications

Strategies to prevent the following complications should be implemented:

- Complications of major blood transfusion – these are similar in the obstetric patient as in the non-obstetric patient and include acid–base disturbance, transfusion-related acute lung injury (TRALI), hypocalcaemia, hyperkalaemia and hypothermia.

- Increased risk of thrombosis – particularly in the early postpartum period, as the risk is exacerbated by lengthy theatre procedures, bed rest associated with ICU admission and following major haemorrhage with an associated massive blood transfusion. Suitable thromboprophylaxis should be considered as soon as feasible.

- Acute kidney injury – irreversible renal failure has been reported as a sequel of acute kidney injury following severe postpartum haemorrhage.[120] Routine monitoring and management of renal impairment is required, keeping in mind that a pregnant patient has a lower urea and creatinine level than non-pregnant patients. Careful titration of fluid for renal purposes is needed because of the increased propensity for pulmonary oedema.

- Rh isoimmunisation – the potential to develop Rh isoimmunisation in Rh-negative women who have experienced antepartum haemorrhage and/or PPH should be considered.[121]

- Sheehan's syndrome – necrosis of the pituitary gland is a very rare complication of severe obstetric haemorrhage. While the syndrome may go undetected for many years, one of the earliest symptoms is a failure to establish lactation, because of the absence of prolactin secretion. Sheehan's syndrome can be prevented by maintaining adequate circulating volume, oxygenation and perfusion.

Use of cell salvage for obstetric haemorrhage

The introduction of cell salvage in obstetrics was delayed in comparison with other surgeries for two key reasons: the theoretical risk of amniotic fluid embolism (AFE) and the risk of rhesus isoimmunisation.[122] Contemporary understanding suggests that AFE is more aligned with an anaphylactic reaction and, in practice, there has been no confirmed case of AFE following the use of cell salvage infusion. Regardless, it is common practice to use a different suction device from the time of amniotic membrane rupture until after delivery (which is not re-used) with blood aspirated from the surgical field collected by the cell salvage device.[123] A leukocyte depletion filter should always be used during the re-infusion of salvaged maternal blood to filter any remaining foreign proteins.[124] While most experience with cell salvage for obstetric haemorrhage has been associated with caesarean birth, there is increasing evidence of its utility following vaginal birth.[125,126] In health services with cell salvage capability, autotransfusion of vaginally shed blood is both safe and feasible.[126] None of the currently available cell saver equipment is able to discern fetal from adult red blood cells and any present fetal cells are transfused to the woman. It is important for Rh-negative women to have a post-infusion Kleihauer–Betke test to quantify the amount of fetal red cells in the maternal circulation in order to ensure that an adequate dose of anti-D immunoglobulin can be given to prevent isoimmunisation.[122]

Amniotic fluid embolism

AFE is a rare and incompletely understood obstetric emergency that usually occurs during labour or pregnancy termination, or shortly after delivery. Traditional understanding of the condition was based around the notion that amniotic fluid entered the maternal bloodstream via the endocervical veins or placental bed, with amniotic fluid, fetal cells, hair or other fetal debris functioning as an embolus, and resulting in the dramatic cardiorespiratory collapse seen with the condition. However, not all women diagnosed with AFE have evidence of fetal squames/amniotic fluid substances in the pulmonary vasculature, while many women who do not develop AFE have fetal cells found in the maternal circulation.[127]

More recently, improved understanding of the mechanics of labour and the interaction of amniotic fluid and maternal blood, as well as the striking similarities between clinical and haemodynamic findings in AFE and both anaphylaxis and septic shock, have led to a belief that a common pathophysiological mechanism is likely to be responsible for all these conditions.[128] As AFE resembles an anaphylactic reaction rather than an embolic event, the term 'anaphylactoid syndrome of pregnancy', instead of AFE, has been proposed.[129] The trigger for AFE is not well understood, although it is thought to be a fetal antigen (which may arise from amniotic fluid). It is possible that all labouring women are exposed to the fetal antigen, with those affected by AFE exhibiting a rare and abnormal maternal immune response.[127] One of the difficulties blocking improved understanding of AFE is the lack of a diagnostic test. A recent contender, insulin-like growth factor binding protein-1, was found to be not useful.[130]

Regardless of the level of understanding, the abnormal mediator release gives rise to acute lung injury, resulting in acute dyspnoea and hypoxia and often the development of acute respiratory distress syndrome.[131] Within 30 minutes of the antigen insult, there is evidence of severe pulmonary hypertension with acute right ventricular failure.[132] It is thought that inflammatory mediators are a more likely cause of pulmonary vasoconstriction, with physical obstruction to the pulmonary vasculature (embolism) not the main mechanism.[133] The left ventricular failure seen in AFE is considered a secondary response due to poor left ventricular filling pressures. Concomitantly, substances in the amniotic fluid trigger a profound consumptive coagulopathy.

Incidence and risk factors

The incidence of AFE is thought to be in the range of 2–8 women per 100,000 deliveries, making it a very rare event.[134] However, the lack of a diagnostic test is a serious limiting factor for accurate determination of incidence and misdiagnosis is common.[135] AFE is more common in North America (1 in 15,200 deliveries) than in Europe (1 in 53,800 deliveries).[133] This may represent a true difference in incidence or reflect differences in clinical diagnosis or methods of case identification. Using similar definitions and case identification, the Australian and New Zealand (ANZ) incidence of AFE was 5.4/100,000 women giving birth, compared with 2.0/100,000 in the UK.[134,136] Similar numbers of women received cardiorespiratory resuscitation and survival rates were also similar, indicating that the higher rate in ANZ is real.

Diagnosis remains one of exclusion and there is a long list of differential diagnoses, including air or thrombotic pulmonary emboli, septic shock, cardiomyopathy, acute myocardial infarction, anaphylaxis, transfusion reaction, aspiration, placental abruption, eclampsia, uterine rupture, local anaesthetic toxicity and primary postpartum haemorrhage.[128] AFE remains a major contributor to maternal death, accounting for 5–15% of all maternal deaths in developed countries.

Although controversy exists, the factors that have been proposed as contributing to an increased likelihood for AFE include:[128,135]

- induction of labour
- caesarean birth
- multiple pregnancy, e.g. twins
- maternal age ≥35 years
- forceps delivery
- placenta praevia
- preeclampsia

- placental abruption
- a history of atopy, or latex, medication or food allergy.

Given the rarity of AFE and the commonality of these potential risk factors, astute clinical assessment and early clinical suspicion based on the clinical presentation of the woman should be the focus for early identification and treatment.

Clinical presentation

The symptoms associated with AFE have been well described and usually comprise premonitory symptoms, such as restlessness, agitation and numbness/tingling, prior to more severe maternal compromise, such as sudden-onset hypotension, dyspnoea, hypoxia, altered mental status and haemorrhage.[137] Collapse of the maternal cardiovascular system leads to fetal distress as the placenta is deprived of maternal oxygen, quickly leading to fetal demise unless the fetus is delivered swiftly. Premonitory symptoms, shortness of breath and fetal distress have been reported as the early signs in the UK and ANZ studies. Overall, haemorrhage and associated coagulopathy, hypotension and shortness of breath were the most commonly recorded symptoms.[137] Cardiac arrest was documented in 40% of cases and seizure in 15%. Haemorrhage and coagulopathy may not be immediately apparent; some women die before it develops. However, these clinical features usually develop in women who survive the initial insult.

Patient management

There is no specific treatment for AFE; all therapy is supportive with the aim of maintaining adequate oxygenation and perfusion, controlling haemorrhage and correcting any coagulopathy. Common interventions include:[138,139]

- urgent delivery of the fetus
- emergency hysterectomy to control postpartum haemorrhage
- admission to the ICU, with associated support such as mechanical ventilation, nitric oxide and extracorporeal membrane oxygenation (ECMO).

Echocardiography may be very helpful for guiding fluid and inotrope management to optimise preload and enhance cardiac output.[140] Mortality ranges from 11% to 44%, and in developed countries a mortality of 15–20% is common.[136,141]

Although it is possible for a woman to experience an AFE in a subsequent pregnancy, repeat AFE is thought to be unlikely as the trigger for AFE is specific to each fetus the woman carries. There have been a number of published case reports of women having a successful subsequent pregnancy and none reporting repeat AFE in the same woman.[142]

Peripartum cardiomyopathy

Peripartum cardiomyopathy, sometimes referred to as postpartum cardiomyopathy, is an idiopathic cardiomyopathy presenting with heart failure secondary to LV systolic dysfunction (left ventricular ejection fraction (LVEF) <45%) towards the end of pregnancy or in the months following delivery, when other causes of heart failure have been excluded.[143] Peripartum cardiomyopathy is considered to be a dilated cardiomyopathy, though there may or may not be dilation of the left ventricle.[144] The incidence of peripartum cardiomyopathy varies widely, from 1:100 in a small region of sub-Saharan Africa to 1:20,000 in Japan, though many studies on peripartum cardiomyopathy were conducted on data that had been gathered retrospectively.[144] A prospective population-based study in the Netherlands found that 1 in 20,000 pregnancies required ICU admission for peripartum cardiomyopathy.[6]

The exact cause of peripartum cardiomyopathy is not well understood and a variety of factors have been implicated, including viral infection, autoimmune mechanisms, cytokine-mediated inflammation, increased myocyte apoptosis, increased oxidative stress, genetic disposition and/or cultural habits and abnormal hormonal regulation.[143] One proposed mechanism is that oxidative stress cleaves the full-length, 23-kDa form of the hormone prolactin into an antiangiogenic, 16-kDa derivative.[145] Notable risk factors are race (African black ancestry), preeclampsia, advanced maternal age and multiple gestation.[144]

Maternal mortality associated with peripartum cardiomyopathy is between 4% and 14%, with lower mortality in developed countries.[146] Studies show that approximately 50–80% of women recover their left ventricular function, usually within 6 months though it may take up to 2 years.[147] Some women never fully recover their cardiac function and require ongoing medical management; a small proportion of women go on to require a mechanical-assist device and heart transplantation.

Patient management

Women with peripartum cardiomyopathy present with varying degrees of left heart failure. Signs and symptoms include dyspnoea, persistent cough, abdominal discomfort, palpitations and oedema and may be mistaken for 'discomforts of pregnancy' and lead to a delayed diagnosis.[144] The diagnosis of peripartum cardiomyopathy is one of exclusion requiring systematic investigation to exclude both cardiac and non-cardiac differential diagnoses such as pulmonary embolism, acute myocardial infarction, severe preeclampsia and pneumonia.[143] Echocardiography is a useful diagnostic tool with a left ventricular end-diastolic diameter >60 mm predictive of poor recovery, as is a LVEF <30%.[143]

The principles of managing acute heart failure in women with peripartum cardiomyopathy are no different to the management of heart failure from any other cause, and aim to reduce preload and afterload and to increase cardiac contractility (see Chapter 10 for a full description). Unfortunately, ACE inhibitors and angiotensin antagonists are contraindicated in pregnancy. Additionally, women with peripartum cardiomyopathy are at risk of arrhythmia and may need treatment/preventative management.[148]

Bromocriptine, a relatively novel treatment for peripartum cardiomyopathy, is associated with increased left ventricular recovery and reduced morbidity and death.[149] Bromocriptine is directly able to reduce oxidative stress by blocking the release of prolactin.[150] However, consensus on the use of bromocriptine for peripartum cardiomyopathy is lacking.[143] For women diagnosed with peripartum cardiomyopathy while pregnant, timing and mode of delivery are two other management decisions to be made. A multidisciplinary team, including cardiologist, obstetrician, anaesthetist and nursing/midwifery staff, should consider and plan for delivery dependent on maternal and fetal condition and the woman's known preferences. Vaginal birth is preferred, with caesarean section indicated for the usual obstetric reasons.[143] Ergometrine-containing drugs, used to contract the uterus post-delivery, are contraindicated because they cause vasoconstriction and the associated increase in afterload may be detrimental for maternal heart function. Synthetic oxytocin preparations are advised instead to prevent postpartum haemorrhage. Early consideration also needs to be given to thromboprophylaxis.[143] Finally, given the postulated role of prolactin in the aetiology of peripartum cardiomyopathy, there is debate about whether women should breastfeed. In cases when bromocriptine is not prescribed, breastfeeding may be possible and, given the many benefits for mother and baby, should be supported according to maternal preference.[143]

Subsequent pregnancy

Family planning counselling is an important part of the care of women as they recover from peripartum cardiomyopathy.[146] After a diagnosis of peripartum cardiomyopathy, women who have recovered their left ventricular function (LVEF >50%) have a 20% risk of relapse in any subsequent pregnancy.[147] Current guidelines recommend against any further pregnancy in women who have not recovered a normal LVEF because of the high risk of mortality.[146]

Exacerbation of medical disease associated with pregnancy

Women with pre-existing medical conditions pose additional challenges during pregnancy. Occasionally, pregnant and postpartum women are admitted to ICU with exacerbation of an underlying medical condition; two of the more common conditions, cardiac disease and asthma, are outlined in this section. Other conditions that result in ICU admission of pregnant or postpartum women include trauma, pneumonia and mental health disorders, and these are reviewed here.

Cardiac disease

Cardiac disease in pregnancy consists of women who have congenital heart disease and women who have acquired heart disease, such as rheumatic heart disease. The physiological adaptations of pregnancy can 'unmask' cardiac disease in women. Notably, only 17% of women who died of cardiac causes during 2009–14 in the UK were known to have pre-existing cardiac problems.[151] Women with cardiac disease who undergo pregnancy need holistic care throughout the pre-pregnancy, pregnancy and post-pregnancy periods.[152]

Congenital heart disease

Congenital heart disease (CHD) refers to defects of the heart, or main vessels connected to the heart, which are present at birth. CHD is the most common serious birth defect, affecting about 1% of births.[153] Largely, the causes are unknown and attributed to factors within the maternal, fetal or placental environment; only 11% have a genetic diagnosis, though this proportion is increasing as advances in genetic testing are made.[154,155] Most develop de novo, and recognised risk factors for the development of CHD in the fetus include maternal obesity,[156] elevated blood glucose levels in the first trimester,[157] and known pre-existing diabetes mellitus,[158] low maternal vitamin D levels[159] and other potentially modifiable lifestyle factors.[160] Some maternal medication also increases the likelihood of offspring CHD, such as selective serotonin reuptake inhibitors.[161]

Increasing numbers of those affected with CHD are surviving into adulthood, with the greatest increase in survival benefit seen in people with severe disease.[162,163] The number of adults living with CHD is predicted to continue to grow, resulting in substantially higher clinical loads for adult CHD centres.[164] The risks women face in the pursuit of motherhood should not be overlooked and include worsening cardiac function, arrhythmias and death.[165] The modified World Health Organization (WHO) classification to predict the likelihood of a cardiac complication associated with pregnancy is the most useful to predict outcomes for women with pre-existing cardiovascular conditions, and provides guidance,[166] pre-conception counselling and care (Table 28.5).[165] Women with very severe disease are choosing to have children, such as those who have undergone Fontan procedures. While many women achieve motherhood, there is an increased likelihood of miscarriage, preterm birth and small babies.[166,167] The combination of cardiovascular and respiratory changes in pregnancy is poorly tolerated by some women, and cardiac disease in pregnancy still remains a leading cause of maternal death in developed nations.[99]

Rheumatic heart disease

Rheumatic heart disease (RHD) is the most frequently acquired heart disease and is a condition normally associated with developing countries.[168] One exception is Australia, where Aboriginal people and Torres Strait Islanders in the Northern Territory have rates of RHD noted to be the highest in the world, and over 30 times higher than those of non-Indigenous Australians.[168] Similarly, in New Zealand, Māori and Pacific Islanders

TABLE 28.5

Predicting risk of pregnancy for women with cardiovascular conditions[165]

MODIFIED WHO RISK CLASS	CARDIOVASCULAR CONDITIONS	RISK OF PREGNANCY BY MEDICAL CONDITION

I	• Uncomplicated small or mild
	   ○ pulmonary stenosis
	   ○ patent ductus arteriosus
	   ○ mitral valve prolapse
	• Successfully repaired simple lesions (atrial or ventricular septal defect, patent ductus arteriosus, anomalous pulmonary venous drainage)
	• Atrial or ventricular ectopic beats, isolated
		No detectable increased risk of maternal mortality and no/mild increase in morbidity.

II	If otherwise well and uncomplicated: • Unoperated atrial or ventricular septal defect • Repaired tetralogy of Fallot • Most arrhythmias	Small increased risk of maternal mortality or moderate increase in morbidity.
II or III	Depending on individual: • Mild left ventricular impairment • Hypertrophic cardiomyopathy • Native or tissue valvular heart disease not considered WHO I or IV • Marfan syndrome without aortic dilation • Aorta <45 mm in aortic disease associated with bicuspid aortic valve • Repaired coarctation	
III	• Mechanical valve • Systemic right ventricle • Fontan circulation • Cyanotic heart disease (unrepaired) • Other complex CHD • Aortic dilation 40–45 mm in Marfan syndrome • Aortic dilation 45–50 mm in aortic disease associated with bicuspid aortic valve	Significantly increased risk of maternal mortality or severe morbidity. Expert counselling required. If pregnancy is decided upon, intensive specialist cardiac and obstetric monitoring is needed throughout pregnancy, childbirth and the puerperium.
IV	• Pulmonary arterial hypertension of any cause • Severe systemic ventricular dysfunction (LVEF <30%, NYHA III–IV) • Severe mitral stenosis, severe symptomatic aortic stenosis • Marfan syndrome with aorta dilated >45 mm • Aortic dilation >50 mm in aortic disease associated with bicuspid aortic valve • Native severe coarctation	Extremely high risk of maternal mortality or severe morbidity; pregnancy contraindicated. If pregnancy occurs, termination should be discussed. If pregnancy continues, care as for Class III.

CHD = congenital heart disease; LVEF = left ventricular ejection fraction; NYHA = New York Heart Association; WHO = World Health Organization.

Source: Adapted from Regitz-Zagrosek V, Roos-Hesselink JW, Bauersachs J, et al. 2018 ESC guidelines for the management of cardiovascular diseases during pregnancy: the task force for the management of cardiovascular diseases during pregnancy of the European Society of Cardiology (ESC). Eur Heart J 2018;39(34):3165–241.

have a much higher incidence of RHD than New Zealanders of European ancestry. Refugee and immigrant women who have migrated from developing countries, such as in sub-Saharan Africa, also have a higher risk for RHD in pregnancy.

RHD is a delayed complication of acute rheumatic fever, and results from an untreated group A streptococcus bacterial throat or skin infection. There is progressive, structural heart damage that occurs after an initial episode of acute rheumatic fever. RHD usually begins with generalised carditis; then, as the disease advances, mitral valve insufficiency develops, although the aortic valve may also be affected. Valvular pathology includes restricted leaflet mobility, valvular prolapse, focal or generalised valvular thickening and abnormal subvalvular thickening, chordae tendineae or papillary muscle rupture and scarring, resulting in regurgitation and, rarely, stenosis.

Serial echocardiography throughout pregnancy by a skilled provider is essential to monitor maternal cardiac function and, specifically, valvular dynamics in women with RHD.[169] Imaging can be technically challenging during pregnancy, and cardiac indices need to be aligned with the normal echocardiography pregnancy reference range. The effect of RHD on pregnancy varies according to the severity of the disease, with episodes of heart failure or arrhythmia leading to hospital admission.[168]

Acute myocardial infarction

Acute myocardial infarction (AMI), once rarely seen in association with pregnancy, is becoming more prevalent.[170] Pregnancy has been reported to increase the risk of AMI 3–4-fold in same-age-matched non-pregnant women,[171] in part because coronary dissection is more common in association with a pregnancy.[172] The increasing incidence of AMI is also thought to be related to the changing demographics of the pregnant population, which now includes higher proportions of older women and women who are obese.[170] Cardiovascular risk factors are prominent in women who present with AMI or acute coronary syndrome during pregnancy.[173]

In the maternity setting, symptoms of AMI or heart failure, such as clamminess, sweating, tachycardia, fatigue, anxiety, breathlessness and chest pain, should not be dismissed without adequate investigation and due consideration of cardiovascular risk factors. Although 'breathlessness' may be a common symptom experienced by pregnant women, nocturnal dyspnoea, or breathlessness at rest, is not normal even in the pregnant context. Similarly, heartburn, fatigue and dependent oedema may also indicate cardiovascular compromise. The UK maternal mortality report emphasises the need to obtain a diagnosis in pregnant women presenting with chest pain, as many women who died at home following an AMI had been sent home with no diagnosis.[151] In particular, ECGs, echocardiography, chest X-rays, cardiac enzymes (troponin) and computed tomographic pulmonary angiography should be attended as clinically indicated and investigations should not be denied to women who need them on the basis that they are pregnant.[151,174] Diagnosis of AMI in pregnancy is the same as for the non-pregnant patient, with troponin levels considered to be both reliable and accurate. However, women with hypertension or preeclampsia may have elevated troponin levels in the absence of myocardial infarction.[175–177] Percutaneous coronary angiography is suggested as the treatment of choice for coronary reperfusion, despite the risk of iatrogenic coronary dissection. There are limited data available to either support or refute the administration of thrombolytics such as tissue plasminogen activator in pregnancy and, because of the increased possibility of coronary dissection, they are not recommended.[178]

Other cardiac conditions

Rarely, spontaneous aortic dissection may occur in pregnant women with no pre-existing cardiac disease.[179]

Signs and symptoms of heart failure and complaints of chest pain must be investigated and not put down to the 'minor discomforts' of pregnancy. Given that the cardiac output is expected to increase by 40–50% in a normal pregnancy, any cardiac condition resulting in poor left ventricular function and/or restricted left ventricular outflow is particularly associated with poor outcomes in pregnancy (see Table 28.5).

Also relevant for the outcome of both mother and baby is whether any valvular disease has been repaired and whether a tissue or mechanical valve has been inserted. Mechanical valves place the mother at high risk in pregnancy because of the risk of valve thrombosis.[169] Use of anticoagulants is of particular concern during pregnancy, with warfarin contraindicated for use in pregnancy. However, the risk of thrombosis is relatively high in pregnant women and some women are advised to remain on warfarin despite the risk of associated congenital anomaly and the increased likelihood of miscarriage.[165]

Practice tip

Congenital and acquired cardiac disease can present for the first time during pregnancy, unmasked by the additional physiological requirements of pregnancy. Women with known pre-existing disease may experience unpredictable deterioration in cardiac function.

Patient management

All women with cardiac disease are considered to have a 'high-risk' pregnancy and should receive maternity care by a multidisciplinary team including, as a minimum, an obstetrician, a midwife, a cardiologist and an anaesthetist.[169,180] The timing and location of delivery, choice of anaesthesia and delivery mode should each be discussed by the team with the woman, and planned well in advance. If a pregnant woman with cardiac disease is admitted to ICU, this multidisciplinary team should be consulted about her care. Priorities of care include:

- *Pre-pregnancy counselling* – this should allow a full and frank discussion about the likely risks of pregnancy for the individual and a discussion of treatment path. This is of particular importance for women who are on potentially teratogenic medication, such as warfarin or ACE inhibitors, and for women who may benefit from surgery or interventional treatment prior to conceiving. Additionally, women with CHD may require genetic counselling to determine the likelihood of CHD in any offspring. The most accurate prediction tool is the modified WHO classification of maternal cardiovascular risk (see Table 28.5).

- *Diagnosis* – standard investigations including chest X-ray, ECG, computed tomography (CT) scan and MRI should be attended to as indicated by the clinical condition. In general, diagnostic imaging of a critically ill woman should not be withheld because of concerns about the fetus, with abdominal shielding used whenever possible. Furthermore, radiation doses should be kept as low as possible, preferably <50 mGy.[165,174]

- *Heart failure* – as was outlined in the section on peripartum cardiomyopathy, the principles of treatment for heart failure in pregnancy are the same as for the non-pregnant population. Due to the slightly higher normal level of B-type natriuretic peptide in pregnancy, a threshold value of 111 pg/mL is indicative of heart failure in pregnant women.[181]

- *Arrhythmias* – commonly used drugs include digoxin, lignocaine (lidocaine), flecainide, verapamil, sotalol, propranolol, adenosine and amiodarone; although limited studies exist in the pregnant population, all have been used safely and effectively during pregnancy.[182] Transient neonatal hypothyroidism has been described in women on amiodarone and monitoring of neonatal thyroid function is recommended.[183] For refractory rhythms or if the woman is haemodynamically unstable, cardioversion is considered a safe procedure during pregnancy.[184]

- *Cardiac surgery and interventional cardiology* – such as valvuloplasty – may be required during pregnancy. Depending on the gestational age of the fetus, elective caesarean section prior to cardiac intervention may be preferable. Open-heart surgery is performed during pregnancy only when the maternal condition is critical, for example coronary artery dissection or severe dysfunctioning valve, because of the high probability of fetal loss, which occurs in about one in three cases.[185] Standard care should be provided to a pregnant woman, with care to nurse the woman ≥20 weeks' gestation with a 15 degrees left lateral tilt or manual left uterine displacement, in order to reduce the negative effects of aortocaval compression. Open-heart surgery and ECMO have been used successfully in pregnant women, with good outcomes for some mothers and babies.[186]

- *Thrombus prevention* – is a priority in women with valvular disease/prosthetic valves, atrial fibrillation or dilated heart chambers at risk of thrombus formation, especially because of the normal hypercoagulopathy associated with pregnancy. Warfarin embryopathy, a recognised collection of developmental anomalies such as nasal hypoplasia and epiphysis stippling, is associated with warfarin use in the first trimester. Despite this, warfarin continues to be used, as pregnant women with mechanical valves experience unacceptably high rates of valve thrombosis and embolism when switched to heparin, and novel oral anticoagulants have not been evaluated for safety in pregnancy. Consequently, many cardiologists consider the risks associated with the continued use of warfarin in pregnancy to be lower than the risks of stopping it.[165] Therefore, a regimen that balances the risk of thrombosis with that of fetal loss or malformation and risk of haemorrhage should be implemented, with some variation of: stopping warfarin for the whole first trimester or from 6–12 weeks' gestation and then resuming until close to delivery, replacing warfarin with low-molecular-weight heparin for the whole pregnancy, or continuing warfarin throughout pregnancy if dosage is ≤5 mg/day and replacing it with heparin for delivery only.[169,187] Appropriate dosing schedules for heparin have not been confirmed with weight-dosed, fixed-dosed and anti-Xa-adjusted dosage schedules used equally effectively.[188]

- *Secondary prevention of RHD* – monthly intramuscular (IM) penicillin, e.g. 1,200,000 units of benzylpenicillin, to minimise repeat acute rheumatic fever and associated further valve degeneration.[168]

Practice tip

When caring for a pregnant woman with cardiac disease or post-cardiac surgery, differences in normal haemodynamic and respiratory parameters in pregnancy must be considered.

Asthma

Asthma is the most common chronic health disease in pregnant women, affecting between 8% and 13% of child-bearing women, with the incidence in Australia one of the highest in the world.[189,190] Although most women have a pre-existing asthma diagnosis, some women develop new-onset asthma during pregnancy.

Course of asthma during pregnancy

The course of asthma during pregnancy is variable, although one-third of women may find their asthma symptoms improve, one-third find their symptoms deteriorate and the other third find there is no change.[191] Asthma exacerbations are not uncommon in pregnancy; however, very severe exacerbation of asthma during pregnancy requiring ICU admission is rare. A persisting problem in pregnant women with asthma is the reluctance to treat (by some doctors) and decreased medication compliance (by some women), based on concerns about the safety of medication during pregnancy, with a substantial number of asthma exacerbations in pregnancy associated with non-adherence to prescribed drugs.[192] There is evidence that prescription practices for asthma change during pregnancy.[193] In an Australian study, fewer than one in five women with asthma had a written asthma plan during pregnancy.[192]

Effect of asthma on pregnancy

The relationship between asthma in pregnancy and adverse maternal and neonatal outcomes, including preeclampsia, gestational diabetes, small-for-gestational-age neonates and preterm birth, is inconsistent. A systematic review suggests women with severe asthma have increased chances of

TABLE 28.6

Summary of management of acute exacerbation of asthma in pregnancy[195]

1	Beta$_2$ agonist bronchodilator with one of the following: • Salbutamol MDI 4–8 puffs every 20 min up to 1 h, then every 1–4 h as needed. • Salbutamol 2.5–5.0 mg nebulised every 20 min for 3 doses, then every 1–4 h as needed. • Salbutamol continuous nebulisation 10–15 mg/h.
2	Add anticholinergic therapy: • Ipratropium bromide nebulised 0.5 mg every 20 min for 3 doses, then as needed, given simultaneously with salbutamol.
3	Oxygen to maintain saturation >95%.
4	Consider fetal monitoring if pregnancy has reached viability (as directed by the obstetrician): • Consult with specialist obstetrician for collaborative management and planning for delivery if relevant.
5	Assess volume status – maintain euvolaemia and adequate maternal cardiac output.
6	Initiate systemic glucocorticoids without delay for patients: • In severe exacerbation. • Who are already on chronic oral glucocorticoids. • Who have mild to moderate symptoms not responsive to steps 1–5 within the first hour. • For those who are critically ill: high-dose IV methylprednisolone 120–180 mg/d (three or four divided doses for 48 h), then 60–80 mg/d, tapered as patient improves.
7	Adjunct therapies for patients not responding to above: • Magnesium sulfate 2 g IV over 20 min (assess baseline serum magnesium level if renal insufficiency present). • Terbutaline 0.25 mg subcutaneously every 20 min for up to 3 doses.
8	Consider intubation and mechanical ventilation: • Plan early and obtain practitioner experienced in pregnant airway management • For patients in severe distress and not responsive to earlier treatment. • When pH <7.35, arterial PaCO$_2$ >normal pregnancy range of 28–32 mmHg, or arterial PaO$_2$ <70 mmHg. • Facilitate avoidance of hyperinflation by using a prolonged expiratory time and monitor intensely for hyperinflation. • Titrate ventilation to achieve normal pH, normal pregnancy PaCO$_2$ 28–32 mmHg and normal PaO$_2$.

MDI = metered dose inhaler.

Source: Adapted from Bonham CA, Patterson KC, Strek ME. Asthma outcomes and management during pregnancy. Chest 2018;153:515–27.

giving birth to small-for-gestational-age babies compared with those with mild asthma, and those suffering exacerbations have higher odds of giving birth to babies with low birth weight or who are small for gestational age. The benefits of women taking their prescribed asthma medication (unless informed not to by their respiratory physician or obstetrician) outweigh any possible risks to their pregnancy.[191]

Patient management

A pregnant woman admitted to ICU with asthma may be experiencing new-onset asthma or an exacerbation of pre-existing asthma. Accurate diagnosis and evaluation of the disease is necessary and should involve the advice of a thoracic medicine specialist and an obstetrician, who will continue the care of the woman once discharged from ICU. Methacholine testing, used as a diagnostic tool for

asthma, is contraindicated in pregnancy.[194] Treatment of severe asthma in pregnancy is no different to the treatment in non-pregnant patients (see Chapter 14), apart from the additional needs to monitor fetal well-being and consider the normal respiratory parameters in pregnancy (Table 28.6).[191,195] Severe hypoxaemia places the fetus at risk and should be avoided; maternal SaO$_2$ should remain ≥95%. Peak-flow measures are recommended to be used during pregnancy to assess and monitor the woman's condition, with the normal values unchanged in pregnancy.[196] The risks associated with current asthma medication use in pregnancy are far less than the risks associated with uncontrolled asthma, and the regular schedule of asthma medications should be prescribed in pregnancy according to asthma symptom level.[191] Likewise, none of the common drug categories, such as inhaled corticosteroids, long-acting beta-agonists and leukotriene-receptor antagonists, is contraindicated during lactation.[191] Influenza, pertussis and COVID-19 vaccination during pregnancy is recommended for all women and is especially important in women with asthma.

Non-obstetric conditions and special considerations for pregnancy

Any health condition resulting in ICU admission may occur in a pregnant woman. The more common of these include physical trauma, acute respiratory infection and mental health disorders, and these are described in detail below. Drug and substance misuse in pregnancy can have harmful effects upon the woman, and her fetus. Substance misuse is complex, and may be interrelated with other factors such as domestic violence and mental health conditions, particularly in pregnancy. Obtaining a health history from a woman in the ICU setting may be challenging. If substance misuse is suspected, a toxicology screen may be useful to ensure the woman receives suitable care, management, support and referral to appropriate services for the remainder of the pregnancy.[197]

Trauma in pregnancy

The term 'trauma' refers to any accidental or intentional event resulting in injury. Blunt trauma accounts for most cases of trauma during pregnancy, with motor vehicle collisions (MVCs) being the most common cause, followed by falls and domestic violence/intimate partner violence.[198] The incidence of trauma in pregnancy is estimated to be in the range of 6–8% of all pregnancies and also includes burns, psychological and sexual abuse, toxicity, homicide and suicide.[199,200]

Violence against women

Violence against women is a complex public health issue. Globally, one in three women experience violence during their lifetime, with the majority resulting from intimate partner violence (IPV) (referred to as domestic abuse in some countries).[201] Rates of IPV are higher in developing countries (37%) than in developed countries (27%).[201] The prevalence of IPV during pregnancy ranges from 1.7% to 13.5%.[202,203] Up to 30% of IPV begins during pregnancy, and healthcare professionals should be trained to identify its signs and symptoms and screen women during routine maternity care.[204] The history regarding any injuries should be considered in relation to the presenting injury and likely mechanism of injury. A potential sign of IPV may be that the woman seems evasive or reluctant to speak in front of her partner. Often, physical violence is directed towards the maternal abdomen.[205] Pregnancy-related violence is associated with low-birth-weight babies, APH, premature labour, fetal trauma, infection, maternal depression, post-traumatic stress disorder, attempted suicide and mortality.[202,206]

Motor vehicle trauma

Women are at increased risk of premature rupture of membranes, preterm labour, placental abruption and death during MVCs.[207] Some pregnant women may believe there is no legal requirement to wear a seatbelt when pregnant and this places them and their fetus at increased risk of injury should they be involved in a MVC.[198] Fetal death rates are reported to be higher for women who are unbelted.[207] Additionally, pregnant women may not be informed on the correct positioning of a seatbelt during pregnancy, and incorrect positioning can increase the likelihood of placental abruption and additional injuries occurring (Fig. 28.2).[198] Uterine rupture has also been reported as a result of MVCs and can lead to fetal and maternal mortality if surgery is not undertaken promptly.[208,209]

Musculoskeletal injuries

Pregnancy hormones affect joints and ligaments, making them laxer and more pliable. This explains why pregnant women are more likely to experience joint injury, pelvic instability, back pain and strained and dislocated joints. A complex interplay of factors including an increase in redistributed body mass impacting on the centre of gravity, a decline in postural stability and changes in gait may go some way to explaining why pregnant women fall more readily.[210]

Trauma management

The order of care should comprise the primary survey, with initiation of resuscitative measures followed by a fetal assessment and secondary survey.[211,212] Trauma in pregnancy presents a number of challenges because of the anatomical and physiological adaptations that occur. For

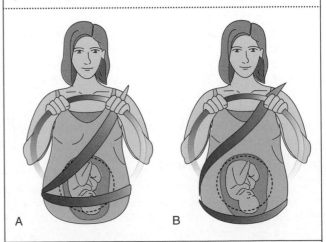

FIGURE 28.2 Positioning of a seatbelt during pregnancy. **(A)** Incorrect positioning. **(B)** Correct positioning.

A   B

Source: Adapted from Brown HL. Trauma in pregnancy. Obstet Gynecol 2009;114(1):147–60. doi: 10.1097/AOG.

example, if a chest drain is necessary to treat a haemothorax, use of the third or fourth intercostal space is recommended to accommodate the raised diaphragm.[212] Moreover, pregnant women may physiologically compensate for significant blood loss and then rapidly deteriorate. There remains some debate over whether a Kleihauer–Betke test is required to detect fetomaternal haemorrhage in all women who experience major/abdominal trauma, or only those who are rhesus negative.[213] Those women who are rhesus negative may require anti-D immunoglobulin.[211]

Potential for perimortem caesarean section

Where a pregnant woman ≥20 weeks' gestation requires CPR, manual displacement of the uterus or left tilt must be employed during CPR and perimortem caesarean section commenced promptly.[29,214] (See section on Modifications to basic and advanced life support below.) If cardiotocography (CTG) monitoring is in progress, all leads must be removed before shocks are delivered.

Obstetric assessment in trauma

Consideration should be given to all women of child-bearing age as to whether they may be pregnant, with pregnancy testing recommended.[211] Where a woman is obviously pregnant, an estimate of gestation can be made by measuring the symphysis fundal height. The height in cm equates approximately to the number of weeks' gestation; for example, 22 cm = 22 weeks' gestation, providing there is a singleton pregnancy and there are no pregnancy complications such as excess amniotic fluid (polyhydramnios) or fetal growth restriction.

All radiological investigations and imaging that are clinically indicated by the maternal condition should be initiated without delay over concerns for the fetus.[212] When possible and appropriate, a pelvic/abdominal lead shield may be used to protect the developing embryo/fetus.

Auscultation of the fetal heart using a handheld Doppler is a quick method of assessing immediate fetal well-being. Subsequently, external CTG may be used to assess fetal well-being where appropriate (see the section on fetal assessment). If there is likelihood of blunt trauma to the abdomen, a continuous external CTG should be undertaken for at least 4 hours, to identify fetal distress resulting from potential placental abruption.[212] An abdominal ultrasound is also usually performed to assess fetal well-being and may be useful in detecting free peritoneal fluid/maternal haemorrhage and placental abruption.[211] The bladder becomes an abdominal organ after 12 weeks of pregnancy and is prone to traumatic injury.

Acute respiratory infections

Pneumonia in pregnancy is one of the more common reasons why a pregnant woman may be admitted to ICU. It is not fully understood why pregnant women may be vulnerable to severe pneumonia, although the adaptations to the mechanics of breathing and changes in the immune response may be contributing factors.[215] Additionally, it

has been postulated that pregnant women are among small children more often and may have an increased likelihood of exposure to infective agents. The treatment and management of pneumonia in pregnancy is no different to pneumonia in non-pregnant women: identify the causative organism and administer appropriate antibiotics or antiviral agents as indicated, maintain oxygenation and prevent complications (see Chapter 15). Assessment of fetal well-being and awareness of the changed respiratory parameters in pregnancy are the additional requirements.

Pregnancy and influenza

WHO has recommended since 2006 that all pregnant women receive the seasonal influenza vaccination, in recognition of the known increased risk that influenza poses during pregnancy and because vaccination during pregnancy is safe and confers immunity to the newborn for the first few vulnerable months. In developed countries, maternal death caused by seasonal influenza is rare. However, the pandemic influenza, H1N1 09 (referred to as 'swine flu'), which swept across the world in 2009, demonstrated how vulnerable pregnant women are to influenza and emphasised the importance of influenza vaccination to prevent severe disease.

The H1N1 2009 flu epidemic killed seven pregnant/postpartum women in Australia and New Zealand in 3 months.[216] Over 60 women were admitted to ICU and a number of their babies died. Women in the second half of pregnancy were over 13 times more likely to be admitted to ICU with H1N1 influenza than non-pregnant women of child-bearing age. Pregnant and postpartum women admitted to ICU with H1N1 influenza were particularly unwell, with 14% of women requiring ECMO.[217]

Pregnancy and COVID-19

The COVID-19 pandemic that became globally established in 2020 affected pregnant women disproportionately. Pregnant women were over twice as likely as non-pregnant women of child-bearing age with COVID-19 to be admitted to ICU, and more than twice as likely to be intubated for mechanical ventilation and to receive ECMO.[218] Pregnant women with COVID-19, compared with pregnant women without COVID-19, were nearly 19 times more likely to be admitted to ICU, and nearly three times more likely to experience a stillbirth or neonatal death.[218] Maternal mortality was also increased in women with COVID-19 infection, with ten women dying in the UK in the first 3 months of the pandemic.[219] The Australian National COVID-19 Clinical Evidence Taskforce COVID-19 living guidelines are a good resource to guide management – available at: https://clinicalevidence.net.au/covid-19/.[220] Other management summaries have been published and most specific COVID-19 treatment (e.g. antivirals, steroids) excluded pregnant women from clinical trials.[221] However, most treatments are unchanged, with the balance of risk versus benefit guiding individual treatment in pregnancy.[222] Although, similarly, pregnant women were excluded from vaccine trials, millions of pregnant women have received novel COVID-19 vaccinations in a 'real world experiment' owing to the high burden of disease. High-quality vaccination surveillance systems have found that there are no adverse events related to pregnancy and the COVID-19 vaccines are safe to be given in all trimesters of pregnancy.[223] COVID-19 vaccination is also safe for breastfeeding women. Vaccine-generated antibodies pass across the placenta and into breast milk, providing the newborn with passive immunity against COVID-19.[224]

Sepsis associated with pregnancy

Maternal sepsis can occur at any time during pregnancy and postpartum and from any cause. Common obstetric-related events include termination of pregnancy, spontaneous miscarriage, prolonged rupture of membranes, caesarean and vaginal birth, and mastitis, and non-obstetric-related events include urinary tract infection and pyelonephritis, and respiratory tract infection. The most common organism responsible for maternal sepsis resulting in death is group A *Streptococcus* (also known as *Streptococcus pyogenes*).[225] Notable in the review of maternal deaths from sepsis is the rapidity with which some women succumbed. The septic course is often insidious and women may appear deceptively well before suddenly collapsing, often with little or no warning.[226] Although there is no research evaluating the Surviving Sepsis Campaign guidelines in the maternity setting, they are recommended for use. The Sepsis Obstetric Score was developed and validated for use in the emergency department to predict likelihood of ICU admission.[227] The Society of Obstetric Medicine of Australia and New Zealand has developed guidelines for the identification and management of sepsis in pregnancy.[228] They recommend use of an obstetric-modified quick Sequential Organ Failure Assessment score. Management of sepsis is described in Chapter 21. The California Maternal Quality Care Collaborative advocate for a two-step approach for the diagnosis of sepsis associated with pregnancy because of the poor performance of routine adult screening systems in pregnancy.[225] In the UK, the 'Sepsis 6' is advocated to guide patient management when sepsis is suspected.[229]

Mental health disorders

Mental health disorders during pregnancy and the postpartum period comprise women with pre-existing disease and those who develop signs and symptoms of mental health disease for the first time and are a significant contributor to maternal deaths.[99] The mental health disorder may be separate from the pregnancy or there may be a relationship between the pregnancy and the development of the disorder, such as antenatal and/or postnatal depression.

Pre-existing mental health disorders

The underlying principles of management of pregnant women with a pre-existing mental health disorder are the same as for non-pregnant women: safety of the woman, stabilisation of the mental illness and empowerment of, and support for, the woman to make her own choices. A considerable additional challenge is maintaining stability of the mental health disorder if changes to medication are required because of potential teratogenesis or contraindication for use during pregnancy. Ideally, pre-conception counselling has occurred, and the woman has commenced and been stabilised on a medication regimen considered safe for pregnancy, prior to becoming pregnant.

Pregnant women with pre-existing mental health disorders may require admission to ICU because of acute deterioration in their mental health. This is most likely to be as a result of cessation or alteration of their regular medications.[230,231] Most relapses occur in the first trimester and many women who initially stop their medication recommence it during the pregnancy.[230] Routine care should be provided as clinically indicated, keeping in mind the additional requirements to monitor fetal well-being, conduct standard antenatal assessment and consider the impact of the physiological adaptations on treatments.

Mental health disorders related to pregnancy

Suicide is highlighted as a leading cause of direct (pregnancy-related) death in the year after pregnancy in the UK.[99] Risk factors for suicide are multifactorial and include unwanted pregnancy in developed countries, especially in adolescents and women from cultures where childbirth outside of marriage is unacceptable, intimate partner violence, fetal or neonatal loss, substance abuse and perinatal depression.[232] Depression may arise during pregnancy (antenatal depression) although it is more likely to present during the postpartum period (postpartum depression). The most severe mental health disorder related to pregnancy is puerperal psychosis.

Puerperal psychosis

Puerperal psychosis is a rare mental health complication of pregnancy, said to occur in 1–2/1000 births.[233] The majority of cases occur in women with pre-existing mental illness, such as bipolar disorder, with just 0.03/1000 deliveries occurring in women with no pre-existing mental health disorder.[234] It usually presents within the first few weeks postpartum and is associated with an increased risk of suicide and infanticide.[235,236] Women with puerperal psychosis are frequently delusional, suffer hallucinations and require acute hospitalisation for treatment.

Postpartum depression

Postnatal depression is defined as a non-psychotic depressive illness; most definitions specify occurrence within 3 months postpartum, although some specify a shorter period of only 1 month.[237,238] Risk factors include prior mental illness, poor social supports, relationship disharmony and recent life events.[237] Depression in the postpartum period raises treatment issues for the nursing mother and the developing infant.

Early diagnosis and effective treatment are indicated. Self-harm in the first 12 months postpartum is a severe concern for women with serious depression.[238] Care in the ICU is no different to that provided to other patients admitted with severe depression. Postnatal depression is not a contraindication to lactation, although some medication may be contraindicated. Women will require appropriate referral for psychological therapies, specialist perinatal mental health support (where available) and discussions regarding the risk versus benefits of pharmacological treatments.[239] Internationally, the most frequently used antidepressants during pregnancy are selective serotonin reuptake inhibitors (SSRIs).[240]

Caring for pregnant women in ICU

Any pregnant woman in ICU is considered to be carrying an 'at-risk' fetus. This means that fetal well-being may be compromised and the fetus is at risk of sustaining injury/ suboptimal growth and development or death in utero. There are circumstances when the woman's clinical status would be improved by delivery of the fetus, and times when the fetus needs to be delivered to increase the likelihood of its survival. Consideration of both the maternal condition and fetal well-being contributes to the decision on when to deliver a fetus. Delivery prior to 22–24 weeks' gestation is an option only if the maternal condition is very critical and considered necessary to potentially save the woman's life; it is likely that the neonate's care in this instance would be palliative. Even though about half of babies born <24 weeks survive, they do so with a far higher risk of permanent disability.[241] Once gestation reaches 28 weeks, the neonate has more than a 95% chance of survival when cared for in a neonatal intensive care unit (NICU).[241]

Childbirth is a highly significant event in many cultures with associated specific practices and beliefs. These practices vary widely and, in particular, may relate to the pregnant woman, the birth event, the placenta, breastfeeding and the postpartum period.[242] For general principles on culturally sensitive care, see Chapter 7.

Obesity in pregnancy is associated with adverse outcomes for both the mother and the baby, with a dose-dependent relationship: the higher the body mass index (BMI), the higher the likelihood of adverse outcomes.[243] This includes a seven-fold increased likelihood of admission to ICU for women with a BMI >50.[243] See Chapter 5 for general principles of caring for bariatric patients. From the maternity perspective, obesity in pregnancy poses difficulties in caring for women including determining fetal well-being, assessment of gestation and monitoring the progress of labour, and increased incidences of preeclampsia and gestational diabetes.[244,245] Lactation also proves more challenging to establish.[246] Additionally, thromboprophylaxis should be considered early, given the increased risk of thrombosis in pregnancy/postpartum,

which is magnified further in obese women. Weight-based dosage for pharmacological options should be considered.[245]

Mechanical ventilation of the pregnant woman

The provision of mechanical ventilation to a pregnant woman occurs rarely and there is little evidence to guide practice. Pregnant women are considered to have a 'high-risk airway', with the reported 'failure to intubate' rate about 1 in 250, approximately eight times more likely than in the non-pregnant population.[247] Nasal intubation is not usually an option for pregnant women owing to the risk of epistaxis. Women with preeclampsia may also have substantial pharyngeal oedema.

The principles of mechanical ventilation in pregnancy are the same as those for the non-obstetric population[248] (see Chapter 15) with additional considerations as follows:

- Ensure target endpoints consider the normal arterial blood gases (ABGs) for pregnancy.
- A small reduction in maternal oxygenation can severely impact on fetal oxygenation because of the left shift in the oxyhaemoglobin dissociation curve associated with fetal haemoglobin.[249]
- Permissive hypercapnia has not been evaluated in pregnancy (fetal carbon dioxide is higher than the maternal level, given the gradient across the placental membrane).
- Normal tidal volumes in pregnancy are increased by up to 40–50% of non-pregnant values, although the mechanical provision of these larger tidal volumes with respect to volutrauma has not been examined; in practice, often the respiratory rate is increased first and then increases in tidal volume are used only when necessary.
- There is no evidence that delivery of the baby will improve the maternal respiratory state.[248]

Other, less common, methods to support gas exchange have been reported in the literature in the form of case studies. Of note, nitrous oxide, hyperbaric oxygen treatment and extracorporeal membrane oxygenators have all been used successfully to treat acute conditions such as pulmonary embolism in pregnant women.[250]

Use of prone ventilation in pregnancy

Prior to the COVID-19 pandemic, there was little experience of using prone ventilation in the ICU setting to manage acute respiratory failure in pregnant women.[251] However, there was evidence that it was safe, having been used for various surgeries,[252,253] and studied in healthy pregnant women and in those with preeclampsia.[254] Furthermore, the prone position was demonstrated to fully resolve the uterine compression of the main vessels if sufficient care was taken in providing padding above and below the uterus to relieve compression, particularly in the third trimester.[255] There has been extensive use of prone ventilation in all trimesters of pregnancy in women with COVID-19.[256] Although commercial padding is available, prone positioning of a pregnant woman can be achieved using pillows and blankets.

Practice tip

Remember that pregnancy is associated with a poor tolerance of short-term apnoea – for example, during induction of anaesthesia and/or intubation – and preoxygenation is important.

Practice tip

Medical staff with experience in managing people with difficult airways should be present when a pregnant woman is intubated.

Fetal assessment

Fetal well-being will be reliant on the critically ill woman receiving the necessary treatment to promote physiological stability.[257] UK data shows the median gestation of pregnant women admitted to ICU is 25 weeks.[258] Fetal mortality in pregnant women admitted to ICU is often as high as 20%[4] and the assessment of fetal well-being in those who are critically ill may be used to guide decision making regarding the optimum timing of birth.

Methods of assessing fetal viability/well-being include maternal monitoring of fetal movements, intermittent auscultation of the fetal heart (FH) rate using a Pinard stethoscope or handheld Doppler, continuous external CTG monitoring and ultrasound and fetal biophysical profiles.[259] The method(s) used will be dependent on the obstetric history and the presence of comorbidities, gestation, reason for admission to and length of stay on the ICU and the presence/absence of labour. Biophysical profiles use real-time ultrasonography to monitor fetal breathing, movements, tone and amniotic fluid volume, but are not utilised in all countries.[260] Uterine artery Doppler flow measurements may be used in specific circumstances – for example, where the fetus is suspected to be small for gestational age.[259] Professionals interpreting fetal surveillance tests in the ICU must take into consideration the medications a woman is receiving, as these may have an impact; for example, some maternal sedative medications may also sedate the fetus.

Cardiotocography

A traditional CTG monitor comprises a Doppler that records the FH rate and a pressure transducer that is placed over the uterine fundus, which detects uterine contractions. The FH and uterine activity are recorded on a timed graph (Fig. 28.3). There have been reports of adverse outcomes where the maternal pulse, or a recorded artefact, has mistakenly been interpreted as the FH.[261] Consequently, it is vital to differentiate between the FH and maternal pulse at commencement of the CTG, and at regular intervals during the CTG.

There is debate regarding the earliest gestation at which a CTG should be done; ranges from 24 to 28 weeks are cited and depend upon the country, legal threshold for fetal viability and the interventions possible if a FH rate abnormality occurs.[262,263] The decision to commence a CTG at very early pregnancy gestations should be made by a senior obstetrician. CTG recordings are not predictive of longer-term fetal well-being and provide information only at the time the trace is recorded.

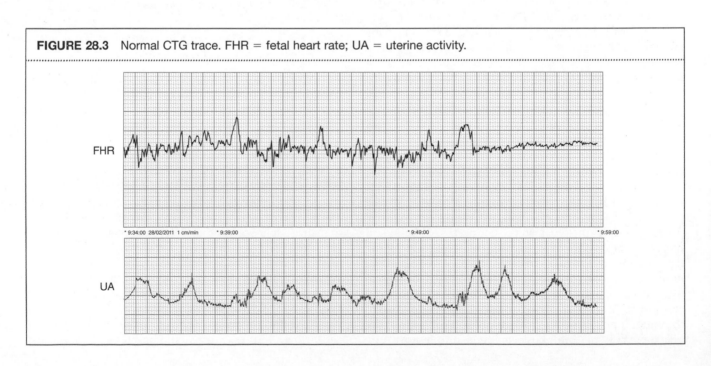

FIGURE 28.3   Normal CTG trace. FHR = fetal heart rate; UA = uterine activity.

A normal FH rate is 110–160 bpm, with variability in the rate of ≤5 bpm.[264] Other features recorded on a CTG include FH rate accelerations and/or decelerations plus the frequency of contractions. A CTG cannot be considered in isolation, but always as part of the overall clinical picture. For example, sedative drugs administered to the mother can affect FH reactivity. Specialist obstetric hospitals may offer a CTG interpretation service for general hospitals without maternity staff to assist with interpretation of CTGs. The required frequency and duration of a CTG recording will vary according to the maternal clinical condition or diagnosis and whether the CTG recording is normal. For example, suspected placental abruption following blunt trauma may require a minimum of 4 hours of continuous monitoring.[211] A CTG will also be recommended during and following elective cardioversion and many other procedures, as advised by the obstetric team.

Ultrasound

An ultrasound scan will measure core components of fetal anatomy, such as head and abdominal circumference and femur length, to assess fetal size as well as to quantify adequacy of amniotic fluid volume. Serial ultrasounds may be used to assess whether fetal growth is adequate in relation to gestational age and can also used for biophysical profiling.[265,266] Doppler velocimetry is also utilised to assess the well-being of the fetus identified 'at risk', with umbilical and uterine artery Dopplers being performed.[266]

Practice tip

The World Health Organization defines a livebirth as:

'The complete expulsion or extraction from its mother of a product of conception, irrespective of the duration of the pregnancy, which, after such separation, breathes or shows any other evidence of life – e.g. beating of the heart, pulsation of the umbilical cord or definite movement of voluntary muscles – whether or not the umbilical cord has been cut or the placenta is attached.'[267]

Whether a stillborn baby needs to be registered as a birth and a death varies according to the jurisdiction. For example, in Australia and New Zealand all births need to be registered if the gestation is ≥20 weeks or, if the gestation is not known, the birth weight is more than 400 g, while in the UK the stillbirth needs to be registered if the gestation is ≥24 weeks.

Recognition of preterm labour

Preterm labour, regular uterine contractions with dilation of the cervix, occurs at a gestation of less than 37 completed weeks.[268] There are many risk factors for preterm labour including urinary tract and vaginal infections, preeclampsia, multiple pregnancy, polyhydramnios and lifestyle factors such as smoking and illegal drug taking.[11] In the critically ill pregnant patient, anaesthesia, mechanical ventilation and the illness itself may be related to the onset of preterm labour. Women may complain of pelvic pain, similar to period pain, or lower back pain, rather than the more typical abdominal pain associated with term labour. The pain has a cyclical pattern though, with complete pain relief in between contractions. For sedated women, be alert to any patient restlessness or increasing sedation requirements and ask for midwifery assistance to assess for the onset of labour. Placing a hand with gentle but firm pressure over the fundus will detect the presence or absence of uterine contraction.

Preparation for preterm birth

Preterm birth occurs at a gestation of less than 37 completed weeks. If it is anticipated that a pregnant woman in ICU is likely to give birth prematurely, cohesive planning between the ICU and the obstetric and neonatal teams is paramount to achieve the best outcomes. In particular, medication administration, as outlined below, aims to prevent respiratory disease in the newborn and to prevent the development of cerebral palsy. Having a neonatologist present at the birth is recommended.

Enhancement of newborn lung function

Ideally, women with threatened or diagnosed preterm labour between 24^{+0} and 34^{+6} weeks' gestation will receive antenatal corticosteroids (e.g. betamethasone 12 mg, 2 doses, 24 hours apart) to promote fetal lung maturity and surfactant production.[269] Antenatal corticosteroids significantly reduce complications related to prematurity including perinatal/neonatal death, respiratory distress syndrome and intraventricular haemorrhage.[269] However, birth should not be delayed to fulfil any time requirement related to steroid administration if the birth circumstances are urgent, as some benefit is seen even if birth occurs <24 hours after a single dose.[269] Antenatal corticosteroids are not contraindicated in women with diabetes, but close monitoring of the blood glucose levels and the need for increased insulin requirements must be taken into consideration.

Fetal neuroprotection

The administration of magnesium sulfate to a woman who is 24^{+0}–29^{+6} weeks' gestation with a viable fetus, in preterm labour (or planned to deliver within 24 hours), has been shown to reduce the likelihood of cerebral palsy developing in the infant.[268] Neuroprotection with magnesium sulfate should also be considered for women up to 33^{+6} weeks' gestation and those between 23^{+0} and 23^{+6} weeks' gestation contingent on the specific circumstances.[270] A common regimen is 4 g IV loading dose over 15 minutes followed by a continuous infusion at 1 g/h for 24 hours or until birth (whichever is sooner).[268] However, the 'best' dosage regimen has not been determined.[271,272] Maternal monitoring must include regular checking of the deep tendon reflexes, pulse, blood pressure and respiration. High doses of magnesium may lead to toxicity, manifesting initially as loss of the deep tendon reflex.

Prevention of rhesus disease

During pregnancy, a small amount of fetal blood can enter the maternal circulation. If the mother is Rh negative and the fetus is Rh positive, the mother produces antibodies against the rhesus D (RhD) antigen on her baby's red blood cells.[121] During this, and subsequent pregnancies, the anti-D antibodies are able to pass across the placenta to the fetus and, if the level is sufficient, cause destruction of RhD-positive fetal red blood cells, leading to the development of haemolytic disease of the fetus and newborn. The disease ranges from mild to severe, and the consequences for the fetus can include varying degrees of anaemia, hydrops fetalis or death. Blood tests for rhesus disease are outlined in Table 28.7.

Haemolytic disease of the fetus and newborn is prevented by treating pregnant women who are RhD negative with anti-D immunoglobulin unless she has received non-invasive prenatal testing (NIPT), which involves testing the maternal blood for fetal DNA to ascertain whether the fetus' genotype is RhD positive or negative.[273] Where women receive NIPT and are found to have a RhD-negative fetus the need for anti-D is negated. Rh-negative women who do not have access to this testing or have an inconclusive NIPT will be given 625 IU of anti-D immunoglobulin at 28 and 34 weeks in Australia and New Zealand,[121] which destroys any RhD-positive fetal red blood cells in their circulation before the immune system recognises them and produces anti-D antibodies. Anti-D is also given when potential sensitising events occur, such as first-trimester miscarriage/ectopic pregnancy and second- or third-trimester APH, MVC and fetal death.[121] Another dose of anti-D is given within 72 hours following birth, if the cord blood of the baby is found to be RhD positive.[121] If anti-D antibodies are produced during pregnancy, haemolytic disease of the fetus and newborn may occur in a subsequent pregnancy.[274]

Practice tip

Ascertain whether NIPT has been performed and, if it has not, check whether anti-D may be required for women who are RhD negative at key points in their pregnancy (28 and 34 weeks and at sensitising events). Anti-D is a blood product and some women may decline it on this basis.

Glucose management in pregnancy

Pregnancy is associated with changes to carbohydrate and fat metabolism in order to provide adequate nutrients to the fetus during pregnancy.[275] Some of the pregnancy hormones, including human placental lactogen, contribute to a progressive insulin resistance as the hormone levels increase throughout the pregnancy. Glucose readily crosses the placenta whereas insulin does not. If the mother has persistently high glucose levels, from either pre-existing diabetes or gestational diabetes, the fetus may be large for gestational age (macrosomic) and develop hyperinsulinaemia.[276] Additionally, hyperglycaemia is associated with poor obstetric and neonatal outcomes including congenital anomalies, birth trauma, caesarean birth, preeclampsia, newborn respiratory distress syndrome and stillbirth.[276] Recommended capillary blood glucose level targets for women with diabetes are <5.3 mmol/L fasting and <6.4 mmol/L 2 hours after a meal.[277] Although hyperglycaemia is associated with adverse obstetric and neonatal outcomes, hypoglycaemia should also be avoided.[277]

Modifications to basic and advanced life support

Generally, all standard basic and advanced life support algorithms can be used with only minor adaptations for the pregnant and postpartum woman (Box 28.6).[278,279] For women over 20 weeks' gestation, left lateral displacement of the uterus is paramount to ensure CPR is as effective as possible (Fig. 28.4).[30] Regardless, it is very difficult to obtain adequate perfusion during CPR of an obviously pregnant woman and arrangements should be made for an emergency caesarean section (termed

---

TABLE 28.7

Tests associated with rhesus disease and haemolytic disease of the fetus/newborn (HDFN)

BLOOD TEST	RATIONALE
Kleihauer–Betke test or flow cytometry	Confirms that fetal blood has passed into the maternal circulation, also estimates the amount of fetal blood that has passed into the maternal circulation.
Indirect Coombs test	Screens maternal blood for anti-D antibodies that may pass through the placenta and cause haemolytic disease of the newborn.
Quantitative analysis of maternal anti-RhD antibodies	An increasing titre level suggests fetal rhesus disease.
Fetal blood (or umbilical cord blood) tests	
Direct Coombs test	Confirms that maternal anti-D antibodies are present in the fetal/newborn circulation.
Full blood count	Haemoglobin level to assess for anaemia.
Bilirubin	Both total and indirect.

BOX 28.6

Maternal modified cardiac arrest algorithm[279]

Anticipate a difficult airway.

Women with an obviously gravid uterus, e.g. >20 weeks' gestation:

- To relieve aortocaval compression and enable more effective CPR, manually displace the uterus towards the left.
- Alternatively, use a wedge to position the woman in a left lateral tilt.
- Call for immediate obstetrician attendance when the arrest is activated.
- Remove any internal or external fetal monitors if present.
- Prepare for a potential emergency caesarean section.
- Aim for delivery within 5 min of onset of resuscitative efforts.
- Continue all elements of resuscitation effort during and after caesarean section.

Consider and treat any possible contributing factors:

- If the woman is on a magnesium infusion, cease and consider administration of calcium chloride 10 mL in 10% solution or calcium gluconate 30 mL in 10% solution to treat hypermagnesaemia.
- Haemorrhage with or without DIC: assess for hypovolaemia and treat appropriately but cautiously.
- Placental abruption/praevia if the woman is in the second half of pregnancy.
- Uterine atony if the woman is postpartum.
- Embolism, e.g. pulmonary, amniotic fluid.
- Anaesthetic complications, e.g. high spinal block.
- Cardiac disease, e.g. pre-existing or new.
- Preeclampsia.
- Sepsis.

Source: Adapted from Vanden Hoek TL, Morrison, LJ, Shuster M, et al. Part 12: Cardiac arrest in special situations: 2010 American Heart Association guidelines for cardiopulmonary resuscitation emergency cardiovascular care. Circulation 2010;122(18 Suppl. 3): S829–61.

---

perimortem caesarean section (PMCS)) or forceps delivery (where appropriate), as soon as resuscitation commences.[280] The general rule is that PMCS should proceed if there is no response to 4 minutes of CPR (the 4-minute rule), with birth of the baby occurring in the next minute, although this timescale is under debate.[30,214,281] A difficult intubation should be anticipated and an experienced individual should be available to intubate the trachea wherever possible.[282] Transfer to an operating theatre for PMCS leads to unnecessary delay and is not advised.[29] The list of obstetric conditions that may have precipitated the arrest should be considered and specific treatment instigated.[15] Cardiac arrest in pregnancy is a rare event (1:36,000 maternities) and the chance of a successful resuscitation will be influenced by factors that include the place of arrest (home versus hospital) and delay in commencing PMCS.[214] Due to the rarity of maternal cardiac arrest, multidisciplinary simulation should be routinely incorporated into resuscitation education.[283]

Medication administration in pregnancy

Many drugs used in the critical care environment have not been researched for safe use in pregnant or lactating mothers. There are two key periods when consideration of drug therapy is paramount: during the first trimester when embryo/fetal malformations may occur and immediately prior to delivery as the newborn baby may be adversely affected (e.g. sedated and unable to breathe spontaneously). The decision to administer various medications is often a balance between the benefit of administering the drug to the pregnant woman and the risk of not administering the drug.[221]

There are a number of anatomical, physiological, cellular and molecular changes in pregnancy that affect the pharmacokinetic and pharmacodynamic mechanisms of drugs administered during pregnancy.[284] These include reduced serum protein levels (altered protein-binding capacity), increased circulating volume (potential for dilution), delayed gut motility (potential for increased gut absorption), increased GFR (potential for increased excretion) and changes to maternal drug-metabolising enzymes (difficult to predict metabolism pattern of regular drugs).[285] Standard adult doses may be inadequate or toxic during pregnancy owing to the adapted physiology of pregnancy. There is a lack of information on efficacy, safety, teratogenicity and pharmacokinetics in pregnancy as drug trials routinely exclude pregnant women.[286]

Potential for teratogenesis

A teratogen is any agent that increases the incidence of a congenital anomaly.[11] The major organs are developed by 10 weeks' gestation; however, the recommendation is to avoid any teratogenic drug throughout the first trimester (14 weeks).[11] Some medications exert an adverse effect in the second or third trimesters of pregnancy, such as ACE inhibitors (fetal anuria and stillbirth), indomethacin (potential premature closure of the ductus arteriosus) and selective serotonin uptake inhibitors (neonatal withdrawal syndrome).[11] Healthcare professionals prescribing and/or administering drugs should each check the potential impact of the medication in pregnancy, and consult a pharmacist when possible.

FIGURE 28.4 Manual displacement of the uterus to the left (one-handed and two-handed).

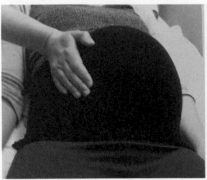 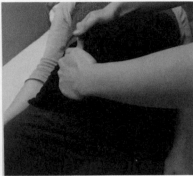

Source: Winter C, Draycott T, Muchatuta N, et al, editors. PROMPT course manual. 3rd ed. Cambridge, UK: Cambridge University Press; 2017, p. 31.

Administered immediately prior to delivery

Apart from effects on the structural development of the fetus in the first trimester, the other key time for consideration of drug administration is immediately prior to delivery. Common sedative agents such as midazolam, morphine, fentanyl and propofol cross the placenta readily and exert an action on the fetus.[287] Consequently, even mature term babies may be born sedated and require assistance with breathing. Planning for delivery of a pregnant woman in ICU should include the involvement of a paediatrician/ neonatologist or the local newborn emergency transport service (NETS) if no paediatrician is on site.

Therapeutic routine drug therapy in pregnancy

For women admitted to ICU for prolonged periods – for example, those with Guillain–Barré syndrome – consideration may be given to routine therapeutic medication in pregnancy. For example, folic acid (400 micrograms daily) is recommended pre-conception and throughout the first trimester to prevent neural tube defects.[11] Similarly, iron and vitamin D supplementation may be indicated depending on blood levels. Vitamin D deficiency is common, yet often unrecognised in critically ill patients.[288] Maternal vitamin D deficiency is associated with childhood asthma and increased risk of osteoporotic fracture in their offspring.[289] Due attention should be paid to a pregnant woman's nutritional status in ICU, as poor nutrition during pregnancy is associated with poor birth outcomes and pregnancy is associated with increased nutritional requirements.[290]

Caring for postpartum women in ICU

Women admitted to ICU during the postpartum period are often separated from their newborn, possibly even

---

BOX 28.7

Routine postnatal observations

- Examination of breasts, looking for signs of engorgement, mastitis, cracked nipples.
- Height, depth and texture of fundus, to ensure involution is happening.
- Lochia, inspection of PV loss.
- Examination of perineum/wound for signs of healing.
- Examination for signs of deep vein thrombosis; thromboprophylaxis is often indicated in a postpartum ICU woman.
- Micturition and bowels; to ensure bowel and urinary pattern returning to normal.

---

transferred to another hospital, and may not see their baby for days, until discharged from ICU.[291] Specific care that should be provided to the postpartum woman includes postpartum observations, assistance to establish lactation as required and support for early nurturing of a mother–infant bond. Finally, attention to the psychological needs of both the woman and her partner is an important part of care.

Routine postpartum observations

Ongoing surveillance of a postpartum woman is essential in addition to any ad hoc visits provided by a midwife. Routine maternity observations include assessment of the fundus, PV loss and perineum, assessment of the breasts and nipples, consideration of deep vein thrombosis and thromboprophylaxis, and evaluation of her psychological well-being and transition to motherhood (Box 28.7).

Uterine involution

Uterine 'involution' is the process by which the uterus returns to its near-normal size, tone and position. The vagina, ligaments of the uterus and muscles of the pelvic floor also return to their pre-pregnant state during the involution process. During this process, the lining of the uterus is cast off in the lochia, more commonly referred to as PV loss, and is later replaced by the new endometrium.[10] Following birth, and post-expulsion of the placenta, the muscles of the uterus constrict the blood vessels, so the blood circulating within the uterus is dramatically decreased.[10] Redundant muscle, fibrous and elastic tissue is disposed of – the phagocytes of the bloodstream deal with this – but the process is usually incomplete, and some elastic tissue remains and the uterus will never fully return to the pre-pregnant state.[11]

The rate of involution is measured by the rate of descent of the uterine fundus (the top of the uterus) in relation to either the umbilicus or the symphysis pubis. Important markers include the following:

- At day 1 postnatal, the height of the fundus is usually at or just below the umbilicus.
- There is a steady decrease in size, of around 1 cm per day.
- By postnatal day 10, the uterus may not be palpable above the symphysis pubis.[11]

The rate of involution varies and may be slower in multiparous women, where there is infection or retained placental tissue and when birth has been by caesarean section.[10] Where deviations from normal have occurred (e.g. caesarean section, atonic postpartum haemorrhage, uterine infection), regular uterine palpation will be required to monitor whether the uterus remains well contracted.[292]

A normally contracted uterus feels firm on palpation; as you palpate the fundus to locate the top and feel the texture of the uterus, you cannot push your fingertips into the tissue of the uterus. A so-called boggy uterus is one that is not contracted properly (atonic) and the fundus does not feel firm on palpation. Reasons for a 'boggy uterus' include uterine atony, retained tissue/membrane/clots or a full bladder that is impeding the uterine nerve stimulus to contract. The uterus responds well to tactile stimulation, and the first treatment for a 'boggy uterus' is to 'rub-up' the fundus. This involves palpating the top of the uterus and literally giving it a rub. The uterus will usually respond and you will feel it tighten and become harder. Such an action may result in a small gush of PV loss. On some occasions, a drug that causes the uterus to contract (uterotonic), such as oxytocin, may be needed to promote uterine contraction. If the uterus does not contract properly, the vessels that supplied the placental bed will not be closed off by the uterine muscle contraction (called the living ligatures) and the woman will continue to bleed.[11]

> ### Practice tip
>
> Uterotonics, drugs that cause the uterus to contract, are usually stored in the refrigerator – for example, Syntocinon, Syntometrine.

> ### Practice tip
>
> Many midwives document fundal height by finger-widths in relation to the belly button. For example, two finger-widths below the belly button would be notated by 2F ↓⊙.

Lochia and perineal care

The changes in the appearance of the lochia are described in three stages: lochia rubra, lochia serosa and lochia alba.[293] Lochia rubra consists of blood coming chiefly from the placental site. Three or four days post-delivery, the lochia changes to a pinky-brownish colour and is called lochia serosa. Seven days post-delivery the lochia changes to yellowish in appearance; this is called lochia alba. Normal lochia is not offensive in odour but the amount and duration of blood loss will vary between women.[294] Offensive lochia with or without maternal pyrexia may indicate a uterine infection (postpartum endometritis). High and low vaginal swabs for culture and sensitivity, and the commencement of antibiotic cover, should be initiated. Offensive lochia coupled with sub-involution of the uterus may require ultrasound to exclude retained placental tissue.

Regular assessment of the PV loss is required in the early postpartum phase. Generally, this includes 1–2-hourly checks if the PV loss is relatively heavy (pad soaked within 1–2 hours) for the first day, progressing to 4-hourly checks on day 2, with further reductions in observation frequency based on clinical condition. Check the fundus and PV loss regularly enough to detect any excessive blood loss or loss of uterine tone. The colour and volume of PV loss is usually documented along with any pad changes. Weighing pads to quantify PV loss is preferable to describing the loss as 'mild', 'moderate' or 'severe'.

The perineum should be examined daily or more frequently as dictated by clinical circumstances. A vulval haematoma/varicosities may be present and require obstetric assessment. For women who have had a vaginal birth, review the medical notes to ascertain whether perineal trauma was sustained or an episiotomy performed. Examine perineal wounds and/or sutures for signs of infection or wound breakdown and ensure the area is kept clean and administer prescribed analgesia, compatible with breastfeeding where appropriate.[292]

Increased potential for deep vein thrombosis

Most postpartum women admitted to ICU are likely to fulfil the criteria that recommend medical thromboprophylaxis.[31,292] Routine postpartum care involves examining the legs for signs of deep vein thrombosis (DVT) and appropriate use of thromboembolic stockings, sequential compression devices and thromboprophylaxis as required.[31]

Breast care and breastfeeding

Breastfeeding provides many health benefits for mothers and their babies and should be facilitated whenever possible in the ICU.[292,295] Exclusive breastfeeding along with many other factors including genetics, the mode of birth (vaginal versus caesarean), intrapartum antibiotics and environmental factors have been identified as influencing the infant gut microbiota, which is strongly linked to health benefits for the neonate in the short term and later in life.[296,297] The complex components in breast milk are responsible for the early colonisation of the gut microbiota and promoting a healthy immune system. There is increased risk of conditions such as asthma and autoimmune conditions like diabetes and inflammatory bowel disease developing later in life where the requisite commensal bacteria in a neonate's gut have been prohibited from developing or there is microbiota dysbiosis.[298] Breast milk is also of great importance for preterm infants as it reduces the likelihood of necrotising enterocolitis developing and may reduce the incidence of late-onset sepsis occurring.[299]

Initiation and establishment of lactation

The establishment and maintenance of lactation are complex hormone-mediated processes termed lactogenesis and galactopoiesis.[10] The physiological trigger for the establishment of lactation is a fall in progesterone combined with maintained levels of prolactin and cortisol.[300] During the initial postnatal period, colostrum is produced and this contains high levels of protein and immunological and growth factors.[301] The normal timing for milk to 'come in' is between 3 and 4 days post-delivery.[302] Of note, the drug dopamine may hinder lactation, as it inhibits prolactin secretion.[303] It is unlikely that the severity of maternal illness plays much of a role in the initial capacity to produce milk; anecdotally, 100 mL of breast milk has been expressed 4-hourly from a postpartum woman on ECMO. The initial regularity of hand expression or breastfeeding and milk removal provide the stimulus to produce milk.

Throughout pregnancy, the breasts develop and are capable of producing colostrum from 16 weeks onwards.[10] Ideally, the first breastfeed should occur within an hour of birth.[304] However, there is some debate regarding how crucial the first 24–48 hours are for the successful establishment of lactation as, in some cultures, colostrum is considered poisonous and breastfeeding is withheld for 2–3 days.[305] These women go on to successfully breastfeed and so too do many women recovering from illness with suboptimal breast expression in the first day or two postpartum. However, for women wanting to breastfeed, early and frequent expression (at least eight times in 24 hours, including during the night) will help to establish lactation.[304]

Hand expression is also used when babies are premature, there are problems with attachment, the mother is ill, or the mother and baby are in different locations.[304] Box 28.8[306] outlines the principles of hand expressions and Fig. 28.5 the process. Frequent, short expression of the breasts is more effective than prolonged infrequent expressing, and night expression is also important because prolactin, the hormone required to stimulate milk secretion, is produced in greater quantities overnight.[307] Breast pumps (hand or electric) may be helpful for women where long-term expression is required. To promote successful milk expression, measures including relaxation, holding or seeing a photograph of the baby and massaging the breasts may be employed.[307] Overall, the two main factors that support the establishment of lactation are breast stimulation (infant suckling or hand/pump expression) and milk removal. In a positive-feedback loop, the more often milk is removed from the breast, the more milk will be produced.[10]

BOX 28.8

Principles of expressing colostrum and breastmilk[306]

How often should I express?
Generally speaking, women are recommended to express 2–3-hourly. This may be challenging to achieve in the ICU environment. Clinicians should aim for 8 times per 24 h including at least once overnight where feasible.

Hand express or machine express?
It is recommended to use hand expression in the first few days with use of a machine reserved for when the milk has come in. When using a pump, the mother is encouraged to be as comfortable as possible and have a picture of the baby beside her if they are separated. The equipment should be cleaned and sterilised prior to each use, in line with local policy. Ideally, the mother will start by gently massaging her breasts/ apply warm cloths as this can assist with the let-down reflex. The breast pump can be used on both breasts in turn and should start with the lowest setting, which can gradually be increased. Expressing by hand or machine should not be painful.

Storage and transport of expressed milk
The most useful container for collection of expressed colostrum is a 2- or 5-mL syringe and a sterile plain specimen container for small volumes of milk. Label the container with the woman's name, date and time of collection. Use a new container for each expression. Breast milk must be stored in a refrigerator and may be frozen according to local policies. A 'cooler bag' with ice packs should be used to transport the milk from the ICU to where the baby is being cared for. The UNICEF website has helpful information on hand expression and storing colostrum/breastmilk by the Breastfeeding Network: (https://www.unicef.org.uk/ babyfriendly/baby-friendly-resources/breastfeeding-resources/expressing-and-storing-breastmilk-bfn/).

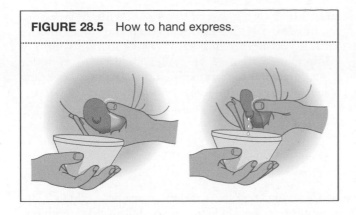

FIGURE 28.5 How to hand express.

If the mother's intention was to formula feed, then the lactation process may be suppressed. In practice, this means providing no stimulation to the breasts (i.e. no hand expression). Although used in the past, medications are rarely prescribed (unless the mother has suffered a stillbirth or late intrauterine fetal death).[308,309] With no breast expression, women may still experience their milk 'coming in' at around days 3–4 postpartum. Comfort measures, although unsubstantiated by evidence, may assist if the breasts become very uncomfortable.[308] Wearing supportive underwear and applying cold compresses may be helpful, and it is important for the critical care nurse to observe for signs like reddened, hot and painful areas on the breast that may be an indication of mastitis.[292] For those women who have suffered a fetal death, cabergoline, a dopamine agonist, may be prescribed to suppress lactation, but is contraindicated in those with hypertensive disorders including pre-eclampsia.[309]

Breast care

A woman's breasts should be assessed at least twice a shift to assess their condition and identify signs of complications, such as mastitis. Assess all women, regardless of whether they are breastfeeding or not. The breasts are usually soft, although as the milk comes in they may become engorged and tender to touch. A localised area that is red and painful may be indicative of mastitis, which results from poor attachment and insufficient emptying of milk from the breast.[310] Mastitis is sometimes accompanied by flu-like symptoms and may require treatment with antibiotics. The nipples should be inspected for cracks and soreness if the woman is using a breast pump or breastfeeding. Good positioning and attachment of the baby at the breast are vital for successful breastfeeding and will minimise the incidence of cracked nipples. Colostrum (or milk once it has come in) may leak from the nipples and can be gently applied over the nipples to promote healing.[311]

Medication administration and lactation

Many drugs are safe to use in breastfeeding, although most common critical care drugs have not been well evaluated.[312,313] Even if the woman is receiving a medication that is contraindicated during breastfeeding, she can still express (and discard) the milk to establish lactation, unless she is likely to stay on the medication long term.

The safety of the expressed milk for the baby depends on three factors: the amount of the medication in the milk, the oral bioavailability of the medication and the ability of the infant to metabolise the medication.[314] The gestation and condition of the infant are relevant, as the function of the gut, liver and kidney varies with maturity and illness. Consequently, advice from the baby's neonatologist or paediatrician can help determine whether the neonate can receive the expressed breast milk, or whether it should be discarded.[315]

Perinatal mental health

Major emotional changes take place in most women during the puerperium, but there is wide variation in the impact these changes have. The 'baby blues' are thought to occur 2–3 days post-birth, and are characterised by emotional lability (mood swings), thoughts of inadequacy and concern for the baby and last up to 2 weeks.[316] It is estimated that the baby blues are experienced by up to 80% of women.[316] It is also recognised that women can suffer post-traumatic stress disorder (PTSD) following childbirth, highlighting the importance of healthcare professionals attending to women's psychological needs during an episode of critical illness.[317]

The family unit

Maternal admission to ICU often separates the mother from her newborn and may also be associated with a period of heavy sedation/loss of consciousness. Hence, the woman may not be able to recollect the birth process and will often not have seen her baby before being transferred to ICU.

Promoting maternal–infant attachment

Promoting maternal–infant attachment depends on the condition of both the mother and her baby, and their physical locations. The best-case scenario is that the baby is able to 'room in' with the mother for periods of time in ICU. Skin-to-skin contact is recommended as it has many benefits for both mother and baby including a calming effect for both, neonatal temperature regulation and stimulation of the lactation hormones.[318] Alternatively, organising for either the baby to visit the mother in the ICU or the mother, if well enough, to visit the baby in the NICU is often feasible. Physically seeing and touching the baby is likely to be an important step for the mother. Digital technologies, like Skype, are used in some ICUs to enable the mother to see her baby in a different hospital and to watch significant events, such as the first bath.

The use of diaries, one about the mother's condition and one about the baby's progress, complete with photos, visitor and clinician entries, is another strategy that may be useful to promote maternal–infant attachment. The first few days following birth are often a blur for the mother, with little recollection of events. It is also common to have photographs of the baby for the mother to look at, and clinicians keep in touch with the nursery where the baby is being cared for and give the mother regular updates on the baby's condition.

Caring for the partner and other family members

The partner is likely to be shocked and distressed by the sudden and severe illness of the mother. The partner may also be torn between two ICUs, with the newborn admitted to a NICU in one hospital and the mother in an ICU in another hospital.[291] This situation is further compounded if there are other children to consider. Usual strategies such as explanations, facilitating visiting wherever possible and social work support are important.

Summary

Intensive care management of pregnant and postpartum women is challenging for a variety of reasons including, but not limited to, the presence of the fetus, physiological adaptations of pregnancy and clinical conditions that are unique to the obstetric population. ICU staff members are often not educationally prepared to provide midwifery care and there may be difficulty in obtaining midwifery and obstetric consultation. Importantly, childbirth is viewed as a normal, healthy event in our society and is usually a cause of celebration. A life-threatening event associated with childbirth may seem more overwhelming because of this context. The best outcomes for both the mother and her baby will result from collaborative and coordinated care between maternity and critical care service providers.

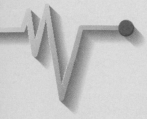

Case study

Julia Kaur presented to hospital with severe breathlessness at 32 weeks' gestation. Her vital signs on arrival were P 115, BP 110/65, RR 28, temperature 37.1°C and SpO_2 92%. Fetal movements were normal and the fetal heart rate was 150. Julia's uterus was not contracting (i.e. she was not in labour). Other symptoms included a new-onset cough and fatigue. Julia tells you that she visited her sister 3 days ago, and has just found out that she tested positive for COVID-19. As Julia was settling into her room, her breathing became more laboured, her respiratory rate increased to 34 and her SpO_2 dropped to 89%. A medical emergency team (MET) call was made, following which Julia was transferred to ICU.

In ICU, an arterial line was inserted along with usual ICU monitoring. The first ABG taken showed PaO_2 65 mmHg, $PaCO_2$ 28 mmHg, pH 7.41, and HCO_3 18. Initially BiPAP was applied to improve Julia's oxygenation. However, she kept taking the mask off and was becoming agitated. The decision was made to intubate Julia to manage her acute respiratory failure. Ventilator settings were synchronised intermittent mandatory ventilation (SIMV) with a mandatory rate set at 8; V_T 480 mL; positive end-expiratory pressure (PEEP) 8 cm; FiO_2 0.6. Her spontaneous breaths of about 8 per minute resulted in a MV of 7.5 L. Over the next few days, Julia received regular periods of prone ventilation, along with specific treatment for COVID-19, as the swab taken on arrival returned a positive result. Her condition improved, she was extubated and transferred to the maternity ward after 5 days of ICU treatment.

CASE STUDY QUESTIONS

1 Besides COVID-19, what other conditions could present in a similar way?
2 Review the physiological adaptations of pregnancy regarding respiratory function and normal ABG parameters.
3 Describe the methods used to assess fetal well-being in a woman 32 weeks pregnant.
4 Explain the specific considerations related to achieving an artificial airway in a woman who is 32 weeks pregnant. What staff and resources do you think you might need?
5 Identify any issues with medication used to enable the intubation and maintain sedation, with regards to the fetus.
6 Outline the process to position Julia for prone ventilation.
7 What support will be feasible to provide Julia's partner? What follow-up will Julia need?

RESEARCH VIGNETTE

Elmir R, Schmeid, V. A qualitative study of the impact of adverse birth experiences on fathers. Women Birth 2022;35:e41–8.[319]

Abstract

Background: Being present during labour and birth can, for some fathers, result in feelings of fear, uncertainty, anxiety and helplessness. Witnessing birth complications or adverse events may cause immediate and long-term anxiety and stress. In turn, this experience can impact on men's sense of self and identity as a man and father and can affect his relationship with his infant and partner. The aim of this study was to explore the immediate and longer-term impact of witnessing a complicated or adverse birth experience on men in heterosexual relationships and their role as a father.

Methods: An interpretive qualitative approach informed the design of this study. A total of 17 fathers, one from New Zealand and sixteen from Australia, participated through face-to-face, telephone and email interviews. The ages of the men were between 24 and 48 years, and the time since the adverse birth experience ranged from 4.5 months to 20.5 years.

Findings: Thematic analysis revealed three major themes representing men's experiences of witnessing a complicated birth or adverse event: 'Worst experience of my life', 'Negotiating my place: communicating with health professionals' and 'Growing stronger or falling apart'. Men were unprepared and feared for the lives of their infants and partners, and they expected and wanted to be involved in the birth and the maternity care journey; instead they were pushed to the side and excluded from the labour and birth during times of emergency. Being excluded from part or all of the birth perpetuated worry and vulnerability as, at times, men were left not knowing anything about what was happening to their partners. Midwives and other health professionals' support was important to the way fathers adjusted and processed the complications of the labour and birth event. This experience impacted on their own mental health and their relationship with their baby and partner.

Conclusion: Findings demonstrate that, following a complicated or adverse birth experience, men questioned their role as a father, their place in the family and their role at the birth. There is a need to include and inform the expectant father that help is available if they experience negative feelings of hopelessness or despair. Maternity services and care providers need to involve fathers so that they feel part of the maternity care system and journey, which may mitigate feelings of helplessness.

Critique

A qualitative methodology was appropriate in order to gain rich in-depth data and the study gained relevant ethical approval before commencing. To uphold the ethical principle of non-maleficence, all participants were provided with 'appropriate referral information' should they need psychological follow-up given the highly sensitive nature of the research topic (Elmir and & Schmied, 2021, p. e42).[319]

Volunteer sampling, a form of non-probability, purposive sampling, was used to gain participants and the sample size was determined when data saturation was achieved, which enhances research rigour.[320] Seventeen fathers comprised the entire sample, which was reached when data saturation was achieved and is appropriate in qualitative research.

A mixture of data collection methods was used based on the preference of the participants; interviews (by telephone or face to face) and email conversations combined with written completion of the interview schedule questions. The two researchers analysed the transcripts in their entirety using thematic analyses to elicit three major themes and used member checking (the returning to two participants to clarify parts of the data), which enhances the study's confirmability and credibility.[321]

The researchers addressed the issue of their personal and interpersonal reflexivity – that is, how their personal and professional experiences might influence the research, thereby enhancing the trustworthiness of the study.[322] The researcher conducting the interviews also acknowledged she held dual roles of midwife and researcher, but clarified her role as researcher with the participants before the interviews commenced so there were no misunderstandings she was present as a midwife, which may have meant the interviews became debriefing sessions.

Findings: The ages of the men ranged from 24 to 48 years and only six were not first-time fathers. The least time since the traumatic birth incident was 4.5 months and the longest was 20.5 years. Only six of the men had witnessed a vaginal birth while the other 11 men's partners had required caesarean births. The first theme was the 'Worst experience of my life' and encompassed the unexpected nature of emergencies for the men, being frightened seeing large numbers of staff coming into a birth room, not knowing what blood loss was normal, and, for some, their partners being transferred to the ICU and fear they may die and concerns they may have to raise a child on their own. The second theme 'Negotiating my place: communication with health professionals' describes how men felt regarding their communications with the healthcare professionals; often excluded through poor communication. The 'Relationships: growing stronger or falling apart' theme encompassed how the men's experiences influenced their relationships with their partners, their babies and how their mental health was sometimes affected after a complex or adverse birth incident. Throughout the findings section, the themes and subthemes are illustrated by the men's own quotes and this enhances the authenticity of the study.[321]

Discussion: This qualitative study highlights that the men were keen to be involved in the birth experience but felt excluded when complexities occurred with their negative feelings at the time of the emergencies linked to suboptimal communication, fear and helplessness. The researchers discuss how a lack or preparedness for birth can lead to unrealistic expectations, which can increase the possibility of men developing postnatal depression, and male postnatal depression rates in Australia are highlighted as equivalent to their female counterparts'.

The researchers discuss how, culturally, childbirth is often seen as the exclusive domain of women, quoting the work of Liamputttong and colleagues (2005).[323] The researchers highlight that, in their study, men from culturally and linguistically diverse (CALD) backgrounds ($n = 3$) felt less able to participate in the birth and less able to talk about their experiences, potentially making them more prone to depression and PTSD.

Implications for practice and conclusions: The researchers acknowledge that information reduced the men's stress and anxiety about their partner and the neonate and state the hospital environment *'provided little support and limits their role in decision making'* (p. 47). Continuity of care models can promote trust and communication and are viewed as a positive way of closing the communication gaps in midwifery and obstetrics. The researchers summarise that men who witness complications around the time of birth question *'their role as a father, their place on the family and their role at the birth'* (p. 47). More research is required to explore the experiences of those in same-sex relationships, first-time parents, older parents and those from CALD backgrounds.

Study limitations: Limitations acknowledged by the researchers include the findings not being generalisable to all fathers experiencing a traumatic birth, although the findings may be *transferable* to those in similar situations, from similar backgrounds and similar healthcare settings, bearing in mind that only three men were from CALD backgrounds.

Learning activities

1   Reflect on what is currently done in your unit to enhance the experiences of partners who have witnessed a traumatic birth/adverse birth incident/its sequelae.

2   On reviewing the Elmir and Schmied (2022) paper, are there any other things you think could be introduced to help partners who visit the critical care unit in terms of reducing their stress and anxiety?

3   What can be done to promote the maternal–infant relationship when a newly delivered mother is a patient in the ICU?

4   Why is it important to promote skin-to-skin contact for both mothers and their partners and what safety aspects (specific for skin to skin) need to be considered?

Online resources

Birth Trauma Associations (BTA), https://www.birthtraumaassociation.org.uk

Health talk.org (women's and partner's experiences of critical care), https://healthtalk.org/conditions-threaten-womens-lives-childbirth-pregnancy/experiences-of-intensive-care-unit-icu-or-high-dependency-units-hdu

MIND Support for women and their partners after a traumatic birth (UK),

https://www.mind.org.uk/information-support/types-of-mental-health-problems/postnatal-depression-and-perinatal-mental-health/partners/

NICE Post-traumatic stress disorder guideline, https://www.nice.org.uk/guidance/ng116

Perinatal Anxiety & Depression Aotearoa (PADA) New Zealand website proving resources for perinatal anxiety and depression, https://www.pada.nz

Perinatal Anxiety & Depression Australia (PANDA), https://panda.org.au/about/about-panda

UNICEF Breastfeeding resources, https://www.unicef.org.uk/babyfriendly/baby-friendly-resources/breastfeeding-resources/

Further reading

Hinton L, Locock L, Knight M. Maternal critical care: what can we learn from patient experience? A qualitative study. BMJ Open 2015;5(4):e006676.

Hollander M, van Hastenberg E, Dillen J, et al. Preventing traumatic childbirth experiences: 2192 women's perceptions and views. Arch Womens Ment Health 2017;20(4):515–23.

Huang X, Chen L, Zhang L. Effects of paternal skin-to-skin contact in newborns and fathers after cesarean delivery. J Perinat Neonatal Nurs 2019;33(1):68–73.

Schobinger E, Stuijfzand S, Horsch A. Acute and post-traumatic stress disorder symptoms in mothers and fathers following childbirth: a prospective cohort study. Front Psychiatr 2022;13:790170. doi: 10.3389/fpsyt.2020.56205.4.

References

1. Pollock W, Rose L, Dennis C-L. Pregnant and postpartum admissions to the intensive care unit: a systematic review. Intensive Care Med 2010;36:1465–74.

2. Maiden M, Finnis M, Duke G, et al. Obstetric admissions to intensive care units in Australia and New Zealand: a registry-based cohort study. BJOG 2020;127(12):1558–67.

3. Jardine J, Gurol-Urganci I, Harris T, et al. Associations between ethnicity and admission to intensive care among women giving birth: a cohort study. BJOG 2022;129(5):733–42.

4. Pollock WE, Harley NS, Nelson SM. Maternal severity of illness across levels of care: a prospective, cross-sectional study. Aust Crit Care 2011;24(4):218–28.

5. Safer Care Victoria (SCV). Victoria's mothers, babies and children 2020. Melbourne, VIC: SCV; 2022. Available from: https://www.safercare.vic.gov.au/publications/victorias-mothers-babies-and-children-2020-report-and-presentations. [Accessed 25 February 2023].

6. Zwart J, Dupuis J, Richters A, et al. Obstetric intensive care unit admission: a 2-year nationwide population-based cohort study. Intensive Care Med 2010;36(2):256–63.

7. Royal College of Anaesthetists (RCOA). Care of the critically ill woman in childbirth; enhanced maternal care. London: RCOA; 2018.

8. Lawton B, MacDonald EJ, Brown SA, et al. Preventability of severe acute maternal morbidity. Am J Obstet Gynecol 2014;210(6):557.e1–6.

9. Bijl R, Valensise H, Novelli G, et al. Methods and considerations concerning cardiac output measurement in pregnant women: recommendations of the International Working Group on Maternal Hemodynamics. Ultrasound Obstet Gynecol 2019;54(1):35–50.

10. Blackburn ST. Maternal, fetal and neonatal physiology: a clinical perspective. St Louis, MO: Elsevier; 2018.

11. Marshall J, Raynor M. Myles textbook for midwives. 17th ed. Edinburgh: Elsevier; 2020.

12. National Institute for Health and Care Excellence (NICE). Postnatal care. Guidance NG194. London: NICE; 2015.

13. Aguree S, Gernand AD. Plasma volume expansion across healthy pregnancy: a systematic review and meta-analysis of longitudinal studies. BMC Pregnancy Childbirth 2019;19(1):508.

14. Churchill D, Nair M, Stanworth SJ, Knight M. The change in haemoglobin concentration between the first and third trimesters of pregnancy: a population study. BMC Pregnancy Childbirth 2019;19(1):359.

15. Paterson-Brown S, Howell C, editors. Managing obstetric emergencies and trauma. The MOET course manual. 3rd ed. Cambridge, UK: Cambridge University Press; 2014.

16. Tanaka KA, Bharadwaj S, Hasan S, et al. Elevated fibrinogen, von Willebrand factor, and Factor VIII confer resistance to dilutional coagulopathy and activated protein C in normal pregnant women. Br J Anaesth 2019;122(6):751–9.

17. Royal College of Obstetricians and Gynaecologists (RCOG). Thrombosis and embolism during pregnancy and the puerperium, acute management. Green-top guideline no. 37b. London: RCOG; 2015. Available from: https://www.rcog.org.uk/media/wj2lpco5/gtg-37b-1.pdf. [Accessed 25 February 2023].

18. Szecsi PB, Jorgensen M, Klajnbard A, et al. Haemostatic reference intervals in pregnancy. Thromb Haemost 2010;103(4):718–27.

19. Murphy N, Broadhurst DI, Khashan AS, et al. Gestation-specific D-dimer reference ranges: a cross-sectional study. BJOG 2015;122(3):395–400.

20. Burrows R, Kelton J. Incidentally detected thrombocytopenia in healthy mothers and their infants. N Engl J Med 1988;319(3):142–5.

21. Yanamandra N, Chandraharan E. Anatomical and physiological changes in pregnancy and their implications in clinical practice. In: Chandraharan E, Arulkumaran S, editors. Obstetric and intrapartum emergencies: a practical guide to management. 2nd ed. Cambridge: Cambridge University Press; 2022, p. 1–9.

22. Sunitha M, Chandrasekharappa S, Brid SV. Electrocardiographic QRS axis, Q wave and T-wave changes in 2nd and 3rd trimester of normal pregnancy. J Clin Diagn Res 2014;8(9):BC17.

23. Mabie W, DiSessa T, Crocker L, et al. A longitudinal study of cardiac output in normal human pregnancy. Am J Obstet Gynecol 1994;170(3):849–56.

24. Lyall F, Robson SC, Bulmer JN. Spiral artery remodeling and trophoblast invasion in preeclampsia and fetal growth restriction: relationship to clinical outcome. Hypertension 2013;62(6):1046–54.

25. Clapp J, Capeless E. Cardiovascular function before, during, and after the first and subsequent pregnancies. Am J Cardiol 1997;80(11):1469–73.

26. Mulder E, de Haas S, Mohseni Z, et al. Cardiac output and peripheral vascular resistance during normotensive and hypertensive pregnancy – a systematic review and meta-analysis. BJOG 2022;129(5):696–707.

27. Green LJ, Mackillop LH, Salvi D, et al. Gestation-specific vital sign reference ranges in pregnancy. Obstet Gynecol 2020;135(3):653–64.

28. Meah VL, Cockcroft JR, Backx K, et al. Cardiac output and related haemodynamics during pregnancy: a series of meta-analyses. Heart 2016;102(7):518–26.

29. Jeejeebhoy FM, Zelop CM, Lipman S, et al. Cardiac arrest in pregnancy: a scientific statement from the American Heart Association. Circulation 2015;132(18):1747–73.

30. Winter C, Crofts J, Draycott T, et al. editors. PROMPT Practical obstetric multi-professional training. 3rd ed. Cambridge, UK: Cambridge University Press; 2017.

31. Royal College of Obstetricians and Gynaecologists (RCOG). Reducing the risk of venous thromboembolism during pregnancy and the puerperium. Green top guideline 37a. London: RCOG; 2015. Available from: https://www.rcog.org.uk/media/qejfhcaj/gtg-37a.pdf. [Accessed 25 February 2023].

32. Yoshida A, Kaji T, Yamada H, et al. Measurement of hemodynamics immediately after vaginal delivery in healthy pregnant women by electrical cardiometry. J Med Invest 2019;66(1.2):75–80.

33. Robson SC, Dunlop W, Moore M, et al. Haemodynamic changes during the puerperium: a Doppler and M-mode echocardiographic study. BJOG 1987;94(11):1028–39.

34. Rankin J, editor. Physiology in childbearing with anatomy and related biosciences. Edinburgh: Elsevier; 2017.

35. Norwitz E, Robinson J. Pregnancy-induced physiologic alterations. In: Phelan JP, Pacheco LD, Foley M, et al, editors. Critical care obstetrics. Oxford: John Wiley & Sons; 2019, p. 41–68.

36. Duvekot J, Peeters L. Maternal cardiovascular hemodynamic adaptation to pregnancy. Obstet Gynecol Surv 1994;48(12):S1–S4.

37. Jensen D, Duffin J, Lam Y-M, et al. Physiological mechanisms of hyperventilation during human pregnancy. Respir Physiol Neurobiol 2008;161(1):76–86.

38. Templeton A, Kelman G. Maternal blood-gases, PAO_2—PaO_2), physiological shunt and VD/VT in normal pregnancy. Br J Anaesth 1976;48(10):1001–4.

39. Prodromakis E, Trakada G, Tsapanos V, et al. Arterial oxygen tension during sleep in the third trimester of pregnancy. Acta Obstet Gynecol Scand 2004;83(2):159–64.

40. LoMauro A, Aliverti A. Respiratory physiology of pregnancy: physiology masterclass. Breathe (Sheff) 2015;11(4):297–301.

41. Boutourline-Young H, Boutourline-Young E. Alveolar carbon dioxide levels in pregnant, parturient and lactating subjects. BJOG 1956;63(4):509–28.

42. Matuszkiewicz-Rowińska J, Małyszko J, Wieliczko M. Urinary tract infections in pregnancy: old and new unresolved diagnostic and therapeutic problems. Arch Med Sci 2015;11(1):67–77.

43. Lopes van Balen VA, van Gansewinkel TAG, de Haas S, et al. Maternal kidney function during pregnancy: systematic review and meta-analysis. Ultrasound Obstet Gynecol 2019;54(3):297–307.

44. Klajnbard A, Szecsi PB, Colov NP, et al. Laboratory reference intervals during pregnancy, delivery and the early postpartum period. Clin Chem Lab Med 2010;48(2):237–48.

45. Mackenzie MJ, Woolnough MJ, Barrett N, et al. Normal urine output after elective caesarean section: an observational study. Int J Obstet Anesth 2010;19(4):379–83.

46. Cheung K, Tan L, Meher S; WHO Intrapartum Care Algorithms Working Group. Clinical algorithms for the management of intrapartum maternal urine abnormalities. BJOG 2022; Apr 12. doi: 10.1111/1471-0528.16726. Online ahead of print.

47. Bouyou J, Gaujoux S, Marcellin L, et al. Abdominal emergencies during pregnancy. J Visc Surg 2015;152(6 Suppl.):S105–15.

48. Baer J, Reis R, Arens R. Appendicitis in pregnancy: with changes in position and axis of the normal appendix in pregnancy. JAMA 1932;98(16):1359–64.

49. Augustin G, Majerovic M. Non-obstetrical acute abdomen during pregnancy. Eur J Obstet Gynecol Reprod Biol 2007;131(1):4–12.

50. Nakai A, Sekiya I, Oya A, et al. Assessment of the hepatic arterial and portal venous blood flows during pregnancy with Doppler ultrasonography. Arch Gynecol Obstet 2002;266(1):25–9.

51. Khatri R, Kulick N, Rementer RJB, et al. Pregnancy-related hormones increase nifedipine metabolism in human hepatocytes by inducing CYP3A4 expression. J Pharm Sci 2021;110(1):412–21.

52. Mor G. The unique immunologic and microbial aspects of pregnancy. Placenta 2017;57:226.

53. Miller EM. Changes in serum immunity during pregnancy. Am J Human Biol 2009;21(3):401–3.

54. Rogerson SJ, Hviid L, Duffy PE, et al. Malaria in pregnancy: pathogenesis and immunity. Lancet Infect Dis 2007;7(2):105–17.

55. Low J. Fetal asphyxia and brain damage. Fetal Maternal Med Rev 2001;12(2):139–58.

56. Jones D, Bhasale A, Bailey M, et al. Effect of a national standard for deteriorating patients on intensive care admissions due to cardiac arrest in Australia. Crit Care Med 2018;46(4):586–93.

57. Nair S, Spring A, Dockrell L, et al. Irish maternal early warning score. Ir J Med Sci 2020;189(1):229–35.

58. Crozier TM, Galt P, Wilson SJ, et al. Rapid response team calls to obstetric patients in a busy quaternary maternity hospital. Aust N Z J Obstet Gynaecol 2018;58(1):47–53.

59. Austin DM, Sadler L, McLintock C, et al. Early detection of severe maternal morbidity: a retrospective assessment of the role of an Early Warning Score System. Aust N Z J Obstet Gynaecol 2014;54(2):152–5.

60. National Institute for Health and Care Excellence (NICE). Hypertension in pregnancy: diagnosis and management. NICE guideline NG133. London: NICE; 2019. Available from: https://www.nice.org.uk/guidance/ng133/chapter/Recommendations#reducing-the-risk-of-hypertensive-disorders-in-pregnancy and ISHP. [Accessed 25 February 2023].

61. Magee LA, Brown MA, Hall DR, et al. The 2021 International Society for the Study of Hypertension in Pregnancy classification, diagnosis & management recommendations for international practice. Pregnancy Hypertens 2022;27:148–69.

62. Lowe SA, Bowyer L, Lust K, et al. SOMANZ guidelines for the management of hypertensive disorders of pregnancy 2014. Aust N Z J Obstet Gynaecol 2015;55(5):e1–29.

63. Druzin ML, Shields M, Peterson N, et al. Improving health care response to hypertensive disorders of pregnancy (v2.0), a California Maternal Quality Care Collaborative quality improvement toolkit. Palo Alto, CA: CMQCC; 2021. Available at: https://www.cmqcc.org/resources-tool-kits/toolkits. [Accessed 25 February 2023].

64. Gu N, Zheng Y, Dai Y. Severe maternal morbidity: admission shift from intensive care unit to obstetric high-dependency unit. BMC Pregnancy Childbirth 2022;22(1):1–7.

65. Say L, Chou D, Gemmill A, et al. Global causes of maternal death: a WHO systematic analysis. Lancet Glob Health 2014;2(6):e323–33.

66. Jardine J, NMPA Project Team. Maternity admissions to intensive care in England, Wales and Scotland in 2015/16: a report from the National Maternity and Perinatal Audit. London: Royal College of Obstetricians and Gynaecologists; 2019.

67. Magee LA, Nicolaides KH, von Dadelszen P. Preeclampsia. N Engl J Med 2022;386(19):1817–32.

68. Chappell LC, Cluver CA, Kingdom J, et al. Pre-eclampsia. Lancet 2021;398(10297):341–54.

69. Plasencia W, Maiz N, Bonino S, et al. Uterine artery doppler at 11 + 0 to 13 + 6 weeks in the prediction of pre-eclampsia. Ultrasound Obstet Gynecol 2007;30(5):742–9.

70. Redman CW, Sargent IL, Staff AC. IFPA senior award lecture: making sense of pre-eclampsia – two placental causes of preeclampsia? Placenta 2014;35:S20–5.

71. Kaitu'u-Lino TJ, Tuohey L, Ye L, et al. Endoglin production. Placenta 2013;34(2):168–73.

72. Han C, Chen Y-Y, Dong J-F. Prothrombotic state associated with preeclampsia. Curr Opin Hematol 2021;28(5):323–30.

73. Rolnik DL, Wright D, Poon LC, et al. Aspirin versus placebo in pregnancies at high risk for preterm preeclampsia. N Engl J Med 2017;377(7):613–22.

74. Mazer Zumaeta A, Wright A, Syngelaki A, et al. Screening for pre-eclampsia at 11–13 weeks' gestation: use of pregnancy-associated plasma protein-A, placental growth factor or both. Ultrasound Obstet Gynecol 2020;56(3):400–7.

75. Abalos E, Cuesta C, Grosso AL, et al. Global and regional estimates of preeclampsia and eclampsia: a systematic review. Eur J Obstet Gynecol Reprod Biol 2013;170(1):1–7.

76. Knight M. Eclampsia in the United Kingdom 2005. BJOG 2007;114(9):1072–8.

77. Pollock W, Peek MJ, Wang A, et al. Eclampsia in Australia and New Zealand: a prospective population-based study. Aust N Z J Obstet Gynaecol 2020;60(4):533–40.

78. Vigil-De Gracia P, Rojas-Suarez J, Ramos E, et al. Incidence of eclampsia with HELLP syndrome and associated mortality in Latin America. Int J Gynecol Obstet 2015;129(3):219–22.

79. Mahran A, Fares H, Elkhateeb R, et al. Risk factors and outcome of patients with eclampsia at a tertiary hospital in Egypt. BMC Pregnancy Childbirth 2017;17(1):435.

80. Schaap TP, Knight M, Zwart JJ, et al. Eclampsia, a comparison within the International Network of Obstetric Survey Systems. BJOG 2014;121(12):1521–8.

81. Weinstein L. Preeclampsia/eclampsia with hemolysis, elevated liver enzymes, and thrombocytopenia. Obstet Gynecol 1985;66(5):657–60.

82. Lisonkova S, Razaz N, Sabr Y, et al. Maternal risk factors and adverse birth outcomes associated with HELLP syndrome: a population-based study. BJOG 2020;127(10):1189–98.

83. Brown MA, Magee LA, Kenny LC, et al. Hypertensive disorders of pregnancy: ISSHP classification, diagnosis, and management recommendations for international practice. Hypertension 2018;72(1):24–43.

84. Knight M; UKOSS. Eclampsia in the United Kingdom 2005. BJOG 2007;114(9):1072–8.

85. Haram K, Svendsen E, Abildgaard U. The HELLP syndrome: clinical issues and management. A review. BMC Pregnancy Childbirth 2009;9(1):8.

86. Woudstra DM, Chandra S, Hofmeyr GJ, et al. Corticosteroids for HELLP (hemolysis, elevated liver enzymes, low platelets) syndrome in pregnancy. Cochrane Database Syst Rev 2010;9:CD008148.

87. Centre for Maternal and Child Enquiries. Saving mothers' lives: reviewing maternal deaths to make motherhood safer: 2006–2008. The eighth report of the confidential enquiries into maternal deaths in the United Kingdom. BJOG 2011;118(Suppl. 1):1–203.

88. Duley L, Meher S, Jones L. Drugs for treatment of very high blood pressure during pregnancy. Cochrane Database Syst Rev 2013;7:CD001449. doi: 10.1002/14651858.CD001449.pub3.

89. National Institute for Health and Care Excellence (NICE). Hypertension in pregnancy. Quality statement 3: antenatal blood pressure targets. London: NICE; 2017 [Available from: https://www.nice.org.uk/guidance/qs35/chapter/Quality-statement-3-Antenatal-blood-pressure-targets. [Accessed 25 February 2023].

90. Young BC, Levine RJ, Karumanchi SA. Pathogenesis of preeclampsia. Annu Rev Pathol 2010;5(1):173–92.

91. Sontia B, Touyz RM. Role of magnesium in hypertension. Arch Biochem Biophys 2007;458(1):33–9.

92. The Magpie Trial Group. Do women with pre-eclampsia, and their babies, benefit from magnesium sulphate? The Magpie trial: a randomised placebo-controlled trial. Lancet 2002;359(9321):1877–90.

93. Dennis AT, Solnordal CB. Acute pulmonary oedema in pregnant women. Anaesthesia 2012;67(6):646–59.

94. Dennis AT, Castro JM. Transthoracic echocardiography in women with treated severe pre-eclampsia. Anaesthesia 2014;69(5):436–44.

95. Royal College of Obstetricians and Gynaecologists (RCOG). Reducing the risk of venous thromboembolism during pregnancy and the puerperium. Green-top guideline no. 37a. London: RCOG; 2015.

96. Bartsch E, Medcalf KE, Park AL, et al. Clinical risk factors for pre-eclampsia determined in early pregnancy: systematic review and meta-analysis of large cohort studies. BMJ 2016;353:i1753.

97. Brown M, Best K, Pearce M, et al. Cardiovascular disease risk in women with pre-eclampsia: systematic review and meta-analysis. Eur J Epidemiol 2013;28(1):1–19.

98. Flood M, McDonald SJ, Pollock W, et al. Incidence, trends and severity of primary postpartum haemorrhage in Australia: a population-based study using Victorian Perinatal Data Collection data for 764 244 births. Aust N Z J Obstet Gynaecol 2019;59(2):228–34.

99. Knight M, Bunch K, Tuffnell D, et al. Saving lives, improving mothers' care - lessons learned to inform maternity care from the UK and Ireland Confidential Enquiries into Maternal Deaths and Morbidity 2017–19. Oxford: National Perinatal Epidemiology Unit, University of Oxford; 2021.

100. Royal College of Obstetricians and Gynaecologists (RCOG). Antepartum haemorrhage. Green–top guideline no. 63. London: RCOG; 2011 (updated 2014).

101. Metcalfe A. Maternal morbidity data in Australia: an assessment of the feasibility of standardised collection. Cat. no. PER56. Canberra, ACT: AIHW; 2012.

102. Varouxaki N, Gnanasambanthan S, Datta S, et al. Antepartum haemorrhage. Obstet Gynaecol Reprod Med 2018;28(8):237–42.

103. Battula SP, Mohammed NHA, Datta S. Antepartum haemorrhage. Obstet Gynaecol Reprod Med 2021;31(4):117–23.

104. Creasy R, Resnik R, Iams J, et al. Creasy and Resnik's maternal-fetal medicine. Principles and practice. 7th ed. Philadelphia: Elsevier Saunders; 2013.

105. Raj S, Kaur A, Grover S, et al. Maternal & perinatal outcome in antepartum hemorrhage-a clinical study. J Adv Med Dent Sci Res 2018;6(8):53–8.

106. Jauniaux E, Collins S, Burton GJ. Placenta accreta spectrum: pathophysiology and evidence-based anatomy for prenatal ultrasound imaging. Am J Obstet Gynecol 2018;218(1):75–87.

107. American College of Obstetricians and Gynecologists; Cahill AG, Beigi R, Heine RP, et al. Placenta accreta spectrum. Obstetric care consensus no. 7. American College of Obstetricians and Gynecologists. Am J Obstet Gynecol 2018;219(6):B2–16.

108. Sentilhes L, Seco A, Azria E, et al. Conservative management or cesarean hysterectomy for placenta accreta spectrum: the PACCRETA prospective study. Am J Obstet Gynecol 2022;226(6):839.e1–24.

109. Thurn L, Wikman A, Westgren M, et al. Massive blood transfusion in relation to delivery: incidence, trends and risk factors: a population based cohort study. BJOG 2019;126(13):1577–86.

110. Ahmadzia HK, Grotegut CA, James AH. A national update on rates of postpartum haemorrhage and related interventions. Blood Transfus 2020;18(4):247.

111. NSW Health. Maternity – prevention, detection, escalation and management of postpartum haemorrhage (PPH). Guideline document no. GL2017_018. Sydney, NSW: NSW Health; 2017.

112. National Blood Authority. Patient blood management guidelines. Module 5. Obstetrics and maternity. Canberra, ACT: National Blood Authority; 2015.

113. Cortet M, Deneux-Tharaux C, Dupont C, et al. Association between fibrinogen level and severity of postpartum haemorrhage: secondary analysis of a prospective trial. Br J Anaesth 2012;108(6):984–9.

114. National Blood Authority. Patient blood management guidelines. Module 1. Critical bleeding/massive transfusion. Canberra, ACT: National Blood Authority; 2011, updated 2022. Available from: https://www.blood.gov.au/pbm-guidelines. [Accessed 25 February 2023].

115. National Blood Authority. Patient blood management guidelines. Module 4. Critical care. Canberra, ACT: National Blood Authority; 2013. Available from: https://www.blood.gov.au/pbm-guidelines. [Accessed 25 February 2023].

116. Amgalan A, Allen T, Othman M, et al. Systematic review of viscoelastic testing (TEG/ROTEM) in obstetrics and recommendations from the women's SSC of the ISTH. J Thromb Haemost 2020;18(8):1813–38.

117. Bell SF, Collis RE, Pallmann P, et al. Reduction in massive postpartum haemorrhage and red blood cell transfusion during a national quality improvement project, Obstetric Bleeding Strategy for Wales, OBS Cymru: an observational study. BMC Pregnancy Childbirth 2021;21(1):377.

118. Shakur H, Roberts I, Fawole B, et al. Effect of early tranexamic acid administration on mortality, hysterectomy, and other morbidities in women with post-partum haemorrhage (WOMAN): an international, randomised, double-blind, placebo-controlled trial. Lancet 2017;389(10084):2105–16.

119. Phillips L, McLintock C, Pollock W, et al. Recombinant activated factor VII in obstetric hemorrhage: experiences from the Aust and New Zealand Haemostasis Registry. Anesth Analg 2009;109(6):1908–15.

120. Wang HY, Chang CT, Wu MS. Postpartum hemorrhage complicated with irreversible renal failure and central diabetes insipidus. Ren Fail 2002;24(6):849–52.

121. National Blood Authority. Prophylactic use of RhD immunoglobulin in pregnancy care. Canberra, ACT: National Blood Authority; 2021. Available from: https://www.blood.gov.au/pbm-guidelines. [Accessed 25 February 2023].

122. Roets M, Sturgess DJ, Wyssusek K, et al. Intraoperative cell salvage: a technology built upon the failures, fads and fashions of blood transfusion. Anaesth Intensive Care 2019;47(3 Suppl.):17–30.

123. King M, Wrench I, Galimberti A, et al. Introduction of cell salvage to a large obstetric unit: the first six months. Int J Obstet Anesth 2009;18(2):111–17.

124. Allam J, Cox M, Yentis SM. Cell salvage in obstetrics. Int J Obstet Anesth 2008;17(1):37–45.

125. Wang R, Luo T, Liu Z, et al. Intraoperative cell salvage is associated with reduced allogeneic blood requirements and has no significant impairment on coagulation function in patients undergoing cesarean delivery: a retrospective study. Arch Gynecol Obstet 2020;301(5):1173–80.

126. Phillips JM, Sakamoto S, Buffie A, et al. How do I perform cell salvage during vaginal obstetric hemorrhage? Transfusion 2022;62(6):1159–65.

127. Clark SL. Amniotic fluid embolism. Obstet Gynecol 2014;123(2, Part 1):337–48.

128. Tuffnell DJ, Slemeck E. Amniotic fluid embolism. Obstet Gynaecol Reprod Med 2017;27(3):86–90.

129. Clark SL, Hankins GD, Dudley DA, et al. Amniotic fluid embolism: analysis of the national registry. Am J Obstet Gynecol 1995;172(4):1158–69.

130. Bouvet L, Gariel C, Charvet A, et al. Contribution of blood detection of insulin-like growth factor binding protein-1 for the diagnosis of amniotic-fluid embolism: a retrospective multicentre cohort study. BJOG 2021;128(12):1966–73.

131. Yang R, Lang M, Li H, et al. Immune storm and coagulation storm in the pathogenesis of amniotic fluid embolism. Eur Rev Med Pharmacol Sci 2021;25(4):1796–803.

132. Shechtman M, Ziser A, Markovits R, et al. Amniotic fluid embolism: early findings of transesophageal echocardiography. Anesth Analg 1999;87(6):1456.

133. Conde-Agudelo A, Romero R. Amniotic fluid embolism: an evidence-based review. Am J Obstet Gynecol 2009; 201(5):e1–13.

134. Knight M, Berg C, Brocklehurst P, et al. Amniotic fluid embolism incidence, risk factors and outcomes: a review and recommendations. BMC Pregnancy Childbirth 2012;12:7.

135. Stafford IA, Moaddab A, Dildy GA, et al. Amniotic fluid embolism syndrome: analysis of the Unites States International Registry. Am J Obstet Gynecol MFM 2020;2(2):100083.

136. McDonnell N, Knight M, Peek MJ, et al. Amniotic fluid embolism: an Australian–New Zealand population-based study. BMC Pregnancy Childbirth 2015;15(1):1–7.

137. Knight M, Tuffnell D, Brocklehurst P, et al, on behalf of the UKOSS. Incidence and risk factors for amniotic-fluid embolism. Obstet Gynecol 2010;115(5):910–27. doi: 10.1097/AOG.0b013e3181d9f629.

138. Combs CA, Montgomery DM, Toner LE, et al. Society for Maternal–Fetal Medicine special statement: checklist for initial management of amniotic fluid embolism. Am J Obstet Gynecol 2021;224(4):B29–32.

139. Pacheco LD, Clark SL, Klassen M, et al. Amniotic fluid embolism: principles of early clinical management. Am J Obstet Gynecol 2020;222(1):48–52.

140. Simard C, Yang S, Koolian M, et al. The role of echocardiography in amniotic fluid embolism: a case series and review of the literature. Can J Anesth 2021;68(10):1541–8.

141. Benson MD. Amniotic fluid embolism mortality rate. J Obstet Gynecol Res 2017;43(11):1714–18

142. Fitzpatrick KE, Tuffnell D, Kurinczuk JJ, et al. Incidence, risk factors, management and outcomes of amniotic-fluid embolism: a population-based cohort and nested case–control study. BJOG 2016;123(1):100–9.

143. Bauersachs J, König T, van der Meer P, et al. Pathophysiology, diagnosis and management of peripartum cardiomyopathy: a position statement from the Heart Failure Association of the European Society of Cardiology Study Group on peripartum cardiomyopathy. Eur J Heart Fail 2019;21(7):827–43.

144. Davis MB, Arany Z, McNamara DM, et al. Peripartum cardiomyopathy: JACC state-of-the-art review. J Am Coll Cardiol 2020;75(2):207–21.

145. Hilfiker-Kleiner D, Struman I, Hoch M, et al. 16-kDa Prolactin and bromocriptine in postpartum cardiomyopathy. Curr Heart Fail Rep 2012;9(3):174–82.

146. Sliwa K, Petrie M, Hilfiker-Kleiner D, et al. Long-term prognosis, subsequent pregnancy, contraception and overall management of peripartum cardiomyopathy: practical guidance paper from the Heart Failure Association of the European Society of Cardiology Study Group on Peripartum Cardiomyopathy. Eur J Heart Fail 2018;20(6):951–62.

147. Honigberg MC, Givertz MM. Peripartum cardiomyopathy. BMJ 2019;364:k5287.

148. Mallikethi-Reddy S, Akintoye E, Trehan N, et al. Burden of arrhythmias in peripartum cardiomyopathy: analysis of 9841 hospitalizations. Int J Cardiol 2017;235:114–17.

149. Hilfiker-Kleiner D, Haghikia A, Berliner D, et al. Bromocriptine for the treatment of peripartum cardiomyopathy: a multicentre randomized study. Eur Heart J 2017;38(35):2671–9.

150. Hilfiker-Kleiner D, Sliwa K. Pathophysiology and epidemiology of peripartum cardiomyopathy. Nat Rev Cardiol 2014;11(6):364–70.

151. Knight M, Nair M, Tuffnel D, et al. Saving Lives, Improving mothers' care – surveillance of maternal deaths in the UK 2012-14 and lessons learned to inform maternity care from the UK and Ireland Confidential Enquiries into Maternal Deaths and Morbidity 2009-14. Oxford: National Perinatal Epidemiology Unit, University of Oxford; 2016.

152. Hutchens J, Frawley J, Sullivan EA. Cardiac disease in pregnancy and the first year postpartum: a story of mental health, identity and connection. BMC Pregnancy Childbirth 2022;22(1):382.

153. van der Linde D, Konings EEM, Slager MA, et al. Birth prevalence of congenital heart disease worldwide: a systematic review and meta-analysis. J Am Coll Cardiol 2011;58(21):2241–7.

154. Hoang TT, Goldmuntz E, Roberts AE, et al. The Congenital Heart Disease Genetic Network study: cohort description. PLoS One 2018;13(1):e0191319.

155. Pierpont ME, Brueckner M, Chung WK, et al. Genetic basis for congenital heart disease: revisited: a scientific statement from the American Heart Association. Circulation 2018;138(21):e653–711.

156. Persson M, Cnattingius S, Villamor E, et al. Risk of major congenital malformations in relation to maternal overweight and obesity severity: cohort study of 1.2 million singletons. BMJ 2017;357:j2563.

157. Helle EIT, Biegley P, Knowles JW, et al. First trimester plasma glucose values in women without diabetes are associated with risk for congenital heart disease in offspring. J Pediatr 2018;195:275–8.

158. Chen L, Yang T, Chen L, et al. Risk of congenital heart defects in offspring exposed to maternal diabetes mellitus: an updated systematic review and meta-analysis. Arch of Gynecol Obstet 2019;300(6):1491–506.

159. Koster MPH, van Duijn L, Krul-Poel YHM, et al. A compromised maternal vitamin D status is associated with congenital heart defects in offspring. Early Hum Dev 2018;117:50–6.

160. Feng Y, Yu D, Yang L, et al. Maternal lifestyle factors in pregnancy and congenital heart defects in offspring: review of the current evidence. Italian J Pediatr 2014;40(1):85.

161. Nembhard WN, Tang X, Hu Z, et al. Maternal and infant genetic variants, maternal periconceptional use of selective serotonin reuptake inhibitors, and risk of congenital heart defects in offspring: population based study. BMJ 2017;356:j832.

162. Silversides CK, Marelli A, Beauchesne L, et al. Canadian Cardiovascular Society 2009 consensus conference on the management of adults with congenital heart disease: executive summary. Can J Cardiol 2010;26(3):143–50.

163. Baumgartner H, De Backer J, Babu-Narayan SV, et al. 2020 ESC Guidelines for the management of adult congenital heart disease: the task force for the management of adult congenital heart disease of the European Society of Cardiology (ESC). Endorsed by: Association for European Paediatric and Congenital Cardiology (AEPC), International Society for Adult Congenital Heart Disease (ISACHD). Eur Heart J 2021;42(6):563–645.

164. Bracher I, Padrutt M, Bonassin F, et al. Burden and impact of congenital syndromes and comorbidities among adults with congenital heart disease. Int J Cardiol 2017;240:159–64.

165. Regitz-Zagrosek V, Roos-Hesselink JW, Bauersachs J, et al. 2018 ESC guidelines for the management of cardiovascular diseases during pregnancy: the task force for the management of cardiovascular diseases during pregnancy of the European Society of Cardiology (ESC). Eur Heart J 2018;39(34):3165–241.

166. Cauldwell M, Steer PJ, Bonner S, et al. Retrospective UK multicentre study of the pregnancy outcomes of women with a Fontan repair. Heart 2018;104(5):401–6.

167. Zentner D, Kotevski A, King I, et al. Fertility and pregnancy in the Fontan population. Int J Cardiol 2016;208:97–101.

168. RHDAustralia (ARF/RHD writing group). The 2020 Australian guideline for prevention, diagnosis and management of acute rheumatic fever and rheumatic heart disease. 3rd ed. Darwin, NT: Menzies School of Health Research.; 2020.

169. Otto CM, Nishimura RA, Bonow RO, et al. 2020 ACC/AHA guideline for the management of patients with valvular heart disease: executive summary: a report of the American College of Cardiology/American Heart Association Joint Committee on Clinical Practice Guidelines. J Am Coll Cardiol 2021;77(4):450–500.

170. Tripathi B, Kumar V, Pitiliya A, et al. Trends in incidence and outcomes of pregnancy-related acute myocardial infarction (from a nationwide inpatient sample database). Am J Cardiol 2019;123(8):1220–7.

171. James AH, Jamison MG, Biswas MS, et al. Acute myocardial infarction in pregnancy: a United States population-based study. Circulation 2006;113(12):1564–71.

172. Elkayam U, Havakuk O. Pregnancy-associated coronary artery dissection: a therapeutic dilemma. J Am Coll Cardiol 2018;71(4):469–70.

173. Baris L, Hakeem A, Moe T, et al. Acute coronary syndrome and ischemic heart disease in pregnancy: data from the EURObservational research programme – European Society of Cardiology registry of pregnancy and cardiac disease. J Am Heart Assoc 2020;9(15):e015490.

174. Brener A, Briller J. Cardiovascular testing and imaging in pregnant women. Cardiol Clin 2021;39(1):21–32.

175. Morton A, Morton A. High sensitivity cardiac troponin I levels in preeclampsia. Pregnancy Hypertens 2018;13:79–82.

176. Dockree S, Brook J, Shine B, et al. Cardiac-specific troponins in uncomplicated pregnancy and pre-eclampsia: a systematic review. PLoS One 2021;16(2):e0247946.

177. Ravichandran J, Woon SY, Quek YS, et al. High-sensitivity cardiac troponin I levels in normal and hypertensive pregnancy. Am J Med 2019;132(3):362–6.

178. van Hagen IM, Cornette J, Johnson MR, et al. Managing cardiac emergencies in pregnancy. Heart 2017;103(2):159–73.

179. De Martino A, Morganti R, Falcetta G, et al. Acute aortic dissection and pregnancy: review and meta-analysis of incidence, presentation, and pathologic substrates. J Cardiac Surg 2019;34(12):1591–7.

180. Pfaller B, Sathananthan G, Grewal J, et al. Preventing complications in pregnant women with cardiac disease. J Am Coll Cardiol 2020; 75(12):1443–52.

181. Malhamé I, Hurlburt H, Larson L, et al. Sensitivity and specificity of B-type natriuretic peptide in diagnosing heart failure in pregnancy. Obstet Gynecol 2019;134(3):440–9.

182. Halpern DG, Weinberg CR, Pinnelas R, et al. Use of medication for cardiovascular disease during pregnancy. J Am Coll Cardiol 2019;73(4):457–76.

183. Bartalena L, Bogazzi F, Braverman LE, et al. Effects of amiodarone administration during pregnancy on neonatal thyroid function and subsequent neurodevelopment. J Endocrinol Invest 2001;24(2):116–30.

184. Canobbio MM, Warnes CA, Aboulhosn J, et al. Management of pregnancy in patients with complex congenital heart disease: a scientific statement for healthcare professionals from the American Heart Association. Circulation 2017;135(8):e50–87.

185. Jha N, Jha AK, Chand Chauhan R, et al. Maternal and fetal outcome after cardiac operations during pregnancy: a meta-analysis. Ann Thorac Surg 2018;106(2):618–26.

186. Carlier L, Devroe S, Budts W, al. Cardiac interventions in pregnancy and peripartum – a narrative review of the literature. J Cardiothorac Vasc Anesth 2020;34(12):3409–19.

187. Voortman M, Roos JW, Slomp J, et al. Strategies for low-molecular-weight heparin management in pregnant women with mechanical prosthetic heart valves: a nationwide survey of Dutch practice. Int J Cardiol Congen Heart Dis 2022;9:100373.

188. Kjaergaard AB, Fuglsang J, Hvas A-M, editors. Anti-Xa monitoring of low-molecular-weight heparin during pregnancy: a systematic review. Semin Thromb Hemost 2021;47(7):824042

189. McLaughlin K, Foureur M, Jensen ME, et al. Review and appraisal of guidelines for the management of asthma during pregnancy. Women Birth 2018;31(6):e349–57.

190. Robijn AL, Bokern MP, Jensen ME, et al. Risk factors for asthma exacerbations during pregnancy: a systematic review and meta-analysis. Eur Respir Rev 2022;31(164):220039.

191. Scottish Intercollegiate Guidelines Network, British Thoracic Society. Sign 158 British guideline on the management of asthma. A national clinical guideline. Revised ed. Edinburgh: Healthcare Improvement Scotland; 2019. Available from: https://www.sign.ac.uk/media/1773/sign158-updated.pdf. [Accessed 25 February 2023].

192. Robijn AL, Jensen ME, Gibson PG, et al. Trends in asthma self-management skills and inhaled corticosteroid use during pregnancy and postpartum from 2004 to 2017. J Asthma 2019;56(6):594–602.

193. Beau A-B, Didier A, Hurault-Delarue C, et al. Prescription of asthma medications before and during pregnancy in France: an observational drug study using the EFEMERIS database. J Asthma 2017;54(3):258–64.

194. Coates AL, Wanger J, Cockcroft DW, et al. ERS technical standard on bronchial challenge testing: general considerations and performance of methacholine challenge tests. Eur Respir J 2017;49(5):1601526.

195. Bonham CA, Patterson KC, Strek ME. Asthma outcomes and management during pregnancy. Chest 2018;153(2):515–27.

196. Jensen ME, Robijn AL, Gibson PG, et al. Longitudinal analysis of lung function in pregnant women with and without asthma. J Allergy Clin Immunol Pract 2021;9(4):1578–85.e3.

197. Steven G, Whitworth M, Cox S. Substance misuse in pregnancy. Obstet Gynaecol Reprod Med 2014;24(10):309–14.

198. Petrone P, Jiménez-Morillas P, Axelrad A, et al. Traumatic injuries to the pregnant patient: a critical literature review. Eur J Trauma Emerg Surg 2019;45(3):383–92.

199. Murphy NJ, Quinlan JD. Trauma in pregnancy: assessment, management, and prevention. Am Fam Physician 2014;90(10):717–22.

200. Huls CK, Detlefs C. Trauma in pregnancy. Semin Perinatol 2018;42(1):13–20.

201. World Health Organization (WHO). Violence against women prevalence estimates, 2018: global, regional and national prevalence estimates for intimate partner violence against women and global and regional prevalence estimates for non-partner sexual violence against women. Geneva: WHO; 2021. Licence: CC BY-NC-SA 3.0 IGO.

202. Devries KM, Kishor S, Johnson H, et al. Intimate partner violence during pregnancy: analysis of prevalence data from 19 countries. Reprod Health Matters 2010;18(36):158–70.

203. National Institute for Health and Care Excellence (NICE). Domestic violence and abuse: multi-agency working. Public health guideline PH50. London: NICE; 2016. Available from: https://www.nice.org.uk/guidance/ph50. [Accessed 25 February 2023].

204. Almeida FSJ, Coutinho EC, Duarte JC, et al. Domestic violence in pregnancy: prevalence and characteristics of the pregnant woman. J Clin Nurs 2017;26(15-16):2417–25.

205. Auger N, Low N, Lee GE, et al. Pregnancy outcomes of women hospitalized for physical assault, sexual assault, and intimate partner violence. J Interpers Violence 2022;37(13-14):NP11135. doi: 10.1177/0886260520985496.

206. Lutgendorf MA. Intimate partner violence and women's health. Obstet Gynecol 2019;134(3):470–80.

207. Amezcua-Prieto C, Ross J, Rogozińska E, et al. Maternal trauma due to motor vehicle crashes and pregnancy outcomes: a systematic review and meta-analysis. BMJ Open 2020;10(10):e035562.

208. Chibber R, Al-Harmi J, Fouda M, et al. Motor-vehicle injury in pregnancy and subsequent feto-maternal outcomes: of grave concern. J Matern Fetal Neonatal Med 2015;28(4):399–402.

209. Brown H. Trauma in pregnancy. Obstet Gynecol 2009;114(1):147–60.

210. Haddox A, Hausselle J, Azoug A. Changes in segmental mass and inertia during pregnancy: a musculoskeletal model of the pregnant woman. Gait Posture 2020;76:389–95.

211. Queensland Clinical Guidelines. Trauma in pregnancy. Document number: MN19.31-V2-R24. Brisbane, QLD: Queensland Health; 2019.

212. Tibbott J, Di Carlofelice M, Menon R, et al. Trauma and pregnancy. TOG 2021;23(4):258–64.

213. Karafin MS, Glisch C, Souers RJ, et al. Use of fetal hemoglobin quantitation for Rh-positive pregnant females: a national survey and review of the literature. Arch Pathol Lab Med 2019;143(12):1539–44.

214. Beckett V, Knight M, Sharpe P. The CAPS Study: incidence, management and outcomes of cardiac arrest in pregnancy in the UK: a prospective, descriptive study. BJOG 2017;124(9):1374–81.

215. Goodnight WHMD, Soper DEMD. Pneumonia in pregnancy. Crit Care Med 2005;33(10 Suppl.):S390–S7.

216. ANZIC Influenza Investigators, Australasian Maternity Outcomes Surveillance System. Critical illness due to 2009 A/H1N1 influenza in pregnant and postpartum women: population based cohort study. BMJ 2010;340:c1279.

217. Webb SA, Pettila V, Seppelt I, et al. Critical care services and 2009 H1N1 influenza in Australia and New Zealand. N Engl J Med 2009; 361(20):1925–34.

218. Allotey J, Stallings E, Bonet M, et al. Clinical manifestations, risk factors, and maternal and perinatal outcomes of coronavirus disease 2019 in pregnancy: living systematic review and meta-analysis. BMJ 2020;370:m3320.

219. Knight M, Bunch K, Cairns A, et al. Saving lives, improving mothers' care rapid report: learning from SARS-CoV-2-related and associated maternal deaths in the UK March–May 2020. Oxford: National Perinatal Epidemiology Unit; 2020.

220. Vogel JP, Tendal B, Giles M, et al. Clinical care of pregnant and postpartum women with COVID-19: Living recommendations from the National COVID-19 Clinical Evidence Taskforce. Aust N Z J Obstet Gynaecol 2020;60(6):840–51.

221. D'Souza R, Ashraf R, Rowe H, et al. Pregnancy and COVID-19: pharmacologic considerations. Ultrasound Obstet Gynecol 2021;57(2):195–203.

222. Lapinsky SE, Al Mandhari M. COVID-19 critical illness in pregnancy. Obstet Med 2022;15(4):220–4.

223. Prasad S, Kalafat E, Blakeway H, et al. Systematic review and meta-analysis of the effectiveness and perinatal outcomes of COVID-19 vaccination in pregnancy. Nature Commun 2022;13(1):2414.

224. Perl SH, Uzan-Yulzari A, Klainer H, et al. SARS-CoV-2–specific antibodies in breast milk after COVID-19 vaccination of breastfeeding women. JAMA 2021;325(19):2013–14.

225. Gibbs R, Bauer M, Olvera L, et al. Improving diagnosis and treatment of maternal sepsis: a quality improvement toolkit. Stanford, CA: California Maternal Quality Care Collaborative; 2020.

226. Knight M, Nair M, Tuffnell D, et al, on behalf of MBRRACE-UK. Saving lives, improving mothers' care – lessons learned to inform maternity care from the UK and Ireland Confidential Enquiries into Maternal Deaths and Morbidity 2013–15. Oxford: National Perinatal Epidemiology Unit; 2017.

227. Albright CM, Has P, Rouse DJ, et al. Internal validation of the sepsis in obstetrics score to identify risk of morbidity from sepsis in pregnancy. Obstet Gynecol 2017;130(4):747–55.

228. Bowyer L, Robinson HL, Barrett H, et al. SOMANZ guidelines for the investigation and management sepsis in pregnancy. Aust N Z J Obstet Gynaecol 2017;57(5):540–51.

229. Daniels R, Nutbeam T, editors. The sepsis manual. 6th ed. United Kingdom Sepsis Trust; 2022. Available from: https://sepsistrust.org/professional-resources/education-resources/. [Accessed 25 February 2023].

230. Cohen LS, Altshuler LL, Harlow BL, et al. Relapse of major depression during pregnancy in women who maintain or discontinue antidepressant treatment. JAMA 2006;295(5):499–507.

231. Kulkarni J. Special issues in managing long-term mental illness in women. Int Rev Psychiatry 2010;22(2):183–90.

232. Chin K, Wendt A, Bennett IM, et al.. Suicide and maternal mortality. Curr Psychiatry Rep 2022;24(4):239–75.

233. VanderKruik R, Barreix M, Chou D, et al. The global prevalence of postpartum psychosis: a systematic review. BMC Psychiatry 2017;17(1):272.

234. Tschinkel S, Harris M, Le Noury J, et al. Postpartum psychosis: two cohorts compared, 1875–1924 and 1994–2005. Psychol Med 2007;37:529–36.

235. Spinelli M. Postpartum psychosis: a diagnosis for the DSMV. Arch Womens Ment Health 2021;24(5):817–22.

236. Sharma V, Mazmanian D, Palagini L, et al. Postpartum psychosis: revisiting the phenomenology, nosology, and treatment. J Affect Disord Rep 2022;10:100378.

237. Howard LM, Molyneaux E, Dennis C-L, et al. Non-psychotic mental disorders in the perinatal period. Lancet 2014;384(9956):1775–88.

238. Wisner KL, Sit DK, McShea MC, et al. Onset timing, thoughts of self-harm, and diagnoses in postpartum women with screen-positive depression findings. JAMA Psychiatry 2013;70(5):490–8.

239. National Institute for Health and Care Excellence (NICE). Antenatal and postnatal mental health: clinical management and service guidance. NICE clinical guideline 192. London: NICE; 2020. Available from: https://www.nice.org.uk/guidance/cg192. [Accessed 25 February 2023].

240. Molenaar NM, Bais B, Lambregtse-van den Berg MP, et al. The international prevalence of antidepressant use before, during, and after pregnancy: a systematic review and meta-analysis of timing, type of prescriptions and geographical variability. J Affect Disord 2020;264:82–9.

241. Chow S, Creighton P, Chambers G, et al. Report of the Australian and New Zealand Neonatal Network 2019. Sydney, NSW: ANZNN 2021.

242. Selin H, Stone PK, editors. Childbirth across cultures: ideas and practices of pregnancy. London, New York: Springer; 2009.

243. Sullivan EA, Dickinson JE, Vaughan GA, et al. Maternal super-obesity and perinatal outcomes in Australia: a national population-based cohort study. BMC Pregnancy Childbirth 2015;15(1):1–10.

244. Martin A, Krishna I, Ellis J, et al. Super obesity in pregnancy: difficulties in clinical management. J Perinatol 2014;34(7):495–502.

245. Creanga AA, Catalano PM, Bateman BT. Obesity in pregnancy. N Engl J Med 2022;387(3):248–59.

246. Catalano PM, Shankar K. Obesity and pregnancy: mechanisms of short term and long term adverse consequences for mother and child. BMJ 2017;356:1.

247. McDonnell NJ, Paech MJ, Clavisi OM, et al. Difficult and failed intubation in obstetric anaesthesia: an observational study of airway management and complications associated with general anaesthesia for caesarean section. Int J Obstet Anesth 2008;17(4):292–7.

248. Lapinsky SE, editor. Management of acute respiratory failure in pregnancy. Semin Respir Crit Care Med 2017;38(2):201–7.

249. Cousins L. Fetal oxygenation, assessment of fetal well-being, and obstetric management of the pregnant patient with asthma. J Allergy Clin Immunol 1999;103(2, Suppl. 1):S343–9.

250. Bhatia PK, Biyani G, Mohammed S, et al. Acute respiratory failure and mechanical ventilation in pregnant patient: a narrative review of literature. J Anaesthesiol Clin Pharmacol 2016;32(4):431–9.

251. Ray B, Trikha A. Prone position ventilation in pregnancy: concerns and evidence. J Obstet Anaesth Crit Care 2018;8(1):7–9.

252. Primrose A, Roy N, Teo M, et al. Prone positioning of pregnant patients for lumbar spinal surgery. Anaesth Cases 2014;2(2):103–6.

253. Casabella AM, Urakov TM, Basil G, et al. Management of foramen magnum meningioma during pregnancy: literature review and case report. World Neurosurg 2017;97:752.e15–18.

254. Dennis AT, Hardy L, Leeton L. The prone position in healthy pregnant women and in women with preeclampsia – a pilot study. BMC Pregnancy Childbirth 2018;18(1):445.

255. Nakai Y, Mine M, Nishio J, et al. Effects of maternal prone position on the umbilical arterial flow. Acta Obstet Gynecol Scand 1998;77(10):967–9.

256. Tolcher MC, McKinney JR, Eppes CS, et al. Prone positioning for pregnant women with hypoxemia due to coronavirus disease 2019 (COVID-19). Obstet Gynecol 2020;136(2):259–61.

257. Gaffney A. Critical care in pregnancy – is it different? Semin Perinatol 2014;38(6):329–40.

258. Intensive Care National Audit & Research Centre (INARC). Female admissions (aged 16-50 years) to adult, general critical care units in England, Wales and Northern Ireland reported as 'currently pregnant' or 'recently pregnant'. Report from the Intensive Care National Audit & Research Centre. London: INARC; 2013.

259. Judd FA, Haran SS, Everett TR. Antenatal fetal wellbeing. Obstet Gynaecol Reprod Med 2020;30(7):197–204.

260. Baschat AA, Galan HL, Lee W, et al. The role of the fetal biophysical profile in the management of fetal growth restriction. Am J Obstet Gynecol 2022;226(4):475–86.

261. Medicines and Healthcare Products Regulatory Agency (MHPRA). Fetal monitor/cardiotocograph (CTG) – adverse outcomes still reported. London: MHPRA; 2010. Available from: https://www.gov.uk/drug-device-alerts/medical-device-alert-fetal-monitor-cardiotocograph-ctg-adverse-outcomes-still-reported. [Accessed 25 February 2023].

262. Afors K, Chandraharan E. Use of continuous electronic fetal monitoring in a preterm fetus: clinical dilemmas and recommendations for practice. J Pregnancy 2011; 2011848794. doi: 10.1155/2011/848794.

263. Grivell RM, Alfirevic Z, Gyte GML, Devane D. Antenatal cardiotocography for fetal assessment. Cochrane Database Syst Rev 2015;2015(9): CD007863.

264. Nageotte MP. Fetal heart rate monitoring. Semin Fetal Neonatal Med 2015;20(3):144–8.

265. Grivell RM, Wong L, Bhatia V. Regimens of fetal surveillance for impaired fetal growth. Cochrane Database Syst Rev 2012;2012(6):CD007113.

266. Lees C, Stampalija T, Baschat A, et al. ISUOG practice guidelines: diagnosis and management of small-for-gestational-age fetus and fetal growth restriction. Ultrasound Obstet Gynecol 2020;56(2):298–312.

267. World Health Organization (WHO). Maternal mortality ratio (per 100 000 live births). Geneva: WHO; n.d. Available from: https://www.who.int/data/gho/indicator-metadata-registry/imr-details/26. [Accessed 25 February 2023].

268. National Institute for Health and Care Excellence (NICE). Preterm labour and birth. NICE guideline NG25. London: NICE; 2015, updated 2022 Available from: https://www.nice.org.uk/guidance/ng25. [Accessed 25 February 2023].

269. Stock SJ, Thomson AJ, Papworth S, the Royal College of Obstetricians and Gynaecologists. Antenatal corticosteroids to reduce neonatal morbidity and mortality. BJOG 2022;129(8):e35–60.

270. De Silva DA, Synnes AR, von Dadelszen P, et al. MAGnesium sulphate for fetal neuroprotection to prevent Cerebral Palsy (MAG-CP) – implementation of a national guideline in Canada. Implement Sci 2018;13(1):8.

271. Bain E, Middleton P, Crowther CA. Different magnesium sulphate regimens for neuroprotection of the fetus for women at risk of preterm birth. Cochrane Database Syst Rev 2012;2:CD009302. doi: 10.1002/14651858.CD009302.pub2.

272. Vilchez G, Dai J, Lagos M, et al. Maternal side effects & fetal neuroprotection according to body mass index after magnesium sulfate in a multicenter randomized controlled trial. J Matern Fetal Neonatal Med 2018;31(2):178–83.

273. National Institute for Health and Care Excellence (NICE). High-throughput non-invasive prenatal testing for fetal RHD genotype. NICE diagnostics guidance DG25. London: NICE; 2016. Available from: https://www.nice.org.uk/guidance/dg25. [Accessed 25 February 2023].

274. Hyland CA, O'Brien H, Flower RL, et al. Non-invasive prenatal testing for management of haemolytic disease of the fetus and newborn induced by maternal alloimmunisation. Transfus Apher Sci 2020;59(5):102947.

275. Zeng Z, Liu F, Li S. Metabolic adaptations in pregnancy: a review. Ann Nutr Metab 2017;70(1):59–65.

276. Wilmot EG, Mansell P. Diabetes and pregnancy. Clin Med 2014;14(6):677–80.

277. National Institute for Health and Care Excellence (NICE). Diabetes in pregnancy: management from preconception to the postnatal period. Clinical guideline NG3. London: NICE; 2015, updated 2020. Available from: https://www.nice.org.uk/guidance/ng3. [Accessed 25 February 2023].

278. Zelop CM, Einav S, Mhyre JM, et al. Cardiac arrest during pregnancy: ongoing clinical conundrum. Am J Obstet Gynecol 2018;219(1):52–61.

279. Vanden Hoek TL, Morrison LJ, Shuster M, et al. Part 12: Cardiac arrest in special situations: 2010 American Heart Association guidelines for cardiopulmonary resuscitation and emergency cardiovascular care. Circulation 2010;122(18 Suppl. 3):S829–61.

280. Lott C, Truhlář A, Alfonzo A, et al. European Resuscitation Council Guidelines 2021: cardiac arrest in special circumstances. Resuscitation 2021;161:152–219.

281. Benson MD, Padovano A, Bourjeily G, et al. Maternal collapse: challenging the four-minute rule. EBioMedicine 2016;6:253–7.

282. Zieleskiewicz L, Chantry A, Duclos G, et al. Intensive care and pregnancy: Epidemiology and general principles of management of obstetrics ICU patients during pregnancy. Anaesth Crit Care Pain Med 2016;35(Suppl. 1):S51–7.

283. Panchal AR, Bartos JA, Cabañas JG, et al. Part 3: Adult basic and advanced life support: 2020 American Heart Association guidelines for cardiopulmonary resuscitation and emergency cardiovascular care. Circulation 2020;142(16 Suppl. 2):S366–468.

284. Dallmann A, Ince I, Coboeken K, et al. A physiologically based pharmacokinetic model for pregnant women to predict the pharmacokinetics of drugs metabolized via several enzymatic pathways. Clin Pharmacokinet 2018;57(6):749–68.

285. Hodge LS, Tracy TS. Alterations in drug disposition during pregnancy. Expert Opin Drug Metab Toxicol 2007;3(4):557–71.

286. Scaffidi J, Mol B, Keelan J. The pregnant women as a drug orphan: a global survey of registered clinical trials of pharmacological interventions in pregnancy. BJOG 2017;124(1):132–40.

287. Littleford J. Effects on the fetus and newborn of maternal analgesia and anesthesia: a review. Can J Anesth 2004;51(6):586–609.

288. Lee P, Eisman JA, Center JR. Vitamin D deficiency in critically ill patients. N Engl J Med 2009;360(18):1912–14.

289. Camargo CA Jr, Rifas-Shiman SL, Litonjua AA, et al. Maternal intake of vitamin D during pregnancy and risk of recurrent wheeze in children at 3 y of age. Am J Clin Nutr 2007;85(3):788–95.

290. Abu-Saad K., Fraser D. Maternal nutrition and birth outcomes. Epidemiol Rev 2010;32:5–25.

291. Ray JG, Urquia ML, Berger H, et al. Maternal and neonatal separation and mortality associated with concurrent admissions to intensive care units. CMAJ 2012; 184(18):e956–62.

292. National Institute for Health and Care Excellence (NICE). Postnatal care. NICE guideline NG194. London: NICE; 2021. Available from: https://www.nice.org.uk/guidance/ng194. [Accessed 25 February 2023].

293. Sherman D, Lurie S, Frenckle E, et al. Characteristics of normal lochia. Am J Perinatol 1999;16(8):399–402.

294. Fletcher S, Grotegut CA, James AH. Lochia patterns among normal women: a systematic review. J Womens Health (Larchmt) 2012;21(12):1290–4.

295. Watson J, Hermann S, Johnson B. Developing a policy to support breastfeeding in women who are hospitalized and acutely ill. Nurs Womens Health 2013;17(3):188–96.

296. Fehr K, Moossavi S, Sbihi H, et al. Breastmilk feeding practices are associated with the co-occurrence of bacteria in mothers' milk and the infant gut: the CHILD cohort study. Cell Host Microbe 2020;28(2):285–97. e4.

297. Ho NT, Li F, Lee-Sarwar KA, et al. Meta-analysis of effects of exclusive breastfeeding on infant gut microbiota across populations. Nature Commun 2018;9(1):1–13.

298. Azad MB, Kozyrskyj AL. Perinatal programming of asthma: the role of gut microbiota. Clin Dev Immunol 2012;2012:932072.

299. Hair AB, Peluso AM, Hawthorne KM, et al. Beyond necrotizing enterocolitis prevention: improving outcomes with an exclusive human milk–based diet. Breastfeed Med 2016;11(2):70–4.

300. Truchet S, Honvo-Houéto E. Physiology of milk secretion. Best Pract Res Clin Endocrinol Metab 2017;31(4):367–84.

301. Ballard O, Morrow AL. Human milk composition: nutrients and bioactive factors. Pediatr Clin N Am 2013;60(1):49–74.

302. Neville MC, Allen JC, Archer PC, et al. Studies in human lactation: milk volume and nutrient composition during weaning and lactogenesis. Am J Clin Nutr 1991;54(1):81–92.

303. Grattan DR. Behavioural significance of prolactin signalling in the central nervous system during pregnancy and lactation. Reproduction 2002;123(4):497–506.

304. UNICEF. Protecting, promoting and supporting breastfeeding: the Baby-friendly Hospital Initiative for small, sick and preterm newborns. Geneva: World Health Organization and the United Nations Children's Fund. Licence: CC BY-NC-SA 3.0 IGO. 2020.

305. Morse J, Jehle C, Gamble D. Initiating breastfeeding: a world survey of the timing of postpartum breastfeeding. Int J Nurs Stud 1990; 27(3):303–13.

306. UNICEF UK and The Baby Friendly Hospital Initiative National Health Service. Off to the best start, important information about feeding your baby. London: Public Health England: 2015.

307. Becker GE, Smith HA, Cooney F. Methods of milk expression for lactating women. Cochrane Database Syst Rev 2016;9:CD006170. doi: 10.1002/14651858.CD006170.pub5.

308. Oladapo OT, Fawole B. Treatments for suppression of lactation. Cochrane Database Syst Rev 2012;2012(9):CD005937.

309. Royal College of Obstetricians and Gynaecologists (RCOG). Late intrauterine fetal death and stillbirth. Green-top guideline No. 55. London: RCOG; 2010.

310. Crepinsek MA, Taylor EA, Michener K, et al. Interventions for preventing mastitis after childbirth. Cochrane Database Syst Rev 2020;9(9): CD007239.

311. Dennis C-L, Jackson K, Watson J. Interventions for treating painful nipples among breastfeeding women. Cochrane Database Syst Rev 2014;12:CD007366. doi: 101002/14651858CD007366pub2.

312. Hotham N, Hotham E. Drugs in breastfeeding. Aust Prescriber 2015;38(5):156–9.

313. American College of Obstetricians and Gynecologists. Committee opinion No. 646: Ethical considerations for including women as research participants. Obstet Gynecol 2015;126(5):e100–7.

314. Hale T. Medications in breastfeeding mothers of preterm infants. Pediatr Ann 2003;32(5):337–47.

315. Miller J, Tonkin E, Damarell RA, et al. A systematic review and meta-analysis of human milk feeding and morbidity in very low birth weight infants. Nutrients 2018;10(6):707.

316. Jones I, Shakespeare J. Postnatal depression. BMJ 2014;349:g4500.

317. de Graaff LF, Honig A, van Pampus MG, et al. Preventing post-traumatic stress disorder following childbirth and traumatic birth experiences: a systematic review. Acta Obstet Gynecol Scand 2018;97(6):648–56.

318. UNICEF UK. The Baby Friendly Initiative. Skin to skin contact. London: UNICEF; 2018. Available from: https://www.unicef.org.uk/babyfriendly/baby-friendly-resources/implementing-standards-resources/skin-to-skin-contact/. [Accessed 25 February 2023].

319. Elmir R, Schmied V. A qualitative study of the impact of adverse birth experiences on fathers. Women Birth 2022;35(1):e41–8.

320. Harvey M, Land L. Research methods for nurses and midwives: theory and practice. Los Angeles, London: SAGE; 2017.

321. Connelly LM. Trustworthiness in qualitative research. Med Surg Nurs 2016;25(6):435–6.

322. Olmos Vega FM, Stalmeijer RE, Varpio L, et al. A practical guide to reflexivity in qualitative research. AMEE Guide no. 149. Med Teach 2022;Apr 7:1–11.

323. Liamputtong P, Yimyam S, Parisunyakul S, et al. Traditional beliefs about pregnancy and child birth among women from Chiang Mai, Northern Thailand. Midwifery 2005;21(2):139–53.

Chapter 29

Organ donation and transplantation

Holly Northam, Bronwyn Levvey

Learning objectives

After reading this chapter, you should be able to:

- discuss why organ donation is a rare opportunity
- describe the physiological characteristics of death
- understand the tests that are used to confirm brain and circulatory death
- differentiate between the different types of living and deceased organ and tissue donation for transplantation practices
- discuss the implications of informed and presumed consent to organ and tissue donation.
- discuss community expectations about donation at the end of life
- describe your advocacy role in the process of potential donor recognition and referral in critical care and emergency settings
- describe the principles of end-of-life care of the dying or deceased person in the critical care setting before and after donation surgery.

Introduction

We had two doctors and a nurse in there telling us about what had happened and what possibilities we had to deal with it. I think we all really trusted and valued their opinions, and they were really good at remaining [separate] that it was our decision not theirs.

(Avril, wife of deceased)[1]

As a critical care nurse you are afforded the extraordinary privilege to enable organ and tissue donation for transplantation. This can be achieved only through collaborative teamwork in the critical care environment linking to a wider national and international network of professionals. The challenge you face is to provide excellence in end-of-life care while, at the same time, maintaining the vision that the work you are involved in is potentially saving and improving the lives of the equivalent of an intensive care unit full of people that you may never meet.

People of all ages wait for this evidence-based and highly regarded treatment including those suffering end-stage organ failure caused by no fault of their own, children in need of bone donation to prevent amputation caused by

KEY WORDS

care of the organ
    donor
cultural safety
death
donation after
    circulatory
    determination of
    death
donation after
    neurological
    determination of
    death
donor
end-of-life care
family
organ donation
tissue donation
transplantation
trauma

cancer, burns patients in need of skin grafts, those who are blind hoping for a corneal graft to enable vision and so many more. Patients, their families and often entire communities that support and care for them are known to be hoping and waiting for lifesaving and transforming gifts of donation.

It needs to be remembered that critical care nurses are at times also the ones providing care to those waiting for transplant and following transplantation surgery – the scope and value of the work is immense.

This chapter seeks to provide a brief overview of the critical care nurse's role in the multidisciplinary team and the care that is required to support the dying/deceased person and their family to enable donation for transplantation; the role of the nurse in successful transplantation; the clinical implications of living and deceased organ and tissue donation and processes and practices required to enable donation for successful transplantation. Every effort has been made to humanise and normalise the language used in this chapter to enable the reader to model language that supports trust, good end-of-life care and organ donation.

In the words of a donor family member keeping a bedside vigil while awaiting the arrival of the surgical transplant team, '*I now understand, nurses are the invisible thread that makes the whole process work*' (Personal communication, Northam, 2009).

Regarded as an experimental procedure until the 1980s, today transplantation is the best lifesaving treatment for end stage organ failure and is performed in 112 countries worldwide.[2] Organs that are transplanted include heart, lungs, liver, kidneys, pancreas and intestine – sometimes in combined approaches. Face and hand transplantation have transformed the lives of people who have suffered mutilating conditions, and uterus transplantation also now offers hope. Organ and tissue transplantation is an established method of lifesaving and cost-effective treatment that offers severely ill people a chance of survival and improved quality of life. The lack of organs and tissue for transplant purposes is a global problem. Many patients never have had the opportunity to be listed on a waiting list for a transplant because of the shortage. Long periods on the waiting list for organ transplantation may result in clinical deterioration, resulting in the removal of desperate patients from the waiting list; others may die because of their condition before a transplant becomes available.

Australia is a world leader in successful transplant outcomes; however, the waiting list for transplantation is increasing by approximately 10% per year and was sitting at 1850 by the end of 2021.[2] This number is not representative of the need, as many people suffering organ failure are never assessed for a transplant or considered for this treatment in Australia.[3–5] In Australia, deaths of people on the waiting list are not published, so it is difficult to quantify the true human impact of the organ shortage.

In the USA, over 106,000 people are waiting for a transplantation, and approximately 20 individuals die each day while waiting.[6] In the member states of the European Union (EU), approximately 35,000 transplants are performed yearly but more than 55,000 patients are waiting for an organ transplantation, and 11 of those die each day because there was no organ available.[6,7]

The potential of organ rejection was one reason that limited the number of transplants performed until the early 1980s when medical advances in the prevention of rejection led to more successful transplants and an increase in demand.[8]

Allografts are transplanted organs or tissues from one person (living or deceased) to another person. The first successful human-to-human transplant of any kind was a corneal transplant performed in Moravia (now the Czech Republic) in 1905. The first successfully transplanted human organ was performed in 1954 at the Peter Bent Brigham Hospital in Boston and was a living kidney donation between identical twins. By the late 1960s, transplantation of the liver, heart and pancreas became successful while transplantation of the lungs and intestines began in the 1980s.[2] Kidney transplantation surgery commenced in Australia in the mid 1960s, followed by liver, heart, lung and pancreas transplantation in the 1980s.[9] It should be noted that, although much was written about the success of this novel intervention, the impact on the donor family was scarcely regarded.[1]

In 1968, Harvard Medical School produced a report on the 'hopelessly unconscious patient', described as having 'no discernible central nervous system activity'.[10] The epidemic of polio and advances in intensive care and ventilation for comatose patients had revealed a group of patients who suffered 'coma impasse' ('beyond coma').[11] To enable certainty in treatment decisions for families and medical teams, an extensive study that involved postmortem examination of the brains of these deceased patients discovered that the brain tissue was necrotic and any recovery or ability to breathe, hear, see and manage cranial nerve responses had been destroyed by the pathophysiological process of hypoxia.[11] This report noted that life (organ) support could be withdrawn from patients diagnosed with 'irreversible coma' or 'brain death' (terms they used interchangeably) and that, with appropriate consent, the organs could be removed for transplantation.[10] The committee's primary concern was to provide an acceptable course of action to permit withdrawal of mechanical ventilator support for the purpose of ending needless suffering for those witnessing the situation, and subsequently also enabling organ donation for human transplantation. It was seen as a moral imperative to enable treatment to be withdrawn from people who were never going to recover; their relative's lives were in limbo knowing their family member was 'gone' but medical staff were unable to stop ventilation and organ supportive interventions waiting until the person went into cardiac arrest and death could be announced.[10]

In 1981, a USA President's Commission declared that individual death depended on either irreversible cessation of circulatory and respiratory functions or irreversible cessation of all functions of the entire brain. The consequent *Uniform Determination of Death Act* referred to 'whole-brain death' as a requirement for the determination of brain death.[12] Similar laws were adopted internationally: in Europe, Spain got their law defining brain death in 1979 and in Sweden the law came in 1988. The law defined brain death and enabled circulation to be maintained until the transplant team were in a position to recover the organs; at this time cardiac standstill occurs when the donation surgery is undertaken. Donation after the confirmation of brain death retrieval was enacted in New Zealand in 1964, and in Australia the first legislation to enable organ donation for transplantation was enacted in the *Transplantation and Anatomy Act* 1978 in the ACT.[13] Legislation heralded the establishment of formal transplant programs. It should be noted that, in each country and setting that enacts transplantation programs, the definition of death remains consistent but the guidelines for determining death may differ.[14] The success of transplantation in the current era as a viable option for end-stage organ failure is primarily due to the growth in understanding of the immune response and the discovery of the immunosuppression agent cyclosporin A, which has been followed by many subsequent significant advances in immunosuppression therapies, reducing rates of acute rejection and graft loss.[15,16]

Vignette: Brian Myerson, memories of waiting for a transplant

When will it be my turn? Every few weeks somebody else at our very large dialysis clinic seems to have died. The mood is very glum today as Robert has not come to his session. We are advised by the nurses that he passed away. Rumours are that he had become disillusioned and had given up. Apparently, he decided to drink a massive amount of fluid along with a large dose of sleeping pills. We all know that that is the way to die for patients on dialysis.

Today's mood is rather unusual as most of the time we all try to overlook our situation on dialysis and try to focus on joking and more pleasant issues. It's pretty difficult going through this process and hiding it from our closest people as we want to protect them as much as we can from the trauma that we all are living through. There is a wonderful camaraderie between us as we try to bolster each other. How lucky are we to have such a great group dialysing together three times every week? And what a fantastic group of nurses! Well, most of them. Some of them are a bit grumpy, but we try to lift their spirits.

How is this going to end? Transplant or death? Which will come first? All we know is that Australia has a very low organ donation rate so the chances are that we will die before a lifesaving organ transplant will be offered to us. Can't think about this as it's just too depressing. My 5-hour session is about to end so time to prepare to 'come off'. Can't wait to get up, go for a walk and focus on the other part of my life away from the dialysis clinic.

Hopefully one day soon I will be a transplant recipient.

Brian received a kidney/pancreas transplant in 1999 that enables him to live a productive life without dialysis or diabetes.

Donation and consent systems

There are currently two general systems of approach to seeking consent for living and deceased organ and tissue donation in operation around the world. Some countries, for example Spain, Singapore, Austria and Wales, have legislated an 'opt out', or presumed consent, system where eligible persons are considered for organ and tissue retrieval at the time of their death if they have not previously indicated their explicit objection.[17,18] Spain leads the world in donation rates that are supported by a strong commitment to donation by families who are asked to decide on behalf of their relative at the time of death by skilled doctors and nurses. Spain does not have a donor register and there is no formal system to record objections or consent to donate.[19] The Spanish approach arose because of community protests with marching in the streets to support patients who were unable to receive transplants. The Spanish government subsequently legislated a 'presumed' consent model because it was evident from the population response that most people supported the idea of donating their organs following death. In 1989, 10 years after the legislative change to 'opt-out', the implementation of a national transplant organisation was the trigger for donation rates to improve.[19]

In Australia, New Zealand, the USA, parts of the UK and many other common-law countries derived from British colonisation, the approach is to 'opt in', with specific consent required from the potential donor's next of kin.[2] In Australia, people can indicate an intent and consent to organ and or tissue donation, selecting what they are comfortable to donate, on the Australian Organ Donor Register (AODR) administered by the Australian Government Department of Human Services.[20] It should be noted that people can donate if not listed on the organ donor register. In practice their family will still be asked for authorisation to donate, and it is important that the question of the person's end-of-life wishes are discussed with the family regardless if it is thought that organ donation is possible; this improves the bereavement experience for family members who, when reflecting on the experience, often regret that donation wasn't discussed, thinking they should have raised the discussion, but failed to do so – overwhelmed by the circumstances. In situations where a person's wishes are known, families are generally more inclined to agree to donate if that was the person's known wish.

In Singapore, the *Human Organ Transplant Act* of 1987 combines a presumed consent system with a required consent system for the Muslim population. The informed consent laws of Japan and Korea are two of the most recent to come into force, in 1997 and 2000 respectively, to allow donation after neurological death; before then, only living donation and donation after cardiac death were possible.[21]

Types of donations

Organ and tissue donation includes retrieval of organs and tissues both after death and from a living person. Donations from a living person include regenerative tissue (blood and bone marrow) and non-regenerative tissue (cord blood, kidneys, liver (lobe/s), lungs (lobe/s), femoral heads). The implications of consent are different for each type of requested tissue. For example, the collection of bone marrow and the retrieval of a kidney, the lobe of a liver or lung are invasive procedures that could potentially risk the health and well-being of the donor. In contrast, donation of a femoral head could be the end-product of a total hip replacement, where the bone is otherwise discarded. Similarly, cord blood from the umbilical cord is discarded if not retrieved immediately after birth. Solid organs can be donated via two pathways: donation after neurological determination of death (DNDD) and donation after circulatory determination of death (DCDD). Solid organs that are able to be donated include heart, lungs, liver, kidneys, pancreas and intestine, and these donors can also donate tissues, including eyes, heart valves, bone and musculoskeletal tissues, if they meet strict criteria.[22]

In many situations where organ donation is not possible, tissue donation may still be possible, in some cases up to 24 hours following the death of the person. This opportunity can provide great comfort to family members who are upset that they cannot do 'more' to help others through organ donation. Tissue donation can be facilitated following deaths in a range of environments in hospital and critical care settings, as well as from the coroner's forensic mortuary and in some cases even after deaths at home.

In 2014, hands and faces were added to the organ transplant list in the USA.[23] Known as vascularised composite allotransplantation (VCA), it is the transplantation of a vascularised body part containing multiple tissue types as an anatomical/structural unit. Protocols for this are determined by individual agencies with no international guidelines yet developed.[24]

Organ donation and transplant networks

The donation and transplantation process in many countries, including Australia and New Zealand, the USA and European countries, is a nationally coordinated network in the healthcare system.[23,24]

International perspectives

From an international perspective, donation and transplantation networks have collaborated to develop consensus on donation and transplantation protocols. As such, the World Health Organization (WHO) guiding principles on human cell, tissue and organ transplantation have been established to apply to both living and deceased donation[22] (Table 29.1).

Many countries internationally, including Australia, have responded with the adoption of reform initiatives to improve organ and tissue donation rates for transplantation, including:

1 An appropriate legal and ethical framework
2 A national coordinating body
3 Hospital-based clinical donation specialists
4 Specialist training for clinical staff in management of the deceased donation process and family donation conversations
5 Implementation of a clinical governance framework that supports quality assurance and audit of hospital clinical practice and governance of the donation process

TABLE 29.1

World Health Organization (WHO) guiding principles on human cell, tissue and organ transplantation

Guiding Principle 1	Cells, tissues and organs may be removed from the bodies of deceased persons for the purpose of transplantation if: (a) any consent required by law is obtained, and (b) there is no reason to believe that the deceased person objected to such removal.
Guiding Principle 2	Physicians determining that a potential donor has died should not be directly involved in cell, tissue or organ removal from the donor or subsequent transplantation procedures; nor should they be responsible for the care of any intended recipient of such cells, tissues and organs.
Guiding Principle 3	Donation from deceased persons should be developed to its maximum therapeutic potential, but adult living persons may donate organs as permitted by domestic regulations. In general, living donors should be genetically, legally or emotionally related to their recipients. Live donations are acceptable when the donor's informed and voluntary consent is obtained, when professional care of donors is ensured and follow-up is well organised, and when selection criteria for donors are scrupulously applied and monitored. Live donors should be informed of the probable risks, benefits and consequences of donation in a complete and understandable fashion; they should be legally competent and capable of weighing the information; and they should be acting willingly, free of any undue influence or coercion.
Guiding Principle 4	No cells, tissues or organs should be removed from the body of a living minor for the purpose of transplantation other than narrow exceptions allowed under national law. Specific measures should be in place to protect the minor and, wherever possible, the minor's assent should be obtained before donation. What is applicable to minors also applies to any legally incompetent person.
Guiding Principle 5	Cells, tissues and organs should only be donated freely, without any monetary payment or other reward of monetary value. Purchasing, or offering to purchase, cells, tissues or organs for transplantation, or their sale by living persons or by the next of kin for deceased persons, should be banned. The prohibition on sale or purchase of cells, tissues and organs does not preclude reimbursing reasonable and verifiable expenses incurred by the donor, including loss of income, or paying the costs of recovering, processing, preserving and supplying human cells, tissues or organs for transplantation.
Guiding Principle 6	Promotion of altruistic donation of human cells, tissues or organs by means of advertisement or public appeal may be undertaken in accordance with domestic regulation. Advertising the need for or availability of cells, tissues or organs, with a view to offering or seeking payment to individuals for their cells, tissues or organs, or, to the next of kin, where the individual is deceased, should be prohibited. Brokering that involves payment to such individuals or to third parties should also be prohibited.
Guiding Principle 7	Physicians and other health professionals should not engage in transplantation procedures, and health insurers and other payers should not cover such procedures, if the cells, tissues or organs concerned have been obtained through exploitation or coercion of, or payment to, the donor or the next of kin of a deceased donor.
Guiding Principle 8	All healthcare facilities and professionals involved in cell, tissue or organ procurement and transplantation procedures should be prohibited from receiving any payment that exceeds the justifiable fee for the services rendered.
Guiding Principle 9	The allocation of organs, cells and tissues should be guided by clinical criteria and ethical norms, not financial or other considerations. Allocation rules, defined by appropriately constituted committees, should be equitable, externally justified and transparent.
Guiding Principle 10	High-quality, safe and efficacious procedures are essential for donors and recipients alike. The long-term outcomes of cell, tissue and organ donation and transplantation should be assessed for the living donor as well as the recipient in order to document benefit and harm. The level of safety, efficacy and quality of human cells, tissues and organs for transplantation, as health products of an exceptional nature, must be maintained and optimised on an ongoing basis. This requires implementation of quality systems including traceability and vigilance, with adverse events and reactions reported, both nationally and for exported human products.
Guiding Principle 11	The organisation and execution of donation and transplantation activities, as well as their clinical results, must be transparent and open to scrutiny, while ensuring that the personal anonymity and privacy of donors and recipients are always protected.

Source: Reprinted from World Health Organization (WHO), Guiding principles on human cell, tissue and organ transplantation. https://apps.who.int/iris/bitstream/handle/10665/341814/WHO-HTP-EHT-CPR-2010.01-eng.pdf?sequence=1. [Accessed November 2022].

6 Financial support to donor hospitals to ensure that costs related to donor management are not a barrier to donation

7 Media engagement and national community awareness and education

8 International cooperation to share best practice through data reporting.[1]

Regulation and management

In Australia, quality processes involved in organ and tissue retrieval and transplant are governed by the Therapeutic Goods Administration, State Government law and professional bodies.[2,26] Other countries have similar agencies that regulate the standards for healthcare products including organ and tissue donation.[21] In Australia, the process of potential donor identification and management in critical care is directed by the Australian and New Zealand Intensive Care Society (ANZICS) (Box 29.1). Donor criteria and organ allocation is regulated by the Transplantation Society of Australia and New Zealand (TSANZ). Donor and recipient data are collated by the Australia and New Zealand Organ Donation Registry (ANZOD Registry) and published on an annual basis.[27] The laws governing organ donation in New Zealand and Australia take the form of legislated Acts covering the use of human tissue both before and after death which differ between states.[2] These laws enable a person to choose to be a donor, and organ donation can proceed unless that wish is reversed or the family does not consent. If the deceased's wishes are not apparent, consent for organ donation rests with the next of kin.

In 1977, the Australian Law Reform Commission addressed the absence of a definition of death in Australian law, recommending that a statutory definition of death should be introduced. They recommended that death be defined as:

1 irreversible cessation of all function of the brain of the person, or

2 irreversible cessation of circulation of blood in the body of the person.[2,27]

Tissue donation is also very tightly regulated in all of Australia and New Zealand. In Australia the Commonwealth statutory body is the Therapeutic Goods Administration (TGA),[26] and in New Zealand the statutory body is the Medicines and Medical Devices Safety Authority (MEDSAFE). Tissue has extraordinary therapeutic benefits when available.

Internationally, a dual approach to consensus has evolved: an international governmental response coordinated by the World Health Assembly and WHO, and a professional response formulated through collaboration with international societies led by The Transplantation Society and the International Society of Nephrology.[23]

In 2014, the Department of Service Delivery and Safety at the WHO consulted with 20 independent experts from all six WHO regions across the world to establish a global agreement on the clinical criteria in the

---

BOX 29.1

Medical management of the potential donor[32]

Referral

- Refer all potential organ donors to the local state DonateLife agency or the regional organ procurement organisation, even if uncertain of medical suitability. Criteria for suitability change over time and may vary according to recipient circumstances (i.e. if someone is on the critical list).

Medical management

- Maintain MAP >70 mmHg: maintain euvolaemia, if required administer vasopressor agents (e.g. noradrenaline (norepinephrine) and/or vasopressin 0.5–2.0 U/h).
- Maintain adequate organ perfusion (monitor UO, lactate); consider invasive haemodynamic monitoring.
- Monitor electrolytes (Na^+, K^+) every 2–4 h and correct to normal range.
- Suspected diabetes insipidus (UO >200 mL/h, rising serum sodium): administer desmopressin (DDAVP) (e.g. 4 micrograms IV in adults) and replace volume loss with 5% dextrose or sterile water for infusion (via CVAD only, observing closely for signs of haemolysis).
- Treat hyperglycaemia (Actrapid infusion): aim for blood glucose 5–8 mmol/L.
- Keep temp >35°C. Pre-emptive use of warming blankets is advised as hypothermia may be difficult to reverse once it has developed.
- Provide ongoing respiratory care (suctioning when needed, positioning/turning, PEEP, recruitment manoeuvres).
- Maintain haemoglobin >80 g/L.

Hormone replacement therapy

The use of hormonal replacement therapy remains controversial and it is infrequently used in Australia. Some centres use it in the setting of persistent haemodynamic instability (despite volume resuscitation and low-dose inotropes) and/or if cardiac ejection fraction <45%. Typical regimens include:

- liothyronine (triiodothyronine) (T3) – 4 micrograms IV bolus, then 3 micrograms/h by IV infusion
- arginine vasopressin (AVP) – 0.5–4.0 U/h to maintain MAP 70 mmHg
- methylprednisolone – 15 mg/kg IV single bolus.

CVAD = central venous access device; IV = intravenous; MAP = mean arterial pressure; PEEP = positive end-expiratory pressure; UO = urine output.

determination of death. As a result, a 'brain death' algorithm was proposed to determine 'neurological arrest', when the traditional cardiocirculatory criteria of death cannot be applied. This algorithm identified the three general components of the process, including:

- the basic requirements that must exist for triggering the algorithm
- the clinical examination and diagnosis
- confirmatory testing to ensure irreversibility.[28]

Professional education

Health professional education in organ and tissue donation has been cited as a key initiative in increasing the donor rate globally.[29,30] The Transplant Procurement Management (TPM) program is an international collaboration that provides training education in organ donation and transplantation for health professionals across over 100 countries, with the aim of increasing the quantity, quality and effectiveness of organ and tissue donation for transplantation through a variety of training initiatives. In Australia, the Australian Organ and Tissue Authority (AOTA) provides funding to each DonateLife Agency across all states and territories in Australia to offer a Professional Education Package (PEP) for all clinicians involved in all aspects of organ and tissue donation and transplantation.[2] The PEP package was developed with collaboration from agencies in both Europe and the USA and has been adopted internationally.

Identification of organ and tissue donors

The four main factors that directly influence the number of multiorgan donations are:

- incidence of neurological (brain) death
- identification of potential donors (both circulatory death and neurological death donors)
- neurological (brain) death confirmation and informed consent for donation
- donor management after neurological (brain) death.

Neurological death

The incidence of neurological death (formerly known as brain death) has traditionally determined the size of the potential organ donor pool. Diagnosis of neurological death is now widely accepted, and most developed countries have legislation governing the definition of death and the retrieval of organs for transplant.[22,31]

The most common cause of neurological death has changed over time from traumatic head injury to cerebrovascular accident, which has implications for the organs and tissues retrieved. Donors are older and often have cardiovascular and other comorbidities. If organs and tissues are not going to be retrieved for transplantation, there is no legal requirement to confirm brain death if treatment is deemed futile.[32]

> **BOX 29.2**
>
> **Conditions associated with neurological death**
> - Hypotension
> - Diabetes insipidus
> - Disseminated intravascular coagulation
> - Arrhythmias
> - Cardiac arrest
> - Pulmonary oedema
> - Hypoxia
> - Acidosis

Neurological death is observed clinically when all cranial nerve reflexes are absent. The patient must be supported with artificial ventilation, as the respiratory reflex lost due to cerebral ischaemia will result in respiratory and cardiac arrest. Artificial (mechanical) ventilation maintains oxygen supply to the natural pacemaker (sinoatrial (SA) node) of the heart, which functions independently of the central nervous system. Neurological death results in hypotension due to loss of vasomotor control of the autonomic nervous system, loss of temperature regulation, reduction in hormone activity and loss of all cranial nerve reflexes. Box 29.2 lists the conditions commonly associated with neurological death, but not all people who have progressed to neurological death exhibit all of the conditions. Irrespective of the degree of external support, cardiac standstill will occur in a matter of hours to days once neurological death has occurred.[32]

Testing methods

The aim of testing for neurological death is to determine irreversible cessation of all function in the brain of the person. Testing does not demonstrate that every brain cell has died but that a point of irreversible ischaemic damage involving cessation of the vital functions of the brainstem has been reached. There are a number of steps in the process, the first being the observation period. With the exception of a hypoxia–ischaemic brain injury that has been treated with therapeutic hypothermia, where an observation period of 24 hours is required following rewarming to 35°C, an observation period of at least 4 hours from onset of observed no response is required.[33] This must be documented before the first set of testing commences, in the context of a patient being mechanically ventilated with a Glasgow Coma Scale score of 3, non-reacting pupils, absent cough and gag reflexes and no spontaneous respiratory effort.[32] The second step is to consider the preconditions (Box 29.3). Once the observation period has passed (during which the patient receives ongoing treatment) and the preconditions have been met, formal testing can occur.

Preconditions of neurological death testing[32]

- Known diagnosis of injury and coma is consistent with progression to neurological death.
- Exclude involvement of drugs, including sedative drug effects.
- Exclude severe metabolic, electrolyte and endocrine causes.
- Exclude hypothermia (core temperature >35°C).
- Adequate blood pressure: MAP >60 mmHg.
- Confirm neuromuscular conduction.
- It is possible to examine the brainstem reflexes.
- It is possible to perform apnoea testing.

Practice tip

Please be aware that family members may have witnessed the trauma causing the death of the patient and may have a good understanding already that death has occurred. It is really important to support the family by determining their understanding of the situation and offering them the opportunity to be present during neurological death testing. A representative from the family may volunteer to be with the patient for this event. It is important to explain to them what is being done and why, what is found and the conclusions. Ideally, a support person that they trust should be with the family to assist in explaining and interpreting the testing process.[34]

The Association of Organ Procurement Organizations in the USA provides information and facts covering the organ donation process (e.g. donor management and declaration of neurological death).[35] The Guide to the quality and safety of organs for transplantation by the Council of Europe provide recommendations on neurological death declaration according to the best practices usually applied at the European level.[36] The guidelines state that the neurological death declaration should be based on scientific and nationally agreed criteria, including that the determination of death and the time of declaration of death stay under the legal responsibility of the physician in charge and address some key points for the clinical diagnosis of neurological death, similar to the ones presented for the Australian context.[32] Formal testing for neurological death, in Australia, is undertaken using either clinical assessment or cerebral blood flow studies.[32] Assessment of the brainstem involves assessment of the cranial nerves and the respiratory centre. The process to test for neurological death is described in Table 29.2. Neurological death is confirmed if there is no reaction to stimulation of these reflexes, with the respiratory centre tested last and only if the other reflexes

are absent. The tests may be done consecutively, but not simultaneously, with no fixed interval between the two sets of clinical tests required, except in specific age-related criteria.

If the preconditions outlined in Box 29.3 are unable to be verified, neurological death can be confirmed using cerebral blood flow imaging to demonstrate absent blood flow to the brain. Both contrast angiography and radionuclide scanning can be used to confirm neurological death. Contrast angiography can be performed by direct injection of contrast into both carotid arteries and one or both of the vertebral arteries, or via the vena cava or aortic arch. Neurological death is confirmed when there is no blood flow above the carotid siphon. A radionuclide scan is performed by administering a bolus of short-acting isotope intravenously, or by nebuliser while imaging the head using a gamma camera for 15 minutes. No intracranial uptake of isotope confirms absent blood flow to the brain.[37] If neurological death is confirmed, the time of death is recorded as the time of certification of the testing result (i.e. at the completion of the second set of clinical tests, or the documentation of the results of the cerebral blood flow scan).[32]

Identification of the potential for a patient to donate and save many people in need of transplants (a multiorgan donor)

The second factor influencing the number of actual organ donors is identification of a potential donor. A potential donor is defined in this situation as a patient who is suspected of, or is confirmed as, being neurologically dead or who will experience cardiac arrest and die within a very short time after being extubated. Inclusion and exclusion criteria for organ and tissue donation are constantly being reviewed and refined and may also be dependent on the critical waiting list of patients.

When considering the medical suitability of potential organ donors, advice can be sought 24 hours a day, 7 days a week, from respective state and territory organ donation agencies in Australia as well as in most countries (see Online resources).

The WHO critical pathway for deceased donation provides a reportable uniformity in the approach to deceased donation. The pathway is a tool for a systematic approach to the organ donation process, and how to assess the potential of deceased donation.[38]

The patient's wishes, talking to the family and seeking their agreement to donate

The third factor influencing the possibility for organ donations is neurological death confirmation and consent for donation.[39] Consent is sought for individual organs and tissues, rather than a 'global' approach. If granted, the

TABLE 29.2

Process for neurological determination of death testing[32]

....

RESPONSIVENESS:

Test:	Apply noxious stimuli in the cranial nerve distribution and all four limbs and trunk, observing for motor responses (e.g. pressure over the supraorbital nerve, sternal rub and deep nail bed pressure).
Response:	There should be no responsiveness. This equates to a GCS of 3. Any motor response within the cranial nerve distribution, or any response in the limbs in response to cranial nerve stimulation: *stop clinical testing as this precludes neurological determination of death.*
Cautionary remarks:	Spinal reflexes may be present in patients with permanent loss of brain function. Spinal reflexes are not to be confused with a pathological flexion or extension response. Throughout this statement, due to the context of intubation, GCS 3 = GCS 2T.

BRAINSTEM REFLEXES:

General remarks:	Testing of the brainstem reflexes comprises examination of the cranial nerves: pupils, eye movements, facial sensation and movement, pharyngeal and tracheal response. These are tested sequentially and bilaterally when possible. Not all cranial nerves have a testable reflex associated with them in the context of severe brain injury. All testable brainstem reflexes must be absent for neurological determination of death.

Pupillary light reflex – cranial nerves II and III

Test	Shine a bright light into the eye and look for a pupillary constrictor response.
Response	No pupillary constriction response: *proceed with testing other brainstem reflexes.* Pupillary light reflex is observed: *stop clinical testing, as this precludes neurological determination of death.*
Cautionary remarks:	The pupils must be at least midsize in diameter. Anticholinergic medications such as atropine can cause pupillary dilation. Cataract or iris surgery does not preclude the test.

Corneal reflex — cranial nerves V and VII

Test	Touch the corneas with sterile soft cotton wool or gauze and examine the eyes for blinking or other response.
Response	No blinking or other response: *proceed with testing other brainstem reflexes.* Blink reflex is observed: *stop clinical testing, as this precludes neurological determination of death.*
Cautionary remarks:	Touching the sclera is not sufficient. Examine the cornea gently, by touching rather than scraping, as it is easily damaged.

Reflex response to pain in the trigeminal distribution – cranial nerves V & VII

Test	Apply pain over the trigeminal distribution, e.g. pressure over the supraorbital nerve.
Response	No facial or limb movement: *proceed with testing other brainstem reflexes.* Facial or limb movement is observed: *stop clinical testing, as this precludes neurological determination of death.*

Vestibulo-ocular reflex – cranial nerves III, IV, VI and VIII

Test	Inspect the external auditory canal with an otoscope to confirm that the eardrum is visible. If the eardrum is not visible, the canal must be cleared before testing can occur. Elevate the head to 30° to place the horizontal semicircular canal in a horizontal position. Instill 50 mL of ice-cold water (less for a child) into the ear canal using a syringe. Hold eyelids open and observe for eye movement for a minimum of 60 seconds.
Response	No eye movement in response to the cold water; the eyes remain in the midline within the socket: *proceed with testing other brainstem reflexes.* Presence of any movement, including tonic deviation or nystagmus: *stop clinical testing, as this precludes neurological determination of death.*

TABLE 29.2

Process for neurological determination of death testing—cont'd

Cautionary remarks:	A ruptured eardrum does not preclude the test. Fractures to the base of the skull or petrous temporal bone may obliterate the response on the side of the fracture. Testing for the oculocephalic reflex (head turning) examines the same reflex pathways but is a submaximal stimulus and is not recommended. It may also aggravate a pre-existing cervical spinal injury.

Gag reflex – cranial nerves IX and X

Test	Touch the posterior pharyngeal wall, on both sides, with a tongue depressor or cotton swab. A laryngoscope or video laryngoscope may assist in obtaining a good view of the pharynx for stimulation.
Response	No gag response: *proceed with testing other brainstem reflexes.* Gag response: *do not proceed with clinical testing, as this precludes neurological determination of death.*
Cautionary remarks:	If the patient is orally intubated, the gag reflex may be difficult to discern. It is important to view the posterior pharyngeal wall and/or uvula.

Cough/tracheal reflex – cranial nerve X

Test	Stimulate the tracheobronchial wall with a soft suction catheter.
Response	No cough response is seen: *proceed with testing other brainstem reflexes.* Cough response is observed: *do not proceed with clinical testing, as this precludes neurological determination of death.*
Cautionary remarks:	The efferent limbs for this reflex are the phrenic nerve and the nerves of the thoracic and abdominal muscles. Therefore, it cannot be assessed in patients with high cervical cord injury.

BREATHING:

	ONLY if all the above reflexes are absent, proceed with testing for apnoea. The apnoea test should be conducted last so that a high pressure of carbon dioxide ($PaCO_2$) could not be potentially confounding if brain perfusion was present.
General remarks:	Apnoeic oxygenation is used to demonstrate lack of ventilatory drive. This involves the supply of 100% O_2 to the trachea, without providing ventilatory assistance. Through gas mass-movement, oxygen reaches the alveoli, allowing for transfer to the blood. In normal circumstances, in the absence of ventilation, $PaCO_2$ rises and pH falls, and associated changes in PCO_2 and pH stimulate the brainstem respiratory centres via peripheral chemoreceptors, or by direct effects on the respiratory centres. Usually $PaCO_2$ rises by ~3 mmHg (0.4 kPa) for every minute of apnoea. As the $PaCO_2$ rises, the ventilatory centre is maximally stimulated by a $PaCO_2$ of ~60 mmHg (a pH <7.30). Attempt at breathing is defined as any respiratory muscle activity that results in abdominal or chest excursions or activity of accessory muscles.

individual organs/tissues are recorded on the consent form or named if the consent is being recorded over the telephone; only those organs/tissues granted will be retrieved. Common practice in Australia and New Zealand is for the treating medical staff and the donation specialist staff to request the family in a collaborative approach after death has been confirmed. It is important to involve the donation specialist staff, as this ensures accurate information on donation and transplantation can be communicated with the family and correct consent processes are undertaken. Contacting the next of kin to seek consent is part of the duty of care to patients who may have indicated their wish to be a donor at the time of their death.[39]

Offering the option of organ donation is also considered part of the duty of care to the family and should be considered as part of routine end-of-life care. The OTA has developed a best practice guideline for offering organ and tissue donation in Australia; this guideline outlines the best practice principles for approaching donation with families. Three elements are involved when approaching a family regarding the option of organ donation:

1 their knowledge, beliefs and attitudes
2 their in-hospital experience
3 any beliefs and biases of health professional/s conducting the approach.

The outcome of an approach cannot be predicted or anticipated. A large UK study demonstrated that clinical staff were incorrect 50% of the time when asked to predict the response of next of kin.[39] Attitudes to organ donation are influenced by spiritual beliefs, cultural background, prior knowledge about organ donation, views on altruism and prior health experiences.[40] Next of kin consider two aspects associated with existing attitudes and knowledge: the decision maker(s)' own thoughts and feelings and the previous wishes and beliefs of the person on whose behalf they are making the decision.[41] There is evidence of a link between consent rates and prior knowledge of the positive outcomes of organ donation.[41] Several other studies found that consent rates improved when conversations about neurological death and organ donation were separated, were held in a private setting and when an organ donation professional/trained requestor was involved.[39,41]

Delivery of relevant information

An important consideration for all health professionals is that family members may have a diminished ability to receive and understand information because of their stress and psychological responses at this time of family crisis. As interviews held with the family are the foundation of the entire organ donation and transplant process, the discussion about neurological death should be clear and emphatic, using language free of medical terminology, and include an explanation of the physical implications.[42] Diagrams, analogies and written materials have been suggested as useful aids for enhancing understanding by next of kin.[39] One approach is to describe neurological death as like a jigsaw puzzle with a piece missing, to illustrate the relationship of the brain to the rest of the body. Opportunities for staff to train and role-play this scenario with programs like TPM and the European Training Program on Organ Donation in Europe (see Online resources) improve the likelihood of meeting the needs of families.[43]

As the time of confirmation of neurological death is the person's legal time of death, multiple family conversations may occur with the family to discuss their options and associated implications. Options are to: (1) cease ventilation and allow cardiac standstill to occur, or (2) maintain ventilation and haemodynamic support to explore and potentially facilitate viable organ and tissue donation. These conversations in Australia are held by the donation specialist staff, ensuring accurate and appropriate information is delivered.[41–43] Table 29.3[2,44] lists some aspects of the organ donation process that are usually by the donation specialist staff in such a discussion. As information given to a family contains information that may be confronting for them, donation specialist staff may sometimes start with the less confronting information such as the benefits of transplantation from donation, the right of the family to refuse consent (legislation differs between countries) and the lack of cost – and then lead into sharing the other critical information such as the reality of the surgical intervention and the lack of

guarantee that the organs will be transplanted.[2] Donation specialist staff members receive specialised training to assist them in understanding and delivering the required information in a manner appropriate for each individual family based on best practice. Families frequently gain solace from the positive aspects of donation, of helping or reducing the suffering of other families. Of note, a best practice approach aims to assist the family members to make the decision that is 'right' for them and does not necessarily result in gaining consent.

Meetings with the family

It is important to build a trusting relationship between the healthcare team and the patient and their family across all stages of care. The transition to end-of-life care and discussions about the dying/deceased person's wishes should be a process that is expected by the family who may have been witness to the events leading to the critical event that has brought about this situation. The family members will identify whom they see as family, and it is important to listen to them and gain an understanding of the relationships prior to having end-of-life discussions about organ donation. It is known that healthcare teams often make decisions about their perceptions of relationships and social situations that are not correct. Cultural humility – the idea of asking the family for their view, the idea of saying that you do not know, when you do not know – is the first step towards building the trust of the family and supporting consent for donation. Identifying who the appropriate family members are to meet with in relation to organ donation is a first consideration, and then the process by which the discussions will be held needs to be considered, especially the location and opportunities to bring spiritual and pastoral support, including cultural aspects, which differ internationally. Meetings with family to discuss organ donation and ascertaining the donor's wishes is a sensitive and potentially difficult conversation; involvement of the donation specialist nursing staff and preparation are critical to these conversations. It is critical that families are provided adequate support and clear, considered information by the healthcare team, which includes the donation specialist nursing staff, about the options that are available once it is clear that death is inevitable or already confirmed. Healthcare professionals aim to balance informational needs, care, compassion and respect for a family's decision regarding organ and tissue donation with the knowledge that there are patients awaiting transplantation while maintaining neutrality and balance as advocates in family discussions.

In Australia the definition of next of kin for adults and children is listed in strict order (Table 29.4).[45] In New Zealand there is no hierarchy of next of kin, with the definition including a surviving spouse or relative.[29] In both countries, the next of kin can override the known wishes of the deceased regarding consent, but experience shows that the family members rarely disagree if the wishes of the deceased are known, regardless of their own

TABLE 29.3

Information about the organ donation process and retrieval to assist in informed decision making[2,44]

INFORMATION	ISSUES
Ensure that the next of kin (NOK) have understanding of:	• Neurological death or impending death via circulatory death. • Time of death. • Eventual organ failure if kept ventilated in intensive care. • The option to consent or decline donation.

If they choose to donate:	• They will not be with the donor at time of circulatory arrest if pursuing donation after neurological determination of death.
	• The potential donor will remain in intensive care, monitored and ventilated until going to theatre for the retrieval surgery.
	• Support the explanation from the donation specialist nurse that the retrieval surgery occurs like any other surgery, including the presence of an anaesthetist to monitor the haemodynamics and ventilation.
	• The donation specialist nurse will discuss which organs and tissue would be potentially medically suitable for retrieval for transplant.
	• The NOK can give specific consent; they are not obliged to grant global consent.
	• Only consented organs and tissues with a suitably matched recipient are retrieved.
	• The donation specialist nurse with communicate with all involved the expected length of process.
	• Work with the donation specialist nurse who will
	  ○ explain reason for bloods being taken and stored
	  ○ explain how the donor will look after the retrieval
	  ○ explain that organ donation will not delay funeral plans
	  ○ explain the consent form
	  ○ provide a copy of the consent form
	  ○ explain privacy implications of the relevant human tissue act, for donor family and transplant recipients
	  ○ explain reasons why donation may not proceed
	  ○ explain that organs may be transplanted some distance away
	  ○ explain that, in the event of an abnormality/diseases, organs will not be retrieved
	  ○ explain consent for research: offer copy of research page
	  ○ explain that the site designated officer (or equivalent) will also sign the consent form.
	• Advise that donation specialist will be present through the entire process.

If a coroner's case:	• Coroner's consent is required and the process required for this including the potential for autopsy. • Police identification is required. • Deceased will go to the coroner's mortuary after retrieval. • Explain contact with coroner's court.
If organs are retrieved and not able to be transplanted:	The donation specialist nurse will talk the family through this and provide: • the information on what can occur in this situation, either returned and placed with donor, or disposed of as medical waste.
Support services:	The donation specialist nurse will: • offer viewing of patient or a telephone call after the retrieval • offer a lock of hair and/or handprint • provide contact details • provide printed information • explain other support services available.
Follow-up information:	The donation specialist nurse will provide the family with the: • outcomes of the retrieval • recipient outcomes • written material and letters • counselling services.

TABLE 29.4

Definition of next of kin for children and adults in Australia[45]

· ·

The Human Tissue Acts in each Australian state and territory provide a priority list of family members (the next of kin) who may be the 'senior available next of kin' consulted about tissue removal. If the first person is not available, then the next person on the list must be approached.

In all states and territories, if the **deceased donor is an adult** (i.e. a person aged over 18 years), the priority order for senior available next of kin is the deceased's:
*   spouse or de facto, domestic or same sex partner
*   adult son or daughter
*   parent
*   brother or sister.

In all states and territories except Western Australia and Queensland, if a **deceased donor is a child**, the priority order for senior available next of kin is:
*   parent
*   adult brother or sister
*   the child's guardian.

In Queensland and Western Australia the domestic partner or spouse of a child will be given priority over a parent, sibling or guardian (however, in Western Australia the spouse or de facto partner must have attained the age of 18).

'Parent' is defined differently in some states and territories. For example, the New South Wales definition includes biological parent, step-parent or adoptive parent. In South Australia, parent includes 'the guardian of the child'. The Australian Capital Territory, Tasmania, Victoria and Western Australia Human Tissue Acts exclude from the definition of 'parent' a guardian or anyone else with parental responsibility. In Queensland, a parent includes a person who under Aboriginal tradition or Island custom, or other cultural traditions, is considered a parent of the child.

Source: Ben White, Lindy Willmott and Penny Neller. End of life law in Australia. Organ donation. Brisbane, QLD: Queensland University of Technology; 2022. Available from: https://end-of-life.qut.edu.au/organ-donation#547407. [Accessed February 2023].

---

personal beliefs. The right to override a known wish to donate or not differs between countries depending on their law. Internationally, there are various cultural differences within populations (including religious perspectives) to consider about the approach for organ donation.[2] Further discussions regarding culturally appropriate communication can be found in Chapter 7.

The timing, location, content and process of discussions with the family are all important considerations. An effective protocol for communicating with the family of a potential donor must include appraising the family's knowledge of the events that led to the catastrophic condition: (1) frequent and honest updates on the patient's prognosis, delivered with compassion, (2) clear explanation of death and the sequence of neurological/circulatory death dependent on the situation and how it is assessed, (3) the decoupling of the death and organ donation conversations until the family accepts that continuing technological interventions to maintain circulation and ventilation is inappropriate because the patient will not recover or is already dead, (4) conversations held in a private and quiet setting and (5) involvement of staff with a trusting relationship with the family and a donation specialist nurse who is introduced as part of the team with a clear definition of roles.[41,43]

There is compelling evidence that the meeting confirming diagnosis of impending death/neurological death should be held separately or decoupled from the conversation about the end-of-life decisions about organ and tissue donation.[41] But this will be determined by the family who may offer donation before the question is raised. Clearly, offers to donate should be accepted with gratitude and every effort should be made to follow up the offer with a discussion about the possibilities, including a formal acknowledgement by the donation team regardless of the outcome. In reality, the pace and flow of discussions should be assessed on a case-by-case basis, as there may be circumstances when the discussion about organ donation is appropriately held prior to the confirmation of death; due to this it is important to involve the donation specialist staff at the point of expected end of life rather than after the end-of-life conversation, as it ensures families have access to accurate information at the time that is appropriate for them.

Staff roles, delineation and involvement

Staff involved in the explanation of death must have a clear understanding of neurological and circulatory death, have practised explaining it themselves to others and feel comfortable with the concept of organ and tissue donation before attempting to explain it to a family. It is recommended for donation to be routine in end-of-life conversation. As a routine end-of-life practice, staff members become much more familiar with speaking to families about the benefits and become more successful in normalising donation. Requestors are donation specialist staff specifically trained in the approach of requesting organ and tissue donation and have completed some form of formal education, for example the OTA's core and practical family donation conversation workshops.

Additionally, having the donation specialist nurse present to answer specific questions raised by the family assists in removing assumptions and 'myths' about donation through providing accurate and contemporary information. The process of organ and tissue donation in critical care environments is significant for all concerned. When death is confirmed, it marks the end of an episode that has been catastrophic for both patients and their loved ones, and a potentially stressful, emotionally conflicting and exhausting experience for many staff members.[46] Approaching the family of a potential donor is a multidisciplinary team effort; however, it should be noted that often the bedside nurse is the first to have a conversation with the family members when they seek information prior to an approach by the medical and donation specialist staff. Best practice is to encourage treating medical and nursing staff to continue their support of the patient and family after neurological death is confirmed as part of the care of the deceased, to provide appropriate respect and compassion for the family and the deceased, for continuity of care.[32] The individual physician's or nurse's willingness to act, to respect, represent and safeguard the (potential) donor's will and wishes in these situations is termed *organ donor advocacy*, and is built on the professional ethics and its demand to make decisions of the best actions for the patient/donor. The concept of *attitudes toward organ donor advocacy*, developed by Flodén, is theoretically anchored in the framework of patient advocacy.[47,48] In the situation of organ donation, participation in the donation process and caring for the potential or actual organ donor can be viewed as advocacy activities (i.e. respecting the potential or actual organ donor's rights, representing or speaking up for his/her wishes as well as the relatives' points of view in the organ donation decision-making process).[47,48] Nursing staff involvement in the care of the deceased throughout and after the process of organ and tissue donation is central and intrinsic to our moral codes and ethical guidelines, including the care of the potential donor and family during the decision-making process and humanisation of the practicalities of the process of preparing for donation surgery. Donor families have identified nurses as being the most helpful health professionals in providing information and emotional support.[1,32,49]

A holistic approach to supporting families in critical care may also include involvement of social workers, pastoral care workers and other allied health professionals. Often these health professionals have been working with the family for several days and act as confidants and a resource for information on issues such as implications of a coronial

enquiry and a religious denomination's stance on organ donation. Most major religions are supportive of organ and tissue donation for transplantation and would instruct the family to make the decision that they felt was correct.

In many countries, there are organ donation coordinators that act as a resource and are invited into critical care when appropriate. In Australia, these are termed donation specialist nurses. They are professionals who are experts in organ and tissue donation, have the time to spend with the family and are the best people to undertake an approach to a potential donor family.

Practice tip

The multidisciplinary team involved in the process of organ donation is not limited to staff within the ICU. In order for the donor's wishes to become a reality and provide organ and tissues for transplantation, the following disciplines are involved:

- medical
- nursing
- pathology
- transportation
- allied health
- pastoral care
- operational services
- administration
- police service
- coroner's and magistrate's office
- designated officer.

Adapted from the DonateLife website, https://www.donatelife.gov.au.

Role of designated specialists

In most countries, senior medical staff eligible to certify neurological death using neurological death criteria must be appointed by the governing body of their health institution, have relevant and recent experience and not be involved with transplant recipient selection. In many countries, the most common medical specialties appointed to the role are intensivists and neurologists.[32] Appointed medical staff confirming neurological death must also act independently, and must be appropriately qualified and suitably experienced in the care of such patients. Medical staff should not be involved in treating the recipient of the organ to be removed but rather be a specialist in charge of the clinical care of the patient.[24]

Role of designated officers

Similarities between Australia and international practice extend to the role of the 'designated officer' whereby an executive level appointment within the institution is afforded the power to authorise a non-coronial postmortem and the removal of tissue from a deceased person for transplant or other therapeutic, medical or scientific purposes,[21] and to protect healthcare consumers. This officer must be satisfied that all necessary inquiries have been made and any necessary consent has been obtained before granting authority. Medical, nursing and administrative staff can be appointed to the role, but they must not act in a case if they have had clinical or personal involvement in the donor's case.[32] International guidelines on ethics, access and safety in tissue and organ transplantation are published by the WHO.[50]

Role of coroner and forensic pathologists

Because of the nature of their death, up to 50% of potential donors are subject to coronial inquiry. In this case, permission to undertake organ and tissue retrieval is sought from the respective forensic pathologist and coroner according to local policy and procedure as part of the consent-seeking process. The coronial system is very supportive of donation for transplant and, in 2021, 52% of the Australian and 41% of New Zealand multiorgan donors were coroner's cases.[51]

Consent indicator databases

The most influential factor to affect family unit decision making is the existence of an advance care directive or prior indication of consent. This information has eased decision making and preserved patient autonomy,[43,52] enabling wishes of the patient to be followed even when family decision makers would have made the opposite decision. This is, however, challenged in countries such as Spain that have the highest donation rates in the world and do not hold a register. The experience of asking the family what they think their loved one would want to do in this situation is often found to be an enabler of a conversation about the qualities of the dying/deceased patient and the hopes to save another's life as a lasting legacy.

Cultural safety

With cultural diversity in many countries, best practice for approaching a family includes creating trust and sharing clear information, transparency and curiosity about the information family member(s) may need to make their decision. As significant differences also exist within every family, population and cultural groups, so expectations of responses cannot be stereotyped. When healthcare professionals are unsure of how a family may perceive a situation, it is best to ask, listen carefully and use an interpreter as appropriate, as acknowledgment of the importance of understanding the family circumstances, expectations and needs can lead to improved communication. Importantly, the most significant differences between potential donor families are socioeconomic and educational factors, especially the approach and relationships with the medical/nursing team rather than cultural or racial background. Therefore, individual relationship building, care and assessment must

guide the approach by health professionals. Cultural aspects of critical care nursing practice are discussed in Chapter 7.

Care of the organ donor

Understanding the physiology of death – the impact of loss of adequate perfusion on the function of organs and tissues, and the importance of time management – is critical in the management of a potential organ donor. Patients who have sustained traumatic brain injuries can suffer organ deterioration rapidly prior to and following neurological death, exhibiting severe physiological instability requiring vigilant monitoring and specialised treatment to stabilise and maintain organ perfusion. This is a time of great distress for families, who see the blood pressure rapidly climbing and falling and seeing evidence of 'storming' – diaphoresis and apparent suffering – despite the neurological evidence of impending death/death. This is a time when it is critical to provide the most expert personal care to the patient that also demonstrates empathy for the family, given the patient's death is usually the result of a sudden, unexpected illness or injury that the family may have witnessed. Therefore, discussion surrounding the care of the patient must be trauma informed, and any discussion about organ and tissue donation must be undertaken in a sensitive manner by skilled staff members who possess a compassionate approach and a sound understanding of the pathophysiology of death and the process required for organ and/or tissue donation.

Ideally, the time between neurological death and organ retrieval should be minimised to ensure an optimal outcome for transplant recipients and the family of the dying/deceased person. Therefore, the focus of medical management changes from ensuring brain perfusion to maintaining good organ perfusion for transplantation. Early referral to donation specialist nurses enables legal processes to be managed, complex tissue typing processes to be planned, application of recognised management protocols and collaboration between the donation, retrieval and transplant teams to be enacted. The care of the potential donor family forms a crucial part of the process, with up-to-date and accurate information essential to ensure that the bereavement experience is managed with compassion and care. Importantly, it should be noted that delays in the process or perceptions of suffering in the patient, or poor quality of care may prompt families to withdraw their consent to donation prior to the donation/retrieval surgery. The onus of responsibility is on the team to continue to provide excellent care to the deceased and their family while waiting for the arrival of the transplant retrieval team.

Referral of potential donor

In Australia, best practice is that referral for donation occurs at the time of expected end of life rather than when the family/next-of-kin is actually asked to consent for donation. The longer the time delay, the more likely that organ failure-related complications may occur, or families decline.[51] The referral process is consistent across international organisations, including North America, Europe and the UK, and begins with donation specialist nurses collating the past and present medical, surgical and social history to determine the suitability of the potential donor. Once suitability is confirmed and consent has been obtained from the family, a full patient medical social history is also collected from the donor family. At a later point in the process this information is relayed to the relevant transplant units to assist in their decision of suitability for the recipients[24,44] (see Table 29.3). Similarly, referral practices through LifeNet in the USA and the NHS referral network in the UK ensure all potential donors are identified and referred early for appropriate management and to ensure the opportunity for organ and tissue donation is honoured[24,44] (see Table 29.3). In Australia, a National Electronic Donor Record was introduced in 2014, enabling secure data collection and rapid relay of information to transplant units. Using this information,

transplant teams determine the organ's suitability and move to determine whether a match with the recipients on their waiting list. If the transplant team does not have a suitable recipient, often based on factors such as blood group or size, the offer is extended to another team in Australia or New Zealand on rotation directed by the joint Australasian Transplant and Donor Coordinators Association (ATCA), Transplant Society of Australia and New Zealand (TSANZ) and the OTA's National standard operating procedure on organ allocation, organ rotation and urgent listings.[35,53]

Tissue typing and cross-matching

A vital component of the assessment and referral process is tissue typing, cross-matching and virology testing of the potential donor's blood. Blood is taken from an arterial or central line of the potential donor and sent to the relevant accredited laboratory (Table 29.5). Tissue typing identifies the human leukocyte antigen (HLA) phenotype from the genes on chromosome 6. The HLA molecules control actions of the immune system to differentiate between 'self' and foreign tissue, and initiate an immune response to foreign matter. As a transplanted organ will always be

---

TABLE 29.5

Blood tests required for organ donation[24,35,50]

MEASUREMENT REQUIRED	TEST
Serology	<ul><li>HIV I and II</li><li>HTLV 1 antibody</li><li>Hepatitis B sAg</li><li>Hepatitis B sAb</li><li>Hepatitis B core Ab</li><li>Hepatitis C sAb</li><li>CMV (IgG)</li><li>EBV</li><li>Syphilis</li><li>Toxoplasma IgG and IgM</li><li>HSV</li><li>COVID PCR testing</li><li>Strongyloides testing</li></ul>
NAT screen (nucleic acid test)	<ul><li>HIV NAT screen</li><li>HCV NAT screen</li><li>HBV NAT screen</li></ul>
Tissue typing	<ul><li>Cross-matching with the blood of potential recipients with relevant ABO – transitioning to HLA genetic typing of potential donor to enable a virtual cross.match (VXM) with potential recipient(s)</li></ul>

Ab = antibody; CMV = cytomegalovirus; EBV = Epstein–Barr virus; HBV = hepatitis B virus; HCV = hepatitis C virus; HIV = human immunodeficiency virus; HLA = human leukocyte antigen; HSV = herpes simplex virus; HTLV = human T-lymphotropic virus; IgG = immunoglobulin G; IgM = immunoglobulin M; NAT = nucleic acid testing; PCR = polymerase chain reaction; sAb = surface antibody; sAg = surface antigen.

identified as foreign tissue by the recipient's body, immunosuppressive drugs are used to suppress the immune response. Cross-matching is routinely used to predict the level of this response. The development of a world-first national organ-matching system in Australia in 2019 called Organ Match, funded by the Australian Government through the OTA, has revolutionised the organ offering and cross-matching process, where computer technology facilitates a virtual cross-match (VXM) that provides a greater level of detail in the compatibility of the donor and potential recipients.[54]

Practice tip

Organ and tissue transplantation is associated with the potential for the transmission of some infectious diseases and malignant conditions. In the process of organ and tissue donation and transplantation, this risk is balanced against the recipients waiting and their urgency.

Source: Adapted from Transplant Society of Australia and New Zealand.

Physiological support for successful transplantation

The fourth factor influencing the number of actual organ donors is the clinical care that the potential donor receives and the communication their family receives after death is confirmed. The processes are clearly different when death is confirmed using neurological death criteria when a patient is ventilated. The aim of the clinical management of the deceased person who is receiving ventilatory and other organ support therapies such as inotropes and fluid management is to optimise organ function until organ retrieval surgery commences to enable successful transplantation. This care must be provided while maintaining dignity and respect for the deceased donor and bereavement support for their family. All aspects of intensive care treatments that support tissue and organ perfusion, apart from brain-oriented therapy, should continue until it is certain that organ donation will not occur. Medical management of potential donors is detailed in Box 29.1.

Retrieval surgery

Organ retrieval surgery occurs in the hospital where the patient has been cared for. The local operating theatre staff are integral to the surgical process. The surgery is listed as urgent and the operating theatre staff including anaesthetics staff are critical to the success of the surgery. Once the specialist transplant retrieval team have confirmed their arrival, the family has said farewell to the deceased donor, and in some centres the staff have a special acknowledgement of the donor when they are transferred to theatre. Routine preoperative checks and documentation is checked, including death certification and consent for organ and tissue retrieval. All documentation, particularly consent, is viewed by all members of the retrieval surgical team and operating theatre staff before surgery commences.[52] Depending on which organs are to be retrieved, the retrieval teams will be specifically tasked to abdominal organs and thoracic organs and will bring most of their specialised equipment with them. An anaesthetist monitors haemodynamics, ventilation and administers medications, which may include a long-acting muscle relaxant given prior to the surgical procedure, to prevent interference in the surgical process by spinal reflexes, only after consultation with the retrieval team. No other anaesthetic agents are administered. The local scrub staff will work with the visiting surgical teams, and the donation specialist nurse coordinator will be present to coordinate the retrieval, document the procedure and outcomes, fulfil any family wishes about theatre, sometimes undertake the abdominal perfusionist role and act as a resource for all staff present.

Surgery may take 4–5 hours depending on the extent of the retrieval. In donation after neurological determination of death, cross-clamp will occur once the surgeons have identified all the various anatomical points. The aorta is cross-clamped with vascular clamps below the diaphragm and at the aortic arch, the heart is stopped and ventilation is ceased. A cold perfusion fluid with an electrolyte mix specific to the organs being retrieved is administered, and removal of the organs from the body occurs. They are then transported to the transplanting hospitals. The donor's surgical wound, from the sternal notch to the pubis, is closed by the surgeons in a routine manner and dressed with a surgical dressing. If the donor is not a coroner's case, the remaining lines, catheter and drains are removed according to local policy, the patient is washed, and arrangements are made to transfer the patient to a location for family viewing or to the mortuary. Musculoskeletal tissue and eye tissue retrieval can occur after the solid organ retrieval in theatre or later in the mortuary.[24]

Donor family care

Supportive care of a donor family begins from the time their family member is admitted to hospital and continues beyond organ retrieval as an expected standard of care in all international organ donation agencies. In addition to personal factors such as cultural background, previous bereavement, family dynamics, coping skills and prior experiences with loss that may influence the grieving process, the family of an organ and tissue donor will be dealing with a number of unique factors. Death of their family member was possibly sudden and unexpected, neurological death can be difficult to understand when people look as if they are asleep rather than dead, having the option of organ donation may mean making a decision on behalf of the person if their wishes were not known, and the process of organ donation following neurological death means they will not be with the person when their heart stops.[1,55] Further information about specific cultural groups and general considerations for tailoring discussions to the family's background can be found in Chapter 7.

Practice tip

Prior to family meetings regarding organ donation, it is beneficial for staff, including the donation specialist nurse, to go over their roles and the potential conversation that might occur. Please make sure you clarify who you are and what your role is in the team, as many families state they did not know who the staff were or whether they were qualified. Providing an opportunity for staff debriefing, operational reviews and documenting staff involved in the donation and retrieval process is also important, particularly in regional or rural settings where cases may be infrequent and the community is smaller, facilitating collaboration with the organ retrieval teams. This is often led by the donation specialist staff of the hospital.

Donor families benefit from emotional and physical support throughout and after the organ donation process. In critical care units, this support can include open visiting times, allocated lounge areas for families to gather, accommodation for families who have travelled from distant locations, privacy for meetings, clear and precise information and regular contact with the attending clinical team, support personnel and the donation specialist nurse. After organ retrieval, ongoing care can include contact with a bereavement specialist, written material, telephone support, private or group counselling and correspondence from recipients.[2] In Australia, this support is provided by the donor family support coordinator based in the DonateLife Agency in each state and territory. Many families comment on the benefit they find in being connected to other donor families through events such as the commemorative services held by the DonateLife Agencies in each state and territory. Internationally, organ donation agencies identify the importance of family support and follow-up in developing trust and providing comfort during and after the donation decision, and the provision of aftercare programs for the families of organ donors through a variety of follow-up support services (see Online resources). Involvement of trained personnel, such as the donation specialist nurses in Australia, with a donor family through this process can positively influence the family's grief journey.

It is highly recommended that the staff caring for the donor and their family meet with the family in the weeks following the death to clarify the cause of death and the processes undertaken, to acknowledge the experience for the family and to express gratitude for their contribution. Donation is not a simple 'sign the form'; it is a process that can be prolonged for families, and they need to be acknowledged for their support to enable the donation. The National Donor Family Support Service operates through the DonateLife Network and is a nationally consistent program of support provided to deceased organ and/or tissue donor families. All families whose next of kin are identified as possible donors are offered end-of-life support including bereavement counselling at the time, whether or not the potential donor proceeds to donation.[2]

Donation after circulatory determination of death

Donation after circulatory determination of death (DCDD), previously known as non-heart-beating donation (NHBD) and in some instances as donation after cardiac death (DCD), provides a solid organ donation option for a patient who has not deteriorated and is not likely to demonstrate neurological death. Prior to neurological death legislation, donation after circulatory death was the source of deceased donor kidneys for transplantation. Four categories of potential DCDD donors, known as the Holland–Maastricht categories, have been identified:

1 dead on arrival (uncontrolled)
2 failed resuscitation (uncontrolled)
3 withdrawal of support (controlled)
4 arrest following brain death (uncontrolled).[56]

The OTA has developed a national DCDD protocol that outlines an ethical process that respects the rights of the patient and ensures clinical consistency, effectiveness and safety for both donors and recipients.[2] Internationally, in some countries, DCDD accounts for a larger number of deceased organ donors compared with donation after neurological determination of death (DNDD) donors. The WHO has estimated that the current transplant rate addresses only 10% of the need globally for organ transplants[57] and several countries now have well-developed protocols in DCDD, including UK, Ireland, Spain and several other European countries.[44] A Donation after Circulatory Determination of Death Registry is maintained by the International Society for Heart and Lung transplantation.[44]

Identification of a potential DCDD donor

The aims of a successful DCDD program are to always maintain dignity for the donor, to provide the donor family with support and information and to limit warm ischaemia time[44] (time from withdrawal of ventilation and treatment to confirmation of death, to commencement of infusion of cold perfusion fluid and/or organ retrieval). Longer warm ischaemia time potentiates the risk of irreparable hypoxic damage to the organ. As noted above, Holland–Maastricht category 3 is the only option that can be controlled and possibly regulate warm ischaemia time. A potential category 3 DCDD donor is a person ventilated and monitored in intensive care about whom a decision has already been made that further treatment is futile, and current interventions are to be withdrawn. Clinical suitability assessment for organ retrieval replicates that for a multiorgan donor, with medical, surgical and social history, virology and organ function information collected; however, in DCDD this occurs before the certification of death. Legal requirements of the consent-seeking process also reflect those of a multiorgan donor. Potential donor families are informed that retrieval may not occur owing to a number of factors, including the length of time from treatment withdrawal to cessation of circulation.[52]

Retrieval process alternatives

Withdrawal of treatment for a potential category 3 DCDD patient can occur in intensive care or in the operating theatre, depending on which organs are planned for retrieval, location of the intensive care unit to the operating theatre and local policy and procedures. Death is determined by cessation of circulation, with recommendations that the ECG is not monitored (electrical activity can persist for many minutes following cessation of circulation), but that an arterial line is used to determine the time of cessation of circulation. The patient is then transferred to theatre for organ retrieval surgery. When withdrawal of treatment occurs in theatre, retrieval may commence after the patient is declared deceased (cessation of circulation for more than 5 minutes).[32] If circulation does not cease during the window of time available for organ retrieval, the patient is transferred back to ICU.[2]

Tissue-only donor

People confirmed as having died using circulatory and neurological criteria can be tissue donors for transplantation and for research. The end-of -life discussion that enables tissue donation can be an extraordinary place of hope for families who were unable to donate a loved ones' solid organs or a patient with end-stage conditions such as cancer who may be able to donate corneal tissue for transplantation. Eyes (whole and corneal button) are retrieved for cornea and sclera transplantation – providing sight to the blind. Musculoskeletal tissue is used for bone grafting (long bones of arms and legs, hemipelvis), urology procedures and treatment of sport injuries (ligaments, tendons, fascia and meniscus). Heart valves (bicuspid, tricuspid valves, aortic and pulmonary tissue) are used for heart valve replacement and cardiac reconstruction. Skin

(retrieved from the lower back and buttocks) is used for the treatment of burns.[2]

Identification of a potential tissue-only donor

The most influential aspect for tissue donation is early notification of the potential donor's death to the relevant tissue bank, ideally within hours of the person's death. All deceased persons can be considered potential donors, with assessment for clinical suitability on a case-by-case basis. As noted earlier, there is no expectation that treating clinicians will be required to make that decision or make the approach to the next of kin; however, good practice would include that discussion as part of quality end-of-life care discussions with the patient and/or family depending on the circumstances. In general, depending on the state and territory, and location, once the death notification has been received by the tissue bank coordinator, the determining factors are age, cause of death, time elapsed since death, virology results and presence of infection. The legal requirements of the consent-seeking process mirror those of the multiorgan donor.

Practice tip

Families should be asked only once about organ and tissue donation. Please ensure that if the care team has spoken to the family it notifies the tissue banks rather than the family receiving additional requests to donate. After organ donation requests this is most often done by the donation specialist nurse, who has specialised knowledge and training on what the tissue banks require for information and the legalities of the consent process.

If there has not been a prior contact with the family, depending on the location, and after checking medical suitability and the relevant consent indicator database, a coordinator from the tissue bank or other trained personnel approaches the next of kin with the option of tissue retrieval.[2] After tissue retrieval, every effort is made to restore anatomical appearance. Wounds are sutured closed and covered with surgical dressings, limbs given back their form, and eye shape is restored with the lids kept closed with eye caps.[2,41] Support requirements for families of tissue donors share many aspects of programs provided for families of organ donors. In truth, the community believes they are the same and the impact of their donations are equally respected and honoured. A sensitive approach, provision of adequate information to assist informed decision making, offers of bereavement counselling and follow-up information of recipient outcomes are evidence-based strategies of successful programs.[2]

Summary

An overview of organ donation has been provided in this chapter. In several countries, including Australia and New Zealand, opt-in systems of giving consent for organ and tissue donation are in place, but in other countries, such as Singapore and Spain, opt-out systems are used. After death has been confirmed, or is impending in the case of DDCD, information from a consent indicator database (such as the AODR in Australia) is sought to determine the wishes of the person and the option of organ and tissue donation should, as a part of routine end-of-life care, be given to the next of kin. Each person is assessed on a case-by-case basis to determine medical suitability for organ and tissue retrieval for transplantation. The treating clinicians are not expected to make this decision, as this is managed best by the donation specialists in consultation with transplant clinicians, but their involvement and care are vital. Support and information are available around the clock from the respective donor agencies and tissue banks. Donor family care commences at the time of the family member's admission and continues as required with structured bereavement programs specific to donor family care. The intent to be an organ and tissue donor can be indicated by people when alive or by the next of kin after death.

Three 'types' of organ or tissue donor are identified: the multiorgan and tissue donor (after neurological death) determination, the multiorgan and tissue donor (after circulatory death determination) and the tissue-only donor. Four factors have been identified that directly influence the number of multiorgan donations internationally and include the incidence of neurological death, the identification of potential donors, neurological death confirmation and gaining consent for donation and, finally, the care and physiological management of the donor after the confirmation of neurological death.

There is evidence to address each factor, but each case needs to be approached on a case-by-case basis. The medical suitability for every potential donor is assessed individually at the time of the person's death, and support and guidance from donor specialist staff and tissue banks are always available. Internationally, priority is given to providing care and support of the potential and actual donor family and, as part of this, regular routine follow-up and debriefing opportunities for all staff involved are important to manage stress reactions or other concerns.

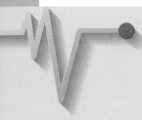

Case study

DAY 1

Peter, a 14-year-old high school student, had been eating breakfast with his mother at 07:20 on a Wednesday morning when he suddenly developed an intensely painful headache, and collapsed in the kitchen. His mother described the event as occurring very rapidly, he called out and collapsed – the entire event lasting less than 5 minutes. She immediately called an ambulance and placed Peter in a recovery position, as he had a pulse and was shallow breathing.

Paramedics arrived on scene in under 7 minutes and immediately intubated and ventilated Peter for transfer to a regional hospital. On arrival at the emergency department 14 minutes later, Peter was assessed by a multidisciplinary team with vital signs documented at 07:48: Glasgow Coma Scale (GCS) score 3, BP 150/120 mmHg, heart rate (HR) 56, SaO_2 94%.

Peter had been intubated at the scene and exhibited no respiratory effort or reaction to painful stimuli. Peter had a single IV line with N/saline at 84 mL/h and a second large-bore IV access was established, and he was escorted to radiology for urgent cerebral computerised tomography (CT), which revealed a grade V subarachnoid haemorrhage (SAH).

Peter was immediately admitted to the ICU at 09:30 for assessment with further line placements of arterial and central lines. Peter's haemodynamic status remained unchanged, with pupils unequal; he was ventilated (synchronised intermittent mandatory ventilation (SIMV), respiratory rate 18, tidal volume 350 mL, positive end-expiratory pressure (PEEP) 5); he received no sedation or paralysing agents and he was an afebrile 35.7°C.

A family interview was conducted to inform Peter's mother (his only kin) of his current condition with the intensive care consultant, registrar, bedside nurse and social worker. Peter's mother was supported by a close friend during the interview and understood her son's poor prognosis. She raised the question of her son's eligibility for organ donation as they had recently discussed this with Peter preparing for his biology test. Peter's mother agreed to talk to the hospital donation specialist nurse.

Initial brainstem death tests were performed at 1:20, just over 4 hours from the first observation of potential neurological death, revealing no reflex responses, fixed dilated pupils and PCO_2 of 70 with apnoea. A second set of testing was performed at 14:30 with confirmed neurological death. A donation specialist nurse led the follow-up family conference with Peter's mother and support person, where Peter's mother gave consent for donation to occur for all organs and tissue, except for eye tissue.

The donation specialist nurse commenced the referral documentation in collaboration with the ICU medical and nursing teams and briefed all staff in the management of the process including family care, physiological management and multidisciplinary involvement, including staff from the emergency department and operational services teams. Coroner's consent was granted following police (deceased person) identification of Peter with Peter's mother, and, with her consent, blood was collected and sent for virology, tissue typing and cross-matching. Peter's full physical, medical and social history and admission documentation were collected as part of the donor work-up and organ offering to the transplant clinicians. Compassionate nursing and medical care of Peter with careful essential care and physiological management continued, with Peter's mother remaining at the bedside throughout, encouraged to be present and help with personal care and any other care needs such as sharing photos and stories with the staff and encouraging his best friend to come and say goodbye with the support of pastoral care teams and the social worker and nurse. The nurses had developed a close therapeutic relationship with Peter's mother.

The donation specialist nursing coordinator advised that transplant teams would arrive on site by 22:00 for retrieval surgery of solid organs including the heart, lungs, liver and kidneys; on arrival they would be oriented to the regional hospital and supported by the operational services staff. Operating theatre staff were aware of the case and had already been shown the certification of death.

The setup commenced with teams providing all the necessary instrumentation and Peter was transferred at 23:20 by the anaesthetist, supported by the operating theatre nurse and donation specialist nurse, who maintained Peter's airways, ventilation and inotropic support to ensure optimal organ function for transplantation. Peter's mother found it very hard to say goodbye at that stage and the nurse in ICU caring for Peter spent time with her, offering a cup of tea, and then providing a stretcher and warm blanket to rest near the bed where Peter would be returned to following surgery to facilitate family viewing, enabling her to say a final goodbye. She was supported throughout by her support person, the bedside ICU nurse and the donation specialist staff. It was after hours and there was no social worker.

DAY 2

At 03:45, retrieval surgery was complete with teams transported to the airport for return to their respective hospitals to complete the transplantation procedure for matched recipients. Peter's body was carefully washed and dressed following surgery, a special teddy that his mother had asked accompany him to theatre was with him, and Peter was returned at 04:30 to a private room in the ICU by the bedside nurse and donation specialist nurse where his mother was waiting

Peter's mother sat with her son over the next 2 hours along with her support person. The donation specialist nurse provided bereavement support contacts and information, and advised that she would be contacted in the next few days to be informed of the transplant outcomes if she wished to know them.

At 06:30 the donation specialist nurse debriefed all staff involved in both the ICU and operating theatre to let them know about the donation surgery outcomes and the care of Peter and his mother, thanked them, and completed all documentation.

DAY 3

At 10:00, as arranged, the donation specialist nursing coordinator rang Peter's mother to let her know the outcomes of the transplant surgery and provided brief recipient information, and followed this with a phone call to the regional donation specialist nurse to enable them to inform hospital staff and advise that they would be receiving follow-up letters within a few days to provide an update. The staff knew that each state and territory do this slightly differently and were delighted for the updates regarding five organ recipients and three tissue recipients.

CASE STUDY QUESTIONS

1   Reflect on the professional responsibility of the bedside nurse for donor advocacy and consider how this applies in the care of a dying patient, the potential organ donor and their family.
2   Identify the priorities of care of the donor in ensuring optimal management for transplantation success.
3   Analyse the effectiveness of healthcare professional attitudes and education in the management of the organ donation process including consent.

RESEARCH VIGNETTE

Witjes M, Jansen NE, van Dongen J, et al. Appointing nurses trained in organ donation to improve family consent rates. Nurse Crit Care 2020;25:200–304

Abstract

Background: One of the most important bottlenecks in the organ donation process worldwide is the high family refusal rate.

Aims and objectives: The main aim of this study was to examine where family guidance by trained donation practitioners increased the family consent rate for organ donation.

Design: This was a prospective intervention study.

Methods: Intensive and coronary care unit nurses were trained in communication about donation (i.e. trained donation practitioners (TDPs)) in two hospitals. The trained donation practitioners were appointed to guide the families of patients with poor medical prognosis. When the patient became a potential donor, the TDP was there to guide the family in making a well-considered decision about donation. The authors compared the family consent rate for donation with and without the guidance of a TDP.

Results: The consent rate for donation with guidance by a TDP was 58.8% (20/34), while the consent rate without guidance by a TDP was 41.4% (41/99, $P = 0.110$) in those patients where the family had to decide on organ donation.

Conclusions: The data suggest that family guidance by a TDP could benefit consent rates for organ donation.

Relevance to clinical practice: Trained nurses play an important role in supporting the families of patients who became potential donors to guide them through the decision-making process after organ donation request.

Critique

This article reports a study that focuses on the practice of organ donation consent in the Netherlands, which has an opt-in national donor registry (DR) currently taken up by only 40% of the population. For the remaining 60% of the population, organ donation is permitted only with the explicit consent of the next of kin (opt-in consent system). The next of kin need to make the very important and difficult decision regarding proceeding with organ donation at a highly stressful time, with a refusal rate up to 68% for potential donors who are not registered on the DR. Evidence from other published articles, and results of previous studies conducted in the Netherlands, suggested higher consent rates for donation occurred if there were specifically trained ICU nurses providing guidance and communication about donation to the next of kin of potential donors.

Funding was obtained to train ICU nurses in some hospitals to provide specific communication about donation and guidance to relatives of potential donors, and the authors compared donation consent rates where TDPs were utilised with consent rates without guidance of a TDP. The results of the study showed that guidance by an ICU nurse trained as a TDP led to a higher consent rate, although this was not statistically significant owing to a lack of power (small sample size) primarily due to a lack of funding for enough trained TDPs to cover 24/7 (including weekends/nights). Other limitations documented were the lack of measurement of potential confounding variables that could influence consent rates (e.g. age, sex, hospital length of stay, known donation wishes of potential donor). Based on their results, the authors of this study see value in continuing with implementing TDP training but highlight the need for further funding to support increased numbers of TDPs. The authors also suggest there is a need to include routine organ donation education for all ICU nurses, so they can provide appropriate support and guidance to families of potential organ donors during the donation request process.

Learning activities

1 Identify factors that might influence a family/next of kin to refuse consent to organ and tissue donation.
2 Describe the differences in existing international donation systems with regard to achieving high consent rates for organ and tissue donation.
3 Outline key benefits in the training of intensive care nurses in the donation request process.
4 Describe other support strategies or personnel that could assist grieving families/next of kin during the organ donation consent process in ICU.

Online resources

Achieving Comprehensive Coordination in Organ Donation throughout the European Union (ACCORD), www.accord-ja.eu

Association of Organ Procurement Organizations (AOPO), https://aopo.org

Australasian Transplant Coordinators Association (ATCA), www.atca.org.au

Australia and New Zealand Dialysis and Transplant Registry (ANZDATA), https://www.anzdata.org.au

Australia and New Zealand Liver Transplant Registry https://www.anzlitr.org

Australia and New Zealand Organ Donation Registry (ANZOD), https://www.anzdata.org.au

Australian and New Zealand Intensive Care Society (ANZICS), www.anzics.com.au/death-and-organ-donation/

Australian Bone Marrow Registry, https://www.abmdr.org.au/

Australian College of Critical Care Nurses (ACCCN), https://acccn.com.au

Australian Corneal Graft Registry, www.flinders.edu.au/medicine/sites/ophthalmology/clinical/the-australian-corneal-graft-registry.cfm

Australian Organ Donor Register (AODR), https://www.servicesaustralia.gov.au/australian-organ-donor-register

DonateLife, https://donatelife.net

Donation and Transplant Institute, https://tpm-dti.com/

Donor Tissue Bank of Victoria, https://dtbv.org.au

European Society for Organ Transplantation, https://esot.org

European Training Program on Organ Donation (ETPOD), http://etpod.eu

Eye Bank Association of Australia and New Zealand, http://www.ebaanz.org/

Eye Bank of South Australia, https://www.flinders.edu.au/medicine/sites/ophthalmology/clinical/eyebank.cfm

Gift of Life, www.giftoflife.on.ca

Global Observatory on Donation and Transplantation (GODT), www.transplant-observatory.org

International Registry in Organ Donation and Transplantation (IRODaT), https://www.irodat.org

Japan Organ Transplant Network, https://www.jotnw.or.jp

Lions Corneal Donation Service, https://www.cera.org.au/community/lions-eye-donation-service/

Lions Eye Bank (WA), https://www.lei.org.au/

MESOT: The Middle East Society for Organ Transplantation, https://www.mesot-tx.org

Multi Organ Harvesting Aid Network Foundation, https://www.mohanfoundation.org

NATCO, The Organization for Transplant Professionals, www.natco1.org

New Zealand National Transplant Donor Coordination Office, https://www.donor.co.nz

Organ Procurement and Transplantation Network, https://optn.transplant.hrsa.gov

Perth Bone and Tissue Bank, https://pluslife.org.au/

Professional Education Package (PEP), https://www.donatelife.gov.au/professional-education-package

Queensland Tissue Bank, https://metrosouth.health.qld.gov.au/news/tissue-banking-an-investment-in-health

The Transplantation Society (TTS), https://www.tts.org

Transplant News Network, https://www.centerspan.org

Transplant Nurses' Association (TNA), https://transplantnurses.org.au

Transplantation Society of Australia and New Zealand (TSANZ), https://tsanz.com.au

United Network for Organ Sharing (UNOS), https://unos.org

World Health Organization (WHO), https://www.who.int/health-topics/transplantation#tab=tab_1

Further reading

Australian and New Zealand Intensive Care Society (ANZICS). Statement on care and decision-making at the end of life for the critically ill. Carlton, VIC: ANZICS; 2014. Available from: https://intensivecareathome.com/wp-content/uploads/2015/05/ANZICS-Statement-on-Care-and-Decision-Making-at-the-End-of-Life.pdf. [Accessed April 2023].

Australian College of Critical Care Nurses (ACCCN). ACCCN Position statement (2012) on organ and tissue donation and transplantation: the roles of critical care nurses and the critical care units and the provision of critical care education. Surry Hills, VIC: ACCCN; 2012. Available from: https://acccn.com.au/wp-content/uploads/Organ-and-Tissue-Donation-and-Transplantation.pdf. [Accessed April 2023].

The National Health and Medical Research Council (NHMRC). Ethical guidelines for organ transplantation from deceased donors. Canberra, ACT: NHMRC; 2016. Available from: https://www.nhmrc.gov.au/research-policy/ethics/ethical-guidelines-organ-and-tissue-donation-and-transplantation. [Accessed April 2023].

References

1. Northam HL. Hope for a peaceful death and organ donation. PhD thesis. Canberra, ACT: University of Canberra; 2015. Available from: https://doi.org/10.26191/8cxf-y648. [Accessed November 2022].

2. Australian Government Organ and Tissue Authority. DonateLife. Organ and Tissue Authority; 2021. Available from: https://www.donatelife.gov.au. [Accessed November 2022].

3. National Indigenous Kidney Transplantation Taskforce (NIKTT). Improving access to and outcomes of kidney transplantation for Aboriginal and Torres Strait Islander People in Australia Performance Report. NIKTT; 2022. Available from: https://tsanz.com.au/committees/niktt.htm. [Accessed March 2023].

4. Chaturvedi S, Ullah S, Lepage A, et al. Rising incidence of end-stage kidney disease and poorer access to kidney transplant among Australian Aboriginal and Torres Strait Islander children and young adults. Kidney Int Rep 2021;6:1704–10. doi: 10.1016/j.ekir.2021.02.040.

5. Scholes-Robertson N, Gutman T, Howell M, et al. Patients' perspectives on access to dialysis and kidney transplantation in rural communities in Australia. Kidney Int Rep 2022;7:591–600. doi: 10.1016/j.ekir.2021.11.010.

6. United Network of Organ Sharing (UNOS). 2021. Available from: https://www.unos.org. [Accessed June 2022].

7. Eurotransplant. Statistics report library. 2021. Available from: https://statistics.eurotransplant.org/. [Accessed June 2022].

8. United Network of Organ Sharing (UNOG). History of transplantation. Richmond, VA: UNOG; 2023. Available from: https://unos.org/transplant/history/#:~:text=In%201954%2C%20the%20kidney%20was,and%20an%20increase%20in%20demand. [Accessed March 2023].

9. McBride M, Chapman JR. An overview of transplantation in Australia. Anaesth Intensive Care 1995;23:60–4.

10. Beecher H, Adams R, Clifford-Berger A, et al. A definition of irreversible coma. JAMA 1968;205(6):85–8.

11. Souter M, Van Norman G. Ethical controversies at end of life after traumatic brain injury: defining death and organ donation. Crit Care Med 2010;38(S9):S502–9.

12. Uniform Determination of Death Act (1980). Available from https://www.uniformlaws.org/committees/community-home?CommunityKey=155faf5d-03c2-4027-99ba-ee4c99019d6c. [Accessed March 2023]

13. Australian Capital Territory Government. Transplantation and Anatomy Act, 1978. Canberra, ACT: Australian Government; 2022. Available from: https://www.legislation.act.gov.au/a/1978-44/. [Accessed March 2023].

14. Arshad A, Anderson B, Sharif A. Comparison of organ donation and transplantation rates between opt-out and opt-in systems. Kidney Int 2019;95:1453–60.

15. Colombo D, Ammirati E. Cyclosporine in transplantation – a history of converging timelines. J Biol Regul Homeost Agents 2011;25(4):493–504.

16. Enderby C, Keller CA. An overview of immunosuppression in solid organ transplantation. Am J Manag Care 2015;21(1 Suppl):S12–23.

17. Madden S, Collett D, Walton P, et al. The effect on consent rates for deceased organ donation in Wales after the introduction of an opt-out system. Anaesthesia 2020;75(9):1146–52. doi: 10.1111/anae.15055.

18. Etheredge HR. Assessing global organ donation policies: opt in vs opt out. Risk Manag Healthc Policy 2021;14:1985–98.

19. Rudge CJ. Organ donation: opting in or opting out? Br J Gen Pract 2018;68(667):62–3. doi: 10.3399%2Fbjgp18X694445.

20. Australian Department of Human Services. Australian Organ Donor Register. Canberra, ACT: Australian Government; 2021. Available from: https://www.servicesaustralia.gov.au/australian-organ-donor-register. [Accessed June 2022].

21. Muthiah MD, Chua MSH, Griva K, et al. A multiethnic Asian perspective of presumed consent for organ donation: a population-based perception study. Front Public Health 2021;9:712584.

22. World Health Organization (WHO). Guiding principles on human cell, tissue and organ transplantation. Geneva: WHO; 2010. Available from: https://apps.who.int/iris/handle/10665/341814. [Accessed April 2023].

23. Human Resources and Services Administration (HRSA). Organ procurement and transplantation network modernization initiative. US Department of Health and Human Services; 2018. Available from: https://www.organdonor.gov. [Accessed November 2022].

24. The Transplantation Society of Australia and New Zealand Inc. (TSANZ). Clinical guidelines for organ transplantation from deceased donors. Sydney, NSW: TSANZ; 2022. Available from: https://tsanz.com.au/storage/documents/TSANZ_Clinical_Guidelines_Version-15_29042021.pdf. [Accessed November 2022]

25. Donatelife. National study of family experiences of organ and tissue donation. Feedback from families. Canberra, ACT: Australian Government Organ and Tissue Authority; Available from: https://www.donatelife.gov.au/about-us/data-and-research/national-study-family-experiences-organ-and-tissue-donation. [Accessed March 2023).

26. Therapeutic Goods Administration. 2022. Available from: https://www.tga.gov.au. [Accessed November 2022].

27. Australia and New Zealand Organ Donation Registry (ANZOD). Registry report. Adelaide, SA: ANZOD; 2022. Available from: https://www.anzdata.org.au/anzod/. [Accessed November 2022].

28. World Health Organization (WHO). Clinical criteria for the determination of death. Licence: CC BY-NC-SA 3.0 IGO. Geneva: WHO; 2017. Available from: https://apps.who.int/iris/bitstream/10665/254737/1/WHO-HIS-SDS-2017.5-eng.pdf. [Accessed March 2023].

29. Barker CF, Markmann JF. Historical overview of transplantation. Cold Spring Harb Perspect Med 2013;3:a014977. Available from: https://perspectivesinmedicine.cshlp.org/content/3/4/a014977.full. [Accessed November 2022].

30. Witjes M, Jansen NE, van der Hoeven JG, et al. Interventions aimed at healthcare professionals to increase the number of organ donors: a systematic review. Crit Care 2019;23(1):227.

31. Shemie SD, Hornby L, Baker A, et al. International guideline development for the determination of death. Intensive Care Med 2014;40(6): 788–97.

32. Australian and New Zealand Intensive Care Society (ANZICS). The ANZICS statement on death and organ donation, ed. 4.1. Melbourne, VIC: ANZICS; 2021. Available from: https://www.anzics.com.au/wp-content/uploads/2022/04/ANZICS-Statement-on-Death-and-Organ-Donation. pdf. [Accessed November 2022].

33. Omairi AM, Pandey S. Targeted temperature management. [Updated 2022 Aug 28]. In: StatPearls [Internet]. Treasure Island, FL: StatPearls Publishing; 2022. Available from: https://www.ncbi.nlm.nih.gov/books/NBK556124/. [Accessed November 2022]

34. Donation Transplant Institute (DTI). 2022. Available from: https://tpm-dti.com/. [Accessed November 2022].

35. Association of Organ Procurement Organizations (AOPO). Who we are. McLean, VA: AOPO; 2022. Available from: https://aopo.org/. [Accessed November 2022].

36. European Directorate for the Quality of Medicines and HealthCare (EDQM). Guide to the quality and safety of organs for transplantation. 8th ed. Strasbourg: EDQM; 2022. Available from: https://www.edqm.eu/en/guide-quality-and-safety-of-organs-for-transplantation. [Accessed November 2022]

37. Escudero D, Valentín MO, Escalante JL, et al. Intensive care practices in brain death diagnosis and organ donation. Anaesthesia 2015;70:1130–9.

38. Domínguez-Gil B, Delmonico FL, Shaheen FA, et al. The critical pathway for deceased donation: reportable uniformity in the approach to deceased donation. Transpl Int 2011;24(4):373–8. doi: 10.1111/j.1432-2277.2011.01243.x.

39. Raza F, Neuberger J. Consent in organ transplantation: putting legal obligations and guidelines into practice. BMC Med Ethics 2022;23:69. doi: 10.1186/s12910-022-00791-y.

40. Escudero D, Valentín MO, Escalante JL, et al. Intensive care practices in brain death diagnosis and organ donation. Anaesthesia 2015;70:1130–9.

41. Hulme W, Allen J, Manara AR, et al. Factors influencing family consent rate for organ donation in the UK. Anaesthesia 2016;71:1053–63.

42. Marck CH, Neate SL, Skinner MR, et al. Factors relating to consent for organ donation: prospective data on potential organ donors. Intern Med J 2015;45(1):40–7.

43. European Training Program on Organ Donation. Barcelona: EDPOD; nd. Available from: www.etpod.eu/etpod.html. [Accessed November 2022].

44. Cypel M, Levvey B, Van Raemdonck D, et al. International society for heart and lung transplantation donation after circulatory death registry report. J Heart Lung Transplant 2015;34(10):1278–82. doi: 10.1016/j.hoalun.2015.08.015.

45. Queensland University of Technology (QUT). End of life law in Australia. Organ donation. Brisbane, QLD: QUT; 2022. Available from: https:// end-of-life.qut.edu.au/organ-donation#547407. [Accessed February 2023].

46. Simonsson J, Keijzer K, Södereld T, et al. Intensive critical care nurses' with limited experience: experiences of caring for an organ donor during the donation process. J Clin Nurs 2020;29:1614–22.

47. Forsberg A, Lennerling A, Fridh I, et al. Attitudes towards organ donor advocacy among Swedish intensive care nurses. Nurs Crit Care 2015;20(3):126–33.

48. Flodén A, Lennerling A, Fridh I, et al. Development and psychometric evaluation of the instrument: Attitudes Towards Organ Donor Advocacy Scale (ATODAS). Open Nurs J 2011;5:65–73.

49. Tawil I, Brown LH, Comfort D, et al. Experiences of the families concerning organ donation of a family member with brain death. Iran J Nurs Midwifery Res 2014;19(3):323–9.

50. World Health Organization (WHO). Clinical criteria for the determination of death WHO technical expert consultation. Geneva: WHO; 2014. Available from: https://apps.who.int/iris/handle/10665/254737. [Accessed April 2023].

51. Australia and New Zealand Organ Donation Registry (ANZOD). Deceased organ donor pathway. Adelaide, SA: ANZOD; 2022. Available from: https://www.anzdata.org.au/wp-content/uploads/2022/05/s03_pathway_2021_ar_2022_v2.0_section_20220521_final.pdf. [Accessed November 2022].

52. Citerio G, Cypel M, Dobb G, et al. Organ donation in adults: a critical care perspective. Intensive Care Med 2016;42(3):305–15.

53. Australasian Transplant Coordinators. National SOP organ allocation organ rotations and urgent listing version 4.0. February 2023. Available from: https://www.atca.org.au/files/TSANZ_OTA_ADTCA_NationalSOP_230223_FINAL.01.pdf. [Accessed April 2023].

54. Australian Government Organ and Tissue Authority. OrganMatch. 2022. Available from: https://www.donatelife.gov.au/for-healthcare-workers/ organmatch/what%E2%80%99s-new. [Accessed November 2022].

55. Sarti AJ, Sutherland S, Meade M, et al. The experiences of family members of deceased organ donors and suggestions to improve the donation process: a qualitative study. CMAJ 2022;194(30):E1054–61. doi: 10.1503/cmaj.220508.

56. Thuong M, Ruiz A, Evrard P, et al. New classification of donation after circulatory death donors definitions and terminology. Transpl Int 2016;29:749–59.

57. Manyalich M, Nelson H, Francis D. The need and opportunity for donation after circulatory death worldwide. Curr Opin Organ Transplant 2018;23(1):1361.

Practice standards for specialist critical care nurses

DOMAIN	NO.	STANDARD	NO.	ELEMENT
Professional practice The standards in this domain relate to the professional, legal and ethical responsibilities of critical care nurses and include knowledge of the legal implications of critical care nursing practice, accountability for practice and the ability to interpret unfamiliar situations in a legal and ethical sense. The standards also include awareness and protection of the rights of patients and their families.	1	Functions within professional and legal parameters of critical care nursing practice.	1.1	Applies a knowledge of relevant legislation, professional standards, policies and procedures to critical care nursing practice.
			1.2	Observant of the legal implications of actions taken within the critical care team and fulfils the duty of care in clinical practice.
			1.3	Recognises and responds to unsafe or unprofessional practices by reporting appropriately.
			1.4	Applies the required legal and ethical framework of recording information in the critical care setting.
			1.5	Contributes to formation of policies and protocols to ensure safe patient outcomes.
	2	Protects the rights of patients and their families.	2.1	Applies knowledge of, and advocates for, the rights of patients and their families in critical care settings.
	3	Demonstrates accountability for nursing practice.	3.1	Accepts responsibility for own actions.
			3.2	Makes complex and informed independent decisions within own level of competence and scope of practice.
	4	Demonstrates and contributes to ethical decision making.	4.1	Demonstrates an accurate knowledge of contemporary ethical issues underpinning critical care nursing practice and complies with the profession's code of ethics and code of conduct.
			4.2	Contributes to multidisciplinary ethical discussion and decision-making processes/ framework within the critical care setting.

DOMAIN	NO.	STANDARD	NO.	ELEMENT
Provision and coordination of care This domain relates to essential nursing practices that establish and sustain a holistic nurse–patient–family relationship that optimises the wellbeing of the patient and family. The standards include an ability to address the physiological, psychological, physical, emotional and spiritual needs of the patient and family, as well as to optimise the physical and non-physical environment.	5	Provides patient- and family-centred critical care.	5.1	Involves the patient and family as active participants in the process of care.
			5.2	Practises with cultural sensitivity and awareness of social factors to enhance patient and family wellbeing.
			5.3	Personalises the patient care environment.
			5.4	Meets the comfort needs of patients and their families.
			5.5	Establishes, maintains and concludes therapeutic interpersonal relationships with patients and their families.
	6	Promotes optimal comfort, wellbeing and safety in a highly technological environment that is often unfamiliar to patients and families.	6.1	Ensures a safe environment for patients, families and staff by identifying, minimising or eliminating risks.
	7	Manages and coordinates the care of a variety of patients.	7.1	Organises workload to meet planned and unplanned patient care needs to ensure optimal patient outcomes.
			7.2	Negotiates and delegates care to optimise matching between nurses' scope of practice and the complexity of care for individual patients.
			7.3	Optimises delivery of care through the effective use of human and physical resource management.
	8	Manages therapeutic interventions.	8.1	Acts on assessment findings to appropriately initiate, monitor and manage therapeutic interventions.
			8.2	Applies specialised knowledge in the use of critical care technologies.
Critical thinking and analysis This domain relates to applying specialised knowledge for clinical problem solving. Integrated clinical decision making provides a foundation for the application of research evidence to practice. The domain reflects the capacity of the critical care nurse to respond to planned and unanticipated changes in patient care and to recognise the need for advanced assessment, planning and application of specialised knowledge to deliver evidence-based care.	9	Applies integrated patient assessment and interpretive skills to achieve optimal patient outcomes.	9.1	Gathers, analyses and integrates data from a variety of sources and acts on the significance of findings to formulate an individualised plan of care.
	10	Develops and manages a plan of care to achieve desired outcomes.	10.1	Formulates and implements an integrated plan of care incorporating specialised knowledge to achieve desired patient outcomes.
			10.2	Assesses effectiveness of nursing care to achieve desired outcomes and reviews plan accordingly.
			10.3	Enables continuity of care in collaboration with other members of the healthcare team.

Continued

DOMAIN	NO.	STANDARD	NO.	ELEMENT
	11	Evaluates and responds effectively to changing situations.	11.1	Initiates pre-emptive interventions in order to avoid complications.
			11.2	Analyses alterations in physiological parameters and intervenes appropriately.
			11.3	Anticipates, evaluates and responds effectively to physiological deterioration and emergency situations.
	12	Engages in and contributes to evidence-based critical care nursing practice.	12.1	Maintains an informed position in relation to current research studies and incorporates evidence-informed practice into critical care setting.
			12.2	Promotes and participates in quality activities to improve critical care patient outcomes.
Collaboration and leadership The standards in this domain relate to the leadership and education role displayed by the specialist critical care nurse and integral part played by experienced critical care nurses in the professional development of peers, students and less experienced staff.	13	Collaborates with the critical care team and other health professionals to achieve desired outcomes.	13.1	Establishes and maintains collaborative and constructive relationships with colleagues in critical care and the broader healthcare team.
			13.2	Acts as an advisor beyond the walls of the critical care environment.
	14	Acts to enhance the professional development of self and others.	14.1	Assesses own abilities and engages in activities to enhance personal and professional development.
			14.2	Identifies and assists in meeting the learning needs of others.
			14.3	Actively participates in promoting the profession of critical care.
	15	Contributes towards a supportive environment for all members of the healthcare team.	15.1	Initiates strategies to support colleagues and facilitates resolution of situations that may impact on the wellbeing of others.

Normal laboratory values

Blood analysis: parameters, applications and normal ranges[1]

PARAMETER	APPLICATION	NORMAL RANGE
Adrenocorticotrophic hormone (ACTH)	Aetiology of corticosteroid abnormality	<10 pmol/L
Albumin	Hydration, nutrition status, protein-related disorders and liver disease	32–45 g/L
Alkaline phosphatase (ALP)	Hepatobiliary or bone disease	Neonates/paediatrics: 0 days to <1 week (80–380) U/L 1 week to <4 weeks (120–550) U/L 4 weeks to <26 weeks (120 650) U/L 26 weeks to <2 years (120–450) U/L 2 years to <6 years (120–370) U/L 6 years to <10 years (120–440) U/L Males: 10 years to <14 years (130–530) U/L 14 years to <15 years (105–480) U/L 15 years to <17 years (80–380) U/L 17 years to <19 years (50–220) U/L 19 years to <22 years (45–150) U/L 22 years to <120 years (30–110) U/L Females: 10 years to <13 years (100–460) U/L 13 years to <14 years (70–330) U/L 14 years to <15 years (50–280) U/L 15 years to <16 years (45–170) U/L 16 years to <22 years (35–140) U/L 22 years to <120 years (30–110) U/L
Alanine aminotransferase (ALT)	Liver damage	Neonate: <50 U/L Adult: <35 U/L
Amylase	Acute pancreatitis	Varies based on age, gender and laboratory analysis method, with normal values generally considered in the range of:[2] Newborn: 6–65 U/L Adults: 30–220 U/L; Note: values may be slightly increased during normal pregnancy and in elderly Values >3 times upper limit of normal are considered critical
Anion gap	Aetiology of metabolic acidosis	8–16 mmol/L (4–13 mmol/L if K not included)

Continued

PARAMETER	APPLICATION	NORMAL RANGE
Aspartate aminotransferase (AST)	Liver damage	Neonates: <80 U/L Adults: <40 U/L
Base excess (arterial blood)	Metabolic component of acid–base disorders	(−3) to (+3) mmol/L
Bicarbonate (HCO_3^-)	Acid–base disorders, particularly metabolic component	Neonates/paediatrics: 0 days to <1 week (15–28) mmol/L 1 week to <2 years (16–29) mmol/L 2 years to <10 years (17–30) mmol/L 10 years to <18 years (20–32) mmol/L Adults: 18 years to <120 years (22–32) mmol/L
Bilirubin	Hepatobiliary disease and haemolysis	Total: <20 micromol/L Direct: <7 micromol/L
Calcium (Ca^{2+})	Hyper/hypocalcaemia	Neonates/paediatrics: 0 days to <1 week (1.85–2.80) mmol/L 1 week to <26 weeks (2.20–2.80) mmol/L 26 weeks to <2 years (2.20–2.70) mmol/L 2 years to <18 years (2.20–2.65) mmol/L Adults: 18 years to <120 years (2.10–2.60) mmol/L Calcium corrected for albumin: 18 years to <120 years (2.10–2.60) mmol/L Ionised calcium: 18 years to <120 years (1.16–1.30) mmol/L
Carboxyhaemoglobin	Carbon monoxide exposure	0.2–2.0% of total haemoglobin normally, up to 8.5% in heavy smokers
Chloride (Cl^-)	Causes of acid–base disturbance	Neonates/paediatrics: 0 days to <1 week (98–115) mmol/L 1 week to <18 years (97–110) mmol/L Adults: 18 years to <120 years (95–110) mmol/L
Cholesterol	Lipid status	Total: ≤4.0 mmol/L (recommended by Australian National Heart Foundation) HDL: 1.0–2.2 mmol/L (females) 0.9–2.0 mmol/L (males) Therapeutic targets: >1.0 mmol/L LDL: 2.0–3.4 mmol/ L Therapeutic LDL targets: <2.5 mmol/L (<1.8 mmol/L for very high risk) Non-HDL: <3.3 mmol/L (<2.5 mmol/L for very high risk) Triglyceride: <2.0 mmol/L (fasting)
Creatinine kinase (CK)	Diagnosis of myocardial damage	Neonate: 70–380 U/L Adult female: 30–180 U/L Adult male: 60–220 U/L
Creatine kinase MB isoenzyme (CKMB)	Diagnosis of myocardial damage	CKMB: 0–10 U/L; 0–5% of the total CK

PARAMETER	APPLICATION	NORMAL RANGE
Creatinine (Cr)	Renal function, particularly glomerular filtration	Neonates/paediatrics: 0 days to <1 week (22–93) micromol/L 1 week to <4 weeks (17–50) micromol/L 4 weeks to <2 years (11–36) micromol/L 2 years to <6 years (20–44) micromol/L 6 years to <12 years (27–58) micromol/L Adult males: 12 years to <15 years (35–83 micromol/L) 15 years to <19 years (50–100 micromol/L) 19 years to <60 years (60–110 micromol/L) Adult females: 12 years to <15 years (35–74 micromol/L) 15 years to <19 years (38–82 micromol/L) 19 years to <60 years (45–90 micromol/L)
Glucose	Hyper/hypoglycaemia	Fasting: 3.0–5.4 mmol/L Random: 3.0–7.7 mmol/L
Haemoglobin A_{1c}	Glycated Hb. Diabetes mellitus: monitoring of glycaemia over previous 3 months. Diagnosis of diabetes	HbA_{1c}: 3.5–6.0% (15–42 mmol/mol) HbA_{1c}: 6.1–6.4% (43–47 mmol/mol) indeterminate HbA_{1c}: ≥6.5% (≥48 mmol/mol) diagnostic of diabetes
Iron	Iron deficiency or overload. Serum ferritin level <30 micrograms/L for an adult is diagnostic of iron deficiency. Levels >310 micrograms/L are associated with liver toxicity	30–300 micrograms/L Values may vary according to laboratory method
L-lactate	Metabolic acidosis	Fasting arterial blood: 0.3–0.8 mmol/L. Fasting venous blood: 0.3–1.3 mmol/L
Lactate dehydrogenase (LDH)	Assessment of liver disease	120–250 U/L (method and age dependent) Normal range for adults
Magnesium (Mg)	Hypomagnesaemia	Neonates/paediatrics: 0 days to <1 week (0.60–1.00) mmol/L 1 week to <18 years (0.65–1.10) mmol/L Adults: 18 years to <120 years (0.70–1.10) mmol/L
Myoglobin (serum)	Detection of muscle damage	<55 micrograms/L[2]
Osmolality	Suspected poisoning with some substances, e.g. alcohol, methanol	Neonates: 270–290 mmol/kg Adults: 275–295 mmol/kg
Phosphate (PO_4)	Renal failure, hyper-/hypoparathyroidism metabolic bone disease	Neonate/paediatrics: 0 days to <1 week (1.25–2.85) mmol/L 1 week to <4 weeks (1.50–2.75) mmol/L 4 weeks to <26 weeks (1.45–2.50) mmol/L 26 weeks to <1 year (1.30–2.30) mmol/L 1 year to <4 years (1.10–2.20) mmol/L 4 years to <15 years (0.90–2.00) mmol/L 15 years to <18 years (0.80–1.85) mmol/L Adults: 18 years to <20 years (0.75–1.65) mmol/L 20 years to <120 years (0.75–1.50) mmol/L

Continued

PARAMETER	APPLICATION	NORMAL RANGE
Potassium (K$^+$)	Hyper/hypokalaemia	Neonates/paediatrics: 0 days to <1 week (3.8–6.5) mmol/L 1 week to <26 weeks (4.2–6.7) mmol/L 26 weeks to <2 years (3.9–5.6) mmol/L 2 years to <18 years (3.6–5.3) mmol/L Adults: 18 years to <120 years (3.5–5.2) mmol/L
Protein	Used in conjunction with albumin to calculate globulin, diagnosis of protein- and nutrition-related disorders	Neonate: 40–75 g/L Child <2 years: 50–75 g/L Adults: 60–80 g/L
Sodium (Na$^+$)	Fluid and electrolyte status	Neonates/paediatrics: 0 days to <1 week (132–147) mmol/L 1 week to <18 years (133–144) mmol/L Adults: 18 years to <120 years (135–145) mmol/L
Troponin I or troponin T	Myocardial infarction	Normally not detected
Urea	Renal function	Neonates: 1.0–4.0 mmol/L Adults: 3.0–8.0 mmol/L

Haematology: parameters, applications and normal values

PARAMETER	APPLICATION	NORMAL VALUE
Activated clotting time (ACT)	Heparin therapy	Varies based on product in use
Activated partial thromboplastin time (APTT)	Coagulopathy and monitoring of heparin therapy	Varies based on laboratory methods, usually 25–35 seconds
Antithrombin III (AT III)	Investigation of venous thromboembolism	Varies based on laboratory method Functional (guide only): 80–120% of activity in pooled normal plasma Immunoassay (guide only): 0.2–0.4 g/L
Bleeding time	Assessment in some bleeding disorders, e.g. von Willebrand's disease	For investigation of bleeding risk, please refer to coagulation profile, platelet function analyser (PFA), platelet aggregometry
D-dimers	Indication of recent or ongoing fibrinolysis, possibly indicating disseminated intravascular coagulation (DIC)	Varies based on laboratory method
Haemoglobin (Hb)	Anaemia	Children 6–59 months: ≥110 g/L Children 5–11 years: ≥115 g/L Children 12–14 years: ≥120 g/L Non-pregnant women (≥15 years): ≥120 g/L Pregnant women: ≥110 g/L Men (>15 years): ≥130 g/L
International normalised ratio (INR)	Oral anticoagulant therapy	Varies according to clinical indication. Target INR will be individualised for each patient. Typical range for atrial fibrillation 2.0–3.0

PARAMETER	APPLICATION	NORMAL VALUE
Packed cell volume (PCV) (also referred to as haematocrit)	Anaemia	Infant (3 months): 0.32–0.44 Child (3–6 years): 0.36–0.44 Child (10–12 years): 0.37–0.45 Adult (female): 0.37–0.47 Adult (male): 0.40–0.54
Plasminogen	Investigation of tendency towards clotting, e.g. venous thromboembolism	50–150%
Platelet count	Excessive or inappropriate bleeding	150–400×10^9/L
Prothrombin time (PT)	Detection of coagulation factor deficiencies due to vitamin K deficiency	Varies based on laboratory Reagent dependent; prothrombin time generally 11–15 seconds
Red cell count (RCC)	Anaemia	Neonate/paediatrics: Term cord blood: 4.0–6.0×10^{12}/L 3 months: 3.2–4.8×10^{12}/L 1 year: 3.6–5.2×10^{12}/L 3–6 years: 4.1–5.5×10^{12}/L 10–12 years: 4.0–5.4×10^{12}/L Adults: Female: 3.8–5.8×10^{12}/L Male: 4.5–6.5×10^{12}/L
Thrombin time (TT)	Acquired or inherited disorders of haemostasis	Varies based on laboratory method, but usually 14–16 seconds
White cell count (WCC)	Infection or inflammatory disease	Neonate: 6.0–22.0×10^9/L Child (1 year): 6.0–18.0×10^9/L Child (4–7 years): 5.0–15.0×10^9/L Child (8–12 years): 4.5–13.5×10^9/L Adult: 3.5–10.0×10^9/L

Blood gases: parameters and normal values

PARAMETER	NORMAL VALUE
Arterial	
pH	7.36–7.44 (36–44 nmol/L)
Partial pressure of oxygen (PaO$_2$)	11.0–13.5 kPa (80–100 mmHg) (varies with age)
Partial pressure of carbon dioxide (PaCO$_2$)	4.6–6.0 kPa (35–45 mmHg)
Oxygen saturation (SaO$_2$)	>94%
Venous	
pH	7.32–7.42
Partial pressure of oxygen (PvO$_2$)	44–69 mmHg
Partial pressure of carbon dioxide (PvCO$_2$)	Male: 39–52 mmHg Female: 36–49 mmHg
Oxygen saturation (SvO$_2$)	>70%

Urine analysis: parameters, applications and normal values

PARAMETER	APPLICATION	NORMAL VALUE
Albumin	Diabetic nephropathy, renal disease	Normal: <30 mg albumin/g creatinine Microalbuminuria: 30–300 mg albumin/g creatinine Macroalbuminuria: >300 mg albumin/g creatinine
Calcium	Renal calculi	2.5–7.5 mmol/24 hours Fasting spot urine: Males: 0.04–0.45 mol/mol creatinine Females: 0.10–0.58 mol/mol creatinine
Chloride	Identification of site of chloride loss in electrolyte disturbance	Dependent on intake, but usually 100–250 mmol/24 hours
Cortisol (free)	Adrenocortical hyperfunction	100–300 nmol/24 hours
Creatinine clearance	Glomerular filtration rate	>70 mL/min in a young adult, typically falling approx. 0.5 mL/min per year at ages over 30 years
Magnesium	Urinary magnesium loss Cardiac arrhythmias	2.5–8.0 mmol/24 hours (related to daily intake) Adults> 18 years 0.70–1.10 mmol/L
Myoglobin	Suspected rhabdomyolysis	Not normally detected
Osmolality	Renal disease, syndrome of inappropriate antidiuretic hormone, polyuric syndromes	50–1200 mmol/kg
Potassium	Differentiation of renal potassium loss from other causes of hypokalaemia	40–100 mmol/24 hours (related to daily intake)
Protein	Renal disease	<150 mg/24 hours During pregnancy: <250 mg/24 hours
Sodium	Causes of hyponatraemia	In hyponatraemia or hypovolaemic shock without acute tubular necrosis, urine sodium should be <20 mmol/L and fractional excretion of sodium should be <1.5% If extracellular fluid volume and plasma sodium are normal, urine sodium should equal intake minus non-renal losses, typically 75–300 mmol/24 hours
Urea	Renal function, occasionally assessment of nitrogen balance in patients receiving parenteral nutrition	420–720 mmol/24 hours

Sources: The Royal College of Pathologists of Australasia. RCPA manual – online. ISSN 1449-821. Available from: https://www.rcpa. edu.au/Manuals/RCPA-Manual. [Accessed 5 March 2023]; Pagana KD, Pagana TJ, Pagana TN. Mosby's diagnostic and laboratory test reference, 12th ed. St Louis, MO: Elsevier; 2015. Rees KL., Koerbin G, Ling L, et al. Reference intervals for venous blood gas measurement in adults. Clin Chem Lab Med 2021;59(5):947–54.

Glossary of terms

actigraph. Used for measuring movement, in particular to measure the quantity of sleep.

action potential. The electrical activity developed in a muscle or nerve cell during activity.

acute coronary syndrome. A broad spectrum of clinical presentations, spanning ST-segment elevation myocardial infarction through to an accelerated pattern of angina without evidence of myonecrosis.

acute respiratory distress syndrome. An acute syndrome of rapid onset in which the patient has evidence of hypoxia and non-cardiogenic pulmonary oedema.

acute respiratory failure. Occurs when there is a reduction in the body's ability to maintain either oxygenation or ventilation, or both.

advance directives. A method to document preferences about an individual's future healthcare should situations arise where they are no longer competent to make decisions.

advanced life support. The provision of effective airway management, ventilation of the lungs and production of circulation by means of techniques additional to those of basic life support. These techniques may include, but are not limited to, advanced airway management, tracheal intubation, intravenous access/drug therapy and defibrillation.

adverse event. An injury or event that is due to healthcare management and results in temporary or permanent harm to patients.

afterload. The load imposed on the muscle during contraction, and translates to systolic myocardial wall tension.

anterior cord syndrome. Spinal cord injury to the motor and sensory pathways in the anterior parts of the spine; thus patients are able to feel crude sensation, but movement and detailed sensation are lost in the posterior part of the spinal cord.

anxiety. A disorder characterised by excessive concern or worry with difficulty controlling the level of concern, and may be accompanied by irritability, restlessness and disturbed sleep.

arterial blood gas. An arterial blood sample taken to assess pH, bicarbonate, oxygen and carbon dioxide levels, and other electrolytes.

asthma. A lower respiratory tract disease characterised by mucosal and immune system dysfunction. The chronic inflammatory process causes narrowing of bronchial airways, obstructing airflow leading to episodes of wheezing, breathlessness and chest tightening.

auscultation. The action of listening to sounds from the heart, lungs or other organs, typically with a stethoscope.

automatic tube compensation. A feature available on some ventilators in which the ventilator employs an algorithm to increase airway pressure to overcome the resistance of the artificial airway during inspiration.

backwards upwards right pressure manoeuvre. A technique where pressure is applied to mobilise the thyroid cartilage in the sequence backwards (towards the spine) and to the right side in order to help visualise the vocal cords and assist with intubation.

beneficence. The doing of good; promoting the well-being of another person.

biphasic. Pattern of electrical flow where the current reverses direction in the middle of the waveform, flowing first from one electrode pad, through the heart, to the second electrode pad, and then from the second pad through the heart to the first.

birth weight. The first weight of the baby (stillborn or live born) obtained after birth.

bronchiolitis. Viral infection causing obstruction and oedema of the small airways, resulting in air trapping and respiratory distress, generally seen in infants 12 months of age and younger.

business case. A management tool used to outline the clinical needs (who, what, when, where and how) and their implications, such as the expected financial return on investment.

caesarean section/birth. Operative birth through an abdominal incision.

capnography. Monitoring of expired carbon dioxide.

cardiac arrest. Cessation of heart action recognised by the absence of response, absence of normal breathing and absence of movement.

cardiac pacing. The delivery of an electrical impulse to either or both the atria and ventricles to initiate or maintain normal cardiac electrical activity.

cardiopulmonary resuscitation. Comprises those techniques used to minimise the effects of circulatory arrest and to assist the return of spontaneous circulation, including the technique of rescue breathing combined with external chest compressions.

care bundle. A set of evidence-based interventions or processes of care, applied to selected patients in order to ensure appropriate, standardised care.

catabolism. The convergent process, in which many different types of molecules are broken down into relatively few types of end-products.

cerebral spinal fluid. An ultrafiltrate of blood plasma composed of 99% water, making it close to the composition of the brain extracellular fluid.

chemoreceptor. A sensor that responds to change in chemical composition in the blood.

chemosis. Conjunctival oedema, often associated with positive-pressure ventilation, positive end-expiratory pressure or prone positioning.

child. 'Young child' is aged between 1 and 8 years and 'older child' is aged between 9 and 14 years inclusive.

chronic heart failure (CHF). Refers to a complex syndrome distinguished by a number of characteristics, particularly shortness of breath or fatigue, that occur at rest or on exertion. It is also characterised by objective evidence of cardiac dysfunction or structured cardiac abnormalities that impair the left ventricle from filling with or ejecting blood to meet the body's demands.

clinical practice guideline. Evidence-based statements outlining appropriate healthcare for specific clinical circumstances.

coagulopathy. Disorder of the clotting mechanism of the blood, which can be caused by pre-existing disease, medications, pathophysiological conditions such as hypothermia and acidosis or current treatment such as massive blood transfusion.

cognitive dysfunction. Associated with problems remembering, solving problems, thinking and making decisions.

coma. A state of unresponsiveness from which the patient cannot be aroused by verbal and physical stimuli to produce any meaningful response; therefore, coma implies the absence of both arousal and content of consciousness.

conduction. The process by which electrical activity is directly transmitted through cells when there is a difference of electrical potential between adjoining regions, without movement of the tissue.

conjunctivitis. An inflammation of the conjunctiva, i.e. the transparent membrane that lines the eyelid and eyeball. Sometimes also called pink eye.

continuous lateral rotation therapy. An intervention in which the patient is rotated continually, on a specialised bed, through a set number of degrees; it helps to relieve pressure areas and can significantly improve oxygenation. It is also known as kinetic bed therapy.

contractility. The force of ventricular ejection, or the inherent ability of the ventricle to perform external work, independent of afterload or preload.

coronary heart disease or coronary artery disease. A narrowing of the small blood vessels that supply blood and oxygen to the heart.

counterpulsation. Rapid inflation of the intra-aortic balloon catheter at the onset of diastole of each cardiac cycle and then deflation immediately before the onset of the next systole.

critical care nursing. Specialised nursing care of critically ill patients who have an immediate life-threatening or potentially life-threatening illness or injury.

critically ill patients. Patients who have an immediate life-threatening or potentially life-threatening illness or injury causing compromise to the function of one or more organs.

croup (laryngotracheobronchitis). A set of symptoms caused by acute swelling causing obstruction in the upper airway (larynx, trachea and bronchi) from inflammation and oedema, most commonly seen in young children during winter months.

cultural safety. Involves effective nursing practice whereby patients and their families determine that their cultural needs have been met and that they feel safe. Effective nursing practice requires nurses to reflect on their own cultural location and how this may influence the way in which they interact with patients from another culture. In addition to ethnically related culture, culture is defined broadly to include age, generation, gender, sexual orientation, socioeconomic status, migrant experience, occupation, religious or spiritual beliefs and disability.

damage-control surgery. A four-stage surgical approach that involves rapid initial control of haemorrhage and contamination, usually with packing and temporary closure, followed by ongoing resuscitation in the ICU and reoperation for definitive repair and reconstruction.

delirium. A reversible cognitive disorder characterised by inattention, disorientation and problems with executive function not explained by another pre-existing, established or evolving other neurocognitive disorder. There are three types of delirium: hyperactive, hypoactive and mixed.

donation after cardiac death. A solid organ donation option for a patient who has not progressed and is not likely to progress to brain death. It is also known as non-heart-beating donor and donation after circulatory death.

depolarisation. The electrical state in an excitable cell where the inside of the cell becomes less negative relative to the outside.

depression. Mental health disorder characterised by feeling sad or low or negative mood. People may experience a lack of motivation and interest in activities, feel slowed down or have difficulties thinking, concentrating or making decisions.

eclampsia. A severe variant of preeclampsia, characterised by tonic–clonic seizures that are not caused by any pre-existing disease or other identifiable causes, e.g. epilepsy, cerebral haemorrhage.

electroencephalography. The recording of electrical activity by sensors attached to the scalp produced by electrical discharge of neurons within the brain.

embolism. Obstruction of an artery, typically by a blood clot or an air bubble.

encephalitis. Inflammation of the brain substance.

endotracheal tube. An artificial airway used in critical care settings to enable delivery of mechanical ventilation and clearance of airway secretions.

enzyme. Substance produced by a living organism that acts as a catalyst to bring about a specific biochemical reaction.

epiglottitis. Inflammation of the epiglottis, frequently involving surrounding structures, with the classic description of a swollen, cherry-red, softened and floppy epiglottis, which tends to fall backwards, obstructing the airway.

ethics. The study of rational processes to inform a course of action in response to a particular situation where conflicting options exist.

evidence-based nursing. The conscientious, explicit and judicious use of research-based information in making decisions about care delivery to individuals or groups of patients.

extracorporeal membrane oxygenation. A therapy in which blood is removed from the patient and oxygenated in an artificial membrane before being returned to the patient, i.e. circulation of blood outside the body providing total artificial support of cardiac and pulmonary function.

family. Those closest to the person in knowledge, care and affection, including the immediate biological family, the family of acquisition (related by marriage or contract), and the family of choice and friends (not related biologically or by marriage or contract).

family-centred care. Incorporates planning, delivery and evaluation of healthcare that is governed by mutually beneficial partnerships among healthcare providers, patients and families.

general anaesthesia. A medication-induced state characterised by muscle relaxation, sedation and unresponsiveness.

gestation. The estimated gestational age of the baby in completed weeks (+/− any part weeks may be written as days) using all available obstetric information (clinical estimation, ultrasound, cycle length, etc.), counting from the first day of the woman's last menstrual period. Commonly recorded as 35+2/40, indicating that the gestation is 35 completed weeks and 2 days.

gravidity. The total number of pregnancies a woman has had, including the index pregnancy, regardless of the outcome (therefore including spontaneous and induced abortions and any stillborn or live born infants).

Guillain–Barré syndrome. An immune-mediated disorder resulting from generation of autoimmune antibodies and/or inflammatory cells that cross-react with epitopes on peripheral nerves and roots, leading to demyelination or axonal damage, or both, and autoimmune insult to the peripheral nerve myelin.

haemodynamic monitoring. The measurement of pressure, flow and oxygenation within the cardiovascular system.

heart failure with preserved ejection fraction. Refers to impaired diastolic filling of the left ventricle. There may or may not be impaired systolic dysfunction.

heart failure with reduced ejection fraction. Refers to inability of the heart to contract in systole.

high-frequency oscillatory ventilation. A mode of ventilation that delivers small breaths at a very high respiratory rate (between 300 and 420 per minute) to maintain alveolar opening and facilitate carbon dioxide elimination.

hypercapnoeic respiratory failure. Also known as type II respiratory failure (or failure to ventilate), presents with a high $PaCO_2$ as well as a low PaO_2.

hypoxaemic respiratory failure. Also known as type I respiratory failure (or failure to oxygenate), presents with a low PaO_2 and a normal or low $PaCO_2$.

icterus. Jaundice.

induction of labour. Procedure performed for the purpose of initiating and stimulating the process of labour. This may include the artificial rupture of the membranes, and/or the use of a balloon catheter, and/or the use of uterine-stimulating medication.

infant. A person up to the first birthday.

intensive care unit-acquired weakness. Generalised weakness that is symmetrical and develops after the onset of critical illness without another identifiable cause. A Medical Research Council – Sum Score of less than 48 (equal to or less than 80% of normal strength) or isometric handgrip dynamometry scores of less than 11 kilograms for males and less than 7 kilograms for females is indicative of ICU-acquired weakness.

intra-aortic balloon pump. Mechanical assistance for a failing heart based on the principles of diastolic augmentation and systolic unloading by counterpulsation of a balloon in the aorta.

intracranial hypertension. A sustained intracranial pressure of >15 mmHg.

intracranial pressure. The pressure exerted by the contents of the brain within the confines of the skull. Normal ICP is 0–10 mmHg.

keratitis. An inflammation of the cornea. May or may not be associated with an infection.

keratopathy. A disease of the cornea.

laryngotracheobronchitis. Also known as croup; a set of symptoms caused by acute swelling causing obstruction in the upper airway (larynx, trachea and bronchi) from inflammation and oedema and is most commonly seen in young children during winter months.

live birth. The birth of an infant, regardless of maturity or birth weight, who breathes or shows any other signs of life after being born.

magnetic resonance imaging. An imaging technique that uses the characteristic of hydrogen protons, which function like tiny spinning magnets, to generate images of the brain and body.

malignant hyperthermia. A severe reaction to anaesthetic agents which can cause muscle rigidity, breakdown of muscle fibres, high temperature, tachycardia and acidosis; if untreated, it can be life threatening.

mechanical circulatory support. Partial or total cardiovascular support devices such as intra-aortic balloon pump, ventricular assist devices and total artificial hearts.

monophasic. Pattern of electrical flow where the current, throughout the pulse, flows in one direction, from one electrode pad through the heart to the other electrode pad.

murmur. A low continuous background noise.

myasthenia gravis. An autoimmune disorder caused by autoantibodies against the nicotinic acetylcholine receptor on the postsynaptic membrane at the neuromuscular junction, which is characterised by weakness and fatigue in voluntary muscles.

myelin sheath. A lipid–protein casing that covers the neuron and provides protection to the axon, speeding the transmission of impulses along the nerve cells.

myocardial infarction. Myocardial cell death due to prolonged ischaemia.

neonate. An infant up to day 28 of life.

neurally adjusted ventilatory assistance. A type of ventilation that uses diaphragmatic movement to trigger gas flow and breath delivery.

neuroglia. The non-neuronal cells of the nervous system that are 10–50 times more prevalent than the number of neurons.

neuron. A specialised cell in the nervous system comprised of a dendrite, a cell body (also known as a soma) and an axon.

neurotransmitter. A chemical messenger used by neurons to communicate in one direction with other neurons.

non-technical skills. Cognitive, social and personal skills that complement technical skills and contribute to safe and efficient task performance.

open disclosure. Telling the truth to the patient or family about what and how an adverse event has occurred.

opioid use disorder. Overuse of opioid medications often resulting in physiological dependency and resulting risk of withdrawal.

patient dependency. An approach to quantify the care needs of individual patients, classifying patients into groups requiring similar nursing care.

patient safety. Reduction of the risk of unnecessary harm to patients to an acceptable level.

person-centred care. Emphasis on the individual with the illness that promotes the perception (and reality) of equal power and a shared partnership between the person and healthcare provider/s.

polysomnography. The continuous non-invasive recording of the physiological parameters brain activity, eye movement and muscle activity during sleep. Other parameters such as respiratory rate may be monitored to diagnose specific sleep disorders.

post-intensive care syndrome. A range of physical and emotional health concerns that patients may experience during recovery after critical illness.

postpartum. After birth. The postpartum period is normally classified as the 6 weeks following birth, when the woman's body returns to the pre-pregnancy state.

postpartum haemorrhage. ≥500 mL blood loss from the genital tract following birth. It is categorised as primary, within the first 24 hours following birth, or secondary, from 24 hours to 6 weeks postpartum.

post-traumatic stress disorder. A response to either experiencing or witnessing a traumatic event. People may present with a range of symptoms including reliving the event, nightmares and/or flashbacks, avoidant behaviours, intrusive thoughts or images and intense distress.

preeclampsia. A multisystem pregnancy disorder resulting from widespread vasospasm that is often characterised by hypertension and proteinuria.

preload. The load imposed by the initial fibre length of the cardiac muscle before contraction (i.e. at the end of diastole).

pulse oximetry. The measurement of peripheral arterial oxygen saturation.

quality monitoring. Measurement of and responses to the incidence and patterns of adverse events.

quality of life. How a person evaluates or views their life. There are many aspects of life that people use to assess its quality such as social, economic, spiritual and psychological health.

rapid response system. System developed to recognise and provide emergency response to patients who experience acute deterioration.

regional anaesthesia. An umbrella term used to describe injection of local anaesthetic in the vicinity of major nerve bundles supplying specific body areas to produce nerve blocks, epidural and spinal blocks.

repolarisation. The process by which the membrane potential of a neuron or muscle cell is restored to the cell's resting potential.

resistive range of motion. The act of actively moving against either an immovable or a resistive object.

resuscitation. Preservation or restoration of life by the establishment and/or maintenance of airway, breathing and circulation, and related emergency care.

return of spontaneous circulation. Resumption of sustained perfusing cardiac activity associated with significant respiratory effort after cardiac arrest.

reverse Trendelenburg position. Head up, feet down. A position in which the patient's hip and knee are not flexed but the head and chest are elevated at 30 degrees from the abdomen and legs.

root cause analysis. A detailed method to investigate an adverse event whereby the system and processes that contributed to the event are examined in an effort to identify system or process improvements to prevent the event from recurring.

safety culture. The product of individual and group values, attitudes, perceptions, competencies and patterns of behaviour that determine the commitment to, and the style and proficiency of, an organisation's health and safety management.

seizure. An abrupt discharge of ions from a group of neurons resulting in epileptic activity. Seizures are classified depending on how they start: as partial or focal seizures, generalised or full-body seizures involving both cerebral hemispheres, or partial seizures with secondary generalisation.

situational awareness. An individual's awareness and understanding of information that is relevant to their current environment and task.

skill mix. The ratio of caregivers with various skills, training and experience in a clinical unit.

sleep. A fully reversible bodily state characterised by specific brain activity, somnolence, eye closure, postural recumbence, and reduced or absent skeletal muscle movement.

somnolence. A state of reduced conscious level from which the patient can be fully aroused.

spontaneous breathing trial. A technique in which the patient is removed from the ventilator to see whether they are able to breathe unassisted by the mechanical ventilator.

spontaneous vaginal birth. When labour starts by itself and the baby is born without any assistance.

status epilepticus. Enduring seizure activity that is not likely to stop spontaneously. Traditionally defined as 30 minutes of continuous seizure activity, this has been changed to 5 minutes or 2 or more seizures without full recovery of consciousness between the seizures.

stupor. A state of unconsciousness from which the patient can be fully aroused but responds inadequately to verbal and physical stimuli.

traumatic brain injury. Heterogeneous pathophysiological process from a mixture of diffuse and focal lesions on the brain because of the mechanism of injury. It can range in severity from concussion through to post-coma unresponsiveness.

values. The beliefs and attitudes that individuals hold about what is important and that therefore influence individual actions and decision making.

venous thromboembolism. A term used to reflect both deep vein thrombosis and pulmonary embolism.

ventilator-associated pneumonia. A form of hospital-acquired pneumonia that occurs in patients who are mechanically ventilated.

ventricular assist device. Full or partial ventricular assistance provided by an implanted device.

visual analogue scale. Psychometric response scale used to measure psychological constructs and other states which are not observable (e.g. pain), on which the respondent marks their level of agreement along a continuous line with an anchor descriptor at each end of the line.

Index

Page numbers followed by "*f*" indicate figures, "*t*" indicate tables, and "*b*" indicate boxes.